THE
MERCK
VETERINARY
MANUAL

SEVENTH EDITION

First Edition   *1955*
Second Edition   *1961*
Third Edition   *1967*
Fourth Edition   *1973*
Fifth Edition   *1979*
Sixth Edition   *1986*
Seventh Edition   *1991*

The Merck Veterinary Manual
is dedicated to the Doctors of Veterinary Medicine
and to their colleagues and associates
in the animal sciences.

OTHER PROFESSIONAL HANDBOOKS OF
MERCK & CO., INC.

THE MERCK INDEX
First Edition, 1889

THE MERCK MANUAL OF DIAGNOSIS AND THERAPY
First Edition, 1899

THE MERCK MANUAL OF GERIATRICS
First Edition, 1990

Professional Handbooks of MERCK & CO., Inc.
are published on a nonprofit basis
as a service to the scientific community.

THE
MERCK
VETERINARY
MANUAL

A HANDBOOK OF DIAGNOSIS, THERAPY, AND DISEASE PREVENTION AND CONTROL FOR THE VETERINARIAN

SEVENTH EDITION

Clarence M. Fraser, B.S.A., D.V.M., M.V.SC., *Editor*
Jan A. Bergeron, V.M.D., *Associate Editor*
Asa Mays, D.V.M., M.M.S., DIP.A.C.L.A.M., *Associate Editor*
Susan E. Aiello, B.S., D.V.M., *Assistant Editor*

EDITORIAL BOARD
Harold E. Amstutz, B.S., D.V.M., DIP.A.C.V.I.M.
James Armour, CBE, PH.D., DR.(H.C.), M.R.C.V.S., F.R.S.E.
Douglas C. Blood, O.B.E., B.V.SC., HON.D.V.SC., F.A.C.V.SC., HON.L.L.D., HON.ASSOC.R.C.V.S.
Cheryl L. Chrisman, D.V.M., M.S.
Franklin M. Loew, B.S., D.V.M., PH.D., DIP.A.C.L.A.M.
Glenn H. Snoeyenbos, D.V.M.

Published by
MERCK & CO., Inc.
RAHWAY, N.J., U.S.A.
1991

MERCK & CO., INC.
WHITEHOUSE STATION, NEW JERSEY, U.S.A.

Merck Human Health Division
Merck Research Laboratories
Merck Manufacturing Division
Merck AgVet Division
Hubbard Farms, Inc.
Merck Vaccine Division
Astra/Merck Group
Calgon Corporation
   Water Management Division
   Calgon Vestal Laboratories
Kelco Division
Merck Consumer Healthcare Group

Library of Congress Catalog Card Number 91-601C7
ISBN Number 911910-55-7
ISSN Number 0076-6542
First Printing   July 1991
Second Printing   June 1993

Foreword

The purpose of The Merck Veterinary Manual is to provide a concise and reliable source of information for those interested in the health and welfare of animals. With the wealth of relevant information that exists, no one can remember it all. While not all of this can be compressed into a handbook, we hope that our efforts will be of real help to practicing veterinarians and their colleagues in the animal sciences. Prevention and control of disease are foremost objectives and, obviously, diagnosis and treatment are essential components of control.

We have noted—with pleasure—that persons other than veterinarians utilize the Manual, and hope that they too find it useful and that this is beneficial to animal health and welfare. However, for any problems with animal health, we recommend consulting a veterinarian, especially before treatment is initiated.

The Manual is divided into 10 parts. Part I, which addresses the diseases of common domestic animals, large and small, is subdivided into 14 sections (*see* the Contents listed on p vii). As we have noted in earlier editions, it is impossible to categorize diseases in a manner that will appeal to all readers, but we hope that the arrangement will be an aid, particularly to those with diagnostic problems. We recommend reading the Guide for Readers (p viii) as well as this Foreword; these should make it easier to utilize the Manual.

Another attempt to assist with diagnosis and with overall comprehension of disease control is the introductory chapter of most of the sections. These introductions are brief reviews of the functions of body systems, and of the consequences of impairment of those functions.

If a reader knows the name of the specific subject on which information is sought, the best first step is to go to the Index. The Index contains bold-faced page entries for major discussions, and standard type for specific but less complete discussions elsewhere in the book. If, however, help is sought with a diagnostic problem, the list of subjects on the opening pages of each section may be more helpful than the Index, particularly if one body system is more obviously involved than are the others. (Those diseases that commonly cause disorders of more than one system are discussed in Generalized Conditions.)

Most of the Manual contents are extensively revised; many are "new" to the Manual. There are, of course, chapters that closely resemble those of the earlier edition(s), but not many in this time of rapidly expanding knowledge.

It is difficult to adequately acknowledge the guidance of the editorial board, and the contributions made by the 501 persons (listed on pp xvi-xxxii) who were so good as to share their expertise; it would be impossible to assemble the book without such help.

Additionally, gratitude is expressed to Viveca Stamper and Fredicia Westbrook, and to Pamela J. Barnes and Gary Zelko (Public Relations) for their help.

As all readers will know, it is increasingly difficult with each edition to maintain our handbook style. One means of reducing the number of pages is our extensive use of abbreviations. For the list of those used throughout the text, *see* pp ix and x. In some chapters, additional abbreviations are used; these are inserted following the spelled out word(s) where the term(s) is first used in the particular chapter.

Great effort has been expended to be accurate, particularly in scientific nomenclature and in therapeutic recommendations. Organisms or drugs likely to be better known to some readers by other names are identified by such names in parentheses following the newer or more widely accepted terms. Recommendations for drug usage are those of the various contributors: mention of a specific remedy does not constitute an implied or expressed warranty, nor does it imply endorsement of any one product over another by MERCK & CO., Inc.

Every effort has been made to select representative drugs or preparations, but this should not be construed as restricting in any way the clinical judgment of the veterinarian in choosing related products or substituting other effective remedies. Careful attention has been given to the quantities and doses of the various agents listed, but personal experience, changes in manufacturers' formulations, or unusual conditions may make it desirable or necessary to depart from those given. No guarantees can be made by the Editors regarding these recommendations. In all cases, current labeling directions should be read and understood.

The veterinarian-client-patient relationship is important in all cases, but especially so if drugs are to be used in dosages or for conditions not on the label. Most drugs are now subject to government regulations. One specific objective of these regulations is the protection of public health and welfare by establishing that it is safe to consume any edible products from treated animals. This necessitates the definition of specific withdrawal times and other warnings and cautions governing the use of certain compounds. Some drugs cannot be used to treat animals that are producing milk or meat for human consumption. Since the regulatory status of any specific drug is subject to change at any time, and tends to vary from country to country, the veterinarian should be informed in detail regarding the conditions and cautions under which such agents are to be used.

C. M. Fraser, *Editor*

Merck Sharp & Dohme Research Laboratories
Rahway, New Jersey, U.S.A.

Contents

Guide for Readers

1. The Table of Contents on p vii shows the title of each section of the Manual, and the corresponding thumb index abbreviation.
2. A list of chapter titles, with subtitles where necessary, is given at the beginning of each section.
3. In most instances, the first statement following a chapter title is a brief definition of the condition to be discussed.
4. A number of abbreviations and symbols are used routinely as space savers throughout the text. (*See also* the Foreword.)
5. Because of the difficulty of listing all proprietary names of drugs, in most instances nonproprietary or generic names are used. When used, proprietary names are capitalized, and on occasions where this does not stand out (eg, at the beginning of a sentence), they are placed within quotation marks.
6. Each page heading on the left-hand page (even page numbers) indicates the title of the first chapter discussed on that page. Each page heading on the right-hand page (odd page numbers) indicates the title of the last chapter discussed on that page.
7. Tables summarizing important data appear throughout the book. A list of these tables appears on pp xi-xv.
8. Locating the specific discussion of a disease, condition, or syndrome for which the name is known can best be done by consulting the Index.

The Manual is arranged into anatomical systems, and specific conditions are located in the system that is primarily affected. Conditions that may affect different systems or more than one system are discussed in Generalized Conditions (GEN). However, the Index will give the specific page.

If confronted with a syndrome, the arrangement of conditions into systems (*see* the Table of Contents) should help to find the discussion, but again, if the name of the condition is known, the Index is likely to provide a more ready access to the appropriate discussion, as well as to discussions of other subjects in which the subject of primary interest is mentioned.

Abbreviations and Symbols

(*See also* READY REFERENCE GUIDES, p 971 for SI units.)

ad lib	as much as desired	IP	intraperitoneal(ly)
ALT	alanine aminotransferase (SGPT)	IU	international unit(s)
		IV	intravenous(ly)
AST	aspartate aminotransferase (SGOT)	kcal	kilocalorie(s)
		kg	kilogram(s)
ATP	adenosine triphosphate	kVp	kilovolt peak
av	average	L	liter(s)
b.i.d.	twice a day	lb	pound(s)
BUN	blood urea nitrogen	lg an	large animal(s), ie, farm animals, horses
C	Celsius (centigrade)		
cal	calorie(s)	m	meter(s)
cm	centimeter(s)	M	molar
CNS	central nervous system	Mcal	megacalorie(s)
CPK	creatinine phosphokinase	ME	metabolizable energy
CSF	cerebrospinal fluid	mEq	milliequivalent(s)
cu	cubic	mg	milligram(s)
dL	deciliter(s)	min	minute(s)
DNA	deoxyribonucleic acid	mL	milliliter(s)
ECG	electrocardiogram	mm	millimeter(s)
eg	for example	mo	month(s)
ELISA	enzyme-linked immunosorbent assay	mOsm	milliosmol(s)
		ng	nanogram(s)
EPG	eggs per gram (of feces)	nm	nanometer(s)
et seq	and the following one(s)	NRC	National Research Council
F	Fahrenheit	oz	ounce(s)
FA	fluorescent antibody	p/pp	page/pages
fL	femtoliter(s)	PCV	packed cell volume
ft	foot, feet	pg	picogram(s)
gal.	gallon(s)	pH	negative logarithm of hydrogen ion activity
g	gram(s)		
GI	gastrointestinal	PO	*per os*, orally
gr	grain(s)	ppb	part(s) per billion
H&E	hematoxylin and eosin (stain)	ppm	part(s) per million
		pt	pint(s)
Hgb	hemoglobin	q4hr	every 4 hours
hr	hour(s)	q.i.d.	four times daily
ie	that is	*qs ad*	quantity sufficient to make
Ig	immunoglobulin (with class following: A, D, E, G, or M)	qt	quart(s)
		qv	which see
		r	roentgen unit(s)
IM	intramuscular(ly)	RBC	red blood cell(s)
in.	inch(es)	RNA	ribonucleic acid

sec	second(s)	tsp	teaspoon(s)
SI units	International System of Units	u	unit(s)
		UK	United Kingdom
sm an	small animal(s), ie, cats, dogs	USA	United States of America
		USSR	Union of Soviet Socialist Republics
sp/spp	species (sing.)/species (pl.)		
SPF	specific pathogen free	viz	namely
sq	square	WBC	white blood cell(s)
subcut.	subcutaneous(ly)	wk	week(s)
tbsp	tablespoon(s)	wt	weight
TDN	total digestible nutrients	yr	year(s)
t.i.d.	3 times a day		

α	alpha	°	degree(s)
β	beta	/	per
δ	delta	%	percent
Δ	delta	~	approximately
ε	epsilon	=	equals
γ	gamma	>	greater than
κ	kappa	≥	greater than or equal to
μ	micro	<	less than
σ	sigma	≤	less than or equal to
		±	plus or minus

Tables

PHM

Contributors

Melvin K. Abelseth, D.V.M., D.V.P.H., PH.D., *Voorheesville, New York.*

William M. Adams, V.M.D., *Albion, Pennsylvania.*

Franklin A. Ahrens, D.V.M., PH.D., *Department of Veterinary Physiology and Pharmacology, College of Veterinary Medicine, Iowa State University, Ames, Iowa.*

Jason S. Albertson, D.V.M., *Irving, Texas.*

D.J. Alexander, B.TECH., PH.D., F.I.BIOL., D.SC., *Central Veterinary Laboratory, Weybridge, Surrey, England.*

T.J.L. Alexander, PH.D., M.V.SC., B.SC., M.R.C.V.S., D.P.M., *Department of Clinical Veterinary Medicine, University of Cambridge, Cambridge, England.*

Mary E. Allen, PH.D., *Allen & Baer Associates, Inc., Olney, Maryland.*

M.B. Allworth, B.V.SC., M.V.S., F.A.C.V.S., *Holbrook, N.S.W., Australia.*

H.E. Amstutz, B.S., D.V.M., DIP.A.C.V.I.M., *Professor Emeritus, Department of Veterinary Clinical Science, Purdue University, West Lafayette, Indiana.*

John F. Anderson, D.V.M., M.S., *Professor, Clinical and Population Sciences, College of Veterinary Medicine, University of Minnesota, Cannon Falls, Minnesota.*

Roy C. Anderson, PH.D., *Professor, Department of Zoology, University of Guelph, Guelph, Ontario, Canada.*

John J. Andrews, D.V.M., M.S., PH.D., *Professor, Veterinary Diagnostic Laboratory, College of Veterinary Medicine, Iowa State University, Ames, Iowa.*

Robert D. Appleman, PH.D., *Extension Animal Scientist, Dairy Management, University of Minnesota, St. Paul, Minnesota.*

James Archibald, D.V.M., M.V.SC., DR.MED.VET., DIP.A.C.V.S., F.R.C.V.S., O.ONT., *Professor Emeritus, University of Guelph, Guelph, Ontario, Canada.*

James Armour, CBE, PH.D., DR.(H.C.), M.R.C.V.S., F.R.S.E., *Professor, Vice Principal, Planning and External Relations, University of Glasgow, Glasgow, Scotland.*

Steven Paul Arnoczky, D.V.M., DIP.A.C.V.S., *Director, Laboratory of Comparative Orthopaedic Research, The Hospital for Special Surgery, New York, New York.*

Lawrence H. Arp, D.V.M., PH.D., *Professor of Veterinary Pathology, College of Veterinary Medicine, Iowa State University, Ames, Iowa.*

A.C. Asbury, D.V.M., *Associate Dean, College of Veterinary Medicine, University of Florida, Gainesville, Florida.*

Matthew A.O. Atilola, D.V.M., M.SC., PH.D., *Assistant Professor, Radiology Unit, Department of Clinical Studies, University of Guelph, Guelph, Ontario, Canada.*

David P. Aucoin, D.V.M., *College of Veterinary Medicine, North Carolina State University, Raleigh, North Carolina.*

John R. August, B.VET.MED., M.S., M.R.C.V.S., *Professor and Head, Department of Small Animal Medicine and Surgery, College of Veterinary Medicine, Texas A&M University, College Station, Texas.*

Lorne A. Babiuk, B.S.A., M.SC., PH.D., D.SC., *Associate Director (Research), University of Saskatchewan, Saskatoon, Saskatchewan, Canada.*

Clell V. Bagley, D.V.M., *Utah State University, Logan, Utah.*

Brian G. Bagnall, D.V.M., PH.D., *West Chester, Pennsylvania.*

Gordon J. Baker, B.V.SC., PH.D., M.R.C.V.S., DIP.A.C.V.S., *College of Veterinary Medicine, University of Illinois, Urbana, Illinois.*

R.M. Barlow, D.SC., D.V.M.&S., M.R.C.V.S., F.R.C.PATH., *Professor of Pathology, Royal Veterinary College, Hawkshead Campus, Hatfield, Hertfordshire, U.K.*

H. John Barnes, D.V.M., PH.D., *Professor, Avian Medicine, College of Veterinary Medicine, North Carolina State University, Raleigh, North Carolina.*

Thomas B.M. Barragry, PH.D. (N.U.I.), M.V.M., M.V.B., M.R.C.V.S., *Senior Lecturer in Veterinary Pharmacology and Therapeutics, Faculty of Veterinary Medicine, University College Dublin, Veterinary College, Ireland.*

Donald W. Bates, B.S., M.S., *Agricultural Engineering, St. Paul, Minnesota.*
Roger M. Batt, B.V.SC., M.SC., PH.D., M.R.C.V.S., *Professor, Department of Small Animal Medicine and Surgery, The Royal Veterinary College, University of London, Hatfield, Hertfordshire, England.*
Louise Bauck, B.SC., D.V.M., M.V.SC., *Ocean County Veterinary Hospital, Lakewood, New Jersey.*
Sandra Ann Baxendell, B.V.SC.(HONS.), PH.D., M.A.C.V.SC., *Gidgegannup, Western Australia, Australia.*
Charles W. Beard, D.V.M., M.S., PH.D., *Athens, Georgia.*
Gary B. Beard, D.V.M., A.V.D.C., *Baton Rouge, Louisiana.*
Val Richard Beasley, D.V.M., PH.D., *Associate Professor of Toxicology, Department of Veterinary Biosciences, University of Illinois, Urbana, Illinois.*
Bonnie V. Beaver, B.S., D.V.M., M.S., *Professor and Chief of Medicine, Department of Small Animal Medicine and Surgery, College of Veterinary Medicine, Texas A&M University, College Station, Texas.*
Jamie R. Bellah, D.V.M., D.A.C.V.S., *Department of Small Animal Clinical Sciences, College of Veterinary Medicine, University of Florida, Gainesville, Florida.*
Malcolm Bennett, B.V.SC., PH.D., M.R.C.V.S., *Department of Veterinary Clinical Science, Veterinary Field Station, "Leahurst", Neston, Wirral, U.K.*
John Bentinck-Smith, D.V.M., *Professor Emeritus, Cornell University, Starkville, Mississippi.*
Herman A. Berkhoff, D.V.M., PH.D., *Professor, Department of Microbiology, Pathology, and Parasitology, College of Veterinary Medicine, North Carolina State University, Raleigh, North Carolina.*
J.D. Bezuidenhout, D.V.SC., *Veterinary Research Institute, Onderstepoort, Republic of South Africa.*
Arthur A. Bickford, V.M.D., M.S., PH.D., *Professor of Clinical Diagnostic Pathology, School of Veterinary Medicine, California Veterinary Diagnostic Laboratory System, University of California, Turlock, California.*
LeRoy G. Biehl, D.V.M., M.S., *College of Veterinary Medicine, University of Illinois, Urbana, Illinois.*
Michael L. Biehl, D.V.M., *College of Veterinary Medicine, University of Illinois, Urbana, Illinois.*
Joseph T. Bielitzki, D.V.M., M.S., *Regional Primate Research Center, University of Washington, Seattle, Washington.*
William Black, D.V.M., M.SC., PH.D., *Professor, Pharmacology and Toxicology, Department of Biomedical Sciences, Ontario Veterinary College, University of Guelph, Guelph, Ontario, Canada.*
Barry R. Blakley, D.V.M., PH.D., *Professor, Department of Veterinary Physiological Sciences, Western College of Veterinary Medicine, University of Saskatchewan, Saskatoon, Saskatchewan, Canada.*
Douglas C. Blood, *Professor Emeritus, University of Melbourne, Veterinary Clinical Centre, Werribee, Victoria, Australia.*
John C. Bloom, V.M.D., PH.D., *Head, Clinical Pathology, Lilly Research Laboratories, Eli Lilly and Company, Greenfield, Indiana.*
Mark S. Bloomberg, D.V.M., M.S., DIP.A.C.V.S., *Professor and Chairman, Department of Small Animal Clinical Sciences, College of Veterinary Medicine, University of Florida, Gainesville, Florida.*
Herman J. Boermans, D.V.M., M.SC., PH.D., *Assistant Professor of Toxicology, Department of Biomedical Sciences, Ontario Veterinary College, University of Guelph, Guelph, Ontario, Canada.*
Dawn Merton Boothe, D.V.M., M.S., PH.D., DIP.A.C.V.I.M., *Assistant Professor, Clinical Pharmacology Laboratory, Department of Veterinary Physiology and Pharmacology, College of Veterinary Medicine, Texas A&M University, College Station, Texas.*
William T.K. Bosu, D.V.M., M.SC., PH.D., *Professor and Chairman, Department of Medical Sciences, School of Veterinary Medicine, University of Wisconsin, Madison, Wisconsin.*
Terry Boundy, B.V.SC., M.R.C.V.S., F.R.AG.S. *Tegfan, Montgomery, Powys, U.K.*
Kenneth C. Bovée, D.V.M., M.MED.SC., *School of Veterinary Medicine, University of Pennsylvania, Philadelphia, Pennsylvania.*
Walter M. Boyce, D.V.M., PH.D., *Assistant Professor of Parasitology, Department of Veterinary Microbiology and Immunology, School of Veterinary Medicine, University of California, Davis, California.*
Gerald R. Bratton, D.V.M., PH.D., *Professor and Head, Department of Veterinary Anatomy and Public Health, College of Veterinary Medicine, Texas A&M University, College Station, Texas.*

Kyle G. Braund, B.V.SC., M.V.SC., PH.D., F.R.C.V.S., D.A.C.V.I.M., *Professor, and Director of Neuromuscular Research and Diagnostic Laboratories, Scott-Ritchey Research Program, College of Veterinary Medicine, Auburn University, Auburn, Alabama.*

Edward B. Breitschwerdt, D.V.M., DIP.A.C.V.I.M., *Professor of Medicine, College of Veterinary Medicine, North Carolina State University, Raleigh, North Carolina.*

Nancy O. Brown, V.M.D., *Plymouth Meeting, Pennsylvania.*

R. Glenn Brown, B.SC., PH.D., *Department of Nutrition, University of Massachusetts, Amherst, Massachusetts.*

Cecil F. Brownie, B.SC., D.V.M., PH.D., D.A.B.V.T., D.A.B.T., *Associate Professor of Pharmacology and Toxicology, College of Veterinary Medicine, North Carolina State University, Raleigh, North Carolina.*

Everett S. Bryant, D.V.M., *Professor of Pathobiology, University of Connecticut, Storrs, Connecticut.*

John H. Bryner, PH.D., F.A.A.M., *National Animal Disease Center, Ames, Iowa.*

William B. Buck, B.S., D.V.M., M.S., *Professor and Director, National Animal Poison Control Center, College of Veterinary Medicine, University of Illinois, Urbana, Illinois.*

John A. Bukowski, D.V.M., M.P.H., *Corporate Epidemiologist, Merck & Co. Inc., Rahway, New Jersey.*

Thomas J. Burke, D.V.M., M.S., *Professor, College of Veterinary Medicine, University of Illinois, Urbana, Illinois.*

Mitchell Bush, D.V.M., A.C.Z.M., *Veterinarian, National Zoological Park, Washington, D.C.*

Robert B. Bushnell, D.V.M., *Roseville, California.*

Edward G. Buss, B.S., M.S., PH.D., *Professor of Agriculture, Emeritus, The Pennsylvania State University, University Park, Pennsylvania.*

Jerry F. Butler, M.S., PH.D., *Professor, Department of Entomology and Nematology, University of Florida, Gainesville, Florida.*

David Buxton, B.V.M.&S., PH.D., M.R.C.PATH., M.R.C.V.S., *Moredun Research Institute, Edinburgh, Scotland.*

Jerry Callis, D.V.M., M.S., D.SC., *Southold, New York.*

Bruce W. Calnek, D.V.M., M.S., *Professor and Chairman, Department of Avian and Aquatic Animal Medicine, College of Veterinary Medicine, Cornell University, Ithaca, New York.*

Clay A. Calvert, D.V.M., DIP.A.C.V.I.M., *Associate Professor, College of Veterinary Medicine, University of Georgia, Athens, Georgia.*

Charles C. Capen, D.V.M., PH.D., *Professor and Chairman, Department of Veterinary Pathobiology, Ohio State University, Columbus, Ohio.*

Clyde S. Card, D.V.M., PH.D., *Assistant Director, Agriculture & Natural Resources, College of Agriculture, University of Arizona, Tucson, Arizona.*

William W. Carlton, D.V.M., PH.D., *Department of Veterinary Pathobiology, School of Veterinary Medicine, Purdue University, West Lafayette, Indiana.*

I.H. Carmichael, B.V.SC., D.V.SC., *Vet Lab, Department of Agriculture, Adelaide, South Australia.*

Vicki R. Carruthers, B.AGR.SC., D.PHIL., *Dairying Research Corporation, Hamilton, New Zealand.*

Gordon R. Carter, D.V.M., M.S., D.V.SC., *Professor Emeritus, Department of Pathobiology, Virginia-Maryland Regional College of Veterinary Medicine, Virginia Polytechnic Institute and State University, Blacksburg, Virginia.*

Sharon A. Center, D.V.M., *Associate Professor, Department of Clinical Sciences, New York State College of Veterinary Medicine, Cornell University, Ithaca, New York.*

Peter R. Cheeke, PH.D., *Department of Animal Science, Oregon State University, Corvallis, Oregon.*

Cheryl L. Chrisman, D.V.M., M.S., *College of Veterinary Medicine, University of Florida, Gainesville, Florida.*

Vern L. Christensen, M.S., PH.D., *Department of Poultry Science, North Carolina State University, Raleigh, North Carolina.*

William B. Christie, B.VET.MED., B.SC., M.R.C.V.S., *Genus, Vallum Farm, Stamfordham, Newcastle-upon-Tyne, England.*

Harold L. Chute, D.V.M., M.S., D.V.SC., *Orono, Maine.*

B.L. Clark, B.V.SC., DIP.BACT., *Bulleen, Victoria, Australia.*

Donald R. Clark, D.V.M., PH.D., DIP.A.C.V.I.M., *Department of Veterinary Physiology and Pharmacology, College of Veterinary Medicine, Texas A&M University, College Station, Texas.*

Keith A. Clark, D.V.M., PH.D., *Marble Falls, Texas.*

L. Kirk Clark, D.V.M., PH.D., *Associate Professor, Department of Veterinary Clinical Sciences, School of Veterinary Medicine, Purdue University, West Lafayette, Indiana.*

T.R. Cline, B.S., M.S., PH.D., *Professor, Department of Animal Sciences, Purdue University, West Lafayette, Indiana.*

Leroy Coggins, D.V.M., PH.D., *Professor and Head, Department of Microbiology, Pathology and Parasitology, College of Veterinary Medicine, North Carolina State University, Raleigh, North Carolina.*

M.S. Collins, B.SC.(HONS.), *Ministry of Agriculture, Fisheries and Food, Central Veterinary Laboratory, Weybridge, Surrey, England.*

Ben H. Colmery III, D.V.M., DIP.A.V.D.C., *Ann Arbor, Michigan.*

Donal P. Conway, M.S., PH.D., *Animal Health Group, Pfizer Inc., New York, New York.*

Jim Corbin, PH.D., *Professor Emeritus, University of Illinois, Urbana, Illinois.*

Charles E. Cornelius, *School of Veterinary Medicine, University of California, Davis, California.*

R.E. Corstvet, M.S., PH.D., *Professor of Veterinary Microbiology, School of Veterinary Medicine, Louisiana State University, Baton Rouge, Louisiana.*

Susan M. Cotter, D.V.M., DIP.A.C.V.I.M., *Professor of Medicine, School of Veterinary Medicine, Tufts University, North Grafton, Massachusetts.*

Geoffrey S. Cottew, M.SC., M.A.S.M., *Burleigh Heads, Queensland, Australia.*

Morris S. Cover, V.M.D., M.S., PH.D., *Foristell, Missouri.*

Rick L. Cowell, D.V.M., M.S., DIP.A.C.V.P., *Associate Professor, Department of Pathology, College of Veterinary Medicine, Oklahoma State University, Stillwater, Oklahoma.*

Timothy A. Cudd, D.V.M., *College of Veterinary Medicine, University of Florida, Gainesville, Florida.*

R.A. Curtis, D.V.M., M.SC., *Professor, Department of Health Management, Atlantic Veterinary College, University of Prince Edward Island, Charlottetown, P.E.I., Canada.*

A.J. DaMassa, PH.D., *Lecturer, Research Associate, Department of Epidemiology and Preventive Medicine, School of Veterinary Medicine, University of California, Davis, California.*

R.C.W. Daniel, B.V.SC., M.SC., PH.D., F.A.C.V.SC., *Reader, Department of Farm Animal Medicine and Production, University of Queensland, Queensland, Australia.*

A.H. Dardiri, D.V.M., B.V.SC., M.SC., PH.D., *Collaborator, U.S. Department of Agriculture, Agricultural Research Service, Plum Island Animal Disease Center, Southold, New York.*

F.G. Davies, M.A., VET.M.B., M.R.C.V.S., *Veterinary Research Laboratory, Ministry of Agriculture, Nairobi, Kenya.*

Richard B. Davis, D.V.M., M.S., *Poultry Disease Research Center, Athens, Georgia.*

Douglas J. DeBoer, D.V.M., DIP.A.C.V.D., *Assistant Professor, Department of Medical Sciences, School of Veterinary Medicine, University of Wisconsin, Madison, Wisconsin.*

Linda J. DeBowes, D.V.M., M.S., DIP.A.C.V.I.M., *Assistant Professor, Department of Clinical Sciences, College of Veterinary Medicine, Kansas State University, Manhattan, Kansas.*

Dominic L. DeGiusti, PH.D., *Professor Emeritus, Department of Immunology and Microbiology, Wayne State University School of Medicine, Detroit, Michigan.*

Antony James Della-Porta, B.SC., PH.D., *C.S.I.R.O., Australian Animal Health Laboratory, Geelong, Victoria, Australia.*

Robert W. Dellers, D.V.M., PH.D., *Wisconsin Animal Health Laboratories, Madison, Wisconsin.*

Walter J. DeLong, M.S., *Research Associate, Caine Veterinary Teaching Center, University of Idaho, Caldwell, Idaho.*

Stanley M. Dennis, B.V.SC., PH.D., F.R.C.V.S., F.R.C.PATH., *Professor, Department of Pathology, College of Veterinary Medicine, Kansas State University, Manhattan, Kansas.*

Robert C. DeNovo, D.V.M., M.S., DIP.A.C.V.I.M., *Associate Professor of Medicine, Department of Urban Practice, College of Veterinary Medicine, University of Tennessee, Knoxville, Tennessee.*

J.B. Derbyshire, B.SC., PH.D., M.R.C.V.S., *Department of Veterinary Microbiology and Immunology, Ontario Veterinary College, University of Guelph, Guelph, Canada.*

D.K. Detweiler, V.M.D., M.S., D.SC., *Professor of Physiology, Emeritus, School of Veterinary Medicine, University of Pennsylvania, Philadelphia, Pennsylvania.*

Joyce A. DeVaney, PH.D., *Melrose, New Mexico.*

W. Jean Dodds, D.V.M., *Director, Laboratory of Comparative Hematology, Wadsworth Center, New York State Department of Health, Albany, New York.*

Nicholas H. Dodman, B.V.M.S., *Professor of Anesthesia, Tufts University School of Veterinary Medicine, North Grafton, Massachusetts.*

Robert E. Dolphin, B.S., D.V.M., *Corona, California.*

Alan R. Doster, D.V.M., PH.D., *Director, Veterinary Diagnostic Center, University of Nebraska, Lincoln, Nebraska.*

J.H. Drudge, D.V.M., SC.D., *Department of Veterinary Science, University of Kentucky, Lexington, Kentucky.*

J.P. Dubey, M.V.SC., PH.D., *Microbiologist, Zoonotic Diseases Laboratory, Livestock and Poultry Sciences Institute, U.S. Department of Agriculture, Agricultural Research Service, Beltsville, Maryland.*

Nicole E. Duffee, D.V.M., PH.D., *Assistant Professor, College of Veterinary Medicine, Oregon State University, Corvallis, Oregon.*

James L. Duncan, B.V.M.S., PH.D., M.R.C.V.S., *Professor, Department of Veterinary Parasitology, Faculty of Veterinary Medicine, University of Glasgow, Bearsden, Glasgow, Scotland.*

Robert W. Dunstan, D.V.M., M.S., DIP.A.C.V.P., *Associate Professor, Department of Pathology, College of Veterinary Medicine, Michigan State University, East Lansing, Michigan.*

J.L. du Plessis, B.V.SC., M.MED.VET.(PATH.), D.V.SC., *Veterinary Research Institute, Onderstepoort, Republic of South Africa.*

Andrew Eales, B.SC., B.V.SC., M.SC., PH.D., M.R.C.V.S., *East Lothian, Scotland.*

Robert A. Easter, B.S., M.S., PH.D., *Professor, Swine Nutrition, Department of Animal Sciences, Unversity of Illinois, Urbana, Illinois.*

Robert J. Eckroade, D.V.M., PH.D., *School of Veterinary Medicine, University of Pennsylvania, Kennett Square, Pennsylvania.*

N. Edington, PH.D., B.V.SC., M.R.C.V.S., *Microbiology, Royal Veterinary College, London, England.*

William C. Edwards, D.V.M., M.S., *Veterinary Toxicologist/Professor, Oklahoma Animal Disease Diagnostic Laboratory, Stillwater, Oklahoma.*

Paul C. Estes, D.V.M., PH.D., *Director of Pathology, Pfizer Inc., Groton, Connecticut.*

A. Konrad Eugster, DR.MED.VET., PH.D., *Texas Veterinary Medical Diagnostic Laboratory, College Station, Texas.*

James F. Evermann, M.S., PH.D., *College of Veterinary Medicine, Washington State University, Pullman, Washington.*

Julius Fabricant, V.M.D., B.S., M.S., PH.D., *Professor Emeritus, Department of Avian and Aquatic Animal Medicine, New York State College of Veterinary Medicine, Cornell University, Ithaca, New York.*

Aly M. Fadly, D.V.M., PH.D., *Veterinary Research Scientist, U.S. Department of Agriculture, Agricultural Research Service, Avian Disease and Oncology Laboratory, East Lansing, Michigan.*

Alicia M. Faggella, D.V.M., *Director, Intensive Care Unit, Angell Memorial Animal Hospital, Boston, Massachusetts.*

Ronald Fayer, PH.D., *Zoonotic Diseases Laboratory, Livestock and Poultry Sciences Institute, U.S. Department of Agriculture, Agricultural Research Service, Beltsville, Maryland.*

John F. Fessler, D.V.M., M.S., *Professor of Large Animal Surgery, School of Veterinary Medicine, Purdue University, West Lafayette, Indiana.*

B.D. Firehammer, M.S., *Professor, Veterinary Research Laboratory, Montana State University, Bozeman, Montana.*

Robert A. Foster, B.V.SC., PH.D., M.A.C.V.SC., DIP.A.C.V.P., *Assistant Professor, Department of Pathology, Ontario Veterinary College, University of Guelph, Guelph, Ontario, Canada.*

James G. Fox, D.V.M., M.S., *Professor and Director, Division of Comparative Medicine, Massachusetts Institute of Technology, Cambridge, Massachusetts.*

Patricia Thomblison Franks, D.V.M., M.S., *Technical Training Manager/Staff Clinician, Hill's Pet Products, Topeka, Kansas.*

Andrew F. Fraser, M.R.C.V.S., M.V.SC., F.I.BIOL., *Professor of Surgery (Veterinary), Faculty of Medicine, Memorial University, Newfoundland, Canada.*

David E. Freeman, M.V.B., M.R.C.V.S., PH.D., *Assistant Professor of Surgery, School of Veterinary Medicine, University of Pennsylvania, Kennett Square, Pennsylvania.*

D.B. Galloway, B.V.SC., F.R.V.C.S., M.A.C.V.SC., V.M.D., *Department of Veterinary Clinical Sciences, University of Melbourne, Werribee, Victoria, Australia.*

Paul C. Gambardella, V.M.D., M.S., DIP.A.C.V.S., *Director of Surgery, Angell Memorial Animal Hospital, Boston, Massachusetts.*

Jack M. Gaskin, D.V.M., PH.D., *Associate Professor, Department of Infectious Diseases, College of Veterinary Medicine, University of Florida, Gainesville, Florida.*

Clive C. Gay, D.V.M., M.V.SC., F.A.C.V.SC., *Professor, Department of Veterinary Clinical Medicine and Surgery, Washington State University, Pullman, Washington.*

Kirk N. Gelatt, V.M.D., *Professor of Comparative Ophthalmology, College of Veterinary Medicine, University of Florida, Gainesville, Florida.*

Jack Gelb, Jr., PH.D., *Associate Professor, Department of Animal Science and Agricultural Biochemistry, College of Agricultural Sciences, University of Delaware, Newark, Delaware.*

E. Paul J. Gibbs, B.V.SC., PH.D., F.R.C.V.S., *College of Veterinary Medicine, University of Florida, Gainesville, Florida.*

Charles D. Gibson, D.V.M., PH.D., *Professor, Department of Large Animal Clinical Sciences, College of Veterinary Medicine, Michigan State University, East Lansing, Michigan.*

Urs Giger, P.D., DR.MED.VET., F.V.H., DIP.A.C.V.I.M., *Associate Professor of Medicine and Medical Genetics, Department of Clinical Studies, School of Veterinary Medicine, University of Pennsylvania, Philadelphia, Pennsylvania.*

John S. Gilmour, B.V.M.&S., F.R.C.V.S., *Moredun Research Institute, Edinburgh, Scotland.*

N.J.L. Gilmour, PH.D., D.SC., B.V.M.S., M.R.C.V.S., *Moredun Research Institute, Edinburgh, Scotland.*

Robert D. Glock, D.V.M., PH.D., *Director, Veterinary Diagnostic Laboratories, Colorado State University, Fort Collins, Colorado.*

W.L. Goff, M.S., PH.D., *Research Microbiologist, Animal Diseases Research Unit, U.S. Department of Agriculture, Agricultural Research Service, Washington State University, Pullman, Washington.*

Robert A. Goodnow, PH.D., *Microbiologist, Rochester, New York.*

Mark A. Goodwin, D.V.M., M.A.M., PH.D., *Veterinary Pathologist, Georgia Poultry Improvement Association, Georgia Poultry Laboratory, Oakwood, Georgia.*

John R. Gorham, D.V.M., PH.D., *Animal Diseases Research Unit, U.S. Department of Agriculture, Agricultural Research Service, Washington State University, Pullman, Washington.*

Rainer Gothe, D.T.V.M., *Professor, Institut for Vergleichende Tropenmedizin und Parasitologie der University Monchen, Munich, Germany.*

R.E. Gough, F.I.M.L.S., M.I.BIOL., *Poultry Department, Central Veterinary Laboratory, Ministry of Agriculture, Fisheries and Food, New Haw, Weybridge, Surrey, England.*

David I. Grant, B.VET.MED., CERT.S.A.D., F.R.C.V.S., *Veterinary Director, R.S.P.C.A., Sir Harold Harmsworth Memorial Animal Hospital, London, England.*

Gregory F. Grauer, D.V.M., M.S., DIP.A.C.V.I.M., *College of Veterinary Medicine and Biomedical Sciences, Colorado State University, Ft. Collins, Colorado.*

Craig E. Greene, D.V.M., M.S., *Professor, Department of Small Animal Medicine, College of Veterinary Medicine, University of Georgia, Athens, Georgia.*

Paul Greenlee, D.V.M., PH.D., DIP.A.C.V.P., *Dallas, Texas.*

Paul R. Greenough, F.R.C.V.S., *Professor, Department of Anesthesiology, Radiology and Surgery, Western College of Veterinary Medicine, University of Saskatchewan, Saskatoon, Saskatchewan, Canada.*

Timothy R.C. Greet, B.V.M.S., M.V.M., CERT.E.O., F.R.C.V.S., *Beaufort Cottage Stables, Newmarket, Suffolk, England.*

Dee Griffin, M.S., D.V.M., *Beef Cattle Veterinarian, University of Nebraska, Great Plains Veterinary Educational Center, Clay Center, Nebraska.*

James E. Grimes, PH.D., *Research Associate, Texas Veterinary Medical Diagnostic Laboratory, College Station, Texas.*

T. Keith Grove, D.D.S., M.S., V.M.D., DIP.A.V.D.C., DIP.A.B.P., *Veterinary Dental Practice, Vero Beach, Florida.*

Frank S. Guillot, PH.D., *Research Leader, Knipling-Bushland U.S. Livestock Insects Research Laboratory, U.S. Department of Agriculture, Agricultural Research Service, Kerrville, Texas.*

Donald P. Gustafson, B.SC., D.V.M., M.S., PH.D., *Leo P. Doyle Professor of Virology, Emeritus, Purdue University, West Lafayette, Indiana.*

Borje K. Gustafsson, D.V.M., PH.D., *Dean and Professor, College of Veterinary Medicine, Washington State University, Pullman, Washington.*

Carlton L. Gyles, D.V.M., PH.D., *Professor, Department of Veterinary Microbiology and Immunology, Ontario Veterinary College, University of Guelph, Guelph, Ontario, Canada.*

William J. Hadlow, D.V.M., *Veterinary Pathologist, Hamilton, Montana.*

Allen W. Hahn, D.V.M., PH.D., *Professor, Veterinary Medicine and Surgery, College of Veterinary Medicine, Adjunct Professor of Computer Science, University of Missouri, Columbia, Missouri.*

David A. Halvorson, D.V.M., *Professor, Department of Veterinary Pathobiology, College of Veterinary Medicine, University of Minnesota, St. Paul, Minnesota.*

Farouk Hamdy, D.V.M., PH.D., *Co-Director, U.S.-Mexico Commission for Prevention of Foot and Mouth Disease and other Exotic Animal Diseases, Mexico D.F., Mexico.*

Robert L. Hamlin, D.V.M., PH.D., DIP.A.C.V.I.M., *Ohio State University, Columbus, Ohio.*

U. Theodore Hammer, B.ED., B.A., M.S., PH.D., *Professor, Department of Biology, University of Saskatchewan, Saskatoon, Canada.*

Lyle E. Hanson, D.V.M., M.S., PH.D., *Professor Emeritus, Department of Veterinary Pathobiology, College of Veterinary Medicine, University of Illinois, Urbana, Illinois.*

Robert M. Hardy, D.V.M., M.S., DIP.A.C.V.I.M., *Department of Small Animal Clinical Sciences, College of Veterinary Medicine, University of Minnesota, St. Paul, Minnesota.*

William H. Harris, D.V.M., M.SC., PH.D., *Department of Biomedical Sciences, Ontario Veterinary College, University of Guelph, Guelph, Ontario, Canada.*

William John Hartley, F.R.C.V.S., F.A.C.V.SC., F.R.C.PATH., M.V.SC., D.SC., *Taronga Zoo, Mosman, N.S.W., Australia.*

Joe Hauptman, D.V.M., M.S., DIP.A.C.V.S., *Associate Professor of Surgery, Department of Small Animal Clinical Sciences, College of Veterinary Medicine, Michigan State University, East Lansing, Michigan.*

W.W. Hawkins, D.V.M., *Dillon, Montana.*

Audrey A. Hayes, V.M.D., DIP.A.C.V.I.M., *The Animal Medical Center, New York, New York.*

K.C. Hayes, D.V.M., PH.D., *Foster Biomedical Research Laboratory, Brandeis University, Waltham, Massachusetts.*

Roger W. Hemken, B.S., M.S., PH.D., *Professor, Animal Science Department, University of Kentucky, Lexington, Kentucky.*

Thomas H. Herdt, D.V.M., M.S., DIP.A.C.V.I.M., *Veterinary Clinical Center, Michigan State University, East Lansing, Michigan.*

David S. Herring, D.V.M., DIP.A.C.V.R., *President, Radiopet, Floral Park, New York.*

Werner P. Heuschele, D.V.M., PH.D., *Director of Research, Center for Reproduction of Endangered Species, Zoological Society of San Diego, San Diego, California.*

Clair M. Hibbs, D.V.M., M.S., PH.D., *Manhattan, Kansas.*

F.W.G. Hill, PH.D., B.VET.MED., M.R.C.V.S., M.A.C.V.SC., *Professor and Dean of Veterinary Science, University of Zimbabwe, Harare, Zimbabwe.*

Howard T. Hill, D.V.M., PH.D., *Veterinary Diagnostic Laboratory, Iowa State University, Ames, Iowa.*

Mark Edward Hitt, D.V.M., DIP.A.B.V.P., DIP.A.C.V.I.M., *Atlantic Veterinary College, University of Prince Edward Island, Charlottetown, P.E.I., Canada.*

Glen F. Hoffsis, D.V.M., M.S., DIP.A.C.V.I.M., *College of Veterinary Medicine, Ohio State University, Columbus, Ohio.*

Peter H. Holmes, B.V.M.S., PH.D., M.R.C.V.S., *Professor, University of Glasgow Veterinary School, Bearsden, Glasgow, Scotland.*

F.D. Horney, D.V.M., DIP.A.C.V.S., *Ontario Veterinary College, University of Guelph, Guelph, Ontario, Canada.*

Carl S. Hornfeldt, M.S., R.PH., *Hennepin Regional Poison Center, Minneapolis, Minnesota.*

Thomas N. Hribernik, D.V.M., DIP.A.C.V.I.M., *Department of Veterinary Clinical Sciences, School of Veterinary Medicine, Louisiana State University, Baton Rouge, Louisiana.*

William T. Hubbert, D.V.M., *Bowie, Maryland.*

K.L. Hughes, M.V.SC., PH.D., DIP.BACT.(LOND.), M.A.C.V.SC., *Dean of Veterinary Science, University of Queensland, Queensland, Australia.*

D. Bruce Hunter, D.V.M., M.SC., *Associate Professor, Department of Pathology, Ontario Veterinary College, University of Guelph, Guelph, Ontario, Canada.*

Mark B. Hurtig, D.V.M., M.V.SC., DIP.A.C.V.S., *Assistant Professor, Department of Clinical Studies, Ontario Veterinary College, University of Guelph, Guelph, Ontario, Canada.*

S.L. Ihle, D.V.M., *Boren Veterinary Medical Teaching Hospital, Oklahoma State University, Stillwater, Oklahoma.*

Dennis E. Jacobs, B.V.M.S., PH.D., M.R.C.V.S., *Department of Veterinary Pathology, The Royal Veterinary College, University of London, England.*

Elliot Jacobson, D.V.M., PH.D., *Professor, College of Veterinary Medicine, University of Florida, Gainesville, Florida.*

Lynn F. James, PH.D., *Research Leader, U.S. Department of Agriculture, Agricultural Research Service, Poisonous Plant Research Laboratory, Logan, Utah.*

Oswald Jarrett, PH.D., B.V.M.S., M.R.C.V.S., *University of Glasgow Veterinary School, Bearsden, Glasgow, Scotland.*

Donald E. Jasper, D.V.M., M.S., PH.D., *Professor Emeritus, Department of Clinical Pathology, School of Veterinary Medicine, University of California, Davis, California.*

L.B. Jeffcott, B.VET.MED., PH.D., F.R.C.V.S., D.V.SC., *Professor of Veterinary Clinical Sciences, and Director, Veterinary Clinic and Hospital, University of Melbourne, Veterinary Clinical Centre, Werribee, Victoria, Australia.*

William L. Jenkins, B.V.SC., M.MED.VET., PH.D., *Dean, School of Veterinary Medicine, Louisiana State University, Baton Rouge, Louisiana.*

Marcus M. Jensen, PH.D., *Department of Microbiology, Brigham Young University, Provo, Utah.*

Cheri A. Johnson, D.V.M., M.S., DIP.A.C.V.I.M., *Associate Professor, Department of Small Animal Clinical Sciences, College of Veterinary Medicine, Michigan State University, East Lansing, Michigan.*

Gareth E. Jones, B.V.SC, PH.D., M.R.C.V.S., D.T.V.M., *Moredun Research Institute, Edinburgh, Scotland.*

J.B. Jones, D.V.M., *Assistant Vice President for Research, Boyd Graduate Studies Research Center, University of Georgia, Athens, Georgia.*

Robert L. Jones, D.V.M., PH.D., DIP.A.C.V.M., *Diagnostic Laboratory, College of Veterinary Medicine and Biomedical Sciences, Colorado State University, Fort Collins, Colorado.*

Richard J. Julian, D.V.M., DIP.PATH., *Ontario Veterinary College, University of Guelph, Guelph, Ontario, Canada.*

Francis A. Kallfelz, D.V.M., PH.D., D.A.C.V.N., *Professor of Veterinary Nutrition, and Director, Veterinary Medical Teaching Hospital, College of Veterinary Medicine, Cornell University, Ithaca, New York.*

Arnold F. Kaufmann, D.V.M., M.S., *Acting Chief, Mycotic Diseases Branch, Division of Bacterial and Mycotic Diseases, Centers for Disease Control, Atlanta, Georgia.*

T.S. Kellerman, B.SC.(AGR.), B.V.SC., *Veterinary Research Institute, Onderstepoort, Republic of South Africa.*

Conrad J. Kercher, PH.D., C.A.S., *Animal Science Department, University of Wyoming, Laramie, Wyoming.*

Ann B. Kier, D.V.M., PH.D., *Associate Professor, Departments of Pathology and Laboratory Animal Medicine, University of Cincinnati Medical Center, Cincinnati, Ohio.*

Robert L. Kilgore, D.V.M., *Fayetteville, Arkansas.*

Cleon V. Kimberling, D.V.M., M.P.H., *Veterinary Teaching Hospital, Colorado State University, Fort Collins, Colorado.*

John M. King, D.V.M., PH.D., *Professor, New York State College of Veterinary Medicine, Cornell University, Ithaca, New York.*

Newton Kingston, B.A., M.SC., PH.D., *Professor of Parasitology, Department of Veterinary Sciences, College of Agriculture, University of Wyoming, Laramie, Wyoming.*

Rebecca Kirby, D.V.M., DIP.A.C.V.I.M., A.C.V.E.C.C., *Director of Education, Veterinary Institute of Trauma, Emergency and Critical Care, Animal Emergency Center, Milwaukee, Wisconsin.*

John H. Kirk, D.V.M., *Large Animal Surgery and Medicine, College of Veterinary Medicine, Auburn University, Auburn, Alabama.*

Carl E. Kirkpatrick, B.S., V.M.D., PH.D., *(Deceased), Urbana, Illinois.*

Allan C. Kirkwood, *Beer, Seaton, Devon, England.*

Mark D. Kittleson, D.V.M., PH.D., *Department of Medicine, School of Veterinary Medicine, University of California, Davis, California.*

Thomas R. Klei, PH.D., *Professor of Parasitology, Department of Veterinary Microbiology and Parasitology, School of Veterinary Medicine, Louisiana State University, Baton Rouge, Louisiana.*

Stanley H. Kleven, D.V.M., PH.D., *Professor, Department of Avian Medicine, College of Veterinary Medicine, University of Georgia, Athens, Georgia.*

Donald P. Knowles, Jr., D.V.M., PH.D., *Veterinary Medical Officer, U.S. Department of Agriculture, Agricultural Research Service, Animal Disease Research Unit, Washington State University, Pullman, Washington.*

Deborah T. Kochevar, D.V.M., PH.D., *Department of Veterinary Physiology and Pharmacology, College of Veterinary Medicine, Texas A&M University, College Station, Texas.*

Erwin M. Kohler, D.V.M., PH.D., *Food Animal Health Research Program, Ohio Agricultural Research and Development Center, Wooster, Ohio.*

Loren D. Koller, D.V.M., PH.D., *College of Veterinary Medicine, Oregon State University, Corvallis, Oregon.*

Lloyd D. Konyha, D.V.M., M.S., *U.S. Department of Agriculture-APHIS, Tampa, Florida.*

Joe N. Kornegay, D.V.M., PH.D., *Professor of Neurology, College of Veterinary Medicine, North Carolina State University, Raleigh, North Carolina.*

Alan L. Kraus, D.V.M., *Professor and Chairman, Division of Laboratory Animal Medicine, Professor of Pathology, and Director of the Vivarium, School of Medicine and Dentistry, University of Rochester, Rochester, New York.*

Donald R. Krawiec, D.V.M., M.S., PH.D., *College of Veterinary Medicine, University of Illinois, Urbana, Illinois.*

Ned F. Kuehn, B.A., D.V.M., M.S., DIP.A.C.V.I.M., *Chief of Staff, Professional Veterinary Hospitals Specialists Center, Allen Park, Michigan.*

S.E. Kunz, PH.D., *Laboratory Director, Knipling-Bushland U.S. Livestock Insects Laboratory, U.S. Department of Agriculture, Agricultural Research Service, Kerrville, Texas.*

J.L. Lancaster, PH.D., *Veterinary Entomologist, Department of Entomology, University of Arkansas, Fayetteville, Arkansas.*

J.G. Lane, B.VET.MED., F.R.C.V.S., *Department of Veterinary Surgery, University of Bristol, Langford House, Langford, Bristol, U.K.*

Thomas J. Lane, B.S., D.V.M., *Extension Veterinarian, University of Florida, Gainesville, Florida.*

Garrick C.M. Latch, M.(AGR.)SC., PH.D., *D.S.I.R. Plant Protection, Palmerston North, New Zealand.*

Michael J. Lees, D.V.M., M.V.SC., *Lecturer, Equine Surgery, Division of Applied Veterinary Medicine, School of Veterinary Studies, Murdoch University, Murdoch, Western Australia.*

Peter Lees, B.PHARM., PH.D., F.I.BIOL., HON.ASSOC.R.C.V.S., *Professor, Department of Veterinary Basic Sciences, Royal Veterinary College, Hawkshead Campus, Hatfield, Hertfordshire, U.K.*

Louis Leibovitz, V.M.D., *Professor Emeritus, Department of Avian and Aquatic Animal Medicine, New York State College of Veterinary Medicine, Cornell University, Ithaca, New York.*

H.W. Leipold, D.V.M., PH.D., *Department of Pathology, College of Veterinary Medicine, Kansas State University, Manhattan, Kansas.*

Norman D. Levine, PH.D., D.SC. *Professor Emeritus, College of Veterinary Medicine, University of Illinois, Urbana, Illinois.*

Karl A. Linklater, B.V.M.&S., PH.D., F.R.C.V.S., *Director, Scottish Veterinary Investigation Service, The Scottish Agricultural College, Perth, Scotland.*

Barry A. Lissman, D.V.M., *Sachem Animal Hospital and Long Island Mobile Veterinary Clinics, Holbrook, New York.*

Peter B. Little, D.V.M., M.S., PH.D., *Professor, Department of Pathology, Ontario Veterinary College, University of Guelph, Guelph, Ontario, Canada.*

Irwin K.M. Liu, D.V.M., PH.D., *Professor, Department of Veterinary Reproduction, School of Veterinary Medicine, University of California, Davis, California.*

John E. Lloyd, PH.D., *Professor of Entomology, Department of Plant, Soil and Insect Sciences, University of Wyoming, Laramie, Wyoming.*

W. Eugene Lloyd, D.V.M., PH.D., *Vet-A-Mix, Inc., Shenandoah, Iowa.*

Ted F. Lock, D.V.M., M.S., DIP.A.C.T., *College of Veterinary Medicine, University of Illinois, Urbana, Illinois.*

Walter F. Loeb, V.M.D., M.SC., PH.D., *Ani Lytics Inc., Gaithersburg, Maryland.*

Jeanne Lofstedt, B.V.SC., M.S., DIP.A.C.V.I.M., *Associate Professor, Department of Health Management, Atlantic Veterinary College, University of Prince Edward Island, Charlottetown, P.E.I., Canada.*

Peter L. Long, D.SC., PH.D., *Department of Poultry Science, University of Georgia, Athens, Georgia.*

Susan L. Longhofer, D.V.M., M.S., *M.S.D.R.L., Rahway, New Jersey.*

Juan Lubroth, D.V.M., M.S., *Comisión México-Estado Unidos para la Prevencion de la Fiebre Aftosa y Otras Entermedades Exóticas de los Animales, Colonia Polanco, Mexico.*

Phil D. Lukert, D.V.M., PH.D., *Department of Medical Microbiology, College of Veterinary Medicine, University of Georgia, Athens, Georgia.*

John H. Lumsden, D.V.M., M.SC., DIP.CLIN.PATH., *Professor, Department of Pathology, Ontario Veterinary College, University of Guelph, Guelph, Ontario, Canada.*

R.L. Lundvall, D.V.M., M.S., *Professor, Veterinary Clinical Sciences, Veterinary Teaching Hospital, Iowa State University, Ames, Iowa.*

George Lust, PH.D., *Professor of Physiological Chemistry, New York State College of Veterinary Medicine, Cornell University, Ithaca, New York.*

Eugene T. Lyons, PH.D., *Professor, Department of Veterinary Science, Gluck Equine Research Center, University of Kentucky, Lexington, Kentucky.*

Gordon K. Macleod, B.S.A., M.S., PH.D., *Professor Emeritus, Department of Animal and Poultry Science, University of Guelph, Guelph, Ontario, Canada.*

Keith T. Maddy, D.V.M., M.P.H., *Pesticide Health and Safety Advisor, California Department of Food and Agriculture, Sacramento, California.*

John E. Madigan, D.V.M., M.S., *Department of Medicine, School of Veterinary Medicine, University of California, Davis, California.*

J.G. Manns, B.S.A., M.SC., PH.D., *University of Saskatchewan, Saskatoon, Saskatchewan, Canada.*

Douglas C. Maplesden, D.V.M., M.S.A., PH.D., *Consultant, Fort Lauderdale, Florida.*

Reuben J. Mapletoft, D.V.M., M.S., PH.D., *Professor, Department of Herd Medicine and Theriogenology, Western College of Veterinary Medicine, University of Saskatchewan, Saskatoon, Saskatchewan, Canada.*

Richard F. Marsh, D.V.M., PH.D., *Professor, Department of Veterinary Science, University of Wisconsin, Madison, Wisconsin.*

A. Edward Marshall, D.V.M., PH.D., *Associate Professor, Department of Anatomy and Histology, College of Veterinary Medicine, Auburn University, Auburn, Alabama.*

Charles L. Martin, D.V.M., M.S., *Director, Veterinary Teaching Hospital, Professor, Small Animal Medicine, College of Veterinary Medicine, University of Georgia, Athens, Georgia.*

Sharron L. Martin, D.V.M., M.SC., *Professor, Department of Veterinary Clinical Sciences, Ohio State University, Columbus, Ohio.*

William J. Mathey, B.S., V.M.D., PH.D., *Nipomo, California.*

Carl Patrick McCoy, D.V.M., M.S., DIP.A.B.V.T., *Associate Professor, College of Veterinary Medicine, Mississippi State University, Mississippi State, Mississippi.*

Leslie E. McDonald, D.V.M., PH.D., *Stillwater, Oklahoma.*

J.B. McFerran, PH.D., D.SC., M.R.C.V.S., F.R.AG.S., *Professor, Veterinary Research Laboratories, Stormont, Belfast, Northern Ireland.*

C. Wayne McIlwraith, B.V.SC., M.S., PH.D., M.R.C.V.S., *Professor, Department of Clinical Sciences, College of Veterinary Medicine and Biomedical Sciences, Colorado State University, Fort Collins, Colorado.*

Quintin A. McKellar, B.V.M.S., PH.D., M.R.C.V.S., *Acting Head, Department of Veterinary Pharmacology, University of Glasgow, Bearsden, Glasgow, Scotland.*

Pauline E. McNeil, B.V.M.S., PH.D., M.R.C.V.S., *Department of Veterinary Pathology, University of Glasgow Veterinary School, Bearsden, Glasgow, Scotland.*

M.S. McNulty, M.V.B., PH.D., M.R.C.V.S., *Veterinary Research Laboratories, Stormont, Belfast, Northern Ireland.*

Charles A. Mebus, D.V.M., PH.D., *Laboratory Chief, U.S. Department of Agriculture-APHIS, Foreign Animal Disease Diagnostic Laboratory, Greenport, New York.*

William Medway, B.S., D.V.M., PH.D., M.A.(HON), *Professor Emeritus, School of Veterinary Medicine, University of Pennsylvania, Philadelphia, Pennsylvania.*

Gavin L. Meerdink, D.V.M., DIP.A.B.V.T., *College of Veterinary Medicine, University of Illinois, Urbana, Illinois.*

Paula I. Menzies, D.V.M., M.P.V.M., *Assistant Professor, Department of Population Medicine, Ontario Veterinary College, University of Guelph, Guelph, Ontario, Canada.*

Michael J. Meredith, M.A., B.SC., B.VET.MED., PH.D., M.R.C.V.S., *Department of Clinical Veterinary Medicine, University of Cambridge, Cambridge, England.*

Donald J. Meuten, D.V.M., PH.D., *Professor of Pathology, College of Veterinary Medicine, North Carolina State University, Raleigh, North Carolina.*

Janice M. Miller, D.V.M., PH.D., *Veterinary Medical Officer, U.S. Department of Agriculture, Agricultural Research Service, National Animal Disease Center, Ames, Iowa.*

Richard B. Miller, B.SC., D.V.M., PH.D., DIP.A.C.V.P., *Chairman and Professor, Department of Pathology, Ontario Veterinary College, University of Guelph, Guelph, Ontario, Canada.*

Frank J. Milne, D.V.M., DR.MED.VET., M.R.C.V.S., *(Deceased), Guelph, Ontario, Canada.*

Karen A. Moriello, D.V.M., DIP.A.C.V.D., *Clinical Assistant Professor of Dermatology, School of Veterinary Medicine, University of Wisconsin, Madison, Wisconsin.*

A.J. Morley, B.V.SC., *Rainbow Chicken Farms (Pty.) Ltd., Hammarsdale, Republic of South Africa.*

Debra Deem Morris, D.V.M., M.S., *Associate Professor, Department of Large Animal Medicine, College of Veterinary Medicine, University of Georgia, Athens, Georgia.*

Mark L. Morris, Jr., D.V.M., PH.D., *Veterinary Clinical Nutritionist, Topeka, Kansas.*

Robert B. Morrison, D.V.M., PH.D., *University of Minnesota, St. Paul, Minnesota.*

W.I. Morrison, PH.D., B.V.M.S., *Agricultural and Food Research Council Institute for Animal Health, Compton Laboratory, Compton, Nr. Newbury, Berkshire, England.*

Raymond L. Morter, D.V.M., PH.D., *West Lafayette, Indiana.*

Edward A. Moser, M.S., V.M.D., DIP.A.C.V.N., *Veterinary Nutritionist, North East, Maryland.*

C. Anne Muckle, D.V.M., M.SC., PH.D., *Assistant Professor, Department of Veterinary Microbiology and Immunology, Ontario Veterinary College, University of Guelph, Guelph, Ontario, Canada.*

Thomas P. Mullaney, M.V.B., PH.D., M.R.C.V.S., *Department of Pathology, Animal Health Diagnostic Laboratory, Michigan State University, East Lansing, Michigan.*

Peter C. Mullowney, M.V.B., M.S., M.R.C.V.S., *Melcomb House, Newport, County Mayo, Ireland.*

Michael J. Murray, D.V.M., M.S., DIP.A.C.V.I.M., *Marion du Pont Scott Equine Medical Center, Leesburg, Virginia.*

Mitchell Durno Murray, B.SC.(VET.SC.), F.R.C.V.S., M.A.C.V.SC., *Pymble, N.S.W., Australia.*

Vinand M. Nantulya, M.D., PH.D., M.R.C.PATH., *International Laboratory for Research on Animal Diseases, Nairobi, Kenya.*

Opendra Narayan, D.V.M., *Professor of Comparative Medicine, Professor of Neurology, The Johns Hopkins University School of Medicine, Baltimore, Maryland.*

Mark P. Nasisse, D.V.M., DIP.A.C.V.O., *College of Veterinary Medicine, North Carolina State University, Raleigh, North Carolina.*

J.M. Ndung'u, B.V.M., PH.D., *Ministry of Research, Science and Technology, Kenya Trypanosomiasis Research Institute, Muguga, Kikuyu, Kenya.*

T. Mark Neer, D.V.M., DIP.A.C.V.I.M., *Associate Professor of Medicine, Department of Clinical Sciences, College of Veterinary Medicine, Louisiana State University, Baton Rouge, Louisiana.*

Christian E. Newcomer, V.M.D., *Clinical Associate Professor, Department of Comparative Medicine, School of Veterinary Medicine, Tufts University, and Director, Division of Laboratory Animal Medicine, Tufts-New England Medical Center, Boston, Massachusetts.*

John A. Newman, D.V.M., PH.D., *Professor, Department of Veterinary Pathobiology, College of Veterinary Medicine, University of Minnesota, St. Paul, Minnesota.*

Paul Nicoletti, D.V.M., M.S., *College of Veterinary Medicine, University of Florida, Gainesville, Florida.*

N. Ole Nielsen, D.V.M. PH.D., *Dean, Ontario Veterinary College, University of Guelph, Guelph, Ontario, Canada.*

R.A.I. Norval, PH.D., D.SC., *International Laboratory for Research on Animal Diseases, Nairobi, Kenya.*

Dennis P. O'Brien, D.V.M., PH.D., *Department of Veterinary Medicine and Surgery, College of Veterinary Medicine, University of Missouri, Columbia, Missouri.*

Joan A. O'Brien, V.M.D., A.C.V.I.M., *(Deceased), Philadelphia, Pennsylvania.*

Michael W. O'Callaghan, B.V.SC., M.SC.V., PH.D., M.R.C.V.S., *Department of Surgery, School of Veterinary Medicine, Tufts University, North Grafton, Massachusetts.*

Frederick W. Oehme, D.V.M., PH.D., *Professor of Toxicology, Medicine and Physiology, and Director, Comparative Toxicology Laboratories, Kansas State University, Manhattan, Kansas.*

J.E. Oldfield, PH.D., *Professor Emeritus, Department of Animal Science, Oregon State University, Corvallis, Oregon.*

N. Bari Olivier, D.V.M., PH.D., *Assistant Professor, Internal Medicine and Physiology, Department of Physiology and Small Animal Clinical Sciences, Michigan State University, East Lansing, Michigan.*

E. Christopher Orton, D.V.M., PH.D., *Associate Professor, Veterinary Teaching Hospital, College of Veterinary Medicine and Biomedical Sciences, Colorado State University, Fort Collins, Colorado.*

Gary D. Osweiler, D.V.M., M.S., PH.D., *Veterinary Diagnostic Laboratory, College of Veterinary Medicine, Iowa State University, Ames, Iowa.*

Richard L. Ott, B.S., D.V.M., *Professor Emeritus, Washington State University, Pullman, Washington.*

Randall S. Ott, D.V.M., M.S., DIP.A.C.T., *Professor, Department of Veterinary Clinical Medicine, College of Veterinary Medicine, University of Illinois, Urbana, Illinois.*

Robert Kenny Page, D.V.M., M.S., *Poultry Disease Research Center, Athens, Georgia.*

N.C. Palmer, D.V.M., M.SC., PH.D., *Veterinary Laboratory Services, Ontario Ministry of Agriculture and Food, Guelph, Ontario, Canada.*

Mary Rose Paradis, D.V.M., M.S., DIP.A.C.V.I.M., *School of Veterinary Medicine, Tufts University, North Grafton, Massachusetts.*

Joane Parent, B.SC., D.V.M., M.VET.SC., DIP.A.C.V.I.M., *Associate Professor, Department of Veterinary Clinical Studies, Ontario Veterinary College, Guelph, Ontario, Canada.*

Alan J. Parker, M.R.C.V.S., PH.D., *Department of Veterinary Clinical Medicine, College of Veterinary Medicine, University of Illinois, Urbana, Illinois.*

Jill E. Parker, V.M.D., DIP.A.C.V.S., *Assistant Professor of Large Animal Surgery, Department of Veterinary Clinical Sciences, Purdue University, West Lafayette, Indiana.*

Robert B. Parker, D.V.M., DIP.A.C.V.S., *Associate Professor and Chief, Small Animal Surgery, College of Veterinary Medicine, University of Florida, Gainesville, Florida.*

Wendy Parker, D.V.M., *Associate Professor, Department of Clinical Studies, Ontario Veterinary College, University of Guelph, Guelph, Ontario, Canada.*

Willis G. Parker, D.V.M., M.SC., *Clinical Theriogenologist, Veterinary Department, American Breeders Service, DeForest, Wisconsin.*

John R. Pascoe, B.V.SC., PH.D., DIP.A.C.V.S., *Associate Professor, Department of Surgery, and Chief, Equine Surgery Service, School of Veterinary Medicine, University of California, Davis, California.*

Nephi M. Patton, D.V.M., PH.D., *Director, Rabbit Research Center, Oregon State University, Corvallis, Oregon.*

Sharon Patton, M.S., PH.D., *Associate Professor, College of Veterinary Medicine, University of Tennessee, Knoxville, Tennessee.*

Robert D. Pechman, D.V.M., *Veterinary Clinical Sciences, School of Veterinary Medicine, Louisiana State University, Baton Rouge, Louisiana.*

Niels C. Pedersen, D.V.M., PH.D., *Professor, Small Animal Internal Medicine, Department of Medicine, School of Veterinary Medicine, University of California, Davis, California.*

Paul W. Pennock, B.S., D.V.M., M.SC., DIP.A.C.V.R., *Professor, Department of Clinical Studies, Ontario Veterinary College, University of Guelph, Guelph, Ontario, Canada.*

Richard H.C. Penny, D.V.SC., PH.D., F.R.C.V.S., D.P.M., *Austrey, Nr. Atherstone, Warwickshire, England.*

Maurice B. Pensaert, D.V.M., PH.D., *Professor, Laboratory of Virology-Immunology, Faculty of Veterinary Medicine, State University of Gent, Gent, Belgium.*

Brian D. Perry, B.V.M.&S., D.T.V.M., M.SC., D.V.M.&S., M.R.C.V.S., *International Laboratory for Research on Animal Diseases, Nairobi, Kenya.*

Tilden Wayne Perry, B.ED., B.S., M.S., PH.D., *Professor of Animal Nutrition, Department of Animal Sciences, Purdue University, West Lafayette, Indiana.*

Mark E. Peterson, D.V.M., *Head, Division of Endocrinology, The Animal Medical Center, New York, New York.*

James E. Phillips, D.V.M.&S., B.SC., M.R.C.V.S., *Department of Veterinary Pathology, Royal (Dick) School of Veterinary Studies, University of Edinburgh, Summerhall, Edinburgh, Scotland.*

Guy L. Pidgeon, D.V.M., DIP.A.C.V.I.M., *Associate Director, Department of Veterinary Affairs, Hill's Pet Products, Topeka, Kansas.*

Carlos Pijoan, D.V.M., PH.D., *College of Veterinary Medicine, University of Minnesota, St. Paul, Minnesota.*

Edwin I. Pilchard, D.V.M., M.S., PH.D., *Silver Spring, Maryland.*

Hugh M. Pirie, B.V.M.S., PH.D., M.R.C.V.S., F.R.C.PATH., *Professor, University of Glasgow Veterinary School, Bearsden, Glasgow, Scotland.*

J.F. Prescott, M.A., VET.M.B., PH.D., *Department of Veterinary Microbiology and Immunology, Ontario Veterinary College, University of Guelph, Guelph, Ontario, Canada.*

John M. Preston, B.V.M.S., PH.D., M.R.C.V.S., *Executive Director, M.S.D. AGVET, Rahway, New Jersey.*

R.K. Prichard, B.SC., PH.D., *Professor, Institute of Parasitology of McGill University, Macdonald College, Ste-Anne de Bellevue, Quebec, Canada.*

Jim E. Proctor, D.V.M., PH.D., *Bristol-Myers Co., Evansville, Indiana.*

George W. Pugh, Jr., D.V.M., PH.D., *National Animal Disease Center, U.S. Department of Agriculture, Agricultural Research Service, Ames, Iowa.*

H. Graham Purchase, B.V.SC., M.R.C.V.S., PH.D., *College of Veterinary Medicine, Mississippi State University, Mississippi State, Mississippi.*

Roger E. Purnell, D.SC., F.I.BIOL., F.R.C.PATH., PH.D., *Technical Services Manager, Animal Health Division, Pfizer Ltd., Sandwich, Kent, England.*

Marc A. Rachofsky, M.S., D.V.M., DIP.A.C.V.D., *Allergy and Dermatology Clinic for Animals, Dallas, Texas.*

O.M. Radostits, D.V.M., M.S., DIP.A.C.V.I.M., *Professor and Head, Department of Veterinary Internal Medicine, Western College of Veterinary Medicine, University of Saskatchewan, Saskatoon, Saskatchewan, Canada.*

William C. Rebhun, D.V.M., DIP.A.C.V.O., DIP.A.C.V.I.M., *Professor of Ophthalmology and Large Animal Medicine, New York State College of Veterinary Medicine, Cornell University, Ithaca, New York.*

Willie M. Reed, D.V.M., PH.D., *Professor of Pathology, Animal Health Diagnostic Laboratory and Department of Pathology, College of Veterinary Medicine, Michigan State University, East Lansing, Michigan.*

Hugh W. Reid, B.V.M.&S., D.T.V.M., PH.D., M.R.C.V.S., *Moredun Research Institute, Edinburgh, Scotland.*

Keith R. Rhoades, D.V.M., PH.D., *Veterinary Medical Officer, National Animal Disease Center, Ames, Iowa.*

James A. Richardson, D.V.M., PH.D., *Assistant Professor, Division of Comparative Medicine, Department of Pathology, University of Texas Southwestern Medical Center at Dallas, Dallas, Texas.*

C. Riddell, D.V.M., PH.D., *Western College of Veterinary Medicine, University of Saskatchewan, Saskatoon, Saskatchewan, Canada.*

Richard B. Rimler, PH.D., *Microbiologist, National Animal Disease Center, Ames, Iowa.*

Ronald J. Roberts, B.V.M.S., PH.D., M.R.C.V.S., F.R.C.PATH., F.I.BIOL., F.R.S.E., *Professor, Institute of Aquaculture, University of Stirling, Stirling, Scotland.*

James T. Robertson, D.V.M., DIP.A.C.V.S., *Veterinary Hospital, Ohio State University, Columbus, Ohio.*

C. Lee Robinette, D.V.M., PH.D., *Associate Professor of Pharmacology and Toxicology, College of Veterinary Medicine, North Carolina State University, Raleigh, North Carolina.*

James F. Roche, M.AGR.SC., PH.D., D.SC., *Department of Animal Husbandry and Production, University College Dublin, Ballsbridge, Dublin, Ireland.*

Barton W. Rohrbach, V.M.D., M.P.H., *Associate Professor, Department of Rural Practice, College of Veterinary Medicine, University of Tennessee, Knoxville, Tennessee.*

R.A. Roncalli, D.V.M., M.S., *M.S.D.R.L., Rahway, New Jersey.*

John K. Rosenberger, B.S., M.S., PH.D., *Professor and Department Chairperson, Department of Animal Science and Agricultural Biochemistry, University of Delaware, Newark, Delaware.*

Robert C. Rosenthal, D.V.M., M.S., PH.D., DIP.A.C.V.I.M., *Veterinary Specialists of Rochester, Rochester, New York.*

James N. Ross, Jr., D.V.M., M.SC., PH.D., DIP.A.C.V.I.M., DIP.A.C.V.E.C.C., *Professor and Chairman, Department of Medicine, Tufts University School of Veterinary Medicine, North Grafton, Massachusetts.*

Linda A. Ross, D.V.M., M.S., DIP.A.C.V.I.M., *Associate Professor, School of Veterinary Medicine, Tufts University, North Grafton, Massachusetts.*

Paul B. Rossiter, B.VET.MED., M.SC., PH.D., M.R.C.V.S., *National Veterinary Research Centre, Kenya Agricultural Research Institute, Muguga, Kikuyu, Kenya.*

Loyd D. Rowe, D.V.M., M.S., DIP.A.B.V.T., *U.S. Department of Agriculture, Agricultural Research Service, Food Animal Protection Research Laboratory, College Station, Texas.*

Stanley I. Rubin, D.V.M., M.S., DIP.A.C.V.I.M., *Professor, Department of Veterinary Internal Medicine, Western College of Veterinary Medicine, University of Saskatchewan, Saskatoon, Saskatchewan, Canada.*

Michael D. Ruff, B.S., M.S., PH.D., *Research Leader, Protozoan Diseases Laboratory, Livestock and Poultry Sciences Institute, U.S. Department of Agriculture, Agricultural Research Service, Beltsville, Maryland.*

George R. Ruth, D.V.M., PH.D., DIP.A.C.V.P., *Professor, Veterinary Diagnostic Laboratory, University of Minnesota, St. Paul, Minnesota.*

J.M. Rutter, B.V.M.&S, B.SC., PH.D., M.R.C.V.S., *Veterinary Medicines Directorate, New Haw, Weybridge, Surrey, England.*

Y.M. Saif, D.V.M., PH.D., *Professor, Food Animal Health Research Program, Ohio Agricultural Research and Development Center, Ohio State University, Wooster, Ohio.*

Tirath S. Sandhu, B.V.SC.&A.H., M.S., PH.D., *Veterinarian, Department of Avian and Aquatic Animal Medicine, New York State College of Veterinary Medicine, Cornell University Duck Research Laboratory, Eastport, New York.*

F.T. Satalowich, D.V.M., M.S.P.H., *Director, Bureau of Veterinary Public Health, Missouri Department of Health, Jefferson City, Missouri.*

Charles M. Scanlan, D.V.M., PH.D., *Department of Veterinary Pathobiology, Texas Veterinary Medical Center, Texas A&M University, College Station, Texas.*

K.A. Schat, D.V.M., PH.D., *Professor, Department of Avian and Aquatic Animal Medicine, New York State College of Veterinary Medicine, Cornell University, Ithaca, New York.*

H. Bruno Schiefer, D.V.M., PH.D., *Director, Toxicology Research Centre, University of Saskatchewan, Saskatoon, Saskatchewan, Canada.*

Donald H. Schlafer, D.V.M., M.S., PH.D., DIP.A.C.V.P., DIP.A.C.V.M., DIP.A.C.T., *Associate Professor, Department of Veterinary Pathology, New York State College of Veterinary Medicine, Cornell University, Ithaca, New York.*

D.G. Schmitz, D.V.M., M.S., *Associate Professor, Department of Large Animal Medicine and Surgery, College of Veterinary Medicine, Texas A&M University, College Station, Texas.*

Norman R. Schneider, D.V.M., M.SC., DIP.A.B.V.T., *Department of Veterinary Science, University of Nebraska, Lincoln, Nebraska.*

Philip J. Scholl, PH.D., *Research Entomologist, Knipling-Bushland U.S. Livestock Insects Laboratory, Kerrville, Texas.*

Edward C. Schroeder, D.V.M., M.S., *College of Veterinary Medicine, University of Tennessee, Knoxville, Tennessee.*

Kevin T. Schultz, D.V.M., PH.D., *Associate Professor, Department of Pathobiological Sciences, School of Veterinary Medicine, and Unit Director Microbiology and Immunology, Wisconsin Regional Primate Research Center, University of Wisconsin, Madison, Wisconsin.*

T. Michael Schwartz, D.V.M., *White House Station, New Jersey.*

Robert M. Schwartzman, V.M.D., M.P.H., PH.D., *Professor of Dermatology, School of Veterinary Medicine, University of Pennsylvania, Philadelphia, Pennsylvania.*

Milton L. Scott, PH.D., *The Jacob Gould Schurman Professor of Nutrition Emeritus at Cornell University, Ithaca, New York.*

Charles J. Sedgwick, D.V.M., DIP.A.C.L.A.M., DIP.A.C.Z.M., *School of Veterinary Medicine, Tufts University, North Grafton, Massachusetts.*

Brad Seguin, D.V.M., M.S., PH.D., DIP.A.C.T., *Professor and Interim Chair, Department of Clinical and Population Sciences, College of Veterinary Medicine, University of Minnesota, St. Paul, Minnesota.*

Robert F. Sellers, SC.D., M.R.C.V.S., F.I.BIOL., F.R.S.E., *Guildford, Surrey, England.*

J.M. Sharp, PH.D., B.V.M.S., M.R.C.V.S., *Animal Diseases Research Association, Moredun Research Institute, Edinburgh, Scotland.*

Nicholas J.H. Sharp, B.VET.MED., M.V.M., M.R.C.V.S., DIP.A.C.V.S., *College of Veterinary Medicine, North Carolina State University, Raleigh, North Carolina.*

Linda G. Shell, D.V.M., DIP.A.C.V.I.M., *Department of Small Animal Clinical Sciences, Virginia-Maryland Regional College of Veterinary Medicine, Virginia Polytechnic Institute and State University, Blacksburg, Virginia.*

J.E. Shelle, B.S., M.S., PH.D., *Associate Professor of Animal Science, Michigan State University, East Lansing, Michigan.*

David M. Sherman, D.V.M., M.S., DIP.A.C.V.I.M., *Associate Professor, Department of Medicine, School of Veterinary Medicine, Tufts University, North Grafton, Massachusetts.*

Chatur S. Sisodia, B.V.SC.&A.H., M.S., PH.D., *Professor, Department of Veterinary Physiological Sciences, Western College of Veterinary Medicine, University of Saskatchewan, Saskatoon, Saskatchewan, Canada.*

J. Owen D. Slocombe, D.I.C.T.A., D.V.M., PH.D., *Department of Pathology, Ontario Veterinary College, University of Guelph, Guelph, Ontario, Canada.*

Alvin W. Smith, D.V.M., PH.D., *Professor, College of Veterinary Medicine, Oregon State University, Corvallis, Oregon.*

Bradford B. Smith, D.V.M., PH.D., *College of Veterinary Medicine, Oregon State University, Corvallis, Oregon.*

Donald F. Smith, D.V.M., *Professor of Surgery, and Associate Dean for Veterinary Education, College of Veterinary Medicine, Cornell University, Ithaca, New York.*

H.J. Smith, B.SC.(AGR.), D.V.M., M.V.SC., *Research Scientist, Health of Animals Laboratory, Health of Animals Division, Agriculture Canada, Sackville, New Brunswick, Canada.*

John M.B. Smith, PH.D., *Associate Professor, Department of Microbiology, University of Otago, Dunedin, New Zealand.*

Joseph E. Smith, D.V.M., PH.D., *Head, Department of Pathology, College of Veterinary Medicine, Kansas State University, Manhattan, Kansas.*

L.L. Smith, D.V.M., M.SC., *Associate Professor, Department of Clinical Studies, Ontario Veterinary College, University of Guelph, Guelph, Ontario, Canada.*

Malcolm Herbert Smith, D.V.M., PH.D., *Professor and Chairman, Department of Veterinary and Microbiological Sciences, North Dakota State University, Fargo, North Dakota.*

Mark M. Smith, V.M.D., *Virginia-Maryland Regional College of Veterinary Medicine, Virginia Polytechnic Institute and State University, Blacksburg, Virginia.*

David R. Snodgrass, B.V.M.S., PH.D., D.SC., M.R.C.V.S., M.R.C.PATH., *Moredun Research Institute, Edinburgh, Scotland.*

Glenn H. Snoeyenbos, D.V.M., *Paige Laboratory, University of Massachusetts, Amherst, Massachusetts.*

Stanley P. Snyder, D.V.M., M.S., PH.D., *Director, Veterinary Diagnostic Laboratory, Oregon State University, Corvallis, Oregon.*

Mark D. Soll, B.V.SC., *M.S.D.R.L., Rahway, New Jersey.*

Josip Spalatin, PH.D., *Lecturer, Department of Veterinary Science, University of Wisconsin, Madison, Wisconsin.*

Glen L. Spaulding, D.V.M., DIP.A.C.V.I.M., *Director, Laboratory Animal Medicine, and Assistant Professor, Department of Environmental Studies and Department of Medicine, School of Veterinary Medicine, Tufts University, North Grafton, Massachusetts.*

Joseph S. Spinelli, D.V.M., *Animal Care and Cell Culture Facility, University of California, San Francisco, California.*

Wilfred T. Springer, B.S., D.V.M., M.S., PH.D., *Department of Veterinary Science, Louisiana State University, Baton Rouge, Louisiana.*

Robert R. Steckel, D.V.M., M.S., DIP.A.C.V.S., *Assistant Professor of Surgery, School of Veterinary Medicine, Tufts University, North Grafton, Massachusetts.*

James H. Steele, D.V.M., M.P.H., *Professor Emeritus, School of Public Health, University of Texas, Houston, Texas.*

George Stein, Jr., B.S., D.V.M., M.S., *Animal Health Laboratory, Maryland Department of Agriculture, Salisbury, Maryland.*

Toby D. St. George, D.V.SC., *C.S.I.R.O., Long Pocket Laboratories, Indooroopilly, Brisbane, Queensland, Australia.*

Margaret E. Stoddart, B.SC., B.VET.MED., PH.D., D.V.R., M.R.C.V.S., *Somerset, England.*

J. Storz, D.V.M., PH.D., *Professor and Head, Department of Veterinary Microbiology and Parasitology, School of Veterinary Medicine, Louisiana State University, Baton Rouge, Louisiana.*

Michael K. Stoskopf, D.V.M., PH.D., DIP.A.C.Z.M., *Professor and Department Head, Department of Companion Animal and Special Species Medicine, College of Veterinary Medicine, North Carolina State University, Raleigh, North Carolina.*

Bert E. Stromberg, PH.D., *Professor, Department of Veterinary Pathobiology, College of Veterinary Medicine, University of Minnesota, St. Paul, Minnesota.*

John David Summers, B.S.A., M.S.A., PH.D., *Department of Animal and Poultry Science, University of Guelph, Guelph, Ontario, Canada.*

G. Sumner-Smith, B.V.SC., M.SC., D.V.SC., F.R.C.V.S., *Professor, Department of Clinical Studies, Ontario Veterinary College, University of Guelph, Guelph, Ontario, Canada.*

T.W. Swerczek, D.V.M., PH.D., *Department of Veterinary Science, University of Kentucky, Lexington, Kentucky.*

Vincent N. Tanya, D.V.M., M.S., *Department of Infectious Diseases, College of Veterinary Medicine, University of Florida, Gainesville, Florida.*

David John Taylor, M.A., PH.D., VET.M.B., M.R.C.V.S., *Department of Veterinary Pathology, University of Glasgow Veterinary School, Bearsden, Glasgow, Scotland.*

Stuart M. Taylor, PH.D., B.V.M.S., M.R.C.V.S., *Senior Veterinary Research Officer, Veterinary Research Laboratories, Stormont, Belfast, Northern Ireland.*

A.B. Thiermann, D.V.M., PH.D., *Deputy Administrator, International Services, Animal and Plant Health Inspection Service, U.S. Department of Agriculture, Washington, D.C.*

Charles O. Thoen, D.V.M., PH.D., *Professor, Department of Microbiology, Immunology and Preventive Medicine, College of Veterinary Medicine, Iowa State University, Ames, Iowa.*

Annette D. Thomas, M.SC., M.A.S.M., *Principal Microbiologist, Oonoonba Veterinary Laboratory, Townsville, Queensland, Australia.*

H. Thompson, PH.D., B.V.M.S., M.R.C.V.S., *Department of Veterinary Pathology, University of Glasgow Veterinary School, Bearsden, Glasgow, Scotland.*

John R. Thornton, B.V.SC., M.SC., PH.D., *Reader in Veterinary Medicine, Department of Companion Animal Medicine and Surgery, University of Queensland, Queensland, Australia.*

Peter J. Timoney, M.V.B., M.S., PH.D., F.R.C.V.S., *Professor, Maxwell H. Gluck Equine Research Center, Department of Veterinary Science, University of Kentucky, Lexington, Kentucky.*

Ian R. Tizard, B.V.M.&S., PH.D., M.R.C.V.S., *Professor, Department of Veterinary Pathobiology, College of Veterinary Medicine, Texas A&M University, College Station, Texas.*

Deoki N. Tripathy, B.V.SC.&A.H., PH.D., DIP.A.C.V.M., *Professor, Department of Veterinary Pathobiology, College of Veterinary Medicine, University of Illinois, Urbana, Illinois.*

Leander Tryphonas, D.V.M., PH.D., *Ottawa, Ontario, Canada.*

Alan Tucker, PH.D., *Professor, Department of Physiology, Colorado State University, Fort Collins, Colorado.*

Harold W. Tvedten, D.V.M., PH.D., DIP.A.C.V.P., *Clinical Pathologist, Department of Pathology, College of Veterinary Medicine, Michigan State University, East Lansing, Michigan.*

David E. Tyler, D.V.M., M.S., PH.D., *Professor, Department of Veterinary Pathology, College of Veterinary Medicine, University of Georgia, Athens, Georgia.*

W.J. Tyznik, PH.D., *Professor of Animal Science, Ohio State University, Columbus, Ohio.*

Norman R. Underdahl, B.A., M.S., *Professor, Lincoln, Nebraska.*

Louis van der Heide, D.V.M., PH.D., *Department of Pathobiology, University of Connecticut, Storrs, Connecticut.*

Kent R. Van Kampen, D.V.M., PH.D., *Chief Executive Officer, Virogenetics Corporation, Troy, New York.*

David C. Van Sickle, D.V.M., PH.D., *Professor and Head, Department of Anatomy, School of Veterinary Medicine, Purdue University, West Lafayette, Indiana.*

John F. Van Vleet, D.V.M., PH.D., *Professor of Veterinary Pathology and Associate Dean of Academic Affairs, Department of Pathobiology, School of Veterinary Medicine, Purdue University, West Lafayette, Indiana.*

Stanley A. Vezey, D.V.M., *Professor, Department of Avian Medicine, College of Veterinary Medicine, University of Georgia, Athens, Georgia.*

Jim C. Vulgamott, D.V.M., DIP.A.C.V.I.M., *Gulf Coast Veterinary Internists, Houston, Texas.*

Dennis P. Wages, D.V.M., *Associate Professor, Avian Medicine, Department of Food Animal and Equine Medicine, College of Veterinary Medicine, North Carolina State University, Raleigh, North Carolina.*

Richard Walshaw, B.V.MS., DIP.A.C.V.S., *Department of Small Animal Clinical Sciences, College of Veterinary Medicine, Michigan State University, East Lansing, Michigan.*

John R. Walton, PH.D. B.V.M.S., DIP.BACT., D.P.M., M.R.C.V.S., *Department of Veterinary Clinical Science, University of Liverpool, Neston, South Wirral, U.K.*

Thomas E. Walton, D.V.M., PH.D., *Research Leader, U.S. Department of Agriculture, Agricultural Research Service, Arthropod-borne Animal Diseases Research Laboratory, Laramie, Wyoming.*

Wallace M. Wass, D.V.M., PH.D., DIP.A.C.V.I.M., *Professor, Department of Veterinary Clinical Sciences, College of Veterinary Medicine, Iowa State University, Ames, Iowa.*

Bruce E. Watkins, PH.D., *Animal Nutrition Consultant, Durango Software/N-Squared Computing, Durango, Colorado.*

Steven H. Weisbroth, M.S., D.V.M., *President, Anmed Biosafe, Inc., Rockville, Maryland.*

G.A.H. Wells, B.VET.MED., M.R.C.V.S., *Central Veterinary Laboratory, Ministry of Agriculture, Fisheries and Food, New Haw, Weybridge, Surrey, England.*

David M. West, B.V.SC., PH.D., F.A.C.V.S.C., *Department of Veterinary Clinical Sciences, Massey University, Palmerston North, New Zealand.*

P.D. Whanger, PH.D., *Professor, Department of Agricultural Chemistry, Oregon State University, Corvallis, Oregon.*

John D. Wheat, D.V.M., *Department of Veterinary Surgery, School of Veterinary Medicine, University of California, Davis, California.*

Stephen D. White, D.V.M., DIP.A.C.V.D., *Associate Professor, Department of Clinical Sciences, College of Veterinary Medicine and Biomedical Sciences, Colorado State University, Fort Collins, Colorado.*

Howard L. Whitmore, D.V.M., PH.D., *Professor and Head, Food Animal Veterinary Medicine and Surgery, College of Veterinary Medicine, University of Illinois, Urbana, Illinois.*

J.C. Williams, PH.D., *Professor, Department of Veterinary Science, Louisiana Agricultural Experiment Station, Baton Rouge, Louisiana.*

Ralph E. Williams, PH.D., *Professor, Department of Entomology, Purdue University, West Lafayette, Indiana.*

M.R. Wilson, B.V.SC., PH.D., M.R.C.V.S., *Department of Population Medicine, Ontario Veterinary College, University of Guelph, Guelph, Ontario, Canada.*

Cedric Michael Wise, B.V.SC., M.S., DIP.A.C.T., M.A.C.V.SC., *Glen Aplin, Queensland, Australia.*

Richard L. Witter, D.V.M., PH.D, *U.S. Department of Agriculture, Agricultural Research Service, Avian Disease and Oncology Laboratory, East Lansing, Michigan.*

Kurt Wohlgemuth, D.V.M., *Extension Veterinarian, Veterinary Science Department, North Dakota State University, Fargo, North Dakota.*

Alice M. Wolf, D.V.M., DIP.A.C.V.I.M., *Associate Professor, Department of Small Animal Medicine and Surgery, Texas Veterinary Medical Center, College of Veterinary Medicine, Texas A&M University, College Station, Texas.*

Richard L. Wood, D.V.M., PH.D., *Veterinary Medical Officer, National Animal Disease Center, U.S. Department of Agriculture, Agricultural Research Service, Ames, Iowa.*

Peter R. Woolcock, PH.D., M.SC., B.SC., *Senior Research Associate, Cornell University, Duck Research Laboratory, Eastport, New York.*

Loveday O. Wosu, B.VET.MED., M.SC., PH.D., *Department of Veterinary Medicine, University of Nigeria, Nsukka, Nigeria.*

Jeffrey D. Wyatt, D.V.M., *Associate Professor, Division of Laboratory Animal Medicine, and Chief, Clinical Medicine, University of Rochester, School of Medicine and Dentistry, Rochester, New York.*

Richard Yamamoto, M.A., PH.D., *Professor of Microbiology, Department of Epidemiology and Preventive Medicine, School of Veterinary Medicine, University of California, Davis, California.*

G.O. Yang, PH.D., *Professor, Chinese Academy of Preventive Medicine, Institute of Nutrition and Food Hygiene, Beijing, China.*

William D.G. Yates, D.V.M., PH.D., *Director, Health of Animals Laboratory, Agriculture Canada, and Adjunct Professor of Veterinary Pathology, Western College of Veterinary Medicine, University of Saskatchewan, Saskatoon, Saskatchewan, Canada.*

Juan Manuel L. Zertuche, M.V.Z., *College of Veterinary Medicine, University of Florida, Gainesville, Florida.*

Dean R. Zimmerman, PH.D., *Professor of Animal Nutrition, Department of Animal Science, Iowa State University, Ames, Iowa.*

Gene M. Zinn, D.V.M., PH.D., *Veterinary Extension Specialist, University of Illinois, College of Veterinary Medicine, Simpson, Illinois.*

PART I

BLOOD, LYMPHATIC, AND CARDIOVASCULAR SYSTEMS

1

BLOOD AND LYMPHATIC SYSTEM, INTRODUCTION

At the cellular level, the hemolymphatic system comprises red blood cells (RBC), platelets, granulocytes (neutrophils, eosinophils, basophils), monocytes/macrophages, and lymphocytes. Organs of the system include the hematopoietic organs (bone marrow and spleen) and the lymphopoietic tissues (bone marrow, thymus, lymph nodes, tonsils, spleen, and Peyer's patches). Because of the functional diversity of the hemolymphatic system, its diseases are best discussed from a functional perspective. Several functional units are present: the erythron (RBC), the thrombon (platelets), the phagocytic system (granulocytes and macrophages), and the specific immune system (lymphocytes). (*See also* IMMUNE SYSTEM, p 421 *et seq.*)

THE ERYTHRON

The function of the erythron is to carry oxygen to the tissues at pressures sufficient to permit rapid diffusion of oxygen from the blood to the metabolizing cells. This is done by 1) a carrier molecule (hemoglobin [Hgb]), 2) a vehicle (RBC) capable of getting the intact carrier molecule to the cellular level, and 3) a metabolism geared to protect both the vehicle cell and the carrier molecule from damage. Interference with Hgb synthesis, RBC production, or RBC metabolism causes diseases of the erythron.

Hgb is a complex molecule, the principal components of which are porphyrin, heme, and globin. Each molecule is formed of 4 heme units attached to 4 globins (2 α and 2 β globins). Since each heme contains an oxygen-carrying iron molecule, each Hgb can carry 4 oxygen molecules to the tissues. Heme synthesis occurs enzymatically on the mitochondria and involves a series of condensation reactions that require pyridoxal phosphate and copper. Iron is added in the last step by the ferrochelatase enzyme. Several of the steps, including the incorporation of iron, are blocked by lead. Globin synthesis is under genetic control and balances heme production.

Interference with the normal production of heme or globin leads to a cytoplasmic-maturation-defect anemia. Causes include deficiencies of copper, iron, and pyridoxal phosphate, and lead poisoning. The thalassemias and hemoglobinopathies, important genetic diseases described in man, have not been observed in other animals. In these conditions the production of globins (α or β, or both) does not balance heme production, and the Hgb is not functional.

Red cell mass, and thus oxygen-carrying capacity, remains constant over time in the normal individual. Mature RBC have a finite life span, and their production and destruction must be carefully balanced, or disease ensues.

Erythropoiesis is regulated by erythropoietin (which stimulates in times of demand, and regulates normal production). Tissue hypoxia is the stimulus for production of erythropoietin, and in most species the kidney is believed to be both the sensor organ and the major site of its production. Erythropoietin acts on the marrow in concert with other humoral mediators to increase the number of stem cells entering RBC production, to shorten RBC maturation time, and to cause early release of reticulocytes. Other factors, many of which are poorly understood, affect erythropoiesis: these include the supply of nutrients (iron, folate, vitamin B_{12}); disorders such as inflammation, infection, malignancy, and renal or endocrine insufficiency; and cell-cell interactions between erythroid precursors, lymphoid cells, and other components of the hematopoietic microenvironment.

Red cell destruction also is regulated. Two mechanisms exist for removal of senescent RBC; both conserve the principal constituents of the cell for reutilization. About 1% of normal aging RBC are removed by intravascular hemolysis, which releases free Hgb; this is quickly converted to Hgb dimers that form complexes with haptoglobin and are transported to the liver. A portion of the free Hgb also may be converted to methemoglobin, which is quickly broken down to heme and globin. The globin protein chains may be recycled immediately; heme is bound to a second serum carrier protein, hemopexin, and carried to the liver and spleen for processing by the fixed monocyte/macrophage system. About 100 g of Hgb/dL can be handled by these transport systems; when this level is exceeded, as in intravascular hemolytic anemias, Hgb (and therefore iron) is excreted in the urine.

Removal of most aged RBC normally occurs by phagocytosis by the fixed macrophages of the spleen. As the cell ages, it loses its flexibility due to impaired ATP production and becomes trapped in the spleen, unable to percolate through the splenic sinusoids. Following phagocytosis, Hgb is converted to heme and globin, and the latter is recycled. Iron is released from the heme moiety and stored by the macrophage as ferritin or hemosiderin, or released into the circulation for transport back to the marrow. The remaining porphyrin is converted to free bilirubin, which is released by the macrophages into the systemic circulation where it complexes with albumin for transport to the hepatocytes. In extravascular hemolytic anemias, RBC have a shortened life span and the same mechanisms occur at an increased rate.

Normal RBC metabolism maintains both structural and functional integrity of the cell. The principal metabolic pathway of RBC is glycolysis, and the main energy source in most species is glucose. Glucose enters RBC by an insulin-independent mechanism, and most is metabolized via the glycolytic scheme, which produces ATP and reduced nicotinamide adenine dinucleotide (NADH). The energy of ATP is used to maintain RBC membrane pumps, which in turn maintain RBC shape and flexibility. The reducing potential of the NADH is utilized via the methemoglobin reductase pathway to maintain the iron in Hgb in its reduced form. The glucose not utilized in glycolysis is metabolized via a second pathway, the hexose monophosphate shunt (HMP). No energy is produced via the HMP; rather, as in the methemoglobin reductase pathway, the principal effect of the HMP is reducing potential, this time in the form of reduced nicotinamide adenine dinucleotide phosphate (NADPH). NADPH, in conjunction with the glutathione reductase/peroxidase system, maintains the sulfhydryl groups of globin in their reduced state. The principal HMP enzyme is glucose-6-phosphate dehydrogenase.

Numerous RBC disorders are the direct result of abnormal RBC metabolism: interference with glycolysis (eg, inherited deficiency of pyruvate kinase, a key glycolytic enzyme) causes ATP deficiency, which leads to reduced RBC life span and hemolytic anemia. Excessive oxidant stress may overload the protective HMP shunt or methemoglobin reductase pathways, and thereby cause Heinz body hemolysis or methemoglobin formation, respectively. Many drug-induced hemolytic anemias, such as phenothiazine hemolysis in horses, or methylene-blue-induced hemolysis in cats, are examples of this mechanism of disease. See also ANEMIA, p 15.

THE PHAGOCYTIC SYSTEM
(The nonspecific immune system)

The principal function of phagocytes is to defend against invading microorganisms by ingesting and destroying them; thus, they constitute an important component of the cellular inflammatory response. There are 2 types of phagocytes: mononuclear phagocytes and granulocytes. Mononuclear phagocytes arise primarily from the marrow and are released into the blood as monocytes where they may circulate for several hours before entering the tissue and differentiating to tissue macrophages. Granulocytes have a segmented nucleus and are classified according to their staining characteristics as neutrophils, eosinophils, or basophils. Five distinct stages in the process of phagocytosis have been identified: 1) attraction of phagocytes (chemotaxis) to microorganisms, 2) attachment to the organism, 3) ingestion, 4) fusion of cell lysosomes with ingested microorganisms and bacterial killing, and 5) digestion.

In addition to their general phagocytic function, many of the cells have other specialized functions. Monocytes form a link to the specific immune system by processing antigen for presentation to lymphocytes. They also are linked to the RBC by the iron, which they store and release for Hgb synthesis. Eosinophils, while they have a role as phagocytes, also have more specific functions that include providing a defense against metazoan parasites and modulating inflammatory processes. They respond chemotactically to histamine, immune complexes, and eosinophil chemotactic factor of anaphylaxis, a substance released by degranulating mast cells. Eosinophilia may be observed with systemic allergic reactions and parasitic disease. Basophils are not true phagocytes, but contain large amounts of histamine as well as other mediators of inflammation, and are important to the normal progression of the acute inflammatory response. As with the RBC, the production and blood levels of phagocytes are tightly regulated and controlled by various humoral factors, including colony-stimulating factors and interleukins. Unlike the RBC, which remain circulating in the blood, the phagocytes use this compartment as a highway to the tissues. Consequently, blood levels of these cells reflect various circumstances in the tissues, such as inflammation (both duration and severity), as well as the ability of the bone marrow to meet the tissue demand for phagocytes. The sensitivity with which blood phagocytes reflect these conditions varies from species to species. Abnormal response of the phagocytes may result in disease. Finally, phagocyte precursors may undergo malignant transformation, which results in leukemia.

THE SPECIFIC IMMUNE SYSTEM

Lymphocytes are responsible for both humoral and cellular immunity. Cells of the 2 branches of the immune system cannot be differentiated morphologically, but they differ in their dynamics of production and circulation. Lymphocyte production in mammals originates in the bone marrow; differentiation then progresses along 2 different pathways. Some of the lymphocytes migrate to the thymus and differentiate further under the influence of thymic hormones; these become "T cells" and are responsible for cellular immunity. Some of the T cells seed the secondary lymphoid organs (spleen and lymph nodes). The remaining lymphocytes migrate directly to the secondary lymphoid organs without undergoing modification in the thymus and become the "B cells", which are responsible for humoral immunity.

Thus, the secondary lymphoid organs have populations of both B and T lymphocytes. In the lymph nodes, follicular centers are primarily B cells, and parafollicular zones are primarily T cells. In the spleen, most of the lymphocytes of the red pulp are B cells, whereas lymphocytes of the periarteriolar lymphoid sheaths are T cells. Close association of T cells and B cells within lymphoid organs is essential to immune function; T cells regulate antibody production by B cells.

Lymphocyte function in the cellular immune system features both afferent (receptor) and efferent (effector) components. Long-lived T cells of the peripheral blood (which account for ~2/3 of the circulating lymphocytes in most species) are the receptors. In response to antigens to which they have been previously sensitized, they leave the circulation and undergo blast transformation to form activated T cells, which in turn cause other T cells to undergo blast transformation, both locally and systemically. Most of the T cells thus stimulated are effector cells and produce effector substances known as lymphokines. Effector lymphokines have a wide range of activities and are named accordingly: macrophage accelerating factor attracts macrophages into areas of antigen localization; migration inhibitory factor prevents macrophage exit; lymphotoxin, a product of killer T cells, can destroy various cell types.

The humoral immune system is composed of B lymphocytes that produce antibodies of several classes; their activation is similar to activation of T lymphocytes. When sensitized B lymphocytes encounter antigen, they undergo blast transformation and divide. Activated B lymphocytes differentiate into plasma cells, the major source of antibody. Therefore, each B lymphocyte initially stimulated produces a clone of plasma cells, all producing the same specific antibody.

Antibody molecules (immunoglobulins [Ig]) fall into several classes: IgG, IgM, IgA, IgD, and IgE. Not all classes have been described in all species. Each class has its own functional characteristics; eg, IgA is the principal antibody of respiratory and intestinal secretion, IgG is the principal antibody of the circulating blood, and IgE is the principal antibody involved in allergic reactions.

Antibodies perform their function by combining with the specific antigens that stimulated their production. Antigen-antibody complexes may be specifically chemotactic for phagocytes, or they may activate complement, a process that produces both cell lysis and substances chemotactic for neutrophils and macrophages. In this manner, the humoral immune system is related to, and interacts with, the nonspecific immune system.

The humoral immune system also is related to both the nonspecific immune system and the cellular immune system in other ways. There is good evidence that one of the principal functions of the cellular immune system is to regulate the humoral immune system. Both "helper" and "repressor" T-cell classes have been described. Helper T cells are required for full expression of a humoral immune response; repressor T cells dampen the production of a given antibody. Killer T cells destroy foreign cell types. Antigen processing by macrophages precedes recognition of an antigen by lymphocytes. These complex processes also are involved in surveillance of neoplastic cells and recognition of "self".

Lymphocyte response in disease may be appropriate (activation of the immune system) or inappropriate (immune-mediated and lymphoproliferative disorders). (See also IMMUNE SYSTEM, p 421 et seq.) One form of immune-mediated disease results from failure of the immune system to recognize host tissues as self. For example, in autoimmune hemolytic anemia, antibodies are produced against the host's own RBC. Another inappropriate response of the immune system is anaphylaxis. In allergic individuals, IgE antibodies to allergens are bound to the surface of basophils and mast cells. When exposure to the allergen occurs, antigen-antibody complexes are formed, and degranulation of the mast cells and basophils releases large amounts of vasoactive amines, which cause shock.

Lymphoproliferative diseases are of several varieties and include lymphosarcoma and the lymphocytic leukemias. While most represent true neoplastic processes, others represent reactive conditions and are benign, eg, persistent lymphocytosis in bovine-leukemia-virus-infected cattle and the large number of atypical lymphocytes sometimes observed in the circulation following vaccinations with modified live virus.

THE THROMBON

Functionally, platelets form the initial hemostatic plug whenever hemorrhage occurs; they also are the source of phospholipid (platelet factor 3 [PF 3]), which is needed for normal coagulation. Platelets play a major role in the inflammatory response by releasing various mediators. They are produced in the bone marrow from megakaryocytes, the regulatory control of which is poorly understood. Actual platelet production occurs with invagination of the megakaryocyte cell membrane and the formation of cytoplasmic channels and islands. The cytoplasmic islands produce platelets by fragmentation from the megakaryocyte.

Mature circulating platelets are densely packed with structures that contain functional substances, including dense granules containing ATP, adenosine diphosphate (ADP), and calcium, as well as serotonin, lysosomes, glycogen, mitochondria, and an intracellular canalicular system formed by invaginations of the platelet external cell membrane. The mitochondria and glycogen are involved in energy production; the dense granules contain the essential chemical substances involved in the regulation and modulation of platelet function (and to some degree inflammation) via the release reaction; and the canalicular system serves both as a transport system for granule components and as a source of PF 3, which is found in high concentration in the membrane lining of the canals.

When vessel walls are damaged, collagen is exposed and circulating platelets adhere and undergo a change in shape with the accompanying release of ADP. ADP stimulates local platelet aggregation with the formation of the primary platelet plug. Change of platelet shape and the release reaction expose PF 3 to the coagulation factors, thereby providing a surface for coagulation and accelerating the clotting process and fibrin formation. The local accumulation of fibrin and platelets is known as hemostatic plug (clot) formation. The clot is consolidated by the action of platelet contractile proteins.

Platelet disorders are either quantitative (thrombocytopenias or thrombocytoses) or qualitative (thrombocytopathies). Thrombocytopenia is one of the most common causes of bleeding disorders in animals. In general, platelet counts must fall to <50,000/μL before there is danger of hemorrhage. Three forms of thrombocytopenia occur: destructive, distributive, and hypoproliferative.

Destructive or consumptive thrombocytopenias are the most important. In these conditions, there is increased removal of platelets as well as increased production by the bone marrow. One common form of consumptive thrombocytopenia occurs with disseminated intravascular coagulation (DIC), secondary to a variety of diseases. A second form is immune-mediated, in which platelets become coated with antiplatelet antibodies and are removed from the circulation by the fixed phagocyte system.

Distributive thrombocytopenias are associated with excessive sequestration of platelets by the spleen, such as occurs in hypersplenism or in canine congestive heart failure. In cases of hypersplenism, it has been estimated that up to 80% of all circulating platelets may be sequestered.

Hypoproliferative thrombocytopenias are characterized by decreased marrow production of platelets. These conditions are often idiopathic, but can be caused by various drugs (eg, thiazide diuretics, gold salts), or be associated with myelophthisic syndromes or myelofibrosis.

Thrombocytosis occurs only rarely and is often idiopathic. It may be associated with primary marrow disease and is a well-documented occurrence in myelofibrosis in both man and dogs. Platelet leukemia (megakaryocytic myelosis or primary thrombocythemia) is also rare but has been documented in man, dogs, and cats.

Thrombocytopathies comprise a poorly defined group of diseases in which platelet numbers are normal, but their function is impaired. Several conditions have been described, most important among which are PF 3 and platelet serotonin deficiencies; drug-induced platelet dysfunction; kidney, thyroid, and liver dysfunction; and thrombasthenia, in which clot retraction is impaired. Von Willebrand's disease, which has been reported in dogs, pigs, and rabbits, is characterized by both a plasma coagulation defect and thrombocytopathy (see also HEMOSTATIC DISORDERS, p 52 et seq).

CARDIOVASCULAR SYSTEM, INTRODUCTION

The cardiovascular system is the transport system that delivers oxygen, substrates, hormones, and regulatory chemicals to all cells; transports carbon dioxide and other waste products of metabolism from the cells to the lungs or kidneys; and redistributes heat from inside the body to the outside, or vice versa. This is accomplished by a closed system of vessels that contain blood, which carries the substances to be transported. Blood moves through the system because of pressure gradients produced by the pumping action of the heart. The left ventricle pumps blood from the pulmonary veins (keeping pulmonary venous pressure low) into the systemic arteries (keeping systemic arterial pressure high), while the right ventricle pumps blood from the systemic veins (keeping that pressure low) into the pulmonary arteries (keeping that pressure high). These pressure gradients (high in the arteries and low in the veins) drive blood through the capillary circulations (systemic and pulmonary), where substances are exchanged between blood and cells. Valves present in the heart and veins insure unidirectional flow.

The amount of blood the heart pumps each minute (cardiac output) is the product of heart rate (beats/min) times the volume of blood (stroke volume) pumped each beat. Normally, the cardiac output is ~100 mL/kg body wt/min. The smaller the animal (eg, dog versus horse), the higher the cardiac output/unit body wt. During exercise, cardiac output may increase almost 10-fold, most (~80%) due to increased heart rate, and a smaller amount due to increased stroke volume.

Various parameters of cardiac function are important to understand disease and its management. Heart rate, contractility, preload, and afterload are 4 major determinants of cardiac performance that should be assessed when heart disease is suspected. The number of beats/min is determined by the rate of discharge of the sinoatrial (SA) node located at the junction of the cranial vena cava and right atrium. Rate of discharge and speed of conduction are determined by a balance between β-adrenergic efferent activity (increases heart rate) and vagal efferent activity (decreases heart rate). Agents that mimic β-adrenergic activity (eg, epinephrine, isoproterenol) increase, and those that mimic vagal efferent activity (eg, edrophonium, acetylcholine) decrease both heart rate and speed of conductance. β-Adrenergic blocking agents (eg, propranolol, atenolol) or vagolytic agents (eg, atropine, glycopyrrolate) decrease or increase heart rate and conductance, respectively. A resting dog's heart rate is normally irregular, increasing during inspiration and decreasing during expiration, in what is termed respiratory sinus arrhythmia. The heart rate becomes regular and faster during excitement, exercise, fever, pain, or many disease states.

The chambers of the heart normally beat in a coordinated, orderly sequence as determined by their electrical activation. After the SA node discharges, the impulse spreads through the atria, produces the P wave of the electrocardiogram (ECG), and initiates atrial contraction (atrial systole). As it spreads through the ventricles, it produces the QRS complex of the ECG and initiates ventricular contraction (ventricular systole). In diastole, the chambers of the heart are relaxed and fill with blood. The atrioventricular (AV) node is the weakest part of the AV conduction system; it conducts slowly and sometimes fails to conduct (AV block).

Force of ventricular contraction depends on 2 major factors: myocardial contractility (inotropism) and volume of blood in the chamber just before it contracts (preload). Inotropism is an inherent property of the muscle, but it increases with increasing levels (either humoral or neural) of catecholamines, and decreases with increased vagal efferent activity and with many disease states (eg, myocardial inflammation, drug intoxication, cardiomyopathy). Preload is determined by the volume of blood within the cardiovascular system, the venous return of blood to the heart, the force with which the atria pump blood into the ventricles, and the stiffness of the ventricular myocardium. The Frank-Starling law states that the greater the preload, the greater the force of contraction, all other factors remaining constant. Of course, the force generated by the ventricle is also affected by the resistance encountered by the ventricle (afterload): if arterial blood pressure is low, the ventricle generates less force, although it may move blood easily from veins to arteries; conversely, if arterial pressure is high, the ventricle may generate great force but move little blood.

This difference between systolic and diastolic arterial pressure (the pulse pressure) is determined by stroke volume, arterial compliance, the interval between heartbeats, and the volume of blood that leaves the arteries during diastole. Diseases that produce a high or "bounding" pulse pressure include arteriosclerosis, aortic insufficiency, patent ductus arteriosus, and other peripheral arteriovenous fistulas. Narrow, weak, pulse pressure is characteristic of a low stroke volume. Reduced stroke volume may be due to reduced preload or inadequate ventricular filling (as in hemorrhage, dehydration, pericardial effusion or tamponade, and tachyarrhythmias), reduced contractility (as in cardiomyopathies, acidosis, and many cardiac diseases), or increased afterload (arterial or pulmonary arterial hypertension—as may occur with renal disease or canine heartworm disease). Ejection fraction (EF) is a useful measure of ventricular function; it is the ratio between stroke volume and end-diastolic volume (preload). EF is normally >0.6, indicating that the ventricle ejects >60% of the preload during each stroke, and that ~40% of the preload remains within the ventricle after it ejects a stroke volume. The remaining volume is called the end-systolic volume.

Afterload, or the impedance to ventricular ejection, results from the need to accelerate blood into the aorta (to overcome its inertia), from the need to overcome the stiffness of the great vessels, and most importantly, from peripheral resistance to blood flow. Resistance is determined primarily by the diameter of the arterioles. Since mean pressure = blood flow × peripheral resistance, mean arterial blood pressure = cardiac output × peripheral resistance. The arterioles or resistance vessels are primary determinants of afterload and thus cardiac performance, as well as blood pressure and blood flow. Arteriolar diameter is controlled by neural, hormonal, and local factors that influence vascular smooth muscle. Regional differences in the relative influence of these factors exist in blood vessels going to and within various organs. Vasoconstriction generally results from any increase in sympathetic activity, specifically α-adrenergic efferent activity. Other agents that cause vasoconstriction include α-adrenergic catecholamines (epinephrine, norepinephrine, phenylephrine), vasopressin (ADH), angiotensin II, prostaglandins A and F, and serotonin (released from platelets). Disease states that cause an increase in these substances increase peripheral resistance. Arteriolar vasodilators include substances that block α-adrenergic receptors (eg, prazosin, phenoxybenzamine), stimulate β_2-adrenergic or dopaminergic receptors (eg, isoproterenol, dopamine), or act directly on vascular smooth muscle to cause its relaxation (eg, hydralazine). Many substances released locally in response to inadequate tissue blood flow, or tissue injury or inflammation cause vasodilation (eg, decreased O_2, increased CO_2, H^+, K^+, adenosine, histamine, bradykinin); there is little resting venous tone. Therefore, while venous smooth muscle can respond similarly to arterial smooth muscle, venodilation occurs only if there is previous venoconstriction.

The concept of myocardial oxygen consumption is important in understanding both heart disease and its treatment. The myocardium always consumes nearly all the oxygen delivered to it by the coronary arteries. The only way for more oxygen to be delivered to the heart (if it needs more to do increased work) is via an increase in coronary blood flow. The coronary arteries therefore dilate in response to vasodilatory substances produced by myocardial metabolism. Diseases that narrow coronary arteries (arteriosclerosis, atherosclerosis) severely limit the ability of the myocardium to meet increased demands. The amount of oxygen required by the myocardium is determined by 3 factors: heart rate, inotropism, and tension in the myocardial wall. Rapid heart rates are most deleterious; they increase myocardial oxygen demand while limiting the period of diastole when cardiac filling occurs and most coronary blood flows. Myocardial wall tension increases when the heart dilates and when it must generate more pressure to eject blood. In general terms, peak tension = preload × arterial blood pressure; it is often given the name afterload. Successful therapy of heart disease should slow heart rate if tachycardia is present, decrease cardiac size if dilatation or increased preload (or both) is present, and reduce afterload if arterial pressure is increased.

For the cardiovascular system to function properly, blood volume and pressure must be controlled within rather narrow limits. Detectors that monitor pressure and flow are located throughout the body, and the limits are normally maintained through neurohumoral reflexes. Examples include pressure receptors in the systemic arteries at the bifurcation of the carotid artery and at the aortic arch, volume receptors in the relatively low-pressure atria, and flow receptors in the kidney at the juxtaglomerular apparatus. These detectors send neural or humoral (or both) signals to the hypothalamus and medulla oblongata, which compare (integrate) the level detected with the level required for optimal function. The integrator, when there is a discrepancy between the desired and the actual level of the variable, sends neural or humoral signals (via vagal and/or sympathetic pathways) to the heart and blood vessels to adjust their function to accomodate the variable to the desired level. For example, if blood pressure is low, the carotid and aortic pressure receptors send fewer neural inhibitory impulses to the brain; the brain then sends neural impulses to the heart that increase its rate and force of contraction, and to the arterioles that make them constrict. These actions elevate systemic arterial blood pressure.

The various neurohumoral controls of the cardiovascular system enable animals to meet widely varying needs, including exercise and the demands of minor injury, tissue repair, inflammation, etc. These controlling mechanisms "compensate for" cardiovascular disease, and the compensatory effects and their consequences frequently can be detected as signs of disease (eg, tachycardia, elevated blood pressure, jugular venous distention, cardiac enlargement, fluid retention).

GENESIS OF SIGNS OF HEART DISEASE

Abnormal structure and function of the heart produce subjective and objective indications of these abnormalities (*see* TABLES 1 and 2, pp 12 and 13). Pharmacological therapy of heart disease usually is restricted to those cases in which signs (eg, cough, ascites, syncope, murmur of patent ductus arteriosus) indicate that either quality or duration of life is compromised.

The severity of signs is graded by functional classification as follows: Class I—no signs, even during strong exertion; II—signs only after strong exertion; III—signs after slight exertion; IV—signs, even at rest. For genesis of specific signs (eg, murmurs, voltage changes on ECG, dimensional changes on echocardiograms or radiographs), a cardiology textbook should be consulted. This discussion is limited to the genesis of those signs indicative of most heart diseases for which therapy can be instituted.

Whether due to weakened systolic force, outflow tract obstruction, a leaking valve, arrhythmia, or increased diastolic stiffness of the ventricle, the heart may fail to adequately empty venous circuits or perfuse arterial circuits, or both. Signs of such inadequate function constitute the clinical entities of heart failure and congestive heart failure. In the former, signs result from inadequate low cardiac output, either absolute or relative to the needs of the organs perfused; in the latter, signs result when capillaries and veins of specific organs are congested with blood. (*See also* HEART DISEASE, p 40.)

Heart Failure: Inadequate perfusion of the brain, skeletal muscles, kidneys, and the heart itself causes serious illness. Inadequate cerebral perfusion leads to a confused state, change in temperament, or, if severe enough, to syncope. Inappropriate perfusion of the kidneys leads to azotemia, sodium retention, oliguria, systemic arterial hypertension, and polydipsia—all may be produced by activation of the renin-angiotensin-aldosterone system. Inadequate perfusion of skeletal muscle leads to weakness (particularly of the hindquarters) and incoordinated movement, usually most pronounced during exertion or excitement when demands are greatest. Inadequate perfusion of the coronary circulation leads to further reduction in systolic and diastolic function or to arrhythmia, or both.

Primary diseases of the central or autonomic nervous systems, kidney, or skeletal muscles can produce similar syndromes.

Congestive Heart Failure (CHF): Signs of CHF result from fluid retention and damming-up of blood in veins and capillaries of organs in which venous effluent is impaired due to a failing ventricle. Two syndromes (or a combination) may occur: damming-up of blood in the lungs due to a failing left ventricle (left-sided CHF), and damming-up of blood in systemic organs due to a failing right ventricle (right-sided CHF). Often, signs of left- and right-sided heart failure occur concurrently because of the likelihood that disease (eg, fibrosis, doxorubicin hydrochloride toxicity) strikes both simultaneously.

Left-sided CHF: Primary failure of the left ventricle, mitral regurgitation, or large left-to-right shunts cause blood volume to increase and may cause damming-up in the left atrium, pulmonary veins, and pulmonary capillaries. This makes the lungs relatively heavy, and the ventral portions may become compressed. Hilar edema, pulmonary congestion, and compression all result in remarkable differences in ventilation of the lungs, ventilation-perfusion mismatch, hypoxia, and cyanosis. If hypoxia is prolonged, polycythemia may develop. The lungs also become stiffer than normal; thus, work of respiration is increased, and minimal exertion may fatigue the animal. The portion of the lungs that is compressed normally during expiration may become so compressed that rales (crackles) are heard as the airways close and again when they open. To aid the primary muscles of ventilation, the affected animal may stand with thoracic limbs abducted and head extended; if the abdominal muscles are used, a "heave line" is produced. Because lying down limits motion of the abdomen and thorax, as well as facilitates venous return to the heart, animals with left-sided CHF often stand or sit to the point of exhaustion. If carried, the animal may become more hypoxic and even faint or die due to restriction of ventilation.

Due to elevation of pulmonary capillary pressure, serum may weep from the pulmonary capillaries into the lungs; if that exceeds the rate at which pulmonary lymphatics can remove the fluid, pulmonary edema develops. This makes the lungs still heavier and may impair diffusion of oxygen between alveolus and capillary. Thus, not only is there a ventilation-perfusion abnormality, but also a diffusion abnormality that produces even greater hypoxemia.

When the left atrium is dilated (especially with mitral regurgitation), it may compress the left mainstem bronchus. This often produces the brassy cough of large-airway disease as well as supraventricular tachyarrhythmias (eg, atrial premature beats or atrial fibrillation) due to stretching and irritation of the left atrial myocardium. Production by atrial cells of atrial natriuretic factor is a signal of atrial distention. This substance promotes loss of sodium and water by the kidneys, but also antagonizes the effects of angiotensin II. Finally, if the left atrium is dilated enough, and the pressure within is high enough, the left atrium may tear, which results in pericardial tamponade and possibly acute collapse and death.

Right-sided CHF: With failure of the right ventricle or with tricuspid regurgitation, fluid is also retained, and blood may dam-up in the right atrium, vena cavae, veins draining into the vena cavae, and capillaries draining into those veins. Thus, systemic organs—including the liver—become congested with blood. If the hepatic capillary hydrostatic pressure is elevated enough, serum may weep from its capillaries faster than it can be absorbed from the abdominal cavity by the lymphatics, and ascites develops. Elevated capillary pressure in other dependent portions of the body (eg, brisket, limbs, prepuce) also can cause edema of those regions. When the liver becomes engorged, it fails to transaminate and manufacture albumin; the lowered serum protein reduces oncotic pressure (hypoproteinemia), and edema becomes even more severe. Since all veins become engorged, distention of the jugular vein and other superficial veins can be seen; in left-sided CHF, distention of the pulmonary veins can be seen radiographically.

Because of elevation of left atrial and pulmonary venous pressures, the ventricle expands to a greater than normal volume during diastole (increased left ventricular preload). Increased preload has both good and bad consequences: the force of ventricular contraction increases, since the fibers are stretched more; however, increased preload causes the ventricular myocardium to consume a disproportionately greater amount of oxygen for the pressure it generates, which may cause a myocardial oxygen debt and further deterioration of ventricular function.

Ventricular gallop detected on cardiac auscultation is a valuable clinical sign of heart failure in small animals. Gallops occur when the ventricle becomes relatively stiff—because it is dilated, hypertrophied, hypoxic, fibrotic, or intoxicated—and diastolic filling is impeded. The filling rate changes from very rapid to slow rather abruptly and, when the sudden deceleration occurs, cardiohemic structures develop oscillations of audiofrequency that produce an extra heart sound either immediately after the second heart sound (S_3 gallop) or immediately before the first (S_4 gallop). S_3 gallops are frequently associated with volume-overloaded ventricles (dilated, congestive cardiomyopathy), whereas S_4 gallops are frequently associated with hypertrophic, stiff ventricles (hypertrophic cardiomyopathy).

Table 1. Classification of Heart Disease

1. Valvular
    Regurgitation (mitral, tricuspid, aortic)
    Stenosis (pulmonic, aortic)

2. Shunts
    Left-to-right (atrial septal defect, ventricular
    septal defect, patent ductus arteriosus)
    Right-to-left (tetralogy of Fallot, Eisenmenger's complex)

3. Decreased Systolic Function
    Arteriolosclerosis—hypoxia
    Dilative cardiomyopathy
    Drug intoxication (halothane, adriamycin)
    Myocardial fibrosis
    Myocarditis

4. Decreased Diastolic Function
    Hypertrophic cardiomyopathy
    Hypoxia
    Myocardial fibrosis
    Pericardial constriction

5. Arrhythmia
    Atrial fibrillation
    Complete heart block
    Sinoatrial syncope
    Ventricular premature depolarizations

6. Miscellaneous
    Electrolyte—acid-base imbalance
    Heartworm infection
    Hypertension—renal
    Hypoadrenocorticism
    Neoplasia (myxoma, chemodectoma, lymphosarcoma)
    Pulmonary (blue bloater, high altitude)
    Thyrotoxic heart disease
    Trauma (hit by car, hardware disease)
    Uremic heart disease

Table 2. Signs of Heart Disease

1. Seen: weakness, disorientation, limb abduction, bulging eyes, neck extension, cyanosis, polydipsia, reluctance to lie down, syncope, ascites, edema, fatigue, dyspnea, jugular venous distention

2. Felt: deviation of precordial heave, venous distention, feeble pulse, waterhammer pulse, hepatomegaly, thrill, tachycardia, bradycardia, arrhythmia

3. Heard: cough, murmur, rub, rales, rhonchi, bronchial sounds, gallops (S_4, S_3), clicks, split S_2

4. Blood Analysis: eosinophilia, basophilia, neutrophilia, hyponatremia, microfilaremia, elevated or depressed thyroxine, elevated BUN or creatinine, polycythemia, decreased oxygen, serology

5. Special Techniques (radiography, ECG, echocardiogram): pulmonary edema, pleural effusion, alveolar pattern, pericardial effusion, dilatation, hypertrophy, high/low voltage, ectopic beats, hypokinesia

Table 3. Arrhythmias and Antiarrhythmics

1. Sinus Tachycardia, Atrial Tachycardia, Atrial Fibrillation
   β-Blockers: propranolol, atenolol
   Digitalis glycosides: digoxin, digitoxin
   Calcium channel blockers: diltiazem, verapamil

2. Ventricular Tachycardia
   Emergency: lidocaine
   Chronic
      a)   Class I antiarrhythmics: procainamide, quinidine, tocainide
      b)   β-Blockers: propranolol, atenolol
      c)   If refractory: amiodarone, bretylium

PRINCIPLES OF THERAPY

The goals of therapy are to regulate cardiac rhythm and rate, restore blood volume, strengthen systolic force, mobilize or remove edema fluids, reduce the regurgitant fraction, and balance myocardial oxygen supply and demand.

Selection of a particular therapeutic approach depends on which features of the cardiovascular system are abnormal. Because of a faulty ignition system or irritation of foci in either the atria (termed supraventricular) or specialized conductile tissue of the ventricles (termed ventricular), the heart may beat too rapidly to permit filling in diastole, too slowly to eject sufficient quantities of blood in systole, or too irregularly to permit either. Such disturbances are termed arrhythmias. Agents that restore a regular rhythm and rate are termed antiarrhythmics (*see* TABLE 3). However, antiarrhythmics may actually produce or exaggerate the very arrhythmias for which they were intended—a proarrhythmic effect. Thus, their potential for benefit must be balanced against that for harm; the proarrhythmic action of antiarrhythmic drugs may be lethal.

Another important strategy in treating heart failure is to strengthen muscles of ventilation; they have been weakened due to poor oxygenation and need to generate greater than normal tension to ventilate congested and/or edematous lungs. Aminophylline and digitalis both increase the strength of contraction of the diaphragm; therefore they exert beneficial effects by 2 routes (ie, by strengthening both heart and diaphragm); aminophylline also causes bronchodilation of small airways.

If blood loss due to hemorrhage, dehydration, or sequestration of blood in certain organs occurs, the amount of blood returning to the heart (and thus the preload) is decreased. Because of the Frank-Starling relationship, the force of contraction and cardiac output are reduced. Agents used to restore blood volume to assure adequate preload are whole blood, plasma, and crystalloid and colloid solutions.

Because of metabolic (eg, depletion of ATP) or structural (eg, faulty valves, myocardial fibrosis) defects, the ventricles may fail to generate a contraction forceful enough to pump adequate quantities of blood. If signs (eg, weakness, fainting, oliguria) result from inadequate blood flow to specific organs, the animal is in heart failure. Systolic force of the heart muscle (myocardial contractility) can be strengthened with positive inotropes (eg, digitalis, dobutamine, milrinone). If the ventricle does not empty blood from the venous compartments, their capillary beds become engorged and serum oozes from the capillaries into the interstices of the organs involved. If the rate of oozing exceeds the rate at which the lymphatics can drain the interstices, the tissues become edematous. If signs are produced by this capillary engorgement and edema, the animal is in CHF.

Large breeds of dogs may develop heart failure because of carnitine deficiency. This amino acid is found in red meat and dairy products. Carnitine is required to transport acetyl coenzyme A into the mitochondria, where it can be used for production of ATP (the energy source for both contraction and relaxation of myocardium). Cats require a great deal of taurine, an amino acid that is often synthesized in inadequate amounts. The precise role of taurine in contraction is not known; however, a deficiency results in decreased myocardial contractility. It is possible that most dilated cardiomyopathies in both dogs and cats result from dietary deficiencies and/or decreased biosynthesis of these 2 amino acids. Animals ill because of these deficiencies often respond dramatically to supplementation. Dietary considerations in both prevention and therapy of heart failure are extremely important.

Edema fluids should be mobilized or removed. This is done with diuretics (eg, furosemide) and a sodium-restricted diet; or if the fluid is "free" within cavities, by paracentesis. If the aperture of the arterioles has decreased and they offer too much resistance to flow of blood into the capillaries; or, if the aorta and other large arteries are too stiff to accommodate easily the left ventricular stroke volume (ie, the afterload is too great), then the ventricle—particularly if it is weakened or afflicted with a diseased valve—may fail to pump adequate quantities of blood. Therapy should reduce this interference to the flow of blood into and through the arterial system, and thus improve peripheral circulation and reduce the strain on the ventricle. Agents that make the aorta more compliant and the aperture of the systemic arterioles greater (eg, captopril, hydralazine, prazosin) are termed afterload reducers.

Mitral regurgitation, a condition in which blood leaks retrograde from the left ventricle into the left atrium, produces dilation, irritation, and possibly rupture of the left atrium, and causes that chamber to compress the left mainstem bronchus. The regurgitant fraction should be reduced. By reducing the afterload on the left ventricle, less force is needed to sustain the forward flow of blood; therefore, less blood flows retrograde across the insufficient mitral valve. This permits decreased size of the left atrium, and reduction in signs attributable to distention of that chamber. Thus, afterload reducers improve forward flow when the left ventricle is failing, and reduce regurgitant fraction (ratio of blood regurgitated to that pumped out that aortic valve) in mitral insufficiency.

Another therapy for pulmonary congestion and edema, and to decrease mitral regurgitation, is preload reducers (eg, furosemide, nitroglycerine). These agents dilate systemic veins, which are then filled with blood from the pulmonary vessels. When fluid shifts from the pulmonary vessels to the peripheral veins, it does little or no harm because of its position in a rather innocuous compartment; and pressure within the pulmonary capillaries is reduced so that pulmonary edema lessens, and weight and stiffness of the lungs decrease. Furthermore, as left atrial volume decreases, the stretching effect of that increased volume on the mitral annulus decreases, the annular dimension decreases, the leaflets of the mitral valve become more competent, and the severity of mitral regurgitation may actually decrease.

Occasionally, because of inadequate lung function due to pulmonary disease (eg, pulmonary fibrosis, pneumonia, neoplasia) or because of disease of the intramural coronary arteries (arteriolosclerosis), portions of the ventricles, usually the left ventricular endocardium, suffer lack of oxygen (ischemia or hypoxia). If the oxygen deficit is severe or prolonged, the ischemic tissue may die or serve as a focus for arrhythmia. Ischemic tissue does not contribute its share to contraction and is stiffer than normal myocardium; consequently, it decreases myocardial contractility and reduces ventricular function. A serious arrhythmia arising from the ischemic tissue may cause sudden death.

The demand for and availability of oxygen must be balanced. Myocardial oxygen demand is determined primarily by heart rate, myocardial contractility, and peak ventricular myocardial tension. These determinants should be adjusted to the minimal levels compatible with adequate ventricular function. Thus, digitalis or propranolol, or both, may be used to slow the heart, and an afterload reducer used to decrease peak tension. Two dilemmas exist, however: 1) while digitalis slows the heart and thus decreases oxygen demand, it also increases contractility, which increases oxygen demand; and 2) when using an afterload reducer that lowers systemic arterial and coronary perfusion pressures, there is a risk of decreasing coronary blood flow and oxygen availability. To increase oxygen supply, pulmonary function must be improved by using bronchodilators (eg, aminophylline, terbutaline), antibiotics, antineoplastics, and increased concentrations of inspired oxygen, as indicated by specific clinical diagnoses.

Failing hearts that have been "driven" by elevated catecholamines of high adrenergic efferent activity have a reduced number of β-adrenergic receptor sites. Thus, if an emergency arises and the heart needs increased drive by a sympathoadrenal influence, the heart cannot respond because there are too few β-adrenergic receptors to which the catecholamines can bind. This is known as "down-regulation" of β-receptors and is a marker of chronic heart failure. β-Receptors can be "up-regulated", quite paradoxically, by using small amounts of substances that block them (eg, propranolol, atenolol). Although these β-blockers may block the receptors and weaken the heart ever so slightly, the net result is to strengthen the heart by increasing the number of β-receptors and the potential to respond to catecholamines. Thus, small doses of β-blockers offer a means of actually reversing the heart failure process. They are also antiarrhythmic and reduce the demand of the myocardium for oxygen, thus restoring a balance between oxygen demand and oxygen availability.

Many specific cardiovascular diseases have straightforward solutions. For abnormal communications (eg, patent ductus arteriosus, ventricular septal defect, atrial septal defect) or for valves that fail to open properly, surgery is best. For animals suffering from decreased preload due to pericardial constriction, removal of the strangulating pericardium is best.

Thus, in some instances (eg, patent ductus arteriosus, constrictive pericarditis, bacterial myocarditis), the goal of therapy is to remove the underlying cause; in other instances (eg, mitral regurgitation, cardiomyopathy, arteriolosclerosis), it is to minimize the consequences. In either case, therapeutic decisions and recommendations should be based on type and severity of the disease process, financial considerations, and quality of life. In general, sodium restriction is advocated to minimize fluid retention. Management is directed toward minimizing cardiac work with restricted physical activity, and normalizing heart rate and ventricular load(s).

ANEMIA

A condition characterized physiologically by insufficient circulating hemoglobin (Hgb) and clinically by reduced exercise tolerance and pale mucous membranes. It is due to decreased production, increased destruction, or loss of red blood cells (RBC); therapy is determined by which of these 3 situations predominates. The polychromatic cell (Wright's stain) or reticulocyte (New Methylene Blue stain) count is the most informative test to determine if the anemia is **responsive** (hemolysis or hemorrhage) or **unresponsive** (hypoproliferative). Anemias are classified to provide a rational basis for treatment.

Table 4. Classification of Anemias

I. Bone Marrow Hypofunction (**unresponsive** anemia)
  A. Decreased RBC production. Nutritional anemia, stem cell injury, myelophthisis (neoplastic infiltration), hematopoietic neoplasia.
  B. Reduction in Hgb synthesis. Deficiency of iron, vitamin E, or vitamin B_6.
  C. Immune-mediated stem cell suppression or destruction.
  D. Viral infections with marrow suppression (eg, retroviruses, parvoviruses).

II. Loss of Abnormal RBC (**responsive** anemia)
  A. RBC with deficient enzyme content. Heinz-body anemia, pyruvate kinase deficiency in Basenji dogs, hereditary anemia and dwarfism in Alaskan Malamutes, phosphofructokinase deficiency in English Springer Spaniels.
  B. Immune-mediated anemias. Isoimmune, idiopathic, and "innocent bystander"; hemolytic disease of the newborn.
  C. Hemolytic anemia due to intravascular fragmentation. Vasculitis of small arteries.

III. Loss of Normal RBC
  A. Hemolysis of normal RBC (**responsive**). Splenomegaly, RBC parasitism, chemical or physical injury.
  B. Loss of normal RBC (**poorly responsive to responsive**). External or internal hemorrhage or parasitism.

Laboratory diagnosis of anemia is based on values of Hgb, packed cell volume (PCV), and RBC. Anemia is characterized further by the RBC indices: mean corpuscular volume (MCV), mean corpuscular hemoglobin (MCH), and mean corpuscular hemoglobin concentration (MCHC). The MCH and MCHC provide similar information, but the MCHC is considered to be more accurate. Therefore, the 2 indices used most commonly are the MCV and MCHC. As rubricytes (RBC precursors) mature in bone marrow, their volume decreases as the Hgb content increases; thus, immature RBC released into the blood in responsive anemias have a higher MCV. Very large RBC (macrocytes) with a high MCV may have a normal total Hgb or MCH, although the percentage saturation (or MCHC) is below normal. These large cells contain RNA and stain blue with Wright's stain (polychromatophilic). They mature in blood in 12-48 hr by completion of Hgb synthesis and loss of their RNA and blue appearance. In 1 wk, they lose sufficient membrane to become normal in size (MCV) and appearance (normocytic). Since polychromasia is short-lived (12-48 hr), the presence of polychromatic RBC is the most sensitive indicator of marrow production. Since RBC indices are mean values, a moderate to marked change in the RBC population is necessary to shift the indices out of the normal range. Therefore, a mild anemia may be regenerative and have normal RBC indices. RBC indices are probably most helpful in recognition of iron deficiency anemia, in which the RBC become smaller (which lowers the MCV) and contain less Hgb (which lowers the MCH and MCHC). Therefore, decreased MCV, MCH, and MCHC indicate iron deficiency anemia.

Evaluation of the marrow erythroid response is most accurate when blood is supravitally stained with New Methylene Blue, and reticulocytes counted as a percentage of total RBC. Their absolute number should be determined to provide an answer that is independent of the degree of anemia; eg, in 1 μL of blood, a normal dog has 6.5×10^6 (6.5×10^{12}/L) RBC with 1% (65,000) reticulocytes; an anemic dog may have 2×10^6 (2×10^{12}/L) RBC with 3% (60,000) reticulocytes. Since the reticulocyte production of both dogs is nearly the same, the response of the anemic dog is poor. A good response is characterized by ≥3×10^5 reticulocytes/μL of blood, eg, 3×10^6 (3×10^{12}/L) RBC with 10% reticulocytes.

A simpler method of evaluating erythroid response is based on counting polychromatic RBC after Wright's or similar staining. The mean number of polychromatic RBC is determined for 10 oil-immersion fields over the length of the monolayer of the blood smear. A normal hemogram or an unresponsive anemia in the dog has 0-1 polychromatic RBC per field; mildly responsive anemias, 5 per field; moderately responsive anemias, 5-10 per field; and highly responsive anemias, 10-20 per field. Much lower numbers (~½ that reported for dogs) are seen in cats, and no polychromasia (or reticulocytosis) is seen in horses.

The cells/μL can be roughly estimated by multiplying the number of responsive cells per oil-immersion field (1000X) by 8000. Thus, if there is a mean of 10 polychromatic RBC per field, there are ~80,000/μL in the blood. Platelets may be enumerated in the same manner. This method consistently underestimates the response as compared to the reticulocyte count.

The normal ranges of RBC values for some domestic species are given below:

Table 5. Red Blood Cell Values: Some Normal Ranges

Species	PCV %	Hgb g/dL	RBC 10⁶/μL (10¹²/L)	MCV μm³ (fL)	MCHC g/dL
Horse					
Light breeds	30-48	11-18	7-11	40-49	35-37
Heavy breeds	25-45	8-14	6-9	37-52	32-38
Cow	25-45	8-15	5-10	30-56	28-36
Sheep	25-50	9-16	8-16	25-50	30-38
Goat	20-37	8-14	8-18	18-34	30-40
Pig	32-50	10-16	5-8	50-68	30-35
Dog	37-55	12-18	5-9	62-70	33-35
Cat	27-45	8-15	5-10	40-55	30-35
Rabbit	35-45	9-15	5-7	60-68	31-35
Chicken	30-40	9-13	3	127	29
Turkey	39	11	2	203	29

Certain signs are characteristic of anemia regardless of the cause or species. Generally, there is pallor of the mucous membranes, weakness, lethargy, reduced tolerance to exercise, anorexia, increased heart and respiratory rates, and there may be a systolic murmur due to reduced blood viscosity. If the anemia is acute or hemorrhagic, or both, there may be hypotension and shock. Anemic animals should be handled and examined carefully since excitement may cause collapse.

ANEMIAS DUE TO BONE MARROW HYPOFUNCTION

DECREASED RBC PRODUCTION

INJURY TO MARROW STEM CELLS

In **hypoplastic** and **aplastic anemias**, the shortage of RBC is not as critical as that of platelets and neutrophils. In total aplasia, death occurs in 10-14 days due to hemorrhage and sepsis. Rarely, there is an immune-mediated RBC aplasia in which granulocytes and platelets are maintained; in these cases, the animals survive longer and benefit from blood transfusions (qv, p 29) and immunosuppression.

Damage to marrow stem cells usually is an individual idiosyncrasy and related to drug or toxic exposure. Chloramphenicol and cyclic hydrocarbons rarely cause marrow aplasia while body irradiation in the 200-500r range regularly does. Bracken fern poisoning (qv, p 1641) in cattle can cause a herd outbreak of marrow aplasia. Panleukopenia virus (qv, p 416) causes aplasia and pancytopenia in Felidae, but death is due to agranulocytosis, dehydration, and thrombocytopenia. Most cases of aplastic anemia are idiopathic. Confirmation is by bone marrow examination.

MARROW DISPLACEMENT BY ABNORMAL CELLS
(Myelophthisis)

Rarely, an animal with chronic infection or in the later (exhaustive) stage of myelogenous leukemia develops myelofibrosis, in which the specialized cells of the marrow are displaced by connective tissue. Much more common is the invasion of marrow by lymphoid tumors and less often by other types of tumors, either myelogenous in origin or metastatic sarcomas and carcinomas. In any case, moderate to marked numbers of rubricytes in the peripheral blood in the absence of polychromasia, especially if the anemia is mild or absent, indicate that the cells may be displaced by tumor growth in the marrow cavity. Peripheral blood and bone marrow should then be examined for tumor cells.

NUTRITIONAL ANEMIA

These anemias are due to a reduction in RBC production as distinguished from a reduction in Hgb synthesis. Vitamin B_{12} and folic acid are required for DNA synthesis; in deficient animals, there are reduced erythroid mitoses, and thus reduced numbers of RBC. The disease in man is macrocytic and normochromic, and characterized by ineffective erythropoiesis, or abnormal cells that are not released into the circulation. No clear counterpart exists in animals; however, a deficiency of cobalt (thus, of B_{12}) occurs with a mild reduction in blood volume but not a marked drop in Hgb. Recently, a B_{12} deficiency was discovered in a family of dogs. Folic acid deficiency anemia in animals is mild, and limited to those with rapidly growing tumors. Anemia due to carbohydrate starvation is mild. Protein deficiency causes a more severe anemia with an accompanying drop in blood volume, which appears to be nonspecific and due to general debility and reduced activity. Recovery is slow, and plasma proteins appear to be replaced before increased erythrogenesis. Thus, plasma volume may increase and the anemia may worsen for a time, even after diets are improved.

Decreased RBC production is the primary cause of the anemia of chronic disease, although some increase in hemolysis usually is present. The reasons for this type of anemia include toxemia of abscessation or uremia, lack of iron utilization, and inadequate nutrition. In chronic diffuse liver disease, there is inadequate detoxification of normal metabolites, altered amino acid supply, and altered fat metabolism. These changes often result in the appearance of "target" RBC in the peripheral blood.

DECREASED HEMOGLOBIN PRODUCTION

DEFICIENT HEME SYNTHESIS

These anemias are due to reductions in heme synthesis, and therefore of Hgb, as distinguished from the macrocytic anemias of reduced cellular multiplication. The result is a microcytic, hypochromic anemia. The most important cause is iron deficiency, which most commonly is secondary to chronic low-grade blood loss due to parasites or GI tumors, ulcers (dog, cat, horse), or lack of dietary iron (neonatal pigs). In absolute iron deficiency, there is no hemosiderin in the bone marrow.

All suckling animals are iron-deficient for a time, but this is regularly critical only in pigs. Pigs should be given iron either parenterally or PO during the first week of life. Care should be exercised before iron is administered by either route to ensure that the pigs are not vitamin-E-deficient; any history of such deficiency in the herd, or previous evidence of iron toxicity is reason to delay iron administration until ≥ 24 hr after the administration of vitamin E (qv, p 1673). A persistent anemia in young pigs that has not responded to previous iron administration should invoke the same precaution. Vitamin E is required for synthesis of heme, and normally there is a large pool of heme present that scavenges any free iron from PO or parenteral administration. Low levels of vitamin E, and therefore heme, allow free iron to circulate, which results in peroxidation of cellular membranes and necrosis, particularly in the heart, liver, and skeletal muscle. (*See* NUTRITIONAL MYOPATHY OF CALVES AND LAMBS, p 548, and HEPATOSIS DIETETICA IN PIGS, p 550.)

Copper deficiency may be absolute or molybdenum-conditioned (qv, p 1197). Copper is required to recharge the ferroxidase enzyme system; deficiency blocks iron utilization, which results in an iron deficiency anemia that is hypochromic and microcytic. In copper deficiency anemias, marrow hemosiderin is adequate or abundant, but serum iron is low. Cobalt and copper usually are added to feeds via a salt block or supplement.

Vitamin B₆ or pyridoxine deficiency reduces heme synthesis and causes anemia, but this is not recognized clinically and is presumed to be rare.

DEFICIENT GLOBIN SYNTHESIS

The synthesis of the α and β chains of globin that combine with heme to form Hgb is controlled genetically. In animals, a globin deficiency has not been recognized, but anemia in some sheep causes a "switching" to alternate globin chains that form Hgb "C", which releases oxygen more readily to the tissues than the normal Hgb A or B; in this respect, it is similar to fetal Hgb and appears to be a protective mechanism that permits more efficient oxygen transport at low Hgb levels.

IMMUNE-MEDIATED MARROW FAILURE

AUTOIMMUNE THYROIDITIS

In the last decade, the frequency of diagnosis of immune-mediated hematological diseases and autoimmune thyroid disease in man and dog has increased. Immune-mediated hemolytic anemia and/or thrombocytopenia are 2 of the sequelae of the systemic polyglandular autoimmune syndrome that often accompanies autoimmune thyroiditis. Most of these immunologic hematopoietic disorders are nonresponsive to therapy, in contrast to the similar but responsive diseases seen before the late 1970's. One explanation of this apparent change is viral infection of the marrow (see below) and/or suppression or destruction of hematopoietic stem cells. Another is that genetic predisposition—in man and dogs—may have increased, eg, some 50 dog breeds are now said to be predisposed to familial autoimmune thyroid disease, and hence to many other immune-mediated disorders.

DRUGS

In man and other animals, various therapeutic compounds are now suspect in an apparently increasing number of immune-mediated hematologic reactions, usually hapten-induced anemias or thrombocytopenias, in which the RBC or platelets are involved as "innocent bystanders" (see also IMMUNE-MEDIATED ANEMIAS, p 20). Most of these disorders seem to be nonregenerative. Many drugs—as many as 30 or more in some estimates—have been associated with such reactions, although a direct cause and effect relationship has not been established. Most of these drugs appear to trigger immunologic reactions only in genetically or otherwise susceptible animals (eg, those with pre-existing immunologic disease, autoimmune thyroiditis, or with a family history of these disorders). Among those associated with such reactions are the sulfonamides, especially when used with trimethoprim, and the nonsteroidal anti-inflammatory agents when used for long periods.

VIRAL INFECTIONS WITH MARROW SUPPRESSION

Some viruses induce immunological deficiencies, usually via effects on the bone marrow. Examples are human immunodeficiency virus (the cause of AIDS in man), simian immunodeficiency virus, feline immunodeficiency virus, and human and canine parvoviruses. Similar viruses are those of feline leukemia and panleukopenia, equine infectious anemia, bovine leukemia, avian leukosis, and caprine arthritis. Bone marrow suppression with transient (21 day) or chronic/latent erythroid dysplasia in the presence or absence of thrombocytopenia and neutropenia, Coombs' positive hemolytic anemia, and immune-mediated thrombocytopenia have been associated with (ie, may prove to be caused by) both retroviral and parvoviral infections in man and other species. Also, modified live parvovirus vaccines in dogs, and killed feline leukemia virus vaccine are suspects as causes (in genetically susceptible animals) of such hematological diseases. Treatment of such animals is with corticosteroids or other immunosuppressive therapy, L-thyroxine to stimulate hematopoeisis and/or treat underlying autoimmune thyroiditis (*see* above), anabolic steroids, supportive antibiotics, or other therapies.

ANEMIAS DUE TO LOSS OF ABNORMAL RBC

RBC WITH DEFICIENT ENZYME CONTENT

Glucose 6-phosphate dehydrogenase (G6PD) deficiency: This enzyme is part of an intraerythrocytic metabolic chain that protects Hgb from oxidative denaturation. In the deficient cells, oxidants cause globin precipitation, which results in formation of Heinz bodies and rapid cell lysis. Old RBC with a lower G6PD level are more susceptible to oxidative denaturation than are young ones. Thus, exposure to an oxidant drug such as phenothiazine, phenylhydrazine, or primaquine causes selective hemolysis of older RBC. In man, low G6PD levels are transmitted genetically, while in animals the susceptibility to oxidant drugs is an acquired defect occurring mainly in debilitated animals. Usually, no treatment is required since the young population of RBC is spared. Blood transfusions should be considered if the PCV drops to <15%. The marrow usually is functional, and spontaneous recovery rapid. A similar condition was observed when dogs were fed large quantities of onions or vitamin K_1; anemias associated with feeding rape, kale, or turnips to herbivores also have a Heinz-body pathogenesis. G6PD or Heinz-body anemia can be diagnosed by incubating 0.1 mL each of heparinized test and control blood in 100 mg/mL of acetylphenylhydrazine in 2 mL of buffer for 2 hr at 37°C. The RBC are then stained with New Methylene Blue and examined microscopically; normal RBC contain few Heinz bodies, and G6PD-deficient RBC contain many.

Pyruvate kinase deficiency in Basenji dogs is a genetically transmitted enzyme deficiency of the RBC similar to that reported in man. The disease is characterized by severe congenital anemia with marked polychromatic RBC response. Similarly, a hereditary anemia characterized by stomatocytes and associated with skeletal dwarfism has been recognized in Alaskan Malamutes.

Phosphofructokinase deficiency in English Springer Spaniels has recently been described and is similar to the analogous human disorder. This inherited disease is characterized by intermittent bouts of severe hemolytic anemia and myoglobulinuria associated with exertion, which induces respiratory alkalosis and enhanced RBC fragility.

IMMUNE-MEDIATED ANEMIAS

See also VIRAL INFECTIONS WITH MARROW SUPPRESSION, p 19, ANEMIAS OF IMMUNE-MEDIATED MARROW FAILURE, p 19, DISEASES INVOLVING CYTOTOXIC ANTIBODIES, p 428, and BLOOD GROUPS AND BLOOD TRANSFUSIONS, p 29.

RBC may become the target of antibodies that coat their surfaces and cause them to be removed from circulation by the reticuloendothelial system (RES). This condition can be diagnosed with reagent antisera specific to the globulin of the species tested. Combination of the reagent antiglobulin with the globulin on the cell membranes constitutes a positive Coombs' or antiglobulin test.

The adsorption of virus to the RBC such as occurs in equine infectious anemia (qv, p 27) may cause a hemolytic crisis because of the attachment of antiviral antibody to the RBC-bound virus. These cells are then destroyed by the RES in what is known as an "innocent bystander reaction". Similarly, the adsorption of drugs to RBC rarely induces an immune hemolysis in man and animals.

Isoimmune hemolytic anemia occurs in horses, cats, dogs, and pigs, and in calves and piglets from vaccinated dams. This is an acute anemia in which RBC of the newborn are agglutinated or hemolyzed by specific isoantibodies produced in their dams.

AUTOIMMUNE HEMOLYTIC ANEMIA (AIHA)

AIHA, also called immune hemolytic anemia (IHA), occurs in cats, horses, and dogs, and is qualitatively similar to the disease in man. AIHA occurs in dogs as part of the uncommon syndrome of canine systemic lupus erythematosus along with thrombocytopenia and rheumatoid arthritis. (*See also* ANEMIAS OF IMMUNE-MEDI-ATED MARROW FAILURE, p 19 and IMMUNE SYSTEM DISEASES, p 421.) The usual form of AIHA, ie, unassociated with lupus, is not rare and is characterized by hemolytic crises with a variable but often very low PCV (<10%), marked polychromasia, spherocytosis, severe rouleaux or RBC aggregations, and frequently, a positive direct Coombs' test or spontaneous autoagglutination of RBC. Recently, the most typical cases in dogs have been marked by a nonregenerative anemia. Some of these have occurred after exposure to parvovirus or modified live parvovirus vaccine, and a few cases progress to a transient or chronic latent erythroid dysplasia (*see also* VIRAL INFECTIONS WITH MARROW SUPPRESSION, p 19).

In chronic cases, icterus is present due to ischemic hepatic damage. If given at all, blood transfusions should be done only with great caution and after matching and typing to avoid further sensitization and exacerbation of the problem. Dexamethasone, prednisone, or prednisolone in high doses, daily for 5-7 days, usually results in a marked rise in the PCV and improved color and condition in dogs. Anabolic steroids given once a week also may be helpful. The dosage of steroid should be decreased to half, or less, of the initial dose in 5-7 days and then to a maintenance dose given daily or every other day, which should be continued for 6-8 wk. Steroids may be required at high levels for up to 3 wk to induce a rise in PCV. An important adjunctive therapy is L-thyroxine to stimulate hematopoiesis and/or treat underlying autoimmune thyroiditis. Vincristine or cyclophosphamide may be used if steroid therapy fails; however, these drugs are myelotoxic, and the WBC count must be monitored at least daily. Recently, steroid-resistant cases have responded well to cyclosporine treatment for 5 consecutive days similar to the regimen used in man. In unresponsive cases, azathioprine has been used in conjunction with cyclosporine and low doses of corticosteroids, and follow-up 5-day courses of cyclosporine at half the initial dosage may be needed. Splenectomy may be indicated as a last resort if steroid or other immunosuppressant therapy fails.

Most therapeutic failures result from discontinuing steroid therapy too soon after remission begins. Some have found dexamethasone superior to either prednisone or prednisolone in treating immune-mediated anemias or thrombocytopenias. Should a hemolytic crisis occur after a steroid-induced remission, even higher levels of steroid may be required to again control the hemolysis. Dogs may develop signs resembling those of Cushing's disease (qv, p 274) during treatment of AIHA, but return to normal as the treatment is decreased or is given every other day. Hematinics usually are not required, and iron is usually not advisable unless iron stores are depleted in cases of chronic marrow failure.

The adsorption of the agent of equine infectious anemia (qv, p 27) to the horse RBC has resulted in a similar syndrome. AIHA also occurs in cats, and probably occurs in other species but is unrecognized.

HEMOLYTIC DISEASE OF NEWBORN CALVES

Spontaneous sensitization of cattle to fetal RBC antigens is rare or does not occur. Vaccines derived from blood and used to prevent babesiosis and anaplasmosis may contain RBC antigens that immunize the dams. If the bull has the same RBC antigens as the vaccine donor, then the calves may share these antigens and develop isoimmune hemolytic anemia when they receive colostrum. Gestation is normal. Antibody eluted from affected calf RBC has been shown to be an IgG and, at least in some cases, hemolytic. A single 2-mL dose of *Babesia* vaccine within a few weeks before calving may result in neonatal isoerythrolysis, and most fatal cases occur when dams have received 4-5 vaccinations within 1 yr. The Coombs' test usually is strongly positive. Owners may note red urine in newborn calves and exacerbate the problem by revaccinating dams on suspicion of neonatal infection.

Clinical Findings: The disease may be mild or peracute with signs occurring 12-48 hr after birth. In peracute cases, death may occur as early as 2 hr after signs of severe dyspnea, and 12-16 hr after birth. Acute cases are characterized by depression, dyspnea, and occasionally, fever that develops 24-48 hr after birth. The calves continue to suck but weaken and have pallor that is masked in 1-2 days by mild to moderate jaundice. Death occurs at 4-5 days. Mildly affected calves show only dullness and reduced activity.

In peracute cases there is hemoglobinuria, hypofibrinogenemia, and high fibrin degradation products, with rapid death, a large spongy spleen, and discoloration of the kidneys. There is an excess of blood-stained pleural fluid, and the lungs are congested and edematous. In the acute form, the PCV drops to 6-7%, and often there is hemoglobinuria. The marrow is responsive but inadequate; 1-2% polychromatophilic RBC and up to 140 rubricytes per 100 WBC are seen. The Coombs' test is positive, the dam's milk agglutinates the calf's RBC, and hemolysis occurs if complement is added. In mild cases, the PCV drops to 18% at 1 wk after birth and rises to 30% by 3 wk. The anemia is normochromic and macrocytic.

Diagnosis: Usually, this is made on clinical findings of a severe anemia in neonatal calves of dams that received a blood-origin vaccine. Confirmation is by agglutination of RBC of the sire and calf by colostrum and maternal serum.

Treatment: Blood usually is not transfused because of donor incompatability. A single transfusion from an unvaccinated cow, or transfusion of saline-washed (3 times) packed RBC of the dam may be used to raise PCV to 25%. Antibiotics and steroids may be helpful.

Prophylaxis: If suspected, the disease can be predicted by determining if cows have a titer against the RBC of the bull. When practical, colostrum from cows with no titer should be used until positive dams have been milked for 24-48 hr.

HEMOLYTIC DISEASE OF NEWBORN FOALS

Affected foals are normal at birth, but can absorb dangerous amounts of isoantibodies from colostrum through their GI tract for up to 36 hr. Clinically recognizable neonatal isoerythrolysis rarely occurs in foals of primiparous mares and generally is not seen until a mare has had her third or fourth foal. Mares are isoimmunized naturally by focal placental breakdown, which permits fetal-placental hemorrhage of incompatible foal blood into the maternal circulation. A fairly large fetal-placental hemorrhage may be required to initially isoimmunize a mare to a significant degree. Restimulation of the mare in subsequent pregnancies requires much less incompatible foal blood of the same type. Also, therapeutic agents such as blood transfusions and incompatible tissue vaccines may contribute to the problem. Neonatal isoerythrolysis can occur only when a foal and its sire possess a blood factor absent in the mare. Certain stallions mated to sensitized mares always sire susceptible foals because they are genetically homozygous for the offending blood factor. Other stallions (heterozygotes) sire such foals only part of the time. Although neonatal erythrolysis may occur in foals of any breed, it is more frequent in Thoroughbreds and mules.

Clinical Findings: The severity of anemia varies considerably, depending on the amount and type of isoantibodies consumed. Hemolytic isoantibodies are the most damaging, and the highest titers exist in the first colostrum; hence, vigorous foals that nurse heartily soon after birth may be affected the most severely.

Signs may appear 8 hr to 5 days after birth. They include lethargy, jaundice, dyspnea, pounding heart, and in severe cases, hemoglobinuria. The foals spend much of their time lying down, and those severely affected often cannot stand. They nurse infrequently and only for short periods. The conjunctiva, sclera, and mucous membranes become progressively icteric in severely affected foals. RBC counts range from ~2 to 4 × 10^6/μL (2-4 × 10^{12}/L), and the RBC tend to autoagglutinate in their own plasma. Foals with RBC counts of this level during the first 24 hr require treatment.

Diagnosis: This can be made clinically. A positive Coombs' test in an anemic foal is strong presumptive evidence, and demonstration of specific antibody against foal RBC in maternal serum or colostrum is definitive. Except for anemia, icterus, and sometimes hematuria, few lesions are regularly seen. Splenomegaly and generalized icterus are often seen in foals dying 24-48 hr after birth.

Treatment: For foals that are not severely affected, ordinary nursing care together with antibiotics and restriction of exercise for the first week usually result in recovery. Blood transfusion is the only known method of saving a severely anemic foal. The whole blood of the dam or the sire cannot be used in transfusions since it contains the hemolytic antibody, but the saline-washed RBC of the mare probably is the treatment of choice. A compatible donor is difficult to find; it should be selected for RBC that are not agglutinated or hemolyzed by the serum or colostrum of the mare, and for serum that contains no demonstrable isoagglutinins or isohemolysins of the foal cells. The RBC count of the foal should be maintained at 3-4 × 10⁶/μL (3-4 × 10¹²/L), or the PCV at ≥15% until recovery. If the dam's RBC are available, 2 or 3 washes in isotonic saline solution are essential; ~2-3 L of mare's blood is sufficient. Alternatively, removal of 3-7 L of the foal's blood and replacement with 4-6 L of the donor's blood will correct the anemia and temporarily relieve the signs. Additional transfusions may be necessary, and supportive therapy is essential. Careful attention should be maintained to detect infection. Affected foals usually have a strong bone marrow response that is characterized by marked anisocytosis of RBC on blood smears and a shift in the MCV from 45-50 to 50-55 mm³ (fL). Spherocytosis is also present but may be difficult to confirm. Polychromatic RBC are seldom found in peripheral blood, and their absence should be recognized as a species characteristic and not marrow failure. Occasionally, rubricytes as well as sideroleukocytes can be seen in severe cases. An accompanying neutrophilic leukocytosis is present. WBC counts increase to 15-25,000/μL (15-25 × 10⁹/ L) with steroid treatment, which should be accompanied by antibiotic therapy.

Prophylaxis: If the mare's serum shows a definite antibody titer (>1:2) near the end of gestation, or if a test of the mare's colostrum with the foal's cells at birth shows an antibody titer of >1:8, the disease can be avoided by separating the foal from its dam immediately at birth for 36 hr. The foal can be nursed by a normal foster mare or bottle-fed on colostrum from nonimmunized mares. Such colostrum can be stored frozen for this purpose. The dam should be milked to remove most of her colostrum. The disease usually can be prevented by mating mares that have already produced one or more affected foals to stallions with RBC that are not agglutinated or hemolyzed by isoantibodies present in the mare's serum. However, in such cases, serum antibody levels should be measured during late gestation to detect the possible appearance of new isoantibodies.

HEMOLYTIC DISEASE OF NEWBORN PIGLETS

Maternal sensitization may occur following use of a crystal-violet-inactivated hog cholera vaccine of blood origin, or by natural transplacental sensitization. The spontaneous disease is primarily an isoimmune thrombocytopenia with lesser effects on the RBC. The piglets are normal at birth, and disease occurs after suckling.

The first signs are due to RBC and platelet destruction in the peripheral blood. The marrow is responsive at first, and the disease is self-correcting for the first week. As antibody continues to be absorbed, marrow precursors are depressed, and the terminal petechiae are associated with decreased platelet production of marrow aplasia. The terminal anemia is due to both hemorrhage and hypoproliferation.

Clinical Findings: Signs occur 1-4 days after birth and consist of pallor, inactivity, dyspnea, and jaundice. These signs gradually subside. After 10-11 days, multiple petechial hemorrhages occur over the ventral areas of the body; most piglets die at this time. The RBC count drops from a normal of 4.5-5.3 × 10^6/μL (4.5-5.3 × 10^{12}/L) at birth to 1-3 × 10^6/μL (1-3 × 10^{12}/L) at 4 days of age. As anemia develops, anisocytosis and polychromasia appear along with some circulating rubricytes. The MCV rises from a normal of 70 μm³ (fL) at birth to 100-120 μm³ at 1-2 wk of age and returns to normal in survivors 4 wk old. The neutrophils rise to 9-10 × 10^3/μL (9-10 × 10^9/L) at 4 days when RBC are lowest, and then decline to normal (3-4 × 10^3/μL [3-4 × 10^9/L]). Platelets have a bimodal response and drop from 300 × 10^3/μL (300 × 10^9/L) at birth to 100 × 10^3/μL (100 × 10^9/L) at day 1, then rise to normal at the first week; however, severe thrombocytopenia follows after 10-14 days. In piglets that die, the bone marrow is hypoplastic and megakaryocytes are absent. RBC are Coombs' positive from day 1-7 and are negative by day 14.

Diagnosis: Usually, this is made on finding anemia, purpura, and mild icterus in neonatal pigs. The anemia is initially hemolytic, macrocytic, normochromic, and responsive; later it becomes hypoplastic. Confirmation is by demonstration of agglutination of sire and piglet RBC and platelets by dam's serum and milk. Leptospirosis can be ruled out by demonstration of thrombocytopenia or by maternal titer.

Treatment and Prophylaxis: Treatment usually is not attempted; a substitute dam may be tried. Sows should not be rebred to the same sire after having affected litters.

HEMOLYTIC DISEASE OF NEWBORN PUPPIES AND KITTENS

Spontaneous sensitization of bitches and queens to fetal RBC antigens from puppies or kittens that share the major blood group antigens of their incompatible sires probably occurs more often than is realized. Of dogs, ~40% carry the DEA 1 antigen, and of cats, ~90% carry the A antigen. Therefore, the random chance of mating an animal carrying that antigen with an animal not carrying the antigen is 40:60 and 90:10 for dogs and cats, respectively. Diagnosis, management, and treatment of puppies or kittens affected with hemolytic disease follow the same principles discussed above for the large animal species.

HEMOLYTIC ANEMIA DUE TO INTRAVASCULAR FRAGMENTATION

Diseases that cause vasculitis activate platelets and the clotting mechanism and cause **disseminated intravascular coagulation** (DIC) of some degree. The passage of RBC at high velocity through damaged arterioles results in fragmentation as they impinge on intraluminal strands of fibrin. The damaged cells are then removed by the reticuloendothelial system. This pathogenesis is referred to as a **microangiopathic hemolytic anemia** (MHA). It is characterized clinically by anemia with marked poikilocytosis and reticulocytosis. MHA occurs in young calves with **hemolytic uremic syndrome**, in which there is severe anemia, poikilocytosis, uremia, hemoglobinuria, and collapse. MHA to a mild or severe degree occurs as a part of the pathogenesis of many other anemias in which there is vasculitis (eg, equine infectious anemia, malignant catarrhal fever, African swine fever, chronic hog cholera), and in thrombotic purpuras. Anemia with marked poikilocytosis may occur in some parasitic diseases, especially when somatic migration is extensive as in *Strongyloides* infection, and in canine heartworm disease. In nonanemic horses, especially with colic, a few highly distorted RBC is likely indicative of MHA due to parasitic vasculitis of the anterior mesenteric artery. MHA occurs in malignancy, especially if there are cavernous and necrotic areas of tumor as in hemangiosarcomas.

ANEMIAS DUE TO LOSS OF NORMAL RBC

HEMOLYSIS

Hemolysis Due to Increased Reticuloendothelial Removal, Splenomegaly, and Hypersplenism: Any condition that causes an enlargement of the spleen results in increased erythrophagocytic activity in that organ. **Splenomegaly** may occur as the result of hyperplasia due to chronic infection, autoimmune disease, or to splenic neoplasia. Diseases of the liver that result in cirrhosis and portal hypertension cause congestive splenomegaly. Stretching of the splenic reticulum in the enlarged spleen stimulates both phagocytosis and fibroplasia. The enlarged spleen pools blood, where an environment of low glucose and cholesterol and high pH results in a premature aging or "conditioning" of RBC, which causes them to become spherocytic and be removed from circulation. Splenomegaly then, for hemodynamic reasons alone, may progress to **hypersplenism**, which is defined as a spleen enlarged from any cause, with marrow hyperplasia and a decrease in one or more of the cellular elements of the blood, which corrects with removal of the spleen. The clinical disease resulting from hypersplenism may be thrombocytopenic purpura, hemolytic anemia, or neutropenia, or any combination of these. If immune factors are added to the congestive pathogenesis, then the disease is more severe, and splenectomy may be the only alternative. There is some danger of thrombotic disease in the immediate postoperative period (1-2 days) due to loss of splenic control of thrombocytosis. This complication is reflected clinically by cold extremities, particularly of the tips of the ears and tail in dogs. If these signs are marked, antiplatelet drugs (eg, aspirin) or anticoagulants (eg, heparin or warfarin) may be needed to control the thrombosis.

Hemolytic Anemia Due to Parasitism: RBC parasitism may result in intravascular hemolysis with hemoglobinemia and hemoglobinuria as in babesiosis (qv, p 69). Alternatively, the parasites can be removed from the RBC by the spleen and the cells returned to the circulation, or the RBC may be removed entirely and destroyed by the cells of the reticuloendothelial system (RES). The latter pathogenesis occurs in haemobartonellosis of cats (qv, p 28), anaplasmosis in cattle and sheep (qv, p 68), eperythrozoonosis (qv, p 72), and malaria in mammals and birds. Ehrlichiosis in horses (qv, p 375), dogs (qv, p 411), and probably cattle, causes anemia with thrombocytopenic purpura because of platelet and WBC parasitism.

Trypanosomes are common in blood of cattle in North America, but generally are nonpathogenic. Rarely, a dog that has returned from South America has trypanosomes in the blood and develops acute hemolytic anemia with marked reticulocytosis. Dogs that have been in the Mediterranean area may become infected with *Leishmania* spp by arthropod vectors. There is epistaxis, but only mild anemia. Biopsy of bone marrow, lymph nodes, or spleen can demonstrate the *Leishmania* organisms in RES cells.

In general, in anemias due to RBC parasitism, the marrow is hyperplastic and there is a marked peripheral blood macrocytosis, polychromasia, and reticulocytosis. If there is hemoglobinuria with iron and protein loss, recovery is slower. The marrow in ehrlichiosis is terminally hypoplastic. Diagnosis is based on titers or demonstration of the organism. Treatment and prevention vary with the disease. The demonstration of *Haemobartonella* in an anemic cat without a marked polychromatic response is cause to look for an RES neoplasm that has lowered normal immunity. A positive Coombs' test has been demonstrated in some of the anemias of RBC parasitism.

Lysis of Normal RBC Due to the Action of Bacterial, Plant, Chemical, or Physical Agents—Bacterial Hemolysins: (See LEPTOSPIROSIS, p 352, and BACILLARY HEMOGLOBINURIA, p 323.) *Bartonella bacilliformis* causes a generally fatal hemolytic anemia in man, dogs, and rodents. The disease is most likely to occur in splenectomized dogs. The disease (Oroya fever) can be diagnosed by demonstrating the intraerythrocytic organisms on stained blood smears. Chloramphenicol at 5-10 mg/lb (11-22 mg/kg), IV, daily for 3-5 days is the treatment of choice.

Plant Hemolysins: Most of the plants that cause hemolytic anemia, such as rape, kale, turnips, and onions, do so because of depletion of glucose 6-phosphate dehydrogenase (G6PD), with Heinz-body production. See RBC WITH DEFICIENT ENZYME CONTENT, above. Direct lysis of the RBC membrane can be caused by saponin from the waxy cuticle of plants, or by ricin from castor beans. Hemolysins are the toxic principles in most spider and snake venoms.

Chemical Hemolysins: A wide range of chemical compounds may produce hemolysis and, in addition, aplastic anemia. The agents most commonly involved with this latter form of anemia are the cyclic hydrocarbons such as benzene, toluene, acetanilide, and phenacetin. Heavy metals such as lead and silver inhibit Hgb synthesis, and arsenicals can cause hemolysis. Phenylhydrazine and other oxidant compounds, including vitamin K_1, produce Heinz bodies and hemolysis as described above (p 20). Anemias of these causes should be treated symptomatically pending specific toxicological diagnosis. Lead poisoning produces nervous signs, usually without anemia. In dogs and man there may be basophilic stippling of RBC, the intermittent release of high numbers of rubricytes and metarubricytes to the peripheral blood, and increased blood levels of lead.

Considerable quantities of copper may be accumulated gradually without apparent harm, but "chronic copper poisoning" (qv, p 1645) occurs congenitally in Wilson's disease of Bedlington Terriers, and with chronic active hepatitis in Doberman Pinschers. It also results when any one of several "stresses" leads to a sudden release of stored copper with subsequent acute hemolytic anemia as occurs in sheep, pigs, and cattle. In sheep, the source of the copper usually is phytogenous, leading to high copper levels in the liver; copper may then be released by hepatic injury of any cause, such as mild pyrrolizidine alkaloid poisoning (qv, p 1698) or forced exercise. In pigs, copper may be included in rations as a growth stimulant. In pigs that are marginally deficient in vitamin E and that develop hepatosis dietetica (qv, p 550), sufficient hepatic necrosis and release of stored copper may occur to cause a hemolytic crisis and icterus.

Excess molybdenum (qv, p 1677), usually phytogenous in origin, inhibits the intermediary metabolism of copper and causes lameness, depigmentation of skin, diarrhea, and hypoplastic anemia that is microcytic and hypochromic. Removal of molybdenum or increased dietary copper is indicated.

Physical Agents That Cause Hemolysis: Intravascular hemolysis may follow full-thickness skin burns and can be expected if >20% of the skin is affected. Excessive ingestion of cold water, especially in calves, may cause hemolysis, likely of osmotic origin, with anemia, dyspnea, and hemoglobinuria. Occasionally, an immune anemia may be triggered by exposure to cold (qv, p 429) if the offending antibody is of the cold agglutinin or IgM type.

HEMORRHAGE AND PARASITISM

Loss Due to External Hemorrhage or External Parasitism: External hemorrhage may occur from wounds, uterine prolapse, and lacerations or surgical trauma, especially dehorning and castration. In acute hemorrhage, there is hypovolemia and hypotension with a normal PCV. In chronic hemorrhage, the PCV is low, usually with an unresponsive marrow due to iron loss. In acute bleeding, IV fluids and blood transfusions are indicated to replace blood volume, platelets, and clotting factors. The marrow usually is responsive, and parenteral iron at 3.4 mg/g of Hgb (estimated loss) and hematinics should be given. In anemias of chronic hemorrhage, transfusions are less likely to be required unless the animal is markedly anemic, especially if the animal is on its feet and bleeding has been stopped. Iron and hematinics should be given as above. Anemic animals should be handled carefully since stress may be fatal.

External parasitism may cause anemia, particularly in young animals. In general, bloodsucking insects such as Tabanidae, black flies, and mosquitoes cause more irritation than blood loss. Calves occasionally become heavily infested with lice and become thin, weak, and mildly to severely anemic. Kittens and puppies can become severely anemic due to heavy flea or louse infestations; in endemic areas, bloodsucking ticks infest a wide variety of hosts. These anemias are primarily of blood loss; the animals should be treated with iron and application of ectoparasiticides. Cattle, especially, suffer marrow depression with heavy louse infestation, and recovery is slow.

Loss of Normal RBC Due to Internal Hemorrhage or Internal Parasitism: Internal hemorrhage may be acute or chronic and occur spontaneously in hemostatic defects or result from surgery, wounds, tumors or abscesses, and GI or urinary tract ulceration. Except for the inherited coagulopathies, in which it is unsafe to do so, diagnosis usually is aided by aspiration of the chest, abdomen, or subcutis. If generalized bleeding is present, peripheral blood should be collected into test tubes with the proper anticoagulant (trisodium citrate) for analysis. Prothrombin time activity is low in anticoagulant rodenticide or sweet clover poisoning (qv, p 1733) and hepatic failure. If urinary or GI bleeding has been mild but very prolonged, iron deficiency may occur, and should be treated as described above. (See HEMOSTATIC DISORDERS, p 52.)

Internal Parasitism—(see also p 237 et seq): Hookworm infection may cause profound anemia in young dogs and cats. In severe cases with collapse, blood transfusions should precede anthelmintic treatment. Iron lost in intestinal parasitism is not reabsorbed, and in chronic cases response may be better to parenteral iron than to an anthelmintic. The marrow usually is productive if iron stores are not exhausted, and peripheral blood reticulocytosis is marked with occasional severe poikilocytosis. In sheep, acute haemonchosis (qv, p 209) may cause death due to anemia without debilitation. Diarrhea occurs with most GI parasitisms of sheep except *Haemonchus*. In calves and yearling cattle, chronic *Ostertagia* infection (qv, p 205) causes cachexia, an anemia with poor reticulocyte response, and occasionally, marked poikilocytosis. Iron may be given parenterally if anemia is severe or serum iron is low.

EQUINE INFECTIOUS ANEMIA
(EIA, Swamp fever)

An acute or chronic viral disease of Equidae, found wherever there are horses. The virus is related to the human AIDS lentivirus, but it is not known to infect man.

Epidemiology and Transmission: In acute cases, the virus is in blood and all tissues and discharges. It persists in WBC of all infected horses for life and is quite stable in serum, but is readily inactivated by common disinfectants that contain detergent.

Transmission is by transfer of blood cells from an infected horse. Insertion and withdrawal of a hypodermic needle may provide adequate inoculum for transmission. Ordinarily, the disease is detected only sporadically, but it may spread in epidemic form from obviously ill horses when bloodsucking flies are abundant or if contaminated needles or surgical instruments are used. Mares may infect their foals *in utero*. The incubation period is 1-3 wk, but may be as long as 3 mo.

Clinical Findings: The disease is characterized by intermittent fever, depression, progressive weakness, weight loss, edema, and progressive or transitory anemia; it tends to become an inapparent infection, but occasionally results in death. In actively diseased horses, PCV and platelet count are decreased and monocytes are increased; in chronic infections, blood may contain WBC with stainable iron and have elevated gamma globulin.

Lesions: In acute cases, the spleen is enlarged and the splenic lymph nodes are swollen. In subacute and chronic cases, necropsy reveals emaciation, pale mucous membranes, subcut. edema (especially along the ventral abdominal wall and limbs), splenomegaly, and enlarged abdominal lymph nodes. Intravascular clotting with emboli is frequently observed in advanced terminal cases.

Microscopically, there is reticuloendothelial cell proliferation in many organs, and periportal and perisinusoidal collections of round cells in the liver with accumulations of hemosiderin in Kupffer's cells. Perivascular lymphoid infiltrations may occur in other organs also. In some horses, there is proliferative glomerulitis with glomerular deposition of immunoglobulins (IgG) and complement (C3).

Diagnosis: Clinical diagnosis should be confirmed by the immunodiffusion or "Coggins" test, a simple and highly accurate serological test to detect infection. Foals nursing infected dams test positive temporarily, and recently infected horses may test negative for ~1 wk until antibody forms.

EIA should be suspected if a horse has a history of weight loss accompanied by periodic fever, or if several horses in a group develop similar signs following introduction of new animals into a herd or death of a horse on pasture.

Treatment and Control: No specific treatment or vaccine is available. General supportive therapy may help in an individual case, but an infected horse, especially one exhibiting clinical signs, should be considered a likely source of infection for other horses. Whenever a diagnosis is established, the infected horse should be promptly isolated from other horses and maintained in isolation, if it is not to be euthanized. Because the horse fly is an important vector, stabling during the fly season helps to prevent spread of infection.

Control of stable flies and mosquitoes by repeated spraying or by screening might also be desirable. Equipment that may cause skin abrasions or absorb secretions or excretions should be avoided or disinfected before use. Hypodermic needles and surgical instruments should be sterilized before each use. Foals born to infected mares, especially if they show clinical illness, should be isolated from other horses until freedom from infection can be established by the disappearance of maternal antibody.

FELINE INFECTIOUS ANEMIA
(FIA, Haemobartonellosis)

An acute or chronic anemia of domestic cats in many parts of the world caused by a rickettsial agent that multiplies within the vascular system.

Etiology: The causative agent, *Haemobartonella felis*, is a small, coccoid, rod-like or ring-like organism, the dimensions of which vary from 0.2 to 1 μm in diameter for the coccoid forms, up to 3 μm in length for the rod forms. The organisms are usually found in varying numbers on the surface of RBC, but are occasionally seen free in the plasma. They appear as dark red-violet bodies in thin blood smears stained with Giemsa stain. The number of RBC affected varies with the severity of infection and the stage in the life cycle of the parasite. The disease can be transmitted experimentally by parenteral or oral transfer of small amounts of infected whole blood into susceptible cats. Intrauterine transmission has been well established, and infections can be transmitted iatrogenically during blood transfusions.

In experimentally induced cases, the incubation period is 1-5 wk, and recovery does not induce immunity to reinfection. Methods of natural transmission have not been established; however, incidence appears to be higher among 1- to 3-yr-old cats, particularly males. Bite wounds may be a mode of transmission. A significant portion of the cat population may carry the infection in a latent form, which becomes exacerbated during debilitating disease or stress. Infected cats may form antibodies to their own RBC, resulting in autoimmune hemolytic anemia (qv, p 21).

Clinical Findings: Any anemic cat may be suspected of having FIA. In acute cases, there is usually a fever of 103-106°F (39-41°C). The temperature may drop to subnormal in moribund cats. Jaundice, anorexia, depression, weakness, and splenomegaly are common. In chronic or slowly developing cases, there may be normal or subnormal temperature, weakness, depression, and emaciation, but there is less likely to be jaundice and splenomegaly. Dyspnea in both instances varies with the degree of anemia. Gross necropsy findings are not distinctive. The spleen and mesenteric lymph nodes may be enlarged, and hyperplasia of the bone marrow may be present.

Diagnosis: Laboratory confirmation depends on identification of the parasite in the peripheral blood or bone marrow. A series of smears stained with Wright's or Giemsa solutions over a period of several days may be required for an accurate diagnosis, since the erythrocytic bodies exhibit periodicity. Certain artifacts such as Howell-Jolly bodies may be mistaken for blood parasites and must be carefully eliminated. The slides should be very clean and stains filtered immediately before use; dirt particles and stain precipitates can mimic the appearance of the organism.

The organisms may be demonstrated in affected cells stained with acridine orange and examined by ultraviolet microscopy.

In the southeastern USA, differentiation from feline cytauxzoonosis (qv, p 72) should be made. *Cytauxzoon felis* appears as an intracellular ring, rod, or coccoid-shaped protozoon 0.5-2 μm in diameter within RBC, while *H felis* tends to form chains on the surface.

Blood cell changes typical of a regenerative anemia are present in positive smears. These include diffuse basophilic granules in the larger cells, nucleated RBC, polychromasia, anisocytosis, Howell-Jolly bodies, and an increased number of reticulocytes. RBC may fall as low as $1 \times 10^6/\mu$L. Hgb values of ≤ 7 g/dL are seen. Mean corpuscular volume increases. There is a moderate increase in WBC counts with monocytosis in acute forms, normal counts in chronic forms, and leukopenia in moribund cases. Because nucleated RBC may be present, a corrected total WBC count must be calculated.

Underlying stress, particularly feline leukemia virus infection, should be investigated, especially with recurrent infection.

Prophylaxis and Treatment: Severely dyspneic cats may require oxygen, and blood transfusion is often indicated, particularly if anemia is acute. Administration of whole blood (30-80 mL, preferably IV) should be repeated as required, perhaps every second or third day.

Oxytetracycline (20 mg/kg, PO) or tetracycline hydrochloride (33-110 mg/kg, PO, t.i.d. or q.i.d.) is effective. To prevent relapses, drug treatments should be continued for 10-20 days. Thiacetarsamide sodium at 0.5 mL/10 lb (0.1 mL/kg), IV on day 1, and repeated on day 3 is reported to be effective. Toxic reactions may occur, and transfusion should precede dosing if the PCV is <20%. Oxyphenarsine hydrochloride has been used successfully, as has prednisolone, to decrease the rate of hemolysis and reverse the depression associated with severe anemia.

In view of limited knowledge about the transmission of this disease, little can be recommended with reference to prophylaxis. Extreme care, however, should be exercised in selecting donor cats for general blood transfusions. Donors should be checked for evidence of latent infection by trial tranfusion into splenectomized cats, or by blood smear examination every other day for ≥ 2 wk following splenectomy.

BLOOD GROUPS AND BLOOD TRANSFUSIONS

Blood groups, as used here, refers to genetically controlled, polymorphic, antigenic components of the RBC membrane. The allelic products of a particular genetic locus are classified as a blood group system. Some of these systems are highly complex with many alleles defined at a locus; others consist of a single defined antigen. Blood group systems, in general, are independent of each other, and their inheritance conforms to Mendelian dominance. For polymorphic blood group systems, an animal usually inherits one allele from each parent and thus expresses no more than 2 blood group antigens of a system. An exception is in cattle, in which multiple alleles or "phenogroups" are inherited. Normally, an individual does not have antibodies against any of the antigens present on its own RBC, nor against other blood group antigens of that species' systems unless they have been induced by transfusion, pregnancy, or immunization. In some species (man, sheep, cow, cat, pig, horse, and dog), so-called "naturally occurring" isoantibodies, not induced by transfusion or pregnancy, may be present in variable but detectable titers. Of randomly selected dogs, ~50% have a naturally occurring cold hemagglutinin, Tr. Also, circulating antibodies to animal blood group antigens may be transfusion-induced. With random blood transfusions in dogs, there is a 30-40% chance of isosensitization of the recipient, primarily to blood group antigen DEA 1 (formerly known as canine A antigen). In horses and cats, possibly in mink, and rarely in pigs and dogs, transplacental immunization of the female by an incompatible fetal antigen inherited from the sire may occur. Immunization also may result when some homologous blood products are used as vaccines, eg, anaplasmosis in cattle.

BLOOD TYPING TESTS

Antisera used to identify blood groups (typing reagents) usually are produced as isoimmune sera, but are termed heteroimmune if produced in another species. Their *in vitro* serological characteristics vary with the species. Many reagents are hemagglutinins; others are hemolytic and require complement to complete the serological reaction, eg, in cattle because RBC do not readily agglutinate, and in horses because RBC rouleaux are a problem. Other typing reagents, neither hemagglutinating nor hemolytic, combine with RBC antigens in an "incomplete" reaction because they lack additional combining sites to agglutinate other RBC. These require addition of species-specific antiglobulin for agglutination.

APPLICATION OF BLOOD GROUPING

The number of major recognized blood group systems varies from species to species: cow, 12; sheep, 7; horse, 9; pig, 16; dog, 7; cat, 2; mink, 5; Rhesus monkey, 6; rat, 4; mouse (C57), 4; chicken, 11; rabbit, 5. Animal blood groups are typed to aid in the matching of donors and recipients, and to identify breeding pairs potentially at risk of producing hemolytic disease in their offspring. Because blood group antigen expression is genetically controlled and the modes of inheritance are understood, these systems also can be utilized to substantiate pedigrees in cattle, horses, and rarely dogs. The increasing use of artificial insemination, cryopreservation, and transfer of embryos has greatly expanded the application of these techniques. Blood typing of semen-donor bulls is widely practiced. Thoroughbred stallions, mares, and foals must be blood-typed before registration.

Table 6. Major Blood Groups of Clinical Interest

Species	Blood Group
Dog	DEA 1.1, 1.2, and 7
Cat	A, B
Horse	A, C, Q
Cattle	B, J
Sheep	B, R

CROSS-MATCHING TECHNIQUES

With appropriate controls, the direct crossmatch procedure is effective for all species. A major crossmatch detects antibodies already present in recipient plasma that could cause a hemolytic reaction when donor RBC are transfused; it will not detect the potential for sensitization to develop. Anticoagulated (EDTA or citrate) blood samples are collected from donor and recipient. The donor RBC are washed 3 times with 0.9% saline, and a 4% saline suspension is made from the washed cells. The major crossmatch consists of combining equal volumes (0.1 mL) of the donor RBC suspension and recipient plasma. The control tube contains recipient 4% RBC suspension and recipient plasma. The samples are incubated at 37°C for 15 min. Following incubation, all tubes are centrifuged at 1000 rpm for 1 min. Hemolysis is evaluated by comparing the color of the supernatant in the test sample with that of the control sample. Each sample is then gently shaken until all cells in the button at the bottom of the tube have returned to suspension. Again, the degree of cell clumping of the test sample is compared to the control sample. The test is negative or compatible when the RBC are readily suspended. A positive or incompatible test can have hemolysis, hemagglutination, or a combination of both. All tests judged macroscopically to be hemagglutination-negative should be confirmed microscopically at low power. This is particularly important in horses because their RBC tend to form rouleaux. All negative tests should then be confirmed by an antiglobulin test: the RBC are washed 3 times with saline, an appropriate antiglobulin (Coombs' serum) is added, the sample is incubated for 15 min at 99°F (37°C), centrifuged at 1000 rpm, and checked for hemagglutination. The minor crossmatch is the reverse of the major crossmatch, ie, recipient cells are combined with the donor plasma.

BLOOD TRANSFUSION

The need for blood transfusions frequently is acute, as for acute hemolysis or hemorrhage. Transfusions are appropriate in treatment of acute or chronic anemias along with efforts to find and treat the cause. Animals with hemostatic disorders often require repeated transfusions of either whole blood, plasma, or platelet preparations. Blood transfusions must be given with care since they have the potential for further compromising the recipient. The diversity of blood groups in animals and the lack of commercially available blood-typing reagents make complete typing and matching difficult but should not preclude the clinical use of transfusions. In horses and dogs, the blood group antigens most commonly implicated in transfusion incompatibilities are known, and by selecting donor animals that lack these groups, the prevalence of recipient sensitization can be decreased. Previously sensitized recipients can be detected by crossmatching, which will preclude administration of incompatible blood. In the USA, >99% of cats are of blood group A, so the risk of incompatible transfusion is low.

Although indicated for acute blood loss, whole blood frequently is not the ideal product to be administered. If the need is to replace the oxygen-carrying capability of the blood, then packed RBC are more appropriate; if replacement of circulatory volume is needed, crystalloid solutions may be used to replace volume, with packed RBC as needed. Platelet numbers rise rapidly after hemorrhage so replacement is not needed. Plasma proteins equilibrate from the interstitial space, so plasma is not needed except in massive hemorrhage (>1 blood volume in 24 hr). Animals that require coagulation factors benefit most from administration of fresh frozen plasma, which significantly reduces the chance of sensitization. Platelet-rich plasma or platelet concentrates may be of value in thrombocytopenia, although immune-mediated thrombocytopenia usually does not respond to administration of platelets, since they are removed rapidly by the spleen.

The amount of RBC to treat anemia is based on the volume necessary to increase the PCV or Hgb concentration to the desired value. All domestic animals have blood volumes of ~7% of the body wt except the cat, which has a blood volume of 4% of the body wt. By determining the recipient's blood volume and knowing the animal's PCV, the required replacement RBC volume can be calculated. For example, a 25-kg dog has a total blood volume of 2000 mL; with a PCV of 15%, the RBC volume is 300 mL; if the PCV is to be increased to 20%, that equals an RBC volume of 400 mL. Therefore, 100 mL of RBC are required to increase the recipient's PCV to the desired level. A similar calculation can determine the amount of blood needed to provide the required volume of RBC, eg, 200 mL of blood from a donor animal with a PCV of 50% would provide 100 mL of RBC. No more than 25% of a donor animal's blood should be collected at one time.

Collection, transfusion, and storage of blood must be done aseptically. Anticoagulants of choice are acid-citrate-dextrose (ACD) or citrate-phosphate-dextrose (CPD), sometimes with adenine added (CPD-A). Commercial blood bags containing the appropriate amount of anticoagulant are less damaging to blood cells than are vacuum collection bottles, and are preferred. Heparin should not be used as an anticoagulant because it has a longer half-life in the recipient and causes platelet activation; also, heparinized blood cannot be stored.

Blood collected in ACD or CPD may be safely stored at 4°C for 3 wk. If the blood will not be used immediately, the plasma can be removed by centrifugation (or gravity) and stored frozen for later use as a source of coagulation factors or albumin for acute reversible hypoalbuminemia. Chronic hypoproteinemia is not helped by plasma because the total body deficit of albumin is so large that it could not be improved by the small amount contained in plasma. Plasma must be frozen at -20° to -30°C within 6 hr of collection to assure that levels of factor VIII are adequate, and will remain so for 1 yr. Concentrated factor VIII, von Willebrand's factor, and fibrinogen can be prepared from fresh frozen plasma as cryoprecipitate.

RISKS OF TRANSFUSION

Although most discussion of transfusion risk centers on acute hemolytic reactions, these are rare in domestic animals. Dogs rarely have clinically significant preformed antibodies so only those that have received repeated transfusions are at risk. The most common hemolytic reaction in multiply transfused dogs is delayed intravascular hemolysis, seen clinically as shortened life span of transfused RBC. A positive Coombs' test will confirm such a reaction. Nonimmune causes of hemolysis include improper collection or separation of blood, freezing or over-warming of RBC, or infusing under pressure through a small needle.

Other complications include sepsis from contaminated blood, hypocalcemia from too much citrate, or hypervolemia especially in animals with pre-existing heart disease or in very small animals. Urticaria, fever, or vomiting are seen occasionally. Transfusions may spread disease from donor to recipient, eg, RBC parasites (eg, *Haemobartonella, Anaplasma,* or *Babesia*) and viruses (eg, retroviruses such as feline or bovine leukemia, equine infectious anemia, or other slow viruses). Other diseases, such as those caused by rickettsia or bacteria, may occur if the donor is infected.

CANINE MALIGNANT LYMPHOMA
(Lymphoma, Lymphosarcoma, Lymphocytic leukemia)

A progressive, fatal disease of dogs characterized by neoplastic transformation and proliferation of lymphoid cells, usually originating in solid lymphoid organs (lymphosarcoma) or bone marrow (lymphocytic leukemia). The variable signs depend on which organs are involved. In contrast to most other domestic species, no viral etiology has been established. The disease is histologically and immunologically heterogeneous, and different morphologic subtypes may behave differently.

It is the most common hematopoietic neoplasm of dogs (reported incidence 24:100,000). All breeds and both sexes are affected, although the incidence is higher in Boxers, Golden Retrievers, and Old English Sheepdogs.

Clinical Findings: The most common early clinical sign is a painless, peripheral lymphadenopathy, often first noticed in lymph nodes about the throat and neck. Subsequently, nonspecific signs, including anorexia, weight loss, anemia, and inactivity, develop gradually as neoplastic cells progressively infiltrate visceral organs. In the alimentary form, signs are associated with GI obstruction or malabsorption; 80% of affected dogs may have diarrhea. Other less commonly encountered types include an anterior mediastinal form with primary involvement of the area of the thymus, an epitheliotropic form (mycosis fungoides), and an extranodal (atypical) form that involves a single organ (eg, kidney).

Hypercalcemia may be seen in 20% of dogs with malignant lymphoma; there are 2 general mechanisms: one is local elaboration of an osteolytic factor that induces resorption of bone and mobilization of calcium when the bone marrow is infiltrated by tumor cells; the other, probably more common, is humoral hypercalcemia in which neoplastic cells produce a substance that acts at a distance. (*See* HUMORAL HYPERCALCEMIA OF MALIGNANCY, p 285.) In both cases, it appears that a bone-resorbing substance is produced that is immunologically distinct from parathyroid hormone, prostaglandin E_2, and 1,25-dihydroxycholecalciferol. Dogs with hypercalcemia suffer polyuria and polydipsia or renal failure. Untreated dogs usually die within 1-2 mo after diagnosis. Urinary excretion of calcium, phosphorus, and hydroxyproline is increased if there is hypercalcemia.

Lesions: Commonly, all superficial and various internal lymph nodes are 3-10 times normal size (multicentric form). Affected nodes are freely movable, firm, gray-tan, bulge on cut surface, and have no cortical-medullary demarcation. Frequently, there is hepatosplenomegaly with either diffuse enlargement or multiple, variable-sized, pale nodules disseminated in the parenchyma. The bone marrow, alimentary tract, kidney, heart, tonsils, pancreas, and eyes may also be involved less commonly.

In the alimentary form, the second most common form of the disease, any part of the GI tract or mesenteric lymph nodes may be affected, but superficial lymph nodes and spleen are rarely involved.

Diagnosis: True lymphocytic leukemia is rare, and must be differentiated from lymphosarcoma because of the different prognosis and response to therapy. This disease is characterized by a normal to elevated WBC count with a predominance of lymphoid cells in peripheral blood and bone marrow. Poorly differentiated, acute lymphoblastic leukemia is an aggressive disease with a poor prognosis, whereas well-differentiated, chronic lymphocytic leukemia is slowly progressive and responds relatively well to therapy. Frequently, there is a diffuse splenomegaly. Most dogs with lymphosarcoma have a normal hematological profile. In the later stages, an absolute neutrophilia may develop.

Most canine lymphomas are high-grade (blast cell) diffuse lymphosarcomas, although ~20% are low-grade (well-differentiated) tumors. The high-grade tumors respond better to chemotherapy and have longer remission and survival times.

The cell of origin is the lymphocyte of either the B- or T-cell lineage, although some are of undetermined origin. Two separate studies have found that >75% of canine lymphomas are of B-cell origin and 10-20% are of T-cell origin. B-cell tumors are associated with better response and longer remission and survival times than T-cell neoplasms. There is a strong correlation between some T-cell neoplasms and hypercalcemia, and these tumors are associated with poorer response rates and shorter survival and remission times.

Microscopical examination of lymphoid tissue is required for positive diagnosis since lymphadenopathy may be caused by non-neoplastic diseases. Examination of peripheral blood or bone marrow usually is not diagnostic except in terminal stages of the disease or in lymphocytic leukemia.

Although cytology of lymph node aspirates or smears of biopsy specimens may provide a diagnosis, histopathological examination of an involved peripheral lymph node is desirable and usually provides a definitive diagnosis. Because the submandibular nodes are often hyperplastic, they are more difficult to evaluate and should be avoided if other nodes are enlarged.

Treatment: Cyclic combination chemotherapy with doses used in man is generally too toxic for use in dogs; however, long-term remission can be achieved at somewhat lower doses. Response rates to chemotherapy of 70-80% and median survival times of 10-14 mo after diagnosis may be expected; 25% may survive ≥2 yr. Most treatment regimens use a combination of cyclophosphamide, vincristine, and prednisone. The addition of asparaginase or adriamycin has improved response rates.

Periodic clinical and laboratory examinations are imperative during the course of all chemotherapeutic regimens since the drugs are toxic. Adverse reactions include bone marrow suppression, increased susceptibility to infection, and hemorrhagic cystitis from cyclophosphamide. Use of antibiotics in an attempt to prevent these occurrences is controversial. Transfusions may be necessary.

Chemotherapy is generally divided into an induction phase, in which a combination of drugs are administered intensively over a short period of time, and a maintenance phase. The following protocol has proved effective:

Induction: Wk 1—vincristine (0.7 mg/m², IV), asparaginase (400 IU/kg, IP), prednisone (30 mg/m², PO); wk 2—cyclophosphamide (200 mg/m², IV), prednisone (20 mg/m², PO); wk 3—doxorubicin (30 mg/m², IV), prednisone (10 mg/m², PO); wk 4-6—as above for wk 1-3, but discontinue asparaginase and prednisone. (For calculation of body surface areas, *see* HEART DISEASE, p 48.)

Maintenance: Continue cyclic administration of the drugs as in wk 4-6, but extend the treatment interval to q2wk for 2 treatment cycles, then q3wk for 2 cycles. Should relapse occur within this time period (as is expected in ~50% of cases), reinduction using asparaginase and prednisone may achieve a second remission. (For asparaginase, all but the first should be given IM or subcut. to reduce chances of inducing anaphylaxis.) Continuous chemotherapy is then reinstituted q2wk, sequentially administering cyclophosphamide, vincristine, and methotrexate (0.5 mg/kg, IV) in combination with prednisone (1 mg/kg, PO, every other day).

Due to delayed cardiac toxicity, the maximal cumulative dose of doxorubicin should be 150-200 mg/m^2. Chlorambucil (1.4 mg/kg, PO, divided into 2 doses) also can be substituted for cyclophosphamide after remission is achieved. The diffuse alimentary form of lymphosarcoma often responds poorly to chemotherapy. However, if the lesion is localized to a segment of the intestine, surgical resection followed by chemotherapy should be performed. In this case, the prognosis is guarded to fair for long-term response.

Well-differentiated lymphocytic leukemia can be treated with chlorambucil at 0.2 mg/kg, PO for 7-10 days, followed by a reduced daily dose of 0.1 mg/kg. Remissions of 1-2 yr can be expected. Treatment of lymphoblastic leukemia has been less successful, with median survival time of <6 mo and a complete response rate of ~30%.

CONGENITAL AND INHERITED ANOMALIES OF THE CARDIOVASCULAR SYSTEM

Improved clinical methods and greater interest in heart disease have increased the number of cases of congenital heart disease recognized, especially in dogs. Certain of these can be corrected surgically. Those of possible clinical significance in veterinary medicine are discussed below. (*See also* HEART DISEASE, p 40.)

In dogs, the types of lesions seen, in approximate order of frequency, are: patent ductus arteriosus, pulmonic stenosis, subaortic stenosis, persistent right aortic arch, interventricular septal defect, atrial septal defect, and tetralogy of Fallot. Cardiovascular malformations occur predominantly in purebred dogs, and certain specific anomalies are seen more often in certain breeds. This evidence, in addition to familial aggregations of affected dogs, indicates that genetic factors are important. Studies indicate that inheritance is complex. The prevalence rate of congenital cardiac defects is much higher in dogs than cats. In cats, the most common reported defects are malformations of the mitral valve complex, dysplasia of the tricuspid valve, ventricular septal defect, aortic stenosis including supravalvular stenosis, persistent common atrioventricular canal, patent ductus arteriosus, and tetralogy of Fallot. In horses and cattle, ventricular septal defects are more common than atrial septal defects; patent ductus arteriosus and tetralogy of Fallot also occur. Aortic stenosis has a heritable basis in pigs.

In mild conditions, such as small interatrial and interventricular septal defects and patent ductus arteriosus, affected animals may reach an advanced age without showing signs of heart disease. When the condition is more serious, neonates may show weakness, dyspnea, cyanosis, and retarded growth. The most severely affected animals die in the early postnatal period. If the condition is not obvious soon after birth, signs of congestive heart failure (CHF) may ensue later, usually before maturity, but occasionally as late as 5-7 yr of age. Signs of CHF in a young or middle-aged animal suggest the possibility of an underlying congenital heart defect.

Early recognition of congenital heart disease may enable the pet owner to reclaim his investment, or the livestock producer to avoid attempting to raise an animal that is destined to die early. Surgical correction of certain defects, notably patent ductus arteriosus, pulmonic stenosis, and persistent right aortic arch, is possible without extensive special equipment. When equipment for extracorporeal circulation or hypothermia is available, correction of other malformations may be attempted.

Signs of CHF (systemic venous congestion, hepatomegaly, ascites, pulmonary congestion, edema) may occur when the underlying congenital malformation severely impairs cardiac function. Animals with such signs may show dramatic improvement when treated with rest, low-sodium diets, diuretics, and cardiac glycosides. Unless the underlying defect is surgically corrected, the response is usually temporary and death eventually results from irreversible CHF.

In dogs, clinical criteria for the common malformations discussed here are well enough developed that a definitive diagnosis often can be based on physical, radiographic, echocardiographic, and electrocardiographic signs. When surgical correction is contemplated, or when more complex anomalies are encountered, additional confirmatory studies such as angiocardiography and cardiac catheterization are often desirable. The clinical features of specific congenital malformations in species other than dogs are not well-known, and in them, accurate diagnosis more often depends on such special studies.

ANOMALIES OF DERIVATIVES OF THE AORTIC ARCHES

Among the embryonic aortic arches that persist in normal mammals are the right and left third, the left fourth, and portions of the right and left sixth arches. The third pair of arches gives rise to the carotid arteries; the left fourth remains as the definitive arch of the aorta; and the sixth arches give rise to the pulmonary artery, its branches, and the ductus arteriosus.

PATENT DUCTUS ARTERIOSUS

During fetal life, an important communication exists between the aorta and pulmonary artery, which is formed by the left sixth aortic arch and known as the ductus arteriosus. Failure of the ductus arteriosus to close shortly after birth leads to an anomaly known as a patent or persistent ductus arteriosus. It is one of the most common clinically recognized congenital cardiovascular anomalies of dogs and may be combined with other cardiac anomalies. It is inherited as a polygenic defect in Miniature and Toy Poodles.

Functional Pathology: During systole, a part of arterial blood is pumped through the patent duct into the pulmonary system (left-to-right shunt) due to the higher pressure in the aorta. If pulmonary resistance remains low, there is increased flow through the lungs, left heart, and ascending aorta, which constitute the path of the shunt; these structures dilate in response to the increased volume of blood they receive. If pulmonary vascular resistance is high, right ventricular hypertrophy and pulmonary hypertension are present, and a right-to-left shunt may occur through the ductus and send venous blood to the descending aorta.

Clinical Findings and Treatment: The so-called "machinery" murmur (*see* p 41) is present during systole and diastole in the left-to-right shunt. The pulse usually is typical—quickly and strongly distending the artery (water-hammer pulse). Electrocardiographic evidence of left ventricular hypertrophy may be present, and thoracic radiographs reveal left atrial and ventricular enlargement, increased pulmonary vascular markings, and dilatation of the ascending aorta.

When pulmonary hypertension with a right-to-left shunt is present, the machinery murmur is absent, and there is accentuation and splitting of the second heart sound, and electrocardiographic and radiographic evidence of right ventricular hypertrophy. Secondary polycythemia is usually present. The visible mucous membranes of the head usually are not cyanotic because the venous blood enters the aorta downstream from where the brachiocephalic trunk and left brachial artery leave the aorta. For this reason, the anomaly may go unrecognized until the affected dog begins to show weakness or collapse of the hindlimbs on exercise owing to inadequate oxygen supply posteriorly.

Ligation or complete surgical division of the patent ductus arteriosus is recommended; however, when right-to-left shunt is present and the pulmonary hypertension is severe, right ventricular failure may follow obliteration of the patent ductus.

PERSISTENT RIGHT AORTIC ARCH

A common vascular anomaly in dogs in which the right fourth embryonic aortic arch persists, displacing the esophagus and trachea to the left. The trachea and esophagus are incarcerated in a vascular ring formed by the arch of the aorta on the right, the pulmonary artery below, the base of the heart ventrally, and the ligamentum arteriosum (or ductus arteriosus) dorsally and to the left.

Persistent right aortic arch is unusually frequent in some German Shepherd and Irish Setter strains. This anomaly has been reported in cattle, horses, and cats.

Other anomalies of the aortic arch system also may result in vascular rings that partially or completely encircle the esophagus and trachea; this may compress these organs and result in dysphagia and regurgitation. Usually, part of the esophagus cranial to the constriction is considerably dilated.

For clinical findings and treatment, *see* DILATATION OF THE ESOPHAGUS, p 110.

AORTIC STENOSIS

In dogs and pigs, stenosis of the outflow tract of the left ventricle is a fairly common congenital lesion. It has been reported chiefly in Boxers and German Shepherd Dogs, and has occurred in familial aggregations in these 2 breeds, and in Newfoundlands. Little is known regarding its prevalence in other species. Usually, the valves are not primarily involved, but rather, the narrowing occurs below them as a fibrous ring (fibrous subaortic stenosis).

Functional Pathology: The chief disturbance is obstruction to emptying of the left ventricle with resultant left ventricular hypertrophy. Often, there is poststenotic dilatation of the ascending aorta.

Clinical Findings and Treatment: In dogs, the systolic murmur of aortic stenosis is ordinarily located in the third or fourth left intercostal space and second to third right intercostal space. It may be transmitted to the neck. Fainting and sudden death are not uncommon. Electrocardiographic evidence of left ventricular hypertrophy may be present, and arrhythmias and conduction disturbances are frequent. Radiographically, left ventricular enlargement and poststenotic dilatation of the aorta are prominent signs. The subvalvular obstruction can be visualized by echocardiography.

Treatment with β-adrenergic blocking drugs decreases myocardial oxygen demand and can be helpful in controlling ventricular arrhythmias. Surgery is not generally done.

PULMONIC STENOSIS

In dogs, valvular, subvalvular, and infundibular pulmonic stenosis have been described. The valvular type is the most common form and involves the valves only. Valvular pulmonic stenosis is hereditary in Beagles.

Functional Pathology: The primary functional disturbance is interference with emptying of the right ventricle, which leads to elevated systolic pressure and right ventricular hypertrophy. Pulmonary arterial pressure is low or normal. Poststenotic dilatation of the pulmonary artery may occur, producing, in advanced cases, rounded enlargement resembling an aneurysm (poststenotic dilatation).

Clinical Findings and Treatment: A harsh, crescendo-decrescendo systolic murmur, frequently accompanied by a thrill, is usually present with its point of maximal intensity located at the third or fourth left intercostal space, slightly below a horizontal line drawn through the point of the shoulder (pulmonic area). The cardiac silhouette shows enlargement of the right ventricular and atrial borders, and poststenotic dilatation of the pulmonary artery may be visible. From abnormally high blood flow velocity recorded by Doppler echocardiography at the site of obstruction, the severity of stenosis can be estimated by calculating the pressure gradient. Electrocardiographically, marked deviation to the right of the mean electrical axis usually occurs and produces an ECG typical of right ventricular enlargement. High subvalvular and valvular stenosis cannot be differentiated without angiocardiography.

Pulmonary valvulotomy is possible for valvular stenosis but should be elected only in severe cases since the results are unpredictable. In principle, the infundibulums should be resected in the subvalvular type.

SEPTAL DEFECTS

ATRIAL SEPTAL DEFECTS

The foramen ovale is an oblique opening in the interatrial septum that normally allows flow from the right atrium to the left atrium during intrauterine life. At birth, it is forced closed by the increase in left atrial pressure, which occurs at the onset of breathing. In dogs, anatomic closure is due to fibrosis, and occurs during the post-natal period (within 1 wk). Closure in horses and cattle is the result of collapse of a vascular-like structure into the foramen ovale, and the foramen may remain patent for some months and may be probe patent for life. A probe-patent foramen ovale may be considered an anatomic defect, but it causes no functional abnormalities as long as the left atrial pressure exceeds that of the right atrium. However, this "one-way valve" may be reopened and allow right-to-left shunting of blood if right atrial pressure becomes abnormally elevated.

True atrial septal defects are those that are consistently open. Defects of the septum secundum type are most common and occur in the thin portion of the inter-atrial septum occupied by the foramen ovale. Septum primum atrial septal defects are situated low in the interatrial septum and usually involve the atrioventricular valves as well.

Functional Pathology: With a large atrial septal defect, blood passes from the left to the right atrium; this additional blood must be pumped as an extra load by the right side, and in time causes dilatation and hypertrophy of this portion of the heart. As a result of the greatly increased blood flow through the pulmonary system, pulmonary hypertension may ensue in horses and cattle, followed by congestive heart failure. Usually, there is no shunting of unoxygenated blood into the systemic circulation. However, a slight cyanosis, indicating a reverse flow of blood from the right to left atrium, may appear, particularly when pulmonary hypertension and conges-tive heart failure are present, or when a coexisting lesion such as pulmonic stenosis causes an increase in right atrial pressure.

Clinical Findings and Treatment: A small patent foramen ovale may be present without producing detectable clinical signs. In large septal defects, dyspnea, palpi-tation, and cyanosis may be observed. Usually, a harsh systolic murmur is noticed over the base of the heart. The second heart sound is increased in amplitude and may be split. The right ventricle and pulmonary outflow tract are enlarged. In-creased pulmonary vascular markings may be evident in the thoracic radiographs. Confirmation of the defect usually requires visualization by echocardiography or tracking blood flow across the septum by angiography.

The atrial wall technique may be used for surgical correction in dogs. Repair under direct vision is facilitated by heart-lung bypass.

INTERVENTRICULAR SEPTAL DEFECTS

These range in size from small openings of little functional importance to almost complete absence of the septum; most occur in the upper membranous part of the septum. They may be combined with other congenital anomalies, such as patent ductus arteriosus, interatrial septal defects, and pulmonic and aortic stenosis.

Functional Pathology: Small, interventricular septal defects transmit blood from the left to right ventricle with considerable force. However, the amount of blood passing through a small opening has little or no effect on the general circulation.

With a large defect without pulmonic stenosis, direction of the shunt depends on the relative resistance to flow through the intrapulmonary vascular bed as compared with that of the systemic vascular bed. In young animals, the resistance in the in-trapulmonary vascular bed is lower than resistance in the systemic circulation, and the shunt is entirely left to right. As a consequence, the load of the right ventricle is increased and leads to hypertrophy and dilatation of the right ventricle and pulmo-nary artery. Subsequently, the resistance to pulmonary blood flow may rise due to obliterative changes in the pulmonary vascular bed in horses and cattle but rarely in dogs. In the earlier stages, when the pulmonary resistance reaches the level of systemic resistance, there may be intermittent shunting in either direction, right-to-left or left-to-right; later, when pulmonary resistance has risen above the systemic level, the right-to-left shunt predominates and cyanosis usually appears.

Clinical Findings and Treatment: An uncomplicated small septal defect often does not result in outward signs of heart disease. Usually, however, there is a distinctive holosystolic, rather harsh murmur, frequently accompanied by a distinct thrill. The murmur and thrill usually are most pronounced in the right second to fourth intercostal spaces near the sternal margin. While the lesion itself may have little functional effect, subacute bacterial endocarditis, which may develop along the margins of the septal defect, is a potential hazard. This uncommon complication has been reported in cattle. Radiographic evidence of right ventricular enlargement and increased pulmonary blood flow is present in defects of moderate to large size. Even small defects can usually be visualized by echocardiography or located by Doppler flow analysis. Animals with a large septal defect and extensive occlusive lesions in the intrapulmonary vascular bed have pulmonary hypertension and a right-to-left shunt. They are cyanotic and have all the associated features of cyanotic congenital heart disease, such as fatigability, anorexia, weakness, and dyspnea.

Surgical correction of interventricular septal defects requires extracorporeal circulation or deep hypothermia. It is usually patched with a nonreactive plastic material. Small defects in which functional changes are minimal may not appreciably shorten life if left untreated.

TETRALOGY OF FALLOT

This complex malformation consists of pulmonic stenosis, usually subvalvular; interventricular septal defect; dextroposition of the aorta, with overriding of the interventricular septum; and right ventricular hypertrophy. Tetralogy of Fallot has been reported in dogs, cattle, sheep, horses, and cats. It is inherited in the Keeshond breed.

Functional Pathology: The combination of pulmonic stenosis and interventricular septal defect is functionally similar to that of a large interventricular septal defect and pulmonary hypertension. Obstruction to outflow from the right ventricle elevates ventricular systolic pressure, resulting in a right-to-left shunt through the ventricular septal defect. The malpositioned aorta partially overrides the septal defect and receives blood from both ventricles, while pulmonary blood flow is diminished. Mixing of arterial and venous blood results in cyanosis.

Clinical Findings and Treatment: Cyanosis is usually present from birth, and is worsened by exercise, which precipitates dyspnea and often collapse. Polycythemia may be present due to chronic hypoxemia. Despite the marked disability that accompanies this defect, dogs have lived for a number of years before dying from congestive heart failure or embolic phenomena.

A loud, harsh systolic murmur usually is heard best in the pulmonic area and right second to third intercostal space, near the sternal margin. A thrill may be palpated in these areas. Right ventricular hypertrophy is indicated by marked right axis deviation in the ECG, accompanied by large S waves in the left precordial leads. Thoracic radiographs reveal right heart enlargement with normal or diminished pulmonary vascular markings. The ascending aorta usually is dilated. The principal defects can be visualized by echocardiography.

Creation of an artificial ductus arteriosus (Blalock-Taussig shunt) may increase pulmonary blood flow and alleviate the cyanosis to some degree. Complete correction by relief of the pulmonary stenosis and closure of the ventricular septal defect is preferable, but requires open heart surgery.

FELINE LYMPHOSARCOMA AND LEUKEMIA
(Feline lymphoma and leukemia, Lymphosarcoma)

Lymphosarcoma is the most frequently diagnosed neoplastic disease of cats. Mediastinal, multicentric, and alimentary forms are recognized. The mediastinal form is common in young cats; involvement of the abdominal organs is more common in older animals. Lymphoid and myeloid leukemia are less frequent.

Etiology and Epidemiology: Feline leukemia virus (FeLV) can be demonstrated in cats with lymphosarcoma in 90% of mediastinal, 70% of multicentric, and 35% of alimentary cases. It is present in the saliva of infected cats, and transmission occurs by cat-to-cat contact and also congenitally. There is no evidence that the disease is transmissible to man. Cats may be infected subclinically and develop immunity to the virus. Alternatively, they may become persistently infected. Most kittens exposed *in utero* or before 8 wk of age become viremic. Older cats are much less susceptible. Viremic cats have a marked predisposition to neoplasia or one of the nonmalignant diseases associated with FeLV infection (*see* below). The incidence of disease is greatest in cats living in households where other cats are viremic.

Clinical Findings: Frequently, the affected cat undergoes a chronic wasting disease marked by anemia, lethargy, and anorexia. Lymphosarcoma of the anterior mediastinum may cause dyspnea or dysphagia. Radiographs may indicate a mediastinal mass with dorsal displacement of the trachea, or the thoracic structures may be obscured by pleural effusion. In the latter case, large numbers of immature lymphocytes are seen in stained smears of aspirated pleural fluids, and differentiate lymphosarcoma from other causes of hydrothorax. The signs of the abdominal form often are those of enteritis or malabsorption. One or more mesenteric lymph nodes frequently are enlarged. The wall of the stomach or intestine may be thickened diffusely, or it may contain a discrete tumor. Uremia can result from extensive infiltration of the kidneys. Hepatic involvement can cause anemia and jaundice. Enlargement of involved viscera may be evident on palpation or in radiographs. In the multicentric form, the superficial lymph nodes may be grossly enlarged. Malignancy of many other sites may also occur, particularly the spinal canal, eye, and skin. In cats with a nonregenerative anemia, persistent leukopenia, or evidence of lymphocytosis or circulating lymphoblasts, a bone marrow aspiration should be performed. In lymphoblastic leukemia, >40% of the nucleated cells in marrow aspirates are lymphoblasts.

In addition to causing neoplasia, FeLV causes nonmalignant diseases. The better characterized of these include nonregenerative anemia and immunosuppression. The latter predisposes the cat to many other infectious diseases, including feline infectious peritonitis and feline infectious anemia. Other diseases that are associated with FeLV infection include enteritis, and fetal resorption or abortion.

Lesions: Lymphosarcoma may originate in the anterior mediastinum. The anterior ventral thorax may be filled with white, lobulated, tumorous tissue surrounding the heart and displacing the lungs dorsally and posteriorly. The abdominal organs affected by lymphosarcoma are intestine (ileum), mesenteric lymph nodes, kidneys, liver, and spleen.

Diagnosis: Lymphosarcoma may be diagnosed by histologic or cytologic examination of tumors in affected organs. Hematological changes in cats with lymphosarcoma are seen frequently, and are useful in the diagnosis of leukemia. The strong association between persistent infection with FeLV and lymphosarcoma makes laboratory testing for the detection of FeLV in blood a useful procedure.

Control: Vaccines are available, but efficacy is controversial. Chemotherapy can extend the life of a cat with lymphosarcoma. Long-term remission (>1 yr) occurs in 10-15% of cases, but median remission time is ~6 mo. The same chemotherapy protocols used in dogs (*see* CANINE MALIGNANT LYMPHOMA, p 32) can be used in cats. Cats tend to tolerate chemotherapy somewhat better than dogs. FeLV may be eradicated from closed households of cats by removing cats that test positive for the virus in the blood. Disinfection of the premises is not necessary since the virus does not survive in the environment.

HEART DISEASE

Heart disease is often a diagnostic problem, although it is infrequently treated, except in dogs and cats. Those aspects of cardiac disease that are of primary interest are discussed below. Recommendations for therapy are limited to those conditions and species in which there has been substantial experience with treatment. (*See also* GENESIS OF SIGNS OF HEART DISEASE, p 10.)

Examination and Diagnosis: A systematic examination is necessary to evaluate cardiac status. This should include palpation of the thorax to detect thrills (low-frequency vibrations that can be felt with the fingertips) and cardiac displacement, careful auscultation, percussion of the area of cardiac dullness, palpation of the arterial pulse, and examination of the pulsations in the jugular vein. Radiographic examination of the cardiac silhouette for distortion and enlargement is important for diagnosis and prognosis in small animals, and is more informative than precordial percussion. An electrocardiogram (ECG) should be obtained whenever feasible. Clinicians that do not have an ECG machine may subscribe to a transtelephonic ECG reading service. In areas where heartworms are found, the blood should be examined for microfilariae.

Heart disease should be considered only when a dependable sign is found, since many other conditions simulate it. Often, animals are brought to veterinarians with a complaint of exercise intolerance. While this by itself is not a dependable sign, heart disease must be considered in the differential diagnosis.

In dogs, heart disease should not be diagnosed unless at least one of the following is detected: 1) a Grade III systolic murmur in the absence of anemia; 2) a diastolic murmur or a diastolic filling sound producing a gallop rhythm; 3) a palpable precordial thrill; 4) generalized venous engorgement; 5) atrial fibrillation or flutter; 6) paroxysmal ventricular tachycardia; 7) atrial or ventricular ectopic beats consistently present and of frequent occurrence; 8) complete atrioventricular (AV) block; 9) left bundle-branch block; 10) electrocardiographic right ventricular enlargement (*see* COR PULMONALE, p 49) pattern; 11) radiographic or echocardiographic evidence of gross heart enlargement, enlargement of one or more chambers, or pericardial effusion; or 12) pronounced and fixed splitting of the second heart sound.

Atrial fibrillation or flutter, complete AV block, pericardial friction rub, loud murmurs, precordial thrills, and generalized venous engorgement are reliable signs of cardiac disease in horses and in most other domestic species including cattle. Signs that are of controversial significance or questionable specificity include: infrequent ventricular ectopic beats, all arrhythmias and conduction disturbances that disappear after exercise, RS-T segment shifts, wandering pacemaker, diastolic murmur (a reliable sign in dogs), and enlargement of the area of cardiac dullness. Systolic murmurs are common in normal horses and, in the absence of other signs, cannot be considered reliable evidence of disease. Diastolic murmurs usually indicate heart disease in horses.

The most common and obvious nonspecific signs in animals with cardiac disease are: systolic murmur, dyspnea, coughing, pulmonary edema and ascites, and ease of fatigability or weakness. While highly suggestive of heart disease, a positive diagnosis should be made only after one or more of the dependable signs have been elicited, or other possibilities eliminated. In certain degenerative diseases of the myocardium, congestive heart failure may be present without abnormal heart sounds or diagnostic electrocardiographic changes.

Echocardiography: Detailed 2-dimensional images and linear time-varying (M-mode) movements of the heart can be obtained with reflected waves of ultrasound (qv, p 957). In addition to these examinations, blood flow velocity can be measured by Doppler echocardiography. Echocardiography complements the other diagnostic procedures by providing quantitation of the dynamic events of the cardiac cycle. With these noninvasive procedures, cardiac chamber and wall dimensions can be determined, the anatomy and motion of valves can be visualized, and pressure gradients and blood flow volumes can be calculated as well as several indexes of cardiac function. It can also identify some changes in myocardial tissue texture indicative of ischemia and fibrosis, masses, valvular vegetations, and many other features previously verifiable only at necropsy.

HEART SOUNDS AND MURMURS

Normal Heart Sounds and Variants: Four heart sounds are frequently audible in **horses.** The first sound (S_1) is associated with closure of the AV valves, the second sound (S_2) with closure of the semilunar valves. The third sound (S_3) occurs in early diastole at the end of the period of rapid ventricular filling. The fourth or atrial sound (S_4) is related to atrial systole. While all these sounds may be heard, often only S_1 and S_2 can be detected.

In **cattle,** only S_1 and S_2 are ordinarily audible. Either S_3 or S_4 is sometimes heard, but less often than in horses. During the IV administration of fluids, such as calcium solutions in cattle with hypocalcemia, either S_4 or S_3, or both, may be accentuated and become audible.

In **dogs,** only S_1 and S_2 are ordinarily heard. Inspiratory splitting of S_2 occurs, but the interval between the 2 components is usually too short to permit auscultation of the splitting. Less commonly S_1 may be split, but this is often an S_4-S_1 complex.

The characteristics of heart sounds in goats, sheep, and pigs have received less attention. In general, only S_1 and S_2 are audible in these species.

Murmurs and other Abnormal Sounds: The intensity of heart murmurs is classified as: Grade I—the murmur of lowest intensity that can be heard, Grade II—a faint murmur restricted to a localized area, Grade III—a murmur that projects widely and is immediately audible when auscultation begins, Grade IV—a murmur immediately heard at the beginning of auscultation and accompanied by a thrill, Grade V—loudest murmur that is still inaudible when the stethoscope chest piece is just removed from the chest, or Grade VI—extremely loud murmur that can still be heard with the stethoscope just removed from the chest wall.

There are 2 general types of systolic murmurs: ejection and regurgitant. **Ejection systolic murmurs** are crescendo-decrescendo in intensity (in the phonocardiogram, they appear diamond-shaped), with the greatest intensity during midsystole. They may be produced by stenosis of the semilunar valves, infundibular stenosis, dilation of the aorta or pulmonary artery, or increased rate of flow through a semilunar valve orifice. **Regurgitant systolic murmurs** are pansystolic and frequently of constant intensity. They can be caused by mitral or tricuspid regurgitation. Pansystolic murmurs can be caused by an interventricular septal defect. These abnormalities do not invariably produce murmurs that can be recognized as either ejection or regurgitant in type.

Diastolic murmurs are caused almost always by aortic or pulmonic insufficiency.

Continuous or machinery murmurs almost always indicate patent ductus arteriosus (qv, p 35). This continuous murmur waxes and wanes in intensity with systole and diastole, being of greatest intensity at the time of S_2.

In horses, presystolic, early systolic, and early diastolic murmurs are frequently audible in the absence of cardiovascular disease or anemia. The early systolic murmurs are most common and are generally heard over the base of the heart (aortic and pulmonic auscultatory areas). A short, high-pitched, squeaking, early diastolic murmur, greatest in intensity near the cardiac apex (mitral area), may occasionally be heard in healthy young horses.

Diastolic gallop rhythms: Triple, 3-beat, or gallop rhythms resemble the cadence of a galloping horse. The "extra" sound is classified as an early diastolic (ventricular), presystolic (atrial), or summation gallop. These sounds represent abnormal accentuations of S_3 and S_4 in animals in which these sounds are normally inaudible. The early diastolic (ventricular) gallop sound (exaggerated S_3) is associated, in dogs and cats, with advanced myocardial disease and congestive heart failure. The presystolic (atrial) gallop sound (exaggerated S_4) becomes audible when the interval between atrial and ventricular systole (PR interval in the ECG) is prolonged. Summation gallop results from fusion of atrial and ventricular gallop sounds and may occur in congestive heart failure with tachycardia. All 3 of these gallop rhythms may be heard in normal horses.

Systolic clicks: Short, sharp, often transient sounds, called clicks, occur during systole but are uncommon in dogs and probably in other domestic species. They usually are single, but may be multiple; they may disappear completely in some cycles. In man, the click or click-murmur syndromes have been associated with prolapsing of the mitral valve into the left atrium during systole. Their clinical significance in other animals is uncertain, but mitral valve abnormalities, such as prolapsing, should be considered.

Splitting of the heart sounds: Audible splitting of either S_1 or S_2 may occur in the absence of other cardiac abnormalities. S_1 may be markedly split when the contraction of the 2 ventricles is asynchronous, as in bundle-branch block and certain ectopic ventricular beats. Splitting is often confused with an S_4-S_1 complex. S_2 may be split during inspiration in dogs and during either inspiration or expiration in horses. Abnormal splitting of S_2 is associated with pulmonary hypertension as in pulmonary emphysema of horses and heartworm infection of dogs. Other causes in dogs (and possibly in other species) include atrial septal defect, pulmonic stenosis, right or left bundle-branch block, and certain ventricular ectopic beats.

Triple rhythms: The various sounds that may produce triple rhythms may be summarized as follows: 1) physiological—S_3 in horses and cattle, S_4 in horses and cattle, and summation gallop in horses during tachycardia; 2) abnormal—systolic click; or 3) pathological—diastolic ventricular gallop, diastolic atrial gallop, and diastolic summation gallop.

Splitting of S_1 or S_2 must be distinguished from triple rhythms in which 2 of the sounds are close together as in certain systolic clicks in dogs, and when S_4 closely precedes S_1 in horses.

Synchronous diaphragmatic flutter: The diaphragm may contract synchronously with the heart to produce loud thumping noises on auscultation and usually visible contraction in the flank area. The syndrome results from stimulation of the phrenic nerve by atrial depolarization and occurs primarily when there is a marked electrolyte or acid-base imbalance, particularly with hypocalcemia. It is most common in horses and dogs, and occurs frequently in eclampsia (qv, pp 448 and 457). It occurs most commonly in dogs in association with electrolyte disturbances induced by GI disease.

ARRHYTHMIAS

Disturbances in heart rate and rhythm arise when there is abnormality in the formation and/or propagation of the electrical impulse through the conducting system of the heart, or when ectopic irritant foci discharge and assume pacemaker activity. They may occur from primary myocardial disease or secondary to increased or decreased myocardial irritability as the result of toxic, anoxic, or drug effects, or of electrolyte imbalance. Ventricular rhythm slightly faster than the sinus rate is a frequent occurrence in trauma cases and, as a result of compromised venous return, in acute gastric dilatation (qv, p 234) in large dogs. This rhythm may evolve into serious arrhythmias that justify treatment with IV lidocaine. Arrhythmia may also occur as the result of normal variation in autonomic traffic to the heart. Arrhythmia (in all species but man) rarely occurs as a normal physiological variation. Respiratory sinus arrhythmia is the normal resting rhythm in dogs, and second degree AV block is normal in quiet, healthy horses. An ECG is required for diagnosis and differentiation of most arrhythmias because success of antiarrhythmic therapy depends on the focus of origin and type of the abnormal rhythm. Clinically, arrhythmias can be divided into bradyarrhythmias, in which the heart rate is too slow, and tachyarrhythmias, in which the heart rate is too fast or too irregular. The former include sinus bradycardia, sinus arrest, SA block, AV block, and premature depolarizations. In horses, atrial fibrillation produces an irregular but not rapid rate at rest, whereas in other species, it usually produces an irregular tachycardia. Pathological tachycardias should always be suspected when the heart rate is elevated beyond that expected for the condition of the animal.

Sinus bradycardia: This is a slow heart rate that may be normal in athletic animals at rest but also occurs in hypocalcemia and with increased intracranial pressure. Bradycardia is considered to be present when sinus rates in dogs are <45-55 beats/min (bpm); in cats, <90 bpm; and in horses, <20 bpm. Bradycardia may also occur with hypothyroidism, digitalis intoxication, hypoxia, hyperkalemia, and adrenocortical insufficiency. Treatment is restricted to correction of the initiating cause.

Respiratory sinus arrhythmia: Sinus arrhythmia is most commonly detected in normal resting dogs. There is a variation in heart rhythm associated with variation in the intensity of vagal tone. Here, R-R intervals vary >10%. The heart rate usually increases with inspiration and decreases with expiration. It is abolished by reduction in vagal tone and increases in heart rate resulting from excitement, exercise, and administration of atropine. It may be associated with a wandering pacemaker within the sinoatrial node, varying PR interval, and P wave amplitide in ECG recordings in dogs.

Sinus arrest and sinoatrial (SA) block: In sinus arrest, there is failure of generation of impulses at the SA node; with SA block, there is failure of propagation from the SA node to the atrium. They cannot be differentiated clinically and are treated similarly. They may result from excessive vagal tone in all species, and reflex effects resulting from firm pressure on the eyes (oculocardiac reflex) and carotid sinus pressure in dogs. In normal horses, an occasional SA block occurs at rest and in the absence of P wave abnormality. In all species, repetitive episodes of SA block involving 2 or more beats and SA block occurring at heart rates above resting normal are suggestive of disease. SA block has been associated with syncope, especially in Doberman Pinschers, young Boxers, Miniature Schnauzers, Dachshunds, and Cocker Spaniels. If syncope is frequent, treatment with atropine or isoproterenol may be therapeutic but is often unsatisfactory. There are some reports of "silent atrium" in English Setters, in which there was no atrial activity (P waves) on the ECG. Echocardiography confirms the lack of contraction of the atrial myocardium.

Atrioventricular (AV) block: Impaired conduction between the atria and the ventricles. In first degree or incomplete AV block, the conduction time is increased and the diagnosis can be made by demonstrating an increased PR interval in the ECG.

In second degree AV block (incomplete block with dropped beats), occasional impulses fail to traverse the AV node and atrial contraction is not followed by ventricular contraction. The block may occur at regular intervals or at random. During the block, there is no S_1 or S_2 and no arterial pulse. In horses, the sound associated with atrial contraction (S_4) is commonly heard, and the occurrence of S_4 not followed by other heart sounds is diagnostic for second or third degree heart block. S_4 may also be audible in dogs. In all species, an atrial jugular wave may be observed during the block. When the PR intervals preceding the dropped beat progressively lengthen, the condition is known as the Wenckebach or Mobitz type I block. If the PR intervals do not change, the condition is known as a Mobitz type II block. Definitive diagnosis is by ECG.

In third degree or complete heart block, none of the impulses are conducted from the atria to the ventricles. The ventricular rhythm is established from an ectopic nodal or ventricular pacemaker that discharges at a slower rate than the SA node, and the atria and ventricles beat independently. The heart and pulse rates are regular, but there is a pronounced bradycardia that is relatively unresponsive to factors (eg, exercise or excitement) that usually increase heart rate. The difference between atrial and ventricular contraction rates produces variation in ventricular filling and varying position of AV valve leaflets with variation in intensity of S_1 and arterial pulse amplitude. Periodically, the atria contract when the ventricle is in systole, which results in large pulsations in the jugular vein (cannon waves). In some animals, the faster atrial contractions can be detected with a stethoscope.

The significance of the AV block varies from species to species. Both first and second degree AV block may be present without outward evidence of cardiac disease. First degree AV block may result from excessive vagal tone and generally is not considered significant in dogs or horses unless other evidence of heart disease is present. In all species, second degree AV block may be indicative of heart disease. However, in horses, it is more commonly the result of high vagal tone. It is detected at resting heart rates of <40 bpm and, as in SA block, may be induced or abolished by maneuvers that decrease vagal tone. Complete AV block is always abnormal, and the prognosis is grave. It is frequently associated with syncope, especially with exercise or excitement.

AV block may be caused by fibrosis, neoplasia, or other injuries to the AV node or may be secondary to toxic, electrolytic, or hypoxic influences on that structure. Treatment is aimed primarily at correcting the underlying cause. Complete heart block is usually associated with irreversible lesions. Antiarrhythmic therapy is generally restricted to animals with complete heart block and is aimed at increasing the heart rate with atropine, probanthine, or isoproterenol. Drug therapy has limited success, and the only reliable treatment for complete heart block is installation of an electronic pacemaker. These devices, when installed correctly, can improve the life of animals that suffer from arrhythmia-related syncope. Only pulse generators that sense the occurrence of a naturally occurring ventricular depolarization should be used. If AV block develops during digitalis therapy, digitalis toxicity should be considered.

Bundle-branch block and the Wolff-Parkinson-White syndrome are rare conduction abnormalities. They have been observed in animals and diagnosis can be confirmed by electrocardiography. Their significance in other animals has not been established, but in man they may predispose to certain ventricular arrhythmias.

Premature beats: Premature or ectopic (misplaced) beats arise from irritated foci within the conducting tissue or working myocardium. Atrial and ventricular ectopic beats may result from primary myocardial disease or occur secondary to toxic, anoxic, or electrolyte effects. These arrhythmias, especially ventricular ectopic beats, are the more common irregularities observed in heart disease. Ectopic beats always indicate myocardial abnormality, but there is some doubt of the clinical significance of the infrequent ectopic beat that is occasionally heard during examination in all species when there is no other evidence of heart disease. Occasional premature beats do not require specific antiarrhythmic therapy, and treatment is directed at correction of the underlying cause. Digitalis glycosides must be used with caution at all times, but special care must be exercised if premature ventricular depolarizations are present. Tachycardias resulting from repetitive discharge may require specific antiarrhythmic therapy. Digitalis toxicity should always be considered as a cause when ectopic beats develop during digitalis therapy.

Supraventricular tachycardias: The pacemaker activity may occur in the sinus node, atrium, or AV node, and an ECG is required for differentiation. The heart and pulse rates are rapid but usually regular. **Sinus tachycardia** occurs normally with exercise or excitement but also occurs with fever, anemia, hyperthermia, toxemia, and shock. **Atrial and junctional tachycardias** occur in atrial myocardial disease. They are often paroxysmal in nature and characterized by periods of rapid, usually regular, contractions that start and stop suddenly. Syncope may occur. Frequently, they are found in conjunction with premature atrial contractions, and in dogs, are most commonly associated with chronic mitral valvular fibrosis leading to left atrial enlargement.

Supraventricular tachycardias may be terminated by factors that increase vagal tone such as digitalis and carotid sinus or ocular pressure, which initiate the oculocardiac reflex. For well-defined indications and under careful monitoring, vasopressors, propranolol, or calcium channel blocking agents (such as diltiazem or verapamil) may be of use in refractory supraventricular arrhythmias. Precise dosages for dogs and cats have not been established.

Ventricular tachycardias: These arise from one or more ectopic pacemakers within the ventricular myocardium. When the discharge is considerably faster than that of the SA node, the ectopic pacemaker dominates, and the heart and pulse rates are fast and are usually regular. When the ectopic pacemaker rate approximates that of the SA node, both pacemakers may influence the heart and there may be a gross irregularity in rhythm. Intensity of the heart sounds, the apex beat, and the arterial pulse vary markedly, and a pulse deficit may be present. Frequently the arrhythmia is paroxysmal. There are characteristic, bizarre QRS complexes on the ECG. Ventricular tachycardias occur with primary myocardial disease and are common in the terminal stages of heart failure. They may also be induced by electrolyte imbalance, acute toxicities, and gastric distention or trauma in dogs. When cardiac function is already compromised by myocardial failure or abnormal valve function, severe dyspnea and weakness, and syncope may be associated with paroxysmal tachycardias. Other signs of acute or chronic heart failure may be present. When contractility is depressed and filling pressure is high, ventricular tachycardias are precursors to ventricular fibrillation. Lidocaine may be used IV for immediate control of a life-threatening tachyarrhythmia while blood levels of quinidine or procainamide are being established. Excitement of the animal should be avoided. In less severe situations, oral quinidine alone may suffice. Treatment directed toward correction of the underlying cause is essential (*see* THE MYOCARDIUM, below).

Atrial fibrillation: This is characterized by a rapid and irregularly irregular cardiac rhythm. Atrial depolarization and repolarization occur over numerous fronts, and there is no coordinated atrial contraction. Stimulation of the AV node occurs frequently but in a random fashion to result in a rapid and grossly irregular heart rate. The irregularity produces variation in the diastolic filling period between beats and, consequently, variation in intensity of the heart sounds and amplitude of the arterial pulse. With exceptionally short diastolic periods, there is insufficient filling of the ventricles to produce an arterial pulse after ventricular contraction. At rapid heart rates, this produces a pulse rate that is considerably lower than the heart rate (pulse deficit). Definitive diagnosis is by the ECG, which shows an absence of P waves, the presence of rapid f waves, and an absolute irregularity in the R-R intervals. In dogs, atrial fibrillation with high heart rates usually indicates severe cardiovascular disease. It occurs in syndromes that produce atrial dilation and hypertrophy and is a common terminal finding in chronic mitral valve fibrosis. It also occurs in idiopathic dilated cardiomyopathy and in hypertrophic cardiomyopathy and is much more common (and occurs with less severe underlying heart disease) in giant breeds. Because this arrhythmia usually does not occur until the late stage of heart disease in dogs, life expectancy is seldom >1 yr. Treatment should be aimed at slowing the ventricular rate, usually with digitalis glycosides, calcium channel blockers, and β-blockers given to slow conduction through the AV node. The purpose is to reduce the heart rate to an acceptably efficient rate and to eliminate the pulse deficit if possible, as well as to increase the efficiency of the myocardium. The doses and combinations of drugs need to be adjusted according to the desired heart rate, and to avoid toxicity. Conversion with quinidine is unlikely to meet with success except in young, large-breed dogs without severe underlying heart disease. Electrical conversion is sometimes successful, but the long-term prognosis is poor due to the underlying and initiating cardiac disease.

In ruminants, atrial fibrillation is sometimes paroxysmal in association with GI tract disorders, but it also may occur as a sequela of cor pulmonale or with cardiac disease.

In horses, atrial fibrillation may occur in conjunction with other cardiac disease such as mitral insufficiency, in which case it establishes as a tachyarrhythmia as in other species. It also can occur in the apparent absence of serious underlying cardiac disease and, in horses with high vagal tone, may occur with a bradycardia. There is gross irregularity of heart rhythm and variation in heart sound intensity and pulse amplitude but no pulse deficit. When the resting rate is 26-48 bpm, there may be few signs of cardiac disability except with heavy exercise. The heart rate will increase in response to moderate exercise. At very slow rates, several seconds may elapse between some beats, and there may be syncope. Atrial fibrillation occurs more commonly in draft and other large horses. It occurs in race horses in association with poor racing performance and may be paroxysmal. Atrial fibrillation with a low, resting heart rate is not incompatible with long life, but affected horses should not be used for riding. Conversion with quinidine can be attempted and is often followed by a return to successful performance in racing animals. Success is greatest when conversion is attempted shortly after the initial onset.

CARDIAC HYPERTROPHY

Any increase in systemic or pulmonary vascular resistance such as systemic hypertension or cor pulmonale leads to left or right ventricular hypertrophy, respectively. Animals suffering from chronic lung disease develop right ventricular hypertrophy due to the increased afterload on the right ventricle. Both left and right ventricular hypertrophy appear to be progressive, but exercise restriction may slow the progression. In horses, progression can also be slowed by avoiding exacerbations of laminitis in the case of left ventricular hypertrophy, and avoiding allergic provocation of cor pulmonale (equine emphysema) in the case of right ventricular hypertrophy.

Avoidance of metabolic, environmental, exercise, or transportation stress in chronic laminitis is important to avoid acute hypertensive episodes, while avoidance of a dusty environment or moldy feeds is essential to management of horses with a sensitized pulmonary tree. In dogs and cats with systemic arterial hypertension due to renal disease, reduction in arterial pressure with antihypertensives may prove useful.

Cardiac hypertrophy in response to congenital anomalies such as pulmonic and aortic stenosis or patent ductus arteriosus and acquired diseases such as heartworm disease in dogs also can be recognized clinically. In dogs, the ECG criteria for right ventricular hypertrophy are fairly well established, while those for left ventricular hypertrophy are far less reliable. Reliable ECG criteria for chamber hypertrophy in other domestic species have not been established.

CARDIAC INSUFFICIENCY AND FAILURE

When cardiac or other disease reduces cardiac reserve, the heart may be unable to meet the requirements of the body in all circumstances. When the reduction in reserve is such that cardiac function is impaired only under extremes of exercise, a state of relative cardiac insufficiency exists. With increasing loss of reserve, increasing grades of severity occur; when the heart cannot fulfill its function in terms of day-to-day activity, cardiac failure exists. Cardiac insufficiency and failure may result from primary myocardial disease reducing the efficiency of myocardial function. It may also result from any factor that increases the work load on the heart and therefore decreases cardiac reserve. Common causes include diseases that produce a pressure load on the heart (eg, stenosis of the outflow valves or pulmonary or systemic arterial hypertension) and abnormalities that cause a volume load on the heart (eg, valvular insufficiency, left-to-right intracardiac shunts [septal defects], or extracardiac shunts such as a patent ductus arteriosus or peripheral arteriovenous shunts). Less common causes of reduction of cardiac reserve and consequent cardiac insufficiency include diseases that produce disorders of filling such as pericardial effusions and stenosis of the AV valves, complete heart block, and reduction in arteriovenous oxygen reserve in severe anemia. In all forms of chronic heart failure, there is usually loss of coronary flow reserve resulting from cardiac hypertrophy or dilation. The failure of the heart to pump blood adequately results in an increase in both end-diastolic volume and venous pressure. Retention of sodium and water also occurs, probably as a result of inadequate renal perfusion and increased renin release, which causes angiotensin elevation, and consequently increased thirst, vasoconstriction, and salt and water retention.

Clinically, cardiac failure can be recognized as left-sided, right-sided, or generalized. Four phases of cardiac decompensation are generally recognized in domestic animals. Phase I, the compensated phase, is asymptomatic; cardiomegaly may be the only sign. In Phase II, some clinical signs are observed after exercise, such as coughing and reduced exercise tolerance. Phase III is decompensation present during minimal activity; pulmonary edema or more subtle radiographic signs are observed, and exercise intolerance is marked. Phase IV is the stage of frank decompensation, marked by signs associated with low cardiac output (such as cachexia), complicated by pulmonary edema and major dyspnea at rest; the animal is usually at risk of sudden death. As **left-sided failure** develops, exercise tolerance decreases and inappropriate dyspnea follows exercise and excitement. Increased pulmonary venous pressure results initially in pulmonary and bronchial congestion and in reflexogenic bronchoconstriction (cardiac asthma). Repetitive coughing after exercise and especially at night is seen in dogs. Orthopnea, with reluctance to lie down, restlessness at night, and paroxysmal attacks of dyspnea are also common. With more severe failure, pulmonary edema with severe dyspnea at rest and rales on auscultation are evident.

Right-sided heart failure is manifest by systemic venous congestion with engorgement of jugular veins. The liver and spleen are enlarged and may be palpable in dogs. In cattle, the liver may become palpable behind the right costal arch, and gross splenic and venous engorgement may be apparent on rectal examination in horses. Fluid retention occurs in all species, but the areas of occurrence vary. In dogs, ascites is most common and usually occurs before development of subcut. edema, hydrothorax, or hydropericardium. In cats, hydrothorax is usually predominant. In large animals, subcut. dependent edema is more common. In cattle, it occurs especially in the submandibular and brisket area, whereas in horses, it tends to initiate in the preputial or mammary area. Limb edema, ascites, and hydrothorax also occur. Hydrothorax should be suspected when there is muffling of the heart and respiratory sounds in the ventral part of the thorax with reduction in resonance on percussion. Hydropericardium produces muffling of the heart sounds and, if severe, produces a defect in filling and low pulse pressure. Both may result in a low-amplitude ECG. Ascites, hydrothorax, or hydropericardium can be confirmed by needle aspiration and subsequent fluid analysis. Radiography and especially echocardiography are useful noninvasive methods of confirming fluid in body cavities, particularly the chest and pericardium. Disturbances in GI function with diarrhea may also result from impaired venous drainage from the intestinal tract.

In **generalized heart failure**, signs of both right-and left-sided failure occur. The findings on auscultation vary, depending on the initiating cause. Radiography is a considerable aid to diagnosis of cardiac enlargement, but a differentiation between cardiac hypertrophy and dilatation is possible only by echocardiography.

Treatment: A primary aim of therapy in congestive heart failure is to eliminate the edema, improve the contractile state of the myocardium, and regulate the rhythm and rate. The aim of conventional therapy has been to reduce the work of the heart (restriction of exercise), reduce the sodium intake, increase the sodium (and water) elimination by use of diuretics, strengthen the heart by means of positive inotropic agents (digitalis glycosides, milrinone, dobutamine, etc), and decrease the load on the ventricle by use of vasodilators.

In dogs, the diet may be regulated to decrease sodium intake; suitable low-sodium diets are available commercially. Many canned dog foods contain excessive sodium (foods of animal origin contain much sodium). Foods low in salt include fresh or frozen vegetables without salt, wheat-based cereals, polished and coated rice, dialyzed milk, and soybean-oil meal. Meat, fish, poultry, and milk and milk-containing foods should be limited, although often these are tolerated as long as no salt is used in their preparation. Public water supplies usually do not contain much sodium, but well water may, and it is nearly always high in softened water. Distilled or deionized water may be helpful in cases reaching the intractable stage of heart failure.

Diuretics to increase sodium (and water) elimination are important and allow liberalization of sodium in the diet so that palatability can be preserved. In dogs, the most effective diuretics are furosemide and the chlorothiazide derivatives. Withdrawal of ascitic fluid by abdominocentesis is indicated only when the volume markedly interferes with breathing, and then only to the extent necessary for comfort. Removal of ascitic fluid results in loss of serum protein, and the abdominal fluid is soon replaced if cardiac compensation and diuresis are not effected by appropriate medical therapy.

Digitalis glycosides slow the heart and increase the strength of myocardial contraction. While rest, sodium restriction, and diuretics are useful adjuncts to the medical therapy of congestive heart failure, digitalis remains the primary therapeutic agent since it acts directly on the failing heart. (*See* NEW POSITIVE INOTROPES, VASODILATORS, AND DIURETICS, below.) Digitalization is seldom done in animals other than dogs and cats. A number of digitalis products are available, but the glycoside digoxin is the most commonly used. Digoxon is supplied in both PO and parenteral dosage forms. The dose depends on the manufacturer, the form (tablet, elixir), and the GI and renal status of the animal.

Digitalization is accomplished when tissue levels are sufficient to produce full therapeutic action. In general, the drug should be given until therapeutic levels are reached, as indicated by amelioration of the clinical signs of congestive heart failure. Since the therapeutic to toxic ratio is near one in dogs and cats, these drugs must be administered with caution. Previous regimes, which strove to achieve rapid tissue concentrations, almost invariably produced toxicity; intensive and rapid administration is not recommended.

Administration of digitalis glycosides: The safest procedure is to digitalize slowly with a daily digoxin maintenance dose of 0.005-0.01 mg/lb (0.01-0.02 mg/ kg), divided b.i.d. Digitalization is usually accomplished in 3-5 days. Larger dogs (>35 lb [16 kg]) require less digoxin, depending on weight/body surface area (BSA) ratio. The BSA in square meters (m^2) is determined by the formula, BSA = $kg^{2/3} \times 0.112$, or it may be found in tables in standard veterinary texts. Using this method, the maintenance dose is 0.22 mg/m^2 of BSA, b.i.d. The therapeutic digoxin serum concentration in dogs should be between 1 and 1.5 ng/mL to reduce likelihood of toxicity yet produce near full inotropic effects; values >2 ng/mL may be toxic. Serum for analyses should be taken 8 hr after the last dose.

In acute fulminating pulmonary edema, furosemide (2-4 mg/kg, IV [dogs]) is the most efficient way to rapidly reduce pulmonary blood volume and ventricular filling pressure since (like nitroglycerine) it acts within ~30 min to shift blood from the lungs to the peripheral veins.

Digitalis toxicity: Since tolerance varies widely, each individual should be observed carefully for signs of toxicity, particularly in the initial period of digitalization. Anorexia and depression are the most common signs. Mild diarrhea is a common early sign of toxicity but does not necessitate discontinuation of the drug; however, anorexia, vomiting, depression, or onset of cardiac arrhythmias signal a need to discontinue it immediately. An increase in PR interval occurs rarely and is a sign of digitalis effect but not necessarily of toxicosis. Worsening of premature ventricular beats may also be seen. When toxicity occurs, digitalis should be withdrawn immediately and 24-48 hr allowed for its excretion and regression of toxic signs; therapy can then be reinstituted at a lower dosage level—usually 50-75% of that used before. Concomitant diuretic therapy, steroid therapy, or GI disturbance may potentiate hypokalemia, which accentuates digitalis toxicity. Severe tachyarrhythmias associated with digitalis toxicity may require specific antiarrhythmic therapy, but fortunately seldom occur.

New positive inotropes, vasodilators, and diuretics: The digitalis glycosides are effective but relatively weak positive inotropes with a low toxic threshold. In acute, severe left-heart failure, cardiac contractility is more effectively and safely supported by IV dobutamine (2-5 μg/lb [4-11 μg/kg]/min). The pressor and chronotropic effects of dobutamine are usually not evident at these dose levels. The most urgent task in treating acute pulmonary edema is to lower left ventricular filling pressure. In addition to a rapid-acting diuretic (eg, furosemide), the IV administration of the vasodilator sodium nitroprusside (2 μg/lb [4 μg/kg]/min, increasing at 15-min intervals by 0.1 μg/lb [0.2 μg/kg]/min) to effect, can be pivotal. The balanced (venous and arterial) dilating effect of this drug reduces filling pressure while facilitating ventricular emptying. If a continuous IV infusion cannot be instituted, nitroglycerin ointment or patches can be applied to the skin to achieve similar but less rapid results. The dose of nitroglycerin ointment is empirical (~1/4-1/2 in./10 lb [~1 cm/5 kg]). If continued, application must be on an alternate-day basis to avoid development of tolerance. Other direct-acting vasodilating agents such as isosorbide dinitrate, hydralazine, minoxidil, or α-adrenergic blocking agents such as phenoxybenzamine, may also be considered as part of the therapy of the failing myocardium.

Treatment of chronic heart failure may be facilitated by the use of orally active balanced vasodilators such as captopril or enalapril (angiotensin-converting-enzyme inhibitors). Increased BUN and creatinine may occur. In the late stages of dilated cardiomyopathy, the heart may be incapable of responding to inotropic stimulation, and modification of loading conditions may be the only way to improve cardiac function. Milrinone (not available commercially), an orally administered analog of amrinone, has combined inotropic and vasodilator properties that make it especially useful for treating animals in heart failure and in sinus rhythm. If atrial fibrillation exists, digoxin is also necessary.

Cor pulmonale is heart disease secondary to pulmonary disease. Pulmonary hypertension leads to right increased pulmonary vascular resistance and ventricular hypertrophy and dilation and, in severe cases, congestive heart failure may occur. Cor pulmonale is common in goats following enzootic pneumonia and in dogs most commonly in association with chronic heartworm disease. In cattle grazing at high altitudes, pulmonary hypertension occurs in some individuals with consequent right-sided heart failure (see HIGH-MOUNTAIN DISEASE, p 632). Cor pulmonale also results from COPD (heaves) or emphysema in horses, and should be considered in the examination of any animal with respiratory disease and right-sided heart failure. Cardiac dilatation may be sufficient to result in tricuspid valve insufficiency.

THE ENDOCARDIUM

Endocarditis, usually of bacterial origin, most commonly involves the valves. Mural endocarditis of the atria occurs in uremia in dogs. Acute mural endocarditis from other causes is occasionally seen at necropsy but is rarely detected clinically. Valvular endocarditis usually follows a prolonged subclinical bacteremia and is often secondary to conditions such as chronic pyemia, mastitis, metritis, and prostatitis. Streptococci, *Erysipelothrix rhusiopathiae*, and *Corynebacterium pyogenes* are the organisms most commonly involved. In horses, migrating strongyles may produce both mural and valvular endocarditis. The mitral, tricuspid, and aortic valves (and rarely the pulmonary) may be affected in all species. In cattle, the tricuspid valve is most frequently involved; in other species, endocarditis of the aortic and mitral valves is more common. Regardless of the valve involved, the result is contraction of the free edges of the valves, and valvular insufficiency. Occasionally, stenosis of some valves and insufficiency of others occur together. Large vegetative lesions are common with endocarditis that involves the AV valves.

The clinical findings in endocarditis relate to those of chronic septicemia and embolism, and to signs resulting primarily from the valvular abnormality. There is often a history of unthriftiness with periods of more severe malaise. The animal may be in poor condition with a rough coat. A low-grade fever is usually present, but during more acute episodes, high fever may occur. There may be evidence of chronic bacteremia and embolism. In cattle, tenosynovitis and arthritis and evidence of renal infarction on urinalysis may be present. Signs relating to valvular damage depend on the valve involved. With tricuspid valve insufficiency, there is a loud pansystolic murmur most audible on the right side over the base of the heart, and usually a jugular pulse. Usually there is a pronounced systolic jugular pulse and right-sided heart failure with generalized venous congestion. Mitral valve endocarditis is associated with a pansystolic murmur heard loudest over the apex of the heart on the left side, and radiating dorsally. Signs of dyspnea and left-sided failure may develop. Aortic insufficiency, occurring most frequently in German Shepherd and larger dogs, produces a diastolic murmur most audible over the base of the heart on the left side. The arterial pulse has a high amplitude. Left-sided failure may develop. With acute bacterial endocarditis, there is usually a pronounced leukocytosis. Blood culture should be attempted. The prognosis is poor, especially when signs of congestive heart failure are present. Prolonged antibacterial therapy is required to control the infection and, when possible, should be based on sensitivity tests. Remission is common. Even when the infection is controlled, there may be severe residual damage to the valve, and continuous treatment for cardiac insufficiency is usually necessary.

Chronic valvular fibrosis (endocardiosis): Chronic fibrosis and nodular thickening of the AV valves with subsequent distortion and defective function is the most common cause of cardiac disease in dogs. The mitral valve is usually affected more often and more severely than the tricuspid valve, and the lesion results in regurgitation. The cause is unknown. The onset of valvular fibrosis occurs relatively early in life (~4-5 yr), and the associated systolic murmur may be detected incidentally during clinical examination for other reasons. In most cases, the lesion produces no outward signs of abnormality until signs of cardiac insufficiency develop during middle age or later. The dog usually has a decreased tolerance for exercise, and there may be a history of coughing after exercise or excitement. Frequently, there is a history of nocturnal coughing that is repetitive and hacking. Less commonly, the owner's initial complaint is that of abdominal distention or acute pulmonary edema. There is a pansystolic murmur, usually grade III or louder, associated with mitral or tricuspid insufficiency, or both, and associated signs of cardiac insufficiency. A third heart sound may be prominent in advanced cases. Radiographic evidence of left atrial and ventricular enlargement and pulmonary congestion or biventricular enlargement may be observed. Clinical features can be similar to dilated cardiomyopathy, but the hyperkinetic left ventricle of mitral regurgitation can easily be distinguished from the hypodynamic myopathic ventricle by echocardiography. There are no typical electrocardiographic changes, but evidence of cardiac enlargement may be present. Left atrial enlargement and vascular lesions predispose to atrial premature beats, which may progress to paroxysmal atrial tachycardia and atrial fibrillation. Ventricular premature beats occur at the advanced stages of heart failure. Untoward sequelae are left atrial rupture with pericardial tamponade, and rupture of the chordae tendineae—both of which produce acute heart failure. Dogs with mild, early signs may respond to salt restriction, diuretic therapy, or afterload reducers, but other forms of therapy may be indicated for treatment and control in severe cases as myocardial failure develops (see CARDIAC INSUFFICIENCY AND FAILURE, above).

Chronic valvular fibrosis is much less common in other species, but lesions on the AV valve occur in older horses and cattle and produce an audible murmur. Occasionally, clinical cardiac insufficiency results.

Valvular blood cysts or hematomas are seen in up to 75% of young calves <3 wk old. The AV valves are most commonly affected. These lesions are also seen in the young of other species; their significance is unknown.

Subendocardial hemorrhages are seen in septicemia and toxemia, and are commonly observed in animals bled to death or following euthanasia with pentobarbital sodium.

THE MYOCARDIUM

Myocardial dysfunction may result from primary myocardial disease or may be secondary to toxic influences or metabolic and electrolyte abnormalities. Degenerative changes occur in lambs, calves, and foals with white muscle disease; in pigs with mulberry heart disease and hepatosis dietetica; and in horses with paralytic myoglobinuria and following snakebites—particularly rattlesnakes. They also occur in severe iron deficiency, copper deficiency, and in toxicity associated with selenium, arsenic, and injectable iron.

Myocarditis may accompany general bacterial, viral, parasitic, and protozoal infections in all species. It is common in septicemic diseases and in pyemic infections in young animals. Significant myocarditis accompanies infection with encephalomyocarditis, foot-and-mouth, and blue-tongue viruses in young animals. Myocarditis may also occur in equine infectious anemia, blackleg, hemorrhagic septicemia, and pullorum disease. It was a frequent sequela of parvoviral infection in young pups before the infection became established in the population, and some lingering cardiomyopathies occurred in dogs, leading to the speculation that these were survivors of puppy parvovirus myocarditis.

Myocardial dysfunction is the cause of death in poisoning with sodium fluoroacetate (1080) and plants such as oleander, foxglove, and phalaris. Myocardial dysfunction also occurs in acute toxemias, severe uremia, diabetic ketoacidosis, adrenocortical dysfunction, and in other diseases with severe electrolyte imbalance, especially those that involve potassium or calcium.

Myocardial infarction is rare in domestic animals, although it may be observed occasionally at necropsy. Gross infarcts of the myocardium, common in people due to coronary atherosclerosis and obstruction of major coronary arteries, are rare in domestic animals. Infarcts from emboli due to vegetative endocarditis have caused clinical signs resembling those of myocardial infarction in man. In dogs, small foci of myocardial necrosis in various stages of resorption and scar formation are found in association with sclerotic narrowing of small intramyocardial arteries.

Many myocardial lesions, if extensive enough, produce typical electrocardiographic changes, such as depression or elevation of the ST segment, depression of the T wave, increased duration of QRS, low voltage, abnormal notching of the QRS complex, and certain arrhythmias (such as atrial fibrillation, ventricular ectopic beats, paroxysmal ventricular tachycardia, and AV block). Clinical diagnosis of myocarditis frequently is difficult or impossible in mild cases. The most frequent diagnostic signs of myocardial inflammation or degeneration are electrocardiographic changes listed above, tachycardia out of proportion to the fever, arrhythmias, cardiac enlargement, and decreased exercise tolerance. Therapy is generally confined to correction or treatment of the initiating cause. Clinical chemistry may aid diagnosis in electrolyte and metabolic disturbances. Lactate dehydrogenase isoenzymes may indicate myocardial damage. When severe arrhythmia occurs, specific antiarrhythmia therapy may be indicated (*see* p 47 *et seq*).

Idiopathic dilated cardiomyopathy characterized by multifocal areas of myocardial necrosis and fibrosis with mononuclear cell infiltration occurs in dogs and cats. In cats, a low plasma level of the amino acid taurine has been associated with cardiomyopathy. Dietary supplementation with taurine increased the plasma levels, and this was associated with a return of left ventricular function toward normal. Most manufacturers have now increased the taurine level of commercial cat food, and the prevalence of the disease has decreased. In a few dogs, l-carnitine deficiency has been associated with reversible dilated cardiomyopathy.

In dogs, dilated cardiomyopathy is most common in giant breeds and in males. Male Doberman Pinschers appear to be highly vulnerable to both canine parvovirus and cardiomyopathy. The developing cardiomyopathy is generally not detected until signs of severe heart disease occur. There is usually atrial fibrillation or premature beats following left atrial hypertrophy. Onset of clinical signs is often rapid, and there is usually a history of a sudden onset of weight loss, exercise intolerance, dyspnea, and abdominal distention. Loss of muscling, especially along the back, is frequently noticeable. Signs are associated with right- and left-sided congestive heart failure. There is frequently biventricular enlargement with dilatation of the valvular annulus to produce a soft pansystolic murmur of AV valve insufficiency. Murmurs are not necessarily present and the degree of AV insufficiency is usually mild. The prognosis is poor, and affected dogs seldom live for more than a few months after onset. Treatment is as for heart failure of other etiologies. Diltiazem and propranolol may also be used when digitalis by itself is not fully effective in reducing the heart rate with atrial fibrillation. The extent of myocardial disease may preclude a significant response to inotropic drugs, and alteration of ventricular loading conditions with vasodilating drugs may be the only effective treatment in the late stages.

In cats, a syndrome of **hypertrophic cardiomyopathy** is common. There is no age incidence, but it is more common in males. In young cats, endomyocarditis of unknown etiology progresses to severe endomyocardial fibrosis in older cats, with left ventricular hypertrophy, left atrial dilatation, and finally cardiomegaly, with aortic and atrial thrombus formation. The disease is insidious, and frequently no abnormality is observed until the onset of heart failure or embolic arterial occlusion. There may be a history of reduced appetite, lethargy, and dyspnea following exertion, or of a mild and poorly defined lameness. Usually, the first sign seen is sudden onset of dyspnea or hindleg locomotor difficulties, or both. Dyspnea is both inspiratory and expiratory and results from left-sided heart failure. Pulmonary congestion and edema, and pleural effusion may be detected radiographically. The heart may be normal on auscultation, but a pansystolic murmur associated with dilation of the mitral valve annulus is common. A gallop rhythm frequently is audible. Radiography and electrocardiography show evidence of marked left atrial enlargement and sometimes left ventricular enlargement. Thromboembolic disease is common. Occlusion of the iliac arteries often results in sudden onset of posterior paresis or paralysis. There is severe pain with cold hindlimbs and tenseness of the gastrocnemius. The femoral pulse may be absent, or variable between the hindlimbs. Thromboembolism may involve other areas, such as the renal arteries to produce renal infarcts or occasionally severe renal disease. The treatment of hypertrophic cardiomyopathy in cats relies on the use of diuretics and negative inotropes. Acepromazine has also been used for embolism to increase collateral blood channels to the limbs. To be effective, surgery to remove aortic emboli must be performed within the first few hours; however, it is generally no more effective than conservative medical therapy. Aspirin and other anticoagulant agents may slow the rate of dangerous thrombus formation, especially at the aortic bifurcation. Recently obtained data suggest that digitalis may be useful for this type of cardiomyopathy because of its ability to improve atrial function and therefore left ventricular preload. Similar clinical signs also occur in cats with the dilated form of cardiomyopathy. A reliable distinction between dilated and hypertrophic cardiomyopathy can be made only by examining left ventricular dimensions and contractile indices with echocardiography.

THE PERICARDIUM AND ITS CONTENTS

The pericardium may be congenitally absent or only partially formed. Such abnormalities are usually of no clinical significance.

Hydropericardium may occur in congestive heart failure and hydremia, eg, in parasitism with associated anemia. Pericarditis with massive sanguineous effusion is a clinical entity that may occur in dogs. Usually the first signs noted are dyspnea, ease of fatigability, and ascites. Diagnostic signs include muffled heart sounds, low electrocardiographic deflection, and a circular and greatly enlarged cardiac silhouette on fluoroscopy; cardiac pulsations cannot be easily discerned, or are absent. Commonly the ECG will show electrical alternation—deflections alternating in amplitude. Even small effusions can be identified by 2-dimensional and M-mode echocardiography, which are the most definitive noninvasive diagnostic procedures for the condition. The technique is equally valuable in farm animals. The fluid closely resembles blood, but does not clot. It is bacteriologically sterile, and its removal results in dramatic alleviation of the clinical signs. The condition may recur.

Similar effusions are sometimes present owing to neoplasms within the pericardial sac (eg, heart-base tumors and hemangiosarcomas). While primary neoplasms of the heart are extremely rare, certain metastatic processes may invade the myocardium and produce ST segment deviations or premature ventricular depolarizations. In cattle, lymphoma may also invade the cardiac structures. This is difficult to differentiate from pericarditis as a sequela of traumatic reticuloperitonitis (qv, p 224). In these cases, removal of the fluid is merely palliative. Blood that clots may be withdrawn in cases of pericardial tamponade due to a fresh left atrial rupture or penetrating wounds. Pericarditis occurs in many infectious diseases in large animals and is associated with traumatic reticuloperitonitis. Clinical detection relies on detecting muffled heart sounds or pericardial friction rubs. If pericardial effusion is marked, there may be venous congestion and a poor pulse amplitude. Echocardiography is especially helpful to establish pericardial effusion or to demonstrate a thickened pericardium. Laboratory examination of aspirated pericardial fluid is of great value in determining the cause.

HEMOSTATIC DISORDERS

Defects in hemostasis may be inherited or acquired. Effective hemostasis requires a normal vessel wall, normal levels of blood coagulation factors, and adequate numbers of functional platelets. Platelets must adhere to the vessel wall at sites of disruption and then stick to each other to form a hemostatic plug. This plug needs to be strengthened by the incorporation of fibrin. A deficiency in vessel response, platelet activity, or fibrin generation leads to defective hemostasis.

INHERITED DISORDERS

Inherited abnormalities of the vessel wall are not often recognized in domestic animals. Connective tissue diseases such as the Ehlers-Danlos syndrome in mink, dogs, and other species may result in vascular thrombocytopenia.

Many types of inherited blood coagulation deficiencies have been reported in domestic animals. Most of these are single factor deficiencies or abnormalities; some have been multiple coagulation defects. Hemophilias A and B are inherited as sex-linked traits and are commonly carried by the female and manifest clinically only in the male, except when hemophilic males are mated to carrier females. Hemophilia A is the most common severe inherited coagulopathy. All other known inherited blood coagulation defects are transmitted as autosomal traits.

The inherited blood coagulation defects that have been reported in domestic animals include: factor I (fibrinogen) deficiency in dogs and goats; factor II (prothrombin) deficiency in Boxers, Otterhounds, and English Cocker Spaniels; factor VII (proconvertin) deficiency in Beagles, English Bulldogs, Alaskan Malamutes and mongrels; factor VIII deficiency (classic hemophilia, hemophilia A) in practically all breeds of dogs and in mongrels, Standardbreds, Thoroughbreds, Quarter Horses, Hereford cattle, and purebred and mixed-breed cats; factor IX deficiency (Christmas disease, hemophilia B) in 16 breeds of dogs and in British Shorthair, Himalayan, and Siamese cats; factor X (Stuart factor) deficiency in American Cocker Spaniels and a mongrel; factor XI deficiency in English Springer Spaniels, Great Pyrenees, Weimaraners, Kerry Blue Terriers, and in Holstein cattle; Fletcher factor (prekallikrein) deficiency in a Poodle; factor XII (Hageman factor) deficiency in cats, Standard Poodles, and German Shorthaired Pointers. Normal marine mammals, birds, and most reptiles lack factor XII but do not bleed as a result.

Von Willebrand's disease is a relatively common inherited defect reported in 54 breeds of purebred dogs, in mongrel dogs, and in cats, rabbits, and pigs. Doberman Pinschers, German Shepherd Dogs, Golden Retrievers, Miniature Schnauzers, Pembroke Welsh Corgis, Scottish Terriers, Shetland Sheepdogs, Basset Hounds, Standard Poodles, and Standard Manchester Terriers have a high prevalence of the disease (10-70%) within their respective breeds. It is characterized by high morbidity, low mortality, and a mild to severe bleeding diathesis that often is exacerbated by physical and physiological stresses as well as by concomitant disease (hypothyroidism, parvovirus infection, autoimmune disease). It is an autosomal trait with 2 forms of clinical and genetic expression: 1) homozygous individuals born of asymptomatic, heterozygous (carrier) parents (seen in Poland-China pigs, Scottish Terriers, Chesapeake Bay Retrievers, and Shetland Sheepdogs), and 2) the more common, incompletely dominant form in which there is variable expression or penetrance (homozygotes and heterozygotes can manifest a bleeding tendency). Homozygosity is usually lethal in this disease.

The defect involves both platelet and coagulation (factor VIII) function. A quantitative decrease in von Willebrand's factor is detected by reduced von Willebrand's factor antigen (VWF:Ag, formerly factor-VIII-related antigen) or coagglutinin cofactor. These are the most diagnostic tests. A functional decrease in the factor is detected by sensitive tests of platelet function, such as the buccal mucosal bleeding time in dogs. The factor is necessary to maintain platelet and vascular function. Decreased coagulant activity (factor-VIII-coagulant [VIII:C]) may be detected occasionally by the activated partial thromboplastin time (APTT), but the APTT is often normal in the disease even though it is the most sensitive clinically available test of the ability of factor VIII to form a clot.

Inherited platelet-function defects (hereditary thrombopathias) have been reported in Otterhounds, Basset Hounds, Simmental cattle, and Fawn-Hooded rats. The basic platelet defect differs. These disorders may produce no clinical signs, or manifest by increased bleeding tendencies, usually due to platelets that react poorly or not at all to stimulation by collagen, adenosine diphosphate, and thrombin, and thus fail to form an adequate hemostatic plug. These bleeding tendencies are often exacerbated by trauma or surgery. Transmission is as an autosomal trait.

ACQUIRED DISORDERS

Acquired disorders of hemostasis may result from a number of diverse causes that affect specific components of the hemostatic mechanism, and except within inbred families of companion animals and for von Willebrand's disease, tend to be more common in domestic animals than are the inherited defects. Vessel wall damage with accompanying petechiation occurs in such conditions as equine purpura (qv, p 58) or in vessel wall hypoxias due to poor circulation or to anemia. Scurvy (vitamin C deficiency) in guinea pigs may result in vascular purpura.

Acquired blood coagulation disorders usually involve multiple factor deficiencies and may result from defective synthesis, excessive utilization, or inhibition of one or more coagulation factors. Certain clotting factors in the circulating blood may be depressed by agents in the feed (*see* SWEET CLOVER POISONING, p 1733), drugs, or various diseases, particularly those causing severe or moderate hepatic damage.

Anticoagulant rodenticides (qv, p 1720), such as warfarin and the newer more potent compounds (brodifacoum, diphacinone, chlorphacinone), or dicumarol depress production of the vitamin-K-dependent coagulation factors (factors II, VII, IX, and X). Since the liver is the major site of coagulation factor synthesis, hepatic damage may result in defective blood coagulation. The low levels of clotting factors in the plasma of newborn animals may predispose to bleeding. Anaphylactic shock, intravascular hemolysis, excessive tissue necrosis (burns, inflammation, neoplasia, trauma, surgery), or bacterial endotoxins can lead to activation of blood platelets and coagulation factors, and result in disseminated intravascular coagulation (DIC, qv, p 24) and thromboembolism. Amniotic fluid contains potent thromboplastins that can be introduced into the maternal circulation during dystocias, leading to intravascular clotting. In addition to depletion of coagulation factors, DIC results in utilization of platelets, enhanced fibrinolytic activity, and the appearance of circulating fibrin degradation products (FDP), all of which contribute to the bleeding tendency that ensues. Increased fibrinolytic activity has been recognized in dogs as a cause of excessive bleeding after trauma or surgery.

The development of inhibitors to coagulation factors has been reported with systemic lupus erythematosus and multiple myeloma in dogs. Inhibitors are antibodies directed against specific procoagulant proteins.

Acquired von Willebrand's disease is now recognized in man and dogs in association with familial autoimmune thyroid disease. Of the 54 dog breeds in which von Willebrand's disease (*see* above) has been reported, 42 also transmit familial hypothyroidism. The prevalence of both conditions appears to have increased rapidly in the last decade. In dogs, von Willebrand's disease is exacerbated by concurrent autoimmune thyroiditis whether or not the disorder has progressed to the stage of clinically overt hypothyroidism. Asymptomatic carriers of inherited von Willebrand's disease may exhibit a bleeding tendency if they subsequently develop thyroiditis or hypothyroidism. Generally, it is impossible to distinguish between inherited and acquired von Willebrand's disease in an individual animal with currently available diagnostic techniques.

Acquired thrombocytopenias can result from various causes (*see* CANINE THROMBOCYTOPENIA, p 56), most of which have an immunologic basis.

In **acquired platelet-function defects** (acquired thrombopathias), the number of platelets may be normal but their function is abnormal. Uremia results in reduced platelet adhesion, abnormal platelet aggregation to adenosine diphosphate and collagen, and a prolonged buccal mucosal bleeding time.

Many drugs, such as aspirin, phenylbutazone, promazine derivatives, and nitrofurantoin, interfere with normal platelet function and thus hemostatic plug formation, although not often to a significant level. Other drugs that may impair hemostasis include sulfonamides, penicillins, estrogens, phenothiazines, antihistamines, anti-inflammatory drugs, and plasma expanders. Qualitative platelet defects may also be associated with hypothyroidism, cirrhosis of the liver, and leukemias. In some acquired platelet function defects, the platelet phospholipid (platelet factor 3) essential for normal blood coagulation is abnormal, or is not released from the platelet.

Diagnosis: Depending on the nature of the hemostatic defect, different signs are seen. The most common signs to be expected with thrombocytopenia include persistent epistaxis and petechial or ecchymotic hemorrhages. The appearance of larger hemorrhages (eg, hematomas), recurrent shifting lameness (hemarthrosis), or bleeding into body cavities tends to indicate a coagulopathy. Exceptions occur with more general signs, eg, excessive bleeding from surgery or trauma.

Vessel wall abnormalities: Defects in the vessel wall are diagnosed by prolonged bleeding times in the absence of other defects in the hemostatic mechanism, or obvious cause such as a ruptured aneurysm or trauma.

Blood coagulation abnormalities: The coagulation system is complex and has many interactions, but for in vitro diagnosis it may be simply divided into the intrinsic, extrinsic, and common pathways to localize the coagulation defect. The activated partial thromboplastin time (APTT) is the most sensitive clinically available test of all coagulation factors except for factor VII. The APTT evaluates the intrinsic and common pathway factors. The prothrombin time (PT or one-stage prothrombin time) evaluates the extrinsic system (clinically, only factor VII) and the common pathway. The Russell's viper venom time (RVVT), less commonly available than the APTT and the PT, evaluates the common pathway factors. The thrombin time (TT) evaluates fibrinogen, and can monitor the effective level of anticoagulants such as heparin, while the modified thrombin time is a standard method to quantitate fibrinogen but too insensitive to monitor anticoagulant therapy.

Use of various combinations of tests can often identify a defect to one of the pathways. A defect in the intrinsic pathway such as hemophilia A (factor VIII) would have a prolonged APTT yet normal PT. Factor VII deficiency would have a prolonged PT and normal APTT. A defect in the common pathway or multiple defects such as the deficiency of factors II, VII, IX, and X in warfarin or warfarin-like rodenticide toxicity would have prolonged PT, APTT, and RVVT, and normal TT.

Specific assays for blood coagulation factors are necessary to determine the particular factor(s) that is deficient, eg, a defect in the intrinsic system could be due to factors VIII, IX, XI, and/or XII.

Disseminated intravascular coagulation (DIC) causes consumption of platelets and coagulation factors and stimulates increased fibrinolysis. A diagnosis may be made with confidence if all the following are present: 1) thrombocytopenia, 2) prolonged bleeding time, 3) increased APTT, 4) increased PT, and 5) increased fibrin degradation products. However, compensatory responses frequently bring one or more of these common hemostatic tests back into the normal range; thus, only 3 of the 5 need be present to diagnose DIC. The combination of thrombocytopenia and evidence of coagulopathy (ie, increased APTT and/or PT) is strong evidence. Some laboratories have more sensitive tests of DIC such as antithrombin 3. Usually, the practitioner is not equipped to perform tests other than platelet counts, platelet estimates (from blood smears), bleeding times, and the activated clotting time. Advice should be sought regarding the laboratory samples and species-specific controls required, since proper type, collection, and processing of the blood are critical.

Platelet abnormalities: An accurate platelet count should be done on fresh whole blood collected by clean venipuncture into EDTA or trisodium citrate anticoagulants. The first blood into the needle should be discarded by using a 2-syringe technique or allowing blood to flow through the needle before attaching the syringe or vacutainer. Estimation of platelets in a stained smear is sufficient to detect marked changes. Normal canine blood has ~8-29 platelets per oil-immersion field. Thrombocytopenia severe enough to cause bleeding signs has 0-3 platelets per field. To best monitor changes with treatment, platelet estimates should be confirmed by platelet counts. The whole blood clot retraction, and toe nail bleeding time are insensitive tests of platelet function. The buccal mucosa bleeding time in dogs is a sensitive test of platelet function; normal dogs stop bleeding in 2.6 ± 0.5 min. In qualitative platelet function defects, assessment of platelets by special tests, such as the aggregation response of platelets to adenosine diphosphate, thrombin, and collagen, and measures of platelet retention (adhesiveness), may be required. In qualitative platelet defects, the buccal mucosa bleeding time is prolonged but the platelet count is normal. Specific measurements of VWF:Ag or the other platelet-related activities of the von Willebrand's factor are necessary for definitive diagnosis of von Willebrand's disease.

Treatment: To help control external bleeding, pressure bandages, hemostatic sponges, topical thrombin, or epinephrine can be applied. Lancing of superficial hematomas may result in hemorrhage that is difficult to control. To reduce the chance of sensitization to RBC antigens and subsequent transfusion reactions, unmatched untyped whole blood transfusions should be restricted to animals that have marked blood loss and signs of severe anemia. A PCV of <13% in dogs and 11% in cats is an indication for transfusion, although rapidly developing anemia causes respiratory distress at a higher PCV than chronic anemias.

In thrombocytopenia and thrombopathia, platelet-rich plasma should be transfused if possible. Such plasma is obtained by slowly centrifuging freshly collected, citrated blood in plastic containers (600-800 rpm or ~150 × gravity for 8-10 min) or by spinning the blood more rapidly for a shorter period of time (1500 rpm or 300 × gravity for 2-5 min).

In blood coagulation factor deficiencies, platelet-poor plasma (fresh citrated blood spun at 3000-5000 rpm or 700-1000 × gravity for 15-20 min) may be used. Since many coagulation factors are labile (eg, factor VIII), plasma should be prepared in sterile plastic containers and used as soon as possible. Alternatively, most of the clotting factor activity of fresh plasma can be preserved for up to 12 mo at -20°C or preferably at lower temperatures (-40 to -70°C) by freezing immediately after collection. Specific clotting factor concentrates have not been commercially available for use in domestic animals, but a canine cryoprecipitate can be made readily from fresh-frozen plasma.

Vitamin K_1 is indicated only in avitaminosis K and prothrombin-complex abnormalities such as rodenticide poisoning, sweet clover poisoning, and hepatic disease. Vitamin K_3 is usually ineffective. Newer rodenticides such as diphacinone require long-term vitamin K_1 therapy. IV administration may cause anaphylaxis. Ascorbic acid may be useful for some vascular purpuras and some liver diseases. Steroids or other immunosuppressant drugs are the medicaments of choice for immune-mediated thrombocytopenia and also have been used to treat coagulation disorders and fibrinolytic states. Their efficacy in the latter 2 situations is questionable. L-thyroxine (b.i.d.) is beneficial because it stimulates thrombopoiesis and increases platelet adhesion. Stilbestrol may enhance capillary resistance but can have a toxic effect in some species, eg, dogs, by causing thrombocytopenia (and bicytopenia or pancytopenia) and thus increased bleeding.

Drugs known to interfere with platelet function are contraindicated or must be used with caution in animals with severe or moderate bleeding tendencies. (*See* pp 53 and 54.) Protamine sulfate has been used to neutralize heparin in cases of heparin overdose or heparinemia. Anticoagulants such as heparin or warfarin have been used in combination with antiplatelet drugs (eg, aspirin) and blood component replacement therapy to treat DIC, but effective management requires identification and alleviation of the underlying cause, when possible.

Animals with severe hemostatic defects, particularly hemophiliacs, should receive drugs PO, subcut., or IV with a small-gauge needle; IM injection may result in hematoma formation at the site of injection.

THROMBOCYTOPENIA

A decrease in the number of platelets. In any species, the same basic causes lead to this, the most common cause of bleeding.

CANINE AND FELINE THROMBOCYTOPENIA

Hemorrhagic disorders are associated with severe thrombocytopenia, usually when platelet numbers are <20,000/μL (20 × 10^9/L). If bleeding occurs with platelet numbers of >50,000/μL, additional causes for bleeding should be considered, eg, von Willebrand's disease with concurrent hypothyroidism, and DIC with circulating fibrin degradation products acting as anticoagulants. Occasionally, bleeding signs are not seen despite severe thrombocytopenia, perhaps due to larger, more active platelets being present. Small hemorrhages such as petechiae and ecchymoses in the skin and mucous membranes, and epistaxis are typical clinical signs.

Etiology: Thrombocytopenia usually occurs due to decreased production due to bone marrow disease, immune-mediated destruction, or consumptive coagulopathy (DIC). Diagnosis of bone marrow disease is by aspirate and biopsy. An absence of, or severe decrease in, megakaryocytes indicates a production defect. Normal to increased numbers of megakaryocytes indicate increased destruction or consumption of platelets by the other 2 general causes. DIC is diagnosed through tests of hemostasis (*see* above). Immune-mediated thrombocytopenia is diagnosed by excluding the other 2 and, in some cases, by association with a particular drug or serologic or morphologic identification of an organism such as *Ehrlichia canis* or *E platys*. The mechanism of thrombocytopenia in dogs with *E canis* is poorly understood: early, the bone marrow is hypercellular, and an immune-mediated removal of platelets is possible, yet not proved. Chronic ehrlichiosis may result in aplastic pancytopenia with irreversible marrow damage. Direct tests of immune-mediated thrombocytopenia such as platelet factor 3 or ELISA tests are not readily available or universally accepted.

Immune-mediated thrombocytopenia may accompany systemic lupus erythematosus (qv, p 430) or immune-mediated hemolytic anemia (qv, p 20). Drug-induced anti-platelet antibodies may be suspected when the thrombocytopenia is associated with drugs such as quinidine, quinine, digitoxin, chlorothiazides, phenytoin, phenylbutazone, penicillins, amphetamine, phenobarbital, and trimethoprim-sulfonamide combinations. About two-thirds of cases of chronic, recurrent thrombocytopenias have an immunological basis; these individuals may develop autoantibodies to their platelets and/or other tissues.

Thrombocytopenia may be due to some viral infections or use of certain modified live virus vaccines (eg, parvovirus, rabies). This may be due to immune-mediated damage to platelets and/or megakaryocytes secondary to antigenic changes related to the virus, or direct cytotoxic effects of the virus.

Bone marrow toxicity in dogs due to estrogen is less common, but estrogen therapy is a potential cause of thrombocytopenia, bicytopenia, or pancytopenia. Other substances toxic to the marrow include cyclophosphamide, 6-mercaptopurine, busulfan, nitrogen mustard, and other chemotherapeutic agents. Leukemic involvement of the marrow may replace normal hematopoietic cells such as megakaryocytes. The original insult may not be known, and only fat or fibrous tissue remains, giving the morphologic diagnosis of aplastic pancytopenia or myelofibrosis.

Gray Collies with cyclic hematopoiesis (qv, p 64) may have cyclic thrombocytopenia. In several acquired disorders (eg, uremia, hepatic disease, neoplasia—including lymphoproliferative disorders with paraproteinemia), quantitative and qualitative platelet defects may coexist.

Clinical Findings and Diagnosis: Petechiae and ecchymoses appear suddenly on visible skin and mucous membranes. These may be accompanied by epistaxis, melena, hematuria, prolonged bleeding from sites of injury, and excessive bruising or hematoma formation following routine clinical palpation. Pallor, weakness, and edema may occur in cases that also have a severe anemia.

Direct platelet counts on fresh blood collected in EDTA or other anticoagulants quantitate the magnitude of the thrombocytopenia. If platelet clumps are noted on the smear, a fresh sample should be obtained. The peripheral blood smear shows a virtual absence (eg, 0-3 platelets per oil-immersion field) of platelets. Large platelets suggest accelerated thrombopoiesis. Platelet function tests such as the bleeding time or clot retraction may detect the thrombocytopenia. A positive direct Coombs' test associated with autoimmune hemolytic anemia, and positive LE preparations or anti-nuclear antibody titer with systemic lupus erythematosus may indirectly suggest immune-mediated thrombocytopenia. The immune-mediated form of thrombocytopenia has been indicated by detection of antiplatelet activity in the plasma or serum using the platelet factor 3 test or other immunological tests, but direct tests such as these are not easily available nor considered reliable.

Treatment: In animals developing thrombocytopenic purpura after prolonged drug therapy or after short-term exposure to a new drug, an iatrogenic cause is a strong possibility; the suspected agent should be discontinued and the animal immediately given corticosteroids (eg, dexamethasone [0.25-0.5 mg/kg body wt], or prednisone or prednisolone [2-4 mg/kg] daily). Drug-induced thrombocytopenia usually is readily reversed by removing the causative agent.

Thrombocytopenia associated with malignancy or myelofibrosis and aplastic pancytopenia is most difficult to treat, since identification or cure of the underlying cause may be impossible.

Remissions of immune thrombocytopenia usually can be achieved by using the same treatment regimen as for immune hemolytic anemia (qv, p 21). Many cases respond to conventional corticosteroid therapy, but relapses can occur after variable periods. Steroid therapy is maintained for 1 wk at the dosages given above, then reduced by ½ for another week. Maintenance doses given daily and then every other day are often needed indefinitely to avoid relapses. Antimetabolite drugs such as vincristine, cyclophosphamide, or cyclosporine have been helpful in steroid-unresponsive cases. L-thyroxine (b.i.d.) tends to stimulate thrombopoiesis and improve platelet adhesion. Splenectomy is usually of only limited or transient benefit, and therefore not recommended.

Whole-blood transfusions are reserved for emergency use to correct severe anemia secondary to blood loss. To replenish platelets with transfusions, freshly collected whole blood or citrated platelet-rich plasma is required. (*See* BLOOD GROUPS AND BLOOD TRANSFUSIONS, p 29.)

BOVINE AND PORCINE THROMBOCYTOPENIA

Thrombocytopenia in cattle and pigs can occur with DIC due to sepsis, be immune-mediated due to drug reactions, or be due to isoimmunization of newborn calves and piglets as discussed under hemolytic disease of the newborn (qv, p 21). In piglets, this reaction primarily results in thrombocytopenia rather than hemolysis, and anemia is a terminal event from bleeding. Bracken fern poisoning in cattle (qv, p 1641) also produces aplastic pancytopenia.

Diagnosis, management, and treatment are similar to those described for small animals (*see* above). Steroids and antibiotics may be effective, but in most cases treatment is impractical.

EQUINE NONTHROMBOCYTOPENIC PURPURA

An acute, frequently fatal, immune-mediated, clinical entity in horses that is not associated with thrombocytopenia. Nonthrombocytopenic purpura is an immune-mediated vasculitis due to immune complex deposition. True thrombocytopenia also occurs secondary to DIC and primary bone marrow disease.

Etiology and Pathogenesis: Equine purpura is a clinical syndrome that may have more than one cause. Characteristically, it occurs as a sequela of upper respiratory *Streptococcus equi* infection (strangles, qv, p 744), 1-3 wk after the initial illness. Viruses are not believed to cause the disease directly, but other pyogenic infections or bacterin injections (especially *S equi*) may do so. The disease is likely a type of Arthus reaction and similar to "serum sickness". (*See* IMMUNE COMPLEX DISEASE, p 424.) The pathogenesis is based on antigen, presumably streptococcal protein, persisting in the circulation. In recovery from the acute infection, antibody is produced that combines with the circulating antigen. Because initially the antigen is in excess, the immune aggregates formed are very small and therefore soluble, which allows them to remain in circulation. Complement is taken up by the antigen-antibody reaction, and these soluble complexes cause vascular endothelial injury throughout the body with resulting edema and purpura. Normally, antibody is in excess; the immune aggregates formed are large and insoluble, and are rapidly cleared from the circulation by the reticuloendothelial system without vascular injury.

Clinical Findings: The characteristic sign is sudden onset of subcut. edema and petechiation of the visible mucous membranes. Urticarial wheals are often observed. The edema is more prominent around the head, eyes, and lips. Dependent edema of the belly (2-8 cm thick) and legs is present. Edema is prominent in the viscera, and is evidenced by pulmonary edema and occasionally diarrhea or colic due to hemorrhage and edema in the gut. There is an inflammatory leukogram with nearly normal platelet counts. Anemia occurs in severe cases, or hemoconcentration may occur if loss of plasma has exceeded loss of RBC. The blood clots normally; fibrinogen should remain at normal levels, but complement levels usually drop. Urine may be scanty, and proteinuria, though not reported, should be expected. The disease lasts 1-2 wk; recovery follows in ~50% of cases. Relapses are common, as are secondary bacterial infections. Death may be rapid due to asphyxia, or due to anemia and toxemia of secondary infection in protracted cases.

Lesions: Marked edema is the most characteristic change; hemorrhages may be sparse or extensive. There may be edematous blockage of the airways of the head, and patchy congestion and edema of both the respiratory and intestinal tracts. Usually, there is blood-tinged edema beneath the hepatic and renal capsules with some degree of ascites, and widely distributed focal lesions in skeletal muscles due to ischemia (pale) or hemorrhage (dark). Deep abscesses or pyogenic cellulitis due to the primary disease is frequently found and often yields *S equi*.

Diagnosis: A history of recent pyogenic infection or immunization with bacterin and the sudden appearance of angioneurotic edema and urticarial wheals that progress to extensive, sharply demarcated, dependent edema, and edema of the head suggest the diagnosis. The purpura is usually more extensive than the petechiae of equine infectious anemia (qv, p 27). In some cases, there may be no history of precipitating disease.

Treatment: Since the disease is likely related to circulating bacterial protein, antibacterial therapy is indicated to clear the inciting antigen from the blood. Penicillin with streptomycin, tetracycline, oxytetracycline, or triple sulfa may be given. The antibiotics, but not the sulfas, may be given in dosage rates up to twice those recommended. Corticosteroids may be indicated in those cases due to bacterin injections, but must be accompanied by high levels of antibiotics. Tracheotomy may be necessary if asphyxia is imminent. Blood transfusion is indicated if the anemia is severe (Hgb <5 g/dL and falling). Bandaging of limbs is helpful, and good nursing is indispensable.

LEUKOCYTIC DISORDERS

LEUKOCYTOSIS AND LEUKOPENIA

Leukocytes, or white blood cells (WBC), in mammalian blood include segmented neutrophils, band (nonsegmented) neutrophils, lymphocytes, monocytes, eosinophils, and basophils. These cells vary in their site of production, duration of peripheral circulation, recirculation, and in the stimuli that affect their release into and migration out of the vascular bed. These factors also vary among species.

Leukocytosis is an increase in the total number of circulating WBC; **leukopenia** is a decrease. Each must be interpreted in light of the species, morphologic appearance of the WBC, and absolute numbers of each WBC type. Differential WBC counts are performed by identifying and classifying the first 100 intact WBC encountered in the monolayer of a blood smear. The absolute number of each WBC type is then determined by multiplying the percentage of a particular WBC in the differential count times the total WBC count. Increases in any of the various cell types are indicated by the suffix "philia" or "cytosis" (eg, neutrophilia, lymphocytosis, monocytosis, eosinophilia, basophilia); decreases are indicated by the suffix "penia" or "cytopenia" (eg, neutropenia, lymphopenia, monocytopenia, eosinopenia, basopenia). An increase in immature (nonsegmented) neutrophils is called a left shift, which may be regenerative or degenerative. If the left shift occurs with a leukocytosis due to a neutrophilia and the absolute number of nonsegmented neutrophils does not exceed the absolute number of segmented neutrophils, it is called a regenerative left shift. A left shift occurring under any other circumstances (eg, lack of a leukocytosis or neutrophilia, nonsegmented neutrophil numbers exceed segmented neutrophil numbers) is called a degenerative left shift. Occasionally, marked peripheral leukocytosis is difficult to differentiate from granulocytic leukemia due to the magnitude of both the left shift and WBC elevation. These reactions are termed leukemoid reactions.

Although nucleated red blood cells (nRBC) are counted as WBC by most counting techniques, they should not be included in the WBC differential count. The total nucleated cell count must be corrected to give an accurate WBC count if >5 nRBC/ 100 WBC are encountered during the WBC differential count. The total WBC count must be corrected for nRBC by the following formula:

$$\frac{100}{100 + (nRBC \text{ per } 100 \text{ WBC})} \times \text{total WBC count} = \text{corrected WBC count}$$

Differential WBC counts may be reported either as total (absolute) cell numbers per volume of blood (μL or L) or in relative percentages of the total. Valid interpretations can be made only by considering the absolute numbers. Reference values for total WBC and differential WBC counts in absolute numbers and in percentages for common domestic species are given in TABLES 8 and 9, pp 967 and 968.

Within blood vessels, WBC occur in 2 subpopulations, the central and the marginal pools, in approximately equal numbers. WBC in venipuncture samples represent only the central pool; venipuncture fails to collect the WBC of the marginal pool along the endothelial surfaces. However, various factors including epinephrine and glucocorticoids can shift cells from the marginal pool to the circulating pool, which increases the measured total WBC count. These and other causes of altered WBC counts are briefly discussed below.

Neutrophils, eosinophils, and basophils are jointly termed **granulocytes** and are produced in the bone marrow from a common progenitor cell, the myeloblast. During maturation, they form granules (second-generation lysosomes), the pH of which determines their staining characteristics. Small numbers of young (band) neutrophils may normally be found in the peripheral blood of some species (pigs, dogs), although this is rare in horses or cattle. Normally, most neutrophils are mature (segmented). Neutrophils enter the peripheral bloodstream, remain for a half-life of ~6 hr, and exit to perform their functions of phagocytosis, killing of bacteria, and enzymatic lysis of phagocytosed bacteria and tissue fragments in the somatic tissues. They do not return to the vascular bed.

Lymphocytes are produced in the lymphopoietic tissues, including the lymph nodes and spleen, but may also originate from the bone marrow. Mature lymphocytes consist of 2 subpopulations, B cells and T cells. B cells (B for bone marrow or bursa equivalent) are the precursors of plasma cells and produce antibodies for humoral immunity. T cells (T for thymus) engage in cellular immunity (eg, histocompatibility and delayed hypersensitivity). A lymphocyte in tissue may return to the vascular bed and recirculate. Some lymphocytes are long-lived and, in some species, may survive for the life of the animal.

Monocytes are formed in the bone marrow, enter the peripheral blood for a short time, and exit to the tissue and become macrophages, Kupffer's cells, etc. Monocytes and macrophages can perform pinocytosis and phagocytosis, and form multinucleated giant cells in the tissue, particularly in response to foreign bodies.

Eosinophils respond to histamine and other mast cell or basophil products released by IgE stimulation. Eosinophils kill parasites, modulate allergic reactions, and may cause tissue injury.

Basophils are rare in all common domestic animals. While they share function with tissue mast cells, basophils do not become mast cells. Also, among species, normal peripheral blood basophil numbers vary inversely with the number of tissue mast cells, eg, in dogs, mast cells are numerous in the tissues, and basophils in the blood are rare.

Morphologic changes in neutrophil cytoplasm (eg, Döhle bodies, toxic granulation, diffuse cytoplasmic basophilia, and cytoplasmic vacuolation) may occur during systemic toxemia and are referred to as "toxic change". While all circulating WBC are exposed to the same systemic toxemia, only neutrophils are evaluated for toxic change. Toxic change is graded subjectively, based on the number of affected neutrophils and the severity of toxic change, as mild, moderate, or marked. Clinical significance is reflected by the type of toxic change and its severity. Bacterial toxins induce the most severe changes. Döhle bodies appear as pale blue, intracytoplasmic inclusions within neutrophils. Even when present in high numbers, Döhle bodies alone never indicate anything more than mild toxic change. They occur so readily in cats that some disregard their presence. More severe toxic change is indicated when toxic granulation, diffuse cytoplasmic basophilia, and/or cytoplasmic vacuolation is present in a moderate to high number of the peripheral blood neutrophils. Toxic granulation is identified by the presence of eosinophilic intracytoplasmic granules within neutrophils; these granules represent the normal nonstaining primary granules of the neutrophil. Diffuse cytoplasmic basophilia and cytoplasmic vacuolation frequently occur together. The cytoplasmic basophilia is thought to be due to increased protein synthesis, and the cytoplasmic vacuolation possibly due to autodigestion of the cell. Many severely toxic neutrophils indicate a poor prognosis.

Typically, in neonates the total WBC count is more variable and often higher than in adults. Age-related reference values should be used to evaluate hemograms in young animals, in which lymphocytes are more numerous (and neutrophils less) than in adults. This may interfere with the identification of lymphopenia. In horses, the highest absolute lymphocyte values are normally present in yearlings. Generally, adult differential WBC patterns are reached at about the age of sexual maturity.

Physiologic leukocytosis may occur as a result of exercise or excitement. It is mediated by increased epinephrine. Epinephrine centralizes the marginal pool; thus, the effect of excitement may double the observed total WBC count within minutes. In addition, splenic contraction releases WBC and RBC into the peripheral circulation.

Glucocorticoid or stress leukogram: Treatment with or endogenous release of glucocorticoids results in a typical leukogram. The net effect on the total WBC count is a function of the species and its normal differential WBC count. In dogs, in which neutrophils are the predominant circulating WBC, glucocorticoids produce leukocytosis, while in cattle, in which lymphocytes predominate, they produce a mild leukopenia. Stress leukograms have a characteristic WBC differential count consisting of a mature neutrophilia, lymphopenia, and eosinopenia. Monocyte numbers are variable; however, a monocytosis often occurs in steroid/stress reactions in dogs and horses.

Although the specific features of **inflammatory leukocytosis and leukopenia** vary with species, there are some generalities. Radiation and radiomimetic drugs (eg, many antineoplastic drugs) produce leukopenia. Lymphocytes are extremely sensitive to radiation. Mature granulocytes, unlike their precursors in the bone marrow, are not particularly radiosensitive. The maintenance of normal numbers of neutrophils in the peripheral blood depends on regular replacement from the bone marrow. Generally, viral infections, particularly acute infections not associated with extensive tissue necrosis, produce leukopenia as neutropenia. This may be associated with mild lymphocytosis. Parvoviral infections may initially produce a severe panleukopenia followed by a leukocytosis. Persistent leukopenia, often associated with anemia, thrombocytopenia, or both, may occur in ehrlichiosis. Leukopenia occurs early in bacterial infections in ruminants due to their low bone marrow neutrophil reserve (storage) pool, and lymphopenia secondary to endogenous glucocorticoid release. A degenerative left shift frequently develops in ruminants with acute inflammatory disease; however, it does not carry the same poor prognosis as in other species unless the WBC count fails to increase in 2-3 days. Leukopenia may occur with overwhelming bacterial infections, especially gram-negative septicemia or endotoxemia in all species. Leukopenia and thrombocytopenia occur in anaphylaxis. Deficits in certain types of WBC, RBC, and/or platelets occur in bone marrow aplasia and in the rare space-occupying lesions of bone marrow (myelophthisis). In viral infections of longer duration (2-3 wk) with secondary bacterial complications, the total WBC count may be elevated or within normal limits due to concurrent neutropenia and lymphopenia.

Leukocytosis as neutrophilia generally characterizes bacterial infections and conditions associated with extensive tissue necrosis, including burns, trauma, extensive surgery, and sometimes, malignant neoplasms. Neutrophilia can be extreme in closed-cavity infections. In pyometra and abscesses, the wall of the cavity inhibits the migration of neutrophils into the site of infection, but does not impair the release of leukotactic chemical substances. The net effect is a high peripheral neutrophil count, which often includes an increased number of bands (regenerative left shift). In bitches with closed pyometra, a total WBC count of $100 \times 10^3/\mu L$ is not uncommon.

Eosinophilia is elicited by histamine and allied substances, and by IgE. These indicate allergy and hypersensitivity, or parasitic diseases, in which the severity of eosinophilia is a factor of the intimacy of contact of parasite chitin with the host tissues. *Trichinella* spp produce a severe eosinophilia. Eosinophilia occurs in ~50% of dogs with dirofilariasis. The severity of eosinophilia produced by fleas depends on the sensitivity of the host and severity of the infestation. Usual techniques of differential WBC counting are not sufficiently sensitive to reliably detect eosinopenia in a single blood count. The absence of eosinophils in repeated hemograms indicates eosinopenia, which is most commonly reported with glucocorticoid (stress) leukograms.

A peripheral basophilia is uncommon; however, it does occur in some animals with heartworm disease (and other causes of systemic antigenemia) or pathologic lipemias. A basopenia is difficult to document and has no diagnostic significance.

A peripheral lymphocytosis may be present for many reasons, including a physiologic (epinephrine) lymphocytosis, lymphocytic leukemia, and immune stimulation. Immune (antigenic) stimulation is associated with chronic inflammation and characterized by the presence of reactive (immunologically stimulated) lymphocytes. These lymphocytes have a more basophilic and slightly more abundant cytoplasm due to increased protein synthesis. Occasionally, these cells become so reactive as to appear plasmacytoid (immunocyte). Reactive lymphocytes may occur in any disease that causes moderate to marked systemic immunostimulation.

Lymphopenia is a common leukogram abnormality. It is most commonly associated with endogenous (stress) or exogenous glucocorticoids. Lymphopenia also occurs due to other causes, such as extravasation of lymph (lymphangiectasia), impaired lymphopoiesis, and immunodeficiency diseases (eg, combined immunodeficiency disease of Arabian foals).

Monocytosis is rarely marked, and may be associated with chronic inflammation, particularly mycotic and other granulomatous infections, or steroid/stress reactions, especially in dogs. Monocytopenias are occasionally observed, but have no diagnostic significance.

The magnitude of neutrophilia induced by inflammation is a function of the size of the bone marrow storage pool of granulocytes, hyperplasia of the marrow, and rate of WBC loss to the tissues. The storage pool is quite large in dogs, and far smaller in cattle; dogs can muster a reactive WBC count of $>100 \times 10^3/\mu L$, while counts of $>30 \times 10^3/\mu L$ are rare in cattle.

In dogs, the normal neutrophil:lymphocyte ratio is ~3.5:1. A variety of infectious and noninfectious diseases can induce changes in the leukogram. Inflammation, glucocorticoid (stress) reactions, and physiologic (epinephrine) response are common causes of leukocytosis. A leukocytosis is typically present at parturition in the bitch. Cyclic hematopoiesis of gray Collies (qv, p 64) produces peripheral neutropenia at 11- to 14-day intervals. Severe panleukopenia with total WBC counts far $<1 \times 10^3/\mu L$ often characterizes parvovirus infection, while in coronavirus infection and in infectious hepatitis, neutropenia may be more moderate. In the later stages of canine distemper with secondary bacterial infection, the total WBC count may be normal with neutrophilia, lymphopenia, and sometimes with increased band neutrophils and toxic changes. Examination of the bone marrow in early stages of ehrlichiosis may reveal an adequately cellular or hypercellular marrow despite peripheral blood thrombocytopenia, anemia, and/or leukopenia.

Cats can muster a strong neutrophilic response, although it is less marked than in dogs. Feline infectious peritonitis generally does not produce a leukopenia, but more commonly a neutrophilia and lymphopenia. Feline leukemia virus has a variable effect on peripheral blood cells. In the absence of lymphoma or leukemia (*see* below), it may produce a panleukopenia with marked neutropenia, toxic changes, and mild lymphopenia sometimes with atypical cells, and resembles feline panleukopenia infection.

In horses, the normal neutrophil:lymphocyte ratio is ~1.1:1. The magnitude of neutrophilic response is much less than in dogs or cats. The total WBC count is rarely $>35 \times 10^3/\mu L$. Total WBC counts $>12 \times 10^3/\mu L$ should be interpreted as leukocytosis. In horses, glucocorticoids induce neutrophilia, lymphopenia, eosinopenia, and frequently, a monocytosis. In equine viral arteritis, an initial leukopenia during the febrile episode is followed by lymphopenia and mild neutrophilia. Leukopenia occurs in equine herpesvirus infection, influenza, and sometimes in the early febrile phase of equine infectious anemia. In equine ehrlichiosis there may be leukopenia, sometimes accompanied by thrombocytopenia and/or anemia.

In cattle, the normal neutrophil:lymphocyte ratio is ~0.5:1, and the neutrophilic response is weaker than in any other common domestic species. Cattle with septic infections, including septic mastitis or peritonitis, characteristically have leukopenia, lymphopenia, and neutropenia the first few days. A return to normal of absolute lymphocyte and neutrophil numbers, or a neutrophilia is a good prognostic sign. Persistent leukopenia or toxic changes in the neutrophils indicates an unfavorable prognosis. Adenovirus infection induces leukopenia, with total WBC counts of 2.5-$4.2 \times 10^3/\mu L$. The initial leukopenia associated with bacterial infections is usually longer and more pronounced in cattle than in other species.

In pigs, the normal neutrophil:lymphocyte ratio is 0.7:1. Pigs are capable of a marked neutrophilic response, possibly more marked than in dogs. The stress of venipuncture may result in a doubling of the circulating neutrophil count in 30 min, which persists for 8 hr; this may impair studies that require frequent serial blood sampling. During parturition, sows manifest neutrophilia, lymphopenia, and eosinopenia, similar to the effect of glucocorticoids. A pronounced leukopenia ($<10 \times 10^3/\mu L$) occurs in hog cholera and African swine fever. Leukopenia also occurs in influenza and herpesvirus suis infection. Lymphopenia may occur in *Hyostrongylus rubidus* infection. In erysipelas, there is an early neutrophilia; band neutrophils increase at 12-36 hr and leukopenia may follow. Eosinophilia characterizes larval parasite migration and lungworm infection.

Leukemia (qv, pp 32, 39, and 391) and lymphoma (qv, p 437) must be considered briefly in conjunction with leukocytosis and leukopenia. In some instances of lymphoma without leukemia, necrosis within the tumor(s) induces neutrophilia. Rarely, lymphomatous or leukemic infiltration of the bone marrow results in leukopenia, generally in association with anemia and thrombocytopenia. Leukemia is defined as malignant neoplastic disease of the WBC or RBC precursors, with neoplastic cells in the peripheral blood and/or bone marrow. Leukemia is recognized generally by identifying moderate to high numbers of blast cells within the peripheral blood. Classifying blast cells (eg, lymphoblasts, rubriblasts, myeloblasts) may be difficult by routine light microscopy, and special stains for cell enzymes (eg, peroxidase, α-naphthol esterase) may be needed to correctly identify the cell line involved. Leukemia and leukocytosis may resemble one another; sometimes the distinction is difficult. Severe leukocytosis (leukemoid reaction) may be confused with leukemia, in particular with chronic myelogenous leukemia, in which a persistent strong leukocytosis exists without the presence of blast cells characteristic of most leukemias.

CHÉDIAK-HIGASHI SYNDROME

A primary immunodeficiency disease, transmitted as an autosomal recessive, that has been described in man, mink, cats, Hereford cattle, mice, and killer whales; all have an increased susceptibility to pyogenic infections, an increased tendency to bleed, and partial oculocutaneous albinism. The beige mouse and the

Aleutian mink exemplify the pigment dilution seen in the syndrome. Abnormal giant granules appear to occur after fusion of smaller lysosomes in many cells of man, mink, cats, and cattle, but in mice, only in the WBC. Staining characteristics of the granules are similar in all species. Disseminated bacterial abscesses have been noted in affected cattle, and an increased susceptibility to viral diseases also occurs. Diagnosis is based on pigment dilution, presence of giant granules, and increased susceptibility to infections. The pigment dilution resembles that associated with canine cyclic neutropenia and hereditary anemia of mice.

CYCLIC HEMATOPOIESIS IN GRAY COLLIE DOGS
(Gray Collie syndrome, Canine cyclic neutropenia)

An autosomal recessive, inherited immunodeficiency characterized by overwhelming recurrent bacterial infections, bleeding, and coat color dilution. The molecular basis is thought to be a cyclic bone-marrow maturation defect at the level of the pluripotential hematopoietic stem cells. Arrest of maturation occurs at regular cycles of 11- to 14-day intervals, and the peripheral neutropenia lasts 3-4 days and is followed by a neutrophilia. All other hematopoietic cells, including lymphocytes, are also cyclic with the same interval but occur at different times compared to the neutropenic phase. Hematopoietic growth factors (eg, erythropoietin) and other hormones (eg, cortisol) also have been demonstrated to have a cyclic pattern.

Affected puppies often die at birth or during the first week, and rarely live >1 yr. Surviving dogs may be stunted and weak, and develop serious recurrent bacterial infections during periods of neutropenia, characterized by fever, septicemia, pneumonia, and gastroenteritis. They also exhibit a bleeding tendency due to a platelet function abnormality and develop amyloidosis of the kidney and other organs. All affected dogs have a diluted coat color, which is known as a pleiotropic effect, with phenotypically black hairs diluted to charcoal gray, and phenotypically brown or sable hairs diluted to silver gray. Diagnosis is based on clinical signs and repeated complete blood counts over a 2-wk period. No new cases have been recognized during the last decade.

Bone marrow transplantation at an early age eliminates the cyclic hematopoiesis and effects a clinical cure. Treatment with lithium carbonate, albeit at toxic levels, has abolished the recurrent neutropenia. Administration of human recombinant granulocyte/monocyte-colony stimulating factors temporarily eliminated the cyclic hematopoiesis until the treated dog produced antibodies against them.

PELGER-HUËT ANOMALY

An inherited condition of man, rabbits, and dogs, characterized by failure of granulocytes to mature from the band form to the segmented form; inheritance appears to be via an autosomal dominant. The cells, particularly the neutrophils, are hyposegmented and the chromatin is condensed; the complete blood count shows an apparent "pseudo" left shift with a normal WBC count. This anomaly is usually an incidental laboratory finding; WBC function is normal, and heterozygotes do not exhibit clinical signs. In rabbits, the homozygous state is lethal and associated with skeletal deformities and increased susceptibility to infection. Pseudo-Pelger-Huët anomaly refers to acquired hyposegmentation of granulocytes and has been reported in rats, dogs, and cattle.

LYMPHADENITIS AND LYMPHANGITIS

CASEOUS LYMPHADENITIS (CLA) OF SHEEP AND GOATS

A caseous abscessation of lymph nodes and internal organs caused by *Corynebacterium pseudotuberculosis*. The disease occurs worldwide and is an important endemic infection in regions with large sheep and goat populations. Economic losses result from reduced weight gain, reproductive efficiency, and milk production, as well as from condemnation of carcasses and devaluation of hides. Although principally an infection of sheep and goats, sporadic disease also occurs in horses and cattle (*see* below), and water buffalo, wild ruminants, primates, pigs, and fowl. It rarely causes regional lymphadenitis in man.

Etiology and Pathogenesis: The small gram-positive rod is a facultative intracellular parasite that is found in soil and manure contaminated with purulent exudate. Two biotypes have been identified: a nitrate-negative group that infects sheep and goats, and a nitrate-positive group that infects horses. Bovine isolates are a heterogeneous group. All strains produce an antigenically similar exotoxin with enzymatic activity (phospholipase D) that appears to be leukotoxic, and can damage endothelial cells and promote spread from the initial site of infection to regional lymph nodes and visceral organs. The chemical composition of its cell wall (high lipid content) enables the organism to resist killing by phagocytes and maintain chronic infection.

Infection may occur after penetration of the organism through unbroken skin or mucous membranes; however, in most cases it probably begins with contamination of superficial skin wounds with purulent material from ruptured abscesses from other sheep and goats. Ruptured superficial and lung abscesses are the primary sources of environmental contamination. Contaminated dipping vats, shearing, handling, and feeding equipment are responsible for spread of the organism. The pus contains large numbers of bacteria that can survive for months in hay, shavings, and soil. The disease is commonly introduced into a flock by entry of an apparently healthy carrier from an infected flock, or by contact on shared pastures.

Clinical Findings: CLA is a chronic, recurring disease. A slowly enlarging, localized, and nonpainful abscess may develop either at the point of entry into the skin or in the regional lymph node (superficial or external CLA), from which it may spread via the blood or lymphatic system and cause abscessation of internal lymph nodes or organs (visceral or internal CLA). Superficial abscesses enlarge and may rupture and discharge infectious pus. In sheep on range, most superficial abscesses occur in the prescapular and prefemoral region, with transmission probably occurring at shearing time. Superficial abscesses occur mainly in the head and neck regions of housed goats and sheep due to transmission by contaminated feed, feeders, and other fomites. Animals show no obvious ill effects unless the location of the abscess interferes with functions, such as swallowing or breathing. Abscessation may recur at the same site. Pulmonary, hepatic, and renal abscesses commonly cause "thin ewe syndrome". Other manifestations include caseous bronchopneumonia, arthritis, abortion, CNS abscessation, scrotal abscessation, and mastitis. The visceral form is usually more extensive in sheep than goats, with a preponderance of pulmonary involvement. The disease incidence steadily increases with age: clinical disease is more prevalent in adults, and up to 40% of animals in a flock can have superficial abscesses.

The typical gross lesion is a discrete abscess distended by thick and often dry, greenish yellow or white, purulent exudate. In sheep, the abscess often has the classically described laminated "onion-ring" appearance in cross section, with concentric fibrous layers separated by inspissated caseous exudate. In goats, the exudate is usually soft and pasty.

Diagnosis: The diagnosis can usually be based on clinical signs and flock history. For definitive diagnosis, an abscess aspirate should be submitted for bacteriological examination; *C pseudotuberculosis* can easily be isolated, although it may be recovered in mixed culture with other pyogenic organisms. Suppurative lymphadenitis and abscesses can also be caused by various other pyogenic organisms, such as *Actinomyces pyogenes, Staphylococcus aureus*, and *Pasteurella multocida*. Scrotal abscesses usually do not involve the epididymis or testicle as with *Brucella ovis*. Emaciated animals also should be examined for ovine progressive pneumonia, paratuberculosis, and parasitism.

Serological diagnosis is not reliable; in infected flocks, kids and lambs develop a titer following contact with infected animals, but the relationship of titer to resistance of infection is not consistent.

Treatment and Control: Treatment of CLA is usually not attempted, although the organism is susceptible to penicillin. The formation of abscesses limits the penetration and effectiveness of antibiotics. Therefore, prophylactic and therapeutic treatment will not eliminate *C pseudotuberculosis* from infected flocks or individuals. Abscesses frequently recur after draining or attempted surgical excision.

Prevention is based on reducing transmission of the organism from infected to susceptible animals. Emaciated animals and those with recurrent abscesses should be culled. When animals are too valuable to cull, those with developing abscesses should be isolated, and the abscesses lanced and flushed with iodine solution. Young animals should be raised in isolation from older, infected animals, keeping in mind that fomites can transmit the disease. Older animals and those with abscesses should be shorn last, and equipment should be disinfected whenever it is contaminated with draining exudate. Skin wounds should be treated topically and sutured if necessary.

Eradication is difficult because diagnostic methods do not detect all infected animals in a flock. Palpation of external lymph nodes does not detect subclinically infected and inapparent carriers, including those with internal abscesses.

A crude bacterin-toxoid vaccine is commercially available, but documentation of its efficacy in the field is limited.

CORYNEBACTERIUM PSEUDOTUBERCULOSIS INFECTION OF HORSES AND CATTLE

In horses, *Corynebacterium pseudotuberculosis* causes **ulcerative lymphangitis**, an infection of the lower limbs, and chronic abscesses in the pectoral region. In cattle, it may cause ventral lymphadenitis, abscesses, and ulcerative dermatitis. Sporadic outbreaks have occurred in cattle in the western USA. Two to 5% of cows may be affected with large, ulcerative skin lesions and lymphangitis. Location on the animal is variable. Healing often occurs without treatment or limited topical treatment. Milk production does not appear to be affected.

Pathogenesis and Clinical Findings: The onset of ulcerative lymphangitis is slow and usually manifests by painful inflammation, nodules, and ulcers, especially in the region of the fetlock; occasionally, the edematous swelling can extend up the entire limb. The exudate is odorless, thick, greenish white, and blood tinged. Usually only one leg is involved. Lesions and swelling progress slowly, and the condition can become chronic with relapses.

In the western USA, *C pseudotuberculosis* infection in horses is seasonal, with a peak incidence in late summer and fall. It results in abscessation of the lower pectoral region or ventral abdominal wall with secondary dissemination to internal organs. Clinical signs include diffuse or localized swellings, ventral pitting edema, ventral midline dermatitis, lameness, draining abscesses or tracts, fever, weight loss, and depression. Leukocytosis and neutrophilia may be present. A marked or prolonged fever indicates untoward sequelae: chronic discharge, multiple or internal abscessation, or systemic infection with abortion. Abscesses can be large, up to 20 cm in diameter before rupturing, and take months to resolve. Weight loss, colic, or ataxia may be the signs of internal abscesses. Dermatitis lesions are painful and mildly pruritic with alopecia, exudation, crusting, and ulceration.

Entry of the bacteria probably occurs via skin wounds, arthropod vectors, and contact of skin by fomites, such as contaminated tack and grooming equipment. Unhygienic and wet conditions predispose animals to infection, particularly of the lower legs and ventral region. However, the disease also occurs under excellent management conditions.

Diagnosis: Isolation of *C pseudotuberculosis* from lesions is necessary for confirmation. In all forms of lymphangitis in horses, samples for culture include abscess aspirates, swabs of purulent exudate beneath crusts associated with folliculitis, and punch biopsies. Differential diagnoses include pyoderma, abscesses, lymphangitis (caused by *Staphylococcus aureus, Rhodococcus equi, Streptococcus,* or *Dermatophilus*), dermatophytosis, sporotrichosis, equine cryptococcosis, North American blastomycosis, and onchocerciasis.

Treatment: Lymphangitis and early abscess swellings are treated with hot packs, poultices, or hydrotherapy. Abscesses are lanced, and flushed with iodine solution. Large abscesses require surgery. Skin lesions and grossly contaminated limbs are scrubbed daily with an iodophor shampoo. Penicillin or trimethoprim-sulfa combinations have been given as antimicrobials; however, antimicrobial treatment may prolong the disease by delaying abscess maturation. Phenylbutazone relieves pain and swelling. General supportive and nursing care is indicated. If treatment is successful, the swelling gradually recedes over days or weeks. Severe or untreated cases often become chronic, and fibrosis and induration of the leg occurs.

STREPTOCOCCAL LYMPHADENITIS OF PIGS
(SLS, Jowl abscess, Cervical abscess)

A contagious disease characterized by abscessation of the cervical or cephalic lymph nodes, or both. Affected pigs are generally thrifty and grow well. SLS can lead to losses from condemnation of affected heads and to "down-time" required for cleanup of the abbatoir when an abscess is accidentally incised.

The only known host for the causative group E streptococcus (GES) is the pig (although GES causes pyogenic infections in man following wound contamination). The organism has been recovered in several areas of the world, but the disease has been economically important only in the USA, where incidence has declined considerably since the mid 1960's.

Transmission, Epidemiology, and Pathogenesis: SLS is endemic; once it occurs on a farm, successive crops of pigs develop abscesses during the growing and finishing period. Pigs may become infected by ingesting GES from draining abscesses; however, recovered carrier pigs are the most common and important source of infection. Recovered pigs harbor GES in their tonsils and readily transmit the agent to susceptible pigs via contact and by contamination of water and feed. Pigs are resistant to infection for the first 3-4 wk of life.

Scattered miliary abscesses develop in lymph nodes within 7 days after infection. By ~21 days, abscesses measuring 5-8 cm in diameter are common; these destroy the internal structure of affected nodes, and may involve adjacent tissue. Incidence may exceed 50% in a given lot of market hogs and sometimes approaches 100%. Developing abscesses may reach the skin, rupture, and drain in 7-10 wk. The drained lesions heal by granulation, leaving a dense, fibrous, subcut. tract that is resolved after several weeks. Deep-seated abscesses may remain undetected until slaughter; they tend not to drain into the pharynx.

Clinical Findings, Lesions, and Diagnosis: Pigs experimentally exposed to GES undergo transient fever, leukocytosis, depression, and anorexia, but these signs are rarely observed in natural infection. Generally, abscesses are the only sign seen by the producer. Abscesses are most common in the mandibular and retropharyngeal lymph nodes, and rarely occur in other nodes. SLS is diagnosed by isolating GES from abscess exudate. Infection also can be detected serologically by an agglutination test.

Treatment and Control: SLS can be controlled in affected herds by weaning piglets at 21 days and rearing the early-weaned pigs in an environment free of older pigs. Oral administration of broad-spectrum antibiotics (tetracyclines at 50 g/ton of feed) is effective prophylactically, and 200-400 g/ton of feed has resulted in a reduction of abscesses.

PARASITIC DISEASES OF THE BLOOD AND CARDIOVASCULAR SYSTEM

ANAPLASMOSIS

A peracute to chronic infectious disease of ruminants, characterized chiefly by anemia, icterus, and fever. It is often endemic in the tropics and subtropics, notably in the Americas and Africa, but also is prevalent in Australia, the South Pacific Islands, and southern Asia. In the USA it has been reported from all the contiguous states, but is most prevalent in the southeast, the intermountain west, and California.

Etiology: The causative rickettsial agent, *Anaplasma marginale*, is a small, spherical body without cytoplasm, and is located in the stroma of the RBC. The form that invades the RBC is an initial body that is 0.2-0.5 μm in diameter. Multiplication appears to be by binary fission within a vacuole, which results in 2 or more initial bodies within inclusions that tend to be found near the margin of the RBC. Inclusions may reach 1 μm in diameter.

Anaplasma centrale, which is more centrally located in the RBC, is a relatively nonpathogenic species found in cattle in some regions of Africa; another species, *A ovis*, occurs in sheep and goats worldwide, and may cause disease in stressful situations. *Anaplasma* spp infections also occur in various wild ungulates such as deer and antelope; their importance as reservoir hosts has not been clearly established.

Transmission and Epidemiology: Anaplasmosis has been transmitted experimentally by at least 20 tick species, but *Boophilus* and *Dermacentor* spp are thought to be the most important vectors. Tick transmission is biological. After a complex developmental cycle, transmission occurs primarily by interhost transfer of adult male ticks, or adult, partially engorged females. Equally important are flies such as horse flies (*Tabanus* spp) and stable flies (*Stomoxys* spp), which are mechanical vectors. Since the infection is easily transmitted by mechanical transfer of infected blood, outbreaks have been traced to mass operations, such as bleeding, dehorning, castrating, ear-tagging, and vaccinating.

Pathogenesis and Clinical Findings: Severity of the disease varies considerably with age. Calves undergo mild infections, with little or no mortality. In yearling cattle, the disease is severe, but most recover. In adult cattle, the disease is more severe; anemia is marked, and mortality is 20-50%. All breeds of cattle are susceptible.

The earliest signs include depression, inappetence, indolence, and fever, commonly to 104-106°F (40-41°C). Milk production in lactating cows falls rapidly. As the disease progresses, marked anemia develops, weight loss is pronounced, and dehydration is noticeable. A marked icterus may develop. Not uncommonly, affected animals succumb from hypoxia when moved or handled for treatment. If the animal survives the period of RBC destruction, it usually recovers gradually; however, recovered animals often remain carriers for life.

Diagnosis: In endemic areas, anaplasmosis should be suspected in mature cattle showing anemia without hemoglobinuria. Icterus is often an important sign. Demonstration of the organisms in Giemsa-stained RBC in blood smears provides a definitive diagnosis. Up to 50-60% of the RBC may be infected. Serology aids diagnosis: the complement fixation and rapid card agglutination tests have been used extensively, and both an indirect FA test and a DNA probe have now been developed.

Necropsy findings are associated with RBC destruction. The blood is thin and watery, and icterus is usually evident. The spleen is enlarged and soft, the liver is turgid and often a mottled mahogany color, the bile is thick and brownish green, and the gallbladder is distended. If death occurs suddenly without anemia or icterus, anthrax might be mistaken for the cause of the gross appearance of the spleen.

Treatment: The most effective treatments for acute anaplasmosis are the tetracyclines, especially if given early in the course of infection during the period of *Anaplasma* multiplication. Long-acting oxytetracycline formulations that contain 200 mg/mL give sustained blood levels. Attempts to clear carrier infections with long-acting oxytetracycline have been variable; some success has been reported with IM administration at 20 mg/kg body wt, 4 times at 3-day intervals, or 3 times at 7-day intervals. Imidocarb dipropionate is used widely for treatment of anaplasmosis and babesiosis (*see* below), but is not approved for use in the USA.

Symptomatic and supportive treatment is important. Transfusion of 4-12 L of normal blood often is indicated, and may be repeated after 48 hr if necessary. Water, given in large volumes by stomach tube, and parenteral administration of dextrose are helpful. Mild laxatives such as mineral oil can be administered, but saline laxatives should be avoided because of the dehydrated state of the animal.

Treatment should be accomplished with as little disturbance to the animals as possible and, in the case of cattle not accustomed to being handled, may be contraindicated since even mild exertion can produce hypoxia and death. Sick and convalescent animals respond well to careful management and good nutrition on pasture, with access to shade and fresh water. Application of suitable insect repellents adds to the comfort of the animals.

Control: Incidence of the disease can be reduced by killing or repelling vectors on the host with chemical dusts and sprays. For these to be effective, cattle must be dipped, sprayed, or dusted at frequent intervals during the vector season. In the USA, large biting flies, particularly horse flies, are believed to be the most serious vectors in the Gulf States, while *Dermacentor* ticks appear to be the most important natural vectors in the intermountain west and on the west coast.

Prophylaxis is by several methods. Inoculation of blood containing *A centrale* (which gives rise to a mild infection that protects against subsequent infection with the virulent *A marginale*) is used in Africa, Asia, Australia, and parts of South America, but is not permitted in the USA. The use of virulent and attenuated *A marginale* isolates to induce premunition or a chronic carrier status in calves is widespread throughout the tropical world where anaplasmosis is endemic. The virulent organisms can be administered to susceptible cattle by inoculating blood from an animal known to be infected, or by using infective frozen blood stabilates. The use of virulent organisms in adult cattle is hazardous, and treatment at the onset of patent infection with oxytetracycline or chlortetracycline is recommended to temper the course of infection. The stabilate vaccine has an advantage in that the incubation or prepatent period usually is predetermined so that the time of treatment is known. Virulent stabilates usually can be given to cattle <1 yr old without treatment.

A vaccine prepared by attenuation of virulent *A marginale* by serial passage in sheep is commercially available in some Latin American countries but is not approved for interstate movement in the USA. A killed vaccine with an adjuvant is approved for use in the USA; this reduces the severity of infection in most cases.

BABESIOSIS

A group of tick-borne diseases caused by protozoa of the genus *Babesia*. Babesiosis is a significant problem in domestic and wild animals wherever suitable tick vectors occur, especially in the tropics. The most important economic losses are caused in cattle by *B bovis* and *B bigemina*, acting either singly or together in the same group of animals. Since these 2 species share tick vectors with *Anaplasma marginale* (*see* above), some or all of them can combine to produce a fatal syndrome known as **tick fever.**

Transmission and Epidemiology: To a large extent, the major *Babesia* spp are both host and vector specific. Thus, *B bovis* and *B bigemina* are found exclusively in cattle, and their distribution coincides with that of their major tick vectors, *Boophilus* spp. Certain other ticks can act as vectors, and mechanical transmission by biting flies can occur. In the Americas and Australia, in areas where *Boophilus* spp are the only tick vectors, the diseases can be controlled by routine acaricidal treatment of the cattle to eliminate this tick. That part of the life cycle occurring in the tick commences when the merozoites (piroplasms), which occur in the RBC of an infected animal, are taken up by a female tick during its final engorgement, and continues when they are passed transovarially to the larval ticks. Development of larvae from eggs occurs on the ground after the engorged female has dropped from its host. The larva attaches to a new host on which it completes its entire life cycle. This development occurs over a 3-wk period and acaricidal treatment of the host during that time may break the cycle. However, *B bovis* is transmitted exclusively by larvae in only a few days, unlike *B bigemina*, which is transmitted by nymphs. In endemic areas, young animals are protected for ~2 mo by colostral antibodies and by a limited innate resistance; there is a reverse-age immunity in susceptible stock. When possible, young animals should be vaccinated with a blood-derived vaccine before turn out onto fresh pastures inhabited by newly hatched infective tick larvae.

Pathogenesis, Clinical Findings, and Lesions: *Babesia* infections may be peracute, acute, chronic, or inapparent. In a typical acute case, the first sign is fever up to 107°F (42°C); this is followed by signs of malaise and inappetence. During tick feeding, parasites in tick saliva pass into the bloodstream and enter the host's RBC, undergo binary fission, and break out into the plasma to invade new cells. This causes the characteristic hemoglobinuria (**redwater**) and also activates the kallikrein system, which increases vasodilation and vascular permeability, which lead to hemoglobinemia, anemia, and anoxia. Anemic anoxia causes changes in heavily vascularized organs dependent on the oxygen-carrying capacity of the blood. Thus, the liver and kidneys become enlarged and dark, and the spleen swollen and pulpy. In *B bovis* infections, vascular congestions exacerbated by the presence of altered fibrinogen can result in formation of a plug that occludes the lumen of the vessel. When the CNS is involved, incoordination, grinding of the teeth, and mania, followed by coma or death may result. Jaundice may occur in protracted cases but less commonly than in anaplasmosis. Death from cerebral babesiosis due to *B bovis* can be diagnosed by detection, in Giemsa-stained cerebral tissue, of capillaries packed with agglutinated infected RBC.

In the case of death due to *B bigemina* infection, the lesions include subcut. and IM edema, icterus, yellow and gelatinous fat, and thin and watery blood. The spleen is markedly enlarged with a soft, dark splenic pulp; the liver is enlarged, pale, and yellowish; and the gallbladder is distended with thick, dark bile. Hemoglobinuria is more common with *B bigemina* than with *B bovis*.

Diagnosis: Definitive diagnosis of babesiosis depends on demonstrating the causative organism in Giemsa-stained, thin blood smears. Although parasites are common in acute cases, particularly immediately before the characteristic hemoglobinuria, it may be necessary to resort to thick blood smears to confirm early cases (eg, with some strains of *B bovis*) or to detect other *Babesia* spp (eg, *B canis*). Various serological tests (complement fixation, indirect hemagglutination, indirect FA) are available for the specific diagnosis of babesiosis. The indirect FA test is the most accurate and sensitive.

Differential diagnosis of *Babesia* spp depends on measurement of the intraerythrocytic piroplasms; the most appropriate stage for measuring is the double pyriform. Although all within the group are pleomorphic, they fall into 2 categories: large and small. *Babesia bigemina*, with pyriform piroplasms of 4-5 × 2 μm, is typical of the former; *B bovis*, with pyriform piroplasms of 2 × 1.5 μm, is a typical small *Babesia*.

Treatment and Control: Acute babesiosis responds well to a variety of treatments if given early, although blood transfusion may be necessary in later stages. Older compounds such as quinuronium sulfate are still used with success, although phenamidine isethionate, amicarbalide di-isethionate, diminazene aceturate, and imidocarb dipropionate are used more widely. For diminazene aceturate, the recommended level for therapy is 1.4-1.6 mg/lb (3-3.5 mg/kg) body wt, IM. In premunition studies, as little as 0.25 mg/lb (0.5 mg/kg) was effective in moderating the clinical course of infection and controlling the parasitemias without eliminating infection. For imidocarb dipropionate, used particularly in Africa, the recommended dosage is 1 mg/lb (2 mg/kg); it is also effective against anaplasmosis at 1.4 mg/lb (3 mg/kg), and can be used prophylactically to give several weeks protection to susceptible animals moved into an endemic area.

Blood-derived vaccines of strains of *B bovis* and *B bigemina* attenuated by passage through splenectomized calves have been used in Australia to immunize cattle against virulent challenge, and are effective if properly prepared. Such vaccines have also been used on a fairly wide scale in Africa and Latin America, and strains from Australia have been largely cross-protective. If fully virulent organisms are used for premunition, as in some countries, the reactions of inoculated animals should be monitored with care, particularly in older animals, and a therapeutic agent should be readily available. An effective control strategy for babesiosis depends on control of the tick vectors by use of acaricides in plunge dips, spray races, or hand-sprays. Regular and frequent use of acaricides in certain ecological situations will eliminate the tick vectors, but this may not be economically appropriate in many situations where animals are widely scattered and ticks have a marked seasonality. Experience in Australia has allowed definition of particular strategies for dipping programs in different climatic conditions; the ideal solution is probably a situation of endemic stability resulting from vaccination of animals at risk, together with a limited dipping program.

OTHER IMPORTANT *BABESIA* SPP

There are >70 recognized *Babesia* spp in domestic and wild animals; the following are important in domestic animals:

Cattle: *Babesia divergens* occurs in Europe. It is small like *B bovis* but is transmitted by *Ixodes ricinus*. Rarely, fatal infections of splenectomized persons have occurred (in the New World a rodent *Babesia*, *B microti*, has been identified in several cases). *Babesia ovata* occurs in the Far East. It is a large *Babesia* and shares the tick vector *Haemaphysalis longicornis* with *Theileria orientalis* (*see* p 77). *Babesia jakimovi*, a large *Babesia*, is the agent of Siberian piroplasmosis, and is harbored by roe deer and transmitted by gadflies and possibly *Ixodes* ticks.

Sheep and Goats: *Babesia motasi* occurs in Europe, northern Africa, and Asia. It is a large *Babesia* transmitted by *Haemaphysalis* ticks. *Babesia ovis* occurs in Europe, northern Africa, and Asia, but is regarded as a serious pathogen only in Romania and Bulgaria. This small *Babesia* is thought to be transmitted by *Rhipicephalus bursa, Ixodes ricinus*, and *Dermacentor reticulatus* ticks.

Horses: *Babesia caballi* has a widespread distribution in the tropics and subtropics, and in the southern USA there is an endemic focus in southeastern Florida. This large *Babesia* is transmitted by *Dermacentor nitens* in the USA, and other *Dermacentor* and *Hyalomma* spp elsewhere. *Babesia equi* has a widespread distribution and has been recorded in mules, donkeys, and zebra (the wildlife reservoir in Africa). It is a small *Babesia* with an unusual developmental cycle: schizonts in lymphocytes have been recorded, and division of piroplasms into 4 daughter organisms is common. *Babesia equi* is able to exist in a wide variety of tick vectors (*Dermacentor, Hyalomma*, and *Rhipicephalus* spp) and ecological niches. The pathogenicity and response to chemotherapy of different strains are quite variable.

Pigs: Pigs harbor a small *Babesia*, *B perroncitoi*, and a large one, *B trautmanni*; both are pathogenic, but their distribution and transmission are unclear. They certainly occur in southern Europe and northern Africa.

Dogs: *Babesia canis* has a widespread distribution but is most troublesome in the southern USA and South Africa. It is a large *Babesia* transmitted principally by *Rhipicephalus sanguineus* in warmer climates, and *Dermacentor marginatus* in cooler ones.

Babesia gibsoni occurs in Asia and northern Africa, where jackals and foxes are significant wildlife reservoirs. It is a small *Babesia* similar to *B equi* and is known to be transmitted by *Haemaphysalis bispinosa*.

CYTAUXZOONOSIS

An acute, usually fatal, protozoal disease of domestic cats, sporadic mostly in rural, often wooded areas of southern USA.

Etiology and Transmission: The clinical and histopathological features resemble those produced by *Cytauxzoon* spp in several species of African ungulates. *Cytauxzoon felis* apparently is a new species with a life cycle that ends in host cats. Ixodid ticks are suspected as vectors.

Clinical Findings and Lesions: Anorexia and depression are followed after 1-3 days by pyrexia ($\geq$104°F [40°C]), and usually by developing anemia and dehydration or icterus, or both. Body temperature falls to subnormal, dyspnea develops, and death follows within 1-3 days.

Gross necropsy findings include generalized pallor and often icterus; marked enlargement of the spleen and occasionally lymph nodes; congestion of mesenteric veins; and sometimes petechial hemorrhages on the lungs, lymph nodes, epicardium, and urinary bladder. Histologically, schizonts appear within mononuclear phagocytes (macrophages) that occlude major venous channels of lung, lymph node, spleen, and other organs.

Diagnosis: The typical clinical picture in an endemic area is suggestive. Demonstration of RBC parasites in Wright's-or Giemsa-stained blood smears, and tissue-phase parasites within mononuclear phagocytes in stained smears of bone marrow or spleen, confirm the diagnosis. *Cytauxzoon* sp must be differentiated from the smaller, denser, chain-forming *Haemobartonella felis* (qv, p 28) and *Babesia felis*. In the case of *Babesia* sp, the blood phase may appear identical, but members of the Babesiidae have no tissue (schizont) phase. In stained blood smears, erythrocytic forms are round to oval bodies (0.5-2 μm in diameter) with a dark red to purple nucleus and pale blue cytoplasm. In stained tissue smears or H&E-stained histological preparations, numerous schizonts (2-75 μm) or merozoites (0.5-2 μm) appear in the cytoplasm of mononuclear phagocytes lining the vascular channels in most organs.

Treatment and Control: Preliminary attempts at treatment have had limited documented success. Parvaquone, 10-30 mg/kg, IM, once daily for 2-3 days resulted in 2 of 18 cats surviving. Sodium thiacetarsamide, 0.1 mg/kg, IV, b.i.d. for 2-3 days, resulted in 1 of 2 cats surviving. Intensive supportive care with fluids and broad-spectrum antibiotics resulted in 1 of 25 cats surviving. Thus, survival with drug therapy or aggressive supportive care is low. General prevention of exposure to ticks or other potential vectors may aid in control.

EPERYTHROZOONOSIS

A sporadic, febrile, hemolytic disease of pigs, sheep, cattle, and other mammals caused by rickettsiae. Most infections are subclinical, and the incidence of overt disease is low. The rickettsiae probably occur in most countries and, in the case of *Eperythrozoon ovis*, serological evidence from Nigeria (36%) and Australia (16.9%) indicates that the incidence of subclinical infection is high; in the USA, serology indicates a 15% incidence of *E suis*. Different species of parasite exist in different hosts (eg, *E suis*, *E ovis*), and each appears to be relatively host specific. Transmission is thought to be chiefly by lice, but surgical instruments and hypodermic needles are also incriminated. Clinical cases have varying degrees of hemolytic anemia, fever, anorexia, weakness, and icterus. Most cases are mild and transient, and usually secondary to other conditions. More severe cases occur in young pigs, and may be associated with stress in sheep and cattle.

Differentiation should be made from nutritional anemias (qv, p 18) and from ictero-anemic conditions due to other infectious agents or toxic substances. Acute eperythrozoonosis may be diagnosed by demonstrating large numbers of rickettsiae in Giemsa-stained blood smears. The parasites may be found free in the plasma, surrounding platelets, or on the surface of RBC.

Tetracycline or oxytetracycline given IM at ≥3 mg/lb (6.6 mg/kg) body wt is effective in single doses against *E suis*. Hematinic drugs (eg, sodium cacodylate and iron dextran) and arsenicals (eg, neoarsphenamine) are indicated. If required, oxytetracycline PO is an effective herd treatment.

HEARTWORM DISEASE

DIROFILARIASIS

A clinical or subclinical disease complex caused by the filarial worm *Dirofilaria immitis*. The disease has a cosmopolitan distribution at sea level in the tropics and subtropics, but is common in many areas at higher elevations and latitudes, including Japan, several parts of Australia, North America, and Europe. In the USA, it occurs frequently in all mosquito-infested areas, particularly in the southeast, in the Atlantic coast states, and the Midwest. Clinical signs are seen primarily in dogs, although cats and ferrets are susceptible to infection.

Etiology and Pathogenesis: Adult females are ~27 cm long, males ~17 cm. The microfilariae, which are ~315 μm long, are discharged into the bloodstream where they remain active for 1-3 yr. Further development occurs when they are ingested by one of several species of mosquitoes. The microfilariae develop into the infective stage within the mosquito in ~2 wk. The infective larvae migrate to the mouthparts and, when the mosquito feeds again, are deposited on the skin of the dog and enter through the bite wound.

The immature stages develop and grow in the subcut. or subserosal tissues for ~2 mo, then begin a 2- to 4-mo migration to the right ventricle. The worms reach sexual maturity after an additional 2-3 mo. Thus, microfilariae first appear in the peripheral circulation ~6-7 mo after infection. Adult worms are found primarily within the pulmonary arteries and right ventricle, although in heavy infections they may also be found in the right atrium, cranial and caudal vena cava, and hepatic veins.

The worms impede blood flow and cause endarteritis, endothelial proliferation, and thrombosis; circulating microfilariae can form immune complexes, notably in the kidneys.

Clinical Findings: The duration and severity of infection, as well as the individual host's reaction to the parasite, determine the severity of clinical signs. The most common clinical findings in dogs are coughing, decreased exercise tolerance, and weight loss. Other signs include dyspnea, fever, and ascites. In the caval syndrome, large numbers of adult worms in the right atrium and vena cava cause sudden weakness, and frequently death. This may be preceded by anorexia and icterus.

The most common signs in cats are anorexia, lethargy, coughing, respiratory distress, and vomiting. Other signs include weight loss and sudden death. Right heart failure and caval syndrome are rare in cats.

Lesions: The most common changes in the pulmonary arteries are endarteritis, subintimal proliferation of smooth muscle cells, and rugose and villous protrusions into the lumen. Thrombosis of smaller arteries may occur as a result of death of worms. The effect of these lesions, in conjunction with obstructing fibrosis, is development of pulmonary hypertension and secondary right heart enlargement. The kidneys may show evidence of glomerulonephritis and hemosiderosis of the convoluted tubules with heme casts in the medulla. In the caval syndrome, enlarged hepatic venules, thickened hepatic veins, and centrilobular necrosis may be seen.

Diagnosis: A provisional diagnosis is based on signs, history, and exposure, and confirmed by presence of *D immitis* microfilariae in a blood sample. The modified

Knott's test and millipore or nucleopore filter tests are common screening tests for microfilariae. Microfilariae of *D immitis* should be differentiated from those of the nonpathogenic filarids *D repens* and *Dipetalonema reconditum* on the basis of morphology and staining characteristics with acid phosphatase. Because many adult infections are asymptomatic, routine screening by serologic tests (ELISA for adult *D immitis* antigens) is often done.

Table 7. Differentiation of Microfilariae of *Dirofilaria immitis* and *Dipetalonema reconditum*

	D immitis	*D reconditum*
Length	>290 μm	<275 μm
Width	>6 μm	<6 μm
Anterior end	Tapered	Blunt
Posterior end	Straight	Sometimes hook-shaped
Body shape	Straight	Crescent

Confirmation of the diagnosis is complicated when animals are amicrofilaremic. Occult infections are seen in ~20% of infected dogs and >80% of infected cats. In these animals, diagnosis is based on a combination of clinical findings plus thoracic radiographs and/or ELISA tests for adult worm antigens. Characteristic radiographic findings in dogs include enlarged and sometimes tortuous lobar pulmonary arteries; increased prominence of the main pulmonary artery; perivascular parenchymal pattern, with a caudal lobar artery distribution; and enlargement of the right ventricle. In cats, the most common radiographic finding is enlargement of the caudal lobar pulmonary arteries.

Echocardiography may aid in the diagnosis of caval syndrome. M-mode echocardiographic evidence of adults in the right atrium with movement into the right ventricle is considered pathognomonic.

Treatment and Control: In dogs, treatment is directed primarily at destruction of the adult worms, followed by microfilaricidal therapy (unless occult infection is present), and subsequent preventive medication to guard against reinfection. Thiacetarsamide is the adulticide commonly used, but it is potentially toxic. Pretreatment laboratory tests are used to identify coexisting problems, but acute thiacetarsamide toxicity is difficulty to predict; most often there is no obvious predisposition. Up to 10-fold increased enzyme activity has not been associated with increased risk. Careful observation of the treated animal for evidence of early toxicity is critical. Each dog should be examined carefully and fed 30 min before each injection. A urine sample should be examined for evidence of bilirubinuria, one of the earliest signs of hepatic toxicity.

Treatment should be discontinued if the animal vomits repeatedly, is depressed, anorectic, or icteric. Gross bilirubinuria after the first or second injection is an indication to proceed with caution only if there are no other signs of toxicity. If treatment is discontinued, activity should be restricted and a low-fat, high-carbohydrate diet fed. The complete adulticide treatment should be re-initiated in ~4-wk, at which time further acute toxicity is uncommon.

Thiacetarsamide should be refrigerated, and discarded if it has an orange discoloration or contains precipitates. Each injection should be given in a different site in a vein as peripheral as feasible. If an indwelling catheter is employed, careful determination of the catheter-vein integrity must be confirmed before each injection. Both the catheter and thiacetarsamide contribute to the risk of phlebitis and vein rupture. If thiacetarsamide is extravasated, the region should be treated with topical dimethyl sulfoxide (DMSO) or DMSO-dexamethasone t.i.d. for several days.

Radiographic evidence of severe pulmonary arterial disease or thromboembolism is an indication to temporarily postpone adulticidal therapy due to the increased risk of treatment complications. During cage confinement, corticosteroids are given for 3-5 days. Adulticidal treatment is reinstituted when there is clinical and radiographic evidence of significant improvement. Dogs with severe pulmonary arterial disease or those in right heart failure appear to benefit from concomitant protracted cage confinement and aspirin therapy before, during, and after thiacetarsamide treatment. Dogs with the caval syndrome should have the worms removed via an emergency jugular venotomy.

Following adulticidal therapy, exercise should be restricted for 4-6 wk. Anorexia, coughing, dyspnea, and fever attributable to worm death, thrombosis, and inflammation may occur within the first 4 wk (most often within 10-17 days) after treatment. Short-term anti-inflammatory treatment with corticosteroids as well as cage rest may be necessary.

Microfilaricidal treatment should follow adulticidal treatment within 3-6 wk. Dithiazanine iodide is the only approved microfilaricide. The American Heartworm Society recommends use of ivermectin as a microfilaricide, but this is not an officially approved usage. Milbemycin oxime, fenthion, and levamisole are also used. When large numbers of microfilariae are present, reaction to their death is common, but is unlikely to be fatal.

Preventive treatment should be initiated as soon as feasible after the treatment of occult infections, or as soon as microfilaricidal treatment is complete. Concentration tests should be performed at the end of the microfilaricidal treatment, and also repeated several weeks later to detect microfilarial recrudescence.

Accepted preventive measures are based on the oral administration of diethylcarbamazine, ivermectin, or milbemycin oxime. These compounds arrest development of tissue-stage larvae, which prevents the parasites from reaching the heart. DEC should be administered daily from 1 mo before the mosquito season until 2 mo after; ivermectin and milbemycin oxime are administered once monthly from 1 mo after the onset of the season until within 1 mo after the end of the season. Regions with continuous mosquito populations require year-round therapy. Preventive products should not be administered to microfilaria-positive dogs.

Treatment in cats is controversial. Acute pulmonary edema and hemorrhage, usually culminating in death, may occur within a few hours after the first or second injection of thiacetarsamide, which is not approved for use in cats. Subclinical infections and those characterized as an intermittent pulmonary infiltrate with eosinophilia syndrome may not require adulticide treatment. There is evidence that experimental infections may be self-limiting. Appropriate symptomatic therapy such as corticosteroids for coughing and pulmonary infiltrates should be administered as indicated.

ANGIOSTRONGYLUS VASORUM INFECTION
(French heartworm)

These smaller heartworms occasionally are found in the pulmonary artery and right ventricle of dogs and foxes in the USA, Europe, and the USSR. The males are ~18 mm and the females ~25 mm long. The eggs hatch in the lungs, and the larvae (~350 μm long) migrate to the pharynx and are passed out in the feces. The life cycle includes a snail or terrestrial slug as an intermediate host.

Eggs entrapped in the lung tissues cause formation of granulomas and perivascular sclerosis. Cardiac hypertrophy and hepatic congestion with ascites have been observed in some severe and chronic cases. Animals may die from cardiac insufficiency. Interference with the blood-clotting mechanism may lead to excess bruising and subcut. swellings. Diagnosis is based on presence of the characteristic larvae (which have a cephalic button and an undulating tail with dorsal appendage) in the feces. Differentiation from *Filaroides* is aided by the fact that larvae are more active and usually much more numerous in *Angiostrongylus* infections. Levamisole subcut. has been effective in treatment.

SCHISTOSOMIASIS
(Blood flukes)

Etiology: Schistosomes are thin, elongated flukes, up to 30 mm long, that live in blood vessels of the final host. The female lies in a longitudinal groove of the male. Various water snails act as intermediate hosts. Schistosomes pathogenic to domestic animals are widely distributed throughout Africa, the Middle East, Asia, and some countries bordering the Mediterranean. In many areas, a high percentage of animals are infected and although many have low burdens and are asymptomatic, severe outbreaks due to heavy infection are reported occasionally. Most pathogenic schistosomes are found in the portal and mesenteric blood vessels, and the principal clinical signs are associated with passage of the spined eggs through the tissues to the gut lumen. One species, *Schistosoma nasale*, is found in the veins of the nasal mucosa of ruminants and horses, where it may cause coryza and dyspnea.

Eggs passed in the feces must be deposited in water if they are to hatch and release the miracidia, which invade suitable water snails and develop through primary and secondary sporocysts to become cercariae. When fully mature, the cercariae leave the snail and swim freely in the water, where they remain viable for several hours. The cercariae invade the final host through the skin and mucous membranes; during penetration, cercariae develop into schistosomula, which are transported via the lymph and blood to their predilection sites. The prepatent period is ~6-9 wk.

In southern and central Africa, *S mattheei* is the predominant species infecting ruminants; in northern and eastern areas, *S bovis* is more common. The latter parasite also occurs in certain areas of southern Europe and the Middle East. In Asia, *S spindale*, *S incognitum*, *S (Ornithobilharzia) turkestanicum*, and *S japonicum* are widespread. The latter is of particular importance because infected ruminants form a reservoir for the disease in man. *Schistosoma nasale* occurs in the Indian subcontinent, Malaysia, and the Caribbean area.

Clinical Findings: The major clinical signs associated with the intestinal and hepatic forms of schistosomiasis in ruminants develop after the onset of egg excretion, and consist of hemorrhagic enteritis, anemia, and emaciation. Severely affected animals deteriorate rapidly and usually die within a few months of infection, while those less heavily infected develop chronic disease and may recover eventually. Many older cattle in endemic areas of Africa have an effective level of immunity against reinfection. Nasal schistosomiasis is a chronic disease of cattle, horses, and occasionally buffalo. In severe cases, there is a copious mucopurulent discharge, snoring, and dyspnea; milder cases frequently are asymptomatic.

Lesions: In the intestinal and hepatic forms, adult flukes are found in the portal, mesenteric, and intestinal submucosal and subserosal veins. However, the main pathological effects are associated with the eggs. In the intestinal form, passage of eggs through the gut wall causes the lesions, while in the less common hepatic form, granulomas or "pseudotubercles" form around the eggs. Other hepatic changes include medial hypertrophy and hyperplasia of the portal veins, development of lymphoid nodules and follicles throughout the organ, and fibrosis in more chronic cases. Extensive granuloma formation also occurs in the GI tract, especially in the small intestine. In severe cases, numerous areas of petechiation and diffuse hemorrhage are seen in the mucosa, and large quantities of discolored blood may be found in the intestinal lumen. Frequently the parasitized blood vessels are dilated and tortuous. Vascular lesions also may be found in the lungs, pancreas, and bladder of heavily infected animals.

In nasal schistosomiasis, adult flukes are found in the blood vessels of the nasal mucosa, but again, the main pathogenic effects are associated with the eggs, which cause abscesses in the mucosa. The abscesses rupture and release eggs and pus into the nasal cavity, which eventually leads to extensive fibrosis. In addition, large granulomatous growths are common on the nasal mucosa, and occlude the nasal passages and cause dyspnea.

Diagnosis: Clinical history and signs are insufficient; the eggs must be identified in the feces, rectal scrapings, or nasal mucus for confirmation. Of the terminal-spined eggs, *S bovis* and *S mattheei* are spindle shaped (150-250 × 40-90 μm), those of *S spindale* are more elongated and flattened on one side (160-400 × 70-90 μm), and the boomerang-shaped eggs of *S nasale* are 300-550 × 50-80 μm. The oval eggs of *S japonicum* are relatively small (70-100 × 50-80 μm) with a small lateral spine. In chronic cases, it may not be possible to find eggs in the feces or nasal mucus, and the diagnosis must be confirmed at necropsy by finding adult flukes in the blood vessels.

Control: Control measures are rarely practiced on a large scale. Most available drugs produce either inconsistent results or have serious side effects. Older remedies include a number of antimonial compounds, but their use requires great care because of toxicity. Various other compounds have schistosomicidal properties, but generally, treatment is uneconomical since a large number of repeated doses at intervals of 2-3 days usually is required. Such drugs include stibophen, lucanthone hydrochloride, hycanthone, and trichlorfon. Praziquantel at 25 mg/kg body wt is effective, although 2 treatments 3-5 wk apart may be required. A vaccine incorporating irradiated *S bovis* schistosomula was highly effective in extensive field trials in the Sudan; however, it is not yet commercially available.

Infection can be reduced by control of the intermediate snail host using molluscicides (eg, copper sulfate, niclosamide, or trifenmorph) or by fencing off contaminated bodies of water and providing clean drinking water. These measures not only help reduce the incidence of schistosomiasis, but they also help control other parasitic trematodes such as *Fasciola gigantica* and *Paramphistomum* spp, which similarly have water snails as intermediate hosts and frequently occur in the same localities as schistosomes.

THEILERIASES

A group of tick-borne protozoal diseases of animals caused by *Theileria* spp. The most important species are *T parva* and *T annulata*, which cause widespread death in cattle in tropical areas of the Old World.

Both *Theileria* and *Babesia* are members of the suborder Piroplasmorina. While *Babesia* are primarily parasites of RBC, *Theileria* utilize, successively, WBC and RBC for completion of their life cycle in the mammalian host. The infective sporozoite stage of the parasite is transmitted in the saliva of infected ticks as they feed. Sporozoites invade lymphocytes (and also monocytes in the case of *T annulata*) and within a few days develop to schizonts. Development of the schizont causes the host WBC to divide; at each cell division the parasite also divides. Thus, the parasitized cell population expands and, through migration, becomes disseminated throughout the lymphoid system. Later in the infection, a portion of the schizonts undergo merogony; the resultant merozoites infect RBC, giving rise to piroplasms. *Theileria parva* piroplasms undergo limited division in RBC, but in other species, notably *T annulata*, *T mutans*, and *T orientalis*, such division represents a second phase of multiplication. Uptake of piroplasm-infected RBC by vector ticks feeding on infected animals is the prelude to a complex cycle of development in which the disease is subsequently transmitted by ticks feeding in their next instar (trans-stadial transmission). There is no transovarial transmission as occurs in *Babesia*. Occurrence of disease is limited to the geographical distribution of the appropriate tick vectors. In some endemic areas, indigenous cattle have a degree of innate resistance. Mortality in such stock is relatively low, but introduced cattle are particularly vulnerable.

EAST COAST FEVER

An acute disease of cattle, characterized usually by high fever, swelling of the lymph nodes, dyspnea, and high mortality, caused by *Theileria parva*. It is a serious problem in East and Central Africa.

Etiology and Transmission: *Theileria parva* sporozoites are injected into cattle by infected vector ticks, *Rhipicephalus appendiculatus*, during feeding. Based on clinical and epidemiological parameters, 3 subtypes of *T parva* are recognized, but these are probably not true subspecies. *Theileria parva parva*, transmitted mainly between cattle, and *T parva lawrencei*, transmitted mainly from buffalo to cattle, are both highly pathogenic, whereas *T parva bovis*, transmitted between cattle, is much less pathogenic.

Pathogenesis, Clinical Findings, and Diagnosis: An occult phase of 5-9 days follows before infected lymphocytes can be detected in Giemsa-stained smears of the local drainage lymph node. Subsequently, the number of parasitized cells increases rapidly throughout the lymphoid system, and from about day 14 onwards, cells undergoing merogony are observed. This is associated with widespread lymphocytolysis, marked lymphoid depletion, and leukopenia. Piroplasms in RBC infected by the resultant micromerozoites assume various forms, but typically they are small and rod-shaped or oval.

The clinical signs vary according to the level of challenge, and range from inapparent or mild to severe and fatal. Typically, fever occurs 7-10 days after the bite of infected ticks, continues throughout the course of infection, and may be >107°F (42°C). Lymph node swelling becomes pronounced and generalized. Lymphoblasts in Giemsa-stained lymph node biopsy smears contain multinuclear schizonts. Anorexia develops and the animal rapidly loses condition; lacrimation and nasal discharge may occur. Terminally, dyspnea is common. Just before death, a sharp fall in temperature is usual, and pulmonary exudate pours from the nostrils. Death usually occurs after 18-24 days. The most striking postmortem lesions are lymph node enlargement and massive pulmonary edema and hyperemia. Hemorrhages are common on the serosal and mucosal surfaces of many organs, sometimes together with obvious areas of necrosis in the lymph nodes and thymus. Anemia is not a major diagnostic sign (as it is in babesiosis) since there is minimal division of the parasites in RBC, and thus no massive destruction of them.

Animals that recover are immune to subsequent challenge with the same strains, but may be susceptible to some heterologous strains. Most recovered or immunized animals remain carriers of the infection.

Treatment and Control: Prospects for survival of cattle with clinical East Coast fever or *T annulata* infection have been increased by the development of parvaquone and its derivative buparvaquone, and the demonstration that the lactate salt of the coccidiostat halofuginone has anti-theilerial activity. Chlortetracycline and oxytetracycline, even when given in large doses as early as possible, are relatively ineffective. However, immunization of cattle using an infection-and-treatment procedure is practical and is gaining acceptance. The components for this procedure are a cryopreserved sporozoite stabilate of the appropriate strain(s) of *Theileria* derived from infected ticks and a single dose of either long-acting oxytetracycline or buparvaquone given simultaneously, or of parvaquone given ~8 days after infection. Cattle should be immunized 3-4 wk before being turned out to infected pasture. Incidence of East Coast fever can be reduced by rigid tick control, but in many areas this means biweekly acaricidal treatment.

OTHER THEILERIASES

Theileria spp in large domestic and wild animals in tick-infested areas of the Old World are almost ubiquitous but, apart from those in cattle, their differentiation into species is unclear. The following species are important: In cattle, *Theileria annulata* is widely distributed in North Africa, the Mediterranean coastal area, the Middle East, India, the USSR, and Asia. It causes **tropical** or **Mediterranean theileriosis** and is transmitted by ticks of the genus *Hyalomma*. *Theileria annulata* can cause mortality of up to 90%, but different strains vary in their pathogenicity. Characteristic signs include fever and swollen superficial lymph nodes; cattle rapidly lose condition and hemoglobinuria may occur. The schizonts and piroplasms are morphologically similar to those of *T parva*. The schizonts can be cultivated *in* *vitro*, and attenuated strains produced by serial passage form the basis of vaccines used in Israel, Iran, and the USSR.

Theileria orientalis (sergenti) occurs in the Far East and to a lesser extent through Asia and the southern USSR, where it may cause a disease syndrome in association with *T annulata*. Transmission is by ticks of the genus *Haemaphysalis*, and mildly pathogenic strains of the parasite exist in Europe and Australasia where *Haemaphysalis* spp occur. The piroplasms are larger than those of *T parva* and *T annulata*, and their intraerythrocytic division is the most important method of multiplication. Mortality, particularly in indigenous cattle, is rare, but a progressive chronic anemia is common.

Theileria mutans occurs in Africa and has been reported from Latin America. Transmission is by ticks of the genus *Amblyomma*, and multiplication is commonly by intraerythrocytic division. The piroplasms are morphologically indistinguishable from those of *T orientalis* and *T taurotragi* (an African parasite of eland and cattle), but the parasites can be differentiated by serological tests such as the indirect FA. Some strains of *T mutans* are pathogenic in their own right. In addition, concurrent infection may add to the pathogenicity of the *T parva* elements of the East Coast fever syndrome.

In sheep and goats, 2 species of *Theileria* have been distinguished, largely based on their relative pathogenicity. Mortality can approach 100% with *T hirci*, which is found in southern Europe, Africa, and throughout Asia. It is transmitted by *Hyalomma anatolicum* ticks in Asia. Schizonts can readily be demonstrated in Giemsa-stained biopsy smears from swollen superficial lymph nodes. Nonpathogenic *Theileria* spp (eg, *T ovis*) are also widely distributed and are mainly transmitted by *R evertsi* ticks in Africa and *Haemaphysalis punctata* ticks in Europe. Piroplasms of these species are polymorphic.

TRYPANOSOMIASES

TSETSE-TRANSMITTED TRYPANOSOMIASIS

A group of diseases caused by protozoa of the genus *Trypanosoma*, which affect all domestic animals. The major species are *T congolense*, *T vivax*, *T brucei*, and *T simiae*.

The animals mainly affected by these tsetse-transmitted trypanosomes are listed in TABLE 8 (below). In order of importance, those affecting cattle, sheep, and goats are *T congolense*, *T vivax*, and *T brucei*. In pigs, *T simiae* is the most important. In dogs and cats, *T brucei* is probably the most important. It is difficult to assign an order of importance for horses and camels.

The trypanosomes that cause tsetse-transmitted trypanosomiasis (sleeping sickness) in man, *T rhodesiense* and *T gambiense*, closely resemble *T brucei* from animals; the animal isolates of *T brucei* are lysed by human serum. There are indications that changes in resistance to human serum occur in some isolates of *T brucei*; therefore, reasonable precautions should be taken when working with such isolates.

TABLE 8 also lists the major geographic areas where tsetse-transmitted trypanosomiasis occurs. The tsetse fly is restricted to Africa from about latitude 15°N to 29°S.

Transmission and Epidemiology: Most tsetse-transmission is cyclical, and begins when blood from a trypanosome-infected animal is ingested by the fly. The trypanosome loses its surface coat, multiplies in the fly, then re-acquires a surface coat and becomes infective. *Trypanosoma brucei* moves from the gut to the proventriculus, to the pharynx, and eventually to the salivary glands; the cycle for *T congolense* stops at the hypopharynx, and the salivary glands are not invaded; the entire cycle for *T vivax* occurs in the proboscis. The animal-infective form in the tsetse salivary gland is referred to as the metacyclic form. The life cycle in the tsetse may be as short as 1 wk with *T vivax*, or extend to a few weeks for *T brucei*.

Tsetses are flies in the genus *Glossina*; the 3 main species inhabit relatively distinctive environments: *Glossina morsitans* usually is found in savanna country,

Table 8. The Most Important Tsetse-transmitted Animal Trypanosomes

Trypanosoma spp	Animals Mainly Affected	Major Geographic Distribution
T congolense	Cattle, sheep, goats, dogs, pigs, camels, horses, most wild animals.	Tsetse region of Africa.
T vivax	Cattle, sheep, goats, camels, horses, various wild animals.	Africa, Central and South America, West India, Mauritius. Note: In non-tsetse areas, transmission is by biting flies.
T brucei	All domestic and various wild animals. Most severe in dogs, horses, cats.	Tsetse region of Africa.
T simiae	Domestic and wild pigs, camels.	Tsetse region of Africa.

G palpalis prefers areas around rivers and lakes, and *G fusca* lives in high forest areas. All 3 species transmit trypanosomes, and all feed on various mammals.

Mechanical transmission can occur through tsetses or other biting flies. In the case of *T vivax*, *Tabanus* spp and other biting flies seem to be the primary mechanical vectors outside the tsetse areas, as in Central and South America. Mechanical transmission requires only blood containing infectious trypanosomes be transferred from one animal to another. Other trypanosomes, eg, *T congolense*, also can be transmitted mechanically and are occasionally found outside the tsetse area of Africa.

Pathogenesis: Infected tsetses inoculate metacyclic trypanosomes into the skin of animals, where the trypanosomes grow for a few days and cause localized swellings (chancres). They enter the lymph nodes, then the bloodstream, where they divide rapidly by binary fission. In *T congolense* infection, the organisms attach to endothelial cells and localize in capillaries and small blood vessels. *Trypanosoma brucei* and *T vivax* invade tissues and result in tissue damage in several organs.

The immune response is vigorous, and immune complexes cause inflammation, which contributes to the signs and lesions of the disease. Antibodies against the surface-coat glycoproteins kill the trypanosomes. However, trypanosomes have multiple genes that code for different surface-coat glycoproteins that are not vulnerable to the immune response; this antigenic variation results in persistence of the organism. The number of antigenic types of glycoprotein that can be made is unknown, but exceeds several hundred. Antigenic variation has prevented development of a vaccine and permits reinfections when animals are exposed to a new antigenic type.

Clinical Findings and Lesions: Severity of disease varies with species and age of the animal infected and the species of trypanosome involved. The incubation period is usually 1-4 wk. The primary clinical signs are intermittent fever, anemia, and weight loss. Cattle usually have a chronic course with high mortality, especially if there is poor nutrition or other stress factors. Ruminants may gradually recover if the number of infected tsetse flies is low; however, stress results in relapse.

Necropsy findings vary and are not specific. In acute, fatal cases, extensive petechiation of the serosal membranes, especially in the peritoneal cavity, may occur. Also, the lymph nodes and spleen are usually swollen. In chronic cases, swollen lymph nodes, serous atrophy of fat, and anemia are seen.

Diagnosis: A presumptive diagnosis is based on finding an anemic animal in poor condition in an endemic area. Confirmation depends on demonstrating trypanosomes in stained blood smears or wet mounts. The most sensitive rapid method is to examine a wet mount of the buffy coat area of a PCV tube after centrifugation.

Other infections that cause anemia and weight loss, such as babesiosis, anaplasmosis, and theileriosis, should be eliminated by examining a stained blood smear.

Various serological tests measure antibody to trypanosomes, but their use is more suitable for herd and area screening than for individual diagnosis; however, tests for detection of circulating trypanosome species-specific antigens in peripheral blood may soon be available for both individual and herd diagnosis.

Treatment and Control: Several drugs can be used, the most common of which are listed in TABLE 9 (below). Most have a narrow therapeutic index, which makes administration of the correct dose essential. Drug resistance occurs and should be considered in refractory cases.

Control can be exercised at several levels, including eradication of tsetses and use of prophylactic drugs. Tsetses can be partially controlled by frequent spraying and dipping of animals, spraying of insecticides on fly-breeding areas, use of insecticide-impregnated screens, bush clearing, and other methods. Animals can be given drugs prophylactically in areas with a high population of trypanosome-infected tsetses. The problem of drug resistance must be carefully monitored by frequent blood examinations for trypanosomes in treated animals.

SURRA
(*Trypanosoma evansi* infection)

This is separated from the tsetse-transmitted diseases because it is usually transmitted by other biting flies that occur within and outside tsetse fly areas. It is essentially a disease of camels and horses. It occurs in North Africa, the Middle East, Asia, the Far East, and Central and South America. The distribution of *T evansi* in Africa extends into the tsetse areas, where it is difficult to differentiate from *T brucei*. All domestic animals are susceptible, and the disease can be fatal, particularly in camels, horses, and dogs. *Trypanosoma evansi* in other animals appears to be nonpathogenic, and these animals serve as reservoirs of infection.

Transmission is primarily by biting flies, probably resulting from interrupted feedings. A few wild animals are susceptible to infection and may serve as reservoirs.

Pathogenesis, clinical findings, lesions, diagnosis, and treatment are similar to those of the tsetse-transmitted trypanosomes (*see* above). Drugs for treatment are listed in TABLE 9.

DOURINE

An often chronic venereal disease of horses, transmitted during coitus, and caused by *T equiperdum*. The disease is recognized on the Mediterranean coast of Africa, the Middle East, southern Africa, and South America; distribution is probably wider.

Classical signs may develop over weeks or months. Early signs include mucopurulent discharge from the urethra in stallions and from the vagina in mares, followed by gross edema of the genitalia. Later, characteristic plaques 2-10 cm in diameter appear on the skin, and the animal becomes progressively emaciated. Mortality in untreated cases is 50-70%.

Demonstration of trypanosomes from the urethral or vaginal discharges, the plaques on the skin, or peripheral blood is difficult unless the material is centrifuged. Infected animals can be detected with the complement fixation test but only in areas where *T evansi* or *T brucei* do not exist, since they have common antigens.

In endemic areas, horses may be treated (TABLE 9). When eradication is required, strict control of breeding and elimination of stray horses has been successful. Alternatively, infected animals may be identified using the complement fixation test; euthanasia is mandatory.

CHAGAS' DISEASE
(*Trypanosoma cruzi* infection)

The common transmission cycle is between opossums, armadillos, rodents, and wild carnivores, with bugs of the Reduviidae family serving as vectors. Distribution is in Central and South America and localized areas of the southern USA. Chagas'

Table 9. Drugs Commonly Used for Trypanosomiases in Domestic Animals
(See also p 1480.)

Drug	Synonyms	Animal	*Trypanosoma*	Main Action
Diminazene aceturate	Berenil, Babesin (as the delactate salt), Ganaseg	Cattle	*vivax, congolense, brucei*	Curative (with the possible exception of *brucei*)
		Dogs	*evansi, congolense, brucei*	
Homidium bromide	Ethidium bromide	Cattle	*vivax, congolense, brucei*	Curative
		Equids	*vivax*	
Homidium chloride	Babidium chloride, Ethidium chloride, Novidium chloride	\multicolumn{3}{c}{As for the bromide salt}		
Isometamidium	Samorin M & B 4180	Cattle	*vivax, congolense*	Curative and prophylactic
Prothidium		Cattle	*vivax, congolense*	Curative and prophylactic
Quinapyramine sulfate	Antrycide sulfate	Cattle	*vivax, congolense, brucei, evansi*	Curative
		Horses	*brucei, evansi, equiperdum*	
		Camels	*evansi*	
		Pigs	*simiae*	
		Dogs	*congolense, brucei*	
Quinapyramine	Antrycide prosalt	Cattle, Pigs	*vivax, congolense, simiae*	Prophylactic
Suramin	Moranyl, Naganol	Horses	*brucei, evansi, equinum*	Curative
	Antrypol	Camels	*evansi*	
	Bayer 205, Naphuride, Germanin	Dogs	*brucei, evansi*	

disease is important in South America. Domestic animals may become infected and introduce the trypanosome into human dwellings where the bugs are present; man then becomes infected by contamination of eye wounds or by eating food contaminated with insect feces that contain trypanosomes. The trypanosome is pathogenic to man, and occasionally to young dogs and cats; other domestic animals act as reservoir hosts.

NONPATHOGENIC TRYPANOSOMES OF DOMESTIC ANIMALS

Trypanosoma theileri or markedly similar trypanosomes have been detected in cultures of peripheral blood from cattle on every continent. Infection with similar trypanosomes also has been detected in domestic and wild buffalo and various other wild ungulates. In the few areas studied, transmission is by contamination following a cycle of development in species of tabanid flies. Although most parasitemias are subpatent, the trypanosomes may be seen in a blood smear being examined for pathogenic protozoa or in a hemocytometer chamber. Pathogenicity has never been proved experimentally.

Trypanosoma melophagium of sheep also has a worldwide distribution and is transmitted by the sheep ked. *Trypanosoma theodori*, reported from goats, may be a synonym for the same trypanosome.

POLYCYTHEMIA

A relative or absolute increase of circulating RBC. The resulting hyperviscosity of the blood may interfere with normal circulation.

Relative Polycythemia: Reduced plasma volume, which results in hemoconcentration, is the most common cause of polycythemia in domestic animals. This usually is a transient state due to dehydration from fluid loss associated with vomiting or diarrhea. A decrease in plasma volume may be due to decreased electrolyte intake (especially if water intake is insufficient), a fluid shift from intra- to extravascular space due to increased vascular permeability, decreased peripheral perfusion associated with endotoxic or anaphylactic shock, or nonspecific factors related to stress. A decrease in plasma water concentration may be accompanied by a temporary increase in plasma protein concentration. Hemoconcentration may mask anemia.

Circulating RBC may increase temporarily as a result of splenic contraction and release of RBC-rich blood into the circulation. The degree of splenic storage and release varies with the species, but is most marked in horses and dogs, in which a 10-40% increase in RBC may occur within minutes.

Splenic contraction is initiated by such factors as excitement, pain, or stress, but plasma protein concentration is unchanged. Other clinical data are necessary to differentiate probable causes of increased RBC concentration.

Absolute Polycythemia: This is an absolute increase in circulating RBC, usually with a normal plasma volume. Definite diagnosis requires direct RBC mass determination and/or plasma volume determination, which usually is not clinically available. Clinical diagnosis is based on a persistent elevation of PCV (thus, not splenic contraction) and a lack of response to fluids (thus, not hemoconcentration).

Absolute polycythemia may be primary or secondary. Primary polycythemia, or **polycythemia vera**, a myeloproliferative disorder of unknown etiology, is rare but has been reported in dogs, cats, and cattle. Increased erythropoiesis with a normal RBC life span results in a persistent marked increase in RBC volume (eg, PCV >60%). Splenomegaly, leukocytosis, and/or thrombocytosis occur frequently in people but are reported infrequently in dogs. Serum erythropoietin concentration and oxygen saturation are not increased.

In **secondary absolute polycythemia**, the increase in RBC concentration develops in response to erythropoietin or an erythropoietin-like substance. Most often this is a result of tissue hypoxia from cardiac or pulmonary diseases or hemoglobinopathy. Appropriate, secondary absolute polycythemia is diagnosed by a decreased arterial oxygen partial pressure and other evidence of cardiopulmonary disease.

Renal carcinoma, non-neoplastic renal abnormalities (renal cysts, hydronephrosis), or nonrenal tumors also may increase erythropoietin production as an inappropriate, secondary absolute polycythemia in the absence of hypoxemia. Plasma erythropoietin concentration is very low in polycythemia vera but increased in secondary absolute polycythemia. The reticulocyte count is helpful in identifying increased erythropoietin production. Reticulocytosis is expected in secondary absolute polycythemia, but not in polycythemia vera.

Treatment of the various polycythemias, if necessary, is directed toward correction of the causative mechanisms. Polycythemia vera may be alleviated by periodic phlebotomy (eg, 10-20 mL/kg, q48hr as required) with or without the use of myelosuppressive agents, eg, hydroxyurea or cyclophosphamide.

THROMBOSIS, EMBOLISM, AND ANEURYSM

A **thrombus** is an intravascular blood clot still at its site of origin; accordingly, it can be classified as venous, arterial, or cardiac (valvular or mural). Venous thrombosis in large animals generally involves the jugular veins or cranial vena cava, and accompanies phlebitis subsequent to prolonged venous catheterization or administration of irritant solutions such as phenylbutazone or calcium salts. Thrombosis of the caudal vena cava occurs in association with hepatic abscessation in cattle, and often results in embolic pneumonia and pulmonary arterial lesions. In dogs, heartworm disease may lead to pulmonary arterial thrombosis; pulmonary embolism is a major secondary effect. Pulmonary thromboembolism is also seen in dogs in association with diseases that result in decreased circulating antithrombin III concentration, eg, renal amyloidosis, hyperadrenocorticism, and membranous glomerulonephropathy. Arterial thrombi often form in association with parasitic arteritis, the most common form of arterial disease in large animals. Septic cardiac thrombi are associated with endocarditis, and nonseptic cardiac thrombi are associated with myocardial disease. All or part of a thrombus may break off and be carried downstream as an **embolus** that lodges distally at a point of narrowing. Nonseptic arterial thrombosis and embolism generally result in ischemia of tissues supplied by the affected artery. Septic emboli result in bacteremia and localized infection as well as ischemia.

An **aneurysm** is a saccular or cylindrical dilatation of an artery due to weakness of a blood vessel wall. Aneurysms may form at the site of degenerative or inflammatory changes, or where the vessel wall has ruptured partially. These changes may disrupt the endothelium as well, and cause overlying thrombus formation with subsequent formation of emboli. Although aneurysm, thrombosis, and formation of emboli may be recognized simultaneously, distinct clinical syndromes involving the separate conditions are recognized in certain species.

The most common type of aneurysm occurs in the cranial mesenteric artery of horses as a result of arteritis caused by migration of *Strongylus vulgaris* larvae. Similar changes in the aorta and iliac arteries can cause iliac thrombosis in horses. Aneurysm of the thoracic aorta occurs in some dogs with esophageal granulomas caused by *Spirocerca lupi*. Nonparasitic aneurysms are seen occasionally in all species. In cattle with thrombosis of the caudal vena cava, aneurysms, in association with pulmonary arteritis from infected emboli, may result in hemorrhage into the airways with resultant epistaxis and death. Rupture of dissecting aortic aneurysms may cause significant losses in rapidly growing, young turkeys (qv, p 1548).

Clinical Findings and Diagnosis: Aneurysms cause no clinical signs unless hemorrhage occurs or an associated thrombus develops. Except for aortic rupture in turkeys (with sudden death), hemorrhage associated with guttural pouch mycosis in horses, or pulmonary arterial aneurysm in cattle, spontaneous aneurysmal hemorrhage is rare, and clinical signs usually are related to thrombosis. The signs vary according to the size and location of the thrombus and whether emboli form. In some horses with verminous aneurysm and thrombosis, emboli develop and partially or completely occlude terminal branches of the mesenteric arteries. Affected intestinal segments show changes ranging from passive congestion to hemorrhagic infarction. Clinical signs are those of colic, constipation, or diarrhea. The colic usually is recurrent, and attacks may be severe and prolonged. Diagnosis is often based on history of recurrent colic, coupled with peritoneal fluid neutrophilia without hematologic evidence of chronic, localized sepsis.

An aneurysm of the abdominal aorta and its branches may be palpated rectally as a fixed firm swelling with a rough irregular surface that pulsates with the heart beat. Fremitus may be present. In excess thrombus formation, the pulse distally may be delayed and have a slow rate of rise in pressure, or may be absent.

Verminous thrombosis with or without aneurysm of the terminal aorta and proximal iliac arteries produces a characteristic syndrome in horses. Although these horses appear normal at rest, graded exercise results in an increasing severity of weakness of the hindlimbs with unilateral or bilateral lameness, muscle tremor, and sweating. Severely affected animals cannot endure exercise; they become lame and then fall or lie down. Following a short rest, the signs disappear and the animal seems normal. Subnormal temperature of the affected limbs may be detectable, along with decreased or absent arterial pulsations and delayed and diminished venous filling. Careful rectal palpation may show variation in pulse amplitude of the internal and/or external iliac arteries and asymmetric vasculature. Atrophy of the hindquarter muscles develops in severe cases, and lameness may become evident with only mild exercise. Complete embolic or thrombotic occlusion of the distal aorta may produce acute bilateral hindlimb paralysis and recumbency in horses. Affected animals are anxious, appear painful, and rapidly go into shock. The hindlimbs are cold, and rectal palpation reveals an absence of pulsation in either iliac artery.

A different syndrome occurs in cats as a result of aortic embolism. In most instances a primary cardiac disorder is present, most commonly cardiomyopathy. Abnormal circulatory dynamics in dilated or hypertrophic cardiomyopathy predispose to intracavitary thrombus formation, usually in the left atrium; the thrombus often dislodges and forms an embolus that obstructs aortic branches. The usual site of embolization is the aortic trifurcation, with obstruction of the internal and external iliac arteries and the median sacral artery. Clinical signs include sudden onset of posterior paresis, severe pain, and muscle spasm. The femoral pulses are weak or absent, and the hindlimbs are cool. If the aortic trifurcation is not completely occluded, the cat may have unilateral paresis or only mild neurologic deficits in both hindlimbs. An embolus may also lodge in other systemic vascular beds or more proximally in the aorta. It has been postulated that factors elaborated by the embolus may inhibit collateral circulation since aortic ligation does not reproduce the clinical signs of aortic thromboembolism, while an experimentally produced thrombus does. Serotonin and thromboxane A_2, both released by activated platelets, cause vasoconstriction and platelet aggregation that likely inhibit collateral circulation and are important in the development of clinical signs.

In unclear cases, or those in which surgery is contemplated, angiocardiography may help to confirm the diagnosis of aneurysm, thrombosis, or embolism, and to assess collateral circulation. Due to the need for general anesthesia, this procedure is often unsafe in cats with underlying dilated cardiomyopathy, and economically unjustifiable in cattle.

Thrombosis of the cranial vena cava produces bilateral jugular engorgement without a jugular pulse. Edema of the head, submandibular area, and brisket, with pronounced oral mucosal hyperemia is common. Significant lingual, pharyngeal, and/or laryngeal edema may occur, and result in dysphagia and dyspnea. Upper respiratory edema may become life threatening, and necessitate tracheostomy. Cranial caval thrombosis may result from embolization of a jugular thrombus or extension of a right atrial endocarditis lesion. Thrombosis of the caudal vena cava may result in pulmonary embolism and secondary pulmonary abscessation, which cause coughing, tachypnea, dyspnea, and abnormal lung sounds. Aneurysms in pulmonary arteries that contain septic emboli may rupture and cause intrapulmonary hemorrhage, or pulmonary abscesses may erode into bronchi and result in hemorrhage into the airways. Epistaxis and hemoptysis may occur. Pulmonary arterial thromboembolism is a frequent complication of right heart endocarditis in cattle, but aneurysms rarely develop.

Treatment: In horses, aneurysms due to *Strongylus vulgaris* rarely rupture, and the chief concern is with thrombosis and formation of emboli. Generally, the arterial wall is sufficiently involved that thrombus removal is impractical, since another would likely form. Antibacterial treatment and anthelmintic dosing to kill the migrating larvae is of considerable value in therapy. The most rational approach to cranial mesenteric and aortic-iliac thrombosis in horses is prevention and control of strongylosis (qv, p 202).

Aortic emboli in cats may be removed surgically; however, cardiac disease and especially heart failure greatly increase the risk of general anesthesia, and acute reperfusion of vascular beds that have accumulated large quantities of hydrogen and potassium can result in acute hyperkalemia and metabolic acidosis severe enough to cause cardiac arrest. Most recommend medical therapy only, which includes judicious administration of fluids (to maintain hydration and blood pressure, but not exacerbate congestive heart failure), analgesics, and heparin. Many cats with aortic thromboembolism die despite treatment, or do not regain hindlimb function. Some paralyzed cats that survive the initial cardiovascular crisis recover the ability to walk after 3-7 wk. The severity of heart disease often determines the long-term prognosis.

Pulmonary thromboemboli in dogs most commonly produce dyspnea. Chest radiographs may be normal, appear underperfused in the affected region, reveal an enlarged main pulmonary artery and right heart, or show evidence of pulmonary hemorrhage/infarction. Blood-gas determination most commonly reveals hypoxemia with low or normal partial pressure of CO_2. Diagnosis can be confirmed with pulmonary angiography or ventilation/perfusion scanning with radionuclide-labeled albumin and gases. Therapeutic recommendations are the same as for aortic thromboemboli in cats. Thrombolytic drugs, eg, streptokinase or tissue plasminogen activator, have not been evaluated sufficiently in cats or horses to justify therapeutic recommendations.

Aspirin (25 mg/kg body wt, PO q72hr) is the most widely used prophylactic therapy for feline thromboembolism. Aspirin inhibits platelet aggregation and preserves collateral circulation by inhibiting thromboxane A_2 formation. Aspirin therapy (17 mg/kg, PO q48hr) also has been recommended as an aid in prevention of equine thromboembolic disease.

Treatment of venous thrombosis is usually limited to supportive care, including hydrotherapy of accessible veins, anti-inflammatory agents, and systemic antimicrobials to control secondary sepsis. Thrombosed jugular veins have been successfully removed surgically in horses. Thrombosis of the cranial or caudal vena cava generally carries a poor prognosis and does not respond to therapy. Measures to minimize trauma to, and bacterial contamination of, veins remain the best means to prevent thrombosis. Anticoagulation therapy with heparin and warfarin has been tried in horses and cats and is rational to control the extent of thrombosis, but is attended by a number of complications such as anemia and fatal hemorrhage. These drugs do not resolve an existing thrombus.

DIGESTIVE SYSTEM

DIG

DISEASES OF THE DIGESTIVE TRACT, Large Animals

DIGESTIVE SYSTEM, INTRODUCTION

The digestive tract includes the oral cavity and associated organs (lips, teeth, tongue, and salivary glands), the esophagus, the forestomachs (reticulum, rumen, omasum) of ruminants and the true stomach in all species, the small intestine, liver, pancreas, the large intestine, rectum, and anus. Gut-associated lymphoid tissue ([GALT], tonsils, Peyer's patches, diffuse lymphoid tissue) is distributed along the GI tract. The peritoneum covers the abdominal viscera and is involved in many GI diseases. Fundamental efforts to manage GI disorders should always be directed toward localizing disease to a particular segment and determining a cause. A rational therapeutic plan can then be formulated.

Function: The primary functions of the GI tract include prehension of feed and water; mastication, ensalivation, and swallowing of feed; digestion of feed and absorption of nutrients; maintenance of fluid and electrolyte balance; and evacuation of waste products. (*See also* pp 1374 and 1387.) The primary functions can be divided into 4 major modes and, correspondingly, 4 major modes of dysfunction: digestion, absorption, motility, and evacuation.

The most important facets of normal GI tract motility are muscle activity, which moves ingesta from the esophagus to the rectum; the segmentation movements, which churn and mix the ingesta; and segmental resistance and sphincter tone, which retard aboral progression of gut content. In ruminants, these movements are of major importance in normal forestomach function.

Pathophysiology: Abnormal motor function usually takes the form of decreased motility. Segmental resistance is usually reduced, and transit rate increases. Motility depends on stimulation via the sympathetic and parasympathetic nervous systems, and thus on the activity of the central and peripheral parts of these systems, and on the GI musculature and its intrinsic nerve plexuses. Debility, accompanied by weakness of the musculature, acute peritonitis, and hypokalemia, produces atony of the gut wall (paralytic ileus). The intestines distend with fluid and gas, and fecal output is reduced. In addition, chronic stasis of the small intestine may predispose to abnormal proliferation of microflora. Such bacterial overgrowth may cause malabsorption by injuring mucosal cells, competing for nutrients, and by deconjugation of bile salts and hydroxylation of fatty acids.

Increased irritability of a particular segment increases that segment's activity, which disrupts the normal progression of ingesta from esophagus to rectum. Not only is the rate of passage of ingesta in that direction increased, but the increased potential activity of an irritated segment may produce a reverse gradient to the anterior segments, which causes the peristaltic waves to be reversed. It is by this means that intestinal contents, even feces, are returned to the stomach, and vomiting occurs.

Vomiting is a neural reflex act that results in ejection of food and fluid from the stomach through the oral cavity. It is always associated with antecedent events such as premonition, nausea, salivation, or shivering, and is accompanied by repeated contractions of the abdominal muscles.

Regurgitation is characterized by passive, retrograde movement of previously swallowed material from the esophagus. In diseases of the esophagus, swallowed material may fail to reach the stomach.

One of the major consequences of subnormal motility is distention with fluid and gas. Much of the accumulated fluid is saliva and gastric and intestinal juices secreted during normal digestion. Distention causes pain and reflex spasm of adjoining gut segments. It also stimulates further secretion of fluid into the lumen of the gut, which exacerbates the condition. When the distention exceeds a critical point, the ability of the musculature of the wall to respond diminishes, the initial pain disappears, and paralytic ileus develops in which all GI muscle tone is lost.

Dehydration, acid-base and electrolyte imbalance, and circulatory failure are major consequences of GI distention. Accumulation of gut fluids stimulates additional secretion of fluids and electrolytes in the anterior segments of the intestine, which can worsen the abnormalities and lead to shock.

Abdominal pain associated with GI disease usually is caused by stretching of the wall of the tract. Contraction of the gut does not of itself cause pain, but does so by causing direct and reflex distention of neighboring segments; spasm, an exaggerated segmenting contraction of one section of intestine, results in distention of the immediately anterior segment when a peristaltic wave arrives. Other factors that may cause abdominal pain include edema and failure of local blood supply, eg, in local embolism or twisting of the mesentery.

Specific diseases cause diarrhea by varied and characteristic mechanisms, the recognition of which is useful in understanding, diagnosing, and managing GI diseases. The major mechanisms of diarrhea are increased permeability, hypersecretion, and osmosis. Hypermotility is often secondary. In healthy animals, water and electrolytes continuously transfer across the intestinal mucosa. Secretions (from blood to gut) and absorptions (from gut to blood) occur simultaneously. In clinically normal animals, absorption exceeds secretion, which results in net absorption. Inflammation in the intestines can be accompanied by an increase in "pore size" in the mucosa, permitting increased flow through the membrane ("leak") down the pressure gradient from blood to the intestinal lumen. If the amount exuded exceeds the absorptive capacity of the intestines, diarrhea results. The size of the material that leaks through the mucosa varies, depending on the magnitude of the increase in pore size. Large increases in pore size permit exudation of plasma protein, resulting in protein-losing enteropathies (eg, lymphangiectasia in dogs, paratuberculosis in cattle, nematode infections).

Hypersecretion is a net intestinal loss of fluid and electrolytes, which occurs independent of changes in permeability, absorptive capacity, or exogenously generated osmotic gradients. Enterotoxic colibacillosis is an example of diarrheal disease due to intestinal hypersecretion: enterotoxigenic *Escherichia coli* produce enterotoxin that stimulates the crypt epithelium to secrete fluid beyond the absorptive capacity of the intestines. The villi, along with their digestive and absorptive capabilities, remain intact. The fluid secreted is isotonic, alkaline, and free of exudates. The intact villi are beneficial because a fluid (administered PO) that contains glucose, amino acids, and sodium is absorbed even in face of hypersecretion.

Osmotic diarrhea occurs when inadequate absorption results in a collection of solutes in the gut lumen, which cause water to be retained by their osmotic activity. It occurs in any condition that results in nutrient malabsorption or maldigestion.

Malabsorption is failure of digestion and absorption due to some defect in the villous digestive and absorptive cells, which are mature cells that cover the villi. Several epitheliotropic viruses directly infect and destroy the villous absorptive epithelial cells or their precursors, eg, coronavirus, transmissible gastroenteritis virus of piglets, and rotavirus of calves. Feline panleukopenia virus and canine parvovirus destroy the crypt epithelium, which results in failure of renewal of villous absorptive cells and collapse of the villi; regeneration is a longer process following parvoviral infection than after viral infections of villous tip epithelium (eg, coronavirus, rotavirus). Intestinal malabsorption also may be caused by any defect that impairs absorptive capacity, such as diffuse inflammatory (eg, lymphocytic plasmacytic enteritis, eosinophilic enteritis) or neoplastic disorders (eg, lymphosarcoma).

Other examples of malabsorption include defects of pancreatic secretion that result in maldigestion. Rarely, because of failure to digest lactose (which, in large amounts, has a hyperosmotic effect), neonatal farm animals or pups may have diarrhea while they are being fed milk. Reduced digestive enzyme secretion activity at the surface of villous tip cells is characteristic of epitheliotropic viral infections recognized in farm animals.

The ability of the GI tract to digest food depends on its motor and secretory functions and, in herbivores, on the activity of the microflora of the forestomachs of ruminants, or of the cecum and colon of horses and pigs. The flora of ruminants can digest cellulose; ferment carbohydrates to volatile fatty acids; and convert nitrogenous substances to ammonia, amino acids, and protein. In certain circumstances, the activity of the flora can be suppressed to the point that digestion becomes abnormal or ceases. Incorrect diet, prolonged starvation or inappetence, and hyperacidity, as occurs in engorgement on grain, all impair microbial digestion. The bacteria, yeasts, and protozoa also may be adversely affected by the oral administration of drugs that are antimicrobial or that drastically alter the pH of the rumen contents.

Clinical Findings: Manifestations of GI tract disease include excessive salivation, diarrhea, constipation or scant feces, vomiting, regurgitation, GI tract hemorrhage, abdominal pain, tenesmus, abdominal distention, shock and dehydration, and suboptimal performance. The location and nature of the lesions that cause malfunction often can be determined by recognition and analysis of the clinical findings. In addition, abnormalities of prehension, mastication, and swallowing usually are associated with diseases of the oral mucosa, the teeth, the mandible or other bony structures of the head, or the esophagus. Vomiting occurs most commonly in single-stomached animals and usually is due to gastroenteritis or nonalimentary disease (eg, uremia, pyometra, endocrine disease). Regurgitation may signify disease of the oropharynx or esophagus and is not accompanied by the premonitory sign of vomiting.

Large-volume, fluid diarrhea usually is associated with hypersecretion, eg, in enterotoxigenic colibacillosis in newborn calves, or with malabsorptive (osmotic) effects. Blood and fibrinous casts in the feces indicate a hemorrhagic, fibrinonecrotic enteritis of the small or large intestine, eg, bovine viral diarrhea, coccidiosis, salmonellosis, or swine dysentery. Black, tarry feces (melena) indicate hemorrhage in the stomach or upper part of the small intestine. Tenesmus of GI origin usually is associated with inflammatory disease of the rectum and anus.

Small amounts of soft feces may indicate a partial obstruction of the intestines. Abdominal distention can result from accumulation of gas, fluid, or ingesta, usually due to hypomotility (functional obstruction, adynamic paralytic ileus) or a physical obstruction (eg, foreign body or intussusception). Distention may, of course, result from something as direct as overeating. A ''ping'' heard during auscultation and percussion of the abdomen indicates a gas-filled viscus. A sudden onset of severe abdominal distention in the adult ruminant usually is due to ruminal tympany. Ballottement and succussion may reveal splashing sounds when the rumen or bowel is filled with fluid. Varying degrees of dehydration and acid-base and electrolyte imbalance, which may lead to shock, occur when large quantities of fluid are lost in diarrhea or sequestered in intestinal obstruction, or in gastric or abomasal volvulus.

Abdominal pain, which is due to stretching or inflammation of the serosal surfaces of abdominal viscera or the peritoneum, may be acute or subacute, and its manifestation varies among species. In horses, acute abdominal pain is common (*see* COLIC, p 168). Subacute pain is more common in cattle and is characterized by reluctance to move, and by grunting with each respiration or deep palpation of the abdomen. Abdominal pain in dogs and cats may be acute or subacute, and is characterized by whining, barking, meowing, and abnormal postures.

Examination of the GI Tract: A complete, accurate history and routine clinical examination will reveal the diagnosis in most cases. In outbreaks of GI tract disease in farm animals, the history and epidemiological findings are of prime importance. If the history and epidemiological and clinical findings are consistent with GI disease, the lesion should be localized within the system, and the type of lesion and its cause determined.

The abnormality may be localized to the large or small bowel by history, physical examination, and fecal characteristics (*see* TABLE 1). The distinction is important because it narrows the differential diagnoses and determines the direction of further investigation.

Table 1. Differentiation of Small-intestinal from Large-intestinal Diarrhea

Clinical Sign	Small Intestine	Large Intestine
Frequency of defecation	Normal or slightly increased	Very frequent
Fecal volume	Large quantity of bulky or watery feces	Small quantities often
Urgency	Absent	Usually present
Tenesmus	Absent	Usually present
Mucus in feces	Usually absent	Frequent
Blood in feces	Dark black (melena)	Red (fresh)
Weight loss	May be present	Rare

The clinical and laboratory techniques and their applications include: visual inspection of the oral cavity, and of the contour of the abdomen for distention or contraction; palpation through the abdominal wall or per rectum to evaluate shape, size, and position of abdominal viscera; abdominal percussion to detect "pings", which suggest gas-filled viscera; auscultation to determine the intensity, frequency, and duration of GI movements, as well as splashing sounds associated with fluid-filled stomachs and intestines, and fluid-rushing sounds associated with diarrheal disease; succussion to reveal fluid-splashing sounds; ballottement to evaluate density and size of abdominal organs by their movement away from and back to the abdominal wall; and gross examination of feces to assess bulk, consistency, color, and for mucus, blood, or undigested food particles.

Digestion of X-ray film or gel can be used to screen for proteolytic enzymes in feces. Microscopical studies include examination for parasites. Examination for the presence of split and neutral fats after Sudan III stain is a sensitive test for steatorrhea in small animals. Cytology of a rectal or colonic mucosal smear stained with New Methylene Blue or Wright's stain for fecal leukocytes is useful to detect inflammatory bowel disease. The following may be useful (or necessary): bacterial culture and virus isolation; endoscopy to visualize the mucosal surface of the esophagus, stomach, colon, and rectum; abdominocentesis to collect fluid from distended viscera or the peritoneal cavity for examination; radiography to diagnose obstructive disease by use of contrast techniques; biopsy to obtain samples for microscopical examination (samples of intestines and liver are useful in diagnosing chronic enteritis and liver disease); tests for digestion and absorption to estimate and differentiate malabsorption and maldigestion. Common absorption tests include the oral fat tolerance (plasma turbidity) test, and glucose and xylose absorption tests. Pancreatic function can be evaluated by the oral bentiromide absorption test and determination of serum trypsin-like immunoreactivity, and by laparotomy to provide biopsy data in cases in which the diagnosis is not clear or that may require surgical correction.

INFECTIOUS DISEASES

Some of the common pathogens that can cause disease of the GI tract are listed below.

VIRUSES

Cattle, Sheep, Goats
>Bovine viral diarrhea
>Rotavirus
>Coronavirus
>Rinderpest
>Malignant catarrhal fever
>Bluetongue

Pigs
>Transmissible gastroenteritis
>Rotavirus
>Coronavirus

Horses
>Rotavirus

Dogs and Cats
>Canine parvovirus
>Canine coronavirus
>Feline panleukopenia virus
>Canine and feline rotaviruses
>Canine and feline astroviruses

RICKETTSIAE

Horses
>Ehrlichiosis (Potomac fever)

Dogs
>Salmon poisoning

BACTERIA

Cattle, Sheep, Goats
>Enterotoxigenic *Escherichia coli*
>*Salmonella* spp
>*Mycobacterium paratuberculosis*
>*Fusobacterium necrophorum*
>*Clostridium perfringens* types B, C, and D
>*Actinobacillus lignieresii*
>*Proteus* spp
>*Pseudomonas* spp
>*Yersinia enterocolitica*

Pigs
>Enterotoxigenic *E coli*
>*Salmonella* spp
>*Treponema hyodysenteriae*
>*Clostridium perfringens* type C

Horses
>Enterotoxigenic *E coli*
>*Salmonella* spp
>*Rhodococcus (Corynebacterium) equi*

Dogs, Cats
  Salmonella spp
  Yersinia enterocolitica
  Campylobacter jejuni
  Bacillus piliformis
  Clostridium spp
  Mycobacterium spp

PROTOZOA

Cattle, Sheep, Goats
  Eimeria spp
  Cryptosporidium spp
Pigs
  Eimeria spp
  Isospora suis
Horses
  Eimeria spp
Dogs, Cats
  Isospora spp
  Sarcocystis spp
  Besnoitia spp
  Hammondia sp
  Toxoplasma sp
  Giardia sp
  Trichomonas spp
  Entamoeba histolytica
  Balantidium coli

FUNGI

Cattle, Pigs
  Candida spp
Horses
  Aspergillus fumigatus
Dogs, Cats
  Histoplasma capsulatum
  Candida albicans
  Phycomycetes

ALGAE

Prototheca spp

PARASITES (HELMINTHS)

These are listed in the discussions of GASTROINTESTINAL
PARASITES OF HORSES, p 201, RUMINANTS, p 205, PIGS, p
219, and SMALL ANIMALS, p 237.

As the list above indicates, the GI tract is subject to infection by many pathogens, which are a major cause of economic loss due to illness, suboptimal performance, and death. These infections spread by direct contact or the fecal-oral route. Many of the pathogens are part of the normal intestinal flora, and disease occurs only following a stressful event, eg, salmonellosis occurring in horses following transportation, extended anesthesia, or surgery. The intestinal flora becomes established within a few hours after birth, which emphasizes the importance of the early ingestion of colostrum to provide protection against septicemia and intestinal infection.

Definitive etiological diagnosis of infectious disease of the GI tract depends on demonstrating the pathogen in the tract or in the feces of the affected animal. In herd epidemics, such as an outbreak of acute undifferentiated diarrhea in newborn calves or piglets, the best opportunity to establish a diagnosis is to select untreated animals in the earliest stage of the disease and submit them for necropsy and detailed microbiological examination of the intestinal flora. When selective necropsy is not an option, a daily series of carefully collected fecal samples must be submitted to the laboratory with a request for special culture techniques, depending on the infectious disease that is suspected.

OVERVIEW OF GASTROINTESTINAL PARASITISM

The GI tract may be inhabited by many species of parasites. Their cycles may be direct, in which eggs and larvae are passed in the feces and stadial development occurs to the infective stage, which is then ingested by the final host. Alternatively, the stages may be ingested by an intermediate host, usually an invertebrate, in which further development occurs; infection is acquired when the intermediate host or free-living stage shed by that host is ingested. Sometimes there is no development in the intermediate host, in which case it is known as a transport or paratenic host, depending on whether the larvae are encapsulated or in the tissues. Clinical parasitism depends on the number and pathogenicity of the parasites, which in turn depend on the biotic potential of the parasites or, when appropriate, their intermediate host and the climate and management practices. In the host, resistance, age, nutrition, and concomitant disease also influence the course of parasitic infection. The economic importance of subclinical parasitism in farm animals is also determined by the above factors, and it is now well established that lightly parasitized animals, which show no clinical evidence of disease, perform less efficiently in the feedlot, dairy, or finishing house.

Feed conversion in light to moderate parasitism is adversely affected and is primarily due to reduced appetite and poor utilization of absorbed protein and energy. Carcass quality and size also are reduced, which further reduce financial returns. Internal parasites of companion animals can cause severe disease or unthriftiness, and are aesthetically undesirable. Furthermore, some of these parasites may also infect man.

Since parasitism is easily confused with other debilitating conditions, diagnosis depends heavily on the seasonal character of parasitic infection, previous farm history, and examination of feces for evidence of oocysts or worm eggs. Elevated serum pepsinogen levels are useful aids to the diagnosis of some abomasal infections, as elevated serum liver enzymes are in liver fluke infection. The ELISA is now in use, and other serological (including monoclonal antibody) techniques are under development; serodiagnosis is likely to become more prevalent as the specificity of the tests improve. They should be particularly useful in companion animals harboring parasites incriminated in zoonoses.

Advances in epidemiology (particularly regarding factors affecting seasonal development of the free-living stages and their survival), coupled with the discovery of highly efficient broad-spectrum anthelmintics, have made successful treatment and control of GI parasites both possible and practical. Response to therapy is usually rapid, and single treatments suffice unless reinfection occurs or the lesions are particularly severe. Prophylactic control in large animals is generally achieved by integrating grassland management with the use of anthelmintics. Improved methods of administering anthelmintics, such as the pour-on technique or sustained or pulsed-release devices have also helped. Strategies to prevent parasitism and related production losses are now part of any modern herd-health, flock, or stud program. Similar preventive programs are equally important in controlling parasitism in pet animals. For estimating parasite load, see p 951. (Control by vaccination is limited to lungworms: vaccine for cattle is available in several European countries; sheep lungworm vaccine is available in parts of eastern Europe, and the Middle East.)

TREATMENT OF INFECTIOUS DISEASES

Antimicrobial agents are used for the treatment of bacterial diseases, and anthelmintics for parasitic diseases. There is no specific therapy for treatment of viral diseases. Antimicrobials are commonly given PO daily for several days until recovery is apparent, but there is little objective evidence for efficacy. Parenteral administration of antimicrobials is indicated when septicemia is apparent or may occur. The choice of antimicrobial agent depends on the suspected disease, previous results, and cost of the drugs. In herd epidemics, antimicrobials may be added to the feed or water supplies at therapeutic levels for several days, followed by prophylactic levels for an extended period, depending on the infection pressure in the population. The feed and water supplies of in-contact animals also may be medicated in an attempt to prevent new cases from occurring.

CONTROL OF INFECTIOUS DISEASES

Effective control of the common infectious diseases of the GI tract depends on sanitation and hygiene, developing and maintaining nonspecific resistance in the animal, and in certain cases, providing specific immunity by vaccinating the pregnant dam or susceptible animal.

Effective sanitation and hygiene is achieved primarily by provision of adequate space for animals, and regular cleaning of pens and efficient removal of manure from the immediate environment. Development and maintenance of nonspecific resistance depends on the genetic selection of animals that have a reasonable degree of inherent resistance, and the provision of adequate nutrition and housing, which minimizes stress and allows the animals to grow and behave normally. The development of infected but clinically normal animals, which can shed pathogens for weeks or months, is a major problem with some infectious diseases of the GI tract, eg, salmonellosis. Ideally, these carrier animals should be identified by microbiological means and isolated from the rest of the herd until free of the infection or culled.

Certain diseases, eg, enterotoxigenic colibacillosis in calves and piglets, can be controlled by vaccination of the pregnant dam several weeks before parturition. This method depends on achieving a protective level of antibodies in the colostrum. There are exceptions, but in most cases, systemic immunity provides little protection against the infectious enteritides; effective immunity against GI disease depends on stimulation of local intestinal immunity after the neonatal period. During the neonatal period, protection can be provided through the local action of maternally derived antibodies. For example, secretory IgA progressively increases in sow's milk from the time of farrowing until weaning, which provides the piglet with daily protection during the nursing period.

NONINFECTIOUS DISEASES

The major causes include: dietary overload or indigestible feeds, chemical or physical agents, obstruction of the stomach and intestines caused by the ingestion of foreign bodies or by any physical displacement or injury to the GI tract that interferes with the flow of ingesta, enzyme deficiencies, abnormalities of the mucosa that interfere with normal function (gastric ulcers, inflammatory bowel disease, villous atrophy, neoplasms), and congenital defects. The equine colics are a special case because of the prevalence of intestinal lesions due to parasitism, which predispose to subacute and acute dysfunction. The causes of several diseases are uncertain; these include abomasal ulcers in cattle, gastric ulcers in pigs and foals, gastric torsion in dogs, and acute intestinal obstruction and displacement of the abomasum in cattle. Within the group of noninfectious diseases of the GI tract, usually only a single animal is affected at one time; exceptions are the diseases associated with excessive feed intake or poisons; in these, herd outbreaks are common.

Some of the common noninfectious diseases of the GI tract are listed below.

ORAL CAVITY

Stomatitis
Diseases of the teeth and peridontium
Neoplasia

ESOPHAGUS

Traumatic esophagitis
Esophageal obstruction
Megaesophagus

SIMPLE STOMACH

Gastritis (chemical and physical agents, chronic inflammatory disease)
Ulceration
Dilatation, torsion
Gastric retention
Neoplasia

RUMINANT STOMACHS

Simple indigestion
Rumen overload (grain overload, ruminal lactic acidosis)
Ruminal tympany (bloat)
Traumatic reticuloperitonitis and sequelae
Left-side displacement of the abomasum
Right-side distention with or without torsion of the abomasum
Abomasal ulcer
Dietary impaction of the abomasum

INTESTINES

Diarrhea due to dietary overload or indigestible diet
Inflammation (eg, eosinophilic or lymphocytic-plasmacytic enteritis)
Neoplasia
Obstruction
Enteritis due to poisonings (copper salts, lead, inorganic arsenic, phosphorus,
    fluoride, molybdenum, petroleum products, poisonous plants, saline and
    alkaline waters)

EQUINE COLICS

Gastric dilatation
Spasmodic colic
Intestinal tympany
Impaction of the large intestine
Acute intestinal obstruction
Thromboembolic colic secondary to verminous mesenteric arteritis

PERITONEUM

Sequela of ischemic necrosis of the stomach(s) or intestines
Traumatic perforation of the stomach(s) or intestines
Postsurgical
Tumors or abscesses

PRINCIPLES OF THERAPY

Although eliminating the cause of the disease is the primary objective, the major
part of treatment is supportive and symptomatic, aimed at relieving pain, correcting
abnormalities, and allowing healing to occur. (*See also* pp 1374 and 1387.) A summary of the principles includes:

Elimination of Primary Cause: This may involve antimicrobials, coccidiostats, antifungal agents, anthelmintics, antidotes for poisons, or surgical correction
of displacements. (*See also* p 98.)

Correction of Abnormal Motility: Correction of excessive or depressed motility appears rational, but often there is uncertainty about the nature and degree of

abnormal motility, and the available drugs may not give consistent results. There is little clinical evidence to recommend the routine use of anticholinergic or opiate drugs to slow intestinal transit. Slowing intestinal transit may be counterproductive to the defense mechanism of diarrhea, which acts to evacuate harmful organisms and their toxins. In general, anticholinergic drugs probably are justified only for short-term symptomatic relief of pain and tenesmus associated with inflammatory diseases of the colon and rectum.

Replacement of Fluid and Electrolytes: This is necessary when dehydration and electrolyte and acid-base imbalance occur as in diarrhea, persistent vomiting, intestinal obstruction, or torsion of the stomach(s), where large amounts of fluid and electrolytes are sequestered. (*See* p 1355.)

Relief of Distention: Distention of the GI tract with gas, fluid, or ingesta may occur at any level due to physical or functional obstruction. The distention may be relieved medically or by stomach tube (as in bloat in ruminants), or surgical intervention may be required (as in acute intestinal obstruction, or torsion of the abomasum in ruminants or of the stomach in monogastric animals).

Relief of Abdominal Pain: Analgesics should be given for relief of abdominal pain that is reflexly affecting other body systems (eg, cardiovascular collapse) or when the pain is causing the animal to injure itself because of violent activity (rolling, kicking, throwing itself). Animals treated with analgesics must be monitored regularly to ensure that the relief of pain does not provide a false sense of security; the lesion may be progressively worsening while under the influence of the analgesic.

Reconstitution of Rumen Flora: In prolonged anorexia or acute indigestion in ruminants, the rumen microflora may be seriously depleted. The flora can be reconstituted by oral administration of ruminal juice from a normal animal (transfaunation), which contains rumen bacteria and protozoa and volatile fatty acids.

AMEBIASIS

An acute or chronic colitis characterized by persistent diarrhea or dysentery that is prevalent in tropical areas worldwide. It is common in man and nonhuman primates, sometimes observed in dogs, but rare in other mammals. Several species of amebae occur in animals, but the only known pathogen is *Entamoeba histolytica*. Man is the natural host for this species and is the usual source of infection for domestic animals.

Clinical Findings: *Entamoeba histolytica* may live in the lumen of the large intestine as a commensal or invade the intestinal mucosa and produce mild to severe, ulcerative, hemorrhagic colitis. In acute disease, fulminating dysentery may develop, which may be fatal, progress to chronicity, or resolve spontaneously. Chronic cases may exhibit weight loss, anorexia, tenesmus, and chronic diarrhea or dysentery, which may be continuous or intermittent. Rarely, amebae may metastasize to other organs, perianal skin, and genitalia. Signs may resemble those of other colonic diseases (eg, trichuriasis, balantidiasis).

Diagnosis: Definitive diagnosis depends on finding *E histolytica* trophozoites in feces by direct saline smears, or in sections of affected colonic tissue. Trophozoites average 20-40 μm in diameter, have a single vesicular nucleus, are slowly motile, and may contain ingested RBC. Fixed and stained fecal smears may be necessary for identification, since fecal leukocytes may be confused for amebae. Nonpathogenic species of amebae and *E histolytica* cysts are rarely seen in canine or feline feces.

Treatment: Scant information on treatment in animals is available. Metronidazole (10 mg/kg, PO, b.i.d. for 1 wk) or furazolidone (2 mg/kg, PO, t.i.d. for 1 wk) has been suggested.

CAMPYLOBACTERIOSIS

Gastrointestinal campylobacteriosis, caused by *Campylobacter jejuni* or *C coli*, is now recognized as a cause of diarrhea in various animal hosts, including dogs, cats, calves, sheep, ferrets, mink, several species of laboratory animals, and man. In man it is a leading cause of diarrhea. *Campylobacter jejuni* and *C coli* are also recovered from feces of asymptomatic carriers. (*See also* OVINE GENITAL CAMPYLOBACTERIOSIS, p 655.) Animals, including dogs and cats (especially those recently purchased from shelters or pounds), and wild animals maintained in captivity can serve as sources of human infection. The agent(s) also is isolated frequently from the feces of chickens, turkeys, pigs, and other species.

The disease occurs worldwide and its prevalence appears to be increasing as proper culture techniques for *C jejuni* and *C coli* are refined and updated. Clinical manifestations may be more severe in younger animals. In studies using monoclonal and polyclonal antibodies, *Campylobacter* spp (probably not *C jejuni*) have been associated with proliferative ileitis in hamsters, porcine proliferative enteritis, and proliferative colitis in ferrets. A cause and effect relationship has not been proved experimentally, however, due to the inability to culture the intracellular *Campylobacter* sp *in vitro*.

Etiology: *Campylobacter* is a gram-negative, microaerophilic, slender, curved, motile bacterium with a polar flagellum. *Campylobacter jejuni* is routinely associated with diarrheal disease; however, *C coli*, distinguished from *C jejuni* on the basis of hippurate hydrolysis, is occasionally isolated from diarrheic animals, and routinely is recovered from asymptomatic pigs. More recently, another intestinal, catalase-negative campylobacter, "*C upsaliensis*", has been isolated from diarrheic dogs as well as asymptomatic dogs and cats. *Campylobacter* (*Vibrio*) sp was once associated with swine dysentery, but this is now recognized as being caused by *Treponema hyodysenteriae*. The relationship between *Campylobacter* sp and porcine proliferative enteritis (qv, p 195) is not clear. A newly discovered gastric campylobacter, *C pylori*, is incriminated as a cause of gastritis and duodenal and gastric ulcers in man, and experimentally, produces gastritis in gnotobiotic piglets. Similar gastric organisms have been isolated in nonhuman primates and ferrets. Further studies are needed to assess their importance.

Because of slow growth and microaerophilic requirements, standard culture methods require selective media that incorporate various antibiotics to suppress competing fecal microflora. *Campylobacter jejuni* and *C coli* grow well at 42°C in an atmosphere of 5-10% carbon dioxide and an equal amount of oxygen. Cultures are incubated 48-72 hr; colonies are round, raised, translucent, and sometimes mucoid. The organism can be identified by a series of biochemical tests readily available in any diagnostic laboratory.

Transmission and Epidemiology: As with most intestinal pathogens, fecal-oral spread and food- or water-borne transmission appear to be the principal avenues for infection. One suspected source of infection for pets, as well as mink and ferrets raised for commercial purposes, is ingestion of undercooked poultry and other raw meat products. Asymptomatic carriers can shed the organism in their feces for prolonged periods and contaminate food, water, milk, and fresh processed meats (including pork, beef, and poultry products). The organism can survive *in vitro* at 41°F (5°C) for 2 mo and can survive in feces, milk, water, and urine. Wild birds also may be important sources of water contamination. Unpasteurized milk has been cited as a principal source of infection in several outbreaks in man.

Clinical Findings: The diarrhea appears to be most severe in young animals. Typical signs in dogs include mucus-laden, watery and/or bile-streaked diarrhea (with or without blood) that lasts 3-7 days; reduced appetite; and occasional vomiting. Fever and leukocytosis may also be present. In certain cases, intermittent diarrhea may persist >2 wk; in some, it may be present for months. Gnotobiotic puppies inoculated with *C jejuni* developed malaise, loose feces, and tenesmus within 3 days of inoculation.

In calves, signs vary from mild to moderate. The diarrhea is thick and mucoid with occasionally visible blood flecks; temperature may be normal. Diarrhea with mucus and blood also has been observed in primates, ferrets, mink, and cats. *Campylobacter mucosalis* and *C hyointestinalis* have been isolated from pigs with intestinal adenomatosis. Diarrhea and wasting disease are also clinically evident in these animals. Organisms with ultrastructure similar to *Campylobacter* spp have been observed in hyperplastic ileal epithelial mucosa of hamsters with proliferative ileitis; *C jejuni* has been isolated from these lesions but has failed to reproduce the syndrome. *Campylobacter* spp also have been associated with proliferative colitis in ferrets and with hyperplastic intestinal lesions in guinea pigs and rats. *Campylobacter*-like organisms have been described in young rabbits with acute typhlitis.

Lesions: In 3-day-old chickens infected with *C jejuni*, the organisms were detected within epithelial cells and mononuclear cells of the lamina propria; the jejunum and ileum were the most severely affected. Congested and edematous colons were found in dogs 43 hr after inoculation; microscopically, there was reduction in epithelial height, loss of brush border, and reduced goblet cells in the colon and cecum. Hyperplastic epithelial glands resulted in a thickened mucosa. Histological changes in calves primarily involve the jejunum, but also can involve the ileum and colon. The lesions can vary from mild changes to severe hemorrhagic enteritis. The mesenteric lymph nodes are edematous. An enterotoxin and cytotoxin have been identified in *C jejuni*; however, their role in production of the disease is not known.

Diagnosis: The standard method for diagnosis is microaerophilic culture of feces at 42°C; a special medium is commercially available. Diagnosis is also possible by using darkfield or phase-contrast microscopy, by which fresh fecal samples are examined for the characteristic darting motility of *C jejuni*. This method is especially useful during the acute stage of diarrhea when large numbers of organisms are more likely to be shed in the feces. Various techniques can detect serum antibodies to various antigens of *Campylobacter* spp. Heat-stabile or heat-labile antigen schemes are being used routinely to serotype various strains. Serial serum samples to demonstrate rising antibody titers are helpful in diagnosis. Intestinal viruses as well as other intestinal bacterial pathogens must be ruled out in animals with *Campylobacter*-associated diarrhea.

Treatment and Control: Isolation of *C jejuni* or *C coli* from the diarrheic feces is not, in itself, an indication for antibiotic therapy. Because *C jejuni* and *C coli* have only recently been recognized as potential intestinal pathogens in animals, efficacy of antibiotic therapy has been reported infrequently. In certain cases in which animals are severely affected or present a zoonotic threat, antibiotic treatment may be indicated. In general, *C jejuni* and *C coli* isolates from animals are similar to those isolates obtained from human populations. Erythromycin, the drug of choice for *Campylobacter* diarrhea in man, is also effective in other animals. Gentamicin, furazolidone, doxycycline, and chloramphenicol also can be used. Also, chloramphenicol has been used to treat proliferative colitis in ferrets. Ampicillin is relatively inactive against most strains of *Campylobacter*. Most strains are resistant to penicillin. Tetracycline and kanamycin resistance in certain *C jejuni* strains is reported to be plasmid-mediated and transmissible within *C jejuni* serotypes. Efficacy of sulfadimethoxine and sulfa combinations is variable. Before therapy is instituted, isolation and sensitivity tests should be done. Some animals continue to shed the organism despite antibiotic therapy. Quinolone antibiotics may be useful in eliminating *C jejuni* and *C coli* in asymptomatic carriers.

COCCIDIOSIS

A usually acute invasion and destruction of intestinal mucosa by protozoa of the genera *Eimeria, Isospora, Cystoisospora*, or *Cryptosporidium*, characterized by diarrhea, fever, inappetence, weight loss, emaciation, and sometimes death. Coccidiosis is a serious disease in cattle, sheep, goats, pigs, poultry (qv, p 1551), and also rabbits, in which the liver as well as the intestine can be affected (qv, p 1063). In dogs, cats, and horses, it is less often diagnosed but can result in clinical illness. Under modern husbandry conditions (off-floor housing), it is rarely a problem in mink. Other species, both as hosts and of protozoa, are involved (*see* SARCOCYS-TOSIS, p 562, and TOXOPLASMOSIS, p 365). **Coccidiasis** is the infection of animals with coccidia but without apparent clinical signs. Coccidiasis is much more prevalent than coccidiosis and is thought to result in poor feed efficiency under intensive rearing conditions.

Etiology and Epidemiology: *Eimeria, Isospora, Cystoisospora,* and *Cryptosporidium* typically require only one host in which to complete their life cycles; *Cystoisospora* (and others) can utilize an intermediate host. Infection results from ingestion of infective oocysts, which enter the environment in the feces of an infected host. At this time, oocysts of *Eimeria, Isospora,* and *Cystoisospora* are unsporulated, and therefore not infective. Under favorable humidity and temperature, oocysts sporulate and become infective in several days. During sporulation, the amorphous protoplasm develops into small bodies (sporozoites) within secondary cysts (sporocysts) in the oocyst. In *Eimeria* spp, the sporulated oocyst has 4 sporocysts, each containing 2 sporozoites; in *Isospora* and *Cystoisospora* spp, the sporulated oocyst has 2 sporocysts, each containing 4 sporozoites; in *Cryptosporidium*, each oocyst contains only 4 sporozoites.

When the sporulated oocyst is ingested by a susceptible animal, the sporozoites escape from the oocyst, invade the intestinal mucosa or epithelial cells in other locations, and develop intracellularly into multinucleate schizonts (also called meronts). Each nucleus develops into an infective body called a merozoite; merozoites enter new cells and repeat the process. After a variable number of asexual generations, merozoites develop into either macrogametocytes (females) or microgametocytes (males). These produce a single macrogamete or a number of microgametes in a host cell. After being fertilized by a microgamete, the macrogamete develops into an oocyst. The oocysts, with their resistant walls, are discharged unsporulated in the feces.

Clinical coccidiosis is most prevalent under conditions of poor nutrition, poor sanitation, or overcrowding, or after the stresses of weaning, shipping, sudden changes of feed, or severe weather.

Of the numerous species of *Eimeria, Isospora,* or *Cystoisospora* that can infect a particular host, not all are pathogenic. Concurrent infections with 2 or more species, some of which may not normally be considered pathogenic, also influence the clinical picture. Within pathogenic species, strains may vary in virulence.

Most animals acquire *Eimeria, Isospora,* or *Cystoisospora* infections of varying degrees when between 1 mo and 1 yr old; *Cryptosporidium* is usually acquired before 1 mo of age. Older animals usually are resistant to clinical disease, but may have sporadic inapparent infections. Such clinically healthy, mature animals usually are sources of infection to young, susceptible animals.

Clinical Findings: The asexual or the sexual stages of the various species destroy the intestinal epithelium, and frequently, the underlying connective tissue of the mucosa. This may be accompanied by hemorrhage into the lumen of the intestine, catarrhal inflammation, and diarrhea. Signs may include discharge of blood or tissue, or both, tenesmus, and dehydration. Serum protein and electrolyte levels may be appreciably altered, but changes in Hgb or PCV are seen only in severely affected animals.

Diagnosis: Finding appreciable numbers of oocysts of pathogenic species in the feces is diagnostic, but because diarrhea may precede the heavy output of oocysts by 1-2 days and may continue after the oocyst discharge has returned to low levels, it is not always possible to find oocysts in a single fecal sample; multiple examinations may be required. The number of oocysts present in feces is influenced by the genetically determined reproductive potential of the species, the number of infective oocysts ingested, stage of the infection, age and immune status of the animal, prior exposure, consistency of the fecal sample, and method of examination. Therefore, the results of fecal examinations must be related to clinical signs and intestinal lesions (macroscopic and microscopic). Furthermore, the species must be identified as those known to be pathogens in that host. The finding of numerous oocysts of a nonpathogenic species concurrent with diarrhea does not constitute a diagnosis of clinical coccidiosis.

Treatment: The life cycles of *Eimeria, Isospora,* and *Cystoisospora* are considered to be self-limiting and end spontaneously within a few weeks unless reinfection occurs. Prompt medication may slow or inhibit development of stages resulting from reinfection, and thus can shorten the length of illness, reduce discharge of oocysts, alleviate hemorrhage and diarrhea, and lessen the likelihood of secondary infections and mortality. Sick animals should be isolated and treated individually whenever possible to guarantee delivery of therapeutic levels of the drug, and to prevent exposure of other animals. Intestinal sulfonamides, eg, sulfaguanidine, or the readily absorbed sulfonamides, eg, sulfamerazine or sulfamethazine, may be used. Sulfaquinoxaline has been reported to give excellent clinical results in beef and dairy calves, sheep, dogs, and cats. Since the soluble sulfonamides may be given PO or parenterally, they are more effective than intestinal sulfonamides. Amprolium has been reported to be effective during outbreaks in calves, sheep, and goats. In outbreaks in feedlots or on lush pastures, prophylactic treatment of healthy exposed animals as a safeguard against additional morbidity should be considered.

Prophylaxis: Prophylaxis is based on limiting the intake of sporulated oocysts by young animals so that an infection is established to induce immunity but not cause clinical signs. Good feeding practices and good management, including sanitation, contribute to this goal. Neonates should receive colostrum. Young susceptible animals should be kept in clean and dry quarters, and feeding and watering devices should be clean and protected from fecal contamination. Stresses, eg, weaning, sudden changes in feed, and shipping, should be minimized.

Prophylactic administration of anticoccidials is recommended when animals under various management regimens can be predictably expected to develop coccidiosis. In virtually all cases, *Eimeria* spp are implicated. Decoquinate, amprolium, and ionophorous antibiotics are effective in cattle. Continuous low-level feeding of amprolium, sulfaguanidine, or ionophorous antibiotics during the first month of feedlot confinement has been reported to have prophylactic value in lambs. Both amprolium and ionophorous antibiotics have been reported to be effective in kids. Sulfas and amprolium have been reported to be effective in pigs.

COCCIDIOSIS OF CATS AND DOGS

About 21 and 22 species of coccidia infect the intestinal tract of cats and dogs, respectively. Except for *Cryptosporidium parvum,* which infects both hosts, all the others are host specific. Cats have species of *Cystoisospora, Besnoitia, Toxoplasma, Hammondia,* and *Sarcocystis.* Dogs have species of *Cystoisospora, Hammondia,* and *Sarcocystis.* Neither dogs nor cats have *Eimeria.*

Cryptosporidium parvum has been found in the feces of healthy kittens and puppies as well as in diarrheal animals, some of which had concurrent viral infections. The clinical significance of *C parvum* infection in kittens and puppies has not been clearly established. No treatment is known.

Besnoitia (qv, p 322), *Sarcocystis* (qv, p 564), and *Toxoplasma* (qv, p 365) are discussed separately. *Hammondia* has an obligatory 2-host life cycle with cats or dogs as final hosts and rodents or ruminants as intermediate hosts, respectively. *Hammondia* oocysts are indistinguishable from those of *Toxoplasma* and *Besnoitia* but are nonpathogenic in either host.

The most common coccidia of cats and dogs are *Cystoisospora.* These were named *Isospora* before it was found that, unlike other isosporans, those of cats and dogs can facultatively infect other mammals and produce in various organs an encysted form that is infective for the cat or dog final host. Two species infect cats: *C felis* and *C rivolta.* Four species infect dogs: *C canis, C ohioensis, C burrowsi,* and *C neorivolta.* In dogs, only *C canis* can be identified by the oocyst structure; the other 3 overlap in dimensions and can be differentiated only by endogenous developmental characteristics. In cats, both species can be identified easily by oocysts.

Clinical coccidiosis, although not common, has been reported in kittens and puppies <1 mo old. The most common clinical signs in severe cases are diarrhea (sometimes bloody), weight loss, and dehydration. Usually, it is associated with other infectious agents, immunosuppression, or stress.

In kennel conditions when the need for prophylaxis might be predicted, amprolium is said to be effective, although it is not approved for use in dogs. In severe cases only, in addition to supportive fluid therapy for dehydration, sulfonamides such as sulfadimethoxine, 50 mg/kg the first day, 25 mg/kg/day for 2-3 wk thereafter, or nitrofurazone at 20 mg/kg/day have been reported to be coccidiostatic. Sanitation is important, especially in catteries and kennels, or where large numbers of animals are housed. Feces should be removed frequently. Fecal contamination of feed and water should be prevented. Runs, cages, and utensils should be disinfected daily. Raw meat should not be fed. Insect control should be established.

COCCIDIOSIS OF CATTLE

CRYPTOSPORIDIOSIS

Infections of calves, usually <1 mo old, with *Cryptosporidium parvum* (*see* p 108) are usually self-limiting, but can be significant, both for the calves, and as sources of infection for others, including man.

EIMERIA INFECTION

Of the 13 species of *Eimeria* that infect cattle, *E zuernii* and *E bovis* are most often associated with clinical disease. Experimentally, other species have been shown to be mildly or moderately pathogenic. Coccidiosis is commonly a disease of young cattle (1-2 mo to 1 yr), and usually is sporadic during the wet seasons of the year. "Summer coccidiosis" and "winter coccidiosis" in range cattle probably result from severe weather stress and crowding around a limited water source, which concentrates the hosts and parasites within a restricted area. Although particularly severe epidemics have been reported in feedlot cattle during extremely cold weather, cattle confined to feedlots are susceptible to coccidiosis at all seasons. Outbreaks usually occur within the first month of confinement. The incubation period is 17-21 days.

In light infections, cattle appear healthy and oocysts are present in normally formed feces, but feed efficiency is somewhat reduced. The most characteristic sign of clinical coccidiosis is watery feces, with little or no blood, and the animal shows only slight discomfort for a few days. Severely affected animals develop diarrhea that may continue for ≥1 wk, which consists of thin bloody fluid, or thin feces with streaks or clots of blood, shreds of epithelium, and mucus. They become anorectic, depressed, and dehydrated; they lose weight, and the hindquarters and tail become soiled with feces. Tenesmus is common. During the acute period some animals die; others die later from secondary complications, eg, pneumonia. Animals that survive severe illness can have significant weight loss that is not quickly regained, or can remain permanently stunted.

The pathogenic coccidia of cattle can damage the mucosa of the lower small intestine, cecum, and colon. The first generation schizonts of *E bovis* appear as white macroscopic bodies in the villi of the small intestine.

For diagnosis, prophylaxis, and treatment, *see* p 104 *et seq.*

COCCIDIOSIS OF GOATS

Ten to 12 species of *Eimeria*, as well as *Cryptosporidium parvum*, are found in goats in North America. The *Eimeria* spp are host specific and are not transmitted from sheep to goats. *Cryptosporidium parvum* (*see* below) infects neonates of numerous species, including goats.

Eimeria arloingi, E christenseni, and *E ninakohlyakimovae* are highly pathogenic in kids. Clinical signs include diarrhea with or without mucus or blood, dehydration, emaciation, weakness, anorexia, and death. Some goats are actually constipated and die acutely without diarrhea. Stages and lesions are confined to the small intestine, which may appear congested, hemorrhagic, or ulcerated and have scattered pale, yellow to white macroscopic plaques in the mucosa. Histologically, villous epithelium is sloughed, and inflammatory cells are seen in the lamina propria and submucosa. Diagnosis is based on finding oocysts of the pathogenic species in diarrheal feces, usually at tens of thousands to millions per g of feces. It is not unusual to find oocyst counts as high as 70,000 in kids without overt disease.

Angora and dairy goats, raised under different management practices, may have similar patterns of exposure for kids. Just after parturition, nursery pens and surrounding areas may be heavily contaminated with oocysts from does; just after shipping, changing rations, introducing new animals, or mixing young with older animals, resistance to infection is decreased. Anticoccidials can be administered to a herd immediately following diagnosis, or as a preventive in those highly predictable situations previously cited.

For diagnosis, prophylaxis, and treatment, *see* p 104 *et seq.*

COCCIDIOSIS OF PIGS

Eight species of *Eimeria* and one each of *Isospora* and *Cryptosporidium* infect pigs in the USA. Piglets 5-15 days old are characteristically infected with only *C parvum* and *I suis,* which produce enteritis and diarrhea. These agents must be differentiated from viruses, bacteria, and helminths that also cause scours in neonatal pigs.

Relatively little is known about *C parvum* in piglets. It is thought to be prevalent but usually of low morbidity and mortality. Infection may result in nonhemorrhagic diarrhea. (*See* CRYPTOSPORIDIOSIS, p 108.)

Isospora suis is prevalent in neonatal pigs. Infection is characterized by a watery or greasy diarrhea, usually yellowish to white and foul smelling. Piglets may appear weak, dehydrated, and undersized; they sometimes die. Oocysts are usually shed in the feces and can be identified by their size, shape, and sporulation characteristics; however, in peracute infections, diagnosis must be based on finding stages of the parasite in impression smears or histological sections of the small intestine because pigs can die before oocysts are formed. Histologically, lesions confined to the jejunum and ileum are characterized by villous atrophy, blunting of villi, focal ulceration, and fibrinonecrotic enteritis with parasite stages in epithelial cells. Prophylactic control has been reported by feeding anticoccidials to sows from 2 wk before farrowing through lactation, or to neonatal pigs from birth to weaning; effectiveness of the latter has not been confirmed. Thorough removal of feces and disinfection of farrowing facilities between litters greatly decreases infection.

Although less commonly associated with clinical coccidiosis, *E debliecki, E neodebliecki, E scabra,* and *E spinosa* have been found in pigs ~1-3 mo of age with diarrhea. Illness may last 7-10 days with pigs remaining unthrifty.

For diagnosis, prophylaxis, and treatment, *see* p 104 *et seq.*

COCCIDIOSIS OF SHEEP

About 15 species of *Eimeria,* as well as *Cryptosporidium parvum,* infect sheep. Historically, some *Eimeria* spp were thought to be infectious and transmissible between sheep and goats, but the parasites are now considered to be host specific. The names of some species of goat coccidia are still erroneously applied to species of similar appearance found in sheep. *Cryptosporidium* sp (*see* below) appears to infect numerous neonates, including lambs <1 mo old. *Eimeria ahsata* and *E ovinoidalis (ninakohlyakimovae)* are pathogens of lambs, usually 1-6 mo old; *E ovina* appears to be somewhat less pathogenic. All other *Eimeria* of sheep are essentially nonpathogenic, even when large numbers of oocysts are present in feces.

Signs include diarrhea (sometimes containing blood or mucus), dehydration, fever, inappetence, weight loss, anemia, wool breaking, and death. The ileum, cecum, and upper colon are usually most affected; they may be thickened, edematous, and inflamed, and sometimes, there is mucosal hemorrhage. Thick, white, opaque patches containing large numbers of *E ovina* oocysts may develop in the small intestine. Because oocysts are prevalent in feces of sheep of all ages, coccidiosis cannot be diagnosed solely by finding oocysts. Peak oocyst counts of >100,000/g of feces have been reported in 8- to 12-wk-old lambs that appeared healthy. However, diarrhea with oocyst counts of a pathogenic species of >20,000/g is characteristic of sheep coccidiosis.

Lambs 1-6 mo old in lambing pens, intensive grazing areas, and feedlots are at greatest risk as a result of shipping, ration change, crowding stress, severe weather, and contamination of the environment with oocysts from ewes or other lambs. Because occurrence of coccidiosis or coccidiasis under these management systems often becomes so predictable, anticoccidials should be administered prophylactically for 28 consecutive days beginning a few days after lambs are introduced into the environment. Therapeutic treatment of affected individuals with anticoccidials once coccidiosis has been diagnosed is not effective, but severity can be reduced if treatment is begun early.

For treatment, *see* p 105.

CRYPTOSPORIDIOSIS

A self-limiting enterocolitis of cosmopolitan distribution caused by the coccidian parasite *Cryptosporidium parvum*. It is common in young ruminants, particularly calves; somewhat less common in man and pigs, and rare in dogs, cats, and horses. Other cryptosporidia cause disease in reptiles and birds. The disease in calves, characterized by weight loss and watery diarrhea, is clinically indistinguishable from many other causes of calf diarrhea. Unless the immune system is compromised, it is self-limiting. There are many reports of infection in man acquired from clinically ill calves.

Etiology and Transmission: *Cryptosporidium parvum* is a minute protozoan that is transmitted by the fecal-oral route. Oocysts shed in the feces are sporulated, hence, they are immediately infective. The mean incubation period is ~4 days.

Clinical Findings and Lesions: Calves 1-3 wk old seem to be most susceptible. Signs—anorexia, weight loss, diarrhea, and tenesmus—resemble those caused by several other intestinal pathogens; however, infections without signs do occur. Uncomplicated cryptosporidiosis is seldom fatal. Although *C parvum* can infect virtually the entire intestinal tract, the distal small intestine usually is most severely affected. Infection in horses is limited to the small intestine. Gross lesions may consist of hyperemic intestinal mucosa and yellowish intestinal contents. Microscopically, mild to severe villous atrophy with spherical organisms in the brush border is evident.

Diagnosis: Organisms can be detected in mucosal scrapings of fresh intestine or by fecal flotation in sucrose or zinc sulfate solutions. Because of their small size and transparency, the oocysts are easily overlooked. They should be sought under high-power magnification, preferably under phase-contrast illumination. Oocysts of *C parvum* measure ~5 μm in diameter. They must be distinguished from oocysts of *C muris* (~6 × 7 μm), which infects the abomasum of calves and is considered either nonpathogenic or responsible for mild diarrhea. Fecal smears may be heat-fixed and stained by an acid-fast technique. *Cryptosporidium* oocysts stain red, whereas yeasts, which are about the same size and shape as the oocysts, stain with the blue or green counterstain. Since oocysts are not shed continuously, repeated sampling may be necessary. Calves usually shed oocysts for a maximum of 2 wk.

Treatment and Control: There is no effective specific treatment; however, since the disease is self-limiting, supportive therapy, such as rehydration, is usually sufficient. The oocysts can be killed in the environment with 5% ammonia solution.

Since *C parvum* has a wide host range, infection in other animal species on the premises should be considered.

CONGENITAL AND INHERITED ANOMALIES OF THE DIGESTIVE SYSTEM

MOUTH

Clefts are the most common congenital abnormality involving the lips of small animals. The mode of transmission is unclear; probably most are hereditary although maternal nutritional deficiencies, stresses, and drug or chemical exposures, and mechanical interference with the fetus are also probable factors. **Cheiloschisis** (cleft lip, harelip) is due to a disturbance of the processes that form the jaws and face during embryonic development. Cleft of the lower lip is rare and usually occurs on the midline. Clefts of the upper lip, usually at the junction of the premaxilla and maxilla, may be unilateral or bilateral, complete or incomplete, and often are associated with clefts of the alveolar process and palate. **Palatoschisis** (cleft palate) is found occasionally in the newborn of all species. The sole cause was long thought to be hereditary, but ingestion of toxic agents, use of steroids, and some viral infections during pregnancy appear to be causes. The defect may involve the palate alone, or may extend from the lip through the alveolar bones of the upper jaw into the palate. It is due to incomplete fusion of the embryonic processes of the upper jaw. Cleft palate may be associated with other less obvious abnormalities.

The initial sign is milk dripping from the nostrils when the newborn attempts to nurse. Respiratory infection due to inhalation of food is common. If untreated, death occurs due to starvation or infection. Examination of the oral cavity readily reveals the defect, except that in foals having only a cleft of the soft palate, this may be difficult to see. It commonly occurs with other defects, such as arthrogryposis, which is inherited in Charolais cattle as a simple autosomal recessive.

Surgical correction is effective only if the defect is small. If attempted, correction should be done before the animal's general health is compromised, and only after ethical considerations have been addressed. Lip clefts cause marked difficulty in nursing, and hand feeding is necessary. Correction of cleft palate is much more difficult; in small animals it is attempted at ~3 mo of age. If unsuccessful at that time, dental acrylic splints can be made when the animal reaches adulthood to temporarily cover the defect for varying periods. Euthanasia is advisable in animals with gross defects, and those treated successfully should not be used for breeding.

Brachygnathia (short lower jaw, parrot mouth) in cattle is inherited as a polygenic factor. It is seen also as a lethal factor associated with impacted molar teeth. It is also associated with impacted molar teeth and osteopetrosis (qv, p 480) in Angus calves, and occasionally in Simmental cattle. Brachygnathia may also be due to an autosomal aberration, or associated with a chromosomal aberration such as trisomy, which is lethal. A range of defects in sheep, from brachygnathia to mandibular aplasia and agnathia, is reportedly inherited as a simple autosomal recessive.

Agnathia, the lack of development of the mandible, has been postulated to be due to homozygosity of a simple autosomal recessive gene in sheep. Sporadic cases occur in cattle. The facial structures, including the maxilla, may reveal a number of defects in all species, but particularly foals and calves. In Angus calves, a facial defect characterized by a broad, short face is accompanied by degenerative joint disease of all major joints. The defect has a complex genetic transmission.

Craniofacial dysplasia in Limousin cattle is suspected to be due to homozygosity of a simple autosomal recessive gene. The defect is characterized by a convex profile of the nose, short lower jaw, deficient ossification of frontal sutures, exophthalmus, and large tongue.

A facial dysplasia, in which the face was short and wide, has been described in Angus cattle. The condition was inherited, most likely as a polygenic. All major joints developed degenerative joint disease soon after birth; affected calves were recumbent and reluctant to get up and walk.

TEETH

Abnormal number of teeth: In most species, a reduction in the number of teeth is rare, although in dogs, molars and premolars may fail to develop or erupt. Supernumerary teeth occasionally are encountered in the incisor or molar regions of horses; in dogs, they usually are unilateral and most often in the upper jaw. Usually, they are removed only if they cause mechanical interference with mastication or, in horses, if irritated by a bit. In horses, they may require periodic rasping or trimming to prevent damage to neighboring soft tissues.

Irregularities of development or shedding of teeth: Eruption of temporary teeth may cause transitory problems. Sometimes, the temporary teeth are shed prematurely, which leaves a depression in the gum surrounded by an inflamed margin; the discomfort of eating may cause a temporary loss of condition. In the case of the premolar teeth, the root of the temporary tooth may be absorbed, but the crown may persist as a covering or "cap" to the erupting permanent tooth; these caps are readily removed with forceps, if they have not separated spontaneously. Delayed shedding of deciduous canine teeth in dogs is common.

Abnormalities in position and direction of individual teeth: In horses, this may affect the incisors. Some of these teeth may be rotated on the long axis, or may overlap adjacent teeth. In dogs, the upper third premolar is the first to rotate in short-muzzled breeds. Later, all upper premolars may rotate; the molars are seldom affected.

Imperfect apposition of the teeth: Overshot jaw, in which the upper jaw overhangs the lower jaw, results in imperfect apposition of the teeth of the upper and lower incisors. **Undershot jaw** (prominent chin, bulldog jaw) is the opposite condition. If a foal is badly affected with either condition, sucking is impossible. Treatment, when feasible, in either case consists of rasping or shearing the offending points and projections. It is possible for the molar arcades to have anterior and posterior projections without being overshot or undershot. Both conditions are common in dogs. In certain breeds (eg, Bulldogs, Boxers), an undershot jaw is a breed characteristic; in others, either condition may be cause for disqualification for show. Since defects in apposition may have a genetic basis, owners should be advised of the ramifications if surgical correction is to be attempted.

Ectopic teeth: The best example of this is the dentigerous cyst or so-called temporal odontoma, which most commonly is located in the mastoid process and is recognized by the presence of a discharging sinus along the edge of the pinna. The only treatment is surgical removal of the teratomatous mass of dental tissue and the associated secretory membrane.

CYSTS AND SINUSES OF THE NECK

These imperfections of fetal development are important in their differentiation from infections, cysts, or fistulas of the salivary gland. **Thyroglossal duct cyst** is the result of postnatal persistence of the early embryonic thyroglossal duct. This rare cyst is always single and found in the middle of the neck, usually at the level of the hyoid bone and larynx. It is smoothly rounded with a well-defined border, anchored to the hyoid bone and deep tissues. Unless infection is superimposed, it is seldom attached to the skin. It is not tender and contains fluid.

A **branchial (or lateral cervical) cyst** develops from branchial apparatus malformation, usually of the second branchial cleft. Unilateral or bilateral branchial cysts occupy a lateral position in the upper neck and usually are only slightly mobile. Their size varies considerably, and an individual cyst may change size periodically as its contents escape through a small opening into the throat or through a small cutaneous fistula (branchial or lateral cervical fistula).

Surgical removal of the cyst(s) is required.

DILATATION OF THE ESOPHAGUS

A generalized or regional increase in the caliber of the esophagus that may follow food retention. (*See also* p 173.) It can result from: 1) constrictive tissue bands that arise from a persistent right aortic arch or from the ligamentum arteriosum associated with the aorta, pulmonary artery, and base of the heart; 2) congenital paralysis of the thoracic esophagus, or similar paralysis in older dogs, considered to be a neuromuscular dysfunction from exogenous or metabolic toxins; or 3) achalasia, in which the terminal esophagus fails to dilate as food approaches the cardia, due to degeneration in the neural plexus or cardiospasm. Secondary dilatation of the cervical esophagus usually follows thoracic esophageal dilatation unless its cause is removed.

ABDOMINAL HERNIAS

A protrusion of abdominal contents into the subcutis through a natural or abnormal opening in the body wall. Protrusion through the diaphragm is termed diaphragmatic hernia (qv, p 711). Herniation as a result of a severe blow that causes the abdominal aponeurosis to tear is frequently called a rupture. The best examples of nontraumatic hernias are the umbilical and inguinal or scrotal hernias, the latter being merely an extension of an inguinal hernia.

Whether to surgically correct **umbilical hernia** in cattle is debatable. Although some cases are hereditary, excess traction of an oversized fetus and cutting the umbilical cord too close to the abdominal wall are other possible causes.

In **scrotal or inguinal hernias** in all species, surgical correction almost invariably involves simultaneous castration. **Perineal hernia** is encountered mainly in mature dogs and differs from the other types of abdominal hernias in that the peritoneal lining of the hernial sac is either absent or thin and degenerate. Although many factors have been cited, the actual cause of perineal hernia is unknown. **Femoral (crural) hernia** is rare in domestic animals, especially in the larger species.

Two types of hernias are recognized: reducible and irreducible. The reducible type is characterized by a noninflammatory, painless, soft, elastic, compressible swelling. It may vary in size from time to time. The swelling can be made to disappear by manipulation or by placing the animal in a suitable position. In dogs, diagnosis of perineal hernia is based on the presence of a swelling at the side of the anus or vulva, between the tail base and the sciatic tuber. The hernia usually can be reduced more easily if the hindquarters are elevated.

Irreducible hernias have the same characteristics as reducible ones, except that the contents cannot be returned to the abdominal cavity. This is due either to adhesions between parts of the hernial contents, to narrowing of the ring, or to distention of a loop of intestine. The contents may be incarcerated or strangulated.

Umbilical abscess may be confused with hernia and the 2 are frequently found together, especially in pigs and cattle. Exploratory puncture is sometimes necessary for differentiation. Hematomas also may be confused with hernias. If the area can be reached by rectal palpation, an inguinal or scrotal hernia can be diagnosed definitely by locating the ring and the contained bowel.

Inguinal hernia in male pigs is common, and it usually extends into the scrotum. Shaking the suspended piglet by the forelegs causes even a small hernial bulge to become visible. In female pigs, this defect is invariably accompanied by arrested genital development; such animals are sterile, and surgery is indicated only when the size of the process is a threat to the growth of the pig to market weight.

Inguinal hernia in male foals often resolves spontaneously during the first year of life. For this reason, early corrective surgery is not indicated unless the hernia is strangulated or of such a magnitude that it interferes with the gait. Strangulated inguinal hernia in stallions is fairly frequent and is characterized by signs of constant and severe abdominal pain. It is readily recognized by rectal palpation. When diagnosed early, the condition often may be relieved by rectal manipulation under general anesthesia of the incarcerated intestine. If this fails, immediate radical surgery is necessary.

Inguinal hernia is rare in cattle; however, it is sometimes encountered in males. When done, surgical correction to conserve the breeding potential of the bull is not always successful.

Perineal hernia (qv, p 132), which may be either unilateral or bilateral, can be surgically corrected. Whether prostatectomy in mature male dogs is indicated at the same time is a matter of debate.

When treatment is elected, umbilical hernias usually are dealt with surgically, preferably at 3-6 mo of age. In calves, some success has been achieved by applying a binder of broad adhesive bandage (10-cm width) for 3-4 wk. The owner should be advised that the weakness may be heritable.

ATRESIA

In horses, in which it is suspected to be a genetic defect, **segmental atresia** of the colon is rare. In cows, pressure on the developing fetus in the longitudinal axis during rectal pregnancy examination between days 37-41 may cause atresia of the colon. However, in Holstein cattle there also seems to be a genetic pattern, possibly a simple autosomal recessive, to account for this defect. Calves affected with atresia of the colon pass little or no meconium, and develop colic soon after birth.

Ileocolonic agangliosis has been reported in white foals out of matings of Overo horses to each other. Although the foals appear normal at birth, they soon develop colic and die on the second day. The affected foals are white and have blue irises. Diagnosis can be confirmed by the lack of ganglia in the colon. Congenital defects of the rectum and anus generally result from arrested embryonic development. Anal atresia results when the dorsal membrane separating the rectum and anus fails to rupture. Clinical signs apparent at birth include tenesmus, abdominal pain and distention, retention of feces, and absence of an anal opening. Surgical removal of the membrane is indicated.

Segmental aplasia (rectal agenesis) occurs when the rectum terminates in a blind pouch before reaching the anus. Surgical correction is difficult because the location of the terminal section varies and iatrogenic damage to nerves in the area may occur.

RECTOVAGINAL FISTULA

A fistulous tract that connects the vagina and rectum, this usually occurs in conjunction with imperforate anus. Passage of feces through the vulva, or signs of colonic obstruction are suggestive. Diagnosis may be confirmed by barium enema, which outlines the extension of the defect into the vagina. Identification of the fistula, surgical correction, and reestablishment of normal anatomic structures are imperative. Prognosis usually is guarded. Complications are common and include fecal and urinary incontinence.

DENTISTRY

DENTAL DEVELOPMENT

Estimation of an animal's age may be aided by the eruption times and appearance of the teeth. Tooth development is subject to variation, and determination of age is only approximate. In young horses and calves, the eruption times are valuable criteria. The deciduous and permanent dental formulas and shape and wear of the incisor teeth also are useful in estimating age. The teeth are designated as incisor (I), canine (C), premolar (P), and molar (M); deciduous teeth are designated Di, Dc, and Dp.

ESTIMATION OF AGE BY EXAMINATION OF THE TEETH

Horses: The age of a horse with a normal mouth and teeth can be estimated; most often this is done by examining the incisor teeth. The deciduous incisors are smaller than the permanent teeth and have a distinct neck. The incisors require ~6 mo from eruption to come into wear. Shape of the teeth also is an aid, as is the "cup" or black cavity in the infundibulum of the incisors. The dental star is a darker dentine that fills the pulp cavity as the tooth wears. Galvayne's groove is a longitudinal groove on the upper corner incisor that is often used in aging horses. The "hook" on the lateral edge of the upper corner incisor develops in many animals at ~7 yr of age, wears off in 2 yr, and reappears at 11 yr of age.

Table 2. Dental Formulas

	Deciduous	Permanent
Horse	$2 (Di \frac{3}{3} Dc \frac{0}{0} Dp \frac{3}{3}) = 24$	$2 (I \frac{3}{3} C \frac{1}{1} P \frac{3\text{-}4}{3} M \frac{3}{3}) = 40\text{-}42$
Cow Sheep Goat	$2 (Di \frac{0}{3} Dc \frac{0}{1} Dp \frac{3}{3}) = 20$	$2 (I \frac{0}{3} C \frac{0}{1} P \frac{3}{3} M \frac{3}{3}) = 32$
Pig	$2 (Di \frac{3}{3} Dc \frac{1}{1} Dp \frac{3}{3}) = 28$	$2 (I \frac{3}{3} C \frac{1}{1} P \frac{4}{4} M \frac{3}{3}) = 44$
Dog	$2 (Di \frac{3}{3} Dc \frac{1}{1} Dp \frac{3}{3}) = 28$	$2 (I \frac{3}{3} C \frac{1}{1} P \frac{4}{4} M \frac{2}{3}) = 42$
Cat	$2 (Di \frac{3}{3} Dc \frac{1}{1} Dp \frac{3}{2}) = 26$	$2 (I \frac{3}{3} C \frac{1}{1} P \frac{3}{2} M \frac{1}{1}) = 30$

Shape of the incisor teeth is often used; the occlusal surface is a long oval in young animals, but as the teeth wear, it becomes round and then triangular, with the apex toward the lingual side. Additionally, the angle of the incisors changes from nearly perpendicular to more or less parallel as the animal ages and the teeth wear.

The more useful signs are arranged chronologically in the following list:

5 yr: I 1 and I 2 level, labial border of I 3 in wear.
6 yr: Cup gone from I 1.
7 yr: All lower incisors level. Cup gone from I 2. Hook in upper I 3. Cement has worn off, changing the color from yellow to bluish white.
8 yr: Dental star appears in I 1. Cup gone from I 3.
9 yr: I 1 round.
10 yr: I 2 round. The distal end of Galvayne's groove emerges from the gum on upper I 3.
13 yr: The enamel spot is small and round in the lower incisors. The dental stars are in the middle of the table surfaces.
15 yr: Dental stars round, dark, and distinct. Galvayne's groove halfway down.
16 yr: I 1 triangular.
17 yr: I 2 triangular. Enamel spots gone from lower incisors.

Cattle: As in horses, signs of wear are much less reliable than eruption for estimation of age. Eruption times of the permanent incisors are often used to estimate the age of calves, particularly show calves. Except for very aged animals, the teeth are rarely used to determine the age of adult cattle.

5 yr: All incisors are in wear. The occlusal surface of I 1 is beginning to level; that is, the ridges on the lingual surface are wearing out and the corresponding border of the occlusal surface is becoming a smooth curve instead of a zigzag line.
6 yr: I 1 is leveled and the neck is visible.
7 yr: I 2 is leveled and the neck is visible.
8 yr: I 3 is leveled and the neck is visible. I 4 may be level.
9 yr: C is leveled and the neck is visible.

Dogs: The data given below were found reliable in ~90% of large dogs. Small dogs (especially ''toy'' breeds) and dogs with undershot or overshot jaws are more variable.

$1^1/_2$ yr: Cusps worn off lower I 1.
$2^1/_2$ yr: Cusps worn off lower I 2.
$3^1/_2$ yr: Cusps worn off upper I 1.

Table 3. Eruption of the Teeth

	Horse	Cow	Sheep, Goat	Pig	Dog	Cat
Di 1	0-1 wk	Before birth	0-1 wk	2-4 wk	4-5 wk	2-3 wk
Di 2	4-6 wk	Before birth	1-2 wk	6-12 wk	4-5 wk	3-4 wk
Di 3	6-9 mo	0-1 wk	2-3 wk	Before birth	5-6 wk	3-4 wk
I 1	2½ yr	1½-2 yr	1-1½ yr	1 yr	2-5 mo	3½-4 mo
I 2	3½ yr	2-2½ yr	1½-2 yr	16-20 mo	2-5 mo	3½-4 mo
I 3	4½ yr	3 yr	2½-3 yr	8-10 mo	4-5 mo	4-4½ mo
Dc	Does not erupt	*0-2 wk	*3-4 wk	Before birth	3-4 wk	3-4 wk
C	4-5 yr	*3½-4 yr	*3-4 yr	6-10 mo	5-6 mo	5 mo
Dp 2	0-2 wk	0-3 wk	0-4 wk	5-7 wk	4-6 wk	Upper: 2 mo / Lower: none
Dp 3	0-2 wk	0-3 wk	0-4 wk	1-4 wk	4-5 wk	4-5 wk
Dp 4	0-2 wk	0-3 wk	0-4 wk	1-4 wk	6-8 wk	4-6 wk
P 1	5-6 mo (wolf tooth)	None	None	5 mo	4-5 mo	None
P 2	2½ yr	2-2½ yr	1½-2 yr	12-15 mo	5-6 mo	Upper: 4½-5 mo / Lower: none
P 3	3 yr	1½-2½ yr	1½-2 yr	12-15 mo	5-6 mo	5-6 mo
P 4	4 yr	2½-3 yr	1½-2 yr	12-15 mo	4-5 mo	5-6 mo
M 1	9-12 mo	5-6 mo	3-5 mo	4-6 mo	5-6 mo	4-5 mo
M 2	2 yr	1-1½ yr	9-12 mo	8-12 mo	6-7 mo	None
M 3	3½-4 yr	2-2½ yr	1½-2 yr	18-20 mo	6-7 mo	None

*The canine tooth of domestic ruminants has commonly been counted as a fourth incisor.

4½ yr: Cusps worn off upper I 2.

5 yr: Cusps of lower I 3 slightly worn. Occlusal surface of lower I 1 and I 2 rectangular. Slight wear of canines.

6 yr: Cusps worn off lower I 3. Canines worn blunt. Lower canine shows impression of upper I 3. (In dogs in which the "tips" of upper and lower incisors meet, ie, do not mesh in a "scissors" bite, the incisors wear down much more rapidly.)

7 yr: Occlusal surface of lower I 1 is elliptical with the long axis sagittal.

8 yr: Occlusal surface of lower I 1 is inclined forward.

10 yr: Lower I 2 and upper I 1 have elliptical occlusal surfaces.

12 yr: Incisors begin to fall out (unless care has been taken to maintain healthy gingival and periodontal tissues).

DENTISTRY, LG AN

Of the common large domestic species, the horse has the most dental problems. In many stables and race track environments, routine dental prophylaxis in horses is handled by nonveterinarians. In the pig industry, removal or amputation of deciduous canine teeth in piglets and tusk amputation in breeding boars may be part of routine management. Exotic species may also have various dental and jaw conditions, eg, impacted tusks in young elephants, or maxillary dental periostitis and actinomycosis in wallabies or kangaroos.

Most large animals are herbivores. Efficient dental function is the key to food intake and maintenance of normal body condition. The teeth of herbivores have evolved to accommodate those forces that result in dental attrition caused by almost continuous grazing (in horses) or rumination. The forces of wear have been matched by development of the hypsodont (high crown) tooth with continuous eruption of the reserve crown. The dental arcades (6 cheek teeth in horses) have regular serrations that expose sharp enamel edges that shred and crush cellulose material. At the same time, the brittle nature of the enamel of the tooth is protected from the forces of dental work by the dentin and cementum.

Signs of Dental Disease: Dental disease (eg, broken teeth, irregular dental arcades) is a common underlying cause of unthriftiness, loss of condition, or poor breeding or nursing performance (eg, broken-mouthed hill sheep), as well as any of the following complaints. Classical signs of dental disease in horses include difficulty and slowness in feeding, and reluctance to drink cold water. During the chewing process, the horse may stop for a few moments and then start again. Sometimes the head is held to one side as if the animal were in pain. Occasionally, the horse may quid, in which it picks up food and forms it into a bolus, but drops the bolus from the mouth after it is partially chewed. Occasionally, the semichewed mass may become packed between the teeth and the cheek. To avoid using a painful tooth, the horse may bolt its food and subsequently suffer indigestion or colic. Unmasticated grain may be noticed in the feces. Other signs include excessive salivation and blood-tinged mucus in the mouth. All of these signs are accompanied by the characteristic, fetid breath of dental decay. There may be a lack of desire to eat hard grain accompanied by a loss of body condition or poor coat condition. Extensive dental decay and accompanying periostitis and root abscessation may lead to empyema of the paranasal sinuses and intermittent unilateral nasal discharge. There may be facial or mandibular swelling and development of a mandibular fistula from a lower cheek tooth apical infection.

Owners may request examinations of horses that are reluctant to take the bit, head shake when being ridden, or resist training techniques. Some of these conditions can be caused by irregularly worn cheek teeth and sharp edges on the maxillary cheek teeth and accompanying buccal mucosal laceration. The presence of "wolf" teeth in horses may or may not be associated with resistance to the bit.

In most cases, there is a correlation between the history, animal's age, and clinical signs. In all cases, a thorough physical examination should precede a detailed oral and dental examination. Examination may be facilitated by sedation and use of an oral gag; however, in most horses, dental examinations can be done with minimal restraint and without a gag. In some cases, a complete oral examination can be done only under general anesthesia; under such circumstances, oral endoscopy or dental radiography may be employed also.

Routine dental prophylaxis is important in the health care of horses. Enamel sharp edges should be removed twice yearly during establishment of the permanent dentition and annually thereafter. Usually this can be done relatively easily without chemical restraint. Major procedures (eg, extractions) require general anesthesia, protection of the airway from debris, and radiographic evaluation. In most instances, repulsion of the decayed tooth is the easiest way to cure this condition. The alveolar socket should be debrided thoroughly, irrigated, and the oral aspect should be packed to protect it from saliva and food. The mandibular or maxillary surgical access wound should be cleaned daily to allow healing by granulation.

Congenital and Developmental Anomalies: In horses, the most common oral congenital deformity is parrot mouth, in which the maxilla is relatively longer than the mandible. In equids and cattle, many forms of dental developmental anomalies may result from exposure to teratogenic toxins; however, an underlying genetic factor should always be considered. Dental irregularities accompany systemic fluorosis in both cattle and sheep. In the milder form of fluorosis, only the dentition may be involved; in extreme fluorosis, eg, 40 ppm in the diet for several years, other skeletal abnormalities may also be seen.

Supernumerary teeth (polyodontia) occur occasionally. This is seen in both horses and cattle, in which double rows of incisor teeth may occur as well as extra cheek teeth.

Abnormal Tooth Eruption: Abnormal eruption of permanent teeth is commonly a sequela of mandibular or maxillary trauma, eg, symphyseal fractures in cattle and horses in which the tooth bud of the permanent tooth is damaged in the fracture or repair process. In horses, delayed eruption or impaction of cheek teeth is a common cause of apical osteitis and subsequent dental decay. This particularly affects the third cheek tooth (premolar 4) and both upper and lower arcades, and is a sequela of a mild degree of dental overcrowding. Medial displacement of the third cheek tooth is another form of maleruption due to overcrowding.

Irregularities of Wear: Except for pigs, most large animals have an intermandibular space that is narrower than the intermaxillary space, ie, anisognathic. In horses, this, together with limited natural movement of the mandible, results in development of enamel points on the buccal edges of the upper arcades and the lingual edges of the lower arcades. In cattle and sheep, because the temporomandibular joint affords greater lateral movement of the mandible, such irregularities do not occur. Extreme forms of such diseases, however, are also influenced by other skeletal deformities of the face, eg, gross shear mouth may result with exaggerated obliquity of the molar tables. It is common in older horses and treatment is usually unsatisfactory.

Enamel points are best treated by regular dental prophylaxis (floating) in horses. This should be done twice annually while the permanent dentition is developing; at the same time retained caps should be removed if they cause oral ulceration or discomfort.

Wave mouth and **step mouth** are irregularities caused by uneven wear of the teeth as a result of local pain. In time, secondary gum and socket disease, ie, periodontitis, develop. Such conditions are best precluded by regular routine dental prophylaxis.

Peridontal disease: In all animals, a degree of inflammatory change occurs during the eruption of both the deciduous and permanent teeth. If, however, malocclusion occurs for any reason, severe peridontal disease is inevitable. In horses this is a common sequela of oral trauma, dental fractures, impactions, and most importantly irregular wear.

In sheep, peridontal disease of the mandibular rostral teeth (incisors) is often referred to as **broken mouth**. Sometimes the viability of grazing sheep is affected dramatically. Many farm-fed sheep have a productive life that is ~2 yr longer than those of range-fed animals. Little can be done to alter the progress of this disease, although some management routines recommend dental prophylaxis and the restoration of occlusal regularity of incisor teeth. This can be done by use of a Drummel tool or a fine-bladed tooth rasp.

Dental Decay: Infection may be introduced into the pulp cavity of the tooth by various routes. In horses, hypoplasia of the enamel of the upper cheek teeth may predispose to caries development, which leads to pulpitis and apical osteitis. If the tooth evolves rostral to the maxillary sinuses, local cellulitis, periostitis, and alveolar periodontitis develop. If, however, the roots and reserve crown of the teeth are found within the maxillary sinuses, paranasal sinus empyema may result. The pathological features of decayed teeth are nonspecific; consequently, the etiology of the apical infection may be obscure. Many cases are not examined until the infection is advanced, and tooth fractures may well be pathological rather than primary. Such conditions are best managed by extraction of the affected tooth, or if surgery is not an economic possibility, the animal should be marketed (eg, sheep, cattle).

DENTISTRY, SM AN

PERIODONTAL DISEASE

A bacterial infection of the tissue surrounding the teeth that causes inflammation of the gingiva, periodontal membrane, cementum, and alveolar bone. Ultimately, teeth are lost due to the loss of their supporting tissues. This is the major reason for tooth loss in dogs.

Etiology: Periodontal disease is caused by gross accumulation of many different bacteria at the gingival margin due in part to a lack of proper oral hygiene. Over a period of weeks, the flora changes from nonmotile, gram-positive, coccoid, aerobic bacteria to more motile, gram-negative, rod-shaped, anaerobic bacteria. Important flora are *Bacteroides asaccharolyticus, Fusobacterium nucleatum, Actinomyces viscosus,* and *A odontolyticus.*

Pathogenesis: As the local bacterial flora increases in mass to 10-20 times normal, gingivitis occurs. The accumulation of bacterial metabolic products increases epithelial permeability in crevicular epithelial desmosomes and allows antigens to contact connective tissue. Metabolic products of bacterial metabolism include hydrogen sulfide, ammonia, endotoxin, hyaluronidase, chondroitin sulfatase, mucopeptides, lipoteichoic acids, acetate, butyrate, isovalerate, and propionate. These bacterial products and host defense mechanisms cause tissue necrosis. Polymorphonuclear leukocytes (PMN) migrate through the sulcular epithelium and form a barrier between the subgingival bacteria and the gingiva. With overwhelming bacterial challenge, PMN die in increasing numbers and release breakdown products. The immune system produces lymphokines that participate in tissue destruction, which follows the path of the local vascular supply. Accelerated tissue destruction and inappropriate repair cause loss of periodontal support. Two forms of periodontal disease are recognized: gingivitis and periodontitis.

Gingivitis: In this inflammation of the marginal gingival tissues (induced by bacterial plaque and not affecting the peridontal ligament or alveolar bone) there is a change from coral-pink to red or purple, swelling of the gingival margin, and a serous or purulent exudate in the sulcus. The gingivae tend to bleed on contact. Fetid breath is common. Gingivitis is reversible with proper tooth cleaning, but if untreated, may lead to periodontitis.

Periodontitis: A destructive inflammatory process of the peridontium, induced and driven by bacterial plaque that contains specific bacteria that destroy the gingiva, peridontal ligament, alveolar bone, and root cementum. This usually occurs after years of plaque, calculus, and gingivitis, and results in permanent loss of tooth support. It is not reversible. There is apical migration of the epithelial attachment and resorption of supporting alveolar bone. Affected teeth may show increased mobility, concurrent gingivitis, and subgingival calculus.

Periodontitis is usually characterized by hyperplasia of the gingival margin in dogs, and recession of the gingival attachment in colony animals. Pet animals also show this tendency; however, infrabony pocket formation (deep isolated areas of bone loss) is more common in pets than in colony-raised animals. Dogs on a hard diet develop fewer problems due to the mechanical cleaning effect of the food. Caudal teeth have more problems than rostral teeth. The maxilla is affected more severely than the mandible, and buccal surfaces have more disease than lingual surfaces. Gingivitis often becomes severe at ~2 yr of age, and if treated, resolves. Periodontitis usually begins at 4-6 yr of age and, if untreated, progresses to tooth loss.

Treatment: The basic principle is that active periodontal disease will not develop around a clean tooth.

Gingivitis usually can be treated by thorough cleaning of the teeth, including below the gingival margin. Cases that do not resolve with treatment should be investigated further for the presence of plaque and calculus, which should be removed in subsequent cleanings. Refractory cases should be investigated for immunocompetence, cellular defects (eg, diminished neutrophil chemotaxis), or systemic disease (eg, diabetes mellitus). Gingivitis reestablishes if the teeth are not kept clean and free of bacteria. Therefore, at-home oral hygiene methods and regular cleanings to prevent gingivitis and its progression to periodontitis should be encouraged.

Periodontitis needs to be treated with thorough cleaning above and below the gum line. In areas of increased subgingival depth (>4 mm), surgical means (usually gingivectomy) should be employed to gain access to the root surface for cleaning. Teeth are generally salvageable until they have lost 75% of their bone support. Radiography of the jaws allows this evaluation and should be performed when periodontal disease is advanced. Bone defects that have an infrabony character (defects below the crest of the alveolar bone) require flap surgery. Defects on the palatal surface of maxillary canine teeth, which are infrabony in character and invade or approximate the nasal cavity, should be treated with infrabony grafting procedures before a decision is made to extract the tooth. Extraction of such teeth frequently leaves oral nasal fistulas (which need to be repaired surgically). Postoperatively, periodontitis cases should be maintained on oral hygiene methods at home and chemoprophylaxis for ≥2 wk with 0.1-0.2% chlorhexidine. Frequent (every 3 mo to 1 yr) prophylactic cleanings should be encouraged to avoid relapse of treated cases into further bone loss.

GINGIVAL HYPERPLASIA
(Fibromatosis gingivae, Fibromatous epulis, Epulis)

See also p 130.

A benign overgrowth of the epithelial and connective tissue of the gums, which usually originates near the gingival margin. The tissue is relatively insensitive and tough and has the density of fibrous connective tissue. The growths usually have a broad base of attachment, are the color of the normal gum or more pale, and may grow large enough to completely cover the surfaces of several teeth. Predisposition may exist among brachycephalic breeds, in which the condition is termed **familial gingival hypertrophy**.

Epulis sometimes refers to giant-cell epulis or tumor of the gum of dogs. This tumor usually is localized to a single tooth. Biopsy is encouraged to assure proper diagnosis, treatment, and prognosis.

Gingival hyperplasia is most common in older dogs and is usually asymptomatic. Hair, food, and debris may collect between the growth and the teeth, and cause irritation and halitosis.

Gingivectomy by electrosurgical techniques is the most satisfactory treatment. Following surgery the mouth should be rinsed daily with 1:1000 benzalkonium chloride solution or 0.2% chlorhexidine until clinically healed (~2 wk).

ENDODONTIC DISEASE

Pulpal Hyperemia: The pulp may become acutely inflamed due to trauma or extension of lesions adjacent to the pulp (eg, caries and resorption). Because this structure is totally confined in dentin, inflammatory swelling may result in pressure necrosis if the insult is prolonged. Severity of the reaction appears to be directly proportional to the extent of injury. Therefore, small injuries that produce transient hyperemia of the pulp may resolve, and a healthy pulp may be reestablished.

Methods to resolve acute pulpal hyperemia are sedative in nature. Cleaning out carious lesions and placing zinc oxide eugenol into resorptions and former carious areas may allow local anesthesia and resolution of hyperemia. A waiting period of several weeks may be required to establish by radiography that pulpitis has not resulted.

Pulpitis: Irreversible inflammation of the pulp with pressure necrosis and abscessation. In general, the abscess cavity is sterile unless the tooth has been opened to the oral environment by trauma, resorption, or caries. Teeth with pulpitis often are acutely painful, and the animal resents manipulation or percussion of the tooth. Such teeth often change to a reddish brown or dark gray color as blood is forced into dentinal tubules as the pulp dies and gas pressure increases in the pulp cavity. Treatment is endodontic therapy and restoration of the tooth structure; as an alternative, teeth that are not vital to the occlusion or function of the dentition may be extracted.

Periapical Lesions: A periapical abscess is a cavitational lesion at the end of the root due to pulpal disease. These areas generally can be seen on radiographs as radiolucent circular areas around the end of the root. Such abscesses can sometimes be palpated over the bony prominence of root ends. Abscesses may extend by pressure drainage into adjacent bone and soft-tissue areas and exit extra-orally into the soft-tissue space between the jaws, beneath the eye, or into the buccal vestibule. Treatment is endodontic therapy (root canal) on the associated tooth, and the abscess and associated fistula usually resolve within a few weeks. When endodontic therapy cannot be done, the offending tooth should be extracted.

Periapical granulomas appear similar radiographically and clinically to periapical abscesses, but signify a greater duration of involvement. Such granulomas generally are not infected and do not have fistulas associated with them. They represent an incomplete attempt at repair. Treatment involves endodontics on the associated tooth or extraction if endodontics is impractical.

DENTAL CARIES

Dental decay is uncommon in dogs and cats, possibly because of differences in oral flora and diets largely free of readily fermentable carbohydrates. Also, the slightly acidic pH of canine saliva makes the mouth more resistant. In dogs, decay usually is seen as pits on the flat surfaces or on the necks of the molar teeth.

"NECK" LESIONS IN CATS

Resorption is a common form of pathology on the surface of any tooth beginning in the area of the "neck" (cemento-enamel junction) of the tooth. Superficially, these teeth may appear normal. Affected cats may hypersalivate viscous mucus, and hesitate to drink or chew. Early diagnosis is facilitated by passing a fine probe along the tooth under the gingiva (under anesthesia) during yearly dental prophylaxis. Affected teeth should be restored or extracted. Teeth with resorption into the pulp need endodontic therapy before restoration with a filling or crown. Those teeth without a palpable apical boundary to the cavitation should always be radiographed to ensure that the root is not severely resorbed. If so, extraction is indicated. "Neck" lesions are common in cats with persistent gingivitis despite cleanings. Such cats often have generalized stomatitis/pharyngitis, and systemic disease should be considered. Defects in normal defense mechanisms due to persistent viral infection (eg, feline leukemia virus, feline immunodeficiency virus, coronavirus), inherited immunoincompetence, or debilitating systemic disease may account for unusually severe gingivitis or stomatitis. Full mouth extractions may be required in anorectic cats that do not respond to repeated prophylaxis.

DEVELOPMENTAL ABNORMALITIES

Malocclusion: Improper relationship of teeth can result from a poor bite because of malposition of the teeth within the jaw. Frequently, it occurs when deciduous teeth are retained and the permanent teeth erupt adjacent to, rather than directly under them; the roots of the deciduous teeth are not resorbed and they tilt the erupting permanent tooth into an abnormal position. Other types of dental malocclusion relate to improper relationships between the size of the teeth and that of the jaws; ie, a jaw may be too small for the size of the teeth developing within it, which causes crowding and subsequent malocclusion. Malocclusion may be treated by early extraction of retained deciduous teeth, selective extraction of permanent teeth, or orthodontics. It is possible in this manner to get a functional bite. Skeletal malocclusions result from an abnormal relationship of the upper and lower jaws to each other, although the teeth may be properly aligned within the jaw. Treatment is much more difficult and should attempt to achieve a functional bite rather than perfect occlusion. Selective extractions, orthodontics, and in severe cases, orthognathic surgery may be necessary.

Enamel Hypoplasia and Intrinsic Stains: During development of the enamel, fevers and deposition of chemicals within the tooth may cause permanent damage. Treatment is unnecessary if the crown of the tooth has normal structural integrity. If the enamel is pitted and irregular, bonding or crowns may be required to prevent debris retention. Use of tetracycline during formation of the enamel of permanent teeth should be avoided if possible.

MAXILLOFACIAL TRAUMA

Fractured teeth should be inspected for damage to the pulp. If fractures extend into the pulp, endodontic therapy is required, or extraction must be performed. Lengthwise fractures that extend below the gingival margin can be difficult to restore; if substantial tooth has been lost, what remains probably should be extracted. Fragmented teeth, especially those with multiple roots, often are left to "see what happens"; extraction is usually better due to poor general healing. Restorative techniques (crowns, bonding, and composite restorations) can restore defects in tooth structure over endodontically treated teeth or teeth with manageable defects limited to the hard structure.

Primary intention closure, when possible, should be used to repair soft-tissue trauma. Results are often good if repaired within a few hours. Thick tissue that has become avascular due to trauma should be removed.

Bone fractures require stabilization by orthopedic techniques. Acrylic splints and arch bars also can be used. In fractures that are not extensively displaced, a gauze tape muzzle that allows a 1-cm opening of the jaws provides adequate fixation in dogs with long muzzles. The animal can eat if the food is reduced to a slurry.

DISEASES OF THE EXOCRINE PANCREAS

Dogs are more commonly affected than other domestic animals. Acute pancreatitis, which occurs as single or recurrent episodes of sudden and severe pancreatic inflammation, occurs most commonly. Chronic pancreatitis refers to recurrent episodes or persistent low-grade inflammation causing progressive loss of pancreatic function. Exocrine pancreatic insufficiency (EPI), a syndrome characterized by maldigestion, occurs most frequently as idiopathic pancreatic atrophy; a high prevalence in German Shepherd Dogs suggests a hereditary predisposition in this breed. Chronic pancreatitis or severe acute pancreatitis can also result in EPI, sometimes with coexistent diabetes mellitus. Acute and chronic pancreatitis and EPI are seldom diagnosed in cats and rarely in horses and pigs. Adenocarcinoma of the acinar or duct epithelium is uncommon, but insidious and devastating in its manifestations. Functional islet-cell tumors (qv, p 269) occur occasionally and cause signs of hypoglycemia. (*See also* DIABETES MELLITUS, p 267).

ACUTE PANCREATITIS

Etiology: The cause is unknown but likely involves multiple etiologies. Nutritional factors believed to contribute to pancreatic acinar-cell injury include obesity, high-fat diets, and hyperlipoproteinemia. Drugs suspected of causing some cases of pancreatitis include thiazides, furosemide, azathioprine, sulfonamides, tetracycline, and corticosteroids. Surgical manipulation, blunt abdominal trauma, biliary tract disease, occlusion of the pancreatic or bile ducts, and duodenal reflux have been implicated. Toxoplasmosis, feline infectious peritonitis, and panleukopenia have been associated with feline pancreatitis.

Pathophysiology: Regardless of the initial insult, pancreatic ischemia is central in the pathogenesis of pancreatitis. The severity of ischemia determines whether mild pancreatic inflammation will progress to a severe, life-threatening, hemorrhagic pancreatitis. Acinar-cell injury results in activation and release of digestive enzymes within the pancreatic interstitium and into surrounding tissues. Pancreatic autodigestion, with endothelial cell damage, edema, ischemia, hemorrhage, and necrosis, occurs. Subsequent activation of complement, vasoactive amines, coagulation and fibrinolysis amplify pancreatic damage and multisystem involvement.

Clinical Findings: Dogs with acute pancreatitis tend to be middle-aged, inactive, and obese; they often eat fat from table scraps or garbage. Females are more commonly affected, whereas working or athletic dogs are rarely affected. Clinical signs are variable, but usually include acute vomiting, anorexia, depression, and sometimes, hemorrhagic diarrhea. Severe disease may cause shock and collapse. Dehydration, fever, and weakness are common. Severe abdominal pain is present in most but not all dogs, and an anterior abdominal mass may be palpable. Less common signs include jaundice, tachypnea, cardiac arrhythmias, and coagulopathy.

Signs of chronic relapsing pancreatitis are nonspecific and less severe. Anorexia, intermittent vomiting, abdominal pain, diarrhea, and weight loss are typical. Voluminous, rancid-smelling, steatorrheic diarrhea may eventually occur from progressive loss of exocrine function. The appetite is typically ravenous despite profound weight loss owing to the maldigestion and subsequent malabsorption of nutrients. Some cases are further complicated by concurrent diabetes mellitus. Chronic pancreatitis occurs infrequently in cats and is usually an incidental finding at necropsy.

Diagnosis: Although there is no diagnostic test for acute pancreatitis, history and clinical signs coupled with results of selected laboratory tests can establish a presumptive diagnosis. Parallel increases of serum amylase and lipase activities are most suggestive of acute pancreatitis; however, marked increases in one enzyme may be accompanied by minimal increases in the other. Occasionally, these enzymes are normal despite active pancreatitis. Leukocytosis, frequently with a left shift, hemoconcentration, and lipemia are common findings. Liver enzyme activities are often increased, and hyperbilirubinemia with clinical icterus occurs in some. Azotemia may occur due to dehydration or primary renal failure, in which case protein and casts may be found in the urine. Hyperglycemia is common and accompanied by glucosuria if overt diabetes mellitus occurs. Mild hypocalcemia may occur but is not associated with clinical signs of tetany. Supportive radiographic findings include increased density and loss of detail in the right cranial abdomen, displacement of the duodenum to the right, and a static gas pattern in the descending duodenum. Differential diagnoses include systemic infections such as parvovirus or infectious canine hepatitis, intestinal obstruction (foreign body or volvulus), hemorrhagic gastroenteritis, acute pyelonephritis or renal failure, pyometra, prostatitis, peritonitis, ketoacidotic diabetes mellitus, and other causes of an acute abdomen.

Treatment: Aggressive fluid therapy is necessary to correct shock and dehydration, thereby restoring pancreatic and systemic perfusion. Balanced electrolyte solutions such as lactated Ringer's should be given IV until dehydration is corrected and vomiting has ceased. Plasma may be necessary if hypoproteinemia is severe. Acid-base and electrolyte imbalances must be corrected. Hypokalemia frequently occurs and serum potassium should be supplemented as needed. Adding 20 mEq of a potassium salt to 1 L of maintenance fluid usually provides adequate potassium if given at 40 mL/kg/day parenterally. Renal function must be adequate, and IV potassium should not exceed 0.5 mEq/kg/hr.

All oral intake should be stopped for 48-72 hr to decrease stimuli for pancreatic secretion. Phenothiazine antiemetics decrease vomiting but are hypotensive. They can be used cautiously for 24-48 hr or until hydration and fluid therapy are adequate. Anticholinergics such as atropine sulfate inhibit the vomiting reflex and pancreatic secretion; their use should be limited to 24-36 hr to avoid ileus. Corticosteroids are indicated only for shock. Antibiotics such as ampicillin or cephalosporins are used if secondary infection or sepsis is suspected. Analgesics such as meperidine can be used for severe abdominal pain. Low-dose heparin (100 u/kg, t.i.d.) subcut. may decrease the tendency for thrombosis and intravascular coagulation. Severe cases that continue to deteriorate despite supportive care may benefit from plasma or whole-blood transfusions. Oral intake should be resumed 24-48 hr after vomiting has stopped, and begin with small amounts of water; if vomiting does not recur, small amounts of baby food or boiled chicken and rice can be added gradually. If vomiting resumes, the animal should have nothing PO for an additional 24-48 hr. Low-fat, high-carbohydrate, high-protein diets are recommended for life-long maintenance.

Prognosis is generally good providing therapy is prompt and aggressive. If exocrine and/or endocrine pancreatic failure occur, management is more difficult. Dietary replacement with pancreatic enzymes and/or insulin is necessary. Persistence or recurrence of fever, abdominal pain or mass, leukocytosis, or jaundice indicates a pancreatic abscess or infected pseudocyst. Surgical drainage or resection is necessary; the prognosis is poor.

EXOCRINE PANCREATIC INSUFFICIENCY (EPI)

Progressive loss of exocrine pancreatic cells results in failure of nutrient absorption due to inadequate synthesis of digestive enzymes. Spontaneously occurring pancreatic acinar atrophy is the most common cause of EPI and occurs predominantly in young adult dogs, especially German Shepherd Dogs, in which predisposition to the condition may be inherited. Less common causes of EPI include chronic pancreatitis, protein-calorie malnutrition, and congenital pancreatic hypoplasia. EPI is seldomly diagnosed in cats. Animals with EPI lose weight despite having a normal to ravenous appetite. Polyphagia may be characterized by pica, coprophagia, and polydipsia. Diarrhea is common, characterized by frequent passage of large volumes of semi-formed feces. Explosive watery diarrhea may occur. A long history of GI signs such as abdominal discomfort, vomiting, borborygmus, and flatulence is not uncommon. Some dogs are very emaciated, with poor coat and muscle wasting. Concurrent diabetes mellitus (qv, p 267) may occur in some.

Diagnosis is confirmed by measurement of serum trypsin-like immunoreactivity (TLI; normal is >5 μg/L, in EPI it is <2.5 μg/L). Microscopical examination of the feces for fat and undigested food, plasma turbidity tests, and measurement of fecal proteolytic activity can be used as simple screening tests; however, they are unreliable. TLI assays require a fasted serum sample.

Most dogs can be successfully managed by dietary supplementation with a powdered, nonenteric-coated pancreatic enzyme preparation. One tsp/10 kg body wt with each meal is usually effective, although dosage varies with the individual. An easily digestible, low-fiber, fat-restricted diet divided into 3 or 4 small meals per day is recommended. Addition of medium-chain triglycerides, which do not require pancreatic lipase for absorption, facilitates fat absorption and provides additional calories. Bacterial overgrowth of the small intestine commonly occurs with EPI and contributes to malabsorption and diarrhea. Animals that do not respond adequately to oral enzymes and dietary modification should be treated with oral antibiotics such as oxytetracycline, metronidazole, or tylosin. Supplementation with parenteral fat-soluble vitamins is advised until weight gain is evident. Prognosis is generally good, provided the owner understands the cost of life-long enzyme replacement. Concurrent diabetes mellitus requires insulin therapy; these cases are more difficult to manage and prognosis is poor.

PANCREATIC NEOPLASMS

Adenocarcinomas of the acinar or duct epithelium of the pancreas can be difficult to diagnose. They occur in older dogs (av 10.8 yr) and are rare in cats. They are highly malignant, and frequently, metastases are widely disseminated, particularly in the liver. Clinical signs are nonspecific and may include weight loss, anorexia, depression, vomiting, and icterus. Addominal pain and occasionally an anterior abdominal mass is detected. There are no specific laboratory tests. Plasma activity of amylase and lipase may be increased. Marked increases in alkaline phosphatase and bilirubin with a lesser increase in ALT (SGPT) are suggestive of obstructive hepatopathy. Definitive diagnosis is made by laparotomy. Prognosis is poor as metastasis has usually occurred by the time of diagnosis.

Functional islet-cell tumors of the pancreas are discussed on p 269.

DISEASES OF THE MOUTH, LG AN

CLEFT PALATE

This condition is found occasionally in the newborn of all species. *See* CONGENITAL ANOMALIES, p 109.

CONTUSIONS AND WOUNDS OF THE LIPS AND CHEEKS

Wounds of the lips and cheeks are most commonly encountered in horses as a result of falls, kicks, inhumane bits, bites, or tears from projecting objects. The vascularity of the region usually means rapid healing, except when a penetrating wound gives rise to a fistula. Treatment is routine: when a laceration involves the border of the lip, suturing should commence at that border to obtain the best cosmetic effect; if penetrating wounds are encountered, deep sutures must be placed in addition to those approximating the skin edges. Skin grafts may be necessary to correct large defects or fistulas.

LAMPAS
(Lampers, Palatitis)

A transient inflammation of the mucosa covering the hard palate. Lampas is not a disease entity, but may occur in young horses during eruption of the permanent incisors, or in horses of any age as a result of stomatitis. It is self-limiting and requires no treatment.

PARALYSIS OF THE TONGUE
(Glossoplegia)

A partial or complete loss of function of the tongue that may be peripheral or central in origin. Rough manipulation and excessive pulling on the tongue during dental examination may cause the peripheral type. Newborn animals may exhibit tongue paralysis following use of an obstetrical snare placed over the mandible and tongue, or from edema of the tongue during dystocias when the head of the fetus has been compressed in the vagina of the dam. Laceration of the tongue by broken glass or other sharp objects in the feed manger as well as various surgical procedures performed on the tongue to prevent self-nursing have also caused tongue paralysis. Glossoplegia of central origin may accompany or follow such conditions as strangles, upper respiratory infection, meningitis, botulism, encephalomyelitis, leukoencephalomalacia, or cerebral abscess in horses. The unilaterally affected tongue is deviated toward the nonaffected side; the bilaterally affected tongue is limp and often protrudes through the relaxed jaws. In mild cases of either central or peripheral origin, a weakness in the muscle power of the tongue is most evident.

The most common cause in cattle is actinobacillosis (qv, p 317). Complete paralysis of the tongue may be accompanied by a variable degree of necrosis of the tip, a condition that has been seen as outbreaks in feedlot cattle, possibly as a result of viral or fungal infection.

Identifying and removing the cause or placing the animals in an environment free of the causative agent are the initial treatment procedures. When a specific disease such as strangles or actinobacillosis is identified, the specific treatment is indicated. Careful nursing, along with providing undamaged toxin-free feed, and adequate potable water aid cases in which spontaneous recovery is likely. Apparent paralysis of the tongue due to edema usually responds to careful massage within a relatively short time. Neonates that are immature or with neonatal maladjustment syndrome (qv, p 610) may have partial paralysis of the tongue and usually regain function if they survive.

When the condition persists >6 wk, the likelihood of regaining normal function is slight.

SLAFRAMINE TOXICOSIS
(Slobber factor)

A noninfectious disease affecting both horses and cattle. Horses are particularly susceptible. The cause is ingestion of forages, particularly clovers, infected with the fungus *Rhizoctonia leguminicola*, which produces the toxic alkaloid slaframine. Clinical signs may be limited to profuse salivation, though increased lacrimation and frequent urination and defecation also may be present. No lesions have been described, and mortality is nil.

Differential diagnoses include bluetongue, vesicular stomatitis, vesicular exanthema, and foot-and-mouth disease. Slaframine toxicosis does not cause mouth, udder, or teat lesions, or laminitis. Removal of infected forages results in rapid recovery.

STOMATITIS

Stomatitis is a prominent sign in many specific diseases. This discussion is of nonspecific inflammation of the oral mucosa caused by trauma or chemical irritants. The most common causes of traumatic injury are awns of barley, foxtail, porcupine grass, and spear grass, and feeding on plants infested with hairy caterpillars. Chemical stomatitis arises most commonly from oral contact with irritant drugs, eg, leg blisters. Consumption of plants of the crowfoot family that contain ranunculin (buttercups, crocus, pasque flower, cowslips), or prolonged medication with mercurials, arsenicals, or iodides may result in stomatitis.

The first clinical sign is excessive frothy salivation, or in the case of plant awns, a reluctance to permit manual examination of the mouth. Animals often exhibit evidence of oral irritation, eg, stand with the mouth open, loll the tongue, or chew with the head turned sideways. They soon develop difficulty in eating. Examination of the oral cavity and tongue reveals local or generalized areas of acute inflammation; the tongue and buccal mucosa may be ulcerated. In chemically induced stomatitis, the buccal mucosa may be edematous and coated with a catarrhal exudate. Usually, the breath has a putrid or sweetish odor. Regional lymph nodes may be enlarged. Actinobacillosis (wooden tongue), foot-and-mouth disease, malignant catarrhal fever, and bovine viral diarrhea must be considered in differential diagnosis in cattle. Epidemic diseases, eg, bluetongue in ruminants and swine vesicular disease, must be considered.

Most animals recover rapidly and uneventfully when the cause is removed. Further treatment is necessary only in severe cases. If inflammation is marked, treatment with a broad-spectrum antibiotic is advisable. Mild antiseptics, eg, a solution of 0.5% hydrogen peroxide, 5% sodium bicarbonate, or 1-3% potassium chlorate, used as a mouthwash may hasten recovery.

"MYCOTIC" STOMATITIS

"Mycotic" stomatitis of cattle was previously believed to be an allergic reaction to fungi and mycotoxins infecting pasture grasses in late summer and fall. Serological tests and virus isolation have proved that the cause is the bluetongue virus (qv, p 390). Vesicular stomatitis (qv, p 372) produces a similar syndrome in cattle, horses, sheep, and pigs.

PAPULAR STOMATITIS

A mild viral disease of cattle from 1 mo to 2 yr old; up to 100% of a susceptible herd may be affected. Lesions occur on the muzzle, inside the nostrils, and on the buccal mucosa, and consist of reddish raised papules (0.5-1 cm in diameter) that appear active for ~1 wk and then regress. Evidence of the healed lesion may be present for several weeks. There is no systemic disturbance; the disease is important chiefly because of the confusion it may cause in the clinical diagnosis of the several forms of stomatitis of cattle.

PHLEGMONOUS STOMATITIS AND CELLULITIS

An acute, deep-seated, diffuse, rapidly spreading inflammation of the oral mucosa, pharynx, and surrounding structures, including the subcut. tissue. It occurs sporadically in cattle of all types and endemically in some of the intensive dairying areas of the midwestern USA. The cause is not completely understood, but hemolytic streptococci or coliform organisms usually can be isolated early in the disease. In cases of moderate duration, a common isolate is *Fusobacterium necrophorum (Sphaerophorus necrophorus)*.

Onset of clinical signs is sudden; an animal may progress from apparently normal to near death in 24 hr. The first sign is excessive salivation, usually associated with excessive lacrimation. These changes are accompanied by a fever of 105-107°F (40.5-41.5°C) and an increase in pulse and respiratory rates. The animal usually refuses to eat or drink. Swelling of tissues around the mouth and nostrils and in the intermandibular space is marked; large pockets of fluid may form in the mandibular region and along the trachea. Breath is foul and large sheets of superficial oral epithelium peel off. A severe toxemia with weakness is characteristic.

Some milder cases recover spontaneously, but the more severely affected animals usually die unless treated.

Sulfonamides administered IV during the acute phase may control the infection; sulfonamide-trimethoprim combinations are superior. Penicillin is less effective. Oral therapy may be employed when the animal can swallow. Endotracheal intubation may be necessary in severely affected animals.

DISEASES OF THE MOUTH, SM AN

CHEILITIS AND LIP FOLD DERMATITIS

An acute or chronic inflammation of the lips and lip folds.

Etiology: Wounds of varying severity are common lip lesions in small animals, the result of fights or chewing on sharp objects. Thorns, plant awns, burrs, and fishhooks may imbed in the lips and cause marked irritation or severe wounds. Irritants such as plastic or plant material may produce inflammation of the lips.

Lip infections may occur secondary to wounds or foreign bodies, or associated with inflammation of adjacent areas. Direct extension of severe periodontal disease or stomatitis can produce cheilitis. Licking areas of bacterial dermatitis or infected wounds may spread the infection to the lips and lip folds. Inflammation of the lips also can be associated with parasitic infections, autoimmune skin diseases, and neoplasia.

Lip fold dermatitis is a chronic moist dermatitis seen in breeds that have pendulous upper lips and lower lip folds (eg, spaniels, English Bulldogs, and St. Bernards) that accumulate food and saliva.

Clinical Findings and Diagnosis: Animals with cheilitis may scratch or rub at their lips, have a foul odor to the breath, and occasionally salivate excessively or be anorectic. With chronic infection of the lip margins or folds, the hair in these areas is discolored, moist, and matted with a thick, yellowish or brown, malodorous discharge overlying hyperemic and sometimes ulcerated skin. The animal may paw at its mouth and drool excessively.

Cheilitis due to extension of infection from the mouth or another area of the body usually is detected easily because of the primary lesion.

Treatment: Cheilitis usually clears up with minimal cleansing, and appropriate antibiotics if a bacterial infection is present. Wounds of the lips should be cleaned and sutured if necessary. Treatment of periodontal disease or stomatitis is necessary to prevent recurrence.

Infectious cheilitis that has spread from a lesion elsewhere usually improves with treatment of the primary lesion, but local treatment also is necessary. With severe infection, hair should be clipped from the lesion and the area gently cleaned and dried. Antibiotics are indicated if the infection is severe or systemic.

Medical management for lip fold dermatitis includes clipping the hair, and cleaning the folds 1-2 times/day with benzoyl peroxide and keeping them dry; however, relapses are to be expected without surgical correction.

EOSINOPHILIC ULCER OF CATS
(Indolent ulcer, Rodent ulcer)

A common oral mucosal lesion of the upper lip in cats, possibly due to hypersensitivity (*see also* p 793). Eosinophilic plaques and granulomas may occur in cats with indolent ulcers, which may be unilateral or bilateral.

The lesions are red, well circumscribed, ulcerated, and have raised edges. The ulcer increases in size gradually and may extend up to the nose. Peripheral eosinophilia is occasionally present. No breed predilection has been observed. It occurs more frequently in females than males.

Diagnosis is based on history, physical examination, and biopsy of the lesion. Histopathology shows chronic ulcerative dermatitis with neutrophils, plasma cells, mononuclear cells, and occasionally some eosinophils.

Corticosteroids are frequently effective: prednisone, 2 mg/lb body wt (4.4 mg/kg), PO once daily until lesions are healed, or methylprednisolone acetate, 20 mg/cat, subcut., q3wk for 3 treatments. Recurrent lesions can be managed with alternate-day oral prednisone (given in the evening), or repeated methylprednisolone acetate injections not to be given more frequently than q2mo. Surgical excision may be effective but distorts the lip. Megestrol acetate has been efficacious for indolent ulcers in cats but is not recommended because of side effects. Other treatments that have been tried with varying success are radiotherapy, cryotherapy, laser therapy, mixed bacterial vaccines, and immunomodulating drugs. Skin testing and hyposensitization have been recommended for cats that become refractory to medical management.

CANINE EOSINOPHILIC GRANULOMA

Rare, idiopathic, nodular to plaque-like lesions in the oral cavity and skin. A hypersensitivity reaction has been suggested as the cause, as has genetics because these tend to occur in Siberian Huskies. The lesions are most common in males <3 yr old.

The oral lesions, ulcerated palatine plaques and vegetative lingual masses, are not painful. Peripheral eosinophilia occurs occasionally. Diagnosis is based on biopsy and the histologic findings, which include collagen degeneration, eosinophilic and histiocytic cellular infiltration, and palisading granuloma.

Glucocorticoid treatment, eg, prednisone (0.25-1 mg/lb [0.5-2.2 mg/kg]/day, PO), frequently causes regression of the lesions in 10-20 days. Lesions may resolve spontaneously.

GLOSSITIS

An acute or chronic inflammation of the tongue due to infectious, physical, or chemical agents; metabolic disease; or other causes. Local causes include irritation from excess tartar and periodontal disease, foreign bodies (penetrating or caught under the tongue), traumatic wounds, burns, and insect stings. Glossitis is especially a problem in long-haired dogs that attempt to remove plant burrs from their coats.

Excessive salivation and a reluctance to eat are common signs, but the cause may go undiscovered unless the mouth is examined closely. Periodontitis may result in reddening, swelling, and occasionally, ulceration of the edge of the tongue. A thread, string, or rubber band caught under the tongue may cause no inflammation of its dorsum but the ventral surface is painful, shows acute or chronic irritation, and frequently is severed by the foreign body. Porcupine quills, plant material, and other foreign materials may become imbedded so deeply that they are not palpable. Insect stings cause an acute swelling of the tongue.

In chronic cases of ulcerative glossitis, a thick, brown, foul-smelling discharge (occasionally with bleeding) may be present. Frequently, the animal is reluctant to allow oral examination.

Foreign bodies and broken or diseased teeth should be removed. Infectious glossitis should be treated with a systemic antibiotic. Debridement and mouthwashes are beneficial in some cases. Lingual curettage may be required if foreign material is embedded in the tongue. A soft diet and parenteral fluids may be necessary. If the animal is debilitated and unable to eat well for a prolonged period, a pharyngostomy or gastrostomy tube should be considered. Acute glossitis due to insect stings may require emergency treatment.

If the glossitis is secondary to another condition, the primary disease should be treated. The tongue tissues heal rapidly after irritation and infection have been eliminated.

MOUTH BURNS

Burns involving the mouth are not uncommon. The tongue, lips, buccal mucosa, and palate are frequently involved with electrical burns. The injuries may be mild, with only temporary discomfort, or may be very destructive with loss of tissue, scar formation, and subsequent deformity or tissue deficits. Chewing on an electrical cord (see BURNS, p 630, and ELECTRIC SHOCK, p 628) is most frequently a problem in puppies.

The owner may have observed the incident, thus providing a history. The animal hesitates to eat or drink, salivates excessively, and resents handling of its mouth or face. If tissue destruction is marked, ulcerative or gangrenous stomatitis may develop, with secondary bacterial infections. If contact with a corrosive chemical is observed and the chemical is alkaline, the mouth may be flushed with mild solutions of vinegar or citrus juice; if the chemical is acidic, a solution of sodium bicarbonate may be used. Copious flushing of the mouth with water may help remove some of the chemical substances. More commonly, the animal is seen too long after the exposure for neutralization to be effective.

Animals showing a reddened oral mucosa without tissue defects require no specific treatment other than a soft or liquid diet until the lesion has healed. If tissue damage is extensive, frequent flushing with isotonic saline solution keeps the burned areas free of necrotic debris and food particles, and hastens healing. If the burn causes extensive tissue destruction, the area may need to be cleaned and debrided under anesthesia. The risk of secondary infection should be minimized with systemic antibiotic therapy for several days.

STOMATITIS

An inflammation of the oral mucosa, which may be a primary disease or secondary to a systemic disease. The inflammation may be localized, eg, gingivitis, or diffuse. The nature and severity of the lesions vary greatly depending on the etiology and duration of disease.

Etiology: The cause may be chemical agents; neoplasia; metabolic, autoimmune, deficiency, or infectious diseases; periodontal disease; trauma; burns; or radiation therapy. Idiopathic stomatitis is the diagnosis when the cause cannot be determined. Infectious agents that have been associated with stomatitis, gingivitis, and oral ulcerations are feline herpesvirus, feline calicivirus, feline leukemia virus, feline immunodeficiency virus, canine distemper virus, *Leptospira canicola, L icterohaemorrhagiae, Nocardia* sp, and *Blastomyces dermatitidis*. Traumatic stomatitis may occur following oral exposure to plant material (embedded plant awns) or fiberglass insulation. *Dieffenbachia* spp may cause oral inflammation and ulcers if chewed on. Thallium is the major heavy metal responsible for oral lesions; incidence of this toxicity is low. Uremia can cause stomatitis and oral ulcers, and the lesions are usually more severe in an acute uremic crisis. Recurrent oral ulcerations occur in silver-gray Collies with cyclic hematopoiesis (qv, p 64).

Clinical Findings: Signs vary widely with the cause and extent of inflammation. Anorexia may occur, especially in cats. Halatosis and excessive salivation are common, and the saliva may be blood tinged. The animal may paw at its mouth and resent any attempt to examine the oral cavity because of pain. Regional lymph nodes may be swollen and tender.

Treatment: Periodontitis should be treated and managed; if appropriate, teeth and remaining teeth roots should be extracted. Radiographs of the oral cavity may be required to locate all roots, especially in cats. Broad-spectrum antibiotics should be administered if primary or secondary bacterial infections are present. Culturing the lesions and performing susceptibility tests are indicated in chronic or recurrent infections. Symptomatic treatment for stomatitis includes dietary changes, antibiotics, debridement, and cautery. Debridement of necrotic tissue may promote healing and can be accomplished mechanically with a gauze sponge. Hydrogen peroxide (3%) assists in cleaning the lesions, and may hasten recovery. Other mouthwash solutions that may be used are 1% gentian violet, 2% potassium permanganate, or 0.2% chlorhexidine. Necrotic and ulcerated areas may be chemically cauterized with 5% silver nitrate solution. Cats with chronic idiopathic oral ulcers and normal thyroid function tests occasionally respond to thyroid hormone supplementation. Animals that are unable or unwilling to eat and drink should be given parenteral or subcut. fluids to prevent dehydration. Placement of a pharyngostomy or gastrostomy tube should be considered in debilitated animals. Frequent feedings of palatable liquids and, later, semisolid foods encourage eating.

MYCOTIC STOMATITIS

A condition in dogs and cats caused by overgrowth of *Candida albicans*, characterized by the appearance of creamy white plaques on the tongue or mucous membranes. The underlying tissue is frequently red and ulcerated. There may be smaller plaques surrounding a larger main plaque. It is usually thought to be associated with other oral diseases, long-term antibiotic therapy, or immunosuppression. The periphery of the lesions is usually reddened. The lesions may coalesce as the disease progresses, and similar lesions may occur in the oral pharynx and at other mucocutaneous junctions. Differential diagnoses include ulcerative stomatitis and bullous autoimmune skin diseases. Diagnosis may be confirmed by culture of the organism from the lesion or by identification of yeast hyphae in biopsies stained with periodic acid-Schiff.

Any existing underlying local or systemic diseases affecting the oral cavity should be treated. Ketoconazole (10 mg/kg, b.i.d.) should be administered until the lesions resolve, after which antibiotic therapy should be discontinued. An adequate level of nutrition should be maintained. The prognosis is guarded if predisposing diseases cannot be adequately treated or controlled.

PLASMA CELL STOMATITIS
(Feline plasma cell gingivitis, Pharyngitis)

A condition characterized by persistent gingivitis-pharyngitis with raised, glistening, erythematous, proliferative lesions in the glossopalatine arches with a cobblestone appearance; the lesions may extend caudally to the palatopharyngeal arch and cranially to involve the gingiva. In severe cases, the gingival margin of the upper canine teeth becomes inflamed and ulcerated. An immune-mediated etiology is suspected.

Halitosis, ptyalism, and dysphagia are especially prominent when the cat attempts to eat hard foods. If the condition is severe and of long duration, weight loss may be evident. The disease is slowly progressive, and if soft palatable foods are being fed, it may be fairly severe before it is recognized that medical attention is needed. Submandibular lymphadenopathy is sometimes present. Frequently, because of pain, the oral cavity cannot be visualized adequately without sedation or anesthesia.

Diagnosis is based on biopsy. Histologically, the lesions are hyperplastic and have an ulcerated mucosa with a submucosal inflammatory cell infiltrate, which is predominantly plasma cells.

Treatment is primarily aimed at achieving and maintaining good oral hygiene. Periodontal disease should be treated and regular dental prophylaxis recommended. If present, fractured tooth roots should be removed (radiography of the oral cavity may be necessary). Treatments that have been tried with various results are hypoallergenic diets, antibiotics, megestrol acetate (not recommended due to potential side effects), levamisole, prednisolone, and mouthwash. Until the etiology can be determined and/or a more successful treatment is found, prognosis is poor.

ULCERATIVE STOMATITIS
(Acute necrotizing ulcerative gingivitis, Necrotizing ulcerative stomatitis, Vincent's stomatitis, Trenchmouth)

A relatively uncommon disease of dogs characterized by severe gingivitis, and ulceration and necrosis of the oral mucosa. Several organisms have been suggested as the primary cause. Fusiform bacilli and spirochetes, normal inhabitants of the mouth, have been suggested as causing this disease after some predisposing factor decreases the resistance of the oral mucosa. *Bacteroides melaninogenicus* has also been suggested as the primary causative agent.

Ulcerative stomatitis appears first as reddening and swelling of the gingival margins, which are painful and bleed easily, and progresses to severe gingivitis and gingival recession. Extension to other areas of the oral mucosa is common, resulting in ulcerated, necrotic mucous membranes, and exposed bone in severe cases. Halitosis is severe, and the animal may be anorectic due to pain. Ptyalism may be present and the saliva may be blood tinged. The infection may spread to cause pneumonia. Differential diagnoses include severe periodontal disease, autoimmune skin disease, uremia, neoplasia, and other systemic disease associated with oral lesions.

Diagnosis is made by exclusion of other etiologies. Organisms commonly cultured from the lesions are staphylococci, *Pseudomonas* spp, and *Pasteurella multocida*. Impression smears of the lesions may show an increased number of spirochetes.

Teeth cleaning, mechanical and chemical (2-5% silver nitrate) debridement of necrotic tissue, antibiotic therapy for 3-6 wk (amoxicillin, ampicillin, clindamycin, or cephalosporins), and mouth rinses (0.2% chlorhexidine or 3% hydrogen peroxide diluted 1:1 with water) are indicated. (*See also* STOMATITIS, p 128).

CANINE ORAL PAPILLOMATOSIS

Papillomas are benign canine tumors caused by a virus. The oral mucosa and commissures of the lip are most frequently involved, but the masses (single or, more frequently, multiple) can involve the palate and oropharynx. It is most common in young animals (*see* PAPILLOMATOSIS, p 854). Signs occur when the papillomas interfere with prehension, mastication, or swallowing. Occasionally, if the papillomas are numerous, the dog may bite them when chewing, and they may bleed and become infected. They may regress spontaneously within a few weeks, and removal is generally not necessary. If necessary, debulking of the tumor mass is best accomplished with electrosurgery. Surgical removal of one or more of the papillomas may initiate regression. The use of commercial or autogenous wart vaccines is usually disappointing. The self-limiting character of the disease makes evaluation of any treatment difficult.

EPULIDES

Tumors of the periodontal ligament, these are the most common benign oral tumors in dogs (*see also* p 118). Cats rarely have benign oral tumors. The 3 types of epulides are fibromatous, ossifying, and acanthomatous.

These tumors may be seen in dogs of any age but generally are found in those >6 yr old. Boxers and English Bulldogs may be predisposed. The tumors may be ulcerated and bleeding. Solitary or multiple fibromatous and ossifying epulides may be present. Both are noninvasive but may become extensive and involve the teeth. An acanthomatous epulis is a more aggressive tumor with invasion of local tissue and bony involvement.

Wide surgical excision of fibromatous and ossifying epulides is recommended if they are causing discomfort. Gingival growths should be biopsied to determine prognosis and behavior of the tumor as all epulides do not behave similarly. Acanthomatous epulis should be excised surgically. To prevent recurrence, surgical excision must remove all involved bone and soft tissue.

MALIGNANT ORAL NEOPLASMS

Tumors of the mouth and pharynx are common and likely to be malignant. In dogs, the 3 most common are malignant melanoma, squamous cell carcinoma, and fibrosarcoma. The gingivae and tonsils are affected most frequently. Incidence of malignant oral tumors is greater in dogs >10 yr old, and Cocker Spaniels and German Shepherd Dogs are predisposed.

Squamous cell carcinomas are by far the most common malignant oral neoplasms in cats; they commonly involve the gingivae and tongue, and are highly invasive and readily metastasize. Fibrosarcomas are the next most common; in cats, they are locally invasive and have a poor prognosis.

Clinical Findings: Signs vary depending on the location and extent of the neoplasm. Halitosis, reluctance to eat, and hypersalivation are common. If the oropharynx is involved, dysphagia may be present. The tumors frequently ulcerate and bleed. The face may become swollen as the tumor enlarges and invades surrounding tissue. Regional lymph nodes often become swollen before oral and pharyngeal tumors are observed.

Diagnosis: A cytological diagnosis from impression smears or a fine needle aspirate is possible in some cases. Biopsy is usually required for definitive diagnosis. Malignant melanomas are variable in appearance, pigmented or nonpigmented, and should be in the differential list for any oral tumor. Squamous cell carcinomas commonly involve the gingivae or tonsils, and lymphosarcoma should be in the differential diagnosis for an enlarged tonsil. Regional lymph nodes and the lungs should be evaluated for metastases.

Treatment: Malignant melanomas are highly invasive and metastasize readily; consequently the prognosis is poor. Surgical resection can extend the survival time by decreasing local recurrence, which is frequent. Nontonsillar squamous cell carcinoma is locally invasive with a low rate of metastasis, and the prognosis is good with aggressive surgical resection and/or radiation therapy. Tonsillar squamous cell carcinomas are aggressive and have a poor prognosis. Fibrosarcomas have a poor prognosis because of their locally aggressive nature. Recurrence of tumor growth following resection is common.

In cats, squamous cell carcinoma has a poor prognosis, and long-term survival is seen only if diagnosed early. Local tumor removal is possible by hemi-mandibulectomy.

DISEASES OF THE RECTUM AND ANUS

ANAL SAC DISEASE

Anal sac disease is the most common disease entity of the anal region in dogs. Small breeds are predisposed; large or giant breeds are rarely affected. It also occurs in cats, most commonly in the form of impaction.

Etiology and Pathogenesis: Anal sac disease may be categorized as impaction, infection, or abscessation. Failure of feces to express the sacs, poor muscle tone in obese dogs, and generalized seborrhea (which produces glandular hypersecretion) lead to retention of sac contents. Such retention may predipose to fermentation, inflammation, and secondary bacterial infection.

Clinical Findings, Lesions, and Diagnosis: Signs are related to pain and discomfort associated with sitting. Scooting, licking, biting at the anal area, and painful defecation with tenesmus are common. Induration, abscesses, and fistulous tracts are common. In impaction, hard masses are palpable in the area of the sacs; with infection or abscessation, severe pain and, often, discoloration of the area are present. Fistulous tracts lead from abscessed sacs and rupture through the skin; these must be differentiated from perianal fistulas.

Diagnosis of impaction, infection, or abscessation is confirmed by digital rectal examination, at which time the sacs can be expressed.

Treatment: Impaction should be treated by gentle manual expression of the sacs. A softening or ceruminolytic agent can be infused into the sac if the contents are too dry to express effectively. Infected sacs should be cleaned with antiseptic; local and systemic antibiotic therapy is recommended. Repeated weekly flushings combined with infusion of a steroid-antibiotic ointment may be needed. If medical treatment is ineffective, or if neoplasia is present, surgical excision is indicated.

Fecal incontinence, which is a common complication of anal sac surgery, may result from damage to the caudal rectal branch of the pudendal nerve and may be complete if bilateral damage occurs. Chronic fistula formation may be seen when sac removal is incomplete or when the sac ruptures. Scar formation in the external anal sphincter may result from surgical trauma and may produce tenesmus.

PERIANAL FISTULA

Perianal fistula is characterized by chronic, purulent, malodorous, ulcerating, sinus tracts in the perianal tissues. It is most common in German Shepherd Dogs, and is also seen in Setters and Retrievers. Dogs >7 yr old are at higher risk.

Etiology and Pathogenesis: The cause is unknown. Contamination of the hair follicles and glands of the anal area by fecal material and anal sac secretions may result in necrosis, ulceration, and chronic inflammation of the perianal skin and tissues. Affected animals may be predisposed to generalized skin problems. The likelihood of contamination is greater in dogs with a broad-based tail; hypothyroidism and poor T-cell function may contribute to susceptibility. Deep anal folds may cause feces to be retained within rectal glands and play a major role. The draining tracts are lined with chronic inflammatory tissue and often extend to the lumen of the rectum and anus. Infection may spread to deeper structures involving the external anal sphincter, and therefore should be treated promptly.

Clinical Findings: In dogs, signs include attitude change, tenesmus, dyschezia, anorexia, lethargy, diarrhea, and attempts to bite and lick the anal area. Signs in cats are similar to those in dogs, but may include matting of fur and sitting in the litter box.

Treatment: Medical treatment is not effective. Surgery should be followed by antibiotics and a low-residue diet. Postoperatively, the anorectal area must be cleaned at least daily. Amputation of the tail at its base has been advocated as an adjunct to other therapy. Fecal incontinence, anal stricture, and relapse may complicate recovery; the probability that these will occur increases with the severity of the initial disease.

PERIANAL TUMORS

See HEPATOID GLAND TUMORS, p 853, and APOCRINE GLAND TUMORS OF ANAL SAC ORIGIN, p 852.

PERINEAL HERNIA

Protrusion of a peritoneally lined hernial sac laterally between the levator ani and either the external anal sphincter muscle or the coccygeus muscle. Intact male dogs, 6-8 yr old, show a disproportionately high incidence, and Welsh Corgis, Boston Terriers, Boxers, Collies, and Pekingese are at higher risk.

Etiology and Pathogenesis: Many factors are involved and include breed predisposition, hormonal imbalance, prostatic disease, chronic constipation, and weakness of the pelvic diaphragm due to chronic straining. The higher incidence among sexually intact males is evidence that hormonal influences probably play a primary role. Prostatic hypertrophy attributed to sex hormone imbalance has been strongly implicated. Both estrogens and androgens have been cited as causative agents.

Clinical Findings and Diagnosis: Common signs include flatulence, pain on defecation, and irregular bowel movements. Tenesmus and perineal swelling, due to rectal deviation and subsequent strangulation, are consistent features. Herniation may be bilateral, but two-thirds are unilateral and >80% of these are on the right side.
   The mass is soft and fluctuant and may be reduced digitally. A firm, painful swelling implies strangulation, which commonly contains the bladder or prostate. Determination of contents is often made by rectal examination. Over 90% of perineal hernias contain a rectal deviation, which must be differentiated from a rectal sacculation or false rectal diverticulum.

Treatment: Rarely is perineal hernia an emergency, except when the bladder has strangulated and the animal is unable to urinate. If catheterization cannot be accomplished, the urine should be removed by cystocentesis and an attempt made to reduce the hernia. An indwelling urinary catheter may be necessary to ensure urethral patency and prevent recurrence of obstruction.
   Surgical correction is always indicated, and concurrent castration to reduce recurrence is recommended. If a rectal sacculation is present, it should be resected or imbricated. The prognosis is guarded because of the high incidence of recurrence (10-46%) and postoperative complications such as infection, rectocutaneous fistula, anal sac fistula, ischiatic and pudendal nerve entrapment, and rectal prolapse.

RECTAL/ANORECTAL STRICTURES

Narrowing of the lumen due to cicatricial tissue. Injury may result from foreign bodies, trauma (eg, bite wounds, accidents), or as a complication of inflammatory disease.
   Neoplasia, enlarged prostate, and scar tissue following perianal fistula or anal sac abscess may all predispose to extraluminal constriction. In small animals, anorectal stricture is more common than rectal strictures, but neither is frequent. Strictures are more common in German Shepherd Dogs, Beagles, and Poodles.

Rectal stricture in cattle may result from trauma, neoplasia, or fat necrosis impinging on or within the lumen, and from defects associated with rectal and vaginal strictures. Rectal strictures in pigs occur secondary to enterocolitis, following repair of rectal prolapse, and as a sequela of salmonella-induced ulcerative proctitis. Treatment is surgical.

RECTAL NEOPLASMS

Malignant rectal neoplasms are usually adenocarcinomas in dogs and lymphosarcomas in cats. Adenocarcinomas are slow growing and infiltrative. Local or systemic metastasis may occur before tenesmus, dyschezia, blood in the feces, or diarrhea is seen. The treatment of choice for adenocarcinomas is surgical, but may be unrewarding since metastasis has usually occurred before the diagnosis. Cats with rectal lymphosarcoma are treated medically with antineoplastic drugs.

RECTAL POLYPS

Rectal adenomatous polyps are an infrequent, usually benign disease, primarily of small animals. The larger the polyp, the greater the potential for malignancy. Signs include tenesmus, hematochezia, and diarrhea. The polyp is usually palpable per rectum, and bleeds easily with surface ulceration. Periodically, the polyp may prolapse through the anal orifice. Surgical excision is usually followed by rapid clinical recovery and lengthy survival time. New polyps may occur following surgery. A biopsy should always be submitted for histopathological diagnosis.

RECTAL PROLAPSE

Protrusion of one or more layers of the rectum through the anus due to persistent tenesmus and associated with intestinal, anorectal, or urogenital disease. Prolapse may be classified as incomplete, in which only the rectal mucosa is everted, or complete, in which all rectal layers are protruded.

Etiology: Rectal prolapse is common in young animals, in association with severe diarrhea and tenesmus. Causal factors include severe enteritis; rectal foreign bodies, lacerations, diverticula, or sacculation; neoplasia of the rectum or distal colon; urolithiasis; urethral obstruction; cystitis; dystocia; colitis; and prostatic disease. Perineal hernia, or other interruption of normal innervation of the external anal sphincter, may also produce prolapse.

Animals of any age, breed, or sex may be affected. Rectal prolapse is probably the most common GI problem in pigs due to diarrhea or weakness of the rectal support tissue within the pelvis. In cattle, it may be associated with coccidiosis or rabies; occasionally, excessive "riding" and associated traumatic injury may be causative in young bulls. It is common in sheep, especially in feedlot lambs, in which high-concentrate rations may be causative. The use of estrogens as growth promotants, or accidental exposure to estrogenic fungal toxins, may also predispose large animals to rectal prolapse.

Clinical Findings, Lesions, and Diagnosis: An elongated, cylindrical mass protruding through the anal orifice is usually diagnostic. However, it must be differentiated from prolapsed ileocolic intussusception by passing a probe, blunt instrument, or finger between the prolapsed mass and the inner rectal wall. In rectal prolapse, the instrument cannot be inserted due to the presence of a fornix.

Ulceration, inflammation, and congestion of the rectal mucosa is common. Early, there is a short, nonulcerated, inflamed segment; later, the mucosal surface darkens and may become congested and necrotic.

Treatment—Small Animals: To identify and eliminate the cause is of primary importance. Treatment includes the prompt replacement of viable prolapsed tissue to its proper anatomical location, or amputation if the segment is necrotic. Small or incomplete prolapses can be manually reduced under anesthesia by utilizing a finger or bougie. Hypertonic sugar solution (50% dextrose or 70% mannitol) applied directly to the mucosa relieves edema and facilitates reduction. The placement of a loose anal purse-string suture for 5-7 days is indicated.

When questionable viability of tissue prohibits manual reduction, rectal resection and anastomosis are required. When rectal tissue is viable but not amenable to manual reduction, celiotomy followed by colopexy is indicated to prevent recurrence. Straining may be prevented by applying a topical anesthetic (1% dibucaine ointment) following reduction or correction. Postoperatively, a moistened diet and a fecal softener (eg, dioctyl sodium sulfosuccinate) are recommended. Diarrhea following surgery may require treatment.

Large Animals: The cause must be identified and eliminated. Reduction and retention with a purse-string suture is recommended. The suture should be loose enough to leave a one-finger opening into the rectum in pigs and sheep, and slightly larger in cattle and horses. Rectal prolapse in mares, if neglected, can lead to prolapse of the small colon. The blood supply to the small colon is easily disrupted and, as a result, replacement of a rectal prolapse followed by purse-string suture of the anus has a poor prognosis. When necrosis is present, submucosal resection or amputation should be performed. Amputation of the rectum should be reserved for severe cases. Complete amputation has a higher incidence of rectal stricture formation. A prolapse ring, syringe case, or plastic tubing may be used as an alternative to complete amputation in pigs and sheep. Postoperatively, the animal should receive antibiotics and fecal softeners. Usually, it is not economically feasible to repair rectal prolapses in lambs ready for market.

RECTAL TEARS

A separation, rent, or tear in the rectal or anal mucosa as a result of a laceration inflicted within the lumen. Foreign bodies, eg, sharp bones, needles, and other rough material, have been implicated. Bite wounds, and in large animals, trauma from rectal palpation are common causes. The tear may involve only the superficial layers of the rectum (partial tear) or penetrate all layers (complete tear).

Clinical Findings and Diagnosis: Constipation and reluctance to defecate are usually attributed to pain. Diagnosis is based on tenesmus and hemorrhage, perineal discoloration, and inspection of rectum and anus; fresh blood found on a glove or on feces following rectal examination is good evidence of a rectal tear. Edema may be present when the injury has persisted. The integrity of the external anal sphincter should be evaluated carefully.

Treatment: In all species, treatment should be initiated immediately. The anorectal area should be cleaned thoroughly and systemic broad-spectrum antibiotics administered. IV fluids and flunixin meglumine may be given for prevention or treatment of septic and endotoxic shock. In small animals, following debridement, lacerations may be sutured through the anal orifice, via laparotomy, or through a combination of both depending on the location and degree of the tear. Antibiotics and fecal softeners should be administered postoperatively.

In cattle and horses, accidental perforation during rectal examination necessitates immediate treatment to reduce the risk of peritonitis and death. Rectal tears in horses have been classified according to the tissue layers penetrated. Grade I tears involve the mucosa or submucosa; grade II tears involve rupture of the muscular layers only; grade III tears involve mucosa, submucosa, and muscular layers, including tears that extend into the mesorectum; grade IV tears involve perforation of all layers of the rectum and extension into the peritoneal cavity.

Grade I tears may be treated conservatively with broad-spectrum antibiotics and IV fluids. Flunixin meglumine may be given to prevent or treat endotoxic shock. Mineral oil is given via stomach tube to soften feces, and the diet should consist of pasture grasses or alfalfa. If near the anus, a grade I tear can be sutured through the anal opening. Grade II and III tears require immediate and more extensive surgery. Grade IV tears carry a grave prognosis; they should be repaired only if the tear is small, and treatment is instituted before the peritoneal cavity is grossly contaminated.

GASTROINTESTINAL ULCERS

In dogs and cats, gastric ulceration can occur spontaneously or secondary to ingestion of spoiled food or foreign bodies, administration of steroidal or nonsteroidal anti-inflammatory drugs, uremia, or neoplasia (mast cell tumors, gastrinoma). Stress ulceration has been reported. Histamine type 2 receptor antagonists (cimetidine, ranitidine, famotidine) and sucralfate have been reported to be effective in controlling gastric ulcers in dogs and cats. Cimetidine has been effective in controlling uremic gastritis. Antacids are useful, but must be administered frequently.

Gastric ulcers are important in pigs, and abomasal ulcers (qv, p 156) in mature cattle and young calves appear to be increasing in importance. In these species, ulcers appear to be associated with feeding practices and the stress of high production and confinement rearing, although the causes have not been determined.

GASTRODUODENAL ULCERS IN HORSES

Etiology: Several syndromes of gastroduodenal ulceration (GDU) affect foals, and vary with age and anatomic location of lesions. Ulceration of the glandular mucosa occurs in 25-40% of young foals with a clinical disorder, and the cause is presumed to be related to stress. Mild ulceration of the squamous mucosa occurs in 50% of neonates, but the cause is unknown. Duodenal ulceration may occur in foals with or without a concurrent clinical problem. Dietary and environmental factors are probably not relevant. Idiopathic, nonobstructive gastroparesis has caused gastric ulceration in some weanlings.

In adult horses, ulcers occur most frequently in the squamous mucosa along the margo plicatus. Prevalence and severity of gastric ulcers is greater in high-performance horses. In both foals and adults, nonsteroidal anti-inflammatory drugs cause gastric ulcers when administered at dosages higher than recommended or concurrently with a stressful condition.

Clinical Findings: Most neonatal foals with mild, squamous mucosal lesions are asymptomatic. Classic clinical signs of GDU in foals include bruxism, abdominal discomfort, diarrhea, interrupted nursing, ptyalism, and dorsal recumbency. Most foals with signs of pain have lesions in the glandular mucosa or duodenum. Diarrhea has been associated with lesions in the squamous mucosa. Gastric ulceration causes unthriftiness and chronic loose feces in weanling foals. Foals with severe ptyalism and/or nasal reflux are likely to have gastric outflow obstruction. Foals with a perforated GDU have abdominal discomfort and may be in shock. Gastric ulceration in adult horses causes poor appetite, weight loss and unthriftiness, abdominal discomfort, and/or attitudinal changes.

Diagnosis and Treatment: Endoscopy is the most accurate means of diagnosis in foals and adult horses. Radiography may assist in diagnosing some cases in foals, and barium contrast can be used to assess gastric outflow. Fecal occult blood analysis may diagnose gastric bleeding in young foals, but is insensitive in older foals and horses. In most cases, laboratory values do not reflect the presence of gastric ulceration. Increases in cells and protein may occur in abdominal fluid of foals with perforated ulcers.

The histamine type 2 receptor antagonists cimetidine and ranitidine are effective in treating GDU in foals and adults. Sucralfate has been suggested for treatment of gastric glandular and duodenal ulceration. Antacids appear to relieve clinical signs, but must be administered frequently to heal ulcers. Surgery is required to correct gastroduodenal outflow obstruction.

ESOPHAGOGASTRIC ULCERS IN PIGS

Ulcers affect the pars esophagea in pigs and cause sporadic cases of acute gastric hemorrhage or unthriftiness due to chronic ulceration.

Etiology: The cause is unknown. It occurs in all ages but is most common in confined growing pigs (100-200 lb [45-90 kg]) fed finely ground rations that may be deficient in fiber, and also in pigs fed large quantities of skimmed milk or whey. Fungi may play a role, especially if the diet is high in sugar. Also, the stress of confinement rearing is thought to promote hyperacidity, which may contribute to development of the lesion. A combination of confinement rearing, stress due to transportation, deprivation of feed, crowding, and mixing with unfamiliar pigs results in a significant increase in the incidence of gastric ulcers in rapidly growing pigs. The disease may be inapparent in a group of rapidly growing feeder pigs or young breeding gilts until some anxiety, tension, or physical stress precipitates the acute illness. This is particularly significant in pigs gathered for slaughter at abattoirs.

Clinical Findings: In the acute form, hemorrhage results in anorexia, weakness, anemia, black tarry feces, and death in hours or days. In the chronic form, unthriftiness, black tarry feces, and anemia are characteristic, but the pig may survive for several weeks. Pigs with the subclinical form may not reach maturity at the expected time. In these, the ulcer usually heals and a scar remains. In some herds, up to 90% of the feeder pigs may be affected; in other herds, it occurs only sporadically. In findings at abattoirs, the incidence of ulcers may be quite high in feeder pigs that have appeared thrifty and have grown normally; clinical disease apparently occurs only following hemorrhage of the ulcer.

Lesions: The typical terminal lesion is found in the gastric mucosa near the esophageal opening in a rectangular area of white, glistening, nonglandular, squamous epithelium. It is common to find a crater 1-2 in. (2.5-5 cm) or more in diameter encompassing the esophagus. The crater appears as a cream or gray, punched-out area and may contain blood clots or debris. In acute hemorrhage, the stomach and upper small intestine contain dark blood. Earlier lesions are characterized by hyperkeratosis and parakeratosis of the squamous epithelium in the area of the esophageal opening into the stomach. Later, the proliferative lesion erodes to form the ulcer. The healed ulcer appears as a stellate scar.

Diagnosis and Treatment: Appearance in a pen of 1 or 2 listless, anorectic pigs that show weight loss, anemia, dark feces, and sometimes dyspnea is suggestive of gastric ulceration, as is the sudden death of an apparently healthy pig. Cimetidine (300 mg/pig, b.i.d.) has been used with some success in treating gastric ulcers in growing pigs, but its use may not be economically feasible. Increasing the fiber content of the diet to 7% and feeding meal rather than pellets may be of value. Reducing stressful conditions such as crowding may minimize the incidence. Growing pigs should be raised in the same pen until marketing.

GIARDIASIS

A chronic, intestinal protozoal disease that occurs worldwide in man, most domestic mammals, and many birds. Infection is common in dogs and cats, sometimes seen in ruminants, and rare in horses and pigs. It has been hypothesized, but not yet proved, that the *Giardia* that infects domestic animals can infect man.

Etiology and Transmission: Flagellate protozoa (trophozoites) of the genus *Giardia* inhabit the mucosal surfaces of the small intestine, where they multiply by binary fission. Transmission occurs in the cyst stage by the fecal-oral route. Incubation and prepatent periods are generally 5-14 days. Earlier classifications have assigned different species names to the *Giardia* of various hosts; it is generally agreed that all the species that infect mammals (except some rodents) are structurally similar.

Clinical Findings: *Giardia* infections in dogs and cats may be inapparent, or produce weight loss and chronic diarrhea or steatorrhea, which can be continuous or intermittent, particularly in puppies and kittens. Calves with clinical giardiasis have been reported. Feces usually are soft, poorly formed, pale, and contain mucus. Watery diarrhea is unusual in uncomplicated cases. Giardiasis must be differentiated from other causes of nutrient malassimilation (eg, exocrine pancreatic insufficiency [qv, p 122], intestinal malabsorption [qv, p 141]). Clinical laboratory findings usually are normal. Gross intestinal lesions are seldom evident, although microscopic lesions, consisting of villous atrophy and cuboidal enterocytes, may be present.

Diagnosis: The motile, piriform trophozoites (av $3 \times 10 \times 15$ μm) are seen occasionally in saline smears of very loose or watery feces. Cysts (av 10×14 μm) are best detected in feces concentrated by the zinc sulfate (specific gravity 1.18) centrifugal flotation technique. Sodium chloride, sucrose, or sodium nitrate flotation media are too hypertonic, and severely distort the cysts. Staining cysts with iodine aids identification. If giardiasis is suspected, several fecal examinations are necessary because the parasites are excreted intermittently. In dogs, duodenal aspiration for trophozoite detection is useful; however, in cats, *Giardia* are more prevalent in the mid to lower small intestine. An ELISA test that detects *Giardia* antigen in the feces is available.

Treatment: No drugs are approved for treating giardiasis in animals. Quinacrine HCl (6.6 mg/kg, PO, b.i.d. for 5-6 days) is effective in dogs, but side effects (eg, emesis, dark urine) are common. Metronidazole (25 mg/kg, PO, b.i.d. for 5-7 days) is more expensive but usually well-tolerated. Metronidazole also is effective in cats (10-25 mg/kg, PO, b.i.d. for 5 days), as is furazolidone (4 mg/kg, PO, b.i.d. for 5 days). Furazolidone is less expensive than metronidazole, and may be easier to administer, since it is available in suspension form. Dogs may also be treated with tinidazole (44 mg/kg, PO, daily for 3 days). Calves may be treated with quinacrine HCl (1 mg/kg, PO, b.i.d. for 7 days), ipronidazole (10 mg/kg, b.i.d. for 5 days), or dimetridazole (50 mg/kg, daily for 5 days). Horses may be treated with metronidazole (5 mg/kg, PO, t.i.d. for 10 days).

INTESTINAL CHLAMYDIAL INFECTIONS

Chlamydiae have been isolated from fecal samples of clinically normal cattle, goats, sheep, and pigs in many parts of the world. Animals with clinically inapparent intestinal infections may shed chlamydiae in the feces for months and possibly years. Accordingly, the GI tract serves as an important reservoir and source for the transmission of these organisms. Chlamydial immunotype 1, which may cause abortions and pneumonia (qv, pp 651 and 710), can readily be isolated from feces of normal sheep or cattle. Immunotype 2 isolates have been recovered from intestinal samples of animals affected with polyarthritis (qv, p 470), encephalomyelitis (qv, p 624), and conjunctivitis (qv, p 301), but not from normal ones. A fecal isolate from pigs represents immunotype 5, but numerous recent isolates are not yet typed. The intestinal infection plays an important role as an initiating event in the pathogenesis of several chlamydia-induced diseases. The intestinal infectious phase also plays an important role in avian chlamydiosis (qv, p 1568).

While most of the intestinal chlamydial infections are clinically quiescent, a primary chlamydia-induced enteritis has been observed under field conditions in newborn calves. Such infections may also lead to a change in the *Escherichia coli* ecology of the GI tract with abnormally high numbers of *E coli* in the abomasum and upper small intestine. Signs are more severe in colostrum-deprived calves or those with only a partial transfer of colostral immunity. Affected newborn calves may have a transient watery to mucoid diarrhea with slight fever and nasal discharge. Many veterinary diagnostic laboratories do not routinely check diarrheic feces for chlamydiae; therefore, such an examination must be requested specifically. Treatments of choice are high doses of parenteral and/or oral tetracyclines.

LIVER DISEASE

Etiology: Some of the more common causes of hepatobiliary disease in different animal species follow:

Cattle: Pyrrolizadine alkaloid poisoning, black disease (*Clostridium novyi* type B), iron toxicity from injectable hematinics, copper toxicity from injectable supplements, zinc toxicity, aflatoxicosis, blue-green algae poisoning (*Microcystis aeruginosa*), fireweed poisoning (*Kochia scoparia*), sawfly larvae toxicosis (*Lophyrotoma interrupta*), herring meal toxicity, hepatic neoplasia, chronic cholangiohepatitis, cholelithiasis, hepatogenous photosensitization (various plants and fungi), hepatic abscesses secondary to rumenitis (*Fusobacterium necrophorum* and *Corynebacterium pyogenes*), fascioliasis, mycotic lupinosis (*Phomopsis* sp growing on lupine seeds), bacillary hemoglobinuria (*Clostridium haemolyticum, C novyi* type D), hepatic lipidosis secondary to ketosis, and bacterial hepatitis secondary to septicemia.

Sheep: Pyrrolizidine alkaloid poisoning, zinc toxicity, copper toxicity from injectable supplements, aflatoxicosis, blue-green algae poisoning (*Microcystis aeruginosa*), black disease, hepatic neoplasia, hepatic abscesses secondary to rumenitis (*Fusobacterium necrophorum* and *Corynebacterium pyogenes*), fascioliasis, mycotic lupinosis (*Phomopsis* sp growing on lupine seeds), bacillary hemoglobinuria (*Clostridium haemolyticum, C novyi* type D), hepatic lipidosis secondary to ketosis, white liver disease (cobalt/vitamin B_{12} deficiency), heritable photosensitivity and jaundice in Southdown sheep, and Dubin-Johnson-like syndrome in Corriedale sheep.

Pigs: Black disease, hepatosis dietetica (vitamin E/selenium deficiency), aflatoxicosis, coal tar toxicity, cyanamide toxicity, blue-green algae toxicity, hepatogenous photosensitization (plants and fungi), ascarid (larvae) migration through the liver, ascarid (adult) bile duct occlusion, mycotic lupinosis, gossypol toxicosis, and bacterial hepatitis secondary to septicemia (*Salmonella* spp).

Horses: Pyrrolizidine alkaloid poisoning, black disease, Tyzzer's disease (*Bacillus piliformis*), iron toxicity from injectable hematinics in foals, neonatal rhinopneumonitis, cholangitis, biliary cirrhosis (alsike clover, *Trifolium hybridum*, and other causes), cholelithiasis, Theiler's disease (acute equine hepatic insufficiency secondary to use of equine-origin biologics), hepatic carcinoma, aflatoxicosis, fasting hyperbilirubinemia, hepatogenous photosensitization (various plants and fungi), hyperlipemia/hepatic lipidosis, equine leukoencephalomalacia (moldy corn poisoning, *Fusarium moniliforme*), and bacterial hepatitis secondary to septicemia.

Cats: Idiopathic hepatic lipidosis, cholangitis-cholangiohepatitis syndrome, common bile duct occlusion (tumors, choleliths), sludged bile syndrome, endotoxemia (toxic hepatopathy), feline infectious peritonitis, occasional infections with *Toxoplasma*, acetaminophen toxicity, neoplasia (lymphosarcoma, myeloproliferative disease, bile duct adenocarcinoma), and portosystemic vascular anomalies.

Dogs: Infectious canine hepatitis; leptospiral hepatitis; occasional infections with *Toxoplasma, Neospora caninum, Salmonella*; portosystemic vascular anomalies; idiopathic chronic active hepatitis; lobular dissecting hepatitis; breed-related chronic active hepatitis (Doberman Pinschers, West Highland White Terriers [possible copper storage disease], Bedlington Terriers [copper storage disease similar to Wilson's disease in man]); chronic active hepatitis associated with idiosyncratic drug reactions (primidone, phenytoin); cholestasis associated with idiosyncratic drug reactions (trimethoprim/sulfa drugs, anabolic steroids); necrosis associated with mebendazole or oxibendazole; glucocorticoid hepatopathy; cholecystitis (possibly with ruptured bile duct); cholelithiasis; severe passive congestion leading to hepatic fibrosis (cardiac insufficiency associated with dirofilariasis); and cirrhosis.

All animals: Bacterial infections (*Actinobacillus, Campylobacter, Clostridium, Corynebacterium, Escherichia, Haemophilus, Listeria, Mycobacterium, Nocardia,*

Pasteurella, Salmonella, and *Yersinia* spp); many mycotoxins produced by *Aspergillus, Blastomyces, Penicillium, Phomopsis,* and *Pithomyces* spp; organic toxins (carbon tetrachloride, arsenicals, dioxin); vitamin D (overdose); and primary tumors (carcinomas) involving both the bile duct and liver, and a variety of other metastatic tumors.

Clinical Findings and Diagnosis: Clinical signs of hepatic disorders result from compromised hepatocellular function due to severe necrosis or atrophy; intra- or extrahepatic cholestasis; diminished hepatic blood flow associated with acquired lesions (fibrosis, cirrhosis), congenital lesions (portosystemic vascular anomalies), or impaired systemic circulation (cardiac decompensation); or reduced hepatic reticuloendothelial system (RES) function. Also, inherited or acquired changes in biochemical function may be present without morphologic lesions. Due to the large reserve and regenerative capabilities of the liver, lesions may exist but not cause clinical signs; disorders are seldom diagnosed early. Any combination of morphologic or functional changes can coexist. Shortly after onset of hepatic necrosis, intrahepatic cholestasis may develop and be followed by an uncomplicated regeneration in a few days, or proceed to a self-perpetuating hepatitis. Chronic hepatitis may progress to bridging fibrosis, the formation of regenerative nodules with or without bile duct hyperplasia. Extensive fibrosis results in cholestasis, reduced hepatic blood flow, portal hypertension, and ultimately, the opening and augmentation of portosystemic vascular communications. Any diffuse severe liver disease can be associated with reduced hepatic RES function. The hepatic RES is the largest supply of fixed macrophages in the body; it removes particulate debris, endotoxins, and bacterial organisms from the portal circulation thereby preventing their entry into the systemic circulation.

Clinical signs of hepatobiliary disease may include: intermittent fever, inappetence, weight loss, polyuria, polydipsia, icterus, photosensitization from phylloerythrin retention (in ruminants and horses), yellow-green urine due to the presence of bile pigments, hepatomegaly or reduced hepatic size, bleeding tendencies due to abnormalities in platelets and coagulation proteins, ascites (due to hypoalbuminemia, sodium retention, and/or portal hypertension), and neurobehavioral abnormalities (hepatoencephalopathy). Hepatoencephalopathy may be characterized by one or more of lethargy, amaurosis, aggression, hysteria, depression, apparent hallucinations, and ptyalism. Such signs develop due to complex biochemical changes in neuronal function and systemic and cerebral metabolism, and to an increased permeability of the blood brain barrier. There are unique species differences in clinical signs associated with liver disease; eg, icterus may be normal in horses and Bolivian squirrel monkeys after an overnight fast; in ruminants, icterus is more common following a hemolytic crisis than in liver disease. Some pathognomonic features of liver disease are inconsistent; eg, fatty, gray to clay-colored (acholic) feces devoid of normal bilirubin pigments, together with the absence of urine urobilinogen, are classically associated with extrahepatic bile duct obstruction. However, fecal pigmentation and urine urobilinogen may be normal if GI hemorrhage (resulting from vitamin K deficiency) is a concurrent problem.

A variety of tests, which must be thoroughly understood for appropriate diagnostic and prognostic approaches, can be used to detect hepatobiliary disorders. (*See also* p 940.) Screening and diagnostic tests are helpful in differentiating the cause of icterus (hemolysis from cholestasis) and can be used as prognostic indicators. In the latter case, regeneration, success of therapy, residual damage, and risk of anesthesia may be appraised. Serum enzyme activities are useful screening tests for the detection of reversible and irreversible permeability changes in hepatocellular membranes. ALT (SGPT), AST (SGOT), sorbitol dehydrogenase (SDH), and arginase can indicate hepatocellular necrosis, enzyme induction, or alterations in membrane permeability. Alkaline phosphatase and γ-glutamyltransferase are useful in detecting cholestasis and enzyme induction. Enzyme induction is especially common in dogs with various medical problems and following exposure to certain drugs (eg, anticonvulsants, glucocorticoids, and phenylbutazone).

True tests of hepatic function include: 1) plasma clearance of organic anions (bilirubin, bromsulfophthalein [BSP], indocyanine green [ICG], or bile acids); 2) the capacity to metabolize carbohydrates, lipids, proteins, ammonia, and uric acid; and 3) measurement of hepatic blood flow (plasma clearance of BSP, ICG, serum bile acids, or ammonia tolerance testing). In dogs and cats, ultrasonography and radiologic contrast techniques can be used to determine hepatic size or distortions, and the presence and location of portosystemic shunts. Liver biopsy is usually required for a definitive diagnosis.

Treatment: Treatment of liver disease is based on providing good nutrition, adequate fluids, and antimicrobials directed at specific infectious agents; and alleviating the retention of bilirubin, bile acids, and other noxious metabolic products. If toxins or causative agents can be removed early, regeneration may occur followed by recovery with little or no residual damage. If the disease is chronic, response to treatment may be curtailed by diffuse fibrosis and a self-perpetuating secondary hepatitis. Anti-inflammatory drugs are appropriate for some forms of chronic self-perpetuating inflammatory disease. Extrahepatic bile duct obstruction usually requires surgery to remove the occlusion and/or create a biliary diversion such as a cholecystojejunostomy.

Since the expense of treatment may make management unfeasible for many large animals, the following discussion focuses on management of liver disease in dogs and cats.

Nutritional support must be tailored to each individual. If hepatic function is adequate, a balanced maintenance feed is recommended. If hepatic function is compromised and encephalopathic tendencies are suspected, a diet with a reduced protein content composed of dairy proteins is best. Most of the calories should be provided in simple, easily digested carbohydrates, eg, boiled white rice. Meals should be frequent and small to maximize digestion and absorption. Because many of the toxins responsible for encephalopathic signs are derived from the GI tract, particularly the colon, a diet resulting in reduced colonic residue is beneficial. Because of the role the liver has in storage, activation, and synthesis of many vitamins and cofactors, a multiple vitamin supplement is recommended, generally at twice the recommended daily dose of the water-soluble component. Lipotropic supplements containing methionine should be avoided, since they can induce an encephalopathic crisis if liver function is severely reduced.

Vitamin K supplementation is recommended (5-15 mg given by deep IM injection, b.i.d.) if bleeding tendencies are detected or coagulation tests are abnormal and the animal is jaundiced. Vitamin K repletion is curtailed when the extrahepatic bile duct is obstructed, and hemorrhagic complications develop within 2 wk due to malabsorption of fat-soluble vitamins. Response to vitamin K_1 is dramatic. Within 12 hr, a >30% correction in the prothrombin and partial thromboplastin times occurs. Often, coagulation tests are normal 24 hr after treatment. In animals with major parenchymal disease associated with a coagulopathy, trial treatment with vitamin K may be used to determine whether supplementation is warranted; the response is less dramatic when parenchymal failure is the underlying problem.

Systemic antibiotics that do not require major hepatic biotransformation or elimination are advised in hepatic disease and suspected compromised hepatic reticuloendothelial system. Ampicillin, amoxicillin, or cephalosporins are commonly used. Metronidazole is especially effective against anaerobic organisms, but a reduced dose should be used when hepatic function is compromised. Specific antibiotic therapy should be based on culture and sensitivity tests on liver tissue or bile.

Animals with encephalopathic signs are treated to reduce the production, availability, or absorption of the many causal gut-derived toxins. Cholestyramine or activated charcoal given PO can be used to trap intestinal endotoxins and bile acids in acute hepatic failure. Lactulose, PO, minimizes the effect of GI ammonia, the largest source of ammonia in the body, by reducing the number of urease-producing bacteria, inhibiting ammonia formation and absorption, and causing catharsis. An initial dose of 0.25 mL/10 lb (4.5 kg) body wt is titrated to yield soft feces 2-3 times/day. Neomycin (22 mg/kg, b.i.d.) can be given PO to modify intestinal flora, which reduces the number of toxin-producing bacteria. Neomycin and lactulose are synergistic. Enemas may also be used to remove or modify colonic contents in a crisis. Mechanical or retention enemas using solutions of 15-20 mL of a 1% neomycin solution, lactulose (1:3 in water), or dilute povidone-iodine (iodine enemas should not be used for retention) have been recommended.

Anorexia and vomiting associated with liver disease may be due to encephalopathy or GI ulceration. In severe liver disease, increased gastrin concentration, reduced visceral blood flow, delayed mucosal turnover, and excess bile acids are ulcerogenic. Cimetidine or ranitidine in combination with sucralfate have been useful for this problem. Appetite stimulants (benzodiazepines) have been recommended, but generally they are unreliable since they promote sedation and may potentiate encephalopathic signs. They require hepatic metabolism for elimination, and may bind to encephalopathy-promoting neuroreceptors in the brain. Forced alimentation is imperative in some cases, eg, feline idiopathic hepatic lipidosis. A nasogastric tube or gastrostomy tube is usually necessary, the latter being preferred. Gastrostomy tubes can be used effectively in the home environment and may make chronic treatment economically feasible.

Anabolic steroids such as oxymethalone or stanozolol have been used as appetite stimulants, to promote weight gain, and to stimulate erythropoiesis. Adequate calories must be provided to allow an anabolic effect. In some animals, cholestasis and jaundice may develop with use of these agents.

Anti-inflammatory drugs are used when chronic persistent hepatic disease is diagnosed and an infectious cause cannot be determined. Glucocorticoids (1-4 mg/kg/day) are used when chronic disease involves round cell (lymphocytes, monocytes, macrophages, plasma cells) infiltrates and developing fibrosis. If response to treatment is inadequate or adverse side effects develop, azathioprine is usually tried. Metronidazole has been used because it provides some inhibition of cell-mediated immunity. Treatment for extensive hepatic fibrosis or cirrhosis may include glucocorticoids, glucocorticoids with azathioprine, colchicine, penicillamine, zinc supplementation, and/or metronidazole. Although each of these medications has beneficial antifibrotic effects, they also have adverse side effects and must be administered judiciously.

If thick, tenacious biliary secretions (sludged bile) are recognized and the biliary outflow tract is patent, a low dose of dehydrocholic acid (10-15 mg/kg, PO, b.i.d. to t.i.d.) may be used as a choleretic. Care is warranted if therapy is chronic, as dehydrocholic acid can be metabolized by intestinal microorganisms to lithocholic acid, an extremely hepatotoxic bile acid. Ursodeoxycholic acid has been used recently in people with cholelithiasis and diseases of the biliary tree leading to hepatic (biliary) fibrosis. Limited information is available for use in animals.

Ascites is a problem in dogs with chronic liver disease but is rare in cats. It is best managed by cage rest, a low-sodium diet, and if necessary, sodium-wasting diuretics. When diuretics are used, dehydration and hypokalemia should be avoided, as these may promote an encephalopathic crisis. Abdominal paracentesis may be necessary to initiate fluid mobilization, but this should be reserved for animals refractory to more conservative treatment.

MALABSORPTION SYNDROMES

The primary functions of the small intestine include mixing and propulsion of luminal contents, absorption of water and ions, digestion and absorption of nutrients, and secretion of hormones. Digestion and absorption of nutrients occur in 3 sequential phases: intraluminal digestion, mucosal digestion and absorption, and delivery of nutrients to the circulation. Many GI diseases cause chronic malabsorption by interfering with these processes. Malabsorptive syndromes in dogs have been studied in most detail; however, basic diagnostic and therapeutic principles are relevant to other species.

Physiology: The normal digestive processes convert dietary nutrients into forms that can cross the brush border of intestinal absorptive epithelial cells, or enterocytes. Main dietary carbohydrates are the polysaccharides starch and glycogen, and the disaccharides sucrose and lactose. Initial intraluminal digestion of starch and glycogen involves hydrolysis by pancreatic amylase to the oligosaccharides maltose, maltotriose, and α-limit dextrins. Oligosaccharides and ingested disaccharides are further hydrolyzed to monosaccharides by enzymes located on the brush border of the intestinal epithelial cell. The final products of mucosal hydrolysis (glucose, galactose, and fructose) are actively transported into the enterocyte by a protein-carrier-mediated process. Once in the cell, monosaccharides diffuse down a concentration gradient through the lamina propria and into the portal venous circulation. Protein digestion and absorption follow a similar pattern. Proteolytic enzymes from the stomach and pancreas degrade protein into short-chain oligopeptides, dipeptides, and amino acids. Oligopeptides are further hydrolyzed by brush border peptidases to dipeptides and amino acids that cross the brush-border membrane on specific carrier proteins.

Fat-soluble molecules do not need specific carriers to cross the phospholipid barrier of the brush border. However, intraluminal degradation of large lipids is essential. Fat in the duodenum stimulates release of cholecystokinin, which, in turn, stimulates secretion of pancreatic lipase. Triglycerides are degraded by lipase at the surface of emulsified lipid droplets to release monoglycerides (MG) and free fatty acids (FFA). Before absorption, these products must be solubilized in the aqueous phase of the lumen contents by combining with aggregates of bile acids called micelles. At the cell membrane, the FFA and MG disaggregate from the micelle and are passively absorbed into the cell. Released bile acids remain within the lumen and are reabsorbed by the ileum. Once inside the cell, FFA and MG are reesterified to triglycerides and incorporated into chylomicrons, which subsequently enter the central lacteals of the villus and are delivered to the venous circulation via the thoracic duct.

Etiology: Malabsorption occurs as a consequence of interference with mechanisms responsible for either the degradation or absorption of dietary constituents. The main potential conditions are summarized in TABLE 4.

Table 4. Conditions Resulting in Malabsorption

Condition	Deficiency	Malabsorption
Exocrine pancreatic insufficiency	α-amylase Proteases Lipase	Starch Protein Triglycerides
Small-intestinal disease (secondary deficiencies)	Disaccharidases Sugar carriers Brush border peptidases Peptide and amino acid carriers Reduced surface area	Disaccharides Monosaccharides Oligopeptides Peptides and amino acids Lipid
Brush-border disease (primary deficiency)	Lactase	Lactose
Bile salt deficiency	Conjugated bile salts	Lipid

Diseases that disrupt the synthesis or secretion of digestive pancreatic enzymes or bile cause maldigestion with subsequent malabsorption. An important cause is exocrine pancreatic insufficiency (EPI, qv, p 122), which occurs when <10-15% of pancreatic mass is functional. This disease is characterized by severe maldigestion-malabsorption of starch, protein, and most notably, fat. EPI is usually complicated by small intestinal bacterial overgrowth (SIBO), which further disrupts nutrient digestion and absorption.

Small-intestinal disease can cause malabsorption by reduction of the number or function of individual enterocytes. Diffuse mucosal or bowel wall diseases reduce brush border enzyme activities, decrease mucosal carrier-protein function, decrease the mucosal absorptive surface area, and interfere with final transport of nutrients into the circulation. Malabsorbed nutrients exert strong intraluminal osmotic effects that diminish intestinal and colonic absorptive surface area, and interfere with final transport of nutrients into the circulation. Malabsorbed nutrients exert strong intraluminal osmotic effects that diminish intestinal and colonic absorption of water and electrolytes. Specific causes include chronic inflammatory bowel diseases such as lymphocytic-plasmacytic enteritis, eosinophilic enteritis, and idiopathic villous atrophy. Histoplasmosis, giardiasis, viral and bacterial enteritis, lymphosarcoma, and amyloidosis typically cause malabsorptive syndromes. Intestinal disease in dogs generally results in malabsorption less marked than that of EPI.

Intraluminal effects of bacteria can also have important consequences. As with EPI, SIBO frequently occurs secondary to diffuse small-intestinal disease. SIBO causes biochemical damage to the intestinal brush border, further diminishing mucosal enzyme and carrier protein activities. Bacterial deconjugation of bile salts interferes with micelle formation, which results in malabsorption of lipid. Deconjugated bile salts and hydroxy fatty acids exacerbate diarrhea by stimulation of colonic secretion. SIBO can also occur in dogs as a primary disease with similar pathologic consequences; the occurrence in other species is unknown.

Fat malabsorption may occur with a deficiency of intraluminal bile salts due to hepatic disease, obstruction to bile flow, or ileal disease that results in defective absorption of conjugated bile salts. Intestinal lymphangiectasia (pathological dilatation of intestinal lymphatic vessels) also causes severe fat malabsorption and intestinal protein loss.

Primary lactase deficiency occurs in dogs and cats; other primary brush-border enzyme defects have not been reported other than in man. Sensitivity to dietary components such as gluten is believed to be an underlying cause of some malabsorptive diseases (wheat-sensitive enteropathy of Irish Setters, idiopathic villous atrophy, inflammatory bowel disease).

Clinical Findings: The duration, severity, and primary cause determine the severity of signs, which typically include chronic diarrhea, and poor weight gain or weight loss. The absence of diarrhea does not exclude the possibility of severe GI disease. Weight loss is usually substantial despite a ravenous appetite, sometimes characterized by coprophagia. Nonspecific signs include dehydration, anemia, ascites, or edema. Thickened bowel loops or enlarged mesenteric lymph nodes may be palpable.

Diagnosis: Chronic diarrhea and weight loss are nonspecific signs common to a variety of intestinal and systemic diseases. Diagnosis begins with a detailed history to determine the duration of the problem. The next step is to exclude dietary or parasitic causes, and localize the disease to the small intestine. Typical features that may help to differentiate between small- and large-intestinal diarrhea are summarized in TABLE 1, p 95. Chronic small-intestinal diarrhea is functionally characterized to determine if maldigestion (eg, EPI) or malabsorption is present. Definitive diagnosis is made with additional laboratory tests, radiographs, endoscopy, biopsy, and/or response to therapy.

The initial data base should include a complete blood count, biochemical profile, urinalysis, fecal examination for parasites, and abdominal radiographs. Hematologic correlates of intestinal diseases include: anemia of chronic blood loss (microcytic-hypochromic), chronic inflammation (normocytic-normochromic), or malnutrition (macrocytic); neutrophilia and/or monocytosis associated with inflammatory bowel diseases or histoplasmosis; eosinophilia associated with parasitism, eosinophilic enteritis, or hypoadrenocorticism; and lymphopenia caused by intestinal lymphangiectasia. Hypoproteinemia frequently occurs secondary to a protein-losing enteropathy; in most cases serum albumin and globulin are low. Enteropathy of Basenjis is an exception, in which hyperglobulinemia occurs with hypoalbuminemia. Biochemical tests and urinalysis will exclude systemic diseases that cause chronic diarrhea, most notably hypoadrenocorticism, renal failure, and liver disease.

Fecal examination should include gross inspection as an aid in localizing disease to the small intestine. Fecal examinations for parasites should include direct saline smears to identify trophozoites of protozoan parasites, especially *Giardia canis*, and fecal flotations to identify metazoan ova. Zinc sulfate centrifugation-flotation is used to identify protozoal cysts such as *Giardia* and coccidia. Frequently, occult giardiasis occurs. Diagnosis in this instance is based on identification of trophozoites in duodenal aspirates, or more simply by response to a therapeutic trial of metronidazole or quinacrine. Microscopical examination of fecal smears prepared with direct and indirect Sudan stain, Lugol's iodine, and New Methylene Blue or Wright's stain are simple screening tests used to identify unabsorbed nutrients, inflammatory cells, and infectious agents. A strongly positive direct Sudan stain (undigested fat) is characterized by numerous fat droplets and is consistent with EPI. Numerous small fat droplets on an indirect Sudan stain (digested fat) with a negative direct Sudan is suggestive of intestinal malabsorption. Lugol's iodine stains for undigested starch; however, this test is unreliable and varies with diet. These screening tests should be done on multiple, fresh fecal samples to improve reliability. Detection of excessive leukocytes on fecal cytology may indicate chronic inflammatory bowel disease or infectious diseases such as salmonellosis or campylobacteriosis, in which case fecal cultures would be indicated. Cytology of colonic scrapings may reveal *Histoplasma* organisms.

Once dietary, parasitic, and infectious causes of chronic small-intestinal diarrhea have been eliminated, EPI must be differentiated from intestinal malabsorption. Numerous tests of exocrine pancreatic function, including qualitative/quantitative fecal fat analysis, plasma turbidity tests, fecal proteolytic activity, and the bentiromide tests, are too inaccurate or impractical to be used to diagnose EPI. Assay of canine serum trypsin-like immunoreactivity (TLI) is a highly sensitive and specific test for the diagnosis of EPI in dogs. This assay quantitates trypsinogen that normally leaks from the pancreas into the blood, thereby providing an indirect assessment of functional pancreatic tissue. In dogs with EPI, functional exocrine tissue is severely depleted and serum TLI concentrations are extremely low, clearly distinguishing EPI from other causes of malabsorption. This test requires a fasted serum sample. A feline serum TLI test is currently unavailable. Assay of multiple fresh fecal samples for proteolytic activity, available through selected reference laboratories, is considered the most reliable test of EPI in cats.

Diagnosis of small-intestinal disease is difficult due to limitations of routine screening procedures, the need for small-intestinal biopsy, and frequently, the absence of diagnostic histological changes. Tests useful to confirm and characterize abnormal intestinal absorption include the xylose absorption test and measurements of serum concentrations of folate and cobalamin (vitamin B_{12}). Oral administration of xylose and timed measurements of blood xylose concentrations (0, 30, 60, 90, 120 min) provide an assessment of proximal small-intestinal function. Normal dogs should have a peak xylose >60 mg/dL at 60-90 min. Decreased xylose absorption indicates severe malabsorption. Delayed gastric emptying and bacterial metabolism of xylose from SIBO can cause false low results. This test is insensitive; it is not uncommon for xylose absorption to be normal in animals with small-intestinal disease.

Folate is absorbed primarily by the proximal small intestine (jejunum), whereas cobalamin is absorbed by the distal small intestine (ileum). As a result, serum folate concentrations can be decreased in proximal small-intestinal diseases, serum cobalamin concentrations can be decreased in distal small-intestinal diseases, and both can be decreased in diffuse enteropathies. Proximal SIBO may cause increased serum folate and/or reduced serum cobalamin concentration, since many enteric bacteria can synthesize folate that is subsequently absorbed in the jejunum, but bind cobalamin, making it unavailable for transport. Normal serum concentrations of these vitamins do not exclude the possibility of small-intestinal disease, since impaired absorption depends on the nature, extent, and duration of a mucosal abnormality, as well as on the type and numbers of organisms present in SIBO. Increased folate and decreased cobalamin also occur frequently in EPI, presumably from secondary SIBO.

Detection of intestinal permeability by measurement of 24-hr urinary excretion of ^{51}Cr-EDTA following oral administration is a sensitive test for small-intestinal damage. Increased mucosal permeability allows increased passage of this probe across the mucosa and into the blood to be excreted by the kidneys. IV administration of ^{51}Cr involves a different principle and is used to document protein-losing enteropathy. The ^{51}Cr quickly attaches to circulating albumin so that 3-day fecal excretion of this tracer provides an estimate of loss of albumin into the intestinal lumen.

Definitive diagnosis of most malabsorptive diseases is best made by intestinal biopsies taken perorally with a suction biopsy capsule or endoscope, or taken at laparotomy. Multiple biopsy samples should be collected from all sections of the small intestine; if a laparotomy is done, mesenteric lymph nodes should be biopsied and other organs examined. Since full-thickness intestinal biopsies do not heal well in animals that are cachexic and/or severely hypoproteinemic, peroral biopsy techniques are recommended. Pre-operative plasma transfusions are advisable.

Obvious morphological abnormalities may be minimal or absent, despite considerable abnormality of intestinal function. Additionally, histological descriptions alone may provide little information on mechanisms of damage to the mucosa; eg, lymphocytic-plasmacytic enteritis (LPE), a feature of many chronic enteropathies, is probably not a distinct entity. This condition likely represents a common response of the mucosa to more than one agent, such as bacterial or dietary antigens in the intestinal lumen. A direct association between LPE and SIBO has been demonstrated, but this is unlikely to be the only cause. Furthermore, some conditions such as SIBO can cause a variety of functional consequences with no obvious histologic damage. Indeed, clinical signs of malabsorption coupled with increased serum folate and decreased serum cobalamin suggest the presence of SIBO, even if intestinal biopsy is normal. Definitive diagnosis of SIBO is made by quantitative aerobic and anaerobic cultures of small-intestinal aspirates. Similarly, dietary sensitivity does not cause pathognomonic lesions, but may be suspected from the history and by eliminating other potential causes of intestinal damage. This can be confirmed only by monitoring response to dietary exclusion and subsequent challenge. Histological changes such as LPE and eosinophilic enteritis have been reported in cats, but little is known about the underlying cause of chronic small-intestinal disease in this species.

Response to therapy is a valid method to diagnose malabsorptive diseases, especially when supported by results from initial screening tests. Giardiasis (qv, p 136) is a common disease in dogs and cats, although diagnosis based on identification of the organism can be difficult. Likewise, response to antibiotic therapy (tetracycline, metronidazole, or tylosin) is a practical method to rule out SIBO. Dietary changes to selectively exclude components such as gluten, meat products, or food additives may be useful in some malabsorptive syndromes.

Treatment: Although specific treatment requires a definitve diagnosis, empirical therapy is beneficial when a specific diagnosis cannot be made. In general, dietary management improves clinical signs in most cases of malabsorptive disease. Diets should be easily digestible, and consist of high biologic value protein with restricted fat, lactose, and additives. Suitable commercial diets, or homemade diets consisting of rice or potato for carbohydrate, cottage cheese, yogurt, boiled chicken or lamb for protein, and supplemented with medium-chain-triglyceride (MCT) oil for calories are recommended. The carbohydrate:protein ratio should be ~4:1. Small portions should be fed frequently. Pancreatic enzyme supplement may be of benefit in malnourished dogs, since protein-calorie malnutrition impairs pancreatic exocrine function. Fat-restricted diets should be supplemented with MCT oil (1-2 mL/kg/day). Additionally, diets should be supplemented with vitamins, particularly A, D, E, and K, and folic acid (5 mg/day for 1-6 mo). Parenteral cobalamin (500 μg/mo) is also recommended.

Gluten-containing grains such as oats, wheat, barley, and rye should be avoided, especially in animals with suspected gluten-sensitive enteropathy. Gluten-free prescription diets are available.

When the underlying cause of malabsorptive disease is not identified, efficacy of drug therapy must be determined by trial and error. Antimicrobials and immunosuppresive drugs indicated for specific diseases are listed in TABLE 5. Corticosteroids are used primarily to treat chronic inflammatory bowel diseases because of their anti-inflammatory and immunosuppressive actions. Corticosteroids also improve absorptive and digestive functions of the intestine by induction of functional proteins in the enterocyte. Because debilitated animals are already in a catabolic and immunosuppressed condition, caution must always be used when treating them with corticosteroids. Metronidazole, in addition to its antiprotozoal action, is effective against anaerobic bacteria that frequently cause SIBO or may be secondarily involved in other chronic enteropathies. Metronidazole also suppresses cell-mediated immune responses in the intestine, which may account for its efficacy in treating some cases of inflammatory bowel disease.

Table 5. Treatments for Selected Malabsorptive Diseases

Disease	Treatment
Exocrine pancreatic insufficiency	Powdered pancreatic enzyme replacement Low-fat diet
Chronic inflammatory bowel disease Eosinophilic enteritis	Prednisone Chicken- or lamb-based diets
Lymphocytic-plasmacytic enteritis	Prednisone (consider azathioprine) alone or in combination with metronidazole, tetracycline, or tylosin High-protein, low-fat diet
Immunoproliferative enteropathy of Basenjis	Same as above
Lymphangiectasia	Low-fat diet, medium-chain triglyceride oil Prednisone
Villous atrophy Gluten enteropathy	Gluten-free diet
Idiopathic	Prednisone, antibiotics, consider gluten-free diet
Bacterial overgrowth	Antibiotics (tetracycline, metronidazole, or tylosin
Giardiasis	Metronidazole or quinacrine
Histoplasmosis	Amphotericin B, ketoconazole, itraconazole
Lymphosarcoma	Vincristine, cyclophosphamide, prednisone (and other chemotherapy drugs)

PERITONITIS

Inflammation of the peritoneum may be acute or chronic, local or diffuse, and most commonly is secondary to contamination of the peritoneal cavity.

Etiology: Primary peritonitis is infrequent. It may be caused by infectious agents such as feline infectious peritonitis virus (qv, p 415), *Nocardia* spp, or *Mycobacterium* spp. Access to the peritoneal cavity is generally by the hematogenous route. Progression of primary peritonitis tends to be chronic (days to weeks).

Secondary peritonitis is often acute, and results in rapid, progressive, systemic illness. It is most commonly associated with GI perforation or dehiscence of visceral wound closure, or with perforation of other infected viscera (eg, prostatic or hepatic abscess, pyometra). Penetrating abdominal injuries may lacerate viscera or inoculate the peritoneal cavity with foreign material and microorganisms. Peritonitis may also occur secondary to chemical irritants (eg, bile, urine) and to other disease processes that allow transmural migration of bacteria (eg, neoplasia, visceral ische-mia). Peritonitis from chemical irritation or foreign bodies (eg, sponge) may be septic or nonseptic. Septic peritonitis may remain localized if the omentum or mes-entery contains the septic process, which sometimes results in formation of an ab-dominal abscess.

Microorganisms associated with septic peritonitis reflect the source of contami-nation. A mixed bacterial population is seen in GI perforation (coliforms, anaer-obes), whereas perforation of nongastrointestinal viscera (eg, gallbladder, uterus, prostate) are usually associated with one organism (*Escherichia coli*). In horses, *Streptococcus equi* and *Rhodococcus (Corynebacterium) equi* may be associated with peritonitis.

Clinical Findings: Signs vary depending on the type of peritonitis (primary or sec-ondary) and the presence of bacterial infection. Abdominal pain may be generalized and severe, so that the animal guards the abdomen, walks with a stiff gait, or is recumbent. Pyrexia is common but may be suppressed by prostaglandin inhibitors. Abdominal distention, which may be inapparent, usually is due to accumulation of peritoneal exudate, and may be accompanied by hemorrhage, septicemia, toxemia, paralytic ileus, shock, and adhesions. Fluid transudation sequesters electrolytes and protein in the abdominal cavity and atonic gut, and venous stasis leads to hypoten-sion, acid-base disturbances, and circulatory collapse. Toxemia and bacteremia contribute to the shock state. Icterus may be present in generalized bile peritonitis. Animals with secondary peritonitis may exhibit signs of the primary illness also.

In small animals, anorexia and depression are often accompanied by vomiting, and feces may not be passed. Dehydration, hypovolemia, and sepsis may result in hypothermia and death due to loss of extravascular fluid volume.

In horses, clinical signs include severe colic, ileus, distended intestines on rectal examination, gastric reflux, and occasionally, diarrhea. The horse is restless and may lie down and roll intermittently. Tachycardia, weak pulse, poor peripheral per-fusion, and pyrexia are common. Septic peritonitis is frequently fatal, despite inten-sive treatment.

In cattle, rumination ceases and milk production drops. Abdominal percussion may detect ruminal tympany.

Diagnosis: History, and physical and rectal examination findings lead to suspicion of peritonitis. Abdominal radiographs may be evaluated for evidence of GI obstruc-tion (bowel dilatation, free abdominal air), ascites, and radiodense foreign material. Loss of serosal detail (a "ground glass" appearance) is indicative of abdominal fluid. Ultrasonography is a valuable adjunctive test to evaluate size, shape, and content of other viscera (eg, gallbladder, prostate gland) suspected to be the source of peritonitis. Abdominal paracentesis should be used in large animals to obtain fluid for cytologic examination and culture, and in small animals to confirm the character of peritoneal fluid. Diagnostic peritoneal lavage is used when small amounts of fluid cannot be obtained by paracentesis. Cytologic examination of ab-dominal fluid may reveal septic or nonseptic suppurative inflammation with one or more bacterial infections. Neutrophils are degenerative in the presence of sepsis. Hypoglycemia and thrombocytopenia may accompany septic peritonitis.

Treatment: Initial treatment must be directed toward stabilization of the metabolic consequences of peritonitis. Replacement fluids, electrolytes, plasma, or whole blood may be necessary to maintain cardiac output. Broad-spectrum antimicrobial therapy (eg, aminoglycoside with penicillin) should be initiated and changed conse-quent to sensitivity testing. Once the animal is stabilized, surgery is done to explore the abdomen, and repair any defects (eg, a ruptured viscus). This is followed by thorough peritoneal lavage with an isothermic, isotonic, balanced electrolyte solu-tion to which nonirritating antimicrobial agents may be added. Abdominal drains to allow postoperative lavage and open peritoneal drainage (small animals) are some-times used to treat severe peritonitis. Parenteral antimicrobial therapy is continued after surgery to assure bioavailability, and food is withheld until the animal's condition improves. Hyperalimentation, or alimentation by feeding-tube gastrostomy and catheter jejunostomy may be needed in anorectic animals.

PHARYNGEAL PARALYSIS

A disorder of central or peripheral origin that most frequently occurs as a sign of encephalitis and is of special clinical significance in rabies in cattle and dogs. It is also an important sign in encephalomyelitis. It is seen in many intoxications, eg, botulism and chronic lead poisoning in horses, probably some fungal poisonings, as well as with the general paralysis of parturient paresis. Peripheral paralysis is infrequent and may result from injury to the glossopharyngeal nerve, pressure from tumors or abscesses, or injury from fracture of the floor of the cranium. Pharyngeal paralysis in horses due to *Aspergillus* infection and erosion of the guttural pouch wall (qv, p 739) is relatively common. (*See also* PHARYNGITIS, p 719.)

Clinical Findings: The animal suddenly loses its ability to swallow; food particles and saliva drop from the mouth and nose, and gurgling sounds emanate from the pharynx. If the interior of the pharynx is palpated, no muscular contractions are produced. Such animals die from aspiration pneumonia or exhaustion. The signs of pharyngeal paralysis of central origin are partially or completely masked by others of the fundamental disease. A ready diagnosis of the fundamental disease often results in the pharyngeal paralysis being ignored.

Diagnosis: It is important to know that in animals, especially dogs and cattle, with pharyngeal paralysis, rabies is a possible cause, which should be considered before beginning the physical examination. It is of primary importance to determine whether the paralysis is of central or peripheral origin. Probing with a stomach tube suffices to differentiate between peripheral paralysis and esophageal obstruction. Foreign bodies in the mouth of the horse may lead to error in diagnosis. Corn cobs and sticks may become wedged between the upper arcades of the cheek teeth.

The prognosis is always guarded. When the paralysis is of central origin, it depends on the fundamental process; when peripheral, on the possibility of removing the cause. There is always the danger of aspiration pneumonia.

Treatment: There is no treatment for local paralysis other than efforts to remove the cause, and none should be attempted before making a complete examination. In peripheral paralysis, or that present in equine encephalomyelitis, the animal should be given feed and water through a stomach tube; dehydration may be life threatening. Allowing the animal to lower the head as much as possible aids in the drainage of accumulating fluids and helps prevent inhalation pneumonia.

SALMONELLOSIS

A disease of all animals caused by many species of salmonellae and characterized clinically by one or more of 3 major syndromes—septicemia, acute enteritis, chronic enteritis. The clinically normal carrier animal is a serious problem in all host species. The disease occurs worldwide and the incidence has increased with the intensification of livestock production. Young calves, piglets, lambs, and foals are all susceptible and usually develop the septicemic form (*see* DIARRHEA IN NEONATAL RUMINANTS, p 181, and DIARRHEAL DISEASES OF FOALS, p 187). Adult cattle, sheep, and horses commonly develop acute enteritis, and chronic enteritis may occur in growing pigs and occasionally in cattle (*see also* INTESTINAL DISEASES IN CATTLE, p 179, IN PIGS, p 190, IN SHEEP AND GOATS, p 180, IN HORSES, p 184, and IN DOGS AND CATS, p 232). The incidence of salmonellosis in man has increased in recent years, and animals have been incriminated as the principal reservoir. Transmission to man occurs via contaminated drinking water, milk, meat, eggs, and foods such as cake mixes that utilize contaminated ingredients; pigs and poultry (qv, p 1596) are also important sources of infection.

Etiology and Epidemiology: While many others may cause disease, the more common *Salmonella* spp are: in cattle—*S typhimurium, S dublin, S newport*; in sheep and goats—*S typhimurium, S dublin, S anatum, S montevideo*; in pigs—*S typhimurium, S choleraesuis*; and in horses—*S typhimurium, S anatum, S newport, S enteritidis, S arizonae*. Although the clinical patterns are not distinct, different species of salmonella tend to differ in their epidemiology. Plasmid profile and drug-resistance pattern are sometimes useful markers for epidemiologic studies. Feces of infected animals can contaminate feed and water, milk, fresh and processed meats from abattoirs, plant and animal products used as fertilizers or feedstuffs, pasture and rangeland, and many inert materials. The organisms may survive for months in wet, warm areas such as in feeder pig barns or in water dugouts. Rodents and wild birds also are sources of infection. The prevalence of infection varies between species and countries and is much higher than the incidence of clinical disease, which is commonly precipitated by stressful situations such as sudden deprivation of feed, transportation, drought, crowding, recent parturition, and the administration of some drugs. The disease is common in hospitalized horses that have been subjected to prolonged surgical procedures. Oral antimicrobial agents are sometimes a risk factor for the disease.

The usual route of infection is oral, and following infection, the organism multiplies in the intestine and causes enteritis. Penetration of bacteria into the lamina propria, and production of cytotoxin and enterotoxin likely contribute to gut damage and diarrhea. Septicemia may follow with subsequent localization in brain and meninges, pregnant uterus, distal aspects of the limbs, and tips of the ears and tails, which can result, respectively, in meningoencephalitis, abortion, osteitis, and dry gangrene of the feet, tail, and ears. The organism frequently also localizes in the gallbladder and mesenteric lymph nodes, and survivors intermittently shed the organism in the feces.

Calves rarely become carriers but virtually all adults do for variable periods—up to 10 wk in sheep and in cattle, up to 14 mo in horses. Adult cattle infected with *S dublin* excrete the organism for years. Infection may persist in lymph nodes or tonsils, with no salmonellae in the feces. Such a latent carrier may begin shedding the organism or even develop clinical disease under stress. A passive carrier acquires infection from the environment but is not invaded, so that if removed from the environment, it ceases to be a carrier.

Cattle and Sheep: In calves and lambs, the disease is usually endemic on a particular farm, with sporadic explosive outbreaks. Subclinical infection with occasional herd outbreaks may occur in adult cattle. Stressors that precipitate clinical disease include deprivation of feed and water, long transportation, recent calving, and mixing and crowding in feedlots.

Pigs: Outbreaks of septicemic salmonellosis in pigs are rare, and usually can be traced to a purchased, infected pig. Purchase of feeder pigs from salmonellae-free herds, and use of the "all-in/all-out" policy in finishing units are effective in minimizing exposure.

Horses: Many horses may be carriers. In adults, most cases occur after the stress of surgery or transport, especially when moved through sales yards, deprived of feed and water, and then overfed at their destination. Salmonellosis in horses hospitalized for other causes is a major problem for equine clinics and stud farms. In these circumstances, carriers are constantly reintroduced, the environment is persistently contaminated, and a large population of vulnerable horses is at risk. Septicemic salmonellosis also is common in foals; it may be endemic on a given premises, or there may be outbreaks.

Clinical Findings: Septicemia is the usual syndrome in newborn calves, lambs, foals, and piglets, and outbreaks may occur in pigs up to 6 mo old. Illness is acute, depression is marked, fever (105-107°F [40.5-41.5°C]) is usual, and death occurs in

24-48 hr. In pigs, a dark red to purple discoloration of the skin is common, especially at the ears and ventral abdomen. Nervous signs may occur in calves and pigs; pigs may also suffer from pneumonia. Mortality may reach 100%.

Acute enteritis is the common form in adults and also in calves, usually ≥ 1 wk old. Initially, there is fever (105-107°F [40.5-41.5°C]), followed by severe watery diarrhea, sometimes dysentery, and often tenesmus. In a herd outbreak, several hours may lapse before the onset of diarrhea, at which time the fever may disappear. The feces vary considerably: they may have a putrid odor and contain mucus, fibrinous casts, even shreds of mucous membrane, and in some cases, large blood clots. Rectal examination causes severe discomfort, tenesmus, and commonly, dysentery. Abdominal pain is common and severe in horses. Affected horses are severely dehydrated and may die within 24 hr of the onset of diarrhea; mortality may reach 100%. A marked leukopenia and neutropenia are characteristic of the acute disease in horses.

Subacute enteritis may occur in adult horses and sheep on farms where the disease is endemic. The signs include mild fever (103-104°F [39-40°C]), soft feces, inappetence, and some dehydration. There may be a high incidence of abortion in cows and ewes, some deaths in ewes after abortion, and a high mortality rate due to enteritis in lambs under a few weeks of age. In cattle, the first signs may be fever and abortion followed several days later by diarrhea.

Chronic enteritis is a common form in pigs and adult cattle. There is persistent diarrhea, severe emaciation, intermittent fever, and poor response to treatment. The feces are scant and may be normal or contain mucus, casts, or blood. In growing pigs, rectal stricture may be a sequela if the terminal part of the rectum is involved. Affected pigs are anorectic and lose weight; the abdomen becomes grossly distended. The lesion is obvious on digital palpation and necropsy.

Dogs and cats rarely develop septicemia from salmonellae, although outbreaks in puppies and kittens have been reported. However, they may be asymptomatic carriers, and many of the types important in other domestic mammals and man have been isolated from dogs and cats.

A number of *Salmonella* spp appear in foxes, especially in kits, and produce a peracute enteritis. Fur-bearing and zoo carnivores may be affected. Contaminated feed is often the source of infection. Several rodents (eg, guinea pigs, hamsters, rats, and mice) and rabbits are susceptible (*see* FLZ, p 976 *et seq*). Rodents commonly act as a source of infection on farms where the disease is endemic. Pet turtles were a common source of infection in man, but that risk virtually has been eliminated by the curtailment of commercial trafficking in turtles.

Diagnosis: This depends on the clinical signs and on the laboratory examination of feces, tissues from affected animals, feed (including all mineral supplements used), water supplies, and feces from wild rodents and birds that may inhabit the premises. The clinical syndromes usually are characteristic but must be differentiated from several similar diseases. **In cattle**: enteric colibacillosis, coccidiosis, cryptosporidiosis, the alimentary tract form of infectious bovine rhinotracheitis, bovine viral diarrhea, hemorrhagic enteritis due to *Clostridium perfringens* types B and C, arsenic poisoning, secondary copper deficiency (molybdenosis), winter dysentery, paratuberculosis, ostertagiasis, and dietetic diarrhea. **In pigs**: enteric colibacillosis of newborn pigs and weanlings, swine dysentery, campylobacteriosis, and the septicemias of growing pigs, which include erysipelas, hog cholera, and pasteurellosis. **In sheep**: enteric colibacillosis, septicemia due to *Haemophilus* sp or pasteurellae, and coccidiosis. **In horses**: septicemia due to *Escherichia coli*, *Actinobacillus equuli*, and streptococci, and colitis-X disease.

The lesions are those of a septicemia or a necrotizing fibrinous enteritis. Culture techniques that involve suppression of fecal *E coli* are usually necessary, and several daily fecal cultures may be necessary to isolate the organism. Blood cultures in septicemic animals may be rewarding but are costly. Serological testing is difficult to interpret.

Treatment: Early treatment is essential for septicemic salmonellosis, but there is controversy regarding the use of antimicrobial agents for intestinal salmonellosis.

Oral antibiotics may deleteriously alter the intestinal microflora, interfere with competitive antagonism, and prolong shedding of the organism. There is also concern that antibiotic-resistant strains of salmonellae selected by oral antibiotics may subsequently infect man. Broad-spectrum antibiotics are used parenterally to treat the septicemia. A mixture of trimethoprim and sulfadiazine is effective for the treatment of salmonellosis in calves. Ampicillin also may be useful for treatment of septicemic salmonellosis in all species. Treatment should be continued daily for up to 6 days. Oral medication should be given in drinking water, since affected animals are thirsty due to dehydration, and their appetite is generally poor. Fluid therapy to correct acid-base imbalance and dehydration is necessary. Calves, adult cattle, and horses need large quantities of fluids. Antibiotic treatment and lysis of the organism releases endotoxin. If endotoxic shock develops, corticosteroids may be beneficial. Horses with acute intestinal salmonellosis are severely acidotic and hyponatremic and may need to be treated initially with 5% sodium bicarbonate given IV at 6-9 qt/1000 lb (5-8 L/400 kg) body wt. This is followed by balanced electrolytes containing potassium to correct the hypokalemia that may follow correction of the acidosis. Septicemic salmonellosis in pigs usually responds favorably if treated early. However, the intestinal form is difficult to treat effectively in all species. Although clinical cure may be achieved, bacteriological cure is difficult, particularly in adult animals, because the organisms become established in the biliary system and are intermittently shed into the intestinal lumen, which causes chronic relapsing enteritis and contamination of the environment.

Control and Prevention: This is a major problem because of carrier animals and contaminated feedstuffs. The principles of control include prevention of introduction and limitation of spread within a herd.

Prevention of Introduction: Every effort must be made to prevent introduction of a carrier; animals should be purchased directly only from farms known to be free of the disease. Ensuring that feed supplies are free of salmonellae depends on the integrity of the source.

Limitation of Spread Within a Herd: Certain procedures should be followed in an outbreak. These include: 1) Carrier animals should be identified and either culled or isolated and treated vigorously. Treated animals must be rechecked several times before there can be confidence that they are not carriers. 2) The prophylactic use of antibiotics in feed or water supplies may be considered (but the hazards have been mentioned above). 3) Movement of animals around the farm should be restricted to limit the infection to the smallest group. Random mixing of animals should be avoided. 4) Feed and water supplies must be protected from fecal contamination. 5) Contaminated buildings must be vigorously cleaned and disinfected. 6) Contaminated material must be disposed of carefully. 7) All persons should be aware of the hazards of working with infected animals and the importance of personal hygiene. 8) Use of a vaccine should be considered, although killed salmonellae are not generally effective. An autogenous vaccine can be made, and some commercial, live, avirulent vaccines are now available. 9) Stress should be avoided or minimized as much as possible, particularly in infected herds.

SALMONELLOSIS IN CALVES

Although salmonellae can infect older cattle (*see* above), most cases occur in calves >1 wk old. The clinical picture in young calves is determined by the level of transferred maternal immunity (as in colibacillosis) and the virulence of the specific salmonellae. Calves are dull, feverish, and usually anorectic. There can be systemic invasion and also diarrhea, which can vary from increased amounts of pasty to fluid, yellow or brown feces to dysentery, characteristically with a fetid odor. Weight loss is marked. At necropsy, there is some petechiation, and the intestine is more congested than in colibacillosis. Salmonellae can be isolated from the tissues.

Therapy is usually unsuccessful. Prophylaxis depends on preventing contact with the causative organisms. Vaccination is of little or no value.

TYZZER'S DISEASE
(*Bacillus piliformis* infection)

An acute bacterial infection of a wide range of animals (*see also* pp 1020 and 1062). It occurs worldwide. Acute fatal epidemics occur in laboratory animals. Sporadic fatal infection of foals is common; the disease is rare in dogs, cats, and calves. It primarily affects young, stressed animals. Immmunosuppressive drugs and some antibacterials, especially sulfonamides, predispose animals to the disease. Some species appear resistant unless stressed or immunosuppressed, while others are susceptible without immunosuppression.

Etiology and Pathogenesis: The cause is *Bacillus piliformis*, a motile, filamentous, gram-negative, spore-forming, obligate intracellular bacterium. It does not grow in cell-free media but can be cultured in the yolk sac of chick embryos. The vegetative phase is very labile; spores may survive in soiled bedding at room temperature for 1 yr and can also survive at 133°F (56°C) for 1 hr.

The pathogenesis is poorly understood. Infection most likely results from oral exposure; possible sources include infective spores from the environment, contact with carrier animals, and in foals, ingestion of horse feces. The primary site of infection is the lower intestinal tract with subsequent dissemination via the blood or lymphatics. The bacterium has an affinity for the intestine (epithelial and smooth muscle cells), hepatocytes, and cardiac myocytes. Stress factors such as capture, overcrowding, shipping, and poor sanitation appear to be predisposing. Sulfonamide administration predisposes rabbits to the disease. Mortality is highest at weaning age except in foals, in which the disease occurs between 1 and 6 wk, with most cases between 1 and 2 wk of age. In some species, the disease has been identified concurrently with other diseases, eg, with feline infectious peritonitis, with distemper and mycotic pneumonia in dogs, and with cryptosporidial and coronaviral enteritis in calves.

Clinical Findings: The incubation period in foals is 3-7 days following experimental infection; under natural conditions, the period is unknown. Signs vary slightly between species. Most foals are found in a coma or dead. Clinical signs, if observed, are of short duration from a few hours to 2 days. Signs are variable; they include depression, anorexia, pyrexia, jaundice, diarrhea, and recumbency. Terminally, there are convulsions and coma. Laboratory animals may show depression, ruffled coat, and varying degrees of watery diarrhea; at the start of an outbreak, they often are found dead.

Clinicopathologic tests are of little value in laboratory animals since they die so rapidly. In foals, the serum enzymes sorbitol dehydrogenase, AST (SGOT), alkaline phosphatase, lactate dehydrogenase, and γ-glutamyltransferase are elevated. There is also hyperbilirubinemia, leukopenia or leukocytosis, hemoconcentration, and terminally, profound hypoglycemia (≤20 mg/dL).

Lesions: Characteristic lesions occur in the liver, myocardium, and intestinal tract. In the liver, white, gray, or yellowish foci of necrosis <2 mm in diameter are few to disseminated. The necrosis is most marked in foals and, in addition, there is marked hepatomegaly. In rabbits, severe lesions occur in the intestines and heart. The terminal ileum, cecum, and proximal colon are diffusely reddened. Diffuse ("paint-brush") hemorrhage is frequently present on the serosa of the cecum. Patchy areas of mucosal necrosis are present in the cecum and colon, together with marked edema of the wall of the cecum. Mesenteric lymph nodes may be enlarged and edematous. White streaks in the myocardium may be present, especially near the apex. Intestinal and heart lesions are generally milder or absent in other animals.

Microscopically, randomly distributed and coalescing foci of necrosis in the liver are associated with scant to moderate infiltration of neutrophils and macrophages. The causative bacteria are found in a criss-cross pattern in viable hepatocytes at the periphery of the necrotic foci. In the cecum and colon of rabbits, patchy areas of necrosis extend as deep as the muscularis externa with associated mucosal and submucosal infiltrates of neutrophils. Organisms may be found in the epithelium, muscularis mucosa, and muscularis externa of affected intestine. When cardiac lesions are present, they consist of foci of fiber fragmentation, vacuolation, loss of cross-striations, and minimal WBC infiltration.

Definitive diagnosis is based on demonstration of organisms in tissue sections with special stains. The organism stains poorly with H&E and Gram's stains. With Giemsa stain, the bacillus stains well in the liver and intestinal epithelium and in smears of infected organs, but poorly in smooth muscles and cardiac muscle cells. The Warthin-Starry or Levaditi silver stains are preferable to other stains since the bacillus stains well in the cytoplasm of all infected cells.

Treatment and Control: The disease most often affects well-nourished animals during periods of stress. Under laboratory conditions, stress is created by immunosuppressive drugs or other factors that can be easily identified. With many experiments, stress may be involved as part of the protocol, and when the disease occurs, it is devastating. When it does occur in a colony, treatment is not recommended since it prolongs the disease and possibly produces carrier animals. It is best to destroy all in the colony and attempt to restock with disease-free animals.

Little is known about the effectiveness of antibiotics for treatment; it is known that some aggravate the disease. The organism is sensitive to tetracycline; partially sensitive to streptomycin, erythromycin, penicillin, and chlortetracycline; and resistant to sulfonamides and chloramphenicol.

In foals, the disease seems to be nearly 100% fatal; although it is likely that some foals survive, this is not known because a definitive clinical diagnosis is difficult to obtain. Once the disease is present on a farm, it may occur sporadically year after year. Suspected cases may be treated initially with 50% dextrose IV, followed by 10% dextrose (slowly IV), other fluid therapy, and antibiotics IV. Most foals respond dramatically to the dextrose therapy, but relapse and die in a few hours. Because the disease in foals is sporadic and not highly contagious, specific preventive measures are usually not indicated. Reducing factors that cause stress and immunosuppression lessens incidence of the disease.

ABOMASAL DISORDERS

Disorders include left and right displacement of the abomasum (LDA, RDA), abomasal volvulus (AV), ulcers, and impaction. Displacement or volvulus occurs commonly in dairy cows, particularly high-producers, but also occurs in bulls, calves, and small ruminants. They are rare in beef cattle. Ulcers are seen in dairy and beef cattle and in calves, and are rarely recognized in small ruminants. Impactions can be primary, which is most frequent in beef, or secondary, which develops most often in dairy cows as a form of vagal indigestion. Impactions may have a hereditary basis in some sheep.

LEFT AND RIGHT DISPLACEMENT OF THE ABOMASUM, AND ABOMASAL VOLVULUS

Because the abomasum is suspended loosely by the greater and lesser omenta, it can be moved from its normal position on the right ventral part of the abdomen to the left or right side (LDA, RDA), or rotate on its mesenteric axis while displaced to the right (AV). It can shift from its normal position to left displacement to right displacement over a relatively short period. AV can develop rapidly or slowly from an uncorrected RDA.

Etiology: Although LDA, RDA, and AV (also referred to as RTA for right torsion of the abomasum) are often considered separately, there is evidence of a common underlying etiology; they may be different manifestations of the same or a similar disease process.

The etiology is multifactorial, although abomasal atony and gas production contribute to development of displacement or volvulus. Atony is related to high-concentrate, low-roughage diets, which result in increased production of volatile fatty acids, high concentrations of which reduce abomasal motility. In addition, high-concentrate diets result in a linear increase in gas production (mostly carbon dioxide, methane, and nitrogen). Other contributing factors include decreased abomasal motility associated with hypocalcemia, concurrent diseases (mastitis, metritis, and ketosis), changes in position of intra-abdominal organs, and genetic predisposition.

Of displacements, ~80% occur within 1 mo of parturition; however, they can occur any time. LDA is much more common than RDA (8:1), and cases of volvulus occur even less frequently (25 LDA:1 AV). In some cows, RDA is a precursor to volvulus.

Pathogenesis—LDA: As a result of abomasal atony and gas production, the partially gas-distended abomasum becomes displaced upward along the left abdominal wall lateral to the rumen. It is primarily the fundus and greater curvature of the abomasum that become displaced, which in turn causes displacement of the pylorus and duodenum. The omasum, reticulum, and liver are also rotated to varying degrees. There is probably some interference with the function of the esophageal groove due to slight clockwise rotation of all the stomach compartments, and this impedes passage of ingesta. The obstruction of the displaced segment is incomplete, and although it contains some gas and fluid, a certain amount can still escape, and the distention rarely becomes severe. Since there is no interference with blood supply, the effects of displacement are entirely due to interference with digestion and passage of ingesta, which lead to chronic inanition. A mild metabolic alkalosis with hypochloremia and hypokalemia are common. The hypochloremic metabolic alkalosis is probably due to abomasal atony, continued secretion of hydrochloric acid into the abomasum, and the partial abomasal outflow obstruction, with sequestration of chloride in the abomasum and reflux into the rumen as a result. Hypokalemia is probably due to decreased intake of feeds high in potassium, and continued renal secretion of potassium. Secondary ketosis is common, and may be complicated by development of fatty liver syndrome (qv, p 444).

RDA and AV: Atony, gas production, and displacement of the partially gas-filled abomasum occurs with RDA as it does with LDA. Mild hypokalemic, hypochloremic, metabolic alkalosis occurs as well. Following this dilatation phase, rotation of the abomasum on its mesentery results in local circulatory impairment and ischemia. The volvulus is usually in a counterclockwise direction when viewed from the rear. The omasum is displaced medially and often is involved in the volvulus with occlusion of its blood supply. The liver and reticulum usually are displaced also. A large quantity of fluid accumulates in the abomasum; chloride is sequestered there as well. Hypochloremic, hypokalemic metabolic alkalosis occurs. Compromise of the blood supply to the abomasum, and often the omasum, eventually results in ischemic necrosis of the abomasum as well as dehydration and circulatory failure. As this progresses, a metabolic acidosis is superimposed on the metabolic alkalosis.

Clinical Findings: The typical history with displacement includes anorexia, most commonly a lack of appetite for grain with a decreased or even normal appetite for roughage, and decreased milk production (usually significant, but not as dramatic as with traumatic reticuloperitonitis or other causes of peritonitis). With AV, anorexia is complete, milk production is more markedly and progressively reduced, and clinical deterioration is rapid. Temperature, heart rate, and respiratory rate are usually normal with abomasal displacement. The caudal part of the rib cage on the side of the displacement may appear "sprung". Hydration appears subjectively normal with displacements except in some long-standing cases. Rumen motility may be normal, but often is reduced in frequency and strength of contraction. Feces are usually reduced in quantity and more fluid than normal.

The most important diagnostic physical finding is a ping on simultaneous auscultation and percussion of the abdomen, which should be performed in the area marked by a line from the tuber coxae to the point of the elbow, and from the elbow toward the stifle. The ping characteristic of an LDA is most commonly located in an area between ribs 9 and 13 in the middle to upper third of the abdomen; however, the ping can be more ventral and/or more caudal. Pings associated with a rumen gas cap or rumen collapse are usually more dorsal, less resonant, and extend more caudally through the paralumbar fossa. Rectal examination can confirm a gas-filled rumen or an extremely empty rumen that correlates with the ping in these cases. Pings associated with pneumoperitoneum typically are less resonant, present on both sides of the abdomen, and inconsistent in location on repeated evaluation. Frequently, secondary ketosis is present, which manifests by ketonuria, ketolactia, or an odor of ketones on the breath or in the milk. Ketosis that occurs in association with abomasal displacement responds only transiently to treatment and recurs (as compared with primary ketosis, which develops early in lactation in high-producing cows and responds to therapy permanently if instituted early).

The ping associated with RDA also most commonly underlies the area between ribs 9 and 13. Differentiation between various causes of a right-sided ping is difficult in some cases. A small ping underlying ribs 12 or 13 and extending as far forward as rib 10 is common in cows with functional ileus from a number of causes. It is most often associated with gas in the ascending colon and resolves with correction of the underlying condition. Cecal dilatation and rotation are characterized by a right-sided ping. The ping extends through the dorsal paralumbar fossa in cecal dilatation, and usually is located more caudally (well into the paralumber fossa) in cecal rotation compared with RDA. Palpation per rectum is helpful in differentiating an RDA from cecal dilatation or rotation. Other right-sided pings are produced by pneumoperitoneum or gas in the rectum, descending colon, duodenum, or occasionally, in the ventral sac of the rumen (with chronic vagal indigestion).

Spontaneous fluid splashing or gas tinkling sounds may be heard on auscultation of the area of the ping or on simultaneous ballottement and auscultation of the abdomen (succussion). The characteristic rectal examination findings with LDA include a medially displaced rumen and left kidney. The abomasum is rarely palpable in LDA, and only occasionally in RDA.

The clinical signs associated with AV are more severe than with simple displacements because of the vascular compromise. However, an early AV is indistinguishable from an RDA except by the anatomic position identified at surgery. In contrast with cases of displacement, an animal with AV has tachycardia proportional to the severity of the condition. The area of the ping is usually larger (extending as far forward as rib 8), and the amount of succussible fluid is greater. The animal is more depressed, and signs of weakness, toxemia, and dehydration develop as the disease progresses. The caudal extent of the abomasum is usually palpable per rectum. Without therapy, the animal often becomes recumbent within 48-72 hr after developing volvulus. Death occurs from shock and dehydration, and is sudden if the ischemic abomasum ruptures.

Diagnosis: For displacement or volvulus, diagnosis is based on the presence of a characteristic ping on simultaneous auscultation and percussion and ruling out other causes of left- or right-sided pings. Recent parturition, partial anorexia, and decreased milk production suggest displacement. A ketosis that is only temporarily responsive to treatment is consistent with abomasal displacement, which may be intermittent. The typical signs on physical examination (in addition to the ping), rectal examination, and laboratory evaluation also support the diagnosis. Melena or signs of peritonitis (fever, tachycardia, localized abdominal pain, pneumoperitoneum) with an LDA may indicate a bleeding or perforated abomasal ulcer, respectively.

Treatment: Although rolling a cow through a 70° arc after casting her on her right side corrects most LDA, recurrence is likely. Surgery (various procedures) is generally successful.

Ancillary treatment of animals with displacements include treating any concurrent disease, eg, metritis, mastitis, and ketosis. Calcium borogluconate subcut. helps restore normal abomasal motility in many cases. In simple displacement, fluid and electrolyte abnormalities correct spontaneously with access to water and a salt block. Providing electrolyte water (2 oz [60 g] sodium chloride and 1 oz [30 g] potassium chloride in 5 gal. [19 L] of water) via stomach tube is helpful in cases of longer duration. Animals with significant dehydration and metabolic derangement require IV therapy. Occasionally, animals with abomasal displacement or volvulus will have atrial fibrillation, thought to be of metabolic or neurogenic origin. It is characterized by an irregularly irregular cardiac rhythm with pulse deficits. Correction of the displacement or volvulus results in correction of the atrial fibrillation, although some cases do not resolve for ≥1 mo.

The prognosis after correction of simple LDA or RDA is good, with reported success of 75-95%. Volvulus has a variable and less favorable prognosis; a large quantity of fluid in the abomasum, a high anion gap, a high heart rate, a low plasma chloride concentration, and metabolic acidosis are associated with a poor prognosis.

Prevention: The incidence of displacements can be decreased by adapting to high-concentrate diets and avoiding lead feeding, feeding a complete ration rather than feeding grain b.i.d., maintaining adequate roughage in the diet, avoiding postparturient hypocalcemia, and minimizing or promptly treating concurrent disease.

ABOMASAL ULCERS

A disease of mature cattle and calves with several different manifestations.

Etiology and Pathogenesis: Except for lymphosarcoma of the abomasum and the erosions of the abomasal mucosa that occur with viral diseases such as bovine viral diarrhea, rinderpest, and bovine malignant catarrhal fever, the causes of abomasal ulceration are not well understood. Many different causes have been suggested. Although the disease can occur any time during lactation, abomasal ulcers are common in high-producing, mature dairy cows within the first 6 wk after parturition, which has led to speculation that the cause is a combination of the stress of parturition, the onset of lactation, and heavy grain feeding.

The acute disease occurs in mature dairy and beef cattle following any prolonged stress such as transportation or illness, and in feedlot cattle on high-concentrate rations. Abomasal ulcers may arise in association with abomasal disorders (displacement, volvulus, or impaction), lymphoma, vagal indigestion, or septic conditions, or appear to be unrelated to other disease.

Abomasal ulcers are common in hand-fed calves after they are weaned from milk or milk replacer and begin to eat roughage. Most of these are subclinical and nonhemorrhagic. They may be due to consumption of dry food. Occasionally, milk-fed calves <2 wk old are affected by acute hemorrhagic abomasal ulcers that may perforate and cause rapid death. Well-nourished suckling beef calves, 2-4 mo old, may be affected by acute abomasal ulcers while on summer pasture. Abomasal trichobezoars are common in these calves, but whether the hair balls initiated the ulcers or developed after them is uncertain. Abomasal ulcers and erosions are also seen in calves in association with septic conditions such as enteritis.

Clinical Findings: The syndrome varies depending on whether ulceration is complicated by hemorrhage or perforation, and with the severity of the hemorrhage or the peritonitis that occurs.

A system of classification is based on the depth of penetration, or the degree of hemorrhage or peritonitis caused by the ulcer: Type I is an erosion or ulcer without hemorrhage, Type II is hemorrhagic, Type III is perforated with acute localized peritonitis, and Type IV is perforated with acute diffuse peritonitis. There may be only a single ulcer, or many acute and chronic ulcers.

Cattle with bleeding abomasal ulcers may be asymptomatic except for intermittent occult blood in the feces, or they can die acutely from massive hemorrhage. Common clinical signs include mild abdominal pain, teeth grinding, sudden onset of anorexia, tachycardia (90-100/min), and fecal occult blood or melena that may be intermittent. Signs of blood loss occur with major hemorrhage, including tachycardia (100-140/min), pale mucous membranes, weak pulse, cool extremities, rapid shallow respirations, and melena. More severe signs include acute rumen stasis, generalized abdominal pain with a reluctance to move and an audible grunt or groan with each breath, weakness, and dehydration. As the condition progresses, body temperature drops, and the animal becomes recumbent and dies within 6-8 hr.

In general, bleeding ulcers do not perforate, and perforating ulcers do not bleed into the GI tract sufficiently to produce melena; however, hemorrhage and perforation are seen together in occasional cases, usually those of long-standing duration and/or associated with abomasal displacement.

Calves with abomasal ulceration and hair balls may have a distended gas- and fluid-filled abomasum that is palpable behind the right costal arch. Deep palpation may reveal abdominal pain associated with local peritonitis due to a perforated ulcer. In calves, perforating ulcers are more common than bleeding ulcers.

Lesions: Ulceration is most common along the greater curvature of the abomasum. Most of the ulcers occur on the ventral part of the fundic region, with a few on the border between the fundic and pyloric regions. The single or multiple ulcers measure from a few mm to 5 cm in diameter. The affected artery is usually visible after ingesta and necrotic tissue are removed from a bleeding ulcerated area. Most cases of perforation are walled off by the omentum, which forms a cavity 12-15 cm in diameter that contains degenerated blood and necrotic debris. Material from this cavity may infiltrate widely through the omental fat. Adhesions may form between the ulcer and surrounding organs or the abdominal wall. Multiple trichobezoars are common in the abomasum of beef calves with abomasal ulcers.

Diagnosis: In cases with only slight bleeding and mild clinical signs, diagnosis may require repeated fecal evaluations for occult blood. Other conditions that can cause partial anorexia and decreased milk production should be ruled out by physical examination and laboratory tests, including abdominocentesis. In cases with melena, the diagnosis can be based on physical examination alone. A PCV can help to determine the degree of hemorrhage. An occult blood test of the feces can confirm melena. Other conditions that result in blood in the feces should be eliminated. Blood from portions of the GI tract distal to the abomasum reacts on fecal occult blood tests; it is usually bright red if produced by the large intestine, or raspberry colored if from the small intestine. Animals with abomasal lymphosarcoma can have a bleeding syndrome similar to that associated with abomasal ulcers, but do not respond to therapy. Occasionally, oral, pharyngeal, and laryngeal lesions bleed, and the blood is swallowed and appears in the feces. Similarly, pulmonary abscesses that form as a sequela of rumenitis by embolization to the lungs and liver can erode blood vessels and result in hemoptysis; if swallowed, this too can result in melena. Fecal occult blood may also be due to abomasal volvulus (AV) or blood-sucking helminths.

Diagnosis of perforating abomasal ulcers is based on physical examination and ruling out other causes of peritonitis. Abomasal ulceration with perforation and local peritonitis may be indistinguishable from chronic traumatic reticuloperitonitis. A magnet in the reticulum (confirmed by use of a compass) or an accurate history of having given the cow a magnet before the onset of signs decreases the likelihood of traumatic reticuloperitonitis. Reticular radiographs may confirm or rule out the presence of radiopaque foreign bodies in the reticulum. In some cases, there is a neutrophilia, possibly with a left shift. Evaluation of peritoneal fluid will confirm peritonitis if total protein and nucleated cell count are elevated. Rarely are intracellular bacteria or degenerate neutrophils seen because, in most cases, the infection is rapidly walled off. The diagnosis of diffuse peritonitis due to perforation is based on physical examination and ruling out of other causes. Rupture of a distended viscus such as AV or cecal rotation produces similar signs. Regardless of the cause of diffuse peritonitis, the prognosis is grave because of overwhelming infection and cardiovascular deterioration. There is neutrophilia with a marked left shift and hemoconcentration. Abdominal fluid is usually readily obtainable in large quantities, and the protein level is elevated; the nucleated cell count may be elevated, or it may be normal due to dilution or utilization.

Treatment: Most cases of abomasal ulcers are treated medically. This includes dietary management, primarily withholding concentrates (eg, high-moisture corn, silage, and concentrates that are finely ground), and providing good-quality roughage, as well as boxstall confinement and elimination of other sources of stress. Broad-spectrum antibiotic therapy (continued for 1-2 wk or until the rectal temperature is normal for 48 hr) is indicated for perforating ulcers. The use of antacids is controversial but seems to be effective in some cases. Because nonsteroidal anti-inflammatory drugs can contribute to ulceration, their use is contraindicated. The prognosis for localized peritonitis associated with perforating abomasal ulcers is good with medical therapy and dietary alteration. Recovery generally takes 1-2 wk, and animals that are fully recovered for 1-2 wk generally do not experience recurrence. Animals in late gestation tend to have a more chronic course, with repeated ulceration and a decreased ability to wall off the perforation. Usually, surgery is indicated for perforating abomasal ulcers only if the abomasum is displaced; however, significant abdominal contamination can occur in the process of breaking down adhesions and resecting or oversewing the ulcer. Cases in which the ulcerated area is resected or oversewn usually recover.

Animals with diffuse peritonitis following perforation of an abomasal ulcer rarely respond to therapy, and the prognosis is grave. Attempts at treatment consist of rapid and continued IV fluid therapy based on the current metabolic status, and IV broad-spectrum antibiotics. Corticosteroids are sometimes used in nonpregnant animals initially to counteract shock, but should not be continued. The few animals that recover from diffuse peritonitis usually have massive abdominal adhesions.

For bleeding ulcers, blood transfusions and fluid therapy may be necessary in addition to dietary management, stall confinement, and oral antacids. If hemorrhage is acute, the PCV may not reflect the severity because equilibration between intravascular and extravascular fluid following blood loss takes ~24 hr. In addition, concurrent dehydration results in a higher PCV. Generally, a transfusion is required if the PCV is <14%. Cross-matching is not usually necessary; a single transfusion of 4-6 L of blood is commonly effective. Some cattle will require more than one transfusion in the course of several days. Complete recovery usually takes 1-2 wk. The prognosis is good if severe anemia has not developed before treatment is started. If treated aggressively, many recover even after developing severe anemia. When the abomasum is displaced in conjunction with bleeding ulcers, the displacement should be corrected as soon as the animal is stable since this usually results in cessation of hemorrhage.

Prevention: Minimizing stress by good management (adequate space, ventilation, access to water, etc), and providing a diet with sufficient roughage and concentrates with larger particle size reduce the incidence.

DIETARY ABOMASAL IMPACTION

Impaction occurs during cold winter months and when cattle are fed poor-quality roughage. The disease is most common in pregnant beef cattle that increase their intake of low-quality roughage during extremely cold weather in an attempt to meet the increased needs. The disease also has occurred in feedlot cattle fed a variety of mixed rations containing chopped or ground roughage (straw, hay) and cereal grains, and in late-pregnancy dairy cows on similar feeds.

Etiology: The cause is considered to be consumption of excess roughage that is low in both digestible protein and energy. Impaction with sand can occur if cattle are fed hay or silage on sandy soils, or root crops that are sandy or dirty. When long roughage without sufficient grain is fed during very cold weather, the cattle cannot eat enough to satisfy energy needs so roughage may then be chopped. The chopped roughage is commonly mixed with some, but frequently not enough, grain to meet energy requirements. Cattle do eat more of these chopped roughage-grain mixtures than long roughage because the smaller particles pass through the forestomachs more rapidly, but impaction of the abomasum, omasum, and rumen may occur because of the relative indigestibility of the roughage. Outbreaks may affect up to

15% of all pregnant cattle on individual farms when the ambient temperature drops to $-14°F$ ($-26°C$) or lower for several days.

Pathogenesis: Chopped roughage and finely ground feeds pass through the forestomachs more quickly than long roughage, and perhaps the combination of low digestibility and excessive intake leads to excessive accumulation in the forestomachs and abomasum. When large quantities of sand are ingested, the omasum, abomasum, large intestine, and cecum can become impacted. The sand that accumulates in the abomasum causes abomasal atony and chronic dilatation. Once impaction of the abomasum occurs, subacute obstruction of the upper GI tract develops. Ions of hydrogen and chloride are continually secreted into the abomasum in spite of the impaction, and atony and an alkalosis with hypochloremia result. Varying degrees of dehydration occur because fluids are not moving beyond the abomasum into the duodenum for absorption. Sequestration of potassium ions in the abomasum results in hypokalemia. Dehydration, alkalosis, electrolyte imbalance, and progressive starvation occur. Impaction of the abomasum may be severe enough to cause irreversible abomasal atony.

Clinical Findings and Lesions: Complete anorexia, scant feces, moderate distention of the abdomen, weight loss, weakness, and recumbency are usually the initial signs. Body temperature is usually normal, but may be subnormal during cold weather. A mucoid nasal discharge tends to collect at the external nares and on the muzzle; usually, the muzzle is dry and cracked due to the failure of the animal to lick its nostrils, and to the effects of dehydration. The heart rate may be increased, and mild dehydration is common.

Most often the rumen is static and distended with dry contents, but it may contain excess fluid if the cow has been fed finely ground feed. The pH of the ruminal fluid is usually normal (6.5-7). Protozoal activity in the rumen ranges from normal to a marked reduction in numbers and activity as assessed on a low-power field. The impacted abomasum is usually in the right lower quadrant on the floor of the abdomen. In feedlot steers and nonpregnant heifers, the impacted abomasum and omasum may be easily palpable on rectal examination, but may not be in the pregnant animal. Deep palpation and strong percussion of the right flank may elicit a "grunt" as is common in acute traumatic reticuloperitonitis, probably because of distention of the abomasum and stretching of its serosa.

Severely affected cattle die 3-6 days after the onset of signs. Rupture of the abomasum occurs in some cases, and death from acute, diffuse peritonitis and shock occurs precipitously in a few hours. In sand impaction, there is considerable weight loss, chronic diarrhea with sand in the feces, weakness, recumbency, and death in a few weeks.

Metabolic alkalosis, hypochloremia, hypokalemia, hemoconcentration, and total and differential WBC count within the normal range are common. At necropsy, the abomasum is commonly enlarged up to twice normal size and impacted with dry rumen-like contents. The omasum may be similarly enlarged and impacted with the same contents. The rumen is usually grossly enlarged and filled with dry contents or fluid. The GI tract beyond the pylorus is characteristically empty and has a dry appearance. Varying degrees of dehydration and emaciation are also present. If rupture of the abomasum has occurred, lesions of acute diffuse peritonitis are present.

Diagnosis: Clinical diagnosis is based on the nutritional history, clinical evidence of impaction, and laboratory results. The disease must be differentiated from secondary abomasal impaction as a form of vagal indigestion, or omasal impaction.

Impaction of the abomasum as a complication of traumatic reticuloperitonitis usually occurs in late pregnancy, commonly only in one animal; a mild fever may or may not be present, and there may be a grunt on deep palpation of the xiphoid. The rumen is usually enlarged and may be atonic or hypermotile. In many cases, it is impossible to distinguish between the 2 causes of impacted abomasum, and a laparotomy may be necessary to explore the abdomen for peritoneal lesions.

Treatment: The challenge is to recognize the cases that will respond to treatment and those that will not, ie, to determine those that should be slaughtered immediately for salvage. Cows with a severely impacted abomasum, that are weak, and have a marked tachycardia (100-120/min) are poor treatment risks and should be slaughtered. Rational treatment consists of correcting the metabolic alkalosis, hypochloremia, hypokalemia, and dehydration, and attempting to move the impacted material with lubricants and cathartics, or surgically emptying the abomasum. Balanced electrolyte solutions are infused IV continuously for up to 72 hr at a daily rate of 1.5-2 oz/lb (100-130 mL/kg) body wt. Some respond well to this therapy and begin ruminating and passing feces in 48 hr.

Dioctyl sodium sulfosuccinate (DSS; docusate sodium) is given by stomach tube at 4-6 oz (120-180 mL) of a 25% solution for a 1000-lb (450-kg) animal mixed with ~5 gal. (20 L) of warm water, and repeated daily for 3-5 days. Alternatively, 2.5 gal. (10 L) of mineral oil mixed with an equal volume of water can be used. The amount of mineral oil can be increased to 3.75 gal. (15 L)/day after day 3 and for a few days until recovery is apparent. Mineral oil and DSS should not be administered simultaneously since DSS may potentiate the absorption of mineral oil. A beneficial response cannot be expected in <24 hr; most cattle that do respond will do so by the end of day 3 after treatment begins.

Surgery may be considered but results are often unsuccessful, probably because of abomasal atony, which appears to worsen following surgery. An alternative may be to do a rumenotomy, empty the rumen, and infuse DSS directly into the abomasum through the reticulo-omasal orifice in an attempt to soften and promote the evacuation of the contents of the abomasum. Secondary impactions that occur as a sequela of traumatic reticuloperitonitis or abomasal volvulus usually show signs of vagal indigestion, and abomasal impaction may be diagnosed at the time of exploratory surgery.

The induction of parturition using dexamethasone (20 mg, IM) may be indicated in affected cattle within 2 wk of term and in which the response to treatment for a few days has been unsuccessful. Parturition may assist recovery because of a reduction in intra-abdominal volume. For sand impaction, affected cattle should be moved off the sandy soil and fed good hay and a grass mixture containing molasses and minerals. Severely affected cattle should be treated with large doses of mineral oil (≥3.75 gal. [15 L]/day).

Control: Prevention is possible by providing the necessary nutrient requirements for wintering pregnant beef cattle. Allowances should be made for cold, windy weather when energy needs may be 30-40% greater than during warm weather. When low-quality roughage is to be used for wintering pregnant beef cattle, it should be analyzed for crude protein and digestible energy. Based on the analysis, grain is usually added to the ration to meet the energy and protein requirements.

The nutrient requirements of beef cattle (qv, p 1171) are guidelines for use under average conditions; higher nutrient levels than those indicated may be necessary, particularly during periods of severe cold stress. Adequate fresh drinking water should be supplied at all times, and the practice of forcing wintering cows to obtain their water requirements by eating snow while on low-quality roughage is hazardous. Whether low-quality roughages should be chopped or ground for wintering pregnant beef cattle is controversial. The daily voluntary intake of low-quality roughage can be increased by chopping or grinding, but neither processing method increases quality or digestibility; in fact, digestibility is usually decreased. If increased consumption during cold weather exceeds physical capacity, impaction of the abomasum may occur.

ABOMASAL BLOAT IN LAMBS

Feeding systems that allow lambs to drink large quantities of milk replacer at infrequent intervals predispose them to abomasal bloat. This situation can occur under *ad lib* feeding when the milk replacer is kept at ~60°F (15°C) or higher, and particularly if it had not been available for several hours, eg, lambs fed warm milk replacer *ad lib* b.i.d. appear to be very susceptible. *Ad lib* feeding of cold milk

replacers that contain few or no insoluble ingredients, and are adequately refrigerated, results in little or no bloating. The cause is thought to be a sudden overfilling
of the abomasum followed by the proliferation of organisms that release an excess
quantity of gas that cannot escape from the abomasum. The severe distention causes
compression of the thoracic and abdominal viscera and blood vessels leading to
them. This results in asphyxia and acute heart failure. Affected lambs become
grossly distended within 1 hr after feeding and die a few minutes after the distention
of the abdomen is clinically obvious. At necropsy, the abomasum is grossly distended with gas, fluid, and milk replacer that usually is not clotted. The abomasal
mucosa is hyperemic.

The addition of formalin (37% formaldehyde) at the rate of 0.1%, to a 20%
solids milk replacer minimizes the incidence of abomasal bloat without adversely
affecting the performance of artificially reared lambs.

ACUTE INTESTINAL OBSTRUCTIONS, LG AN

Intestinal obstructions occur in all large animal species but are most common in
horses. Cattle are the most commonly affected ruminants; diagnosis in sheep and
goats is rare. Those other than inguinal hernias are infrequently recognized in pigs.
In general, obstructions are mechanical or functional, and occur in any part of the
intestinal tract. They can interrupt flow of ingesta with or without vascular compromise (strangulating or simple obstruction, respectively).

Etiology and Pathogenesis: The inciting cause of an intestinal obstruction often is
not determined. Functional obstructions are associated with altered intestinal motility, often due to dietary or management factors, parasite infection, enteritis, or peritonitis. Mechanical obstructions (physical blockage of ingesta) occur due to
abnormalities in the bowel lumen, in the wall, or outside the tract.

Specific causes in cattle include cecal dilatation and rotation, intussusception,
volvulus of the small intestine, and volvulus at the root of the mesentery. Decreased
motility caused by accumulation of volatile fatty acids, possibly related to high-
concentrate rations or abrupt increase in the concentrate:forage ratio, have been suggested as causes of cecal dilatation and rotation in cattle. They also are associated
with advanced pregnancy and ileus from concurrent disease. Intussusceptions are
thought to be the result of irregular peristaltic movements related to enteritis, intestinal parasites, dietary disorders, and bowel tumors. Altered intestinal motility may
also cause intestinal volvulus. Obstructions of the small intestine can occur due to a
variety of fibrous bands (eg, adhesions, parovarian bands, falciform ligament), mural thickening (eg, intestinal adenocarcinoma), extramural masses (eg,
lymphosarcoma, fat necrosis, abdominal abscesses), or herniation (inguinal or umbilical). Adhesions and abdominal abscesses can form subsequent to peritonitis, IP
injections, or previous abdominal surgery.

In horses, transient functional obstructions are common, as are feed impactions,
which usually involve the pelvic flexure. Parasite infection and/or migration, dental
abnormalities, and dietary or management factors are often implicated. Impactions
and other luminal obstructions can result from coarse feeds, reduced water intake,
enteroliths, or ingested foreign material. Sites of impaction other than the pelvic
flexure are the small colon, transverse colon, right dorsal colon, cecum, and ileum.
Other causes of intestinal obstruction in horses are volvulus (twist on the mesenteric
axis), torsion (twist along the long axis of the bowel), and displacement of the
ascending (large) colon; and volvulus of part or all of the small intestine. Altered
motility and possibly strenuous exercise and rolling may be initiating causes.
Broodmares may be predisposed to volvulus, torsion, or displacement of the ascending colon during gestation and shortly after parturition. Obstruction occurs due
to incarceration of the intestine (usually small) by herniation through the umbilicus,
inguinal canal, diaphragm, mesenteric defects or epiploic foramen; or because of
fibrous bands (adhesions, mesodiverticular bands, or stalks of pedunculated lipomas). Standardbred stallions and colts develop inguinal and scrotal hernias more

commonly than other breeds. Diaphragmatic hernias and mesenteric defects may be congenital or traumatically induced. Adhesions in horses are most often the sequela of parasite migration, and also occur frequently after abdominal surgery; however, most adhesions are clinically silent. Pedunculated lipomas are common in older horses. Ileocecal, cecocecal, cecocolic, and small-intestinal intussusception also occur. Lymphosarcoma and other abdominal neoplasms as well as abdominal abscesses can cause intestinal obstruction.

Clinical Findings: Intestinal obstruction in horses is generally manifest as abdominal pain (see COLIC, p 168). Signs of abdominal pain in cattle include treading, stretching, and kicking at the abdomen, and less commonly rolling and bellowing. These signs are generally more subtle than in horses and are usually referable to small-intestinal distention, tension on the intestinal mesentery (by the weight of distended bowel), or vascular impairment. Although seen in only a small percentage of cases, the most common cause in cattle, usually referred to as indigestion, is a functional obstruction that results from abrupt change in the diet. Signs of pain are relatively consistent but often transient with intussusceptions, and are seen in some cases of cecal rotation. Cattle with volvulus of the small intestine at the root of the mesentery are severely affected.

Usually, cattle with intestinal obstruction are anorectic and pass little or no feces, and lactating cows produce less milk. The feces that are passed may be covered with mucus, or mixed or coated with blood. Thick, raspberry-colored blood mixed with scant feces is characteristic of small intestinal bleeding, particularly that associated with intussusception. It can also occur with severe indigestion. Blood from the colon or rectum is generally a brighter red color. Melena is typical of abomasal bleeding.

Abdominal distention, usually with a ping on simultaneous auscultation and percussion, in the upper right abdominal quadrant occurs with cecal rotation. Cecal dilatation does not produce abdominal distention, but a ping is generally present in the dorsal paralumbar fossa. In cecal dilatation and rotation, the cecum is palpable per rectum either with the apex pointed toward the pelvic inlet (dilatation) or as a curved, inner-tube-shaped structure (rotation). Rumen motility is usually present, and metabolic and cardiovascular derangements tend to be mild except in cecal rotation of long duration.

Abdominal distention in the lower right abdominal quadrant is sometimes seen with small intestinal distention. Distended loops of bowel may be palpable on rectal examination, and fluid may be heard when the abdomen is simultaneously balloted and auscultated. Small areas of tympanic resonance may be heard on simultaneous auscultation and percussion. Intussusceptions and fibrous bands that cause small intestinal obstruction can be palpated rectally in some cases.

Profound changes in cardiovascular parameters, such as tachycardia, abnormal mucous membrane color, prolonged capillary refill time, and dehydration, are most commonly associated with strangulating obstructions, such as volvulus of the small intestine. Volvulus of the small intestine or volvulus at the root of the mesentery is characterized by acute onset and rapid cardiovascular deterioration. This is in contrast with cecal dilatation or rotation or with intussusceptions that can continue for several days.

Metabolic derangements range from hypokalemic, hypochloremic metabolic alkalosis in long-standing small-intestinal and duodenal obstructions, to severe metabolic acidosis with strangulating obstructions. Usually, there are no metabolic derangements in mild functional obstructions and early (simple) mechanical obstructions, particularly if a relatively distal part of the intestinal tract is involved. Hypocalcemia can develop, presumably due to decreased calcium absorption from the duodenum.

Peritoneal fluid changes reflect the degree of peritonitis and may aid in the diagnosis in both cattle and horses, although the results seem to be more variable in cattle. Strangulating obstructions are characterized by an increase in RBC, with subsequent elevations in total protein and nucleated cell counts due to extravasation through the bowel wall. Neutrophils become degenerative, and intracellular gram-positive and gram-negative bacteria are seen as the integrity of the bowel wall is lost. Plant material in the peritoneal cavity is indicative of bowel rupture or inadvertent enterocentesis. Simple obstructions with severe dilatation of the bowel can be associated with elevations of total protein and, less commonly, nucleated cell counts. Peritoneal fluid analysis is normal with most simple mechanical and functional obstructions. When neoplasms are present, neoplastic cells are sometimes identified in peritoneal fluid.

Treatment: For treatment of obstruction in horses, *see* COLIC, p 168. Treatment of functional obstructions in cattle is generally symptomatic and supportive after identifying and eliminating the inciting cause (eg, excessive grain intake), and allowing time for normal intestinal motility to return. Some cases require correction (PO or IV) of dehydration and electrolyte imbalances. Lactating cows often benefit from calcium borogluconate administered subcut., and secondary ketosis should be treated if present. Occasionally, cases of functional obstruction require surgical decompression.

Mechanical obstructions almost always require surgery. Prophylactic antibiotic therapy should be started preoperatively; supportive therapy such as fluids, electrolytes, and calcium should be administered if needed. The prognosis with most functional obstructions is good with appropriate supportive therapy, particularly if the inciting cause is identified and eliminated.

Horses that require exploratory celiotomy to correct an intestinal obstruction have an overall survival rate of 50%. Strangulating obstructions have a lower survival rate compared with simple obstructions, but early surgical intervention can improve the prognosis.

In cattle, cecal dilation and rotation have a good prognosis, although 10% of cases recur, and cases with cecal rotation of long-standing duration can develop ischemic necrosis. Cases of small-intestinal obstruction amenable to resection and anastomosis have a fair to good prognosis. Cows with volvulus of the small intestine or at the root of the mesentery have a poor prognosis unless they are diagnosed and surgically corrected within a few hours of onset.

Prevention: Abrupt changes in feeding and management, inadequate water intake, parasite infection, dental abnormalities, and access to coarse feeds and foreign material should be avoided or corrected.

BLOAT IN RUMINANTS
(Ruminal tympany)

An overdistention of the rumenoreticulum with the gases of fermentation, either in the form of a persistent foam mixed with the ruminal contents, or in the form of free gas separated from the ingesta. Predominantly a disorder of cattle, it may also occur in sheep.

Etiology—Primary Ruminal Tympany (Frothy Bloat): The cause of frothy bloat is entrapment of the normal gases of fermentation in a stable foam. It occurs mainly on legume pasture and on high-level grain diets, but individual susceptibility may be influenced genetically. Coalescence of the small gas bubbles is inhibited and intraruminal pressure increases because eructation cannot occur. Susceptible animals have a higher concentration of small feed particles suspended in the rumen, and the contents contain small yellow bubbles before feeding. The immediate effect of feeding is probably to supply nutrients for a burst of microbial fermentation. However, the major factor that determines if bloat will occur is the nature of the ruminal contents. Plant proteins are the primary foaming agent. Protein content and rate of digestion reflect the forage's potential for causing bloat. Over a 24-hr period, the bloat-causing forage and unknown animal factors combine to maintain an elevated concentration of small feed particles and enhance the susceptibility to bloat. Legume forages such as alfalfa and clover have a higher percentage of protein and are digested more quickly. In cattle fed alfalfa, the small feed particles contain

~50% protein. Other legumes, such as sainfoin and birdsfoot trefoil, are high in protein but do not cause bloat, probably because they contain condensed tannins, which precipitate protein, and are digested more slowly than alfalfa or clover. Leguminous bloat is most common when cattle are placed on lush pastures, particularly those dominated by rapidly growing leguminous plants, but can also occur when high-quality hay is fed.

The cause of the foam in feedlot bloat is uncertain but is thought to be either the production of insoluble slime by certain species of rumen bacteria in cattle fed high carbohydrate diets, or the entrapment of the gases of fermentation by the fine particle size of ground feed. Fine particulate matter, such as in finely ground grain, can markedly affect foam stability. Feedlot bloat is most common in cattle that have been on a grain diet for 1-2 mo. This timing may be due to the increase in the level of grain feeding, or the time it takes for the slime-producing rumen bacteria to proliferate to large enough numbers.

Secondary Ruminal Tympany (Free Gas Bloat): Physical obstruction of eructation occurs in esophageal obstruction caused by a foreign body, stenosis, or pressure from enlargement outside the esophagus (as from lymphadenopathy). Interference with esophageal groove function in vagal indigestion and diaphragmatic hernia may cause chronic ruminal tympany. This also occurs in tetanus. Tumors and other lesions of the esophageal groove or the reticular wall are less common causes of obstructive bloat. There also may be interference with the nerve pathways that maintain the eructation reflex. Lesions of the wall of the reticulum (which contains tension receptors and receptors that discriminate between gas, foam, and liquid) may interrupt the normal reflex that is essential for escape of gas from the rumen.

Ruminal tympany also can be secondary to the acute onset of ruminal atony that occurs in anaphylaxis and in grain overload; this causes a reduction in rumen pH and possibly an esophagitis and rumenitis that can interfere with eructation. Chronic ruminal tympany is relatively frequent in calves up to 6 mo old without apparent cause; this form usually resolves spontaneously.

Unusual postures, particularly lateral recumbency, are commonly characterized by secondary tympany; ruminants may die of bloat if they become accidentally cast in dorsal recumbency or other restrictive positions in handling facilities, crowded transportation vehicles, or irrigation ditches.

Clinical Findings: Bloat is a common cause of sudden death: cattle not observed closely, such as pastured and feedlot cattle and dry dairy cattle usually are found dead; in lactating dairy cattle, which are observed regularly, bloat commonly begins within 1 hr after being turned onto a bloat-producing pasture. Bloat may occur on the first day after being placed on the pasture, but more commonly on the second or third days.

In primary pasture bloat, obvious distention of the rumen occurs suddenly, and distention of the left flank may be so severe that the contour of the paralumbar fossa protrudes above the vertebral column, and the entire abdomen is enlarged. As the bloat progresses, the skin over the left flank becomes progressively more taut and in severe cases cannot be "tented". Dyspnea and grunting are marked and are accompanied by mouth breathing, protrusion of the tongue, and extension of the head. Occasionally, vomiting occurs. Rumen motility does not decrease until the animal is severely bloated. If the tympany continues to worsen, the animal will collapse and die. Death may occur within 1 hr after grazing began but is more common ~3-4 hr after onset of clinical signs. In a group of affected cattle, there are usually several with clinical bloat and some with mild to moderate distention of the abdomen.

In secondary bloat, the excess gas is usually free on top of the solid and fluid ruminal contents, although frothy bloat may occur in vagal indigestion when there is increased ruminal activity. In free-gas bloat the passage of a stomach tube or trocarization releases large quantities of gas and alleviates distention.

Lesions: Necropsy findings are characteristic. There is marked congestion and hemorrhage of the lymph nodes of the head and neck, epicardium, and upper respiratory tract. The lungs are compressed, and intrabronchial hemorrhage may be present. The cervical esophagus is congested and hemorrhagic, but the thoracic portion of the esophagus is pale and blanched—the demarcation known as the "bloat line" of the esophagus. The rumen is distended but the contents usually are much less frothy than before death. The liver is pale due to expulsion of blood from the organ.

Diagnosis: Usually, the clinical diagnosis of frothy bloat is obvious. The causes of secondary bloat must be ascertained by clinical examination to determine the cause of the failure of eructation.

Treatment: In life-threatening cases, an emergency rumenotomy may be necessary; it is followed by an explosive release of ruminal contents, and marked relief for the cow. Recovery is usually uneventful with only occasional minor complications.

A trocar and cannula may be used for emergency relief, although the standard-sized instrument is not large enough to allow the viscous, stable foam in peracute cases to escape quickly enough. A larger bore instrument (1 in. [2.5 cm] in diameter) is necessary, but an incision through the skin must be made before it can be inserted through the muscle layers and into the rumen. If the cannula fails to reduce the bloat and the animal's life is compromised, an emergency rumenotomy should be performed. If the cannula provides some relief, the antifoaming agent of choice can be administered through the cannula, which can remain in place until the animal has returned to normal, usually within several hours.

When the animal's life is not immediately threatened, passing a stomach tube of the largest bore possible is recommended. A few attempts should be made to clear the tube by blowing and moving it back and forth in an attempt to find large pockets of rumen gas that can be released. In frothy bloat, it may be impossible to reduce the pressure with the tube, and an antifoaming agent should be administered while the tube is in place. If the bloat is not relieved quickly by the antifoaming agent, the animal must be observed carefully for the next hour to determine if the treatment has been successful, or if an alternative therapy is necessary.

A variety of antifoaming agents are effective, including vegetable oils (eg, peanut, corn, soybean) and mineral oils (paraffins), at doses of 80-250 mL. Dioctyl sodium sulfosuccinate, a surfactant, is commonly incorporated into one of the above oils; sold as proprietary anti-bloat remedies, these are effective if administered early.

Control—Pasture Bloat: Prevention of pasture bloat can be difficult. Management practices that have been used include feeding hay before turning cattle on pasture, maintaining grass dominance in the sward, or using strip grazing to restrict intake. For hay to be effective, it must comprise at least one-third of the diet. Feeding hay or strip grazing may be reliable when the pasture is only moderately dangerous, but these methods are less reliable when the pasture is in the pre-bloom stage and the bloat potential is high. Mature pastures are less likely to cause bloat than immature or rapidly growing pastures.

The only satisfactory method available for preventing pasture bloating is strategic administration of an antifoaming agent. This is widely practiced in grassland countries such as Australia and New Zealand. The most reliable method is b.i.d. drenching, eg, at milking times, with an antifoaming agent. Spraying the agent onto the bloat-potent pasture is equally effective, provided that the animals have access only to treated pasture. This method is ideal for strip grazing but not when grazing is uncontrolled. The antifoaming agent may be added to the feed or water, but success with this method depends on adequate individual intake. The agent also may be incorporated into blocks or painted on the flanks of the animals from which it is licked during the day. These methods are wasteful, and some animals will not lick and thus will not be protected.

Available antifoaming agents include oils and fats and synthetic nonionic surfactants. Oils and fats are given at 2-4 oz (60-120 mL)/head/day; doses up to 8 oz (240 mL) are indicated during most dangerous periods. Poloxalene, a synthetic polymer, is a highly effective nonionic surfactant given at 10-20 g/head/day and up to 40 g in high-risk situations. It can be added to water, feed grain mixtures, and mineral blocks. Alcohol ethoxylate detergents are equally effective and are more palatable than poloxalene.

The ultimate aim in control is development of a pasture that permits high production, yet causes a low incidence of bloat. Current research centers on developing strains of legumes that have low bloat potential. On a practical basis, the use of pastures of clover and grasses in equal amounts comes closest to achieving this goal. Alternatively, animals with bloat-prone dams or sires should not be kept as replacements. Research in this area centers on identifying the genetically predisposed animal and eliminating it from breeding programs.

Feedlot Bloat: Feedlot rations should contain at least 10-15% cut or chopped roughage mixed into the complete feed. Preferably the roughage should be a cereal, grain straw, grass hay, or equivalent. Grains should be rolled or cracked, not finely ground. Pelleted rations made from finely ground grain should be avoided. The addition of tallow (3-5% of the total ration) may be successful occasionally, but it was not effective in controlled trials. The nonionic surfactants such as poloxalene have been ineffective in preventing feedlot bloat.

BOVINE VIRAL DIARRHEA (BVD), MUCOSAL DISEASE COMPLEX

An infectious disease of cattle caused by a pestivirus (family Togaviridae). The infection is usually subclinical or mild with high morbidity and low mortality, but severe disease with high mortality also occurs. BVD virus is immunosuppressive and may predispose to, or exacerbate, outbreaks of concurrent disease.

Epidemiology: The disease has been recognized in many parts of the world. Cattle of all ages are susceptible, but it is most common in animals 8-24 mo old. Although calves may receive antibodies in colostrum, antibody levels decline by 3-8 mo of age, and calves can then become infected. Infection of the fetus with noncytopathic strains of BVD virus before the fetus achieves immunocompetence (~120 days gestation) may result in persistent infection and immunotolerance. Such calves may be born alive and survive for varying periods up to adulthood; they are persistent carriers and shedders of BVD virus and are seronegative. As such, they are important in perpetuation of the disease and can be a source of infection when introduced into a herd. Seroprevalence surveys indicate that infection is common. The virus is present in high titer in the secretions and excretions of infected animals, and transmission is by direct contact or by contaminated feed or other materials; however, persistent shedders are seronegative. The incubation period is variable but is generally ~5-10 days.

Clinical Findings: Severe cases are characterized by fever, anorexia, depression, erosions and hemorrhages of the GI tract, diarrhea, and dehydration. In mild cases, diarrhea may not be prominent. Most BVD infections are subclinical, and the course of the disease varies from 2-3 days up to 3 wk; however, this results in measurable increases in antibody levels. Cattle with acute BVD can die in 48 hr. Most affected cattle are anorectic and exhibit oral lesions and mild diarrhea for 2-4 days. Calves with clinical BVD are dull, depressed, and anorectic, and mild bloat may occur. Temperatures are 104-106°F (40-41°C) early, but usually return to normal or below in 1-2 days and before diarrhea occurs. Diphasic temperature elevation has been detected in experimental infection, but seldom is observed in field cases. Heart and respiratory rates are generally increased. The feces may contain mucus or blood and have a foul odor; watery diarrhea can occur and lead to rapid dehydration. If the diarrhea is profuse, the prognosis is grave.

Oral lesions are present in ~75% of clinical cases when the animals start to scour. Typically, there is diffuse reddening of the oral mucosa, then mottling of the mucosa with pinpoint lesions that enlarge to 1-2 cm, shallow, epithelial erosions. Sites of erosions include the hard and soft palates, dorsum and sides of the tongue, gums, and commissures of the mouth. In early cases, the cheek papillae are hyperemic and their tips slough, leaving blunt shortened papillae as the disease progresses.

Additional signs occur sporadically in individual animals. These include mucopurulent nasal discharge, hyperemic encrusted external nares, erosions of the coronary band and interdigital cleft, and corneal opacity. In some outbreaks, oral lesions and diarrhea are minimal, and the prominent signs may suggest respiratory disease. (The respiratory signs may be due to the activity of other microbial agents, and BVD infection has been implicated in the "shipping fever complex".) Leukopenia with relative lymphocytosis is common early in the disease. Leukocytosis may occur with secondary bacterial infection. The occasional animal that survives the acute disease usually is so debilitated as to be an economic liability.

Infection during pregnancy can result in embryonic death or abortion, birth of undersized weak calves, or calves with congenital infections. Such an infection often is clinically inapparent in the dam; effects on the fetus vary with the strain of the virus and the age and immunocompetence of the fetus. Fetal death, with resorption or mummification, or abortion may occur following infection in early to mid-gestation up to ~120 days. When a large portion of dams are susceptible, the initial evidence of BVD may be herd infertility or an abortion storm. Infection at mid-gestation (~120-150 days) can result in calves with congenital defects. These include cerebellar hypoplasia, cataracts, retinal degeneration, microphthalmia, hypoplasia of the optic tracts, hydrocephalus, and tight curly coats. Congenital BVD infection may be a factor in the "weak calf" syndrome. Acute mucosal disease may be provoked in congenitally infected yearling or adult cattle when they are exposed to either antigenically related or antigenically different cytopathic strains of BVD virus or by various unknown factors. The syndrome of mucosal disease is as described for severe BVD above, but it is invariably fatal. When infection (with cytopathic or noncytopathic BVD virus) of the dam occurs in late gestation (>150 days), there may be fetal infection with antibody formation but no adverse effects on the fetus.

Lesions: Gross lesions are primarily confined to the alimentary tract. Microscopically, foci of degenerate epithelial cells comprise the basic lesions. These develop with edema and vasculitis immediately below epithelial surfaces, which results in erosions of the esophagus, forestomachs, abomasum, and intestine. Epithelial necrosis is more prominent in mucosal disease when ulceration is marked, especially in the oronasal areas. Catarrhal enteritis may be severe in more chronic forms of the disease.

Necrosis of lymphoid tissues occurs, particularly in those associated with the intestine. In chronic mucosal disease, the affected Peyer's patches are hemorrhagic, dark red, and necrotic. Microscopically, destruction of the epithelial lining of crypts of Lieberkühn in the lower small intestine, cecum, and colon is a characteristic lesion. Animals with mucosal disease die with a febrile systemic infection and circulatory collapse.

Diagnosis: Because diseases such as rinderpest and malignant catarrhal fever can cause similar syndromes, diagnosis of BVD-like disease is important. Diagnosis of severe cases of BVD infection usually can be based on history, clinical findings, and postmortem lesions. Unfortunately, in most cases, clinical signs are less obvious, and arriving at an accurate diagnosis can be difficult. Due to the prevalence of infection in the general cattle population, a single positive serum titer is of no diagnostic significance; paired serum samples should be taken to demonstrate seroconversion or a rising titer. Clinical (lesion material, blood, nasopharyngeal and ocular discharges) or postmortem samples (spleen, mesenteric lymph nodes, Peyer's patches) should be submitted for virus isolation or FA examination. Diagnosis of abortion and congenital infection associated with BVD requires laboratory assistance. Appropriate samples should be submitted for histology and virus isolation along with a precolostral serum sample. Diagnosis in persistently infected cattle requires isolation of the virus from blood, serum, or buffy coat.

Control: There is no specific treatment for BVD, but supportive therapy is indicated. Modified live virus and inactivated virus vaccines are available and can provide significant protection. In general, vaccines are administered at 6-10 mo of age when colostral immunity has waned: manufacturers' recommendations as to use and inoculation schedule should be strictly followed. There is evidence that vaccination of immunotolerant, persistently infected cattle with an attenuated cytopathic BVD virus vaccine can result in severe mucosal disease; however, this does not always occur and such animals can develop neutralizing antibody to the vaccine virus. Inactivated BVD vaccines are also available, and their use may overcome the problems sometimes attributed to the use of attenuated vaccines. Since persistently infected animals can act as a continuing source of infection within a herd, in theory, they should be detected and culled. However, this is expensive, since it requires a serological survey of the herd and virus isolation from the blood of seronegative animals. The use of nucleic acid (gene) probes to detect BVD viruses in buffy coat samples may reduce the cost of the test. Pregnant sheep should not be run with cattle since infection with BVD virus may result in border disease (qv, p 334).

COLIC IN HORSES

A potentially fatal syndrome, manifest by peracute to chronic onset, mild to severe abdominal pain, and depression.

Etiology and Pathogenesis: Visceral pain usually emanates from a GI tract disorder, but some urogenital tract abnormalities can cause identical signs. Other conditions that must be considered are causes of parietal abdominal pain (eg, peritonitis, uterine torsion, pyelonephritis) or of signs that mimic abdominal pain (eg, generalized myositis or tetany, laminitis, or pleurisy). Myriad disease processes that cause altered (or cessation of) ingesta flow, which results in gastric and/or intestinal luminal distention, mural swelling, transmural ischemia or infarction, or acute or chronic bowel inflammation (from infectious enteritis or mucosal ulcerative conditions), may cause signs of abdominal pain in varying degrees. The major inciting conditions are divided into simple (functional) or strangulating obstructions.

Improper husbandry practices, such as rapid dietary alterations (a "feeding accident"), can cause a change of the ingesta pH, a shift in intestinal flora, fermentation with resultant gas production, and transient ileus that causes bowel tympany and pain. Simple intraluminal bowel obstructions that slow or stop the movement of ingesta may occur at any level of the GI tract, but typically are found at the ileum, ileocecal junction, cecum, pelvic flexure of the great (ascending) colon, transverse colon, or even the small (descending) colon. Simple impaction is common and may be caused by relative dehydration due to water deprivation and excess drying of ingesta (usually seen in winter), a diet of particularly coarse roughage, or prolonged retention of meconium in foals. Ingested foreign bodies (fibrous material, eg, ropes, haynets, or fencing) accrete mineral salts from the ingesta and gradually increase in size, intermittently or acutely obstructing at the transverse colon or pelvic flexure. Enteroliths form spontaneously over years, concentrically around a small nidus by the same accretion process, and obstruct the bowel at the transverse or proximal small colon.

Anatomic displacements (usually the left branches of the great colon) mimic simple intraluminal obstruction by slowing or stopping ingesta and gas flow. Extramural disease processes, such as organizing adhesions from previous surgery or peritonitis, may locally slow ingesta flow due to inflammation or "kink" bowel loops. Abdominal abscesses may be painful and enlarge to cause generalized inflammatory peritonitis, interluminal adhesions, or extramural collapse of the bowel. Vascular accidents due to intra-abdominal trauma (eg, dystocia), or coagulopathies may cause mural or mesenteric hematoma formation with extraluminal bowel compression, local ischemia, or both.

Strangulation obstructions cause acute circulatory compromise of the affected bowel (while simultaneously obstructing flow of ingesta), acute nonseptic peritonitis, and concomitant ileus. Intra-abdominal causes include volvulus of the small intestine or large colon; intussusception of the small intestine, cecum, or large colon; mesenteric rents; mesodiverticular bands; gastrosplenic hernias; and epiploic foramen incarcerations of the small intestine. Mesenteric lipomas on long, string-like pedicles occur in older horses, and may become tied around a loop of intestine (usually small), acutely occluding the bowel extraluminally, resulting in fulminant signs of colic. Acute umbilical, inguinal (scrotal), or diaphragmatic hernias cause strangulation obstruction of the bowel outside the abdominal cavity.

Nonstrangulating infarction of a segment of bowel or a portion of organ wall is usually due to migration of strongyle larvae, and associated mesenteric arteritis and thromboembolism. Other causes include partial incarceration of the bowel (parietal hernia) or avulsion of the supplying mesenteric vessels (eg, during dystocia). Occasionally, peracute infectious enteritis of the large or small intestine may be fulminant enough (eg, peracute salmonellosis) to cause transmural necrosis of portions of the cecum, large colon, small colon, or occasionally, the duodenum and proximal jejunum. Severe acute intestinal inflammatory conditions, while initially causing fluid feces and increased peristalsis, progress to GI tract ileus, cessation of ingesta flow, retention of fluid and gas, and often, severe pain due to tympany.

Ulceration of the GI tract appears to cause no signs in some; in others, particularly foals and those being exercised regularly and strenuously, signs range from vague indications of discomfort to colic. Endoscopy may permit specific diagnosis.

Pain from a urogenital tract lesion is infrequent, but most typical in pre- or postparturient mares. Primary uterine injuries (eg, a uterine vessel rupture prepartum, or wall perforation during parturition) can result in moderate to severe abdominal pain. Renal cortical or pelvic disease, although rare, can cause mild signs of colic, usually in adults. Lower tract disease, most commonly urolithiasis, causes hematuria and associated abdominal pain, usually in males. Spontaneous bladder rupture may occur in the first few days of life of colts.

Cessation of ingesta flow with a buildup of fluid and gas that results in bowel distention is one source of pain in simple obstructive diseases. Ischemic tissue itself is exquisitely painful until tissue death occurs. Both components contribute to signs of colic in cases of strangulation obstruction.

Obstruction of ingesta flow, whether due to simple or strangulation obstruction, regional infarction, or inflammatory enteritis, invariably disrupts the normal sequence of small intestinal tract fluid secretion and cecum and colon reabsorption, and results in a net circulatory volume loss. The rapidity of circulatory fluid loss, and resultant hemoconcentration and eventual hypovolemic shock syndrome, is generally determined by the location of the lesion along the tract and the amount of tissue involved in the injury. Upper tract obstructions prevent cecal reabsorption of GI secretions and therefore induce a rapid onset of hypovolemia, whereas lesions distal to the cecum are generally slow to produce cardiovascular shock (excepting colonic volvulus). The magnitude of the lesion, eg, complete mesenteric volvulus of the small intestine or complete colonic volvulus, intensifies the onset of hypovolemic shock because of massive blood loss into the strangulated tissue as well as interference with recovery of GI secretory fluid. Changes in the luminal flora due to stasis of ingesta flow and resultant release of gram-negative endotoxin compound the effect of hypovolemia on cardiovascular fluid dynamics.

The cause of death in severe cases is cardiovascular shock, alone or in combination with gram-negative endotoxemia. Most causes are complicated by net fluid loss from the circulation.

Clinical Findings and Diagnosis: Evaluation and interpretation of all physical and laboratory findings must be considered, fully cognizant that the horse may already be in or eventually experience cardiovascular shock. Manifestation of pain is variable regardless of the inciting problem, although signs generally correlate with the severity of the GI tract insult. Severe unrelenting pain should be interpreted as potentially life-threatening.

In most cases, regardless of cause, the initial signs are similar but vary in severity. The animal may exhibit discomfort by one or several of pawing, kicking at the abdomen, getting up and down, rolling, flank-watching, and abnormal postures, eg, dog-sitting, adopting a "sawhorse" stance, or lying in dorsal recumbency. Bouts of pain may be intermittent (and subacute), especially in medically treatable cases and early in the course of more severe cases. Self-inflicted trauma can result from violent activity during bouts of severe pain. Other signs referable to pain, eg, sweating, tachycardia, hyperpnea, and relative polycythemia, may be early indications of impending cardiovascular shock.

The horse's cardiovascular status should be assessed on the first and subsequent examinations (if they become necessary), since hypovolemic and endotoxic shock are eventual sequelae of net circulatory volume loss and obstruction of ingesta flow. A small blood sample should always be taken for PCV and total protein measurement. An initial reading is important should the condition become protracted. Blood pressure can be measured indirectly at the coccygeal artery by ultrasonic and oscillometric devices. Systemic hypotension in the standing horse corresponds to a coccygeal systolic pressure up to 80 mm Hg. Palpable arterial pulse amplitude is diminished proportionally. Other findings in acute circulatory failure include tachycardia; discolored and tacky oral mucosa, with a prolonged capillary refill time; poor jugular filling rate; palpably cold ears and limbs; relative polycythemia and hyperproteinemia; prerenal azotemia; metabolic acidosis, seen as a decreased blood pH and bicarbonate (or "total CO_2") concentration, increased blood lactate concentration, and an increased anion gap; and moderate to marked depression, which can mask the amount of discomfort exhibited. The more severely compromised the circulatory system, the more these deviate from normal and the greater the urgency in providing therapy for shock.

A thorough physical examination, including abdominal auscultation, rectal palpation, passage of a nasogastric tube, and abdominocentesis, is essential. Written notes should be kept and the examination repeated q2hr. Gut sounds (borborygmi) may be loud in spasmodic colic, high-pitched in flatulent colic, increased in frequency in spasmodic and flatulent colic and enteritis, and vary from normal to decreased in frequency and amplitude in other conditions. Absence of intestinal sounds is not proof of, but frequently occurs in, serious intestinal disorders.

The amount, consistency, color, and odor of the feces should be noted. An absence of feces in the rectum of an adult is unusual and significant. Scant fecal balls or the complete absence of them, and a dry mucus-filled rectum are consistent with a simple obstruction of the descending colon (eg, enterolithiasis). Watery or occasionally blood-tinged feces suggest impending enterocolitis as the cause of abdominal pain. Sand particles palpable in fecal balls are consistent with chronic ingestion of sand and probable impaction. Occasionally, adult small strongyles may be found on the examiner's arm when it is withdrawn, indicating severe parasitism.

A rectal examination may provide an etiologic diagnosis, but more often it is helpful only in determining the general location and type of obstruction, eg, small intestine versus small colon, cecum versus large colon. A fluid- and/or gas-filled segment of bowel occurs proximal to impaction or dislocation. Any distention of bowel should be noted and interpreted as a sign of possible obstruction or displacement. The type, size, and location of bowel loops are important in monitoring the progression of signs on subsequent examinations. In some cases, markedly tympanic loops of small intestine may be palpable; in others, a taut band of mesentery may be within reach, pulled away by a fluid-distended loop of bowel deeper in the abdomen. A tympanitic large bowel may obstruct palpation beyond the pelvic inlet. Tympany of the large intestine is often severe enough to cause obvious abdominal distention (bloat) in adults; in foals, and occasionally in adults, tympany of the small intestine may be similarly evident.

The primary problem can be definitively palpated in some cases, eg, intraluminal obstructions of the ileocecal valve, cecum, and large and small colon; some intussusceptions and volvulae; incarceration through the inguinal ring; rectal constriction (as with a pedunculated lipoma); and nephrosplenic entrapment of the left colon. Flatulent colic can cause some intestinal tympany. No abnormalities are palpable in spasmodic colic or early in the course of dislocations. If cranial mesenteric verminous arteritis is the problem, the enlarged knobby artery may be palpated on the midline, caudal to the pole of the left kidney.

Gastric distention may be primary, but more frequently it is secondary to small intestinal obstruction, and sometimes to obstruction of the duodenum due to severe tympany of the large intestine. It causes signs of severe discomfort and is not palpable. Passage of a nasogastric tube may allow spontaneous gastric decompression, which usually ameliorates clinical signs. The volume of evacuated fluid should be noted. Its color varies with the last food ingested, but a green, foul-smelling fluid is typical. The pH of the fluid should be strongly acidic; alkaline fluid is typical with upper small bowel obstruction and/or ileus. Blood in the gastric reflux may be observed with primary gastritis (ulcers), proximal duodenojejunitis, or strangulation obstruction of the proximal small intestine. Distention secondary to grain engorgement is difficult to relieve by stomach tube. Vomiting or spontaneous nasogastric regurgitation is usually accompanied by dramatic signs of pain immediately before gastric rupture.

Ventral midline abdominocentesis is diagnostically important. The sample should be collected without peripheral blood contamination by using a blunt cannula. Enteritides, simple obstruction, displacements, or small infarcted lesions produce few changes in peritoneal fluid. A strangulating intestinal obstruction causes hemorrhagic diapedesis of RBC into the peritoneal cavity. Concomitantly, the acute inflammation causes a variable exudation of WBC and protein. Thus, fluid is frequently readily obtainable, and discolored and turbid (in proportion to the number and type of cells present). Cytologically, free and phagocytosed RBC may be present, while neutrophils are usually the predominant nucleated cell. Macrophages and mesothelial cells also may be present.

Lactate concentration in the peritoneal fluid increases in proportion to the degree and amount of intestinal ischemia. Phagocytosed and/or free bacteria are seen with complete bowel wall necrosis, and usually indicate a poor prognosis. Differentiation from primary, septic peritonitis (without bowel necrosis) can be difficult. The presence of mixed microorganisms plus blood and plant fibers are pathognomonic of an acute bowel rupture. Accidental enterocentesis can be distinguished from a bowel rupture in that bacteria are not phagocytosed, ciliates may be present, and WBC morphology is normal; in a ruptured bowel, some bacteria may be phagocytosed and many WBC are markedly degenerate.

Unconjugated bilirubin concentration in the blood may be increased in many colic cases; however, in cholelithiasis, both unconjugated and conjugated bilirubin concentrations are increased. Consequently, in cholelithiasis, the horse may have icteric mucosae, sclera, plasma, and peritoneal fluid, with bilirubinuria and increased serum alkaline phosphatase and γ-glutamyltransferase activities.

Treatment: Analgesia and/or mild sedation should be used as necessary to allow a thorough, proper examination and/or medical therapy or treatment for shock. Horses showing vital signs consistent with hypovolemic shock (including heart rate >80/min) should have an IV jugular catheter inserted and IV fluid volume replacement therapy initiated based on a clinical assessment of the degree of dehydration. A nasogastric tube should be passed to check for and relieve gastric tympany and fluid distention. Mild impactions may be dispersed with mineral oil (2-4 L for an adult) or dioctyl sodium sulfosuccinate (7.5-30 g) by stomach tube. Magnesium sulfate (0.5-1 g/kg body wt by stomach tube) acts as an osmotic cathartic and is useful in some sand colics. IV fluid volume replacement in excess of the daily maintenance requirement (overhydration), in combination with the above medicaments, effectively relieves impaction of the cecum and colon. For either impaction colic or sand colic, the treatment should be followed with correction of the diet, including, for the latter, removal of the horse from the source of sand. Ready access to water is also required. A markedly tympanitic large bowel may require decompression by trocharization through the upper flank. Horses with signs referable to verminous arteritis may benefit from treatment with ivermectin (200 μg/kg body wt); however, the causal lesions take weeks to regress.

Atropine is contraindicated in all colic cases because of its potential to produce ileus. Dipyrone (11 mg/kg, IV and IM) is useful for analgesia in spasmodic colics. Horses exhibiting severe pain require potent analgesic therapy to prevent self-injury. Useful drugs include xylazine (0.25-0.5 mg/lb [0.5-1 mg/kg], IV or IM), flunixin meglumine (0.5 mg/lb [1 mg/kg], IV or IM), meperidine (0.5-1 mg/lb [1-2 mg/kg], IM), pentazocine (0.15-0.2 mg/lb [0.3-0.4 mg/kg], IV or IM), and chloral hydrate (3.5-7 g, IV, or 15-16 g by stomach tube to an adult). Promazine tranquilizers, while possibly useful for mild colics, are contraindicated when cardiovascular status may be compromised because of their hypotensive side effects. Horses on analgesic therapy must be monitored closely lest their clinical condition deteriorates. Horses with decreased circulatory function or in shock require aggressive IV therapy, with isotonic polyionic fluids and possibly bicarbonate supplementation. Flunixin meglumine (0.5 mg/lb [1 mg/kg], IV or IM) and massive doses of corticosteriods (1 g prednisolone sodium succinate, IV, or 100 mg dexamethasone, IV) may be useful to prevent or treat shock. However, flunixin meglumine is best reserved for use in cases that have been diagnosed definitively; otherwise, continuing general clinical deterioration may be masked by its powerful analgesic property.

Medical therapy is adequate for most colic cases; however, 6-10% of cases have obstruction that requires surgery. Indications for surgery include acute colic unresponsive to analgesic and medical therapy, "positive" rectal findings (eg, intussusception, obstruction, markedly distended loops of bowel), declining circulatory status, and history of chronic recurrent colics. For pedunculated mesenteric lipomas, early diagnosis and surgical correction are essential.

Prognosis for survival is greatest if surgery is performed before development, or at least in the early stages, of cardiovascular shock; advanced shock generally precludes a successful outcome after surgery. The most reliable early clinical indicator of the need for surgical therapy is severe and/or unrelenting pain. Manifestation of severe pain precedes a decline in the cardiovascular parameters. Additionally, the manifestation of pain generally correlates with the severity of the GI injury. Horses exhibiting severe pain should be considered as candidates for surgery even on the first examination.

Weanling horses may exhibit colic within a day of their first deworming due to an adult ascarid impaction, which usually occurs at the ileum; exploratory surgery is the definitive treatment. Other young horses habitually chew and occasionally ingest fibrous (wood, rope) or synthetic (nylon) materials that can cause a simple obstruction of the ascending, transverse, or descending colon and necessitate surgical removal. The same criteria used to gauge the need for surgery in adults, except for a rectal examination, are applicable to neonatal or weanling horses. Likewise, timely cardiovascular supportive therapy and decisive action regarding surgery increase a favorable prognosis.

When appropriate, dental attention and advice on feeding, exercising, and husbandry (including parasite control) should be provided.

COLIC IN FOALS

A variety of lesions (see above) are seen in young horses with colic, although with less overall frequency. Colic and abdominal distention in the first few days of life are usually due to rupture of the bladder, but volvulus of the small intestine or colon have been observed infrequently. Again, manifestation of pain is the discriminating clinical sign. In young foals, the most common cause of colic that requires surgical therapy is jejunal intussusception.

Retention of meconium is a common cause of impaction of the large or small colon in neonates, particularly in colts. Initial signs are not dramatic, but recurring bouts of pain may be evident, and any feces passed tend to be scant, hard, and covered with mucus. Severe cases may require use of blunt forceps or, especially if the retention is higher in the tract, even surgery to remove the impacted mass. Usually, however, enemas carefully introduced with a foot-long flexible tube will suffice. Mild soapy water, or water containing a surface-tension-reducing agent, given at ~4-hr intervals is recommended. Small doses of mineral oil, PO, also at intervals, may be helpful. Many advise administering a mild enema to every foal soon after birth, and to continue until the meconium passes.

DISEASES OF THE ESOPHAGUS, LG AN

CHOKE

An obstruction of the esophagus by food masses or foreign objects.

Etiology: Horses choke most frequently on greedily eaten dry grains; less often on ears of corn, potatoes, or a bolus of hay; and occasionally on medicinal boluses. Choke in horses often is a complication of stenosis or diverticulosis, as well as of esophagitis. Ruminants usually choke on solid objects, eg, apples, pears, beets, plums, potatoes, turnips, or ears of corn. On rare occasions, cattle choke on foreign objects in the feed. In large animals, obstruction occurs more frequently in the cervical than in the thoracic portion of the esophagus.

Clinical Findings—Horses: The affected horse exhibits anxiety, an arched neck, and retching. Salivation is profuse, and food and saliva are regurgitated through the nostrils. Coughing is pronounced, and the animal may paw at the ground, get up and down, and show other signs of distress. Milk runs from the nostrils of nursing foals as they attempt to swallow, and this sign must be differentiated from that caused by cleft palate. After ~1 hr, the forced or spasmodic efforts at swallowing become less frequent and the animal may become quiet.

   Cattle: Bloat (qv, p 163) and salivation are characteristic signs. The degree of tympany varies with the completeness of esophageal stenosis and the length of time that it has existed. Chewing movements, protrusion of the tongue, extension of the head and neck, dyspnea, grunting, and coughing are also seen.

Diagnosis: The history and clinical signs are very suggestive. An obstructing object in the cervical esophagus can be located by external palpation or passage of a stomach tube. Thoracic obstructions may be diagnosed by careful passage of a stomach tube. In any animal with dysphagia, the possibility of rabies should be considered.

Treatment—Horses: Obstructions from grain and hay tend to resolve spontaneously as the bolus is softened by saliva. The course may be a few hours to several days; however, pressure necrosis or esophagitis may occur and ultimately cause stenosis with dilatation. Inhalation pneumonia may occur. Hasty procedures are to be avoided. Controlling the pain with sedatives, confining the animal, and allowing it access to water, but not to feed, may result in spontaneous recovery. Passage of a stomach tube to the obstruction and repeated pumping and siphoning may relieve grain choke. Pentazocine, xylazine, acepromazine, or methampyrone are used to control the pain and the spasms. In some cases, solid thoracic obstructions may be gently pushed into the stomach with a large stomach tube or probang, if the horse is tractable or anesthetized.

   Cattle: Relief of tympany is the first consideration, and in acute bloat the rumen should be trocarized promptly. Solid objects in the cervical portion of the esophagus may be massaged upward and removed through a mouth speculum, or a steel wire (No. 9) may be made into a loop, passed through the mouth speculum until beyond the object and then slowly withdrawn. When other methods fail, a probang may be tried. Stiff stomach tubes of large caliber work well for this purpose. The disadvantage of this method is the risk of tissue damage and subsequent esophagitis. If the obstruction is near the diaphragm, a rumenotomy may be performed to remove the object.

   Esophagotomy may be elected in cervical choke in either species, but should be resorted to only when usual methods of treatment fail; often it is followed by an esophageal fistula, which may not heal, or if it does, may result in esophageal stricture.

ESOPHAGEAL DIVERTICULUM (DILATATION)

   This condition is of greatest importance in horses. It most often complicates stenosis, and thus may be indirectly associated with esophagitis or chronic choke. In foals, gastroesophageal reflux secondary to functional or mechanical gastric outflow obstruction can cause dilatation of the distal esophagus. Most diverticula are found in the low cervical or thoracic esophagus. The important signs usually are seen after feeding and are similar to those of choke. (*See also* p 110.)

Diagnosis is based on history and clinical signs. Some cervical dilatations can be palpated and even observed by visual examination. Esophagoscopy allows direct visualization of the dilatation, as well as any associated stenotic region. Contrast radiography has been used in diagnosis. Surgical exposure of the diverticulum and careful apposition of the esophageal musculature without penetrating the esophageal mucosa is the only effective treatment.

ESOPHAGEAL SPASM
(Esophagism)

A condition occurring in horses, most commonly in the young. Although the exact etiology is unknown, it has been observed in nursing foals when they begin to take solid food; in young animals convalescing from debilitating acute infections; in horses with acute esophagitis, such as that induced by the breaking of a capsule that contains some irritant drug; following routine use of a stomach tube, which may have injured the mucosa; and following the injection of large doses of morphine. Esophagism may also occur in tetanus and rabies.

Clinical signs resemble those of esophageal obstruction but are not necessarily related to the intake of food. Sometimes they are brought on by drinking cold water. The chin is pulled down and backward; some animals make convulsive efforts to vomit, and place their feet under their body and extend their head. Frothy saliva is discharged from the mouth and nostrils, and coughing is frequent. Periods of spasm may occur several times a day, or only at intervals of several days. Sometimes there is interference with passage of a stomach tube. The spasms are symptomatic and cease once the primary cause is removed. Atropine seems to control the spasms. Severe spasm may be relieved by morphine, or by use of spasmolytic agents, eg, dipyrone. Tranquilizers may control signs in nervous individuals.

ESOPHAGEAL STENOSIS

Etiology: Stenosis may be caused by cicatricial tissue or by compression. Cicatricial tissue in horses may follow esophageal obstruction that damages the wall, or irritation to the wall from rough handling in attempts to remove the obstruction. Aged horses may develop stenosis of the terminal esophagus due to fibrosis of the muscular wall. On rare occasions, caustic chemicals may cause esophagitis and subsequent scarring. Compression of the esophagus occurs occasionally in cattle with lymphosarcoma and from adhesions and traumatic reticulitis near the esophageal hiatus. Compression of the esophagus by a persistent right aortic arch (qv, p 35) also has been reported. In sheep, compression from caseous lymphadenitis (qv, p 64) involving the mediastinal lymph nodes is a rare cause. In horses, stenosis is often accompanied by a diverticulum, or the diverticulum may cause stenosis.

Clinical Findings: Stenosis in horses results in repeated occurrences of choke. Repeated obstruction leads to weakened walls and eventual dilatation. The clinical signs of choke, described above, occur intermittently. Water is swallowed with no difficulty. Chronically affected animals tend to remain thin. Afflicted cattle tend to be chronic bloaters and may show a tendency to choke.

Diagnosis: Habitual choke in large animals suggests stenosis and esophageal diverticulum. Passage of a fairly large stomach tube reveals the narrowing. Tubes of gradually increasing diameter may be used to determine the degree of stenosis. Contrast radiography may be used in cervical choke to ascertain the area involved.

Treatment: Feeding on thin mashes and fine-cut hay helps to prevent obstruction, but is palliative only, and euthanasia may have to be considered. In some cases, use of bougienage has been effective. The procedure is performed on several occasions, resulting in breakdown of fibrous connective tissue and restoration of the esophageal lumen. If the primary cause is a diverticulum, it may be possible to correct it surgically.

ESOPHAGITIS

Esophagitis is rarely diagnosed as a clinical entity in large animals. It may occur occasionally in horses, usually because of trauma from foreign bodies or injudicious use of stomach tubes; infrequently, irritating chemicals may be involved. Esophagitis in foals, and occasionally in adult horses, results from gastroesophageal reflux, which occurs secondary to gastric outflow obstruction. In cattle, it may be secondary to infectious diseases, eg, bovine viral diarrhea, infectious bovine rhinotracheitis, or malignant catarrhal fever.

In severe cases, dysphagia, salivation, spasms of the esophageal and cervical musculature, vomiting, and extension of the head and neck may be seen.

Withholding feed and water for 2 days often relieves the condition. Electrolytes, methampyrone, and corticosteroids should be administered as supportive therapy and to control spasms. Water is then given and if this is tolerated, moistened mashes may be tried. Sulfonamides or antibiotics should be used to control infection.

DIGESTIVE DISORDERS OF THE RUMEN

See also GASTRITIS, LG AN, p 199.

GRAIN OVERLOAD
(Lactic acidosis, Carbohydrate engorgement, Rumen impaction)

An acute disease of ruminants characterized by indigestion, rumen stasis, dehydration, acidosis, toxemia, incoordination, collapse, and frequently death.

Etiology and Pathogenesis: The disease is most common in cattle that accidentally gain access to large quantities of carbohydrates, particularly grain. It also is common in feedlot cattle when they are introduced to heavy grain diets. Less common causes include engorgement with apples, grapes, bread, batter's dough, sugar beets, mangels, or sour wet brewer's grain that was incompletely fermented in the brewery. The amount of a feed required to produce acute illness depends on the kind of grain, previous experience of the animal with that grain, the nutritional status and condition of the animal, and the nature of the microflora. Cattle accustomed to heavy grain diets may consume 30-45 lb (15-20 kg) of grain and develop only moderate illness, while others may become acutely ill and die after eating 20 lb (10 kg) of grain.

Ingestion of toxic amounts of highly fermentable carbohydrates is followed within 2-6 hr by a change in the microbial population in the rumen. There is a marked increase in the number of gram-positive bacteria (*Streptococcus bovis*), which results in the production of large quantities of lactic acid. The rumen pH falls to ≤5, which destroys protozoa, cellulolytic organisms, and lactate-utilizing organisms, and impairs rumen motility. The low pH allows the lactobacilli to utilize the carbohydrate and to produce excessive quantities of lactic acid. The superimposition of lactic acid and its salt, lactate, on the existing solutes in the rumen liquid causes a substantial rise in osmotic pressure, which draws fluid into the rumen and causes dehydration.

The lactic acid causes a chemical rumenitis, and its absorption results in lactic acidosis. In addition to acidosis and dehydration, the pathophysiological consequences are hemoconcentration, cardiovascular collapse, renal failure, muscular weakness, shock, and death. Animals that survive may develop mycotic rumenitis in several days, or have hepatic necrobacillosis several weeks or months later, or chronic laminitis, and evidence of ruminal scars at slaughter.

Clinical Findings: Overload results in conditions ranging from simple indigestion (*see* below) to a rapidly fatal acidosis. The interval between overeating and onset of signs is shorter with ground feed than with whole grain, and severity increases with the amount eaten. A few hours after engorgement, the only detectable abnormality may be a full rumen and possibly some abdominal pain (belly kicking). In the mild form, the rumen movements are reduced but not entirely absent, the cattle are anorectic but bright and alert; diarrhea is common. Eating usually begins again on day 3 or 4 without any specific treatment.

Within 24-48 hr of onset of severe overload, some animals will be down, some will be staggering, and others will be standing quietly by themselves. All will be completely off feed. Immediately after consuming large quantities of dry grain, cattle may engorge themselves on water, but once ill they usually do not drink at all.

Body temperature is usually below normal, 98-101°F (36.5-38.5°C), but in animals exposed to the sun in hot weather, may be increased to 106°F (41°C). Respirations tend to be shallow and rapid, up to 60-90/min. The heart rate usually is increased in accordance with severity of the acidosis; prognosis for those with rates of 120-140/min is poor. Diarrhea is common and usually profuse; the feces are soft to watery, light colored, and have an obvious sweet-sour odor. The feces frequently contain undigested fragments of the feed that has induced the overload. In mild cases, dehydration equals 4-6% body wt; with severe involvement, up to 10-12% of body wt.

In severe overload, the primary contractions of the rumen are completely absent, although the gurgling sounds of gas rising through the large quantity of fluid are usually audible on auscultation. The ruminal contents, as palpated through the left paralumbar fossa, may feel firm and doughy in cattle that were previously on a roughage diet and have consumed a large amount of grain. In cattle that have become ill on smaller amounts of grain, the rumen will not necessarily feel full, but rather will feel resilient because of the excessive fluid. Severely affected animals stagger and may bump into objects; their palpebral reflex is sluggish or absent; the pupillary light reflex is usually present but slower than normal. They commonly lie quietly, often with the head turned into the flank, and their response to any stimulus is much decreased so that they resemble cases of parturient paresis.

Acute laminitis may be present and is most common in those animals that are not severely affected; chronic laminitis may occur weeks or months later. Anuria is a common finding in acute cases, and diuresis following fluid therapy is a good prognostic sign.

Death may occur in 24-72 hr and rapid development of acute signs, particularly recumbency, indicates the need for urgent radical treatment. A reduction in heart rate, rise in temperature, return of ruminal movement, and passage of large amounts of soft feces are more favorable signs. However, some animals appear to improve temporarily but become severely ill again on days 3 or 4, probably because of severe fungal rumenitis; in these, death from acute diffuse peritonitis usually follows in 2-3 days. In pregnant cattle that survive the severe form of the disease, abortion may occur 10-14 days later.

Diagnosis: The diagnosis is usually obvious if the history is available. It may be confirmed by the clinical findings, a low ruminal pH, and examining the microflora of the rumen. When only one animal is involved and there is no history of engorgement, the diagnosis is less obvious, but the clinical signs—a static rumen with gurgling fluid sounds, diarrhea, ataxia, and a normal temperature—are characteristic.

Although parturient paresis (qv, p 451) may simulate rumen overload, diarrhea and dehydration are not typical, the intensity of heart sounds is reduced, and the response to calcium injection is usually dramatic. Peracute coliform mastitis and acute diffuse peritonitis may also resemble overload, but usually a careful examination will reveal the cause of the toxemia.

To avoid an increase in pH on exposure to air, rumen fluid obtained by stomach tube or paracentesis should be checked promptly. Normally, the pH in cattle on roughage is 6-7, in those on a grain diet, 5.5-6. Values below those ranges are strongly suggestive of overload, and a pH <5 indicates severe acidosis. Wide-range (2-11) pH indicator paper is suitable for field use. Ruminal fluid may be examined microscopically; under low power, 5-7 protozoa are normally present; in acidosis, the protozoa are virtually absent. A Gram's stain of the fluid will reveal a change from predominantly gram-negative bacteria in the normal animal to predominantly gram-positive bacteria in acidosis.

Additional changes are present, eg, increased blood lactate and inorganic phosphate levels, mild hypocalcemia, and reduced urinary pH, but it is seldom necessary to check such values to make a firm diagnosis. The diagnostic problem is to properly assess which animals require vigorous therapy (or slaughter), which require supportive therapy, which have only a mild indigestion that will correct itself if water and grain intake are restricted and hay and exercise are provided, and which need nothing beyond their routine care and ration.

If the cattle are found while still eating, it is possible that some of the group will fall into each category, and close monitoring is necessary to minimize the losses. Cattle found while engorging or shortly thereafter should be allowed no more concentrate or water, but plenty of good hay for up to 24 hr, and forced to exercise periodically. Those that appear normal at the end of the first day are probably in good health, although if even one is ill, all should be monitored closely for 48 hr. Most of those that have eaten enough concentrate to be affected seriously show signs within 6-8 hr.

Treatment: For all cattle suspected of having eaten toxic quantities of concentrate, it is important to restrict water intake for the first 18-24 hr. If overload is serious, slaughter should be considered; in feeders nearing the end of their feeding period, it may well be the most economical choice. Mortality is high in severely affected animals unless vigorous therapeutic measures are initiated early. In such animals, removal of rumen contents and replacing them with ingesta taken from healthy animals is necessary. In animals that are still standing, emptying may be accomplished with a large stomach tube if sufficient water is available. A large bore tube (1 in. inside diameter, 10 ft long [2.5 cm × 3 m]) is used, enough water is added to distend the left paralumbar fossa, and gravity flow is allowed to empty out what it will. Repeating this 15-20 times achieves the same results (and requires about as much time) as using rumenotomy to empty and wash out the rumen with a siphon.

This must be followed by rumen inoculation (qv, p 1390) and, if not accomplished before severe signs of toxicosis are evident, by rigorous fluid therapy to correct the acidosis and dehydration and to restore renal function. Initially, over a period of ~30 min, 5% sodium bicarbonate solution should be given IV (5 qt/1000 lb [5 L/450 kg]). During the next 6-12 hr, a balanced electrolyte solution, or a 1.3% solution of sodium bicarbonate in saline, may be given IV, up to as much as 15 gal./1000 lb (60 L/450 kg) body wt. (Urination should resume during this period.) Usually, it is unnecessary and even undesirable to give antacids PO (or intraruminally) in addition to the therapy outlined above.

In less severe cases, emptying the rumen is unnecessary. In these, magnesium hydroxide (500 g/1000 lb [450 kg] body wt) should be added to warm water, pumped into the rumen, and mixed therein via kneading of the flank. This may be all that is necessary if the rumen pH is >5 and the animal is still standing and reasonably alert several hours after the engorgement. A heart rate of 70-85/min, weak ruminal contractions, a normal body temperature, and especially, a willingness to eat are additional reassurances that this therapy will suffice. If any question remains, additional fluids should be given. During the convalescent period, which may last 2-4 days, good-quality hay and no grain should be given, and the grain then reintroduced gradually. Return of good appetite within 3 days allows a good prognosis. However, if treatment has not been initiated early enough to prevent acidification of the ruminal contents, and mycotic infection of the rumen wall ensues, relapse of the clinical condition is likely within 3-5 days; if this occurs, the prognosis is grave.

Prevention: Accidental access to concentrates for which the cattle have developed an appetite, in quantities to which they are unaccustomed, should be avoided. Feedlot cattle should be introduced gradually to concentrate rations over a period of ~3 wk, beginning with a mixture of ≤50% concentrate in the milled feed containing roughage.

RUMINAL PARAKERATOSIS

A disease of cattle and sheep, characterized by hardening and enlargement of the papillae of the rumen, that is most common in animals fed a high-concentrate ration during the finishing period. It also occurs in cattle fed rations of heat-treated alfalfa pellets. It does not appear to be related to the feeding of antibiotics or protein concentrates. Incidence in a group may be as high as 40%. It is thought that the lesions are caused by the lowered pH and the increased concentration of volatile fatty acids (VFA) in the rumen juice (*see also* "SIMPLE" INDIGESTION, below). The lesions usually do not occur in cattle fed unprocessed whole grain (on which animals gain weight as readily), which may be related to the higher pH and higher concentration of acetic acid compared to the longer chain VFA in the rumen juice.

Many of the papillae are enlarged and hardened and several may adhere together to form bundles. The papillae of the anterior ventral sac are commonly affected. In cattle, the roof of the dorsal sac may show multiple foci of parakeratosis, each being 2-3 sq cm in area. In sheep, abnormal papillae may be visible and palpable through the wall of the intact rumen. Affected papillae contain excessive layers of keratinized epithelial cells, particles of food, and bacteria. The rumens of affected cattle are difficult to clean in the preparation of tripe. The abnormal epithelium, by interfering with absorption, may reduce efficiency of feed utilization and rate of gain, although there is little evidence to support this theory.

Ruminal parakeratosis may be prevented by finishing animals on rations that contain unground ingredients in the proportion of one part of roughage to 3 parts of concentrate. At present, the necessity and economics of prevention are not well defined.

"SIMPLE" INDIGESTION
(Mild dietary indigestion)

A minor disturbance in ruminant GI function that occurs in cattle and rarely in sheep. It is usually related to a change in the quality or quantity of the diet.

Etiology: Almost any dietary factor that can alter the ruminal environment can cause simple indigestion. The disease is common in hand-fed dairy and beef cattle because of variability in the quality and quantity of their feed. Dairy cattle may suddenly eat excessive quantities of highly palatable feeds such as corn or grass silage; beef cattle may eat excessive quantities of relatively indigestible, poor-quality roughage during winter. During drought, cattle and sheep may be forced to eat large quantities of poor-quality straw, bedding, or scrub. A sudden change in feed, using spoiled or frozen feeds, introducing urea to a ration, turning cattle onto a lush cereal grain pasture, or ingestion of placentas by postparturient cows can result in simple indigestion, as can introduction of feedlot cattle to a high-level grain ration.

Simple indigestion is primarily ruminal atony, and may follow a sudden change in the pH of the ruminal contents caused by excessive fermentation or putrefaction of ingested feed. The simple accumulation of excessive quantities of relatively indigestible feed may physically impair rumen function for 24-48 hr.

Clinical Findings: The signs depend on the type of animal affected and cause of the disorder. Silage overfeeding causes anorexia and a moderate drop in production in dairy cattle. The rumen is usually full, firm, and doughy, and primary contractions are absent, but secondary contractions may be present. Temperature, pulse, and respiration are normal. The feces are normal to firm in consistency but reduced in amount. Spontaneous recovery usually occurs in 24-48 hr.

Simple indigestion due to excessive feeding of grain results in anorexia and ruminal stasis; the rumen is not necessarily full and may contain excessive fluid. The feces are usually soft and foul smelling. The affected animal is bright and alert and usually begins to eat within 24 hr. A more severe upset from the same cause is described under grain overload (*see* above).

Diagnosis: This is based largely on the elimination of other possibilities and a history of a change in the nature or amount of the diet. The systemic reaction and painful responses to percussion seen in traumatic reticuloperitonitis are not observed. The absence of ketonuria, and the history, help eliminate ketosis from consideration. Displaced abomasum usually can be eliminated by auscultation. Vagal indigestion and abomasal torsions become more readily detectable as they progress because they have a longer course, but initial differentiation may be difficult. Grain overload is distinguishable by its greater severity and the pronounced fall in the pH of the rumen contents. Phytobezoars cause partial or complete anorexia and scant feces; on rectal examination, distended loops of intestine and the firm phytobezoar masses are palpable.

Treatment: Treatment is aimed at correcting the suspected dietary factors. Spontaneous recovery is usual. Administration of 5-10 gal. (20-40 L) of warm water or saline via a stomach tube, followed by vigorous kneading of the rumen, may help restore rumen function. Magnesium hydroxide PO seems to be useful when excessive amounts of high-energy feeds have been ingested. If too much urea (*see* p 1693) or protein has been ingested, acetic acid or vinegar may be administered PO. If the activity of the ruminal microbes is reduced, administration of 1-2 gal. (4-8 L) of ruminal fluid from a healthy cow will help. (*See* RUMINAL FLUID TRANSFER, p 1390.)

VAGAL INDIGESTION

Lesions that involve the vagus nerve of the forestomach and abomasum cause varying degrees of paralysis of those organs, and cause syndromes characterized by delayed passage of ingesta, distention of the abdomen, anorexia, and passage of small quantities of soft pasty feces. It is common in cattle and has been recorded in sheep. In cattle, traumatic reticuloperitonitis (qv, p 224) is the most common cause of lesions of the vagus nerves. In some cases, vagal nerve injury cannot be demonstrated. Damage to the tension receptors in the right wall of the reticulum, which reflexly control vagal activity, may explain such cases. It is most common in late pregnancy but can occur in nonpregnant cattle. Onset is insidious, and most cattle have been ill for several days or weeks when first seen by the veterinarian. The temperature is usually normal; the heart rate may be slower than normal in the early stages, but later is 84-100/min. The rumen usually is distended with fluid and may be atonic or hypermotile. This can be confirmed by rectal examination except during advanced pregnancy when palpation of the rumen is difficult. Auscultation of the left flank may reveal resonant sounds similar to those heard in left abomasal displacement. The abomasum may be impacted and palpable externally through the abdominal wall behind the right costal arch or the right side of the ventral floor of the abdomen. The rectum is usually empty except for sticky mucus. Most affected cattle die of secondary starvation, dehydration, and acid-base and electrolyte imbalances.

Response to treatment is unsatisfactory. Valuable cows that are near parturition (1-2 wk) can be maintained on continuous IV fluid therapy using balanced electrolytes and glucose. Rumenotomy provides only temporary relief, and the use of cathartics, GI stimulants, and lubricating substances has been unreliable. Fluid therapy and rumen lavage with a large-bore stomach tube are indicated. Parturition may be induced in animals that have been pregnant >8 mo (*see* INDUCED ABORTION AND PARTURITION, p 650).

INTESTINAL DISEASES IN RUMINANTS

INTESTINAL DISEASES IN CATTLE

The intestinal diseases of neonates are discussed separately below, although some of the causes affect older animals as well. Infection with *Salmonella* spp (qv, p 148) can produce diarrhea in animals of all ages, especially those that are stressed, closely stocked, or exposed to a heavily contaminated feed or water supply. The disease in older animals is manifest by dysentery and toxemia, and mortality can be significant. Rotavirus and coronavirus (qv, p 181) occasionally cause outbreaks of diarrhea in suckling calves 2-3 mo old. The feces are voluminous and may contain mucus. Toxemia is not evident and mortality is negligible, but production is decreased. Bovine viral diarrhea (BVD, qv, p 166) is most common in young cattle (6-24 mo old) and generally is accompanied by typical mucosal lesions; it must be distinguished from other viral diseases that produce diarrhea and mucosal lesions. These include bovine malignant catarrhal fever (qv, p 397), which usually is a sporadic disease in more mature cattle, and rinderpest (qv, p 404), which can occur in outbreak form but is exotic in most countries. Coccidiosis (qv, p 103) usually occurs in cattle <1 yr old, especially in situations of heavy stocking density and overgrazing. It is characterized by dysentery and tenesmus and may be accompanied by nervous signs. Intestinal helminthiasis, particularly ostertagiasis (qv, p 205), occurs in cattle of the same age group. Type I ostertagiasis occurs in cattle on pasture, but Type II ostertagiasis may occur in housed animals. Explosive outbreaks of diarrhea in mature cattle are most commonly associated with winter dysentery (qv, p 226) but also can be associated with salmonellosis when there is heavy contamination of feed or water. Chronic diarrhea with unthriftiness and wasting, and occurring as a sporadic disease, most commonly is associated with paratuberculosis (qv, p 399), but also may be caused by chronic salmonellosis and chronic BVD infections. Diarrhea with wasting also may be seen in individual cattle with congestive heart failure, uremia, or chronic infections of the peritoneal cavity. Persistent diarrhea with unthriftiness, and occasionally wasting in yearling and mature cattle, can be associated with a secondary copper deficiency due to excess molybdenum in the pastures (qv, p 1197), and diarrhea may also accompany selenium-responsive ill-thrift syndromes in growing cattle.

Individual cases or outbreaks of diarrhea may be associated with dietary indiscretions. Diarrhea may follow cases of simple indigestion and is common in rumen overload (qv, p 175). It also follows ingestion of toxic amounts of chemicals (eg, arsenic, copper, zinc, and molybdenum) or certain poisonous plants, and with dipyridyl and organophosphate poisoning. Cattle may also harbor *Campylobacter jejuni* in the intestine; although this is rarely associated with clinical disease in cows, fecal contamination of milk may lead to outbreaks of gastroenteritis in people who consume unpasteurized milk or cheese products. Intestinal adenocarcinoma occurs in some geographic areas, commonly in association with bovine enzootic hematuria, and is believed to result from the interaction of a carcinogen in bracken fern (*Pteridium* spp) and papilloma virus (*see* p 1641).

Determination of the cause of intestinal disease in cattle is based on clinical, epidemiological, and laboratory findings. Nonspecific therapy includes replacement of fluid and electrolyte loss. Specific therapy and prevention are detailed under the individual disease headings.

INTESTINAL DISEASES IN SHEEP AND GOATS

The causes and circumstances of diarrhea in neonatal lambs and kids are similar to those in newborn calves. Intensive lambing practices and shed-lambing increase the potential for disease and buildup of infectious agents, and can be associated with serious outbreaks of diarrhea. The serotypes of enteropathogenic *Escherichia coli* that cause secretory diarrhea in calves (qv, p 181) also do so in lambs, and the approach to diagnosis, treatment, and control is similar. Similarly, rotavirus (qv, p 181), coronavirus (qv, p 181), and cryptosporidia (qv, p 108) also cause outbreaks of diarrhea in lambs. Lamb dysentery caused by *Clostridium perfringens* type B (qv, p 325) is a distinct intestinal disease of lambs in the first week of life. It occurs principally in hill breeds of sheep in the UK and is characterized by sudden death or diarrhea, dysentery, and toxemia. In the USA, *C perfringens* type C (qv, p 325) causes a similar syndrome. Coccidiosis (qv, p 103) and GI helminthiasis (qv, p 209), except for haemonchosis, are important causes of diarrhea in older nursing and weaned sheep.

GI helminthiasis is the most common cause of diarrhea in pastured sheep. Coccidiosis occurs in association with overstocking or intensive indoor housing and poor sanitation. Salmonellosis (qv, p 148) can cause diarrhea in all ages; the circumstances in young lambs are similar to those in calves. It also can cause outbreaks of diarrhea late in pregnancy and is frequently accompanied by abortion. Salmonellosis is more common when sheep or goats are congregated intensively or stressed, particularly by shipping. Diarrhea may be present in bluetongue in sheep (qv, p 390) and is accompanied by typical mucosal lesions. In goats, diarrhea is often prominent in enterotoxemia associated with *C perfringens* type D (qv, p 326). This is not a feature of the clinical disease in sheep but may be present in flockmates of affected sheep. In feedlot sheep, diarrhea most commonly is associated with grain overload, salmonellosis, or coccidiosis.

Other intestinal diseases of adult sheep may manifest with diarrhea. Infection with *C perfringens* type C (struck, qv, p 325) manifests with abdominal pain, straining to defecate, and rapid death. Sheep with paratuberculosis (qv, p 399) usually show progressive emaciation without diarrhea. Progressive emaciation also is the primary sign in adult sheep with intestinal adenocarcinoma, which can be prevalent in certain geographic areas, associated with ingestion of bracken fern (*Pteridium* sp—*see* p 1641).

DIARRHEA IN NEONATAL RUMINANTS
(Scours)

Diarrhea is common in newborn calves, lambs, and kids. The acute disease is characterized by progressive dehydration and death, sometimes in as few as 12 hr. In the subacute form, diarrhea may persist for several days and result in malnutrition and emaciation. This discussion emphasizes the disease in calves, but the principles of pathophysiology and treatment apply to lambs and kids as well.

Etiology: Several enteropathogens are associated with neonatal diarrhea, and their relative importance varies geographically. *Escherichia coli* is the most common bacterial cause of diarrhea in calves; many varieties exist and there are at least 2, and probably 3, distinct types of diarrhea caused by different strains of this organism. Strains that can invade the gut wall and survive in serum commonly cause septicemia, which may or may not be accompanied by diarrhea. Strains that produce enterotoxin and possess the K99 fimbrial antigen cause severe diarrhea without septicemia. Usually, only calves <3 days old are affected by these first 2 types of *E coli*. A third and much less common type is known as "attaching-and-effacing" or "verotoxin-producing". This type of infection appears to occur in calves >3 days old and may be accompanied by blood and inflammatory products in the feces. *Salmonella* spp, especially *S typhimurium* and *S dublin*, cause diarrhea in calves 2-6 wk old (*see also* p 148). *Clostridium perfringens* types A, B, C, and E can cause hemorrhagic enteritis and rapid death in calves and lambs. *Campylobacter jejuni* may be present in the feces of diarrheic calves, but also may be found in the feces of healthy calves.

Rotavirus and coronavirus are common causes of calf diarrhea, usually in calves 5-15 days old. Other viral and chlamydial agents cause diarrhea in calves, but appear to be less prevalent than rotavirus and coronavirus. The viruses of bovine viral diarrhea and infectious bovine rhinotracheitis are reported to cause calf diarrhea, but this is not a common manifestation of these infections. *Cryptosporidium* spp are protozoa that commonly cause diarrhea in calves 5-35 days old (*see* p 108).

Diarrhea also can be caused by feeding excessive milk or using inappropriately formulated milk replacers. Also, there is evidence that vitamin C deficiency is a factor in diarrhea in neonates in some herds.

Enteropathogens associated with diarrhea in calves can commonly be found in the feces of healthy calves, and whether intestinal infection leads to diarrhea depends on a number of determinants. Several epidemiological determinants include: insufficient transfer of colostral immunoglobulins, lack of specific colostral antibodies in dams that have not been exposed to specific pathogens, stress caused by a poor indoor environment or inadequate protection from the weather, insufficient or inappropriate diet, inadequate hygiene, and a poor overall level of management.

Pathogenesis: Diarrhea in neonatal ruminants is usually associated with disease of the small intestine and can be caused by either hypersecretion or malabsorption. Hypersecretory diarrhea occurs when an abnormal amount of fluid is secreted into the gut, and exceeds the resorptive capacity of the mucosa. In malabsorptive diarrhea, the capacity of the mucosa to absorb fluid and nutrients is impaired to the extent that it cannot keep pace with the normal influx of ingested and secreted fluids. Malabsorptive diarrhea may be aggravated by the colonic fermentation of nutrients that would normally have been absorbed in the small intestine. Fermentation products, especially lactic acid, appear to draw water into the colon osmotically, which contributes to the severity of diarrhea. Most infectious forms of diarrhea probably have both hypersecretory and malabsorptive components, although one or the other usually predominates. Both lead to rapid loss of body water, electrolytes, and bicarbonate, which results in severe dehydration and acidosis.

Enterotoxigenic *E coli* (those possessing an attachment factor, such as the K99 antigen, and producing an enterotoxin) stimulate marked hypersecretion. Other forms of *E coli*, and salmonellae as well, may also produce hypersecretion-inducing enterotoxins, but these have not been chemically identified. In addition to the production of specific enterotoxins, bacteria might also induce diarrhea secondarily due to the hypersecretory actions of various products of inflammation. Salmonellae usually cause septicemia, in addition to diarrhea. Pathogenic *C perfringens* produce necrotizing toxins.

Viruses usually produce a malabsorptive diarrhea by destroying the absorptive cells of the mucosa, thus shortening the intestinal villi. The mechanism by which cryptosporidia produce diarrhea is not completely understood, but it appears to have a malabsorptive component.

Inappropriately formulated milk replacers produce diarrhea by 2 mechanisms, both associated with malabsorption. Vegetable (especially soybean) products are commonly used as protein sources in the manufacture of milk replacers. Depending on the degree of refinement, these products may contain carbohydrates that are indigestible in young calves. Such carbohydrates are not absorbed in the small intestine and may contribute to diarrhea via colonic fermentation. In addition, most calves <3 wk old appear to have an allergic reaction to soy proteins that results in villous atrophy, leading to diarrhea that is probably malabsorptive.

Clinical Findings: The major signs are diarrhea, dehydration, profound weakness, and death within one to several days of onset. Usually, it is difficult to make a definite etiological diagnosis based solely on clinical findings. However, the history, age of the animal(s) affected, and clinical signs may permit a presumptive diagnosis.

Diarrhea due to enterotoxigenic (K99-bearing) *E coli* occurs in calves <3-5 days old, rarely later. Onset is sudden. Profuse amounts of liquid feces are passed, and the calves rapidly become depressed and recumbent. Circulatory collapse and death may occur in 12-24 hr. Body temperature may be elevated, but is commonly normal or subnormal. Response to fluid and electrolyte therapy is usually good, if administered early. Diarrhea due to *Salmonella* spp usually does not occur in calves <14 days old. It is characterized by feces that are foul smelling and contain blood, fibrin, and copious amounts of mucus; a fever is common. Calves with salmonellosis usually lose weight rapidly and often die in spite of vigorous therapy. Hemorrhagic enterotoxemia due to *C perfringens* type B or C is characterized by acute onset of depression, weakness, bloody diarrhea, abdominal pain, and death within a few hr. It usually occurs in vigorous calves that are just a few days old that have large appetites and a ready source of milk. Calves affected with *C perfringens* usually die before treatment can be instituted.

Diarrhea due to rotavirus, coronavirus, and other viruses usually occurs in 5- to 15-day-old calves. Affected calves are only moderately depressed and often continue to suck or drink milk. The feces are voluminous, soft to liquid, and often contain large amounts of mucus. Diarrhea commonly persists for 3 to several days, with some cases of coronaviral diarrhea becoming chronic. Cases of viral diarrhea that are uncomplicated by other pathogens commonly respond within a few days to fluid and electrolyte therapy and adequate nutritional support.

Cryptosporidiosis occurs in calves 5-35 days old and is characterized by persistent diarrhea that does not respond to therapy. Diarrhea due to *Cryptosporidium* spp alone is often mild and self-limiting, although the severity may be related to the general strength of the calf and the intensity of exposure to the organism. Combination infections with cryptosporidia and rota- and/or coronavirus are common and result in persistent diarrhea that is often characterized by emaciation and death.

Dietary diarrheas occur in calves <3 wk old and are characterized by voluminous feces with pasty to gelatinous consistency. Initially, the calves are bright and alert and have good appetites. Eventually, however, they become weak and emaciated if the diet is not corrected. Infectious forms of diarrhea are often complicated by poor-quality diets and/or insufficient nutritional intake.

Laboratory Diagnosis: Fecal samples can be submitted for isolation and characterization of the common enteropathogens. Special techniques are necessary for the demonstration of viruses, cryptosporidia, and K99-bearing *E coli*. Demonstration of viruses requires fecal samples from calves in the early stages of diarrhea. The interpretation of fecal microbiology can be difficult because of mixed infections. When outbreaks of diarrhea occur, the best diagnostic information is usually obtained by submitting untreated, acutely affected animals for necropsy. This allows examination of intestinal mucosa for evidence of diagnostic lesions and the physical presence of enteropathogens such as cryptosporidia. The diagnostic value of a necropsy diminishes quickly with time after death; important lesions can disappear within minutes due to autolysis. It is important to submit live animals when attempting to diagnose severe herd problems. In all cases, information on total milk or milk replacer consumption should be gathered. When milk replacer is being fed, the composition of the diet should be evaluated. Nonspecific immunity should be assessed by determining immunoglobulin and vitamin A concentrations in serum.

Treatment: Many of the factors involved in disease resistance are nonspecific; thus, important preventive measures can be taken and therapy can be initiated before an etiological diagnosis has been established. Treatment includes fluid and electrolyte replacement, alterations of the diet, antimicrobial and immunoglobulin therapy, and use of antidiarrheal drugs and adsorbents. Vitamin C may warrant at least a trial in outbreaks. Fluid and electrolyte therapy is most important and should be instituted as soon as possible. Calves that are still able to stand, and are willing and able to suck can often be treated with oral electrolytes alone. Many commercial preparations containing sodium, glucose, and other ingredients are available and are formulated to promote sodium and water absorption across the gut wall. These can be administered by nipple bottle or, if necessary, by stomach tube. The solutions should be used liberally until the animal is rehydrated. Whether or not milk should be fed during the rehydration period is controversial. Feeding milk may increase fecal volume, but it provides energy to the calf and may promote gut healing. Calves have large energy requirements and little reserve. Electrolyte solutions do not meet calf energy requirements; therefore, if milk is withheld, it should not be for more than 24-36 hr.

Calves that are recumbent and weak, and show evidence of water loss ≥8% of their body wt require IV fluid and electrolyte therapy. These calves are usually acidotic, and the fluid and base deficits can be corrected initially by administering an isotonic (13 g/L) solution of sodium bicarbonate. Ideally, 100 mL/kg body wt of this solution should be administered over 4-6 hr. The calves are frequently hypoglycemic; addition of 25-50 g of dextrose to the bicarbonate solution is often beneficial. The bicarbonate solution should be followed by continuous IV fluid therapy with a physiologically balanced electrolyte solution administered at 5-8 mL/kg/hr for the next 20 hr; higher rates may be necessary depending on the severity of diarrhea. Oral electrolyte solutions can, and probably should, be used concurrently with IV therapy.

The use of antimicrobials is controversial and not supported by clinical trials. Several drugs, such as opiate derivatives, which affect intestinal secretion and motility in some species, are available but not of established efficacy in neonatal ruminants. Intestinal gels and adsorbents, such as kaolin and pectin, are in general use, but their only established effect is to increase fecal consistency.

Prevention and Control: Because of the complex nature of diarrhea in neonates, it is unrealistic to expect total prevention—economical control is the major objective. The incidence of clinical disease and the case fatality rate depend on the balance between the level of exposure to infectious agents and the level of resistance in the calf. Differences in herd size; availability of facilities, land and labor; and general management objectives make it impossible to recommend specific management procedures that are applicable to all situations. However, 3 broad principles apply in all herds: 1) reduce the degree of exposure of neonates by isolating diseased animals, or by moving calving and calf rearing to a separate area, and by practicing good general hygiene; 2) provide maximal nonspecific resistance by providing good nutrition to the dam and neonate and assuring that newborn calves consume ≥5% of their body wt of high-quality colostrum within 6 hr of birth; and 3) increase the specific resistance of the newborn by vaccination of the dam or the newborn. A significant portion of both naturally sucking dairy calves and calves hand-fed colostrum fail to acquire adequate amounts of immunoglobulin because of delayed sucking or feeding and/or the ingestion of an inadequate volume. (*See* DISEASE-MANAGEMENT INTERACTION: CATTLE, p 1108, and MANAGEMENT OF REPRODUCTION: CATTLE, p 1127.)

Immunization of calves against colibacillosis by vaccination of pregnant dams can control enterotoxigenic colibacillosis. The pregnant dam is vaccinated 6 and 2 wk before parturition to stimulate antibodies to strains of enterotoxigenic *E coli*; these antibodies are then passed on to the newborn through the colostrum (provided the calf ingests the colostrum).

A monoclonal K99 *E coli* antibody is now commercially available for oral administration to calves immediately after birth. It is an effective substitute for the K99-specific antibody in the colostrum of vaccinated cows, although calves that receive this product should also receive colostrum for its nonspecific protection. Rotaviral and coronaviral vaccines are used in a similar manner; however, the concentration of antibodies that is stimulated in colostrum or milk by currently available commercial vaccines may not be protective.

INTESTINAL DISEASES IN HORSES

Intestinal disease in horses is suggested by diarrhea, weight loss, hypoproteinemia, and abdominal pain (*see* COLIC, p 168).

DIARRHEAL DISEASES OF ADULT HORSES

Diarrhea in adult horses can be acute or chronic. Known causes of acute diarrhea include bacteria such as salmonellae, *Ehrlichia risticii*, and clostridia. An acute, fatal diarrheal disease of unknown etiology is classified as colitis-X. Diarrhea that persists >1 mo is considered chronic, and is often a perplexing diagnostic problem. Differential diagnoses include parasitism, sand enteropathy, and infiltrative lesions. Allergy to components of feed may also play a role in chronic diarrhea.

SALMONELLOSIS

Clinical manifestations range from asymptomatic (carrier) to acute, severe diarrhea. The disease most commonly occurs sporadically but may become an epidemic depending on the virulence of the specific serotype. Infection can occur via contamination of feed or water, or by contact with active shedders of the bacteria. Stress appears to play an important role in pathogenesis; a history of surgery, transportation, and concurrent disease often precedes the diarrhea by 2-7 days. *Salmonella typhimurium, S enteritidis, S agona, S anatum, S heidelberg,* and *S newport* are the most common serotypes associated with diarrhea in adults. Knowledge of the serotype may aid in developing an accurate prognosis. Some serotypes, eg, *S typhimurium,* appear to be more pathogenic than others.

Clinical Findings: Three forms have been recognized in adult horses. One is the asymptomatic carrier, which may or may not be actively shedding the organism, but has the potential of transmitting it to susceptible animals. If stressed, the carrier may also develop clinical disease. Multiple fecal cultures may be necessary to identify this form because the organism is shed intermittently and in small numbers.

The second form is a mild disease, with signs of depression, fever, anorexia, and soft but not watery feces. The horses have an absolute neutropenia. Clinical disease may last 4-5 days and usually is self-limiting. Salmonellae can be cultured from the feces. Recovered animals may continue to excrete the organism in their feces for a few weeks; therefore, isolation and thorough disinfection of the contaminated area are recommended.

The third and most common form is characterized by an acute onset of severe depression, anorexia, profound neutropenia, and frequently, abdominal pain. Diarrhea occurs in 6-24 hr. Feces are fluid, foul smelling, and may contain mucosal elements and rarely, frank blood. These animals dehydrate rapidly. Acidosis and electrolyte losses (Na^+, K^+, Cl^-) occur as the condition deteriorates. Severe salmonellosis is also a protein-losing enteropathy. Plasma protein levels may become dangerously low after a few days of diarrhea. Occasionally, these animals become bacteremic. If untreated, this form is usually fatal.

Diagnosis: This is made on clinical signs, a severe neutropenia, and positive cultures of feces or blood. Culturing small amounts of feces has been more successful in identifying carriers of salmonellae than culturing rectal swabs. Because salmonellae cannot be consistently cultured from active shedders, it is necessary to submit multiple samples collected at different times. Additional culturing of rectal mucosal biopsies increases the probability of isolating the organism. Samples should be placed in selenite broth at the time of collection to minimize growth of other lactose-fermenting bacteria.

Treatment: Treatment for the severe form of salmonellosis is based on IV fluid and electrolyte replacement. A balanced electrolyte solution, eg, lactated Ringer's, is good for volume replacement. Because fluid is actively being secreted into the lumen of the intestine, volumes of 40-80 L may be necessary. Electrolyte and acid-base deficiencies can be corrected by use of fluids enriched with potassium chloride and sodium bicarbonate.

Specific antimicrobial therapy is questionable. Multiple antibiotic resistances have developed; resistance appears to be increased to ampicillin, chloramphenicol, and gentamicin. Sensitivity patterns can change over the course of an outbreak. Selection of antibiotic should be determined by the sensitivity pattern of the organism isolated.

The use of GI protectants, eg, bismuth subsalicylate and activated charcoal, may be beneficial, but this has not been proved. Low doses of flunixin meglumine given systemically help counteract the effect of endotoxins that are released.

Owners should be made aware of the zoonotic nature of *Salmonella* spp. Strict hygienic practices should be maintained when dealing with infected animals.

POTOMAC HORSE FEVER
(Equine ehrlichial colitis, Equine monocytic ehrlichiosis)

(See also EQUINE EHRLICHIOSIS, p 375.)

An acute diarrheal syndrome first described in horses in close proximity to the Potomac River in Maryland and Virginia, and the Susquehanna River Valley in Pennsylvania. The causative agent was identified as *Ehrlichia risticii*. Subsequently, antibodies to *E risticii* have been found in horses in 18 states and Canada. The disease has not been recorded outside North America. It occurs sporadically, frequently with only one animal being affected on a farm.

Because of the seasonal nature of the disease (high incidence during summer and autumn) and because it can be transmitted by blood inoculation, an arthropod vector is suspected. Most rickettsiae are transmitted by ticks, fleas, or lice. To date, no particular species has been incriminated as a vector for *E risticii*.

Clinical Findings: The first signs following a 9- to 15-day incubation period are depression, anorexia, fever, mucous membrane injection, and ileus. Diarrhea may then be seen within 24 hr after the first signs. In fully susceptible populations, mild diarrhea develops in ~30% of affected horses, and severe watery diarrhea in ~50%. Colic and laminitis may occur in up to 30% of cases.

The WBC count is variable; a marked leukopenia followed by leukocytosis is common. Lymphopenia and a mild neutrophilic left shift commonly occur at the onset of fever and depression.

Severity varies considerably, but in the absence of treatment, mortality approaches 30%, with death occurring primarily from dehydration and hypovolemic shock, or because laminitis necessitates euthanasia. Postmortem findings include fluid contents of the cecum and large colon. Intestinal lesions vary from patchy areas of hyperemia and petechiation to diffuse enterocolitis.

Diagnosis: This can be made on the clinical signs, a transient leukopenia (specifically lymphopenia) in the early clinical disease, failure to culture *Salmonella* spp, and perhaps the presence of a high serum titer for *E risticii* measured by immunofluorescent antibody (IFA) and ELISA tests. Unfortunately, IFA titers are near their maximum by the time of the onset of diarrhea; therefore, no change in titer may occur between acute and convalescent samples. Another complicating factor is that titers may remain high (>1:320) for >1 yr. For these reasons, clinical interpretation of titer results may not be valid on an individual case basis.

Isolation of *E risticii* is the most accurate method of diagnosis but is difficult. Rarely, the causative organism can be seen within monocytes on a Giemsa- or Wright's-stained blood smear.

Treatment: The therapeutic regimen for Potomac horse fever is similar to that of acute salmonellosis, which is the principal differential diagnosis. It should include aggressive IV fluid and electrolyte replacement. *Ehrlichia risticii* appears to be most sensitive to oxytetracycline in both *in vivo* and *in vitro* studies.

CLOSTRIDIOSIS

Clostridium perfringens type A, by production of an enterotoxin, can cause acute diarrhea and toxemia in horses. The incidence is sporadic, and animals of all ages can be affected. Prognosis depends on severity of the intoxication.

Signs are similar to those of other cases of peracute to acute watery diarrhea. Depression, dehydration, and discolored mucous membranes are prominent. Heart rates may be >100 beats/min. Leukopenia may be followed by leukocytosis. An elevated AST (SGOT) indicates liver damage, which can be confirmed on biopsy.

Postmortem findings include hemorrhagic or necrotizing typhlitis and colitis. The small intestine may also be involved. Myocardial degeneration may be evident microscopically. Pulmonary hyperemia, edema, hemorrhage, and over-inflation are seen consistently. Fecal culture and quantitation of bacteria are necessary for confirmation. A *C perfringens* count of $\geq 10^2$ colony-forming units/g of feces is considered diagnostic. This organism is rarely isolated from normal feces.

Supportive therapy (IV) with a balanced electrolyte fluid is important. In Sweden, affected animals are treated with a milk product that is produced from a lactic-acid-producing strain of streptococci; it appears to be effective, although the pharmacologic action is unknown. Some therapeutic success has been reported with the use of *C perfringens* types C and D antitoxin, 250 mL diluted in 2 L of lactated Ringer's solution and administered IV, slowly. Once the animal has recovered from the acute disease, it should be rested ≥ 1 mo to allow the possible myocardial lesions to heal.

COLITIS-X

A peracute, fatal disease of unknown etiology, characterized by sudden onset of profuse watery diarrhea and development of hypovolemic shock. Many affected horses have a history of stress.

Clinically, there may be a short febrile period, but the temperature soon returns to normal or subnormal. Tachypnea, tachycardia, and marked depression are present. An explosive diarrhea develops, followed by extreme dehydration. Hypovolemic and probably endotoxic shock are manifested in poor capillary refill time, purplish mucous membranes, and cold extremities. Death may occur within 3 hr of onset or, in less acute cases, within 24-48 hr. Most horses remain standing until the terminal stage. At necropsy, there is pronounced edema and hemorrhage in the wall of the large colon and cecum, and the intestinal contents are fluid and blood-stained.

Typically, the PCV is >65% even only shortly after the onset. The leukogram ranges from normal to neutropenia with a degenerative left shift. Metabolic acidosis and electrolyte disorders that are associated with the diarrhea are also present.

Disease onset is often closely associated with stress, such as surgery and transport. Peracute salmonellosis may cause signs identical to those of colitis-X, but in these horses, *Salmonella* spp cannot be cultured from the feces or organs. Other diarrheal diseases that may mimic colitis-X are enterotoxemia caused by *C perfringens* type A, Potomac horse fever, experimental endotoxic shock in ponies, and anaphylaxis. A similar condition may be seen following use of tetracycline or lincomycin.

Treatment for colitis-X is similar to that of salmonellosis (*see* above). Large volumes of IV fluid are needed to counter the severe dehydration, and electrolyte and bicarbonate replacement is necessary. Flunixin meglumine may help block the endotoxin effects.

PARASITISM

Both large and small strongyles have been incriminated as a cause of chronic diarrhea. *See* GASTROINTESTINAL PARASITES OF HORSES, p 201.

Giardiasis (qv, p 136) has been reported as a possible cause of intermittent diarrhea in horses.

SAND ENTEROPATHY

Consumption of large amounts of sand can produce GI irritation or obstruction. Sand is ingested when the horse grazes on sandy pasture or is fed hay and grain on the ground. The mucosal irritation may cause diarrhea before an obstruction is noted. A diagnosis can be made on the history of a sandy environment and the presence of sand in the feces. Treatment involves use of a hemicellulose product that can be administered via nasogastric tube or added daily to the feed at 125-175 g.

INFILTRATIVE DISEASE

Any process that causes a thickening of the walls of the large colon may interfere with absorption of water, and thus result in chronic diarrhea. This includes neoplasia, inflammation, and scar formation from previous acute colitis. Rectal examination may help detect neoplasia. A rectal biopsy may be beneficial in diagnosis, but a surgically obtained colonic biopsy is more reliable.

DIARRHEAL DISEASES OF FOALS

Diarrhea is fairly common in foals <6 mo old. Many episodes are mild and self-limiting, but some can be fatal if the foal is septic or dehydrated. Foal heat diarrhea, as well as bacteria and viruses are the most frequent causes of diarrhea in foals.

FOAL HEAT DIARRHEA

Between 4 and 14 days postpartum, foals often develop a mild, self-limiting diarrhea. During this time the dam is usually undergoing her first estrous cycle, hence the name foal heat diarrhea. Though the cause is still unclear, it may be associated with alterations in the foal's microbial flora or an increase of roughage being introduced to the large colon. It does not appear to be infectious or parasitic.

The foal remains active and alert, and appetite is unaffected. Vital signs remain within normal limits. Fecal consistency can range from soft to watery. Observation to ensure that the animal's condition does not deteriorate is important.

Specific treatment is not necessary, but application of zinc oxide around the perineum helps prevent scalding. Bismuth subsalicylate PO may be beneficial in some prolonged cases.

BACTERIAL DIARRHEA

Bacterial enteritis/colitis in neonatal foals is often a component of neonatal septicemia. Organisms that may be involved include *Salmonella, Escherichia coli,* and *Klebsiella.* Intensive antimicrobial therapy, fluid and electrolyte correction, and nursing care are needed. Because most affected foals have not received adequate colostrum, plasma transfusions may be indicated (*see* SEPTICEMIA IN FOALS, p 378).

An acute, fulminant, hemorrhagic diarrhea with high mortality occurs in young foals associated with *Clostridium perfringens* types B and C. Infections may be sporadic or widespread on a farm. Severe depression and rapid deterioration of cardiovascular status is followed by death in 24-48 hr. Intraluminal hemorrhage and extensive mucosal necrosis of the small intestine is found on necropsy.

Other bacteria that have been associated with foal diarrhea are *Bacteroides fragilis, Clostridium difficile,* and *Rhodococcus (Corynebacterium) equi.* The first 2 occur in foals <2 wk old and require intensive supportive care. Although *R equi* is primarily a respiratory infection, both acute and chronic enteritis can be seen; diarrhea is seen in 1- to 4-mo-old foals. The diagnosis is easier if pneumonia is present. The bacteria can be cultured from a tracheal wash. A positive fecal culture is not helpful because *R equi* is normally found in the feces of healthy foals. Erythromycin combined with rifampin is the treatment of choice.

VIRAL DIARRHEA

Rotavirus is the main viral cause of diarrhea in foals. It is highly contagious and may spread to all foals on a farm within 3-5 days. It is characterized by depression, anorexia, and profuse watery diarrhea. It is usually seen in foals <2 mo old and affects the younger ones more severely. The diarrhea usually last 4-7 days, though it can persist for weeks.

The virus destroys the absorptive enterocytes in the small intestine, which causes malabsorption. Lactase also becomes deficient, which results in lactose passing into the large intestine and inducing an osmotic diarrhea.

Diagnosis is made by viral identification in the feces by electron microscopy or ELISA. The ELISA test is rapid and convenient.

Treatment is generally supportive. Use of a commercial lactase preparation added to the foal's milk may benefit persistently infected foals.

MISCELLANEOUS

Nutritional diarrhea can result from overfeeding, such as occurs when a foal is reunited with the mare after a period of separation; and improper nutrition, such as in orphan foals fed calf milk replacer, or foals given sucrose. Lactose intolerance in foals is recorded, but is rare and can be determined by lactose tolerance challenge tests. Diarrhea in foals may also be associated with *Strongyloides westeri* and cryptosporidiosis. Intestinal disease may be seen in Arabian foals with combined immunodeficiency syndrome.

WEIGHT LOSS AND HYPOPROTEINEMIA

The causes for weight loss in horses are numerous and can involve any of the general body systems. This discussion is confined to diseases of the GI tract. Protein loss may or may not be associated with weight loss. The disorders that are commonly associated with either of these signs are GI neoplasia, inflammatory bowel disease, and phenylbutazone toxicity.

GASTROINTESTINAL NEOPLASIA

Squamous cell carcinoma of the stomach and the alimentary form of lymphosarcoma are the most common forms of GI neoplasia in horses. Chronic weight loss may be the only complaint. Chronic diarrhea and hypoalbuminemia may be seen in horses with lymphosarcoma that has infiltrated the wall of the intestine.

Because the incidence of GI neoplasia is low, other causes of weight loss should be investigated first. Diagnosis is usually made through exclusion of these other causes, and necropsy. Squamous cell carcinoma of the stomach can be diagnosed by gastroscopy; a 2-3 m fiberoptic endoscope is necessary to examine the gastric mucosa of adult horses. In lymphosarcoma, rectal palpation may detect enlarged lymph nodes or thickened bowel. An exploratory laparotomy with intestinal biopsy can provide a definitive diagnosis.

No specific treatment is available to treat GI neoplasia in horses. Prognosis is grave.

INFLAMMATORY BOWEL DISEASE

Granulomatous enteritis and chronic eosinophilic gastroenteritis should be considered in the differential diagnosis of weight loss and hypoproteinemia. Both conditions involve the infiltration of the small and large intestine and regional lymph nodes with inflammatory cells. This results in malabsorption and a protein-losing enteropathy. Diarrhea may or may not be a clinical feature.

Diagnosis of either of these syndromes is made on clinical signs, the presence of thickened bowel on rectal palpation, low serum protein, and intestinal or rectal biopsy. An oral glucose-tolerance test or a D-xylose absorption test may verify the presence of malabsorption.

The pathophysiology of these syndromes in horses is not fully understood. Tuberculosis, parasitic migration, and immune-mediated causes have been suggested.

Various medical therapies have been tried with limited success. Corticosteriods, metronidazole, and the antimetabolite azathioprine have been used with variable efficacy. Supportive nutritional care should involve frequent feeding of good-quality, high-energy feeds. Force feeding with a nasogastric tube may be needed in horses that are anorectic. (The use of human alimentation formulas in horses is under investigation.) The prognosis is grave.

PHENYLBUTAZONE TOXICOSIS

Phenylbutazone can cause a protein-losing gastroenteropathy in horses when administered at >8.8 mg/kg body wt. Ponies and foals appear more sensitive to the toxic effects of this drug than adults. Signs may include oral ulceration, anorexia, depression, weight loss, and ventral edema. Hypoproteinemia occurs due to protein leakage through the intestinal wall; this can occur without visible ulceration of the large or small intestine. However, gastric ulceration is often a sequela of phenylbutazone toxicosis. Renal papillary necrosis may also occur.

Diagnosis can be made on the history of phenylbutazone administration, clinical signs, and presence of hypoproteinemia. Gastric ulceration can be confirmed by gastroscopy using a 2-3 m fiberoptic endoscope.

Use of phenylbutazone or any nonsteroidal anti-inflammatory drug should be discontinued. Anti-ulcer medications, such as cimetidine, ranitidine, and sucralfate, may be beneficial in treating gastric ulcers. A convalescent period of several months may be necessary before the hypoproteinemia resolves.

PROXIMAL ENTERITIS
(Anterior enteritis, Duodenitis-jejunitis)

A syndrome characterized by moderate to severe abdominal pain, ileus, and gastric distention. Affected horses are usually tachycardic and may have a mild increase in body temperature. If untreated, these animals develop shock and possibly gastric rupture. The PCV and serum proteins may be increased, indicative of dehydration. The peripheral WBC count varies between cases. Abdominal paracentesis samples generally have a normal WBC count, but frequently peritoneal protein levels are >3 g/dL.

This syndrome should be differentiated from small-intestinal obstruction, which has many of the same clinical signs. Important differences are found on rectal palpation and response to gastric emptying. In a small-intestinal obstruction, rectal palpation generally reveals grossly distended loops of small bowel; in proximal enteritis, a slightly distended or thickened small intestine may be felt, but the rectum may also be normal.

Passage of a nasogastric tube in either syndrome may result in large amounts of gastric reflux. Horses with proximal enteritis are greatly relieved by this treatment, while horses with small-intestinal obstruction continue to deteriorate.

Horses with proximal enteritis may continue to reflux large amounts of fluid into the stomach for several days. Treatment involves repeated or continuous nasogastric decompression. Because of the large volume of fluid loss, 40-60 L of IV fluids may be required daily. Nonsteroidal anti-inflammatory drugs may be needed to relieve pain and provide protection from endotoxins. Though no etiologic agent has been identified, broad-spectrum antibiotics may be beneficial.

Possible complications include aspiration pneumonia and laminitis. Prognosis is guarded, but with intensive care, many of these animals survive.

INTESTINAL DISEASES IN PIGS

Pigs of all ages are susceptible to intestinal diseases. Diarrhea is the sign common to nearly all such disorders. Transmission of infectious enteropathies is by the fecal-oral route. At least 12 different etiological agents, including bacteria, viruses, and parasites, can cause primary intestinal disease. Diarrhea in a herd may be due to a single agent, but concurrent infections are common. Because some diseases are age-dependent, differential diagnosis is best considered by age group (*see* TABLE 6).

Table 6. Age Distribution of Diarrheal Diseases in Pigs

	Age Group		
	Nursing	Weaning	Growing-Finishing, Breeding
Bacterial Diseases			
Clostridium perfringens type C enteritis	+ +	—	—
Enteric colibacillosis	+ + +	+ + +	—
Porcine proliferative enteritis	—	+	+ + +
Salmonella enteritis	+	+	+ + +
Swine dysentery	+	+	+ + +
Parasitism			
Cryptosporidium sp	+	+	—
Isospora suis	+ + +	+	—
Strongyloides ransomi	+	+	+
Trichuris suis	—	—	+ +
Viral Diseases			
Porcine epidemic diarrhea	+	+ +	+ + +
Rotaviral enteritis	+ + +	+ + +	+
Transmissible gastroenteritis	+ + +	+ + +	+ +
Other (adeno-, entero-, pararotavirus)	+	+	—

   — Rare, or does not occur
   + Uncommon
  + + Common
+ + + Very common

CLOSTRIDIUM PERFRINGENS TYPE C ENTERITIS

A highly fatal, necrohemorrhagic enteritis caused by infection of the small intestine by type C strains of *C perfringens (welchii)*. It most commonly affects 1- to 5-day-old piglets, but may occur in pigs up to 3 wk old (and in other species, *see also* p 325).

Etiology and Pathogenesis: The organism penetrates between the absorptive cells of the upper jejunum, and elaborates β toxin, a potent, heat-labile, trypsin-sensitive exotoxin that causes necrosis of all structural components of the villi. Necrotizing inflammation usually extends to the mucosal crypts. The infection may continue caudally and involve the ileum, but it rarely affects the colon. Necrosis of the mucosa is accompanied by blood loss into the intestinal wall and lumen.

Clinical Findings: Sudden onset of hemorrhagic diarrhea followed by collapse and death is characteristic in 1- to 3-day-old piglets. In less acute cases, brownish liquid feces develops at 3-5 days. Infrequently, 1- to 3-wk-old pigs develop a persistent, pasty, gray diarrhea and become progressively emaciated. In peracute cases, the perineal region is blood stained.
    Lesions: The small intestines are dark red, hemorrhagic, and filled with hemorrhagic liquid; less acute cases at 3-5 days may have gas bubbles in the wall of the jejunum, and necrosis of the mucosa of the jejunum and ileum. More chronic cases have a thickened small intestine that is lined by a pale yellow or gray necrotic membrane tightly adhered to the submucosa.

Diagnosis: Necropsy is usually sufficient to establish the diagnosis in the peracute hemorrhagic form and in the acute form with jejunal emphysema. A rapid presumptive diagnosis can be made by demonstrating coccidial forms in gram-stained mucosal impression smears. Histological observation of villous necrosis with mucosal colonization by numerous large gram-positive rods is adequate for confirmation. Subacute and chronic forms of the disease in pigs 6-14 days old are easily confused at necropsy with *Isospora suis* enteritis, but diagnosis is usually possible by histological examination of the jejunum and ileum, or by observing clostridia or coccidia in mucosal smears stained with Gram's or Giemsa stain.

Treatment and Control: Treatment of pigs with clinical signs is of little benefit because lesions usually are irreversible at the onset of diarrhea. In an acute outbreak, prophylactic administration of type C antitoxin and/or antibiotic parenterally or PO is protective if given to piglets within 2 hr of birth. The disease tends to recur on infected premises. Vaccination of gestating sows at 6 and 3 wk before parturition with type C bacterin-toxoid confers some passive lactogenic immunity to subsequent litters, provided piglets consume colostrum soon after birth. Once immunized with 2 doses of bacterin-toxoid, sows should receive one dose ~3 wk before each subsequent farrowing.

EDEMA DISEASE
(*Escherichia coli* enterotoxemia)

An acute, highly fatal, neurological disorder (qv, p 598) that usually occurs 5 days to 2 wk after weaning, and may be accompanied by diarrhea.

ENTERIC COLIBACILLOSIS

A common disease of nursing and weanling pigs caused by colonization of the small intestine by enterotoxigenic strains of *Escherichia coli*.

Etiology and Pathogenesis: Certain strains of *E coli* possess fimbria or pili that allow them to adhere to or colonize the absorptive epithelial cells of the jejunum and ileum. The common antigenic types of pili associated with pathogenicity are K88, K99, 987P, and F41. Pathogenic strains produce enterotoxins causing fluid and electrolytes to be secreted into the intestinal lumen, resulting in diarrhea, dehydration, and acidosis. Infection in neonates is commonly caused by K88 and 987P strains, whereas postweaning colibacillosis is nearly always due to the K88 strain.

Clinical Findings: Profuse watery diarrhea with rapid dehydration, acidosis, and death is common. Rarely, pigs may collapse and die before diarrhea commences.
Lesions: Dehydration and distention of the small intestine with yellowish, slightly mucoid fluid is characteristic. The colon contains similar fluid. The fundic portion of the gastric mucosa is often reddened. Pigs dying suddenly may have patchy cutaneous erythema. Histologically, the villa are usually of normal length and have many small bacterial rods adhered to the absorptive enterocytes.

Diagnosis: Confirmation is based on histological observation of villous colonization; demonstration of K88, K99, 987P, or F41 pilus antigens in intestinal scrapings by immunofluorescence or other immunological procedures; and isolation of the organism from the small intestine. Since *E coli* is a common secondary agent, the possibility of involvement of other agents such as viruses or coccidia should be considered.

Treatment and Control: Therapy includes prompt treatment with antibacterials and restoration of fluid and electrolyte balance. Bacterial antibiotic sensitivity testing is helpful to identify effective medication. Prevention includes reducing predisposing factors such as dampness and chilling; improving sanitation, such as by replacing solid or slatted concrete flooring with wire-mesh flooring; and vaccinating gestating sows with pilus-specific vaccines. Stimulation of active intestinal immunity by oral feeding of pilus-specific antigens is helpful to prevent late nursing and postweaning colibacillosis.

INTESTINAL SALMONELLOSIS

Enteropathogenic salmonellae cause inflammation and necrosis of the small and large intestine, resulting in diarrhea that may be accompanied by generalized sepsis. All ages are susceptible, but the disease is most common in weaned and growing-finishing pigs.

Etiology and Pathogenesis: *Salmonella choleraesuis* var *kunzendorf* is the most common salmonella species affecting pigs. It sometimes produces necrotizing enterocolitis, but far more common is a septicemic disease characterized by hepatitis, pneumonia, and cerebral vasculitis. *Salmonella typhimurium, S typhisuis,* and several other species affect the GI tract primarily. Infection of the intestine results in necrotizing, nonsuppurative inflammation of the mucosa-submucosa of the ileum, cecum, and colon; frequently the mucosa is ulcerated. Usually, there is extension to regional lymph nodes and, occasionally, generalized septicemia. Sources of infection include carrier pigs, rodents, and contaminated feed and premises. (*See also* SALMONELLOSIS, p 148.)

Clinical Findings: Nursing pigs may develop diarrhea but usually succumb to generalized septicemia. Weaning or growing-finishing pigs are febrile and have liquid feces that may be yellow and contain shreds of necrotic debris.
Lesions: Pigs infected with *S typhimurium* have inflamed, slightly thickened ileums and colons, usually with necrotic debris on the mucosal surface. Mesenteric lymph nodes are enlarged, edematous, and sometimes red. Mucosal ulceration may or may not be evident. A small amount of hemorrhage may be seen in acute cases. Occasionally, rectal strictures may develop (*see* below). Other enteropathogenic salmonellae, except for *S typhisuis,* produce lesions similar to those of *S typhimurium,* but less severe. Lesions of *S typhisuis* enteritis are distinctive, typically yellow, round (button) ulcers in the colon, cecum, and less commonly, the ileum.

Diagnosis: Culture of feces or intestinal mucosa in a selective medium may yield the organism; however, *Salmonella* spp often are isolated (and more reliably) from enlarged mesenteric lymph nodes by direct streaking on selective medium such as brilliant green agar or by inoculation of enrichment media. Histological examination of affected intestine and liver to differentiate salmonellosis from proliferative enteritis and swine dysentery is a valuable supplemental procedure.

Treatment and Control: Parenteral administration of antibacterials to acutely ill pigs, and medication of the affected group via water or feed may decrease severity of the outbreak. Neomycin and the nitrofurazones are the most often used water medications. Generally, treatment does not produce dramatic improvement, and recovery often is slow. Susceptibility testing of the isolated organism is useful in selecting an appropriate antibacterial. Thorough cleaning and disinfection of contaminated facilities and elimination of the source of the organism decrease the likelihood of repeated epidemics.

MESENTERIC TORSION OF THE SMALL INTESTINE

A cause of sporadic, sudden, unexpected death in pigs up to market weight.

Etiology and Pathogenesis: No specific cause of this condition has been identified. Predisposing factors may include vigorous exercise, handling, fighting, piling, or irregular feeding. Long-loined pigs may be more likely to develop mesenteric torsion than shorter pigs. Rotation of the entire intestine, including the posterior part of the duodenum and the anterior part of the rectum, around the root of the mesentery obstructs venous outflow of blood while allowing arterial supply to continue. This causes blood to pool and stagnate in the intestine and soon results in infarction. Rotation may be only partial and difficult to demonstrate at necropsy, which makes diagnosis more difficult.

Clinical Findings: Sudden, unexpected death with abdominal distention usually is all that is observed. Pigs exhibit abdominal distress shortly before death. The entire clinical course is ~2 hr. Sometimes only one pig of a group is affected, but it is not uncommon for several growing pigs from a pen to die over 2-3 wk.
    Lesions: Affected pigs usually are well nourished. There is patchy cutaneous erythema, and the abdomen is distended. The small and large intestines are dark red and filled with unclotted hemorrhagic fluid. The stomach usually is filled with feed, and the anterior duodenum is unaffected. The colon is displaced cranioventrally and the wall is hyperemic. Palpation of the root of the mesentery reveals the torsion.

Diagnosis: Necropsy findings are sufficient to establish the diagnosis. Histological examination of the jejunum and ileum reveals massive engorgement of the vasculature and hemorrhage throughout the mucosa and submucosa. Agonal and postmortem deterioration of the mucosa results in detachment of most of the mucosal epithelium.

Control: There is no treatment. Regular feeding, providing adequate feeder space, and reducing unusual physical stress may help minimize losses.

PARASITOSES

See also pp 103, 108, and 219.
    Ascaris suum: The most common intestinal nematode of pigs, adults in the intestine reduce feed efficiency, and heavy infections cause emaciation; larval migration incites inflammation in the liver and lungs.
    Cryptosporidium sp: A coccidium that attaches to the mucosal epithelium of the intestine of pigs $\geq$10 days old, causing villous atrophy in the lower small intestine that may result in malabsorption and diarrhea.

Eimeria spp: Coccidia of this genus are common in pigs, but overt disease is seldom seen. Heavy infections may cause significant enterocolitis in young growing pigs.

Hyostrongylus rubidus: The common stomach worm found in pasture-raised pigs, this parasite usually causes little harm.

Isospora suis: A common and important cause of coccidiosis in pigs 6 days to 3 wk old. Infection causes necrosis and villous atrophy of the ileum and jejunum. Secondary bacterial infection of the injured intestinal mucosa is common. Mortality often is 20-25%, and many pigs are stunted. Diagnosis can be based on identification of immature coccidial forms in the intestinal mucosa by direct mucosal smear stained with Giemsa stain, or by histological examination of the affected intestine. Successful prevention most commonly depends on thorough cleaning of farrowing facilities to minimize the number of oocysts. After cleaning, thorough disinfection with 50% bleach has been useful. Coccidiostats are sometimes fed to sows 2 wk before farrowing or administered PO to pigs from birth to 3 wk of age.

Oesophagostomum spp: Adult nodular worms in the large intestine cause little harm, but heavy infection by larvae encysted in the intestinal wall may lead to emaciation.

Strongyloides ransomi: Larvae of intestinal threadworm can be transmitted via colostrum or acquired from contaminated skin of the dam. Heavily infected piglets develop severe diarrhea when 10-14 days old, with high mortality. Diagnosis may be based on direct microscopical observation of mucosal scrapings.

Trichuris suis: Whipworms penetrate the mucosa of the cecum and colon, and cause multifocal inflammation; heavy infections cause diarrhea and emaciation. The feces may be hemorrhagic; therefore, heavy whipworm infections may be confused clinically with swine dysentery or proliferative enteritis. Diagnosis may be based on direct observation of whipworms in the large intestine, or fecal flotation.

PORCINE EPIDEMIC DIARRHEA (PED)

A coronaviral diarrhea (not yet recognized in the Western Hemisphere) that affects pigs of all ages and clinically resembles transmissible gastroenteritis (TGE, *see* below) in several respects.

Etiology and Epidemiology: The porcine epidemic diarrhea virus (PEDV) is not related to any other member of the Coronaviridae. Pigs are the only host known to be infected. Antibodies to PEDV have not been found in wild pigs or in other animal species. Infections occur in most European countries and in China. Large epidemics occurred in Europe in 1969; no antibodies have been found in sera collected before 1969. Since then, the virus has become widespread and endemic in several European countries, and acute outbreaks have become rare. On large breeding farms, the virus persists in consecutive litters of pigs after weaning and after they lose their lactogenic immunity. On these farms, PEDV may be associated with weaning diarrhea. In Belgium, PEDV is most frequently associated with diarrhea in feeder pigs occurring shortly after they are gathered from different breeding farms and assembled in large fattening units. The virus was demonstrated in fecal material in 80% of these groups. Epidemiological data from other countries are scarce. Virus spread mainly occurs directly through infected pigs, and indirectly through virus-contaminated fomites and also via transport trucks.

Pathogenesis: The pathogenesis and immunity mechanisms are similar to those reported for TGE. Oral infection results in viral replication in the epithelial cells covering the small intestinal villi. Cells on colonic villi also become infected. No other tissue tropisms have been shown. Virus is excreted in the feces.

Clinical Findings: Diarrhea is the only direct virus-induced clinical sign observed. An acute outbreak on a susceptible breeding farm resembles a TGE outbreak and is characterized by watery diarrhea in pigs of all ages. However, as compared to TGE, the incubation period is longer (3-4 days), not all the litters of suckling pigs may become sick, and the mortality in neonatal pigs is lower (av 50%). Also, spread of the disease within the farm occurs more slowly. In all outbreaks, signs are most consistently observed in feeders, finishers, and adults—they appear to be most susceptible since outbreaks often start in these age groups. With PED, older animals are more lethargic and depressed than with TGE. Sick animals appear to have colics.

Acute outbreaks in susceptible finishing pigs are characterized by watery diarrhea, but a markedly increased number of acute deaths may be observed, particularly in animals infected toward the end of the finishing period and in stress-sensitive breeds. Death may even occur during the incubation period.

Lesions: Macroscopic lesions are confined to the small intestine with villous shortening as the main characteristic. These lesions closely resemble those observed with TGE. No lesions have been described in the colon. A consistent finding is acute back muscle necrosis.

Diagnosis: Clinical differentiation from TGE is difficult. TGE in its typical epidemic form causes a rapidly spreading diarrhea in animals of all ages with high mortality in neonates. With PED, spread of the diarrhea occurs at a slower rate, and although diarrhea is seen in most of the litters, some litters may remain healthy even in the absence of immunity. Morbidity is 100% in older animals, and they are severely sick. Acute deaths observed in adults and finishing pigs due to muscle necrosis and occurring during an outbreak of diarrhea are typical for PED, and are not seen with any other infectious diarrhea.

Laboratory diagnosis in neonates is made by direct immunofluorescence on cryostat sections of small intestine or colon. ELISA to detect viral antigens in feces or intestinal contents is more useful for older animals. Antibodies can be detected in paired serum samples through ELISA-blocking.

Control: No specific treatment is available. Measures taken during a PED outbreak are of a general nature. Animals with diarrhea should have free access to water, and finishing pigs should be deprived of feed for 1-2 days.

On breeding farms, in the face of an outbreak, spread of virus to the farrowing house can be prevented temporarily by sanitary measures. If performed together with a deliberate infection of pregnant sows, losses in neonates may be lowered. No vaccine is available.

PORCINE PROLIFERATIVE ENTERITIS
(Porcine intestinal adenomatosis, Proliferative hemorrhagic enteropathy)

A common diarrheal disease of growing-finishing and young breeding pigs characterized by hyperplasia and inflammation of the ileum and colon. It often is mild and self-limiting, but sometimes causes persistent diarrhea, severe necrotic enteritis, or hemorrhagic enteritis with high mortality.

Etiology and Pathogenesis: The etiology is obscure, but *Campylobacter sputorum* or *C hyointestinalis* is consistently present in the cytoplasm of mucosal epithelial cells in affected areas of the intestine. The disease is assumed to be spread by contact with infected pigs, but the mechanism that triggers its onset is unknown. (*See also* CAMPYLOBACTERIOSIS, p 102.)

Clinical Findings: The more common, nonhemorrhagic form of the disease often affects 40- to 80-lb (18- to 36-kg) pigs and is characterized by sudden onset of diarrhea. The feces are watery to pasty, brownish, or faintly blood stained. After ~2 days, pigs may pass yellow fibrinonecrotic casts that have formed in the ileum. Most affected pigs recover spontaneously, but a significant number develop chronic necrotic enteritis with progressive emaciation. The hemorrhagic form is characterized by cutaneous pallor, weakness, and passage of hemorrhagic or black, tarry feces. Pregnant gilts may abort.

Lesions: Lesions may occur anywhere in the lower half of the small intestine, cecum, or colon but are most frequent and obvious in the ileum. The wall of the intestine is thickened, and the mesentery may be edematous. The mesenteric lymph nodes are enlarged. The intestinal mucosa appears thickened and rugose, may be covered with a brownish or yellow fibrinonecrotic membrane, and sometimes has petechial hemorrhages. Yellow necrotic casts may be found in the ileum or passing through the colon. Diffuse, complete mucosal necrosis in chronic cases causes the intestine to be rigid, resembling a garden hose. Proliferative mucosal lesions often are in the colon but are detected only by careful inspection at necropsy. In the profusely hemorrhagic form, there are red or black, tarry feces in the colon and clotted blood in the ileum.

Diagnosis: Confirmation is based on histological observation of characteristic proliferation and inflammation of mucosal crypts. Intracellular *Campylobacter* organisms can usually be demonstrated by silver stains. Bacterial culture of intestine and lymph nodes to exclude *Salmonella* infection, together with histological examination and culture of cecum and colon to exclude swine dysentery, are essential additional procedures. The colon also should be examined for whipworms.

Treatment and Control: Various antibacterials administered parenterally to acutely affected animals and by feed or water to the remainder of the group help reduce severity of the enteritis and prevent development of chronic, irreversible, necrotic enteritis. Methods to detect carrier animals are not available.

RECTAL STRICTURES

In growing pigs, rectal strictures are sequelae of severely traumatized rectal prolapses (qv, p 133) or infections that interfere with rectal blood supply. The former cause sporadic cases; the latter may be epidemic. One cause is *Salmonella typhimurium* infection (*see* above), which produces an ulcerative proctitis that heals in such a manner that normal function is not restored. The stricture is reportedly the result of fibrosis of the rectal tissue due to persistent ischemia caused by infection in an area of limited blood supply.

Clinical Findings: Several bloated pigs in varying stages of emaciation are generally observed in a group of growing pigs. Other clinical signs, including prior outbreaks of severe debilitating diarrhea, are common but not always reported. An index finger rarely can be passed into the rectum without considerable resistance.

Lesions: At necropsy the colon is grossly distended, and the intestine is filled with gas and green feces. The predominant lesion is a narrowed rectal canal, due to annular fibrotic ulcers or rectal strictures, found 2-5 cm cranial to the anus.

Diagnosis: An epidemic of rectal strictures without prior rectal prolapses is indicative. Culture of feces and regional lymph nodes usually yields *S typhimurium*. However, it is not possible to determine whether the lesion or the infection occurred first.

Treatment and Control: Early diagnosis and treatment of diarrhea is imperative for control. Good housing, management, and sanitation, with "all-in/all-out" movement of pigs is the best method to prevent further outbreaks. Surgery is not thought to be economically feasible.

ROTAVIRAL ENTERITIS

A common disease of the small intestine of pigs. All ages are susceptible, but significant diarrheal disease usually occurs in nursing or postweaning pigs.

Etiology and Pathogenesis: The causal rotavirus infects and destroys villous enterocytes throughout the small intestine, but lesions are most severe in the middle third of the intestine. Loss of villous epithelium results in partial villous atropy, malabsorption, and osmotic diarrhea. Multiple antigenic types of rotavirus affect pigs. They are easily spread by direct contact. Healthy carrier sows may be fecal shedders during the periparturient period, thereby exposing their litters to infection.

Clinical Findings: If neonatal pigs do not receive protective levels of maternal antibody, they are likely to develop profuse watery diarrhea when 12-48 hr old. More commonly, the infection is endemic in a herd, and sows have varying levels of antibody in the colostrum and milk, which provide varying degrees of passive protection to nursing pigs. Diarrhea often begins in pigs 5 days to 3 wk old, or immediately after weaning. The feces of nursing pigs often are yellow or gray and pasty in the early stages, and progress to gray and pasty after ~2 days. Diarrhea persists for 2-5 days. Diarrheic pigs become gaunt and rough-haired, but mortality usually is low. Weaned pigs have watery feces that contain poorly digested feed. Weaners become inappetent and noncompetitive, which results in emaciation, stunting, and probably predisposition to pneumonia and other diseases.

Lesions: The small intestine appears thin-walled, and the cecum and colon contain liquid feces.

Diagnosis: Laboratory procedures are required. Confirmation is based on histological demonstration of villous atrophy in the jejunum, electron microscopical demonstration of virions in the intestinal contents, and immunodiagnostic procedures to demonstrate viral antigen in the intestinal mucosa or feces. Differential diagnoses include endemic transmissible gastroenteritis, *Isospora suis* enteritis, and enteric colibacillosis.

Treatment and Contol: There is no specific treatment. Minimizing heat loss and providing adequate water to maintain hydration are helpful. Vaccination of sows may be useful. Concurrent infection by enterotoxigenic *E coli* is common; therefore, antibiotic therapy may reduce mortality. Providing diarrheic weaned pigs with a warm, dry, draft-free environment, and frequent limited feedings help prevent starvation, secondary diseases, and permanent stunting.

STREPTOCOCCUS DISPAR ENTERITIS

A diarrheal disease of nursing piglets usually 5-10 days old has been associated with colonization of the small intestine with *S dispar*. Diagnosis may be aided by observation of gram-positive cocci adhered to the villous epithelial cells. Antibacterials such as penicillin should be useful in treatment.

SWINE DYSENTERY
(Bloody scours)

A common, mucohemorrhagic diarrheal disease of pigs, which affects the large intestine.

Etiology and Pathogenesis: The essential causal agent is *Treponema hyodysenteriae*, an anaerobic spirochete that produces a hemolysin, although other organisms may contribute to the severity of lesions. It proliferates in the large intestine, causing degeneration and inflammation of the superficial mucosa, hypersecretion of mucus by mucosal epithelium, and multifocal bleeding points on the mucosal surface. The organism does not penetrate beyond the intestinal mucosa. Decreased ability of the mucosa to reabsorb endogenous secretions from the unaffected small intestine results in diarrhea.

Clinical Findings: The first signs are partial anorexia with or without fever, and passage of soft feces. The course is variable. Some animals die peracutely. More commonly, a mucoid diarrhea with flecks of blood and mucus develops and progresses to a watery mucohemorrhagic diarrhea. After several days, the feces are brown and contain flecks of fibrin and debris. Diarrheic pigs are dehydrated, profoundly weak, gaunt, and emaciated.

Lesions: The diffuse lesions are confined to the cecum, spiral colon, and rectum. The affected mucosa is covered with a layer of transparent or gray mucus, often with suspended flecks of blood in early stages; a mixture of blood, fibrin, and necrotic debris in more advanced cases; and a yellow, necrotic debris late in the course.

Diagnosis: Clinical signs and necropsy findings are usually sufficient for a presumptive diagnosis. Confirmation is based on demonstration of typical histological lesions in the large intestine and isolation of *T hyodysenteriae* by anaerobic culture. Concurrent diseases are not uncommon. Differential diagnoses include proliferative enteritis, salmonellosis, and heavy whipworm infections.

Treatment and Control: Therapeutic use of antibacterials is effective if started early. Water medication is preferred at first. Because drug-resistant strains are prevalent, it is essential to choose a drug to which the organism is sensitive. Bacitracin, carbadox, lincomycin, nitroimidazoles, tiamulin, and virginiamycin are commonly used. The disease may be eradicated from infected premises by a persistent and carefully planned program that includes treatment of carrier pigs with bactericidal drugs and thorough cleaning and disinfection of vacated facilities.

TRANSMISSIBLE GASTROENTERITIS (TGE)

A common viral disease of the small intestine that causes vomiting and profuse diarrhea in pigs of all ages.

Etiology and Pathogenesis: The causal coronavirus infects and destroys villous epithelial cells of the jejunum and ileum, which results in severe villous atrophy, malabsorption, osmotic diarrhea, and dehydration. The incubation period is ~18 hr. The infection spreads rapidly by aerosol or contact exposure. Recovered pigs may carry the virus in their respiratory tract for ≥4 mo. Severe epidemics are more common during winter due to survival of the virus in colder temperatures.

Clinical Findings: In nonimmune herds, vomiting often is the initial sign; this is followed by profuse watery diarrhea, dehydration, and excessive thirst. Feces of nursing pigs often contain curds of undigested milk. Mortality is nearly 100% in piglets <1 wk old, whereas pigs >1 mo old seldom die. Gestating sows occasionally abort and lactating sows often exhibit vomiting, diarrhea, and agalactia. Diarrhea in surviving nursing piglets continues for ~5 days, but older pigs may be diarrheic for a shorter period.

In large herds with endemic TGE, clinical signs are variable, depending on the level of immunity and magnitude of exposure. Lactogenic immunity usually is sufficient to protect pigs until they 4-5 days old. As the antibody level in milk decreases, infection and mild disease may occur. Depending on the level of immunity and exposure, diarrhea may be mild in some litters but severe in others. If passive protection is sufficient to protect pigs throughout the nursing period, diarrhea often develops during the first few days after weaning.

Lesions: Piglets dying of TGE are severely dehydrated, and the skin is soiled with liquid feces. The stomach usually contains mild curd but may be empty. The small intestine is thin-walled, and the entire intestine contains greenish or yellow watery fluid and clumps of undigested milk. Older pigs have few remarkable lesions except that the colon contains liquid rather than formed feces. Villous atrophy can be observed by examining the mucosa of the small intestine with a hand lens.

Diagnosis: Clinical signs in the epidemic form of TGE usually justify a presumptive diagnosis. In the mild endemic form, laboratory procedures are required. Histological and immunofluorescent examination of the small intestine to demonstrate typical lesions and the presence of TGE viral antigen provide confirmatory evidence. In some outbreaks, coronaviral encephalomyelitis (qv, p 388) may cause similar signs.

Treatment and Control: There is no specific treatment. Increasing farrowing room temperature to minimize body heat loss and providing electrolyte solutions to combat dehydration are helpful. Weaning older nursing pigs that are consuming creep feed may reduce mortality.

Protective immunity depends on presence of antibody in the small intestine. Passive protection of piglets is provided by continuous nursing of immune sows. Active protective immunity develops after TGE infection of the intestinal mucosa. Parenteral injection of sows with TGE vaccine elicits high levels of antibody in the colostrum but only low levels of antibody in the postcolostral milk. Oral and parenteral administration of vaccine offers somewhat better protection because infection of the intestine elicits a secretory IgA response. Active infection of the intestine with virulent virus provides protective immunity for 6-18 mo. Vaccination of naturally immune sows boosts immunity sufficiently to protect neonates, and is particularly useful in endemically infected herds.

Planned infection of pregnant sows in herds known to be infected with virulent virus at least 2-4 wk before farrowing usually provides adequate immunity. This may be accomplished by mixing ground, TGE-virus-infected intestine and feces in the gestation ration. Because of the obvious hazards associated with this procedure, it should be undertaken only if a later epidemic in the farrowing house seems inevitable. The infectious material should be used only in the same herd from which it was collected, and the tissues should be as free as possible from other pathogens of pigs.

Because TGE virus is easily spread during an epidemic by persons, animals, and fomites, special care should be taken to prevent spread to unexposed groups of pigs and to neighboring herds.

OTHER INTESTINAL VIRUSES OF PIGS

Adenovirus: Infection of the intestine of nursing pigs with porcine adenovirus causes formation of intranuclear inclusion bodies in the dome epithelial cells overlying the organized lymphoid tissue of the ileum. Gnotobiotic piglets with experimental adenoviral infections develop rather severe diarrhea, but there is little evidence that this disease is of economic significance to the pig industry.

Enterovirus: Enteroviruses are commonly present in the intestine. Diarrhea has been produced in pigs infected experimentally, but there is little evidence to suggest that intestinal infection by enteroviruses is of much practical significance.

Pararotavirus: Pararotaviruses are morphologically similar to, but antigenically distinct from, rotaviruses. Pararotaviruses produce lesions and diarrhea similar to rotaviral infection in young pigs (*see* p 196).

GASTRITIS, LG AN
(Gastric catarrh)

Etiology: Gastritis may occur with or without involvement of other parts of the GI tract. It may be caused by ingestion of caustic or irritating chemicals, but in such cases usually is accompanied by stomatitis and enteritis. Gastric disturbance with accompanying gastritis may follow overeating; abrupt dietary changes; ingestion of spoiled, moldy, or excessively hot/cold feed; or the ingestion of sand or other foreign material. Gastritis is a common sequela of enterogastric reflux, secondary to mechanical or functional intestinal obstruction. Chemical rumenitis may occur with grain overload in cattle, and frequently is followed by a fungal or bacterial rumenitis. (*See* p 175 *et seq* for discussions of rumenitis.)

Ruminal drinking occasionally occurs in milk-fed veal calves due to failure of the reticular groove reflex; rumenitis develops and there is an associated villous atrophy in the duodenum and jejunum. Abomasal ulceration and abomasitis are common in calves, and often are associated with ingestion of straw or other poorly digestible roughage, or with other types of nutritional stress. In all species, GI parasitic infections are a common cause of inflammatory reaction.

Abomasal ulcers occur in braxy and in pasteurellosis in sheep, and gastric venous infarction is common in acute septicemic and toxemic disease in pigs. Gastritis is common in the erosive and vesicular viral diseases of ruminants and occurs in conjunction with many intestinal infections in all species.

Clinical Findings: The syndrome is indistinct and varies with the cause. In horses, acute gastritis usually results from enterogastric reflux. Acute gastritis also occurs in severely septic horses and foals. Laminitis may accompany these conditions.

Acute gastric dilatation in horses most often results from enterogastric reflux secondary to mechanical obstruction of the small intestine. Overeating, ingestion of highly fermentable feedstuffs, excess water consumption, and gastric ulceration also have been implicated in gastric dilatation.

Severe pain is characteristic of acute gastric dilatation in horses. Dehydration and shock develop rapidly. Initial depression of cardiac and respiratory function is followed by increased respiratory and cardiac rates as toxic products are absorbed. The prognosis is guarded. Gastric rupture is a possible sequela.

In pigs, vomiting is the cardinal sign of gastritis, with depression, inappetence, and evidence of abdominal pain.

In ruminants, abomasitis is manifest by depression, inappetence, and a fall in production. Body temperature and pulse rate usually are elevated mildly, and rumination is depressed. Occasionally, a pain response is elicited by percussion over the abomasum. Acute rumen overload produces a characteristic syndrome (qv, p 175). Abomasal ulceration in calves may cause unthriftiness, but usually is clinically inapparent unless perforation is sufficient to produce local peritonitis. Rumenitis in calves due to ruminal drinking causes bloat, inappetence, abdominal distention, clay-like feces, and reduced growth rate.

Most parasitic infections of the stomach produce a protein-losing gastropathy with unthriftiness and diarrhea without evidence of abdominal pain. However, haemonchosis may manifest as a severe anemia without diarrhea, and hyostrongylosis in adult pigs may simply produce a syndrome of chronic wasting.

Treatment: For acute gastric dilatation in horses, passage of a nasogastric tube to remove excess fluid and gas is of primary importance. Otherwise, first and most important is to remove the cause. Feed should be withheld until the cause of gastritis and/or dilatation has been resolved, and function and patency of the GI tract have been confirmed. While feed is withheld, oral fluids may be administered, although if the function and patency of the GI tract is uncertain, fluids should be given IV. Feed should be reintroduced gradually, and consist of small amounts of easily digested feeds such as green grass, mashes of grain, or pelleted feed. If the condition is due to spoiled or irritating feeds, evacuation of the GI tract with a mild laxative (eg, mineral oil) is indicated. If infection is suspected, oral sulfonamides or antibiotics should be administered. To provide protection to the irritated gastric mucosa, protective agents, eg, kaolin, bismuth subnitrate, or sucralfate, may be given. Sedatives are indicated for acute gastritis or gastric dilatation in horses. Nonsteroidal anti-inflammatory agents are useful in preventing subsequent development of laminitis. Antispasmodic drugs give dramatic relief in some cases of functional hypermotility, but their use should be avoided in cases of gastritis or gastric dilatation because of the danger of producing atony of the gut. Gastric lavage with isotonic saline solution should be attempted in cases of chemical gastritis and when impaction has occurred. Fluid therapy (IV) and other measures to combat shock (qv, p 1369) should be initiated.

With severe impactions or overload in cattle or sheep, removal of the food mass is indicated (*see* p 177). Following cessation of signs, the animal should be returned slowly to a normal diet. In cattle, gastritis often results in disturbance of the normal rumen flora. Rumen inoculation (qv, p 1390) with fresh rumen contents may aid recovery.

See GI PARASITES OF HORSES, below, RUMINANTS, p 205, and PIGS, p 219, for treatment of parasitic gastritis.

GASTROINTESTINAL PARASITES OF HORSES

GASTEROPHILUS INFECTION

Horse bots, which are found in the stomach, are the larvae of bot flies, *Gasterophilus* spp. Three major species are distributed worldwide, and a number of minor species occur in parts of Europe, Africa, and Asia. The adult flies are not parasitic and cannot feed; they die as soon as the nutrients remaining from the larval stage are used, usually in ~2 wk. The 3 important species can be differentiated in any stage of their development. The eggs of *G intestinalis* (the common bot) are glued to the hairs of almost any part of the body, but especially the forelegs and shoulders. The larvae hatch in ~1 wk when stimulated, usually by the animals' licking. The eggs of *G haemorrhoidalis* (the nose or lip bot) are attached to the hairs of the lips. The larvae emerge in 2-3 days without stimulation and crawl into the mouth. *Gasterophilus nasalis* (the throat bot) deposits eggs on the hairs of the submaxillary region. They hatch in ~1 wk without stimulation.

The larvae of all 3 species apparently stay embedded in the tongue or in the mucosa of the mouth for ~1 mo, after which they pass to the stomach where they attach themselves to the cardiac or pyloric portions and, in the case of *G nasalis*, to the mucosa of the first part of the small intestine. After development for ~8-10 mo, they pass out in the feces and pupate in the soil for 3-5 wk. The adult emerges after ~1 mo. The main pathogenic effect is caused by larvae, which attach by oral hooks to the lining of the stomach. This induces erosions and ulcerations at the site of attachment and a hyperplastic reaction around it.

Clinical Findings and Diagnosis: Bots cause a mild gastritis, but large numbers may be present with no clinical signs. The first instars migrating in the mouth can cause stomatitis and may produce pain on eating. The adult flies are responsible for much annoyance when laying their eggs during the summer. Specific diagnosis of *Gasterophilus* infection is difficult and can be made only by demonstrating larvae as they pass in the feces. Infection is often assumed in the fall. History of the individual animals, knowledge of the local seasonal cycle of the fly, and observation of the cream-white bot eggs (1-2 mm) on the animal's hairs are all helpful.

Treatment: In temperate areas, it is assumed that most animals are infected by the end of summer. The traditional single treatment in late fall or early winter after the flies have disappeared is usually adequate. However, trichlorfon, dichlorvos, and ivermectin are effective against all stages of bots and, when used as part of a routine parasite control program, provide effective bot control throughout the season. Although there is no satisfactory method for protecting exposed animals from attack by the adult flies, bot control programs, when applied on a regional basis to all horses, markedly reduce fly numbers and larval infections.

HABRONEMA INFECTION

Adults of the widely distributed stomach worms, *Habronema muscae*, *H microstoma (majus)*, and *Draschia (Habronema) megastoma*, are 6-25 mm in size. *Draschia* occurs in tumor-like swellings in the stomach wall. The other species are free on the mucosa. The eggs or larvae are ingested by larvae of house or stable flies, which serve as intermediate hosts. Horses are infected by ingesting flies that contain infective larvae or by free larvae that emerge from flies as they feed around the lips. (*See also* CUTANEOUS HABRONEMIASIS, p 806.)

A catarrhal gastritis with excess mucus production may result from heavy infections with adult worms. *Draschia* produces the most severe lesions—tumor-like enlargements up to 10 cm in diameter. These are filled with necrotic material and a large number of worms, and are covered by intact epithelium, except for a small opening through which the eggs pass. These nodules rarely rupture and cause fatal peritonitis. Larvae of *Habronema* spp and *Draschia* have been found in the lungs of foals associated with *Rhodococcus equi* abscesses (qv, p 743). Clinical signs usually are absent except when granulomas associated with *Draschia* infection lead to mechanical obstruction or rupture.

Antemortem diagnosis is difficult since the thin-shelled eggs or larvae are easily missed in fecal examinations. Worms and eggs may be found by gastric lavage. Most anthelmintics have not been tested against *Habronema* spp or *Draschia* sp, although ivermectin is effective against their cutaneous larvae and adults of *Habronema muscae*.

OXYURIS INFECTION

Adult pinworms, *Oxyuris equi*, are found mainly in the large intestine. The females are 7.5-15 cm long; males are smaller and fewer in number. The gravid females pass toward the rectum to lay their eggs and cement them to the perineum around the anus. Masses of eggs and cement around the anus appear as a white to yellow, crusty mass. The eggs, which are flattened on one side, become embryonated in a few hours and are infective in 4-5 days.

Adult pinworms are of little significance in the intestine, but cause perineal irritation following egg laying. Rubbing of the tail and anal regions, with resulting broken hairs and bare patches around the tail and buttocks, is characteristic and suggests the presence of pinworms. Fecal examination may or may not disclose a pinworm infection. Samples collected around the perineal region may contain dried female worms or eggs. Application of cellophane tape to the skin of the perineum or scraping the area with a tongue depressor may recover ova for microscopical examination.

Most of the broad-spectrum drugs recommended for the strongyles (*see* below) are effective against pinworms.

PARASCARIS INFECTION

Adults of the equine ascarid, *Parascaris equorum*, are stout, whitish worms, up to 30 cm long, with 3 prominent lips. The life cycle is similar to that of the porcine ascarid, with a prepatent period of 10-12 wk. Infective eggs can remain viable for years in contaminated soil. Adult animals usually harbor very few worms. The principal source of infection for young foals is contamination of pasture, paddock, or stall with eggs from foals of the previous year.

In heavy infections, the migrating larvae may produce respiratory signs ("summer colds"). In heavy intestinal infections, foals show unthriftiness, loss of energy, and occasionally, colic. Intestinal obstruction and perforation have been reported. Diagnosis is based on demonstration of eggs in the feces. If disease due to prepatent infection is suspected, diagnosis may be confirmed by administration of an anthelmintic, after which large numbers of immature worms may be observed in the feces.

On farms where the infection is common, most foals become infected soon after birth. As a result, most of the worms are maturing when the foals are ~4-5 mo old. Treatment should be started when foals are ~8 wk old and repeated at 6- to 8-wk intervals until they are yearlings. Piperazine or piperazine-thiabendazole is effective against the adult worms and has considerable activity against the immature stages, and all of the broad-spectrum equine anthelmintics are effective; therefore, ascarids are readily controlled by an appropriate worm control program.

LARGE-STRONGYLE INFECTION

The large strongyles of horses are also known as blood worms, palisade worms, sclerostomes, or red worms. The 3 major species and their respective lengths are: *Strongylus vulgaris*, up to 25 mm; *S edentatus*, up to 40 mm; and *S equinus*, up to 50 mm. (*See also Triodontophorus* spp, p 204.) Under favorable conditions, the larvae develop to the infective stage within 1-2 wk after the eggs are passed. Infection is by ingestion of infective larvae, which exsheath in the intestine and migrate extensively before developing to maturity in the large intestine. The prepatent period is 6-11 mo. The larvae of *S vulgaris* migrate extensively in the cranial mesenteric artery and its branches, where they may cause parasitic thrombosis and arteritis. Larvae of the other 2 species may be found in various parts of the body, including the liver, perirenal tissues, flanks, and pancreas. These species do not produce lesions in the mesenteric arteries. Mixed infections of large and small strongyles are the rule.

Clinical Findings: Adult large strongyles have large buccal capsules and are active feeders, ingesting plugs of mucosa as they move about in the intestine. The attendant blood loss may lead to anemia. Weakness, emaciation, and diarrhea also are common. *Strongylus vulgaris* is especially important because of the damage it does to the cranial mesenteric artery and its branches. As a result of the interference with the flow of blood to the intestine and thromboembolism, any of several conditions may follow: colic; gangrenous enteritis; or intestinal stasis, torsion or intussusception, and possibly rupture. Cerebrospinal nematodiasis (qv, p 604) can cause a variety of lesions depending on the part of the CNS affected.

Diagnosis and Treatment: Diagnosis of mixed strongyle infection is based on demonstration of eggs in the feces. Differential diagnosis can be made by identifying the infective larvae after fecal culture. When colic due to verminous arteritis is suspected, a painful enlargement at the root of the mesentery may be palpable per rectum. Serological diagnosis based on a rise in β globulins has been recommended but is not specific for *S vulgaris*. Parasitic arterial lesions have been demonstrated using arteriography.

Colic due to arterial lesions has been successfully controlled with large doses of thiabendazole. Ivermectin at its standard dose is effective against the larval stages of *S vulgaris*; fenbendazole and oxfendazole, at doses higher than for the adult parasite, are also effective against larval infections. A number of anthelmintics including the benzimidazoles, dichlorvos, pyrantel, and ivermectin are active against adult large and small strongyles.

Parasite control programs assume that grazing horses are infected; hence, treatments are administered to minimize the level of pasture contamination and reduce the risks associated with migrating larvae.

Routine or interval treatments are traditional, and the interval between treatments depends on the length of time a particular drug keeps the feces clear of eggs (generally 4-8 wk). The frequency of treatment is influenced also by the value of the animals, and varies with access to pasture and management practices. However, frequent treatments can lead to strongyles that are resistant to anthelmintics. Fewer treatments are effective control procedures when given strategically. In northern temperate areas, when mature animals are given 2-3 treatments in spring to summer, pasture contamination and transmission of the parasites are markedly reduced. Removal of feces from paddocks and pastures manually or by mechanical means also aids in control.

In parasite control programs, all horses on a farm should be treated, and those that run together on the same pasture or paddock should be treated at the same time. Boarded horses or horses returning after having been off the premises for an extended time should be quarantined, or isolated and dewormed before admittance to the farm proper. In administering the anthelmintic, it is important that all horses receive the proper dose. The issue of rotating or not rotating different classes of anthelmintics whether in a fast rotation scheme (every few weeks) or slow rotation scheme (annually, in temperate climates) to prevent development of resistant strains of parasites is being debated. Whatever program is used, fecal samples should be examined periodically to maintain surveillance of the effectiveness of the program.

Colic may be associated with the use of anthelmintics. Special precautions are necessary when organophosphorous products (trichlorfon and dichlorvos) are used: concurrent use of other organophosphates and phenothiazine compounds (including tranquilizers) may have untoward effects; succinylcholine should not be used <1 mo after administration of organophosphates.

SMALL-STRONGYLE INFECTION

Many species in several genera of "small strongyles" are found in the cecum and colon. Most of them are appreciably smaller than the "large strongyles", but some may be almost as large as *Strongylus vulgaris*, eg, *Triodontophorus* spp, which by some are classified as nonmigratory large strongyles. One species, *T tenuicollis*, produces rather severe ulcers in the wall of the colon. Most of the small strongyles feed superficially on the intestinal mucosa. There is apparently no extraintestinal migration of the larvae in the host; larvae develop in the wall of the large intestine. Larvae may undergo hypobiosis and remain dormant in the intestinal wall over prolonged periods. In temperate areas, an acute syndrome of diarrhea and death in young ponies and horses in late winter and spring has been reported. This is associated with the mass emergence of larvae from the intestinal wall and may have some similarity to Type II ostertagiasis in young cattle. Response to treatment is variable, and the condition is best prevented by adopting a good worm control program. For treatment and control, *see* LARGE STRONGYLES, above.

Several species of small strongyles are resistant to many of the benzimidazoles. Resistance in small strongyles is a heritable trait and not reversible. Benzimidazole-resistant small strongyles are susceptible to piperazine, pyrantel, dichlorvos, and ivermectin. Drug efficacy may be determined by comparing the worm egg count at the time of treatment and 10-14 days later. An effective drug reduces the egg count to 0 or to very low levels.

STRONGYLOIDES INFECTION

Strongyloides westeri is found in the small intestine. Larvae are passed in the milk, and diarrhea can be seen in foals from 10 days of age. The life cycle of the worm in horses is not known to differ significantly from that of *Strongyloides* in pigs (qv, p 221). Thiabendazole, cambendazole, and ivermectin are effective, as are some of the modern benzimidazoles at increased dose rates.

TAPEWORM INFECTION

Three species of tapeworms are found in horses: *Anoplocephala magna*, *A perfoliata*, and *Paranoplocephala mamillana*. They are 8-25 cm long (the first usually being the longest, and the last the shortest). *Anoplocephela magna* and *P mamillana* usually are in the small intestine, but may also be in the stomach; *A perfoliata* occurs mostly in the cecum, but may occur in the small intestine. The life cycle is similar to that of *Moniezia* spp in ruminants and involves free-living orbatid mites as intermediate hosts. Diagnosis is by demonstration of the characteristic eggs in the feces, but because the discharge of proglottids is sporadic, a single fecal examination may not disclose a tapeworm infection. In light infections, no signs of disease are present; in heavy infections, GI disturbances may occur. Unthriftiness and anemia have been reported. Ulceration of the mucosa occurs quite commonly in the area of attachment of *A perfoliata*, and this has been suggested as one cause of intussusception. Pyrantel pamoate at twice the label dose is effective against *A perfoliata*. Niclosamide and dichlorophen also have been recommended.

TRICHOSTRONGYLUS INFECTION

The small stomach worm (hairworm) of horses, *Trichostrongylus axei*, is also found in ruminants. The adults are slender and measure up to 8 mm long. Details of the cycle in Equidae have not been carefully studied, but it is known that the larvae penetrate the mucosa. These worms produce a chronic catarrhal gastritis and may result in weight loss. The lesions comprise nodular areas of thickened mucosa surrounded by a zone of congestion and covered with a variable amount of mucus. The lesions may be rather small and irregularly circumscribed, or may coalesce and involve most or all of the glandular portion of the stomach, and erosions and ulcerations may be seen.

Definite diagnosis based on fecal examination is difficult because the eggs are similar to strongyle eggs. The feces can be cultured and, in ~5 days, the infective larvae identified. Some of the benzimidazoles and ivermectin are effective against *T axei*.

GASTROINTESTINAL PARASITES OF RUMINANTS

GASTROINTESTINAL PARASITES OF CATTLE

HAEMONCHUS, OSTERTAGIA, AND *TRICHOSTRONGYLUS* INFECTIONS

The common stomach worms of cattle are *Haemonchus placei* (barber's pole worm, large stomach worm, wire worm), *Ostertagia ostertagi* (medium or brown stomach worm), and *Trichostrongylus axei* (small stomach worm). In some tropical countries, *Mecistocirrus digitatus*, a large worm up to 40 mm long, is present. *Haemonchus placei* is primarily a parasite of tropical regions, whereas *O ostertagi* and to a lesser extent, *T axei*, prefer temperate climates. Adult male *Haemonchus* are up to 18 mm long, females up to 30 mm. *Ostertagia* adults are 6-9 mm long, and *Trichostrongylus*, ~5 mm.

The preparasitic life cycles of the 3 groups are generally similar. With favorable temperatures, larvae hatch shortly after the eggs are passed in the feces, and reach the infective stage in ~2 wk under optimal temperatures (~75°F [24°C]). Development to the infective stage is delayed during cold weather. In areas with narrow diurnal temperature variations, those months with a mean maximum temperature of 65°F (18°C) and with rainfall >2 in. (5 cm) are favorable for development of the free-living stages of *H placei*, but where wide fluctuations occur, the mean minimum temperature of 50°F (10°C) is a more accurate criterion. The preparasitic forms of *O ostertagi* and *T axei* develop and survive better in cooler conditions, but their upper limits for survival are lower. If the temperature is unfavorable or drought conditions exist, infective larvae may remain dormant in the feces for weeks until conditions become favorable again, after which large numbers of infective larvae emerge.

The prepatent period of *O ostertagi* is normally 18-25 days. Ingested larvae enter the lumen of the abomasal glands and molt by the fourth day; they remain there during the prepatent period, growing and undergoing a final molt before emerging to the lumen of the abomasum as young adults. Larvae in gastric glands cause cellular hyperplasia and result in nodules, which may be discrete or confluent. Severe epithelial cytolysis may occur when the larvae emerge. At this time, the parietal cells are replaced by undifferentiated, rapidly dividing cells. As a consequence, in heavy infections, the pH in the abomasum rises from 2 to >6. A protein-losing gastroenteropathy results and, together with anorexia and impaired protein digestion, leads to hypoproteinemia and weight loss. Diarrhea is persistent. Disease resulting from recent infections is defined as **Type I ostertagiasis**; in this infection, most of the worms present are adults and the condition responds well to anthelmintic treatment. Type I disease occurs primarily in calves 7-15 mo old. It is most common from time of weaning and ensuing months in warm temperate regions, and in young cattle during summer and early autumn in cool temperate regions.

In **Type II ostertagiasis**, large numbers of larvae, which had become dormant or inhibited in development at the early fourth larval stage, emerge from the glands. This occurs primarily in 12- to 20-mo-old cattle. In warm temperate regions, inhibition-prone larvae are acquired in spring, and disease may result when large numbers of larvae resume development to the adult stage in late summer/autumn. In cold temperate regions, acquisition of inhibition-prone larvae occurs during late autumn, and maturation during late winter/early spring. Larval inhibition (hypobiosis) in *O ostertagi* and other nematodes is thought to be analogous to diapause in insects. It has been interpreted as a survival mechanism in which the preparasitic stages on pasture avoid the adverse conditions of winter in cool regions, and hot and dry or hot and alternately wet and dry conditions of many warm regions. The factors that cause inhibition are not completely known, but experimental cold conditioning of infective larvae was found to be important in a cool temperate region. In warm regions of both Northern and Southern Hemispheres, conditioning of preparasitic stages to inhibition occurs principally during spring before the hot and dry conditions of summer. Factors involved in maturation are even less well defined, but may include effects of parturition, nutrition, concurrent infection, host immune response, or simply lapse of time.

Haemonchus placei also may become dormant over winter, and resume development in the spring and infect the pastures with eggs at a time suitable for their development. Both the larval and adult stages are pathogenic due to their blood-sucking ability. Trichostrongylus axei causes gastritis with superficial erosion of the mucosa, hyperemia, and diarrhea. Protein loss from the damaged mucosa and anorexia cause hypoproteinemia and weight loss. Hypobiosis does not occur to the same degree with T axei.

Clinical Findings: Young animals are more often affected, but adults not previously exposed to infection frequently show signs and succumb. Ostertagia and Trichostrongylus infections are characterized by profuse, watery diarrhea that usually is persistent. In haemonchosis and Mecistocirrus infection, there may be little or no diarrhea but possibly intermittent periods of constipation. Anemia of variable degree is a characteristic sign of both these infections.

Concurrent with the diarrhea of O ostertagi and T axei infections, and the anemia of heavy Haemonchus infection, there is often hypoproteinemia and edema, particularly under the lower jaw (**bottle jaw**) and sometimes along the ventral abdomen. Heavy infections can produce death before clinical signs appear. Other variable signs include progressive weight loss, weakness, rough coat, and anorexia.

Lesions: Worms can readily be seen and identified in the abomasum, and small petechiae may be seen where the worms have been feeding. The most characteristic lesions of Ostertagia infection are small, umbilicated nodules 1-2 mm in diameter throughout the abomasum. These may be discrete, but in heavy infections they tend to coalesce and give rise to a "cobblestone" or "morocco leather" appearance. Nodules are most marked in the fundic region but may cover the entire abomasal mucosa. If the pH rises to 6-7, surplus pepsinogen may be reabsorbed and high levels can be found in the plasma. There is also evidence that presence of adult Ostertagia can cause direct secretion of pepsinogen. Edema is often marked and, in severe cases, may extend over the abomasum and into the small intestine and omentum.

In T axei infections, the mucosa of the abomasum shows slight to medium congestion, but superficial erosions, sometimes covered with a fibrinonecrotic exudate, may be seen.

Diagnosis, Treatment and Control: See p 211 et seq.

COOPERIA INFECTION

Several species of Cooperia occur in the small intestine of cattle; C punctata, C oncophora, and C pectinata are the most common. The red, coiled adults are 5-8 mm long, and the male has a large bursa. They may be difficult to observe grossly. Their life cycle is essentially the same as that of other trichostrongylids. These worms apparently do not suck blood. Most of them are found in the first 10-20 ft (3-6 m) of the small intestine. The prepatent period is 12-15 days.

The eggs usually can be differentiated from those of the common GI nematodes by their practically parallel sides, but a larval culture of the feces is necessary to definitively diagnose Cooperia infection in the living animal. In heavy infections with C punctata and C pectinata, there is profuse diarrhea, anorexia, and emaciation, but no anemia; the upper small intestine shows marked congestion of the mucosa, with small hemorrhages. The mucosa may show a fine lace-like superficial necrosis. Cooperia oncophora produces a milder disease but can be responsible for weight loss and poor productivity. It is usually necessary to make scrapings of the mucosa to demonstrate *Cooperia* spp, which must be differentiated from *Trichostrongylus, Strongyloides papillosus*, and immature *Nematodirus*.

For diagnosis, treatment and control, *see* p 211 *et seq*.

BUNOSTOMUM INFECTION

The adult male *Bunostomum phlebotomum* is ~15 mm, and the female ~25 mm long. Hookworms have well-developed buccal capsules into which the mucosa is drawn; cutting plates at the anterior edge of the buccal capsule are used to abrade the mucosa during feeding. The prepatent period is ~2 mo. Infection is by ingestion or skin penetration; the latter is more common.

Larval penetration of the lower limbs may cause uneasiness and stamping, particularly in stabled cattle. Adult worms cause anemia and rapid weight loss. Diarrhea and constipation may alternate. Hypoproteinemic edema may be present, but "bottle jaw" is rarely as severe as in haemonchosis. During the patent period, a diagnosis may be made by demonstrating the characteristic eggs in the feces.

On necropsy, the mucosa may appear congested and swollen, with numerous small hemorrhagic points where the worms were attached. The worms are readily seen in the first few feet of the small intestine, and the contents are often blood stained. As few as 2000 worms may cause death in calves. Local lesions, edema, and scab formation may result from penetration of larvae into the skin of resistant calves.

For diagnosis, treatment and control, *see* p 211 *et seq*.

STRONGYLOIDES INFECTION

The intestinal threadworm, *Strongyloides papillosus*, has an unusual life cycle. Only females occur in the parasitic phase of the cycle. These are 3.5-6 mm long and are embedded in the mucosa of the upper small intestine. Small, embryonated eggs are passed in the feces, hatch rapidly, and may develop directly into infective larvae or free-living adults. The offspring of these free-living adults may develop into another generation of infective larvae or free-living adults. The host is infected by penetration of the skin or by ingestion; transmission of infective larvae in colostrum may occur as in other species of the genus. The prepatent period is ~10 days.

Infections are most common in young calves, particularly dairy stock. Although signs are rare, they may include intermittent diarrhea, loss of appetite and weight, and sometimes, blood and mucus in the feces. Large numbers of worms in the intestine produce catarrhal enteritis with petechiae and ecchymoses, especially in the duodenum and jejunum.

For diagnosis, treatment and control, *see* p 211 *et seq*.

NEMATODIRUS INFECTION

Although several others, eg, *Nematodirus spathiger* and *N battus*, can infect cattle, *N helvetianus* is generally recognized as the most common species in cattle. The adult males of *N helvetianus* are ~12 mm, and the females 18-25 mm long. The eggs develop slowly; the infective third stage is reached within the egg in 2-4 wk and may remain within the egg for several months. Eggs may accumulate on pastures and hatch in large numbers after rain to produce heavy infections over a short period. The eggs are highly resistant, and those passed by calves in one season may remain alive and infect calves the next season. After ingestion of infective larvae, the adult stage is reached in ~3 wk. Worms are most numerous 10-20 ft (3-6 m) from the pylorus.

Signs include diarrhea and anorexia. They usually develop during the third week of infection, before the worms are sexually mature; clinical infections may be seen in dairy calves from 6 wk onward. During the prepatent period, diagnosis is difficult; during the patent period, diagnosis is easily made on the basis of the characteristic eggs. Relatively small numbers of eggs are produced. Resistance to reinfection develops rapidly. Necropsy may show only a thickened, edematous mucosa.

For diagnosis, treatment and control, *see* p 211 *et seq*.

TOXOCARA INFECTION

The ascarid *Toxocara vitulorum* is a stout, whitish worm (males 20-25 cm, females 25-30 cm) that occurs in the small intestine of calves <6 mo old; older calves are resistant. Larvae hatching from ingested eggs pass to the tissues and, in pregnant cows, are mobilized late in pregnancy and passed via the milk to the calves. Eggs appear in the feces of calves from 3 wk of age and are easily recognized by their thick, pitted shells. In some parts of the world the infection is considered serious, particularly in buffalo calves.

For diagnosis, treatment and control, *see* p 211 *et seq.*

OESOPHAGOSTOMUM INFECTION

Adults of *Oesophagostomum radiatum* (nodular worm) are 12-15 mm long, and the head is bent dorsally. The eggs are very similar to those of *Haemonchus placei*, and often are grouped with them on routine fecal examination. The life cycle is direct. The larvae penetrate primarily into the wall of the lower 10-20 ft (3-6 m) of the small intestine, but also into the cecum and colon, where they remain for 5-10 days and then return to the lumen as fourth-stage larvae. The prepatent period in susceptible animals is ~6 wk. However, in subsequent reinfections, larvae become arrested for some time and many may never return to the lumen (host encystment).

Young animals suffer from the effects of adult worms, whereas in older animals, the effect of the nodules plays a more important part. Infection causes anorexia; severe, constant, dark, fetid diarrhea that persists; weight loss; and death. In older, resistant animals the nodules surrounding the larvae become caseated and calcified, thus decreasing the motility of the intestine. Stenosis or intussusception occasionally occurs. Nodules can be palpated per rectum, and the worms and nodules can be seen readily at necropsy.

For diagnosis, treatment and control, *see* p 211 *et seq.*

CHABERTIA INFECTION

Adults of the large-mouth bowel worm, *Chabertia ovina,* are ~12 mm long and bent ventrally at the anterior end. There is a typical direct life cycle. The larvae penetrate the mucosa of the small intestine shortly after ingestion, and later emerge and pass to the colon. The prepatent period is ≥7 wk. Larvae and adults may cause small hemorrhages with edema in the colon and passage of feces coated with mucus. Clinical chabertiasis is seldom if ever seen in cattle.

For diagnosis, treatment and control, *see* p 211 *et seq.*

TRICHURIS INFECTION

Trichuris spp infections are common in young calves and yearlings, but numbers of worms are seldom large. The eggs are resistant, and infections are likely to persist on problem premises. Clinical signs are unlikely, but in occasional heavy infections, dark feces, anemia, and anorexia may be observed.

For diagnosis, treatment and control, *see* p 211 *et seq.*

TAPEWORM INFECTION

The anoplocephalid tapeworms *Moniezia expansa* and *M benedeni* are found in young cattle. The worms of this group are characterized by the absence of a rostellum and hooks, and the segments usually are wider than they are long. The eggs are triangular or rectangular and are ingested by free-living oribatid mites, which live in the soil and grass. After 6-16 wk, infective cysticercoids are present in the mites. Infection occurs by ingestion of the mites; the prepatent period is ~5 wk. *Moniezia* are commonly considered nonpathogenic in calves, but intestinal stasis has been reported.

For diagnosis, treatment and control, *see* p 211 *et seq.*

GASTROINTESTINAL PARASITES OF SHEEP AND GOATS

A number of species of nematodes and cestodes cause parasitic gastritis and enteritis in sheep and goats. The most important of these are *Haemonchus contortus, Ostertagia circumcincta, Trichostrongylus axei*, intestinal species of *Trichostrongylus, Nematodirus* spp, *Bunostomum trigonocephalum*, and *Oesophagostomum columbianum*. *Cooperia curticei, Strongyloides papillosus, Trichuris ovis*, and *Chabertia ovina* may also be pathogenic in sheep; these and related species are discussed under helminths of cattle (*see* above).

HAEMONCHUS, OSTERTAGIA, AND TRICHOSTRONGYLUS INFECTIONS

The principal stomach worms of sheep and goats are *Haemonchus contortus, Ostertagia circumcincta, O trifurcata*, and *Trichostrongylus axei*, and in some tropical regions, *Mecistocirrus digitatus*. Cross-transmission of *Haemonchus* between sheep and cattle can occur, but not as readily as transmission between homologous species. Sheep are more susceptible to the cattle species than are cattle to the sheep species. For descriptions and life cycles, *see* GI PARASITES OF CATTLE, above.

Haemonchus is most common in tropical or subtropical areas or in those areas with summer rainfall, while *Ostertagia* and *T axei* are more common in winter rainfall areas. The latter species also predominate in temperate zones.

Ovine haemonchosis may be classified as hyperacute, acute, or chronic. In the hyperacute disease, death may occur within 1 wk of heavy infection without significant signs. The acute disease is characterized by severe anemia accompanied by generalized edema; anemia is also characteristic of the chronic infection, often of low worm burdens, and is accompanied by progressive weight loss. Diarrhea is not a sign of haemonchosis; the lesions are those associated with anemia. The abomasum is edematous and, in the chronic phase, the pH becomes elevated, which causes gastric dysfunction. Mature sheep may develop heavy, even fatal infections, particularly during lactation.

The lesions, pathogenesis, and signs of *Ostertagia* and *T axei* infections are similar to those found in cattle. Even subclinical infection depresses appetite, impairs gastric digestion, and reduces utilization of metabolizable energy and protein. *Ostertagia* is the principal genus involved in the periparturient rise in fecal egg counts in sheep, and heavy infections may cause diarrhea and depress milk production in ewes. This output of eggs serves as the main source of contamination for the lambs. The same type of inhibited development (hypobiosis) observed in cattle has been seen with both *Ostertagia* and *Haemonchus* in sheep.

For diagnosis, treatment and control, *see* p 211 *et seq*.

INTESTINAL TRICHOSTRONGYLOSIS

The life cycle of intestinal *Trichostrongylus (T colubriformis, T vitrinus, T rugatus)* is direct; the developing larvae burrow superficially in the crypts of the mucosa and develop to egg-laying adults in 18-21 days.

Anorexia, persistent diarrhea, and weight loss are the main signs. Villous atrophy occurs and results in impaired digestion and malabsorption; protein loss occurs across the damaged mucosa. There are no diagnostic lesions; a total worm count should be done to demonstrate the worms and evaluate the condition.

For diagnosis, treatment and control, *see* p 211 *et seq*.

BUNOSTOMUM AND GAIGERIA INFECTIONS

Adult *Bunostomum trigonocephalum* (hookworm) are found in the jejunum. The life cycle and clinical findings are essentially the same as for the cattle hookworm. As few as 100 worms may cause clinical signs. *Gaigeria pachyscelis* is found in Africa and Asia, and resembles *Bunostomum* in size and form (2-3 cm). Larvae of *G pachyscelis* infect the host only by skin penetration. It is a voracious bloodsucker and probably the most pathogenic hookworm.

For diagnosis, treatment and control, *see* p 211 *et seq*.

NEMATODIRUS INFECTION

The species of *Nematodirus* that occur in the small intestine of sheep are similar in morphology and life cycle to *N helvetianus* (qv, p 207). Clinical *Nematodirus* infections are of considerable importance in the UK, New Zealand, and Australia, where death losses of 20% of the lambs in affected flocks have been reported. The parasites are endemic in some parts of the Rocky Mountain states of the USA where they occasionally cause clinical disease in lambs.

In those areas where clinical infections are common, the disease often has a characteristic seasonal pattern. Many of the eggs passed by affected lambs lie dormant through the remainder of the grazing season and the winter, with large numbers of larvae appearing during the early grazing period of the following year. Thus, the lambs of one season contaminate the pastures for the next season's lambs, and the life cycle can be broken if the same area is not used for lambing each year. Most clinical infections occur in lambs 6-12 wk old.

Nematodirus battus occurs in the UK and other parts of Europe and recently has been reported in North America. It appears to be more pathogenic than other species; because of the management techniques used in those areas and because the eggs do not hatch until they have been exposed to cold conditions, the disease occurs regularly in the spring. Because the eggs are very resistant and do not hatch except in moist conditions, they accumulate in periods of dry weather and hatch in large numbers after rain, with disease outbreaks occurring 2-4 wk later. *Nematodirus* spp often occur in low-rainfall regions (eg, the Karroo in South Africa and inland Australia) where other parasites rarely occur.

The disease is characterized by sudden onset, "loss of bloom", unthriftiness, profuse diarrhea, and marked dehydration, with death as early as 2-3 days after an outbreak begins. Nematodirosis is commonly confined to lambs or weaner sheep, but in low-rainfall country where outbreaks are sporadic, older sheep may experience heavy infections. The lesions usually consist of dehydration and a mild catarrhal enteritis, but acute inflammation of the entire small intestine may occur. Counts of ≥10,000 worms, together with characteristic signs and history, are indicative of clinical infections. Affected lambs may pass large numbers of eggs, which can be identified easily; however, since the onset may precede the maturation of the female worms, this is not a constant finding.

For diagnosis, treatment and control, *see* p 211 *et seq.*

OESOPHAGOSTOMUM INFECTION

The nodular worm of sheep, *Oesophagostomum columbianum*, is similar morphologically and in its life cycle to the nodular worm of cattle (qv, p 208).

Diarrhea usually develops during the second week of infection. The feces may contain excess mucus as well as streaks of blood. As the diarrhea progresses, the animals become emaciated and weak. These signs often subside near the end of the prepatent period, but the continuing presence of numerous adult worms may result in a chronic infection in which signs may not develop for several months. The animals become weak, lose weight despite a good appetite, and show intermittent diarrhea and constipation.

As resistance develops, nodules form around the larvae and these may become caseated and calcified. Nodule formation usually is more pronounced in sheep than in cattle. Affected sheep walk with a stilted gait and often have a humped back. Stenosis and intussusception may occur in severe cases. Diagnosis is difficult during the prepatent period, at which time it must be based largely on clinical signs, although the nodules often can be palpated per rectum.

For diagnosis, treatment and control, *see* p 211 *et seq.*

CHABERTIA INFECTION

Adult worms cause severe damage to the mucosa of the colon with resulting congestion, ulceration, and small hemorrhages. Infected sheep are unthrifty; the feces are soft and contain much mucus, and may be streaked with blood.

Immunity develops quickly, and outbreaks are seen only under conditions of severe stress.

For diagnosis, treatment and control, *see* below.

STRONGYLOIDES INFECTION

Heavy infections with adult worms cause a disease resembling trichostrongylosis. Infection is usually by skin penetration but can also occur via the milk. Damage to the skin between the claws, produced by skin-penetrating larvae, resembles the early stages of foot rot and may aid the penetration of the causal agents of foot rot. Most infections are transitory and inconsequential.

For diagnosis, treatment and control, *see* below.

TRICHURIS INFECTION

Heavy infections with whipworms are not common, but may occur in very young lambs or during drought conditions where sheep are fed grain on the ground. The eggs are very resistant. Congestion and edema of the cecal mucosa, accompanied by diarrhea and unthriftiness are seen.

For diagnosis, treatment and control, *see* below.

TAPEWORM INFECTION

The pathogenicity of *Moniezia expansa* in sheep has long been debated. Many earlier observations, which associated this infection with diarrhea, emaciation, and weight loss, did not accurately differentiate between tapeworm infections and infection with certain of the small nematodes (eg, *Trichostrongylus colubriformis*). It is now recognized that tapeworms are relatively nonpathogenic, but heavy infections may result in mild unthriftiness and GI disturbances. Diagnosis may be made by finding yellowish to pearl-white, bell-shaped proglottids in the feces or protruding from the anus, or by demonstrating the characteristic eggs on fecal examination. The life cycle involves an oribatid mite that lives in the mat of pastures. The prepatent period is 6-7 wk. Lambs develop resistance quickly and infections are unusual after ~4-5 mo.

Thysanosoma actinioides, the "fringed tapeworm", inhabits the small intestine, as well as the bile and pancreatic ducts. It is commonly found in sheep from Rocky Mountain areas of the USA. Although it has not been associated with clinical disease, it is of economic importance because livers are condemned when tapeworms are found in the bile duct.

For diagnosis, treatment and control, *see* below.

DIAGNOSIS OF GASTROINTESTINAL PARASITISM IN RUMINANTS

The clinical signs associated with GI parasitisms are shared by many diseases and conditions; however, presumptive diagnosis based on signs, grazing history, and season is often justified. Infection usually can be confirmed by demonstrating eggs on fecal examination (*see* ESTIMATING INTERNAL PARASITE LOAD, p 951). In clinical evaluation of fecal examinations, 2 points should be remembered: 1) an EPG count is not always an accurate indication of the number of adult worms present, and 2) specific identification of eggs is impractical except in specialized laboratories. EPG counts may be negative or deceptively low in the presence of large numbers of immature worms; even when many adult parasites are present, the count may be low if egg production has been suppressed by immune reaction or previous anthelmintic treatment. Variations in the egg-producing capacity of different worms (significantly lower for *Trichostrongylus, Ostertagia,* and *Nematodirus* than for *Haemonchus*) also may distort the true picture. The ova of *Nematodirus, Bunostomum, Strongyloides,* and *Trichuris* are distinctive, but reliable differentiation of the more common species of ruminant nematode ova is difficult. Fecal cultures can produce distinctive third-stage larvae if antemortem differentiation is important.

The advent of safe and effective broad-spectrum anthelmintics has largely reduced the need for differentiating the genera and species of these parasites. In areas where *Ostertagia* spp predominate, the examination of sera for elevated plasma pepsinogen levels is a useful diagnostic aid. Generally, tyrosine levels >3 IU are associated with clinical signs. Problems of interpretation may arise in immune animals under challenge, in which there are no clinical signs but the pepsinogen levels may be elevated because of the immune reaction. Where *Haemonchus* spp predominate, a PCV estimate on heparinized blood provides a quick guide to the degree of anemia. In some countries, serological diagnosis (ELISA) of important species such as *Ostertagia* and *Cooperia* infections in cattle is employed. As yet, there is insufficient information on the correlation between serological titers and parasite load.

In many management situations, high levels of infection can be expected, particularly after favorable temperatures and rainfall conditions in certain seasons. "Diagnostic drenching" is recommended when eggs are few or absent, yet history and signs suggest infections. A clinical response to a broad-spectrum anthelmintic permits a retrospective diagnosis, but the animals should be placed on "clean" pastures after treatment to avoid reinfection.

Necropsy is the most direct method to identify and quantitate GI parasitisms. Death of one or more animals can provide valuable parasitological data about the status of the rest of the herd or flock. Routine postmortem examinations are invaluable to diagnosis and are recommended.

On necropsy, *Haemonchus*, *Bunostomum*, *Oesophagostomum*, *Trichuris*, and *Chabertia* adults (or advanced immature worms) can be seen easily. *Ostertagia*, *Trichostrongylus*, *Cooperia*, and *Nematodirus* are difficult to see except by their movement in fluid ingesta. Clinically important infections are easily overlooked with these genera, and the total contents and all washings should be combined to a known volume and a worm count done to evaluate the severity of the infection. Measured samples of GI contents and scrapings of the mucosa should be examined microscopically under low power. These smaller nematodes can be stained (5 min) with a strong iodine solution. After the background ingesta and tissue are decolorized with 5% sodium thiosulfate, the small nematodes are easily seen. The significance of the numbers of worms present varies according to species of worms and host species, eg, only 100 *Haemonchus* are of clinical significance in lambs, whereas 5000-10,000 *Ostertagia* probably are required to be significant. When the animals have been diarrheic for a few days, worms may have been shed, and the type and severity of gross lesions may also be of considerable diagnostic value.

Multifactorial causation should be considered in evaluating clinical, laboratory, and necropsy findings. Mixed parasite infections are the rule. Shipping fever, nutrition-related GI disorders, salmonellosis, paratuberculosis, viral diarrhea, trace-element deficiencies, fascioliasis, lungworm, etc, are differential diagnoses.

Diagnosis of ostertagiasis in cattle during the period of larval inhibition (pretype II) presents technical problems, particularly for the feedlot industry in the USA. Fecal egg counts and plasma pepsinogen analysis do not provide useful information, and immunological methods of detecting inhibited larvae have not been developed. Predisposing factors for inhibition are important to consider and include geographical source of cattle, time of year or season of arrival, age of cattle, previous grazing history and management, weather conditions prevailing during last grazing period, and prevalence of *O ostertagi* in the source region.

Information on such factors usually is not available for feedlot cattle. If they have arrived following spring grazing in the south or autumn grazing in the north of the USA, they could have heavy burdens of inhibited larvae. Lighter calves from areas of high parasite prevalence may also have such a problem. It is becoming more widely accepted that one of the significant causes of clinical disease or feed efficiency problems in feedlot cattle is parasitism, possibly ostertagiasis. For those who receive their cattle from a suspect area and at a suspect time of year, it may be advisable to treat the new arrivals promptly with an anthelmintic effective against inhibited larvae.

TREATMENT OF GASTROINTESTINAL PARASITISM IN RUMINANTS

Effective worm control cannot always be achieved by drugs alone; however, anthelmintics play an important role. They should be used to reduce pasture contamination, particularly at times critical for survival of the preparasitic stages. Coordination with other methods of control, such as alternate grazing of different host species, integrated rotational grazing of different age groups within the one species (including creep grazing), and alternation of grazing and cropping, are other management techniques that can provide safe pasture and give economic advantage when combined with anthelmintic treatment.

The "ideal anthelmintic" should be safe, highly effective against adults and immature stages (including hypobiotic larvae) of the important worms, rapidly and completely metabolized, available in a variety of convenient formulations, economical to use, and compatible with other commonly used compounds. Several drugs now satisfy all or most of these requirements. (*See also* p 1481.) Thiabendazole was the forerunner of the modern anthelmintics and set a new standard in efficacy and safety. Despite ineffectiveness against hypobiotic *Ostertagia* larvae in cattle and 1 or 2 other worm species, it is still widely used. Following thiabendazole and mebendazole, other benzimidazoles (such as fenbendazole, oxfendazole, and albendazole) and the pro-benzimidazoles (thiophanate, febantel, and netobomin) were developed; these compounds are effective against most of the major GI parasites of ruminants, including varying levels of activity against hypobiotic larvae. Levamisole and the pyrantel group also are highly effective, safe, wide-spectrum anthelmintics except against hypobiotic larvae in cattle. Ivermectin is highly effective against adults and larval stages, including hypobiotic larvae of all the common GI nematodes of ruminants, and some of the important ectoparasites.

Routes of administration other than drenching or injection (eg, incorporating into feed, drinking water, and mineral or energy blocks) are used to reduce labor costs, and may be useful under drylot conditions or when grazing animals are being given supplemental feed. Another advantage of these "in-feed" routes is that continuous low-level administration of a drug can be achieved and pasture contamination reduced during periods that are optimal for free-living development of the parasites. The disadvantages include erratic consumption of anthelmintic, unacceptable tissue residues, and possible encouragement of drug resistance by continuous exposure. Another labor-saving route of administration is the "pour-on" dermal treatment developed for some of the organophosphates, eg, trichlorfon, and now used for levamisole and ivermectin. The morantel sustained-release bolus has been particularly effective in prevention of parasitism from spring into summer in cool temperate regions.

Lead arsenate, niclosamide, and the newer benzimidazoles (albendazole, fenbendazole, and oxfendazole) are effective against tapeworms (*Moniezia* spp) in cattle and sheep. Treatment of *Thysanosoma actinioides* has presented problems, but niclosamide was reported to be effective at 250 mg/kg. Additionally, bithionol (200 mg/kg) has been used, and praziquantel is likely to be effective.

Consideration should be given to the following when treating clinically affected animals: 1) providing adequate nutrition, 2) treating all animals in the group as a preventive measure and to reduce further pasture contamination, and 3) moving stock to "clean" pastures to minimize reinfection. The definition of safe pastures varies in different climates and depends on local knowledge of the seasonal mortality of infective larvae.

Finally, development of drug resistance by populations of *Haemonchus contortus*, *Trichostrongylus* spp, and *Ostertagia* spp in sheep and goats to thiabendazole and other benzimidazoles, levamisole, and ivermectin has been demonstrated. While such resistance is currently a problem only in certain areas, it should be considered when response to therapy is suboptimal and other factors can be ruled out, eg, improper dosage, rapid reinfection, poor nutrition, or some disease state other than parasitism. Drug resistance in parasites of cattle has not yet been demonstrated definitively, but overuse and otherwise indiscriminate treatment should be avoided.

GENERAL CONTROL MEASURES FOR GASTROINTESTINAL PARASITISM IN RUMINANTS

The word "control" generally implies the suppression of parasite burdens in the host below that level at which economic loss occurs. To do this effectively requires a comprehensive knowledge of the epidemiological and ecological factors that govern pasture larval populations and the role of host resistance to infection.

The goals of control are to: 1) prevent heavy exposure in susceptible hosts (recovery from heavy infection is always slow), 2) reduce overall levels of pasture contamination, 3) minimize the effects of parasite burdens, and 4) encourage the development of immunity or resistance.

Strategic use of anthelmintics is designed to reduce worm burdens and, thereby, the contamination of pastures; timing of administration is based on knowledge of the seasonal changes in infection and the regional epidemiology of the various helminthoses. Tactical use is based on prompt recognition of circumstances likely to favor development of parasitic disease, eg, weather, grazing behavior, and loss of weight and condition.

For example, in the UK, where the pattern of disease caused by *Nematodirus* infection in sheep is clearly defined, strategic treatments with 2-3 doses of anthelmintic at 3-wk intervals, beginning just before the disease characteristically appears, are recommended. Similarly, in the northern USA, Canada, or western Europe, pasture levels of *Ostertagia* and other parasites increase substantially after mid-July, ie, the general pattern of infectivity is minimal in spring, but increases rapidly to peak levels in late summer and early autumn. Current practices in these areas indicate the effectiveness of 2 or more anthelmintic treatments (usually at intervals of 3-5 wk) given when cattle first go to grass in spring. Single treatments and subsequent transfer of animals to safe pasture, and treatment associated with delayed spring turn out also have been effective.

In other countries of either cool or warm temperate climate, similar controls may be used if the seasonal pattern of the disease is known, but in most regions a tactical use of anthelmintics is employed, eg, during warm, moist conditions.

CATTLE—SPECIAL CONSIDERATIONS

Worm problems occur most frequently in young beef cattle from time of weaning and several months thereafter, and in segregated groups of dairy calves during the first season at grass. Immunity to the GI nematodes is acquired slowly and usually requires 2 grazing seasons before a significant level is attained. In endemic areas, cows may continue to harbor low burdens and these may be the cause of suboptimal production. GI parasitism in young stock may be controlled by use of broad-spectrum anthelmintics in conjunction with pasture management to limit reinfection; the latter includes a move to "clean" pastures (eg, grass conservation areas) or newly established winter annual pastures, alternate grazing with other host species, or integrated rotational grazing in which susceptible calves are followed by immune adults. Simple pasture rotation is not effective because the bovine fecal mass may protect larvae for several months from adverse environmental conditions and, therefore, rotating calves could be subject to reinfection at a later date.

In beef herds, anthelmintic treatment at weaning is of value, particularly if the young cattle are to be retained, eg, as replacement heifer stock or as steers to be fed. Cattle finished on grass should receive treatment at weaning and at intervals during the next 12 mo, and if possible, should be moved to safe pastures.

When cattle cannot be moved readily to other pastures, strategic treatments may be given at vital times to limit contamination of pastures and rapid reinfection. In the northern USA or western Europe, eg, these would be given on 2 or 3 occasions in the spring and early summer. Alternatively, rumen boluses containing morantel tartrate (continuous release over 60-90 days), or oxfendazole, albendazole, or levamisole (pulse-released at intervals of 21-30 days) may be used in countries where they are approved. In warm temperate regions of the world, such as Australia and New Zealand, the southern USA, and the large cattle-raising regions of southern Brazil, Uruguay, and Argentina, young cattle may be given ≥2 treatments from late summer and into autumn for prevention of large increases in pasture contamination and infection during winter and spring. Application of 2-3 close-interval, strategic treatments from the time of weaning in such regions could be just as effective as those administered at spring treatment in cool temperate regions. However, survival of infective larvae on pasture from the time of autumn weaning in warm temperate regions is most often persistent, and longer intervals between treatments (eg, at weaning, during winter, and in late spring) may be more applicable. However, in many areas, anthelmintics are simply given at regular intervals after weaning. Intervals between treatments must necessarily vary according to the local epidemiology. When Type II ostertagiasis is a problem, treatment with an anthelmintic effective against hypobiotic larvae is recommended before the expected time of outbreak.

SHEEP—SPECIAL CONSIDERATIONS

A special strategic treatment is required in most regions to counter the postparturient relaxation of resistance (periparturient rise, etc) seen in ewes. The precise timing of such treatment varies between regions and for different species of parasites, but in general, treatment within the month before and again within the month after parturition appears desirable. A treatment 2 wk before breeding, as part of a "flushing" program, is another strategic application of anthelmintics. Supportive management after treatment includes movement of sheep from contaminated pastures to cattle pastures, grass conservation areas, root crops, or pasture not grazed by sheep for several months. The latter period varies according to the seasonal pattern of larval mortality in different countries and may be as long as 1 yr in some temperate countries.

Sheep are more consistently susceptible to the adverse effects of worms than other livestock. Clinical disease is more common. Resistance is not strong and frequent treatments may be required, particularly during the first year of life.

FLUKE INFECTIONS IN RUMINANTS

Fasciola hepatica, the most important trematode of domestic ruminants, is the most common cause of liver fluke disease in temperate areas of the world. In the USA, it is endemic along the Gulf Coast, the West Coast, the Rocky Mountain region, and other areas. It is present in eastern Canada, British Columbia, South America, and is of particular economic importance in the British Isles, western and eastern Europe, Australia, and New Zealand. *Fasciola gigantica* is economically important in Africa and Asia, and is found in Hawaii. *Fascioloides magna* has been reported in at least 21 states (USA) and in Europe. In North America, *Dicrocoelium dendriticum* is confined mainly to New York, New Jersey, Massachusetts, and the Atlantic provinces of Canada. It is also found in Europe and Asia. *Eurytrema* spp, the pancreatic flukes, parasitize sheep, pigs, and cattle in Brazil and parts of Asia. Several species of paramphistomes or rumen flukes are found throughout much of the world.

FASCIOLA HEPATICA
(Common liver fluke)

Etiology: *Fasciola hepatica* (30 × 12 mm and leaf-shaped) has a worldwide distribution and a broad host range. Economically important infections occur in cattle and sheep in 3 forms: **chronic**, which is rarely fatal in cattle but often fatal in sheep; **subacute or acute**, primarily in sheep and often fatal; and in conjunction with "**black disease**", almost exclusive to sheep and usually fatal.

Eggs passed in the feces develop into miracidia in ~2-4 wk, depending on temperature, and hatch in water. Miracidia infect lymnaeid snails, in which development and multiplication occur through the stages of sporocysts, rediae (sometimes daughter rediae), and cercariae. After ~2 mo (or longer if temperatures are low), cercariae emerge from snails and encyst on aquatic vegetation. Snails may extend the period by hibernating during the winter. Encysted cercariae (metacercariae) may remain viable for many months unless they become desiccated.

After ingestion by the host, usually with herbage, young flukes are released in the duodenum, penetrate the intestinal wall, and enter the peritoneal cavity. The young flukes penetrate the liver capsule and wander in the parenchyma for several weeks, growing and destroying tissue. They enter the bile ducts and mature, and begin to produce eggs. The prepatent period is usually 2-3 mo depending on the fluke burden. The adult fluke may live in the bile ducts of sheep for years; most are shed from cattle within 5-6 mo. Prenatal infections have been reported in cattle.

Clinical Findings: Fascioliasis in ruminants ranges in severity from a devastating disease in sheep to an asymptomatic infection in cattle. The course usually is determined by the numbers of metacercariae ingested over a short period. In sheep, acute fascioliasis occurs seasonally and is manifest by a distended, painful abdomen, anemia, and sudden death. Deaths can occur within 6 wk of infection. The acute syndrome must be differentiated from "black disease", infectious necrotic hepatitis (INH, qv, p 327). In subacute disease, survival is longer (7-10 wk), even in cases with great damage to livers, but deaths occur due to hemorrhage and anemia. Chronic fascioliasis occurs in all seasons; signs may include anemia, unthriftiness, submandibular edema, and reduced milk secretion, but even heavily infected cattle may show no clinical signs. Heavy chronic infection is fatal in sheep.

Sheep do not appear to develop resistance to infection, and chronic liver damage is cumulative over several years. In cattle, there is evidence of reduced susceptibility following fibrosis of liver tissues and calcification of bile ducts.

Lesions: Immature, wandering flukes destroy liver tissue and cause hemorrhage. Extensive damage leads to acute fascioliasis in which the liver is enlarged and friable with fibrinous deposits on the capsule. Migratory tracts can be seen, and the surface has an uneven appearance. In chronic cases, cirrhosis develops. Mature flukes damage the bile ducts, which become enlarged, or even cystic, and have thickened fibrosed walls. In cattle, the duct walls become greatly thickened and often calcified. Flukes may be found in aberrant sites, eg, lungs. Mixed infections with *F magna* can occur in cattle.

Tissue destruction by wandering flukes may create a microenvironment favorable to activation of clostridial spores.

Diagnosis: The oval, operculated, golden brown eggs, 130-150 × 65-90 μm, must be distinguished from those of paramphistomes (rumen flukes), which are larger and clear. Eggs of *F hepatica* cannot be demonstrated in feces during acute fascioliasis. In subacute or chronic disease, the number varies from day to day and repeated fecal examination may be required. At necropsy, the nature of the liver damage is diagnostic. Adult flukes are readily seen in the bile ducts, and immature stages may be squeezed or teased from the cut surface.

Control: Control measures for *F hepatica* infections are designed to reduce the number of flukes in the host animal, the snail population in the environment, and exposure of livestock to snail-infested ground. Routine treatments of livestock in autumn and spring are advisable; additional treatments are determined by local epidemiological factors; eg, in the Gulf Coast States (USA), cattle should be treated before the fall rainy season begins (which reduces pasture contamination) and again in the late spring. In northwestern USA, cattle should be treated at the end of the pasture season (November-December) and again in late January or February. Animals brought into feedlot may require treatment on arrival and again in 8 wk. When drug safety permits, pregnant animals should be treated a few weeks before parturition to ensure that they are not anemic during lactation. Certain products are prohibited in lactating dairy cows.

Recently, a number of compounds such as oxyclozanide, diamphenethide (not active in cattle), rafoxanide, nitroxynil, albendazole, closantel, triclabendazole, netobimin, and clorsulon have become available. (Only albendazole and clorsulon are currently approved for use in the USA.) Some of these (diamphenethide, 100 mg/kg; nitroxynil, 15 mg/kg; closantel, 10 mg/kg; triclabendazole, 10 mg/kg; clorsulon, 7 mg/kg) are active against immature flukes.

The selection of a fasciolicide should be based on the disease situation, host animal, and local environmental conditions and regulations; contraindications should be observed and use precautions followed. Vaccination of sheep against INH is essential in some countries.

The snail intermediate host may be controlled by drainage of land, suitable management, and use of molluscicides. The ideal compound would kill snails and their eggs when used in low concentration and be harmless to mammals and fishes. Routine treatment of an area several times a year may be necessary for adequate control. Copper compounds, sodium pentachlorphenate, and trifenmorph, are the commonly used molluscicides and are effective if applied correctly.

Suitable management and fencing may be used to exclude grazing animals from snail habitats. Control is complicated by reservoir infections in horses and wildlife, such as deer and rabbits. When sheep and cattle graze together, it is necessary to treat both in a control plan.

FASCIOLA GIGANTICA
(Giant liver fluke)

Fasciola gigantica is similar in shape to *F hepatica* but is larger (75 mm), with less clearly defined shoulders. It occurs in warmer climates (Asia, Africa) in cattle and buffalo, in which it is responsible for chronic fascioliasis, and in sheep, in which the disease is frequently acute and fatal. The life cycle is similar to that of *F hepatica* except for species of snail intermediate hosts. The pathology of infection, diagnostic procedures, and control measures are similar to those for *F hepatica*.

FASCIOLOIDES MAGNA
(Large American liver fluke, Giant liver fluke)

Fascioloides magna is up to 100 mm long, thick, and oval; it is distinguished from *Fasciola* spp by the lack of an anterior projecting cone. It occurs in domestic and wild ruminants; deer are the normal hosts. The life cycle resembles that of *Fasciola* spp.

The life cycle is not completed in cattle. In this host, pathogenicity is low, and losses are confined primarily to liver condemnations. In sheep and goats, a few parasites can produce death due to extensive fluke migration in the liver parenchyma. In deer, there is little tissue reaction and the parasites are enclosed in thin fibrous cysts that communicate with bile ducts. In cattle, *F magna* cause severe tissue reaction, resulting in thick-walled encapsulations that do not communicate with bile ducts. In sheep, encapsulations do not develop and the parasites migrate in the liver and other organs, causing tremendous damage. On section, infected livers of cattle, sheep, and deer show black tortuous tracts formed by migrations of young flukes.

While the eggs of *F magna* resemble those of *F hepatica*, this is of limited use; eggs usually are not passed in cattle and sheep. Recovery of the parasites at necropsy and differentiation of *F hepatica* and *F gigantica* is necessary for definite diagnosis. When domestic ruminants and deer share the same grazing, the presence of disease due to *F magna* should be kept in mind. Mixed infections with *F hepatica* occur in cattle.

Oxyclozanide has been reported to be effective against *F magna* in white-tailed deer, and rafoxanide has been used successfully against natural infections in cattle. Albendazole (7.5 mg/kg), clorsulon (15 mg/kg), and closantel (15 mg/kg) have shown efficacy against this fluke in sheep. Currently no products are approved for use against this fluke in the USA. Deer are required for completion of the life cycle; if they can be excluded from the areas grazed by cattle and sheep, control may be effected. Control of the intermediate host (lymnaeid snails) may be possible once it has been identified in a region and the nature of its habitat examined.

DICROCOELIUM DENDRITICUM
(Lancet fluke, Lesser liver fluke)

The lancet fluke is slender and 6-10 mm long. It is widely distributed in many countries and infects a wide range of final hosts, including domestic ruminants. Another species, *D hospes*, is common in Africa. The first intermediate host is a terrestrial snail (*Cionella lubrica*, in the USA), from which cercariae emerge and are aggregated in a mass of sticky mucus (slime-ball). The cercariae are ingested by the second intermediate host, which are ants (*Formica fusca*, in the USA), and encyst in the abdominal cavity. One or 2 metacercariae in the subesophageal ganglion of the ant cause abnormal behavior in which the ants attach themselves to the herbage, which in turn increases the probability of ingestion by the final host. The young flukes migrate to the liver via the bile duct and begin egg-laying ~10-12 wk after infection.

There appears to be no immunity, and heavy infections may accumulate (up to 50,000 flukes in a mature sheep). Cirrhosis occurs and the bile ducts may be thickened and distended. Economic loss is due primarily to condemnation of livers. Clinical signs are not obvious, but may be seen in massive infections. The eggs are very small (40 × 25 μm), lopsided, yellowish brown, and contain a miracidium.

The complex life cycle makes attack on the intermediate hosts difficult unless aggregations of snails and ants can be located and eliminated. Against the flukes, hetolin (19-22 mg/kg), albendazole (20 mg/kg), fenbendazole (50 mg/kg), netobimin (20 mg/kg), and praziquantel (50 mg/kg) have reported efficacies ≥90%, but their use is not approved in all countries.

EURYTREMA SPP
(Pancreatic fluke)

These flukes are 8-16 mm long, 6 mm wide, and have a thick body. They are parasites of the pancreatic ducts and occasionally of the bile ducts of sheep, pigs, and cattle in Brazil and Asia. Three species, *E pancreaticum*, *E coelomaticum*, and *E ovis*, are recognized. The first intermediate hosts are terrestrial snails (*Bradybaena* spp), and the cercariae encyst in grasshoppers (*Conocephalus* spp), the second intermediate host. After ingestion of a grasshopper, the immature flukes are released and migrate to the pancreatic duct where they mature and produce eggs in ~11-14 wk.

There are no obvious clinical signs. *Dicrocoelium*-like eggs can be demonstrated in feces. Light infections cause proliferative inflammation of the pancreatic duct, which may become enlarged and occluded. In heavy infections, fibrotic, necrotic, and degenerative lesions occur. Losses are reported due to condemned pancreas, but the pathogenesis suggests an additional loss of production.

As for *Dicrocoelium*, the control of intermediate hosts may not be practical. Treatment with praziquantel (20 mg/kg, for 2 days) has been reported to be effective.

PARAMPHISTOMES
(Amphistomes, Rumen flukes, Conical flukes)

There are numerous species (*Paramphistomum, Calicophoron, Cotylophoron*) in ruminants worldwide. The adult parasites are pear-shaped, pink or red, up to 15 mm long, and attach to the lining of the rumen. Immature forms occur in the duodenum and are 1-3 mm long.

Eggs are passed in the feces, and miracidiae hatch in the water and infect planorbid or bulinid snails. Development in the snail is similar to that of *Fasciola hepatica*, with the snail shedding cercariae that encyst on the herbage. In the ruminant host, the young flukes excyst and remain in the small intestine for 3-5 wk before migrating forward through the reticulum to the rumen. Eggs are produced 7-14 wk after infection.

Adult flukes do not cause overt disease and large numbers may be encountered. The immature worms attach to the duodenal and, at times, the ileal mucosa by means of a large posterior sucker and cause severe enteritis, possibly necrosis, and hemorrhage. Affected animals exhibit anorexia, polydipsia, unthriftiness, and severe diarrhea. Extensive mortality may occur, especially in young cattle and sheep. Older animals can develop resistance to reinfection but may continue to harbor numerous adult flukes.

The large, clear, operculated eggs are readily recognized, but in acute paramphistomiasis there may be no eggs in the feces. Known occurrence in the area and examination of the fluid feces may reveal immature flukes, many of which are passed in these cases. Diagnosis is commonly made at necropsy.

The snail hosts may be attacked as described in the control of fascioliasis (qv, p 217). The immature flukes in sheep are susceptible to niclosamide, niclofolan, bithional, oxyclozanide, and rafoxanide, but resorantel and oxyclozanide are considered the anthelmintics of choice with efficacies >90% and activity against both immature and adult rumen flukes in cattle and sheep. Not all of these compounds are approved for use in all countries.

GASTROINTESTINAL PARASITES OF PIGS

Periparturient Relaxation of Immunity in Sows: During the periparturient period (2 wk before parturition to 6 wk after), a relaxation of immunity occurs in sows; if they harbor a strongyle infection, the fecal egg count increases markedly. At weaning, fecal egg output drops abruptly and many worms, particularly *Oesophagostomum*, are eliminated. This phenomenon is less constant than the corresponding occurrence in sheep, but has considerable epidemiological importance since the environment of the young is contaminated.

Worm Control: Apart from good basic hygiene in pig houses, which should be emphasized, control is based on anthelmintics. In-feed products include benzimidazoles, levamisole, and dichlorvos. A simple anthelmintic program is as follows: treat sows and gilts ~10 days before breeding and again before farrowing; treat weaners/feeders before entering clean pens; treat boars at 6-mo intervals. Alternatively, an injection of ivermectin, also effective against lice and mange mites, may be given in a similar program.

ASCARIS INFECTION

Adults of the large roundworm, *Ascaris suum*, are found principally in the small intestine, but may migrate into the stomach or bile ducts. They are ≥30 cm long and quite thick. Large numbers of eggs are produced (as many as 250,000/day); they can develop to the infective stage in 2-3 wk and are resistant to chemical agents. When the eggs are ingested, the larvae hatch in the intestine, penetrate the intestinal wall, and enter the portal circulation. After a period in the liver, they are carried by the circulation to the lungs, where they pass through the capillaries into the alveolar spaces. About 9-10 days after ingestion, the larvae pass up the bronchial tree, return to the GI tract, and then mature in the small intestine. The first eggs are passed 2-2½ mo after infection.

Clinical Findings: Adult worms may significantly reduce the growth rate of young animals; if sufficiently numerous, they may cause mechanical obstruction of the intestine, or migrate into and occlude the bile ducts, producing icterus.

Migration of larvae through the liver causes hemorrhage and fibrosis that appears as "white spots" under the capsule. In heavy infections, the larvae can cause pulmonary edema and consolidation, and exacerbate swine influenza and endemic pneumonia. Affected pigs show abdominal breathing, commonly referred to as "thumps". In addition to the respiratory signs, marked unthriftiness and weight loss are seen. Permanent stunting may result in pigs up to 4-5 mo old.

Diagnosis: During the patent period, diagnosis may be made by demonstrating the typical eggs in the feces. However, many young pigs show signs (especially respiratory) during the prepatent period. A presumptive diagnosis can be made based on history and signs, and can be confirmed by demonstrating immature worms on necropsy. In acute cases in which no worms are found in the intestine, it may be possible to recover larvae from affected lung tissue.

Treatment: Supportive therapy, including treatment for secondary bacterial invaders, may be necessary during the respiratory phase of infection. Many drugs have been used to remove adult ascarids. Piperazine preparations have low toxicity and are moderately priced, and for many years were the drug of choice. The benzimidazoles and probenzimidazoles, dichlorvos, ivermectin, levamisole, and pyrantel are effective and have a broader spectrum of activity than piperazine.

Hygromycin is active against ascarids when administered as a low-level additive to the feed. Many drugs have been tested for efficacy in destruction of the migratory stages; pyrantel shows greatest promise. The beneficial effects of reduced lung and liver damage deserve close study.

MACRACANTHORHYNCHUS INFECTION

Adult *M hirudinaceus* (thorny headed worm) usually are in the small intestine. They may be 30 cm long and 3-9 mm wide, slightly pink, and have a transversely wrinkled outer covering. The anterior end bears a spiny, retractable proboscis or rostellum used for firm attachment to the intestinal wall. The eggs are ingested by the grubs of various beetles that serve as intermediate hosts.

Signs are not specific; antemortem diagnosis is difficult, since the ova do not float reliably in salt solutions. The site of attachment may have a necrotic center surrounded by a zone of inflammation. These lesions usually can be seen through the serosa. The rostellum may perforate the intestinal wall and cause peritonitis and death.

Levamisole is effective for treatment. Control depends on avoiding use of contaminated hog lots or pastures.

OESOPHAGOSTOMUM INFECTION

Oesophagostomum spp are prevalent worldwide; *O dentatum* is the most common species. The adults are found in the lumen of the large intestine; they are 8-12 mm long, slender, and white or gray. The life cycle is direct; infection results from ingestion of larvae. These penetrate the mucosa of the large intestine within a few hours of ingestion, and return to the lumen in 6-20 days. Sows may have a periparturient rise in worm-egg output, which is an important source of infection for piglets. Most infections are asymptomatic, but heavily infected animals may show anorexia, emaciation, and GI disturbances. The serosa shows small nodules, their size reflecting species and previous exposure. In severe cases, the intestinal wall may be thickened and necrotic. In patent infections, typical strongyle eggs are found in feces, often in large numbers. These can be differentiated from those of *Hyostrongylus* by larval culture. At necropsy, the worms and lesions are readily seen. The benzimidazoles, levamisole, piperazines, dichlorvos, pyrantel tartrate, and ivermectin are effective.

STOMACH WORM INFECTIONS

Three types of stomach worms occur in pigs: a thin worm, *Hyostrongylus rubidus* (the red stomach worm), and 2 thick stomach worms, *Ascarops strongylina* and *Physocephalus sexalatus*. The thin stomach worm is ~6 mm long, slender, and has a direct life cycle. The thick stomach worms are ≥12 mm long, much stouter, and have coprophagous beetles as intermediate hosts.

Clinical Findings: These worms are more common in grazing pigs. When present in large numbers or when the host's condition is reduced by poor nutrition or other factors, they may cause variable appetite, anemia, diarrhea, or weight loss. *Hyostrongylus* sp characteristically is found under a heavy catarrhal or mucous exudate and may produce mucosal lesions similar to those of *Ostertagia* spp in ruminants, except that hemorrhages are more common. Retarded development of larval stages in the mucosa is analogous to that of *Ostertagia*. In sows, inhibited larvae resume development near parturition and may cause severe gastritis and, in addition, contaminate the environment of the young pigs.

Diagnosis and Treatment: Clinical signs other than unthriftiness are not obvious. Fatal hemorrhages have been reported in hyostrongylosis. Fecal examinations may show the distinctive ova of *Physocephalus* and *Ascarops*—small (35-40 × 20 μm), thick-shelled eggs that each contain an active larva. *Hyostrongylus* ova resemble those of other strongyle worms (*Oesophagostomum, Globocephalus*), and fecal cultures are required to obtain infective larvae for differential diagnosis.

At necropsy, adult worms, especially *Physocephalus* and *Ascarops*, are readily seen. Mucosal scrapings for microscopical examination are essential for detection of immature *Hyostrongylus*.

Thiabendazole, levamisole, and dichlorvos are effective against *Hyostrongylus*. The newer benzimidazoles, probenzimidazoles, and ivermectin are highly effective and also remove retarded stages. Carbon disulfide, or the complex with piperazine, which is active in the stomach, is recommended against *Physocephalus* and *Ascarops*, but precise data are lacking.

STRONGYLOIDES INFECTION

The life cycle of *Strongyloides ransomi* (intestinal threadworm) is apparently similar to that of *S papillosus* of cattle (qv, p 207). Transmission of *S ransomi* larvae in the colostrum is the most common route of infection in neonatal pigs and explains the serious nature of the infection. The adult worms (only females in the parasitic cycle) burrow into the wall of the small intestine. In light and moderate infections, the animals usually show no signs. In heavy infections, diarrhea, anemia, and emaciation may be observed, and death may result.

Demonstration of the characteristic small, thin-shelled, embryonated eggs in the feces or of the adults in scrapings from the intestinal mucosa is diagnostic. *Strongyloides* ova must be differentiated from the larger *Metastrongylus* (swine lungworm) ova, which also are embryonated in fresh feces. At necropsy, immature worms may be recovered from minced tissues placed in a Baermann isolation apparatus.

The benzimidazoles are effective against intestinal infections. If administered in the feed for several days before and after parturition, they reduce infections in suckling piglets. Ivermectin is effective against adults and, if given to the sow 1-2 wk before farrowing, controls transmission to the piglets.

TRICHURIS INFECTION

Trichuris suis is 5-8 cm long and has a slender anterior portion and a thickened posterior third. Infection is by ingestion of embryonated ova. Heavy infections may cause inflammatory lesions in the cecum and adjacent large intestine, and be accompanied by diarrhea and unthriftiness. The double-operculated eggs are diagnostic. Dichlorvos, levamisole, and some benzimidazoles are effective.

LIVER ABSCESSES IN CATTLE

Secondary to rumenitis, liver abscesses occur in all ages and breeds of cattle, and wherever cattle are raised, but are most common in feedlots: up to 95% of a group of fattened cattle may be affected. Abscesses reduce efficiency of feed conversion, and affected livers are condemned.

Etiology and Pathogenesis: *Fusobacterium necrophorum*, a gram-negative, obligate anaerobic bacterium, and a component of normal rumen microflora, is the primary etiological agent. Of the 3 biotypes (A, B, and C), only A and B have been implicated. Type A strains are isolated from ~85% of the abscesses and are usually found in pure culture. Type B strains are isolated from ~15% of the abscesses and are always found in mixed culture, being present with type A or other bacterial species. *Corynebacterium pyogenes*, streptococci, staphylococci, and *Bacteroides* spp are most frequently recovered from mixed cultures.

Rumenitis is usually the result of rapid intraruminal fermentation of dietary carbohydrate with subsequent increased acidity of the ruminal fluid. Rations with high levels of carbohydrate are the principal cause, but texture of the feed can be contributory. The incidence of rumenitis in feedlot cattle is significantly higher when they are transferred directly from a roughage ration to a finishing ration. *Fusobacterium necrophorum*, alone or with other bacteria, colonizes the ulcerated rumen wall. Bacterial emboli from the lesions invade the hepatic portal venous system and are transported to the liver, where they can establish infectious foci of necrobacillosis that eventually develop into abscesses.

Clinical Findings, Lesions, and Diagnosis: Cattle with liver abscesses seldom exhibit clinical signs. Feedlot cattle with abscessed livers have reduced feed efficiency, and those severely abscessed gain 5-15% less per day than abscess-free cattle. Most liver abscesses are occult lesions that regress to a sterile scar; a few rupture and drain into the peritoneal cavity, the hepatic blood vessels, or the caudal vena cava. Sudden death and vague GI and respiratory disturbances are associated with such ruptured abscesses.

The ruminal lesions are characterized by a marked inflammatory reaction and necrosis. Occasionally, abscesses are observed in the deeper layers of the rumen wall. Hepatic necrobacillosis lesions of <6 days duration are pale yellow and spherical with irregular outlines, and are characterized by coagulation necrosis of the hepatocytes. Older abscesses have a core that is progressively encapsulated by fibrous connective tissue. Abscesses are usually 4-6 cm in diameter. Affected livers usually have 3-10 abscesses but may have up to 100.

Liver abscesses are found in ~10% of cattle slaughtered in the USA. Culture is seldom done to confirm the diagnosis. Occasionally, liver abscesses due to *F necrophorum* must be distinguished from those resulting from traumatic reticuloperitonitis (qv, p 224).

Treatment and Control: Chlortetracycline fed continuously at 70 mg/head/day during the finishing period significantly reduces the number of liver abscesses and increases feed efficiency and weight gain, but has little, if any, effect on prevalence of ruminal lesions. Fewer ruminal lesions develop when the ratio of concentrate to roughage is decreased, and when the transition period from a roughage to a finishing ration is increased. Increased roughage in the ration and multiple daily feedings increase the time of mastication and saliva flow; this increases buffer to the rumen and provides a continuous and uniform fermentation that reduces intraruminal pH, which, in turn, lowers the number of ruminal lesions, and indirectly the number of liver abscesses.

PERITONEAL FAT NECROSIS

Occurs in cattle ≥2 yr old after prolonged grazing of tall fescue infected with *Acremonium coenophialum* (*see also* SUMMER FESCUE TOXICOSIS, p 1688). The condition is seen throughout the USA where tall fescue is used as the primary pasture plant. Over 90% of such pastures are infected. Hard masses of necrotic fat form in the omentum, mesentery, and perirenal fat and may cause clinical disease when they compress the intestine, obstruct the birth canal, or compress ureters. Rectal examination is useful in diagnosis and in determining prevalence in a herd. Removal of cattle from endophyte-infected pastures or dilution of intake by supplying legume or other grass pasture promotes slow reduction in the size of masses.

A second form, less well defined, appears to be related to pancreatic problems. Although not associated with a clinical syndrome, this is not a rare finding at necropsy; the lesions (discrete or confluent masses of necrotic adipose tissue) may be found throughout the abdomen.

A third form, a focal necrosis of abdominal and retroperitoneal fat, is seen most often in sheep, but also in pigs, horses, and others.

"RATTLE BELLY" IN LAMBS
(Watery mouth, Slavery mouth, Slavers)

A disease in intensive lambing flocks throughout the UK that can cause serious loss in newborn lambs. It occurs most commonly in lambs 12-72 hr old. Morbidity in a flock can be as high as 30% and, if untreated, most affected lambs die. An apparently similar condition can occur in older lambs but almost certainly has a different etiology.

Etiology: Watery mouth has been induced in lambs by oral infection with a variety of strains of *Escherichia coli* that in most situations would be expected to be nonpathogenic. It is thought that rapid multiplication of these bacteria in the gut results in production of endotoxin that causes the disease. Passage of orally ingested bacteria to the gut would be facilitated by the lack of acidity in the abomasum of newborn lambs; rapid multiplication within the gut would be enhanced by depressed gut motility, which is characteristic in the first 48 hr of life. Furthermore *E coli* are commonly recovered from field cases. Other bacteria may be involved. Despite the apparent bacterial etiology, there is no evidence of contagion. The condition is most common in twins and triplets, in lambs out of ewes in poor condition, and in lambs from either very young or very old ewes. Ingestion of adequate colostrum (50 mL/ kg) in the first hour of life considerably reduces susceptibility.

Clinical Findings and Pathogenesis: Early signs include dullness, a loss of sucking drive, lacrimation, and excessive salivation (watery mouth). Within a few hours the abomasum becomes distended with gas, and gut motility is depressed or absent. Increased pressure within the abdomen may embarrass breathing. Bacteremia develops. If untreated, death follows within 12-24 hr due to hypoglycemia, hypothermia, and toxemia.

Lesions: In the early stages, there is patchy inflammation of the small or large intestines, or both. In fatal cases, the abomasum is enlarged and may contain copious amounts of fluid, the intestines are inflamed, there are signs of toxemia, and fat reserves are exhausted.

Diagnosis: A confident diagnosis can be made only by clinical examination of the lamb in the early stages before the secondary effects of starvation, toxemia, and abdominal tympany supervene. Differential diagnoses include primary starvation and infectious enteritis.

Treatment: Supportive treatment is essential. Parenteral antibiotics should be given daily. A minimum of 50 mL of an electrolyte and 10% glucose solution containing a water-soluble, oral antibiotic preparation (neomycin and/or streptomycin) should be fed by stomach tube t.i.d.; if the lamb is not sucking, the volume of each feeding should be increased to 100-200 mL. Treatment should be continued until the signs resolve and the lamb is sucking again.

Control: Good management practices are important. Ewes should be well nourished to ensure a plentiful supply of colostrum. Lambing pens should be kept clean to reduce bacterial contamination. Lambs should ingest adequate colostrum (50 mL/ kg) in the first hour of life, and should not be castrated with rubber rings in the first

24 hr, since this depresses colostrum intake. If these measures fail, antibiotics (oral or injectable) given in the first hour of life have been effective.

TRAUMATIC RETICULOPERITONITIS
(Traumatic gastritis, Hardware disease)

A disease of cattle resulting from perforation of the reticulum. It is important in the differential diagnosis of diseases marked by stasis of the GI tract because its signs are similar to those of other such diseases. It is most common in mature dairy cattle, occasionally observed in beef cattle, and rarely reported in other ruminants.

Cattle commonly have foreign objects in their stomach because they do not discriminate against hard materials in feed, and do not completely masticate feed before swallowing. The disease is common when greenchop, silage, and hay are made from fields that contain old rusting fences and baling wire, and when pastures are on such areas or sites where buildings have recently been constructed, burned, or torn down. The grain ration may also be a source due to accidental or felonious addition of metal.

Etiology: Swallowed metallic objects, such as nails or pieces of wire, fall directly into the reticulum or pass into the rumen, and are subsequently carried over the ruminoreticular fold into the cranioventral part of the reticulum by ruminal contractions. The reticulo-omasal orifice is elevated above the floor, which tends to retain heavy objects in the reticulum, and the honeycomb-like reticular mucosa traps sharp objects. Contractions of the reticulum promote penetration of the wall by the foreign object. Compression of the ruminoreticulum by the uterus in late pregnancy, straining during parturition, and mounting during estrus increase the likelihood of an initial penetration of the reticulum and may also disrupt adhesions caused by an earlier penetration.

Perforation of the wall of the reticulum allows leakage of ingesta and bacteria, which causes contamination of the peritoneal cavity. The resulting peritonitis is generally localized and frequently results in adhesions. Less commonly, a more severe peritonitis develops. Diffuse peritonitis is rare. The object can penetrate the diaphragm and enter the thoracic cavity (causing pleuritis and sometimes pneumonitis) and the pericardial sac (causing pericarditis, sometimes followed by myocarditis, endocarditis, and septicemia). Occasionally, other organs (liver, spleen) may be pierced and become infected.

Clinical Findings: The initial attack is characterized by sudden onset of ruminoreticular atony and a sharp fall in milk production. Fecal output is decreased. The rectal temperature is often mildly elevated, and the heart rate is normal or slightly increased. Respiration is usually shallow and rapid. Initially, the animal exhibits an arched back, an anxious expression, a reluctance to move, and an uneasy careful gait. Forced sudden movements and defecating, urinating, lying down, getting up, and stepping over barriers may be accompanied by groaning. A grunt may be elicited by applying pressure to the xiphoid, or by elevating this area firmly and then pinching the chine, which causes extension of the thorax and lower abdomen. The grunt can be detected by placing a stethoscope over the trachea. Tremor of the triceps and abduction of the elbow may be observed. In more chronic cases, feed intake and fecal output are reduced, and milk production remains low. Signs of cranial abdominal pain become less apparent, and the rectal temperature usually returns to normal as the acute inflammation subsides and peritoneal contamination is walled off. Some cattle develop chronic vagal indigestion, possibly due to the adhesions that form after foreign body perforation, particularly those on the ventromedial reticulum.

Animals with pleuritis or pericarditis due to foreign body perforation usually are depressed, and have tachycardia (>90 bpm) and pyrexia (104°F [40°C]). Pleuritis is manifest by fast shallow respiration, muffling of lung sounds, and possibly pleuritic friction rubs. Thoracentesis may yield several liters of fluid. Traumatic pericarditis usually is characterized by muffled heart sounds possibly with pericardial friction rubs, and occasionally by gas and fluid splashing sounds on auscultation. This has been described as a washing machine murmur. Jugular vein distention with a pronounced jugular pulse is present early in the course, and congestive heart failure with marked submandibular and brisket edema is a frequent sequela. Prognosis is grave with these complications. Penetration through the myocardium usually produces extensive hemorrhage into the pericardial sac and sudden death.

Diagnosis: This can be based on history (when available) and clinical findings if the animal is examined when signs initially appear. Without an accurate history and when the condition has been present for several days or longer, diagnosis is more difficult. Other causes of peritonitis, particularly perforated abomasal ulcers, can be difficult to distinguish from traumatic reticuloperitonitis. Differential diagnoses should include conditions that can produce variable or nonspecific GI signs, eg, indigestion, lymphosarcoma, or intestinal obstruction. Abomasal displacement or volvulus should be ruled out by simultaneous auscultation and percussion. Pleuritis or pericarditis of nontraumatic origin produces signs similar to those associated with foreign body perforation. Although not always necessary, laboratory tests may be helpful. In many cases, there is an increase in neutrophils with a left shift. Fibrinogen and, in chronic cases, total plasma protein concentrations may be high. The acid-base status and serum electrolyte levels are typically normal since abomasal and small-intestinal absorption can remain normal. However, marked hypokalemic, hypochloremic metabolic alkalosis can occur, presumably because adynamic ileus from peritonitis can affect abomasal and GI motility and resorption of abomasal secretions. The metabolic alkalosis can be created or exacerbated by treatment with alkalinizing agents such as magnesium hydroxide used as a laxative.

Peritoneal fluid analysis can be helpful in determining if peritonitis is present. However, the nucleated cell count and the protein level return to normal as the contamination is walled off.

Radiographs may detect metallic material in the reticulum. To determine whether perforation of the reticulum has occurred, the foreign body must be visible beyond the border of the reticulum, or an abscess must be identified. Portable radiographic units cannot penetrate the reticular area of standing adult cattle, and the cow may need to be transported to where there is equipment with sufficient power. The area can be radiographed using portable equipment if the systemic condition does not preclude placing the animal in dorsal recumbency. A perforating foreign body will remain in the ventral aspect of the reticulum and be surrounded by gas.

Electronic metal detectors will identify metal in the reticulum, but do not distinguish between perforating and nonperforating foreign bodies.

Ultrasonography of the heart and thorax is useful in the diagnosis of pleuritis and pericarditis.

Treatment: Treatment of the typical case seen early in its course may be surgical or medical. Either approach seems to improve the chances of recovery from ~60% in untreated cases to 80-90%. Surgery involves rumenotomy with manual removal of the object or objects, and if an abscess is adhered to the reticulum, it should be aspirated (to confirm that it is an abscess), and then drained into the reticulum. Antibiotics should be administered perioperatively. Medical treatment involves antibacterials to control the peritonitis, and administration of a magnet to prevent recurrence. Because of the mixed bacterial flora in the lesion, a broad-spectrum antimicrobial agent such as oxytetracycline (6.6-11 mg/kg) should be used. Penicillin (22,000 IU/kg, IM, b.i.d.) is used widely and is effective in many cases despite its limited spectrum. Affected animals should be confined for 1-2 wk, and placing them on an inclined plane with the front end elevated may limit further penetration of the foreign object. Supportive therapy, such as oral or occasionally IV fluids and subcut. calcium borogluconate, should be administered as needed. Rumen inoculation is beneficial in some cases with prolonged ruminal stasis and loss of normal flora. The use of flexible magnetic metal retrievers introduced orally or through an incision in the flank to aid in removal of the objects has been described.

More advanced cases, those with obvious secondary complications, or those that do not respond to initial medical or surgical therapy should be evaluated from an economic perspective: if the animal is of limited value, slaughter should be considered if the carcass is likely to pass inspection.

Prevention: Avoiding the use of baling wire, passing feed over magnets to remove metallic objects, keeping the animals away from sites of new construction, and completely removing old buildings and fences are preventive steps. Additionally, bar magnets may be administered PO, preferably after fasting for 18-24 hr. Usually the magnet remains in the reticulum and holds any ferromagnetic objects on its surface. There is good evidence that giving magnets to all herd replacement heifers and bulls at ~1 yr of age minimizes the incidence of traumatic reticuloperitonitis.

WINTER DYSENTERY
(Winter scours)

An acute, highly contagious disease of cattle characterized by a brief attack of severe diarrhea or dysentery and by high morbidity but low mortality. It can lead to dehydration, loss of weight and condition and, in lactating animals, a moderate to severe drop in milk production. The disease occurs in several countries but the reported incidence is higher in northern USA, Canada, and Europe.

Etiology and Epidemiology: Coronaviruses, closely related to the Nebraska calf diarrhea virus strain, have been detected in feces of cattle clinically ill with winter dysentery and appear to be causally associated with the disease.

In the Northern Hemisphere, the disease occurs from November through March. The incubation period is short, and usually the disease spreads rapidly within the herd; 100% of susceptible cattle may show illness within 4-5 days of the onset of the outbreak. All ages can be affected, but disease is more common and severe in adults, especially postparturient dairy cows. Outbreaks of winter dysentery may occur within an area or a community over a short period of time, and the disease does not generally recur for 3-4 yr.

Clinical Findings: In most outbreaks, several cows develop profuse watery diarrhea with a slightly fetid or musty odor the first day, and the remainder of the herd is involved rapidly. The diarrhea may be preceded by slight fever, nasolacrimal discharge, and a moist cough. The feces are dark brown to greenish black and often contain mucus and blood. Unless complications occur, the temperature is normal when clinical signs are apparent, as are the pulse and respiration rates. Appetite may be slightly depressed, but thirst is increased. Severely affected animals may show evidence of abdominal pain. Lactating cows have a moderate to severe decrease in milk production, and those that have recently calved are most affected. Full herd production may not be regained for several weeks to months after the outbreak. The course in individual animals is 3-4 days, and deaths are uncommon.

Lesions: The predominant lesion is catarrhal inflammation of the GI tract, primarily the jejunum and ileum, characterized by edematous intestinal walls, injected serosal blood vessels, and swollen and congested mucosa. Intestinal contents are dark and fluid and may contain mucus and blood. Peyer's patches and mesenteric lymph nodes may be swollen and edematous. Microscopically, there is focal necrosis and degeneration of crypt epithelium in the colon.

Diagnosis: The seasonal incidence of the disease, the age and number of animals affected, and the acute onset are helpful in diagnosis. Bovine viral diarrhea, coccidiosis, other parasitoses, salmonellosis, rinderpest, dietary changes, and toxic agents should be considered in the differential diagnosis.

Prophylaxis and Treatment: Newly introduced animals should be kept in isolation for 2 wk. Any animal suffering from acute diarrhea, regardless of cause, should be separated from the main herd until recovered. Access to the premises should be restricted, and all persons having contact with the cattle should always make sure of the cleanliness of their footwear, clothing, and equipment. No specific vaccine is available.

Most cattle with winter dysentery do not require treatment since they recover spontaneously within a few days. Severely affected animals can be given oral astringents along with fluid and electrolyte therapy.

COLITIS

A common, acute or chronic cause of diarrhea in dogs and cats, characterized by colonic inflammation.

Etiology and Pathogenesis: Acute colitis may occur following ingestion of garbage or other irritating foreign material. Chronic large-bowel diarrhea may result from: inflammatory diseases of the large intestine (lymphocytic-plasmacytic, histiocytic ulcerative, eosinophilic, granulomatous, suppurative), or parasitic (*Trichuris*, *Giardia*, *Ancylostoma*, *Uncinaria*, *Entamoeba histolytica*, *Balantidium coli*), infectious (*Histoplasma capsulatum*, *Salmonella*, *Campylobacter*, *Yersinia enterocolitica*, *Prototheca*, *Clostridium difficile*), noninflammatory (irritable bowel syndrome, cecal inversion, ileocolic intussusception, secondary to small bowel malassimilatory disorders), or neoplastic (polyp, leiomyoma, adenocarcinoma, lymphosarcoma, leiomyosarcoma, plasmacytoma, mast cell tumor) conditions. Chronic diarrhea may also accompany metabolic disorders such as uremia, hypoadrenocorticism, hypothyroidism, and recurrent pancreatitis.

Colitis results in altered colonic motility, decreased absorption of water and electrolytes, and excess secretions. Loss of normal rhythmic segmentation contractions allows the normal peristalsis to move feces more rapidly aborally. Heightened sensitivity to the defecation reflex results in increased frequency of defecation. Tenesmus results from a direct stimulation of the defecation reflex by the inflammatory process. Impaired sodium and water absorption results in increased fecal volume. Mucosal irritation stimulates mucus secretion. Denudation of the superficial epithelium can cause ulceration and hemorrhage and result in fresh blood in the feces.

Clinical Findings: Signs of acute colitis are a sudden onset of severe, watery, sometimes bloody, mucoid diarrhea, and occasional vomiting. The animal may be depressed, dehydrated, and febrile with abdominal pain. Rectal examination may reveal bloody feces and foreign material, eg, bone, plastic, wood, or aluminum foil.

Animals with chronic colitis defecate more frequently, but pass small volumes of feces each time. Defecation is often associated with a sense of urgency, and tenesmus may be present. The feces may be semi-formed to liquid; fresh blood and mucus may be present. Weight loss, vomiting, lethargy, and anorexia are infrequent. Physical examination is usually unremarkable except for weight loss in severe cases. Abdominal palpation may reveal an abdominal mass, sublumbar lymphadenopathy, or colonic thickening. Rectal examination may reveal the character of the feces, rough and corrugated rectal mucosa, or a rectal mass or stricture.

Diagnosis: The signs are indicative of colitis (*see also* EXAMINATION OF THE GI TRACT, p 95). Routine laboratory tests may rule out other causes of chronic diarrhea, eg, noninflammatory colonic diseases. Repeated fecal flotation and direct saline smears may be necessary to identify or rule out parasitic causes; feces should be cultured for bacterial pathogens. Proctoscopy, usually performed following a 24-48 hr fast, or endoscopy is valuable. Enemas with warm water or an oral GI lavage solution that contains polyethylene glycol should be given before examination. Sedation or general anesthesia is usually desirable. The normal colonic mucosa is easily distended with air, smooth, glistening, pale pink, and has visible submucosal vessels. Animals with colonic disease display increased mucosal granularity, and no submucosal vessels can be seen. The mucosa may be excessively friable and bleed after contact with the endoscope. The colonic wall may be less distensible than normal. Erosions, ulcers, hemorrhage, parasites, strictures, tumors, and excess mucus may be observed. A mucosal biopsy is necessary for a definitive diagnosis. A barium enema may be useful when cecocolic or ileocolic intussusception, stricture, or neoplasia is suspected.

Treatment: If possible, treatment should be directed at the primary causes. Acute nonspecific colitis should be treated symptomatically with fluids and parenteral antibiotics. Antispasmodics (propantheline, diphenoxylate, imodium, codeine) may be given if tenesmus or abdominal pain are present. The animal should be fasted for 24-48 hr to rest the gut.

Dietary management is one of the most important steps in treatment of chronic colitis. Small, multiple meals of a bland hypoallergenic diet, eg, rice mixed with cottage cheese or lamb, or a commercial hypoallergenic diet, are fed initially. When a dietary allergy is suspected, an elimination diet may be necessary to determine the offending antigen. Animals that respond well to the hypoallergenic diet may eventually be switched back to a regular commercial diet. For animals that exhibit a partial response to dietary management, fiber can be added to the diet as plain bran or psyllium.

Antimicrobials useful for chronic colitis include sulfasalazine, tylosin, and metronidazole. Motility modifiers may be useful during acute exacerbations of the diarrhea and when the condition is thought to be stress-related (eg, irritable bowel syndrome). Motility modifiers include the anticholinergic drugs (propantheline bromide, isopropamide/prochlorperazine), narcotic analgesics (tincture of opium, paregoric, codeine, loperamide, diphenoxylate), and combinations of CNS depressants and antispasmodics (chlordiazepoxide/clidinium, isopropamide/prochlorperazine). Immunosuppressive drugs such as prednisone, or azathioprine may be useful in animals refractory to other medical therapies.

CONSTIPATION/OBSTIPATION

Constipation is a condition in which bowel movements are infrequent or absent: the feces are excessively hard or dry, and there is a reduced fecal volume and tenesmus. Obstipation is a state of intractable constipation in which defecation has become impossible. Uncorrected obstipation may lead to megacolon, a condition of extreme dilatation of the colon with fecal impaction.

Etiology: Either condition may result from ingestion of bones, foreign material, or hair; disruption of normal defecation patterns due to a change in the environment; painful anorectal lesions (anal sacculitis, rectal strictures, perianal fistulas, rectal tumors); intraluminal or extraluminal obstruction (foreign body, perineal hernia, rectal diverticulum, pelvic fracture, prostatic enlargement, pseudocoprostasis, or a colonic, rectal, anal, pelvic, or prostatic tumor); neurogenic disease (spinal cord disease, congenital neuromuscular dysfunction); metabolic and endocrine disease (hypothyroidism, hyperparathyroidism, hypokalemia); drug-induced (anticholinergics, barium sulfate, diuretics, opiates); and congenital anomalies (imperforate anus).

Clinical Findings: Tenesmus, usually preceding defecation, is noted in chronic constipation. Hard, brittle feces occasionally streaked with blood may be passed. Soft feces of a narrow diameter ("ribbon-like") are suggestive of a constrictive lesion. If constipation persists, the animal becomes depressed, inappetant, weak, dehydrated, and may vomit occasionally. Watery, brown, putrid feces may be passed as fluid passes around the hardened fecal mass. Abdominal palpation reveals hard feces in the colon. A grossly enlarged colon impacted with feces may be diagnostic for megacolon. Digital examination of the rectum is resented.

Diagnosis: A history of difficult, painful, or infrequent passage of feces, and palpation of the impacted fecal mass in the colon is pathognomonic. Plain abdominal radiographs reveal a distended colon. Because of the technical difficulty of performing a barium enema, proctoscopy/endoscopy of the colon is preferred to visualize obstructive masses or strictures. Exploratory celiotomy may be necessary for accurate evaluation.

Treatment and Control: For simple constipation, an enema (warm water or saline), small quantities of lubricant or surfactant (mineral oil, dioctyl sodium sulfosuccinate [DSS]) given PO, or suppositories (bisacodyl, DSS) are effective. In severely constipated animals, fluid and electrolyte balance should be restored by IV administration of a balanced solution. Treatment can then proceed with oral laxatives (bisacodyl), surfactants (DSS), and enemas, and/or manual removal of the impacted fecal material under general anesthesia. Surfactant laxatives such as DSS may also be added to the enema fluid. Gentle breaking of the mass by hand or, in more severe cases, judicious manipulation with forceps may be required. Daily removal of portions of a stubborn impaction will allow medical treatment between manipulations. Surgery may be necessary for conditions refractory to enemas and mechanical breakdown. Sodium phosphate retention enemas should not be used in small dogs with moderate to severe constipation, or in cats; they have been associated with hyperphosphatemia, hypernatremia, hypocalcemia, and death. Successful long-term treatment requires identification and removal or amelioration of the underlying cause. Long-term management includes dietary manipulation and medication. Psyllium or bran can be mixed with food. Surfactant laxatives (eg, DSS) or lubricants (eg, mineral oil) or more palatable commercial petrolatum-vitamin preparations are helpful when administered routinely.

Persistent impaction in cats can lead to megacolon; subtotal or total colectomy may be required.

CORONAVIRAL GASTROENTERITIS

A highly contagious GI disease of dogs of any age, characterized by vomiting and diarrhea. Clinical signs are less severe in adults than in the young. Only dogs, coyotes, and foxes are known to develop the disease; however, the virus replicates in cats, and probably additional carnivores are susceptible. The disease has been reported from Europe, North America, and Australia. It probably occurs worldwide.

Etiology, Transmission, and Pathogenesis: Canine coronavirus (CCV) is an enveloped, single-stranded RNA virus antigenically related to the feline coronaviruses (feline infectious peritonitis virus and feline enteric coronavirus) and to transmissible gastroenteritis virus of pigs. It is sensitive to lipid solvents and most disinfectants.

Ingestion of fecal material from infected animals is the main route of infection. After ingestion, the virus infects epithelial cells of the villi in the small intestine. Viremia and infection of other visceral organs have not been reported. Some asymptomatic carrier dogs may shed virus for extended periods.

Clinical Findings: Generally, the signs are milder than those of canine parvoviral (CPV) infection (qv, p 249), but anorexia, diarrhea, vomiting, fever, and depression, often of sudden onset, can occur. The feces are liquid or loose and may contain blood and mucus and often have a particularly fetid odor. Dehydration may be severe. The WBC count is normal. Experimental infections by CCV cause only mild disease; the incubation period is 24-36 hr. Dual infections with CCV and CPV are likely to be severe.

Lesions: Lesions in experimental infections usually are not severe, consisting of dilated loops of intestine filled with watery, green-yellow material. Naturally occurring cases, especially those with mixed infections, can have severe lesions with frank hemorrhage in the intestinal mucosa and enlarged, congested mesenteric lymph nodes.

Diagnosis: A history of a contagious gastroenteritis in a kennel suggests viral enteritis. Although isolation confirms the diagnosis, CCV is generally difficult to culture *in vitro*. Therefore, observation of coronavirus structures in fresh (not frozen) feces or intestinal contents by electron microscopy is the primary method of diagnosis. Histopathology on sections of fresh small intestine may reveal atrophy and fusion of intestinal villi and deepening of crypts, increase in cellularity of the lamina propria, and flattening of epithelial cells.

Treatment and Control: There is no specific treatment, but supportive fluid therapy and antibiotic treatment as described for canine hemorrhagic gastroenteritis or canine parvoviral infection should be used. Vaccines are available. Prevention should focus on avoiding contact with infected animals and their excretions, improving sanitation, and vaccinating high-risk dogs, eg, kennel and show dogs.

DISEASES OF THE ESOPHAGUS, SM AN

CRICOPHARYNGEAL ACHALASIA

A disease of unknown cause characterized by inadequate relaxation of the cricopharyngeal muscle, which leads to relative inability of the animal to swallow food or liquids. It occurs primarily in puppies and occasionally in middle-aged dogs. Repeated attempts to swallow are followed by gagging and regurgitation; aspiration pneumonia is a common complication. An accurate diagnosis requires fluoroscopic evaluation of swallowing after oral administration of contrast material (alone or mixed with food). Abnormal function (lack of relaxation) of the cricopharyngeal muscle results in retention of barium in the posterior pharyngeal region.

Treatment consists of cricopharyngeal myotomy; normal swallowing occurs immediately after surgery. Aspiration pneumonia, if present, should be treated aggressively with a systemic antibiotic, based on culture and sensitivity if possible.

DILATATION OF THE ESOPHAGUS
(Megaesophagus)

Esophageal dilatation in young animals may be the result of a vascular ring anomaly or due to an unknown cause. Idiopathic megaesophagus may also occur in adult dogs, and the esophagus may dilate secondary to systemic diseases such as myasthenia gravis, systemic lupus erythematosus, polymyositis, distemper, hypoadrenocorticism, heavy metal toxicity, hypothyroidism, CNS neoplasia, or trauma. Esophageal dilatation has been produced experimentally by chronic administration of cholinesterase inhibitors; it may also occur anterior to an esophageal stricture, neoplasia, or extraesophageal compression.

The cardinal sign is regurgitation. A puppy with congenital megaesophagus characteristically begins to regurgitate when it begins to eat solid food. Initially, regurgitation occurs soon after swallowing; as the condition progresses, the esophagus enlarges and food is retained longer. Affected pups are generally unthrifty and smaller than their littermates. Pressure applied to the abdomen may cause ballooning of the esophagus at the thoracic inlet. Aspiration pneumonia is a common complication, and the associated signs are fever, cough, and nasal discharge. Adults with megaesophagus regurgitate and, generally, have lost weight. Respiratory signs may predominate, with little or no history of regurgitation. Thoracic radiographs reveal air, fluid, or food in a dilated esophagus. The thoracic esophagus is usually uniformly dilated, and a large ventral deviation may be present anterior to the heart. The cervical esophagus may also be dilated. Strictures, foreign bodies, or a vascular ring anomaly should be ruled out with an esophagogram or esophagoscopy.

In adult dogs, associated diseases (eg, myasthenia gravis) should be treated. Surgery is indicated for a vascular ring anomaly. Medical managment is indicated for congenital or acquired idiopathic megaesophagus. The consistency of the diet that best prevents regurgitation varies from dog to dog; a soft gruel works well in many, but dry food works better for some. A feeding schedule of frequent small meals is preferred. Feeding from an elevated dish (which requires the dog to eat with forelimbs higher than hind) or holding the dog in an upright position for 10-15 min after eating allows gravity to assist food passage into the stomach. Surgery at the gastroesophageal junction generally does not improve the signs of idiopathic megaesophagus; the overall prognosis is poor, and many die from aspiration pneumonia.

ESOPHAGEAL STENOSIS
(Esophageal stricture)

A pathological narrowing of the lumen may occur after trauma, esophagitis, surgery, or tumor invasion. Most strictures occur at the thoracic inlet. Esophageal tumors are rare, but the association of esophageal sarcoma and *Spirocerca lupi* infection (qv, p 237) requires consideration in areas where this parasite is prevalent.

Clinical signs are similar to those associated with foreign bodies. Contrast radiography may show dilatation of the esophagus anterior to the stricture. An esophagogram is important for evaluating the number of strictures, and their length and location.

Treatment with balloon catheter dilation has been successful; bougienage is another available technique but is more traumatic. Surgical resection, although not always successful, may be necessary. Any treatment is likely to induce some degree of esophagitis, which must be treated to decrease the chance of the stricture reforming.

ESOPHAGITIS

Inflammation of the esophagus, a more frequent problem in dogs than cats, is usually caused by gastric reflux. Gastric reflux esophagitis is associated with anesthesia, drugs that decrease lower esophageal sphincter tone (eg, atropine, acepromazine), and acute or chronic vomiting. Other causes include trauma due to ingestion or lodging of foreign bodies, ingestion of irritating or caustic substances, or complications of megaesophagus. Cardioplasty, irritation caused by instruments or pharyngostomy tubes, neoplasms, and *Spirocerca lupi* infection (qv, p 237) may also cause esophagitis. Calicivirus in cats rarely causes esophagitis.

Regurgitation is the classical sign of esophageal disease; however, mild esophagitis may have no associated clinical signs. Moderate to severe esophagitis may be painful, and result in depression and anorexia. Other signs are dysphagia, excess salivation, repeated swallowing attempts, and extension of the head and neck.

Endoscopy allows visualization of esophageal foreign bodies and direct assessment of esophageal damage. Plain radiographs and esophagograms are of little or no benefit in diagnosing esophagitis. Fluoroscopy may be used to identify decreased motility secondary to esophageal inflammation. Histopathological evaluation of a punch biopsy will confirm the clinical diagnosis, and is essential in the rare cases that have no grossly visible pathology.

Mild esophagitis usually requires no treatment. If clinical signs are present, medical therapy should be initiated. H_2-receptor blockers (eg, cimetidine, ranitidine) decrease gastric acid production. Metoclopramide increases lower esophageal sphincter tone and esophageal contractions.

Soft food, low in fat, should be fed 3-4 times daily. If esophagitis is severe, a gastrostomy tube may be used to rest the esophagus. In severe esophagitis, administration of glucocorticoids for 2-3 wk may decrease the chance of stricture formation. A broad-spectrum antibiotic is usually given to prevent bacterial complications.

FOREIGN BODIES IN THE ESOPHAGUS

Esophageal foreign bodies are more common in dogs than cats. Bones are the most common, but needles, fishhooks, wood, metal objects, etc, may be found. Usually such an object lodges at the thoracic inlet, base of the heart, or in the caudal esophagus just above the diaphragm; occasionally it may lodge at the upper esophageal sphincter.

Salivation, gagging, and dysphagia are signs of cervical foreign bodies. A complete obstruction causes regurgitation after food or water intake; partial obstruction permits the passage of liquids and possibly soft foods. The signs depend on the location and composition of the foreign body, and the degree and duration of esophageal obstruction. Anorexia and weight loss may be predominant signs in chronic obstruction.

Perforation of the cervical esophagus may result in local abscessation or, in the thoracic portion, pleuritis, mediastinitis, pyothorax, pneumothorax, or bronchoesophageal fistula. Esophagitis, mucosal laceration, esophageal stricture, and esophageal diverticulum are other potential secondary problems. Aspiration pneumonia can be a serious complication of regurgitation. Many esophageal foreign bodies are radiopaque, but a contrast esophagogram may be required to evaluate mucosal tears or radiolucent foreign bodies. If a perforation is suspected, an aqueous iodinated contrast medium should be used instead of barium sulfate suspensions. Esophagoscopy permits direct examination of both the foreign body and the esophageal wall. Cervical esophageal bodies occasionally can be localized by external palpation.

When possible, the object should be removed *per os* with either a flexible endoscope and forceps, or a rigid scope and alligator forceps. In small to medium dogs and cats, a rigid proctoscope may be used; in large dogs, a rigid esophagoscope. Care should be taken to avoid lacerating or perforating the esophagus. If the foreign body is smooth, a Foley urethral catheter can be inserted and distended aboral to the foreign body, then removed orally, bringing the foreign body with it.

If a foreign body cannot be removed *per os*, it may be pushed into the stomach where it can be digested (eg, smooth bones), passed, or removed via a gastrotomy. When an object is embedded in the esophagus or has a sharp point, if the first 2 methods are unsuccessful, if the esophagus is necrotic or perforated, or if it is unlikely that the foreign body can be moved without lacerating or perforating the esophagus, surgery is indicated; however, the prognosis is poor.

Esophagitis should be managed medically following removal of the foreign body (*see* ESOPHAGITIS, above). Antibiotics and, if thoracic involvement is significant, chest drains should be used.

ENTERITIS

An acute or chronic inflammation of the small intestine. Enteritis can exist as an isolated disease involving only the small intestine, or more commonly as part of a more generalized process involving the stomach or colon.

Etiology: Acute enteritis is caused by a variety of disorders, including dietary indiscretion or intolerance to specific foods (eg, gluten), intestinal parasites, infectious agents (viral, bacterial, fungal), drugs, and toxins. In general, enteritis caused by parasites, medications, or ingestion of decaying or contaminated foods tends to be mild and self-limiting; infectious diseases are more severe and life-threatening. Specific causes of chronic enteritis are less defined; recognized syndromes include lymphocytic-plasmacytic enteritis, eosinophilic enteritis, villous atrophy, wheat-sensitive enteropathy, immunoproliferative enteropathy of Basenjis, small intestinal bacterial overgrowth, lymphangiectasia, and lymphosarcoma. These disorders frequently cause intestinal malabsorption (*see* p 141 *et seq*).

Enteritis is frequently caused by intestinal parasites, especially with *Ancylostoma caninum, Giardia canis,* and coccidia. Viral infections are important causes of acute, severe or fatal enteritis in dogs and cats. Canine enteric viruses include parvo-, corona-, rota-, astro-, and distemper virus. Feline parvo- (panleukopenia), corona-, and rotavirus as well as feline infectious peritonitis, feline leukemia virus, and feline immunodeficiency virus can cause severe enteritis. Bacteria are not frequently diagnosed as the primary cause of enteritis in dogs and cats. Bacterial pathogens that can cause enteric disease either by invading the enterocytes or by producing toxins are enteropathogenic *Escherichia coli, Salmonella, Yersinia, Campylobacter, Clostridium perfringens, Bacillus piliformis,* and *Mycobacterium.* Of particular importance are *Salmonella, Campylobacter,* and *Yersinia,* which are significant human pathogens. Mycotic pathogens include *Histoplasma capsulatum* and rarely *Aspergillus* spp, *Pythium* spp, and *Candida albicans.* Rickettsial infection with *Neorickettsia helminthoeca* or *N elokominica* causes severe and frequently fatal enteritis in dogs that have ingested raw salmon that harbor the fluke vector; the Pacific Northwest is an endemic area. Several drugs including antibiotics, nonsteroidal anti-inflammatories, antineoplastics, and insecticides and toxins such as heavy metals, herbicides, and fungicides can cause enteric disease.

Clinical Findings: Acute watery diarrhea is the most common clinical sign. Inappetence, lethargy, and vomiting occur in most, especially if the proximal intestine and stomach are involved. Tenesmus, frequency, and mucoid feces are characteristic of large-intestinal involvement. Dark green to black feces occur from upper GI bleeding, whereas hemorrhage from the large intestine results in feces streaked with fresh blood. Fever, abdominal distention and pain, pale mucous membranes, and dehydration indicate serious disease. The severity and duration of clinical signs varies with etiology and with the animal's age; in general, immature animals have more severe clinical signs. Chronic disease may have no signs other than recurrent diarrhea and weight loss.

Diagnosis: Presumptive diagnosis is readily made from the history, clinical signs, and physical examination; establishing the cause may require extensive laboratory work. The history should review vaccination status, medications, diet, and environment. Fecal examination of direct saline smears, and flotations and sedimentation (for ova, larvae, cysts, and trophozoites) should be accompanied by visible inspection for tapeworms and foreign material. Animals with severe hemorrhagic diarrhea accompanied by systemic signs of fever, dehydration, weakness, lethargy, or abdominal pain warrant an expanded data base. A complete blood count, biochemical profile, electrolytes, and urinalysis should be done. Plain abdominal radiographs should be taken; contrast studies are indicated if a mechanical or obstructive lesion is suspected. Virologic tests should be considered, as well as fecal cultures for *Salmonella* and *Campylobacter*; selective culture techniques are necessary.

Treatment: All food should be withheld for ≥24 hr after onset. Dehydration and electrolyte imbalance should be treated by parenteral administration of fluids. The type of fluid depends on the severity of vomiting that has occurred relative to that of the diarrhea. If vomiting is predominant, a hypochloremic alkalosis tends to develop; 0.9% saline (NaCl) solution should be used to replace deficits. If diarrhea predominates, metabolic acidosis is more common; lactated Ringer's solution is recommended. Fluids should be supplemented with potassium salts, provided renal function is adequate. In general, 20 mEq of potassium salt added to 1 L of fluid provides a solution that can safely be given parenterally based on a total fluid volume of 40 mL/kg/day. The rate of IV potassium supplementation should not exceed 0.5 mEq/kg/hr, and serum potassium should be closely monitored. Dextrose may be added to the IV fluids to make a 2½% solution to treat hypoglycemia, which frequently is seen in parvovirus enteritis and septicemia.

In general, antiemetics should be used symptomatically in situations in which the underlying disorder has been diagnosed or when vomiting is so profuse that fluid, electrolyte, and acid-base balance are difficult to control. Indiscriminate use of these drugs may mask the primary disease and delay diagnosis. The centrally acting phenothiazines (chlorpromazine or prochlorperazine) are most effective. These drugs are hypotensive; they should not be used until dehydration is corrected. Metoclopramide has central antiemetic effects as well as having a prokinetic effect on the distal esophagus, stomach, and proximal small intestine. It is most useful to control vomiting caused by acute viral enteritis and by chemotherapy. Antiemetic therapy should be limited to 24-36 hr.

Narcotic analgesics are most effective for symptomatic control of diarrhea. Paregoric, diphenoxylate, and loperamide relieve abdominal pain and cramping in addition to decreasing the frequency and volume of diarrhea. Their use should be limited to 48 hr. These motility-modifying drugs are contraindicated with infectious diarrheas. Preparations containing bismuth subsalicylate decrease fecal water loss and have antimicrobial and anti-inflammatory actions in the gut. Use is recommended in acute enteritis, especially when bacterial infection is suspected. Bismuth compounds will turn the feces dark brown to black, which could be misinterpreted as melena.

Antibiotics should be used in animals with hemorrhagic diarrhea (hemorrhagic gastroenteritis, parvovirus) and in cases of enterocolitis with systemic involvement (fever, congested mucous membranes, leukocytosis, or leukopenia). Aggressive treatment with parenteral antibiotics effective against gram-positive anaerobes and gram-negative bacteria is recommended. A combination of ampicillin with an aminoglycoside is effective and safe, providing that hydration and renal function are adequate. Therapy for specific infections should be based on culture-sensitivity results. In general, *Salmonella* is susceptible to trimethoprim-sulfa, cephalothin, and chloramphenicol; *Campylobacter* to erythromycin, furazolidone, chloramphenicol, and aminoglycosides; *Yersinia* to trimethoprim-sulfa, tetracycline, chloramphenicol, and aminoglycosides. Metronidazole and quinacrine are effective against *Giardia* sp. Metronidazole is also effective against anaerobes and may be useful in some cases of nonspecific inflammatory bowel disease. Sulfasalazine is specifically indicated for ulcerative and granulomatous colitis.

Once vomiting has ceased, a bland diet of soups, broths, baby food, rice, softboiled eggs, cottage cheese, and small portions of lean meat can be started. The animal should gradually be weaned back to a normal diet.

Enteritis that accompanies infectious diseases or uremia is managed by treating the primary disease in addition to the above treatments. The outcome of poisoning with heavy metals may be favorable if an early diagnosis has been made and treatment with a specific antidote is instituted. Parenteral fluid therapy and antidiarrheic drugs should be used.

GASTRIC DILATATION-VOLVULUS
(GDV, Gastric torsion, Bloat)

Dilatation of the stomach caused by aerophagia, food, GI secretions, and gas from fermentation. Distention occurs as simple dilatation or, more commonly, as dilatation with volvulus. GDV is a life-threatening emergency that begins as a mechanical alteration of normal anatomy and progresses to a severe metabolic disease. GDV has been identified primarily in large and giant breed dogs (deep chested), but has been reported in smaller breeds such as the Dachshund, and in other species.

Etiology and Pathogenesis: GDV has been associated with many possible causes. In dogs, these include anatomy (large, deep-chested dogs with pendulous stomachs that are subject to chronic stretching of the hepatogastric and hepatoduodenal ligaments), paraprandial exercise, and hereditary predisposition. Additional factors associated with GDV are cereal- versus meat-based diets, pyloric dysfunction, and elevated serum gastrin levels. It is unclear whether the primary abnormality is gastric dilatation as a result of gastric retention, or gastric volvulus as a result of gastric ligamentous laxity. In at least some cases, volvulus is present before dilatation.

Ingestion of food and water, and aerophagia initiate gastric dilatation. Vigorous exercise or altered body position appears to escalate the process. Gastric volvulus prevents effective vomiting, but still allows air to be swallowed (and an orogastric tube to be passed). The pylorus is also obstructed. Gastric dilatation leads to increased intra-abdominal pressure, which significantly reduces caudal vena caval and portal venous blood flow. Cardiac output diminishes because of decreased venous return. As the dilatation and volvulus progress, gastric arterial blood flow may be compromised. Stasis of blood and tissue hypoxia result in sequestration of fluid and endotoxin accumulation in the splanchnic organs. Arterial hypotension causes decreased coronary blood flow, and myocardial hypoxia. Hence, cardiogenic, hypovolemic, and endotoxic forms of shock all contribute to the physiologic derangements seen in GDV. Additional complications include production of myocardial depressant factor from the hypoxic pancreas, hypoxemia due to reduced diaphragmatic excursion (hypoventilation) and altered pulmonary gas exchange, multiple acid-base abnormalities, and disseminated intravascular coagulation (DIC).

Clinical Findings and Diagnosis: History is variable. Simple gastric dilatation may have occurred previously. Simple acute gastric dilatation cannot be differentiated from dilatation with volvulus by physical examination alone. Acute onset of restlessness, abdominal discomfort, localized epigastric pain, retching, and excessive ptyalism are reported frequently. The cranial abdomen is markedly distended and tympanic on percussion. Passage of an orogastric tube does not rule out volvulus. Radiography demonstrates a large, gas-filled stomach. The right lateral recumbent view often shows displacement of the gas-filled pylorus dorsocranial to and to the left of the fundus. Barium may also be used to evaluate the position of the stomach. Splenomegaly and gas distention of the small intestine may be seen. Gastric volvulus may also be identified at laparotomy. As the condition worsens, shock and marked depression develop. Dyspnea and tachypnea are common. Chronic forms of gastric dilatation and gastric volvulus do occur.

Lesions: The stomach is large and atonic. Gastric volvulus usually occurs in a clockwise pattern when viewed caudal to cranial. Engorgement and discoloration of the splanchnic organs is common. The gastric wall along the left greater curvature is often compromised, varying from hyperemic to blackened. Gastric mucosal injury is often severe. Distention and gastric wall necrosis occasionally result in gastric perforation and peritonitis.

Treatment: Emergency treatment is required. Gastric decompression is accomplished preferably by passage of an orogastric tube of appropriate diameter. Elevation of the cranial end of the dog and gentle manipulation of the tube and animal may facilitate passage. If this fails, decompression can be performed with a 16-18 gauge, 1.5 in. (3.8 cm) needle via the right paracostal area, after which the stomach tube can often be passed. Warm water gastric lavage to remove stomach contents may be performed. Sedation usually is not required, but if needed, demerol or oxymorphone is recommended. Preparations for emergency endotracheal intubation should be in place before sedation is effected. Temporary gastrostomy can be performed if necessary via the right paracostal area with a local "L" block using lidocaine. Decompression can be maintained by gastrostomy or pharyngostomy tubes, until surgery can be performed.

Shock should be assessed and treated quickly. One or 2 large-gauge IV catheters and a urinary catheter should be placed, and fluid therapy with an isosmotic polyionic fluid begun at initial volumes of 70-90 mL/kg body wt. Urine and blood samples should be obtained for data base, electrolytes, and acid-base status. A water-soluble and rapid-acting corticosteroid (prednisolone sodium succinate, 30 mg/kg; or dexamethasone sodium phosphate, 2 mg/kg) should be given IV, as well as ampicillin or sodium penicillin G. Sodium bicarbonate is not currently recommended without blood-gas and acid-base analyses: numerous counterbalancing acid-base abnormalities often leave the animal with a normal pH, and possible overcorrection and hyperosmolality from use of sodium bicarbonate can cause decompensation. Pulse, ECG, PCV, total protein, and urine production must be monitored throughout treatment.

Laparotomy is required to correct gastric volvulus. Gastropexy to the right abdominal wall is always indicated following GDV. Without fixation of the stomach, the recurrence rate is 60-80%; with surgery, the recurrence rate is 2-4%. Splanchnic ischemic necrosis (usually gastric) and endotoxemia appear to be the largest determinants of survival after treatment is initiated. The need for partial gastrectomy due to ischemic necrosis is associated with increased severity and higher mortality. Splenectomy is indicated only if splenic thrombosis or infarction is present.

Postoperative management is critical. Irreversible shock, cardiac arrhythmia, DIC, acute renal failure, and surgical complications are common. Cardiac dysrhythmias include paroxysmal ventricular tachycardia, premature ventricular contractions, and atrial fibrillation. Use of lidocaine at 1-2 mg/kg, IV bolus and then 60-100 μg/kg/min, IV constant rate infusion is recommended when ventricular tachyarrhythmias are >150 beats/min or are multiformed. Concurrent or subsequent use of quinidine or procainamide may be useful. Quinidine may also be useful in converting atrial fibrillation. Monitoring should be continued ≥72 hr. Cimetidine (10 mg/kg, IM, b.i.d. to t.i.d.) may decrease production of gastric hydrochloric acid, and thereby lessen gastric mucosal injury and metabolic acidosis. Metoclopramide (0.2-0.4 mg/kg, subcut., t.i.d.) may be used to enchance gastric emptying and accelerate the return of gastric motility. Management of DIC is controversial; however, whole blood transfusion and low-dose heparin therapy (loading dose 100 u/kg, maintenance dose 20 u/kg, subcut., q.i.d.) are often recommended.

Currently suggested methods that may prevent or reduce the recurrence of GDV in susceptible dogs include: feed 2-3 smaller meals each day, observe for early signs of GDV, avoid vigorous exercise 1 hr preprandial and 2 hr postprandial, and avoid abrupt dietary changes.

GASTRITIS

A low-grade inflammation with shallow erosions of the gastric mucosa caused by overeating, ingestion of spoiled food or indigestible material (eg, bones, hair, paper, toys), administration of irritant drugs (eg, aspirin), or as a sequela of gastric torsion. Gastritis is also associated with infectious diseases (eg, distemper, viral hepatitis, leptospirosis, and pyelonephritis), chronic renal failure, acute pancreatitis, and GI parasites. Ingestion of caustics, arsenic, mercury, lead, thallium, or phenol may produce acute corrosive gastritis.

Subacute gastritis occurs when acute gastritis has been improperly treated or when ingestion of irritant materials is continuous. Chronic vomiting may be present in gastric neoplasia, hypertrophic gastritis, or infiltrative gastritis.

Clinical Findings: Vomiting, depression, and abdominal pain are the cardinal signs. Animals may exhibit excessive thirst, but vomit shortly after ingestion of water. If mucosal damage is extensive, vomiting may be repetitive regardless of food intake. If corrosive agents have caused the gastritis, the vomitus may contain blood and shreds of gastric mucosa. Animals may refuse food or exhibit a depraved appetite (licking concrete, chewing dirt). Pain may cause restlessness, and the animal may object to palpation of the anterior abdomen. Animals may assume a crouched position or stretch out on a cool surface. When the gastritis is severe, there often is an accompanying enteritis. Subacute gastritis is manifest by continued vomiting and weight loss, dehydration, and electrolyte imbalance.

Diagnosis: In most cases of acute gastritis, diagnosis is based on history, clinical signs, and response to therapy. If signs persist, radiograms of the stomach may reveal foreign bodies or abnormalities in position or contour of the stomach. Because it is difficult to visualize ulcers and neoplasms on plain films, it may be necessary to distend the stomach with contrast media or use a double-contrast technique. Hypertrophy of the gastric rugae is not a constant radiographic finding. Endoscopy and histopathologic evaluation of mucosal biopsies provide the most reliable means of diagnosis.

Treatment: In acute gastritis, food should be withheld ≥24 hr. If the vomiting is persistent, water intake should be restricted by giving the animal only ice cubes to lick. If the gastritis is secondary to foreign bodies, gastric torsion, or a similar lesion, the underlying cause must be corrected. If fluid losses are significant, parenteral fluid therapy with a balanced electrolyte solution must be instituted to offset dehydration and electrolyte imbalance. Because prolonged vomiting may cause metabolic alkalosis, hypokalemia, and hypochloremia, appropriate laboratory evaluations should be employed in severe cases.

Meperidine may be used in corrosive gastritis to minimize pain. A centrally acting antiemetic (eg, chlorpromazine or prochlorperazine) may be required until specific therapy for the underlying condition becomes effective. If a poison has been ingested, an emetic (eg, apomorphine) should be administered soon after ingestion unless the substance swallowed is corrosive. For poisoning, the antidote should be administered immediately, or gastric or GI lavage may be employed to remove the irritant foreign material from the stomach.

After the first 24 hr, small amounts of water may be given, followed by broth, soup, or boiled milk. The following day, a bland diet (high carbohydrate, low fat) can be instituted, eg, pabulum and milk, oatmeal, grits, cooked rice, or milk puddings. This diet should be fed in small amounts 3-4 times daily and gradually modified to a normal diet.

GASTROINTESTINAL PARASITES, SM AN

SPIROCERCA LUPI INFECTION
(Esophageal worm)

Adult *Spirocerca lupi* are bright red worms 40 mm (male) to 70 mm (female) long, generally located within nodules in the esophageal, gastric, or aortic walls. Infections are encountered in southern areas of the USA as well as most tropical regions worldwide. Dogs are infected by eating an intermediate host (usually dung beetle) or a transport host (eg, chickens, reptiles, or rodents). The larvae migrate via the wall of the thoracic aorta, where they usually remain for ~3 mo. Eggs are passed in feces ~5-6 mo after infection.

Clinical Findings: Most dogs with *S lupi* infection show no clinical signs. When the esophageal lesion is very large (usually when it has become neoplastic), the dog has difficulty in swallowing and may vomit repeatedly after trying to eat. Such dogs salivate profusely and eventually become emaciated. These clinical signs, especially if accompanied by spondylitis or enlargement of the extremities characteristic of osteopathy, are strongly suggestive of spirocercosis with associated neoplasia, particularly in regions where the parasite is prevalent. Occasionally, a dog will die suddenly as the result of massive hemorrhage into the thorax following rupture of the aorta damaged by the developing worms.

Lesions: The characteristic lesions are aneurysm of the thoracic aorta, reactive granulomas of variable size around the worms, and often deformative ossifying spondylitis of the posterior thoracic vertebrae. Esophageal sarcoma, often with metastases, is sometimes associated (apparently causally) with *S lupi* infection, particularly in hound breeds. Dogs with *Spirocerca*-related sarcoma often develop hypertrophic pulmonary osteopathy (qv, p 489).

Diagnosis: Diagnosis can be made by demonstrating the characteristic elongated eggs containing larvae in the feces (*see* p 951), although eggs are sporadically voided in feces and often missed. Gastroscopy occasionally reveals a nodule or an adult worm. A presumptive diagnosis can be made by radiographic examination when it reveals dense masses in the esophagus. Barium helps define the lesion.

Most infections are not diagnosed until necropsy. The granulomas vary greatly in size and location in the esophagus, but usually are so characteristic as to be diagnostic, even if the worms are no longer present. Worms and granulomas may be present in the lungs, trachea, mediastinum, wall of stomach, or other abnormal location. Healed aneurysms of the aorta persist for the life of the dog and are diagnostic of previous infection. When sarcomas are associated with the infection, the esophageal lesion usually is larger and often contains cartilage or bone; metastases frequently are present in the lungs, lymph nodes, heart, liver, or kidneys.

Control: In endemic areas, dogs should be prevented from eating dung beetles, frogs, mice, lizards, etc, and not fed raw chicken scraps. Treatment is not practical, although preliminary studies have shown that levamisole, disophenol, and albendazole may be useful. Surgical removal usually is unsuccessful because of the large areas of the esophagus involved.

PHYSALOPTERA INFECTION
(Stomach worm)

Several species of these stomach nematodes of dogs and cats occur throughout the world. They are usually attached to the gastric or duodenal mucosa by 2 strong lips. The males are ~30 mm and the females ~40 mm long. The eggs are oval, 32 × 55 μm, thick-shelled, and larvated.

Encysted infective larvae of *Physaloptera* spp have been found in several species of beetles, cockroaches, crickets, and flour beetles. Mice and frogs may be paratenic carriers. Following infection through ingestion of the intermediate or paratenic host, development of the larva to adult is direct. These parasites cause gastritis or duodenitis, or both, which often results in vomiting, anorexia, and dark feces. Bleeding, ulcerated areas remain on the gastric mucosa when the parasites move to other locations; in heavy infections, anemia and weight loss may develop. Gastroscopy and identification of the characteristic eggs in the feces are used for diagnosis. Treatments using pyrantel pamoate and carbon disulfide are effective.

Ollulanus tricuspis is a minute worm, ≤1 mm long, that infects several animal species and occasionally provokes a mild erosive or catarrhal gastritis in cats. The females are viviparous, so large infections can build up endogenously. Transmission is via vomitus, and diagnosis is by microscopical demonstration of worms in the vomitus. Treatment with fenbendazole or pyrantel could be attempted.

STRONGYLOIDOSIS

Strongyloides stercoralis is a small, slender nematode that when fully mature is buried in the mucosa of the anterior half of the small intestine of dogs. The worms are almost transparent and all but impossible to see grossly at necropsy. Usually, infections are associated with warm, wet, crowded, unsanitary housing. Some evidence suggests that the species most often found in dogs is identical with that found in man. Other species in dogs include *S planiceps* and *S fuelleborni*; *S cati* and *S tumefaciens* are found in cats.

The parasitic worms are all females. The eggs embryonate rapidly, and most larvae hatch before being passed in the feces. Under appropriate conditions of warmth and moisture, extracorporeal development is rapid. The third larval stage may be reached in little more than a day. Some of these larvae develop into infective filariform larvae; others develop into free-living worms that mate and produce progeny similar to that of the parasitic female. The filariform larvae penetrate the skin, but also may infect a host via the oral mucosa. Transmammary transmission is highly suspected but not proved. Progeny may be shed in the feces 7-10 days after infection.

Clinical signs indicate a heavy infection that has been building up for some weeks. A blood-streaked, mucoid diarrhea, usually seen in young animals during hot humid weather, is characteristic. Emaciation is prominent, and reduced growth rate may be one of the first signs. The appetite usually is good, and the animal is normally active in the earlier stages of the disease. In the absence of concurrent infections, there is little or no fever. Usually in advanced stages, there is shallow rapid breathing and pyrexia, and the prognosis is grave. At necropsy, there is evidence of verminous pneumonia with large areas of consolidation in the lungs, and marked enteritis with hemorrhage, mucosal exfoliation, and much mucus secretion.

Poor sanitation and mixing of susceptible with infected animals lead to a rapid buildup of the infection in all animals in a kennel or pen. Animals with diarrhea should be promptly isolated from asymptomatic dogs. Direct sunlight, elevated soil or surface temperatures, and desiccation are deleterious to all free larval stages. Thorough washing of wooden and impervious surfaces with concentrated salt or lime solutions, followed by rinsing with hot water, effectively destroys the parasite in these areas. Since the disease in man can be serious, caution should be exercised in handling infected dogs.

A single dose of ivermectin or multiple doses of thiabendazole can give good results, but only at dosages that may be toxic. Otherwise, diethylcarbamazine or dithiazanine may be attempted. Lower doses of thiabendazole can be fed continuously to prevent mature infection.

ASCARIASIS

The large roundworms (ascaridoid nematodes) of dogs and cats are common, especially in puppies and kittens. Of the 3 species, *Toxocara canis, Toxascaris leonina*, and *Toxocara cati*, the most important is *T canis*, not only because its larvae may migrate in man, but because fatal infections may occur in young pups. *Toxascaris leonina* occurs most often in adult dogs, less often in cats. These species also occur in wild carnivores.

In puppies, the usual mode of infection with *T canis* is transplacental transfer; if pups <6 wk old ingest embryonated eggs, the hatched larvae, on reaching the lungs, are coughed up, swallowed, and mature to egg-laying adults in the small intestine. However, when embryonated infective eggs of *T canis* are swallowed by older dogs, the larvae hatch, penetrate the intestinal mucosa, and migrate to the liver, lungs, muscles, connective tissue, kidneys, and many other tissues. In the pregnant bitch, these dormant larvae are mobilized and migrate into the developing fetus, and can be found in the intestine of the pup as early as 1 wk after birth. Some larvae migrate to the mammary gland, so that pups may be reinfected via the milk. During this perinatal period, the immunity of the bitch to ascarid infection is partially suppressed, and substantial numbers of eggs may be passed.

Larvae of ascaridoid nematodes may migrate into the tissues of many animals and thus provide an alternative source of infection, particularly for cats and wild carnivores. Such migration also occurs if eggs are swallowed by man. Most human infections are asymptomatic, but fever, persistent eosinophilia, and hepatomegaly (sometimes with pulmonary involvement) may occur, producing a condition known as **visceral larva migrans**. Rarely, a larva may settle in the retina causing impaired vision (**ocular larva migrans**).

The life cycles of *T cati* and *T leonina* are similar except that, in the former, no prenatal infection occurs, while in the latter, migration is restricted to the intestinal wall so that neither prenatal nor transmammary transmission occurs.

Clinical Findings and Lesions: The first indication of infection in young animals is lack of growth and loss of condition. Infected animals have a dull coat and often are "pot-bellied" Worms may be vomited and are often voided in the feces. In the early stages, pulmonary damage due to migrating larvae may occur; this may be complicated by bacterial pneumonitis, so that respiratory distress of variable severity may supervene. Diarrhea with mucus may be evident.

In severe infections of puppies, verminous pneumonia, ascites, fatty degeneration of the liver, and mucoid enteritis are common. Cortical kidney granulomas containing larvae are frequent in young dogs.

Diagnosis: Infection in dogs and cats is diagnosed by detection of eggs in feces. It is important to distinguish the spherical, pitted-shelled eggs of *Toxocara* spp from the oval smooth-shelled eggs of *T leonina*, owing to the public health significance of the former.

Treatment: Piperazine salts are still widely used. Broader-spectrum compounds include dichlorvos, febantel, fenbendazole, flubendazole, mebendazole, nitroscanate, oxfendazole, and pyrantel pamoate. Diethylcarbamazine and dithiazanine are also employed.

Control: Eggs on the ground and somatic larvae in the bitch are the main reservoirs of infection. Perinatal transmission of infection is greatly reduced by daily doses of fenbendazole given to bitches from day 40 of pregnancy to day 14 after whelping. Otherwise, to minimize egg output, pups should be treated as early as possible; ideally, treatment should be given 2 wk after birth and repeated at 2- to 3-wk intervals to 3 mo of age. Nursing bitches should be treated at the same times. Prophylactic programs for heartworm disease using styrylpyridine or oxibendazole combined with diethylcarbamazine also help to control intestinal ascarid infection. Because the eggs adhere to paws, hair, skin, and other surfaces, and become mixed in soil and dust, strict hygiene should be observed by people, particularly children, exposed to potentially contaminated animals or localities.

HOOKWORM INFECTION

Ancylostoma caninum is the principal cause of canine hookworm disease in most tropical and subtropical areas of the world. *Ancylostoma tubaeforme* of cats has a similar but more sparse distribution. *Ancylostoma braziliense* of cats and dogs is sparsely distributed from Florida to North Carolina in the USA. *Uncinaria stenocephala* is the principal canine hookworm in cooler regions; it is the canine hookworm in Canada and the northern fringe of the USA, where it is primarily a fox parasite. *Ancylostoma caninum* males are ~12 mm long, females, 15 mm; the other species are somewhat smaller. The infective larvae of canine hookworms, particularly of *A braziliense*, may penetrate and wander under the skin of man and cause **cutaneous larva migrans**.

The elongate (>65 μm), thin-walled, hookworm eggs in the early cleavage stages (2-8 cells) are first passed in the feces 15-20 days after infection; they complete embryonation and hatch in 24-72 hr on warm, moist soil. Transmission commonly results from ingestion of infective larvae from the environment or, with *A caninum*, from the colostrum or milk of infected bitches. Intestinal infections with either *A caninum* or *A braziliense* can also occur from larval invasion through the skin, but this route is of little significance for *U stenocephala*. Skin penetration in young pups is followed by migration of the larvae through the blood to the lungs, where they are coughed up and swallowed to mature in the small intestine. However, in animals >3 mo old, *A caninum* larvae, after migration through the lungs, are arrested in the somatic tissues. These arrested larvae are activated during pregnancy and accumulate in the mammary glands.

Clinical Findings: An acute normocytic, normochromic anemia followed by hypochromic, microcytic "iron deficiency" anemia in young puppies is the characteristic, and often fatal, clinical manifestation of *A caninum* infection. Surviving puppies develop some immunity and show lesser clinical signs. Nevertheless, debilitated and malnourished animals may continue to be unthrifty and suffer from chronic anemia. Mature, well-nourished dogs may harbor a few worms without showing signs. These are of primary concern as the direct or indirect source of infection for pups. Diarrhea with dark, tarry feces accompanies severe infections. Hydremia, emaciation, and weakness develop in chronic disease.

Lesions: Anemia results directly from the blood sucking and the bleeding ulcerations when *A caninum* shift feeding sites. The amount of blood loss due to a single worm in 24 hr has been estimated to be up to 0.1 mL. There is no interference with erythropoiesis in uncomplicated hookworm disease. The liver and other organs may appear ischemic with some fatty infiltration of the liver. Neither *A braziliense* nor *U stenocephala* is an avid blood feeder, and anemia does not occur. However, hypoproteinemia is characteristic, and serum seepage around the site of attachment in the intestine may reduce blood protein by >10%. Hemorrhagic enteritis with swollen intestinal mucosa that shows red bite-marks and small ulcers and attached worms is usually seen in acute fatal cases.

Dermatitis due to larval invasion of the skin may occur with any of the hookworms but has been observed most frequently in the interdigital spaces with *U stenocephala*. Pneumonia and lung consolidation may occur with overwhelming infections in pups.

Diagnosis: The characteristic thin-shelled, oval eggs are easily seen on flotation of fresh feces from infected dogs. Acute anemia and death from lactogenic infections may be observed in young pups before eggs are passed in their feces.

Treatment and Control: The bitch should be free of hookworms before breeding and kept out of contaminated areas during pregnancy. The bitch should whelp and the pups should be suckled in sanitary quarters. Concrete runways that can be washed at least twice a week in warm weather are best. Sunlit clay or sandy runways can be decontaminated with sodium borate (10 lb/100 sq ft [1 kg/2 sq m]). Chemical prophylaxis with styrylpyridinium or oxibendazole usually is in combination with diethylcarbamazine to prevent both hookworm and heartworm infection; milbemycin oxime also controls both infections. Fenbendazole given to pregnant bitches from day 40 of pregnancy to day 14 after whelping greatly reduces transmammary transmission to the pups.

Single-dose treatments include dichlorvos, pyrantel pamoate, and nitroscanate, which are administered PO alone or with food, and butamisole and disophenol, given by injection. The latter have relatively narrow safety margins. Butamisole must not be used concurrently with bunamidine, while repeat treatments with disophenol are contraindicated. Other drugs are more effective if given in divided doses. These include dithiazanine, febantel, fenbendazole, flubendazole, mebendazole, and thenium. Label recommendations and precautions should always be heeded. When anemia is severe, chemotherapy may have to be supported by blood transfusion or supplemental iron, or both, and followed by a high-protein diet until the Hgb level is normal.

WHIPWORM INFECTION
(Trichuriasis)

Adult *Trichuris vulpis* are 40-70 mm long, and consist of a long, slender anterior portion and a thick posterior third. They commonly inhabit the cecum where they are firmly attached to the wall, with their anterior end embedded in the mucosa. Thick-shelled eggs with bipolar plugs are passed in the feces and become infective in 2-4 wk in a warm, moist environment. Although eggs may remain viable in a suitable environment for up to 5 yr, they are susceptible to desiccation. The life cycle is direct. Following the ingestion of infective eggs, larval development occurs in the jejunal wall, and the adults mature in the cecum in ~11 wk. They may remain for up to 16 mo.

No signs are seen in light infections, but as the worm burden increases and the inflammatory (and occasionally hemorrhagic) reaction in the cecum becomes more pronounced, weight loss and diarrhea become evident. Fresh blood may accompany the feces of heavily infected dogs, and anemia occasionally follows.

In addition to regular anthelmintic treatment of dogs, advantage should be taken of the susceptibility of the eggs to desiccation. By maintaining cleanliness and eliminating moist areas, the infection in dogs can be reduced considerably, although *T vulpis* infections can be difficult to control. Effective compounds include dichlorvos, febantel, fenbendazole, flubendazole, mebendazole, and oxantel pamoate, which are administered PO alone or with the feed. Butamisole is given by injection but has a relatively narrow safety margin and must not be used in heartworm-infected dogs, or concurrently with bunamidine. Phthalofyne and glycobiarsol also have been used.

ONCICOLA CANIS INFECTION

These acanthocephalid parasites have been found rarely in the small intestine of dogs and cats in the Western Hemisphere. They are white, ~12 mm long, and their thorny heads are embedded in the mucosa. The females lay brown, thick-shelled, embryonated, wide oval eggs (45 × 65 μm). The life cycle is not completely known, but it is thought to include an arthropod intermediate host and paratenic hosts such as turkeys or armadillos. Most infections cause no clinical signs.

CESTODE INFECTIONS
(Tapeworm infections)

Most urban dogs and cats eat prepared foods and have restricted access to natural prey. Such animals may acquire *Dipylidium caninum* from fleas. Cats with access to infected house (or outdoor) mice and rats also acquire *Taenia taeniaeformis*. Suburban, rural, and hunting dogs have more access to various small mammals and raw meat and offal from domestic and wild ungulates. A number of cestodes can be expected in such dogs (*see* TABLE 7). On sheep ranges and wherever wild ungulates (particularly Cervidae) and wolves are common, dogs may acquire *Echinococcus granulosus*. Sylvatic *E multilocularis*, previously known only from arctic North America, now occurs in midwestern and western USA and Canada, but thus far, infections in cats or dogs are rare. Association with infected dogs may result in human infection with metacestodes of *E granulosus*, *E multilocularis*, *T multiceps*, *T serialis*, or *T crassiceps* in various tissues, or adult *D caninum* in the intestine. The presence of metacestodes in livestock may limit commercial use of such carcasses or offal meats. Thus, cestodes of dogs and cats may be of public health importance (*see* TABLE 8).

Adult cestodes in the intestine of dogs and cats rarely cause serious disease, and clinical signs, if present, may depend on the degree of infection, age, condition, and breed of host. Clinical signs vary from unthriftiness, malaise, irritability, capricious appetite, and shaggy coat to colic, mild diarrhea, and rarely, emaciation and seizures. Diagnosis is based on finding proglottids or eggs in the feces. The eggs of *Taenia* spp and *Echinococcus* spp cannot be reliably differentiated by microscopical examination.

Control of intestinal tapeworms of dogs and cats requires therapy and prevention. Animals that roam freely usually become reinfected by metacestodes available in carrion or animals they kill. *Dipylidium caninum* is different since it can cycle through fleas that may be associated with confined infected animals; therefore, an accurate diagnosis is necessary for effective advice on preventing reinfection.

Effective treatment of infected animals should remove the attached scolices from the small intestine. Bunamidine compounds are effective against mature *Echinococcus* spp and *Taenia* spp, but they are less effective against immature *Echinococcus* spp and *Dipylidium* spp. Bunamidine also is effective against *Spirometra* sp in cats. Niclosamide and its piperazine salt are reasonably effective against *Taenia* spp in dogs and cats, but much less so against *Dipylidium* spp and *Echinococcus* spp; vomiting and diarrhea may occur. Dichlorophen and quinacrine hydrochloride also are used, although neither is as effective as some of the other drugs listed above. Mebendazole may be used in removing most adult *Taenia* spp from the intestine of infected animals, as can febantel, fenbendazole, and flubendazole, but these are not as effective against *E granulosus*. Praziquantel is most efficacious against both larvae and adults of most tapeworms of dogs and cats, but it is not active against the eggs.

FLUKE INFECTIONS

INTESTINAL FLUKES

Nanophyetus (Troglotrema) salmincola, the "salmon poisoning" fluke, is a small (0.5 × 0.3 mm), oval fluke found in the small intestine of dogs, cats, and many wild carnivores in the northwestern USA, southwestern Canada, and Siberia. The eggs, which pass with the feces of infected hosts, are light brown, 55 × 45 μm, and indistinctly operculated with a small knob at one pole. The life cycle includes an extended period (3 mo) of oval embryonation. The first intermediate hosts are snails found in endemic locations (eg, *Oxytrema silicula* in the USA). The cercariae of these snails penetrate the skin of young salmonid fishes and encyst (metacercariae) in their muscles and organs. Dogs and other animals become infected by eating raw or improperly prepared infected fish.

Because these flukes embed deeply between the villi of the intestine, infection with a large number of them may cause enteritis. Most infections, however, are

Table 7. Cestodes of Dogs and Cats of North America
(In order of importance)

Cestode[1]	Definitive Host	Intermediate Host and Organs Invaded[2]	Diagnostic Features of Adult Worm	Remarks
Dipylidium caninum (Double-pored dog tapeworm)	Dog, cat, coyote, wolf, fox, other animals.	Fleas and more rarely lice; free in body cavity.	Strobila 15-70 cm long and up to 3 mm in maximum width. 30-150 rostellar hooks of rose-thorn shape in 3 or 4 circles; large hooks 12-15 μm, smallest 5-6 μm long. Segments shaped like cucumber seeds with pore near middle of each lateral margin.	Probably most common tapeworm of dogs, less common in cats; cosmopolitan. Occasionally infects man, particularly infants.
Taenia taeniaeformis[3]	Cat, dog, lynx, wolf, other animals.	Various rats, mice, other rodents; in large cysts in liver.	Strobila 15-60 cm long, 5-6 mm in maximum width. 26-52 rostellar hooks in double row; large hooks 380-420 μm, small hooks 250-270 μm long. No neck. Sacculate lateral branches of uterus difficult to count.	Common cestode of cats, rare in dogs; cosmopolitan.
Taenia pisiformis	Dog, cat, fox, wolf, coyote, lynx, other animals.	Rabbits and hares, rarely squirrels and other rodents; in pelvic or peritoneal cavity attached to viscera.	Strobila 60 cm to 2 m long, 5 mm in maximum width. About 34-48 rostellar hooks in double row; large hooks 225-290 μm, small hooks 132-177 μm long. 5-10 lateral branches on each side of gravid uterus.	Particularly common in suburban, farm, and hunting dogs that eat rabbit and rabbit viscera.
Taenia hydatigena	Dog, wolf, coyote, lynx, rarely cat.	Domestic and wild cloven-hooved animals, rarely hares and rodents; in liver and abdominal cavity.	Strobila to 5 m long and 7 mm in maximum width. About 26-44 rostellar hooks in double row; large hooks 170-220 μm, small hooks 110-160 μm long. 5-10 lateral branches on each side of gravid uterus.	In farm dogs, more rarely hunting dogs; cosmopolitan.
Diphyllobothrium spp[4]	Man, dog, cat, other fish-eating animals.	Encysted in various organs, or free in body cavity of various fish.	Strobila to 10 m long, 20 mm in maximum width, but usually smaller. Scolex with 2 grooves (bothria) and no hooks. Genital pores ventral on midline of segment.	Canada, Alaska and various other states of the USA, USSR, and other areas.

(continued)

Table 7. Cestodes of Dogs and Cats of North America (continued)
(In order of importance)

Cestode[1]	Definitive Host	Intermediate Host and Organs Invaded[2]	Diagnostic Features of Adult Worm	Remarks
Echinococcus granulosus (Hydatid tapeworm)	Dog, wolf, coyote, possibly fox, and several other wild carnivores.	Sheep, goats, cattle, pigs, horses, deer, moose, some rodents, occasionally man and other animals; commonly in liver and lungs, occasionally in other organs and tissues.	Strobila 2-6 mm long with 3-5 segments. 28-50, usually 30-36, rostellar hooks in double row; large hooks 27-40 μm, small hooks 21-25 μm long.	Foci, especially among North American range sheep and dogs associating with them, are known; sylvatic moose-wolf cycle where these animals occur; probably cosmopolitan.
Echinococcus multilocularis (Alveolar hydatid tapeworm)	Arctic, red, and gray foxes; coyote, cat, dog.	Microtine rodents, occasionally in man; in the liver.	Strobila 1.2-2.7 mm long with 2-4 segments; along with above species smallest tapeworm in dogs. 26-36 rostellar hooks in double row; large hooks 23-29 μm, small hooks 19-26 μm.	Eastern Europe, USSR, Alaska and midwestern USA, and Canada; thus far, significant cycle in cats and dogs in North America not recognized.
Echinococcus vogeli	Dog, bush dog.	Picas and other rodents.	Strobila 4-5.5 mm long with 3 segments. 28-36 rostellar hooks in double rows; large hooks 49-57 μm, small hooks 30-47 μm. Uterus in gravid segment has no lateral branches.	Central and northern South America.
Mesocestoides spp	Many wild canids, felids, mustelids; other animals, including dog and cat.	Complete life cycle unknown; arthropod intermediate hosts are suspected; juvenile tetrathyridia in abdominal cavity and elsewhere of various mammals, birds, and reptiles; tetrathyridia from body cavity of dogs may enter intestine through intestinal wall.	Strobila 10 cm long and 2-5 mm wide. Scolex with 4 suckers, but no rostellum or hooks. Genital pore ventral in midline of worm. Gravid segments with paruterine organ.	Reported from dog and cat in midwest and west; in wild animals elsewhere in USA and Canada; probably cosmopolitan.

Species	Definitive hosts	Intermediate hosts	Description	Remarks
Taenia multiceps	Dog, coyote, fox, wolf.	Sheep, goats, and other domestic or wild ruminants, rarely man; usually in brain and spinal cord.	Strobila 40-100 cm long and up to 5 mm wide. Scolex with 4 suckers and 22-32 hooks in double row; large hooks 150-170 μm, small hooks 90-130 μm long. Vagina with reflexed curve near lateral excretory canal. 9-26 lateral branches on gravid uterus.	Rare in domestic carnivores in western North America; more common in wild animals; probably cosmopolitan.
Taenia serialis	Dog, coyote, fox, wolf.	Rabbit, hare, squirrel, rarely man; in subcut. connective tissue or retroperitoneally.	Strobila 20-72 cm long and 3-5 mm wide. 26-32 hooks in double row; large hooks 110-175 μm, small hooks 68-120 μm long. Vagina with reflexed curve near lateral excretory canal. 20-25 lateral branches on gravid uterus.	Primarily in wild canids; considered by some authorities as not distinct from T. multiceps.
Taenia crassiceps	Dog, coyote, fox, wolf.	Various rodents, perhaps other animals, one record in man; subcut. and in body cavities.	Strobila 70-170 mm long and 1-2 mm wide. Scolex with 30-36 hooks in double row; large hooks 126-132 μm, small hooks 121-140 μm long. 16-21 lateral branches on uterus, sometimes becoming diffuse.	Reported from Canada and northern USA, including Alaska.
Taenia krabbei	Dog, coyote, wolf, bobcat.	Moose, deer, reindeer; in striated muscle.	Strobila ~20 cm long and up to 9 mm wide. Scolex small with 26-36 hooks in double row; large hooks 146-195 μm, small hooks 85-141 μm long. 18-24 straight and narrow lateral branches on gravid uterus.	Reported from Canada and northern USA, including Alaska; considered by some a subspecies of T. ovis.
Taenia ovis	Dog, cat (rarely).	Sheep and goat; in musculature, rarely elsewhere.	Strobila 45-110 cm long and up to 4-8.5 mm wide. Scolex with 32-38 hooks in double row; large hooks 160-202 μm long. 20-25 lateral branches on gravid uterus. Vagina crosses ovary on poral side of segment.	Occasionally from farm dogs in western North America; cosmopolitan.

[1]Taenia polyacantha, recorded rarely from dogs in Alaska, is excluded here.

[2]In all cases in which the life cycle is known, cats and dogs become infected by ingesting tapeworm eggs (except in Mesocestoides spp and Diphyllobothrium spp. which have an extra stage in the life cycle), which are passed in the feces of the definitive host. These intermediate hosts become infected by eating animals, or parts therefrom, that contain the infective metacestode.

[3]Several other large-hooked Taenia spp occur in the larger wild cats, but most use lagomorphs and ungulates as intermediate hosts, so domestic cats rarely are exposed.

[4]Several species of Diphyllobothrium have been recorded from North American dogs and cats; they require extensive study before they can be identified with certainty.

Table 8. Cestodes of Public Health Importance[1]

	Taenia saginata	*Taenia solium*	*Diphyllobothrium* spp[2]	*Echinococcus granulosus*	*Echinococcus multilocularis*
Host of adult worm	Man only	Man only	Man, dog, cat, and other fish-eating mammals and birds	Dog, wolf, fox, and several other wild carnivores	Canidae and the domestic cat
Name or metacestode intermediate	Cysticercus "beef measles"	Cysticercus "pork measles"	Procercoid in copepod, plerocercoid in fish	Hydatid cyst	Multilocular or alveolar "cyst" or hydatid
Measurements of metacestode	9 × 5 mm	6-10 × 5-10 mm	2-25 × 2.5 mm	Diameter 50-100 mm, sometimes ≥150 mm	Variable, penetrates like neoplastic tissue
Principal intermediate hosts	Cattle	Pig, dog (man may be both definitive and intermediate host)	Copepod first host, then fish	Sheep, cattle, pigs, moose, deer, rarely dog, cat, man	Field mice, voles, lemmings, sometimes domestic mammals and man
Site of metacestode	Skeletal and cardiac muscle	Skeletal and cardiac muscle, occasionally nervous system	Mesenteric tissues, testes, ovary, muscles	Commonly in liver and lungs, occasionally in other organs and tissues	Various organs and tissues

[1]Human infections with the metacestodes of *Taenia crassiceps*, *T multiceps*, *T serialis*, *Mesocestoides* sp, and other cestodes occur rarely.
[2]Since several species of *Diphyllobothrium* infect man in North America, it is no longer advisable to refer to all such infections as due to *D latum*.

complicated through development of the salmon poisoning complex (qv, p 414) caused by rickettsial organisms, which the fluke transmits. Praziquantel is an effective treatment.

Alaria alata, A canis, and other *Alaria* spp are small (0.5 mm) flukes usually found in the small intestine of the dog, cat, fox, and mink in the Western Hemisphere, as well as in Europe, Australia, and Japan. The anterior part of the body is flat and the posterior part is conical. The eggs are oval, light brown, and fairly large (120 × 65 μm). The life cycle includes fresh water snails (*Planorbis* spp) as first intermediate hosts. Cercariae emerge from the snails and penetrate frogs; dogs and other definitive hosts become infected by feeding on the frogs. Metacercariae may encyst again in birds, snakes, and rodents when these animals feed on frogs, and dogs also may become infected by feeding on these animals. The young flukes migrate through various viscera of the definitive host before reaching the small intestine. Although generally considered to be nonpathogenic, large numbers of flukes may cause enteritis. These flukes may infect man. Infections may be treated with bithionol, praziquantel, albendazole, or niclosamide.

Other species of flukes, usually not pathogenic, have been found occasionally in the intestine of dogs, cats, and other carnivores; these include *Heterophyes heterophyes* in some north African and Asian countries; *Metagonimus yokogawai* in Asia; *Cryptocotyle lingua* in the USA, Canada, Japan, Siberia, and Europe; and *Apophallus donicum* in North America and eastern Europe. Their life cycles include snails as first intermediate hosts and fish as second intermediate hosts in which metacercariae become encysted.

Heterobilharzia americanum has been found in the mesenteric veins of dogs and wild animals in southern USA. The spined eggs pass through the tissues of the intestine to the lumen and pass with the feces. From the snail intermediate host, the cercariae escape into the water and penetrate the skin of dogs and other definitive hosts, migrate to the liver, mature, and move to the mesenteric vessels. Granulomas around the eggs are formed in the wall of the intestine and other parts of the body. Enteritis may develop in heavy infections. "Water dermatitis" is sometimes produced when cercariae penetrate the skin. Praziquantel may be effective for treatment.

HEPATIC DISTOMIASIS

Flukes in the bile ducts and gallbladder cause mild to severe fibrosis. Many species of distome trematodes have been reported from the liver of dogs and cats in most parts of the world. Mild infections may pass unnoticed; however, in severe infection, dogs may develop progressive weakness, ending in complete exhaustion, coma, and death. The following are some of the most commonly encountered of these trematodes.

Opisthorchis tenuicollis (felineus) is parasitic in the bile duct, pancreatic duct, and small intestine of dogs and cats in eastern Europe and parts of Asia. *Opisthorchis viverrini* occurs in dogs as well as domestic and wild cats in southeast Asia. They are small (9 × 2 mm) and elongate. Their life cycle includes certain snails (*Bithynia* sp) and certain cyprinid fishes as intermediate hosts. A related species, *Clonorchis sinensis,* the oriental liver fluke of man, also has been found in the bile ducts and pancreatic ducts of dogs and cats as well as other animals. It is larger than *Opisthorchis* spp. The operculated eggs of these parasites may be identified in the feces of infected animals.

Long-term presence of these flukes in the bile duct causes adenomatous thickening and fibrosis of the duct wall. Carcinomas in the liver or pancreas have been observed in chronic and severe cases.

Platynosomum fastosum (conicum) is a small fluke (6 × 2 mm) found in the bile ducts of Felidae in southeastern USA, Puerto Rico and other Caribbean Islands, South America, some of the Pacific islands, and parts of Africa. Its life cycle includes the snail *Sublima octona* as intermediate host, and certain lizards as paratenic hosts. Cats acquire the parasite by feeding on infected lizards. In mild cases, vague chronic signs of unthriftiness may be observed. Severe infections, however, may cause the "lizard poisoning" syndrome characterized by anorexia, persistent vomiting, diarrhea, and jaundice leading to death. Praziquantel and nitroscanate treatments have been used with some success.

Metorchis albidus and *M conjunctus* are 2 minute flukes (5 × 1.5 mm) that have been found in the bile ducts and gallbladder of dogs, cats, and other carnivores in North America, Europe, and the USSR. They seldom cause any recognizable clinical signs. The life cycle includes certain freshwater snails and cyprinid fish as intermediate hosts. Their eggs are small (27 × 15 μm).

HEMORRHAGIC GASTROENTERITIS (HGE)

A syndrome characterized by acute onset of vomiting, bloody diarrhea, collapse, a rapid course, and death of untreated dogs.

Etiology: The cause is unknown; however, culture of intestinal contents from affected dogs have yielded large numbers of *Clostridium perfringens*, which suggests that this organism (or its toxins) is the primary cause. In addition, similar clinical signs have been observed in experimental models of endotoxic shock, anaphylaxis, and immune-mediated bowel disease in dogs. There is no direct evidence that such mechanisms are operative in HGE. Toy and miniature breeds are predisposed, particularly Schnauzers and Toy Poodles, although any breed may be affected.

Clinical Findings: Sudden onset of shock, partial collapse, vomiting, and dysentery, the latter often of a jam-like consistency and with a characteristic odor, are the common signs. Rectal temperature is normal or subnormal. Abdominal pain is usually absent. Hemoconcentration is not reflected by loss of skin turgor.

Barium may pass slowly, if at all; the small intestine may have ileus. An elevated PCV, RBC count, and Hgb concentration are characteristic. The WBC count may be low, normal, or elevated. In most cases, the platelet count is low or low normal. A PCV >70% is a sign of serious illness.

Diagnosis: Diagnosis is based on the clinical findings and elevated PCV. Parvoviral infection, GI foreign body, intussusception, volvulus, adrenocortical insufficiency, and acute pancreatitis are differential diagnoses.

Treatment: Vigorous fluid volume replacement is the mainstay of therapy and usually results in rapid recovery. A balanced, multiple electrolyte solution such as lactated Ringer's should be given IV. In severe cases, the infusion rate should be 90 mL/kg/hr until return of capillary refill time to normal and the PCV to <50%. IV fluids are then continued at a more moderate rate, as needed to keep the PCV <50% and to support adequate circulation. Glucocorticoids, eg, methylprednisolone sodium succinate or dexamethasone sodium phosphate, may be necessary for animals in hypovolemic shock. Antibiotics effective against both aerobic and anaerobic bacteria should be administered parenterally. An antiemetic such as metoclopramide may be helpful if vomiting is severe. Food and water are withheld until the vomiting and diarrhea have ceased. Small amounts of bland food can then be fed.

INTESTINAL DISEASE OF THE NEWBORN

Although the kitten and puppy obtain a small portion of their transferred maternal immunity transplacentally, colostrum is the primary source. Providing that the pups and kittens suckle as soon as possible after birth and certainly within 8 hr, infectious neonatal intestinal disease usually is not a problem. However, a reaction to the dam's milk, or to any therapeutic agent the dam has received and that is secreted into the milk, may cause diarrhea. Antibiotics secreted in the dam's milk may adversely affect the normal development of the newborn's intestinal microflora. Most cases of diarrhea respond to supportive fluid and electrolyte therapy. Antibiotics (ampicillin, trimethoprim/sulfa, cephalothin) should be administered parenterally in cases of bloody diarrhea because the blood-mucosal barrier may be broken and there is risk that the infection will become systemic.

PARVOVIRAL INFECTION

An enteritis of acute onset and varying morbidity and mortality, caused by a parvovirus that was first recognized in 1978; it is now found worldwide. Although dogs of all ages have been affected, puppies appear to be more susceptible. Only members of the Canidae (dogs, wolves, coyotes) are known to be susceptible to natural infection.

Etiology and Pathogenesis: Canine parvovirus, a nonenveloped single-stranded DNA virus, is closely related to but different from feline panleukopenia virus, mink enteritis virus, and raccoon parvovirus. A sodium hypochlorite (household bleach) solution is an effective disinfectant after organic material such as feces is removed, but the virus is very resistant in the environment; it remains viable outside the host for years. Ingestion of fecal material from infected animals is the major route of infection. Infected dogs shed virus in feces for ~2 wk.

After ingestion, tonsillar crypts and Peyer's patches are infected first, followed by a viremia and then infection of intestinal crypts. Collapse of intestinal villi is the result of crypt cell necrosis. Death may follow due to dehydration, electrolyte imbalance, endotoxic shock, or secondary septicemia.

Clinical Findings: Canine parvovirus produces 2 different disease forms, myocarditis and enteritis. Myocarditis with sudden death in puppies predominantly 4-8 wk old was commonly seen when the infection first appeared; immune bitches and maternal antibody in newborn puppies prevent this form of disease today. The incidence of enteritis has been greatly reduced, but it still prevails. Death is infrequent, but mortality among pups 8-12 wk old may be quite high. The incubation period is 5-11 days. Anorexia, lethargy, and rapid dehydration are other signs. Vomiting is often the initial sign, and can be severe and protracted. Diarrhea is usually seen within 24-48 hr. The feces are either streaked with blood or frankly hemorrhagic and remain fluid until recovery or death. Some dogs are febrile, especially during the early phase of disease. Lymphopenia, but not always leukopenia, can be found in most affected dogs. Sudden "shock-like" death may occur as early as 2 days after the onset of illness. Prolonged illness is uncommon. Dogs either die or recover quickly.

Lesions: The small intestines are primarily affected. Intestinal congestion is variable, although in young pups the intestine can be blanched. The intestines are thickened or inelastic, and the serosal surface has a granular appearance. The mucosa is ragged, and the contents are fluid with floccules of epithelial debris or frank blood. There is thymic atrophy.

In the myocardial form of the disease, pulmonary edema is the main finding. Microscopy reveals a diagnostic myocarditis with fiber loss, edema, and intranuclear basophilic inclusions. Extensive lymphocytic infiltration and fibrosis are found in chronic cases.

Diagnosis: Vomiting, hemorrhagic diarrhea, temperature rise, and lymphopenia are not restricted to parvoviral enteritis. Virus isolation from feces or demonstration of virus by electron microscopy confirms the diagnosis. At necropsy, crypt cell necrosis, crypt dilatation, intestinal villous collapse, and intranuclear inclusions (not always present) confirm the diagnosis. Demonstration of virus-specific IgM in serum indicates parvoviral infection if dogs have not been vaccinated within 3 wk.

Treatment: Prompt intensive care, including fluid therapy, atropine, and antibiotics has been successful. Treatment may have to continue for 72 hr. The IV route of fluid therapy is preferred. In severe cases, potassium and bicarbonate supplementation may be necessary.

Prophylaxis: Modified live canine parvovirus, feline panleukopenia virus, and inactivated canine parvovirus vaccines are available. All protect dogs from the disease if maternal antibody does not prevent immunization; however, not all dogs become immunized with modified live feline parvovirus unless the virus titer in the vaccine is extremely high. Older dogs respond less to parvovirus vaccination than do young, growing dogs.

Puppies with low levels of maternal antibody are susceptible to virulent virus, yet will not respond to vaccine virus. Since a period of susceptibility cannot be avoided, weaned puppies should be vaccinated q2-3wk until 18 wk old. Annual revaccination is recommended for all dogs.

Diseased dogs should be kept in isolation.

SALIVARY DISORDERS, SM AN

PTYALISM
(Sialosis)

Hypersecretion of saliva characterized by profuse drooling. Pseudoptyalism occurs when there is a normal quantity of saliva, but increased drooling because of dysphagia. Ptyalism and pseudoptyalism are discussed together as ptyalism.

Ptyalism may result from: 1) drugs, eg, organophosphates or poisons; 2) local irritation or inflammation associated with stomatitis, glossitis (especially in cats), oral foreign bodies or neoplasms, injuries, or other mucosal defects; 3) infectious diseases, eg, rabies, the nervous form of distemper, or other convulsive disorders; 4) motion sickness, fear, nervousness, and excitement; 5) reluctance to swallow from irritation of the esophagus or stimulation of GI receptors with gastritis or enteritis; 6) sublingual salivary mucocele; 7) tonsillitis; 8) administration of medicine in some species (particularly cats); 9) conformational defects; 10) metabolic disorders, eg, hepatic encephalopathy, uremia; 11) abscess or other inflammatory blockage or condition of the salivary gland.

The possibility of rabies should be eliminated before examination.

The underlying cause, local or systemic, should be determined and treated. For treating poisonings, *see* TOXICOLOGY, p 1632 *et seq*. For treating stomatitis, glossitis, *see* DISEASES OF THE MOUTH, SM AN, p 125. Sedatives, anti-motion-sickness drugs, or tranquilizers may be helpful in nervous and reflex disturbances. If necessary, an anticholinergic agent may be given to suppress salivation until the cause is determined.

Acute moist dermatitis of the lips and face may develop if the skin is not kept as dry as possible. Cleansing with a dilute chlorhexidine solution may be helpful. If a superficial pyoderma (qv, p 828) develops, a topical antibiotic cream may be applied.

SALIVARY FISTULA

A rare problem following trauma of the mandibular, zygomatic, or sublingual salivary glands. Wounds of the parotid gland are more likely to develop a fistula. A draining tract discharging saliva from the glands is caused most commonly by a wound that penetrates the gland, spontaneous rupture of a gland abscess, or prior surgery in the area with iatrogenic rupture. Parotid gland fistulas may occur following a lateral ear resection. The constant flow of saliva prevents healing and a fistula develops.

History of injury in the gland area, location of the fistula, and nature of the discharge are characteristic. A salivary fistula must be differentiated from a draining sinus (due to a penetrating foreign body) in the neck region, or from sinuses arising from congenital defects.

Complete surgical removal of the gland and fistulous tract is the only satisfactory treatment.

SALIVARY GLAND TUMORS

Rare in dogs and cats, there is no breed or sex predilection; most are in those ≥10 yr old. Most are malignant, and adenocarcinoma occurs with the greatest frequency.

Metastasis to regional lymph nodes is common, and local recurrence following surgical excision is high. Radiation is possibly an effective adjunct therapy.

SALIVARY MUCOCELE
(Sialocele)

An accumulation of mucoid saliva in the tissue, which has collected after damage to the salivary duct or gland. This is the most common salivary gland disorder of dogs and cats. While any of the salivary glands may be affected, the sublingual gland is involved most commonly. Usually the saliva collects at the intermandibular or cranial cervical area (cervical mucocele). It may also collect in the sublingual tissues on the floor of the mouth (ranula). A less common site is in the pharyngeal wall.

The cause may be traumatic or inflammatory blockage or rupture of the duct of the sublingual, mandibular, parotid, or zygomatic salivary gland. Usually the cause is not determined.

Signs depend on the site of saliva accumulation. In the acute phase of a cervical mucocele, the area is swollen and painful. Frequently, this stage is not observed by the owner, and the first noticed sign may be a nonpainful, slowly enlarging, fluctuant mass in the cervical region. A ranula may not be seen until it is traumatized and bleeds. A pharyngeal mucocele may obstruct the airways and result in moderate to severe respiratory distress.

A mucocele is detectable as a soft, fluctuant, painless mass that must be differentiated from abscesses, tumors, and other retention cysts of the neck. Pain or fever may be present if the mucocele becomes infected. A salivary mucocele usually can be diagnosed by palpation and aspiration of the characteristic golden or blood-tinged, stringy saliva. Usually, careful palpation with the animal in dorsal recumbency can determine the affected side; if not, sialography may be helpful.

Surgery is recommended to remove the damaged salivary gland and duct, which usually involves removal of the mandibular-sublingual gland complex. Cervical mucoceles can be managed with periodic drainage if surgery is not an option. Drainage, marsupialization, or gland removal has been recommended for treatment of ranulas and pharyngeal mucoceles.

SIALADENITIS
(Salivary gland inflammation)

Acute or chronic inflammation of a salivary gland may be associated with mucocele formation or abscesses of the head and neck. It can also occur as a separate entity.

The cause may be trauma, commonly from penetrating wounds such as bites, or infection of the salivary gland or surrounding tissue. Sialadenitis as a component of systemic disease has been reported with rabies, distemper, and the paramyxovirus that causes mumps in people.

Signs include fever, depression, and painful, swollen salivary glands. Rupture of an abscessed gland discharges pus into the surrounding tissue or the mouth. Rupture through the skin may cause formation of a salivary fistula. Swelling of the parotid gland is most prominent below the ear, swelling of the mandibular gland at the angle of the jaw, and swelling of the zygomatic gland just caudal to the eye. Zygomatic gland involvement may result in retrobulbar swelling, divergent strabismus of the affected eye, exophthalmos, excess tearing, and reluctance to open the mouth or eat. Abscesses of the zygomatic and parotid glands are acutely painful; the animal may hold its head rigidly and resent any manipulation involving the head or neck.

Radiographs and laboratory tests are usually not helpful, although evaluation of fluid in an abscess can lead to a diagnosis. Histopathology of salivary gland tissue can reveal acute or chronic inflammatory changes or necrosis.

Mild sialadenitis requires no treatment, and recovery is usually rapid and complete. A developed abscess should be drained through the overlying skin or, if involving the zygomatic gland, drained behind the last upper molar on the affected side. Systemic antibiotics should be administered.

Lack of resolution or recurrence necessitates surgical removal of the affected gland.

XEROSTOMIA
(Aptyalism)

Decreased secretion of saliva, characterized by a dry mouth; uncommon in dogs and cats.

Decreased salivary secretion may result from use of certain drugs (eg, atropine), extreme dehydration or pyrexia, or anesthesia. It is seen in some dogs with keratoconjunctivitis sicca, and may be immune-mediated. Occasionally, decreased secretion of saliva is due to disease of the salivary gland.

Determination and treatment of the underlying cause is of primary importance. Physiologically balanced mouthwashes relieve the discomfort that results from xerostomia. Fluids may be administered to correct dehydration, if present.

SMALL-INTESTINAL OBSTRUCTION, SM AN

Etiology: Partial or complete obstruction of the small bowel can be caused by indigestible foreign material, masses of parasites, postoperative adhesions, neoplasms, granulomas, and abscesses. In addition, volvulus, intussusception, and hernial incarceration can cause complete obstruction of the small intestine and occlusion of its vascular integrity. Paralysis or stasis of a segment of small bowel caused by local or generalized peritonitis, enteritis, or pancreatitis, or following laparotomy may cause signs of intestinal obstruction.

Mesenteric **volvulus** is rare in small animals while **intussusception** is more common, particularly in young animals with severe enteritis or a heavy parasite infection. Intussusception occurs commonly in the jejunum or proximal ileum, or at the ileocecal junction. Ingestion of foreign bodies is most common in young dogs and cats but may occur at any age. Toys, rubber balls, stones, bones, cloth, fishhooks, and needles are ingested frequently. Cats are especially likely to swallow linear foreign objects (eg, string). Cats also may swallow large amounts of hair, which may form a mass in the stomach or intestines.

Clinical Findings: Signs of foreign body obstruction are extremely variable. Some animals vomit intermittently, with a normal appetite and little or no weight loss. Foreign bodies (depending on their surface characteristics and size) may cause acute gastritis, or gastric outflow obstruction with frequent vomiting unassociated with eating, or vomiting several hours after a meal. Hair balls (trichobezoars) in the stomach of cats can cause retching and gagging, vomiting, inappetence, and loss of condition. Signs of intestinal foreign bodies depend on the location, duration, and extent of obstruction; most consistent are vomiting, depression, and anorexia. Abdominal distention, diarrhea, and abdominal pain may also occur. Frequently, the foreign object can be outlined or the typical firm "sausage-shaped" intussusception palpated. Signs of complete duodenal obstruction are nausea, vomiting of bile, abdominal pain, anorexia, dehydration, depression, and weakness. Electrolyte and water loss is rapid. Intestinal rupture, peritonitis, and endotoxic shock are complications of small-bowel obstruction.

Obstruction in the distal small bowel may be tolerated longer than proximal obstruction. The vomitus is feces-like and the onset of dehydration and weakness may be delayed. Abdominal distention develops slowly. Gas- and-fluid-filled loops of bowel or a tender abdominal mass may be palpated.

Partial intestinal obstruction causes prolonged or intermittent signs similar to distal small bowel obstruction. The animal exhibits reduced food and water intake and chronic weight loss, yet remains alert. The feces are reduced in volume, fluid, bloody, and putrid. Transient response to previous antibiotic therapy may have been noted.

Diagnosis: A history of chewing foreign objects, anorexia, vomiting, dehydration, and constipation, and palpation of dilated gut loops or foreign objects suggest intestinal obstruction. If abdominal tenderness prevents palpation, use of meperidine may cause sufficient relaxation. Normal peristaltic sounds cannot be auscultated, but borborygmi can be heard in the dilated loops of gut. Radiopaque foreign objects, empty loops of gut dilated with gas, or gas-capped fluid at different levels of the dilated intestine are seen anterior to the obstruction on radiographs. The increased soft-tissue density of an intussusception may be seen. Radiolucent foreign bodies may be demonstrated by use of contrast media. Endoscopy is an excellent method for confirming the presence of a gastric foreign body.

Treatment: Intestinal obstruction can be a surgical emergency. Apomorphine may be given in a few selected cases to induce vomiting of small smooth foreign objects, but vomiting should not be induced if there is a chance the foreign body will lacerate, perforate, or obstruct the esophagus. Small objects can sometimes be removed during endoscopy using forceps or snares; care must be taken to avoid injuring the esophagus. Small sharp objects, such as needles, pins, or tacks, may pass safely through the GI tract. If this approach is taken, the animal should be observed carefully and fed a high-fiber diet and lubricants. Intestinal foreign bodies, especially if not passed within 48 hr, usually require surgical removal. Surgical removal of gastric foreign bodies is required if they will not pass or cannot be removed during gastroscopy. Fluid therapy and correction of electrolyte and acid-base imbalances should be done before surgery.

Medical treatment includes meperidine to relieve pain, and IV administration of fluids and electrolytes before and during surgery. Electrolyte and acid-base disturbances are not predictable, and appropriate laboratory tests are recommended. If blood-gas and pH data are not available, a balanced electrolyte solution with broad-spectrum antibiotics should be administered IV and continued postoperatively. When circulatory shock coexists, whole blood or plasma may be needed. Oral fluids and a bland, low-residue diet are gradually introduced after 1-3 days; a regular diet can be given in 5-7 days.

Hair balls in cats are usually passed with the feces after the administration of petrolatum or another petroleum-based product; 2-3 days of therapy may be required. Rarely, surgical removal is necessary.

ENDOCRINE SYSTEM

ENDOCRINE SYSTEM, INTRODUCTION

Endocrine glands are collections of specialized cells that synthesize, store, and release their secretions directly into the bloodstream. These sensing and signalling devices are located in the extracellular fluid and are capable of responding to changes in the internal and external environments to coordinate activities that maintain homeostasis. Endocrine secretions are proteins, peptides, steroids, catecholamines, or iodothyronine hormones that are transported by the blood to influence the functional activity of target cells elsewhere in the body. Other populations of cells are concerned with degradation of hormone after it has exerted its physiologic function. Degradation is accomplished by peptidases on the cell surface, by lysosomal enzymes after uptake by cells, or by excretion in the bile or urine after conjugation with glucuronide or sulfate.

Endocrine glands are small compared with other body organs; they are richly supplied with blood, and there is a close anatomical relationship between the endocrine cells and the capillary network.

TYPES OF HORMONES

Polypeptide Hormones: The primary site of action for polypeptide hormones is the outer surface of the plasma membrane of target cells, which contains receptor proteins for the hormone. These hormones are water soluble, have a short half-life in blood (usually measured in minutes), and usually lack specific plasma-binding proteins. The hormone receptors perform 2 key functions: 1) they recognize minute quantities of active hormone and bind this to the receptor site to form a reversible hormone-receptor complex, and 2) they convey the message to the inside of the target cell. The magnitude of this signal depends on the hormone concentration, the affinity of the receptor for the hormone, and the concentration of receptors on the target cell.

Once attached to the receptor, the polypeptide hormones transmit their signal across the cell membrane and cause a second messenger, often cyclic adenosine monophosphate (cAMP), to be released inside the cell. This second messenger normally has effects that are unique to the cell because the target cells have very specific functions.

Cells that produce polypeptide hormones have a well-developed endoplasmic reticulum with many attached ribosomes where the hormone is assembled, and a prominent Golgi apparatus for packaging hormones into granules for intracellular storage and transport. Secretory granules are unique to polypeptide-hormone- and catecholamine-secreting endocrine cells, and provide a mechanism for intracellular storage of substantial amounts of preformed active hormone. Hormone synthesized in excess of the body's requirement is degraded by fusion of the hormone-containing granules with lysosomes.

Steroid Hormones: Steroid-hormone-secreting cells are characterized by large lipid bodies in the cytoplasm that contain cholesterol and other precursor molecules. Continued biosynthesis is necessary to maintain the normal secretory rate of steroid hormones.

Steroid hormones have a long half-life in blood (typically measured in hours) and bind reversibly to high-affinity, specific binding proteins in plasma. They are lipid soluble, and therefore move readily through the cell membrane; their primary site of action is the nucleus of target cells.

Catecholamine and Iodothyronine: These hormones are tyrosine derivatives. They include the catecholamines (epinephrine, norepinephrine) secreted by the adrenal medulla, and the iodothyronines (thyroxine, triiodothyronine) produced by the thyroid gland. Catecholamines share similar mechanisms of action with polypeptide hormones, whereas iodothyronines more closely resemble the characteristics of steroid hormones.

PROLIFERATIVE LESIONS IN ENDOCRINE GLANDS

Neoplasms derived from hormone-secreting endocrine cells usually consist of one predominant cell type and may be associated with the hypersecretion of one or more hormones. However, immunocytochemical and electron microscopical investigations suggest that some endocrine tumors are composed of more than one type of neoplastic cell and are capable of synthesizing multiple hormones.

The histological classification between focal (nodular) hyperplasia, adenoma, or carcinoma often is difficult in endocrine glands since in many (especially thyroid C-cells, secretory cells of the adrenal medulla, and specific tropic-hormone-secreting cells of the adenohypophysis), there appears to be a continuous spectrum of proliferative lesions between diffuse or focal hyperplasia and adenomas derived from a specific population of cells. Prolonged stimulation of a population of secretory endocrine cells appears to predispose to subsequent development of a higher than expected incidence of tumors. Long-term stimulation may lead to development of clones of cells within the hyperplastic endocrine gland, which grow more rapidly than the rest, and are more susceptible to neoplastic transformation when exposed to the right combination of carcinogens or are more likely to undergo spontaneous mutations.

Many neoplasms derived from endocrine glands are functionally active, secrete excess hormone either continuously or episodically, and cause dramatic clinical syndromes of hormone excess. Classical examples include the hypoglycemia of insulin-secreting neoplasms of the pancreatic islets in dogs, hyperthyroidism associated with adenomas and nodular hyperplasia of thyroid follicular cells in cats, hypercalcitoninism in bulls with thyroid C-cell tumors, and hypercortisolism in dogs associated either with adrenocorticotropic hormone (ACTH)-secreting pituitary adenomas or neoplasms of the adrenal cortex. Quantitation of hormone levels in serum or plasma in the basal, suppressed, or stimulated state, and the measurement of hormonal metabolites in the urine over a 24-hr period of excretion are essential to confirm that an endocrine tumor is functional.

MECHANISMS OF ENDOCRINE DISEASE

Disorders of the endocrine system are encountered in many animal species and are challenging diagnostic problems. The following examples are the major mechanisms responsible for disturbances of endocrine function that result in clinically important diseases in animals. For each category, several specific disease problems are used to illustrate the response of a particular endocrine gland to the disruption of function.

Many diseases of the endocrine system are characterized by dramatic functional disturbances and characteristic clinicopathologic alterations affecting one or several body systems. These changes may involve primarily the skin (hair loss caused by hypothyroidism), nervous system (seizures caused by hyperinsulinism), urinary system (polyuria caused by diabetes mellitus, diabetes insipidus, or hypercortisolism), or skeletal system (fractures induced by hyperparathyroidism or hypercortisolism). If the underlying endocrine problem is recognized early in the course of the disease, it often is amenable either to surgical removal of the source of excess hormone production, or to supplementation of the specific hormone secreted in inadequate amounts by the diseased gland.

Primary Hyperfunction of an Endocrine Gland: This is one of the most important and common pathological mechanisms. A neoplasm derived from endocrine cells often synthesizes and secretes hormone at an autonomous rate in excess of the body's ability to utilize and subsequently degrade the hormone, thereby resulting in functional disturbances of hormone excess. Several examples that occur in different animal species are summarized in TABLE 1, below.

The autonomous secretion of parathyroid hormone (PTH) results in progressive and generalized demineralization of the skeleton, leading to hypercalcemia, which results in soft-tissue mineralization and development of renal calculi. The accelerated osteoclastic resorption of bone results in marked thinning and tunneling of cortical bone, and predisposes bone to pathological fractures.

The autonomous hypersecretion of thyroxine (T_4) and triiodothyronine (T_3) is being recognized with increasing frequency in cats (*see* HYPERTHYROIDISM, p 284), and is associated with a spectrum of proliferative lesions of follicular cells. Functional thyroid lesions in cats are potentially malignant because a low percentage are adenocarcinomas that may metastasize to regional lymph nodes.

Table 1. Examples of Primary Hyperfunction of Endocrine Glands

Disease	Hormone Secreted in Excess	Species Most Frequently Affected	Principal Lesion or Functional Disturbances
Chief cell adenoma or carcinoma	Parathyroid hormone	Dog	Generalized osteitis fibrosa
Thyroid C-cell adenoma or carcinoma	Calcitonin	Bull	Vertebral osteosclerosis
β-Cell adenoma or carcinoma (Pancreatic islets)	Insulin	Dog	Hypoglycemia
Sertoli cell tumor (Testis)	Estrogens	Dog	Feminization of the male
Pheochromocytoma (Adrenal medulla)	Norepinephrine, epinephrine	Dog	Hypertension, hyperglycemia
Thyroid follicular cell adenoma or multinodular hyperplasia	Thyroxine, triiodothyronine	Cat	Increased metabolic rate, weight loss
Adrenal cortical adenoma or carcinoma	Cortisol	Dog	Cushing's syndrome

The functional disturbances of hyperactivity, weight loss despite increased appetite, hyperthermia, and tachycardia reflect chronic stimulation of multiple populations of target cells by the abnormally elevated blood levels of thyroid hormones.

Secondary Hyperfunction of an Endocrine Gland: A lesion in one organ results in the secretion of an excess of a tropic hormone that leads to chronic stimulation and hypersecretion of hormone by a target endocrine organ. The classical example is the ACTH-secreting tumor derived from pituitary corticotrophs in dogs (qv, p 274). The clinical signs and lesions in the animal result primarily from elevated blood cortisol levels associated with the ACTH-stimulated hypertrophy, and hyperplasia of the adrenal cortex. The syndrome of cortisol excess in dogs is characterized by progressive alopecia, hyperpigmentation, and muscle wasting caused by the protein catabolic effects of glucocorticoids. In some dogs, particularly Poodles, that have a similar marked adrenocortical enlargement and clinical evidence of cortisol excess, there is no evidence of a tumor in the pituitary gland. These dogs appear to have a change in their "set point" to the negative feedback signal (blood cortisol). This can be caused by an abnormal accumulation of certain neurotransmitter substances near neurons in the hypothalamus that secrete corticotropic-hormone-releasing factor. The end result is corticotroph hyperplasia, elevated ACTH levels in the blood, and chronic stimulation of the adrenal cortex, which result in hyperplasia of the adrenal cortex and the clinical syndrome of cortisol excess.

Primary Hypofunction of an Endocrine Gland: Hormone secretion is subnormal because of extensive destruction of secretory cells by a disease process, the failure of an endocrine gland to develop properly, or the result of a specific biochemical defect in hormone synthesis.

Immune-mediated injury causes hypofunction of several endocrine glands in animals, including the parathyroid, adrenal cortex, and thyroid. Thyroiditis caused by this mechanism is characterized by marked infiltration of lymphocytes and plasmacytes, and deposition of electron-dense immune complexes along the follicular basement membranes with progressive destruction of secretory parenchyma (*see* DISEASES INVOLVING IMMUNE COMPLEXES, p 430).

Failure of development also results in primary hypofunction of an endocrine gland. The classical example of this mechanism in animals is the failure of oropharyngeal ectoderm to differentiate completely into tropic-hormone-secreting cells of the adenohypophysis in dogs, resulting in pituitary dwarfism and a failure to attain somatic maturation. A large, multicompartmented cyst is present on the ventral aspect of the brain in the pituitary region of these dogs. The cyst compresses the normally developed neurohypophysis and results in disturbances of water metabolism. (*See also* THE PITUITARY GLAND, p 273).

Another form of primary hypofunction is a failure of hormone synthesis caused by a genetically determined defect in a biosynthetic pathway or lack of a specific enzyme. A well-documented example of this is vitamin-D-dependent rickets in pigs. It is caused by the lack of an enzyme in the proximal convoluted tubules of the kidney, which is needed to synthesize the hormonal form of vitamin D. Blood calcium and phosphorus levels progressively decrease due to the subnormal ability of the pig to produce the biologically active, hormonal form of vitamin D (1,25-dihydroxycholecalciferol) in the kidney. The lowered blood concentrations of calcium and phosphorus lead to failure of mineralization of osteoid, overgrowth of cartilage in the physes, and associated severe skeletal deformities.

Congenital dyshormonogenetic goiter in sheep, goats, and cattle is another example of primary hypofunction caused by failure of hormone synthesis. The low blood T_4 and T_3 levels and clinical evidence of severe hypothyroidism in these animals are due to an inability of follicular cells to synthesize thyroglobulin. The molecular defect is due to defective processing of the primary transcripts for thyroglobulin messenger ribonucleic acid (mRNA) and aberrant transport of mRNA from the nucleus to the ribosomes. This results in subnormal amounts of thyroglobulin mRNA in follicular cells, particularly mRNA that is attached to membranes of the endoplasmic reticulum in the cytoplasm.

Secondary Hypofunction of an Endocrine Gland: A destructive lesion in one organ, such as the pituitary, interferes with secretion of tropic hormone. This results in hypofunction of the target endocrine glands. Large, endocrinologically inactive, pituitary neoplasms in adult dogs, cats, and other species may interfere with the secretion of the several pituitary tropic hormones and result in clinically detectable hypofunction of the adrenal cortex, follicular cells of the thyroid, and gonads. The adrenal cortex of animals with a large pituitary neoplasm of this type has marked atrophy and degeneration of the ACTH-dependent inner zones; however, the aldosterone-secreting zona glomerulosa, which is not under direct ACTH control, remains intact. Thyroid function may be subnormal due to a lack of thyrotropin and atrophy of follicular cells, but the calcitonin-secreting C-cells function normally since they are not controlled by pituitary tropic hormones.

Endocrine Hyperactivity Secondary to Diseases of Other Organs: The best characterized example of this is the hyperparathyroidism that develops secondary to chronic renal failure or nutritional imbalances. In the renal form, the early retention of phosphorus and subsequent progressive destruction of cells in the proximal convoluted tubules interfere with the metabolic activation of vitamin D by an enzyme in the kidney. This rate-limiting step in the metabolic activation of vitamin D is tightly controlled by PTH and several other factors. The impaired intestinal absorption of calcium results in development of progressive hypocalcemia, which leads to chronic parathyroid stimulation and subsequent development of generalized demineralization of the skeleton. Many bones, particularly the cancellous bone of the skull, become weakened and more susceptible to fractures.

Nutritional hyperparathyroidism (*see also* p 483) develops in animals fed abnormal diets that are low in calcium, high in phosphorus, or (for certain nonhuman primates) deficient in cholecalciferol (vitamin D_3). Unsupplemented all-meat diets fed to carnivores fail to supply the daily requirements for calcium, leading to progressive hypocalcemia that stimulates parathyroid gland activity. The normal kidneys in these animals respond to the increased PTH by increasing phosphorus excretion and lowering the blood phosphorus level.

Hypersecretion of Hormones or Hormone-like Substances by Nonendocrine Tumors: The hypersecretion by nonendocrine tumors of "hormone-like humoral substances" that share chemical or biological (or both) similarities with the native hormone secreted by the endocrine gland has been recognized in animals including man. Most of these humoral factors secreted by nonendocrine tumors are peptides. Steroids and iodothyronines require more complex biosynthetic pathways and do not appear to be secreted by nonendocrine tumors. A classical example of this disease mechanism is the adenocarcinoma derived from apocrine glands of the anal sac in dogs. This tumor produces a humoral substance termed "PTH-related peptide" that stimulates target cells in bone and kidney. The resulting accelerated mobilization of calcium from bone by osteoclasts leads to development of persistent hypercalcemia, even though the parathyroid glands are smaller than normal and composed of inactive chief cells, and circulating PTH levels are subnormal. This neoplasm develops predominantly in older female dogs, is composed of solid and glandular areas, and is distinct from the commonly occurring perianal gland tumor in male dogs.

Following surgical removal of the apocrine adenocarcinoma, the serum calcium and phosphorus levels return to normal, immunoreactive PTH levels increase rapidly, and the active vitamin D metabolite levels in blood decrease.

Endocrine Dysfunction Due to Failure of Target Cell Response: Steroid and iodothyronine hormones penetrate the cell membrane, bind to cytosolic receptors, and are transported to the nucleus where they interact with the genetic information in the cell to increase new protein synthesis. Polypeptide and catecholamine hormones bind to receptors on the surface of target cells and activate a membrane-bound enzyme that generates an intracellular messenger (cAMP) to elicit the physiological response.

Failure of target cells to respond to hormone may be due to a lack of adenylate cyclase in the cell membrane or to an alteration in hormone receptors on the cell surface. Hormone is secreted in normal or increased amounts by cells of the endocrine gland. Certain forms of insulin-resistance associated with obesity result from a decrease in the number of receptors on the surface target cells. This develops in response to the chronic increased insulin secretion stimulated by the hyperglycemia resulting from excess food intake. Secretory cells in the corresponding endocrine gland (pancreatic islets) undergo compensatory hypertrophy and hyperplasia in an attempt to secrete additional insulin. The normal pancreatic islets contain predominantly granulated β cells, whereas the β cells in the enlarged islets from an obese diabetic animal are markedly hyperplastic and depleted of insulin-containing secretory granules.

Failure of Fetal Endocrine Function: Subnormal function of the fetal endocrine system, especially in ruminants, may disrupt normal fetal development and result in prolonged gestation. In some breeds of cattle, a genetically determined failure of the adenohypophysis to develop (although the neurohypophysis develops normally) results in a lack of fetal pituitary tropic hormone secretion during the last trimester and hypoplastic development of target endocrine organs, such as adrenal cortex, gonads, and follicular cells of the thyroid gland. Fetal development is normal up to ~7 mo, but subsequently ceases, irrespective of how long the viable fetus is retained in the uterus.

Gestation in sheep is prolonged after maternal ingestion early in gestation of a plant that results in extensive malformations of the CNS and hypothalamus in the lamb. Although the adenohypophysis is present, it lacks the necessary fine control derived from the releasing hormones of the hypothalamus to be able to secrete normal amounts of tropic hormones (eg, adrenocorticotropin). (*See* PROLONGED GESTATION IN CATTLE AND SHEEP, p 694.)

The concepts that have emerged from the study of these 2 syndromes are: 1) fetal hormones are necessary for final growth and development *in utero* in certain animals, and 2) normal parturition at term in these species requires an intact fetal hypothalamic-adenohypophyseal-adrenocortical axis working in concert with trophoblasts of the placenta.

Although the presence or absence of functional adenohypophyseal tissue determines whether the fetus continues to grow *in utero*, the pathogenesis of prolongation of gestation is similar in these 2 examples. The subnormal development of the fetal adrenal cortex in calves and lambs results in an inadequate secretion of cortisol and a failure of induction of the 17-hydroxylase in the placenta that converts precursor molecules, such as progesterone, to estrogens. As a result, the circulating progesterone levels in the dam remain high, and the marked increase in estrogens necessary for parturition and normally seen at term does not occur. The normal estrogen surge at parturition stimulates the synthesis of prostaglandins in the uterus, which cause smooth muscle contractions and biochemical changes in collagen along the birth canal that permit delivery of the fetus.

Endocrine Dysfunction Resulting from Abnormal Degradation of Hormone: In animals with abnormal degradation of hormone, the secretion of hormone by an endocrine gland is normal but blood levels are elevated persistently. A decreased rate of degradation simulates a state of hypersecretion. Chronic renal disease in animals may be associated with subnormal, normal, or elevated blood concentrations of calcium. The hypercalcemia associated with certain forms of renal disease may be related, in part, to diminished degradation of PTH along with decreased urinary excretion of calcium by the diseased kidney. Biologically active PTH is degraded in the kidney either by peptidases on the surface of tubular cells or by lysosomal enzymes after uptake of the hormone from the glomerular filtrate.

Iatrogenic Syndromes of Hormone Excess: The administration of large doses of exogenous hormone, either directly or indirectly, can influence the activity of target cells and result in clinical disturbances. Prolonged daily administration of potent preparations of adrenal corticosteroids at inappropriate doses in the symptomatic treatment of various diseases will reproduce most of the functional disturbances associated with endogenous hypersecretion of cortisol. These disturbances include muscle weakness, marked hair loss, and thinning of and mineral deposition in the skin. The elevated blood levels of exogenous cortisol result in marked atrophy of the adrenal cortex.

The administration of certain progestogens has been reported to result indirectly in a syndrome of hormone excess. The injection of medroxyprogesterone acetate for the prevention of estrus in dogs stimulates increased secretion of growth hormone, resulting in many of the clinical manifestations of acromegaly. The excess skin folds, expansion of interdental spaces, and abdominal enlargement in dogs with iatrogenic acromegaly are related to the protein anabolic effects of growth hormone on connective tissues.

THE ADRENAL GLANDS

The adrenal glands of mammals are located near the cranial pole of the kidneys, and consist of 2 distinct parts that differ in morphology, function, and origin. Because of their close structural relationship, the outer cortex and inner medulla of the adrenal gland are considered parts of one organ.

ADRENAL CORTEX

The adrenal cortex is subdivided into 3 layers or zones, although the demarcation between zones often is not distinct. The zona glomerulosa (multiformis) is the outer cortical zone. It is responsible for the secretion of mineralocorticoid hormones. The zona fasciculata, the middle zone, comprises ~70% of the cortex and is composed of cells that contain abundant cytoplasmic lipid and the glucocorticoid hormones. The zona reticularis accounts for the remaining 15% of the cortex; this inner layer is responsible for the secretion of sex steroids by the adrenal gland.

Mineralocorticoids, of which the most potent naturally occurring one is aldosterone, are adrenal steroids that have their principal effects on ion transport by epithelial cells, resulting in a loss of potassium and conservation of sodium. Sweat glands and the enzymatically controlled electrolyte "pumps" in epithelial cells of the renal tubule respond to mineralocorticoids by conserving sodium and chloride, and by excreting potassium. In the distal convoluted tubule of the mammalian nephron, a cation-exchange mechanism resorbs sodium from the glomerular filtrate, and secretes potassium into the lumen. These reactions are accelerated by mineralocorticoids, and proceed more slowly in their absence. A lack of secretion of mineralocorticoids (eg, in the Addison's-like disease of dogs) may result in a lethal retention of potassium and loss of sodium.

Cortisol and lesser amounts of corticosterone are the most important glucocorticoid hormones secreted by the adrenal gland in many species. In general, the actions of glucocorticoids on carbohydrate, protein, and lipid metabolism result in sparing of glucose, and a tendency to hyperglycemia and increased glucose production. In addition, they decrease lipogenesis and increase lipolysis in adipose tissue, which results in release of glycerol and free fatty acids.

Glucocorticoids also suppress both inflammatory and immunologic responses and thereby attenuate the associated tissue destruction and fibroplasia. However, high levels of glucocorticoids reduce resistance to bacteria, viruses, and fungi, and favor the spread of infections. Glucocorticoids may impair the immunologic response at any stage from the initial interaction and processing of antigens by cells of the reticuloendothelial system, through the induction and proliferation of immunocompetent lymphocytes and subsequent antibody production. Inhibition of a number of lymphoid cell functions forms part of the basis for immunosuppression.

Glucocorticoids can exert a profound negative effect on wound healing. High therapeutic levels of adrenal corticosteroids or the syndrome of hypercortisolism may cause wound dehiscence after surgery. The basic mechanism involved is an inhibition of fibroblast proliferation and collagen synthesis, leading to a decrease in scar tissue formation.

Progesterone, estrogens, and androgens are adrenal sex hormones. Excess secretion may be associated with a neoplasm of the zona reticularis. The manifestation of virilism, precocious sexual development, or feminization depends on which steroid is secreted in excess, sex of the individual, and age of onset.

HYPERADRENOCORTICISM
(Cortisol excess, Cushing's syndrome, Cushing's disease)

The clinical signs and lesions associated with hyperadrenocorticism result primarily from chronic elevation of cortisol. Cortisol excess is one of the most frequent endocrinopathies in adult to aged dogs but is infrequent in other domestic animals. Affected dogs develop a spectrum of functional disturbances and lesions from the combined glyconeogenic, lipolytic, protein catabolic, and anti-inflammatory effects of the glucocorticoid hormones on many organ systems. The disease is insidious and slowly progressive.

Etiology and Pathogenesis: The elevation in circulating cortisol levels in dogs may result from one of several pathogenic mechanisms; the most common is a functional corticotroph (adrenocorticotropic hormone [ACTH]-secreting) adenoma of the pituitary gland (pars distalis or pars intermedia), which causes bilateral adrenal cortical hypertrophy and hyperplasia. Hypercortisolism associated with idiopathic adrenal cortical hyperplasia occurs more frequently in Poodles than in other breeds. The cortex of both adrenal glands is thickened considerably. Functional adrenal neoplasms are an infrequent (10-15% of cases) cause of the Cushing's-like syndrome of cortisol excess in dogs. Many of the signs and lesions of naturally occurring hyperadrenocorticism can be induced by long-term, daily administration of large doses of corticosteroids for the treatment of other diseases. To differentiate between the pathogenic mechanisms that can result in the syndrome of cortisol excess, plasma cortisol levels must be evaluated in the basal (resting) state and in response to dexamethasone (high or low dose) and exogenous ACTH stimulation.

Clinical Findings and Lesions: Appetite and food intake often are increased either as a direct result of the hypercortisolism, or the involvement of hypothalamic appetite centers by a large pituitary tumor. The muscles of the extremities and abdomen are weakened and atrophied, with gradual abdominal enlargement, lordosis, muscle trembling, and a straight-legged skeletal-braced posture. Hepatomegaly due to increased fat and glycogen deposition may contribute to the distended, often pendulous, abdomen. The muscular asthenia and wasting is the result of increased catabolism and structural proteins, combined with diminished protein synthesis under the influence of chronic cortisol excess.

Skin lesions occur frequently in dogs with hyperadrenocorticism, initially observed over points of wear (eg, neck, flanks, behind the ears, and over bony prominences). These spread bilaterally and symmetrically to involve a significant portion of the body surface. There is atrophy of the epidermis and pilosebaceous apparatus, combined with loss of collagen and elastin in the dermis and subcutis. The skin is of fine texture, and most of the hair follicles are inactive. The epidermis is markedly thinned and consists of only 1-2 cell layers. However, the stratum corneum is considerably thickened owing to the accumulation of multiple layers of keratin on the surface; these keratin aggregations may become extensive and appear as large interlapping plates.

Cutaneous mineralization is a characteristic lesion in dogs (~30-40%) with hypercortisolism. Although mineral deposition may occur anywhere in the skin, the dorsal midline, ventral abdomen, and inguinal region are affected most frequently. Numerous mineral crystals are deposited along collagen and elastin fibers in the dermis and outer subcutis, and may protrude through the atrophic and thinned epidermis. The epidermis remains intact in less severe cases and appears irregularly elevated by the firm, opaque, white deposits of mineral. A narrow rim of hyperemia and foreign-body granulomatous inflammation often surrounds the areas of mineralization. The mineral deposits occur despite normal blood calcium and phosphorus levels, probably because of the glyconeogenic and protein catabolic action of cortisol. Severe mineralization also occurs in several other tissues of the body, most frequently the lungs and sometimes active skeletal muscles and the stomach wall.

In addition to corticotroph (ACTH-secreting) adenomas in the pituitary, cortisol excess may result from an adrenal cortical tumor.

Adenomas of the adrenal cortex are seen most frequently in old dogs and sporadically in horses, cattle, and sheep. Cortical adenomas are well-demarcated, usually single nodules in one adrenal gland, but may be bilateral. Larger cortical adenomas are yellow to red, distort the external contour of the affected gland, and are partially or completely encapsulated. Adjacent cortical parenchyma is compressed, and the tumor may extend into the medulla.

Adrenal cortical carcinomas occur less frequently than adenomas and have been reported most often in adult to older cattle and dogs, and with no apparent breed or sex prevalence. Adrenal carcinomas are larger then adenomas and more likely to be bilateral. In dogs, they are composed of a variegated, yellow-red, friable tissue that incorporates the affected adrenal gland. They often are fixed in location because of extensive invasion of surrounding tissues and into the posterior vena cava (forming a large tumor-cell thrombus). Carcinomas may attain considerable size in cattle (up to 10 cm or more in diameter), have multiple areas of mineralization or ossification, and usually completely obliterate the affected adrenal.

Some carcinomas and adenomas of the adrenal cortex in dogs are functional and secrete excess cortisol. They may compress adjacent organs, invade the aorta or posterior vena cava leading to intra-abdominal hemorrhage, and metastasize to distant sites (eg, liver, kidneys, mesenteric lymph nodes, and lungs). Functional cortical adenomas and carcinomas are associated with profound atrophy of the contralateral cortex because of inhibition of pituitary ACTH secretion by the elevated blood cortisol levels. The adrenal medulla appears expanded and is relatively more conspicuous because of the lack of cortical parenchyma.

Diagnosis: Several laboratory procedures are available to assist in the diagnosis of hypercortisolism. Involution of lymphoid tissue results in a significant lymphopenia. There is intravascular destruction of eosinophils and sequestration of circulating eosinophils in the lungs and spleen, which lead to eosinopenia. In many dogs, the total WBC count is elevated moderately, and the percentage of neutrophils is increased. Because the life span of neutrophils in the circulation is prolonged, the nuclei may become hypersegmented.

Dogs with hyperadrenocorticism usually have normal serum concentrations of sodium, potassium, and chloride, although a consistent finding is the excretion of large volumes of dilute urine with a low specific gravity (≤ 1.007). Because cortisol excess stimulates the synthesis and release of an isoenzyme of alkaline phosphatase, markedly elevated levels of alkaline phosphatase are usually observed. Blood glucose is moderately elevated and, occasionally, marked hyperglycemia develops. The serum concentration of cholesterol may be elevated to 250-400 mg/dL.

The most direct and sensitive test for diagnosis and elucidation of the pathogenesis is measurement of plasma cortisol levels by accurate and sensitive radioimmunoassay techniques. Resting levels of cortisol in normal dogs are 1-5 $\mu g/dL$; however, because baseline levels in dogs with cortisol excess often fall within this range, stimulation and suppression tests are essential to make an accurate diagnosis. If the adrenal cortices are hyperplastic or have benign neoplasms that remain under tropic control, plasma cortisol levels increase markedly within 90 min of ACTH administration.

Another diagnostic test is the dexamethasone suppression test in combination with ACTH stimulation. In normal dogs and in those with idiopathic adrenal cortical hyperplasia, plasma cortisol is reduced to <1 $\mu g/dL$ 8 hr after IM injection of dexamethasone at 0.01 mg/kg body wt. Only partial suppression of plasma cortisol occurs in dogs with adrenal cortical hyperplasia associated with functional pituitary tumors following administration of dexamethasone; no significant suppression of plasma cortisol levels occurs in dogs with functional adrenal cortical tumors. A high-dose dexamethasone suppression test (1 mg/kg, IM) may be helpful in separating questionable cases of cortisol excess in dogs caused by functional pituitary tumors from those caused by an adrenal cortical tumor. Cortisol levels in most dogs with pituitary tumors become depressed at this higher dose of dexamethasone, whereas there is no depression in dogs with functional adrenal cortical tumors.

Treatment: Dogs with laboratory confirmed hyperadrenocorticism can be treated medically or surgically. Dogs with the syndrome of cortisol excess caused by diffuse cortical hyperplasia (corticotroph adenoma of pituitary or idiopathic adrenal hyperplasia) can be managed medically by the oral administration of the drug mitotane (o,p'DDD). The recommended treatment schedule involves initial administration at 50 mg/kg/day for 5-10 days. If the dog has polydipsia, monitoring the water consumption is helpful in regulating the dosage. When water intake decreases markedly, the daily administration of the drug is stopped, and a maintenance dose of 50 mg/kg is administered once a week to prevent recurrence of clinical signs.

There is a considerable range of individual sensitivity to mitotane in dogs; owners should be warned of the possibility of overt hypoadrenocorticism developing after several months of treatment so they will be alert for suggestive signs, eg, vomiting and diarrhea. Some dogs require gradually increasing doses of the drug to maintain adequate clinical remission, but others appear to become progressively more sensitive with long-term administration. Thus, dogs should be closely monitored during therapy. The use of baseline cortisol measurements in combination with ACTH stimulation is helpful in establishing that the drug has destroyed a sufficient portion of the cortisol-secreting cells.

Clinical signs of cortisol excess are reversed rapidly in dogs treated with mitotane. Reduction in water consumption, frequency of urination, and appetite are the initial responses to therapy. Muscle strength and physical activity increase within a few weeks and substantial hair regrowth usually occurs in 1-3 mo. The levels of plasma cortisol decline progressively. The exaggerated increase in plasma corticosteroids as a response to ACTH stimulation in dogs with adrenal cortical hyperplasia is eliminated after treatment with mitotane. The weekly doses of mitotane must be continued for the life of the dog to prevent recurrence of the functional disturbances and lesions of hypercortisolism. If the intermittent doses of mitotane are discontinued, small nests of viable cortical cells will regenerate, and the functional disturbances and the biochemical alterations will return.

Side effects of mitotane at the recommended dose levels are usually mild. Clinical signs of GI irritation, including vomiting and anorexia, are encountered in some dogs. CNS disturbances, mild hypoglycemia, and a moderate increase in serum alkaline phosphatase levels have been observed. If signs such as depression or ataxia develop, dividing the daily dose into 2 equal parts and administering at 8- to 12-hr intervals usually alleviates these side effects.

Dose levels of mitotane that are effectively cytotoxic to hyperplastic adrenal cortices will not destroy functional adrenal cortical adenomas and carcinomas in dogs. Higher dose levels of the drug are toxic to several parenchymal organs.

When there is evidence of an adrenal cortical tumor, the recommended treatment is removal of the affected gland. Both glands should be visualized at surgery to eliminate the possibility of bilateral tumors. Careful medical management before, during, and after surgery is of major importance. Even if a unilateral adrenalectomy is performed, the dog will have functional adrenal cortical insufficiency after surgery because of long-term adrenal cortical atrophy of the contralateral adrenal gland. A corticosteroid with high mineralocorticoid activity (such as desoxycorticosterone acetate [DOCA]) and prednisolone are administered for 24-48 hr before surgery. During surgery, IV administration of prednisolone sodium succinate dissolved in 5% dextrose and 0.9% saline solution should be administered. Serum sodium and potassium levels are monitored carefully after surgery, and DOCA is continued if necessary to maintain a normal sodium:potassium ratio. The dog should be monitored closely for shock after surgery and treated appropriately with cortisol or prednisolone. The continual use of glucocorticoids or mineralocorticoids probably is not necessary after the acute postsurgical stage unless bilateral adrenalectomy was performed.

HYPOADRENOCORTICISM
(Addison's disease)

A deficiency in adrenocortical hormones is seen most commonly in young to middle-aged dogs and occasionally in horses. The cause of primary adrenocortical failure usually is not known, although most cases probably result from an autoimmune process. Other causes can be destruction of the adrenal gland by granulomatous disease, metastatic tumor, hemorrhage, infarction, or overdose of mitotane.

Clinical Findings: Many of the functional disturbances of chronic adrenal insufficiency are not highly specific and include recurrent episodes of gastroenteritis, a slowly progressive loss of body condition, and failure to respond appropriately to stress. Although hypoadrenocorticism occurs in dogs of any breed, sex, or age, idiopathic adrenocortical insufficiency occurs most frequently in young adults. This may be related to its suspected immune-mediated pathogenesis.

A reduction in secretion of aldosterone, the principal mineralocorticoid, results in marked alterations of serum levels of potassium, sodium, and chloride. Potassium excretion by the kidneys is reduced, which results in a progressive rise in serum potassium levels, and less sodium and chloride are reabsorbed from renal tubules, which leads to a decline in their blood levels. The severe hyperkalemia causes a slow and irregular heart rate with alterations in the ECG. In some dogs, a pronounced bradycardia develops (heart rate ≤50/min), which is not responsive to exercise and predisposes to weakness or circulatory collapse after minimal exertion.

Although the development of clinical signs often is insidious and not readily apparent, frequently it leads to acute circulatory collapse and evidence of renal failure. A progressive decrease in blood volume contributes to hypotension, weakness, and microcardia. Peripheral circulatory collapse may result from the progressive hemoconcentration. Increased excretion of water by the kidneys, due to decreased reabsorption of sodium and chloride, results in progressive dehydration and hemoconcentration. Emesis, diarrhea, and anorexia are common and contribute to the animal's deterioration. Weight loss is frequently severe.

A decreased production of glucocorticoids results in several characteristic functional disturbances. Decreased gluconeogenesis and increased sensitivity to insulin contribute to the development of moderate hypoglycemia. Hyperpigmentation of the skin occurs in some dogs due to the lack of negative feedback on the pituitary gland and increased release of ACTH (and possibly melanocyte-stimulating hormone). The plasma cortisol levels in dogs with hypoadrenocorticism are 0.1-1.5 µg/dL, and there is little or no increase in blood cortisol levels following administration of ACTH.

Lesions: The most frequently observed lesion in dogs with hypoadrenocorticism is bilateral idiopathic adrenocortical atrophy, in which all layers of the cortex are markedly reduced in thickness. The adrenal cortex is reduced to one-tenth or less its normal thickness and consists primarily of the adrenal capsule. The adrenal medulla is relatively more prominent, and with the capsule, makes up the bulk of the remaining adrenal glands.

All 3 zones of the adrenal cortex are involved, including the zona glomerulosa (which is not under ACTH control), but no obvious pituitary lesions have been observed in dogs with idiopathic adrenal cortical atrophy.

A destructive pituitary lesion that decreases ACTH secretion is characterized by severe atrophy of the inner 2 cortical zones of the adrenal gland; the zona glomerulosa remains intact.

Diagnosis: For diagnosis, definitive evaluation of adrenal function is required. After obtaining a baseline blood sample, 1 u ACTH gel/lb body wt is administered IM and a second blood sample obtained 1-2 hr later. Affected dogs have low baseline cortisol levels, and there is little response to ACTH administration. This test can be completed in most animals before replacement hormone therapy is started.

A preliminary diagnosis and treatment of Addison's disease is based on the history and the presence of supportive, although not specific, laboratory abnormalities. These include hyponatremia, hyperkalemia, a sodium:potassium ratio of <25:1, azotemia, mild acidosis, and normocytic normochromic anemia. Occasionally, mild hypoglycemia is present. The hyperkalemia results in ECG changes as evidenced by an elevation (spiking) of the T wave, a flattening or absence of the P wave, a prolonged PR interval, and a widening of the QRS complex. Ventricular fibrillation or asystole may occur with potassium levels >11 mEq/L.

Differential diagnoses include primary GI disturbances, renal failure, acute pancreatitis, and ingestion of toxins.

Treatment: An adrenal crisis is an acute medical emergency. An IV catheter should be inserted and 0.9% saline infusion begun. If the dog is hypoglycemic and not dehydrated, the saline can include 5% dextrose. If the animal is dehydrated, 50% dextrose (0.45 mL/lb [1 mL/kg]) can be given separately over a 10-min period. If the animal is hypotensive, fluids should be given at 9-18 mL/lb/hr (20-40 mL/kg/hr) for the first 1-2 hr. Urine output should be assessed to be sure the dog is not anuric. Fluids should be continued at a rate of 23-27 mL/lb/day (50-60 mL/kg/day) until blood electrolytes, BUN, and hydration return to normal.

Prednisolone sodium succinate (2-10 mg/lb body wt [4.4-22 mg/kg]) or dexamethasone (1-2 mg/lb body wt [2.2-4.4 mg/kg]) should be given IV as soon as possible and prednisolone or prednisone continued (0.45 mg/lb [1 mg/kg], b.i.d., IM) for the next several days. The dose subsequently can be reduced to 0.11-0.22 mg/lb (0.25-0.5 mg/kg), b.i.d. The signs are mainly related to electrolyte imbalances, water loss, and the resultant circulatory problems. Therefore, it is essential that the mineralocorticoid desoxycorticosterone acetate (DOCA, 1-2 mg/10 lb [0.22-0.44 mg/kg]) be given IM early in the course of therapy and continued daily. Electrolytes should be monitored to prevent hypokalemia from developing due to the mineralocorticoid administration.

In cases of severe nonresponsive hyperkalemia, 10% glucose (2-5 mL/lb [4.4-11 mL/kg]) can be given over 30-60 min in the saline infusion to increase potassium movement into the cells. Regular insulin (0.125-0.5 u/lb [0.28-1.1 u/kg]) may be administered IM to enhance glucose and potassium uptake, but should be given with 20 mL (IV) of 10% glucose/unit insulin to avoid hypoglycemia. The acidosis in severely ill dogs can be treated by replacing 25% of the calculated deficit or administering 1 mEq sodium bicarbonate/lb (2.2 mEq/kg), IV, over the first 6 hr. Treatment of chronic Addison's disease is less intensive and may require only DOCA and prednisolone treatment. If the adrenal insufficiency is secondary to rapid withdrawal of glucocorticoid therapy, steroid treatment should be reinitiated and withdrawn in tapering doses after which no further treatment is necessary.

For long-term maintenance therapy, the mineralocorticoid fludrocortisone acetate is administered PO at 0.1-0.5 mg/day, depending on the size of the dog. Serum electrolytes should be monitored weekly until the proper dose is determined. Salt (NaCl) tablets (1-5 g) should be given once daily. Some dogs also require oral glucocorticoid treatment daily for optimal well-being. The dose for cortisone acetate is 0.45-0.9 mg/lb (1-2 mg/kg) body wt, and for prednisolone 0.09-0.18 mg/lb (0.2-0.4 mg/kg). Dogs with chronic hypoadrenocorticism should be reexamined q3-6mo.

Treatment of horses with the disease should take the same approach: aggressive replacement of fluids, steroids, and glucose if needed in an adrenal crisis. Supportive therapy and rest are indicated in cases of chronic Addison's disease.

ADRENAL MEDULLA

The adrenal medulla, although apparently not essential to life, plays an important role in response to stress or hypoglycemia. It secretes epinephrine and norepinephrine, which increase cardiac output, elevate blood pressure and blood glucose, and reduce GI activity.

Pheochromocytomas may develop in domestic animals, most often in cattle and dogs. These secrete either or both epinephrine and norepinephrine, and have caused increased heart rate, edema, and enlarged hearts in the few reported cases. Other tumors, such as neuroblastomas and ganglioneuromas, may arise in the medulla from cells of the sympathetic nervous system. Tumors arising elsewhere have also been reported, either from metastic or direct invasion. (*See also* p 288.)

THE PANCREAS

The endocrine function of the pancreas is performed by small groups of cells (islets of Langerhans) that are completely surrounded by acinar (exocrine) cells that produce digestive enzymes. A close relationship exists between the endocrine and exocrine portions (qv, p 120) of the pancreas during development. Evidence suggests that islet, acinar, and ductal cells arise from a common multipotential precursor cell.

Pancreatic islets of normal animals contain α, β, and δ cells, each of which synthesize a unique polypeptide hormone. β cells are the predominant secretory cells and synthesize insulin, α cells are less numerous than β cells and secrete glucagon, and δ cells secrete somatostatin. F-cells are present in islets of the uncinate process of dogs, but not in all animal species.

The pancreatic islets function as discrete microendocrine organs, and are embedded throughout the pancreas with a characteristic pattern of cellular interrelationships to assure an appropriate balance of hormones. In some species, the insulin-secreting β cells, which account for 60-70% of the islet-cell population, are located in a relatively homogeneous central mass. The glucagon-producing α cells are located primarily at the periphery of the islet in an external mantle. The somatostatin-secreting δ cells are interspersed between the outer layer of α cells and inner core of β cells. Afferent vessels and nerves enter the islet in this peripheral tricellular region. The close anatomic relationship of α, β, and δ cells in this heterogeneous cortical region may function as a local "glucose sensor", permitting a coordinated output of insulin and glucagon in response to fluctuations in blood glucose. Specialized tight junctions between membranes of adjacent endocrine cells tend to partition the intercellular space and may permit somatostatin to exert a direct local ("paracrine") restraint on glucagon secretion by α cells.

Insulin is formed initially as a single polypeptide chain of 81-86 amino acid residues. This prohormone (proinsulin) contains the A and B chains of the insulin molecule, plus a connecting peptide. Proinsulin is converted enzymatically to insulin before storage in membrane-limited secretory ("storage") granules, which are stored until there is an appropriate stimulus for secretion.

The major physiologic stimulus for the release of insulin from β cells is glucose. Specific "glucoreceptors" that bind with glucose exist on the plasma membrane of β cells. An appropriate level of extracellular fluid calcium ion is a requirement for insulin secretion. In certain hypocalcemic disorders (eg, parturient hypocalcemia in cows), insulin secretion may be inhibited owing to the low extracellular fluid calcium, and this can result in hyperglycemia.

Although change in the concentration of glucose in extracellular fluid is the principal physiologic stimulus for insulin release, other sugars (fructose, mannose, ribose), amino acids (leucine, arginine), hormones (glucagon, secretin), drugs (sulfonylurea, theophylline), short-chain fatty acids, and ketone bodies may also stimulate insulin secretion under certain conditions. Pancreatic β cells have the unique property of being able to respond to a specific physiologic stimulus with release of stored hormone in a modulated fashion, rather than releasing all of the stored hormone at once.

Insulin affects, either directly or indirectly, the function of every organ in the body. Tissues that are especially responsive to insulin include skeletal and cardiac muscle, adipose tissue, fibroblasts, liver, WBC, mammary glands, cartilage, bone, skin, aorta, pituitary gland, and peripheral nerves. The main function of insulin is to stimulate anabolic reactions involving carbohydrates, fats, proteins, and nucleic acids. It catalyzes the formation of macromolecules used in cell structure and energy stores, and it regulates many cell functions. Liver, adipose cells, and muscle are 3 principal target sites for insulin. In general, insulin increases the transfer of glucose and certain other monosaccharides, some amino acids and fatty acids, and potassium and magnesium ions across the plasma membrane of target cells; enhances glucose oxidation and glycogenesis; and stimulates lipogenesis and the formation of ATP, DNA, and RNA. Insulin also decreases the rate of lipolysis, proteolysis, ketogenesis, and gluconeogenesis.

Glucagon is secreted in response to a reduction in blood glucose. It promotes mobilization of stores of energy-yielding nutrients by increasing glycogenolysis, gluconeogenesis, and lipolysis. At physiologic concentrations, glucagon increases both hepatic glycogenolysis and gluconeogenesis, thereby elevating blood glucose.

Insulin and glucagon acting in concert function to maintain the concentration of glucose in extracellular fluids within relatively narrow limits. A "glucose sensor" in the pancreatic islets controls the relative amounts of insulin and glucagon secreted from the α and β cells. Glucagon controls glucose release from the liver into the extracellular space, and insulin controls glucose transport from the extracellular space into insulin-sensitive tissues such as fat, muscle, and liver.

DIABETES MELLITUS

A chronic disorder of carbohydrate metabolism due to relative or absolute insulin deficiency. Diabetes mellitus is a common endocrinopathy in dogs (reported incidence 1:200). Most cases of spontaneous diabetes occur in mature dogs, about twice as often in females as males. Incidence appears to be increased in certain small breeds of dogs such as Miniature Poodles, Dachshunds, Schnauzers, Cairn Terriers, and Beagles, but any breed can be affected.

Etiology and Pathogenesis: The pathogenic mechanisms responsible for the diminished available insulin are multiple, but usually they are related to destruction of islets secondary to severe pancreatitis or to selective degeneration of islet cells. In dogs, the pancreatic islets are often destroyed secondary to an inflammatory disease of the exocrine pancreas. Chronic relapsing pancreatitis with progressive loss of both exocrine and endocrine cells and their replacement by fibrous connective tissue is a frequent cause of diabetes mellitus; the pancreas becomes firm, multinodular, and often has scattered areas of hemorrhage and necrosis. Later in the course of disease, a thin fibrous band or nodule near the duodenum and stomach may be all that remains of the pancreas. Selective infiltration of islets with amyloid, glycogen, and collagen with destruction of islet cells are less frequent causes of diabetes mellitus in dogs than in cats. In other cases, the numbers of β cells are decreased, vacuolated, and if chronic, the islets are difficult to find. Insulin resistance and secondary diabetes mellitus are also seen in many dogs with hyperadrenocorticism, and chronic administration of glucocorticoids or progestogen can predispose to diabetes mellitus. Obesity also predisposes to insulin resistance in both dogs and cats.

Cats with diabetes mellitus usually have specific degenerative lesions localized selectively in the islets of Langerhans, whereas the remainder of the pancreas appears to be normal. The selective deposition of amyloid in islets, with degenerative changes in α and β cells, is the most common pancreatic lesion in cats with diabetes; however, scattered amyloid deposits in the pancreatic islets occur in many cats without development of overt clinical diabetes mellitus. Another common islet lesion in cats is hydropic vacuolar degeneration of the α and β cells. The cytoplasmic area of β cells is expanded by massive accumulation of glycogen, which displaces secretory organelles to the periphery of the β cell. This selective islet lesion has been observed in cats that were resistant to large doses of exogenous insulin. Vacuolar degeneration with glycogen accumulation in cats appears to develop in β cells as a response to chronic overstimulation (exhaustion) because of insulin resistance. Obese cats are particularly prone to this phenomenon.

Infection with certain viruses may cause selective islet damage or pancreatitis, and has been suggested to be responsible for certain cases of rapidly developing diabetes mellitus. The selective degeneration and necrosis of β cells is accompanied by infiltration of the islets by lymphocytes and macrophages. Stress, obesity, and administration of corticosteroids or progestogens may increase the severity of clinical signs.

Clinical Findings: The onset of diabetes is often insidious, and the clinical course chronic. Signs frequently associated with diabetes mellitus in dogs include polydipsia, polyuria, increased food consumption but loss of weight, bilateral cataracts, and weakness. The disturbances in water metabolism develop primarily due to an osmotic diuresis. In dogs with persistent hyperglycemia, the kidneys are unable to reabsorb all the glucose filtered, and consequently there is a glycosuria and exessive urine production.

Diabetic animals have diminished resistance to bacterial or fungal infections and often develop chronic or recurrent infections, such as suppurative cystitis, prostatitis, bronchopneumonia, and dermatitis. This increased susceptibility to infection may be related in part to impaired chemotactic, phagocytic, and microbicidal functions with decreased adherence of polymorphonuclear WBC. Radiographic evidence of emphysematous cystitis (rare) is suggestive of diabetes mellitus because of infections with glucose-fermenting organisms such as *Proteus* sp, *Aerobacter aerogenes*, and *Escherichia coli*, which result in gas formation in the wall and lumen of the bladder. Emphysema also may develop in the wall of the gallbladder in diabetic dogs.

Hepatomegaly due to lipid accumulation is common in diabetic dogs. The fatty liver results from increased fat mobilization from adipose tissue. Individual liver cells are greatly enlarged by the accumulation of multiple droplets of neutral lipid.

Cataracts develop frequently in animals with poorly controlled diabetes mellitus. The lenticular opacities appear initially along the suture lines of lens fibers and are stellate ("asteroid") in shape. Cataract formation in diabetic animals is related to the unique sorbitol pathway by which glucose is metabolized in the lens, which leads to lens edema and disruption of normal light transmission.

Other extra-pancreatic lesions associated with diabetes mellitus such as chronic renal disease, blindness, and gangrene of extremities are the result of chronic microangiopathy with thickening of the capillary basement membranes. These lesions occur in dogs and cats but are rarely of clinical importance.

Complete expression of the complex metabolic disturbances in diabetes mellitus appears to be the result of a bihormonal abnormality. Although a relative or absolute deficiency of insulin action in response to a rising extracellular glucose concentration has been long recognized as the major pathogenic factor, the importance of an absolute or relative increase of glucagon secretion has been appreciated more recently. Hyperglucagonemia in diabetes may be the result of increased secretion of pancreatic glucagon, enteroglucagon, or both. Increased blood glucagon appears to contribute to development of the severe endogenous hyperglycemia by mobilizing hepatic stores of glucose and to development of ketoacidosis by increasing the oxidation of fatty acids in the liver. The major glucoregulatory consequence of insulin deficiency is reduced glucose entry into insulin-dependent tissues (eg, fat and muscle) coupled with an increase in hepatic glucose production, resulting in marked hyperglycemia.

Diagnosis: Diabetes mellitus is diagnosed clinically by finding fasting hyperglycemia, glycosuria, and often a ketonemia in an animal with typical clinical signs. The normal fasting value for blood sugar in dogs is 75-120 mg/dL. Blood sugar levels consistently >120 mg/dL in fasting animals are present in diabetes mellitus, with >500 mg/dL having been reported.

Treatment: Long-term success depends on the understanding and cooperation of the owner. Mild diabetes is uncommonly recognized but may be controlled by a combination of weight reduction and a diet that is high in complex carbohydrates and fiber. Intact females should be neutered. A search should be made for drugs or diseases that predispose to diabetes. If diet and weight reduction do not control the disease, either protamine-zinc, ultralente, NPH, or lente insulin should be given, adjusting the dose until the disease is brought under control and the urine contains only intermittent traces of sugar. Maintenance doses are ~0.5-1 u/kg/day. Approximately 25% of the total daily calories is fed at the time of insulin administration, and the remaining 75% is fed 1-2 hr before the maximum insulin effect. If the administered insulin results in hypoglycemia, 5-20 g of glucose should be given PO or parenterally and the daily insulin dose reduced. Oral hypoglycemic agents rarely have value in the treatment of canine diabetes mellitus due to the presence of degenerative changes in β cells.

Ketoacidosis is a serious complication of diabetes mellitus and should be regarded as a medical emergency. The objectives of therapy include: correction of dehydration by the administration of IV fluids, such as 0.9% sodium chloride or lactated Ringer's solution; reduction of hyperglycemia and ketosis by the administration of crystalline zinc (regular) insulin; careful maintenance of serum electrolyte levels, especially potassium, through supplemental administration of appropriate electrolyte solutions; and identification and treatment of underlying and complicating diseases, such as acute pancreatitis or infections.

Numerous methods of managing the insulin therapy have been used in treatment of ketoacidotic diabetes mellitus. One method is an intermittent insulin regimen, in which 0.2 u/kg (0.1 u/lb) of regular insulin is administered IM as the initial dose, followed by the hourly administration of 0.1 u/kg (0.05 u/lb). Once the serum glucose is <250 mg/dL, the insulin is injected subcut. at a dosage between 0.1 and 0.4 u/kg, q4-6hr, with careful monitoring of the serum glucose q1-2hr. During aggressive treatment with insulin, blood glucose levels may fall rapidly, and require the addition of 2.5-5% dextrose to the IV fluids.

When insulin therapy has been instituted, the blood glucose should be checked frequently until an adequate maintenance dose has been determined. Once the animal is on maintenance therapy and its condition stable, it should be reassessed 2 or 3 times yearly.

FUNCTIONAL ISLET CELL TUMORS

The most frequent pancreatic islet tumor is an islet cell carcinoma derived from insulin-secreting β cells. These neoplasms frequently are endocrinologically active and secrete insulin inappropriate for the blood glucose concentration, which leads to hypoglycemia. Other pancreatic tumors appear to be derived from multipotential ductal epithelial cells, with differentiation into one of the several other cell types of the pancreatic islets that do not secrete insulin. β-Cell neoplasms of pancreatic islets are seen most frequently in dogs 5-12 yr old. They also are reported to occur in older cattle and may be associated with periodic convulsions.

Clinical Findings: The clinical alterations observed with functional β-cell tumors result from excessive insulin secretion, which leads to an increased rate of transfer of glucose from the extracellular fluid to body tissues, and thus to severe hypoglycemia. The clinical signs are a reflection of the hypoglycemia and are not specific for hyperinsulinism associated with β-cell neoplasms. Initial signs include posterior weakness, fatigue after exercise, generalized muscular twitching and weakness, ataxia, mental confusion, and changes of temperament. The dogs are easily agitated, and there are intermittent periods of excitability and restlessness. Periodic tonic-clonic convulsions occur later in the disease and increase progressively in frequency and intensity.

The disturbances with functional β-cell neoplasms characteristically are episodic and occur initially at widely spaced intervals, but become more frequent and prolonged as the disease progresses. Hypoglycemic attacks may be precipitated by physical exercise (increased glucose utilization) or fasting (decreased availability), as well as by ingestion of food (stimulation of insulin release). Administration of glucose rapidly alleviates the signs.

The predominance of clinical signs relating to the CNS demonstrates the primary dependence of the brain on the metabolism of glucose for energy. When the brain is not supplied with glucose, cerebral oxidation decreases and manifestations of anoxia appear.

Because dogs with functional islet cell tumors have clinical signs compatible with primary disease of the CNS, they may be misdiagnosed as having idiopathic epilepsy, brain tumors, or other organic neurological disease. Repeated episodes of prolonged and severe hypoglycemia may result in irreversible neuronal degeneration throughout the brain. Permanent neurologic disability probably accounts for the terminal coma, unresponsiveness to glucose, and eventual death of some dogs.

Lesions: Adenocarcinomas of the pancreatic islets, so-called insulinomas, usually appear as single, yellow to dark red, spherical, small (1-3 cm) nodules visible from the serosal surface. They are of similar consistency to, to slightly firmer than, the surrounding pancreatic parenchyma. Functional islet cell adenocarcinomas occur singly or occasionally as multiple nodules in the same or different lobes of the pancreas. A thin layer of fibrous connective tissue separates the neoplasm from the adjacent parenchyma. Islet cell adenocarcinomas frequently metastasize to regional lymph nodes and/or the liver before diagnosis. True benign adenomas of islet cells are rare.

Diagnosis: A blood glucose determination should be done on all older dogs with a history of periodic convulsions. The finding of fasting hypoglycemia (≤ 60 mg/dL) in a middle-aged to older dog is strong support for a probable "insulinoma". Serum insulin concentrations taken at the time of hypoglycemia typically are >30 μu/mL. Differential diagnoses include hypoadrenocorticism, hepatic failure, large extrapancreatic neoplasms, sepsis, polycythemia, overdosage with insulin, and laboratory error. Ruling out other causes for hypoglycemia and exploratory surgery are often the most cost-effective measures to confirm the diagnosis.

Treatment: Although β-cell adenocarcinomas are usually single in dogs, the entire pancreas should be examined carefully for multiple tumors. Complete excision of solitary islet cell adenocarcinomas ameliorates the hypoglycemia and associated neurologic signs, unless there have been irreversible changes in the CNS or nonvisable metastases are present. Even though the potential for malignancy of "insulinomas" is high, prolonged quality survival (>1 yr) can be obtained in many dogs by debulking all visible tumors at surgery. Dogs with inoperable tumors may be managed fairly well with multiple feedings/day and glucocorticoid administration

(0.5-1 mg/kg/day). The drug diazoxide (20-80 mg/kg/day, t.i.d.) may also alleviate clinical signs in some dogs.

GASTRIN-SECRETING NON-β ISLET CELL TUMORS

These tumors of the pancreas have been reported in man, dogs, and a cat. Hypersecretion of gastrin in man results in the well-documented Zollinger-Ellison syndrome, consisting of hypersecretion of gastric acid and recurrent peptic ulceration in the GI tract. The tumors, derived from ectopic APUD (amine precursor uptake decarboxylase) cells in the pancreas, produce an excess of the hormone gastrin, which normally is secreted by cells of the antral and duodenal mucosa.

Clinical Findings: The incidence of these tumors in dogs and cats is rare; they occur less frequently than the insulin-secreting β-cell neoplasms. In the few documented cases, dogs and cats have had anorexia, hematemesis, intermittent diarrhea (usually with dark blood present), progressive weight loss, and dehydration. The prominent functional disturbances appear to result from multiple ulcerations of the GI mucosa that develop from gastrin hypersecretion.

Lesions: Animals studied with the Zollinger-Ellison-like syndrome have had single or multiple tumors of varying size in the pancreas. They often were firm on palpation due to an increase of fibrous connective tissue in the stroma, and all had evidence of metastasis before diagnosis.

Diagnosis: Serum gastrin levels have been evaluated in a limited number of dogs with non-β islet cell tumors. Gastrin levels in a dog with a Zollinger-Ellison-like syndrome varied from 155-2780 pg/mL, whereas the mean serum gastrin in clinically normal (control) dogs (N = 17) was 70.9 pg/mL. The finding of recurrent gastric/duodenal ulcers in dogs with no identified cause warrants exploratory surgery and careful inspection of the pancreas.

Treatment: Excision of the gastrin-secreting mass in the pancreas should be attempted. The gastrin-secreting tumors of the pancreas that have been studied in dogs have all had evidence for local invasion into adjacent parenchyma and had metastasized to regional lymph nodes and liver. The dogs have either single or multiple ulcerations in the gastric and/or duodenal mucosa associated with free blood in the lumen. Medical management with H_2-receptor antagonists (cimetidine or ranitidine) or the new "proton-pump" inhibitor, omeprazole, may allow for temporary alleviation of clinical signs in animals with inoperable disease.

THE PARATHYROID GLANDS

The parathyroid glands secrete parathyroid hormone (PTH, parathormone), which increases blood calcium (Ca) and enhances renal excretion of phosphorus (P). Calcium ion level regulates the release of calcitonin (CT, thyrocalcitonin) from a second endocrine cell population in the thyroid, which favors Ca homeostasis. PTH maintains ionized Ca concentrations in extracellular fluid by increasing bone resorption, GI absorption of Ca in the presence of vitamin D, and by reducing urinary Ca excretion. Secretion of PTH is regulated by changes in the concentration of blood Ca.

Since aberrant Ca and P metabolism is reflected in the skeletal system, specific syndromes are presented in that section (*see* DYSTROPHIES ASSOCIATED WITH CALCIUM, PHOSPHORUS, AND VITAMIN D, p 481). *See* also HUMORAL HYPERCALCEMIA OF MALIGNANCY, p 285.

CALCIUM-REGULATING HORMONES

The concentration of Ca in the blood of mammals is ~10 mg/dL, with some variation due to species (eg, in horses and rabbits up to 13 mg/dL is normal), age, dietary intake, and analytic method. The blood Ca is composed of protein-bound and diffusible fractions. Diffusible Ca consists of Ca complexed to anions, such as phosphate and citrate, plus biologically active free (ionic) Ca.

The Ca ion plays a key role in muscle contraction, blood coagulation, enzyme activity, neural excitability, secondary messengers, hormone release, and membrane permeability, and is an essential structural component of the skeleton. Precise control of Ca ion in extracellular fluids is vital to health. Three major hormones (PTH, CT, and vitamin D) interact to maintain a constant concentration of Ca, despite variations in intake and excretion; other hormones, such as adrenal corticosteroids, estrogens, thyroxine, somatotropin, and glucagon, may also contribute to the maintenance of Ca homeostasis.

PARATHYROID HORMONE (PTH)

PTH is synthesized and stored in the chief cells of the parathyroid glands. Synthesis is regulated by a feedback mechanism involving the level of blood Ca (and to a lesser degree, magnesium). In addition, biological amines, peptides, steroids, and several classes of drugs can influence PTH secretion.

The primary function of PTH is to control Ca concentration in the extracellular fluid, which in turn is a function of the rate of transfer of Ca into and out of bone, resorption in the kidneys, and absorption from the GI tract. The effect on the kidneys is the most rapid, and causes reabsorption of Ca and excretion of P. The major initial effect on bone is to mobilize Ca from the bone to the extracellular fluid; later, bone formation may be enhanced. PTH does not directly affect Ca absorption from the gut; rather, its effect is mediated indirectly by regulation of synthesis of the active metabolite of vitamin D.

CALCITONIN
(CT, Thyrocalcitonin)

A polypeptide hormone secreted by the parafollicular cells of the thyroid in mammals and by ultimobranchial tissue in avian and other submammalian species.

The concentration of Ca ion in extracellular fluids is the principal stimulus for the secretion of CT by C-cells. It is secreted continuously in normocalcemia, but in hypercalcemia its rate of secretion is increased greatly by rapid discharge of stored hormone from C-cells into interfollicular capillaries. Hyperplasia of C-cells occurs in response to long-term hypercalcemia. When blood Ca is lowered, the stimulus for CT secretion is diminished and numerous secretory granules accumulate in the cytoplasm of C-cells. The storage of large amounts of preformed hormone in C-cells and rapid release in response to moderate elevations in blood Ca probably reflect the physiological role of CT as an "emergency" hormone to protect against development of hypercalcemia. CT secretion is increased in response to a high-calcium meal, often before a significant rise in plasma Ca can be detected, which suggests that GI hormones may trigger the early release of CT.

The administration of CT or stimulation of endogenous secretion results in development of varying degrees of hypocalcemia and hypophosphatemia. These effects are most evident in animals with increased rates of skeletal remodeling. CT exerts its function by interacting with target cells, primarily in bone and kidney. The action of PTH and CT are antagonistic on bone resorption but synergistic on decreasing the renal tubular reabsorption of P. The hypocalcemic effects of CT are primarily the result of decreased entry of Ca from the skeleton into plasma due to a temporary inhibition of PTH-stimulated bone resorption. The hypophosphatemia develops from a direct action of CT, by increasing the rate of movement of P out of plasma into soft tissue and bone, as well as from inhibiting bone resorption. One action of CT is inhibition of the bone resorption stimulated by PTH and other factors.

CHOLECALCIFEROL (VITAMIN D)

The third major hormone involved in the regulation of Ca metabolism and skeletal remodeling is cholecalciferol, or vitamin D_3. Although this compound has long been designated as a vitamin, evidence suggests it can also be considered a hormone. Cholecalciferol is ingested in small amounts but, in addition, is synthesized in the epidermis from a percursor molecule (7-dehydrocholesterol) through a previtamin D_3 intermediate form. This reaction is catalyzed by ultraviolet irradiation.

Vitamin D must be metabolically activated before it can function physiologically. The first metabolite of cholecalciferol is produced in the liver and transported to the kidneys, where it undergoes further hydroxylation under the influence of an enzyme in cells of the proximal convoluted tubules to form the biologically active (hormonal) form, 1,25-dihydroxycholecalciferol. This conversion in the kidneys is the rate-limiting step in vitamin D metabolism, and is partly responsible for the delay between vitamin D administration and expression of its biological effects. PTH and conditions that stimulate its secretion, as well as low blood P, increase the formation of the active vitamin D metabolite. High blood P has the opposite effect. Under certain conditions, prolactin, estradiol, placental lactogen, and possibly somatotropin have a similar enhancing effect. Increased secretion of these hormones, either alone or in combination, appears to be important in the efficient adaptation to the major Ca demands of pregnancy, lactation, and growth.

THE PITUITARY GLAND

The pituitary gland (hypophysis) has 2 distinct parts, viz, the neurohypophysis (posterior lobe) and the adenohypophysis (anterior lobe).

Adenohypophysis: In adults, the pituitary gland is completely separated from the oral cavity. The adenohypophysis, which surrounds the pars nervosa of the neurohypophyseal system to varying degrees in different species, consists of 3 portions, viz, the pars distalis, pars tuberalis, and pars intermedia. The pars distalis is the largest and contains multiple populations of endocrine cells. The pars tuberalis functions primarily as a scaffold for the capillary network of the hypophyseal portal system. The pars intermedia forms the junction between the pars distalis and pars nervosa. It contains 2 populations of cells in dogs, one of which synthesizes adrenocorticotropic hormone (ACTH).

A specific population of endocrine cells in the pars distalis (and in the pars intermedia for ACTH in dogs) synthesizes and secretes each of the pituitary tropic hormones. Pituitary cells have a secretory cycle and enter an actively synthesizing phase in response to increased demand for a particular hormone. Secretory cells in the adenohypophysis are often subdivided into chromophils (acidophils, basophils) and chromophobes based on interaction of the secretory granules with pH-dependent histochemical stains.

Acidophils are further subdivided into somatotrophs that secrete growth hormone (GH, somatotropin) and lactotrophs that secrete prolactin. Basophils include both gonadotrophs that secrete luteinizing hormone (LH) and follicle-stimulating hormone (FSH), and thyrotrophs that secrete thyrotropic hormone (TSH). Chromophobes include the endocrine cells involved in the synthesis of ACTH and melanocyte-stimulating hormone (MSH), nonsecretory follicular cells, and undifferentiated stem cells.

Endocrine cells in the adenohypophysis are under the control of corresponding hypothalamic-releasing hormones. These releasing hormones are conveyed by the hypophyseal portal system to specific cells in the adenohypophysis, where they stimulate the rapid release of preformed tropic hormones.

There are separate hypothalamic-releasing hormones that regulate the rate of secretion of each tropic hormone from the adenohypophysis. For most pituitary tropic hormones, negative feedback control is accomplished by a feedback loop involving the blood concentration of the hormone produced by the target endocrine gland (eg, thyroid gland, adrenal cortex, ovary, and testis). Hormones such as prolactin, GH, and MSH have more complex feedback mechanisms; eg, prolactin effects primarily the mammary gland, and GH has its principal effect on the liver—both nonendocrine tissues. The negative feedback in such cases includes metabolites and other messengers (eg, insulin-like growth factor I produced by the liver). In the case of GH, there is an inhibitory (somatostatin) as well as stimulatory (GH-releasing hormone) hypothalamic regulator.

Neurohypophysis: The neurohypophysis (pars nervosa, posterior lobe) has 3 anatomic subdivisions. Secretion granules that contain the neurohypophyseal hormones, ie, oxytocin and antidiuretic hormone (ADH, vasopressin), are synthesized in the hypothalamus but are released into the bloodstream in the pars nervosa. The infundibular stalk joins the pars nervosa to the overlying hypothalamus.

ADH, an octapeptide synthesized in the hypothalamus, is packaged into membrane-limited granules with a corresponding binding protein (neurophysin) and transported to the pars nervosa, where it is released into the circulation. ADH binds to specific receptors in the distal part of the nephron and collecting duct of the kidney; it increases the renal tubular reabsorption of water from the glomerular filtrate.

The output of ADH is directly related to the degree of hydration of the body. Hydration of the body inhibits release of ADH, which in turn causes less water resorption from glomerular filtrate, thereby removing excess water from the body. Dehydration of the body or injection of hypertonic electrolyte solutions favors release of ADH, which in turn causes increased water resorption from the glomerular filtrate, which results in dilution and decreased osmolarity of body fluids. Other factors, such as barbiturates, ether, chloroform, morphine, acetylcholine, nicotine, and pain, increase ADH release, which leads to less urine formation. Ethanol inhibits ADH release, which leads to diuresis.

The pressor effect of ADH is less prominent than the antidiuretic effect. At a dosage several hundred times larger than the antidiuretic dosage, ADH has a pronounced pressor effect, which may also lead to coronary constriction. The contractile mechanism of the capillaries, as well as GI and uterine muscle, is stimulated, and a rather prolonged elevation of blood pressure follows. Oxytocin has specific effects on the smooth muscle of the uterus and the myoepithelial cells of the mammary gland. It has no established physiological function in the male, although there are suggestions that it may affect sperm transport.

ACTH-SECRETING TUMORS ASSOCIATED WITH HYPERCORTISOLISM

Functional tumors arising in the pituitary gland most frequently are derived from corticotroph (ACTH-secreting) cells in either the pars distalis or the pars intermedia. They cause a clinical syndrome of cortisol excess (Cushing's disease). These neoplasms develop most frequently in adult to aged dogs and have been reported in a number of breeds, chiefly Boxers, Boston Terriers, and Dachshunds. They are infrequent in other animals. Chronic overproduction of glucocorticoid hormones by hyperplastic adrenal cortices result in combined gluconeogenic, lipolytic, protein catabolic, and anti-inflammatory actions on many organ systems.

Clinical Findings: A number of distinctive clinical and functional alterations develop. Centripetal redistribution of adipose tissue leads to prominent fat pads on the dorsal midline of the neck, giving the neck and shoulders a thick appearance. Food intake may increase either as a direct stimulation of the appetite center by the cortisol excess or as a result of destruction of the "satiety center" in the hypothalamus by the adenoma.

Muscles of the extremities and abdomen are weakened and atrophied. The loss of tone of abdominal muscles and muscles of the abaxial skeleton results in gradual development of a "pot-bellied" appearance, lordosis, muscle trembling, and a straight-legged skeletal-braced posture to support the body weight. Profound atrophy of the temporal muscles may result in concave indentations and readily palpable prominences of the underlying skull bones. Hepatomegaly due in part to increased fat and glycogen deposition and vacuolation of liver cells may contribute to the development of the distended, often pendulous, abdomen.

Lesions: The pituitary gland is enlarged in dogs with corticotroph adenomas. Neither occurrence nor severity of disturbances appears to be related directly to the size of the neoplasm. Growth of the pituitary tumor may incorporate the second, third, and fourth cranial nerves, leading to corresponding functional disturbances.

There is bilateral enlargement of the adrenal glands in dogs with functional corticotroph adenomas. This enlargement often is striking and is due entirely to increased cortical parenchyma. Nodules of yellow-orange cortical tissue often are found outside the capsule in the periadrenal fat as well as extending down into the adrenal medulla. The secretion of excess cortisol in these dogs can be diminished by administration of the adrenocytotoxic drug mitotane (o,p'-DDD).

Adenomas derived from corticotroph cells of the pars intermedia develop less often in brachycephalic breeds than in other dogs. Adenomas of the pars intermedia in dogs may be associated with secretion of excess ACTH, leading to bilateral adrenocortical hyperplasia and the syndrome of cortisol excess. The clinical signs of functional corticotroph adenomas arising in the pars intermedia are similar to those of an adenoma arising in the pars distalis.

Pituitary tumors arising in the pars intermedia of dogs frequently invade the pars nervosa and infundibular stalk, and result in disturbances of water metabolism early in their development.

NONFUNCTIONAL PITUITARY TUMORS

These occur in dogs, cats, laboratory rodents, and parakeets but are uncommon in other species. Although chromophobe adenomas appear to be endocrinologically inactive, they may cause compression atrophy of adjacent portions of the pituitary gland, and extend into the overlying brain. Clinical disturbances occur either because of a lack of secretion of pituitary tropic hormones and diminished target organ function (eg, adrenal cortex), or dysfunction of the CNS. Affected animals often are depressed, incoordinated, and weak, and may collapse with exercise. (*See also* ADULT-ONSET PANHYPOPITUITARISM, below.)

Endocrinologically inactive pituitary adenomas often attain considerable size before they cause obvious signs (or death). The proliferating tumor cells incorporate the remaining structures of the adenohypophysis and infundibular stalk. The entire hypothalamus may become compressed and replaced by the tumor.

HIRSUTISM ASSOCIATED WITH ADENOMAS OF THE PARS INTERMEDIA
(Hypertrichosis)

A disease that develops in older horses, more often in mares, hirsutism (hypertrichosis) usually is associated with a pituitary adenoma derived from cells of the pars intermedia. Such adenomas often severely compress the overlying hypothalamus. The hypothalamus is the primary center for homeostatic regulation of body temperature, appetite, and cyclic shedding of hair.

Clinical Findings and Lesions: Signs are polyuria, polydipsia, ravenous appetite, weakness, somnolence, intermittent hyperpyrexia, and generalized hyperhidrosis. Hirsutism often becomes evident because of failure of the cyclic seasonal shedding of hair. The hair over most of the trunk and extremities is long (up to 4-5 in. [10-12 mm]), abnormally thick, wavy, and often matted.

Horses with larger tumors may have hyperglycemia (insulin-resistant) and glycosuria, probably because of a down-regulation of insulin receptors on target cells induced by the chronic overeating and hyperinsulinemia.

These are the most common pituitary tumors in horses; they are yellow to white, multinodular, and incorporate the pars nervosa. Plasma cortisol and immunoreactive adrenocorticotropin levels are modestly elevated; the cortisol levels lack the normal diurnal rhythm, and are not suppressed by either high or low doses of dexamethasone.

Diagnosis: Hyperglycemia and some insensitivity to insulin are highly suggestive of pituitary adenoma in horses. Other nonspecific findings include an absolute or relative neutrophilia, and eosinopenia and lymphopenia; lipemia; hypercholesterolemia; and a mild, normochromic, normocytic anemia. Liver enzymes may be elevated. Electrolytes are usually normal. The urinalysis is normal except for occasional glycosuria and a low to normal specific gravity.

The definitive diagnosis is based on response to tests to stimulate the pituitary-adrenal axis. Baseline cortisol is in the high-normal to modestly elevated range. The response to ACTH (1 u/kg, IV) may be exaggerated (>2 times the increase normally seen at 2 hr) in some horses. Dexamethasone (40 μg/kg, IM) often will not suppress cortisol levels to at least 30% of baseline or to <1 μg/dL, as it does in normal horses 6 hr after administration.

Differential diagnoses include syndromes resulting in chronic debilitation, eg, poor management and nutrition, parasitism, and chronic systemic diseases. The polyuria/polydipsia must be differentiated from that due to chronic renal disease or diabetes insipidus. The hyperglycemia, glycosuria, and polyuria/polydipsia must be differentiated from primary diabetes mellitus. Pheochromocytomas may cause hyperhidrosis, hyperglycemia, and tachypnea, although they usually are nonfunctional and only found incidentally at necropsy.

Treatment: Few horses have been treated successfully, but daily cyproheptadine (0.13-0.26 mg/kg, PO) has helped some. This dose is maintained for 3 mo, after which alternate-day therapy can be tried. A decrease in the polyuria/polydipsia should be seen within 1-2 mo if the therapy is successful. Pergolide, a dopaminergic agonist, also has been used successfully in a few horses at a daily dose of 4-11 μg/kg, PO. Although they have not been observed, potential side effects are those related to the drug's vasoconstrictive effects.

ADULT-ONSET PANHYPOPITUITARISM

Endocrinologically inactive, nonfunctional pituitary tumors occur frequently in dogs, cats, and parakeets, but are uncommon in other species. They develop most commonly in the adult to aged animal; there is no apparent breed predisposition. The most common cause is a chromophobe adenoma arising in the pars distalis. Other infrequent causes include: extensive inflammatory destruction of pituitary tissue, ischemic necrosis of the pituitary due to infarction from invasion of tumor cells, parasitic or septic emboli, diffuse necrosis associated with toxemia, invasion by neoplasms arising in adjacent structures (eg, meninges, sphenoid bone, nasal cavity, etc), and widespread hemorrhage and subsequent scarring following traumatic injury. Dogs and cats with nonfunctional adenomas develop clinical disturbances related to a lack of secretion of pituitary tropic hormones and diminished target organ function, or dysfunction of the CNS.

Clinical Findings: Affected dogs often are depressed, incoordinated, and collapse with exercise, and occasionally exhibit a change in attitude. They may become unresponsive to people and develop a tendency to hide at the slightest provocation. In chronic cases, there may be evidence of blindness with dilated and fixed pupils due to compression and disruption of optic nerves by dorsal extension of the pituitary tumor. Affected dogs often have a progressive loss of weight with muscle atrophy due to a lack of protein anabolic effect of growth hormone. Compression of the cells that secrete gonadotropic hormones or the corresponding releasing hormone from the hypothalamus results in atrophy of the gonads. Disturbances of water balance are the result of an interference with the synthesis of antidiuretic hormone or its release into capillaries of the pars nervosa. The posterior lobe, infundibular stalk, and hypothalamus are compressed or disrupted by neoplastic cells. Animals with panhypopituitarism appear to be dehydrated, despite increased water consumption. Dogs and cats with large nonfunctional pituitary tumors usually excrete large volumes of dilute urine with a low specific gravity (≤1.007), and may break housetraining. Clinical signs are not highly specific and can be confused with other CNS disorders (eg, brain tumors or encephalitis) or chronic renal disease.

Hypopituitarism caused by pituitary tumors should be included in the differential diagnosis of diseases characterized by incoordination, depression, polyuria, blindness, and a sudden behavioral change in adult or aged animals. Because the blindness is central in origin, ophthalmoscopic examination usually fails to reveal significant lesions. There is no effect on body stature associated with compression of the pars distalis and probable interference of growth hormone secretion, because these neoplasms usually arise in dogs that have already completed their growth. Parakeets with chromophobe adenomas often develop exophthalmos due to extension of neoplastic cells along the optic nerve.

Lesions: Endocrinologically inactive pituitary adenomas usually reach considerable size before they cause obvious signs or death. The proliferating tumor cells incorporate the remaining structures of the adenohypophysis and infundibular stalk. The entire hypothalamus may be compressed and replaced by tumor.

Thyroid glands in dogs and cats with large pituitary adenomas often are smaller than normal, though to a much lesser degree than the adrenal cortex. The adrenal glands are small and consist primarily of medullary tissue surrounded by a narrow zone of cortex. Seminiferous tubules are small and show little evidence of active spermatogenesis.

The atrophy of the skin and loss of muscle mass may be related to a lack of protein anabolic effects of growth hormone in an adult dog or cat. Interference with the secretion of pituitary tropic hormones often results in gonadal atrophy resulting in either decreased libido or anestrus, and hypoglycemia from atrophy of the adrenal cortex.

JUVENILE-ONSET PANHYPOPITUITARISM

Pituitary dwarfism occurs most frequently in German Shepherd Dogs, in which it often occurs in littermates and related litters, suggesting a simple autosomal recessive mode of inheritance. It has been reported in other breeds such as the Spitz, Miniature Pinscher, and Karelian Bear Dogs (from Denmark).

It usually is associated with a failure of the oropharyngeal ectoderm of the cranial pharyngeal duct (Rathke's pouch) to differentiate into tropic-hormone-secreting cells of the pars distalis. Consequently, the adenohypophysis is not completely developed. The second most common cause is a craniopharyngioma, a benign tumor derived from the oropharyngeal ectoderm of Rathke's pouch. Compared with all other types of pituitary neoplasms, craniopharyngiomas develop in younger dogs. They cause panhypopituitarism and dwarfism in young dogs through subnormal secretion of somatotropin and other tropic hormones beginning at an early age, before closure of the growth plates.

Clinical Findings: The dwarf pups are indistinguishable from normal littermates up to ~2 mo old. Subsequently, the slower growth rate compared with littermates, retention of puppy coat, and lack of primary guard hairs gradually become evident in dwarf pups. German Shepherd Dogs with pituitary dwarfism appear coyote- or fox-like owing to their size and soft, woolly coat. A bilaterally symmetrical alopecia develops gradually and often becomes complete except for the head and tufts of hair on the legs. Permanent dentition is delayed or completely absent. Closure of the epiphyses is delayed as long as 4 yr, depending on the severity of the hormonal insufficiency. The testes and penis are small, calcification of the os penis is delayed or incomplete, and the penile sheath is flaccid. The ovarian cortex is hypoplastic, and estrus irregular or absent. The life span of these dogs is shortened because of the panhypopituitarism and the resulting secondary endocrine dysfunction, such as hypothyroidism and hypoadrenocorticism.

Lesions: Pituitary cysts fill with mucus, and eventually occupy the entire pituitary area and severely compress the pars nervosa and infundibular stalk.

Craniopharyngiomas are large, solid, cystic areas that extend into the overlying hypothalamus. They also may grow along the ventral aspect of the brain, where they incorporate several cranial nerves that result in specific nerve function deficits.

Diagnosis: Levels of thyroxine, triiodothyronine, and cortisol are reduced or in the low-normal range. In those animals with an equivocal change in basal hormone level, the responses to challenge by exogenous thyrotropin or adrenocorticotropin are subnormal, owing to the hypoplasia of the thyroid gland and adrenal cortex. Other useful diagnostic aids include comparison of height with littermates, radiographs of open epiphyseal lines, and skin biopsy. Cutaneous lesions include hyperkeratosis, follicular keratosis, hyperpigmentation, adnexal atrophy and a loss of elastin fibers, and a loose network of collagen fibers in the dermis. Hair shafts are absent, and hair follicles are primarily in the telogen stage of the growth cycle.

The activity of somatomedin (a cartilage growth-promoting peptide produced in the liver from somatotropin) is low in dwarf dogs. Intermediate somatomedin activity is present in the phenotypical normal ancestors suspected to be heterozygous carriers. Assays for somatomedin provide an indirect measurement of circulating growth hormone activity in dogs with suspected pituitary dwarfism. Basal levels of circulating canine growth hormone are reported to be detectable but low (normal range: 1.75 ± 0.17 ng/mL) in pituitary dwarfs, and fail to increase following a provocative test for growth hormone secretion provided by clonidine injection (30 µg/kg, IV) as in normal dogs. Insulin hyprsensitivity has been demonstrated in pituitary dwarf dogs, probably due to a change in insulin receptor numbers or affinity of binding in response to the low growth-hormone levels.

DIABETES INSIPIDUS (DI)

A condition due to reduced secretion of antidiuretic hormone (ADH), or to target cells in the kidney that lack the biochemical machinery necessary to respond to the secretion of normal or elevated circulating levels of hormone. It occurs in dogs, cats, laboratory rats, and infrequently in other animals.

Etiology: The hypophyseal form develops as a result of compression and destruction of the pars nervosa, infundibular stalk, or supraoptic nucleus in the hypothalamus. The lesions responsible for the disruption of ADH synthesis or secretion in hypophyseal DI include large pituitary neoplasms (endocrinologically active or inactive), a dorsally expanding cyst or inflammatory granuloma, and traumatic injury to the skull with hemorrhage and glial proliferation in the neurohypophyseal system.

Clinical Findings and Lesions: Affected animals excrete large volumes of hypotonic urine, and drink equally large amounts of water. Urine osmolality is decreased below normal plasma osmolality (~300 mOsm/kg) in both hypophyseal and nephrogenic forms of DI, even if water is deprived. The elevation of urine osmolality above that of plasma in response to exogenous ADH in the hypophyseal form, but not in the nephrogenic form, is useful in the clinical separation of the 2 forms of the disease.

The posterior lobe, infundibular stalk, and hypothalamus are compressed or disrupted by neoplastic cells. This interrupts the nonmyelinated axons that transport ADH from its site of production (the hypothalamus) to its site of release (the pars nervosa).

Diagnosis: This is based on chronic polyuria that does not respond to dehydration and is not due to primary renal disease. To evaluate the ability to concentrate urine, a water deprivation test should be done if the animal is not dehydrated and does not have renal disease. The bladder is emptied, and water and food are withheld (usually 3-8 hr) to provide a maximum stimulus for ADH secretion. The animal should be monitored during this period to prevent a loss of >6% body wt and severe dehydration. Urine and plasma osmolality should be determined; however, these tests are not readily available to most practitioners, and urine specific gravity (SG) frequently is used instead. At the end of the test, urine SG is >1.025 in those animals with only a partial ADH deficiency or with antagonism to ADH action as in hypercortisolism. There is little change in SG in those animals with a complete lack of ADH activity, whether it be from a primary loss of ADH or unresponsiveness of the kidneys.

An ADH response test should follow to differentiate DI from other conditions that may result in large volumes of urine that is chronically low in SG but otherwise normal. These include nephrogenic DI (an inability of the kidneys to respond to ADH), psychogenic DI (a polydipsia in response to some psychological disturbance but a normal response to ADH [qv, p 927]), and hypercortisolism (which results in a partial deficiency of ADH action due to cortisol antagonism of ADH action in the kidneys). This test also can be used to evaluate animals in which a water deprivation test could not be performed. Urine SG is determined at the start of the test; vasopressin tannate in oil is injected IM (2.5 u for cats and small dogs, 5 u for larger dogs); the bladder is emptied at 2 hr; and urine SG measured 4, 8, 12, 18, and 24 hr after ADH administration. The SG peaks at >1.026 in animals with a primary deficiency in ADH, is significantly increased above the level induced with water deprivation in those with a partial deficiency in ADH activity, and shows little change in those with nephrogenic DI.

If osmolality is measured, the ratio of urine to plasma osmolality following water deprivation is >3 in normal animals, 1.8-3 in those with moderate ADH deficiency, and <1.8 in those with severe deficiency. The ratio of urine osmolality after ADH administration as compared to water deprivation is >2 in animals with primary ADH deficiency, between 1.1 and 2 in animals with inhibitors to ADH action, and <1.1 in animals unresponsive to ADH.

DI also needs to be distinguished from other diseases with polyuria. The most common are diabetes mellitus with glycosuria and high urine SG, and chronic nephritis with a urine SG that is usually high and shows evidence of renal failure (protein, casts, etc).

Treatment: Polyuria should be controlled. Two drugs can be used: vasopressin tannate in oil (2-5 u, IM as needed, usually every 2-4 days) and desmopressin acetate, a synthetic analog of ADH. The initial dose of the latter is 2 drops applied to the nasal mucosae or conjunctivae; this is gradually increased until the minimal effective dose is determined. Maximum effect usually occurs in 2-6 hr and lasts for 10-12 hr. Water should not be restricted. Treatment needs to be continued once or twice daily for the life of the animal.

THE THYROID GLAND

All vertebrates have a thyroid gland. In mammals, it is usually bilobed and located just caudal to the larynx, adjacent to the lateral surface of the trachea. The 2 lobes may be connected by a fibrous isthmus (eg, in ruminants, horses), or a connecting isthmus may be indistinct (eg, in dogs, cats). The gland is extremely vascular. In birds, it is found within the thoracic cavity; both lobes are located near the syrinx, adjacent to the carotid artery near the origin of the vertebral artery.

Ectopic or accessory thyroid tissue is relatively common in most species, especially dogs and cats. It may be located anywhere from the larynx to the diaphragm, and may be responsible for maintenance of normal thyroid function following surgical thyroidectomy. In addition, ectopic thyroid tissue occasionally is the site of hyperplasia or neoplasia.

Physiology: Thyroid hormones are the only iodinated organic compounds in the body. Thyroxine (T_4) is the main secretory product of the normal thyroid gland. However, the gland also secretes 3,5,3'-triiodothyronine (T_3), reverse T_3, and other deiodinated metabolites. Triiodothyronine is ~3-5 times more potent than T_4, while reverse T_3 is thyromimetically inactive.

Although all T_4 is secreted by the thyroid, a considerable amount of T_3 is derived from T_4; therefore, T_4 has been called a prohormone. Its activation to the more potent T_3 is a step regulated individually by peripheral tissues.

Thyroid hormone secretion is regulated primarily via negative-feedback control through the coordinated response of the hypothalamic-pituitary-thyroid axis: thyrotropin-releasing hormone (TRH) binds to the thyrotroph cell in the pituitary and stimulates secretion of thyrotropin (thyroid-stimulating hormone, TSH), which binds to the follicular cell membrane and stimulates thyroid hormone synthesis and secretion.

Thyroid hormones are water-insoluble lipophilic compounds that are bound to plasma proteins (thyroxine-binding protein, thyroxine-binding prealbumin [transthyretin], and albumin). The major function of the thyroid-hormone-binding proteins is probably to provide a hormone reservoir in the plasma and to "buffer" hormone delivery into tissue. In the healthy euthyroid animal, ~0.1% of total serum T_4 is free (not bound to thyroid-hormone-binding proteins), whereas ~1% of circulating T_3 is free. Most evidence suggests that the fractions of circulating free T_4 and free T_3 determine the amount of hormone that is available for uptake by tissues.

Action of Thyroid Hormones: Thyroid hormones act on many different cellular processes; however, no single reaction or metabolic event can be equated with their action. Although both T_4 and T_3 have intrinsic metabolic activity, T_3 is 3-5 times more potent in binding to the nuclear receptors and similarly more potent in stimulating oxygen consumption.

Effects of thyroid hormones generally are divided into 2 categories: 1) those that manifest within minutes to hours after hormone receptor binding and do not require protein synthesis, and 2) those that manifest later (usually >6 hr) and require synthesis of new proteins. About half the increase in oxygen consumption produced by thyroid hormones is related to activation of the plasma-membrane-bound Na^+/K^+ ATPase; thyroid hormones also stimulate mitochondrial oxygen consumption. These changes are linked directly to the calorigenic effect of thyroid hormones. More chronic effects invariably are related to the cellular actions that require interaction with nuclear T_3 receptors followed by an increase in protein synthesis crucial to physiological processes such as growth, differentiation, proliferation, and maturation.

Thyroid hormones, in physiological quantities, are anabolic. In conjunction with growth hormone and insulin, protein synthesis is stimulated and nitrogen excretion is reduced. However, in excess (hyperthyroidism), they can be catabolic, with increased gluconeogenesis, protein breakdown, and nitrogen wasting.

HYPOTHYROIDISM

Impaired production and secretion of the thyroid hormones result in a decreased metabolic rate. This disorder is most common in dogs, but also develops rarely in other species, including cats and large domestic animals.

Etiology: Although dysfunction anywhere in the hypothalamic-pituitary-thyroid axis may result in thyroid hormone deficiency, >95% of clinical cases of canine hypothyroidism appear to result from destruction of the thyroid gland itself (primary hypothyroidism). The 2 most common causes of adult-onset primary hypothyroidism in dogs include lymphocytic thyroiditis and idiopathic atrophy of the thyroid gland. Lymphocytic thyroiditis, probably immune-mediated, is characterized histologically by a diffuse infiltration of the gland by lymphocytes, plasma cells, and macrophages, and results in progressive destruction of follicles and secondary fibrosis. Idiopathic atrophy of the thyroid gland is characterized histologically by loss of thyroid parenchyma and replacement by adipose tissue. *See also* AUTOIMMUNE THYROIDITIS, p 433.

In dogs, the most common cause of secondary hypothyroidism is destruction of pituitary thyrotrophs by an expanding, space-occupying tumor. Because of the nonselective nature of the resulting compressive atrophy and replacement of pituitary tissue by such large tumors, deficiencies of other (one or more) pituitary hormones also usually occurs.

Other rare forms of canine hypothyroidism include neoplastic destruction of thyroid tissue and congenital (or juvenile-onset) hypothyroidism. Congenital primary hypothyroidism may result from one of various forms of thyroid dysgenesis (eg, athyreosis, thyroid hypoplasia) or may result from dyshormonogenesis (usually an inherited inability to organify iodide). Congenital secondary hypothyroidism has been documented only in German Shepherd Dogs, with pituitary dwarfism associated with a cystic Rathke's pouch. However, the degree of TSH deficiency in these dogs is variable, and clinical signs are usually caused primarily by deficiency of growth hormone (rather than thyroid hormone).

In cats, iatrogenic hypothyroidism following treatment for hyperthyroidism with radioiodine, surgical thyroidectomy, or use of an antithyroid drug is the most common cause of hypothyroidism.

Clinical Findings: Although onset is variable, hypothyroidism is most common in 4- to 10-yr-old dogs. It usually affects mid- to large-size breeds and is rare in toy and miniature breeds. Breeds reported to be predisposed include the Golden Retriever, Doberman Pinscher, Irish Setter, Miniature Schnauzer, Dachshund, Cocker Spaniel, and Airedale Terrier. There does not appear to be a sex predilection, but spayed females appear to display a higher risk of developing hypothyroidism than intact females.

A deficiency of thyroid hormone affects the function of all organ systems, and as a result, clinical signs are diffuse, variable, often nonspecific, and rarely pathognomonic. While the disorder should be highly suspect, overdiagnosis should be avoided, because many diseases, especially those of the skin, can easily be misdiagnosed as hypothyroidism.

Many of the clinical signs associated with canine hypothyroidism are directly related to slowing of cellular metabolism. This results in development of mental dullness, lethargy, intolerance of exercise, and weight gain without a corresponding increase in appetite. Mild to marked obesity develops in some dogs. Difficulty in maintaining body temperature may lead to frank hypothermia; the "classic" hypothyroid dog is a heat-seeker. Alterations in the skin and coat are common; dryness, excessive shedding, and retarded regrowth of hair are usually the earliest dermatologic changes. Nonpruritic hair thinning or alopecia (usually bilaterally symmetric in distribution), which may involve the ventral and lateral trunk, the caudal surfaces of the thighs, dorsum of the tail, ventral neck, and the dorsum of the nose, occurs in about two-thirds of dogs with hypothyroidism. Such hair thinning or alopecia, sometimes associated with hyperpigmentation, often starts initially over points of wear. Occasionally, secondary pyoderma (which may produce pruritus) is observed.

In moderate to severe cases, thickening of the skin secondary to accumulation of glycosaminoglycans (mostly hyaluronic acid) in the dermis is observed. In such cases, myxedema is most common on the forehead and face, resulting in a puffy appearance and thickened skin folds above the eyes. This puffiness, together with slight drooping of the upper eyelid, gives some dogs a "tragic" facial expression. These changes also have been described in the GI tract, heart, and skeletal muscles.

In intact dogs, hypothyroidism may cause various reproductive disturbances: in females, failure to cycle (anestrus) or sporadic cycling, infertility, abortion, or poor litter survival; and in males, lack of libido, testicular atrophy, hypospermia, or infertility.

Myxedema coma, a rare syndrome, is the extreme expression of severe hypothyroidism. The course can develop rapidly; lethargy progresses to stupor and then coma. The common signs of hypothyroidism (eg, hair loss) are usually present but other signs of hypoventilation, hypotension, bradycardia, and profound hypothermia are usually observed as well.

During the fetal period and in the first few months of postnatal life, thyroid hormones are crucial for growth and development of the skeleton and CNS. Therefore, in addition to the well-recognized signs of adult-onset hypothyroidism, disproportionate dwarfism and impaired mental development (cretinism) are prominent signs of congenital and juvenile-onset hypothyroidism. In primary congenital hypothyroidism, enlargement of the thyroid gland (goiter) also may be detected, depending on the cause of the hypothyroidism. Radiographic signs of epiphyseal dysgenesis (underdeveloped epiphyses throughout the long bones), shortened vertebral bodies, and delayed epiphyseal closure are common.

In dogs with congenital hypopituitarism (pituitary dwarfism), there may be variable degrees of thyroidal, adrenocortical, and gonadal deficiency, but clinical signs are primarily related to growth hormone deficiency. Signs include proportionate dwarfism (rather than the disproportionate form of dwarfism characteristic of congenital hypothyroidism), loss of primary guard hairs with retention of the puppy coat, hyperpigmentation of the skin, and bilateral symmetric alopecia of the trunk.

The classic hematological and serum biochemical findings associated with hypothyroidism are a normocytic, normochromic, nonregenerative anemia and hypercholesterolemia. Serum triglyceride concentrations are less consistently increased.

Diagnosis: The determination of basal serum total T_4 concentration by radioimmunoassay techniques may provide important information to rule out hypothyroidism. Since T_4 is produced only from the thyroid gland, hypothyroid dogs can, in most cases, be distinguished from normal dogs based on a low resting serum T_4 concentration. However, many nonthyroidal illnesses and certain drugs may also "falsely" lower baseline serum T_4 concentrations in dogs. Even when historical and physical findings do not suggest other factors that would lower serum T_4, the diagnosis of hypothyroidism should be confirmed with a dynamic thyroid function test (eg, TSH stimulation test).

Because T_3 is the most potent thyroid hormone at the cellular level, it would seem logical to measure its concentration for diagnostic purposes. However, serum T_3 concentrations may be low, normal, or (occasionally) high in dogs with documented hypothyroidism. The diagnostic value of a serum T_3 determination appears particularly weak during early thyroid failure because the "failing thyroid" tends to increase the relative synthesis and secretion of T_3 over T_4. In the hypothyroid dog in which values for serum T_3 are high, anti-T_3 antibodies, which produce spurious results in most T_3 radioimmunoassays, should be suspect.

Administration of exogenous bovine TSH followed by the measurement of serum T_4 provides important diagnostic information because it tests thyroid secretory reserve. The TSH stimulation test is the most definitive noninvasive test to diagnose primary hypothyroidism. A widely used protocol is to collect a baseline blood sample for serum T_4 determination, administer TSH at 0.1 u/kg, IV (up to a maximum dose of 5 u), and then collect a serum sample for T_4 determination 6 hr after injection.

In primary hypothyroidism, the post-TSH serum T_4 concentration remains below the normal range for basal T_4 (<1 μg/dL, <10 nmol/L) and rarely increases more than 0.2 μg/dL (2.5 nmol/L) above the baseline value. With TSH stimulation testing, primary hypothyroidism can be distinguished from other causes of depression of basal serum T_4 concentrations (eg, drugs and nonthyroidal illness), in which the serum T_4 response may be suppressed but the slope of the increase is similar to that of normal. To rule out a diagnosis of hypothyroidism, the post-TSH T_4 concentration should generally either increase by at least 2 μg/dL (25 nmol/L) over the basal serum T_4 value or exceed the normal range of basal T_4 concentrations by 6 hr after injection of TSH. Dogs that fail to meet these criteria can be considered to have hypothyroidism, and their response to thyroid hormone replacement therapy should be evaluated.

Biopsy of the thyroid gland is a useful and reliable means of diagnosing and differentiating the primary and secondary forms of hypothyroidism.

Treatment: Thyroxine (T_4) is the thyroid hormone replacement compound of choice in dogs. With few exceptions, thyroid hormone replacement therapy is necessary for the remainder of the dog's life; careful initial diagnosis and tailoring of treatment is essential. The reported replacement doses for T_4 in dogs range from a total dose of 0.01-0.02 mg/lb (0.02-0.04 mg/kg), daily, given once or divided b.i.d.

The most important indicator of the success of thyroid replacement therapy is clinical improvement. Reversal of changes in coat and body weight should be assessed only after 1-2 mo of therapy. When clinical improvement is marginal or signs of thyrotoxicosis are seen, the clinical observations can be supported by therapeutic monitoring of serum thyroid hormone concentrations ("post-pill testing"). With once-daily T_4 administration, the peak serum concentrations of T_4 generally should be in the slightly high to high-normal range 4-8 hr after dosing and should be low-normal to normal 24 hr after dosing. Animals on b.i.d. administration probably can be checked at any time, but peak concentrations can be expected at the middle of the dosing interval (4-8 hr) and the nadir just before the next dose. When the dog's dose is stabilized, 1-2 checks per year of serum T_4 (with or without T_3) concentrations are recommended.

If clinical signs of hypothyroidism remain despite the use of reasonable doses of thyroid hormone, the following must be considered: 1) the dose or frequency of administration is improper; 2) the owner is not complying with instructions or is not successfully administering the product; 3) the animal is not absorbing the product well, or is metabolizing and/or excreting it too rapidly; 4) the product is outdated; or 5) the diagnosis is incorrect.

NON-NEOPLASTIC ENLARGEMENT OF THE THYROID GLAND
(Goiter)

Non-neoplastic and noninflammatory enlargements of the thyroid gland develop in all domestic mammals as well as birds. The major causes of goiter include iodine deficiency, goitrogenic substances, dietary iodine excess, and inherited enzyme defects in the biosynthesis of thyroid hormones. Many animals with goiter appear to remain euthyroid, but clinical signs of hypothyroidism may develop in some, especially in newborns.

Iodine Deficiency: Iodine deficiency resulting in thyroid hyperplasia was common in many goitrogenic areas throughout the world before the widespread supplementation of iodized salt to animal diets. Although outbreaks of iodine-deficient goiter are now sporadic with fewer animals being affected, iodine deficiency is responsible for most goiters seen in large domestic animals.

Insufficient iodine reduces the ability of the thyroid to make thyroid hormone. With reduced circulating thyroid hormone levels, the pituitary secretes more TSH, which acts as a stimulus for hyperplasia of the thyroid gland and goiter. The hyperplastic gland may, and usually does, compensate for the reduced availability of iodine; therefore, goiter is in no way synonymous with hypothyroidism. However, animals born to females on iodine-deficient diets are more likely to develop severe thyroid enlargement and have clinical signs of hypothyroidism.

Goiter caused by iodine deficiency is most common in newborn pigs, lambs, calves, and foals in iodine-deficient territories. The thyroid lobes of the young animal usually are at least twice normal size, soft, and dark red. In severe cases, there is an accompanying lack of hair (especially in pigs) or wool (lambs). The neck is usually grossly enlarged and the skin and other tissue may be thickened, flabby, and edematous. In mildly affected animals, treatment with iodized salt (containing ≥0.007% iodine) may resolve the goiter and associated clinical signs, but many die before or soon after birth. Prophylaxis is more effective than treatment. The use of stabilized iodized salt is recommended in all areas known or suspected to be iodine deficient.

Goitrogenic Substances: Feeding of certain plants may produce goiter when ingested in sufficient amounts, especially in the absence of adequate iodine intake. Soybeans are most notable, but cabbage, rape, kale, and turnips all contain less potent goitrogens. Cooking or heating (and the usual processing of soybean meal) destroys the goitrogenic substance in these plants. All of the goitrogenic substances act by interfering with production of thyroid hormone. As with iodine deficiency, the pituitary responds to the reduced circulating thyroid hormone levels by increasing its secretion of TSH, which results in thyroid gland enlargement. In adult animals, the disease is usually not significant, but severe thyroid enlargement and hypothyroidism may develop in newborns.

Iodine Toxicity: Foals of dams fed excess iodine may develop extreme thyroid enlargement, and may die before birth or shortly thereafter. Clinical signs may include general weakness, long hair, and marked limb abnormalities.

Familial Dyshormonogenetic Goiter: This has been reported in sheep, cattle, goats, and pigs, and appears to be inherited as an autosomal recessive. Essentially, it is a genetic enzyme defect in the biosynthesis of thyroid hormones. As with iodine deficiency, reduced thyroid hormone production leads to secretion of increased levels of TSH and subsequent goiter. Clinical signs may include subnormal growth rate, absence of normal wool development or a sparse coat, myxedematous swelling of subcut. tissues, and weakness. Many affected animals die shortly after birth or are very sensitive to adverse environmental conditions.

HYPERTHYROIDISM

Excessive secretion of the thyroid hormones, thyroxine (T_4) and triiodothyronine (T_3), results in signs that reflect an increased metabolic rate and produces clinical hyperthyroidism. It is most common in middle-aged to old cats, but also develops rarely in dogs.

Functional thyroid adenoma (adenomatous hyperplasia) is the most common cause of feline hyperthyroidism; in ~70% of cases both thyroid lobes are enlarged. Thyroid carcinoma, the primary cause of hyperthyroidism in dogs, is rare in cats (1-2% of hyperthyroidism cases).

Clinical Findings and Diagnosis: The most common signs include weight loss, hyperexcitability, increased appetite, polydipsia, polyuria, and palpable enlargement of the thyroid gland. GI signs are also common and may include vomiting, diarrhea, and increased volume of feces. Cardiovascular signs include tachycardia, systolic murmurs, dyspnea, cardiomegaly, and congestive heart failure. Of hyperthyroid cats, ~10% exhibit apathetic signs (eg, anorexia, lethargy, and depression); weight loss is common.

Elevated serum concentrations of T_4 and T_3 confirm the diagnosis; however, they are subject to a wide degree of fluctuation, and more than one basal measurement may be necessary.

Treatment: Spontaneous hyperthyroidism can be treated by thyroidectomy, radioiodine therapy, or chronic administration of an antithyroid drug. With unilateral thyroid tumors, hemithyroidectomy corrects the hyperthyroid state, and thyroxine supplementation usually is not necessary. For bilateral thyroid tumors, complete thyroidectomy is indicated, but parathyroid function must be preserved to avoid postoperative hypocalcemia. Thyroxine supplementation should be initiated 1-2 days following complete thyroidectomy. If iatrogenic hypoparathyroidism develops, treatment with vitamin D and calcium is also indicated.

Radioactive iodine provides a simple and safe treatment: radioiodine is concentrated within the thyroid gland and selectively irradiates and destroys hyperfunctioning thyroid tissue. The main disadvantage of such therapy is that most practitioners do not have access to radioiodine.

Treatment with methimazole, an antithyroid drug, controls hyperthyroidism by blocking thyroid hormone synthesis. Propylthiouracil, another antithyroid drug, is not recommended for use in cats because of the high incidence of serious side effects (especially hemolytic anemia and thrombocytopenia). The recommended initial daily dose of methimazole is 10-15 mg in 2 or 3 divided doses. The dose is adjusted to maintain circulating thyroid hormone concentrations within the normal range, and the drug is given daily. Adverse side effects, the more serious of which are agranulocytosis and thrombocytopenia, develop in <5% of treated cats. If this occurs, methimazole should be discontinued and supportive therapy instituted; these adverse reactions should resolve within 2 wk. To maintain normal levels of thyroid hormone, and to monitor for adverse reactions during the first 3 mo of treatment (when the most serious side effects associated with methimazole therapy develop), complete blood counts and serum thyroid hormone determinations should be repeated at 2- to 4-wk intervals, and the drug dose adjusted as necessary. Subsequently, serum T_4 concentrations should be measured at 3- to 6-mo intervals to monitor dosage requirements and response to treatment.

HUMORAL HYPERCALCEMIA OF MALIGNANCY
(HHM, Pseudohyperparathyroidism)

A metabolic disorder in which peptides resembling parathyroid hormone (PTH) or other bone-resorbing substances are secreted in excess amounts by malignant tumors of nonparathyroid origin.

Hypercalcemia and hypophosphatemia develop in dogs, cats, horses, and man, with several malignant neoplasms in the absence of bone metastases and functional lesions in the parathyroid glands. Neoplasms associated with this syndrome in animals include adenocarcinomas derived from apocrine glands of the anal sac, squamous cell carcinoma of the stomach, malignant lymphoma, and adenocarcinoma of the mammary gland.

Etiology and Pathogenesis: Evidence suggests that the hypercalcemia and hypophosphatemia are the result of secretion of bone-resorbing substances by tumor cells. Tumor cells can produce several humoral substances that induce calcium mobilization from bone. These include PTH-like protein, prostaglandins, interleukin-1 (osteoclast-activating factor), and transforming growth factors. Other growth factors, such as platelet-derived growth factor and epidermal growth factor, have been reported to directly stimulate bone resorption *in vitro*.

PTH-like factors bind to the PTH receptors of bone and kidney, but do not cross-react immunologically with native PTH. These factors stimulate adenylate cyclase in bone and kidney cells by binding to PTH receptors, and stimulate bone resorption. Interleukin-1 stimulates bone resorption *in vivo* and *in vitro* and acts synergistically with PTH. Transforming growth factors α and β can stimulate bone resorption *in vitro* and have been found in certain tumors associated with HHM.

Purification of PTH-like activity from the canine anal sac adenocarcinoma and multiple human tumors associated with HHM has resulted in the identification of novel proteins designated PTH-related proteins (PTHrP). It is likely that PTHrP are important in the pathogenesis of the clinical manifestations of HHM, in calcium (Ca) metabolism of the mammary gland and fetus, and in the differentiation of epidermal cells.

Canine lymphosarcoma is associated with hypercalcemia in 20-40% of the cases. Some dogs with lymphosarcoma and hypercalcemia have HHM. The affected dogs have increased fasting and 24-hr Ca excretion, increased fractional phosphorus excretion, increased nephrogenous cyclic adenosine monophosphate (cAMP), and no change in serum PTH or 1,25-dihydroxycholecalciferol levels. Increased osteoclastic resorption is present in bones without evidence of tumor metastasis. Hypercalcemia may be induced by circulating PTH-like factors in canine lymphosarcoma, which may be related to or the same as PTHrP.

Some human patients with lymphosarcoma and hypercalcemia have increased serum levels of 1,25-dihydroxycholecalciferol, which may be responsible for the induction of hypercalcemia. It is uncertain if this mechanism results in hypercalcemia in other animals with lymphosarcoma, but clinical data has identified a few dogs with lymphosarcoma, hypercalcemia, and increased serum 1,25-dihydroxycholecalciferol concentrations.

Clinical Findings: The best characterized example of HHM in animals occurs in association with adenocarcinoma derived from apocrine glands of the anal sac (qv, p 852), a syndrome characterized by persistent hypercalcemia and hypophosphatemia. Serum Ca values are 11.4-24 mg/dL (av ~16 mg/dL).

Functional disturbances in dogs with HHM are primarily due to severe hypercalcemia, and include generalized weakness, anorexia, vomiting, bradycardia, depression, polyuria, and polydipsia. Anorexia, vomiting, and constipation result from the decreased excitability of GI smooth muscle. Generalized weakness of skeletal muscle develops as a result of decreased neuromuscular excitability, which also may cause depression of lower motor neuron reflexes (eg, hyporeflexia of patellar, gastrocnemius, and triceps reflexes). Behavioral changes, depression, stupor, coma, seizures, and muscle twitching have been observed in dogs with hypercalcemia. Cardiac arrhythmia, shortening of the Q-T interval, and prolongation of the P-R interval (first degree heart block) may be detected on an ECG. Ventricular fibrillation can develop in extreme hypercalcemia.

Polydipsia and polyuria are encountered early in the course of diseases characterized by hypercalcemia. Initially, the polyuria and polydipsia are independent of uremic signs from primary renal failure; however, uremia may develop as a result of the toxic effects of persistent hypercalcemia on the kidneys. Severe dehydration often occurs from the combined effects of polyuria, emesis, and lack of water intake.

Lesions: Apocrine adenocarcinomas develop as firm masses in the perirectal area, ventrolateral to the anus, in close association with the anal sac but not attached to the overlying skin. It is histologically distinct from the more common perianal (circumanal) gland tumor (qv, p 853) that occurs predominantly in male dogs. Parathyroid glands of the affected dogs are small and difficult to locate or not visible macroscopically. The apocrine adenocarcinomas do not produce a substance that stimulates PTH secretion, but rather the parathyroid glands undergo atrophy in response to the persistent hypercalcemia. Thyroid C-cells often respond to the persistent elevation in blood Ca by undergoing diffuse or nodular hyperplasia.

Skeletal demineralization in dogs with HHM is mild in comparison with those of other causes of hypercalcemia, eg, primary hyperparathyroidism, and usually undetectable by conventional radiographic methods. Neoplastic cells from the perirectal adenocarcinomas rarely metastasize to bone and cause localized osteolysis. Variable numbers of osteoclasts are detected on bone surfaces in dogs with marked hypercalcemia, possibly reflecting different states in the course of the disease and phases of bone remodeling. Trabecular bone volume seems to be significantly decreased as compared to age-matched control dogs. Total resorptive surface is increased significantly, as are the numbers of osteoclasts.

Diagnosis: Criteria for the diagnosis include: 1) persistent hypercalcemia and hypophosphatemia, 2) absence of radiographic or pathological evidence of tumor metastases in bone, 3) atrophy of parathyroid glands and C-cell hyperplasia in the thyroid gland, 4) remission of hypercalcemia when the tumor is destroyed or excised, 5) demonstration of biologically active peptides or other bone-resorbing substances in tumor tissue, and 6) exacerbation of hypercalcemia if the tumor recurs following therapy.

Signs are referable primarily to the persistent hypercalcemia (≥ 12 mg/dL) and a mass in the perineum. Perirectal adenocarcinomas often require careful rectal palpation to confirm their presence, since their size ranges from 7 mm to ≥ 8 cm in diameter. In addition, dogs with this tumor have moderate hypophosphatemia (<3 mg/dL), decreased serum levels of immunoreactive PTH, normal serum levels of a major metabolite of prostaglandin E_2, and increased urinary excretion of Ca, phosphorus, and cAMP.

Affected dogs have inappropriate levels (maintenance of levels in normal range) of 1,25-dihydroxycholecalciferol for the degree of hypercalcemia. This suggests that the humoral factor produced by the neoplastic cells is capable of stimulating the renal 1-α-hydroxylase and increasing the formation of the active metabolite of vitamin D (1,25-dihydroxycholecalciferol), even in the presence of marked hypercalcemia.

Lymphosarcoma (malignant lymphoma) is the most common neoplasm associated with hypercalcemia in dogs and cats, and thus must be considered in differential diagnosis of HHM. (*See* CANINE LYMPHOMA, p 32, and FELINE LYMPHOSARCOMA, p 39.) The prevalence of hypercalcemia in lymphoma is estimated to be 10-40% in dogs. Peripheral lymph node enlargement may or may not be detected, but there usually is evidence of anterior mediastinal or visceral involvement. It is not completely resolved whether the hypercalcemia develops from the production of humoral substances by neoplastic cells or from physical disruption of trabecular bone due to frequent bone marrow involvement, or both.

Other sporadic causes of hypercalcemia in animals include solid tumors metastasizing widely to bone, hematologic malignancies in bone marrow, hypoadrenocorticism, renal failure in horses and dogs, hypervitaminosis D (from excess dietary supplementation, ingestion of vermicides, consumption of calcinogenic plants containing the active metabolite of vitamin D, or granulomatous diseases associated with 1,25-dihydroxycholecaliferol overproduction by macrophages), hemoconcentration with hyperproteinemia, immobilization, and osteomyelitis.

Treatment: Surgical removal of the tumor in the perirectal area results in a rapid return to normal of serum Ca, phosphorus, immunoreactive PTH, and 1,25-dihydroxycholecalciferol. However, sublumbar metastases occur in >90% of dogs with this tumor and are associated with a recrudescence of the biochemical alterations in serum and urine.

Dehydration exacerbates many of the severe effects of hypercalcemia; disturbances in fluid balance should be corrected. Replacement fluids such as isotonic solutions, lactated Ringer's, or 0.9% sodium chloride should be administered IV; calciuresis may be enhanced by administering 0.9% sodium chloride IV, because the additional sodium presented to the renal tubules diminishes Ca reabsorption. If the serum concentration of Ca is only moderately increased (12-14 mg/dL), these measures alone may result in adequate initial lowering of serum Ca. Additional measures may be necessary when the clinical signs and Ca elevation are more severe (>15 mg/dL). Furosemide and sodium sulfate are calciuretic agents that may be used. Adequate extracellular fluid volume must be maintained by proper administration of IV fluids while using these diuretics. Furosemide given to dogs with experimental hypercalcemia at 5 mg/kg, IV, has been reported to reduce the serum Ca concentration. Thiazide diuretics reduce the urinary excretion of Ca and are contraindicated in cases of hypercalcemia. Peritoneal dialysis is an alternative method of removing Ca from the body, particularly in uremic animals.

Glucocorticoids may lower serum Ca concentration, probably by inhibiting its intestinal absorption and increasing its urinary excretion. In addition, direct antitumor activity may be responsible for reduction of serum Ca concentration, most notably in lymphosarcoma. For hypercalcemic crises, IV administration of sodium bicarbonate may temporarily reduce the toxic effects via diminution in the level of ionized Ca associated with alkalosis.

Since prerenal factors are commonly associated with hypercalcemia, fluid therapy also helps to maintain renal perfusion, thereby minimizing progressive ischemic damage to nephrons. No therapy eliminates the renal lesions already present; however, tubular lesions may be repaired by regeneration and functional adaptation if the hypercalcemia can be controlled, and the animal kept alive long enough. Mineral deposits may dissolve, although this is a slow process.

NEUROENDOCRINE TISSUE TUMORS

Neuroendocrine tissues derived from the embryonic neural crest are widely dispersed throughout the body. In mammals, they are in the center of the adrenal gland, and are concerned with the synthesis and secretion of the catecholamine hormones (epinephrine and norepinephrine). C-cells in the mammalian thyroid gland also are derived from the neural crest, and during early embryonic development are incorporated into the last (ultimobranchial) pharyngeal pouch, which subsequently fuses with each thyroid lobe. C-cells are concerned with the biosynthesis of calcitonin, a hormone involved in the regulation of calcium homeostasis and skeletal turnover.

Tumors develop occasionally from neuroendocrine cells in the adrenal medulla, thyroid, and aortic and carotid bodies. They are of clinical significance both from physical disruption of adjacent normal tissues by the enlarging mass, and possibly by autonomous secretion of excess hormone.

ADRENAL MEDULLA

Adrenal Medullary Hyperplasia: Diffuse or nodular adrenal medullary hyperplasia appears to precede the development of pheochromocytoma in bulls with C-cell tumors of the thyroid gland. This diffuse proliferation of chromaffin cells is nonencapsulated but compresses the surrounding adrenal cortex. In bulls with prominent diffuse medullary hyperplasia, there are often a few small foci of intense nodular proliferation of medullary cells.

Neuroblastomas and Ganglioneuromas: Neuroblastomas arise from primitive neuroectodermal cells, often in younger animals, and form a large intra-abdominal mass. They differ from pheochromocytomas in that they are composed of small tumor cells with a hyperchromatic nucleus and a scant amount of cytoplasm. They often resemble lymphocytes and tend to form pseudorosettes. Neurofibrils or unmyelinated nerve fibers can be demonstrated in neuroblastomas.

Ganglioneuromas are usually well-differentiated, small tumors that have multipolar ganglion cells and neurofibrils. They are benign tumors in the medulla, composed of multipolar ganglion cells and neurofibrils with a prominent fibrous connective tissue stroma. The surrounding adrenal cortex is severely compressed. Neoplastic cells in medullary tumors occasionally differentiate in 2 directions resulting in adjacent pheochromocytomas and ganglioneuromas in the same adrenal gland.

Pheochromocytomas: These are tumors of chromaffin cells and are almost always located in the adrenal glands. They are the most common tumors in the adrenal medulla of animals, and develop most often in cattle, laboratory rats, and dogs, and infrequently in other domestic animals. In bulls and rats, pheochromocytomas develop concurrently with calcitonin-secreting C-cell tumors of the thyroid gland. This may represent a neoplastic transformation of multiple types of endocrine cells of neuroectodermal origin in the same individual. Malignant pheochromocytoma designates a medullary tumor that invades through the adrenal capsule and into adjacent structures (eg, posterior vena cava) and/or metastasizes to distant sites (eg, liver, regional lymph nodes, or lungs). Functional pheochromocytomas are reported infrequently in animals; however, several dogs and horses with pheochromocytomas have had tachycardia, edema, and cardiac hypertrophy attributed to excess catecholamine secretion.

Although size varies considerably, they often are large (≥ 10 cm in diameter) and incorporate most of the affected adrenal. A small remnant of the adrenal gland often can be found at one pole. Smaller tumors are well encapsulated by a thin, compressed rim of adrenal cortex. Large pheochromocytomas are multilobular and variegated, and light brown to yellow-red, due to areas of hemorrhage and necrosis; they may exert pressure on and invade adjacent tissues, particularly the vena cava and aorta, which may be partially occluded. In dogs, metastases to the liver, regional lymph nodes, spleen, and lungs occur in ~50% of pheochromocytomas.

THYROID C-CELL TUMORS

Tumors derived from C-(parafollicular, ultimobranchial) cells of the thyroid gland are most common in adult to aged bulls and horses, and certain strains of laboratory rats. A high percentage of aged bulls has been reported to develop C-cell tumors ($\geq 30\%$) or hyperplasia of C-cells and ultimobranchial derivatives (≥ 15-20%). These have not been observed in cows fed similar diets. The incidence increases with advancing age in bulls and is often associated with development of increased vertebral density. Multiple endocrine tumors, especially bilateral pheochromocytomas and occasionally pituitary adenomas, are detected coincidentally in bulls (and people) with C-cell tumors. A high frequency of thyroid C-cell tumors and pheochromocytomas has been reported in a family of Guernsey bulls, which suggests an autosomal dominant pattern of inheritance. A diffuse or nodular hyperplasia of secretory cells in the adrenal medulla often precedes the development of pheochromocytoma.

Adenomas: C-cell adenomas appear in one or both thyroid lobes as discrete, single or multiple, gray to tan nodules. Adenomas are smaller ($\sim$1-3 cm in diameter) than carcinomas and are separated from the thyroid parenchyma by a thin, fibrous, connective tissue capsule. The adjacent thyroid is compressed but not invaded by the tumor. In horses, C-cell adenomas may result in a palpable enlargement in the anterior cervical region. Larger C-cell adenomas incorporate most of the thyroid lobe, but a rim of dark brown-red thyroid often is present on one side.

Focal and/or nodular hyperplasia of C-cells often precedes development of C-cell neoplasms. Nodular hyperplasia of C-cells consists of foci less than the size of a colloid-filled follicle, whereas a thyroid C-cell adenoma is a discrete, expansive mass of cells, greater in size than a colloid-distended follicle. Calcitonin immunoreactivity has been localized to the cytoplasm of hyperplastic C-cells.

Carcinomas: Thyroid C-cell carcinomas cause extensive multinodular enlargements of one or both thyroid lobes, and may incorporate the entire thyroid gland. Multiple metastases in anterior cervical lymph nodes usually are large and have areas of necrosis and hemorrhage. Pulmonary metastases are infrequent and appear as discrete tan nodules throughout all lobes of the lung.

The chronic stimulation of C-cells by long-term dietary intake of excess calcium may be related to the high incidence of these tumors in bulls; adult bulls frequently were fed diets with 3.5-6 times the amount of calcium normally recommended for maintenance, and a significant decline in incidence of the tumors has been reported when they were switched to a reduced calcium intake.

Syndromes associated with abnormalities in the secretion of calcitonin are recognized much less frequently than disorders involving parathyroid hormone (PTH). A hypersecretion of calcitonin has been reported in people, bulls, and laboratory rats with medullary (ultimobranchial) thyroid neoplasms derived from C-cells. The syndrome often involves many individuals in a human family. In adults with a chronic excess secretion of calcitonin, serum calcium and phosphorus levels usually remain in the low-normal range owing to the relatively slow turnover rate of bone and compensatory increase in PTH secretion. Osteosclerotic changes have been reported in bulls with this syndrome, but the relationship of long-term excess calcitonin secretion to the pathogenesis of the skeletal lesions and their occurrence in other species is unclear.

CHEMORECEPTOR ORGANS

Sensitive barometers of changes in the carbon dioxide and oxygen content and pH of the blood, these aid in the regulation of respiration and circulation. Although chemoreceptor tissue appears to be widely distributed in the body, tumors develop principally in the aortic and carotid bodies, more frequently in the former in animals, but more frequently in the latter in man. These tumors occur primarily in dogs, and rarely in cats and cattle. Brachycephalic breeds of dogs, such as the Boxer and Boston Terrier, are predisposed to tumors of the aortic and carotid bodies.

Aortic body tumors appear most frequently as single masses or as multiple nodules within the pericardial sac near the base of the heart. They vary considerably in size (0.5-12.5 cm), with carcinomas, in general, being larger than adenomas. Solitary, small adenomas either are attached to the adventitia of the pulmonary artery and ascending aorta, or are embedded in the adipose connective tissue between these major vascular trunks. They have a smooth external surface and on cross-section are white and mottled, with red to brown areas. Larger adenomas may indent the atria or displace the trachea, are multilobular, and partially surround the major arterial trunks at the base of the heart.

In dogs, malignant aortic body tumors occur less frequently than adenomas. Carcinomas may infiltrate the wall of the pulmonary artery to form papillary projections into the lumen or invade through the wall into the lumen of the atria. Although tumor cells often invade blood vessels, metastases to the lungs and liver occur infrequently in dogs with aortic body carcinomas.

Tumors of the aortic bodies in animals are not functional (ie, they do not secrete excess hormone into the circulation), but as space-occupying lesions may result in various functional disturbances. These include manifestations of cardiac decompensation due to pressure on the atria, vena cava, or both, associated with larger aortic body adenomas and carcinomas. Aortic body tumors tend to be more benign than tumors of the carotid body. They grow slowly by expansion and exert pressure on the vena cava and atria. Aortic body carcinomas may invade locally into the atria, pericardium, and adjacent large thin-walled vessels.

A **carotid body tumor** arises near the bifurcation of the common carotid artery, and usually appears as a unilateral slow-growing mass. Adenomas are ~1-4 cm in diameter, well encapsulated, and have a smooth external surface. The bifurcation of the carotid artery is incorporated in the mass, and tumor cells are firmly adherent to the tunica adventitia. Adenomas are firm, white with scattered areas of hemorrhage, and extremely vascular. Complete excision or biopsy often is difficult due to the high degree of vascularity and intimate relationship with major arterial trunks in the neck.

Malignant carotid body tumors are larger and more coarsely multinodular then adenomas. Although carcinomas appear to be encapsulated, tumor cells invade the capsule and penetrate into the walls of adjacent vessels and lymphatics. The external jugular vein and several cranial nerves may be incorporated by the neoplasm. Metastases of carotid body tumors occur in ~30% of cases and have been found in the lung, bronchial and mediastinal lymph nodes, liver, pancreas, and kidneys. Multicentric neoplastic transformation of chemoreceptor tissue occurs frequently in brachycephalic breeds of dogs.

The histologic characteristics of chemoreceptor tumors ("chemodectomas") are essentially similar whether derived from the carotid or aortic body.

Although the etiology of carotid and aortic body tumors is unknown, it has been suggested that a genetic predisposition aggravated by chronic hypoxia may account for the higher risk in certain brachycephalic breeds. Carotid bodies of several mammalian species, including dogs, have undergone hyperplasia when subjected to chronic hypoxia by living in a high-altitude environment.

EYE AND EAR

EE

OPHTHALMOLOGY

PHYSICAL EXAMINATION OF THE EYE

The initial ocular examination should assess symmetry, conformation, and gross lesions; the eye should be viewed from 2-3 ft (≤ 1 m) away, in good light, and with minimal restraint of the head. The anterior segment of the eye and pupillary light reflexes are examined in detail with a strong light and under magnification in a darkened room. Schirmer's tear testing, fluorescein staining, corneal and conjunctival cytology and cultures, intraocular pressure measurement (tonometry), eversion of lids for examination, and flushing the nasolacrimal duct are ancillary procedures for evaluating diseases of the adnexa and anterior segment of the eye. Diseases of the vitreous and ocular fundus are detected or evaluated by ophthalmoscopy, usually performed after inducing mydriasis, and vision testing (obstacle course).

Schirmer's tear test and corneoconjunctival cultures should be performed before instillation of topical anesthetic. Fluorescein staining and eversion of the eyelids do not require topical anesthesia, but intraocular pressure measurement (tonometry), examination of the posterior face of the nictitating membrane, conjunctival and corneal cytology, gonioscopy, and lavage of the nasolacrimal duct usually do.

Special examinations such as slit-lamp biomicroscopy or electroretinography may require sedation or local, regional, or general anesthesia.

EYELIDS

CONFORMATIONAL ABNORMALITIES

Entropion: An inversion of all or part of the lid margins that may involve one or both eyelids and the canthi. Entropion is usually associated with inherited eyelid defects in many canine and ovine breeds, cicatrix formation, or severe blepharospasm due to ocular or periocular pain. Inversion of the cilia or facial hairs creates further discomfort, conjunctival and corneal irritation, and if protracted, causes corneal scarring, pigmentation, and perhaps ulceration. Early spastic entropion may be reversed if: 1) the inciting cause is removed, or 2) further pain is alleviated by everting the lid hairs away from the eye with mattress sutures in the lid, injections (eg, of procaine penicillin) into the lid adjacent to the entropion, or palpebral nerve blocks. Established entropion may require surgical correction.

Ectropion: A slack everted lid margin, usually with a large palpebral fissure, is a common bilateral conformational fault in a number of dog breeds; contracting scars in the lid or facial nerve paralysis may produce unilateral ectropion in any species. Conjunctival exposure results in chronic or recurrent conjunctivitis from environmental irritants and bacterial infection. Topical antibiotic-corticosteroid preparations may temporarily control intermittent infections, but surgical correction is indicated in many instances. Mild cases can be controlled by repeated periodic lavage with mild decongestant solutions.

Lagophthalmos: Inability to fully close the lids and protect the cornea from drying and trauma may result from extremely shallow orbits, exophthalmia due to a space-occupying orbital lesion, or facial nerve paralysis. Corneal scarring, pigmentation, and ulceration usually result. Unless the cause can be corrected, the therapy is topical lubricants and surgical shortening or closure of the fissure(s) either permanently or temporarily, depending on the cause. Excessive nasal skin folds and facial hair may aggravate the damage caused by lagophthalmos.

Abnormalities of the Cilia: Extra or misdirected cilia on the lid margin can produce epiphora or corneal scarring and ulceration. In many instances, anomalous cilia are very fine and produce neither clinical signs nor damage. However, misdirected cilia protruding through the palpebral conjunctiva can cause profound pain. If the signs correlate with the extra cilia, excision or cryothermy of the cilia follicle is indicated. Anomalies of the cilia are common in some dog breeds and probably are inherited.

INFLAMMATION

Blepharitis (inflammation of the eyelids) can result from extension of a generalized dermatitis, conjunctivitis or local infections, or irritants such as plant oils or solar exposure. The lids can be the original site of involvement for agents that progress to a generalized dermatitis. Dermatophytes, *Demodex canis*, and bacteria such as staphylococci often are involved. The mucocutaneous junction of the skin and conjunctiva can be the site for immune-mediated diseases such as pemphigus. Local glandular infections may be acute or chronic (stye and chalazion). In generalized blepharitis, systemic therapy often is indicated in addition to topical treatment. Supportive therapy of hot packing and frequent cleansing often is indicated in acute cases. Nonophthalmic preparations can be used to treat the eyelids, but caution in application is indicated to avoid corneal irritation. Skin scrapings, cultures, and biopsies may be required for an accurate diagnosis.

LACRIMAL APPARATUS

Hypertrophy and prolapse of the gland of the nictitating membrane (**cherry eye**) is common in young dogs. In the acute stages, the large red mass swells and protrudes over the edge of the nictitans, and there is a mucopurulent discharge. Although the swelling may recede for short periods, it eventually remains prolapsed, but rarely produces detrimental signs in the chronic stages. Since it is a major tear gland, it should be preserved by anchoring sutures to the orbital rim or by partial excision. Complete excision may predispose to keratoconjunctivitis sicca (*see* below).

Dacryocystitis (inflammation of the lacrimal sac) usually is caused by obstruction of the proximal nasolacrimal duct by inflammatory debris, foreign bodies, or masses pressing on the duct. It produces epiphora and secondary conjunctivitis refractory to treatment.

Abscessation of the lacrimal sac may occur. Irrigation of the nasolacrimal duct will reveal an obstruction of the duct or reflux of mucopurulent discharge from the puncta, or both. Radiographs of the skull after injection of contrast material into the duct may be necessary to establish the site and cause of the obstruction. Therapy consists of maintaining patency of the duct and instilling topical antibiotic solutions. Polyethylene tubing temporarily implanted in the duct may be necessary to maintain patency.

Atresia of the lacrimal puncta is a cause of epiphora in dogs and cats, while atresia of the nasal end of the nasolacrimal duct is a cause of dacryocystitis in young horses and cattle. Therapy consists of surgically opening the orifice and maintaining its patency.

Keratoconjunctivitis sicca (KCS) is due to a tear deficiency and usually results in persistent, mucopurulent conjunctivitis and corneal scarring and ulceration. The syndrome is common in dogs, in which it often is associated with autoimmune adenitis. Distemper infection, chronic sulfonamide therapy, and trauma are less frequent causes of KCS. The disease is infrequent in cats and rare in horses. Topical therapy consists of artificial tears and, if there is no ulceration, antibiotic-steroid combinations. Lacrimogenics such as pilocarpine mixed in food may be useful (a 20-30 lb [10-15 kg] dog should be started on 2-4 drops of 2% pilocarpine b.i.d.). Topical 2% cyclosporin (although not available as a commercial ophthalmic preparation) b.i.d. increases tear production in many dogs. Mucolytic agents, eg, 10% acetylcysteine, lyse excess mucus and restore the spreading capability of other topical agents. In chronic KCS, medical therapy is usually inadequate to control the progression of corneal scarring, and parotid duct transplantation is indicated.

CONJUNCTIVA

Subconjunctival hemorrhage may arise from trauma or blood dyscrasias; it does not require therapy, but close inspection is warranted to determine if more important intraocular alterations have occurred. If definite evidence or history of trauma is not present, then systemic examination is indicated to determine the cause.

Chemosis, or **conjunctival edema**, occurs to some degree with all cases of conjunctivitis, but the most dramatic examples are seen with allergic reactions, trauma, and insect bites. The latter are treated with topical corticosteroids and usually resolve rapidly. Specific therapy for the etiological agent is indicated.

Conjunctivitis is common in all domestic species; the etiological agent(s) varies from infectious to environmental irritants. The signs are hyperemia, chemosis, ocular discharge, follicular hyperplasia, and mild ocular discomfort. The appearance of the conjunctiva usually is not sufficiently distinctive to suggest the etiological agent, and specific diagnosis depends on history, physical examination, conjunctival scrapings and culture, Schirmer's tear test, and occasionally, biopsy. Unilateral conjunctivitis indicates a condition unique to one eye, such as a foreign body, dacryocystitis, or KCS (*see* above). In cats, mycoplasma or *Chlamydia cati* may produce conjunctivitis that begins in one eye and becomes bilateral after ~1 wk. Specific diagnosis is made most rapidly by demonstrating the inclusions or the agent in conjunctival scrapings. Bilateral conjunctivitis is common in a variety of viral infections in all species. Herpesviruses produce conjunctivitis in cats, cattle, horses, and pigs, and transiently in dogs. Purulent discharge indicates a bacterial component, but this may be opportunistic due to debilitation of the mucous membrane. Environmental irritants and allergens are common causes for conjunctivitis in all species. If a mucopurulent exudate is present, topical antibiotic therapy is indicated, but may not be curative if other predisposing factors are involved. Mechanical factors such as foreign bodies, environmental irritants, parasites, and conformational defects should be removed or corrected. Topical tetracycline is indicated for chlamydial infection; topical antiviral preparations, such as idoxuridine, are indicated for herpesvirus infections.

CORNEA

Superficial keratitis is common in all species and is characterized by corneal vascularization and opacification, which may be due to edema, cellular infiltrates, pigmentation, or fibroplasia. If ulceration is present, pain, manifest by epiphora and blepharospasm, is an outstanding sign. Unilateral keratitis frequently is traumatic in origin. Mechanical factors, such as lid conformational defects and foreign bodies, should always be eliminated as possible causes since improvement will not occur until they are resolved. Ulcerative keratitis may be complicated by secondary invasion by bacteria, and, in horses, by saprophytic fungi. Bilateral superficial keratitis may be immune-mediated or associated with a lack of tears, conformational defects, or infectious agents.

A specific **chronic superficial keratitis** (Uberreiter's disease, pannus) is a bilateral, progressive, proliferative, superficial keratitis that begins laterally at the limbus and eventually extends from all quadrants to cover the cornea. It is most common in German Shepherd Dogs. Specific therapy for superficial keratitis consists of topical antibiotics, antiviral or antimycotic agents when appropriate, removal of mechanical irritants when present, tear replacement when deficient, and corticosteroids when immune-mediated. The latter may have to be continued indefinitely and the frequency varied depending on the response.

Interstitial keratitis is a deep involvement of the stroma and is present with all chronic and many acute cases of anterior uveitis. The corneal neovascularization is deeper and less branching than in superficial keratitis; if the endothelium has been disrupted, corneal edema is often marked. Systemic diseases, such as infectious canine hepatitis, malignant catarrhal fever, systemic mycoses, and septicemias that localize in the eye, are causes for bilateral or unilateral interstitial keratitis. Therapy is directed at the anterior uveitis, the systemic infection, or both.

Ulcerative keratitis may be superficial, deep, deep with descemetocele, or perforating. Pain, corneal irregularity, edema, and eventually, neovascularization are signs of ulceration. A dense, white infiltrate at the ulcer margin indicates strong leukotaxis and bacterial involvement. To detect small ulcers, topical sodium fluorescein may be required. In dogs and horses, most ulcers are mechanical in origin; in cattle and sheep, infectious agents and mechanical causes are important; and in cats, herpesvirus. All ulcers have the potential for secondary bacterial contamination or endogenous enzymatic "melting" of the stroma. Therapy for superficial ulcers is usually medical, and consists of topical antibiotic(s), topical atropine for iridocycloplegia, and correction of any mechanical factors. Slow-healing superficial ulcers occur in dogs, cats, and horses; in cats, herpesvirus should be suspected; in dogs, they may be due to basement membrane disease, and may recur. Multiple punctures or cross-hatching of the basement membrane with a 25-gauge needle stimulates most indolent ulcers to heal within 7-10 days. Nictitating membrane flaps (or a soft contact lens) act as a pressure bandage and often are therapeutic. Deep ulcers are treated medically similarly to superficial ulcers, but in addition, most require surgery to rapidly strengthen the cornea.

Dermoids are fleshy, hair-covered masses that may involve the cornea, limbus, conjunctiva, nictitating membrane, and eyelids in all species. Present at birth and usually detected shortly thereafter, local excision is curative.

Inflammatory nodules of the cornea and conjunctiva, such as nodular fasciitis in dogs and proliferative keratoconjunctivitis in Collies, may mimic neoplasms by their fleshy appearance and recurrence. Treatment is topical corticosteroids, local excision, cryothermy, or azothioprine. In cats, eosinophilic keratitis has similar clinical signs and is treated by topical corticosteroids, oral megestrol acetate, or local excision.

ANTERIOR UVEA

Persistent pupillary membranes are remnants of a congenital vascular network that filled the pupillary region. Persistence of pigmented strands across the pupil from one area of the iris to another, or to the lens or cornea, is not uncommon in dogs, and occurs occasionally in other species. In the Basenji, the condition is inherited.

Atrophy of the iris is common in dogs and may involve the pupillary margin or the stroma. Atrophy of the pupillary margin creates a scalloped border and a weakening of the sphincter muscle, which is manifest as a dilated pupil(s) or by sluggish pupillary light reflexes. Stromal atrophy results in dramatic holes in the iris, and often, displacement of the pupil. Neither form of atrophy appears detrimental to visual function. Animals lacking a functional iridal sphincter may have blepharospasm in bright light.

Iridic cysts in dogs usually are free-floating, pigmented spheres in the aqueous humor. In cats, the cysts frequently are attached at the pupillary margin; in horses, they are present in the stroma of the iris. Therapy is rarely necessary, but aspiration can be performed. Transillumination demonstrates their cystic nature and differentiates them from neoplasms.

Anterior uveitis or **iridocyclitis**, when acute, is manifest by miosis, increased protein and cells in the anterior chamber, hypotonia, bulbar conjunctival vascular injection, iridal swelling, photophobia, and blepharospasm. Glaucoma, cataract, and corneal opacification may be complications of anterior uveitis. Causes of anterior uveitis can be separated into exogenous and endogenous. Penetrating and nonpenetrating trauma, infectious systemic disease, and rarely, intraocular neoplasms or intraocular helminths are causes of unilateral uveitis. Systemic infectious diseases and immune-mediated diseases are the most common causes of bilateral uveitis. Examples of the former are infectious canine hepatitis, feline infectious peritonitis, feline leukemia, toxoplasmosis, systemic mycoses, canine brucellosis, leptospirosis, malignant catarrhal fever, infectious bovine rhinotracheitis, equine viral arteritis, hog cholera, canine ehrlichiosis, and neonatal bacterial infections (joints, navel, and gut) of calves. Recurrent uveitis that is at least in part immune-mediated affects horses (equine uveitis, qv, p 302) and dogs (panuveitis with dermal depigmentation). A thorough history, examination of the cornea for injuries, physical examination, and aqueous centesis for culture and cytology are diagnostic aids.

Nonspecific therapy consists of topical atropine 2-4 times/day, topical corticosteroids (if nonbacterial) 4-6 times/day, a darkened environment, and prostaglandin inhibitors (such as aspirin, flunixin meglumine, and phenylbutazone). If bacterial in origin, topical, systemic, and perhaps intraocular antibiotics are indicated. Immune-mediated processes may require systemic or subconjunctival as well as topical corticosteroids.

GLAUCOMA

A group of diseases manifest by an increase in intraocular pressure that damages the retina and optic nerve. Accompanying signs are dilated, fixed, or sluggish pupil; selective conjunctival injection; corneal edema; and a firm globe. Enlargement of the globe may result in lens displacement and breaks in Descemet's membrane. Pain usually is manifest by behavioral changes rather than blepharospasm. The condition is classified as primary or secondary, and as to whether the anterior chamber angle is open or obstructed (closed). Primary glaucomas, which are suspected of having a genetic predisposition, eventually become bilateral; primary open angle glaucoma in Beagles is inherited as a simple autosomal recessive. American Cocker Spaniels and Basset Hounds also are afflicted commonly. Secondary glaucomas are associated with acquired intraocular diseases that interfere with aqueous outflow. Intraocular inflammation is the most common cause, but neoplasms, hyphema, and lens displacements are additional causes.

Since high intraocular pressure can permanently damage the eye within a few days, acute glaucoma is an emergency. Therapy consists of IV mannitol, oral carbonic anhydrase inhibitors, and topical pilocarpine or timolol. Many animals with primary glaucoma are candidates for surgery or cyclocryothermy, since normal ocular pressures cannot be consistently maintained medically for longer than 2-3 days. Therapy for secondary glaucoma varies with the response to medication and whether the secondary cause can be removed surgically. Blind glaucomatous eyes may be treated by enucleation, intraocular prosthesis, cyclocryothermy, or injection of 10-25 mg of gentamicin into the vitreous.

LENS

Cataracts are an opacity of the lens or its capsule, and should be differentiated from the normal increase in nuclear density (nuclear sclerosis) that occurs in older animals. Cataracts usually are classified by their age of onset (congenital, juvenile, senile), location, cause, degree of opacification (incipient, immature, mature, hypermature), and shape. Most cataracts can be detected by dilating the pupil and examining the pupillary region against the retroillumination of the tapetal fundus. Dogs suffer from cataracts (often inherited) more commonly than other species. Other etiologies include diabetes mellitus, malnutrition, inflammation, and trauma. In cats and horses, most cataracts are secondary to inflammation. In general, the only therapy for cataracts that are severe enough to produce blindness is surgical removal of the lens. Juvenile cataracts may undergo sufficient resorption to regain sight; congenital nuclear cataracts may reduce in size with growth of the lens. Animals with immature (incomplete) cataracts may benefit from atropine 2-3 times/wk, which allows vision around a central density.

Lens displacement is seen in all species, but is common as a primary inherited defect in several terrier breeds. Complete displacement into the anterior chamber produces acute signs and frequently is accompanied by glaucoma and corneal edema. Treatment is surgical removal. Posterior displacement into the vitreous cavity is asymptomatic or associated with ocular inflammation or glaucoma. Subluxated lenses are recognized by an aphakic crescent and trembling of the iris (iridodonesis). The decision to remove subluxated lenses is based on the severity of signs, and judgment as to the role of the lens in producing the signs. Lens displacements also can be produced by trauma, enlargement of the globe, and degenerative zonular changes with chronic cataracts.

OCULAR FUNDUS

Diseases of the ocular fundus (retina, choroid, optic disk) may be isolated to the eye, or may be manifestations of systemic diseases. Inherited abnormalities may be congenital or appear later, and are important in the pathogenesis of retinopathies in dogs. Trauma, metabolic disturbances, systemic infections, neoplasms, blood dyscrasias, and nutritional deficiencies are possible underlying causes for retinopathies in all species.

INHERITED RETINOPATHIES

Collie eye anomaly is a congenital, recessively inherited, ocular defect with variable expression. The basic lesion is an area of chorioretinal hypoplasia lateral to the optic disk. More severely affected dogs have additional colobomatous lesions of the papilla or peripapillary region, and retinal detachments. Retinal vascular tortuosity is common and intraocular hemorrhage may occur. Vision is not appreciably affected unless a retinal detachment is present.

Progressive retinal atrophy (PRA) is a group of degenerative retinopathies consisting of several inherited photoreceptor diseases that have a similar clinical appearance. It is a recessive trait in various dog breeds, and a similar disease has been described in cats. The age of onset of clinical signs varies with the type of PRA, from 4-6 mo in Irish Setters and Collies, to 3-5 yr in Miniature Poodles and other breeds. Night blindness is noted early and progresses to total blindness over months to years. Ophthalmoscopic lesions are a bilateral symmetrical increase in reflectivity of the tapetal fundus, decreased pigmentation of the nontapetal fundus, attenuation and a decrease in the number of retinal vessels, and eventually, atrophy of the optic papilla. Progressive cortical cataracts are common later in the course of PRA and may mask the underlying retinopathy. No effective therapy is available.

A second type of retinal degeneration in dogs is **central progressive retinal atrophy** (CPRA) that primarily involves retinal pigment epithelium dystrophy. Breeds most often affected are the Labrador Retriever, rough and smooth Collies, Border Collie, Shetland Sheepdog, and Briard. CPRA is inherited in Labrador Retrievers as a dominant trait with variable penetrance. Early ophthalmoscopic findings are small foci of irregular pigmentation in the tapetal fundus, which eventually coalesce and fade as its reflectivity increases. The nontapetal fundus becomes mottled, retinal vessels disappear, and the optic nerve head atrophies. Progressive impairment of vision occurs gradually over several years. There is no effective treatment.

Retinal dysplasia is a congenital, local or generalized maldevelopment of the retina that may arise from trauma, genetic defect, or intrauterine damage, such as viral infection. Focal areas of retinal maldevelopment may be asymptomatic or interfere with central vision. Severe dysplasia is manifest as complete retinal detachment. Cataracts may accompany the syndrome, and in Labrador Retrievers may be associated with skeletal dysplasia (shortening) of the forelegs.

Optic nerve hypoplasia may be inherited in Miniature Poodles; in cats, it may be a result of *in utero* panleukopenia infection. The condition may be unilateral or bilateral. Bilateral involvement is manifest as blindness in the neonate; unilateral involvement is often an incidental finding later in life, or becomes manifest if a disease process affects the other eye.

CHORIORETINITIS

Chorioretinitis frequently is a manifestation of systemic infectious disease; it is a convenient diagnostic clue and a prognosticator of visual function. Unless the lesions are generalized or involve the optic nerve, they often are "silent". Scars may be differentiated from active lesions by the haze and ill-defined borders of the latter. Chorioretinitis may be present with canine distemper, systemic mycoses, prototheocosis, toxoplasmosis, tuberculosis, bacterial septicemias, feline infectious peritonitis, thromboembolic meningoencephalitis, malignant catarrhal fever, hog cholera, leptospirosis in horses, and onchocerciasis. Therapy usually is directed at the systemic disease.

ORBIT

The signs of **orbital cellulitis** are acute pain on opening the mouth, unilateral prolapse of the nictitating membrane, forward displacement of the globe, and conjunctivitis. Keratitis may develop from lagophthalmos (qv, p 292). The condition is seen predominantly in large breeds of dogs; in small dogs, it usually is due to a tooth abscess. Foreign bodies such as migrating grass awns, and zygomatic sialadenitis are additional causes. Orbital hemorrhage and neoplasia mimic inflammation except that opening the mouth is not painful. In acute cases, systemic broad-spectrum antibiotics are usually curative, but if swelling behind the last molar is present, drainage of this area is indicated. Relapses may occur, and radiographs are indicated to detect abscessed teeth. Warm compresses and topical lubricants to protect the cornea are also indicated.

PROLAPSE OF THE EYE

Acute prolapse is a result of trauma and is most common in dogs and cats. The globe should be replaced if the animal's physical condition allows general anesthesia. The lateral canthus is incised and the globe manually retropulsed. Eyelid and nictitating membrane sutures prevent recurrence. The traumatic injury is treated by a systemic route. The prognosis is guarded for retention of vision, but good for retention of the globe.

OPHTHALMIC ONCOLOGY

The eye and associated structures can develop neoplasms from the different tissues within the orbit; they also can be metastatic sites. Ophthalmic neoplasms vary in frequency and importance in different species.

BOVINE OPHTHALMIC ONCOLOGY

The most frequent ophthalmic neoplasms in cattle are the squamous cell carcinoma complex and the orbital infiltration associated with lymphosarcoma. The latter, with extensive invasion of the orbital structures, results in progressive exophthalmia, reduced ocular mobility, exposure keratitis, and corneal ulcerations that can perforate.

Bovine ocular squamous cell carcinoma (cancer eye) may affect the eyelids, conjunctivae, and nictitating membrane, but most frequently the medial and lateral limbal regions (corneoscleral junction). The cancerous or precancerous lesions are bilateral or multiple in the same eye in ~28% of cases. It occurs most often in Herefords, less often in Simmentals and Holstein-Friesians, and rarely in other breeds.

Ocular squamous cell carcinoma is the most common neoplasm of cattle; it results in significant economic loss due to condemnation at slaughter and a shortened productive life. The peak age incidence is 8 yr. The etiology is multifactorial with heritability, sunlight, nutrition, and perhaps viral involvement. The manifestations on the eyelid have been related to a lack of pigmentation; those on the globe have not, but they also have a heritable basis. Ultraviolet radiation and a high plane of nutrition are contributing influences. The viruses of infectious bovine rhinotracheitis and papilloma have been isolated from the neoplasms, but their significance is unknown.

The lesions usually begin as benign, smooth, white plaques on the conjunctival surfaces that may progress to a papilloma and then a squamous cell carcinoma, or go directly to the malignant stage. The lid lesions usually begin as either an ulcerative or a hyperkeratotic lesion (cutaneous horn). While in this benign stage, ~30% may spontaneously regress. The tumor may get quite large without invading the globe, but invasion into the eye and orbit, and metastasis to regional lymph nodes are late stages of the disease. Diagnosis usually is made by the typical clinical appearance, but can be confirmed rapidly by cytological examination of impression smears. The intraocular tumor invasion must be differentiated from severely disorganized eyes after trauma and infectious bovine keratoconjunctivitis.

Squamous cell carcinomas have responded to medical therapy, excision, cryotherapy, hyperthermia, radiation therapy, and immunotherapy. Both cryotherapy and hyperthermia have yielded excellent short-term results, but recurrence at the same or a different site is ~25%.

For advanced lesions confined to the globe, enucleation is recommended. When adjacent tissues are affected also, exenteration (removal of the globe and all orbital contents) should be performed. Immunotherapy is still experimental and the tumor regression may be temporary. Radiation therapy is not practical in the field, but may be an option for valuable animals referred to institutions.

Owners of problem herds should be advised of the heritability factor, and affected animals and their offspring culled to decrease the incidence.

CANINE OPHTHALMIC ONCOLOGY

Orbital neoplasms are exhibited as progressive space-occupying masses that produce exophthalmia, conjunctival and eyelid swelling, strabismus, exposure keratitis, and inability to retropulse the globe. Usually, there is no pain. Because 90% of the neoplasms are malignant and 75% arise within the orbit, the prognosis for long-term survival is poor. The neoplasm type should be ascertained by biopsy, and the extent of the mass determined by physical examination, skull radiographs including special contrast procedures, and ultrasonography before treatment by surgical excision or radiation.

Eyelid neoplasms are the most frequent group of ophthalmic neoplasms in dogs. Adenoma and adenocarcinoma of the meibomian gland are the most common lid neoplasms; local disfigurement and irritation associated with the mass necessitate local excision, which is usually successful. Sebaceous adenocarcinomas are locally invasive and histologically malignant, but are not known to metastasize. Lid melanomas, exhibited as spreading pigmented masses on the eyelid margins, should be widely excised. Other frequent eyelid neoplasms include histiocytoma, mastocytoma, and papilloma.

Corneal and limbal neoplasms are uncommon in dogs, and can be confused with nodular fasciitis and proliferative keratoconjunctivitis in Collies. Limbal malignant melanomas are focal, usually superficial, pigmented masses that extend both onto the cornea and caudally toward the globe's equator. After close intraocular examination, including gonioscopy, to detect possible penetration of the sclera, full-thickness surgical excision with scleral grafts is frequently successful. If intraocular extension occurs, enucleation should be performed.

Malignant melanomas, the most common uveal neoplasm, are usually pigmented and most frequently involve the iris and ciliary body. Clinical signs of anterior uveal melanomas may include an obvious mass, persistent iridocyclitis, hyphema, glaucoma, and pain. Adenoma and adenocarcincoma are the most frequent epithelial neoplasms of the anterior uvea. Signs may include hyphema, glaucoma, and usually a nonpigmented mass behind the iris and in the pupil. Neoplasms of neuroectodermal origin are rare. Treatment is usually enucleation. Secondary uveal adenocarcinomas are relatively infrequent and originate from a number of distant sites. Other neoplasms such as the transmissible venereal tumor and hemangiosarcoma may metastasize to the anterior uvea. Lymphosarcoma is the most frequent secondary ocular tumor, and usually manifests as anterior uveitis and secondary glaucoma.

EQUINE OPHTHALMIC ONCOLOGY

In equids, tumors of the skin, eye, and genital systems are the most frequent, and ~80% of the eye neoplasms are malignant. Neoplasms of the eyelids and conjunctivae are the most frequent ophthalmic tumors in horses; most are either squamous cell carcinoma or sarcoid. Orbital neoplasms are rare and are usually extensions of eyelid, conjunctiva, or sinus tumors. Intraocular neoplasms are rare.

Squamous cell carcinoma occurs most frequently in older horses (av 9.8 yr) and may occur more frequently in those with lightly or nonpigmented eyelids. The eyelids, conjunctivae, nictitating membrane, and limbal regions can be affected; one or both eyes are usually involved. Squamous cell carcinoma of the nictitans is more likely to invade the orbit than are those from other sites. Treatment of ophthalmic squamous cell carcinoma in horses is similar to cattle, although presentation for treatment is usually earlier, and greater emphasis is placed on cosmetic appearance after therapy.

The equine sarcoid generally affects young horses (av 3.8 yr) and represents ~40% of all neoplasms in horses. Because sarcoids are locally destructive and have a high recurrence rate after surgery, effective treatment when the periocular tissues are involved presents cosmetic and functional problems. Sarcoids appear initially as subcut. masses in the eyelids or canthi; they usually enlarge rapidly and may invade the skin, appearing as red fleshy masses. Treatment by surgery, hyperthermia, cryotherapy, and chemotherapy has limited success. After attempts to remove surgically, recurrence may be rapid, and precede the wound healing. Radiation therapy for equine sarcoids also has limited success. Immunotherapy using BCG (bacillus Calmette-Guérin) as potentiator of the cellular immune system offers considerable promise. After surgical debulking of large sarcoids, the BCG preparation (7.5 mg purified cell-wall extract suspended in 10 mL saline solution) is injected directly into the remaining mass (2 mL/site). The injections may be repeated at 2- to 4-wk intervals until the mass disappears. Systemic corticosteroids and antiprostaglandins before and after treatment may be indicated since anaphylactic reactions can occur.

FELINE OPHTHALMIC ONCOLOGY

Ophthalmic neoplasms in cats are less frequent than in dogs. Eyelid and conjunctival tumors are the most frequent primary ophthalmic neoplasms. In contrast to dogs, these neoplasms in cats are usually malignant and invasive and more difficult to treat. Squamous cell carcinomas, which are more common in white cats with nonpigmented eyelid margins, can involve the eyelids, conjunctivae, and the nictitating membrane; they are white, roughened, irregular masses, or thickened ulcerations. Other neoplasms include adenocarcinomas, fibrosarcomas, neurofibrosarcomas, and basal cell carcinomas. Treatment varies with the tumor type, location, and size, and includes surgical excision, radiation therapy, and cryothermy.

The most common primary intraocular neoplasm in cats is malignant melanoma. Clinical signs and treatment are the same as for dogs (see above). Intraocular sarcoma in cats may be associated with previous ocular trauma.

Feline lymphosarcoma-leukemia complex (FeLLC) is the most common secondary ocular neoplasm. Cats with ocular FeLLC exhibit a range of clinical signs from isolated ocular lesions to severe systemic illness; one or both eyes may be affected. Corneal abnormalities may include keratitis, edema, neovascularization, corneal infiltrates, and hemorrhages within the stroma. Ulcerative keratitis may result. Masses may occur in the conjunctivae and eyelids. Pupillary abnormalities including mydriasis, anisocoria, pupil irregularities, and lack of light-induced pupillary reflexes occur. Anterior uveitis is the most common clinical finding in FeLLC. Other findings include hypotonia, changes in iridal pigmentation, keratic precipitates, hyphema, anterior and posterior synechiae, miosis, and aqueous flare. Posterior segment changes include retinal hemorrhages, tortuous dilated vessels, perivascular cuffing, retinal detachments, and degeneration.

CHLAMYDIAL CONJUNCTIVITIS

A significant infectious disease of cats, lambs, goats, and guinea pigs.

Etiology and Epidemiology: Different strains of *Chlamydia psittaci* cause eye infection in animals. These infections are occasionally transmitted to man. (*See also* INTESTINAL CHLAMYDIAL INFECTIONS, p 137.) The organisms causing trachoma and inclusion conjunctivitis in man are of the species *C trachomatis*.

The disease in cats is also known as feline pneumonitis. This is largely a misnomer since chlamydiae rarely cause pneumonia in cats; the infection usually involves the eye and mucosa of the upper respiratory tract (rhinitis, sinusitis, pharyngitis). Serological surveys indicate that 2-12% of cats, depending on age and geographic location, have complement-fixing chlamydial antibodies.

Chlamydial keratoconjunctivitis in lambs and goats can have significant economic impact, particularly in confinement flocks, in which up to 90% can become affected. Concurrently, lambs often have chlamydial polyarthritis (qv, p 470). Also, chlamydial abortions (qv, p 653) have been observed in a goat herd affected simultaneously with chlamydial keratoconjunctivitis.

Conjunctival chlamydial infections, sometimes asymptomatic, are common in guinea pig herds (*see* p 1027). Conjunctivitis is usually observed in 4- to 8-wk-old animals. Genital infections cause salpingitis and cystitis in female guinea pigs, and urethritis in males.

Chlamydial keratoconjunctivitis has been reported in dogs, cattle, horses, and pigs, and can be produced experimentally in these species.

Clinical Findings: Signs in cats range from serous to mucopurulent conjunctivitis and rhinitis. Early signs are unilateral, reddened, slightly swollen conjunctivae. The incubation period after exposure to an infected cat is 3-10 days. Bilateral conjunctivitis develops after a few days, and the conjunctivae become hyperemic and chemotic, with prominent follicles on the inside of the third eyelid in more severe cases. The signs are most severe 9-13 days after onset and then subside over 2-3 wk. Some cats develop, with or without secondary bacterial or mycoplasmal infections, vascular keratitis, pannus, and corneal scarring. In some cats, clinical signs can last for weeks despite treatment, and recurrence is not uncommon.

Similar eye lesions occur in sheep and goats. Secondary infections in lambs and goats are also common which, if untreated, can lead to severe complications.

Lesions: Inflammatory reactions in the conjunctivae are prominent, and various cells such as neutrophils, lymphocytes, plasma cells, and macrophages infiltrate early in the disease course. These cells, together with conjunctival epithelial cells containing chlamydial inclusions, are found in smears made from conjunctival scrapings. Gastric epithelial cells of cats are also infected. Ulcerative keratitis with resultant penetration of the anterior chamber can also be found in severely affected cats or those with secondary infections.

Diagnosis: Diagnosis can be confirmed by demonstration of chlamydial inclusions of exfoliative cytological preparations or by isolation of the chlamydial organism. Scrapings are prepared by lightly but firmly moving a spatula or sharp teaspoon over the conjunctiva and smearing the scraped material onto a glass slide; the preparation is air-dried and stained. The elementary bodies appear basophilic or purple if stained with Giemsa, and reddish if stained with Gimenez. Scrapings may also be submitted for isolation of chlamydiae in chicken embryos or cell cultures. A serological diagnosis is difficult and requires paired samples taken during the acute and convalescent phases of the disease to compare antibody levels; false seronegative results occur occasionally.

Chlamydial conjunctivitis in cats needs to be differentiated from herpes- and calicivirus infections, and in lambs and goats from mycoplasmal and other bacterial infections (eg, "pinkeye").

Prophylaxis and Treatment: Vaccines are available for chlamydiosis in cats but not for other species. The feline chlamydial vaccine does not completely protect the cat, but significantly reduces severity and infection rates.

All *C psittaci* isolates are susceptible to tetracyclines. In cats, ophthalmic ointments that contain tetracycline may be the only therapy necessary. However, in severe or recurring cases, oral or parenteral treatment with tetracyclines is advisable. Cats that are pregnant or have kidney disease should be treated with erythromycin.

Systemic rather than ophthalmic treatment with oxytetracycline (20 mg/kg/day) or tylosin starting early in the course of the disease is advisable in lambs and goats. Daily feeding of 150-200 mg of chlortetracycline to affected lambs in feedlots also reduces the incidence of conjunctivitis and polyarthritis.

To reduce recurrence, treatment regimes in cats as well as lambs and goats should be extended for 7-10 days after clinical signs disappear.

EQUINE UVEITIS
(Periodic ophthalmia, Recurrent iridocyclitis, Moon blindness)

Recurrent episodes of inflammation in one or both eyes of Equidae. Incidence varies geographically, but it is reported worldwide. Inflammation of the uveal tract (iris, ciliary body, choroid) is responsible for the clinical signs and sequelae that make this disease the leading cause of blindness in horses.

Etiology: Of the many proposed causes, few have been verified. Leptospirosis and *Onchocerca cervicalis* microfilariae have considerable supportive evidence. Other bacterial, viral, genetic, nutritional, and lunar influences have been suggested but are not supported by scientific data, although recent work suggests that the Appaloosa breed may have a genetic predisposition. Apparently, most cases are due to immune-mediated inflammatory reactions in the uveal tract. This is consistent with uveitis in many other species, including man. Other causes of equine uveitis have been confirmed, but treatment is similar, regardless of specific cause.

Clinical Findings: Acute signs include varying degrees of blepharospasm, lacrimation, photophobia, conjunctival and ciliary injection, peripheral corneal edema and vascularization, aqueous flare, hypopyon or hyphema, miosis, a swollen dull iris, hypotonia, vitreal inflammation, and retinal vasculitis or peripapillary inflammation. No single case shows all these signs. Some cases are low grade or insidious, and can be missed by the owner for a long period; others are painful and obvious.

Subacute, chronic, or recurrent cases have some of the same lesions and may also have sequelae (anterior and posterior synechiae, cataracts, lens luxation, pigment changes in the iris, vitreal debris, peripapillary retinal scars, or retinal detachments) in addition to acute lesions. Cataracts and pupillary seclusion or occlusion are the most frequent causes of blindness in horses suffering from uveitis. Occasionally, glaucoma with buphthalmos develops secondary to lens luxation, anterior synechiae, or pupillary seclusion. Fibrosis of the uveal tract ends in phthisis bulbi. Any combination of sequelae is possible in chronic cases. In many instances, vitreal or retinal lesions cannot be appreciated due to severe inflammation of the anterior segment, or sequelae. In multiple attacks, lesions usually are bilateral.

Diagnosis: Ophthalmic signs suffice for diagnosis. Ulcerative diseases of the cornea should be ruled out by fluorescein staining. In addition to ophthalmic signs, serum may be submitted for leptospiral titration and any other organisms (viruses, *Toxoplasma* spp) that might be suspected. If *O cervicalis* microfilariae (qv, p 808) are suspected as a cause of keratoconjunctivitis at the temporal quadrant of the cornea, or of conjunctival granulomas, conjunctival biopsies or wet mounts are indicated. *Leptospira pomona* antibody titers >1:1600 on the microagglutination test suggest recent or chronic infection (*see also* p 356). These 2 pathogens must be considered when uveitis is endemic within a stable or band of horses. Recent confirmation of Lyme disease (qv, p 359) as a potential cause of uveitis in horses may necessitate serology for diagnosis of this disease. Horses with Lyme disease generally have systemic illness as well as uveitis.

Treatment: Treatment must be aggressive to reduce ocular inflammation quickly, prevent as many sequelae as possible, and reduce the likelihood of chronic active inflammation or rapidly recurring episodes. High-quality, high-potency, topical corticosteroids are indicated since lesser steroids are not effective in reducing inflammation in the uveal tract. Topical products should contain 0.1% dexamethasone or 1% prednisolone acetate, and should be administered 4-12 times/day, depending on severity of the inflammation and on the preparation. Topical atropine is also essential; it not only dilates the pupil but also provides analgesia through its cycloplegic action, which prevents painful ciliary spasm. Atropine (1%) should be used 4-8 times daily until the pupil dilates, and then decreased to b.i.d. or t.i.d.

Subconjunctival (bulbar) injections of depot corticosteroids, eg, methyl-prednisolone acetate (0.5-1 mL) or betamethasone, are helpful. Systemic nonsteroidal anti-inflammatories, eg, phenylbutazone, aspirin, or flunixin meglumine, may be used to provide activity against the prostaglandin-mediated portion of the ocular inflammation and to provide analgesia. Systemic corticosteroids are seldom indicated except in severe cases or when *Onchocerca* microfilariae have been identified as the cause, and should be used judiciously to avoid inducing other medical problems.

Systemic antibiotics usually are not indicated unless the uveitis appears to be septic, the horse is febrile, or leptospirosis or Lyme disease has been identified as the cause. In *O cervicalis*-induced uveitis, larvicidal medication is indicated **after** the active inflammation has been controlled. Ivermectin (200 μg/kg, once) or a daily dose of diethylcarbamazine (2-3 mg/lb [4.4-6.6 mg/kg], PO for 21 days) has been used for this, although ivermectin may not be completely effective; with either drug, the eyes should also be treated topically with corticosteroids during the course of larvicidal therapy to prevent inflammation associated with the dying microfilariae. The microfilaricidal effect of ivermectin lasts for days, and the steroid therapy should be prolonged accordingly. Frequency of topical treatment can be reduced as clinical improvement occurs but should continue at least 3-4 wk. This is long after apparent clinical improvement, but considers histological evidence of continued low-grade inflammation and may prevent the rather rapid recurrence seen in some horses that have had short courses of therapy.

Prognosis and Prevention: Prognosis varies directly with duration of signs before institution of adequate therapy; if several days have elapsed, permanent sequelae such as synechiae and blindness may develop. Also, in chronic low-grade uveitis, the problem may not be discovered until permanent sequelae already exist. In peracute cases, if therapy is prompt, intensive, and prolonged, the prognosis for preserving vision is fair to good. This also requires educating the owner to anticipate future attacks in one or both eyes at unpredictable intervals. With repeat attacks or chronic active inflammation, sequelae are inevitable.

In any evaluation of soundness, present or past evidence of uveitis should be recorded and judged.

When *L pomona* has been identified as the cause of endemic uveitis in a band of horses, vaccination of the resident animals with bacterin has successfully controlled further cases. All horses (including affected ones) should be vaccinated twice to establish primary immunity, and given boosters q6-12mo.

EYEWORM DISEASE
(Thelaziasis)

EYEWORMS OF LARGE ANIMALS

Etiology and Epidemiology: Eyeworms (*Thelazia* spp) are common parasites of horses and cattle in many countries, including several areas of North America. Horses are infected primarily by *T lacrymalis*; cattle mainly by *T gulosa*, *T skrjabini*, and *T rhodesii*. The latter is the most common and harmful to cattle in many countries, but it has been conspicuously absent in recent reports on cattle from eastern North America. *Thelazia* spp are also found in pigs, sheep, goats, deer, water buffalo, dromedaries, rabbits, dogs and cats (*see* below), birds, and man.

Several species of muscid flies serve as intermediate hosts. The face fly, *Musca autumnalis*, is a common vector. Feeding habits of this fly include a proclivity for eye secretions, which provides an ideal relationship for transmission. Details of the life cycle of *Thelazia* spp are sparse: female worms are ovoviviparous and discharge larvae, which extend themselves in their egg shells and enter the ocular secretions; the larvae are ingested by the fly and become infective in <2 wk to >4 wk. Infective larvae are mechanically deposited in the host's eye by the fly during feeding. Development of sexually mature worms takes 3-4 wk for *T rhodesii* and 6 wk for *T gulosa* in cattle, and 10-11 wk for *T lacrymalis* in ponies. Infections are found year-round, but clinical disease outbreaks, particularly in cattle, usually are associated with the warm season activities of the flies. Young stock are relatively more susceptible.

Pathogenesis: The lacrimal gland and its ducts are common sites for *T lacrymalis* and *T gulosa*; the glands of the nictitating membrane and the nasolacrimal ducts, less so. Superficial locations on the cornea, in the conjunctival sac, and under the eyelids and nictitating membrane are more typical for *T skrjabini* and *T rhodesii*, but *T lacrymalis* and *T gulosa* are often in these sites too. Worms are also found on the periorbital hair or skin during anesthesia or following migration after death of the host. Conjecture has blamed the irritation and inflammation on the serrated cuticle of the worms, especially of *T rhodesii*. Invasion of the lacrimal gland and excretory ducts may cause inflammation and necrotic exudation; occlusion of the ducts reduces tear production. Inflammation of the lacrimal ducts and sac has been reported in horses. Mild to severe conjunctivitis and blepharitis are common. Also, keratitis, including opacity, ulceration, perforation, and permanent fibrosis, may develop in severe cases, particularly with *T rhodesii* infections in cattle.

Clinical Findings and Diagnosis: Asymptomatic infections in both horses and cattle appear to be typical of thelaziasis in North America. Infection may be encountered incidentally during surgery, and recent reports indicate a surprisingly high prevalence when a specific search is made at necropsy. In Europe and Asia, thelaziasis is commonly associated with severe clinical manifestations, including conjunctivitis, photophobia, and keratitis. Characteristically, there is chronic conjunctivitis with lymphoid hyperplasia and a seromucoid exudate.

A clinically feasible technique for reliable detection of adult eyeworms is lacking. Gross inspection of the eyes may reveal the worms, and is generally recommended for *T rhodesii*, commonly found in the conjunctival sac. However, *T gulosa* and *T skrjabini* in cattle, and *T lacrymalis* in horses tend to be more invasive and are less apt to be observed. Topical anesthetics are helpful for detection and recovery of the latter species by fostering their release and movement to more superficial sites. Microscopical examination of lacrimal fluids for larvae may be tried. Clinical signs may be helpful in differential diagnosis. Thelaziasis tends to be a chronic conjunctivitis. In cattle, infectious keratoconjunctivitis (*see* below) is an acute, rapidly spreading infection of the cornea. In horses, infective larvae of the stomach worms *Draschia* and *Habronema* spp may produce lesions near the medial canthus of the eyelid that are raised, ulcerative granulomas, often containing characteristic yellow plaque-like "sulfur granules" 1-2 mm in diameter. Microfilariae of *Onchocerca* sp invade the eye and may result in a variety of manifestations. Small (<1 mm), raised, white nodules in the pigmented conjunctiva adjacent to the temporal limbus are pathognomonic of *Onchocerca* infection. Depigmentation of the bulbar conjunctiva in this area also frequently occurs. Other lesions of onchocerciasis involve the cornea, and include edema and punctate or streaking types of opacities of the stroma, superficial erosions, and a wedge-shaped sclerosing keratitis emanating from the temporal limbus. Intraocular structures also may be affected by microfilariae of *Onchocerca* sp (qv, p 808).

Treatment and Control: Mechanical removal with forceps following instillation of a local anesthetic is useful for *T rhodesii* in cattle. This also may be feasible for the more invasive *T gulosa* or *T skrjabini* in cattle, or *T lacrymalis* in horses. Irrigation of the eyes with 50-75 mL aqueous solution of 0.5% iodine and 0.75% potassium iodide has been recommended for *T gulosa* and *T skrjabini*. This also may be effective for *T lacrymalis* in horses. Topical application of 0.03% echothiophate iodide or 0.02% isoflurophate has been successful for *T lacrymalis* in horses. Concurrent use of an antibiotic-steroid ointment for the inflammation and secondary invaders is recommended. These topical agents should also be useful for *T gulosa* and *T skrjabini* in cattle. Certain systemic anthelmintics have exhibited activity against eyeworms, although none are approved in the USA for *Thelazia* spp in either cattle or horses. However, in cattle, levamisole at various dose levels and ivermectin at 0.2 mg/kg have shown activity against all 3 species of *Thelazia*. For *T lacrymalis* in horses, single doses of the commonly used anthelmintics, including ivermectin at 0.2 mg/kg, have limited, if any, effect on eyeworms; whereas, the multi-dose regimen of fenbendazole (10 mg/kg, daily for 5 days) is efficacious against *T lacrymalis*. Fly control measures, directed especially against the face fly, aid in the control of thelaziasis in both cattle and horses.

EYEWORMS OF SMALL ANIMALS

Thelazia californiensis and *T callipaeda* are found in dogs, cats, and other animals including man in the western USA and other areas of the world. They are whitish, 7-19 mm long, and move in a rapid serpentine motion across the eye. Up to 100 eyeworms may be seen in the conjunctival sac, tear ducts, and on the conjunctiva under the nictitating membrane and eyelids. Filth flies (*Musca* spp, *Fannia* spp) apparently serve as intermediate hosts, and deposit infective larvae on the eye while feeding on ocular secretions.

Clinical signs include excessive lacrimation, conjunctivitis, corneal opacity and ulceration, and rarely blindness. Following local anesthesia, diagnosis and treatment are readily accomplished by observing and removing the parasites with forceps. Ocular solutions (2% levamisole) or ointments (1% levamisole or 4% morantel) also may be effective.

INFECTIOUS KERATOCONJUNCTIVITIS
(Pinkeye, Infectious ophthalmia)

Infectious diseases of cattle, sheep, and goats characterized by blepharospasm, conjunctivitis, lacrimation, and varying degrees of corneal opacity and ulceration. The clinical syndromes in the 3 species are distinct and apparently are caused by species-specific agents.

In cattle, *Moraxella bovis* is the most common cause, although infectious bovine rhinotracheitis (IBR) virus and a *Mycoplasma* have produced conjunctivitis and transient corneal opacity; the latter 2 agents may potentiate *M bovis* disease. In sheep, *Neisseria ovis*, rickettsiae, and mycoplasmas have been associated with keratoconjunctivitis. Although much of the syndrome in young goats is caused by

Mycoplasma agalactiae (*see* CONTAGIOUS AGALACTIA, p 658), it also is caused by *Moraxella capri* and *Mycoplasma conjunctivae*.

Clinical Findings: The disease usually is acute and tends to spread rapidly. One or both eyes may be affected. In cattle, dry dusty environmental conditions, shipping stress, bright sunlight, and irritants such as pollens, grasses, and flies tend to predispose to and exacerbate the disease. Flies also serve as vectors. In cattle and goats, young animals are affected most frequently; in sheep only adults are involved, and outbreaks often follow closed herding at or about lambing. The initial signs are photophobia, blepharospasm, and excessive lacrimation; later, the ocular discharge may become mucopurulent. Conjunctivitis, with or without varying degrees of keratitis, is always present. Usually, appetite is only slightly depressed in affected animals. The clinical course varies from a few days to several weeks unless complicated by other diseases.

Lesions: Lesions vary in severity. In cattle, one or more small ulcers occur near the center of the cornea (but occasionally near the limbus) without corneal opacities. Initially, the cornea is clear around the lesion, but within a few hours a faint haze appears that subsequently becomes more dense. Lesions may regress in the early stages, or may continue to progress. After 48-72 hr in severe cases, the entire cornea may be opaque, and the animal is blind in that eye. About 1 wk after the lesion first appears, blood vessels begin to invade the cornea (adventitious vascularization) from the limbus toward the ulcer. Rarely, continued active ulceration may cause rupture of the cornea. In sheep and goats, disease rarely advances beyond a mild corneal opacity, with the accompanying ulcer and conjunctivitis. Relapse may occur at any stage of recovery, but late lesions are not as severe as initial lesions.

Diagnosis: Care must be taken to ensure that the lesions are not due to foreign bodies or parasites. (*See* EYEWORMS OF LG AN, above.) In IBR, upper respiratory signs and conjunctivitis predominate, while keratitis accompanied by ulceration is rare. In bovine malignant catarrh, respiratory signs are prominent and keratitis resolves from the center of the cornea; in infectious bovine keratoconjunctivitis, the corneal lesions resolve from the limbus toward the center. Lesions caused by mycoplasmas alone do not involve the cornea in cattle. In sheep and cattle, diagnosis usually is based on clinical signs. Involvement of the sclera has been considered pathognomonic in sheep. Isolation and identification of the causative agents in all 3 species also is helpful in differential diagnosis.

Prophylaxis and Treatment: Recovered cattle appear to be immune, although they may remain carriers of *M bovis*. Vaccines prepared from *M bovis* antigens appear to offer some protection but have not yet proved reliable. Vaccines against IBR confer ocular immunity. *Moraxella bovis* infections may be controlled by many antibiotics (penicillin, nitrofurazone, tetracycline, or gentamicin) unless resistant strains have developed. They may be administered either topically as solutions or ointments, or by subconjunctival injection; repeated ocular application may be necessary, and affected animals should be placed in a shaded area. Corticosteroids injected subconjunctivally with antibiotics may be effective. Subconjunctival injections and blepharorrhaphy involving both the eyelids and nictitating membranes are effective in many cases of severe corneal ulceration. In sheep and goats, antibiotics effective against mycoplasmas and chlamydiae (tetracycline), as well as penicillin, streptomycin, and nitrofurazone, are recommended. Treatment usually is restricted to those animals with obvious corneal involvement.

DEAFNESS

Acquired deafness can be due to occlusion of the external ear canal as in chronic otitis externa, or to destruction of the middle or inner ear. Other causes include trauma to the petrous temporal bone, loud noises (eg, gunfire), demyelinating conditions, ototoxic drugs (eg, aminoglycoside antibiotics [gentamicin, kanamycin, neomycin, streptomycin] or salicylates), neoplasms involving the ear or brain stem, and the consequences of old age. Unilateral deafness and/or partial hearing loss is possible in some of these instances.

Congenital deafness can occur from a heritable trait or from damage (toxic or viral) to the developing fetus. An autosomal gene in cats causes white fur, blue eyes, and deafness; it is dominant with complete expression for white fur and incomplete expression for deafness and the blue iris. Deafness in this instance is due to cochleosaccular degenerative changes that are expressed in the first week of life. Merle and white coat colors are associated with congenital deafness in dogs and other animals. Dog breeds commonly affected include the Dalmatian, Australian Heeler, English Setter, Australian Shepherd, Boston Terrier, Old English Sheepdog, Great Dane, and Boxer. The list of affected breeds changes with time due to breed popularity and elimination of the defect through selective breeding; eg, Cocker Spaniels were known to have hereditary deafness, but the trait is no longer common in the breed.

Diagnosis requires careful observation of the animal's response to sound. It is helpful to consider the owner's description of behavior and to ask appropriate questions. The response to visual, tactile, and olfactory stimuli must be differentiated from the response to sound. In the young animal or animals kept in groups, deafness may be difficult to detect, since the suspect individual will follow the response of the others in the group. If the animal is observed as an individual after an age when responses to auditory stimuli are predictable (~3-4 wk for dogs and cats), then the deafness may be detected. The primary sign is failure to respond to an auditory stimulus. An example of this is failure of noise to awaken a sleeping dog or failure to alert to the source of a sound. Other signs include unusual behavior such as excessive barking, unusual voice, hyperactivity, confusion when given vocal commands, and lack of reflex-alerting and attention movements of the pinnae. An animal that once could hear but has gradually become deaf, as in old age, may become unresponsive to the surroundings, and refuse to answer the owner's call. Unilateral deafness is difficult to detect, except by astute observation or by electrodiagnostic procedures. Otoscopic examination of the external ear, radiography of the tympanic bullae, and neurologic examination may reveal the cause, especially in cases of acquired deafness. In congenital deafness, these procedures usually reveal normal structure but not signs of hearing, except in cases of unilateral deafness. Brain stem auditory evoked responses (BAER, an electrodiagnostic test) can be used to determine the presence and level of an auditory defect from either or both ears. Impedence audiometry can evaluate the integrity of the middle ear and the conduction system.

Deafness due to occlusion of the external ear canal usually responds to appropriate surgical or medical treatment. Deafness due to bacterial infections of the middle and internal ear may respond to appropriate antibiotic treatment. Recovery from deafness due to intense noise, trauma, or viral infections may be complete, partial, or nil. Any recovery depends on time. Recovery from deafness caused by ototoxic drugs is rare. Hereditary deafness may be eliminated from a breed by removal of identifiable carriers from the breeding program. The mode of inheritance of the deafness trait may be determined by study of pedigrees or by test mating. More recently, BAER have been used to identify both unilaterally and bilaterally affected dogs, which can then be eliminated from the breeding program.

DISEASES OF THE EXTERNAL EAR

DISEASES OF THE PINNA

Several ectoparasitic diseases cause pinnal lesions. Canine and feline scabies are associated with crusting and excoriations of the pinnal margins and extreme pruritus. Fly-bite dermatitis of dogs is caused by the stable fly, *Stomoxys calcitrans*, which feeds on the ear tips of prick-eared dogs in summer. Signs include headshaking and scratching. Lesions consist of hemorrhagic crusts and excoriations on the tips of the pinnae. Treatment consists of keeping the dog inside during the day or applying insect repellent frequently to the ear tips.

Aural plaques of horses (a variant of equine papillomatosis, qv, p 854) are thought to be associated with a chronic hypersensitivity response to salivary antigens of black flies that feed on the inner surface of the pinnae. The lesions consists of nonpruritic, well-circumscribed, flat, gray-white plaques that are usually covered with a pale keratinous crust.

Marginal auricular dermatosis affects Dachshunds. The cause is unknown, but it may be associated with abnormal microcirculation in the pinnae. Early lesions consist of alopecia, crusts, and scales around the margins of the pinnae. In chronic cases, the whole pinna may become alopecic, and painful ulceration, fissuring, and lichenification may occur around the margins.

Several immune-mediated diseases, including pemphigus foliaceous, pemphigus erythematosus, bullous pemphigoid, systemic lupus erythematosus, discoid lupus erythematosus, cold aggulutinin disease, and drug eruptions cause pinnal alopecia, crusting, and ulceration. Pinnal inflammation and pruritus are frequent in canine atopy and food hypersensitivity.

Frostbite may cause discoloration and sloughing of the ear tips. Actinic lesions of the pinnae may occur in white cats that are chronically exposed to strong sunlight. Lesions first appear as erythema and scaling on the sparsely haired tips of the ears. Crusting, exudation, and ulceration may develop as the actinic keratosis undergoes transformation into a squamous cell carcinoma. During early stages of the disease, treatment consists of reducing exposure to ultraviolet light through confinement indoors or use of topical sunscreens. Squamous cell carcinomas of the pinnae are treated with surgical excision, alone or in combination with radiation therapy.

AURICULAR HEMATOMA

Fluid-filled swellings that develop on the concave surface of the pinna in dogs, cats, and pigs. The lesions may develop following rupture of blood vessels within the pinna, as a result of head-shaking or ear-scratching due to otic pruritus. The condition is most common in dogs with pendulous pinnae. It has also been proposed that the lesion results from an autoimmune disease of the pinnal tissues, rather than from pinnal trauma. In pigs, sarcoptic mange, pediculosis, and meal in ears (from overhead feeders) have been implicated as causes of head-shaking that has lead to aural hematomas. Bites from other pigs also may be at fault (*see also* NECROTIC EAR SYNDROME, below).

Treatment is surgical to allow drainage and debridement. Underlying causes of otic discomfort, such as parasites or hypersensitivity diseases, should be identified and treated to prevent recurrence.

NECROTIC EAR SYNDROME, SWINE
(Ear necrosis, Necrotic auricular dermatitis)

A condition characterized by unilateral or bilateral necrosis of the pinnae that occurs sporadically in weaned and growing pigs under all management systems. Affected pigs are unthrifty and commonly develop septic arthritis or die from secondary bacterial septicemia.

Etiology, Transmission, and Pathogenesis: The causes have not been determined conclusively. Circumstantial evidence strongly suggests that the disease is due to trauma (fighting) and subsequent bacterial invasion of the damaged tissue.

The lesions evolve through mild superficial dermatitis to severe deep inflammation with exudation, ulceration, thrombosis, and necrosis. In mild cases, resolution occurs with no loss of ear tissue; in severe cases, the margins, tips, or even the entire pinna may be lost. Histological and microbiological findings suggest that the aggressive erosive lesion is due to secondary bacterial infection. In the early phases of the disease, large numbers of *Staphylococcus hyicus* and low to moderate numbers of β-hemolytic streptococci are found in the surface exudate; later, during the ulcerative and necrotic stage, large numbers of the streptococci are found deep in the lesion. It has been hypothesized that *S hyicus* colonizes the traumatized tissue, which prepares the way for the highly invasive streptococci that induce the changes that lead to ulceration and necrosis. Efforts to reproduce the disease by experimental inoculation of the 2 organisms have been unsuccessful.

Clinical Findings, Lesions, and Diagnosis: The nature and extent of clinical signs depend on the severity of the local lesion and the development of secondary bacterial septicemia. Thus, a spectrum of signs, including unthriftiness, inappetence, fever, septic arthritis, collapse, and death, may be seen.

Mild lesions consist of superficial scratches covered with thin, dry, brown crusts. Mild edema or erythema may be present near the scratches. In more severe cases, thick, brown, moist scabs cover deep ulcers. In the most severe cases, there is extensive necrosis.

Diagnosis is made on the appearance of the affected ears.

Control: Tincture of iodine, applied topically b.i.d. for 1 wk, has reduced the incidence and severity of the disease. Antibacterial drugs administered in the feed are effective in some herds, but not in others. Lack of effectiveness could be due to drug resistance. In cases of antibacterial ineffectiveness, specimens should be collected aseptically from the deep aspect of the ulcerative lesions and cultured, and their antimicrobial sensitivity determined. Traumatizing events should be minimized. Management (ventilation, location and functioning of waterers, pen design, group size, mixing) and nutritional (protein and salt intake) factors have been suggested as contributing to the incidence of ear biting. (*See also* DISEASE-MANAGEMENT INTERACTION: PIGS, p 1120.)

OTITIS EXTERNA

An acute or chronic inflammation of the epithelium of the external auditory meatus, sometimes involving the pinna, and characterized by erythema, increased discharges or desquamation of the epithelium, and varying degrees of pain and pruritus. It is the most common disease of the ear canal in dogs and cats, and usually has a multifactorial etiology. It is uncommon in large animals, and is occasionally seen in rabbits, in which it is usually due to the mite *Psoroptes cuniculi*.

Etiology: By determining whether the causes are primary, predisposing, or perpetuating, a more accurate prognosis can be provided and a specific and safe therapeutic plan formulated.

Primary Causes: Internal and external factors may directly induce inflammation and pruritus in the external ear canal. External factors are usually easily identified, and prompt removal often results in a cure. Unfortunately, however, many refractory cases are due to primary causes that may be lifelong metabolic problems. Primary causes include parasites, foreign bodies, hypersensitivity diseases, disorders of keratinization, and autoimmune diseases.

Predisposing Causes: Small changes in the otic microclimate may alter the delicate balance of normal secretions and microflora and result in opportunistic infections. Causes include conformation, maceration of the ear canal, treatment errors, obstructive ear disease, pyrexia, and systemic disease.

Perpetuating Factors: Once the environment of the ear canal has been altered by a combination of primary and predisposing factors, opportunistic infections and pathologic changes occur, which prevent resolution of the disease. Factors include bacteria, yeasts, otitis media, and progressive pathologic changes.

Clinical Findings and Diagnosis: Unless all the causes are identified and treated, recurrence may be expected. Chronic pathologic changes in the ears may also reflect a generalized systemic or skin disease.

A thorough dermatological history can provide much information and may be suggestive of other problems, eg, hypersensitivity disease or disorders of keratinization. Signalment is important; certain breeds of dogs are predisposed to conformational disorders of the ear canal, hypersensitivity diseases, and disorders of keratinization.

A thorough physical and dermatological examination should precede in-depth examination of the ears. Hormonal, endocrine, and immune disorders may be apparent at other sites on the body and affect the ear. Skin scrapings, a Wood's lamp examination, and dermatophyte culture may provide information about a generalized dermatosis that has spread to the ear canals.

The pinnae and periauricular regions should be inspected for evidence of self-trauma, erythema, and primary and secondary skin lesions. Pinnal deformities suggest chronic otic discomfort and head-shaking.

For animals with unilateral signs, the unaffected ear should be examined first: 1) the problem may, in fact, be bilateral, with one side being affected more severely; 2) the animal may be more amenable to close inspection of the affected ear later; 3) this may prevent iatrogenic contamination of the unaffected ear with organisms, eg, *Pseudomonas aeruginosa* or *Proteus mirabilis*, that may be present in the diseased ear.

Sedation or anesthesia may be needed for a thorough otoscopic examination if the ear is painful, or if the canal is obstructed with exudate or proliferative inflammatory tissue. Similar recommendations should be made for all animals with recurring signs since deep otic foreign bodies, low-grade infections with *Otodectes cynotis*, and ruptured tympanic membranes may be missed during a more cursory examination.

During an otoscopic examination, the ear canal should be inspected for changes in diameter, pathologic changes in the skin, quantity of cerumen, quantity and type of exudate, parasites (especially *Otobius megnini* [spinose ear tick of large animals], *Otodectes cynotis*, and occasionally *Psoroptes cuniculi* or others), foreign bodies, neoplasms, and changes in the tympanic membrane.

Stained smears taken from the horizontal ear canal may provide immediate diagnostic information. Cytologic smears, and microbial cultures when indicated, are taken before otoscopy is completed. In large dogs, swabs should be taken when the sterile otoscope cone is first inserted into the horizontal canal. The tympanic membrane should be examined for evidence of disease or rupture before the swab is introduced, since the swab may push debris up the canal and obscure the membrane. It may be impossible to pass a swab through a cone used for small dogs and cats; it may be preferable to remove the cone and gently thread a small swab into the canal to retrieve samples.

Cytologic smears are made by rolling the swab onto clean glass slides, which are allowed to air dry. Modified Wright's stains are suitable for these preparations. Following examination under low-power magnification, smears should be evaluated under high power (preferably utilizing immersion oil) for numbers and morphology of bacteria, yeasts, and WBC; evidence of phagocytosis of microorganisms; parasites; cerumen; foreign bodies; fungal hyphae; and neoplastic cells.

The external ear canals of most dogs and cats harbor small numbers of commensal and potentially pathogenic bacteria; however, stained smears can quickly determine if microbial overgrowth is present. Coccal organisms are usually staphylococci or streptococci. Rod-shaped organisms are usually *Pseudomonas aeruginosa* or *Proteus mirabilis*, and their appearance in large numbers should prompt bacterial culture and sensitivity testing, due to their known resistance to many antimicrobial agents. The presence of many neutrophils phagocytizing bacteria confirms the pathogenic nature of the organisms.

The yeast *Mallassezia canis* is found in low numbers in the ear canals of many normal dogs and cats. Because yeasts colonize the surface of the ear canal, they are most easily found adhered to clumps of exfoliated squamous cells. No more than 2-3 organisms should be present on any aggregate of cells from a normal animal. Concurrent bacterial infections, especially with gram-positive cocci, are common.

Cytologic smears should be examined for eggs, larvae, or adults of the ear mite *Otodectes cynotis* since a small population of mites may be missed on otoscopic examination. Similarly, cytologic smears from rabbits' and goats' ears should be examined for *Psoroptes cuniculi*. Rarely, refractory ceruminous otitis externa may be associated with localized proliferation of *Demodex* spp in the external ear canals of dogs and cats. Large numbers of adult mites may be observed in smears of cerumen.

Culture and sensitivity testing aids selection of systemic antimicrobial agents when chronic otitis externa is complicated by opportunistic bacterial infections. Some believe that failure to use systemic antimicrobial therapy is an important predisposing and perpetuating cause of chronic ear disease in dogs. Findings to prompt microbial culture and sensitivity testing include a deep bacterial infection in the skin of the external ear canal, a history of therapeutic failures with topical antimicrobial agents or chronic recurring ear infections, the presence of many rod-shaped or gram-negative organisms on cytologic smears, and otitis media. Swabs for culture should be taken from the horizontal canal, the region where most infections arise and a convenient site to collect exudates from the middle ear in cases of tympanic rupture.

Fungal cultures rarely provide more information than cytologic smears. *Mallassezia canis* is identified readily on microscopical examination and its numbers easily assessed; when unidentified yeasts or hyphal organisms are seen in significant numbers in cytologic smears, the species should be identified through culture.

Although the histopathologic changes associated with chronic otitis externa are often nonspecific, biopsy may be indicated for animals with pruritus confined to the ear canals, particularly when other diagnostic tests fail to reveal a cause. Histopathologic evidence of a hypersensitivity response supports a recommendation for intradermal allergy testing or a hypoallergenic diet trial. Additionally, biopsies from animals with chronic, obstructive, unilateral otitis externa may reveal whether neoplastic changes are present.

Radiography of the osseous bullae is indicated when cerumen, exudates, or proliferative tissues prevent adequate visualization of the tympanic membrane; when otitis media is suspected as a cause of relapsing bacterial otitis externa; and when neurologic signs accompany otitis externa. Fluid densities and proliferative or lytic osseous changes provide evidence of middle ear involvement.

Treatment: The following principles apply when treating otitis externa:

1) Identify and correct underlying primary, predisposing, and perpetuating factors. When the otitis externa is secondary to poor ventilation and drainage of the external auditory meatus, the periauricular area should be clipped, and hair plucked from the ears. Maceration of the ear canal should be minimized by use of topical astringents in dogs that swim frequently, and by preventing water from entering the ear canals during shampooing.

2) Clean and dry the ears before treatment is started. Topical therapy is ineffective if exudates and cerumen prevent medications from reaching the epithelium or infectious agents, and less effective if large numbers of bacteria or yeasts remain in the infected ear canal. In animals with chronic or painful acute otitis externa, proper cleaning of the ear canals requires general anesthesia. The ears may be flushed with an antibacterial cleansing solution such as chlorhexidine or polyhydroxydine, or with a ceruminolytic solution such as dioctyl sodium sulfosuccinate (DSS). If the tympanic membrane is ruptured, detergents and DSS are contraindicated; milder cleansers (eg, carbamide peroxide, urea, propylene glycol) should be used to flush the ear. Thorough rinsing must always follow. After all debris has been removed, the canal should be flushed with sterile saline to prevent chemical irritation to the outer and middle ears from the cleansing solution, and then dried.

3) Keep therapy specific and simple. Contributing causes should be treated specifically and aggressively. In general, topical medications that contain combinations of drugs should be used only for specific problems: a) Antibacterial agents in combination with corticosteroids should be used in the treatment of acute bacterial otitis externa. The corticosteroids reduce exudation, pain, and swelling, and decrease glandular secretions. Resolution may be accelerated if the topical corticosteroids are withdrawn after 4-7 days, unless the animal has an underlying hypersensitivity disorder. b) Bacterial superinfections develop in some animals treated with fungicidal

agents, and fungal overgrowth develops in some treated with antibacterial agents; treatment should be with antibacterial and antifungal drugs when such infections arise. c) Animals with recurring bacterial otitis externa and a history of infection with *Otodectes cynotis* should be treated with a topical product that contains antibacterial and antiparasitic agents to ensure that undetected low-grade parasitic infections are eliminated.

4) Select topical therapy based on the stage of the disease. Properly applied, the ideal medication coats the epithelium of the external ear canal as a thin film. Nonocclusive solutions or lotions should be used for acute or chronic exudative otitis externa. Occlusive oil-based ointments should be reserved for dry, scaly lesions within the ear canals. Changes in the skin of the ear canals during treatment may require a different vehicle or base.

5) Treat for an adequate time. Topical therapy for bacterial infections should be administered for ≥2 wk, that for yeast infections for ≥3 wk. Animals with *Otodectes cynotis* or *Psoroptes cuniculi* should receive appropriate parasiticide treatment in the ears and on the whole body, for ≥4 wk. *Otobius megnini* infestations are best treated by manual removal of the ticks, followed by a acaricide/corticosteroid otic preparation.

6) Incorporate systemic therapy when indicated. For example, allergic otitis externa resolves more quickly when systemic corticosteroid or antihistamine therapy is incorporated with systemic antibacterial agents.

7) Avoid irritating medications. They cause swelling of the lining of the ear canal and an increase in glandular secretions, which predispose to opportunistic infections. Powders form irritating concretions within the ear canal.

8) Keep the ear canals dry and well ventilated. Chronic maceration impairs the barrier function of the skin, which predisposes to opportunistic infection. Additionally, chronic moisture in the ear canal stimulates glandular secretions. Prophylactic otic astringents may decrease the frequency of bacterial or mycotic infections in moist ear canals. Clipping hair from the inside of the pinna and around the external auditory meatus, and plucking it from hirsute ear canals, improves ventilation and decreases humidity in the ears.

TUMORS OF THE EAR CANAL

Relatively uncommon compared to cutaneous tumors elsewhere on the body, these may arise from any of the structures lining or supporting the ear canal, including the squamous epithelium, the ceruminous or sebaceous glands, or the mesenchymal tissues. They are more likely to arise in the external ear canal and auditory meatus than in the middle and inner ear cavities.

Signs include chronic otic discharges and odors, swelling or abscesses around the ears, deafness, and signs of middle or inner ear involvement, including head tilt, ataxia, nystagmus, or Horner's syndrome. Because the signs associated with tumors of the ear canal often mimic those seen in chronic otitis externa, lesions may be advanced by the time a definitive diagnosis is made.

Squamous cell carcinomas are most frequent on the pinnae, and are the most common tumor of the middle and inner ear. The lesions are usually ulcerated. When present in the middle and inner ears of cats, signs include facial paralysis, ataxia, head tilt, nystagmus, and Horner's syndrome. Prognosis is poor. Treatment consists of early surgical intervention combined with radiation therapy to slow the progress of local disease.

For ceruminous gland tumors, *see* p 852.

OTITIS MEDIA AND INTERNA

Inflammation of the middle and inner ear structures. Otitis media is usually due to extension of infection from the external ear canal or penetration of the tympanic membrane by a foreign object. It occurs in all species, but is more common in dogs, cats, and rabbits. Extension of infection through the auditory tube occurs in dogs, cats, and pigs. Hematogenous spread of infection to these areas is possible but rare. Otitis media can lead to otitis interna, and may result in loss of equilibrium and deafness on the affected side.

Clinical Findings and Diagnosis: The signs of otitis media and otitis externa (*see* above) are somewhat similar. Head shaking, rubbing the affected ear on the floor, rotating the head to the affected side, a painful ear, and a discharge and inflammatory changes in the ear canal usually are present. Because the facial and sympathetic nerves course through the middle ear, a facial nerve palsy and/or a Horner's syndrome (miosis, ptosis, enophthalmos) may be present on the same side as the otitis media. If otitis interna is superimposed, head rotation to the affected side is more pronounced. Additionally, the animal circles and falls to the affected side, and has generalized incoordination—if incoordination is severe enough, it may be unable to rise. Nystagmus may also be seen with otitis interna, and characteristically, is a spontaneous, horizontal to rotary type, with the fast phase away from the affected side. Rarely, the infection ascends the vestibulocochlear and facial nerves to the brain stem, and results in meningitis, a brain-stem abscess, and death.

Otitis media should be suspected in cases of severe purulent otitis externa, or whenever the tympanic membrane has been penetrated by a foreign object or has ruptured secondary to chronic otitis externa. The diagnosis can be confirmed by bulging, discoloration, or rupture of the tympanic membrane. Fluid in the tympanic cavity or sclerotic changes of the tympanic bullae may be detected radiographically. Cytological examination (Gram stain and Wright's stain) and culture and sensitivity of the exudate may be beneficial.

Otitis interna should be strongly suspected if the previously mentioned vestibular signs are present. Otoscopic examination and radiographs of the tympanic bulla may confirm a concurrent otitis media.

Treatment and Prognosis: Because of the possibility of impairment of hearing and damage to the vestibular apparatus, long-term (3-6 wk) systemic antibacterial therapy should be instituted as soon as the diagnosis is made. Chloramphenicol, ampicillin, trimethoprim-sulfa combinations, or tetracyclines should be used until the results of bacterial sensitivity tests are known. If the eardrum is ruptured, the tympanic cavity should be carefully cleaned using an otoscope, long alligator forceps, and flushes of warm saline. Small perforations of the eardrum will heal in time. Any associated otitis externa should be treated carefully. Additionally, anti-inflammatory doses of glucocorticoids used for the first 5-7 days of treatment may decrease the inflammatory changes in the vestibulocochlear, facial, or sympathetic nerves.

In otitis media and interna with a clean, normal external ear, but a bulging or discolored tympanum, it may be advantageous to incise the tympanum to permit culture of the fluid, relieve the pressure (thus the pain), and permit removal of the inflammatory exudate, which could cause a permanent hearing deficiency. Systemic antibiotic therapy based on sensitivity testing should be continued 3-4 wk, and possibly ≥6 wk in otitis interna. In chronic otitis media with radiographic changes of osteomyelitis or fluid in the tympanic bulla, a bulla osteotomy may be necessary.

Otitis media with an intact tympanum responds well to systemic antibiotic therapy, but when chronic otitis externa and a ruptured tympanum are present, the chances of successful treatment are reduced. When facial and sympathetic nerve deficits develop, these may persist even after the infection has been cleared. Otitis interna usually responds well to long-term antibiotic therapy, but some neurological deficits (such as incoordination, head tilt, and deafness) may persist for life. Animals recovering from otitis interna should be given adequate time to adapt to any persistent neurological deficiencies.

GENERALIZED CONDITIONS

GENERALIZED INFECTIONS OF HORSES

GEN

ACTINOBACILLOSIS

A disease that most often affects soft tissues and lymph nodes, although bony structures also may be involved by direct extension; it is similar to actinomycosis (*see* below). The several species of causal agents relate to the various host species and to their biochemical characteristics: *Actinobacillus lignieresii* (cattle and sheep), *A equuli* and *A suis* (horses and pigs, especially young animals), *A capsulatus* (rabbits—arthritis), and *A (Haemophilus) pleuropneumoniae* (pigs—pleuropneumonia). *Actinobacillus seminis* (rams—epididymitis) may not be a valid member of the genus.

In cattle, classical actinobacillosis usually affects the tongue ("wooden tongue") and rumen and reticulum and, less frequently, other tissues such as skeletal muscles and liver. Small abscesses with a diffuse, extensive connective tissue proliferation are a prominent feature. The spread via lymphatics and invasion of local lymph nodes helps to distinguish *A lignieresii* infection from that of actinomycosis. In sheep, actinobacillosis is a purulent disease of the skin, lymph nodes, lungs, and soft tissues of the head and neck. Epididymitis is common in rams. In pigs, septicemia, suppurative joint lesions, endocarditis, osteomyelitis, pneumonia, and infections of the mammary glands and soft tissue of the head have been recorded. Septicemia and crippling infections, especially of the joints, occur in foals.

Pus from lesions may contain grayish white granules or "rosettes" <1 mm in diameter, which are smaller than the "sulfur granules" of actinomycosis. Such granules, which are found only in lesions in cattle and sheep, contain club-like bodies that emanate radially from the center, which is made up of gram-negative bacilli and cell deposits. Clubs may be weakly acid-fast. The absence of gram-positive filaments distinguishes this disease from actinomycosis.

Circumscribed lesions may be treated by complete excision. The response to iodides is usually dramatic. Sulfonamides, and a number of broad-spectrum antibiotics are effective as well. Streptomycin or gentamicin is possibly the drug of choice. Chronic lesions may be polymicrobial and contain other bacteria, eg, *Actinomyces bovis*.

ACTINOMYCOSIS

A local or systemic, chronic, suppurative, granulomatous disease that affects a wide variety of domestic animals and, rarely, wild animals. Causative agents include *Actinomyces bovis, A viscosus* (first isolated from gingival plaques of hamsters with periodontal disease, but now known to be an important pathogen of dogs and, to a lesser extent, pigs and goats), *A hordeovulneris*, and *A suis*. The exact taxonomic classification of this latter species is undecided. *Actinomyces bovis* has been confirmed only from bovine infections. Predominantly human types, such as *A israelii*, may occasionally be recovered from lesions in other animals. Several species (*A denticolens, A howellii*, and *A slackii*) have been recovered from bovine dental plaque, but their pathogenic potential is undetermined.

ACTINOMYCOSIS IN CATTLE
(Lumpy jaw)

A chronic disease of the mandible, maxilla, or other bony tissues of the head; it seldom involves soft tissue. Actinomycosis of the mandible and maxilla is characterized by swelling, abscesses, fistulous tracts, extensive fibrosis, osteitis, and granulomas. Distortion of the affected bone due to laying down of new bone is characteristic. The teeth loosen, and mastication is difficult. Swelling of the nasal cavity may cause dyspnea. There is gradual emaciation. Incision of the lesion reveals coalescence of abscesses that contain viscid, mucoid, yellow pus and "sulfur granules", 2-5 mm in diameter. Fistulous tracts extend through the skin, discharge pus for a period, and then indurate, leaving indented fibrotic scars.

Diagnosis: A history of a slow-developing swelling on the maxilla or mandible with fluctuating abscesses or fistulous tracts suggests actinomycosis. For confirmation, pus should be collected in a tube and shaken with saline to dissolve the mucus. The contents then are poured into a Petri dish, and "sulfur granules" are picked out, crushed on a glass slide, and gram stained. The "sulfur granule" shows as a central mass of gram-positive bacteria surrounded by a peripheral rosette of "clubs", which stain gram-negative. Under oil immersion, *A bovis* appears as long gram-positive filaments (some older cells may be gram-negative), rods, and cocci. In liquid media, short branching rods (diphtheroid-type morphology) are the rule. The presence of these structures confirms *A bovis* and differentiates the organisms from those of actinobacillosis (*see* above) and staphylococcosis, which also produce pus that contains yellow granules. Further confirmation of the diagnosis can be obtained by bacteriological and histological laboratory techniques.

Treatment: Actinomycotic lesions are always chronic over a course of many months. Infection of the maxilla or mandible seldom can be arrested, except when diagnosed and vigorously treated at its onset. When the lesions are small and circumscribed, surgery is the treatment of choice; if the lesions are not circumscribed, or if the abscesses are advanced, the fistulas and abscesses should be curetted. In either case, the wound should be packed with tampons soaked in tincture of iodine.

Actinomyces bovis is sensitive to penicillin. However, since it is often protected by its location deep in sinus tracts and bones, or surrounded by exudates and granulation tissue, prolonged therapy is indicated. Iodides are no longer recommended. The value of antibiotics active against anaerobes, eg, clindamycin and imipenem, in treating actinomycosis in lower animals is unknown. In contrast to actinobacillosis (with which *A bovis* infection has been confused), the aminoglycosides are not recommended. However, the possibility of concurrent *A bovis* and *Actinobacillus lignieresii* infection in chronic oral lesions cannot be ignored.

Once rarefying osteitis becomes extensive, treatment prolongs the life of the animal, but complete recovery should not be expected. Radiation therapy will temporarily reduce the size of the lesions, but does not destroy the infection and must be repeated.

ACTINOMYCOSIS IN OTHER SPECIES

Pigs: *Actinomyces suis* (and *A bovis*?) cause primary chronic granulomatous and suppurative mastitis. Small abscesses in the udder contain cohesive, viscid, yellow pus surrounded by a wide zone of dense connective tissue. As in cattle, yellow mineralized granules are scattered throughout the pus. Some of the deepseated abscesses rupture and discharge exudate through fistulas. Large, irregular, granulating skin ulcerations can be seen at the opening of the fistulas. Granulomatous nodules or abscesses also are seen under the skin of the abdomen. Occasionally, *A suis* causes generalized infection with pyogranulomatous nodules throughout the lungs, spleen, kidneys, and other viscera.

The prognosis is poor since one or more mammae are destroyed and the infection does not respond favorably to chemotherapy. Often, the infected mammary gland must be excised to save the life of the sow and make her acceptable for slaughter.

Horses: An anaerobic *A bovis*-like microbe, synergistic with *Brucella abortus* or *B suis*, is an apparent cause of fistulous withers or poll evil (qv, p 469). The anaerobe alone causes abscesses with fistulous tracts in the submaxillary, pharyngeal, and cervical region. The lymph nodes of the region contain nodules, abscesses, and discharging fistulas.

Dogs: *Actinomyces viscosus* causes a chronic, granulomatous pleuritis. Frequently, subcut. lesions (abscesses, fistulous tracts), which may follow bites, are present as well. The prognosis is poor since the infection usually is noticed too late. Granules with filamentous and coccal bacteria, but without the surrounding clubs, occur.

Actinomyces hordeovulneris, a recently described and clearly distinct species, has been recovered from thoracic, abdominal, and recurrent localized canine infections that are sometimes associated with foxtail awns (*Hordeum* sp).

AMYLOIDOSIS

Amyloid is the name given to certain proteins deposited in tissues as a result of chronic inflammation or a plasma cell tumor (myeloma). (*See also* p 880.) All amyloid proteins consist of β-pleated sheets of amino acids, a structure that makes them almost totally refractory to enzymatic breakdown; thus, when deposited in tissues, they are not removed. There are 2 major amyloid proteins. One, called AA, is released from hepatocytes under the influence of interleukin 1. Since interleukin 1 is released by stimulated macrophages, chronic infections lead to prolonged interleukin 1 production and release of excess AA from hepatocytes. The second, AL, is composed of partially degraded immunoglobulin light chains produced by malignant plasma cells. Several other minor types occur in old animals and in certain metabolic diseases. Thus, amyloid is deposited in tissues in animals that have chronic infections such as arthritis, traumatic reticulitis, or osteomyelitis, and in animals with myelomas or other monoclonal gammopathies.

Disease is caused by displacement of normal cells with amyloid deposits, chiefly in the liver, spleen, brain, and kidneys. Because of this diffuse deposition and its insidious onset, amyloidosis is difficult to diagnose clinically, although it is seen not infrequently at necropsy. If, however, it damages the glomeruli and tubules of the kidneys, clinical signs of renal failure may be apparent. Amyloidosis should be suspected if renal failure occurs in animals with chronic infections or inflammation. Amyloidosis of the liver leads to signs of hepatic failure. There is no effective treatment.

ANTHRAX
(Splenic fever, Charbon, Milzbrand)

An acute, febrile disease of virtually all warm-blooded animals, including man, caused by *Bacillus anthracis*. Most commonly, it is a septicemia characterized principally by a rapidly fatal course. It occurs worldwide, and is irregularly distributed in districts where repeated outbreaks occur. In the USA, there are recognized areas of infection in South Dakota, Nebraska, Arkansas, Mississippi, Louisiana, Texas, and California; small areas exist in a number of other states.

Etiology and Epidemiology: *Bacillus anthracis* is a gram-positive, nonmotile, spore-forming bacterium (4-8 × 1-1.5 μm). After discharge from an infected animal or when bacilli from an opened carcass are exposed to free oxygen, they form spores that are resistant to extremes of temperature, chemical disinfectants, and desiccation. For this reason, the carcass of an animal dead of anthrax should not be necropsied.

Outbreaks of anthrax commonly are associated with neutral or alkaline, calcareous soils that serve as "incubator areas" for the organisms. In these areas, the spores apparently revert to the vegetative form and multiply to infectious levels when optimal environmental conditions of soil, moisture, temperature, and nutrition occur. Cattle, horses, mules, sheep, and goats may readily become infected when grazing such areas. Outbreaks originating from soil-borne infection occur primarily in seasons when the minimal daily temperature is >60°F (16°C). Epidemics tend to occur in association with marked climatic or ecologic change, such as heavy rainfall, flooding, or drought. Even in endemic areas, anthrax occurs irregularly, often with many years between occurrences. During an epidemic, flies and other biting insects may mechanically transmit the disease from one animal to another, but this mode of transmission is of little importance. Infection also may be caused by consumption of contaminated natural or artificial feedstuffs, such as oil cake and tankage. Occasionally, crops such as hay raised on contaminated soil have caused small outbreaks. Pigs, dogs, cats, mink, and wild animals in captivity have acquired the disease from consumption of contaminated meat.

Man may develop localized cutaneous lesions (malignant carbuncle) from contact of broken skin with infected blood or tissues, acquire a highly fatal hemorrhagic mediastinitis (woolsorters' disease) from spore inhalation when handling contaminated wool or hair, or intestinal anthrax from consumption of undercooked meat.

Clinical Findings: Typically, the incubation period is 3-7 days (range 1 to ≥14 days). The clinical course ranges from peracute to chronic. The peracute form is characterized by sudden onset and a rapidly fatal course. Staggering, dyspnea, trembling, collapse, a few convulsive movements, and death may occur in cattle, sheep, or goats without any previous evidence of illness.

In acute anthrax of cattle and sheep, there is an abrupt rise in body temperature and a period of excitement followed by depression, stupor, respiratory or cardiac distress, staggering, convulsion, and death. The body temperature may reach 107°F (41.5°C), rumination ceases, milk production is materially reduced, and pregnant animals may abort. There may be bloody discharges from the natural body openings.

Chronic infections are characterized by localized, subcut., edematous swelling that can be quite extensive. Areas most frequently involved are the ventral neck, thorax, and shoulders.

The disease in horses is acute. They may show fever, chills, severe colic, anorexia, depression, weakness, bloody diarrhea, and swellings in the region of the neck, sternum, lower abdomen, and external genitalia. Death usually occurs within 2-3 days of onset.

Some pigs in a group may die of acute anthrax without having shown any previous signs. Others may show rapidly progressive swelling about the throat, which may cause death by suffocation. Many of the group may develop the disease in a mild chronic form and recover gradually. However, some of these, when slaughtered as normal animals, may show evidence of anthrax infection in the cervical lymph nodes and tonsils.

Lesions: *Rigor mortis* is frequently absent or incomplete. Dark blood may ooze from the mouth, nostrils, and anus with marked bloating and rapid body decomposition. If the carcass is inadvertently opened, septicemic lesions are observed. The blood is dark and thickened, and fails to clot readily. Hemorrhages of various sizes are common on the serosal surfaces of the abdomen and thorax as well as on the epicardium and endocardium. Edematous, red-tinged effusions commonly are present under the serosa of various organs, between skeletal muscle groups, and in the subcutis. Hemorrhages frequently occur along the GI tract mucosa, and ulcers, particularly over Peyer's patches, may be present. An enlarged, dark red or black, soft, semifluid spleen is common. The liver, kidneys, and lymph nodes usually are congested and enlarged.

In pigs with chronic anthrax, the lesions usually are restricted to the tonsils, cervical lymph nodes, and surrounding tissues. The lymphatic tissues of the area are enlarged and are a mottled salmon to brick-red color on cut surface. Diphtheritic membranes or ulcers may be present over the surface of the tonsils. The area around involved lymphatic tissues generally is gelatinous and edematous.

Diagnosis: A diagnosis based on clinical signs may be difficult, especially when the disease occurs in a new area. Therefore, a confirmatory laboratory examination should be done. A small amount of blood collected aseptically from a superficial vessel such as the jugular vein is the preferred specimen. Since pigs with localized disease are rarely bacteremic, a small piece of affected lymphatic tissue that has been collected aseptically should be submitted. Before submission, the laboratory should be contacted to determine appropriate shipping procedures.

Anthrax must be differentiated from other conditions that cause sudden death. In cattle and sheep, clostridial infections, bloat, and lightning stroke may be confused with anthrax. Also, acute leptospirosis, bacillary hemoglobinuria, anaplasmosis, and acute poisonings by bracken fern, sweet clover, and lead must be considered in cattle. In horses, acute infectious anemia, purpura, the various colics, lead poisoning, lightning stroke, and sunstroke may resemble anthrax. In pigs, acute hog cholera, African swine fever, and pharyngeal malignant edema are diagnostic considerations. In dogs, acute systemic infections and pharyngeal swellings due to other causes must be considered.

Treatment and Control: Since anthrax is often fatal, early treatment and vigorous implementation of a preventive program are essential. When a soil-borne outbreak occurs, it is best to use antibiotics for the sick animals and immunize all apparently well animals in the herd and on surrounding premises. If the outbreak is associated with a discrete source, such as contaminated bone meal, antibiotic treatment of exposed animals and removal of the source may be more effective than vaccination in reducing losses. Domestic livestock respond well to penicillin if treated in the early stages of the disease. Oxytetracycline given daily in divided doses also is effective. Other antibacterials, eg, erythromycin or sulfonamides, also can be utilized, but their effectiveness in comparison to penicillin and the tetracyclines has not been evaluated under field conditions.

Anthrax of livestock can be controlled largely by annual vaccination of all grazing animals in the endemic area and implementing control measures during outbreaks. The nonencapsulated Sterne-strain vaccine is used almost universally for livestock immunization. Vaccination should be done 2-4 wk before the season when outbreaks may be expected. Animals should not be vaccinated within 2 mo of anticipated slaughter. Because this is a live vaccine, antibiotics should not be administered within 1 wk of vaccination. Before vaccination of dairy cattle during an outbreak, the procedures required by local laws should be determined.

Specific control procedures, in addition to therapy and immunization, are necessary to contain the disease and prevent its spread. These include: 1) notification of the appropriate regulatory officials; 2) rigid enforcement of quarantine; 3) prompt disposal of dead animals, manure, bedding, or other contaminated material by cremation or deep burial; 4) isolation of sick animals and removal of well animals from the contaminated areas; 5) disinfection of stables, pens, milking barns, and equipment used on livestock; 6) use of insect repellents; 7) control of scavengers that feed on animals dead of the disease; and 8) observation of general sanitary procedures by persons who contact diseased animals, for their own safety, and to prevent spread of the disease.

BESNOITIOSIS

A protozoan disease of the skin, subcutis, blood vessels, mucous membranes, and other tissues.

Etiology and Transmission: The causal agent of the cutaneous disease in cattle is *Besnoitia besnoiti* and that in horses and burros, *B bennetti. Besnoitia jellisoni* and *B wallacei* have been described from rodents; *B tarandi* from reindeer; *B darlingi* from lizards, opossums, and snakes; and *B sauriana* from lizards. Viscerotropic strains of *B besnoiti* have been isolated from African antelope; an unidentified *Besnoitia* sp has been found in goats. *Besnoitia besnoiti* has been reported from southern Europe, Africa, Asia, and South America, but has not been reported in cattle in North America. These *Toxoplasma*-like organisms multiply in endothelial, histiocytic, and other cells, and produce characteristic large, thick-walled cysts filled with bradyzoites.

Experimental cyclic transmission with intestinal sexual stages in a definitive host, the cat, has been reported for *B besnoiti, B wallacei*, and *B darlingi*. Transmission of *B besnoiti* from cattle to cats has not been substantiated by subsequent studies. Biting flies or ticks may transmit *B besnoiti* mechanically from chronically infected cattle; some *Besnoitia* spp can be transmitted artificially to suitable hosts by needle inoculation of tissues that contain cysts.

Clinical Findings: Infected cattle often show no clinical signs other than a few cysts in the scleral conjunctiva. Illness commences with fever followed by anasarca. Inappetence, photophobia, rhinitis, swollen lymph glands, and orchitis also are seen. Anasarca gives way to sclerodermatitis. The skin becomes hard, thick, and wrinkled, and develops cracks that allow secondary bacterial infection and myiasis to develop; movement is painful. There is loss of hair and epidermis. Severely affected animals become emaciated. Cysts appear in the scleral conjunctiva and nasal mucosa. Although mortality is low, convalescence is slow in severe cases. Severely affected bulls can become permanently sterile. Affected animals remain carriers for life.

Signs in horses are similar to those in cattle.

Prophylaxis and Treatment: In some countries, cattle are immunized with a live, tissue-culture-adapted vaccine. Affected animals should be isolated and treated symptomatically. In limited studies of *B besnoiti* in rabbits, both antimony and sulfanilamide complex prevented cyst development.

CLOSTRIDIAL DISEASES

Members of the genus *Clostridium* are relatively large, anaerobic, spore-forming, rod-shaped organisms. The spores are oval, sometimes spherical, and are central, subterminal, or terminal in position. The vegetative forms of clostridia in tissue fluids of infected animals occur singly, in pairs, or rarely in chains. Differentiation of the various pathogenic and related species is based on cultural characteristics, spore shape and position, and the serological specificity of the toxin or the somatic antigens. The natural habitats of the organisms are the soil and intestinal tract of animals, including man. Pathogenic strains may be acquired by susceptible animals either by wound contamination or by ingestion. Diseases thus produced are a constant threat to successful livestock production in many parts of the world.

Clostridial diseases can be divided into 2 categories: 1) those in which the organisms actively invade and reproduce in the tissues of the host with the production of toxins that enhance the spread of infection and are responsible for death, and which are sometimes referred to as the gas-gangrene group; 2) those characterized by toxemia resulting from the absorption of toxins produced by organisms within the digestive system (the enterotoxemias), in devitalized tissue (tetanus), or in food or carrion outside the body (botulism). If treatment of the first group is attempted, large doses of antibiotic are indicated to establish effective levels in the center of necrotic tissue where clostridia are found.

BACILLARY HEMOGLOBINURIA
(Red water disease)

An acute, infectious, toxemic disease, primarily of cattle, caused by *Clostridium haemolyticum (C novyi* type D). It has been found in sheep and rarely in dogs. It occurs in the western part of the USA, along the Gulf of Mexico, in Venezuela, Chile, Great Britain, Turkey, and probably other parts of the world.

Etiology: *Clostridium haemolyticum* is a soil-borne organism that may be found naturally in the alimentary tract of cattle. It may survive for long periods in contaminated soil or in bones from carcasses of animals that had been infected. Following ingestion, latent spores ultimately become lodged in the liver. The incubation period is extremely variable, the onset depending on the occurrence of a locus of anaerobiosis in the liver. Such a nidus for germination is most often caused by fluke infection, much less often by high nitrate content of the diet, accidental liver puncture, liver biopsy, or any other cause of localized necrosis. When favorable conditions of anaerobiosis occur, the spores germinate, and the resulting vegetative cells multiply and produce β toxin (phospholipase C), which causes an acute hemolytic anemia.

Clinical Findings: Cattle may be found dead without premonitory signs. Usually, there is a sudden onset of severe depression, fever, abdominal pain, dyspnea, dysentery, and hemoglobinuria. Varying degrees of anemia and jaundice are present. Edema of the brisket may occur. Hgb and RBC levels are quite low. The duration of clinical signs varies from ~12 hr in pregnant cows to ~3-4 days in other cattle. The mortality in untreated animals is ~95%. Some cattle suffer from subclinical attacks of the disease and thereafter act as immune carriers.

Lesions: After death, *rigor mortis* sets in more rapidly than usual. Dehydration, anemia, and sometimes subcut. edema are present. There is bloody fluid in the abdominal and thoracic cavities. The lungs are not grossly affected, and the trachea contains bloody froth with hemorrhages in the mucosa. The small intestine, and occasionally the large, are hemorrhagic and their contents often contain free or clotted blood. An anemic infarct in the liver is virtually pathognomonic; it is slightly elevated, lighter in color than the surrounding tissue, and outlined by a bluish red zone of congestion. The kidneys are dark, friable, and usually studded with petechiae. The bladder contains purplish red urine.

Diagnosis: The general clinical picture usually permits a diagnosis. The most striking sign is the typical port-wine-colored urine, which foams freely when voided or on agitation. The presence of the typical liver infarct is sufficient for a presumptive diagnosis. The normal size and consistency of the spleen serve to exclude anthrax and anaplasmosis. Bracken fern poisoning and leptospirosis also should be considered. Diagnosis may be confirmed bacteriologically by isolating *C haemolyticum* from the liver infarct, but the organism is difficult to culture. Rapid and accurate diagnosis may be achieved by demonstrating the organism in the liver tissue by FA test, or demonstrating the toxin in the fluid in the peritoneal cavity or in a saline extract of the infarct.

Control: Early treatment with penicillin or broad-spectrum antibiotics is essential. Whole blood and fluid therapy also are helpful.

Clostridium haemolyticum bacterin prepared from whole cultures confers immunity for ~6 mo. In areas where the disease is seasonal, one preseasonal dose is usually adequate; where the disease occurs throughout the year, semiannual immunization is necessary. Cattle that are in contact with animals from areas where this disease is endemic should be immunized, since the latter may be carriers.

BIG HEAD

An acute, infectious disease, caused by *Clostridium novyi, C sordellii,* or rarely, *C chauvoei,* characterized by a nongaseous, nonhemorrhagic, edematous swelling of the head, face, and neck of young rams. This infection is initiated in young rams by their continual butting of one another. The bruised and battered subcut. tissues provide conditions suitable for growth of pathogenic clostridia, and the breaks in the skin offer an opportunity for their entrance. Treatment is with broad-spectrum antibiotics or penicillin.

BLACKLEG

An acute, febrile disease of cattle and sheep caused by *Clostridium chauvoei (feseri)* and characterized by emphysematous swelling, usually in the heavy muscles. The disease is found worldwide.

Etiology: *Clostridium chauvoei* occurs naturally in the intestinal tract of animals. It probably can remain viable in the soil for many years, although it does not actively grow there. Outbreaks of blackleg have occurred in cattle on farms in which recent excavations have occurred, which suggests that disturbance of soil may activate latent spores. The organisms probably are ingested, pass through the wall of the digestive tract, and, after gaining access to the bloodstream, are deposited in muscle and other tissues.

In cattle, blackleg infection is endogenous, in contrast to malignant edema (*see* below). Lesions develop without any history of wounds, although bruising may precipitate some cases. Commonly, the animals that contract blackleg are of the beef breeds, in excellent health, gaining weight, and usually the best animals of their group. Outbreaks occur in which a few new cases are found each day for several days. Most cases occur in cattle from 6 mo to 2 yr old, but thrifty calves as young as 6 wk and cattle as old as 10-12 yr may be affected. The disease usually occurs in summer and fall and is uncommon during the winter. In sheep, the disease is not restricted to the young, and most cases follow some form of injury such as shearing cuts, docking, crutching, or castration. Endogenous blackleg in sheep is uncommon in the USA; it is much more common in New Zealand where blackleg is seen more frequently in sheep than in cattle.

Clinical Findings and Lesions: Usually, onset is sudden and a few cattle may be found dead without premonitory signs. Acute lameness and marked depression are common. Initially, there is a fever but, by the time clinical signs are obvious, the temperature may be normal or subnormal. Characteristic edematous and crepitant swellings develop in the hip, shoulder, chest, back, neck, or elsewhere. At first, the swelling is small, hot, and painful. As the disease rapidly progresses, the swelling enlarges, there is crepitation on palpation, and the skin becomes cold and insensitive as the blood supply to the area diminishes. General signs include prostration and tremors. Death occurs in 12-48 hr. In some cattle, the lesions are restricted to the myocardium and the diaphragm, with no reliable antemortem evidence of the localized lesion.

Diagnosis: A rapidly fatal febrile disease in well-nourished young cattle, particularly of the beef breeds, with crepitant swellings of the heavy muscles suggests blackleg. The affected muscle is dark red to black, dry and spongy, has a sweetish odor, and is infiltrated with small bubbles, but with little edema. The lesions may be in any muscle, even in the tongue or diaphragm. In sheep, since the lesions of the spontaneously occurring type are often small and deep, they may be overlooked. Occasionally, the tissue changes caused by *C septicum, C novyi, C sordellii,* and *C perfringens* may resemble those of blackleg; at times, both *C septicum* and *C chauvoei* may be isolated from blackleg lesions, particularly when the carcass is examined ≥24 hr after death, which allows time for postmortem invasion of the tissues by *C septicum.* Field diagnoses are confirmed by laboratory demonstration of *C chauvoei* in affected muscle. The samples of muscle should be taken as soon after death as possible. The FA test for *C chauvoei* is rapid and reliable.

Control: A bacterin containing *C chauvoei* and *C septicum* is safe and reliable for both cattle and sheep. Calves should be vaccinated twice, 2 wk apart, between 2 and 6 mo of age; in high-risk areas, revaccination may be necessary at 1 yr and q5yr thereafter. When outbreaks are encountered, all susceptible cattle should be vaccinated and treated prophylactically with penicillin to prevent new cases, which may develop for up to 10 days, when the bacterin provides protection. In some areas, multi-component clostridial vaccines are warranted. Treatment of clinical cases with parenteral and multiple local injections of penicillin may be attempted, but is frequently unsuccessful.

ENTEROTOXEMIAS
(*Clostridium perfringens* infection)

Clostridium perfringens is widely distributed in the soil and the alimentary tract of animals, and is characterized by its ability to produce potent exotoxins, some of which are responsible for specific enterotoxemias. Six types (A, B, C, D, E, and F) have been identified on the basis of the toxins produced, but only 3 (B, C, and D) are important. However, type A, although present in the gut of many clinically normal animals, has been suspected as the cause of hemorrhagic enteritis in cattle, horses, and sheep.

ENTEROTOXEMIA CAUSED BY *C PERFRINGENS* TYPES B AND C

Infection with types B and C causes severe enteritis, dysentery, toxemia, and high mortality in young lambs, calves, pigs, and foals. Type C also causes enterotoxemia in adult cattle, sheep, and goats. The diseases are listed below, categorized as to cause and host. (*See also* INTESTINAL DISEASES IN HORSES, p 184.) *Clostridium perfringens* also has been associated with hemorrhagic enteritis in dogs.

Lamb dysentery: *C perfringens* type B in lambs up to 3 wk of age. **Calf enterotoxemia:** types B and C in well-fed calves up to 1 mo. **Pig enterotoxemia:** type C in piglets during the first few days of life. **Foal enterotoxemia:** type B in foals in the first week of life. **Struck:** type C in adult sheep. **Goat enterotoxemia:** type C in adult goats.

Clinical Findings: Lamb dysentery is an acute disease of lambs <3 wk old. Many may die before signs are observed, but some newborn animals stop nursing, become listless, and remain recumbent. A fetid, blood-tinged diarrhea is common, and death usually occurs within a few days.

In calves, there is acute diarrhea, dysentery, abdominal pain, convulsions, and opisthotonos. Death may occur in a few hours, but less severe cases survive for a few days and recovery over a period of several days is possible. Pigs become acutely ill within a few days of birth and there is diarrhea, dysentery, reddening of the anus, and a high fatality rate; most affected piglets die within 12 hr. In foals, there is acute dysentery, toxemia, and rapid death. Struck in adult sheep is characterized by death without premonitory signs.

Lesions: Hemorrhagic enteritis with ulceration of the mucosa is the major lesion in all species. Grossly, the affected portion of the intestine is deep blue-purple and appears at first glance to be an infarction associated with mesenteric torsion. Smears of intestinal contents can be examined for large numbers of gram-positive rod-shaped bacteria, and filtrates made for detection of toxin and subsequent identification by neutralization with specific antiserum.

Control: Treatment is usually ineffective because of severity of the disease, but if available, specific hyperimmune serum is indicated and oral administration of antibiotics may be helpful. The disease is best controlled by vaccination of the pregnant dam during the last third of pregnancy: initially, 2 vaccinations a month apart, and annually thereafter. When outbreaks occur in newborn animals from unvaccinated dams, antiserum should be administered immediately after birth.

TYPE D ENTEROTOXEMIA
(Pulpy kidney disease, Overeating disease)

An enterotoxemia of sheep, less frequently of goats, and rarely of cattle. This is the classic enterotoxemia of sheep. It is worldwide in distribution and may occur in animals of any age. It is most common in the young, either <2 wk of age or in weaned lambs in feedlots, on a high-carbohydrate diet or, less often, on lush green pastures. The disease has been suspected in well-nourished beef calves nursing high-producing cows grazing lush pasture, and in sudden death syndrome in feedlot cattle, but supportive laboratory evidence in the latter is lacking.

Etiology: The causative agent is *C perfringens* type D. However, predisposing factors also are essential; the most common of these is the ingestion of excessive amounts of feed or milk in the very young, and grain in feedlot lambs. In young lambs, the disease usually is restricted to the single lambs, for seldom does a ewe with twins give enough milk to allow enterotoxemia to develop. In the feedlot, the disease usually occurs in lambs on high-grain diets. As the starch intake increases, it provides a suitable medium for growth of the causative bacteria, which produce ε toxin. A major effect of the toxin is to cause vascular damage, particularly of capillaries in the brain. Many sheep carry strains of *C perfringens* type D as part of the normal microflora of the intestine, and serve as the source of organisms to infect the newborn. Most such carriers show non-vaccinal antitoxin in their sera.

Clinical Findings: Usually, sudden deaths in the best-conditioned lambs are the first indication of enterotoxemia. In some cases, excitement, incoordination, and convulsions occur before death. Opisthotonos, circling, and pushing the head against fixed objects are common signs of CNS involvement; frequently, hyperglycemia or glycosuria is observed. Diarrhea may or may not develop. Occasionally, adult sheep are affected; they show weakness, incoordination, and convulsions, and die within 24 hr. Acutely affected calves not found dead show mania, convulsions, blindness, and death in a few hours. Subacutely affected calves are stuporous for a few days and may recover. In goats, diarrhea and nervous signs are seen, and death occurs in several weeks.

Lesions: Necropsy may reveal only a few hyperemic areas on the intestine and a fluid-filled pericardial sac. This is particularly the case in young lambs. In older animals, hemorrhagic areas on the myocardium, and petechiae and ecchymoses of the abdominal muscles and serosa of the intestine may be found. Bilateral pulmonary edema and congestion frequently occur, but usually not in young lambs. The rumen and abomasum contain an abundance of feed, and undigested feed often is found in the ileum. Edema and malacia can be seen microscopically in the basal ganglia and cerebellum of lambs. Rapid postmortem autolysis of the kidneys has lead to the popular name, pulpy kidney disease, although pulpy kidneys are by no means always found in young lambs, and are seldom found in goats or cattle.

Diagnosis: A presumptive diagnosis of enterotoxemia is based on sudden, convulsive deaths in lambs on carbohydrate-rich feed. Smears of intestinal contents reveal many gram-positive, short, thick bacilli. Confirmation requires demonstration of ε toxin in the small intestinal fluid. Fluid, not ingesta, should be collected in a sterile vial within a few hours after death, and sent under refrigeration to a laboratory for toxin identification. Chloroform, added at one drop for each 10 mL of intestinal fluid, will stabilize any toxin present.

Control: The method of control depends on the age of the lambs, the frequency with which the disease appears on a particular property, and the method of husbandry. If the disease occurs consistently in young lambs on a property, ewe immunization probably is the most satisfactory method of control. The breeding females should be given 2 injections of type D toxoid their first year and one injection, 4-6 wk before lambing, each year thereafter.

Enterotoxemia in feedlot lambs can be controlled by reducing the amount of concentrate in the diet. However, this may not be economical, in which case immunization of all animals with toxoid when they first enter the feedlot probably will reduce losses to an acceptable level. Two injections, 2 wk apart, will protect them through the feeding period. When alum-precipitated toxoids or bacterins are used, the injection should be given at such a site that the cold abscesses, which commonly develop at the site of injection, can be removed easily during normal dressing and not blemish the carcass.

INFECTIOUS NECROTIC HEPATITIS
(INH, *Clostridium novyi [oedematiens]* infection, Black disease)

An acute, infectious disease of sheep, sometimes of cattle, and rarely of pigs and horses.

Etiology and Pathogenesis: The etiological agent, *Clostridium novyi* type B, is soil-borne and frequently present in the intestines of herbivores; it may be present on skin surfaces and is a potential source of wound infections. Fecal contamination of pasture by carrier animals is the most important source of the infection. The organism multiplies in areas of liver necrosis caused by the migration of liver flukes, and produces a powerful necrotizing toxin. The disease is worldwide in distribution, wherever sheep and liver flukes coincide.

Clostridium novyi has been suspected but not yet confirmed as a cause of sudden death in cattle and pigs fed high-level grain diets, and in which pre-existing lesions of the liver were not detectable. The lethal and necrotizing toxins (primarily α toxin) damage hepatic parenchyma, thereby permitting the bacteria to multiply and produce a lethal amount of toxin.

Clinical Findings: Usually, death is sudden with no well-defined signs. Affected animals tend to lag behind the flock, assume sternal recumbency, and die within a few hours. Most cases occur in the summer and early fall when liver fluke infection is at its height. The disease is most prevalent in 1- to 4-yr-old sheep and is limited to animals infected with liver flukes. Differentiation from acute fascioliasis may be difficult, but peracute deaths of animals that show typical lesions on necropsy should arouse suspicion of black disease.

Lesions: The most characteristic lesions are the grayish yellow necrotic foci in the liver that often follow the migratory tracks of the young flukes. Other common findings are an enlarged pericardial sac filled with straw-colored fluid, and excess fluid in the peritoneal and thoracic cavities. Usually, there is extensive rupture of the capillaries in the subcut. tissue, which causes the adjacent skin to turn black, hence the common name.

Control: The incidence may be lowered by reducing the numbers of snails, usually *Lymnaea* spp, that act as intermediate hosts for the liver flukes, or by otherwise reducing the fluke infection of sheep. However, these procedures are not always practical, and active immunization with *C novyi* toxoid is more effective. Long-term immunity is produced by one vaccination. Following this, only new introductions to the flock (lambs and sheep brought in from other areas) need to be vaccinated. This is best done before the late summer.

MALIGNANT EDEMA

An acute, generally fatal toxemia of cattle, horses, sheep, goats, and pigs usually caused by *Clostridium septicum* and often accompanied by other clostridial species. A similar infection in man is not uncommon. The disease occurs worldwide. Other clostridia implicated in wound infections include *C chauvoei*, *C perfringens*, *C novyi*, and *C sordellii*.

Etiology: *Clostridium septicum* is found in soil and intestinal contents of animals (including man) throughout the world. Infection ordinarily occurs through contamination of wounds containing devitalized tissue, soil, or some other tissue-debilitant. Wounds caused by accident, castration, docking, insanitary vaccination, and parturition may become infected.

Clinical Findings and Diagnosis: General signs, such as anorexia, intoxication, and high fever, as well as local lesions, develop within a few hours to a few days after predisposing injury. The local lesions are soft swellings that pit on pressure and extend rapidly because of the formation of large quantities of exudate that infiltrate the subcut. and IM connective tissue of the affected areas. The muscle in such areas is dark brown to black. Accumulations of gas are uncommon. Severe edema of the head of rams occurs following infection of wounds inflicted by fighting. Malignant edema associated with lacerations of the vulva at parturition is characterized by marked edema of the vulva, severe toxemia, and death in 24-48 hr. Similarity to blackleg (*see* above) is marked, and differentiation made on necropsy is unreliable; laboratory confirmation is the only certain procedure. Horses and pigs are susceptible to malignant edema, but not to blackleg. (*Clostridium septicum* also causes **braxy** in sheep, a highly fatal infection characterized by toxemia and inflammation of the abomasal wall. This disease seems to be confined mostly to European sheep fed on "frosted" pasture.)

Diagnosis can be confirmed rapidly on the basis of FA staining of *C septicum* from a tissue smear. However, *C septicum* is an extremely active postmortem invader from the intestine, and its presence in a specimen taken from an animal that has been dead for ≥24 hr is not significant.

Control: Bacterins are used for immunization. *Clostridium septicum* usually is combined with *C chauvoei* in a blackleg-malignant edema vaccine, and is available in multi-component vaccines. In endemic areas, animals should be vaccinated before they are castrated, dehorned, or docked. Calves should be vaccinated at ~2 mo of age. Two doses 2-3 wk apart generally give protection. In high-risk areas, annual vaccination is indicated as is revaccination following severe trauma.

Treatment with high doses of penicillin or broad-spectrum antibiotics is indicated early in the disease. The injection of penicillin directly into the periphery of the lesion may minimize spread of the lesion, but usually the affected tissues still slough.

BOTULISM
(Lamziekte)

A rapidly fatal motor paralysis caused by the ingestion of the toxin of *Clostridium botulinum*; the organism proliferates in decomposing animal tissue and sometimes in plant material.

Etiology: Botulism is an intoxication, not an infection, and results from ingestion of toxin in food. There are 8 types and subtypes of *C botulinum*, differentiated on the serological specificity of the toxins: A, B, C_α, C_β, D, E, F, and G. Types A, B, and E are of most importance in human botulism; C_α in wild ducks, pheasants, and chickens; C_β in mink, cattle, and horses; D in cattle. Only 2 outbreaks, both in man, are known to have been caused by type F. Type G, which was isolated from soil in Argentina, is not known to have been involved in any outbreak of botulism either in man or other animals. The usual source of the toxin is decaying carcasses or vegetable materials such as decaying grass, hay, grain, and spoiled silage. Toxins of all types have the same pharmacologic action.

The incidence of botulism in animals is not known with accuracy, but it is relatively low in cattle and horses, probably more frequent in chickens, and high in wild waterfowl. Probably 10,000-50,000 birds are lost in most years, with losses reaching one million or more during the great outbreaks in the western USA. Most affected birds are ducks, although loons, mergansers, geese, and gulls also are susceptible. (*See also* BOTULISM [POU], p 1608.) Dogs, cats, and pigs are comparatively resistant to all types of botulinum toxin when it is administered by mouth.

Most botulism in cattle occurs in South Africa, where a combination of extensive agriculture, phosphorus deficiency in soil, and *C botulinum* type D in animals creates conditions ideal for the disease. The phosphorus-deficient cattle chew any bones with accompanying tags of flesh that they find on the range; if these came from an animal that had been carrying type D strains of *C botulinum*, intoxication is likely to result. A gram or so of dried flesh from such a carcass may contain enough toxin to kill a mature cow. Any animal eating such material also ingests spores, which germinate in the intestine and, after death of the host, invade the musculature, which in turn becomes toxic for other cattle. Type C strains also cause botulism in cattle in a similar fashion. This type of botulism in cattle is rare in the USA, although a few cases have been reported from Texas under the name of **loin disease**, and a few cases have occurred in Montana. Botulism in sheep has been encountered in Australia, not associated with phosphorus deficiency as in cattle, but with protein and carbohydrate deficiency, which results in sheep eating carcasses of rabbits and other small animals found on the range.

Toxicoinfectious botulism is the name given the disease in which *C botulinum* grows in tissues of a living animal and produces toxins there. The toxins are liberated from the lesions and cause typical botulism. This has been suggested as a means of producing the **shaker foal syndrome**. Gastric ulcers, foci of necrosis in the liver, abscesses in the navel and lungs, and wounds of the skin and muscle are predisposing sites for development of toxicoinfectious botulism. This disease of foals and adult horses appears to resemble "wound botulism" in man.

Botulism in mink usually is caused by type C$_\beta$ strains that have produced toxin in chopped raw meat or fish. Type A and E strains are seldom involved.

Clinical Findings: The signs of botulism are caused by muscle paralysis and include progressive motor paralysis, disturbed vision, difficulty in chewing and swallowing, and generalized progressive weakness. Death is usually due to respiratory or cardiac paralysis. The toxin prevents synthesis or release of acetylcholine at motor end-plates. Passage of impulses down the motor nerves and contractility of muscles are not greatly hindered; only the passage of impulses from nerves to motor end-plates is affected. No characteristic lesions develop, and pathological changes may be ascribed to the general paralytic action of toxin, particularly in the muscles of the respiratory system, rather than to the specific effect of toxin on any particular organ.

Epidemics have occurred in dairy herds in which up to 65% of adult cows developed clinical botulism and died 6-72 hr after the onset of recumbency. Major clinical findings included drooling, inability to urinate, dysphagia, and sternal recumbency, which progressed to lateral recumbency just before death. Skin sensation is usually normal, and withdrawal reflexes of the limbs are weak. Initially, clinical signs resemble second-stage milk fever, but the cows do not respond to calcium therapy.

In the shaker foal syndrome, foals are usually <4 wk old. They may be found dead without premonitory signs; most often, they exhibit signs of progressive symmetrical motor paralysis. Stilted gait, muscular tremors, and the inability to stand for longer than 4-5 min are salient features. Other clinical signs include dysphagia, constipation, mydriasis, and frequent urination. As the disease progresses, dyspnea with extension of the head and neck, tachycardia, and respiratory arrest occur. Death occurs most often 24-72 hr after the onset of clinical signs. The most consistent necropsy findings are pulmonary edema and congestion and excessive pericardial fluid, which contains free-floating strands of fibrin.

Diagnosis: Although sporadic cases of botulism often are suspected because of the characteristic motor paralysis, it is sometimes difficult to establish the diagnosis by demonstrating the toxin in animal tissues or sera, or in the suspect feed. Commonly, the diagnosis is made by eliminating other causes of motor paralysis. Filtrates of the stomach and intestinal contents should be tested for toxicity in mice, but a negative answer is unreliable. Primary supportive evidence is provided by feeding suspect material to susceptible animals. In peracute cases, the toxin may be detectable in the blood by mouse inoculation tests but usually is not detectable in the average field case in farm animals. In toxicoinfectious botulism, the organism may be cultured from tissues of affected animals.

Control: Any dietary deficiencies should be corrected, and carcasses disposed of if possible. Decaying grass or spoiled silage should be removed from the diet. Immunization of cattle with types C and D toxoid has proved successful in South Africa and Australia. Toxoid is also effective in immunizing mink and has been used in pheasants.

Botulinum antitoxin has been used for treatment with varying degrees of success, depending on the type of toxin involved and the species of host. Treatment of ducks and mink with type C antitoxin is often successful; however, such treatment is rarely used in cattle. Treatment with guanidine hydrochloride, 5 mg/lb (11 mg/kg) body wt, has been reported to overcome some of the paralysis caused by the toxin; however, its use has not been extensive enough to determine its value.

TETANUS

A toxemia caused by a specific neurotoxin produced by *Clostridium tetani* in necrotic tissue. Almost all mammals are susceptible to this disease, although cats seem much more resistant than any other domestic or laboratory mammal. Birds are quite resistant; the lethal dose for pigeons and chickens is 10,000-300,000 times greater (on a body weight basis) than for horses. Horses are the most sensitive of all species, with the possible exception of man. Although tetanus is worldwide in distribution, there are some areas, such as the northern Rocky Mountain section of the USA, where the organism is rarely found in the soil and where tetanus is almost unknown. In general, the occurrence of *C tetani* in the soil and the incidence of tetanus in man and horses is higher in the warmer parts of the various continents.

Etiology and Pathogenesis: *Clostridium tetani*, an anaerobe with terminal, spherical spores, is found in soil and intestinal tracts. In most cases, it is introduced into the tissues through wounds, particularly deep puncture wounds, which provide a suitable anaerobic environment. Often in lambs, however, and sometimes in other species, it follows docking or castration. Sometimes, it is not possible to find the point of entry since the lesion itself may be minor or healed.

The spores of *C tetani* are unable to grow in normal tissue, or even in wounds if the tissue remains at the oxidation-reduction potential of the circulating blood. Suitable conditions for multiplication occur when a small amount of soil or a foreign object causes tissue necrosis. The bacteria remain localized in the necrotic tissue at the original site of infection and multiply. As bacterial cells undergo autolysis, the potent neurotoxin is released. Usually, toxin is absorbed by the motor nerves in the area and passes up the nerve tract to the spinal cord, where it causes ascending tetanus. The toxin causes spasmodic, tonic contractions of the voluntary muscles by interfering with the release of neurotransmitters. If more toxin is released at the site of the infection than the surrounding nerves can take up, the excess is carried off by the lymph to the bloodstream and thus to the CNS, where it causes descending tetanus. Even minor stimulation of the affected individual may trigger the characteristic muscular spasms.

Clinical Findings: The incubation period varies from one to several weeks, but usually averages 10-14 days. Localized stiffness, often involving the masseter muscles and muscles of the neck, the hindlimbs, and the region of the infected wound is seen first; general stiffness becomes pronounced ~1 day later, and tonic spasms and hyperesthesia become evident.

The reflexes are increased in intensity and the animal is easily excited into more violent, general spasms by sudden movement or noise. Spasms of head muscles cause difficulty in prehension and mastication of food, hence the common designation, **lockjaw**. In horses, the ears are erect, the tail stiff and extended, the anterior nares dilated, and the third eyelid prolapsed. Walking, turning, and backing are difficult. Spasms of the neck and back muscles cause extension of the head and neck, while stiffness of the leg muscles causes the animal to assume a "sawhorse" stance. Sweating frequently occurs. General spasms disturb circulation and respiration, which results in increased heart rate, rapid breathing, and congestion of mucous membranes. Sheep, goats, and pigs often fall to the ground and have opisthotonos when startled. Consciousness is not affected.

Usually, the temperature remains slightly above normal, but it may rise to 108-110°F (42-43°C) toward the end of a fatal attack. In mild attacks, the pulse and temperature remain nearly normal. Mortality averages ~80%. In animals that recover, there is a convalescent period of 2-6 wk; protective immunity usually does not develop following recovery.

Control: Active immunization can be accomplished with tetanus toxoid. If a dangerous wound occurs after immunization, another injection of toxoid to increase the circulating antibody should be given. If the animal has not been immunized previously, it should be treated with 1500-3000 IU or more of tetanus antitoxin, which usually provides passive protection for up to 2 wk. Toxoid should be given simultaneously with the antitoxin and repeated in 30 days. Yearly booster injections of toxoid are advisable. Mares should be vaccinated during the last 6 wk of pregnancy and the foals vaccinated at 5-8 wk of age. In high-risk areas, foals may be given tetanus antitoxin immediately after birth and q2-3wk until they are 3 mo old, at which time they can be given toxoid. The decision to vaccinate lambs or calves depends on the prevalence of the disease in the area.

All surgical procedures should be conducted with the best possible techniques. After such surgery, animals should be turned out on clean ground, preferably grass pastures. Only the oxidizing disinfectants such as iodine or chlorine can be depended on to kill the spores.

When administered in the early stages of the disease, curariform agents, tranquilizers, or barbiturate sedatives, in conjunction with 300,000 IU of tetanus antitoxin q12hr, have been effective in the treatment of horses. Good results have been obtained in horses by injecting 50,000 IU of tetanus antitoxin directly into the subarachnoid space through the cisterna magna. Such therapy should be supported by drainage and cleaning of wounds and administering penicillin or broad-spectrum antibiotics. Good nursing is invaluable during the acute period of spasms. The animal should be placed in a quiet, darkened box-stall with feeding and watering devices high enough to allow their use without lowering the head. Slings may be useful in cases where standing or rising is difficult.

CONGENITAL AND INHERITED ANOMALIES

Structural and functional defects have been described in neonatal animals ranging from variant through blemish, imperfection, and deviant, to malformation and monstrosity. Defective development may be expressed by embryonic mortality, fetal death, abortion, stillbirth, or a nonviable or viable neonate. (*See also* discussions of CONGENITAL ANOMALIES in the sections BLC, NER, REP, SKN, URN; many of the diseases mentioned below are discussed more fully elsewhere in the MANUAL, and may be located via the index.)

Susceptibility to injurious environmental or genetic agents varies with the stage of development and species, and decreases with fetal age. The zygote is resistant to teratogens, but susceptible to genetic mutations and chromosomal aberrations. The embryo is highly susceptible to teratogens, but this lessens as the embryo ages and the critical developmental periods of various organs or organ systems are passed. The fetus becomes increasingly resistant to teratogenic agents, except for later-differentiating structures such as the cerebellum, palate, and urogenital system.

Many congenital defects have no clearly established cause; others are caused by environmental, nutritional, or genetic factors, or from environmental/genetic interaction.

Environmental Factors: Teratogenic factors include toxic plants, viruses, drugs, trace elements, and physical agents such as irradiation, hyperthermia, and pressure during rectal examination.

Crooked calf disease, characterized by joint contractures, torticollis, scoliosis, or kyphosis, and various degrees of cleft palate and combinations of these defects is due to ingestion of either *Lupinus caudatus, L sericeus,* or *L nootkatensis.* Cows fed lupines between days 40 and 70 of gestation produced calves with these deformities. The alkaloid anagyrine was identified as the teratogen. Fetal development is at greatest risk when pregnant cows graze lupine early in the plant growth or during seed formation. Similar deformities have been reproduced by feeding *Conium maculatum* to cows between days 50 and 75 of pregnancy. Other plants suspected of causing similar defects in calves include *Senecio, Cycadales, Blighia, Papaveracea, Colchicum,* and *Vinca* spp; *Indigofera spicata*; loco plants; tobacco; and related plants.

Epidemics of cyclopian defects in lambs occurred in bands of sheep in southcentral and southwestern Idaho while grazing on *Veratrum californicum* on certain alpine ranges. Epidemics of arthrogryposis on Kentucky farms occurred when sows ingested tobacco stalks during pregnancy.

Sudan grass pasture (*Sorghum vulgare*) has been incriminated as a cause of arthrogryposis in horses, and *Sorghum sudanense* may have caused arthrogryposis in calves.

Locoweed poisoning by plants of the genera *Oxytropis* and *Astragalus* in all types of range livestock (most commonly cattle, sheep, and horses) resulted in various clinical signs such as emaciation, visual impairment, neurological signs, habituation, abortion, and congenital defects. Locoweed produced musculoskeletal defects in calves and lambs, and hypoplastic testicles and enlarged seminal vesicles in rams. *Swainsonia* and locoweed poisoning in growing cattle may have similarities to genetic mannosidosis in Angus cattle since the alkaloid indolizidine-1, 2, 8-triol is a potent and specific inhibitor of the hydrolytic enzyme α-mannosidase.

Ronnel (fenchlorphos) given PO in therapeutic doses to pregnant blue foxes (*Alopex lagopus*) for treating parasitism reduced litter size to 1.2 whelps per vixen (compared to 9.5 in gray vixen controls) and caused incomplete ossification of cranial bones, palatoschisis, and hydrocephalus.

Atresia of the gut, particularly the colon, may be caused by external pressure on the amnion during rectal palpation between days 35 and 40 of gestation.

Prenatal viral infections may be teratogenic in cattle, sheep, goats, pigs, dogs, and cats, but have not been incriminated in the common equine defects. Intrauterine Akabane virus infection (*see* below) in cattle, sheep, and goats has caused abortions, premature births, and congenital defects (arthrogryposis and hydranencephaly).

Bovine viral diarrhea (BVD) virus may cause defects such as cerebellar dysplasia, brachygnathia, alopecia, dysmyelinogenesis, internal hydrocephalus, optic neuritis, dysmaturity (intrauterine growth retardation), and impaired immunocompetence. Different strains of BVD virus may have different effects on the developing fetus, and the resulting lesion depends on the stage of pregnancy when the susceptible cow was exposed.

Bluetongue (BT) virus causes hydranencephaly, porencephaly, and arthrogryposis in sheep. Prenatal infection with BT virus in calves may result in abortions, stillbirths, and congenital defects such as arthrogryposis, campylognathia, and prognathia with a domed cranium. Hydranencephaly and a "dummy-calf" syndrome (inactivity, dullness, behavioral disturbances) also have been seen.

Wesselsbron disease virus reportedly has caused congenital porencephaly and cerebellar hypoplasia in calves in South Africa.

Prenatal infection with the togavirus of hypomyelinogenesis congenita in lambs ("hairy shaker" or "fuzzy" lambs) or Border disease (*see* below) is manifest by embryonic and fetal death, which lead to abortion or full-term stillbirths, and/or dysmorphogenesis of CNS, skeleton, and skin/fleece, and birth of small, weak lambs with poor growth and viability. There is defective myelinogenesis due to retardation of the myelinating process that is partially reversible if the lamb survives. The hairy fleece is due to a fall in the ratio of secondary to primary wool follicles and increased size and altered structure of primary wool fibers.

Hog cholera virus, a togavirus, is teratogenic in piglets, and causes micrencephaly, internal hydrocephalus, and cerebellar hypoplasia. Common associated findings are ascites, cirrhosis, kidney defects, severe pulmonary hypoplasia, and defects of the snout, ear, and limb.

Congenital tremor syndrome of piglets consists of several etiologically and pathologically distinct developmental defects of the brain and spinal cord.

Porcine fetuses, experimentally infected with swine influenza virus, developed pulmonary hypoplasia.

Natural and experimental infection of pregnant cats with feline panleukopenia virus has caused cerebellar hypoplasia in newborn kittens. Injection of pregnant ferrets *in utero* with this same virus also resulted in cerebellar hypoplasia.

Nutritional Factors: Deficiency of one or more nutrients during pregnancy may cause congenital defects in the newborn. Severe deficiencies may interrupt pregnancy or result in weak or nonviable young. Iodine deficiency is endemic in certain areas and may cause goiter or cretinism in all species. Copper deficiency causes enzootic ataxia in lambs; a deficiency of manganese causes limb deformities in calves. Vitamin deficiency may cause neonatal rickets (vitamin D), or eye defects or harelip (vitamin A). Experimentally, teratogenic effects have been induced by deficiencies of choline, riboflavin, pantothenic acid, cobalamin, and folic acid, and by hypervitaminosis A.

AKABANE DISEASE

An insect-transmitted viral disease that causes congenital abnormalities of the CNS in ruminants. It has been recognized in Australia, China, Israel, Japan, Korea, and South Africa; antibodies to it have been found in Cyprus. The clinical disease affects fetuses of cattle, sheep, and goats. Asymptomatic infection has been demonstrated serologically in horses, buffalo, deer, and dogs (but not in man or pigs) in endemic areas.

Etiology, Transmission, and Epidemiology: The causal agent, Akabane virus, is a member of the Simbu serogroup of Bunyaviridae. It has been isolated from mosquitoes and *Culicoides* in Australia, Japan, and Kenya. It also has been isolated from the blood of healthy sentinel cattle and from fetuses of ewes that seroconverted naturally. The disease has been reproduced experimentally.

Akabane virus is common in many tropical and subtropical areas between ~35°N and 35°S. In these endemic areas, herbivores are bitten by the vectors, become infected at an early age, and develop a solid immunity by the time of breeding; thus, congenital abnormalities are seldom seen. However, if for any reason, such as an extended humid summer, the vector (hence the virus) spreads into new areas, outbreaks of congenital infection may be expected. These outbreaks usually occur at the northern or southern limits of normal distribution of the insect vectors, or in areas of higher altitude. Similarly, pregnant ruminants from disease-free areas moved to virus-infected areas are at risk.

Clinical Findings and Lesions: Pathogenesis and clinical signs depend on the species of animal and time of infection. Calves infected late in pregnancy may be born alive but unable to stand, or be incoordinated and on necropsy show a disseminated encephalomyelitis. Those infected earlier (during the second trimester) have rigid fixation of limbs, usually in flexion (arthrogryposis) and sometimes also torticollis, kyphosis, and scoliosis with associated neurogenic muscle atrophy due to loss of spinal motor neurons. (These calves usually cause dystocia.) Calves affected earlier still (late in the first trimester) are usually born alive, but walk poorly and are depressed and blind. These calves have varying degrees of cavitation of cerebral hemispheres; usually extreme hydranencephaly is present. Some calves may be affected with both arthrogryposis and hydranencephaly. Cerebellar cavitation occurs occasionally.

In lambs and kids, there may be similar lesions of arthrogryposis and hydranencephaly. However, in Australia, affected lambs die shortly after birth, or show neurological signs and have extreme to mild micrencephaly with dilated lateral ventricles.

Abortion with or without CNS developmental abnormalities also occurs.

Diagnosis: A presumptive diagnosis can be made on the gross CNS lesions, but the disease must be differentiated from other infectious and genetic conditions. Confirmation of infection can be made by testing sera from unsuckled, affected offspring and their dams for serum neutralizing antibodies against Akabane virus.

Two additional viruses that cause similar signs have recently been reported. Aino virus, another Simbu serogroup virus, has been isolated from mosquitoes and *Culicoides* in Japan and Australia, where it has been associated with some cases of bovine arthrogryposis and hydranencephaly. Antibodies have been found in cattle, sheep, buffalo, and man. In Japan, Chuzan virus, a reovirus, is transmitted by *Culicoides oxystoma* and causes congenital infection in calves similar to Akabane virus.

Treatment and Control: There is no treatment. Introduction of stock from nonendemic to endemic areas should be done well before first breeding.

BORDER DISEASE
(Hairy shaker disease)

Border disease (Britain) or hairy shaker disease (Australia and New Zealand) is a congenital disorder of lambs characterized by low birth weight and viability, poor conformation, tremor, and an excessively hairy birth coat in normally smooth-coated breeds. Kids may also be affected, and a similar condition occasionally occurs in calves. The disease has been recognized in most sheep-rearing areas of the world, including western USA.

Etiology, Pathogenesis, and Epidemiology: Border disease (BD) is caused by infection of the fetus in early pregnancy with a pestivirus (Togaviridae) closely related or identical to the virus of bovine viral diarrhea/mucosal disease (qv, p 166). Surviving lambs are persistently viremic, and the virus is present in their excretions and secretions, including semen. Ruminants and possibly also pigs can be readily infected by contact with these persistent excretors or with acutely infected sheep. Acute infections in immunocompetent animals usually are transient and subclinical, and result in immunity to challenge with homologous but not heterologous strains of virus.

Virus acquired in early pregnancy by previously unexposed animals crosses the placenta and invades the fetus. Placentitis occurs 10-30 days after infection and may cause fetal death with expulsion, resorption, or mummification. Abortion may occur at any stage of pregnancy and may pass unnoticed since there is little maternal malaise.

In sustained pregnancies, the virus becomes widely distributed in fetal tissues, but pathological changes are most obvious in skin, skeleton, and CNS. Affected lambs may be born 2-3 days early, and many die before or at weaning. In survivors, the clinical signs gradually regress, but such animals remain infected and excrete virus for the remainder of their lives, which constitutes a liability to their progeny and flockmates. Death from a syndrome similar to bovine mucosal disease may occur in these "recovered" hairy-shaker sheep at any time.

In flocks in the first season of a new infection, up to 50% or more of lambs born may be affected with BD. Thereafter, prevalence declines, although the disease may become endemic when "recovered" lambs are retained for breeding.

Clinical Findings: Affected flocks probably are recognized first at lambing time by an increase in the number of barren ewes and the birth of undersized lambs with excessively hairy and sometimes excessively pigmented fleece. Some lambs exhibit involuntary muscular tremors, particularly of the trunk and hindlegs. The tremors are reduced at rest and exacerbated by purposive movement. In others, skeletal defects such as dropped pasterns and mandibular brachygnathia may predominate. Affected lambs have a poor survival rate. In survivors, nervous signs gradually disappear within 3-4 mo. Even in the absence of typical hairy-shaker lambs, outbreaks of low fertility in ewes, and poor viability and illthrift in lambs are becoming associated more often with BD virus infection.

Lesions: In severe cases, cavitation of the cerebrum may be seen at necropsy. Otherwise, the characteristic lesions are microscopic and involve the white matter of the CNS. There is a deficiency of myelin and an increase in intrafascicular glial cells, in which myelin-like lipid droplets may accumulate. These changes are most obvious in the newborn and gradually resolve.

Diagnosis: Clinical findings usually allow a diagnosis, although in rough-coated breeds of sheep, abnormal hairiness of the birth coat may not be apparent. The diagnosis must be confirmed by histological demonstration of the pathognomonic lesions in the CNS. In typical hairy-shaker lambs, the virus may be recovered readily in tissue culture from blood clots and tissues. Precolostral serum does not contain virus-neutralizing antibody, but maternal serum contains such antibody at high titer, unless the dam is a persistently infected survivor of an early fetal infection. Antigenic differences between strains of pestivirus may cause difficulties in serodiagnosis.

Other causes of ovine abortion, eg, *Chlamydia* sp, *Salmonella* spp, *Campylobacter* spp, *Toxoplasma gondii*, and *Rickettsia* spp, should be considered in the differential diagnosis. In the live-born lamb, BD must be differentiated from swayback (enzootic ataxia), bacterial meningoencephalitis, focal symmetrical encephalomalacia, and "daft lamb" disease.

Control: There is no effective treatment. Serology should be done on the dams of affected lambs. Most should have high levels of antibody and be immune to further challenge with the same strain of virus in subsequent pregnancies. Any that do not have antibody titers may be persistent excretors of virus and should be culled. Recovered animals should not be retained for breeding, but should be mixed with replacement stock well before breeding season to maximize opportunities for the latter to become infected and develop immunity before subsequent matings.

ERYSIPELAS

Erysipelothrix rhusiopathiae (insidiosa) has a widespread distribution and is capable of living in water, soil, decaying organic matter, slime on the bodies of fish, and in carcasses, even after processing. The bacterium has a variable survival time in soil, but not usually >35 days; however, carrier pigs (or other hosts) may cause recontamination. It causes swine erysipelas in its various forms; nonsuppurative arthritis in lambs and less frequently in calves and kids; post-dipping lameness in sheep; uncommonly, joint-ill in goats (qv, p 505); and acute septicemia in turkeys, ducks, and occasionally, geese and other birds (*see* p 1571). In man, the infection is usually localized and is termed erysipeloid. (It should not be confused with erysipelas in man, a superficial cellulitis caused by group A β-hemolytic streptococci.)

In acute disease, *E rhusiopathiae* usually occurs as a slender, gram-positive rod, ~1-2 μm long. In chronic lesions and old cultures, it often appears as a mixture of rods and filaments up to 20 μm long. It is resistant to certain commonly used antiseptics, such as formaldehyde, phenol, hydrogen peroxide, and alcohol, but is readily destroyed by caustic soda and hypochlorites. It is very sensitive to penicillin and less so to the tetracyclines. The many strains vary markedly in pathogenicity.

SWINE ERYSIPELAS

An infectious disease mainly of growing pigs, common in many areas of the world. Although acute septicemic swine erysipelas causes death, the greatest economic loss probably occurs from the chronic, nonfatal forms of the disease.

Etiology: On farms where the organism is endemic, pigs are exposed naturally to *E rhusiopathiae* when they are young; their maternal antibodies provide a degree of active immunity without visible disease. The organism is excreted by infected animals and survives for short periods in most soils. Recovered animals and those chronically infected may be carriers of the organism, possibly for life. *Erysipelothrix rhusiopathiae* was thought to cause an allergic reaction in the joints of sensitized pigs that resulted in chronic, sterile lesions similar to those observed in rheumatoid arthritis in man; this belief is now questioned.

Clinical Findings: Acute septicemia, the skin (subacute) form, chronic arthritis, and vegetative endocarditis may occur in sequence, or separately. Pigs with acute septicemia may die suddenly without previous signs. This occurs most frequently in finishing pigs (100-200 lb [45-90 kg]). Acutely infected animals are febrile (104-108°F [40-42°C]), walk stiffly on their toes, and lie on their sternums separately rather than piling in groups. They squeal plaintively when handled and may shift weight from foot to foot when standing. Skin discoloration may vary from widespread erythema and purplish discoloration of the ears, snout, and abdomen, to diamond-shaped skin lesions almost anywhere on the body, but particularly the lateral and dorsal parts. The lesions may occur as pink or light-purple areas of varying size that become raised and firm to the touch within 2-3 days of illness. They may disappear or progress to a more chronic type of lesion such as diamond-skin disease. If untreated, necrosis and separation of large areas of skin can occur, but more commonly, the tips of the ears and tail may become necrotic and slough.

Clinical disease is usually sporadic, and affects individuals or small groups, but sometimes larger outbreaks occur. Mortality is 0-100%, and death may occur up to 6 days after the first signs of illness. Acutely affected pregnant sows may abort, probably due to the fever, and suckling sows may show agalactia. Untreated animals may develop chronic arthritis or vegetative valvular endocarditis; such lesions may also occur in pigs with no previous signs of septicemia. Valvular endocarditis is most common in mature or young adult pigs and is frequently manifest by sudden death, usually from embolism. Chronic arthritis, the most common form of chronic infection, produces mild to severe lameness; the affected joints may be difficult to detect, but tend to become visibly enlarged and firm. Mortality in chronic cases is low, but growth rate is retarded.

Lesions: In acute infection, in addition to skin lesions, lymph nodes are usually enlarged and congested, the spleen swollen, and the lungs edematous and congested. Petechiae may be found in the kidneys, heart, and occasionally elsewhere.

In cases of valvular endocarditis, embolisms and infarctions may occur. Arthritis may involve joints of one or more legs, or the intervertebral articulations; the joint enlargement is proliferative but nonsuppurative, and tags of granulation tissue form in the articular cavity. In chronic cases, there may be erosion of the articular cartilage, and ankylosis may result.

Diagnosis: Acute erysipelas is difficult to diagnose in pigs showing only fever, poor appetite, and listlessness; however, since erysipelas responds extremely well to penicillin, a marked improvement within 24 hr supports the diagnosis. The typical diamond-shaped skin lesions are diagnostic. Arthritis and endocarditis are difficult to diagnose in the live animal since other agents can cause similar syndromes (*see* LAMENESS IN PIGS, p 532). At necropsy, demonstration of the organism in stained smears or cultures confirms the diagnosis, although in chronic arthritis cases, organisms may not be cultured. The organism can be isolated readily on blood agar plates from spleen, kidney, and long bones of acutely sick pigs (and from the tonsils and other lymph nodes of many apparently normal ones). Serology can prove unreliable, although a rising titer in an agglutination test (with controls) is helpful, as is the complement fixation test.

Prophylaxis and Treatment: Killed bacterins or, in some countries, live-culture immunizing strains of low virulence for pigs are used. The formalin-killed, aluminum-hydroxide-adsorbed bacterin confers an immunity that, in most instances, protects the growing pig from acute disease until it reaches market age. An oral vaccine of low virulence is also used. Young breeding stock, including boars, should be vaccinated twice at the recommended interval, and then revaccinated q6mo or after each litter. Vaccination of heavily pregnant animals is not advisable.

Vaccination raises the level of immunity, but does not provide complete protection. Acute cases may occur following stress, and protection may not be provided against the arthritic or cardiac forms of the disease. Antigenic variation occurs between bacterial strains, so a vaccine may not be equally effective against all wild strains.

If acute cases suddenly occur in an unvaccinated herd, antiserum, if available, may be administered to in-contact pigs, or they may be given penicillin or tetracyclines. Penicillin is the drug of choice in acutely affected pigs, and has been used concurrently with antiserum. Treatment of chronic infection is ineffective, and such animals should be culled.

Elimination of carriers, good sanitation, and a regular vaccination program should be effective, even in herds that have had recurring and serious problems.

NONSUPPURATIVE POLYARTHRITIS IN LAMBS

An acute or, more commonly, chronic arthritis of one or more of the joints, usually of the limbs. Calves and kids also are affected sometimes.

Etiology: The infective agent, *Erysipelothrix rhusiopathiae*, usually enters the body through wounds in young lambs, sometimes through the navel but more commonly after docking and castration. After a transient septicemia, the organism localizes in joints, without leaving evidence of infection at the site of entry. Poor condition of the lambs at the time of surgery, or adverse weather afterwards, may predispose to a high infection rate.

Clinical Findings: In the acute form, the characteristic lesion is a nonsuppurative arthritis manifest by heat and pain, but only slight swelling of the joint tissues. The joints most commonly involved are the hock, stifle, elbow, and knee. Affected lambs are reluctant to move, and growth is often severely depressed, but complete recovery may occur in 2-3 wk. In ~10-15% of cases, however, the infection persists, and chronic arthritis with permanent enlargement of the joint develops. Mortality is usually low, but some lambs die from acute septicemia or complications arising from recumbency.

In outbreaks following docking and castration, the incubation period is remarkably constant; the first cases appear 9-19 days after the operation, and practically all subsequent cases develop within 5 days. The incidence may reach 50%, but in most outbreaks it is <10%.

In the chronic form, signs usually are not observed until lambs are 2-6 mo of age. Typically, several joints are affected, and cause the lambs to have a stiff gait.

Diagnosis: In outbreaks following docking and castration, a presumptive diagnosis can be made from the history and clinical signs. In sporadic cases, isolation and identification of the organism from affected joints should be attempted. The disease must be distinguished from polyarthritis due to other bacteria (eg, streptococcal joint-ill), white muscle disease, and other causes of lameness.

Prophylaxis and Treatment: The adoption of strict antiseptic techniques and the maintenance of hygienic conditions for docking and castration are recommended, but cannot be relied on for prevention. The so-called "bloodless" methods of performing both operations may reduce the chances of wound contamination, but outbreaks are known to follow all of the common methods. Vaccination should be considered where the disease is a recurring problem. Penicillin given early in acute disease is the best therapy, but is of no value in the chronic form.

POST-DIPPING LAMENESS IN SHEEP

A cellulitis and laminitis arising from an extension of a focal cutaneous infection, caused by the penetration of *Erysipelothrix rhusiopathiae* through small skin abrasions in the region of the hoof. The condition, which normally occurs in outbreaks, has been described in most large sheep-raising countries.

Etiology: With time and repeated use, dipping solutions or suspensions of insecticidal agents, which have little or no bacteriostatic activity, become heavily charged with various species of bacteria. *Erysipelothrix rhusiopathiae* is a common contaminant, and its presence in the vat, sometimes in enormous numbers, leads to infection of skin wounds during dipping. Small skin abrasions in the region of the hoof and fetlock joint are a common portal of entry. Lesions extending from these leg wounds to the laminae of the hoof cause the acute post-dipping lameness. Outbreaks may also occur when sheep must walk through muddy areas heavily contaminated with the organism.

Clinical Findings: Two to 4 days after dipping, a variable number (up to 90%) of sheep in the flock may be lame in one or more legs. Affected legs appear normal except for the hoof and pastern regions, which are hot and painful. Later, there is a variable degree of hair loss, sometimes extending as far as the carpus or tarsus. Most sheep recover spontaneously in 2-4 wk with nothing more serious than a slight loss of body weight. In some outbreaks, however, mortality may reach 5% and, in young sheep particularly, much body condition may be lost. Acute and chronic arthritis are rare sequelae.

Prophylaxis and Treatment: The addition of copper sulfate to the dip (0.04%) should provide effective control, although dips heavily contaminated with organic matter are best discarded. Penicillin is the antibiotic of choice, and early treatment should speed recovery.

FOOT-AND-MOUTH DISEASE (FMD)

An acute, highly contagious, viral infection of domestic and wild cloven-hooved animals. Morbidity and mortality are highest in the young. Initially, it is characterized by vesicular lesions; subsequently, by erosions of the epithelium of the mouth, nares, muzzle, feet, teats, udder, and rumen pillars. The natural hosts are cattle, pigs, sheep, goats, water buffalo, bison, deer, antelope, wild pigs, reindeer, llamas, chamois, alpacas, vicunas, giraffes, elephants, elk, camels, capybaras, moles, voles, rats, and hedgehogs. Experimentally, FMD virus (FMDV) may be transmitted to mice, guinea pigs, rabbits, hamsters, embryonating chicken eggs, chickens, chinchillas, muskrats, grizzly bears, armadillos, and peccaries. Horses are resistant. The virus will replicate when inoculated into monkeys, turtles, frogs, and snakes, but these species do not normally develop lesions.

FMD is endemic in Asia, Africa, parts of Europe, and most of South America. North and Central America, the Caribbean, Australia, New Zealand, and many of the islands of Oceania are free of FMD. Great Britain and many other western European countries, such as Denmark, Norway, and Sweden, are free most of the time. Ireland has been free since 1941, and it has not occurred in Japan for decades.

Etiology: FMD is caused by an enterovirus of the family Picornaviridae. At least 7 immunologically distinct types of FMDV have been identified by complement fixation as A; O; C; South African Territories (SAT) 1, 2, 3; and Asia 1. Within the 7 types, >60 subtypes were identified before the World Reference Laboratory (Pirbright, England) stopped classifying on a sequential basis. Since ~1980, new subtypes have been identified on a geographic basis. Many of the subtypes are sufficiently different antigenically to warrant preparation of subtype vaccines. The virus is inactivated rapidly by low or high pH, sunlight (although it may survive for long periods in tissue fragments), and high temperatures. The virus lacks a lipid-containing envelope, and therefore is resistant to ether and chloroform. The most commonly used disinfectants are sodium hydroxide, sodium carbonate, and acetic acid.

Transmission and Epidemiology: Most transmission is via aerosols, usually when animals are in close proximity, although there is increasing evidence that, under certain conditions, the virus may be spread by the wind for up to 30 mi (50 km). It has been demonstrated that when man inhales the respiratory aerosols of FMD-infected animals, the virus may persist in the respiratory tract for as long as 24 hr. During this time, it is possible to transmit the virus to other people and animals via the respiratory route. (There are cases of FMD in man on record; however, it is not a public health problem.)

Esophageal fluids from FMD-infected animals may contain virus before signs and lesions appear—and after lesions disappear. Cattle may retain the virus in tonsillar cells for as long as 3 yr after recovery. There is circumstantial evidence that such carrier animals may transmit the infection when introduced into a FMD-free herd, but this has never been demonstrated experimentally.

FMDV may be found in large quantities in the milk of infected animals. Pasteurization temperatures do not destroy the virus in such samples because the virus is afforded protection by cell debris, fat, and other components of milk. Vestigial virus also survives processing of casein, caseinate, and some cheeses, but in the case of casein and cheese, there is virus decay after relatively short periods of storage. Experimentally, FMDV may be transmitted by artificial insemination. Meat scraps and bones from infected animals often have been the source of infection in pigs, which can then readily transmit the infection to cattle and other animals. Several outbreaks in the USA were traced to pigs that had been fed uncooked garbage from ships that had taken on provisions in countries where FMD existed. Outbreaks have also been traced to the use of contaminated biological products, such as vaccinia and hog cholera vaccines and pituitary extract. Since the virus is present in much of the skin, salting, drying, or surface disinfection of hides from infected animals does not preclude virus survival. Outside the animal body, variable conditions affect its viability.

Pigs tend to excrete more virus than do cattle or sheep. The clinical manifestations vary with the strains of virus. The disease may be difficult to detect in sheep, but they can readily transmit the virus to other species.

Pathogenesis: The usual primary site of infection and initial replication is in the cells of the mucous membrane of the throat. From there, the virus spreads to adjacent cells, enters the circulatory system, and then infects other susceptible cells and organs throughout the animal. After 24-48 hr the animal develops a fever, and vesicles appear in the buccal cavity, between the claws, and elsewhere. The vesicles rupture within another 48 hr, often leaving a raw, denuded area. At the end of viremia, the fever subsides and healing begins with gradual disappearance of lesions and virus except from the tissues of the throat where, in cattle, sheep, goats, and other ruminants, the virus may persist for as long as 3 yr.

Clinical Findings: Initially, animals may show dullness, inappetence, fever, and shivering followed by smacking of the lips, drooling, and shaking or kicking of the feet. The characteristic signs of FMD are drooling, and vesicles on the nares, in the buccal cavity, and between the claws; however, these same signs may be seen in other vesicular diseases. After vesicle formation, there is pronounced salivation and lameness. Pregnant animals may abort and young animals may die, especially piglets nursing an infected sow. Lesions in sheep and goats are the same as those in cattle but are less pronounced. Secondary lesions, especially on the feet, may be caused by bacteria.

Chronic secondary lesions of oral, nasal, or pedal lesions may develop. Hoof deformation may result in permanent lameness. Mammary gland involvement may result in mastitis and permanent impairment of milk production. Prolonged unthriftiness and failure to gain weight is common.

Lesions: Vesicles or blisters may be found on the tongue, dental pad, gums, cheek, hard and soft palate, lips, nostrils, muzzle, coronary bands, teats, and udder, as well as on the snout of pigs, corium of dewclaws, and interdigital spaces. Lesions may be found on all feet, but sometimes only 1 or 2 are involved. In sheep, the dental pad is the most common site for lesions. At necropsy, lesions may be seen on the rumen pillars, in the myocardium, and in skeletal muscles. Type C virus seems to have a predilection for heart muscle.

Diagnosis: In cattle, sheep, goats, and pigs, the clinical signs of FMD are indistinguishable from those of vesicular stomatitis (qv, p 372). The same is true of vesicular exanthema (qv, p 388) and vesicular disease (qv, p 386) in pigs, and with the diseases caused by caliciviruses of marine mammals (qv, p 1045). Differential diagnosis by one of several laboratory methods including complement fixation, virus neutralization, agar-gel precipitation, and ELISA is essential. The measurement of physical and chemical properties and ribonuclease T-1 "fingerprinting" are used increasingly to track the movement of virus strains. DNA probes, labelled with avidin-biotin, have recently been developed and may be useful for detecting virus in products from infected animals.

Treatment and Control: There is no known cure, and while treatment may alleviate signs, it does not prevent spread of the infection. The most effective preventive measure is to prohibit introduction of animals or animal products into FMD-free countries from countries that have the disease, except when it is known that product processing has destroyed the virus.

Individual countries have different policies for the control of FMD. Because of the ability of the virus to spread, control is best approached on a regional, national, and continental basis. In FMD-free areas, rapid diagnosis is essential, followed by quarantine of the premises (including movement of persons and vehicles), followed by slaughter and disposal of the carcasses by burning or burial, and decontamination of the premises. After 30 days, the premises are restocked with susceptible sentinel animals that are carefully monitored for 30 days before the owner is permitted to restock.

In countries where the disease is endemic, slaughter of infected animals is not always possible for economic or social reasons. In these instances, vaccines are administered. In some countries, cattle are vaccinated 1-3 times/yr. In many western European countries, annual vaccination of cattle has been vigorously applied for >30 yr and, when outbreaks occur, the same eradication procedures utilized as in FMD-free countries. Whenever an outbreak occurs in a country where vaccines are used, the virus from the outbreak must be isolated and typed to determine whether the vaccine that is being used contains antigen that is homologous to that of the field virus. In other countries where the vaccines are not applied as routinely, eg, in South America, infected animals are usually quarantined until they have recovered and the entire herd has been revaccinated.

In Europe, outbreaks have been traced to improperly prepared vaccines or escape of the virus from the site of vaccine production. If it is possible to develop subunit vaccines they will be much safer; such products have been developed experimentally against several types and subtypes of the virus.

FUNGAL INFECTIONS
(Mycoses)

Most agents of systemic mycoses exist as saprophytes in soil, decaying vegetation and dung, and on keratinized animal tissues. The soil reservoir is the primary source of most infections, which can be acquired by inhalation, ingestion, or traumatic introduction of fungal elements. (*See also* DERMATOPHYTOSIS, p 789.)

Pathogenic fungi establish infection in apparently normal hosts, and such diseases as histoplasmosis, coccidioidomycosis, and blastomycosis are regarded as primary systemic mycoses. Opportunistic fungi usually require a host that is debilitated (eg, by such stresses as captivity, metabolic acidosis, malnutrition, or neoplasia) to establish infection. Prolonged exposure to antimicrobials or immunosuppressive substances appears to increase the likelihood of infection by the opportunistic fungi that cause diseases such as aspergillosis, mucormycosis, cryptococcosis, and candidosis, which may be focal or systemic. Cryptococcosis has been recorded in apparently normal animals; in these cases, it is possible that some subtle host defect (possibly in cell-mediated immunity) was overlooked.

Clinical findings and gross lesions are not definitively diagnostic of systemic mycoses; microscopical or cultural studies, or both, are required. Identification of the fungus and the tissue reaction via microscopical examination of exudates and biopsy material is adequate for diagnosis of histoplasmosis, cryptococcosis, blastomycosis, coccidioidomycosis, and rhinosporidiosis. Other diseases, such as candidosis, aspergillosis, and mucormycosis, require both cultural isolation and microscopical evaluation for a definitive diagnosis. These fungi are also common contaminants of cultures; thus, tissue invasion and reaction must be demonstrated to make the cultural isolation significant. Serology and skin testing with specific antigens may be useful for diagnosis (and prognosis) of some mycotic diseases such as histoplasmosis and coccidioidomycosis.

No available chemotherapeutic agent consistently gives satisfactory results against systemic mycoses. Amphotericin B is used most frequently, but it is nephrotoxic; cats are less tolerant than dogs. Miconazole, ketoconazole, and flucytosine (5-fluorocytosine) also are used. The latter is used infrequently as a single agent, but it is thought to be synergistic in combination with amphotericin B against some fungal infections.

ASPERGILLOSIS

A disease induced by a number of *Aspergillus* spp, especially *A fumigatus*. It is found worldwide and in almost all domestic animals and birds as well as many wild species. It is primarily a respiratory infection that may become generalized; however, tissue predilection varies among animal species. The most common forms are pulmonary infections in poultry and other birds, mycotic abortion in cattle, guttural pouch mycosis in horses, and infections of the nasal and paranasal tissues of dogs. Pulmonary and intestinal forms have been described in domestic cats, with most of the intestinal cases associated with feline infectious enteritis.

Clinical Findings and Lesions: In birds, aspergillosis (qv, p 1613) is primarily bronchopulmonary, with dyspnea, gasping, and polypnea accompanied by somnolence, anorexia, and emaciation. Torticollis and disturbances of equilibrium are observed when infection disseminates to the brain. Yellow nodules of varying size and consistency or plaque lesions occur in the respiratory passages, lungs, air sacs, or membranes of body cavities. Fur-like growth of fungus may be found on the thickened walls of air sacs. Other species with bronchopulmonary aspergillosis may have nodular lesions in the lungs, or an acute pneumonia accompanied by serosanguineous fluid in the pleural cavity and a fibrinous pleuritis.

In ruminants, aspergillosis may be asymptomatic, occur in a bronchopulmonary form, or cause placentitis and abortion. Mycotic pneumonia may be rapidly fatal. Signs include pyrexia; rapid, shallow, stertorous respiration; nasal discharge; and a moist cough. The lungs are firm, heavy, and mottled, and do not collapse. In subacute to chronic mycotic pneumonia, the lungs contain multiple discrete granulomas and the disease grossly resembles tuberculosis.

In the absence of pneumonia, infected cows generally have no signs except for abortion; a dead fetus is aborted between months 6 and 9, and the fetal membranes are retained. Lesions are found in the uterus, fetal membranes, and often the fetal skin. In the uterus, the intercaruncular areas are grossly thickened, leathery, dark red to tan, and contain elevated or eroded foci covered by a yellow-gray adherent pseudomembrane. Maternal caruncles are dark red to brown, and the adherent fetal cotyledons are markedly thickened. Cutaneous lesions in aborted fetuses consist of soft, red to gray, elevated, discrete foci that resemble ringworm.

In horses, epistaxis and dysphagia are common complications of gutturomycosis (*see also* p 739). It is characterized by a necrotizing inflammation of the guttural pouch, which is thickened, hemorrhagic, and covered by a friable pseudomembrane. Locomotor and visual disturbances, including blindness, may occur when the infection spreads to the brain and optic nerve.

In dogs, aspergillosis is generally caused by *A fumigatus*; it affects the nasal chambers and paranasal sinuses, but lesions may occur in several organs, including the eye. It occurs mainly in dolichocephalic breeds, and commences in the posterior region of the ventral maxilloturbinate with signs of lethargy, sneezing, uni- or bilateral sero- to mucopurulent nasal discharge, and frequently, epistaxis. Dogs with ocular aspergillosis have funduscopic findings consistent with endophthalmitis. Gross lesions vary considerably with site of infection, but the mucosa of the nasal and paranasal sinuses may be covered by a layer of gray-black necrotic material and fungal growth. The mucosa and the underlying bone may be necrotic with loss of bone definition on radiographs.

Disseminated disease in dogs, without apparent respiratory tract involvement, is increasingly reported. Most cases have been in German Shepherd Dogs and have involved unusual aspergilli (eg, *A terreus* and *A deflectus*).

Diagnosis: Since aspergilli are ubiquitous and often isolated from nonaspergillic lesions, diagnosis by culture is difficult; positive results should be supported by demonstration of narrow, hyaline, septate, branching hyphae within lesions. The agar-gel double-diffusion test for serum antibody is a reliable technique for diagnosis; improved sensitivity may be possible with techniques such as ELISA. Immunofluorescent procedures can be used to identify hyphae in tissue sections.

Treatment: Several surgical techniques and drug regimens have been used with varying success. Surgical exposure and curettage have been used in canine nasal aspergillosis and equine gutturomycosis. Drugs used have included thiabendazole, flucytosine, and amphotericin B.

CANDIDOSIS

A localized mucocutaneous disease distributed worldwide in a variety of animals, caused by species of the yeast-like fungus, *Candida* spp, most commonly *C albicans*. The fungus is a common inhabitant of the oral mucosa and is part of the flora of the GI tract. The organism most frequently infects birds (qv, p 1562), in which it involves the oral mucosa, esophagus, and crop. Infections are rare in dogs, cats, and horses. However, *Candida* spp have been considered a cause of bovine mastitis and abortion, and oral, GI, cutaneous, and vaginal infections are described in most domestic animals and in nonhuman primates. Dissemination may occur to other organs. Infections are more common in young animals, and often follow some predisposing cause or debilitating factor such as malnutrition, or extended immunosuppressive or antibacterial therapy.

Clinical Findings and Lesions: Signs are variable and nonspecific and may be associated more with the primary or predisposing conditions than with the candidosis itself. Calves with forestomach candidosis have watery diarrhea, anorexia, and dehydration, with gradual progression to prostration and death. Affected chicks are listless and have reduced feed intake and growth rate. Porcine candidosis affects the oral, esophageal, and gastric mucosa, with diarrhea and emaciation the most consistent signs.

Gross lesions of the skin and mucosae are generally single or multiple, raised, circular, white masses covered with scabs. The organism can penetrate keratinized epithelium and cause marked keratinous thickening of the mucosae of the tongue, esophagus, and rumen. In birds, the crop and esophageal lesions are white, circular ulcers with raised surface scabs that produce thickening of the mucosa; an easily removed pseudomembrane is common.

Diagnosis: Fungal organisms are numerous in proliferating epithelial tissue, and diagnosis can be made by examination of scrapings or biopsy specimens from mucocutaneous lesions. *Candida albicans* are ovoid, budding, yeast cells (2-4 μm in diameter) with thin walls, or occur in chains that produce pseudohyphae when the blastospores remain attached after budding division. Filamentous, regular, true hyphae also may be visible. The fungal cells generally are limited to epithelial tissue and rarely extend deeper.

Treatment: Nystatin ointment or topical application of amphotericin B or 1% iodine solution may be useful in the treatment of oral or cutaneous candidosis. Some imidazoles (eg, miconazole, ketoconazole) may be superior to nystatin.

CHROMOMYCOSIS

A chronic, cutaneous, or subcut. infection caused by one of several genera and species of brown or black fungi of the family Dematiaceae. The infections may be grouped into clinicopathological syndromes: superficial chromomycosis, chromoblastomycosis, and chromohyphomycosis (phaeohyphomycosis). Superficial chromomycosis, infection of the stratum corneum by pigmented fungi, has not been described in domestic animals. Chromoblastomycosis is characterized by the presence of spherical septate forms of the fungus (muriform cells) in the dermis. In chromohyphomycosis, the pigmented fungal forms are hyphal without obvious muriform cells. Dematiaceous fungi have also been associated with mycetomas (*see* p 348).

Fungi of chromomycosis are saprophytic, widely distributed organisms found in soil, water, and decaying vegetable matter. Infection may result from fungal implantation into tissue at the site of an injury. The list of recorded pathogens is increasing rapidly; taxonomic aspects of the causal fungi are in a constant state of flux.

Clinical Findings and Lesions: Chromohyphomycosis has been described in cows, cats, horses, and dogs from which such fungi as *Bipolaris spicifera* (*Drechslera spiciferum*), *Exophiala jeanselmi*, and *Phialophora verrucosa* have been isolated. Slowly enlarging, subcut. masses are found about the head, nasal mucosa, limbs, and chest. The nodules may ulcerate and have draining fistulous tracts. These pyogranulomas contain pigmented, septate hyphae with irregular enlargements and thin-walled, budding yeast-like forms and, with some fungi, chlamydospores. *Xylophypha bantiana* (*Cladosporium trichoides*) has been isolated from more deepseated lesions (CNS, kidney) in cats and a dog.

Chromomycosis involving both cutaneous and deeper tissue has also been described in frogs, tortoises, lobsters, and several species of fish—more common causal fungi are *Cladosporium* spp, *Exophiala* spp (eg, *E pisciphila* and *E salmonis*), *Phoma herbarum*, and *Scolecobasidium humicola* (possibly a *Dactylaria* sp). CNS disease in various avian species has been attributed to *Dactylaria constricta* (*gallopava*).

Diagnosis: The clinical features of chromomycosis are such that the differential diagnosis should include neoplasia, other granulomas, and epidermoid cysts. In histological sections, it has been confused with eumycotic mycetomas caused by dematiaceous fungi. In chromoblastomycosis, clusters of muriform cells are seen both within giant cells and extracellularly. Chromohyphomycosis can be diagnosed by microscopical examination of exudate and biopsy specimens, which reveals pigmented or hyaline filamentous hyphae (2-6 μm in diameter) with terminal and intercalated vesicles (chlamydoconidia [6-12 μm]), and spores. The several causative fungi cannot be identified by their histological features in tissues; cultural isolation is required. Organisms can be identified in tissue sections stained with fluorescein-isothiocyanate-conjugated immunoglobulins specific for the particular fungal agent.

Treatment: In most cases, the infection is confined to the skin and subcut. tissues. In a favorable location, cure may be effected by wide excision of the lesion. Combination chemotherapy with local administration of amphotericin B and systemic use of fluorocytosine may be considered for treatment. In the laboratory, many agents of chromomycosis appear resistant to amphotericin B; ketoconazole, which has been used with benefit in man, may be of value in such cases.

COCCIDIOIDOMYCOSIS

A dust-borne, noncontagious infection caused by the dimorphic fungus *Coccidioides immitis*. Infections are limited to arid regions of southwestern USA and to similar areas of Mexico and Central and South America. While many species of animals, including man, are susceptible, only dogs are affected significantly. Ruminants and pigs may have subclinical infections with lesions restricted to foci in the lungs and lymph nodes of the thorax. Inhalation of fungal spores is the only established mode of infection, and spores may be carried on dust particles. Most bovine infections are contracted in dusty feedlots.

Clinical Findings and Lesions: The disease varies from inapparent or benign (cattle, sheep, pigs, dogs, cats) to progressive, disseminated, and fatal (dogs, nonhuman primates, rarely cats and man). Coccidioidomycosis is primarily a chronic respiratory disease, but canine infections disseminate to many tissues, including the eye and bone. Thus, clinical signs can vary greatly, depending on organ involvement and severity of infection. Dogs with disseminated disease may have chronic cough, anorexia, cachexia, lameness, enlarged joints, fever, and intermittent diarrhea. Dissemination to the skin with draining ulceration may occur, but primary infection through the skin is rare.

Gross lesions may be limited to the lungs, mediastinum, and lymph nodes of the thorax, or be disseminated to various organs. Lesions are discrete, variable-sized nodules with a firm, gray-white cut surface, and resemble those of tuberculosis. The nodules are pyogranulomas composed of epithelioid and giant cells, and the center of some foci may contain purulent exudate and fungal organisms. Some lesions may have mineralized foci.

Diagnosis: In endemic areas, coccidioidomycosis should be considered in dogs with chronic bronchopulmonary disease, and when pulmonary nodules and enlarged lymph nodes are found on thoracic radiographs. The lesions are pyogranulomas that contain *C immitis* free in the exudate, and in epithelioid and multinucleate giant cells. The organisms vary in size and appear as relatively large (20-80 μm, up to 200 μm) spherules with a double-contoured wall. The mature spherules (sporangia) contain endospores (sporangiospores) 2-5 μm in diameter. Diagnosis is established by demonstrating the spherules in tissues. A positive coccidioidin skin test (swelling with edema or induration present at the test site 48 hr after injection) indicates exposure. For the test, 0.1 mL of undiluted coccidioidin is injected intradermally into the lower edge of the skin of the flank. Attempts to culture the fungus should be restricted to those laboratories equipped to handle such dangerously infective cultures.

Treatment: Amphotericin B is the drug of choice. Ketoconazole has been used in man and may be of value in other species.

CRYPTOCOCCOSIS

A systemic fungal disease that may affect the lungs, CNS, and skin, particularly of the face and neck of cats and dogs. The causal fungus, *Cryptococcus neoformans* (teleomorph: *Filobasidiella neoformans*), exists in the environment and in tissues in a yeast form. Although infection occurs worldwide, there are no known endemic areas, veterinary or human. The fungus is found in the soil and fowl manure, especially in pigeon droppings. Transmission is by inhalation of spores or contamination of wounds. In avian droppings, it may occur in a noncapsulated form as small as 1 μm, which can be inhaled into the deeper portions of the lungs. Cryptococcosis is most common in dogs and cats but also occurs in cattle, horses, sheep, goats, birds, and wild animals. In man, many cases are associated with a defective cell-mediated immune response; probably the same is true in lower animals.

Clinical Findings and Lesions: Infection often becomes disseminated, and the variable and nonspecific signs depend on organ involvement. Lesions are common in the lungs, CNS, and facial regions, especially the oral and nasal mucosa, but also may occur in the pharyngeal mucosa and cranial sinuses. These lesions are accompanied by a cough, sneezing, nasal and ocular discharges, and the presence of expanding masses. With infection of the CNS, signs include ataxia, changes in behavior, circling, locomotor dysfunction, and blindness, the latter due to lesions in the brain or globes, or both. Cutaneous lesions are nodular, usually ulcerated, and accompanied by soft-tissue swelling. Bovine cryptococcosis has been found only in cases of mastitis, and many cows in a herd may be infected. Affected cows have anorexia, decreased milk flow, swelling and firmness of affected quarters, and enlarged supramammary lymph nodes. The milk becomes viscid, mucoid, and gray-white, or may be watery with flakes. The disease in horses almost invariably is a respiratory ailment with obstructive growths in the nasal cavities.

The lesions in the skin, lungs, and CNS usually are grossly slimy, lytic, and cystic, and numerous cryptococcal blastospores are seen microscopically. Severely affected meninges appear thickened. Often, there is little tissue response with few to moderate numbers of mononuclear WBC, but some lesions are granulomas. In tissue, especially the brain and meninges, the fungus multiplies to form cysts occupied by fungal cells and their mucoid capsules.

Diagnosis: Cryptococcosis should be considered in dogs and cats with respiratory and CNS disease, especially when cutaneous ulcerations and nodular swellings are present. The slimy, mucoid, and lytic nature of the lesions is highly suggestive; diagnosis can be confirmed by microscopical examination of tissues, body fluids, and CSF. The organisms are pale, round to oval, 5-20 μm in diameter with buds, a thin wall, and a wide mucin-rich capsule that is unstained in H&E sections. The organisms may be present in tissues as elongated pseudohyphae as well. In India-ink preparations the wide, mucinous capsule appears as a clear, unstained sphere on a black background. The encapsulated yeast can be identified by FA reagent specific for *C neoformans*.

Treatment: Treatment is of little value in disseminated infections, especially those with bronchopulmonary and meningeal and cerebral involvement. Focal cutaneous lesions without dissemination may be removed surgically. Amphotericin B and 5-fluorocytosine may be used in combination in dogs or cats. Treatment of feline cryptococcosis confined to the nasal passages and skin with oral flucytosine or prolonged high doses of ketoconazole has been successful.

ENTOMOPHTHOROMYCOSIS
(Basidiobolomycosis, Conidiobolomycosis)

This is primarily an infection of the nasal mucosa and subcut. tissue of horses and rarely other animals by *Conidiobolus coronatus (Entomophthora coronata)* or *Basidiobolus ranarum (haptosporus)*. These ubiquitous fungi are present in soil and decaying vegetation and, in the case of basidioboli, the GI tracts of amphibians, reptiles, and macropods. *Conidiobolus coronatus* is an important insect pathogen. Infection has been described in which ulcerative granulomatous lesions contained cores of necrotic tissue (kunkers).

Clinical Findings and Lesions: Ulcerative granulomas of the mucous membrane of the nostril or mouth, or nodular growths of the nasal mucosa and the lips caused by *C coronatus* may cause mechanical blockage, resulting in dyspnea and nasal discharge. Lesions caused by *B ranarum* are large, usually single, circular, ulcerative, and pruritic nodules of the skin of the upper body. Fistulous tracts discharge a serosanguineous fluid from the lesions, which frequently are traumatized. Extension to regional lymph nodes results in swelling of the nodes and development of yellow necrotic foci. Lesions may contain a creamy, yellow, central core of necrotic tissue. Disseminated basidiobolomycosis is rare, but has been described in dogs and a mandrill.

In excised tissues or necropsy specimens, a thickened fibrotic dermis has scattered, red or creamy white areas. The lesions, which contain hyphal forms, a heavy infiltrate of eosinophils, and sequestered areas of necrosis, have histologic features of infectious granulomas.

Diagnosis: Clinically, entomophthoromycosis may be confused with cutaneous habronemiasis (qv, p 806) and oomycosis (qv, p 349), but can be differentiated by microscopical examination of tissues. In H&E sections, the fungus appears as holes and elongated channels, and many hyphae have an eosinophilic cuff; in sections stained for fungi, the organism consists of large, branching, sometimes septate, 4-8 μm hyphae. Cultural examination is required to identify the causative fungus. Entomophthoromycosis is differentiated from oomycosis by differences in anatomic distribution, and by the slow growth of the lesion, shallower penetration, and the smaller number and size of the necrotic foci in the former.

Treatment: Surgical excision, immunotherapy, or both, have been successful. The immunotherapy consisted of intradermal injections of 0.02-0.1 mL particulate fungal material. Localized mycotic disease has been treated with amphotericin B given systemically or locally, or both. Ideally, treatment includes early surgical removal of the lesion followed by administration of amphotericin B. Ketoconazole has been active *in vitro* against the causative fungi.

EPIZOOTIC LYMPHANGITIS

A chronic granulomatous disease of the skin, lymph vessels, and lymph nodes of the limbs and neck of Equidae, caused by the dimorphic fungus *Histoplasma farciminosum*. The disease occurs in the Orient and Mediterranean areas but is unknown in the USA. The fungus forms mycelia in nature and yeast forms in tissues, and has a saprophytic phase in soil. Infection probably is acquired by wound infection or transmission by blood-sucking insects.

Clinical Findings and Lesions: Clinically, the disease is characterized by freely movable cutaneous nodules. These nodules originate from infected superficial lymph vessels and nodes, and tend to ulcerate and undergo alternating periods of discharge and closure. Affected lymph nodes are enlarged and hard. The skin covering the nodules may become thick, indurated, and fused to the underlying tissues. Lesions also may be present in the lungs, conjunctiva, cornea, nasal mucosa, and other organs. The nodules are pyogranulomas that have a thick fibrous capsule, and contain thick creamy pus and the causative organisms.

Diagnosis: The clinical features are highly suggestive, and diagnosis can be confirmed by microscopical examination of exudates and biopsy specimens. The yeast forms of the organisms distend the cytoplasm of macrophages and appear in H&E sections as 3-4 μm globose or oval bodies with a central basophilic body surrounded by an unstained zone. The organism closely resembles *H capsulatum*.

Treatment: No completely satisfactory treatment is known. Surgical excision of lesions combined with antifungal drugs (amphotericin B) could be used.

GEOTRICHOSIS

A rare mycosis due to infection with *Geotrichum candidum*, a ubiquitous saprophyte in soil and decaying organic matter. The organism has caused systemic disease in dogs, bovine abortion and mastitis, caseous nodules in the lymph nodes of pigs, and has been isolated from feces of animals with enteritis, skin lesions in various animals and birds, and the respiratory system of horses, penguins, chickens, and man.

Clinical Findings and Lesions: Clinical signs vary with organ involvement and may be nonspecific. A dog with disseminated geotrichosis had fever, nonproductive coughing, respiratory distress, anorexia, and vomiting. Radiograhic findings include nodular densities with confluence in some regions of the lungs. Lesions are found in various organs in disseminated geotrichosis, and are multiple, yellow-gray, firm, fleshy nodules, which microscopically are well-defined granulomas.

Diagnosis: Definitive diagnosis is based on cultural and microscopical characteristics. Fungal elements may be abundant, both free and in macrophages and multinucleated giant cells, as ovoid yeast-like cells (3-7 μm in diameter) and as short, jointed chains of round yeast cells forming pseudohyphae. In histologic sections of tissues stained with H&E, *G candidum* resemble *Candida albicans* and *Histoplasma capsulatum*.

Treatment: Nystatin given as an oral suspension was effective in treatment of gorillas with watery diarrhea associated with isolation of *G candidum* from fecal wet mounts.

HISTOPLASMOSIS

A chronic, noncontagious, disseminated, granulomatous disease of man and other animals caused by the dimorphic fungus *Histoplasma capsulatum*. The fungus inhabits the soil, in which it reproduces asexually; it is commonly found in soil that contains bird and bat manure. It produces mycelial growth in the soil and in culture at room temperature; it grows in a yeast form in tissues and in cultures at 37°C.

Histoplasmosis is found throughout the world. Endemic areas in the USA include the Mississippi and Ohio River valleys and the Appalachian Mountain range. Infection has been described in many animal species, but disease is uncommon to rare in all but dogs and cats. Infection is commonly via aerosol contamination of the respiratory tract (rarely orally); and the lungs and lymph nodes of the chest are the sites of primary infection. The organisms enter the bloodstream from a primary focus and become disseminated throughout the body; they may localize in the eye and produce chorioretinitis or endophthalmitis.

Clinical Findings and Lesions: The signs vary and are nonspecific, reflecting the various organ involvement. Many dogs have a protracted course of weight loss to emaciation, chronic cough, persistent diarrhea, fever, anemia, hepatomegaly, splenomegaly, lymphadenopathy, and nasopharyngeal and GI ulceration. Obstructive respiratory difficulty due to tracheobronchial lymphadenopathy also has been found in dogs. Dissemination may involve the skin, in which weeping, ulcerated, nodular lesions develop. Acute histoplasmosis may be fatal after 2-5 wk.

Gross lesions include enlargement of the liver, spleen, and mesenteric lymph nodes; ascites; yellow-white, variable-sized nodules in the lungs; and enlargement of bronchial lymph nodes. The enlarged liver may have multiple, scattered, irregular-shaped, pale yellow foci of granulomatous inflammation. Pale foci may be present in the myocardium, and the small intestine may have thickened, gray walls and ulceration of the mucosa.

Diagnosis: Histoplasmosis and other fungal infections should be considered when the clinical signs include respiratory distress, diarrhea, enlarged bronchial lymph nodes, and pulmonary nodules. Additional diagnostic information may be obtained by injecting 0.1 mL histoplasmin into the skin of the lower edge of the flank. An area of edema or induration (≥ 5 μm) at the test site at 48 hr is considered a positive reaction. Diagnosis may be confirmed by microscopical examination of fluids or exudates from cutaneous lesions and of biopsy specimens. Yeast forms in macrophages and giant cells are round to ovoid (1-4 μm) structures with a pink (H&E),

thin cell wall and a thin, clear zone between the cell wall and cellular cytoplasm. Organisms are readily visualized by stains for glycogen.

Treatment: Treatment can be symptomatic or more specific, using amphotericin B or ketoconazole. Acute and disseminated histoplasmosis usually is fatal.

MUCORMYCOSIS

A category of infections by fungi of the order Mucorales, genera *Mucor, Absidia, Rhizopus*, and *Mortierella*. The most pathogenic thermotolerant *Mucor* spp are now classified in a "new" genus, *Rhizomucor*. These ubiquitous monomorphic fungi are common inhabitants of soil, manure, and rotting vegetation. Infections are often opportunistic, secondary to disorders such as metabolic acidosis and immunosuppression. The fungi cause granulomatous lesions in several organs of various species, including cattle, pigs, sheep, horses, dogs, cats, various wild animals (including nonhuman primates, rodents, and birds), and man. Lesions may be focal, involving body surfaces, lymph nodes, and portions of the GI tract; or the disease may be disseminated with lesions in several organs. Mucormycosis is particularly important as a cause of placentitis and abortion in Bovidae.

Clinical Findings and Lesions: Signs generally are nonspecific and reflect organ involvement. Some animals with focal or disseminated lesions may be asymptomatic. Others, with pneumonia, may have rapid, shallow, stertorous respiration; nasal discharge; pleural effusion; and pleuritis. Systemic mucormycosis can cause anorexia, pyrexia, and persistent diarrhea; neurologic disturbances have followed brain involvement.

Nodular lesions in lymph nodes, liver, lungs, and kidneys (pigs and cattle) are white to yellow, and solid to cavitated. Affected lymph nodes in older cattle appear tuberculous: nodes are yellow, grossly enlarged, caseocalcareous, and fibrotic. In another form of the disease, circular to oval ulcers are found in the forestomachs and abomasum of cattle and in the GI tract of pigs.

Diagnosis: Antemortem diagnosis is uncommon; many cases are asymptomatic or the signs are nonspecific. Mucormycosis can be diagnosed microscopically by demonstrating broad, branching, aseptate, irregular hyphae (10-20 μm in width) and the expected tissue reaction with angioinvasion, thrombosis, and necrosis. Fungi can be identified in tissue sections by FA techniques using fluorescein antiglobulins specific for each genus of the Mucorales. Cultural studies are required to identify the infecting fungus to species, and the same fungus should be recovered from several specimens of the carcass. Serology is useful in the diagnosis of bovine abortion caused by *Mortierella wolfii*.

Treatment: Surgical excision of focal superficial lesions may be combined with local administration of amphotericin B. However, no completely satisfactory treatment is known.

MYCETOMAS

Two different types of microbes—actinomycetes and fungi—cause granulomatous tumors of the subcut. tissues, which may spread locally to involve bone. The causal agents of eumycotic (fungal) mycetomas include a variety of saprophytic geophilic fungi, including *Acremonium* spp, *Curvularia geniculata*, *Madurella grisea*, and *Scedosporium (Monosporium) apiospermum* (the asexual state of *Pseudallescheria [Petriellidium, Allescheria] boydii*).

In lesions, the fungal mycelia proliferate and organize into aggregates known as granules or grains. In these granules, the mycelium is compact and frequently bizarre and distorted in form. Chlamydospores are frequent, especially at the periphery, and the mycelium may or may not be embedded in an amorphous cement-like substance. Histologically, the granules are frequently surrounded by eosinophilic deposits. Granules may be of various colors and sizes, depending on the species of fungus involved.

Confirmed cases of mycetomas in nonhumans have been rare. The dog has been the prime victim with the dematiaceous *C geniculata*, the principal etiologic agent. *Scedosporium apiospermum* may be an underestimated causal agent. Treatment is primarily limited to surgery; chemotherapy with drugs has not been effective.

NORTH AMERICAN BLASTOMYCOSIS

A disease caused by the dimorphic fungus, *Blastomyces dermatitidis*, character-ized by pyogranulomatous lesions in various tissues. It is most common in man and dogs, but is described in cats and horses and in such widely divergent species as an African lion, a bottle-nosed dolphin, and a sea lion. It appears not to be a disease of cattle, sheep, or pigs. Blastomycosis is generally limited to North America, and most cases have occurred in the Mississippi River system and around the Great Lakes. Its pathogenesis is not clearly defined, but the primary portal of entry is the respiratory tract via inhalation of spores from a site of saprophytic fungal growth. Cutaneous lesions may result from a primary entry through the skin or, more com-monly, by dissemination from a pulmonary focus.

Clinical Findings and Lesions: The signs vary with organ involvement and are not specific. Wasting may be accompanied by coughing, anorexia, dyspnea, fever, and a nasal exudate. Small cutaneous pustules covered with yellow scabs or subcut. nodules may occur. The subcut. pyogranulomas, often multiple, ulcerate through the skin and discharge a purulent exudate. Commonly, the bronchial lymph nodes are greatly enlarged and appear in radiographs as dense masses. In thoracic blasto-mycosis, the predominant radiographic patterns are those of nodular interstitial den-sities and a mixed lung pattern. Hematuria, nocturia, and dysuria with tenesmus may occur with urogenital blastomycosis. In dogs, the obvious signs may be ophthalmic.

Gross lesions consist of few to numerous, variable-sized, irregular, firm, gray to yellow areas of pulmonary consolidation and nodules in the lungs and lymph nodes of the thorax. Dissemination may result in nodular lesions in various organs, but especially the skin, eye, and bone. Cutaneous lesions are single or multiple papules, or chronic draining nodular pyogranulomas.

Diagnosis: Blastomycosis should be considered in dogs with draining cutaneous nodules and signs of respiratory disease. Radiographic findings in the lungs include noncalcified nodules or consolidation, and enlargement of the bronchial and medias-tinal lymph nodes. Diagnosis can be made from biopsy tissue or aspirated speci-mens from cutaneous lesions, and at necropsy by the presence of the yeast form of the fungus. These round to ovoid, pale pink (H&E) blastospores measure 8-25 μm and have a refractile, double-contoured wall. They may be empty or contain baso-philic nuclear material and have single broad-based buds. An antibody response detected by gel immunodiffusion test usually occurs. The organism can also be identified by FA techniques.

Treatment: Rare primary cutaneous disease may persist for months; these lesions should be removed surgically since blastomycosis responds poorly to therapy. Am-photericin B is considered the drug of choice, but treatment is of little avail once the disease is disseminated. The combination of amphotericin B and ketoconazole has been suggested to reduce the rate of relapse.

OOMYCOSIS

Diseases caused by fungi of the class Oomycetes. Organisms of veterinary sig-nificance include various species of *Saprolegnia* and *Achyla* (eg, *S diclina*), which are the common agents of cutaneous mycoses in fishes, and *Pythium insidiosum* (*Hyphomyces destruens*), the cause of dermal mycosis of horses (bursatti, swamp cancer, leeches). *Pythium* sp, considered by some not to be a fungus, also has been isolated from cases of cutaneous, oral, and GI mycosis in dogs, and pulmonary lesions in a horse. Natural disease also has been recorded in cattle (cutaneous) and man, and probably cats and sheep. Pythiosis, as the disease has been called, is a common disease of domestic animals in some tropical and subtropical countries of the world.

Clinical Findings and Lesions: In horses, lesions are large, roughly circular, granulomatous, ulcerated, fistulated nodules, or subcut. swellings with yellow-gray necrotic masses or cores. The lesions are pruritic, discharge a mucosanguineous exudate, often are self-traumatized, and contain yellow, irregularly branching "coagula" either free within sinuses or firmly attached to surrounding tissue. The sinus tracts contain thick sanguineous to mucopurulent material. The lesions are most common on the legs (especially the lower limbs), abdomen, chest, and genitalia. Distribution of lesions is attributable to the aquatic nature of the organism.

Specimens removed at surgery or necropsy consist of fibrous tissue with irregularly spaced, firm, focal areas of necrosis that vary in size and color. Microscopically, alterations vary from foci of acute exudative inflammation with numerous eosinophils to a granulomatous reaction with sequestered areas of necrosis and a framework of hyphae that are thick walled, branching, and slightly irregular in width.

Diagnosis: The equine lesions of oomycosis are similar to those of entomophthoromycosis (qv, p 345) and may be confused with cutaneous habronemiasis (qv, p 806). In oomycosis, the necrotic cores are distinct from the surrounding tissue, and a seropurulent discharge from the sinus tracts is prominent. The lesions contain irregular, branching, sometimes septate hyphae, 4-8 μm in diameter.

Treatment: Surgical excision, immunotherapy, or a combination of both have been effective. Immunotherapy consists of the intradermal injection of 0.02-0.1 mL of particulate material of the causative fungus. Osteitis or deep-seated laminitis may be a significant complication of such therapy. Surgical removal plus systemic or local administration of amphotericin B is a satisfactory treatment if the disease is localized.

PAECILOMYCOSIS

Systemic (mainly pulmonary) mycoses caused by *Paecilomyces* spp have been described in man and various lower animals, especially those with lowered body temperatures. Infection in captive reptiles and amphibians is probably fairly common—other hosts include dogs, horses, cats (nasal granuloma), and goats (mastitis). More significant causal fungi are *P lilacinus* and *P variotii*. The fungi, usually considered nonpathogenic, are widely distributed in soil and decaying organic matter. Infection usually has been secondary to debilitation, immunosuppression, and/or alteration of normal microbial flora by prolonged administration of antibiotics.

Clinical Findings and Lesions: Signs vary and are not specific, but may reflect tissue or organ involvement. Involved organs are enlarged and contain raised gray-white nodules. Granulomatous lesions (multiple, pale foci) that contain septate pseudohyphae (2-3 μm in diameter), oval conidia, and spherical to oval, thin-walled spores (3-6 μm) are found in many tissues (eg, lungs) in disseminated cases, and are closely associated with small and medium-sized arterioles.

Diagnosis: The gross lesions can be confused with those of other systemic mycoses. However, the septate hyphae, conidia, and spores of this fungus differ from common pathogenic fungi such as *Aspergillus* sp and those of mucormycosis. Diagnosis can be made by cultural isolation of the fungus from multiple specimens of lesions. With most species, growth may be absent or restricted at 37°C, but good at 5-30°C.

Treatment: No treatment regimens have been described. *Paecilomyces* spp vary greatly in sensitivity to antifungal agents—*P lilacinus* appears highly resistant to amphotericin B and flucytosine but sensitive to ketoconazole, while *P variotii* is sensitive to the first 2 drugs.

PENICILLIOSIS

Infections with *Penicillium* spp are rare in domestic animals, but the agent has been isolated from a case of feline dermatosis, from orbital cellulitis and sinusitis with pneumonia in another cat, from invasive destructive disease of nasal tissues in dogs, and from systemic disease in bamboo rats (in these cases the fungus was *P marneffei*) in southeast Asia. *Penicillium* spp are widely distributed in nature and are found in soils, grains, and various foods and feeds.

Clinical Findings and Lesions: Dogs with nasal penicilliosis have chronic sneezing and an acute to chronic nasal discharge that varies from intermittent hemorrhagic to intermittent or continuous mucoid or mucopurulent. Radiographic findings include areas of turbinate destruction with increased radiolucency. Grossly, the nasal mucosa has foci of necrosis and ulceration; microscopically, fungal hyphae may form a thick mat over an intact mucosa adjacent to these foci.

Diagnosis: Diagnosis is based on fungal culture, character of the lesions and presence of fungal hyphae, and a positive agar-gel double-diffusion test. Cultural isolation of a *Penicillium* sp must be accompanied by demonstration of tissue invasion by the fungus for confirmation. In tissues, *P marneffei* closely resembles the yeast phase of *Histoplasma capsulatum*.

Treatment: Surgical turbinectomy with curettage has been combined with flushing of the nasal cavity with 1% tincture of iodine or (10:1) povidone-iodine and oral thiabendazole. Thiabendazole combined with flucytosine has been a suggested treatment.

RHINOSPORIDIOSIS

A chronic, nonfatal, pyogranulomatous infection, primarily of the nasal mucosa and occasionally of the skin of Equidae, cattle, dogs, and aquatic birds, caused by the fungus *Rhinosporidium seeberi*. Uncommon in North America, it is seen most often in India, Africa, and South America. The organism has not been cultured and its natural habitat is unknown. Trauma may predispose to infection, which is not considered transmissible.

Clinical Findings and Lesions: Infection of the nasal mucosa is characterized by polypoid growths that may be soft, pink, friable, lobulated with roughened surfaces, and large enough to occlude the nasal passages. The cutaneous lesions may be single or multiple, sessile or pedunculated. The nasal polyps and cutaneous lesions have a granulomatous fibromyxoid inflammatory component and contain the fungal organism.

Diagnosis: Rhinosporidiosis may be confused with other granulomatous lesions of the nasal mucosa and skin, including aspergillosis, entomophthoromycosis, "nasal granuloma", and cryptococcosis. Microscopical demonstration of spherules (sporangia) of *R seeberi* in biopsy specimens confirms the diagnosis. The spherules may be numerous, vary in size (up to 300 μm), have thick periodic-acid-Schiff-positive walls, and contain endospores 4-19 μm in diameter. Developing stages of varying size without spores are distributed throughout the lesion.

Treatment: Surgical excision of the lesions is considered standard, but recurrence is not uncommon.

SPOROTRICHOSIS

An uncommon and sporadic chronic granulomatous disease of man and various domestic and laboratory animals caused by *Sporothrix (Sporotrichum) schenckii*. The dimorphic fungus is distributed worldwide and is a saprophyte found in vegetable matter (eg, straw and sphagnum moss), animal excreta, and soil. Infection occurs when spores gain entrance via cutaneous wounds.

Clinical Findings and Lesions: The head, thorax, ear, nose, and limbs of affected animals have firm, raised, sometimes crusted and alopecic cutaneous nodules that are disseminated along local lymph vessels and nodes. The superficial lesions ulcerate and discharge a brownish red exudate. The infection may, on rare occasions, become generalized with lesions in the thoracic and abdominal viscera and in the brain and eye. A creamy yellow, odorless exudate may be obtained on incision of the nodules. Several cases have been described in horses, in which it resembles epizootic lymphangitis (qv, p 346). The nodules, microscopically, are pyogranulomatous lesions composed of macrophages, giant cells, and various other cell types, including neutrophils.

Diagnosis: Diagnosis can be made by cultural (samples obtained from unopened lesions) or microscopical examination of the exudate or biopsy specimens. In tissues and exudate, the organism is present as few to numerous, cigar-shaped, single cells within macrophages. The fungal cells are pleomorphic and small (2-10 × 1-3 μm); buds may be present and give the appearance of a ping-pong paddle. An FA technique has been used to identify the yeast-like cells in tissues. In cultures, a true mycelium is produced, with fine, branching, septate hyphae bearing pear-shaped conidia on slender conidiophores.

Treatment: Iodides (potassium or sodium) have been used with some success; therapy is continued until signs of iodism develop and for several weeks after apparent recovery to prevent recurrence. Amphotericin B and griseofulvin also may be of value, especially when combined with flucytosine. Surgical incision, excision, and cauterization of the cutaneous lesions are not recommended. These procedures are often followed by an increase in the severity of the lesions.

LEPTOSPIROSIS

A contagious disease of animals, including man, caused by infection with various immunologically distinct leptospiral serovars, most of which are regarded as subgroups of *Leptospira interrogans*. Infections may be asymptomatic or result in various disease conditions, including fever, icterus, hemoglobinuria, infertility, abortion, and death. Following acute infection, leptospires frequently localize in the kidneys or reproductive organs and are shed in the urine, sometimes in large numbers for months or years. The disease is often water-borne, since the organisms survive in surface waters for extended periods.

Infection is commonly acquired by contact of skin or mucous membrane with urine, and to a lesser extent by intake of urine-contaminated feed or water. Infections can be readily established via the conjunctiva, vaginal mucosa, or skin abrasions. If shedder animals are introduced into a herd previously free of the disease, leptospires are rapidly disseminated, and abortions and stillbirths may occur, most frequently during the middle or last third of gestation. Clinical signs may be severe, mild, or inapparent. Generally, recovery from acute signs is associated with the appearance of circulating antibodies and disappearance of leptospires from the blood. Leptospiral abortions may be followed by retention of fetal membranes, and fertility may be impaired. Disease outbreaks in small herds are often self-limiting. However, control of endemic infections in large herds generally requires immunization, chemotherapy, fencing the herd from surface waters, and limiting contact with rodents and other wildlife carriers.

Of >175 antigenically distinct pathogenic leptospiral serovars, only 7 have been isolated from domestic animals in the USA, although others have been isolated from wildlife. Cross-immunity between serovars is only moderate, and double and even triple infections have been reported. Agglutinating antibodies usually appear 6-12 days after infection; titers rise rapidly, then generally decline over several months to moderate levels that may persist for weeks to years. A single seropositive test is of limited diagnostic significance since it can be the result of a recent vaccination, passive immunity in calves, or a current or past infection. Diagnosis can be confirmed by a rising titer in paired serum samples, if the first is taken during the acute stage, and the second after 7-10 days. Vaccination with bacterins can stimulate significant concentrations of agglutinins but, without previous exposure, the microscopic agglutination titers decrease in 2-3 mo. Some carrier or shedder animals in which the infection has localized do not have diagnostic titers. The serological methods commonly used include the microscopic agglutination test, the microtiter agglutination test, and occasionally, the ELISA and complement fixation tests.

Primary isolations are made during the acute state of infection by inoculating 0.5 mL of blood, collected aseptically, into laboratory animals or suitable laboratory media. A series of inoculum dilutions should be made to reduce the probability of contamination. Similarly, urine may be examined by darkfield microscopy or cultured 2-4 wk or longer after acute infection. Negative results do not rule out infection since leptospires often are shed intermittently in the urine.

Clinical diagnosis may also be confirmed by demonstrating the organism in sections of kidney and liver stained by the silver-impregnation method of Levaditi or the Warthin-Starry technique. Leptospires do not stain with the common aniline dyes. Fresh tissue scrapings from liver or kidney, or the centrifuged deposit from freshly collected urine may also be examined with specific fluorescent conjugates or by darkfield microscopy, but such procedures require considerable experience. Characteristic motility under darkfield microscopy must be observed to provide positive identification.

Man is susceptible to all the pathogenic serovars found in domestic animals, and wildlife transmission generally occurs when contact is made with tissues of infected animals or surface waters contaminated by urine from infected animals. Because of these origins, the disease in man often is occupationally related. As in other animals, the disease varies from inapparent to severe and can be fatal when renal failure occurs. The most common signs are fever, headaches, rash, myalgia, and malaise; laboratory techniques are necessary for a definitive diagnosis. Animal owners should be informed of the potential zoonotic risk of leptospirosis.

LEPTOSPIROSIS IN CATTLE
(Redwater of calves)

In the USA, the disease is primarily due to *hardjo, pomona*, and *grippotyphosa* serovars. However, *canicola* and *icterohaemorrhagiae* serovars also have been isolated.

Clinical Findings: Hemolytic icterus and hemoglobinuria occur in ≥50% of young calves infected with the *pomona* serovar. Mortality is 5-15%. The acute clinical syndrome occurs in <10% of adults, and deaths are rare. Morbidity may be >75% in older stock, and usually approaches 100% in calves.

Calves usually show fever, prostration, anorexia, and dyspnea, and in *pomona* infections, icterus, hemoglobinuria, and anemia. Body temperature may rise suddenly to 105-106°F (40.5-41°C). Hemoglobinuria rarely lasts longer than 48-72 hr. Icterus clears rapidly and is followed by anemia. The RBC begin to increase in number by 4-5 days and return to normal 7-10 days later. Most affected cattle show leukocytosis. Some degree of albuminuria is common during the febrile peak. However, *hardjo* infections seldom cause icterus, hemoglobinuria, and anemia, which makes diagnosis more difficult.

In older cattle, signs vary greatly and diagnosis is more difficult. Endemic *hardjo* infections, which usually cause production of abnormal milk, are more obvious in dairy than in beef cattle. Signs usually are restricted to lowered milk and calf production; a hemolytic crisis is not seen. The milk is thick, yellow, and blood-tinged, although there is little evidence of mammary inflammation. Milk production returns to normal within 10 days, even in the absence of treatment. Abortion and stillbirths, which are common with *pomona* and sporadic with *hardjo*, generally occur 3-10 wk following initial infection. The abortions are more common during the third trimester. An abortion storm in a breeding herd is often the first indication that leptospirosis exists, since the mild initial signs often pass unnoticed. In endemically infected herds, abortions occur mostly in younger animals and are sporadic, not manifested as abortion storms. Calves reared by previously infected cows are protected by colostral antibodies for up to 6 mo. The calves generally have an antibody titer similar to that of their dams.

Lesions: Anemia and icterus are prominent features of *pomona* infections. The urine is a clear-red or port-wine color. The kidneys show the most significant lesion in the form of red or white infarcts that cause mottling of the cortex, often sufficiently pronounced to be visible through the capsule. The liver may be swollen, with minute areas of focal necrosis. Petechiae in the epicardium and lymph nodes are seen in fulminating cases; however, in the more prevalent *hardjo* infections, the lesions are primarily restricted to the kidneys.

Diagnosis: Serology with paired serum samples, direct culture in special media, or animal inoculation techniques are usually necessary to confirm clinical and post-mortem findings. In herd evaluation, sera should be obtained from various age groups. Isolation of the causative agent constitutes the most reliable diagnostic tool. Gross physical changes in the milk in the absence of mammary inflammation are suggestive of leptospirosis. Similarly, elimination of brucellosis, campylobacteriosis, and trichomoniasis as the cause of an abortion outbreak point to leptospirosis. Agglutination titers often reach their peaks before abortion since the acute infection occurred several weeks previously. Abortion due to *hardjo* often occurs in the absence of serological titers.

Treatment: Streptomycin, chlortetracycline, and oxytetracycline have been reported to be successful if given early. Dihydrostreptomycin is recommended for treatment of the carrier or shedder state, although recent work indicates that carriers are not eliminated by antibiotic therapy. For valuable animals, IV transfusion of washed RBC may prove beneficial if the anemia approaches the critical level. Treatment has limited effect on the course of disease once a renal crisis has developed. Management of infected herds merits special consideration. When leptospirosis is diagnosed in pregnant beef cows during the early epidemic phase, further abortions can be prevented by prompt vaccination of the entire herd and simultaneous treatment of all animals with appropriate antibiotics. The antibiotic reduces the number of leptospires in the kidneys and other tissues, at least during treatment, and provides a measure of protection until immunity is induced by vaccination. In dairy herds, generally only the sick animals should be treated with antibiotics since the loss of market milk after treatment must be considered.

Prophylaxis: Cattle owners rely on annual vaccinations, confinement rearing, and chemoprophylaxis for control. Bacterins generally confer protection against abortions and death, and significantly reduce renal infections, although some infections do occur. Management methods to reduce transmission include rat control, fencing cattle from potentially contaminated streams and ponds, separation of cattle from pigs and wildlife, selection of replacement stock from herds that are seronegative for leptospirosis, and chemoprophylaxis and vaccination of replacement stock.

LEPTOSPIROSIS IN DOGS
(Canine typhus, Stuttgart disease, Infectious jaundice)

Infection usually is due to serovars *canicola* or *copenhageni*, a member of the *icterohaemorrhagiae* serogroup, although *pomona, grippotyphosa,* and *ballum* also have been isolated from dogs in the USA. Infections with *canicola* or *copenhageni* are prevalent in some dog populations. The *copenhageni* serovar has frequently been the cause of the so-called hemorrhagic and icteric type of leptospirosis. Brown rats are the primary reservoir of *copenhageni* in the USA, while dogs are the reservoir of *canicola*.

Clinical Findings: Dogs of all ages may be affected, and the incidence is much greater in males. The incubation period is 5-15 days. In severe cases, onset is sudden and characterized by slight weakness, anorexia, vomiting, a fever of 103-105°F (39.5-40.5°C), and often a mild conjunctivitis. At this stage, clinical diagnosis is difficult. Within several days, the temperature drops sharply, depression is more pronounced, breathing is labored, and thirst is marked. In some dogs, icterus of varying intensity may be the first manifestation of illness. The dog may be reluctant to rise from a sitting position, and may exhibit signs of pain if the lumbar region or anterior dorsal abdomen is palpated. The oral mucosa may at first show irregular hemorrhagic patches resembling abrasions or burns, which later become dry and necrotic and slough in sections. A tenacious salivary secretion around the gums may be tinged with blood. Swallowing is difficult. Animals with more advanced disease show profound depression and muscular tremors, with the temperature dropping gradually to as low as 97°F (36°C). Bloody vomitus and feces may be seen, which indicate hemorrhagic gastroenteritis. Frequent urination with albumin and casts in the urine indicates acute nephritis. The eyes become sunken and the vessels of the conjunctiva are injected. The pulse becomes thready and, in severe cases, uremia develops. Mortality is seldom >10%; deaths, usually caused by renal failure, generally occur 5-10 days after onset. Chronic, progressive nephritis frequently follows acute *canicola* infections. In such cases, death may not occur until long after the initial illness has subsided.

The WBC count may rise to 35,000; the BUN also may be elevated. Other laboratory findings are variable, depending on the severity and stage of the disease.

Lesions: Hemorrhagic gastroenteritis often is the predominant lesion. In such cases, the tissues may be uniformly bile-stained, the liver engorged, and the lymph nodes hemorrhagic. The myocardium may be diffusely hemorrhagic. The organs may have a uremic odor. The kidneys become enlarged in the acute phase and have red foci. As the disease develops, subacute interstitial nephritis results in gray foci or mottling at the corticomedullary junction. Oral ulcers and tongue sloughs may occur in the uremic animal. Chronic cases have varying degrees of interstitial nephritis. Diagnosis is based on clinical and necropsy findings; histological demonstration of leptospires in the kidney, liver, or urine; and serology.

Treatment: Tetracycline, doxycycline, and streptomycin are recommended for acute infections; dihydrostreptomycin in heavy doses for 1 wk is suggested for reduction of the carrier/shedder state. Doxycycline rather than tetracycline should be used when acute nephritis is present. Dehydration and acidosis can be treated by giving 0.17M lactate solution, alone or with saline-dextrose solution, and high doses of B vitamins. In the anuric phase of the disease, excessive fluid volume must not be administered; the fluid volume should be adjusted so that a 40-lb (18-kg) dog loses ~0.2 lb (90 g) per day. Peritoneal dialysis can be lifesaving in uremic cases.

Prophylaxis: To reduce the chances of exposure, owners are advised to engage in rodent control and keep their dogs leashed. During epidemics, confinement to the owner's premises should be recommended. Bivalent bacterins are available and should be administered q6-8mo to maintain a protective titer for dogs at high risk, eg, show, stud, or hunting dogs. If leptospirosis is diagnosed in a kennel, treatment and vaccination of all dogs in the kennel should be considered. Dogs in contact with wildlife should receive bacterins containing *grippotyphosa* and *pomona* antigens.

LEPTOSPIROSIS IN HORSES

During investigations of the etiology of equine uveitis (qv, p 302), serology revealed that many affected horses had high titers to *pomona*, and the organism has been isolated from eyes of horses. Chronic uveitis has been induced experimentally with leptospiral infections. Acute leptospirosis in horses is characterized by fever of 103-105°F (39.5-40.5°C) for 2-3 days, depression or dullness, anorexia, icterus, and neutrophilia. Abortion may occur several weeks after the fever, and chronic uveitis months later. In Europe, *pomona, hardjo, icterohaemorrhagiae,* and *bratislava* have been isolated from aborted equine fetuses. The incidence of leptospirosis in horses is unknown; however, serological evidence indicates a higher incidence than is apparent clinically.

Many cases of leptospirosis undoubtedly occur without being recognized because of the mild, transient course, which leaves only the later apparent eye lesions as visible evidence. Measures for control and treatment are similar to cattle and pigs, but specific bacterins have not been developed for horses.

LEPTOSPIROSIS IN PIGS

Although *pomona* was the serovar most commonly encountered in pigs, recent serosurveys indicate *bratislava* is the most widespread. Infection usually is from contact with the urine of other pigs or wildlife. Pigs may also be infected with the *grippotyphosa, canicola,* and *icterohaemorrhagiae* serovars. Pigs apparently can excrete large numbers of organisms in their urine up to 1 yr following recovery from an acute infection. They often transmit the disease to man, and in Europe, it has been known as "swineherd's disease". Acute leptospirosis, which occurs in young pigs due to *pomona* or *grippotyphosa,* is characterized by fever, icterus, hemorrhages, and death. Infections with *bratislava* have been associated primarily with reduced breeding efficiency.

Acute porcine leptospirosis often is not a clearly defined entity. In some pigs, infection may be inapparent; others show only fever and anorexia lasting 3-4 days. More severe clinical signs include poor weight gain, anorexia, GI disturbances, and occasionally, meningitis with rigidity, spasms, and circling. Leptospires have been isolated frequently from aborted porcine fetuses. Abortions late in pregnancy, stillbirths, or weak neonates represent the most recognizable signs of leptospirosis in a herd. Early in an outbreak, abortions can be reduced by treatment and vaccination of all breeding animals in the herd. Rodent control is important in reducing transmission of some serovars.

LEPTOSPIROSIS IN SHEEP

Prevalence in sheep is lower than in cattle, possibly due to less intensive husbandry methods and their tendency to avoid contact with surface water. In the USA, *pomona* and *hardjo* have been the most common serovars isolated from sheep. Clinical features, diagnosis, and management of the disease are essentially as described above for mature cattle and calves.

LISTERIOSIS
(Listerellosis, Circling disease)

A sporadic bacterial infection with worldwide distribution that occurs more in temperate and colder climates. It affects a wide range of animals and birds, including man. There is a high incidence of intestinal carriers, and the disease occurs more commonly than it is diagnosed. Encephalitis or meningoencephalitis in adult ruminants is the most frequently recognized form.

Etiology and Epidemiology: *Listeria monocytogenes* is a small, motile, gram-positive, nonspore-forming, extremely resistant, diphtheroid coccobacillus that grows under a wide temperature range, 39-111°F (4-44°C). Its ability to grow at 4°C is an important diagnostic aid (in the "cold enrichment" method) for isolation of the organism from brain tissue (but not from placental or fetal tissues). Primary isolation is enhanced under microaerophilic conditions. It is a ubiquitous saprophyte that lives in a plant-soil environment and has been isolated from ≥42 species of domestic and wild mammals and 22 of birds, as well as fish, crustaceans, insects, sewage, water, silage and other feedstuffs, milk, cheese, meconium, feces, and soil.

The natural reservoirs of *L monocytogenes* appear to be soil and mammalian GI tracts, both of which contaminate vegetation. Grazing animals ingest the organism and further contaminate vegetation and soil. Animal-to-animal transmission occurs via the fecal-oral route.

Listeriosis is primarily a winter-spring disease of feedlot or housed ruminants. The alkaline pH of spoiled silage enhances multiplication of *L monocytogenes*. Outbreaks may occur ≥10 days after feeding poor-quality silage. Corn silage has been implicated more commonly in sheep than cattle. Removal or change of silage in the ration often stops the spread of listeriosis; feeding the same silage months later may produce new cases.

Pathogenesis: *Listeria* that are ingested or inhaled tend to cause septicemia, abortion, and latent infection. Those that gain entry to tissues have a predilection to localize in the intestinal wall, medulla oblongata, and placenta; or to cause encephalitis via minute wounds in buccal mucosa, or via inhalation or the conjunctiva.

The various manifestations of infection occur in all susceptible species and are associated with characteristic clinical syndromes: encephalitis or meningoencephalitis in adult ruminants, abortion and perinatal mortality in all species, septicemia in monogastric and neonatal ruminants, and septicemia with myocardial and/or hepatic necrosis in poultry (*see* p 1578). Most infections are subclinical or latent but, when stressed, clinical listeriosis may occur.

Listeric encephalitis affects sheep, cattle, goats, and occasionally, pigs. It is essentially a localized infection of the brain stem that occurs when *L monocytogenes* ascends the cranial nerves. Clinical signs vary according to the function of damaged neurons, but often are unilateral and include facial paralysis and circling.

Septicemic or visceral listeriosis is most common in monogastrics, including pigs, dogs, cats, domestic and wild rabbits, and many other small mammals. These animals may play a role in transmission of *L monocytogenes*. This form is found also in young ruminants before the rumen is functional. Though rare, septicemia has been reported in older domestic ruminants and deer. The septicemic form affects organs other than the brain, the principal lesion being focal hepatic necrosis.

The uterus of all domestic animals, especially ruminants, is susceptible to *L monocytogenes* at all stages of pregnancy, which can result in placentitis, metritis, fetal infection and death, abortion, stillbirths, neonatal deaths, and possibly, viable carriers. The metritis has little or no effect on subsequent reproduction; however, listeria may be shed ≥1 mo via the vagina and milk.

Oral infections tend to localize in the intestinal wall and result in inapparent infection and prolonged fecal excretion. It has been postulated that listeria-contaminated silage results in numerous latent infections, often approaching 100% of the exposed herd or flock, but clinical listeriosis in only a few animals.

Clinical Findings: Encephalitis is the most readily recognized form of listeriosis in ruminants. It affects all ages and both sexes, sometimes as an epidemic in feedlot cattle or sheep. The course in sheep and goats is rapid; death may occur 4-48 hr after onset of signs, and recovery is rare. In cattle it is less acute, with most surviving for 4-14 days. Spontaneous recovery may occur, but survivors often have permanent CNS injury. Lesions are localized in the brain stem, and the signs indicate dysfunction of the third to seventh cranial nerves.

Initially, affected animals are depressed, febrile, disoriented, and indifferent to their surroundings, and usually separate themselves. They tend to crowd into corners or lean and push their head against stationary objects. If they walk, they stumble and move in a circle, always in the same direction. Marked nasal discharge, anorexia, strabismus, and conjunctivitis are common, and they appear to be blind. Facial paralysis with drooping ear, dilated nostril, and lowered eyelid on the affected side often develops, more commonly in cattle. There may be intermittent twitching and paralysis of facial and throat muscles and tongue, which interferes with swallowing and results in profuse salivation. Terminally affected animals fall, and unable to rise, lie on the same side; involuntary running movements are common.

Listeric encephalitis may recur on the same premises in successive years. The number of animals clinically involved in an outbreak usually is small, but may reach 30% in a flock of sheep or goats and 10% in cattle; mortality is high. Deaths cease suddenly when sheep are turned out to pasture.

Listeriosis is relatively uncommon in pigs, with septicemia occurring in those <1 mo old, and encephalitis in older pigs; it has a rapid fatal course of 3-4 days.

Listeric abortion usually occurs in the last trimester without premonitory signs. Fetuses usually die *in utero*, but stillbirths and neonatal deaths occur. The abortion rate varies and has been up to 20% in sheep flocks. Fatal septicemia of the dam secondary to metritis is rare. Encephalitis and abortion usually do not occur simultaneously in the same herd or flock. However, the clinical pattern in sheep in England has been changing: abortions, encephalitis, and diarrhea are increasing, and outbreaks of abortions and encephalitis occur together in the same flock.

Lesions: In listeric encephalitis, there are few gross lesions apart from some congestion of meninges. Microscopic lesions are confined primarily to the pons, medulla oblongata, and anterior spinal cord.

In septicemic listeriosis, small necrotic foci may be found in any organ, especially the liver. In calves that die when <3 wk old, in addition to focal hepatic necrosis, there is frequently marked hemorrhagic gastritis and enteritis.

In aborted fetuses, there is slight to marked autolysis, clear to blood-tinged fluid in the serous cavities, and numerous small necrotic foci (0.5-2 μm) in the liver, especially in the right half. Necrotic foci may be found in other viscera such as lung and spleen. Shallow erosions, 1-3 mm, may be present in abomasal mucosa. Autolytic changes may mask these lesions. Gram-stained smears of abomasal contents reveal numerous gram-positive, pleomorphic coccobacilli.

Diagnosis: There is no satisfactory antemortem diagnostic test. Listeriosis can be confirmed only by isolation and identification of *L monocytogenes*. Specimens of choice are brain from animals with CNS involvement, and aborted placenta and fetus. If primary isolation attempts fail, ground brain tissue should be held at 39°F (4°C) for several weeks and recultured weekly. Occasionally, *L monocytogenes* has been isolated from spinal fluid, nasal discharge, urine, feces, and milk of clinically ill ruminants. Serology is not used routinely for diagnosis because many healthy animals have high listeria titers. Immunofluorescence is effective for rapidly identifying *L monocytogenes* in smears from animals dead or aborted from listeriosis, and from milk, meat, and other sources.

It may be difficult to distinguish between listeriosis and pregnancy toxemia in ewes (qv, p 456) or ketosis in cattle (qv, p 446), but in pregnancy toxemia or ketosis, facial and ear paralysis are less likely, and ketonuria is common. In cattle, the localizing signs of listeriosis, if present, help to differentiate it from thromboembolic encephalitis (qv, p 602), polioencephalomalacia (qv, p 614), sporadic bovine encephalomyelitis (qv, p 624), and lead poisoning (qv, p 1674). Rabies (qv, p 619) must always be considered in the differential diagnosis of listeriosis. Other causes of brain abscesses, while rare, and coenurosis (qv, p 604) may be clinically indistinguishable from listeriosis.

Treatment and Control: *Listeria monocytogenes* is susceptible to penicillin, erythromycin, chloramphenicol, and tetracyclines; the drug of choice is penicillin. High doses are required because of the difficulty of maintaining therapeutic levels in the brain. Recovery depends on early treatment. If signs of encephalitis are severe, death usually occurs in spite of treatment.

Penicillin G should be given at 44,000 u/kg body wt, IM, daily for 1-2 wk, the first injection to be accompanied by the same dose IV.

Chlortetracycline, 10 mg/kg body wt, IV, daily for 5 days, is reported to be effective for meningoencephalitis in cattle but less so for sheep. Supportive therapy, including fluids and electrolytes, is required for animals having difficulty eating and drinking.

Results with vaccines have been inconclusive. In an outbreak, affected animals should be segregated. If silage is being fed, use of the particular silage should be discontinued on a trial basis. Spoiled silage should be avoided routinely. Corn ensiled before being too mature is likely to have a more acid pH, which discourages multiplication of *L monocytogenes*.

Zoonotic Risk: The concept that animals serve as a reservoir of infection for man may be questioned since *Listeria* have been isolated from feces of a significant number of apparently normal people as well as animals. However, despite this and the apparently low invasiveness of *L monocytogenes*, all suspected material should be handled with caution. Aborted fetuses and necropsy of septicemic animals present the greatest hazard. People have developed fatal meningitis, septicemia, and papular exanthema on the arms after handling aborted material. In cases with encephalitis, *L monocytogenes* is usually confined to the brain and presents little risk of transmission unless the brain is removed. Pregnant animals (including women) should be protected from infection because of danger to the fetus.

Listeria monocytogenes can be isolated from milk of mastitic, aborting, and apparently normal cows. Excretion in milk is usually intermittent but may persist for many months. Infected milk is a hazard because *Listeria* may survive certain forms of pasteurization. *Listeria* also have been isolated from milk of sheep, goats, and women.

LYME DISEASE
(Borreliosis)

A tick-borne, immune-mediated inflammatory disease of dogs, cats, horses, cows, wild animals, and man. In the USA, it is endemic along the northeastern seaboard, and in Minnesota and Wisconsin; it has been reported in 44 states, including the southeast, west, and midwest. It also has been reported in Canada, Europe, and Australia. It has a significant zoonotic impact, and human cases parallel animal cases geographically. Veterinarians should be aware of the potential transmission to man posed by handling infected ticks, blood, urine, and synovial fluid.

Etiology and Transmission: The causative agent is the spirochete *Borrelia burgdorferi*. It is transmitted principally by the ticks *Ixodes dammini, I pacificus, I ricinus,* and *I scapularis.* Other hard ticks, such as *Dermacentor variabilis* and *Amblyomma americanum,* probably serve as vectors of secondary importance. Infection usually occurs during summer and fall, when tick activity is at its peak. Nymphs and adults may transmit the organism to the host, but because the nymphs are only 1-2 mm long, they may not be observed. The primary host for the larval and nymphal stages is the white-footed mouse, and for the adult stage, the white-tailed deer. Non-vector transmission may occur transplacentally, or through infected urine.

Clinical Findings and Diagnosis: Lameness and fever are the predominant clinical signs, but anorexia, fatigue, and lymphadenopathy are common. The lameness is caused by arthritis, which can involve one or several joints. The arthritis is often episodic, but may become chronic. Joints of the forelimb seem to be affected most frequently, and are often painful, warm, and swollen. However, radiographs and routine blood profiles are usually normal. Neurological, cardiac, renal, and reproductive signs have also been observed.

Isolation or demonstration of *B burgdorferi* from blood, urine, or synovial fluid is diagnostic, but so technically difficult as to be of little clinical value. Diagnosis is usually via serology using indirect immunofluorescence or an ELISA test. Results may be obscured by early use of antibiotics, and chronic disease may still occur. High antibody levels may persist for many months, even after treatment. Synovial and/or CSF fluid from animals showing arthritis or neurological signs may also have high antibody titers.

Treatment and Control: Tetracycline, penicillin, erythromycin, and ceftriaxone have all proved beneficial in treating human cases, and even chronic disease has responded to high dose, IV penicillin therapy. Although species-specific therapeutic regimens have not been fully evaluated in domestic animals, it is likely that the same classes of drugs are of value. Dogs have responded to tetracycline, amoxicillin, or ampicillin at standard dosages, given for 21-28 days. Seropositive, asymptomatic animals probably should be treated because reactivity may be a prediction of future disease.

Because ticks do not transmit the spirochete immediately after attachment, the most effective preventive is to examine animals daily or more frequently, and remove ticks immediately. Treating animals frequently with acaricidal dips and tick repellents (such as pyrethrin products) is helpful. Environmental control measures, such as brush clearing and yard spraying are also useful parts of a complete control program. A killed vaccine is available for use in dogs ≥12 wk old. Two 1-mL doses (IM) should be given 3 wk apart, followed by annual revaccination.

MELIOIDOSIS

A bacterial infection characterized by suppurative or caseous lesions in lymph nodes and viscera. Macroscopically, the lesions have no characteristic feature; microscopically, there is a mixed purulent and granulomatous response.

Etiology and Epidemiology: It is caused by *Pseudomonas pseudomallei* (*Bacillus whitmori*, *Loefflerella pseudomallei*, *Malleomyces pseudomallei*), an oval, motile, gram-negative bacillus with bipolar staining. The organisms are found in lesions and discharges, eg, nasal mucus when the respiratory tract is infected, and urine when the kidneys are involved. Originally thought to be restricted to water and moist soils in tropical and subtropical areas, *P pseudomallei* has been isolated from temperate regions (southwest Australia and France). Infection apparently is transmitted from the environment rather than from animal to animal. Outbreaks originating from soil-borne infection occur primarily during or after heavy rainfall or flooding in regions with high humidity or temperature. The organism is an opportunistic pathogen, especially in immunologically depressed hosts. It can be killed easily by heat but can survive for many months in soil and water.

Infections have been recorded in sheep, goats, pigs, cattle, horses, dogs, birds, dolphins, tropical fish, various wild animals, and man. In the laboratory, hamsters, guinea pigs, and rabbits are highly susceptible. Since melioidosis has been recognized frequently in primates imported for research, it is likely that the disease could also occur in primates sold as pets.

Clinical Findings: Signs vary with the site of the lesions; because of this, melioidosis has been called the "mimic" disease. Differential diagnoses include pneumonia, tuberculosis, cholera, malaria, and various arthritides. In domestic animals, it is usually chronic and progressive. In sheep and goats, lung abscesses are common and pneumonia is evident. Nasal discharge occurs if the nasal septum is ulcerated. Sometimes, joints are affected and the animal is lame. Signs of encephalitis may be associated with microabscesses in the CNS. Mastitis can occur in goats, and *P pseudomallei* can be isolated from the milk.

Melioidosis in horses has been reported as nervous disorders, respiratory distress, or colic and diarrhea. In pigs, abscesses in the spleen are commonly found at slaughter. One or more infected abscesses have often been found in clinically normal sheep, goats, and pigs. Death occurs when the abscesses are extensive or when a vital organ is involved.

Diagnosis: Diagnosis is by isolation and identification of the organism and should include agglutination with antiserum. It grows readily on routine diagnostic media and has a characteristic colony form and odor, especially on glycerol-based agar. Some organisms with many of the bacteriological features of *P pseudomallei* are not agglutinated by specific antisera and are not pathogenic to guinea pigs. The complement fixation and indirect hemagglutination tests on serum are useful diagnostic aids in most species, including man. Enzyme immunoassays and immunofluorescent tests are becoming more widely used.

Treatment and Control: Treatment is costly and generally unsatisfactory, because animals can relapse when treatment is discontinued. The organism is sensitive to kanamycin, novobiocin, tetracycline, sulfonamides, and trimethoprim-sulfamethoxazole. Some strains are not sensitive to chloramphenicol. Recently, the β-lactams, imipenem and ceftazidime, have proved active *in vitro* against *P pseudomallei*. The disease can be controlled in intensive farming by raising the animals off the soil and providing clean drinking water (filtered and/or chlorinated). When diarrhea occurs, stables need to be disinfected and carcasses, bedding, and manure disposed of safely. Control in extensive farming is limited to careful surveillance and vaccination. However, vaccines are not effective against a heavy challenge.

NEOSPOROSIS

A recently recognized protozoal infection of dogs and, experimentally, of rodents and cats.

Etiology: *Neospora caninum* is an obligate intracellular parasite that has been confused previously with *Toxoplasma gondii*. Only asexual stages are known, and they resemble *T gondii*. The complete life cycle of *N caninum* is unknown, but it can be transmitted transplacentally in dogs, and subsequent litters may be affected. Tachyzoites are 5-7 × 1-5 μm, depending on the stage of division. They divide by endodyogeny. Tachyzoites are found in myocytes, neural cells, dermal cells, macrophages, and other cells. They are often located directly in the host cell cytoplasm, without a vacuole. Tissue cysts up to 100 μm in diameter are found in neural cells; the cyst wall is amorphous and up to 4 μm thick. Cysts have no septa, and enclose slender 7 × 1.5 μm bradyzoites.

Clinical Findings: Both pups and older dogs are affected. Not all littermates are affected. Most severe infections are in young pups, and typically evident as ascending paralysis of limbs, particularly hindlimbs. The paralysis is often progressive and results in rigid contracture of the muscles of affected limbs. In some dogs, only neural signs are observed. The syndrome of polyradiculoneuromyositis appears typical of neosporosis. Ulcerative dermatitis, hepatitis, pneumonia, and encephalitis may also occur.

Lesions: Nonsuppurative encephalomyelitis, polyradiculoneuritis, acute necrotizing myositis, phlebitis, multifocal/coagulative hepatic necrosis, and atrophy of muscles are predominant findings.

Diagnosis: Serum CPK, AST (SGOT), and ALT (SGPT) levels are elevated. Occasionally, parasites are observed in biopsy specimens. An immunoperoxidase test using specific antibodies can identify *N caninum* in tissue sections or biopsy smears; an indirect FA test can be used to detect antibodies.

Treatment: Treatment is not known, but drugs used to treat toxoplasmosis (sulfadiazine, daraprim, clindamycin) may be tried.

NOCARDIOSIS

A chronic infection resulting from soil-borne organisms of the genus *Nocardia*, and characterized by generalized, purulent, and granulomatous nodular lesions. Etiological agents are *N asteroides, N brasiliensis*, and *N otitidis-caviarum (caviae)*. Cattle appear to be affected most frequently, although the disease is seen in dogs, horses, cats, sheep, goats, and birds, as well as fish and various wild and captive animals, including marine mammals. The histological picture of suppuration and granulation is remarkably similar in different animal species, different anatomical sites, and with the various pathogenic nocardiae. Debate still surrounds the taxonomic classification of *N farcinica*, apparently a chimera of mycobacteria and true nocardiae. *Nocardia asteroides* is now the type species of the genus.

Clinical Findings—Dogs: Signs include fever, soreness, lameness, dyspnea, empyema, enlarged abdomen, lymphadenitis, and fluctuating subcut. or salivary gland abscesses. Granulomatous swellings that resemble actinomycotic lesions are seen, frequently on the extremities. Superficial abscesses rupture and discharge pus that contains flakes of necrotic tissue. The lungs and bronchial lymph nodes nearly always contain suppurative and granulomatous lesions. Well-defined microcolonies are seen in pleural exudates.

Cattle: Mastitis has been the predominant nocardial infection reported in cattle. Systemic illness—prolonged fever, anorexia, loss of condition, increased lacrimation, and salivation—may or may not be evident. Affected mammary glands may become enlarged and firm. The whitish, viscid exudate contains discrete blood clots and small (1 μm) whitish clumps (microcolonies) of bacteria. Sulfur granules are never present. Small draining sinuses are often formed; in severe cases, the gland may rupture. Metastasis to lungs and supramammary lymph nodes may occur. Bovine farcy (a purulent lymphadenitis and lymphangitis), abortion, and pulmonary and generalized infections also have been recorded. Both true nocardiae and mycobacteria (eg, *Mycobacterium farcinogenes*) appear capable of inducing bovine farcy.

Diagnosis: Nocardiosis should be suspected in dogs with unexplained pulmonary disease, with subcut. and salivary gland nodules, or with abscesses. Chest radiographs have revealed diffuse, noncalcified, soft nodules in several lobes of the lungs.

For diagnostic purposes, pus, sputum, or a biopsy specimen is collected from a lesion, and smears are prepared, dried, gram-stained, and examined under oil immersion. The organisms appear as beaded, gram-positive, thin (≤ 1 μm), branching filaments and bacillary forms. They possess a certain degree of acid-fastness, but this is difficult to demonstrate in formalin-fixed material. *Nocardia* spp are easily cultured on blood or brain-heart infusion agar plates incubated at 37°C for ≥ 3 days.

Specific diagnosis of mastitis in cattle depends on culture of clumps in fresh, unrefrigerated milk from the affected quarter. Complement-fixing antibodies and precipitins have been demonstrated in sera of infected cattle. Cutaneous hypersensitivity reactions have proved of diagnostic value.

Treatment: Nocardiosis is frequently fatal despite vigorous chemotherapy. The ability of nocardiae to convert to, or exist in, a cell-wall deficient form may be a factor in the pathogenesis of some infections. Prolonged (6-12 wk) use of cotrimoxazole appears to be the best treatment for dogs. Adjuncts include excision of subcut. abscesses or nodules.

Bovine nocardial mastitis has been treated successfully with udder infusion of 500 mg of novobiocin combined with 25-40 mL of 0.2% nitrofurazone b.i.d. for 3-5 days. However, as with dogs, the treatment of choice is co-trimoxazole. Sanitation and good milking practices are possibly more important than chemotherapy in the control of nocardiosis in a herd. The veterinary role of antibiotics (eg, imipenem, amikacin) effective in human nocardiosis is as yet unknown.

PLAGUE

A disease affecting mainly the lymphatics and lungs, caused by *Yersinia (Pasteurella) pestis*. Although plague is a historic scourge of man, wild rodents, and rabbits, cases associated with cats and dogs are now recognized as hazards to man. Experimental infection in 5 cats resulted in acute illness within 24-48 hr in all. Fever was as high as 106°F (41°C), and 3 of the 5 died (on days 4, 6, and 20). Temperature of the 2 survivors returned to normal by day 6. All of 10 dogs infected experimentally showed transient signs of illness with fever as high as 105°F (40.5°C) persisting for as long as 72 hr, but all recovered and were clinically normal by day 7 after exposure.

Endemic foci of sylvatic plague exist in the western USA and several other areas of the world. Fleas are the vectors that are the primary means of spreading *Y pestis* from these reservoirs, although contact with infected rabbit carcasses has been a significant source of infection for man during winter.

In endemic areas, plague should be suspected in cats as well as wild Felidae (eg, bobcats) that exhibit fever, pneumonia, and lymphadenitis. Diagnosis can be confirmed by blood culture or FA test of lymph node aspirate. Since plague in cats often can be rapidly lethal, therapy should be initiated immediately. Streptomycin and tetracycline in combination are effective and, based on human cases, should be continued for ≥5 days after temperature returns to normal to avoid relapse. Prevention involves eliminating contact with infected wild rodents or rabbits, and their fleas.

Q-FEVER

A rickettsial infection, usually inapparent, but able to cause abortion in sheep, goats, and cattle, and an influenza-like disease in man that may result in chronic endocarditis. The risk of infection is greatly increased for people (veterinarians, livestockmen, abattoir workers, and laboratory personnel) in occupations that bring them in direct or indirect contact with infected, parturient sheep, goats, or cattle, or with products (wool or hides) of infected animals. Several episodes of Q-fever have occurred in personnel and human patients in medical institutions where latently infected sheep were used for research. Human infection apparently was acquired by inhalation of airborne infectious agents.

Etiology and Epidemiology: The causative organism, *Coxiella burnetii*, is distributed worldwide and has been found in various wild and domestic mammals, arthropods, and birds. Domestic cattle, sheep, goats, dogs, and cats are susceptible to infection, and the disease is found in most areas where cattle, sheep, and goats are kept. Ixodid and argasid ticks can be reservoirs of the organism.

The epidemiology is complex because there are 2 major patterns of transmission; in one, the organism circulates between wild animals and their ectoparasites, mainly ticks; the other occurs in domestic ruminants, independent of the wild animal cycle. The organism is disseminated through infected milk, placentas, and postpartum discharges, which provide potential sources of infection for man and other animals.

Coxiella burnetii can survive weeks to years in the environment, and can be spread through aerosolization of infected particles, by direct contact, or by ingestion of reproductive discharges or milk. Based on epidemiological evidence, tick transmission may occur among domestic ruminants. The most important mode of transmission from domestic ruminants to man is through airborne transmission of dust particles from desiccated reproductive fluids; however, obstetrical procedures and raw milk are also involved. High-temperature pasteurization effectively kills the organism. Ticks may occasionally transmit the disease to man.

Clinical Findings and Diagnosis: Infection is usually subclinical, but can cause anorexia and abortion in sheep and goats. Recent reports implicate *C burnetii* as a cause of infertility and sporadic abortion in cattle. Once a domestic ruminant is infected, the organism can localize in mammary glands, supramammary lymph nodes, placenta, and uterus, from which it may be shed in subsequent parturitions and lactations.

Gross lesions are nonspecific in domestic ruminants. The complement fixation test is done most commonly, but agglutination and immunofluorescence tests and microscopy of stained tissues also may be diagnostic. Recovery of the organism poses a threat to laboratory personnel. In domestic ruminants, a differential diagnosis should include infectious and noninfectious agents that cause abortion.

Treatment and Control: A vaccine for animals, although not currently available in the USA, has prevented infection when administered to uninfected sheep and cattle. Tetracycline is the drug of choice for treatment, but it is not as effective as in treatment of other rickettsioses. Segregation of pregnant animals and burning or burying reproductive offal can greatly reduce spread of the organism. *Coxiella burnetii* is highly resistant to physical and chemical agents.

SWEATING SICKNESS

An acute, febrile, tick-borne toxicosis characterized mainly by a profuse, moist eczema and hyperemia of the skin and visible mucous membranes. It is essentially a disease of young calves, although adults also are susceptible. Sheep, pigs, goats, and a dog have been infected experimentally. It occurs in eastern, central, and southern Africa, and probably in Sri Lanka and southern India.

Etiology: The cause is an epitheliotropic toxin produced by females of certain strains of *Hyalomma truncatum*. The toxin develops in the tick, not in the vertebrate host. The potential to produce toxin is retained by ticks for 20 generations, and possibly more. Attempted experimental transmissions between affected and normal animals by contact or inoculations of blood have been unsuccessful.

Graded periods of infestation of a susceptible host by "infected" ticks have different effects on the host. A very short period has no effect; the animal remains susceptible. A period just long enough to produce a reaction may confer an immunity, but if the exposure is >5 days, severe clinical signs and death may result. Recovery confers a durable immunity, which may last ≥4 yr. Other closely related forms of *H truncatum* toxicoses have been described.

Clinical Findings, Lesions, and Diagnosis: After an incubation period of 4-11 days, signs appear suddenly and include hyperthermia, anorexia, listlessness, watering of the eyes and nose, hyperemia of the visible mucous membranes, salivation, necrosis of the oral mucosa, and hyperesthesia. Later, the eyelids stick together. The skin feels hot, and a moist dermatitis soon develops, starting from the base of the ears, the axillae, groin, and perineum, and extending over the entire body. The hair becomes matted, and beads of moisture may be seen on it. The skin becomes extremely sensitive and emits a sour odor. Later, the hair and epidermis can be readily pulled off, exposing red raw wounds. The tips of the ears and the tail may slough away. Eventually, the skin becomes hard and cracked, and predisposed to secondary infection or screwworm infestation. The animal is sensitive to handling, shows pain when moving, and seeks shade.

Often, the course is rapid, and death may occur within a few days. In less acute cases, the course is more protracted and recovery may occur. Mortality in affected calves is 30-70% under natural conditions. Morbidity in endemic areas is ~10%. The severity of infection is influenced by the number of ticks as well as the length of time they remain on the host.

Emaciation, dehydration, diphtheroid stomatitis, pharyngitis, laryngitis, esophagitis, vaginitis or posthitis, edema and hyperemia of the lungs, atrophy of the spleen, and congestion of the liver, kidneys, and meninges are found in addition to the skin lesions described above.

For diagnosis, it is essential to determine the presence of the vector. Typically, there is a generalized hyperemia with subsequent desquamation of the superficial layers of the mucous membranes of the upper respiratory, GI, and external genital tracts, and profuse moist dermatitis followed by superficial desquamation of the skin.

Prophylaxis and Treatment: Control of tick infestation is the only effective prophylactic measure. Removal of ticks, symptomatic treatment, and good nursing are indicated. Non-nephrotoxic antibiotics and anti-inflammatory agents are useful to combat secondary infection. Immune serum can be used to good effect as a specific treatment.

TOXOPLASMOSIS

Toxoplasma gondii is a protozoan that infects most species of warm-blooded animals, including birds and man, in most parts of the world.

Etiology: The entire life cycle is completed in the epithelium of the small intestine of members of the cat family; asexual and sexual stages develop endogenously, and oocysts are shed in the feces. Three forms or stages of *T gondii* can initiate infection in cats or other vertebrates: 1) The trophozoite or tachyzoite is the actively proliferating form seen in acute disseminated infections and can be present in blood, urine, tears, saliva, semen, feces, or body fluids, and in a wide range of tissues. It is crescent-shaped, 4-8 × 2-4 μm, and stains well with Giemsa. It survives in the environment or in dead animal tissues for only a few hours. 2) The cystozoite or bradyzoite is the resting form of *Toxoplasma* and is present in congenital and acquired, chronic, or asymptomatic infections. It is found in cysts, mainly in the brain, eye, liver, and skeletal and cardiac musculature. Individual cysts are 50-150 μm in diameter, and each has an argyrophilic, elastic cyst wall that encloses many hundreds of closely packed periodic-acid-Schiff-positive zoites. This form can survive in tissues for several days after death, but is readily destroyed by cooking to ≥151°F (66°C). 3) The oocyst is passed in the feces of susceptible cats following ingestion of any of the 3 infective forms (tachyzoites, bradyzoites, oocysts). Following ingestion of encysted *Toxoplasma* bradyzoites, oocysts (10 × 12 μm) appear in the feces after 4-5 days and continue to be excreted, often in enormous numbers, for 3-20 days. These oocysts sporulate in 2-4 days and are then infective for virtually all vertebrates. Oocysts are resistant and may survive >1 yr under favorable conditions. They are destroyed by dry heat at 158°F (70°C), boiling water, strong iodine, and strong ammonia solutions.

Clinical Findings: Most infections by *Toxoplasma* are latent or asymptomatic. High serum IgG titers are common in sheep, pigs, and cats; less common in dogs and horses; and even less common in cattle. Clinical infection is relatively uncommon in most species, but sporadic cases and occasional epidemics are seen, particularly in young and stressed animals, and outbreaks of congenital infection have been reported. Generally, the clinical infection runs a similar course in most species. In the young, the infection is usually acute and generalized; in adults, it is often associated with chronic CNS involvement alone. In young animals, particularly puppies, kittens, and piglets, signs include fever, anorexia, cough, dyspnea, diarrhea, jaundice, and CNS dysfunction. Lesions include pneumonitis, lymphadenitis, hepatitis, myocarditis, and encephalomyelitis.

Toxoplasmosis is an important cause of abortions and stillbirths, particularly in sheep and sometimes in pigs and goats. In sheep and goats, lesions in the fetal cotyledons consist of multiple white foci of necrosis up to 2 mm in diameter; in the fetus, there may be extensive areas of leukoencephalomalacia and glial nodules, some of which may show central necrosis and mineralization.

Diagnosis: Demonstration of the characteristic lesions and *Toxoplasma*-like organisms in tissue sections should be supported by isolation of the organism and serological testing. Isolation consists of IP injection of suspect material into mice free of natural *Toxoplasma* infection. Some strains of *Toxoplasma* are lethal to mice in 5-12 days and Giemsa-stained smears of peritoneal exudate show many intracellular and free forms of *Toxoplasma* trophozoites. Most strains of *Toxoplasma* are not lethal to mice but produce a chronic infection with tissue cysts. Mice can be bled after 4-6 wk and their serum *Toxoplasma* antibody titer measured. Also, wet "squash" preparations of brain can be made and examined for *Toxoplasma* cysts.

Several reliable serological tests are available for the detection of *Toxoplasma* antibodies, although *Hammondia* antibody from intermediate hosts reacts with *Toxoplasma* antigen and must be ruled out in such tests. The Sabin-Feldman dye test (DT), and the complement fixation, indirect fluorescent antibody (IFA), indirect hemagglutination (IHA), ELISA, and agglutination (AG) tests are some of the serological tests used for diagnosis. Kits that contain all reagents needed for IFA, IHA, ELISA, and AG are commercially available. The IFA and IHA tests are less sensitive than the DT.

A 4-fold rise in IgG antibody titers in samples taken 2-3 wk apart is required to confirm active infection. High IgG titers reflect past infection and continued presence of encysted *Toxoplasma*; in cats, they indicate immunity to oocyst shedding. High IgM titers in cats indicate active infection and correlate well with recent shedding of oocysts or disease (which means that such cats [with high IgM titers] are potential public health risks).

Some of the reported cases of toxoplasmosis in cattle diagnosed by histological methods probably were due to other protozoan parasites, eg, the schizont stage of *Sarcocystis*. Similarly, infections in calves, puppies, and kittens may have been confused with infections caused by *Neospora caninum* (qv, p 361) or closely related protozoa.

Treatment: For animals other than man, treatment is seldom warranted. Sulfadiazine (73 mg/kg body wt) acts synergistically with pyrimethamine (0.44 mg/kg) in the treatment of acute, severe toxoplasmosis in laboratory animals and man. Since these drugs seem to affect only the free organisms (not cysts), treatment should be instituted as early as possible. This therapy can produce a reversible toxic depression of the bone marrow, which can be prevented by B vitamins and folinic acid. Clindamycin is the drug of choice for treatment of *Toxoplasma* infections of dogs and cats. Total dosages (oral or parenteral) are 10-40 and 25-50 mg/kg, respectively, for dogs and cats. Treatment is continued for ≥2 wk. Side effects of anorexia, vomiting, or diarrhea are alleviated by reducing or dividing the daily dosage.

Transmission and Prophylaxis: A previously unexposed pregnant animal can develop parasitemia with spread of the infection to the uterus; a latent or overt congenital infection can result. In several species of laboratory rodents, asymptomatic congenital infections have been transmitted vertically for several generations.

Probably most *Toxoplasma* infections are acquired after birth. In strict carnivores, infection is thought to follow ingestion of fresh, infected (and uncooked) meat or carcasses from a wide range of intermediate hosts. In herbivores, most infections are thought to result from ingestion of herbage contaminated by *Toxoplasma* oocysts derived from cat feces. In omnivores, including man, infection seems to result both from ingestion of undercooked meat and from accidental ingestion of oocysts.

In any host species, latent toxoplasmosis can become active and cause an overt generalized infection. This has resulted from concurrent infections (eg, viruses, protozoans), neoplastic diseases, environmental stresses, or immunosuppression. At any given time, ~1% of all cats in the USA are shedding *Toxoplasma* oocysts in their feces. Reshedding oocysts infrequently follows reinfection by *Toxoplasma* cysts, and rarely (if ever) occurs if the cat develops enteritis, becomes infected with other coccidia, or is immunosuppressed.

To minimize oocyst transmission, cats should not be fed raw meat nor permitted to kill birds or rodents; litter should be disposed of daily (before sporulation of oocysts), preferably by incineration. Pregnant women should avoid contact with cats and cat litter. Laboratory personnel working with cats or handling cat feces should avoid contamination of laboratory benches and instruments, and should wear gloves and protective clothing.

A vaccine is not available.

TUBERCULOSIS (TB)

An infectious disease caused by acid-fast bacilli of the genus *Mycobacterium*. Although commonly defined as a chronic, debilitating disease, TB occasionally assumes an acute, rapidly progressive course. The disease affects practically all species of vertebrates, and before control measures were adopted, was a major disease of man and domestic animals. Signs and lesions are generally similar in the various species.

Etiology: Three main types of tubercle bacilli are recognized: human, bovine, and avian; respectively, *M tuberculosis, M bovis,* and *M avium* complex (*M avium-intracellulare-scrofulaceum*). The 3 types differ in cultural characteristics and pathogenicity. The 2 mammalian types are more closely related to each other than to the avian type. More than 30 serovars of *M avium* complex are recognized; however, only serovars 1 and 2 are pathogenic for birds (*see also* p 1601).

All 3 types may produce infection in host species other than their own. *Mycobacterium tuberculosis* is most specific; it rarely produces progressive disease in the lower animals other than nonhuman primates and occasionally dogs and parrots. *Mycobacterium avium* complex (serovars 1 and 2) is the only species of consequence in birds, but it is also pathogenic for pigs, cattle, sheep, mink, dogs, cats, and some cold-blooded animals. *Mycobacterium bovis* can cause progressive disease in most warm-blooded vertebrates, including man. Mycobacteria other than tubercle bacilli (qv, p 370) are infrequently isolated from exotic and domestic animals.

Pathogenesis: Disease commences with formation of a primary focus, which in man and cattle, usually is in a lung, and, in poultry, nearly always in the intestinal tract. Lymphatic drainage from the primary focus in mammals leads to formation of caseous lesions in adjacent lymph nodes; these lesions, together with the primary focus, are known as the "primary complex". This primary complex seldom heals in animals, but may progress slowly or rapidly.

When the lesion localizes, a tumor-like, granulomatous mass called a tubercle results. Continued growth of organisms causes enlargement of the granuloma with subsequent central necrosis, caseation, and a tendency to mineralize. In mammals, tubercles may become enclosed by dense, fibrous, connective tissue, and the disease becomes arrested. Lymphatogenous and hematogenous spread of bacilli from primary foci result in tubercles in other organs and tissues, the number and extent of which are related to the number of circulating bacilli. These generalized lesions may become encapsulated and remain small for long periods, usually causing no detectable clinical signs; however, an acute form of generalization, known as miliary TB, is often rapidly fatal.

Clinical Findings: Signs depend on the extent and location of lesions. Enlarged superficial lymph nodes provide a useful diagnostic sign; however, lesions in deep lymph nodes are of little or no value in establishing a clinical diagnosis. The general signs are weakness, anorexia, dyspnea, emaciation, and low-grade fluctuating fever. In *M bovis* infections in mammals, the thoracic organs usually are involved. When lungs are extensively involved, an intermittent, hacking cough is common. The principal sign of TB commonly is chronic wasting or emaciation, which occurs despite good nutrition and care. In pigs, lesions due to *M avium* are most often observed in lymph nodes associated with the GI tract; however, generalized disease does occur.

Diagnosis: Clinical diagnosis is usually possible only after the disease is advanced. Most infected animals have become shedders of tubercle bacilli by this time and a menace to other animals. Radiography is used in nonhuman primates and small domestic animals. The most reliable and practical method of reaching a tentative diagnosis in large domestic animals is the tuberculin skin test. Animals infected with mycobacteria develop a delayed hypersensitivity reaction, characterized by inflammation and swelling, where tuberculin was injected intradermally.

Animals infected with either *M bovis* or *M tuberculosis* react about equally to tuberculin prepared from a culture filtrate of either organism. Because birds or mammals with avian TB react less, or not at all, to mammalian tuberculin, avian tuberculin must be used in those cases.

The dose used in an intradermal tuberculin test is 0.1 mL (0.1 mg protein) in mammals and 0.05 mL in chickens. In larger mammals in the USA, tuberculin is usually injected in a skin fold near the base of the tail or in skin of the cervical region. In pigs, the injection is in the skin on the dorsal surface of an ear or the vulva; in chickens, in the skin of a wattle. Injection sites are observed and palpated for characteristic swelling 48 hr after injection in pigs and chickens, and 72 hr in cattle and most exotic and wild animals except primates. (*See also* p 1032.)

Nearly all countries currently use a strain of *M bovis* for preparation of mammalian tuberculin for veterinary use. Heat-concentrated, synthetic-medium tuberculin (old tuberculin [OT]) is still used in some countries, but a majority (including the USA) are now using a purified-protein-derivative (PPD) tuberculin at a protein concentration of 1 mg/mL. The PPD tuberculins are preferable because they are easier to standardize and more specific than OT. PPD tuberculins also are particularly useful in the comparative-cervical (c-c) tuberculin test used to differentiate responses caused by mammalian tubercle bacilli and by other mycobacteria. The c-c test in cattle is performed by injecting *M avium* and *M bovis* PPD tuberculins intradermally into separate sites on the neck. The difference in size of the 2 responses usually indicates whether tuberculin sensitivity is caused by infection with *M bovis* rather than *M avium* complex, *M paratuberculosis*, or a transient sensitization from saprophytic mycobacteria (eg, *M terrae*, *M nonchromogenicum*) in the environment. These organisms are responsible for some of the false-positive tuberculin reactions that are a major problem in areas where TB has been nearly eliminated. The incidence of reactors with no gross lesions can be greatly reduced by use of the c-c test applied by experienced personnel; however, the c-c test should not be used in herds in which *M bovis* has been diagnosed. To confirm a diagnosis of TB, the etiological agent must be isolated and identified. Culture results usually require 4-8 wk.

Control: The main reservoirs of infection are man and cattle; however, badgers, bison, opossums, kudu, deer, llamas, elk, and domestic and feral pigs have been found infected with *M bovis*. The prevalence of the disease in such reservoirs influences the incidence of disease in other species.

The 3 principal approaches to the control of TB are test and slaughter, test and segregation, and chemotherapy. In the test-and-slaughter method, reactors to the tuberculin test are slaughtered. This method has been used widely in the UK, USA, Canada, New Zealand, and Australia. In most European countries, where test and slaughter would have been impractical, varying forms of test and segregation have been used, with test and slaughter employed only in the final stages of eradication. Isoniazid (INH) can be used for chemotherapy, but the disadvantages are so great (up to 25% refractory cases, emergence of drug-resistant strains, presence of INH in the milk, and danger of relapse when the drug is withdrawn) that treatment of bovine TB is not allowed in the USA or in most other countries.

While BCG (bacillus of Calmette-Guérin) vaccine is an immunizing agent used in man in some high-risk areas, it does not completely prevent infection in cattle or captive exotic animals. Moreover, vaccinated animals react to the tuberculin skin test. Countries that attempted to use vaccination as the basis of a control program for bovine TB ultimately abandoned the procedure in favor of the test-and-slaughter method.

TUBERCULOSIS IN CAPTIVE, EXOTIC, HOOFED ANIMALS

Numerous species, including bison, elephants, rhinoceri, kudu, camels, llamas, giraffes, and oryx are susceptible to *M bovis*. Lesions usually involve the lungs and thoracic lymph nodes. A tentative diagnosis can usually be made by conducting tuberculin skin tests. Isoniazid therapy has been used. Because of public health significance, infected animals should be maintained in isolation.

TUBERCULOSIS IN CATS

Cats, unlike dogs, are resistant to infection with *M tuberculosis*. Most natural infections with *M bovis* arise from ingestion of contaminated milk, and primary lesions are found in the GI tract. However, respiratory infection does occur. Infected wounds sometimes give rise to tuberculous sinuses. At one time, up to 12% of cats necropsied in parts of Europe were tuberculous, but with elimination of tubercle bacilli from the milk supply, the disease has become rare.

Lesions in cats generally resemble those in dogs. Few isolated primary foci have been recorded, and it appears that infection is followed by rapid dissemination. Lesions and discharges usually contain large numbers of bacilli.

The tuberculin skin test is considered unreliable in cats, and radiographic diagnosis is often difficult. Isolation of acid-fast bacilli provides evidence of infection, but negative culture results are of questionable value. Because of the public health significance, affected animals should be euthanized, as should cats on premises being depopulated because of bovine TB.

TUBERCULOSIS IN CATTLE

Once widespread, particularly in dairy cattle, control programs have so reduced the incidence that several countries have virtually eliminated it. A few infected herds continue to be identified in diverse areas of the USA. The source of infection is usually other infected cattle, although in some countries, pulmonary or genitourinary TB in man, or bovine TB in wild animals are sources of infection.

Tuberculous animals with nonencapsulated lung lesions expel infected droplets into the air by coughing, and contaminate pasture via the feces. Adult animals are infected by inhalation of airborne dust particles as well as by ingestion of contaminated feed or water. Calves may become infected by drinking contaminated milk.

Acute lesions are usually found in the thorax and sometimes in the lymph nodes of the head or intestines. Lesions may be found in many organs in advanced stages of the disease and in tissues that seldom are primarily affected; thus, infection of the udder, uterus, various lymph nodes, kidneys, and the meninges occurs with varying frequency. The skeletal muscles are seldom affected, even in advanced cases. TB of the udder is of special significance because of the contamination of milk with viable tubercle bacilli.

TUBERCULOSIS IN DOGS

Dogs may be infected by *M tuberculosis*, *M bovis*, and rarely by *M avium* complex or *M fortuitum*. Dogs may be infected from a human source and may in turn infect man, especially children. The short-nosed breeds appear to be more susceptible, and males are affected more commonly than females.

Tuberculous lesions in dogs often resemble neoplasms, and calcification is rare. The lesions are usually grayish white and circumscribed. Liver lesions are large and yellowish with depressed centers and hemorrhagic edges. Some of these lesions have soft, purulent centers; others appear as ragged bloody cavities or may take the form of multiple, small, gray nodules scattered throughout the liver.

Lung lesions usually consist of grayish red bronchopneumonic areas; some disseminate to form cavities. These may open into the pleural cavity or communicate with a bronchus. Pulmonary and pleural lesions are invariably exudative, and a large quantity of straw-colored liquid may be in the thorax. Some lesions may cause collapse of the lower portions of lung.

False-negative tuberculin tests are common in dogs; radiographs and history of exposure are useful in diagnosis. Because of the public health significance, affected dogs should be euthanized, as should dogs on premises being depopulated of cattle infected with bovine TB.

TUBERCULOSIS IN NONHUMAN PRIMATES

Monkeys and large apes are susceptible to *M bovis*, *M tuberculosis*, and *M avium*. Epidemics have been reported in several primate colonies. Control and eradication are difficult to achieve, since pulmonary disease commonly occurs. New World monkeys appear to be more resistant to infection than Old World monkeys. Isoniazid has been used to treat animals infected with *M tuberculosis* or *M bovis*; however, monkeys may continue to shed bacilli in urine. Tuberculin skin tests have been widely used in detecting infected animals. Tuberculins prepared for veterinary use should be utilized in testing monkeys. PPD tuberculins prepared for use in man are not sufficiently potent to elicit delayed-type hypersensitivity responses in these species. (*See also* p 1032.)

TUBERCULOSIS IN PIGS

Pigs are susceptible to infection with all 3 types of tubercle bacilli. Infection is most often contracted by ingestion of infected materials; hence, the primary lesions are in the GI tract and associated lymph nodes, particularly the mesenteric, cervical, or submaxillary.

Dissemination is often severe and rapid with *M bovis*, but infection with *M avium* or *M tuberculosis* is usually limited to the lymph nodes of the head and to the GI tract and associated lymph nodes. Lesions caused by *M avium* or *M tuberculosis* generally are not invasive, whereas *M bovis* usually causes a rapidly progressive disease with caseation and liquefaction of the lesions. Differentiation of type of infection must be confirmed by isolation and identification of the organism.

TUBERCULOSIS IN SHEEP AND GOATS

TB is rare in sheep and goats, but when it occurs, *M bovis* causes a condition similar to that in cattle; the avian bacillus may cause disseminated lesions. A tentative diagnosis may be made by injecting *M bovis* and *M avium* PPD tuberculin at separate sites in the cervical region.

MYCOBACTERIAL INFECTIONS OTHER THAN TUBERCULOSIS

Mycobacteria found in soil and water have been isolated from tissues of animals. *Mycobacterium fortuitum*, a rapidly growing organism that is highly resistant to penicillin G, streptomycin, ampicillin, sulfamethoxazole, and chloramphenicol, has been associated with mastitis in cows, pulmonary infections in dogs, lymph node lesions in pigs and certain exotic animals, and cutaneous lesions in cats and dogs. Drug susceptibility tests indicate the organism is inhibited by capreomycin and by ethionamide. *Mycobacterium chelonei*, another rapidly growing mycobacterium similar to *M fortuitum* in biochemical reactions, has been isolated from contaminated wounds and injection abscesses. These organisms must be distinguished from *M parafortuitum*, *M phlei*, *M smegmatis*, and *M vaccae*, which are rarely if ever pathogenic.

Fish and other cold-blooded animals can be infected with a photochromogenic acid-fast organism, *M marinum*, which has been recognized as a human pathogen. Another photochromogenic organism, *M kansasii*, has been isolated from pigs, cattle, and nonhuman primates. These organisms can be differentiated on biochemical and seroagglutination tests.

Mycobacterium scrofulaceum, a scotochromogen, has been isolated from lymph node lesions in pigs, cattle, and certain nonhuman primates. *Myobacterium xenopi*, a slowly growing scotochromogen, has been isolated from pigs, seafowl, and amphibians. These organisms should be differentiated from *M gordonae* and *M flavescens*, and other slowly growing scotochromogenic mycobacteria that are common contaminants of water.

Numerous nonpathogenic, nonphotochromogenic mycobacteria that closely resemble potential pathogens can be isolated from water and soil: *M nonchromogenicum*, *M gastri*, *M triviale*, and *M terrae*, which closely resemble strains of the *M avium* complex, may be differentiated by *in vitro* laboratory examinations.

Although opportunistic mycobacteria usually fail to produce progessive disease, they may be important in inducing transient tuberculin skin sensitivity in animals. The application of c-c skin tests, using biologically balanced PPD tuberculins prepared from culture filtrates of *M bovis* and *M avium*, provides useful information on the possible cause of tuberculin skin sensitivity. Tuberculins prepared for veterinary use, containing ~5000 tuberculin units per test dose, should be used for skin tests in domestic, wild, and exotic animals.

Mycobacterium lepraemurium, a nonphotochromogenic, slow-growing, acid-fast bacillus, causes a disease in cats and rats similar in some respects to leprosy in man. The organism can be grown on media containing cytochrome C and α-ketoglutarate. The cause of leprosy in man, *M leprae*, has been found in spontaneously occurring disease in armadillos. This organism has not been grown on artificial culture medium.

TULAREMIA

A bacterial septicemia that affects >100 species of wild and domestic mammals, birds, reptiles, and fish, as well as man. The primary domestic animal host is the sheep, but clinical infection has been reported in dogs, cats, pigs, and horses. Cattle appear to be resistant. Little is known of the true incidence and spectrum of clinical disease in domestic animals. Important wild animal hosts include cottontail and jack rabbits, beaver, muskrat, meadow voles, and sheep in North America, and other voles, field mice, and lemmings in Europe and Asia.

Natural foci of infection exist in North America and Eurasia, where the organism circulates between arthropod vectors and various mammals, birds, reptiles, and fish.

Etiology: The causative organism, *Francisella tularensis*, is a nonsporulating, gram-negative rod that is antigenically related to brucellae. It is killed rapidly by heat and proper disinfection, but survives for weeks or months in a moist environment. It is fastidious in growth, but can be cultured readily; laboratory personnel are at high risk of infection. The organisms occur in 2 types, based on their biochemistry and virulence. Type A has been found only in North America and is more virulent; in man, the mortality rate may be 5-7% if untreated. Type B is less virulent and is most commonly isolated from aquatic animals and water-associated infections. Both types have been isolated from arthropod vectors.

Transmission and Epidemiology: Tularemia is a classic zoonosis, capable of being transmitted by aerosol, direct contact, ingestion, or arthropods. Inhalation of infectious aerosols (or organisms, as in the laboratory) can produce a pneumonic form. Direct contact with, or ingestion of, infected carcasses of wild animals (eg, cottontail rabbit) can produce the ulceroglandular, oculoglandular, or oropharyngeal form (local lesion with regional lymphadenitis), or the typhoidal form. Immersion in or drinking contaminated water can produce infection in aquatic animals. Ticks can maintain infection transstadially and transovarially, which makes them an efficient reservoir as well as a vector. Recognized vectors in the USA include *Dermacentor andersoni*, the "wood tick"; *Amblyomma americanum*, the "lone star tick"; *Dermacentor variabilis*, the "dog tick"; and *Chrysops discalis*, the "deerfly".

The most common source of infection for man and herbivores is the bite of an infected tick, but persons who dress, prepare, or eat improperly cooked wild game are also at increased risk. Dogs, cats, and other carnivores may acquire infection from ingestion of an infected carcass.

Clinical Findings and Lesions: Tularemia has an incubation period of 1-10 days. In sheep and most mammals, it is characterized by sudden onset of high fever, lethargy, anorexia, stiffness, reduced mobility, or other signs associated with septicemic disease. Pulse and respiration rates are accelerated; coughing, diarrhea, and pollakiuria may develop. Prostration and death may occur in a few hours or days. Sporadic cases in any species are best recognized by signs of septicemia. Mortality may be up to 15% in outbreaks in untreated lambs. Subclinical cases may be common.

The most consistent lesions are miliary, whitish foci of necrosis in the liver, and sometimes in the spleen and lymph nodes. Enlargement of the liver, spleen, and lymph nodes is common. Organisms can be readily isolated from necropsy specimens by use of special media. Risk of infection during necropsy or to laboratory personnel is significant; special procedures and facilities are essential.

Diagnosis: Tularemia must be differentiated from other septicemic diseases (especially plague) or acute pneumonia. When large numbers of sheep exhibit typical signs during periods of heavy tick infestation, tularemia or tick paralysis (qv, p 624) should be suspected.

Diagnosis of acute infection is confirmed by culture and identification of the bacterium, indirect FA test, or a 4-fold increase in antibody titer between acute and convalescent serum specimens. A single titer of $\geq$1:80 by the tube agglutination test is presumptive evidence of prior infection.

Treatment and Control: Streptomycin, tetracyclines, gentamicin, and doxycycline are effective at recommended dose levels. Early treatment should prevent death loss. Control is difficult and is limited to reducing tick infestation and to rapid diagnosis and treatment. Persistent treatment may be necessary since many organisms are intracellular. Vaccines are available for high-risk personnel; recovery confers long-lasting immunity.

VESICULAR STOMATITIS

A viral disease characterized by fever and vesicles on the mucous membranes of the mouth, epithelium of the tongue, teats, soles of the feet, coronary band, and occasionally other parts of the body. Cattle, horses, and pigs are naturally susceptible; sheep and goats are infected occasionally. The agents have a wide host range, including deer, bobcats, raccoons, and monkeys; many rodents and cold-blooded animals have been infected experimentally. An influenza-like disease has occurred in people working with affected animals or the virus. Vesicular stomatitis has been confirmed only in North and South America.

Etiology and Epidemiology: The rod-shaped viruses belong to the rhabdovirus group, members of which parasitize not only mammals, but also fish, insects, and plants—a diversity of hosts unknown for any other group of viruses.

There are 2 distinct serotypes: the New Jersey and Indiana, with 3 subtypes of the latter. There is no cross-immunity between the 2 serotypes or between the viruses of vesicular stomatitis, foot-and-mouth disease, vesicular exanthema, and swine vesicular disease. It is not as contagious as foot-and-mouth disease. In a herd, up to 90% of the animals show clinical signs, and nearly all develop antibodies. The virus is found in abundance in the clear vesicular fluid and vesicular coverings; it is most infective when the vesicles rupture or shortly thereafter. However, the lesions may be innocuous 5 or 6 days later.

Vesicular stomatitis usually occurs epidemically in temperate regions and endemically in warmer regions. Insect vectors and movement of animals probably are responsible for its spread. The Indiana serotype is transmitted by phlebotomine sandflies. It can spread rapidly, often affecting many animals in 1 wk. In endemic regions, it occurs during the warm season, often during or at the end of the rainy season. A persistent phase of the virus also is probable.

The primary route of infection is unknown but may be through the skin or respiratory tract. Generalized lesions occur, but viremia is unusual.

Clinical Findings: The incubation period is 2-8 days, or possibly longer. Frequently, excessive salivation is the first sign. Examination of the mouth may reveal blanched, raised vesicles. The lesions vary in size; some are no larger than a pea, while others may involve the entire surface of the tongue. In horses, the lesions are principally confined to the upper surface of the tongue but may involve the inner surface of the lips, angles of the mouth, and the gums. In cattle, the lesions may also occur on the hard palate, lips, and gums, and sometimes extend to the muzzle and around the nostrils. Secondary lesions involving the feet of horses and cattle are not exceptional. Teat lesions are found in dairy herds. In natural infections of pigs, foot lesions are frequent, and lameness often is the first sign observed. Body temperature may rise immediately before, or simultaneously with, the appearance of vesicles. Ordinarily, there are no complications and the disease is self-limiting, with recovery in ~2 wk. In dairy herds, loss of production may be serious and mastitis may be a sequela. Serum antibodies persist for life, but recrudescence of disease or reinfection may occur.

Diagnosis: Vesicular stomatitis, while economically important, is of particular significance because of its similarity to foot-and-mouth disease, vesicular exanthema, and swine vesicular disease. Because of this, outbreaks must be diagnosed accurately. When vesicular stomatitis affects horses under natural conditions, there is no serious diagnostic problem because horses are not susceptible to foot-and-mouth disease. Diagnosis is made on the distribution and character of the lesions, and the disease may be differentiated from horse pox by the absence of papules and pustules. In cattle and pigs, diagnosis is by complement fixation or ELISA using a suspension of the epithelial lesion as antigen. If this is negative, the material is passaged in mice, embryonating eggs, or tissue cultures, and then complement fixation, ELISA, and virus neutralization tests are performed. Antibodies in the sera of recovered animals also can be detected by these tests. Electron microscopy may be performed on the original sample or passaged material.

Treatment and Control: Suspected cases should be brought immediately to the attention of state or federal authorities. There is no specific treatment. Secondary infection of the abraded tissue and other sequelae should be treated symptomatically. Vaccines are available in some Latin American countries. Movement of animals should be restricted, and trucks and fomites disinfected.

AFRICAN HORSE SICKNESS (AHS)

An acute or subacute, insect-borne, viral disease of Equidae, endemic to the African continent, and characterized by clinical signs and lesions associated with respiratory and circulatory impairment.

Etiology and Epidemiology: AHS is caused by an orbivirus, 55-70 nm in diameter, of the family Reoviridae. There are 9 immunologically distinct types. Extracts of mouse brain infected with AHS virus hemagglutinate horse RBC. The virus is inactivated at a pH of <6 or ≥12, or by formalin, β-propiolactone, acetylethyleneimine derivatives, or radiation.

Appearance of AHS is preceded by seasons of heavy rain that alternate with hot and dry climatic conditions. Outbreaks in Central and East Africa have extended to

Egypt, the Middle East, and southern Arabia. In 1950-1960, a major epidemic extended from India to the Near Eastern countries; an estimated 300,000 Equidae were destroyed. A second outbreak in 1966 occurred in northeast Africa and southern Spain. In 1987, the disease entered Spain via imported zebra from Namibia. Both these outbreaks in Spain were controlled, but another occurred in 1988, and sporadic cases occurred through early 1989. In a survey in Egypt, antibodies to AHS virus were detected in sheep, goats, camels, buffaloes, and dogs.

Transmission: *Culicoides* spp are the principal vectors of transmission. AHS occurs during rainy warm seasons, which favor propagation of the vectors, and disappears after frost. The virus has been isolated from blood of clinically healthy street dogs, the dog tick *Rhipicephalus sanguineus sanguineus*, and the camel tick *Hyalomma dromedarii* during winter in the Aswan region in southern Egypt where the disease is endemic. It has been transmitted experimentally by mosquitoes. Limited studies in Egypt using dogs that had recovered from experimental infection revealed that 3 successive daily attacks by groups of *Culex pipiens* activated latent AHS virus and initiated viremia and fever. It was suggested that the virus may overwinter in dogs with persistent infection. However, the full role of arthropods in transmission of the disease is unknown.

Clinical Findings and Lesions: Mortality depends on virulence of the isolate and susceptibility of the host, and may reach 90% in epidemics. The acute respiratory form is characterized by an incubation period of 3-5 days, interlobular edema, and hydropericardium; death occurs in ~1 wk. A fever of 40-40.5°C (104-105°F) for 1-2 days is followed by dyspnea, spasmodic coughing, and dilated nostrils; the animal stands with its legs apart and head extended. The conjunctiva is congested and the supraorbital fossa may be swollen. Recovery is rare, and the animal dies of anoxia. At necropsy, there is pulmonary edema, which is especially visible in the intralobular spaces. The lungs are distended and heavy, and frothy fluid may be found in the trachea, bronchi, and bronchioles. There may be pleural effusion. Thoracic lymph nodes may be edematous, and the gastric fundus congested. There may be an increase in pericardial fluid. Cardiac lesions usually are not outstanding. The abdominal viscera may be congested. A frothy exudate may ooze from the nostrils. The pulmonary form is the usual form in dogs.

The cardiac form is subacute, and the incubation period is 1-2 wk. The febrile reaction of <1 wk is followed by swelling of the supraorbital fossa, which is pathognomonic. Swelling usually extends to the eyelids, facial tissues, neck, thorax, brisket, and shoulders. Death usually occurs within 1 wk and may be preceded by colic. Mortality rate is ~50%. Petechiae and ecchymoses on the epicardium and endocardium are prominent. The lungs are usually flaccid or slightly edematous. There are yellow, gelatinous infiltrations of the subcut. and IM tissues, especially along the jugular veins and ligamentum nuchae. Other lesions include hydrocardium, myocarditis, hemorrhagic gastritis, and petechiae on the ventral surface of the tongue and peritoneum. A mixed pulmonary and cardiac form is usually found in outbreaks, with signs and lesions of one type predominating.

Diagnosis: In endemic areas, clinical signs and lesions may lead to provisional diagnosis. However, laboratory confirmation is essential for definitive diagnosis and determination of the serotype; the latter is important for control measures. Blood specimens should be obtained at the peak of fever, preserved in OCG solution (50% glycerol, 0.5% potassium oxalate, 0.5% phenol), and transported (at 4°C) to the laboratory. Spleen samples collected from freshly dead animals should be preserved in 10% buffered glycerin. For virus isolation, infant mice or cell cultures are used. Infected mice may develop nervous and paralytic signs and should be observed for 3 wk. To obtain a high-titered antigen from mouse brains for the complement fixation (CF) test, 2 or 3 subpassages may be necessary. Brains from paralyzed mice only are harvested for antigen preparation. The CF test is useful for disease diagnosis; virus neutralization and/or hemagglutination-inhibition tests are used for serotyping.

Prevention and Control: Surviving Equidae develop solid immunity to the particular serotype but remain susceptible to other serotypes. There are vaccines for all 9 serotypes. These are either cell-culture adapted or mouse-brain attenuated, and provide long-lasting protection. Inactivated vaccines are available; 2 doses are required to provide adequate immunity. These vaccines induce local reaction at the site of inoculation and a short protection period.

When the disease first appears in an area, affected horses should be eliminated immediately, and the noninfected Equidae should be vaccinated with polyvalent vaccine and rested for 2 wk. When the virus isolate has been typed, animals that received polyvalent vaccine should be revaccinated with the homologous vaccine. Vector control is also initiated by using insecticides and repellents. Vaccinated horses should be kept in insect-proof housing since vaccine failure may occur. Aircraft flying from endemic areas to countries free of the disease should be sprayed with insecticides on arrival. In the USA, equids from African countries are quarantined for 2 mo and then tested for the virus. Presence of antibodies does not interfere with importation of Equidae into countries free of the disease.

EQUINE EHRLICHIOSIS

An infectious, noncontagious, seasonal disease seen chiefly in northern California but also recognized in Colorado, Illinois, Florida, Arkansas, Washington, and Pennsylvania. (*See also* POTOMAC HORSE FEVER, p 185.)

Etiology: The causal rickettsial agent, *Ehrlichia equi*, resembles the etiological agents of tick-borne fever and bovine petechial fever. *Ehrlichia equi* is present in cytoplasmic vacuoles of neutrophils and, occasionally, eosinophils during the acute state. Giemsa- or Wright-Leishman-stained blood smears reveal one or more loose aggregates (morulae or inclusion bodies, 1.5-5 μm in diameter) of blue-gray to dark blue coccoid, coccobacillary, or pleomorphic organisms within the cytoplasm of neutrophils. The vector, reservoir, incubation period, and mode of transmission of *E equi* are unknown, although tick transmission is suspected. The infection can be experimentally transmitted to susceptible horses by whole blood; incubation is 1-2 wk.

Clinical Findings and Lesions: Severity of signs varies with age of the animal and duration of the illness. Signs may be mild. Horses <1 yr old may have a fever only. One- to 3-yr-olds develop fever, depression, mild limb edema, and ataxia. Adults show the characteristic signs of fever, partial anorexia, depression, limb edema, petechiation, icterus, and reluctance to move. The fever is highest during the first 1-3 days of infection, fluctuating between 103-104°F (39.5-40°C). Fever of 102-104°F (39-40°C) persists for 6-12 days. Signs become more severe over several days. Rarely, myocardial vasculitis may cause transient ventricular arrhythmias. Exacerbation of any concurrent infection such as a leg wound or respiratory infection can occur. Cytoplasmic inclusion bodies are few during the first 48 hr and increase to 30-40% of circulating neutrophils at days 3-5 of infection. The disease is seasonal in California, occurring in the late fall, winter, and spring.

Gross petechiation, ecchymoses, and edema occur in the subcutis and fascia. Vasculitis is regional, with the subcutis and fascia of the legs being affected predominantly.

Diagnosis: Demonstration of the characteristic cytoplasmic inclusion bodies in a standard blood smear is diagnostic. An indirect FA test has been described. Differential diagnoses include viral encephalitis, primary liver disease, equine infectious anemia, purpura hemorrhagica, and viral arteritis.

Treatment: Oxytetracycline is extremely effective against *E equi*. Penicillin, chloramphenicol, and streptomycin have no inhibitory effect. Tetracycline IV, 7 mg/kg, once daily for 8 days, has eliminated the infection. Horses with severe ataxia and edema may benefit from short-term corticosteroid treatment (20 mg dexamethasone, once daily). Recovered horses are solidly immune for at least 2 yr, and are not carriers.

EQUINE VIRAL ARTERITIS
(Equine typhoid, Epizootic cellulitis, Pinkeye)

An acute, contagious, viral disease characterized by fever, nasal and ocular discharges, edema, and abortion.

Etiology and Epidemiology: The etiologic agent has been classified as an arterivirus, family Togaviridae. Although, based on serological tests, the virus appears to be widely distributed throughout the world, the disease is not diagnosed commonly. It occurs in sporadic outbreaks that are often associated with movement of horses. Transmission occurs primarily by the respiratory and venereal routes during the acute phase of the infection; in short- or long-term carrier stallions, it is spread venereally only. Clinical signs are more severe in young, old, and debilitated animals. Mares may abort at various stages of pregnancy. Epidemics may occur where horses are congregated, eg, sales, shows, breeding farms. Exposure to the virus may result in clinical or inapparent infection, depending on the strain of virus. Mortality is rare in natural infection and has been seen only in neonates; recoveries are complete. A significant number of recovered stallions are carriers, and they play a major role in dissemination and perpetuation of the virus. Carrier mares have not been detected.

Clinical Findings: After an incubation period of 1-8 days, fever and leukopenia may be accompanied by lacrimation, conjunctivitis, nasal congestion and discharge, weakness, depression, anorexia, and limb edema (especially of the hindlimbs). Less consistent findings include periorbital/supraorbital edema; edema of the ventral body wall, including the scrotum, prepuce, and mammae; photophobia; skin rash most commonly on the neck but sometimes generalized; colic; dyspnea; myalgia and arthralgia; diarrhea; icterus; and ataxia. Abortion occurs late in the febrile phase or early in the convalescent phase of the disease. Most commonly, many animals with acute infection are asymptomatic or develop only mild signs of fever, variable limb edema, conjunctivitis, and rhinitis. Severity of clinical signs varies greatly.
   Lesions: The virus affects the endothelial and muscle cells, primarily of the small arteries throughout the body; panvasculitis can result. Lesions include endothelial swelling and degeneration, thrombus formation, and characteristic degeneration and necrosis of the media of arteries and venules, especially the small ones. Gross lesions seen in fatal cases of experimental infection with the unattenuated Bucyrus strain of the virus include: edema; petechiae, especially in the subcutis of the limbs and abdomen; excess peritoneal and pleural fluid; and edema and hemorrhage of the intra-abdominal lymph nodes as well as the small and large intestine, especially the cecum and colon. Enteritis, hemorrhage and infarcts in the spleen, pulmonary edema and emphysema, and interstitial pneumonia are seen in naturally infected neonatal foals, few of which die. Aborted fetuses are frequently partly autolyzed. Edema and petechiae are widespread, and an excess of fluid is found in the body cavities. There are no pathognomonic lesions in infected fetuses.

Diagnosis: While equine viral arteritis can be provisionally differentiated from equine herpesvirus 1 infection (EHV-1, qv, p 734) and equine influenza (qv, p 737) based on clinical signs, the diagnosis cannot be confirmed without virus isolation and/or serology or histopathology. The clinical syndrome may be confused with that seen in Getah virus infection or African horse sickness in countries in which these infections occur. Sporadic cases must be differentiated from equine infectious anemia (qv, p 27) and purpura hemorrhagica (qv, p 431).

Abortion during or just following an illness is a valuable, but not invariable, diagnostic feature: abortion rarely accompanies influenza, and the mare usually displays no clinical signs before EHV-1 abortion. Fetuses aborted due to EHV-1 frequently have characteristic lesions, while those aborted due to equine arteritis virus have neither specific lesions nor inclusion bodies.

Appropriate specimens for virus isolation include nasopharyngeal and conjunctival swabs, citrated blood samples, and semen. Specimens should be collected as soon as possible after the onset of illness. In putative cases of equine arteritis virus abortion, placental and fetal fluids and a wide range of placental, lymphoreticular, and other tissues can be productive sources of virus. Since few work with this virus, it is advisable to seek advice from a qualified laboratory before collecting specimens for serology or virology.

Prophylaxis and Treatment: There is no specific treatment; antibacterial drugs and symptomatic therapy are indicated, and good nursing and absolute rest with gradual return to activity are desirable. Equine viral arteritis can be prevented and controlled by sound management practices and selective use (where authorized) of a commercial, modified live virus vaccine.

GLANDERS
(Farcy)

A contagious, acute or chronic, usually fatal disease of Equidae, caused by *Pseudomonas mallei* and characterized by serial development of ulcerating nodules that occur most commonly in the upper respiratory tract, lungs, and skin. Man, Felidae, and other species are susceptible, and infections usually are fatal. Glanders is one of the oldest diseases known and once was prevalent throughout the world. It has now been eradicated or effectively controlled in many countries, including the USA.

Etiology: *Pseudomonas mallei* is present in exudates of the nose and ulcerative skin of infected animals, and the disease is commonly contracted by ingesting food or water contaminated by the nasal discharge of carrier animals. The organism is susceptible to heat, light, and disinfectants, and is unlikely to survive in a contaminated area for >6 wk.

Clinical Findings: Following an incubation period of ~2 wk, affected animals usually exhibit septicemia and high fever (up to 106°F [41°C]) and, subsequently, a thick, mucopurulent nasal discharge and respiratory signs. Death occurs within a few days. The chronic disease is common in horses and occurs as a debilitating condition with nodular or ulcerative cutaneous and nasal lesions. Animals may live for years while disseminating the organism. The prognosis is unfavorable. Recovered animals may not develop immunity.

Nasal, pulmonary, and cutaneous forms of glanders are recognized, and an animal may be affected by more than one form at a time. In the **nasal form**, nodules develop in the mucosa of the nasal septum and lower parts of the turbinates. The nodules degenerate into deep ulcers with raised irregular borders. Characteristic star-shaped cicatrices remain after the ulcers heal. In the early stage, the submaxillary lymph nodes are enlarged and edematous, and later become adherent to the skin, or deeper tissues.

In the **pulmonary form**, small tubercle-like nodules, which have caseous or calcified centers surrounded by inflammatory zones, are found in the lungs. If the disease process is extensive, consolidation of the lung tissue and pneumonia may be present. The nodules tend to break down and may discharge their contents into the bronchioles, resulting in extension of the infection to the upper respiratory tract.

In the **cutaneous form** ("farcy"), nodules appear along the course of the lymph vessels, particularly of the extremities. These nodules undergo degeneration, and form ulcers that discharge a highly infectious, sticky pus. The liver and spleen also may show typical nodular lesions.

Diagnosis: The typical nodules, ulcers, scar formation, and debilitated condition may provide sufficient evidence for a clinical diagnosis. However, since these signs usually do not develop until the disease is well advanced, specific diagnostic tests should be applied as early as possible. In addition to the mallein test, which is the procedure of choice, complement fixation is the most accurate of several serological tests that may be used, although the latter occasionally gives a false positive. Culture of exudate from lesions reveals the presence of the causative organism.

Prophylaxis and Treatment: There is no vaccine. Prophylaxis and control depend on early detection and elimination of affected animals, as well as complete quarantine and rigorous disinfection of the area involved. Treatment is given only in endemic areas. Antibiotics are not very effective. Sulfadiazine given daily for 20 days has been successful.

SEPTICEMIA IN FOALS

Septicemia may occur *in utero* but is more commonly acquired from environmental sources after birth. Failure of ingestion or absorption of adequate colostrum increases susceptibility to bacterial infection, the most common causes of which are gram-negative organisms, eg, *Escherichia coli, Klebsiella* sp, and *Actinobacillus* sp. The subtle clinical signs of sepsis, lethargy, weakness, loss of suckle reflex, and inability to stand without assistance can be present at birth or may develop over the first few days of life. The foals may be hypo- or hyperthermic. Tachycardia and tachypnea develop with shock and metabolic acidosis.

Fulminant neonatal sepsis in horses is a multisystemic disease. The more obvious signs of septicemia vary with the organ system involved and the degree of failure present. Hematogenous spread of bacteria commonly results in pneumonia and polyarthritis-polyosteomyelitis, although bacterial localization can occur at almost any site. If the bacteria localize in the GI tract, then enteritis/colitis results in abdominal distention and diarrhea. When meningitis is present, the foal may be comatose or in convulsions.

Laboratory evaluation is also variable, but the most common findings are an IgG level of <800 mg/dL, an abnormal leukogram, and elevated serum fibrinogen. Neutropenia or neutrophilia can be present depending on the stage of the disease. An increase in immature neutrophils is seen, and evidence of toxic changes in the neutrophils is common. Affected foals are often hypoglycemic. A metabolic or a mixed metabolic and respiratory acidosis may be present.

Definitive diagnosis is based on a positive blood culture. Differential diagnoses include neonatal maladjustment syndrome (qv, p 610), isoimmune hemolytic anemia (qv, p 22), congenital white muscle disease (qv, p 548), uroperitoneum (qv, p 894), retained meconium (*see* p 172), and equine herpesvirus-1 infection (qv, p 734). Prognosis is poor if the diagnosis is not made early. Intensive neonatal care is indicated, and survivors can become successful athletes.

Therapy includes broad-spectrum parenteral antibacterials such as a combination of penicillin/ampicillin with gentamicin/amikacin. Plasma transfusions and IV fluids should be given to combat the immunoglobulin deficiency, septic shock, and metabolic acidosis. Dextrose should be administered if hypoglycemia is suspected. Seizures can be controlled with phenobarbital or diazepam. Adequate warmth and nutrition must be provided.

Preventive measures include hygiene at foaling and in the foaling environment. The most important aspect is assurance of adequate absorption of colostral immunoglobulin. A serum sample taken from the foal at 24 hr of age should be tested for immunoglobulin concentration. If the IgG levels are <800 mg/dL, a prophylactic plasma transfusion is indicated.

AFRICAN SWINE FEVER (ASF)

A highly contagious viral disease with signs and lesions resembling those of hog cholera (qv, p 381). Before 1957, it was restricted to Africa and appeared as a highly virulent infection of domestic pigs in contact with endogenous wild pigs. The warthog, bushpig, and giant forest hog are frequently infected, inapparent carriers of the virus. The first extensions of ASF outside Africa occurred in Portugal in 1957 and in Spain in 1960. There were numerous outbreaks in France and Italy over the next 20 yr; it spread to the Caribbean and South America in the 1970's, and to Belgium and Holland in the 1980's. In contrast to the severe clinical manifestations of the African isolates, less virulent forms emerged during epidemics on the Iberian peninsula, which has made the clinical diagnosis much more difficult. It has been eradicated from the Western Hemisphere but continues to exist in domestic pigs in Portugal and Spain, and in wild pigs on Sardinia and in several countries in Africa.

Etiology and Epidemiology: Although ASF virus is classified as an iridovirus, it has some properties of poxviruses. This DNA virus replicates primarily in cells of the monocyte-macrophage system and is found in nearly all fluids and tissues of acutely infected pigs. Virus can be isolated from tissues of carrier animals for up to 3 yr after infection. It is exceptionally hardy, and retains infectivity for ≥18 mo at room temperature, for ≥1 hr at 56°C, and in commercially processed hams for 6 mo. Blood smears remained infectious after 24 hr exposure to 1% sodium hydroxide, but not to 2%. It is relatively resistant to trypsin and acids but sensitive to ether. It has been passed in rabbits, goat kids, embryonating eggs, and tissue cultures. Neither attenuated viral strains nor killed virus products have provided significant protection from challenge with virulent heterologous virus, although some protection from challenge to closely related isolates has been reported. The absence of a reliable vaccine is a critical factor in control efforts. An unusual aspect of the immune response to ASF virus is the absence of readily demonstrable neutralizing antibody. Antibodies are produced, and their passive transfer offers some protection as measured by delayed onset, reduction in amounts of circulating virus, and modification of severity of clinical signs.

Only Suidae appear naturally susceptible to ASF, which can be transmitted by direct and indirect contact. In the Western Hemisphere, the initial outbreaks appear to have been caused by feeding infected pork scraps in garbage from international aircraft.

Ornithodoros sp ticks can act as vectors for up to 8 yr after exposure to the virus. In some ticks, ASF virus can survive a complete tick cycle by transovarial passage, thus making them extremely effective vectors. It has recently been shown that ≥6 species of *Ornithodoros* are capable of transmitting ASF, including 2 (*O coriaceus* and *O turicata*) from the USA.

Infection usually occurs by oronasal exposure. Virus initially replicates in macrophages in the tonsils and regional lymph nodes. This is closely followed by viremia, which is detectable 2-4 days after exposure and lasts 2-4 wk.

Clinical Findings: The first sign is fever; temperatures of 105-108°F (40.5-42°C) occur 5-15 days after natural infection. There is an early leukopenia and thrombocytopenia. With virulent isolates, after ~4 days of fever or ~24-48 hr before death, animals usually stop eating and become listless, incoordinated, and cyanotic. The pulse and respiration rates are increased. Vomiting, diarrhea, and eye discharges are sometimes observed. Death often occurs 4-7 days after the onset of fever. Pregnant sows may abort. With virulent strains of the virus, mortality in domestic pigs frequently approaches 100%. Survivors usually are carriers for life, although the virus is not continuously present in the excretions.

Lesions: Gross lesions in the acute stage of infection with virulent isolates include pronounced hemorrhages of lymph nodes, petechial hemorrhages of the renal cortex, and congestive splenomegaly. Hairless portions frequently exhibit edematous areas of cyanosis. Cutaneous ecchymoses occur on the legs and abdomen. Pleural, pericardial, and peritoneal fluids are excessive. Petechiae occur in the mucous membranes of the larynx and bladder, in the renal cortex, and on visceral surfaces of organs. Edema often is prominent in the mesenteric structures of the colon and adjacent to the gallbladder. In the chronic form, focal caseous necrosis and mineralization of the lungs may be seen.

Diagnosis: Any hog-cholera-like disease should be reported immediately to state and federal authorities. The gross lesions of hog cholera and ASF are too similar to allow certain differential diagnosis; however, there are minor differences that may be somewhat helpful. Infarcts in the spleen and "button ulcers" of hog cholera rarely occur in acute ASF. Severe edema of the lungs and walls of the gallbladder, and excessive pericardial, pleural, and peritoneal fluids are common in ASF but rare in hog cholera.

For laboratory diagnosis, samples of blood, spleen, and gastrohepatic lymph nodes should be taken. The suspect virus can be replicated in swine bone marrow or buffy coat cultures. Swine RBC adsorb to WBC that are infected with virulent ASF virus, causing a hemadsorption reaction, and later, the virus causes lysis of the WBC. Hemadsorption does not occur with hog cholera virus. Serum antibodies to ASF virus in chronically infected animals may be identified by immunoelectro-osmophoresis, indirect immunofluorescence, indirect immunoperoxidase, or ELISA tests. Pigs immunized with hog cholera virus become infected if challenged with ASF virus. Infected cells in tissue can be detected by direct and indirect immunofluorescence, immunoperoxidase, or nucleic acid probe hybridization procedures.

Control: The spread of ASF to Europe, the Caribbean, and Brazil, and the absence of a vaccine, intensify the international hazard. Cooperative international efforts to prohibit the movement of infected animals, products, or vectors are necessary. All veterinarians must be alert to recognize ASF, and should utilize state or federal diagnostic services. A positive diagnosis of ASF should be followed by strict quarantine and slaughter.

ENCEPHALOMYOCARDITIS (EMC) VIRUS INFECTION

An infection of man and other animals, principally pigs and nonhuman primates, caused by the EMC group of the picornaviruses. Although subclinical infection is common in many species, sporadic death or epidemics have occurred most frequently in pigs. EMC viruses have caused little human illness; sporadic individual human cases, particularly in adolescents, have been manifested as aseptic meningitis, poliomyelitis-like disease, or Guillain-Barré syndrome.

Epidemiology: Serological studies indicate that EMC viruses occur worldwide. Reports of disease in pigs have originated from the Americas, Australasia, and South Africa. Rodents, principally rats, are the main asymptomatic reservoir. Disease outbreaks are usually associated with increased contact with rodents or their excreta. The susceptibility of various zoo animals, including orangutans, chimpanzees, baboons, cynomologous monkeys, lemurs, llamas, sloths, certain antelope species, black rhinoceri, and African elephants has been demonstrated in the USA by recovery of virus from animals dying with consistent gross and histologic findings. EMC virus has been isolated from fetal and stillborn piglets, indicating that transplacental infection may occur.

Clinical Findings, Lesions, and Diagnosis: Most affected animals are found dead or die suddenly when excited through handling or other means. A brief period of depression, inappetence, ataxia, vomiting, or dyspnea may precede death. The clinical findings are consistent with acute heart failure.

Lesions of acute heart failure, including liver enlargement, pulmonary edema, mesenteric edema, and ascites may be present. The heart is usually dilated, particularly on the right side. The ventricular myocardium frequently has multiple, discrete white areas or ill-defined pale zones. Histologically, myocardial necrosis with infiltration by lymphocytes and macrophages is typically present. Vasculitis and endocarditis are not found.

The gross lesions must be differentiated from those of vitamin E/selenium deficiency, heart infarcts due to septic emboli, the cardiac form of foot-and-mouth disease, and gut edema. Virus may be recovered in acute cases from many organs, but especially heart and spleen. Antibodies are detectable as early as 5-7 days after infection.

Control: Vaccines are not commercially available, but an experimental, killed, adjuvanted vaccine is being used to protect zoo animals in the USA. Rodent control is indicated. The virus is comparatively stable in the environment, and chlorine-, iodine-, or aldehyde-based disinfectants are useful.

GLÄSSER'S DISEASE
(Porcine polyserositis, Infectious polyarthritis)

A fibrinous, occasionally fatal, polyserositis, polyarthritis, and meningitis of pigs. This syndrome is now considered to be due to *Haemophilus parasuis* (*suis*), but possibly *H parainfluenzae* may cause a similar disease. Stress factors, such as weaning or transport, predispose to the disease, and similar conditions have been reported due to *Mycoplasma* spp, notably *M hyorhinis* in young piglets (*see* LAMENESS IN PIGS, p 532). *Mycoplasma hyosynoviae* commonly causes arthritis but not polyserositis in young adults. Glässer's disease probably occurs worldwide, although most reports come from Europe.

Clinical Findings: The disease is usually mild with low morbidity, but it may be severe with high morbidity and mortality when infection enters a susceptible herd. The incubation period is 1-5 days, disease occurring 2-7 days after the precipitating stress. Young pigs (weaning to 4 mo) are usually affected. A temperature of 104-107°F [41-42°C] develops, and there is anorexia, depression, and sometimes mild rhinitis and dyspnea with cough. Some pigs become lame with painful, warm, swollen, and fluctuating joints. Chronic arthritis, and occasionally meningitis and convulsions, may develop. Pigs may die during the acute stage, or recovery or partial recovery may occur.

Lesions: The classic lesion is a serofibrinous or fibrinopurulent pleurisy, pericarditis, and peritonitis with or without bronchopneumonia and fibrinopurulent meningoencephalitis. The joint fluid is turbid with greenish fibrin deposits, and the periarticular tissues are inflamed.

Diagnosis: The provisional diagnosis, based on history, clinical signs, and necropsy, is confirmed by culture of the organism from joint fluids, cardiac blood, or CSF. Serology, based on precipitation or complement fixation tests at titers of >1:80, may help differentiate this condition from other causes of polyserositis and arthritis.

Treatment and Control: Response to injections of penicillin, streptomycin, tetracyclines, trimethoprim, or sulfamethazine is usually good. Control measures should aim at removing stresses, and in-feed or water medication of pigs at risk may be of value. A formalin-killed bacterin is used in some countries with apparent success. The mycoplasmal infections respond better to drugs such as tylosin, lincomycin, or erythromycin; this may help in differentiation.

HOG CHOLERA
(Swine fever, Classical swine fever)

A highly contagious viral disease of pigs. Disease due to virulent viral strains has a sudden onset, and affects pigs of all ages with high morbidity and mortality, although adults are least affected. Less virulent strains cause chronic or mild disease, reproductive failure, and neonatal losses. Inapparent infection can also occur.

Hog cholera is endemic in many South American, African, and Asian countries. It is absent from Canada, Australia, and New Zealand, and has been eradicated from the USA and a number of European countries.

Etiology and Pathogenesis: The cause is a pestivirus, family Togaviridae. It has some antigens in common with bovine viral diarrhea virus (BVDV), but neutralization tests distinguish them as separate species. Hog cholera virus strains are host-specific under natural conditions; generally, they form a more compact antigenic group than do BVDV strains, but serological variants, of low virulence and low antigenicity, can cause diagnostic difficulties. The virus replicates in cell cultures of pig origin and most strains do not produce a cytopathic effect. In pig houses, excreta and bedding may remain contaminated for days to weeks depending mainly on prevailing temperatures. The virus survives in frozen pork for ≥ 4 yr and in chilled meats or preserved carcasses for 3-6 mo or more.

Direct contact is the most common mode of transmission. Infected pigs shed virus in all body excretions and secretions in amounts relative to virulence of the viral strain. Pigs persistently viremic after transplacental or postnatal infection can infect healthy stock. The feeding of unprocessed, or inadequately processed, waste food that contains infected meat can also be an important means of spread. Tissues from infected pigs are potentially infective even before onset of detectable disease or, in recovery, after development of serum neutralizing antibodies. Other routes of spread, though far less important, include numerous mechanical vectors, but airborne spread seems unlikely.

The most common route of viral entry is ingestion, and the tonsil is the primary site of replication. Lymphatic spread and viremia ensue 24 hr after infection. Secondary replication of virus in circulating WBC, endothelial cells of blood vessels and lymphatics, visceral lymphoid tissue, spleen, and bone marrow contributes further to viremia by 5-6 days. Spread to epithelial structures after 3-4 days results in shedding of virus in excretions and secretions. Pigs surviving infection for 6 wk have a generalized depletion of lymphoid tissue and are susceptible to concurrent infections.

Clinical Findings: The disease may be acute, chronic, mild, or clinically inapparent in relation to the virulence of the virus and host response. After a 5-10 day (range 2-20) incubation period, acutely affected pigs are lethargic, anorectic, and have a fever, commonly persisting at 106°F (41°C). Multifocal hyperemia of the skin, conjunctivitis, transient constipation, and then diarrhea, occasionally with vomiting, follow. Dyspnea is common. Nervous signs are ataxia, paresis, and convulsions. Pigs pile up or huddle together. Mortality in young pigs can approach 100%. In acute cases, signs persist until the comatose pig dies 5-15 days after onset of illness. Preterminal cyanosis of the skin may be observed, especially ventrally, at the base of the ears, and on the snout.

In chronic cases, signs of dullness, capricious and sometimes depraved appetite, pyrexia, and diarrhea persist for >1 mo. There is a phase of apparent recovery, with eventual relapse and death. In mild disease, resulting from infection with viral strains of low virulence, signs may be confined to transient pyrexia and inappetence, or reproductive losses due to transplacental infection may occur. Such losses include fetal death, resorption, abortion, mummification or stillbirth, or piglets born weak and trembling. Hog cholera virus is a recognized infectious cause of congenital tremor syndrome (qv, p 583). Congenitally infected piglets, if they survive (sometimes apparently healthy), usually are viremic for several months before "late-onset" clinical disease.

Lesions: In acute cases, most of the lesions result from viral damage to blood vessel endothelium, but there is also bone marrow depression, which results in leukopenia and profound thrombocytopenia. The latter could be associated with the hemorrhagic diathesis. Petechiae and ecchymoses are widespread and often prominent in the skin, larynx, bladder, ileocecal junction, brain, and kidney pelvis and cortex. In the latter, they produce the so-called "turkey egg" appearance. Multifocal infarction of the margin of the spleen is characteristic but inconstant. In the large intestine, similar blood vessel damage and consequent necrosis produce raised circular "button ulcers". Enlarged hemorrhagic lymph nodes are common. Histology of the brain shows a nonsuppurative encephalitis with severe vasculitis in a high portion of acute fatal cases. In chronic cases, hemorrhagic inflammatory lesions are often absent, but there is generalized depletion of lymphoid tissue. Transplacental infection can produce central dysmyelinogenesis, cerebellar hypoplasia, microencephaly, and pulmonary hypoplasia.

Diagnosis: The history, clinical signs, and gross lesions support a tentative diagnosis in acute outbreaks. Widespread petechiation, involving larynx, bladder, and kidney; splenic infarction; "button ulcers"; skin erythema; and pneumonia are strongly indicative. Leukopenia and thrombocytopenia are frequent findings, but WBC counts should be determined in $\geq$6 pigs.

Differential diagnoses include African swine fever, septicemic salmonellosis, pasteurellosis, streptococcosis, leptospirosis, erysipelas, purpura, coumarin poisoning, and mulberry heart disease. Nervous signs of hog cholera cannot be differentiated from those due to other encephalitides, or from some noninfectious nervous disorders. Confirmation of the diagnosis in any of its clinical forms requires laboratory methods.

Laboratory diagnosis is currently based on direct examination by immunofluorescence (for viral antigen) of fresh tissues (preferably submitted on ice) and of cell cultures. Preferred tissues are tonsil, pharyngeal lymph nodes, spleen, kidney, and distal ileum. Immunoperoxidase may also be used for antigen labelling. Monoclonal antibodies can be used to distinguish hog cholera from other pestivirus isolates. Serological detection of antibody to hog cholera and its differentiation from BVDV antibody is based on neutralization tests or ELISA. Histological examination of the brain has been a useful diagnostic adjunct. WBC and thrombocyte counts may be helpful, and viral isolation or animal transmission experiments may be attempted. In countries with a statutory policy toward control of hog cholera, regulatory authorities should be notified immediately of suspected cases.

Treatment and Control: Hyperimmune serum is the only available treatment and may be effective in the early stages of disease or for protection of in-contact animals. Control is essentially by eradication or vaccination. Eradication by slaughter of all in-contact pigs and disposal of carcasses has been successful. Infected premises are disinfected and not repopulated for a period. Pig movements in affected areas are strictly controlled. Waste-food feeding in countries with an eradication policy is strictly regulated. In countries where the disease is endemic, attenuated virus vaccines are mainly employed. While vaccination can reduce the prevalence of endemic disease, it should cease when eradication by slaughter is introduced, and is prohibited in areas "officially" free of the disease.

STREPTOCOCCAL INFECTIONS IN PIGS

STREPTOCOCCUS SUIS INFECTIONS

Streptococcus suis (Lancefield group D) is a common cause of meningitis and arthritis in large intensive pig farms; in some countries, including the USA and Canada, it is also associated with pneumonia, endocarditis, myocarditis, and diseases of the sow's genital tract. In man, *S suis* type 2 can cause arthritis, fever, meningitis, and permanent hearing loss. Although fewer than 100 human cases have been reported worldwide, it is wise to take precautions, particularly when performing necropsies.

Etiology and Epidemiology: *Streptococcus suis* usually appears in lesions as oval diplococci or short chains. It is a gram-positive, facultative aerobe that forms small colonies overnight on blood agar. The colonies are surrounded by a narrow zone of clear hemolysis on horse-blood agar and partial (green) hemolysis on calf- or sheep-blood agar. *Streptococcus suis* is subdivided into at least 9 serotypes based on specific polysaccharide capsular antigens. Typing by biochemical tests only can be misleading because other streptococci have similar spectra of activity. Clinical disease is usually associated with types 1 and 2. Poor ventilation, high levels of slurry gases, overcrowding, and other stresses predispose to outbreaks of meningitis caused by type 2. Isolates of high and low virulence have been reported. There is little information on the causal relationship of other serotypes to disease. In the USA, serotype 7 seems to be isolated from lesions more frequently than other serotypes.

Type 1 is endemic in most herds but only sporadically affects pigs up to ~8 wk of age. Virulent strains of type 2 are less widespread and tend to occur most in large intensive herds. Type 2 affects pigs up to market weight. Both types 1 and 2 are carried subclinically in the tonsillar crypts for long periods and sometimes can be detected in the nose.

Type 2 is spread between herds mainly by movement of subclinical carrier pigs but also appears to spread in other ways. One possible method is by flies, which readily travel 1-2 miles between farms. Flies can carry the infection for up to 5 days. Within herds, the main spread is between weaned pigs, particularly when they are housed intensively. Subclinical carriers readily transmit it to other pigs in close contact; the carrier rate may be high (60-100%). The organism appears to be less readily transmitted from carrier sows to their piglets, at least during the neonatal period. The environment probably also plays a role in spread since the organism survives long periods in feces, dust, and dead carcasses. Fortunately, it is readily killed by detergents and common disinfectants.

Clinical Findings: *Streptococcus suis* type 1 causes sporadic cases of polyarthritis and sometimes meningitis in suckling piglets but is of minor importance.

Streptococcus suis type 2 causes acute, often fatal, meningitis in weaners and growing pigs. Incidence in endemic herds may fluctuate between 2 and 15%, and remain a constant problem. Meningitis, which may occur when a pig is first infected or arise when carriers are stressed, is manifested as depression, fever, tremors, incoordination, opisthotonus, convulsions, blindness, and deafness.

In some countries, *S suis* type 2 is associated more frequently with bronchopneumonia than with meningitis, although there is no evidence that it is primary. Sudden death due to endocarditis and/or myocarditis and diseases of the genital tract of sows, including abortion, are reported to occur sporadically in some countries. Polyarthritis and lameness are common.

Lesions: The skin may be reddened in patches. Lymph nodes are often enlarged and congested, and fibrinous polyserositis is common. Joint capsules may be thickened, and joints may contain excess clear or cloudy fluid. Often the meninges and brain appear normal, but there may be congestion, edema, and excess clear or cloudy CSF. Histologically, changes are typical of acute bacterial meningitis. Affected lungs may show varying degrees of consolidation and fibrinopurulent bronchopneumonia.

Diagnosis: History and clinical signs may suggest *S suis* infection, and histology and FA tests may provide additional evidence, although FA tests are not specific. Definitive diagnosis depends on isolation and identification of the causative organism, otherwise the disease can be confused with other streptococcal infections; other bacterial infections such as erysipelas, salmonellosis, or acute Glässer's disease; water deprivation; or possibly pseudorabies.

Treatment and Control: Control of *S suis* type 2 meningitis is the main concern. Attempts to prevent introduction of carrier pigs from endemic herds are not completely reliable since the organism can be subclinical, and there are no reliable tests to monitor its presence. Furthermore, it may be introduced in other ways (eg, by flies). Another possibility when new outbreaks occur is that mild strains already endemic have mutated to become more virulent. Once in a herd, it tends to remain endemic; neither vaccination nor blanket therapy will eliminate it. Although killed vaccines are used, their efficacy is unproved. Good husbandry reduces environmental stress and decreases clinical disease. Prophylactic/strategic medication is commonly used, usually in feed or water but sometimes by injection of long-acting antibiotics. The organism tends to become resistant to tetracyclines and sulfonamides. Most isolates are sensitive to penicillin, but it is rapidly inactivated in feed and therefore may fail to control disease.

GROUPS C AND L AND OTHER STREPTOCOCCAL INFECTIONS

Septicemia, arthritis, endocarditis, and other sporadic conditions of pigs are sometimes associated with *Streptococcus equisimilis* (Lancefield group C), or less commonly Group L or other ungroupable streptococci.

Etiology and Epidemiology: *Streptococcus equisimilis* and Group L streptococci appear in lesions as gram-positive elongated cocci in pairs or short chains. They produce small colonies overnight on blood agar surrounded by distinct zones of complete hemolysis. Identification is based on Lancefield grouping and sugar reactions.

Groups C and L streptococci are commonly present in many body locations, including excretions and secretions in normal pigs in most herds. Contamination is also possible from non-pig sources. The organisms are opportunists and usually gain entry to the young pig's body via injuries, including clipped needle teeth, docked tails, or floor abrasions. They cause a bacteremia or septicemia usually followed by arthritis or endocarditis.

Clinical Findings: Arthritis with warm swollen joints is frequently observed in suckling pigs and is accompanied by fever, depression, anorexia, and other indications of septicemia. Similar clinical findings may also occur in pigs in the postweaning period. Endocarditis is not uncommon in older pigs but is usually diagnosed only at necropsy.

Streptococci are also occasionally associated with cutaneous abscesses, mastitis, and pneumonia, and appear to be involved along with other causative factors in ear necrosis (qv, p 308). These organisms are frequently isolated from female reproductive tracts, including vaginal discharges, but they have probably been overrated as a cause of reproductive failure.

Lesions: The most common lesions are associated with arthritis in young pigs and include increased amounts of turbid synovial fluid frequently accompanied by periarticular swelling. Endocarditis in older pigs is frequently caused by streptococci, which may be observed microscopically as coccoid organisms in vegetative heart valve lesions.

Diagnosis: Clinical signs are often suggestive of infections with group C or L streptococci, but definitive identification should be based on bacterial isolation and identification.

Treatment and Control: Young pigs are almost certain to encounter group C or L streptococci, but incidence of clinically significant infections can be reduced through good sanitation with regard to housing and during minor surgical procedures. Housing modifications to reduce skin abrasions and trauma are also very helpful. Specific therapy usually involves penicillin and related antibiotics.

GROUP E STREPTOCOCCAL INFECTIONS

Group E streptococci used to be a common cause of jowl abscess (lymphadenitis, swine strangles) in feeder pigs in the USA, and resulted in carcass trimming and condemnation at slaughter. It is less common now. The organism occurs in chains of 3 to ~15 capsulated, gram-positive cocci that produce small colonies surrounded by zones of complete hemolysis. It ferments sugars, but definitive identification is by Lancefield grouping. There are at least 6 serotypes, but serotype IV is the main one causing jowl abscess. The organism is carried in the tonsillar crypts and spreads by nasal and oral secretions. The disease occurs repeatedly on some farms.

Signs are pronounced swelling of the cervical lymph nodes, sometimes accompanied by pyrexia and anorexia. Abscessed cervical lymph nodes, with enlarging areas of liquefaction become encapsulated after ~1 wk; secondary abscesses may occur in other organs. Diagnosis is based on the typical clinicopathological syndrome, and confirmed by culture and identification of the causal organism.

Large abscesses may be lanced. In advanced cases, antibiotics are usually ineffective. Live attenuated vaccines have been produced but are used little. The widespread use of medicated feeds and changes in husbandry systems have probably been responsible for the reduced incidence.

SWINE VESICULAR DISEASE (SVD)

Typically, a transient disease of pigs in which vesicular lesions appear in the mouth and on the feet. The lesions are similar to those of foot-and-mouth disease (FMD, qv, p 378), vesicular exanthema of swine (VES, qv, p 388), and vesicular stomatitis (VS, qv, p 372), but the pig does not lose condition, and the lesions heal rapidly. Nervous signs have been described but rarely observed in the field. The disease does not cause severe production losses but is of major economic importance because it must be differentiated from FMD, eradication is costly, and embargoes on pork are often imposed on nations not free of SVD.

Although infection in laboratory workers has occurred, and the virus may be present in sheep or cattle, pigs are said to be the only natural host. The disease was first identified in Italy in 1966 and subsequently in Hong Kong, Japan, and a number of countries in western Europe. It has been eradicated from some countries (eg, Britain and Switzerland).

Etiology: The causal agent is an enterovirus of the Picornaviridae family. It is transmitted by direct or indirect contact or by feeding infected pork or pork products. Infection gives rise to viremia and generalized vesicles that contain large amounts of virus.

Clinical Findings and Diagnosis: The primary signs are vesicular lesions in the mouth, on the lips or snout, and on the feet, especially the coronary band. The lesions may be mild or inapparent, especially when pigs are kept on soft bedding.

Diagnosis is based on laboratory tests on epithelial samples or serum. Complement fixation and ELISA are the tests of choice, but passage in swine tissue culture may often be required. Serum neutralization and agar-gel diffusion are also used. Differentiation from other vesicular diseases depends on complement fixation, ELISA, susceptibility of tissue cultures, range of pH susceptibility, and electron microscopy.

Control: Countries free of the disease can remain so by banning the import of pigs and pork products, or ensuring that pork products are treated (heat or otherwise) to kill the virus. Any suspected outbreak should be reported to the proper authorities. If disease does appear, important control measures are thorough cooking (according to regulations) of all garbage fed to pigs, and control of pig movement. The virus remains infective for long periods; thus, disinfection of premises, trucks, and equipment must be thorough. The most effective disinfectants are strong alkalies, although hypochlorites or acid-containing iodophors can be used when organic material is not present.

TRICHINOSIS

A parasitic disease of public health importance. Human infections are established by consumption of insufficiently cooked infected meat, usually pork or bear, although other species have been implicated. Natural infections occur in wild carnivores; it has also been found in horses, rats, beavers, opossums, walruses, whales, and meat-eating birds. Most mammals are susceptible.

Etiology and Epidemiology: A number of species or subspecies of the causative nematode are now recognized. Since these have few distinct morphological differences, other characteristics such as reproductive isolation, infectivity to certain hosts, and resistance to low temperatures are used in differentiation. A trinomial nomenclature is currently being used to differentiate them: *Trichinella spiralis spiralis (domestica)*—high infectivity for rats, mice, and pigs, and low resistance to freezing; *T spiralis nativa*—found in arctic carnivores, low infectivity for rats and pigs, and resistant to freezing; *T spiralis nelsoni*—found in Africa and Europe up to ~50th or 60th parallel, low infectivity for mice, rats, and pigs, and low virulence; *T spiralis pseudospiralis*—lacks cyst in muscle stage, small size, primarily a parasite of birds.

Infection occurs by ingestion of larvae encysted in muscle. The cyst wall is digested in the stomach, and the liberated larvae penetrate into the duodenal and jejunal mucosa. Within ~4 days, the larvae develop into sexually mature adults. The females (3-4 μm) penetrate deeper into the mucosa and discharge living larvae by day 5 or 6; one adult generally produces 500-1000 larvae over 2-6 wk. Following reproduction, the adult worms die and usually are digested. The minute larvae (0.1 μm) migrate to the muscle, and follow the lymphatic and portal systems to the peripheral circulation; those that reach striated muscle enter individual muscle cells. They grow rapidly (to 1 μm) and begin to coil within the cell, usually one per cell. Capsule formation is initiated ~15 days after infection, and is completed by 4-5 wk. Calcification occurs at different rates in various hosts, even among individuals within a given species. Larvae may remain viable in the cysts for years and continue their development if ingested by another suitable host. The diaphragm, tongue, masseter, and intercostal muscles are among those most heavily involved.

If larvae pass through the intestine and are eliminated in the feces before maturation, they are infective to other animals.

Clinical Findings and Diagnosis: Most infections in domestic and wild animals go undiagnosed. In man, heavy infections produce serious illness with 3 clinical phases (intestinal, muscle invasion, convalescent) and occasional deaths.

Although antemortem diagnoses in animals other than man are rare, trichinosis may be suspected if there is a history of eating rodents or raw infected meat. Microscopical examination of a muscle biopsy sample will confirm but not necessarily rule out trichinosis. The ELISA is a reliable test to detect anti-*Trichinella* antibodies, although seroconversion may not occur until ~18 days after infection.

Control: Treatment is generally impractical in animals. The objective is to prevent ingestion, by any animal including man, of viable *Trichinella* cysts in muscle. In pigs, this may be accomplished with good management, including rodent control and cooking of garbage (fed to the pigs) for 30 min at 212°F (100°C), and prevention of access to wildlife carcasses.

Inspection of meat for viable trichinae at the time of slaughter (by trichinoscopic or digestion methods) is effective in preventing human infection in many countries. In North America, the assumption is that pork may be infected, so that those products that appear as "ready to eat" must be processed by adequate heating, freezing, or curing to kill trichinae before marketing. Other pork should be cooked to assure that all tissue is heated to a temperature of ≥136°F (58°C). Freezing pork at an appropriate temperature for an appropriate time is also effective (5°F [-15°C] for 20 days, -9.4°F [-23°C] for 10 days, or -22°F [-30°C] for 6 days). The assumption has been that infections in pigs are *T spiralis spiralis*. Freezing does not reliably kill trichinae in meat other than pork.

VESICULAR EXANTHEMA OF SWINE
(VES, San Miguel sea lion virus [SMSV] disease)

An acute, highly infectious disease characterized by fever and formation of blisters on the snout, oral mucosa, soles of the feet, between the toes, and on the coronary band. Many immunologically distinct types of the causal calicivirus have been demonstrated (13 types of VESV from pig populations and ≥20 of SMSV from marine sources). Marine mammals, fish, snakes, cattle, mink, horses, primates, and man are susceptible to one or more serotypes of the virus.

In pigs, the clinical disease is indistinguishable from foot-and-mouth disease (qv, p 338), vesicular stomatitis (qv, p 372), or swine vesicular disease (qv, p 386). Originally confined to California, the disease became widespread in the USA during the 1950's, but a vigorous campaign to eradicate the disease was successful. In 1959, the country was declared free of VES, and the disease was designated a Foreign Animal Disease; it has never been reported as a natural infection of pigs in any other part of the world.

Since 1972, a virus indistinguishable from vesicular exanthema of swine virus (VESV), designated as San Miguel sea lion virus (SMSV), has been isolated from throat and rectal swabs from premature and 4-mo-old California sea lion pups, dead and weanling northern fur seal pups, and nursing northern elephant seal pups; and from vesicular lesions on marine mammals, commercial seal meat produced in Alaska, and perch-like fish collected from tidal pools off the southern California coast. SMSV isolated from both fish and marine mammals are capable of producing VES in pigs. In addition, caliciviruses isolated from throat and rectal swabs from dairy calves cause clinical vesicular exanthema in exposed pigs. One calicivirus-type has been recovered from vesicular lesions on the palms and soles of a researcher working with the virus.

Presumptive diagnosis in pigs is based on fever and the presence of typical vesicles, which break within 24-48 hr to form erosions. Diagnosis can be confirmed by complement-fixation tests and electron microscopy on epithelial tissue, or after passage in swine tissue cultures. Serum neutralization tests and immunoelectron microscopy are also used. Suspected cases of vesicular exanthema should be reported immediately to regulatory authorities. Garbage and fish should be cooked before being fed to pigs.

VOMITING AND WASTING DISEASE
(VWD, Hemagglutinating encephalomyelitis, Coronaviral encephalomyelitis)

A viral disease of young pigs characterized by vomiting, constipation, and anorexia that results either in rapid death or chronic emaciation (vomiting and wasting disease). Motor disorders due to acute encephalomyelitis (hemagglutinating encephalomyelitis) also may be observed during some outbreaks.

Etiology and Epidemiology: The causal coronavirus, hemagglutinating encephalomyelitis virus (HEV), is of a single antigenic type, and it grows in several types of porcine cell cultures, in which it causes syncytia. It agglutinates RBC of several animal species. Pigs are the only natural host. The virus is spread via aerosol.

Infection appears to be widespread in North America, western Europe, and Australia. It usually remains subclinical. The virus is endemic in most breeding herds, and a herd immunity exists. Immune sows transfer maternal antibodies to their litters, which are protected until they have developed an age resistance; thus, clinical outbreaks are rare. However, if the virus enters a susceptible herd with neonatal piglets, morbidity and mortality may be high.

Pathogenesis: Replication first takes place in the nasal mucosa, tonsils, lungs, and to a very limited extent, in the small intestine. From these sites of entry, the virus invades defined nuclei of the medulla oblongata via the peripheral nervous system and subsequently spreads to the entire brain stem, and possibly to the cerebum and cerebellum. Vomiting is thought to be caused by viral replication in the vagal sensory ganglion. Wasting is due to vomiting and delayed emptying of the stomach, which is the result of virus-induced lesions in the intramural plexus. Infection of cerebral and cerebellar neurons may cause motor disorders which are, however, rarely observed during an outbreak.

Clinical Findings and Lesions: Both clinical syndromes, the VWD and the encephalitic forms, are confined almost exclusively to pigs <4 wk old. The VWD form has an incubation period of 4-7 days. Repeated retching and vomiting are seen. Pigs start suckling but soon stop, withdraw from the sow, and vomit the milk they have ingested. They dip their mouths into water bowls but drink little, possibly indicative of pharyngeal paralysis. The persistent vomiting results in a rapid decline of condition. Neonatal pigs become dehydrated, cyanotic, and comatose, and die. Older pigs, however, continue to vomit, although less frequently than in the early stage of the disease. They lose appetite and become emaciated. A large distention of the cranial abdomen can develop. This "wasting" state may persist 1-6 wk until the pigs die of starvation. Mortality approaches 100% within the litter, and survivors remain permanently stunted.

The encephalomyelitis form also starts with vomiting, usually 4-7 days after birth. Vomiting continues intermittently for 1-2 days, but it is rarely severe and does not result in dehydration. After 1-3 days, generalized muscle tremors and hyperesthesia are observed. The pigs tend to walk backwards, often ending in a dog-sitting position. They soon become weak, are unable to rise, and paddle their limbs. Blindness, opisthotonus, and nystagmus also occur. After a few days, they become dyspneic, comatose, and die.

From onset to disappearance, an outbreak on a farm lasts 2-3 wk. Disappearance of disease coincides with the development of immunity in highly pregnant sows, which subsequently protects pigs through maternal antibodies.

Cachexia and abdominal distention are seen in chronically affected pigs. Their stomachs are dilated and filled with gas. Microscopically, perivascular cuffing, gliosis, and neuronal degeneration are found in the medulla in 70-100% of pigs with nervous signs, and in 20-60% of pigs showing the VWD syndrome. Neuritis of peripheral sensory ganglia, particularly the trigeminal ganglia, is observed regularly. Degeneration of the ganglia of the stomach wall and perivascular cuffing are found in 15-85% of pigs with VWD. The lesions are most pronounced in the pyloric gland area.

Diagnosis: A laboratory diagnosis can be made routinely by virus isolation from the brain stem if the pigs are euthanized within 2 days after clinical signs appear. It is difficult to isolate the virus from pigs that have been affected for >2 days.

A significant rise in antibody titer can be demonstrated in paired serum samples. The acute serum sample must be collected immediately after the start of disease, since pigs may already have built-up a low antibody titer when the first signs appear.

Differential diagnoses include Teschen-Talfan disease (qv, p 616) and pseudorabies (qv, p 617). Respiratory signs in older pigs and abortions in sows are part of a pseudorabies outbreak. With Teschen, older pigs are usually involved.

Control: There is no treatment. Once signs are evident, the disease runs its course. Spontaneous recoveries are rare. Piglets born from nonimmune sows during an outbreak can be protected by injecting, at birth, either hyperimmune serum or serum from sows randomly selected at slaughter. However, the time lapse between diagnosis and cessation of the disease is usually too short to gain much profit from this procedure. Maintaining the virus on the farm and thus keeping naturally induced immunity in the sows avoids outbreaks in piglets.

BLUETONGUE

A noncontagious, insect-transmitted, viral disease of sheep, cattle, goats, and wild ruminants. The disease occurs widely on the African continent and to a lesser extent in North America, Asia, and Europe. The virus has been isolated from biting insects (*Culicoides* spp) and cattle in Australia; however, there is no clinical evidence that bluetongue disease exists in ruminants on that continent. Serological evidence of widespread infection in ruminants in the Caribbean and some countries in South and Central America exists, but clinical disease has not been confirmed.

Etiology and Transmission: Bluetongue virus is an orbivirus, family Reoviridae; 24 antigenic serotypes have been identified in the world, 5 in the USA. Under natural conditions, the virus is biologically transmitted by *Culicoides* spp. Cattle are an important reservoir for sheep and other susceptible ruminants; some wild ruminant species also may be reservoirs.

Clinical Findings: The usual incubation period in sheep is 5-10 days. In sequence of appearance, clinical signs include: dyspnea with panting; hyperemia of the muzzle, lips, and ears; pyrexia (up to 107.5°F [42°C]); depression; and inflammation, ulceration, erosion, and necrosis of the mucosa of the mouth, especially the dental pad. Signs that may appear, depending on disease severity, include a swollen and less frequently cyanotic tongue, lameness due to coronitis, torticollis, vomiting, pneumonia, conjunctivitis, and occasionally, alopecia. Bluetongue in sheep in the USA is much milder than in Africa, with mortalities of 0-30%. Cattle are commonly inapparently infected, but some may develop clinical signs similar to those in infected sheep. If cattle become infected during gestation, they may abort or give birth to abnormal calves (arthrogryposis, hydranencephaly, and ataxia). Also, the virus has been found in semen of infected bulls, but amounts are usually low and occur only during the viremic stage of infection. In white-tailed deer and pronghorn antelope, the virus often causes a peracute fatal hemorrhagic disease.

Diagnosis: Clinical diagnosis can be confirmed by direct isolation of the virus in chicken embryos inoculated intravascularly, certain cell cultures, or susceptible sheep. The virus also can be grown (less readily) in suckling mice and hamsters inoculated intracerebrally. Viruses isolated can then be identified by FA or serum neutralization tests. An indirect presumptive diagnosis can be made on a rise in antibody titer in paired sera from recovered animals. Serological tests include complement fixation, agar-gel diffusion, ELISA, and serum neutralization.

Viremia is primarily associated with RBC, and the virus can coexist in infected animals with high concentrations of its specific neutralizing antibody. Therefore, washed RBC are often necessary for virus isolation.

Bluetongue is often misdiagnosed (depending on the species involved) as photosensitization, "mycotic" stomatitis, bovine viral diarrhea and its mucosal form, infectious bovine rhinotracheitis, malignant catarrhal fever, vesicular stomatitis, epizootic hemorrhagic disease of deer, contagious ecthyma, grub in the head, or foot-and-mouth disease.

Prevention and Control: A monovalent (serotype 10), modified live vaccine of cell culture origin is available only for use in sheep in the USA. Modified live vaccines with other serotypes found in the USA, and killed vaccines are being developed. The live vaccine should not be used in nonendemic areas during the vector season since it is infectious to the insect vector, and passage of the vaccine virus through the insect increases its pathogenicity for sheep. Pregnant ewes should not be vaccinated in early gestation since this frequently results in hydranencephalus and other deformities in lambs. Passive immunity in lambs lasts ~6 mo, and during this time may interfere with development of active immunity from vaccination. In an outbreak, the decision to vaccinate depends on existing circumstances. Measures to reduce insect bites on susceptible ruminants by reducing insect populations in the area should help to minimize the extent of the disease.

BOVINE LEUKOSIS

(Lymphosarcoma, Malignant lymphoma, Leukemia)

The term leukosis indicates a malignant proliferation of leukocyte-forming tissue. Because lymphoid tumors predominate in cattle, lymphosarcoma and malignant lymphoma are synonymous. Sometimes, the disease is called leukemia, but the presence of malignant cells in blood is not a consistent finding.

Four clinicopathologic syndromes are recognized: calf, thymic, skin, and adult. The first 3 forms are called sporadic leukosis because there is no evidence that they are contagious. The adult syndrome, also known as enzootic leukosis, is caused by the bovine leukosis virus (BLV). Sporadic leukosis occurs worldwide, whereas the geographic distribution of enzootic leukosis is directly related to BLV prevalence.

Sheep and goats can be infected experimentally with BLV, and most infected sheep develop lymphosarcoma. There have been a few reports of naturally infected flocks, but the source and mechanism of infection for these are unknown. All evidence indicates that BLV does not spread from sheep to cattle or from cattle to sheep by normal contact. Epidemiological and serological studies have failed to show any evidence of human infection or disease associated with exposure to BLV.

Transmission, Epidemiology, and Pathogenesis: Transmission of BLV occurs primarily by transfer of blood lymphocytes between animals. Virus is rarely present in nasal secretion, saliva, urine, or semen, except when those fluids are contaminated by blood or cellular exudate. Insects may act as mechanical vectors of blood, but trauma, use of common bleeding needles, and surgical procedures probably are more common mechanisms of transmission.

The BLV can be transmitted to fetuses *in utero*, but usually <10% of calves from infected dams carry the virus at birth. When embryos from BLV-infected cows are transferred to BLV-negative cows, the calves produced are routinely free of infection. Transmission of BLV to calves through colostrum or milk is rare due to the protection conferred by colostral antibody.

Most BLV infections are asymptomatic and can be recognized only by a serological test that detects viral-specific antibody. The animal becomes seropositive 4-12 wk after viral exposure. Of infected cattle, ~30% develop persistent lymphocytosis, but this response to infection is not associated with any clinical sign of disease.

The development of leukosis is a rare manifestation of BLV infection. The incidence of tumor cases varies considerably from herd to herd; the average annual rate in infected cattle is estimated to be 0.3%.

Clinical Findings: In the **calf form** of leukosis, which affects animals <6 mo old, generalized lymphadenopathy and widespread tumor metastasis involve most organ systems and bone marrow.

Thymic cases typically occur in animals 6-8 mo old. The tumor is usually confined to the thymus and results in a diffuse swelling of the ventral neck. Neoplastic tissue may also extend into the thorax, and metastasis to local lymph nodes is not uncommon. Lesions posterior to the diaphragm are unusual.

Skin leukosis, the only nonfatal lymphoid tumor in cattle, is seen in young adults. The superficial cutaneous tumors are present only a few weeks, and after lesions regress, recurrence is rare.

Enzootic leukosis is a disease of mature cattle, and most cases occur in animals that are 4-8 yr old. The distribution of tumor is unpredictable, but tissues most commonly affected include lymph nodes, abomasum, heart, spleen, kidneys, uterus, spinal meninges, and retrobulbar lymphatic tissue.

Diagnosis: A presumptive diagnosis of leukosis can be made if there is clinical evidence of lymphadenopathy or tumor in a commonly affected tissue. Sometimes, leukemia can be demonstrated in the calf form, but thymic and skin cases are usually aleukemic. Blood examination is seldom useful in the diagnosis of enzootic leukosis because so many clinically normal BLV-infected cattle have persistent lymphocytosis. A seronegative test for BLV infection is informative when enzootic leukosis is suspected; in that case, the disease can be ruled out. However, a positive result indicates only BLV infection and is not meaningful for differential diagnosis. The serological test is not appropriate for calf, thymic, and skin leukosis, since the sporadic forms are not caused by BLV.

A definitive diagnosis of leukosis requires histological examination of affected tissues because the gross appearance of lymphoid tumor can be similar to that of other types of neoplasia or other proliferative disease.

Control: There is no treatment for leukosis or for BLV infection in individual animals. Virus can be eliminated from a herd if all cattle are tested serologically at 2- to 3-mo intervals and positive animals removed immediately. The length of time required to obtain a BLV-free herd varies, depending on the initial prevalence of infection, but in most herds the virus can be eradicated within 1 yr. If the prevalence of infection is too high to permit removal of all BLV reactors, spread of the virus can be reduced by segregating them to prevent direct contact with the BLV-negative cattle. Calves from infected dams also should be isolated until they are ≥6 mo old, at which time they can be serologically tested without interference from colostral antibody. Although the segregation procedure may be useful to reduce BLV prevalance in a herd, the ultimate goal of serological surveillance is total elimination of the virus.

BOVINE PETECHIAL FEVER
(Ondiri disease)

An infectious disease of cattle characterized by hemorrhage and edema. It has been confirmed only in Kenya at altitudes of >5000 ft (1500 m), although it may occur also in neighboring countries of similar topography. The organism can multiply after experimental infection in cattle, sheep, goats, bushbuck, impala, Thomson's gazelle, and wildebeest, and hence, probably in most domestic and wild ruminants.

Etiology and Epidemiology: The causative agent is a rickettsia-like organism, *Ehrlichia (Cytoecetes) ondiri*. It can be observed in circulating granulocytes and monocytes while cattle are ill, and in the spleen at necropsy. It is believed to multiply initially in the spleen, with subsequent spread to other organs. Latent infections occur after recovery in some animals. Immunity lasts several years.

The disease is restricted to scrub or forest edge areas that have heavy shade, a thick litter layer, and high relative humidity. It occurs sporadically throughout the year in imported breeds of cattle. An arthropod vector is suspected, but extensive attempts to incriminate ticks, biting insects, and mites have failed. Bushbuck (*Tragelaphus scriptus*) are reservoirs of *E ondiri* in endemic areas, and other wild ruminants may be potential reservoirs.

Clinical Findings: The disease ranges from inapparent to fatal, and is characterized by fever, apathy, and petechiation of mucous membranes. After an incubation period of 4-14 days, animals develop a high fever; 2-3 days later, most animals appear dull, and petechiae appear on mucous membranes, particularly the lower surface of the tongue and the vaginal mucosa. These hemorrhages enlarge over several days, and then regress. Marked conjunctival edema and hemorrhage ("poached egg eye") are characteristic in some severe cases. Typically there is total eosinopenia and marked lymphopenia, followed by an equally pronounced neutropenia. At necropsy, widespread hemorrhage and edema are accompanied by lymphoid hyperplasia. No characteristic histological abnormalities have been described. The organism has been observed by electron microscopy in cytoplasmic vacuoles in capillary endothelium, damage to which may account for the characteristic hemorrhages and edema.

Diagnosis: In areas where the disease is endemic, a history of movement to rough grazing areas, coupled with clinical and postmortem signs, allows a presumptive diagnosis. In other areas, demonstration of the causal organism is necessary, either in Giemsa-stained blood or spleen smears, or by inoculation of tissue suspensions into susceptible cattle or sheep. Blood smears from the recipient animal should be taken daily for 10 days and examined for *E ondiri*. *Ehrlichia ondiri* stains blue with Giemsa, and in natural and experimental infections can be observed as small bodies (0.4 μm), larger bodies (1-2 μm), groups of small and large bodies, and groups or morulae of small bodies. They occur in cytoplasmic vacuoles and are most commonly seen in neutrophils.

Treatment and Control: Dithiosemicarbazone has been used successfully to treat early experimental cases. In endemic areas, avoidance of areas associated with previous cases is practiced where possible.

CAPRINE ARTHRITIS AND ENCEPHALITIS (CAE)

A disease syndrome most often manifest in adult dairy goats as chronic, nonresponsive arthritis and mastitis, and in young goats as encephalitis (leukoencephalomyelitis). Serology suggests that the virus is widely distributed among dairy goats in most industrialized countries but rare among indigenous goats of developing countries. The disease has been described in North America, Europe, Australia, and New Zealand. Sheep have been infected experimentally. Currently, there is no evidence that CAE virus (CAEV) will infect man; however, pasteurization of goat milk for human consumption is recommended since it contains high levels of the virus and is a potential source of organisms of zoonotic concern, such as *Coxiella burnetii* and *Salmonella* spp.

Etiology and Pathogenesis: CAEV is a nononcogenic retrovirus in the subfamily Lentivirinae and is antigenically related to the virus of ovine progressive pneumonia and maedi-visna. Monoclonal antibodies can distinguish the viruses of CAE and ovine progressive pneumonia; however, a commercial test to do so is not yet available. The virus usually does not infect the fetus, and most transmission occurs through milk and colostrum. Some transmission may occur during the birth process. Horizontal transmission among nonlactating goats appears to be limited, requiring months or years of contact in most instances. However, infected does that are lactating are considered a relatively potent source of horizontal infection.

Serological surveys indicate an infection rate of >60% among dairy goats in industrialized countries; however, the prevalence of clinical disease is 9-38%. Serology indicates that the older the population of goats, the greater the infection rate.

Most goats are infected while young, carry the virus for life, and develop disease months or years later due to as yet undefined factors.

Clinical Findings: Leukoencephalomyelitis is usually seen in kids 2-4 mo old; it may develop in adults, albeit more insidiously. It usually begins with inability of the kid to adduct one or both hindlegs, often progresses as an ascending paralysis, and ends with seizures and death. Before seizures, the kid is afebrile, alert, and able to eat and drink. Death does not always occur, but regression of paralysis is rare.

The arthritis usually has a long clinical course, but acute exacerbations of pain, lameness, and swelling of joints are common. It most often affects adults but may be seen as early as 4 mo of age. Poor physical condition is typical in chronic cases. Although any joint may be affected, carpi, hocks, stifles, elbows, shoulders, and bursae are involved most commonly. Synovial fluid cells are predominantly mononuclear during all but the most acute stages of the disease. Radiography of chronic cases reveals soft-tissue mineralization around joints and bursae.

Lesions: Kids with the encephalitic form may have grossly visible light brown areas in the white matter of the brain and spinal cord, but histology is necessary to adequately demonstrate the characteristic perivascular cuffs, demyelination, and malacia. On necropsy of a goat with the arthritic form, the carcass is often in poor condition due to inappetence or inability to eat in the later stages of the disease. The joints and bursae are enlarged due to excessive synovial fluid production, fibrous connective tissue proliferation, inflammatory cell infiltrates, and necrotic debris. Open joints reveal thickened, tan synovial membranes; necrosis of connective tissue; and chalky material that is calcium phosphate. The mastitis is characterized by a diffusely swollen, firm udder. The firmness is due to dense periductal to diffuse infiltrations of lymphocytes, plasma cells, and histiocytes. Interstitial pneumonia affecting the cranioventral lobes has been associated with CAEV infection.

Diagnosis: Diagnosis of the encephalitic form of CAE is based on clinical and postmortem findings. Histology is often necessary for a definitive diagnosis. Precipitating antibody against the virus probably indicates persistent infection but is not pathognomonic for any form of the disease since encephalitis, arthritis, mastitis, or pneumonia may have other causes in seropositive animals. Differential diagnoses include various bacterial and parasitic encephalitides, enzootic ataxia (swayback), toxicoses, and trauma.

Diagnosis of CAE arthritis is based on a history of chronic arthritis that is resistant to any form of treatment, and the necropsy findings. Seropositive findings are helpful, but should be considered only as an adjunct to the diagnosis. Differential diagnoses include joint-ill of young goats, trauma, mineral imbalance, chlamydial polyarthritis, mycoplasmal arthritis, and erysipelas.

Diagnoses of CAE mastitis and pneumonia are based on clinical and postmortem findings. Differential diagnoses include various bacterial causes (in mastitis) and viral or bacterial causes (in pneumonia).

Treatment and Control: The course of the encephalitic form cannot be altered by any known therapy. Palliative measures may be helpful in all forms of the disease, and phenylbutazone has been recommended to reduce pain and inflammation in the arthritic form.

The rate of infection of newborn goats can be reduced by >90% by removing kids from infected does as they pass from the birth canal, providing them with colostrum that has been heated to 132°F (56°C) for 1 hr, pasteurizing the milk, and raising them in isolation from infected goats. Serological tests such as the agar-gel immunodiffusion can be used to monitor infection.

CRIMEAN-CONGO HEMORRHAGIC FEVER
(CCHF, Congo virus disease)

A severe, often fatal, viral disease of man transmitted by ticks; infections in domestic animals and adult mammalian wildlife may produce a poorly defined febrile illness that lasts a few days. Although birds are resistant, they may disseminate infective ticks over wide areas. The agent, CCHF virus (a nairovirus, Bunyaviridae), is found in southern China and the USSR, southeastern Europe, India, the Near East, and throughout Africa. CCHF virus is associated with ≥30 tick species of 8 genera, chiefly ixodids (hard ticks). It is probable that the virus is widespread in all countries in Africa and Eurasia that are within the limits of the world distribution of *Hyalomma* ticks. Epidemics occur when *Hyalomma* population densities explode owing to natural climatic cycles or environmental changes; at other times, human cases are sporadic. The virus is maintained in the tick population from the larval to the nymphal and adult stages, and is transmitted transovarially. It is transmitted to man and other animals in the saliva of biting ticks, by contact with infected carcasses or infected bloody discharges, and also by laboratory accidents. CCHF can be diagnosed by virus isolation in suckling mice and tissue culture or by ELISA. Neither vaccine nor treatment is available.

EPHEMERAL FEVER
(Three-day sickness)

An arthropod-transmitted disease of cattle and water buffalo that occurs in Africa, Australia, and Asia, except the USSR. Inapparent infections occur in cape buffalo, hartebeest, waterbuck, wildebeest, and deer.

Etiology and Epidemiology: Ephemeral fever virus is classified as a rhabdovirus (single-stranded RNA). It is best isolated from infected cattle by inoculation of mosquito (*Aedes albopictus*) tissue cultures with defibrinated blood and transfer to baby hamster kidney (BHK 21) or monkey kidney (Vero) cell cultures after 15 days. Both BHK 21 and Vero cell lines may be used to grow the virus and conduct serological tests. Suckling mice may also be used for primary isolation by intracerebral inoculation.

The disease can be transmitted from infected to susceptible cattle by IV inoculation only; as little as 0.005 mL of blood collected during the febrile stage is infective. Although the virus has been recovered from some *Culicoides* and mosquito species (anopheline and culicine) collected in the field, the vectors during major epidemics are not proved. Transmission by contact or fomites does not occur, and the virus does not appear to persist in recovered cattle. Most recovered cattle have life-long immunity.

The prevalence, extent, and severity of the disease vary from year to year, and epidemics occur periodically. During epidemics, onset is rapid, affecting many animals within days or 2-3 wk. It is most prevalent in the wet season in the tropics and in summer to early autumn in the subtropics or temperate regions (when conditions favor multiplication of biting arthropods), and disappears abruptly in winter. Morbidity may be as high as 50-80%, but overall mortality usually is 1-2%, although it is higher in well-conditioned cattle.

Clinical Signs, Lesions, and Diagnosis: Signs, which occur suddenly and vary in severity, include biphasic or polyphasic fever, shivering, inappetence, lacrimation, serous nasal discharge, drooling, dyspnea, atelectasis, atony of forestomachs, depression, stiffness and lameness, and a sudden decrease in milk yield. Affected cattle may become recumbent and paralyzed for 8 hr to ≥1 wk. Lesions include polyserositis affecting joint, pleural, and peritoneal surfaces; some lung edema; and atelectasis. Following recovery, milk production often fails to return to normal levels until the next lactation. Abortion, with total loss of season's lactation, occurs in ~5% of cows pregnant for 8-9 mo. Bulls, other heavy cattle, and heavily producing dairy cows are the most severely affected, but even so, spontaneous recovery usually occurs within a few days.

Diagnosis is based almost entirely on clinical signs in an epidemic. Confirmation is by serology, rarely by virus isolation. All clinical cases have neutrophilia with band forms.

Treatment and Control: Complete rest is the most effective treatment. Anti-inflammatory drugs given early and in repeated doses for 2-3 days are effective. Oral dosing is to be avoided unless the swallowing reflex is functional. Signs of hypocalcemia are treated as for milk fever. Attenuated virus vaccines appear to be effective but should be used only in endemic areas. Inactivated virus vaccines have not produced long-term protection against experimental challenge with virulent virus, and cannot guarantee lasting immunity.

HEARTWATER
(Cowdriosis)

An infectious, noncontagious, rickettsial disease of ruminants in areas infested by ticks of the genus *Amblyomma*, which include regions of Africa south of the Sahara, and the islands of Madagascar, Reunion, Mauritius, and the Caribbean. Many ruminants, including antelopes, are susceptible; others, such as the blesbok and wildebeest become subclinically infected and may act as reservoirs. *Bos indicus* indigenous breeds of cattle appear more resistant than imported breeds.

Etiology and Transmission: The causative organism, *Cowdria ruminantium*, an obligate intracellular parasite, is transmitted under natural conditions by "bont" ticks belonging to the genus *Amblyomma*. These 3-host ticks become infected during either larval or nymphal stages and transmit the infection during one of the subsequent stages. The progeny of an infected female tick are not infective.

The heartwater agent can be propagated experimentally by serial passage either by inoculating infective blood into, or by feeding infected larval and nymphal stages of the tick on, susceptible animals. At room temperature, blood loses its infectivity within a few hours, but the organisms may be preserved in liquid nitrogen. *Cowdria ruminantium* can also be propagated in endothelial-cell tissue culture.

There is no, or only partial, cross-protection between the different strains of *C ruminantium*. Most of them are infective for, but cannot be serially passaged in, mice; however, a few strains are pathogenic to mice infected by the IV route. One of these, the Kümm strain, is highly pathogenic to mice and can be passaged in them even if they are infected IP. The peritoneal macrophages of mice infected with this strain serve as antigen in the indirect FA test.

Clinical Findings and Pathogenesis: The signs are dramatic in the peracute and acute forms. In peracute cases, the animals develop fever, which is followed rapidly by hyperesthesia, lacrimation, and convulsions. In the acute form, the animals show anorexia and nervous signs such as depression, a high-stepping stiff gait, exaggerated blinking of eyes, and chewing movements, which terminate in convulsions and prostration. Diarrhea is occasionally seen. In subacute cases, the signs are less marked, and CNS involvement is inconsistent.

The causative organism initially reproduces in the reticuloendothelial cells, particularly in macrophages, and then invades and multiplies in the vascular endothelium. During the febrile stages, and for a short while thereafter, the blood is infective to susceptible animals. Signs and lesions are associated with injury to the vascular endothelium, which results in increased vascular permeability and extensive tissue hemorrhages. These conditions precipitate a fall in the arterial pressure and general circulatory failure. The lesions in peracute and acute cases are hydrothorax, hydropericardium, edema and congestion of the lungs, splenomegaly, petechiae and ecchymoses on the mucosal and serosal surfaces, and occasionally, hemorrhage into the GI tract.

Diagnosis: In acute forms, diagnosis can be based on clinical signs. Demonstration of colonies of the organism in the cytoplasm of capillary endothelial cells is necessary for definitive diagnosis. This is done with Giemsa-stained "squash" smears of cerebral gray matter. An indirect FA test is used to detect antibodies in the serum of animals that have recovered from clinical or subclinical natural or artificial infection. In sheep and goats these antibodies persist for several years, and their presence correlates well with resistance to natural or artifical challenge. Seropositive cattle are resistant to challenge, although antibodies are no longer detectable 9-12 mo after infection. Immunity in heartwater appears to be chiefly, if not exclusively, cell-mediated.

Treatment and Control: Control of tick infestation is a useful prophylactic measure in some instances, but may be difficult and expensive to maintain in others. Excessive reduction of tick numbers, however, interferes with the maintenance of an adequate immunity through regular challenge and may result in heavy losses.

Infected sheep blood is used as a vaccine in combination with antibiotic treatment at the time of reaction. Young calves (<6 wk) and lambs and kids (<1 wk) are fairly resistant and may recover spontaneously from natural and experimental infections. Tetracyclines at 10 mg/kg body wt usually effect a cure if administered early. In sheep, goats, and susceptible cattle breeds, a higher treatment level (10-20 mg/kg) may be required, particularly late in the febrile reaction or when clinical signs appear. A second or third treatment may be necessary.

MALIGNANT CATARRHAL FEVER
(MCF, Malignant head catarrh, Snotsiekte, Catarrhal fever, Gangrenous coryza)

An acute, sporadic, infectious disease of cattle and some other Bovidae and Cervidae, characterized by low morbidity and extremely high mortality, although on occasions, morbidity can be high, particularly in susceptible species such as Pere David's deer and Bali cattle. MCF has become an important disease of farmed deer.

Etiology: While MCF is a single clinicopathological entity, there are at least 2 distinct but related agents that can cause the disease naturally. One, alcelaphine herpesvirus 1 (AHV-1), which is carried inapparently by wildebeest (*Connochaetes taurinus*), is prevalent in Africa and in zoological parks, and is responsible for "wildebeest-derived" MCF (WD-MCF). The other principal cause is the "sheep-associated" (SA) agent of MCF. While the SA-MCF agent has not been isolated, molecular and serological evidence indicate it is similar to AHV-1. It occurs worldwide and is thought to infect most domestic sheep, usually without causing disease. Experimentally, both MCF agents can be transmitted to cattle, deer, rabbits, and hamsters with blood or lymph node cells from affected animals. WD-MCF can also be transmitted to guinea pigs and rats with infected lymph node cells. In addition, viruses similar to AHV-1 isolated from 2 other species of alcelaphine antelope, topi, and hartebeest have caused MCF following experimental inoculation in cattle. Herpesviruses isolated from these 2 species are distinct from AHV-1 and have been designated AHV-2.

Transmission and Epidemiology: AHV-1 is transmitted vertically and horizontally in populations of wildebeest. Some wildebeest calves, infected *in utero*, later spread virus in nasal and ocular secretions and feces to others, most being infected by 6 mo of age. Fomites, particularly those contaminated at calving, are thought to be able to carry infection to susceptible ruminants. It seems likely that a similar scenario occurs with the SA agent at lambing time, but the evidence to support this hypothesis is circumstantial. Under farm conditions, MCF usually occurs in adults. In zoos, juveniles may also be affected. Deer farms can experience a 1% annual mortality. Susceptibility to MCF among deer varies: wapiti and red deer are much more susceptible than cattle; Pere David's and, apparently, sika and whitetail deer are highly susceptible. Disease has not been reported in fallow deer, which suggests they are resistant. Susceptible ruminants are "end hosts", which develop clinical MCF following an incubation period of 3 wk to 6 mo. In such animals the virus is cell-associated, and lateral transmission is rare.

Pathogenesis: The most plausible current hypothesis is that development of the disease hinges on infection of immunoregulatory, large, granular lymphocytes, with "natural-killer" (NK) activity. The normal MCF reaction has the characteristics of a T-lymphocyte hyperplasia, a polyclonal response resulting from deregulation of the T lymphocytes. It is suggested that the necrotizing process of the terminal phase of the disease is an autoimmune phenomenon arising through the expression of NK-like activity of certain immune system cells.

Clinical Findings: MCF can take acute (especially in deer), subacute ("head and eye"), or chronic forms. Acute cases may be seen as sudden deaths, but usually, death is preceded by fever, depression, enlarged lymph nodes, serous nasal and ocular discharges, erosions of the buccal papillae, ophthalmia, and diarrhea (sometimes hemorrhagic). Deer may have prominent intestinal hemorrhage and evidence of disseminated intravascular coagulation (qv, p 24). Dyspnea also may be present. Death occurs in 1-3 days. The "head and eye" syndrome is the most common form in cattle. Additional signs include inflammatory and erosive lesions in the mucosa of the upper respiratory tract that lead to profuse mucopurulent nasal discharge with encrustation of the muzzle, ulceration of the oral mucosa, salivation, and mucopurulent conjunctivitis with corneal opacity that begins at the corneoscleral junction and progresses centripetally. Hypopyon may be present. Patchy exanthema with matting of the hair, and ulceration of the perineum, vulva, coronet, interdigital skin, and teats may occur. Some animals show CNS signs such as excitability, hyperesthesia, and muscular tremors. Occasionally, these may progress to convulsions or an aggressiveness suggestive of rabies. The course of the "head and eye" form can last for up to 2 wk. In chronic MCF, inanition develops. Recovery is rare. The hemogram may show lymphocytosis followed by lymphopenia. Neutrophilia may occur if tissue damage is extensive.

Lesions: These are widespread and usually affect all organs, but their severity and nature vary considerably. The principal changes that characterize MCF are epithelial necrosis (GI, respiratory, or urinary) associated with mucosal and/or dermal lymphoid inflammation, lymphoproliferation, interstitial infiltration of nonlymphoid tissues, and vasculitis. In deer, hemorrhage into the lumen of the ileum, cecum, and colon may be prominent, together with ecchymoses in the colonic serosa. Most lymph nodes are hyperplastic with prominent development of the paracortex, but hemorrhage and necrosis may occur terminally. A prominent feature is interstitial infiltration of organs by lymphocytes, especially heart, liver, adrenal gland, meninges, CNS perivascular spaces, and kidney. In the kidney it can be detected grossly as white, raised foci under the capsule. Vascular lesions can occur in most body systems and vary in intensity from a mild infiltration of the adventitia by lymphocytes to transmural lesions comprising fibrinoid necrosis, lymphoid infiltration, and occasionally thrombosis. In chronic cases, proliferative changes in the walls of affected vessels may lead to their enlargement and prominence. The rete mirabilis is a tissue of choice to demonstrate vascular lesions.

Diagnosis: MCF is a clinicopathological entity and, while it may be suspected clinically, confirmation relies on histological examination, especially the demonstration of degenerative epithelial lesions, multisystemic lymphoid infiltration, and vasculitis. When AHV-1 is the cause, virus isolation from the buffy coat of ante- and postmortem blood samples collected at necropsy can confirm a diagnosis. Antibody that reacts with this virus can be detected by indirect immunofluoresence in serum from wildebeest, sheep, and some clinically affected animals. Virus neutralization and ELISA tests may also provide evidence of infection. MCF antibodies may cross-react with other bovine herpesviruses in the immunofluorescence and ELISA tests, but not by virus neutralization. Differential diagnoses include rinderpest, bluetongue, vesicular diseases, East Coast cattle fever (*Theileria parva*), infectious bovine rhinotracheitis, bovine viral diarrhea-mucosal disease, and shipping fever and, when there are nervous signs, rabies and the tick-borne encephalitides. When farmed red deer are affected, yersiniosis must be excluded.

Treatment and Control: Survival is rare, but antibiotics or sulfonamides to control secondary bacterial infection and supportive therapy (fluids) may be worthwhile in valuable animals. The separation of susceptible animals from the source of infection, viz wildebeest and sheep, is essential to prevent the disease.

NAIROBI SHEEP DISEASE

A tick-borne viral disease of sheep and goats characterized by fever and gastroenteritis. It occurs in Kenya, Uganda, Tanzania, Somalia, Ethiopia, and Zaire. Although man is susceptible, human infections are rare.

Etiology and Transmission: The causal nairovirus, family Bunyaviridae, is possibly the most pathogenic virus known for sheep and goats. It is closely related to Ganjam virus, a tick-borne infection in India of sheep, goats, and man; to Dugbe virus, another tick-borne infection; and Crimean-Congo hemorrhagic fever virus (qv, p 394). It is transmitted transovarially and transtadially by the brown ear tick, *Rhipicephalus appendiculatus*, in which it can survive for ~2½ yr. Other *Rhipicephalus* and *Amblyomma* ticks also may transmit the disease. The virus is shed in the urine and feces, but the disease is not spread by contact.

Clinical Findings: A prodromal fever lasting 1-3 days follows an incubation period of 4-15 days. Sometimes, the fever is diphasic. Illness is manifest by depression; anorexia; mucopurulent, blood-stained, nasal discharge; and fetid dysentery that causes painful straining. Pregnant animals frequently abort. Death may occur in the early febrile viremic phase or follow ~2 days after remission of the fever. Mortality in sheep is 30-90%. Native sheep are more susceptible than Merinos. The disease in goats is usually less severe, although 80% mortality has been reported.

    Lesions: The main lesions are hyperplasia of lymphoid tissues and hemorrhages of the GI (particularly the abomasum) and respiratory tracts, gallbladder, spleen, and heart. However, these hemorrhages are not invariably seen, particularly when death occurs early in the viremic stage. The fetus has dermal hemorrhages. Additional histological lesions are glomerulonephritis and myocardial necrosis.

Diagnosis: The occurrence of a disease in sheep or goats with high mortality, accompanied by a tick infestation is suggestive, especially if it follows movements into endemic areas or changes in tick populations that have been induced by heavy and prolonged rainfall. Confirmation of suggestive signs and lesions requires isolation and serological identification of the virus. The preferred specimens are blood, mesenteric lymph nodes, and spleen.

Control: In endemic areas, clinical signs are not seen unless susceptible animals are introduced. Such animals should be vaccinated, as should those exposed when the range of the tick vector extends. Tick control is not practical.

PARATUBERCULOSIS
(Johne's Disease)

    A chronic, contagious enteritis characterized by persistent and progressive diarrhea, weight loss, debilitation, and eventually, death. It affects cattle, sheep, goats, llamas, camels, farmed deer, and other domestic and wild ruminants. Distribution is worldwide. The zoonotic risk has been considered minimal, but the isolation of similar organisms from some people with Crohn's enteritis makes this less certain.

Etiology and Pathogenesis: Cultivation of *Mycobacterium paratuberculosis* *(johnei)*, the causative organism, requires incorporation of mycobactin, a growth factor derived from mycobacteria, into the media. The organism is quite resistant and can survive in feces and soil for >1 yr. It is shed in large numbers in feces of infected animals, and infection is acquired by ingestion of contaminated feed and water. Introduction of the disease into a clean herd is usually by subclinically infected carriers.

    Infection is acquired early in life, but clinical signs rarely develop in cattle <2 yr old. Resistance increases with age and cattle first exposed as adults are unlikely to become infected. Most calves are infected soon after birth by nursing udders contaminated with feces from infected animals, or when they are housed in contaminated pens. The organism can also be present in colostrum and milk of infected cows. After ingestion, the bacteria localize in the mucosa of the lower small intestine and in associated lymph nodes. If not eliminated, the organisms multiply and initiate development of the intestinal lesions that result in overt clinical signs. However, fecal shedding begins before clinical signs are apparent. *Mycobacterium paratuberculosis* can be isolated from feces, mesenteric and ileocecal lymph nodes, thickened intestinal wall, and less frequently, the udder and the reproductive tracts of both sexes.

Clinical Findings: The disease is characterized by weight loss and diarrhea, but initial signs are variable and often vague. Over weeks or months the diarrhea becomes more severe, there is further weight loss, coat color may fade, and ventral and intermandibular edema may develop. In dairy cattle, milk yield may drop or fail to reach expected levels. Animals are alert, and temperature and appetite are usually normal, although thirst may be increased. The disease is progressive and ultimately terminates in emaciation and death. Most cases occur in 2- to 6-yr-old cattle. The disease in sheep and goats is similar, but diarrhea is less marked than in cattle. In deer, the course of the disease can be more rapid.

Lesions: A granulomatous response characterized by progressive accumulation of epithelioid cells in the mucosa and submucosa occurs in the lower small intestine. This results in diffuse hypertrophy of the lower jejunum, ileum, and ileocecal valve and adjacent cecum, with the formation of thick transverse folds. The lesions are characterized by absence of inflammation or ulceration. Lymphangitis with varying involvement of adjacent lymph nodes is common. Often, there is no correlation between clinical signs and severity of lesions. Sheep and goats may develop foci of caseation with calcification in the intestinal wall and lymph nodes, and intestinal thickening is usually less marked than in cattle.

Diagnosis: Fecal culture is the most reliable method of detecting animals shedding *M paratuberculosis*, but requires 12-16 wk incubation before results are available. Positive tests are significant, but because shedding may be intermittent, negative results mean little, and testing of additional samples is required. Fecal culture detects ~20-50% of the infected animals on initial herd tests. The organism can also be detected in fecal samples by means of gene probes that identify nucleic acid sequences to *M paratuberculosis*. Procedures that amplify the desired nucleic acid sequences make it possible to detect infection even when only low numbers of organisms are present. At necropsy, the organism may be detected in the intestinal epithelium and adjacent lymph nodes, either histologically or by culture.

Serologic tests provide more rapid results than fecal culture, but have some deficiencies. The complement-fixation test is cumbersome and relatively insensitive, and is seldom used. The agar-gel-immunodiffusion test, while easy to perform, has low sensitivity and is used primarily to confirm infection in animals with clinical signs. The ELISA has good sensitivity with somewhat lower specificity, and is useful when applied as a herd test rather than to individual animals.

Tests of cell-mediated immunity (eg, Johnin test, lymphocyte transformation, and leukocyte-migration-inhibition tests) are of little practical diagnostic value.

Control: No satisfactory treatment is known. Control requires good sanitation and management. Herds with confirmed cases should be tested to determine the extent of infection, and positive animals sent to slaughter. Retesting, at 6-mo to 1-yr intervals, should be continued until ≥3 negative tests are obtained. Calves should be removed from cows immediately after birth, bottle-fed colostrum that has been pasteurized or obtained from negative cows, and then reared completely segregated from adults until >1 yr old. Because intrauterine infection can occur, calves from dams that have or develop signs of the disease should be culled. Even if replacements are from herds believed to be free of the disease, they should be tested before and after purchase.

In many countries, use of vaccines is subject to approval by regulatory agencies, and restricted to infected herds. Calfhood (<1 mo of age) vaccination can be effective in reducing disease incidence, but does not eliminate infection. Cattle inoculated with inactivated whole-cell, mineral-oil vaccine develop granulomas, one to several inches in diameter, at the site of inoculation (brisket) and may react positively on subsequent tuberculin tests. Accidental self-inoculation can result in severe acute reactions with sloughing and chronic synovitis and tendinitis. Vaccination does not eliminate the need for good management and sanitation.

PASTEURELLOSIS OF SHEEP

There are 2 distinct syndromes depending on the biotype of *Pasteurella haemolytica* involved (*P multocida* rarely causes endemic disease, at least in temperate climates). Biotype A strains (12 serotypes) cause pneumonia in flocks and sporadically in individuals as well as septicemic infections in young lambs. Biotype T strains (4 serotypes) cause peracute disease of a different pathogenesis. Untypable strains are isolated from ~10% of cases. Pneumonic pasteurellosis has been reported from most of the principal sheep-rearing countries. The distribution of biotype T disease is unclear, but it does occur in the UK, USA, and Hungary.

PNEUMONIC PASTEURELLOSIS (ENZOOTIC PNEUMONIA)

A variable portion of healthy sheep carry biotype A strains in the upper respiratory tract. The factors that predispose sheep to active lung infections are poorly understood. Environmental stress and infectious agents, eg, parainfluenza virus type 3 and adenovirus, are among those that have been incriminated. A flock outbreak usually starts suddenly with sheep dying or acutely ill with respiratory disease. Other sheep in the flock show less severe signs, such as coughing and mild oculonasal discharge. Mortality is rarely >10%. In lambs <2 mo old, the disease is more often septicemic than pneumonic.

In the acute disease, there is fibrinous pericardial effusion and a clear pleural exudate with fibrin clots. The lungs are enlarged, edematous, and bright purplish red, usually with distinct consolidation in the anteroventral areas. In sheep that have survived longer, the lesions are more sharply demarcated and darker red, and there are adhesions between the pleurae. Diagnosis depends on the recovery of large numbers of *P haemolytica* biotype A from the lesions. Biotype T strains are rarely isolated under these circumstances.

In acute cases, the clostridial diseases appropriate to the age group affected must be considered in differential diagnosis.

Oxytetracycline (20 mg/kg of the long-acting preparation) every 3-4 days is appropriate for therapy and for prophylaxis in in-contact sheep. Multivalent vaccines, including a range of the more common serotypes, generally give protection when used according to the manufacturers' instructions. Antibody titer has been demonstrated in ewe colostrum and in serum of lambs suckled on ewes vaccinated with biotype A antigens.

SYSTEMIC PASTEURELLOSIS

The systemic form of pasteurellosis is caused by biotype T strains, which are carried in the tonsils, spread to and multiply in the lungs, and then spread further to other organs. The epidemiology is poorly understood. The disease often manifests itself a few days after the plane of nutrition has been increased or after the stress of transport; this is especially true in sheep ~6 mo old. Deaths often occur in those in good condition, and continue for a few days with mortality of ~5%. Affected sheep usually are found dead. Those seen alive are dull, unwilling to move, and have dyspnea, a frothy discharge from the mouth, and unless in the terminal stages, a fever. At necropsy, there is evidence of systemic infection. Hemorrhagic, exudative inflammation of the abomasal mucosa and petechiae on the visceral peritoneum, in the neck, and beneath the parietal pleura are prominent. The kidneys may show cortical softening as in pulpy kidney disease. Pure cultures of *P haemolytica* biotype T may be recovered from the organs and cardiac blood. Acute toxicoses, metabolic disorders, and septicemias caused by organisms other than pasteurellae are differential diagnoses. Antibiotic therapy often is not possible because of the sudden onset of the disease. Gradual introduction to feed of increased nutritive value should be practiced, and prophylactic vaccination should be considered.

Pasteurella haemolytica also causes sporadic cases of mid-lactation mastitis, meningitis, and arthritis.

PESTE DES PETITS RUMINANTS (PPR)

PPR is also known as pseudorinderpest of small ruminants, pest of small ruminants, pest of sheep and goats, Kata, stomatitis-pneumoenteritis syndrome, contagious pustular stomatitis, and pneumoenteritis complex. It is an acute or subcute viral disease of goats and sheep characterized by fever, necrotic stomatitis, gastroenteritis, and pneumonia. It was first reported as a clinical entity in the Ivory Coast in 1942, and subsequently in Senegal, Ghana, Togo, Benin, and Nigeria. Sheep are less susceptible than goats; cattle are only subclinically infected. Man is not at risk.

Etiology and Epidemiology: The causal virus, a morbillivirus of the family Paramyxoviridae (*see also* RINDERPEST [RP], p 404), has a particular affinity for lymphoid tissues and epithelial tissue of the GI tract, in which it produces characteristic lesions.

PPR is prevalent in West and Central Africa and the Middle East. Outbreaks that affect only a few animals frequently are not reported; epidemics occur when the population of susceptible animals increases. Such an epidemic may eliminate the goats and sheep in an area. Transmission is by close contact, and confinement seems to favor outbreaks. Secretions and excretions of sick animals are the sources of infection. As in RP, it is generally accepted that there is no carrier state; however, subclinical cases may spread the infection during their incubation phase. White-tailed deer are fully susceptible; these and other wild ruminants may play a role in the epidemiology of the disease. Although subclinical infections can be experimentally induced in pigs, they do not transmit the disease to susceptible pigs or goats; therefore, pigs may have no role in PPR epidemiology. Although cattle are susceptible to infection, they usually do not exhibit clinical signs or transmit the disease.

Clinical Findings: The acute form of PPR is accompanied by a sudden rise in body temperature to 104-106°F (40-41.3°C). Affected animals appear ill and restless and have a dull coat, dry muzzle, congested mucous membranes, and depressed appetite. Early, the nasal discharge is serous; later, it becomes mucopurulent and gives a putrid odor to the breath. The incubation period is usually 4-5 days. Small areas of necrosis may be observed on the mucous membrane on the floor of the nasal cavity. The conjunctiva is frequently congested, and the medial canthus may exhibit a small degree of crusting. Some affected animals develop a profuse catarrhal conjunctivitis with matting of the eyelids. Necrotic stomatitis affects the lower lip and gum and around the insertions of the incisor teeth; in more severe cases, it may involve the dental pad, palate, cheeks and their papillae, and the tongue. Diarrhea may be profuse and is accompanied by dehydration and emaciation; hypothermia and death follow, usually after 5-10 days. Bronchopneumonia, characterized by coughing, may develop later. Pregnant animals may abort. In young animals, morbidity and mortality rates are higher than in adults. Latent infections may be activated and complicate the clinical picture.

Lesions: Emaciation, conjunctivitis, and stomatitis are seen; necrotic lesions are inside the lower lip and on the adjacent gum, the cheeks near the commissure, and on the ventral surface of the tongue. In severe cases, the lesions may extend to the hard palate and pharynx. The erosions are shallow, with a red raw base and later become pinkish white; they are bounded by normal epithelium that provides a sharply demarcated margin. The rumen, reticulum, and omasum rarely are involved. The abomasum exhibits regularly outlined erosions that have a red raw floor, and ooze blood.

Severe lesions are less common in the small intestine than in the mouth, abomasum, or large intestines. Streaks of hemorrhages, and less frequently erosions, may be present in the first portion of the duodenum and terminal ileum. Peyer's patches are severely affected; entire patches of lymphoid tissue may slough. The large intestine is usually more severely affected, with lesions occurring around the ileocecal valve and at the cecocolic junction and rectum. The latter exhibits streaks of congestion along the folds of the mucosa resulting in the characteristic "zebra-striped" appearance.

Petechiae may appear in the turbinates, larynx, and trachea. Patches of bronchopneumonia may be present.

Diagnosis: A presumptive diagnosis is based on clinical, pathological, and epidemiological findings, and may be confirmed by virus isolation and identification. The specimens required are unclotted blood, lymph nodes, tonsils, spleen, and whole lung. Detection of viral antigens by complement fixation or agar-gel precipitin tests does not differentiate the disease from RP. Detection of virus-neutralizing antibodies with a rising titer in surviving animals is diagnostic. PPR must be differentiated from other acute GI infections (eg, RP), from respiratory infections (eg, contagious caprine pleuropneumonia), and from such other diseases as contagious ecthyma, heartwater, coccidiosis, and mineral poisoning.

Control: When PPR is suspected, state and federal authorities should be notified. Eradication is recommended when the disease appears in previously PPR-free countries; RP eradication methods are useful. There is no specific treatment; however, treatment for bacterial and parasitic complications decreases mortality in affected herds. An attenuated vaccine has been prepared in embryonic caprine kidney cell culture; it affords protection from natural disease for ~1 yr. RP cell culture vaccine also has been used successfully for immunization against PPR.

RIFT VALLEY FEVER
(Infectious enzootic hepatitis of sheep and cattle)

A mosquito-borne viral disease of animals, including man, characterized by a short incubation period, fever, hepatitis, abortion, and death in young animals. Most domestic animals are affected except for pigs, guinea pigs, rabbits, and chickens. Young lambs, kids, calves, and puppies are highly susceptible. Sheep and man are more susceptible than cattle and dogs. Significant morbidity and mortality occur in sheep, cattle, and man. The disease has been diagnosed in many African countries; recent outbreaks have occurred in Egypt, Senegal, and Mauritania.

Etiology and Epidemiology: The causal agent is a phlebovirus, family Bunyaviridae; it is rapidly inactivated at a pH of <6.2. Explosive epidemics have occurred at 5- to 15-yr intervals and are normally associated with periods of heavy rainfall in generally dry areas. In the interepidemic periods, the virus is believed to be in dormant eggs of the mosquito *Aedes lineatopennis* in the dry soil of grassland depressions (dambos). With adequate rainfall, the infected mosquitoes develop and infect ruminants, which amplify the virus. The virus is spread by many species of mosquitoes. Man is also readily infected through aerosols from infected animals, their tissues, aborted fetuses, and laboratory procedures, and has the potential to introduce the disease (via mosquitoes) to other animals in uninfected areas.

Clinical Findings: The incubation period in sheep and cattle is 12-96 hr. In young lambs, kids, calves, and puppies, the onset is rapid, with fever of 104-107°F (40-41.5°C), listlessness, anorexia, weakness, and death. In lambs <1 wk old, mortality may be >90% in 36 hr; in lambs and calves >1 wk old, it is ~20%. In adult sheep, there may be fever, listlessness, anorexia, unsteady gait, vomiting, mucopurulent nasal discharge, diarrhea, and abortion, or abortion may be the only sign; mortality is seldom >30%. In adult cattle, there may be fever, anorexia, salivation, drop in milk production, abortion, and diarrhea, or abortion may be the only sign; mortality is usually <10%.

Lesions: The primary lesion in all species is a focal hepatic necrosis, which may or may not be grossly visible. Lambs dying of the disease have enlarged, soft, friable, yellowish brown to dark red livers with gray, necrotic foci and petechiae. Widespread cutaneous, visceral, and serosal hemorrhages occur. Adult sheep and cattle may have scattered, pale, necrotic foci in the liver; visceral and serosal hemorrhages; and hemorrhagic enteritis. In lambs, there is a focal to diffuse coagulative necrosis of hepatocytes. Intranuclear inclusion bodies have been observed. In adult sheep and cattle, the focal areas of hepatic necrosis are smaller and fewer than in lambs.

Diagnosis: Rift Valley fever should be suspected when the epidemiologic pattern includes: short incubation period, high mortality in animals <1 wk old (particularly lambs, calves, kids, and puppies), illness and abortions in sheep and cattle, liver lesions, hemorrhagic or influenza-like disease in man, and the presence of an arthropod vector. Differential diagnoses include bluetongue, enterotoxemia, Wesselsbron disease, and ephemeral fever. Confirmation of a suspected diagnosis requires isolation and serological identification of the virus using mice and/or cell cultures. Serological surveys are complicated by cross-reactions between Rift Valley fever virus and other phleboviruses.

Control: Moving stock from low-lying, mosquito-infested regions to higher altitudes, or stabling plus spraying is recommended. Inactivated vaccine requires 2 injections and must be repeated annually. An attenuated neurotropic vaccine produced in mice stimulates rapid and long-lasting immunity but is abortogenic and teratogenic. A recently developed and tested mutagenized vaccine produces rapid protection, has no adverse effect on newborn lambs, is safe for pregnant animals, and produces a low viremia that is not a source of virus for mosquitoes.

RINDERPEST
(Cattle plague)

A disease of cloven-hoofed animals characterized by fever, necrotic stomatitis, gastroenteritis, lymphoid necrosis, and high mortality. In epidemic form, it is the most lethal plague known in cattle. Susceptibility varies among species: it is high in African buffalo, giraffes, wild Suidae, Tragelaphinae, and breeds of cattle such as Ankole, Channel Islands, and Japanese Black; moderate in wildebeest and East African zebus; and mild in gazelles and small domestic ruminants. Rinderpest is subclinical in European pigs and hippopotami. It is endemic in India and Africa. Lack of control in bordering countries has recently led to epidemics in west, east, and north Africa; the Near East; and parts of Asia.

Etiology, Epidemiology, and Pathogenesis: The infectious agent is a morbillivirus, closely related to the viruses of peste des petits ruminants (qv, p 402), canine distemper (qv, p 408), and measles. Strains of virus vary markedly in host range and virulence. Sera from recovered or vaccinated cattle cross-react with all strains in neutralization tests, but minor antigenic differences have been demonstrated.

Virus is present in small amounts in nasal secretions 1-2 days before fever; levels are high in secretions and excretions during the first week of clinical disease and decrease rapidly as animals develop antibody and begin to recover. Transmission requires direct or close indirect contact; infection is via the nasopharynx. The virus is fragile and rapidly inactivated by heat and light, but remains viable for long periods in chilled or frozen tissues. There is no carrier state; the virus maintains itself by continuous transmission among susceptible animals. In endemic areas, young cattle become infected after maternal immunity disappears and before vaccine immunity begins, with possible auxiliary cycles in sheep, goats, and wild ungulates. In epidemic areas, the virus infects most susceptible animals and tends to limit itself unless the population is large enough to support endemicity.

Following primary growth in lymph nodes associated with the nasopharynx, the virus proliferates throughout the lymphoid tissue and spreads via the blood to the mucosae of the GI and upper respiratory tracts. Tissue damage is caused by viral cytopathology. Viral antigens induce a potent immune response that controls the infection and allows recovery if tissue damage is not too severe.

Clinical Findings: An incubation period of 3-15 days is followed by fever, anorexia, and depression; oculonasal discharge develops 1-2 days later. Within 2-3 days, pinpoint necrotic lesions, which rapidly enlarge to form cheesy plaques, appear on the gums, buccal mucosa, and tongue. The hard and soft palates are affected often. The oculonasal discharge becomes mucopurulent, and the muzzle dry and cracked. Diarrhea, the final clinical sign, may be watery and contain blood, mucus, and mucous membrane. Animals show severe abdominal pain, thirst, and dyspnea, and may die from dehydration. Convalescence is prolonged and may be complicated by concurrent infections due to immunosuppression. In endemic areas, morbidity is low and clinical signs often mild, whereas in epidemics, morbidity is often 100% and mortality up to 90%.

Lesions: Gross pathological changes are evident throughout the GI and upper respiratory tracts, either as areas of necrosis and erosion, or congestion and hemorrhage, the latter causing classical "zebra striping" in the rectum. Lymph nodes may be enlarged and edematous, with white necrotic foci in the Peyer's patches. Histological examination reveals lymphoid and epithelial necrosis with viral syncytia and intracytoplasmic inclusions.

Diagnosis: Clinical and pathological findings may be sufficient for diagnosis in endemic areas and after initial laboratory confirmation of an epidemic. In areas where the disease is uncommon or absent, laboratory tests must be used to differentiate it from bovine viral diarrhea in particular, and East Coast fever, foot-and-mouth disease, infectious bovine rhinotracheitis, and malignant catarrhal fever. Virus isolation and detection of specific viral antigens in affected tissues are standard tests, and demonstration of rising antibody titers is useful. Simple, rapid tests for antigen detection (immunodiffusion or counter immunoelectrophoresis) are valuable in the field.

Specimens for the laboratory must be collected from several animals during the early stages of clinical disease, preferably before onset of diarrhea. Whole blood, lymphoid tissue, spleen, and gut lesions should be collected aseptically and transported swiftly at 25°F (4°C) or on ice.

Control: Treatment usually is not attempted, but nursing care with supportive fluid and antibiotic therapy may aid recovery of valuable animals. Active immunity is usually lifelong; maternal immunity lasts 6-11 mo. Control in endemic areas is by immunization of all cattle and domestic buffalo >1 yr old with attenuated cell culture vaccine. In these areas, outbreaks are controlled by quarantine and "ring vaccination" and sometimes slaughter. In epidemic areas, the disease is best controlled by slaughter and quarantine. Control of animal movement is paramount since most outbreaks are due to introduction of infected cattle. Countries free of the disease and that border endemic areas must be extremely vigilant or vaccinate as a precaution.

TICK-BORNE FEVER (TBF)

A disease of ruminants transmitted by *Ixodes ricinus* in Europe and *Rhipicephalus haemaphysaloides supino* in India. It has been identified in sheep and cattle in the UK, Eire, Norway, Finland, and India. It has also been described in goats and deer.

Etiology: The causative agent is generally accepted to be a member of the order Rickettsiales, although its final classification remains unresolved. Formerly called *Rickettsia phagocytophila*, it is now commonly referred to as *Ehrlichia phagocytophila* or *Cytoecetes phagocytophila*. The agent primarily parasitizes neutrophils and is visible as grayish blue bodies in the cytoplasm under light microscopy of Romanowsky-stained blood smears.

Several morphological forms of the agent have been described; they range from small rounded or rod-shaped bodies of 0.5 μm diameter to larger rounded bodies of up to 3 μm in diameter. Groups of bodies (called morulae), 2-4 μm in diameter, also have been described.

Trans-stadial transmission in *I ricinus* has been demonstrated, although transovarial has not. Lambs and calves on tick-infested pastures pick up a tick burden soon after birth, and are infected within the first 2-3 wk of life. Although not all ticks carry the agent of TBF, a high portion of adult and nymphal ticks appear to be infected since even a light tick infestation on pasture is sufficient to transmit and maintain the disease.

Transmission may also occur by contaminated needles.

Clinical Findings: Following an incubation period of 2-6 days, the most common and often the only clinical signs are pyrexia, dullness, and anorexia, which last ~5-8 days. Thereafter, the animals recover and, although largely immune to subsequent infection, many remain as carriers and act as reservoirs of infection for new generations of ticks. Several more severe effects have been noted. These include a growth check or weight loss in lambs, and a marked but temporary drop in milk yield in cows. Abortion has been reported in ewes and cows, and rams and bulls may show greatly reduced semen quality. Variations in the severity of the clinical effects may be related to differences between strains of TBF or in host susceptibility.

Perhaps the most significant effect of TBF infection is its serious impairment of humoral and cellular defense mechanisms, which predisposes the host to secondary infections, eg, tick pyemia, pneumonic pasteurellosis, and louping-ill infection.

Lesions: A series of distinct though transient hematological changes follow infection with TBF. Two to 4 days after infection a modest neutrophilia develops, followed by a marked neutropenia for 4-8 days. Eosinophil and lymphocyte numbers may decrease in parallel with the fall in neutrophils. In sheep and cattle, the neutrophil is the main WBC parasitized, and at the peak of the reaction ≥90% of circulating neutrophils may contain rickettsial bodies.

The severe neutropenia and heavy parasitism of the remaining neutrophils greatly impair the functional capacity of these cells. Concurrently, a lymphocytopenia develops and reduces the ability of the animal to produce antibodies and mount a cell-mediated response. These changes may last 2-3 wk; then, the animal shows greatly increased susceptibility to secondary infections.

At necropsy of uncomplicated cases, gross abnormalities are restricted to an enlarged spleen.

Diagnosis: Clinical history and the presence of the tick vector are useful aids. Clinical disease usually occurs only in young animals born in tick-infested areas or in older animals newly introduced to such areas. Diagnosis should be confirmed by microscopical examination of stained (commonly Leishman's or Giemsa) blood smears for the presence of TBF organisms in the cytoplasm of circulating WBC, chiefly neutrophils.

Control: There are 3 aspects of control: vector control, immunity, and chemotherapy. Effective control can be achieved by eliminating or markedly reducing contact with the tick vector, by grazing cattle and sheep on tick-free pastures in lowland areas, or by use of acaricides. In sheep practice, this commonly involves keeping the ewe and lamb in a fenced, relatively tick-free pasture until the lamb is ~6 wk old. The lamb also benefits from improved nutrition of the ewe. Dipping of lambs within 1-2 wk of birth is not commonly practiced because of difficulties of gathering the lambs on widely dispersed hill farms, the risks of mis-mothering, and the relatively short duration of protection provided by the acaricide, possibly because of the short fleece and rapid growth rate of the lamb. However, dipping twice with a 2- to 3-wk interval does reduce the incidence of infection. Studies have also demonstrated the benefit of pour-on acaricides in lambs.

Several aspects of the immunity remain controversial, but it is generally accepted that sheep and cattle are immune to challenge following recovery from 1 or 2 clinical reactions to TBF. The immunity may last for up to 1 yr, although it apparently wanes more rapidly if the animals are removed from tick-infested pasture. Some residual immunity may persist even when animals become reinfected since secondary reactions are commonly milder than the initial one. Different strains of TBF exist, usually with a significant degree of cross-immunity between them. Ruminants with acquired immunity are usually carriers, ie, small numbers of organisms persist in their bodies, and most that graze tick-infested pasture act as continual sources of tick infection.

A number of drugs have been used to suppress or prevent TBF. Oxytetracycline used in outbreaks in dairy cattle has reduced pyrexia and restored milk yield. Treatment is particularly effective if given within a few days of infection, although relapses may occur. Sulfamethazine has also proved useful, and its effects are similar to those of oxytetracycline. Long-acting tetracycline administered to lambs in the first 2-3 wk of life has resulted in protection that lasts ~2 wk; it also effectively reduces the incidence of secondary infections such as tick pyemia and leads to improved growth rate.

TICK PYEMIA

An endemic staphylococcal disease of lambs between 2 wk and 3 mo old, associated with infestations of *Ixodes ricinus*. It is characterized by pyemic abscesses commonly found in joints, although they may be present in virtually any organ. The disease is an important cause of economic loss through debilitation and death of lambs. It has been described in all the tick-infested areas of the UK and Eire.

Etiology: *Staphylococcus aureus* is consistently isolated from the pyemic abscesses. There is evidence that the staphylococci are inoculated by the tick during feeding, thus bypassing the cutaneous defenses. However, it also seems likely that the bacteria gain entrance from any wound or from an infected umbilicus, and produce pyemia because of the severe leukopenia associated with tick-borne fever (TBF, *see* above).

Incidence of tick pyemia varies from year to year, although the cause of this unpredictability is not known: in some years, up to 25% of lambs on tick-infested pasture may become pyemic, but the incidence rarely is >10%.

Clinical Findings: Tick pyemia is most commonly recognized as crippled lambs. Various lesions may be found in affected lambs; staphylococci localize in the joints and cause abscesses and lameness. Other lambs may be paraplegic or have other nervous signs as a result of lesions in the CNS, while abscess formation in the internal organs is commonly associated with loss of condition and ill-thrift. In addition to this chronic or pyemic syndrome, an acute or septicemic form of staphylococcal infection has been described.

Lesions: At necropsy, abscesses are most common in the liver, joints, lungs, and kidneys. They are also found in the meninges of the brain or spinal cord, and in the pericardium and myocardium; less commonly in the diaphragm, thymus, and adrenal glands.

Ticks are usually found in the groins of affected lambs, and frequently the sites of attachment are inflamed.

Diagnosis: History and clinical signs are valuable indicators, and the strict geographical restriction of the disease and its relation to tick infestation are diagnostic features. Tick pyemia may resemble other suppurative infections of the newborn, including infection caused by streptococci, but the lesions are more extensive and *S aureus* can be isolated.

Control: Control of tick infestation is the most effective measure and, as in control of TBF, may be achieved by restricting lambs and ewes to low ground tick-free pastures for the first few weeks of life, or administering acaricides as dips or smears to the lambs. Use of cypermethrin as a pour-on has indicated that this may be the best tick-control method in young lambs.

Use of long-acting tetracycline can help prevent both TBF and tick pyemia when administered in the first weeks of life. Although not a substitute for the use of acaricides and other methods of tick control, it is best regarded as a useful adjunct in controlling lamb morbidity and mortality. A single injection at double the standard dose at 3 wk of age can significantly reduce mortality and morbidity in young hill lambs on tick-infested pasture, and improve weight gains and condition in the remainder. The antibiotic may prevent development of TBF, possibly for 3 wk, with freedom from pyrexia and immunosuppression so that the incidence of tick pyemia and other infections such as pasteurellosis and colibacillosis are reduced. When the lambs eventually develop TBF, they are several weeks older and apparently less susceptible to secondary infection.

Treatment of clinical cases with penicillin or oxytetracycline can be effective, provided the lesions are not too advanced.

WESSELSBRON DISEASE

An arthropod-borne viral infection of sheep, cattle, goats, horses, and pigs. The virus also has been isolated from man. Sheep are affected most severely; signs are fever, depression, anorexia, abortion, and death. Mortality is high in newborn lambs and pregnant ewes. Postmortem findings include hepatitis, hepatomegaly, icterus, hepatic congestion, and subcut. edema. The histological lesions include necrosis of the hepatocytes, Kupffer's cell proliferation, and WBC infiltration of the portal triads.

The epidemiology is similar to that of Rift Valley fever (RVF, qv, p 403), but the 2 viruses are unrelated and there is no cross-protection. Wesselsbron virus, a flavivirus, is widely distributed in the warmer and moister parts of Africa. Infection is common but disease is rare. Disease outbreaks have been limited to countries in southern Africa. Transmission is by various species of *Aedes* mosquitoes. There may also be mechanical transmission by biting flies.

The virus can be isolated by intracerebral inoculation of newborn mice. Weaned mice are not susceptible to Wesselsbron virus (as they are to RVF virus). Hemagglutination inhibition, complement fixation, and virus neutralization are commonly used for diagnosis.

Control involves the use of an attenuated virus vaccine, but due to possible teratogenic effects, vaccination of pregnant ewes is not recommended. It is often combined with RVF vaccine. Control also can be attempted by controlling the mosquito vectors.

CANINE DISTEMPER
(Hardpad disease)

A highly contagious, systemic, viral disease of dogs seen worldwide; it is characterized by a diphasic fever, leukopenia, GI and respiratory catarrh, and frequently, pneumonic and neurological complications. The disease occurs in Canidae (dogs, foxes, wolves), Mustelidae (eg, ferret, mink, skunk), most Procyonidae (eg, raccoon, coati mundi), and some Viveridae (binturong). Although it has been speculated that canine distemper virus causes multiple sclerosis in man, there is no supportive evidence. Unjustified concern has been expressed over human contact with dogs vaccinated with measles virus. Attenuated measles virus is used to protect dogs against distemper, but dogs do not shed the virus after vaccination.

Etiology and Pathogenesis: Canine distemper is caused by a paramyxovirus closely related to the viruses of measles and rinderpest. The virus is sensitive to lipid solvents and most disinfectants, and is unstable outside the host. The main route of infection is via aerosol droplet secretions from infected animals. Some infected dogs may shed virus for several months.

Virus replication initially occurs in the lymphatic tissue of the respiratory tract. A cell-associated viremia results in infection of all lymphatic organs, which is followed by infection of respiratory, GI, and urogenital epithelium, as well as the CNS. Disease follows virus replication in these organs.

Clinical Findings: A fever usually occurs 3-6 days after infection. There also may be a leukopenia (especially lymphopenia) at this time. These signs may go unnoticed. The fever subsides for several days before a second fever occurs, which lasts ≥1 wk. This may be accompanied by serous nasal discharge, mucopurulent ocular discharge, and anorexia. GI and respiratory signs may follow, and are usually complicated by secondary bacterial infections. CNS signs may accompany or follow the systemic disease, or occur after subclinical infection. Hyperkeratosis of the footpads ("hardpad" disease) and epithelium of the nasal plane may be observed. Neurological signs frequently are observed in dogs with hyperkeratosis. CNS signs include: 1) localized twitching of a muscle or group of muscles (chorea, flexor spasm, hyperkinesia), such as in the leg or facial muscles; 2) paresis or paralysis, often beginning in the hindlimbs evident as ataxia, followed by ascending paresis and paralysis; and 3) convulsions characterized by salivation and chewing movements of the jaw (petit mal, "chewing-gum fits"). The seizures become more frequent and severe, and the dog may then fall on its side and paddle its legs; involuntary urination and defecation (grand mal seizure, epileptiform convulsion) often occur. A dog may exhibit any, or all 3, of these nervous manifestations in the course of the disease. The consequences of infection vary from a mild, inapparent infection to severe disease manifest by most of the above signs. The course of the disease may be as short as 10 days, but may be prolonged for several weeks or months. In exceptional cases, there may be intervening periods of abatement followed by relapse. Often, when recovery seems imminent, permanent neurologic sequelae, as noted above, appear.

Old-dog encephalitis (ODE), a rare condition marked by ataxia, compulsive movements such as head pressing or continual pacing, and incoordinated hypermetria, may occur in the adult dog without a prior history of canine distemper virus (CDV)-related clinical signs. Convulsions and neuromuscular twitching (chorea) do not seem to occur with ODE. Although CDV antigen has been detected in the brain of dogs with ODE by FA staining, dogs with ODE are not infectious and replication-competent virus has not been isolated. The pathophysiology of ODE is not known.

Lesions: Thymus atrophy is a consistent postmortem finding. Hyperkeratosis of the nose and foot pads may be present. Depending on the degree of secondary bacterial infection, bronchopneumonia, enteritis, and skin pustules may also be present. Histologically, CDV produces necrosis of lymphatic tissues, cytoplasmic and intranuclear inclusion bodies in respiratory, urinary, and GI epithelium, and an interstitial pneumonia. Lesions found in the brain of dogs with neurological complications include neuronal degeneration, gliosis, demyelination, perivascular cuffing, nonsuppurative leptomeningitis, and intranuclear inclusion bodies predominately within glial cells.

Diagnosis: Distemper should be considered in the diagnosis of any febrile condition in puppies. While the typical clinical case is not difficult to diagnose, sometimes the characteristic signs fail to appear until late in the disease. The clinical picture may be modified by superimposed toxoplasmosis, coccidiosis, ascariasis, and numerous viral and bacterial infections. Distemper is sometimes confused with leptospirosis, infectious canine hepatitis, or lead poisoning. A febrile catarrhal illness with neurologic sequelae justifies a diagnosis of distemper. At necropsy, clinical diagnosis is best confirmed by histological lesions and/or by immunofluorescent assay of viral antigen in tissues. In living animals, conjunctival, tracheal, vaginal or other epithelium, or the buffy coat of the blood, can be examined with these procedures. These samples are usually negative when circulating antibody is present in the diseased dog. The diagnosis can then be made by demonstration of virus-specific IgM.

Treatment: Treatments are directed at limiting secondary bacterial invasion, supporting the fluid balance and overall well-being of the dog, and controlling nervous manifestations. These include antibiotics, electrolyte solutions, protein hydrolysates, dietary supplements, antipyretics, nasal preparations, analgesics, and anticonvulsants. No one treatment is specific or uniformly successful. Good nursing care is essential, and despite intensive care, some dogs fail to make a satisfactory recovery. Although treatments for chorea and other neurologic manifestations of distemper are usually unsuccessful, antispasmodics and sedatives may lessen the severity of signs.

Prophylaxis: Successful immunization of pups with canine distemper modified live virus vaccines depends on the absence of interfering maternal antibody. The age at which pups can be immunized can be predicted from a nomograph if the serum antibody titer of the mother is known; this service is available in many diagnostic laboratories. Alternatively, pups can be vaccinated with modified live virus vaccine when 6 wk old and at 2- to 4-wk intervals until 16 wk old. A modified live virus measles vaccine and a combination of modified live measles and modified live canine distemper vaccine are available. These vaccines must be administered IM. The measles or combination vaccine should be administered to pups 6-7 wk old. Measles virus induces immunity to CDV in the presence of maternal distemper antibody. The pup so vaccinated should receive a modified live virus distemper vaccine when 12-16 wk old. Many varieties of attenuated distemper vaccine are available and should be used according to manufacturer's directions. Annual revaccination is suggested.

CANINE HERPESVIRAL INFECTION

A fatal, viral infection of puppies worldwide. The virus also may be associated with a vesicular vaginitis in adult female dogs. Only members of the Canidae (dogs, wolves, coyotes) are known to be susceptible.

Etiology: The disease is caused by an enveloped DNA canine herpesvirus (CHV), which is sensitive to lipid solvents and most disinfectants. It is relatively unstable outside the host.

Transmission usually occurs by contact between susceptible puppies and the infected oral-nasal or vaginal secretions of their dam or oral-nasal secretions of dogs allowed to commingle with puppies during the first 3 wk of life. *In utero* transmission may occur.

Infection of newborn susceptible puppies results in replication of CHV in the surface cells of nasal mucosa, pharynx, and tonsils, followed by viremia and viral invasion of visceral organs.

Clinical Findings: Deaths due to CHV infection usually occur at 1-3 wk, but occasionally occur in puppies up to 1 mo old; they are rare in pups as old as 6 mo. Typically, onset is sudden, and death occurs after an illness of ≤24 hr. Older dogs exposed to or experimentally inoculated with CHV may develop a mild rhinitis or a vesicular vaginitis. Some investigators have linked CHV with abortions, stillbirths, and infertility. There is little evidence of association of CHV with infectious tracheobronchitis.

Lesions: The characteristic lesions consist of disseminated focal necrosis and hemorrhages. The most pronounced lesions are seen in the lungs, cortical portion of the kidneys, adrenal glands, liver, and GI tract. All lymph nodes are enlarged and hyperemic, and the spleen is swollen. Lesions may also occur in the CNS. The basic histological lesion is necrosis with hemorrhage in the adjacent parenchyma. Most often there is no inflammatory reaction. Single, small, basophilic, intranuclear inclusion bodies are most common in areas of necrosis in the lung, liver, and kidneys. Occasionally, they occur as faintly acidophilic bodies located within the nuclear space.

Diagnosis: CHV infection may be confused with infectious canine hepatitis (qv, p 418), but it is not accompanied by the thickened, edematous gallbladder often associated with the latter. The focal areas of necrosis and hemorrhage, especially those that occur in the kidneys, distinguish it from hepatitis and toxoplasmosis. CHV causes serious disease only in very young puppies. The rapid death and characteristic lesions distinguish it from canine distemper (*see* above). The virus can be isolated from fresh lung, liver, kidney, and spleen by cell culture techniques. The tissues should be submitted to the laboratory refrigerated, but not frozen.

Control: No vaccine is available. Infected bitches develop antibodies, and litters subsequent to the first infected litter receive maternal antibodies in the colostrum. Puppies that receive maternal antibodies may be infected with the virus, but disease does not result.

Removal of puppies from affected bitches by cesarean section and rearing them in isolation has prevented deaths under experimental conditions. However, infections have been noted even in cesarean-delivered puppies. Deaths may be reduced when infected puppies are reared in incubators at elevated temperatures (95°F [35°C], 50% relative humidity). Puppies so reared must be given adequate fluids and supportive therapy. The prognosis of puppies that survive neonatal infections of CHV is guarded, since damage to lymphoid organs, kidneys, and liver may be irreparable.

CANINE RICKETTSIAL DISEASES

CANINE EHRLICHIOSIS

An acute to chronic disease, caused by *Ehrlichia canis*. It is endemic in many parts of the USA, and occurs worldwide. To date, 46 cases of human infection with *E canis* have been reported, although there is no evidence of direct transmission from dogs to man. Human illness mimics Rocky Mountain spotted fever.

Etiology: The causative agent is seen rarely as colonies of coccoid bodies in the cytoplasm of WBC. Monocytes are affected most frequently, although some strains may affect only neutrophils or eosinophils, or both. The brown dog tick (*Rhipicephalus sanguineus*) is the primary vector and reservoir, and may transmit the disease for up to 5 mo after engorgement. Blood transfusions, or other means by which infected WBC are transferred, also transmit the disease. In some areas, ~50% of infected animals also have a titer to *E platys*, the agent of infectious cyclic thrombocytopenia (*see* below), but the clinical relationship between the 2 organisms is unknown.

Clinical Findings: Signs arise from the involvement of the hemic and lymphoreticular systems, and commonly progress from acute to chronic, depending on the strain of organism and immune status of the host. In acute cases, there is reticuloendothelial hyperplasia, fever, generalized lymphadenopathy, splenomegaly, and thrombocytopenia. Variable signs of anorexia, depression, loss of stamina, stiffness and reluctance to walk, edema of the limbs or scrotum, and coughing or dyspnea may occur. Most acute cases occur in the spring, summer, and early fall, coincident with the greatest activity of the tick vector.

The hemogram is usually normal, but may reflect a mild normocytic, normochromic anemia, leukopenia or mild leukocytosis. Thrombocytopenia is common, but petechiae may not be evident, and platelets may not be obviously decreased on a blood smear. Infrequently, thrombocytopathia contributes to hemorrhage. Aspiration cytology reveals reactive lymph nodes and, usually, marked plasmacytosis.

Mortality in the acute stage is rare: spontaneous recovery may occur, the dog may remain asymptomatic, or chronic disease may ensue. In chronic cases, the bone marrow becomes hypoplastic, and lymphocytes and plasmacytes infiltrate various organs. Depending on which organs are affected, and to what degree, signs are variable and appear without regard to season. Clinical findings may include marked splenomegaly, glomerulonephritis, renal failure, interstitial pneumonitis, anterior uveitis, cerebellar ataxia, depression, paresis, and hyperesthesia. Severe weight loss is a prominent finding.

The hemogram is usually markedly abnormal in the chronic state. Frequently, severe thrombocytopenia may cause hemorrhagic diathesis. In dolichocephalic breeds, epistaxis is common; hematuria, melena, and petechiae and ecchymoses of the skin and mucous membranes occur in all breeds. Variably severe pancytopenia (mature leukopenia, nonregenerative anemia, thrombocytopenia, or any combination thereof) may occur. Frequently, polyclonal, or occasionally monoclonal, hypergammaglobulinemia occurs.

Lesions: During the acute stage, lesions generally are nonspecific, but splenomegaly and heavy, discolored lungs are common. Histologically, there is lymphoreticular hyperplasia, and lymphocytic and plasmacytic perivascular cuffing. In chronic cases, these lesions may be accompanied by widespread hemorrhage and increased mononuclear cell infiltration of organs.

Diagnosis: Clinical diagnosis is confirmed by demonstrating the organisms within WBC, or by a combination of clinical signs, positive indirect FA titer, and response to treatment. Low numbers of organisms make demonstration difficult, except in the acute phase before treatment. The antibody response may be delayed up to 28 days; thus, an antibody titer may not be a reliable diagnostic tool early in the course of the disease. Since thrombocytopenia is a relatively consistent finding, a platelet count is an important screening test.

Differential diagnoses during the acute stage include other causes of fever and lymphadenopathy (eg, Rocky Mountain spotted fever, brucellosis, blastomycosis, endocarditis); immune-mediated diseases, especially thrombocytopenia and systemic lupus erythematosus; and lymphosarcoma. Differential diagnoses during the chronic stage include estrogen toxicity, myelophthisis, immune-mediated pancytopenia, and other diseases associated with specific organ dysfunction (eg, glomerulonephritis).

Treatment: The drug of choice for all forms of ehrlichiosis is tetracycline (22 mg/kg, PO, t.i.d.) for a minimum of 2 wk in acute cases, 1-2 mo in chronic cases. Doxycycline (5-10 mg/kg, PO or IV, daily for 10-14 days) is effective in some cases in which tetracycline fails. Two doses of imidocarb dipropionate (5-7 mg/kg, IM), 2 wk apart, are variably effective against both ehrlichiosis and babesiosis; however, the drug is not approved for use in the USA. In all forms of the disease, the temperature returns to normal within 24-48 hr after treatment, and the dog becomes more active and begins to eat. In chronic cases, the hematological abnormalities may persist for 3-6 mo. Supportive therapy may be necessary to combat wasting and specific organ dysfunction; platelet or whole-blood transfusions may be required if hemorrhage is extensive. The *E canis* antibody titer should be measured again within 6 mo of illness to confirm a seronegative status indicative of successful therapy.

Prophylaxis: Prevention is enhanced by controlling ticks and using indirect FA-negative blood donors. Tetracycline (6.6 mg/kg, PO, daily) is an effective preventive in kennels where ehrlichiosis is endemic.

CANINE INFECTIOUS CYCLIC THROMBOCYTOPENIA

The etiological agent is *Ehrlichia platys*. It is morphologically similar to *E canis* but affects only platelets. Distribution of the organism parallels that for *E canis* (see above).

Dogs generally show no signs of *E platys* infection despite the presence of the organism in the platelets. The primary finding is cyclic thrombocytopenia, recurring at 10-day intervals. Generally, the cyclic nature diminishes and the thrombocytopenia becomes mild and slowly resolves.

Morulae can be demonstrated in platelets with any Romanowski stain. However, parasitemia is rare or absent when platelet numbers are low, and the portion affected decreases with each successive cycle; therefore, direct demonstration may be difficult. Seroconversion occurs 13-19 days after inoculation, and is reliably detected by an indirect FA test. Positive titers confirm previous exposure, but their significance must be correlated with clinical findings. Frequently, dogs positive for *E canis* also are positive for *E platys*.

Treatment is as for *E canis*.

ELOKOMIN FLUKE FEVER

A fluke-transmitted disease of canids, bears, raccoons, and ferrets. It is seen alone or as a complicating agent in salmon poisoning disease (SPD, *see* below). It utilizes *Nanophyetus salmincola* in the same manner as described for SPD. The elokomin fluke fever agent (*Neorickettsia elokominica*) resembles *N helminthoeca*, but differs antigenically and has a wider host range.

The incubation period (9-12 days) is longer than for SPD. Unlike SPD, the fever generally plateaus and persists for 4-7 days. Bloody diarrhea is absent, as is the severe dehydration seen with SPD. Generalized lymphadenopathy is striking and usually greater than that caused by *N helminthoeca*. Although mortality in untreated cases is usually <10%, many dogs exhibit severe, persistent lymphadenopathy and weight loss for weeks after recovery from other signs. Occasionally, ataxia and meningoencephalitis are observed. Fluke eggs are seen on fecal examination. The lesions of uncomplicated elokomin fluke fever resemble those of SPD, except that the severe GI lesions are absent. Diagnosis, treatment, and prophylaxis are as for SPD.

ROCKY MOUNTAIN SPOTTED FEVER
(RMSF, Tick fever)

A disease of man, dogs, and other small mammals, which is caused by *Rickettsia rickettsii*. Because *Dermacentor andersoni* and *D variabilis* transmit the disease, >80% of the cases occur in dogs that frequent the outdoors. Because of their susceptibility, dogs are an excellent sentinel of *R rickettsii*. Seroprevalence has ranged from 4.3 to 63.4%, but these values do not accurately reflect infection rates due to the detection of cross-reacting antibodies to other spotted-fever-group rickettsiae. Since rickettsemia may occur during the acute stages, blood and tissue specimens should be handled with care.

Although direct transmission from dogs to man does not occur, there is a risk when rickettsiae in tick hemolymph or excreta contact abraded skin or conjunctiva during removal of engorged ticks from pets.

Clinical Findings: Early signs may include any combination of fever (up to 105°F [40.5°C]), anorexia, lymphadenopathy, polyarthritis, coughing or dyspnea, abdominal pain, and edema of the face or extremities. Petechiation occurs later, if at all, and is generally confined to the mucous membranes. Neurologic manifestations are common, and may include altered mental states, vestibular dysfunction, and nuchal rigidity. Focal retinal hemorrhage is a consistent finding during the early course of disease.

Thrombocytopenia is common but generally mild enough to be overlooked on a peripheral blood smear. Leukopenia occurs during the early stages of infection and is followed by progressive leukocytosis. Generally, serum biochemical abnormalities are mild, but may include hypoproteinemia, hypoalbuminemia, azotemia, hyponatremia, hypocalcemia, and increased liver enzyme levels.

Lesions: Vascular endothelial damage is due to direct cytopathic effects of the rickettsiae. Severity of the necrotizing vasculitis can be directly correlated to the infective dose. Vascular endothelial damage and thrombocytopenia contribute to development of petechiae and ecchymoses.

Diagnosis: Indirect FA titer is the most sensitive test. However, because of the high incidence of cross-reacting antibodies, demonstration of a 4-fold rise in titer should be documented in conjunction with a compatible clinical syndrome. Differential diagnoses include other causes of fever of unknown origin. The therapeutic response is generally dramatic, as it is in other canine rickettsial diseases. Following natural infection, immunity appears to be lifelong; therefore, recurrent episodes of tick fever should not be attributed to RMSF.

Treatment: The tetracyclines at 22 mg/kg, PO, t.i.d. for 2 wk are effective. Supportive care for dehydration and hemorrhagic diathesis may be necessary. Due to alterations in vascular integrity, conservative rates of fluid administration are advised. There is no prophylactic treatment.

SALMON POISONING DISEASE (SPD)

An acute, infectious disease of canids in which the infective agent is transmitted through the various stages of a fluke in a snail-fish-dog life cycle. The name of the disease is misleading since no toxin is involved.

Etiology: SPD is caused by *Neorickettsia helminthoeca*. The disease is sometimes complicated by a second agent (*see* ELOKOMIN FLUKE FEVER, above). The vector is a small fluke, *Nanophyetus salmincola*. The dog becomes infected by ingesting trout, salmon, or Pacific giant salamanders that contain encysted metacercariae of the rickettsia-infected fluke. In the dog's intestine, the larval flukes excyst, embed in the duodenal mucosa, and introduce the rickettsiae. The fluke infection itself produces little or no clinical disease.

The life cycle is maintained by the passage of infected fluke ova in the feces of the host. Miracidia develop from these ova and infect the snail *Oxytrema plicifer* to form rediae. Rediae develop into cercariae that are released from the snail, penetrate the salmon or trout, and develop into infective, encysted metacercariae. The cycle is completed when a dog eats the fish and becomes infected with the rickettsiae. Transmission by cage-to-cage contact, rectal thermometers, or aerosols is rare.

It appears that age, sex, and breed do not influence the pathogenesis of the disease, which may appear at any time, but the incidence is higher when the availability of fish is greater. Infected fish are found in the Pacific Ocean from San Francisco to the coast of Alaska, but SPD is more prevalent from northern California to Puget Sound. It is also seen inland along the rivers of fish migration. Apparently, the snail is the geographically limiting factor.

Clinical Findings: Signs appear suddenly, usually 5-7 days after eating infected fish, but may be delayed as long as 33 days, and persist for 7-10 days before culminating in death in up to 90% of untreated animals; body temperature peaks at 104-107.6°F (40-42°C) 1-2 days later, then gradually declines for 4-8 days and returns to normal. Frequently, animals are hypothermic before death. Fever is accompanied by depression and complete anorexia in virtually all cases. Persistent vomiting usually occurs by day 4 or 5. Diarrhea develops by day 5-7; it often contains blood, and may be severe. Dehydration and extreme weight loss occur. When severe, the GI signs are clinically indistinguishable from those of canine parvoviral infection (qv, p 249). Generalized lymphadenopathy occurs in ~60% of cases. Nasal or conjunctival exudate may be present and mimic distemper. Neutrophilia is common, but a marked, absolute leukopenia with a degenerative left shift may occur. Thrombocytopenia is reported in 94% of the cases. Serum chemistry values are normal.

Lesions: SPD appears to affect chiefly the lymphoid tissues and intestine. There is enlargement of the GI lymph follicles, lymph nodes, tonsils, thymus, and to some extent, the spleen, with microscopic necrosis, hemorrhage, and hyperplasia. A variable, but often severe hemorrhagic enteritis, which seems to arise from damaged lymph follicles, is seen throughout the intestine. Microscopic foci of necrosis also appear apart from the follicles. Flukes embedded in the duodenum account for little tissue damage. Nonsuppurative meningitis or meningoencephalitis has been identified in some dogs.

Diagnosis: Fluke ova are found on fecal examination in ~92% of cases, which lends support to the diagnosis. The ova are oval, yellowish brown, rough-surfaced, and ~87-97 × 35-55 μm, with an indistinct operculum amd a small blunt point on the opposite end. During the first day or 2, few ova may be passed. Intracellular organisms have been demonstrated via lymph node aspiration in ~70% of the cases. Other causes of fever of unknown origin, generalized lymphadenopathy, vomiting, and diarrhea are differential diagnoses. When diarrhea and exudative conjunctivitis occur, distemper should be considered.

Prophylaxis and Treatment: Currently, the only means of prophylaxis is to prevent the ingestion of uncooked salmon, trout, steelhead, and similar freshwater fish. In recovered cases, a profound humoral immune response persists, but there is no cross-resistance between *N helminthoeca* and *N elokominica*. Various sulfonamides given PO or parenterally are effective, as are chlortetracycline, oxytetracycline, and chloramphenicol. Animals usually succumb because of dehydration, electrolyte and acid-base imbalances, and anemia. Therefore, general supportive therapy to maintain hydration and acid-base balance, while meeting nutritional requirements and controlling diarrhea, is often essential. Judicious use of whole blood transfusions may be helpful.

FELINE INFECTIOUS PERITONITIS AND PLEURITIS
(FIP, Feline coronaviral infection)

A contagious viral infection of domestic and wild Felidae worldwide; it affects both sexes and all ages, occurring most commonly in those 6 mo to 2 yr old. The incidence of infection decreases in cats 5-13 yr old, followed by an increase in those 14-15 yr old. FIP is characterized by an insidious onset and development of a wet (effusive) or dry (noneffusive) form. Mortality approaches 100%.

Etiology and Epidemiology: FIP is caused by one or more coronaviruses, which are related antigenically to porcine transmissible gastroenteritis virus, canine coronavirus, human bronchitis virus 229E, and feline enteric coronavirus (FECV). The exact relationship between the multiple strains of FIPV and FECV has yet to be fully elucidated. FIPV is shed in both saliva and feces following oral inoculation of virus grown in tissue culture, which suggests that the natural route of infection is primarily oral following exposure to contaminated saliva or feces. Forty to 50% of field cases of FIP occur in cats also infected with feline leukemia virus (FeLV). This relationship may have an immunological basis.

Clinical Findings: The acute infection may be asymptomatic, but fever of unknown origin, transient conjunctivitis, signs of respiratory tract infection, or diarrhea may occur. This prodromal period may last days or weeks before the clinical signs of wet or dry FIP occur.

Wet FIP is the more common form of the disease and is characterized by development of ascites and/or pleural effusion. Pericardial effusion has also been reported. In dry FIP, granulomatous lesions occur without the development of fluid, and may be found in any organ, including the CNS and eye. The wide range of clinical signs seen depends on which organ is predominantly affected, which makes dry FIP more difficult to diagnose than the effusive form.

In the final stages of both forms, the cat becomes moribund, and it is thought that disseminated intravascular coagulation favors multiplication of the virus and its dissemination across cell walls, which result in rapid organ failure and death.

Lesions: The primary lesion is an acute, immune-mediated, perivascular necrosis, which progresses to a chronic pyogranulomatous lesion. Lesions may appear in various tissues, but omentum, peritoneal serosa, liver, kidney, pleurae, lung parenchyma, pericardium, meninges, brain, and uvea are common sites.

Diagnosis: Presumptive diagnosis is based on the history of a persistent antibiotic-resistant fever, anorexia, weight loss, progressive lethargy, chronic diarrhea, and debilitation, as well as various other signs associated with specific organ involvement. Characteristic fluid exudates in body cavities are highly suggestive. Homogeneous "ground glass" fluid density may obscure detail in thoracic or abdominal radiographs. Progressive, nonregenerative anemia, relative mature neutrophilia, and mild lymphopenia are common. A shift in the albumin/globulin ratio, caused by hyperglobulinemia, is found in most cases. Serum protein electrophoresis has shown the hyperglobulinemia results from increased amounts of both α_2 and γ globulins and reflects the active (α_2) and chronic (γ) inflammatory stages of the disease. The ascitic and/or pleural effusion also contains increased amounts of α_2 and γ globulins, is of high specific gravity, contains relatively few cellular elements but much coarse granular material, and may clot on standing.

Immunofluorescent or ELISA tests generally indicate moderate to high coronaviral antibody titers in infected cats. However, some cats with FIP have exhibited no or low titers, and some healthy cats with no clinical signs of disease have had high titers (over time, the titers of the latter group may decrease). Biopsy of affected organs not only confirms the diagnosis, but also reveals the extent and stage of the disease.

Treatment and Control: Treatment is generally ineffective. Reports of possible benefits from various immune modulators need to be evaluated further. Since confirmed cases of FIP are usually associated with high FECV antibody titers, nonspecific immunostimulators do not appear to be indicated. Combinations of anti-inflammatories and immunosuppressives in conjunction with supportive care may make the cat more comfortable, thereby increasing survival time by several months.

The presence of circulating antibodies against FIPV, and probably anti-FECV antibodies, sensitizes a cat so that subsequent exposure to virulent FIPV may produce an anamnestic antibody response, resulting in a rapid onset of acute, fulminating disease. Consequently, a vaccine has not been developed. Healthy cats should be prevented from contacting cats with a confirmed diagnosis of FIP.

Unlike FeLV tests, which identify the FeLV group-specific antigen in the blood or body fluids of infected cats, no test is available to screen large numbers of cats for FIP viral antigen.

A control program based on the presence of serum antibodies to coronaviruses is not warranted. No healthy animal should be destroyed on the basis of this antibody test.

FELINE PANLEUKOPENIA
(Feline infectious enteritis, Feline distemper, Feline agranulocytosis)

A highly contagious viral disease of cats, characterized by sudden onset, pyrexia, anorexia, depression, dehydration, vomiting and diarrhea, profound leukopenia, hypothermia late in the disease, and high mortality.

Etiology and Epidemiology: The causal parvovirus attacks all members of the cat family (Felidae), and the raccoon, coati mundi, Palm civet, and kinkajou in the raccoon family (Procyonidae). It is closely related antigenically to canine parvovirus type 2, and antigenically identical to mink enteritis virus. Most free-roaming cats are exposed to the virus during their first year. Virus may be shed in the urine and feces for up to 6 wk after recovery, and it is in all secretions and excretions of affected animals. Infection spreads by direct contact or fomites. The virus may survive for years in a contaminated environment, but can be destroyed by a dilution of household bleach (sodium hypochlorite). The virus requires actively dividing cells for effective replication. Tissues undergoing the most rapid mitotic activity are damaged the most severely.

Clinical Findings, Lesions, and Diagnosis: The incubation period is 2-10 days. With the onset of pyrexia, animals become anorectic, depressed, and weak. Diarrhea and vomiting may occur 1-2 days after the initial temperature rise. Extreme dehydration occurs rapidly, although affected cats seem thirsty. Leukopenia develops shortly before the onset of pyrexia. In most acute cases, the leukopenia is due to an absolute neutropenia. Severely affected cats may have an absolute lymphopenia. Total WBC counts of <2000 cells/μL indicate a poor prognosis. A gradual leukocytosis may occur, characterized by a marked left shift and many bizarre immature neutrophils. The course of the disease seldom is >5-7 days. Kittens with peracute panleukopenia may die within 12 hr of the onset of clinical signs. Mortality is high, especially in young cats; losses of 60-90% are reported. Infection of kittens *in utero* or during the neonatal period destroys the external granular layer of the cerebellum, which is manifest by incoordination that is first noted when the kitten begins to walk (feline cerebellar ataxia). Mild or subclinical infections are common in some outbreaks, especially in unvaccinated adult cats.

Dehydration and emaciation are marked except in peracute cases in which gross changes may be negligible. The first changes are hyperplasia, edema, and necrosis of the mesenteric lymph nodes and thymus. The bone marrow may appear semifluid and fatty. The bowel wall is usually thickened and turgid; gas is in some bowel loops. The serosal surface of severely affected areas may be hyperemic, with ecchymotic or petechial hemorrhages. The intestinal crypts are usually dilated and contain debris consisting of sloughed necrotic epithelial cells. Blunting and fusion of villi may be present. The liver, kidneys, and spleen may appear slightly swollen. Degeneration of hepatic cells and renal tubular epithelial cells is noted. Eosinophilic intranuclear inclusion bodies may develop transiently in tissues in which viral replication occurs.

Confirmatory diagnosis requires use of one or more of serum neutralization, hemagglutination, hemagglutination-inhibition, or ELISA, and even these are not always reliable.

Prophylaxis and Treatment: Inactivated and modified live vaccines are available. Attenuated vaccines should not be given to pregnant, immunosuppressed, or sick cats, or to kittens <4 wk of age. Kittens should be vaccinated first at 8-10 wk of age, again at 12-14 wk, and annually thereafter. In high-risk areas, a third vaccination may be recommended at 16-18 wk. The initial vaccination series should never be terminated before 12 wk of age. Immunization should be complete 2 wk before possible exposure.

Homologous antiserum provides rapid passive immunity for 7-10 days, but may interfere with vaccination for 2-3 wk. Antiserum (2-4 mL/kg body wt, subcut.) may be used in susceptible cats that have been exposed to feline parvovirus or in colostrum-deprived kittens.

Therapy depends on supportive management and nursing care until natural defenses return. Cats that survive for 5-7 days will probably recover. Food and water should be withheld until antiemetics are no longer needed. Phenothiazine-derivative antiemetics are preferred. A balanced electrolyte solution, such as lactated Ringer's, should be administered through an indwelling IV catheter. Early treatment with plasma or whole blood from healthy immune donors is indicated for cats that are moribund, or severely anemic or hypoproteinemic.

A parenteral antimicrobial, eg, gentamicin, should be administered to the hydrated cat for 5 days to prevent gram-negative bacterial sepsis and endotoxemia. Anticholinergic antidiarrheal-antiemetic agents are contraindicated since they may cause sustained ileus. A hot-water blanket or heating pad (with care, to avoid burns) should be used for hypothermia. After vomiting has subsided, frequent small amounts of bland, easily digestible foods may be offered. The return to a normal diet and feeding schedule should be gradual to avoid inducing gastroenteritis. Affected cats should be isolated from susceptible ones for 6 wk after recovery.

INFECTIOUS CANINE HEPATITIS (ICH)

A worldwide, contagious disease of dogs with signs that vary from a slight fever and congestion of the mucous membranes to severe depression, marked leukopenia, and prolonged bleeding time. It also occurs in foxes, wolves, coyotes, skunks, and bears; other carnivores may become infected without developing disease.

Etiology and Pathogenesis: ICH is caused by a nonenveloped DNA virus, canine adenovirus 1 (CAV-1), which is antigenically related only to CAV-2 (one of the causes of infectious canine tracheobronchitis [qv, p 769]). CAV-1 is resistant to lipid solvents and survives outside the host for weeks or months, but a 1-3% solution of sodium hypochlorite (bleach) is an effective disinfectant.

Ingestion of urine, feces, or saliva from infected animals is the main route of infection. Recovered dogs shed virus in urine for ≥6 mo. Initial infection occurs in the tonsillar crypts and Peyer's patches followed by viremia and infection of endothelial cells in many tissues, which initiates infection of visceral organs. Liver, kidneys, spleen, and lungs are the main target organs. Chronic kidney lesions and corneal clouding ("blue eye") result from immune-complex reactions following recovery from acute disease.

Clinical Findings: The disease varies from a slight fever to a fatal illness. The mortality rate is highest in very young dogs. The incubation period is 4-9 days. The first sign is a fever of >104°F (40°C), which lasts 1-6 days and is usually biphasic. Tachycardia out of proportion to the fever may be observed. On the day after the initial temperature rise, leukopenia develops and persists throughout the febrile period. The degree of leukopenia varies and seems to be correlated with the severity of illness. If the fever is of short duration, leukopenia may be the only sign, but if it persists for >1 day, acute illness develops.

Signs are apathy, anorexia, thirst, conjunctivitis, serous discharge from the eyes and nose, and occasionally, abdominal pain. Intense hyperemia or petechiae of the oral mucosa, as well as enlarged tonsils, may be seen. Vomiting also may be observed. There may be subcut. edema of the head, neck, and trunk.

Clotting time is directly correlated with the severity of illness, and it may be difficult to control hemorrhage, which is manifest by bleeding around deciduous teeth and by spontaneous hematomas. However, disseminated intravascular coagulation is common, and may be significant in the pathogenesis of the disease. Respiratory signs usually are not seen in dogs with ICH; however, CAV-1 has been recovered from dogs with signs of infectious tracheobronchitis and from dogs with the respiratory signs induced by exposure to the nebulated isolate. Foxes may have intermittent convulsions during the course of illness, and terminal paralysis may involve one or more limbs or the entire body. Although CNS involvement is unusual, the severely infected dog may have a terminal convulsion, and brain-stem hemorrhages are common.

On recovery, dogs eat well but regain weight slowly. Seven to 10 days after the acute signs disappear, ~25% of recovered dogs develop bilateral corneal opacity, which usually disappears spontaneously. In mild cases of ICH, transient corneal opacity may be the only sign of disease.

Chronic hepatitis may develop in dogs having low levels of passive antibody when exposed. Simultaneous infection with CAV-1 and distemper virus is sometimes seen.

Lesions: Endothelial damage results in "paint brush" hemorrhages on the gastric serosa, lymph nodes, thymus, pancreas, and subcut. tissues. Hepatic cell necrosis produces varying color changes in the liver, which may be normal in size or swollen. The gallbladder wall may be edematous and thickened; edema of the thymus may be found. Grayish white foci may be seen in the kidney cortex.

Diagnosis: Usually, the abrupt onset and prolonged bleeding time suggest ICH. Clinical evidence is not always sufficient to differentiate ICH from distemper (qv, p 408). The diagnosis is confirmed by virus isolation, immunofluorescence, or characteristic intranuclear inclusion bodies in the liver.

Treatment: Blood transfusions may be necessary in severely ill dogs. In addition, 5% dextrose in isotonic saline should be given, preferably IV. In dogs with prolonged clotting time, subcut. administration of fluids may be dangerous. A broadspectrum antibiotic should be administered. Since use of tetracyclines during tooth development (late prenatal, neonatal, and early postnatal periods) may discolor the teeth, they should not be used in puppies before their permanent teeth erupt. Although the transient corneal opacity (which may occur during the course of ICH or be associated with vaccination with attenuated CAV-1 vaccines) usually requires no treatment, atropine ophthalmic ointment may alleviate the painful ciliary spasm that may be associated with it. The dog should be protected against bright light when the problem occurs. Corticosteroids are generally contraindicated for treatment of corneal opacity associated with ICH.

Prophylaxis: Modified live virus vaccines are available. These are often combined with other vaccines. Immunization against ICH is recommended at the time of canine distemper immunizations. Attenuated CAV-1 vaccines have produced transient unilateral or bilateral opacities of the cornea and may be shed in urine. A CAV-2 attenuated live virus is now available that protects dogs against CAV-1 and CAV-2 infection. This vaccine does not produce corneal opacities or uveitis, and the virus is not shed in urine. It is available in the same combinations as CAV-1 vaccine. Annual revaccination against ICH is recommended.

Maternal antibody from immune bitches interferes with active immunization until puppies are 9-12 wk old.

VISCERAL LEISHMANIASIS

A chronic, ultimately fatal, protozoal disease of man, dogs, and certain rodents characterized by intermittent fever, hepatomegaly, splenomegaly, lymphadenopathy, anemia, and hyperproteinemia.

Infection in dogs is prevalent in Brazil, China, and the Mediterranean region, and a focus has been described in Oklahoma, USA. Cats are rarely infected and do not show signs of visceral disease, although they occasionally have cutaneous ulcers due to infection with dermotropic *Leishmania* spp.

Etiology and Transmission: *Leishmania donovani* is the causative agent in the Eastern Hemisphere, and *L chagasi* in the Western Hemisphere. The parasites are transmitted as promastigotes by the bite of several species of phlebotomine flies (sandflies). In mammalian hosts, promastigotes are engulfed by macrophages in which they transform into, and divide as, amastigotes.

Clinical Findings and Diagnosis: Amastigotes may be found in macrophages in almost any tissue of the body, but the organs most severely affected are the bone marrow, spleen, liver, and lymph nodes. The latter 3 enlarge due to lymphoid hyperplasia. In dogs, the incubation period may be months or years. Signs include cachexia, alopecia, onychogryphosis, lymphadenopathy, hepatomegaly, and splenomegaly. Fever may be present. Laboratory findings often include anemia, lymphopenia, and hypergammaglobulinemia. Proteinuria may be present.

Occasional findings are anterior ocular lesions, skin lesions, interstitial pneumonitis, and amyloidosis. Differential diagnoses include lymphosarcoma, myeloma, ehrlichiosis, and systemic fungal infections. Definitive diagnosis requires demonstration of the organisms in methanol-fixed, Giemsa-stained, impression smears or aspirates of affected lymphoid tissue, culture of tissue samples or aspirates in special media, or subinoculation of infected material into golden hamsters. Blood may contain low numbers of parasites, and examination of lymphoid tissues is more reliable. Serum antibody testing is not routinely available. Amastigotes appear as 5 μm, spherical inclusions in macrophages, usually in foci of granulomatous inflammation. They resemble *Histoplasma capsulatum*, but *Leishmania* spp amastigotes contain both a nucleus and a kinetoplast.

Treatment: Pentavalent antimonial compounds (sodium stibogluconate and meglumine antimoniate) are used in man, but are not officially approved for use in dogs. Several weeks of treatment (30-50 mg/kg body wt/day, IV or IM) with these drugs may be necessary in dogs, although toxic effects are likely, and relapses following treatment are common. Attempted treatment of dogs imported into nonendemic areas is probably unwise, owing to public health considerations.

IMMUNE SYSTEM

IMM

IMMUNOPATHOLOGICAL MECHANISMS

Normal immune responses are vital in protecting the host against invasion by foreign organisms, tissues, and substances. Under certain circumstances, however, these usually protective responses can have a deleterious effect on the host; all such adverse responses are called allergies or hypersensitivities. Autoimmune diseases occur as a result of tissue injury caused by a specific immune reaction of the host to its own tissues. There are 4 situations in which the host's immune system damages its own tissues: 1) Type I or anaphylaxis, 2) Type II or cytotoxic antibodies, 3) Type III or immune complex diseases, and 4) Type IV or cell-mediated immune reactions. In addition to the 4 classical categories of hypersensitivity, other disorders of the immune system can occur, including immunodeficiencies, tumors, and gammopathies (*see* pp 433-438).

TYPE I REACTIONS
(Anaphylaxis)

These are caused by pharmacologically active chemical mediators released from basophils or mast cells. The mediators include histamine, the leukotrienes, prostaglandins, bradykinins, and eosinophil chemotactic factors. The release of chemical mediators by mast cells is triggered when antigen (allergen) binds to specific antibody molecules (reagins) that are present on the mast-cell membrane.

Antibodies that mediate Type I reactions usually are of the immunoglobulin (Ig) E class and less commonly IgG. These antibodies are produced mainly by mucosal-associated lymphoid tissue. IgE antibodies also are called reaginic or homocytotropic antibodies because of their propensity to bind to mast cells and basophils. Many types of antigens can induce reaginic antibodies (eg, serums, hormones, enzymes, venoms, pollens, complex polysaccharides, iodinated X-ray contrast media, antibiotics, and other drugs). Reaginic antibodies, while often detrimental, probably evolved as a specialized defense mechanism against parasitic infections. Unfortunately, certain individuals overreact to nonparasite antigens by producing high levels of reaginic antibodies. The genetic predisposition to produce high levels of such antibodies is known as **atopy**.

The nature of the clinical disorder that occurs following the interaction of allergen and cell-bound IgE varies with the dose of allergen, the route by which the allergen enters the body, and the location of IgE-coated mast cells. Allergic reaction may affect the respiratory system (rhinitis, bronchial spasms, laryngeal edema), GI tract (nausea, cramps, vomiting, diarrhea), cardiovascular system (intestinal and hepatic vasodilatation), or skin (hives, urticaria).

TYPE II REACTIONS
(Antibody-mediated cytotoxicity)

Cytotoxic reactions occur as a result of the binding of IgG, IgM, or IgA antibodies to antigens on the surface of body cells or associated structures (myoneural receptors, intracellular cement substance, etc). Complement also may participate in the reaction. Many types of cells can be damaged, but blood cells appear to be particularly susceptible to immune-mediated lysis and phagocytosis.

It is still unclear why an animal produces "autoantibodies" that react against its own tissues. It is thought that clones of autoantibody-producing cells are normally produced during an animal's lifetime, but are suppressed by lymphocytes. In some "autoimmune" disorders, there appears to be a deficiency of suppressor lymphocytes. Suppressor lymphocytes are important in the regulation of the normal immune response, and one of their functions might be to suppress autoantibody production. There is strong evidence that many autoimmune disorders have a genetic predisposition. External factors (eg, viral infections) may trigger the production of autoantibodies, but such factors are important only in genetically predisposed individuals.

Acute viral infections may induce transient changes in immunoregulation, perhaps by destroying suppressor T lymphocytes or changing the relative balance of various regulatory lymphocyte subpopulations, thus allowing formation of autoantibodies. Postviral autoimmune hemolytic anemia and thrombocytopenia are seen in man, and occasionally dogs. Chronic viral infections, such as feline leukemia virus and feline immunodeficiency virus infections of cats, also may be associated with a higher than expected incidence of autoimmune phenomena. Similarly, diseases of the lymphoid system, lymphoreticular neoplasms in particular, may alter normal immunoregulation. Autoimmune phenomena in such cases often precede other signs of the tumor.

Some tissue antigens are hidden deep in the cell membrane or in other areas inaccessible to the host's lymphoid cells. Because of their sequestered nature, the host's immune system may not recognize them as "self" during embryonic development. If these antigens are unmasked or released during postembryonic life, the host may recognize them as foreign and make antibodies against them. As RBC age, a "new" surface antigen is exposed, and they are destroyed by autoantibodies.

This could explain the transitory appearance of autoantibodies to cell constituents following myocardial infarcts or liver disease in man.

Cross-reacting antibodies also may damage host tissues. Certain microbial proteins and drugs are antigenically similar to host antigens or can react with and antigenically alter host proteins, eg, streptococcal-M antigens that stimulate production of antibodies that cross-react with normal glomerular or vascular basement membranes. Neoplasms can elaborate embryonic antigens or neoantigens, which can stimulate cross-reacting antibodies. Host cells also may be damaged as a result of immunologic reactions occurring in other sites: the first component of complement binds to the antigen-antibody complex, but for unexplained reasons the rest of the complement components may bind to normal host tissues, which are then destroyed by complement-mediated lysis or phagocytosis.

Microbial agents may infect certain tissues, and thus focus the immune response of the host on that tissue. *Babesia and Haemobartonella* spp can parasitize RBC, and cell destruction and anemia may result from the host's immune attack on parasitized cells.

TYPE III REACTIONS
(Immune complex disease)

These reactions occur when antigen-antibody complexes localize in tissues, usually vessel walls. The prerequisites of such diseases are a continuous source of circulating antigen and a continuous production of antibody. When the level of circulating antigen and antibody reaches critical concentrations, antigen-antibody complexes of intermediate size are produced. Smaller complexes are soluble and pass through the vessel walls, while larger complexes are removed by the reticuloendothelial system. Complexes of intermediate size tend to pass through endothelial cell spaces, but become trapped around the basement membrane. Complement that is bound to the complexes chemotactically draws polymorphonuclear cells or macrophages into the area; these ingest the complexes, and as a result, inflammatory mediators are released and damage the surrounding tissues.

A number of conditions can lead to immune complex disease: 1) Infections—chronic, persistent, low-grade, viral, bacterial, fungal, protozoal, or parasitic. 2) Malignancy—neoplasms, particularly lymphoreticular neoplasms. 3) "Autoimmune" disorders—eg, immune complex disease is an important part of systemic lupus erythematosus (SLE). 4) Serum sickness—the result of therapeutic use of heterologous serum. 5) Drug reactions—several drugs, eg, lincomycin, erythromycin, sulfonamides, trimethoprim-sulfonamide, and some hormones appear to induce immune-complex diseases in a small portion of treated animals. The drugs or their metabolites appear to do this by acting as antigens or haptens (small antigenic molecules that can induce an antibody response when combined with larger host proteins). The haptens may combine with host substances to produce new antigens; the antibodies produced react not only with the hapten complex, but also with the associated body substance. Drugs such as propylthiouracil sometimes alter normal immunoregulation and induce a disease resembling SLE. 6) Idiopathic—in many cases the origin of the antigen, and therefore the cause of the disease, is not identifiable.

Clinical manifestations of immune complex disease are extremely variable. The Arthus reaction results from local formation of immune complexes; if the complexes are deposited mainly in the glomeruli, glomerulonephritis is the primary clinical presentation. Synovitis is a result of synovial deposition. Pneumonitis occurs if the complexes are deposited in the alveoli. Dermal eruptions result from deposition in dermal vessels. Vasculitis results from deposition in the walls of small arteries. Meningitis, myopathy, myelopathy, neuropathy, or localized hemorrhages can be additional sequelae of immune complex disease. In any individual, immune complex disease may involve any one or a combination of the above major organ systems.

TYPE IV REACTIONS
(Cell-mediated immune reactions, Delayed hypersensitivity)

The most familiar example is the tuberculin reaction induced in the skin of sensitized individuals by the intradermal injection of a protein derivative of mycobacteria. The skin reaction occurs from the interaction of sensitized thymus-derived lymphocytes with the sensitizing antigen. The tissue reaction is a result of lymphokines elaborated by the sensitized lymphocytes. Lymphokines can be cytotoxic to specific target cells, activate macrophages to become cytotoxic, inhibit the movement of macrophages out of the area, and cause small lymphocytes to transform into large basophilic blast cells. This type of reaction focuses macrophage activity at the site of antigen invasion, and therefore is extremely effective in combating many microbial infections. It is also important in destruction of some tumors and foreign-tissue grafts. A persistent and uncontrolled Type IV reaction, usually to intracellular pathogens or foreign material, may cause extensive granulomas.

SPECIFIC DISEASE ENTITIES OF AN IMMUNOPATHOLOGICAL NATURE

Specific disease entities with an immune basis have been best characterized in companion and laboratory animal species. Except for the relative frequencies of these various disorders among species, the clinical manifestations and treatment usually are similar regardless of the species.

DISEASES INVOLVING ANAPHYLACTIC REACTIONS
(Type I reactions, Atopic disease)

Type I reactions are either systemic or localized. Injection of the sensitizing antigens (allergens) directly into the bloodstream can result in anaphylactic shock or more focal reactions (hives, urticaria, facial-conjunctival edema). If the sensitizing allergen enters through the mucous membranes or the skin, more localized reactions usually occur.

SYSTEMIC ANAPHYLAXIS
(Generalized anaphylactic reactions)

Anaphylactic shock occurs in sensitized animals following parenteral injection of vaccines or drugs, ingestion of foods, or after insect bites. Clinical signs occur within seconds after the allergen enters the circulation. This latent period is the time required for the allergen to bind to sensitized mast cells, and for vasoactive mediators to be released. In man and most domestic animals, lungs are the primary target organ, and the portal-mesenteric vasculature is secondary; this is reversed in dogs. Mast cell degranulation in the pulmonary vasculature causes constriction of bronchial airways or pulmonary veins and pooling of blood in the pulmonary vascular bed, which results in severe respiratory distress. Mast cell degranulation in the portosystemic vasculature causes venous dilatation and pooling of blood in the intestines and liver, with resultant shock, agitation, colic, nausea, hypersalivation, dyspnea, cyanosis, and in severe cases, death.

Anaphylactic shock is treated with an IV injection of epinephrine to counteract bronchial constriction and portal-mesenteric vasodilation. Ancillary support of blood pressure and respiration may be necessary. Because of the peracute onset of signs, antihistamines are of little therapeutic benefit. Antihistamines are more effective in treating urticarial infections and facial-conjunctival edema, but even in those cases, they are more effective when used to prevent attacks in animals with a known allergic predisposition.

Urticarial reactions (hives or angioedematous plaques) of the skin and subcut. tissue, and acute edema of the lips, conjunctiva, and skin of the face (facial-conjunctival angioneurotic edema) are less severe manifestations of a systemic allergic reaction. Hives are the least severe reaction and are seldom associated with other clinical abnormalities. Facial-conjunctival edema is more severe, and can be associated with mild to moderately severe systemic anaphylaxis. These reactions usually follow administration of vaccines or drugs, ingestion of certain foodstuffs, or insect bites. (*See* SWEET ITCH IN HORSES, p 804; DERMATITIS, p 786; and URTICARIA, p 867.) Urticarial reactions and facial-conjunctival edema occur in most species, and usually resolve spontaneously within 24 hr.

Milk allergy occurs occasionally in cows, and less frequently in mares, when delayed milking or rapid weaning increases intramammary pressure to a point that normally sequestered milk components, notably casein, gain access to the circulation; these "foreign" proteins induce a type I hypersensitivity that can be localized or systemic. Recovery usually is prompt once the gland is emptied.

LOCALIZED ANAPHYLACTIC REACTIONS

Allergic rhinitis, manifest by serous nasal discharge and sneezing, is less common in other animals than in man. Often, it is seasonal, correlating with pollen exposure. Nonseasonal rhinitis may be associated with exposure to ubiquitous allergens, such as molds, danders, bedding, and feedstuffs. Chronic obstructive pulmonary disease in horses (qv, p 733) may be a sequela of low-grade respiratory allergies. Summer snuffles is a seasonal allergic rhinitis occurring commonly in Guernsey or Jersey cattle placed on certain types of flowering pastures in late summer and early autumn. Allergic rhinitis can be diagnosed tentatively by identifying eosinophils in the nasal exudate, a favorable response to antihistamines, disappearance of signs when the offending allergen is removed, or occasionally by its seasonal nature. Unlike in man, skin testing is not an accurate means to diagnose nasal allergies in animals.

Chronic **allergic bronchitis** has been best characterized in dogs. A dry, harsh, hacking cough that is easily precipitated by exertion or by pressure on the trachea is seen. The disease may be seasonal or occur year-round. Usually, it is not associated with other signs of illness. The bronchial exudate is rich in eosinophils and free of bacteria. Chest radiographs are normal, and there may or may not be a low-grade peripheral eosinophilia. The condition is treated with preparations that contain bronchial dilators and expectorants (aminophylline and potassium iodide or guaifenesin), which aid in the removal of thick, tenacious mucus. Glucocorticoids are dramatically effective, especially when their use can be limited to certain seasons or to low-dose, alternate-day therapy. Avoidance of the offending allergen(s) usually is not possible because only rarely is it identifiable.

Allergic bronchiolitis is most common in cats. It is manifest by a low-grade cough, wheezing, some dyspnea, and increased peribronchiolar density on radiographs, and may be mistaken for other conditions (allergic asthma or lungworm disease). It responds well to moderate to high dosages of corticosteroids, but cures are uncommon. The offending allergen usually is not identified.

Pulmonary infiltration with eosinophilia (PIE syndrome) occurs most frequently in dogs but has been recognized in all species. It is associated with diffuse inflammatory infiltrates in the lungs and a pronounced peripheral eosinophilia; frequently, the serum globulins are elevated. Unlike in allergic bronchitis, affected animals are often dyspneic or tire easily with exercise. Diffuse bronchial exudate contains numerous eosinophils. The specific offending allergen usually is not discovered. Glucocorticoids are the treatment of choice. A PIE-like syndrome is also associated with resident or migratory parasitic infections of the lungs in young animals.

Allergic asthma is less common in other animals than in man. Among animals it is most frequent in cats, in which the signs are similar to those in man. It occurs more frequently in summer and after going outdoors; individual attacks can be transient and mild, or protracted and severe (status asthmaticus). Mild attacks may manifest as wheezing and coughing, while in severe attacks there may be expiratory dyspnea, hyperinflation of the lungs, aerophagia, cyanosis, and frantic attempts to obtain air.

Intestinal allergies (food allergies) are relatively common in dogs and cats, particularly kittens. Allergic gastritis is manifest by vomiting, which occurs 1 to >12 times weekly, within 1-2 hr of eating. The vomitus may be bile-tinged. Dogs may also have loose feces intermittently; in cats, vomiting may be the sole sign. Cats and dogs with allergic gastritis are usually normal except for vomiting, although in severe cases there can be loss of weight and coat condition. Allergic enteritis is associated with a mild inflammation of the small intestine but with little or no eosinophilia. The feces usually are normal in volume and frequency, but consistency varies from semiformed to watery. The feces may be extremely odorous, especially in cats. Affected animals may be excessively thin despite good appetite. Skin lesions and poor coat are commonly associated with food allergies in cats, but less commonly in dogs. The allergy often follows bouts of viral, bacterial, or protozoal enteritis (a phenomenon known as allergic breakthrough). Food allergy may be a cause of diarrhea in newly weaned piglets, although the supporting evidence is not clear; the diarrhea is usually treated as an infection rather than an allergy. Eosinophilic enteritis is the most severe form of allergic bowel disease. It manifests by moderate to severe inflammation of the intestines and a pronounced eosinophilia. Diarrhea, weight loss, and poor coat condition are usually evident. Allergic colitis is uncommon in dogs, but common in cats; in dogs, it is often associated with frequent defecation and soft, mucus-laden and sometimes bloody feces; in cats, it most frequently manifests by more normal feces coated or spotted with fresh blood.

Both diagnosis and treatment of intestinal allergies is by a strictly controlled diet. In dogs, this means low-protein feeds that contain as few ingredients as possible. A basic diet of rice, cottage cheese (or tofu), and mutton, supplemented with vitamins and minerals is a good starting diet. When the signs (usually diarrhea) have disappeared, additional foods can be introduced one at a time into the diet. Suitable commercial prescription diets are also available. Low doses of glucocorticoids given daily or every other day also can provide excellent relief for dogs that are not helped by dietary changes. Allergic enteritis in cats is treated by feeding exclusively meat protein. Ground, cooked turkey and lamb are good hypoallergenic foods for cats. If the cats are not also allergic to these foods, feces, weight, coat quality, and skin lesions improve dramatically within 1-2 wk. Once a response occurs, new foods are introduced one at a time at 2-wk or longer intervals. Kittens with food allergies often grow out of them, while older animals may need hypoallergenic diets for life.

Atopic dermatitis is a pruritic, chronic skin disorder that occurs in many species, but has been studied mostly in dogs. Animals with atopic dermatitis have a genetic predisposition that leads to excessive production of reaginic (IgE) antibodies. It has been estimated that ~10% of all dogs suffer from atopy, but the incidence is higher in terriers and Dalmatians. Atopic dermatitis of dogs often is due to inhaled allergens, eg, pollens, molds, danders. Unlike man (in whom the respiratory and conjunctival mucous membranes are the usual target tissues), in dogs, the skin is the target tissue. In cats, food allergens probably are a more common cause of skin lesions than are inhaled allergens. Sweet itch (qv, p 804) is a seasonal allergic dermatitis of horses associated with certain insect bites, especially night-feeding *Culicoides*. Intensely pruritic lesions appear along the dorsum from the ears to tail head and perianal area. Similar allergic skin reactions to insect bites can be observed about the ears and face of cats and dogs.

Atopic dogs often chew at their feet and axillae. Excessive sweating is especially noticeable in the hairless areas. The skin lesions are greatly increased in severity by licking, scratching, and secondary bacterial infection. Atopic skin lesions in cats are either miliary (small scabs) and widespread, or larger and more localized. Localized lesions are often pruritic.

Treatment consists of identifying the offending allergens by intradermal skin testing and their elimination (or avoidance) whenever possible. Skin testing (qv, p 778) is much less reliable for detecting the offending allergen in cats than in dogs. The "wheal and flare" reaction seen when the offending allergen is injected into the dermis is a focal manifestation of the allergic state. Hyposensitization is effective in ~60% of dogs with atopic dermatitis; this consists of injecting an appropriate amount of the offending allergen IM at monthly intervals until improvement is noted. If hyposensitization fails, or is not utilized, alternate-day glucocorticoid therapy is beneficial. Antihistamines have been of minimal effectiveness.

DISEASES INVOLVING CYTOTOXIC ANTIBODIES
(Type II reactions)

Autoimmune hemolytic anemia (AIHA, qv, p 21) and **thrombocytopenia** (qv, p 56) are the most common type II reactions. They can be associated with systemic lupus erythematosus (SLE [more common in dogs]) or with lymphoreticular malignancies (more common in horses and cats). Drugs, vaccinations, or infections also can precipitate attacks of hemolytic anemia or thrombocytopenia in most species. More often than not, however, the triggering cause is unknown. The condition has 4 basic forms: peracute, acute or subacute, chronic, and pure red cell aplasia. Most forms are treatable, and relapses are uncommon.

Peracute AIHA is seen mainly in middle-aged, larger breeds of dogs. Affected dogs are acutely depressed, and within 24-48 hr there is a fulminating decrease in the PCV with bilirubinemia and variable icterus, and sometimes hemoglobinuria. Initially the anemia is nonresponsive, but it becomes responsive within 3-5 days. Thrombocytopenia and thrombotic phenomena may be accompanying features. The Coombs' test is often negative, spherocytes may or may not be present, but in-tube or slide agglutination of RBC is marked. The autoagglutination is not dispersed by saline dilution, hence the term hemolytic anemia with in-saline agglutinins. The serum usually contains autoantibodies that cause agglutination of most donor RBC (including heterospecies). The prognosis of peracute AIHA is poor even with prompt and vigorous therapy. The most effective therapy has been to begin immediately with high dosages of glucocorticoids plus cyclophosphamide. Incompatible blood transfusions should be avoided if possible. If incompatible blood must be used, the animal should first be heparinized and maintained on heparin for the first 10 days. Even without transfusion, heparinization may be beneficial for the first 2 wk or more.

Acute AIHA is the most common form of the disease, with a breed predilection in Cocker Spaniels. Initial signs usually are pallor and fatigue, and less commonly, icterus. Hepatosplenomegaly is prominent, and the anemia is usually responsive initially. The WBC count often is elevated due to bone marrow hyperplasia. Autoagglutination of RBC is uncommon, and the Coombs' test is generally positive. These animals usually respond well to glucocorticoid therapy. If a favorable response is not seen within 7-10 days, cytotoxic drugs (cyclophosphamide or azathioprine) should be added to the regimen.

Chronic AIHA differs from the acute form in that the PCV falls to a constant level and remains there for weeks or months. Usually, the anemia is responsive early in the course but responds minimally or not at all by the time it becomes severe. The bone marrow is either normal or hyperresponsive, and the Coombs' test is often negative. Chronic AIHA is relatively more common in cats than dogs. The animals are treated initially with glucocorticoids; if there is no response within 2 wk, cytotoxic drugs are added to the regimen.

Pure red cell aplasia is a variant of the above disorders and is most common in dogs. It occurs in 2 forms, one in post-weanling to adolescent puppies and the other in adults. Unlike AIHA, the bone marrow shows a selective depression of erythroid elements; granulocytes and platelets are unaffected. Therefore, the peripheral anemia is unresponsive. The immune attack apparently is directed at RBC precursors, and the Coombs' test is usually negative. However, there is often some difficulty in identifying compatible donors. Treatment is usually as for chronic AIHA.

Autoimmune thrombocytopenia is common, especially in dogs. It is more common in females than males. The most frequent clinical signs are hemorrhages of the skin and mucous membranes. Melena, epistaxis, and hematuria may be accompanying features, and can cause profound anemia. Hemolytic anemia and thrombocytopenia sometimes occur together. Autoimmune thrombocytopenia usually is diagnosed on the basis of low peripheral platelet counts in the face of a pronounced megakaryocytosis in the marrow. Occasionally, however, megakaryocytes may be selectively absent from the marrow. This condition is analogous to pure red cell aplasia. Tests for antiplatelet antibodies are difficult to conduct and may be positive in only 70% or fewer cases. The diagnosis is usually made on clinical appearance and response to therapy, rather than antiplatelet antibody tests.

Animals with autoimmune thrombocytopenia that show only petechial and ecchymotic hemorrhages, with no significant blood loss and megakaryocytes in the marrow, are usually treated initially with glucocorticoids alone. The clinical signs should abate and the platelet count begin to rise after 5-7 days. If the platelet count has not increased significantly by days 7-10, either cyclophosphamide, azathioprine, or vincristine can be added to the glucocorticoid regimen. In animals with megakaryocytes in the marrow and severe blood loss, a more rapid response to therapy is desirable. Such animals are treated with a single injection of vincristine combined with daily glucocorticoids; a favorable response usually occurs after 3-5 days. If the blood loss is life-threatening, platelet-rich whole blood should be administered. If the platelet count has risen by day 7, a second dose of vincristine is not given, and remission is maintained on glucocorticoids alone. If there is no response after 7 days, a second dose of vincristine is given. If the platelet count is still low after 2 wk, vincristine is discontinued and either cyclophosphamide or azathioprine is added. Animals with thrombocytopenia and no megakaryocytes respond much more slowly to glucocorticoids, or glucocorticoids and vincristine. Preferred treatment for these animals is with prednisolone and cyclophosphamide, and a response should not be expected much earlier than 1-2 wk after beginning therapy. Therapy can be discontinued in most animals with autoimmune thrombocytopenia 1-3 mo after the platelet count returns to normal. Some animals have more or less persistent thrombocytopenia in the face of drug therapy, or can be maintained in remission only with chronic high-dose treatment. The alternatives in such instances are to allow the animals to live with the thrombocytopenia if signs are minimal, or to use long-term combination drug therapy with glucocorticoids and either vincristine, azathioprine, or cyclophosphamide. Splenectomy may be helpful; it is seldom curative by itself but may allow use of lower and safer dosages of immunosuppressive drugs.

Cold agglutinin (hemolytic) disease is an AIHA that has been recognized most often in dogs and horses. It is often idiopathic, but can be secondary to a chronic infection, other autoimmune diseases, or a neoplastic process. The IgM autoantibodies can be agglutinating or nonagglutinating. Complete agglutination is not seen at body temperature, but rather at some lower temperature. The disease is more frequent in colder climates and during colder seasons. Initial signs may be of a hemolytic disease; or in the agglutinating type, there also may be microcapillary stasis with subsequent acrocyanosis and necrosis of the nose, tips of the ears and tail, digits, scrotum, and prepuce. Diagnosis is based on a reversible autoagglutination that occurs only at a cool temperature. The direct Coombs' reaction is usually negative for IgG, frequently positive for C3, and usually positive for IgM if the reaction is performed in the cold. Associated mortality is high. In the absence of precipitating disorders, eg, infection or neoplasia, the disease is best controlled with high doses of glucocorticoids used in combination with cyclophosphamide. Cyclophosphamide is withdrawn when the anemia disappears and cold agglutinins are no longer detected.

Autoimmune skin disorders—pemphigus vulgaris and the variant condition, pemphigus foliaceus, are immunologic skin disorders that involve antibodies directed against intracellular cement substances at the basal cell layer, which result in separation of the epidermal cells (acantholysis). Pemphigus vulgaris is relatively uncommon, but has been described in dogs. It is characterized by bullous lesions along the mucocutaneous junctions of the mouth, anus, prepuce, and vulva, and in the oral cavity. Other areas of the skin are only mildly involved. Because the epidermis of animals is relatively thin (compared to human skin), the bullae rupture rapidly and form erosions; consequently, characteristic bullae are seldom seen. The bullae occur as a result of suprabasilar acantholysis. Secondary bacterial infection often complicates the lesions, and if untreated, the disorder is often fatal. It is treated with high doses of glucocorticoids alone or in combination with other drugs such as cyclophosphamide, azathioprine, or gold salts. The disease is difficult to maintain in remission, and the long-term prognosis is fair to poor.

Pemphigus foliaceus is more common in dogs than in cats and horses. It is characterized clinically by erosions, ulcerations, and thick encrustations of the skin and mucocutaneous junctions. The absence of lesions in the mouth, and the widespread thick, crusty nature of the skin lesions, tend to differentiate it from pemphigus vulgaris. As in pemphigus vulgaris, autoantibodies are present in the skin and react with intracellular cement substance. These autoantibodies cause a separation of the cornified from uncornified cell layers. High doses of glucocorticoids are used initially, but low-dose, alternate-day therapy is used once the disease is under control. More potent immunosuppressive drugs such as cyclophosphamide or azathioprine are used with glucocorticoids in cases unresponsive to steroids. Gold salts, in conjunction with low doses of glucocorticoids, are sometimes helpful in maintaining remission in animals in which steroids alone are ineffective. Animals that respond poorly to initial therapy, or require high dosages of drugs to control lesions, have a poor long-term prognosis.

Bullous pemphigoid has been recognized in dogs, most often in Collies and Doberman Pinschers. Lesions are often widespread, but tend to be concentrated in the groin. The involved skin resembles a severe scald. Bullae also may be seen; they are subepidermal and may be full of eosinophils. Autoantibodies to the basal lamina proteins are seen in FA-stained sections. The treatment of choice is prednisolone and azathioprine used in combination; remission is frequent, but continuous drug therapy at relatively high dosages may be required to keep the disease under control. The long-term prognosis is poor.

Myasthenia gravis (acquired form) occurs in dogs, and less commonly in goats and cats. Affected animals produce autoantibodies to the acetylcholine receptors, which bind to the receptor and reduce acetylcholine; the clinical manifestations mimic those produced by curare. Extreme generalized muscle weakness, accentuated by mild exercise, is common in myasthenia gravis. Megaesophagus is a common primary or accompanying complaint in dogs. Thymomas are often associated with myasthenia gravis in man, but this is uncommon in other animals. Administration of a short-acting anticholinesterase (edrophonium chloride) produces a dramatic increase in muscle strength. Treatment is with a long-acting anticholinesterase. Chronic immunosuppressive drug therapy for this disease is logical and should be investigated. Autoantibodies to the acetylcholine receptors can be detected in the serum of affected animals using an indirect FA procedure with normal muscle as a substrate.

DISEASES INVOLVING IMMUNE COMPLEXES
(Type III reactions)

Immune complex disorders are among the most common of the immunologic diseases. They may be idiopathic or of secondary origin. The site of deposition of the immune complexes determines the nature of the disease.

Glomerulonephritis (qv, p 880) is caused by deposition of antigen-antibody complexes in the subendothelial or subepithelial surface of the glomerular basement membrane. Secondary glomerulonephritis occurs as a side effect of chronic infectious, neoplastic, or immunologic disorders. Animals with idiopathic glomerulonephritis (>50% of cases) usually have signs of renal disease, whereas secondary glomerulonephritis is often a relatively minor part of a more serious disease.

Hypersensitivity pneumonitis is caused by deposition of immune complexes in the alveoli; it is most common in large animals that are exposed to antigenic dusts. The most potent antigens of this type are those contained in the spores of thermophilic actinomycetes from moldy hay. Inhalation of these spores causes farmer's lung in man and an atypical pneumonia in cattle (qv, p 725). It is characterized by the onset of respiratory distress 4-6 hr after exposure to moldy hay. The most effective treatment is removal of the source of the antigen. Otherwise, steroid therapy may help.

Systemic lupus erythematosus (SLE) occurs in dogs, less commonly in cats, and rarely in large animals. It has 2 immunological features; immune complex disease and a heightened antibody responsiveness with a tendency to produce autoantibodies. Therefore, it is a combination of Types II and III diseases. Antibodies to nucleic acid are the hallmark of SLE, but in some individuals, antibodies to RBC, platelets, lymphocytes, clotting factors, immunoglobulin (rheumatoid factors), and thyroglobulin also may be present. These autoantibodies, in particular those to nucleic acids, are not always pathogenic by themselves. Rather, they should be considered markers of the disease. Although combinations of autoantibodies and self-antigens may contribute to the total pool of immune complexes, they are not the sole source of immune complexes. Usually, either the immune complex or the autoantibody aspect of the disease predominates in a given animal. Immune complex deposition around small blood vessels leads to synovitis, dermal reactions, oral erosions and ulcers, myositis, neuritis, meningitis, arteritis, myelopathy, glomerulonephritis, and pleuritis. Glomerulonephritis is one of the major life-threatening complications of SLE in man and cats, but not dogs. Psychosis, a major sign of SLE in man, is seen mainly in cats. Autoimmune hemolytic anemia and/or thrombocytopenia are the most common autoantibody manifestations of SLE in animals.

SLE is characterized by the presence of antinuclear antibodies (ANA), and tests for these or the associated LE cells may help in diagnosis. However, some healthy animals may have ANA, and not all animals with SLE have detectable ANA in their blood. Diagnosis of SLE should be based on the entire clinical syndrome, and not just on the presence or absence of ANA.

SLE usually can be treated with glucocorticoids. Initially, they are used in high daily doses, and when remission occurs, alternate-day, low-dose therapy is used. Drug treatment should be continued for at least 2-3 mo after all clinical signs have disappeared. Cyclophosphamide, azathioprine, or both are used in combination with glucocorticoids in animals with SLE that is difficult to control with glucocorticoids alone.

Vasculitis mediated by immune complexes is common in animals, especially dogs and horses. Lesions are most prevalent in the dermis of the distal limbs and mucous membranes of the mouth, particularly the palate and tongue (dogs) and lips (horses). Involvement of the nose, ears, eyelids, cornea, and anus are less common. Early lesions are reddened areas that raised rapidly from shallow erosions. A scab quickly forms over dermal erosions. Edema of the limbs is common in horses, and a less frequent but equally flamboyant sign in dogs. Vasculitis is a feature of SLE in some animals, but most often is idiopathic. Drug-induced vasculitis has been well recognized in dogs. The vasculitis is detected on histopathological and immunohistopathological examination of superficial and deep biopsies taken from the margins of lesions.

Vasculitis is treated by withdrawal of offending drugs (if implicated in the cause) or by immunosuppressive drug therapy. Glucocorticoids used alone or in combination with other agents such as azathioprine or cyclophosphamide are usually used to treat nondrug-induced cases. (*See also* PERIARTERITIS NODOSA, below.)

Purpura hemorrhagica of horses is a form of nonthrombocytopenic purpura (qv, p 58) that often is a sequela of an earlier *Streptococcus equi* respiratory infection; it is mediated by immune complexes of IgA and streptococcal M antigen in vascular basement membranes.

Anterior uveitis (qv, p 295) often involves immune-complex-mediated reactions; it frequently occurs in the recovery stage of infectious canine hepatitis (qv, p 418) due to the reaction of serum antibodies with uveal endothelial cells that contain canine adenovirus 1. Similarly, equine uveitis (qv, p 302) or anterior uveitis of horses may be associated with immunologic reactions to *Leptospira* or *Onchocerca* spp. Uveitis caused by *Toxoplasma* and feline infectious peritonitis virus infections of cats also has an immunologic basis.

Canine rheumatoid arthritis (*see also* ARTHRITIS AND RELATED DISORDERS, SM AN, p 472) manifests initially as a shifting lameness with soft-tissue swelling around involved joints. Within weeks or months the disease localizes in individual joints, and characteristic radiographic changes develop. The earliest radiographic changes consist of soft-tissue swelling and a loss of trabecular bone density in the area of the joint. Lucent, cyst-like areas frequently are seen in the subchondral bone. The prominent lesion is a progressive erosion of cartilage and subchondral bone in the area of synovial attachments, which results in loss of articular cartilage and collapse of the joint space. Angular deformities often occur, and luxation of the joint is a frequent sequela. Deformities are most frequent in the carpal, tarsal, and phalangeal joints, and less frequent in the elbow and stifle. Synovial fluid changes indicate a sterile, inflammatory synovitis, with elevated total cell count and a high proportion of neutrophils in the synovial fluid cell population. It is believed to be due to deposition of immune complexes in the synovia.

A rheumatoid arthritis also has been recognized in cats. It tends to occur in older male cats and frequently is associated with feline leukemia virus infection. The development of disease in cats is much more insidious than in dogs.

Plasmacytic-lymphocytic synovitis, possibly a variant of rheumatoid arthritis, is common in medium and large breeds of dogs. Although multiple joints often are involved, the disease has a predisposition for the stifles. The most common complaint is hindlimb lameness and anterior drawer motion of the stifles. Lymphocytes and polymorphonuclear neutrophils predominate in the synovial fluid, although in some cases the fluid is essentially normal. Gross inspection of the joint reveals a yellowish proliferation of the synovial membrane and stretching or rupture of the cruciate ligaments.

Canine rheumatoid arthritis and plasmacytic-lymphocytic synovitis respond poorly to systemic glucocorticoids alone. Cyclophosphamide and azathioprine frequently are used with glucocorticoids to treat these disorders; nonsteroidal anti-inflammatory drugs, eg, aspirin, may help bring relief.

In **idiopathic polyarthritis**, a common disorder of dogs, there is no evidence of a primary chronic infectious disease process or systemic lupus erythematosus; joint disease is often the sole manifestation. It is most common in large dogs, particularly German Shepherd Dogs, Doberman Pinschers, retrievers, spaniels, and pointers. In toy breeds, it is most frequent in Toy Poodles, Yorkshire Terriers, and Chihuahuas, or mixes of these breeds. Diagnosis is made based on the history of cyclic antibiotic-unresponsive fever, malaise, and anorexia, with stiffness or lameness. Bony changes are not seen on radiographs until the disease is well established. Even then, radiographic changes are mild and can mimic degenerative joint disease. Synovial fluid is inflammatory in nature but sterile. The disease may be controlled with daily high-dose glucocorticoids followed by low-dose, alternate-day therapy. Treatment usually can be discontinued after 3-5 mo. Dogs that do not respond well to such therapy (>50%) are treated with more potent immunosuppressive drugs such as azathioprine or cyclophosphamide in addition to glucocorticoids. Gold salts may be helpful in augmenting glucocorticoid therapy in some animals.

Periarteritis nodosa (polyarteritis nodosa, necrotizing polyarteritis) is a rare, idiopathic disease of domestic animals that occurs usually as a secondary immunological manifestation caused by deposition of immune complexes and inflammation in walls of small and medium-sized arteries. Among farm animals, it is most common in pigs, usually associated with erysipelas and streptococcal infections, and is attributed to a hypertensive arterial reaction to these bacteria or to their vaccines. It has been reported in cats, although it has often been mistaken for the noneffusive form of feline infectious peritonitis.

Immune-mediated meningitis is believed to occur in dogs. The condition also has been called periarteritis nodosa, although its relationship to the human syndrome is uncertain. A steroid-responsive meningitis is particularly common in adolescent or young adult Beagles, Boxers, German Shorthaired Pointers, Akitas, and much less common in other pure and mixed breeds. The clinical signs in Beagles, Boxers, and German Shorthaired Pointers consist of cyclic bouts of fever, severe neck pain and rigidity, reluctance to move, and depression. Each attack lasts 5-10 days, with intervening periods of complete or partial normalcy lasting ≥1 wk. During attacks, protein and neutrophils in the CSF are elevated. The lesion is an arteritis, primarily of the meningeal vessels, but occasionally of other organs as well. The disease is often self-limiting over several months; attacks become milder and less frequent. Glucocorticoid therapy reduces the severity of attacks. In some animals, the disease becomes chronic and only partially amenable to therapy.

A more severe form of this type of meningitis has been reported in a litter of young Bernese Mountain Dogs. The disease in this litter was somewhat cyclical, but the resolution in intervening periods was less than in the disorder of Beagles, German Shorthaired Pointers, and Boxers. CSF abnormalities resembled those of the disease in other breeds. The condition was less self-limiting and required long-term high-dose glucocorticoid therapy to keep the animals comfortable.

A syndrome of meningitis, often associated with polyarthritis, is seen in Akitas as young as 12 wk old. The animals show severe (but somewhat cyclical) bouts of fever, depression, cervical pain and rigidity, and generalized stiffness. Affected animals grow at a slower rate and often appear unthrifty. The condition responds poorly to glucocorticoid and combination immunosuppressive therapy, and most animals are euthanized as young adults. In older Akitas, a milder and more drug-responsive form of the disease is seen, which may be associated with pemphigus foliaceus, uveitis, and plasmacytic-lymphocytic thyroiditis.

DISEASES INVOLVING CELL-MEDIATED IMMUNITY
(Type IV reactions)

Granulomatous reactions to microorganisms such as mycobacteria, *Coccidioides, Blastomyces,* and *Histoplasma* spp, and possibly feline infectious peritonitis virus, may be due to chronic cell-mediated immune reactions. Although cell-mediated immunity effectively controls these types of infections in most individuals, for poorly understood reasons, these same mechanisms are only partially effective in others, and a granulomatous reaction occurs.

In **lymphocytic choriomeningitis** virus infection of mice (qv, p 1024), CNS damage is due to the destruction of virus-infected cells by thymus-derived lymphocytes. **Old-dog encephalitis** (qv, p 409) also may result from cell-mediated immune mechanisms directed against cells persistently infected with canine distemper virus. The initiating canine distemper virus infection is usually clinically inapparent and may precede the encephalitis by years.

In **contact hypersensitivity**, chemicals react with dermal proteins, and new antigenic proteins are produced. The host's cell-mediated immune response against these chemically altered dermal proteins damages the skin, eg, poison oak and poison ivy reactions in man. It has been described in both dogs and horses, and usually occurs as a result of contact with sensitizing chemicals incorporated in plastic food dishes, plastic collars, and in drug compounds placed on the skin.

Autoimmune thyroiditis has been recognized in dogs and is characterized by destruction of the thyroid gland by an autoimmune process that has both humoral (type II) and cell-mediated components (type IV). The disease is particularly prevalent in breeds such as the Doberman Pinscher, Beagle, Golden Retriever, and Akita. Hypothyroidism (qv, p 280) may be the sole manifestation of the disease, or may be a clinical or subclinical component of a broader autoimmune disorder such as systemic lupus erythematosus, idiopathic polyarthritis, immune-mediated meningitis (periarteritis nodosa), panendocrinopathy, and rheumatoid arthritis.

Autoimmune adrenalitis has been reported in dogs. The adrenal glands are slowly destroyed by a plasmacytic-lymphocytic infiltrate. When sufficient glandular tissue is destroyed, the animals develop Addison's syndrome (adrenocortical insufficiency). The condition is sometimes associated with a similar immune attack against other endocrine glands, in particular the thyroids.

Keratitis sicca occurs in dogs, with a genetic predisposition in Cocker Spaniels. It can occur in a primary form, or secondary to chronic use of sulfonamides. The disorder is associated with an immune-mediated destruction of the lacrimal glands. It is somewhat analogous to Sjögren's syndrome of man, which is caused by disease of the salivary glands and a lack of saliva. Of affected dogs, ≥50% respond favorably to cyclosporine-containing eyedrops. Cyclosporine selectively inhibits T-lymphocyte-mediated disorders.

IMMUNE-DEFICIENCY DISEASES

Deficiencies in Phagocytosis: Phagocytosis is an essential feature of the host's immune system. Phagocytes are found underlying the mucous membranes and skin, and in the bloodstream, spleen, lymph nodes, meninges, synovial membrane, bone marrow, and around blood vessels throughout the body. Phagocytes are either in the tissue (histiocytes, synovial macrophages, Kupffer's cells, etc) or in the blood (polymorphonuclear leukocytes, monocytes). Phagocytosis involves recognition by the phagocytes of foreign, noxious, or damaged materials; chemotaxis of the phagocyte to the material; adherence of the material to the plasma membrane of the phagocyte; incorporation of the material into a pinocytotic vesicle; formation of a phagosome; and activation of the respiratory burst and lysosomal enzymes in the phagosome. Deficiencies in phagocytosis can involve acquired or congenital defects in any of these steps, or in the available number of phagocytes. Phagocytes have immunoglobulin and complement receptors on their surfaces that assist in the engulfment (opsonization) of foreign material coated with specific antibody (opsonins) or complement, or both.

Deficiencies in the phagocytic process often manifest as an increased susceptibility to bacterial infections of the skin, respiratory system, and GI tract, which respond poorly to antibiotics. Acquired phagocytic deficiencies include disorders that lead to profound and chronic depressions of WBC. Feline leukemia virus infection, feline panleukopenia virus infection, feline immunodeficiency virus infection, tropical canine pancytopenia, idiopathic granulocytopenias, drug-induced granulocytopenias (anticancer drugs, estrogens, anticonvulsants, sulfonamides, etc), and myeloproliferative disorders are a few conditions in which secondary infections can develop as a life-threatening complication.

A cyclic decrease of all cellular elements, most notably neutrophils, occurs in the peripheral blood and lowers the resistance to infection of gray Collies and Collie crosses. (*See* CYCLIC HEMATOPOIESIS IN GRAY COLLIE DOGS, p 64.)

Congenital abnormalities that lead to impaired phagocytosis are well documented in man. Deficiencies of opsonins, complement factors, chemotactic abilities, myeloperoxidase, and lysosomal enzyme activation have been recognized, but not in animals other than man. Chronic granulomatous disease has been recognized as an X-linked defect in some Irish Setters (canine granulocytopathy syndrome). Some lines of Weimaraners suffer from bacterial septicemias (usually manifest by bone and joint infections) as puppies. The underlying cause for this phenomenon is unknown; some of the affected animals have lower than normal levels of IgM and IgG, and preliminary research indicates that WBC have a bactericidal defect.

Leukocyte Adhesion Deficiency in Irish Setters (Canine Granulocytopathy Syndrome): A primary immunodeficiency disorder that is an autosomal recessive has been described in man and Irish Setters with a deficient expression of leukocyte surface glycoproteins. Clinically, it is characterized by recurrent, severe bacterial infections, impaired pus formation, and delayed wound healing. Infected animals usually have severe pyrexia, anorexia, and weight loss, and respond poorly to antibiotic therapy. Extreme, persistent leukocytosis may occur (>100,000 WBC/μL), and consists predominantly of a mature neutrophilia.

Deficiencies in Immunoglobulins: These may be acquired or congenital. Acquired deficiencies occur in neonates that do not receive adequate maternal antibodies (failure of passive transfer), or in older animals from conditions that decrease active immunoglobulin synthesis. Failure of passive transfer of immunoglobulin occurs occasionally in all species that have colostrum as the major source of maternal antibodies. It is commonly associated with clinical problems in calves, lambs, and foals. Failure of passive transfer can occur when the young fail to nurse properly during the first several days of life, or when the dam's colostrum contains low levels of specific antibodies. Theoretically, problems with the intestinal absorption of immunoglobulin in the milk also can occur. Immunoglobulin levels <400 mg/dL in a postnursing serum sample indicate a failure of passive transfer in foals. Removing calves from their dams too soon is a frequent problem in dairy herds. Newborn animals that fail to obtain adequate maternal antibodies often succumb to fatal bacterial or viral infections of the GI and respiratory tracts.

Idiopathic (essential) hypogammaglobulinemia has not been described in animals other than man, but undoubtedly it occurs. In man, it is associated with excessive suppressor cell activity that depresses antigen-stimulated immunoglobulin synthesis by B lymphocytes.

Hypogammaglobulinemia of clinical significance can be associated with any disorder that interferes with immunoglobulin synthesis. Tumors, such as plasma cell myelomas or lymphosarcomas that occasionally secrete large amounts of monoclonal antibody, can be associated with profound deficiencies of normal beneficial antibodies. This may be because the tumor cells are competing for necessary substrate substances with normal immunoglobulin-producing cells, or because of thymus-derived suppressor lymphocytes in the blood that nonselectively attempt to inhibit the abnormal immunoglobulin production. Animals with monoclonal-antibody-producing tumors can have severe secondary infections. Some viral infections, eg, canine distemper and canine parvovirus, may damage the lymphoreticular system so severely that normal antibody production is virtually halted.

Congenital hypogammaglobulinemia has been recognized either by itself, or in combination with deficiencies in cell-mediated immunity (combined immunodeficiency, *see* below). Deficiencies in IgG subclass synthesis have been seen in some breeds of cattle; IgM deficiency has been described in horses; and IgA deficiencies have been described in Beagles, German Shepherd Dogs, and Shar-Peis. Cattle with IgG subclass deficiency are usually asymptomatic, while older foals with IgM deficiencies suffer from respiratory infections. Dogs with IgA deficiency, like their human counterparts, suffer mainly from eczema, chronic respiratory infections, and possibly allergies. The IgA deficiency of Beagles appears to be due to a defect in the secretion of IgA, since IgA-positive cells are present in normal numbers. Some German Shepherd Dogs seem to have lower IgA levels than other breeds and a higher incidence of GI allergies. IgA deficiency in Shar-Peis is highly variable; some have negligible serum and secretory levels, and some have normal serum levels and low or negligible secretory levels. Like the German Shepherd Dogs, affected Shar-Peis have more problems than expected with allergies.

Transient hypogammaglobulinemia has been recognized most frequently in foals and puppies. It may be more common in Spitz-type puppies than in other breeds. It is congenital and manifest by a delay in development of active immunity. Affected foals frequently develop clinical signs of hypogammaglobulinemia (usually respiratory infections) at ~6 mo of age when their maternal antibody reaches a very low level. After another 3-5 mo, they begin to produce immunoglobulin. Puppies with this condition also developed recurrent respiratory infections at 1-6 mo of age, but recovered and were essentially normal by 8 mo of age.

Deficiencies in Cell-mediated Immunity: Pure deficiencies in cell-mediated immunity are relatively rare in man, and have not yet been described in other animals. In general, deficiencies in cell-mediated immune responses are associated with **thymic aplasia**, an absent or very small thymus. This is seen in some inbred lines of dogs and cattle; they were deficient in cell-mediated immune functions, such as lymphocyte blastogenesis, as well as having pituitary dysfunction.

Combined Immunodeficiency Disease: An autosomal recessive type of this disease has been identified in Arabian foals and Basset Hounds. Sporadic cases of combined immunodeficiency, probably heritable, have also been seen in Toy Poodle, Rottweiler, and mongrel puppies. Affected animals are frequently asymptomatic during the first several months of life, but become progressively more susceptible to microbial infections as maternal antibody wanes. Arabian foals with the disorder frequently succumb to adenovirus pneumonia or other infections when ~2 mo old. The foals are persistently lymphopenic. Precolostral serum samples have no detectable IgM antibody. Immunoglobulin levels are normal following nursing, but progressively decrease after that time compared to normal foals. At necropsy, the thymus gland is difficult to identify and is architecturally abnormal. There is a pronounced depletion of lymphoid elements in lymph nodes, Peyer's patches, and spleen. Puppies with combined immunodeficiency disease generally are normal until 6-12 wk old. The most common cause of death from this condition is canine distemper as a consequence of routine immunization with modified live virus distemper vaccine.

Complement Deficiencies: A congenital deficiency of C3 has been described in an inbred line of Brittanys. These animals suffered from recurrent bacterial infections, especially skin diseases and pneumonias. Although complement is necessary for opsonization and neutrophil chemotaxis, many persons or laboratory animals with these deficiencies do not always suffer from bacterial infections. This is mainly because the existence of 2 pathways provides a way of activating the system even if one pathway is blocked.

Congenital deficiency in the C1 inhibitor has been recognized in man and much less commonly in dogs. Affected animals suffer from recurrent bouts of facial edema.

Selective Immunodeficiencies: Rottweiler puppies have a breed predilection for severe and often fatal canine parvovirus infections. Their resistance to other diseases is essentially normal, and the basis of this selective immunodeficiency is unknown.

Persian cats have a predilection toward severe, and sometimes protracted, dermatophyte infections. In some Persian cats, the fungal infections invade the dermis and cause granulomatous disease (mycetomas).

Mink with the Aleutian coat color mutation are susceptible to chronic parvovirus infection and develop a disorder called Aleutian mink disease (qv, p 1053). Other strains of mink are susceptible to infection with this virus but do not develop clinical disease.

Focal and systemic aspergillosis (and mycoses due to related fungi) affect certain types of dogs. Long-nosed breeds, in particular German Shepherd Dogs and shepherd-crosses, are prone to develop focal aspergillosis in the nasal passages. Systemic aspergillosis is seen almost exclusively in German Shepherd Dogs, and more commonly in Western Australia than elsewhere. It is characterized by fungal pyelonephritis, osteomyelitis, and diskospondylitis. The organism can be isolated readily from blood and urine.

Viral-induced Immunodeficiencies: These have been caused by a number of agents in animals. Canine distemper virus causes a profound combined immunodeficiency in affected puppies. The infection is associated with a progressive decline in levels of antibody globulin and increased susceptibility to agents normally contained by cellular immunity, eg, toxoplasmosis, nocardiosis.

Parvoviral infection in both dogs and cats causes a profound and transient depression in the numbers of neutrophils and lymphocyte responsiveness. This has led to an increased incidence of fungal infections (aspergillosis, mucormycosis, candidiasis) in the immediate postrecovery period. A severe parvoviral-induced immunodeficiency syndrome has also been observed in mice.

Retroviral-induced immunodeficiency has received increased scrutiny since appearance of the acquired immunodeficiency syndrome (AIDS) in man. Feline leukemia virus (FeLV) infection is associated with acquired immunodeficiency and increased incidence of secondary and opportunistic infections. Acquired immunodeficiency in FeLV infection is multifactorial and broad in nature. Infected cats can have deficiencies of neutrophils, decreased synthesis of antibodies (especially to bacterial antigens), decreased cellular immunity, and variable levels of complement. Immune responses to FeLV infection also appear to inhibit ongoing feline infectious peritonitis (FIP) virus immunity specifically, which leads to reactivation of quiescent FIP.

Simian type D retrovirus (types 1-5 and Mason-Pfizer monkey virus) infection of macaques has a similar pathogenesis to that of FeLV infection of cats, but induces even more severe immunodeficiency. Each serotype tends to be found in specific species of macaques in the wild and within defined geographical areas. Type-D retrovirus infection of macaques can cause severe disease in adolescent animals from zoos and in primate centers with large breeding groups. Although the infection rate in the wild may be high, these viruses cause a less severe syndrome in wild than in captive populations. Affected macaques either die within several months with fever, lymphadenopathy, and opportunistic infections of the CNS, respiratory tract, and intestines; become lifelong asymptomatic carriers; or recover fully. A progressive retroperitoneal fibrosis is a feature with some serotypes. Healthy monkeys can be antibody positive and have virus in their blood and saliva (asymptomatic carriers), or antibody positive without isolatable virus (immune). Animals with clinical signs are always viremic, but may or may not have serum antibodies, depending on disease severity.

Simian immunodeficiency virus (SIV) is a lentivirus with considerable genetic homology to human immunodeficiency virus (HIV), the cause of AIDS in man. Many strains of SIV exist in nature. The common hosts are African primates such as African Green Monkeys, Sooty Mangabeys, Mandrills, Baboons, and other guenons. Transmission between infected and noninfected monkeys is probably by bites and *in utero* exposure. It is not present in native populations of Asian primates. It rarely causes disease in the host African species. If animals are under heavy stress, as in captivity, some infected animals may develop AIDS-like disease. SIV, especially of Sooty Mangabey origin, causes severe disease in macaques (rhesus, stumptail, pig-tail, bonnet, etc). Most affected macaques have come from zoos and primate centers where contact is allowed between African and Asian species, and tissues and body fluids are often exchanged between animals for research purposes. The immunosuppression associated with SIV can last for weeks or years. Encephalitis (usually asymptomatic except for wasting) and lymphomas are frequent sequelae of SIV infection in macaques. Infected animals, whether healthy or diseased, carry the infection for life. Monkeys that are infected with SIV usually make serum antibodies detectable by a number of procedures. Since the infection is lifelong, the presence of serum antibodies to SIV indicates the presence of virus in the body.

Feline immunodeficiency virus (FIV, originally feline T-lymphotropic lentivirus) is a related lentivirus that has been recently discovered in domestic cats. The infection is endemic in cats throughout the world. It is shed mainly in the saliva, and the principal mode of transmission is through bites. Free-roaming (feral and pet), male, and aged cats are at the greatest risk of infection. FIV infection is uncommon in closed purebred catteries. Following infection, there is a transient period of fever, lymphadenopathy, and neutropenia. Most cats recover from this stage and appear normal for months or years before immunodeficiency occurs. The percentage of infected cats that enter the terminal phase of the illness is unknown. Cats with FIV-induced acquired immunodeficiency suffer from chronic secondary and opportunistic infections of the respiratory, GI (including mouth), and urinary tracts, and the skin. FIV-infected cats have a higher than expected incidence of FeLV-negative lymphomas, usually of the B-cell type, and myeloproliferative disorders (neoplasias and dysplasias). Of affected cats, ~5% have neurological signs referable to cerebral cortex disease (behavioral abnormalities, psychomotor disturbances, dementia, convulsions). Cats remain infected for life; the presence of serum antibodies is directly correlated with the ability to isolate virus from blood cells and saliva.

A lentivirus has been recently isolated from cattle, and has been called **bovine immunodeficiency-like virus** (BIV). The virus was originally isolated from bovine leukemia virus (BLV)-negative cattle with persistent lymphocytosis and hemolymphadenopathy. It also has been isolated from cattle with BLV-negative lymphosarcomas. The overall incidence in cattle appears to be ~1%, although in some herds it may be ≥15%. Preliminary evidence indicates that the virus is not a major cause of immunodeficiency in cattle. Some infected cattle can be detected by serologic tests for viral antibodies. Virus isolation from blood appears to be the most accurate way to detect infected animals.

TUMORS OF THE IMMUNE SYSTEM

The normal immune responses require a burst of rapid proliferation of lymphocytes. On occasion however, this proliferation may be uncontrolled, and lymphoid neoplasms result. Lymphomas may be either T cell or B cell in origin.

Most cases of canine lymphosarcoma, Marek's disease, calf leukosis, and feline leukemia are of T-cell origin, as are thymomas. Thymomas, which are relatively uncommon in domestic animals, generally cause loss of condition and respiratory distress. They are commonly confirmed by radiography. In man, thymomas may be associated with signs of myasthenia gravis. While this association has been reported in dogs, it is uncommon. Many T-cell lymphomas are associated with a simultaneous immunosuppression as shown by a predisposition to recurrent infections.

Adult bovine and ovine leukosis, alimentary feline leukemia, and avian leukosis are usually of B-cell origin. Under some circumstances, neoplastic B cells may develop into plasma cells. Plasma-cell tumors are known as myelomas. Because neoplastic plasma cells can secrete immunoglobulin products, they give rise to gammopathies.

GAMMOPATHIES

Gammopathies are conditions in which serum immunoglobulin levels are greatly increased. They can be classified as either polyclonal, which involves an increase in all major immunoglobulin classes, or as monoclonal if they involve only a single homogeneous immunoglobulin.

Polyclonal gammopathies in animals are seen in chronic pyodermas; chronic viral, bacterial, or fungal infections; granulomatous diseases; abscessation; chronic parasitic infections; chronic rickettsial diseases, such as tropical canine pancytopenia (TCP); chronic immunologic diseases, such as systemic lupus erythematosus, rheumatoid arthritis, and myositis; or with neoplasia. They also may be idiopathic. In some animals, the gammopathy may appear initially to be monoclonal because of a predominance of one immunoglobulin class (usually IgG). Examples of this phenomenon have been seen in cats with noneffusive feline infectious peritonitis and dogs with chronic TCP.

Monoclonal gammopathies are characterized by the presence in the serum of a homogeneous immunoglobulin protein. Uninvolved immunoglobulin classes are usually depressed. Monoclonal gammopathies are either benign (ie, associated with no underlying disease), or they may be associated with immunoglobulin-secreting tumors. In man, benign gammopathies may become malignant at a later date; in other animals, they are rare and are not associated with a demonstrable tumor or clinical illness.

Monoclonal-antibody-secreting tumors originate either from plasma cells (myeloma) or lymphoblasts (lymphosarcoma). Plasma-cell myelomas can secrete intact proteins of any immunoglobulin class, or immunoglobulin subunits (light chains or heavy chains). Myeloma proteins in dogs are commonly IgG or IgA types, and less commonly IgM. Myelomas of the IgA type are particularly common in Doberman Pinschers. Monoclonal immunoglobulin produced by lymphosarcoma are often of the IgM class, regardless of species. Myeloma proteins in cats and horses usually are IgG, and uncommonly, IgM, IgG(T) (horses), or IgA.

Clinical signs depend on the location and severity of the primary neoplasm, and on the amount and type of immunoglobulin secreted. Plasma-cell myelomas frequently develop in marrow cavities of flat bones of the skull, ribs, and pelvis, and in the vertebrae. Pathologic fractures of diseased bone can lead to CNS or spinal disorders, or pain and lameness. Lymphosarcomas frequently involve parenchymatous organs; therefore, clinical signs are more diverse.

Clinically evident illness can result from the presence of the monoclonal protein itself. Amyloidosis (qv, p 319) can be due to increased immunoglobulin catabolism. Hyperviscosity syndrome, especially with IgM or IgA monoclonal proteins, can occur if the protein levels in blood are high. In this syndrome, plasma viscosity can be many times normal, which leads to profound vascular disturbances, thrombosis, and bleeding diathesis. Depression, blindness, and neurological manifestations can be due to hemorrhage in the nervous system and retina. Some IgM monoclonal proteins act as cryoglobulins and aggregate *in vitro* and *in vivo* when the plasma is cooled. Animals with cryoglobulinemia often develop gangrenous sloughs of the ear tips, eyelids, digits, and tip of the tail, especially during cold weather. (*See also* COLD HEMOLYTIC DISEASE, p 429.) Myelomas that produce autoantibodies to various tissues have been identified in man, but not in animals. Finally, animals with monoclonal gammopathies may have greatly depressed levels of normal immunoglobulin, and therefore may suffer from serious secondary infections.

Immunoglobulin-secreting tumors usually are treated with glucocorticoids and alkylating drugs. The prognosis for remission following therapy is much better in dogs than cats. Even in dogs, however, the long-term prognosis is poor, and relapse is common after 6-12 mo. Plasmapheresis may be needed to lower serum viscosity in animals with clinical signs of hyperviscosity syndrome. Antibiotics and globulin injections may be needed to help prevent secondary infections.

METABOLIC DISTURBANCES

METABOLIC DISTURBANCES, INTRODUCTION

Metabolic diseases may be inherited or acquired, the latter being more important. Metabolic diseases are of clinical significance because they affect energy production or damage tissues critical for survival.

INHERITED METABOLIC DISEASES

Inborn errors of metabolism are rare genetic disorders that affect many animals, most commonly dogs and cats. Disease results from the partial or complete absence of an enzyme critical in intermediary metabolism. Most documented disorders primarily affect the CNS, the so-called "storage diseases". Disease results because abnormal quantities of enzyme substrate are "stored" within lysosomes of neurons, which impairs their function. Generally, animals are normal at birth but manifest clinical signs within the first few weeks or months of life. These diseases are progressive and usually fatal, and no specific treatment currently exists for any of them. The gangliosidoses, GM_1 and GM_2, occur in Siamese, Korat, and domestic cats; and Beagles, German Shorthaired Pointers, and Japanese Spaniels. Sphingomyelinosis occurs in Siamese and domestic cats. Ceroid lipofuscinosis occurs in English Setters, Cocker Spaniels, Dachshunds, Chihuahuas, and Salukis, and in domestic cats. Mannosidosis occurs in domestic and Persian cats. Glycogenosis type II occurs in Lapland dogs, and type III in German Shepherd Dogs. Globoid cell leukodystrophy (Krabbe's) disease occurs in Cairn Terriers, West Highland White Terriers, Bluetick Hounds, Beagles, Poodles, Pomeranians, and Basset Hounds. Mucopolysaccharidosis type VI, a disease primarily associated with lameness, occurs in Siamese cats; type I occurs in dogs and cats. Diseases associated with decreased RBC survival and anemia include pyruvate kinase deficiency in Basenjis and Beagles, and phosphofructokinase deficiency in English Springer Spaniels. Horses have no recorded metabolic disease except possibly congenital methemoglobinemia and Quarterhorse episodic tremor.

In farm animals, the number of such diseases is small, and most of those that do occur have a low incidence. Mannosidosis of Angus, Galloway, and Murray Grey cattle, and of goats is probably the most common. Other identified diseases that are manifest by nervous signs and in most instances appear to be inherited defects are GM_1 and GM_2 gangliosidoses in cattle and pigs, respectively; ceroid lipofuscinosis of sheep; generalized glycogenosis of cattle and sheep; citrullinemia and maple syrup urine disease of cattle; and globoid cell leukodystrophy in sheep.

Other inherited diseases in which basic errors of metabolism of specific tissues occur are goiter of sheep and goats, inherited parakeratosis (edema disease) of cattle, osteogenesis imperfecta of sheep and cattle, and possibly cardiomyopathy of cattle, the hypotrichoses, baldy calves, photosensitization of sheep, dermatosis vegetans and porcine stress syndrome of pigs, and dermatosparaxia and Ehlers-Danlos syndrome of cattle. Many other inherited defects, especially those based on abnormal growth of collagen, cartilage, and bone also are likely to have basic errors of metabolism of structural tissues.

PRODUCTION-RELATED DISEASES
(Acquired metabolic diseases)

"True metabolic disease" usually results from an inherited excess or deficiency of catalyst(s) or enzyme(s). However, most of the diseases discussed in this section are primarily production- or management-related, although metabolism is a critical factor in the pathogenesis of each disease. Their cause in many cases is not an inborn error in metabolism, but rather an increased demand for a particular nutrient, the supply of which becomes adequate under select conditions. These diseases, such as hypocalcemia, hypomagnesemia, and hypoglycemia, are fostered by management practices that are aimed at greater production. Therefore, they are most aptly entitled production diseases. However, they are also metabolic diseases because the management of the animal demands a production output which, at its peak, is beyond the capacity of the animal's metabolic reserves to sustain the particular nutrient at physiologic concentrations. Thus, parturient paresis of cows occurs when the mammary secretion of calcium is greater than what either the diet or bone reserves can supply. There are parallel situations with glucose and magnesium, and with phosphorus in relation to postparturient hemoglobinuria.

Not all production-induced "metabolic diseases" are due to a simple negative balance of a particular nutrient. In some situations, dietary intake of a nutrient is suddenly reduced in the face of a high, continuing metabolic need, eg, pregnancy toxemia of ewes and beef cows, fat cow syndrome in dairy cows, and probably hyperlipemia in pony mares. Because a financially dictated decision not to supplement an animal with a rapidly falling nutritional plane precipitates these diseases, they are still classified as production-induced.

Paralytic myoglobinuria of horses is another production-induced metabolic disease. In this case, the production output—the physical activity of draft or racing—is being maintained by a particular level of nutritive intake. A management decision not to work or race the animal without a concomitant decrease in food intake may result in accumulation of muscle glycogen to a dangerous level. The

MET

disease is produced when work is resumed and the production of lactate exceeds its metabolism.

The difference between production-related metabolic disease and nutritional deficiency is often subtle. In general terms, nutritional deficiencies are long-term, steady states, corrected only by supplementation of the diet. Metabolic diseases are acute states that respond dramatically to the systemic administration of the needed metabolite, although the animal may require subsequent dietary supplementation to avoid recurrence.

The most important aspect of dealing with production-induced metabolic diseases is accurate and rapid diagnosis. If possible, the same tests should be used to predict the likely occurrence of the disease before its clinical onset to avoid the financial losses that they generate. A particular diagnostic system that does this is the Compton Metabolic Profile Test. The test is based on examining several sample groups of animals, and comparing the biochemical status of animals within the subject herd that is in a state of metabolic stress with those that are not. A deviation of the stressed group from the normal group is taken as an indication of impending disease. The system has the disadvantage of being expensive. An extension of the system to predict developing disease in individual animals is not favorably regarded for the same reason.

BODY TEMPERATURE

In homeotherms, normal cellular function depends on a relatively constant body temperature. This temperature is the sum of heat production and heat loss or conservation, and is regulated by a central mechanism within the hypothalamus that activates both physiological and behavioral activities. Heat production is increased by shivering, nonshivering thermogenesis, exercise, food intake, metabolic rate, and secretion of certain hormones. In herbivores, bacterial fermentation in the GI tract is an additional source of heat. Heat conservation results from peripheral vasoconstriction and behavioral responses that reduce the surface area from which heat can be lost. Animals exposed to excessive heat seek a cooler environment where heat loss is accelerated.

Heat is lost from the body by radiation, conduction, and vaporization of water from the respiratory passages and the skin; small amounts are lost in the feces and urine. Losses are accelerated by exposing more surface area, a cooler environment, peripheral vasodilation, panting, and sweating. Since fur reduces the ability to lose heat, heavily coated animals and those with dark fur are vulnerable to high temperatures. Ruminants possess a limited sweating mechanism; hence, their evaporative loss is inefficient.

In warm-blooded or homeothermic animals, the actual temperature at which the body is maintained varies from species to species and sometimes between individuals (see TABLES 3 and 4, pp 965 and 966); normal temperature may vary from as low as 95°F (35°C) to as high as 110°F (43°C). Peripheral parts of the body are at different temperatures, largely due to the environmental temperature and amount of insulation. The rectal temperature is representative of the core body temperature, which varies less. Basal temperature may be obtained early in the morning after a period of rest, without exciting the animal.

Normal Variation: The body temperature of healthy animals is subject to slight diurnal variations. The temperature rises during the day and falls during the night. Large animals, eg, horse, cow, and elephant, show small diurnal variations of ~1°F (0.5°C). Certain animals, eg, the camel, that are adapted to large variations in environmental temperature and restricted availability of water, have diurnal fluctuations of body temperature of as much as 11°F (5°C).

Hyperthermia of several degrees may result from exertion, excitement, or prolonged exposure to warm or humid environments. Hyperthermia due to reduced heat loss may seriously affect normal functions, eg, cows subjected to excessively high environmental temperatures reduce their food intake and lose weight, and milk production falls. Heat loss is associated with water loss. Teratogenic effects have been demonstrated in embryos when the dam has been subjected to hyperthermia during pregnancy. When water is not available, dehydration leads to inhibition of sweating; this may lead to hyperthermia, which can be treated readily by administration of water. (*See also* MALIGNANT HYPERTHERMIA, p 448.)

Seasonal variations in body temperature are related to environmental stresses and the reproductive cycle. In cold weather, the rectal temperature may be 1-2°F (1°C) below the summer levels. Before ovulation, the basal temperature may be 1°F below the level of the preceding days. During estrus, the level is somewhat higher. It is slightly above normal during the first half of pregnancy. Young animals have more labile temperature levels than older animals, with somewhat greater diurnal fluctuations.

Fever is produced by a bacterial, viral, or chemical pyrogen. It is the result of a "resetting" of the thermoregulatory mechanisms to function above the normal level. In many animals, prostaglandins are responsible for the readjustment; this accounts for the effectiveness of aspirin in reducing fever. Immediately after birth, neonates do not exhibit fever during infection, but within a few days, young animals respond to infection with a much higher fever than do mature animals. In old animals, even severe infection may produce little or no change in body temperature. In diurnal fever, which may indicate chronic infection, the temperature may rise several degrees during the day and return to normal each night. Many infections cause fever by inducing production of endogenous pyrogen (interleukin-1) from polymorphonuclear WBC, which constitutes a protective mechanism. This pyrogen crosses the blood-brain barrier to reset the thermoregulatory centers in the brain. In acute infections, the temperature may remain several degrees above normal for a few days, sometimes with a superimposed diurnal fluctuation. The relapsing fever of some chronic infections (eg, brucellosis) is characterized by several days of elevated body temperature, followed by several days of normal temperature.

A **chill** usually heralds a febrile episode and represents a period of heat production and conservation. The episode begins with extreme irritability, shivering, seeking a warm environment, and reducing body surface area (as by "curling up") from which heat can be lost. At the time of the chill, the body temperature is already rising; the mechanisms mentioned above generate more heat and cause the temperature to rise further.

Metabolic disturbances occur as a result of fever. The most striking of these is due to excessive loss of water. Severe dehydration may produce a rise in body temperature, which resolves with administration of fluids. Persistent fever can lead to a loss of sodium chloride and brain damage. During hot weather and after fever, horses and cattle should have salt available to replenish losses.

Acid-base and electrolyte imbalances, associated with prolonged fever or hyperthermia, may lead to acidosis. If fever persists, convulsions may ensue and lead to excessive heat production, brain damage, and possibly death. The fever may be treated by cooling the animal with cold soaks or dips, or in smaller animals, alcohol sponge baths. Convulsions may be controlled by sedation or anesthetic doses of barbiturates. The maximum body temperature compatible with life is 10°F (5°C) above the normal level of the animal.

Hypothermia: (*See also* p 627.) When the skin or blood is cooled enough to lower the body temperature in nonhibernating animals, metabolic and physiological processes slow. Respiration and heart rate are slow, blood pressure is low, and consciousness is lost. At a rectal temperature of <82°F (28°C), the ability to regain normal temperature is lost, but the animal will continue to survive and, if external heat is applied, the temperature returns to normal. These findings have been adapted and used extensively in heart and brain surgery in man. In hypothermic states, the oxygen need of cells, particularly neurons, is greatly reduced, and the circulation can be stopped for relatively long periods.

A lowered body temperature is seen in moribund states. It is a poor prognostic sign in infectious diseases. In accidental hypothermia, the animal should be brought into a heated environment and allowed to warm slowly to its normal temperature.

CONGENITAL ERYTHROPOIETIC PORPHYRIA
(Porphyrinuria, Pink tooth)

A rare hereditary disease of cattle, pigs, cats, and man, in which defective Hgb formation results in production of an excess of Type I porphyrins in the nuclei of developing normoblasts.

The defect in cattle is inherited as a simple recessive, and usually is confined to herds in which inbreeding or close line-breeding is practiced. The disease has been recognized in the USA, Canada, Denmark, Jamaica, England, South Africa, Australia, and Argentina. The heterozygous animal seems to be normal, but the homozygous recessive animal is affected at birth with reddish brown discoloration of the teeth, bones, and urine. The urine contains an excess of coproporphyrin I and uroporphyrin I, but the discoloration of teeth and bones is due primarily to uroporphyrin I. Bones, urine, and teeth (especially the deciduous teeth) fluoresce pink when irradiated with near-ultraviolet light. Prolonged exposure to sunlight causes typical lesions of photosensitization with superficial necrosis of unpigmented portions of the skin. A normochromic, hemolytic anemia with macrocytes and microcytes and marked basophilic stippling develops. Splenomegaly eventually occurs, and the bones have increased fragility due to a diminished cortex. The animal becomes progressively unthrifty and may die unless protected from sunlight. A similar disease (qv, p 784) causes photosensitivity only in Limousin cattle and man.

The defect in pigs and cats is extremely rare and differs from the disease in cattle in that photosensitization is not a feature; it is transmitted as an autosomal dominant. The disease in pigs has been reported only from Denmark and New Zealand; in cats it has been recognized only in the USA.

Diagnosis should be based on the excretion of abnormal uroporphyrins and on the brown discoloration of the teeth, which fluoresce when irradiated with near-ultraviolet light. Affected animals and their heterozygous sires and dams should be excluded from the breeding program, because there is no definitive laboratory test for detection of clinically normal heterozygotes.

FAT COW SYNDROME
(Fatty liver disease of cattle)

This disease of fat dairy cows that have calved recently has much in common with pregnancy toxemia (qv, p 456) and is often bracketed with it; however, their epidemiologies are different. Fatty liver disease occurs after calving rather than before, and usually in cows that are being challenge fed, ie, their intake is planned to be greater than their nutritional demands for lactation. Because the cows are actually in negative energy balance during the sudden demand for energy after calving, there is a high mobilization of fat from body depots, which results in deposition in the liver. Only fat cows develop the disease. Clinically, there is severe ketonuria, anorexia, weakness, recumbency, and terminally, tachycardia and coma. Usually, death occurs in 7-10 days. No specific treatment can be recommended. General supportive measures are usually adopted: high-quality, palatable roughage; injection of anabolic steroids; IV infusion of combined electrolyte solutions or glucose, or both; insulin; and cud transfers or intraruminal infusion of large volumes of rumen juice. The results are poor. Because this is a disease of high-producing cows in intensively managed herds, prevention has a high priority. Avoidance of obesity and assiduous treatment of periparturient disease are critical.

HYPOMAGNESEMIC TETANY IN CATTLE AND SHEEP
(Grass tetany, Grass staggers)

A metabolic disturbance characterized by hypomagnesemia. It is most common in adult cows and ewes, especially those in heavy lactation and on lush grass pastures. It also occurs in cattle of any age or condition, particularly beef cattle, that are grazing on wheat or other cereal crops, or that are undernourished and exposed to changeable, cold weather. It is manifest by irritability, tetany, and convulsions, and has a high mortality rate.

Etiology: The rate of onset depends on the degree of deficiency; it is rapid in lactating cows allowed lush pasture after being housed over the winter, and slow in undernourished beef cows. The low levels of magnesium and high levels of potassium and nitrogen in grass and wheat pastures combine to limit magnesium absorption. Excitement, milking, transport, and adverse weather are all possible triggers. Hypocalcemia is a consistent concurrent finding, possibly secondary to hypomagnesemia.

Although serum magnesium levels <1.5 mg/dL are suspicious and levels <1 mg/dL are diagnostic, they may return to almost normal (1.7-3 mg/dL) during the convulsive stage. Serum calcium levels are usually moderately depressed (5-8 mg/dL). The levels of magnesium in the CSF are low, and this is thought to cause characteristic convulsive episodes.

Clinical Findings: In the most acute form, affected cows, which may be grazing in an apparently normal manner, suddenly throw up their heads, bellow, gallop in a blind and frenzied manner, fall, and undergo severe paddling convulsions. These convulsive episodes may be repeated at short intervals, and death usually occurs within a few hours. In many instances, animals at pasture are found dead without illness having been observed. In less severe cases, the cow is obviously ill at ease, walks stiffly, is hypersensitive to touch and sound, urinates frequently, and may progress to the acute, convulsive stage after a period as long as 2-3 days. Because hypocalcemia occurs consistently with hypomagnesemia, it may be difficult to determine which is the primary problem; grass tetany may accompany parturient paresis, and the classical signs of the latter be obscured by the tetanic convulsions. In all cases of grass tetany, the loudness of the heart sounds and tachycardia are characteristic signs.

The disease in sheep occurs under essentially the same conditions and has the same clinical signs as in cattle.

Treatment: Affected animals require treatment immediately. Usually, this includes administration of magnesium and calcium compounds, and sometimes sedatives if the convulsions and tetany are severe. An IV injection of calcium and magnesium may be used, but it must be given slowly and the heart monitored carefully. A less risky alternative is to give the calcium IV (*see* PARTURIENT PARESIS, p 451) and the magnesium sulfate subcut. (200 mL of a 50% solution/cow). Unless the animal is removed from the tetany-producing pasture, and fed hay and concentrate, the blood magnesium level is likely to fall again to dangerously low levels 24-36 hr after therapy. To prevent this, follow-up treatment using 2 oz (60 g) of magnesium oxide PO daily for ≥1 wk should be started and gradually withdrawn.

Prophylaxis: Prevention is largely a combination of increasing the intake of magnesium in danger periods and of management. Daily oral supplements of magnesite or magnesium oxide (2 oz [60 g] to cattle and ⅓ oz [10 g] to sheep) can be incorporated in the concentrate feed or in licks containing molasses; unpalatability effectively precludes free-choice consumption. Magnesium alloy "bullets" have been developed for cattle and sheep to give a slow release of magnesium in the rumen. Fertilization with magnesium limestone or magnesium oxide to increase herbage

magnesium is successful only with certain soil types. Dusting of herbage with powdered magnesium oxide (110 lb/acre [125 kg/hectare]) or spraying with a 2% solution of magnesium sulfate at intervals of 2 wk gives good short-term prevention
against grass tetany under suitable weather conditions.

Out-wintered stock should be protected from wind and cold and provided with
supplementary food. Potassium and nitrogen fertilization reduces the content and
availability to the animal of magnesium in herbage and should be avoided in the
spring before the first grazing. Sheep and cattle should have access to hay or dry
pasture. Changing the calving date so that cows are not in early lactation when the
weather is inclement is an effective preventive measure, but may be economically
impractical.

HYPOMAGNESEMIC TETANY IN CALVES

Tetany in calves is clinically identical to grass tetany in adult cattle; it is characterized by hypomagnesemia and, commonly, hypocalcemia. Because of its occurrence in 2- to 4-mo-old calves being fed milk only, or in younger calves on milk
replacer or with chronic scours, the disease is considered to be due to inadequate
absorption of magnesium from the gut. The inadequacy may be due to a primary
deficiency of magnesium in the diet, or to rapid passage of the ingesta through the
intestines. In the latter case, the chronic diarrhea must be stopped. Affected calves
require prompt treatment with a 10% solution of magnesium sulfate (100 mL subcut.) followed by 10-15 g magnesium oxide PO, daily. This level of oral dosing
with magnesium oxide is also an effective prophylactic. Supplementation of the diet
with hay or pasture is also recommended.

KETOSIS IN CATTLE
(Acetonemia, Ketonemia)

A metabolic disease of lactating cows that occurs within a few days to a few
weeks after calving. It is characterized by hypoglycemia, ketonemia, ketonuria, inappetence, either lethargy or excitability, weight loss, depressed milk production,
and occasionally incoordination. In most areas, the incidence is highest in high-
producing cows that are being stall-fed.

Etiology: Any factor that reduces intake or absorption of dietary carbohydrate precursors in early lactation can cause primary ketosis. Although, theoretically, factors
that affect the metabolism of absorbed carbohydrates may similarly cause hypoglycemia and primary ketosis, no such factors have been identified. The theory that a
primary cause of ketosis is dysfunction of the adrenal cortex has not been substantiated. Ketosis is commonly secondary to depressed appetite due to a primary disease
such as metritis, mastitis, or abomasal displacement.

The carbohydrate deficiency hypothesis is based on the observation that, of the
various forms of carbohydrate ingested by ruminants, little is absorbed as glucose.
The animal's principal sources of energy are acetic, propionic, and butyric acids
produced by microbial fermentation in the rumen; of these, propionic acid is
generally accepted as the major carbohydrate precursor and the only one that has
antiketogenic properties. If this is so, the lactating cow receives little or no carbohydrate beyond that required for synthesis of the lactose secreted in the milk. Caloric
intake can be inadequate when the food is insufficient or unpalatable, or when the
balance of ketogenic and antiketogenic substances in the diet is disturbed, eg, by the
feeding of certain silages with high butyric acid content. The composition of the
diet similarly can modify the microbial population of the rumen, and thus influence
the relative proportions of the volatile fatty acids (VFA) produced by fermentation.
If the predisposition is to the production of ketogenic VFA, ketosis is likely to result.

In dairy cows during heavy lactation, demands for glucose for lactose production are great; if the demand for a direct supply cannot be met from the hepatic

stores of glycogen, tissues are raided for fats, the metabolism of which promotes ketogenesis.

Clinical Findings: Signs include inappetence, constipation, mucus-covered feces, depression, a staring expression, a drop in milk production, sometimes a humpback posture suggestive of mild abdominal pain, and in a short time in untreated cases, an obvious weight loss. Most cases are of this wasting, lethargic type, but a few show signs of frenzy and aggression. Clinical signs include circling, staggering, licking, chewing, bellowing, hyperesthesia, compulsive walking, and head pressing. These occur in episodes that last ～1 hr and recur at intervals. The breath has an acetone odor. Hypoglycemia, ketonuria, and ketonemia are always present. The disease is self-limiting because the reduction of food intake eventually causes a cessation of milk flow, and glucose drain. Subclinical ketosis is the diagnosis in cows that have ketonuria after calving but are clinically normal. These cows have a small reduction in milk yield but a significant level of reproductive inefficiency associated with endometritis.

Diagnosis: While a negative urine or milk test (Rothera or "Acetest") rules out ketosis, the presence of hypoglycemia, ketonemia, and ketonuria is not sufficient for a positive diagnosis of primary ketosis. Any abnormality that causes a cow in early lactation to go off feed, eg, metritis, pneumonia, or mastitis, produces some degree of secondary or fasting ketosis. Such conditions, of course, may accompany the pure ketotic syndrome. One of the most common causes of secondary ketosis is left abomasal displacement (qv, p 153). Persistent subclinical hypomagnesemia (qv, p 445) also has been identified as a precursor of acetonemia, and as is cobalt deficiency (qv, p 1197), is an identifiable predisposing factor in pastured cattle. In secondary ketosis, the positive reaction to "Acetest" tablets by urine is often neither as rapid nor as pronounced as in the primary disease. Sometimes, judgment on the diagnosis should be reserved until the response to treatment has been observed. Failure of a definite and continuing response to glucose or hormone therapy is cause for reconsideration of the signs and possible complications.

Treatment: In thin cows that obviously have been undernourished, replacement of carbohydrate is recommended. In fat cows, in which nutritional imbalance is more likely to be the cause, glucocorticoids are as effective. The IV injection of glucose is not sufficiently effective, even when repeated daily for 3-4 days, to be recommended as the sole treatment. However, it is commonly used as an adjunct to either parenteral glucocorticoids or oral propylene glycol. An injection of glucose results in a prompt increase in blood glucose that is followed by a decrease within the next several hours to a value usually below normal, but still greater than the pretreatment level; the blood glucose may not return to normal for several days, even in cows that show a good response.

Following the IM injection of glucocorticoids, blood glucose usually returns to normal within 8-10 hr and may rise to a value considerably above normal within 24 hr, especially when the cause is inadequate caloric intake. In such cases, appetite and general behavior usually improve markedly within 24 hr, and blood ketone levels return to normal by the third to fifth day. Milk production may decrease during steroid therapy but increases rapidly 2-3 days after treatment. Anabolic steroids are currently being used as treatment, but are not officially approved in all countries.

Propylene glycol (225 g b.i.d. for 2 days followed by 110 g daily for 2 days) or ammonium lactate (200 g daily for 5 days) given PO effect recovery in many cases. However, compared with other treatments, the response is slower and treatment must be extended over a longer period. These substances appear to be of greatest value when used as supportive treatment following use of glucocorticoids or glucose. Sodium acetate given PO is less effective. Chloral hydrate sometimes is used in conjunction with other treatments and is especially helpful if hyperexcitability is exhibited. When the appetite is regained following any of the above treatments, good feeding is required to restore the animal to full health and production.

Since it is often difficult to distinguish between primary and secondary ketosis when the cow exhibits signs of other diseases, it is advisable to treat for both ketosis and the complicating condition.

Prophylaxis: Animals susceptible to ketosis should be maintained on a relatively high energy intake before calving, and the level should be increased substantially after parturition. A good guide to optimal feeding is the cow's body condition, which must be maintained so as to avoid being overfat or overthin. The protein content of the ration should be moderate ($\sim16\%$), and the amount of concentrate fed to stall-fed cows should be ~1 kg/3 kg of milk produced.

Daily intake of hay to maintain body condition should be ~3 kg/100 kg body wt. The roughage must be of good quality, palatable, digestible, and nutritious. Wet silage and moldy, dusty hay are common precursors to acetonemia in high-producing cows. Rations that induce a high production of propionic acids in the rumen may contribute materially to the prevention of ketosis when fed for a few weeks before and after calving; eg, a ration of finely ground and pelleted alfalfa hay plus a steam-heated cereal (flaked corn, barley, etc), in which the ratio of hay to steamed cereal may be as great as 8:1, effects a high production of propionic acid. For this ration to be effective, the animal must not have access to long hay, straw, shavings, or other unground roughage. When large amounts of silage are being fed, its replacement by hay may be advantageous. Addition of sodium propionate to the feed reduces the incidence.

LACTATION TETANY IN MARES
(Transit tetany, Eclampsia)

A condition associated with hypocalcemia and sometimes with alterations in blood magnesium levels. It occurs most often in mares ~10 days after foaling or 1-2 days after weaning, or in nursing mares on lush pasture. Occasionally it is seen in nonlactating horses, usually following some stress, eg, prolonged transport. Extremely rare since the "passing" of the draft horse, it is characterized by incoordination, tetany, sweating, muscle tremors, rapid and violent respiration, and a thumping sound from within the chest, considered by many to be a spasmodic contraction of the diaphragm. Handling may exacerbate signs, but affected horses are not hypersensitive to sound, and there is no prolapse of the third eyelid as in tetanus. However, stiffness of gait and a high tail carriage are apparent. The body temperature remains close to normal, and the appetite appears unimpaired, but during an attack the animal is unable to eat, urinate, or defecate. Mildly affected animals may recover spontaneously; severely affected ones go down in ~24 hr, develop tetanic convulsions, and usually die the next day.

Response to IV injections of calcium solutions given very slowly is generally good. If the tetany is associated with transport, it may be advisable to incorporate magnesium in the solution. Sedation is often indicated for excitable mares.

MALIGNANT HYPERTHERMIA
(MH, Porcine stress syndrome [PSS], Pale soft exudative pork [PSE], Back muscle necrosis, Transport myopathy)

A shock-like, hypermetabolic, genetically transmitted myopathy triggered by stress, volatile anesthetic agents, or depolarizing muscle relaxants. Pigs are the principal animals involved, but cases have been reported in horses, dogs, cats, deer, chickens, rabbits, cattle (double muscling syndrome, qv, p 477), and man. Capture myopathy of wild animals (qv, p 553) is similar in many respects. In pigs, the leaner, more heavily muscled, fast-growing breeds, such as Pietrain, Landrace, Poland China, and crossbreeds of these strains, are the most susceptible.

Etiology: Although MH was thought to be transmitted by means of a single autosomal dominant gene with incomplete or variable expression, more recent evidence suggests that it is inherited as an autosomal recessive. A number of different phenotypes have been identified, which suggests that inheritance may vary from strain to strain or even from herd to herd.

The primary defect is an abnormality in skeletal muscle calcium kinetics. Increased concentration of myoplasmic and mitochondrial calcium occurs in malignant hyperthermic episodes. Elevated myoplasmic calcium levels stimulate excitation-contraction coupling, and increase muscular glycogenolysis and heat production. Under natural conditions, MH is initiated by stress, eg, handling, managing, transport, mating, excitement, and exercise. Experimentally, the syndrome can be induced by inhalation of anesthetic agents, eg, halothane, methoxyflurane, chloroform, enflurane, fluroxene. Depolarizing muscle relaxants, such as succinylcholine, and α-adrenergic agonists also may initiate or potentiate the syndrome.

Clinical Findings: The initial sign is fine, rapid muscle tremors of the tail, back, and legs. Tremors progress to muscle rigor, and the animal becomes unable to move. Blanching and erythema followed by cyanosis are evident in white-skinned pigs due to peripheral vasoconstriction. Tachycardia (~200 beats/min), cardiac arrhythmias, open-mouth breathing, hyperventilation, fever, and hypercapnia are followed by carbon dioxide narcosis, apnea, and death. Body temperature may increase by as much as 2°F (1°C) q5-7min and may reach 113°F (45°C) before death.

After death, rigor mortis develops within a few minutes. Muscle temperature is elevated, and the high levels of lactic acid cause a low muscle pH (≤ 5); however, the muscle pH rises rapidly as the body cools. Muscles of the back, thigh, loin, and shoulder are affected most frequently. Muscles with a high portion of type 2 fibers, such as the semitendinosus and psoas, are affected most extensively and should be examined grossly and histologically at necropsy. Affected muscles from an animal that dies acutely are pale and wet, and ooze fluid at necropsy. Repeated episodes may produce dry and dark foci in affected muscles. Histologic changes in muscles are nonspecific and may include a variation in the cross-sectioned diameter of muscle fibers and hyaline degeneration.

Diagnosis: A history of stress or exposure to stressor drugs and genetic susceptibility are important considerations, combined with acute shock-like clinical signs, muscle tremor, rapid rise in temperature, tachypnea, and rigidity. Blood pH is decreased (<6), and blood lactate and pyruvate levels are increased. Blood lactic acid levels may reach 425 mg/dL. Partial pressure of carbon dioxide is elevated in arterial blood, and oxygen consumption is increased. Plasma catecholamine concentration is increased and is responsible for concurrent hyperglycemia. The main plasma electrolyte changes are increases in potassium and phosphate.

Differential diagnoses include: 1) heatstroke, which is due to confinement or forced exercise in a hot environment; 2) hypocalcemic (puerperal) tetany with muscular contractions and increased body temperature; 3) capture myopathy in wild animals (if this is a different diagnosis); and 4) azoturia or tying-up syndrome, characterized by myoglobinuria, which develops following exercise in horses, draft oxen, sheep, and racing Greyhounds.

PSS, MH, and PSE are considered as one syndrome by some, and as 3 syndromes by others. Experimental evidence indicates that these syndromes are similar clinically and all are genetically determined. However, different genes appear to control the susceptibility to particular stressors, eg, all pigs that develop PSE do not appear to be susceptible to the stress of halothane anesthesia. The susceptibility to different stressors may have been the main factor in differentiating the 3 syndromes.

Treatment: Since MH is genetically determined, it is essential to screen breeding stock for susceptibility; however, desirable genetically controlled characteristics such as muscularity and growth rates must be maintained. Several screening tests have been used. In the halothane-challenge test, pigs are exposed to halothane anesthesia (3-6% v/v) for ~5 min, and pre- and postanesthesia levels of serum CPK are measured; an increase of 20- to 100-fold is found in susceptible pigs. Recent evidence indicates a combination of halothane and succinylcholine provides a more sensitive test to detect MH. Another test that has been used is an exercise test, in which an increased CPK level following exercise indicates susceptibility to MH. Resistance (and susceptibility) to MH also has been linked with certain blood groups and RBC osmotic fragility.

Treatment consists of removing the animal from the impending stress or inhalation anesthetic, IV administration of tranquilizers, bicarbonate, fluid therapy to correct the lactic acidosis, surface cooling, and hyperventilation with oxygen. An experimental intracellular muscle relaxant, dantrolene (a phenytoin derivative), has been demonstrated experimentally to inhibit and control episodes of MH in pigs. Reported doses were 3-5 mg/kg body wt, IV. Tachyarrhythmia may be treated with procainamide.

OBESITY

The storage of excess fat that results when there is an imbalance between intake and expenditure of calories. Obesity occurs when body weight is ≥15% above optimum. *See* MHN section, p 1088 *et seq* for nutritional requirements of various species. *See also* APPETITE, p 1093 and BEHAVIOR, p 895 *et seq.*

Etiology: The principal cause is excessive food intake combined with inadequate exercise. It is the most common nutritional disorder in dogs, and incidence increases with age (up to 50%), probably because of a reduction of both basal metabolic rate and physical activity. It is more common in females than in males, and in neutered than in non-neutered dogs of either sex. Some breeds of dogs tend to be more obese, including Labradors, Dachshunds, and Beagles. Dogs fed home-cooked meals, table scraps, and snacks have a greater tendency to be overweight than those on an exclusive diet of commercial pet food. In contrast to dogs, cats are better able to regulate food intake according to caloric need, and obesity is less common. However, obesity appears to be increasing in frequency in cats, probably due to improved palatability of commercial cat foods. Pathological conditions that may be associated with obesity include hypothyroidism, hyperadrenocorticism, diabetes mellitus, and insulinoma.

The point at which fat accumulation in food animals becomes excessive is somewhat subjective. Invariably it is the result of abnormal feeding patterns imposed on the animals.

Clinical Findings: The thickness of the fat layer over the rib cage is a good indicator of obesity if the optimal body weight for that animal is not known. Normally, the ribs should be easily felt but not seen, whereas the ribs cannot be easily palpated in the obese animal. A pendulous abdomen, a waddling gait, and sluggish behavior are other features of some obese animals. Obesity may predispose to many problems including joint or locomotion disorders, dyspnea and fatigue, hepatic lipidosis, impaired reproductive efficiency and dystocia, and increased anesthetic and surgical risk.

Management: The caloric intake must be reduced and a regular exercise program developed to expend energy and possibly reduce appetite. Ideally, daily caloric intake should be decreased to ~60-70% of that required for maintenance. This may be achieved most effectively by feeding a nutritionally complete, but low-calorie, high-fiber, reducing diet. Commercial or homemade reducing diets are preferable to feeding smaller quantities of the normal diet. Small meals may be fed frequently during the day, and snacks and table food should be eliminated. The rate of weight loss should be ~3%/wk for the first 6 wk but less later in the program. Progress should be monitored by weighing weekly, and dietary modifications made if necessary. Frequent monitoring also helps the owner maintain enthusiasm for a weight-loss program.

Dramatic weight reduction can be achieved in dogs when food intake is almost completely restricted. This should not be attempted in obese cats. Ideally, the animal should be hospitalized during this time and examined daily; vitamin-mineral supplements should be fed, and water given *ad lib.* Metabolic acidosis and ketosis are generally not clinical problems in dogs when fat is mobilized. However, when changes in fluid balance have been calculated, loss of adipose tissue occurs at similar rates on weight-reducing and starvation diets. Drugs such as amphetamines have proved ineffective in dogs, and surgical procedures such as jejunoileal bypass are not necessary or recommended.

PARTURIENT PARESIS IN COWS
(Milk fever)

An afebrile disease of mature dairy cows that occurs most commonly at or soon after parturition; it is manifest by circulatory collapse, generalized paresis, and depression.

Etiology: The disease, usually associated with the sudden onset of profuse lactation, is an acute hypocalcemia in which the serum calcium level drops from a normal of ~10 mg/dL to 3-7 mg/dL (av 5 mg/dL). Serum magnesium may be depressed and result in tetany, or elevated and result in flaccid paralysis and somnolence. The disease may occur in cows of any age but is most common in dairy cows 5-9 yr old. There is a higher incidence in the Jersey breed.

Clinical Findings and Diagnosis: Parturient paresis usually occurs within 72 hr after parturition, but occasionally before, during, or even some months thereafter. The disease is sometimes the cause of dystocia that arises from inadequate expulsive efforts, and prolapse of the uterus may be a complication.

Early in the onset, the cow may exhibit some unsteadiness as she walks. More frequently, she is in sternal recumbency and unable to rise; the head may be displaced to one side or turned into the flank. The eyes are dull and staring and the pupils dilated. Anorexia is complete, the muzzle tends to be dry, and the extremities are cool. The pulse rate usually is elevated, and the temperature normal or subnormal. The GI tract is atonic with suppressed defecation and a relaxed anus. If treatment is delayed many hours, the dullness gives way to coma, which becomes progressively deeper, and death ensues. With approaching coma, the animal assumes lateral recumbency, which predisposes to bloating, regurgitation, and aspiration pneumonia. Treatment in the early stages is more successful, and fewer relapses occur. Animals affected at or within a few hours of parturition appear to develop more severe signs more rapidly than animals affected at other times. Differential diagnoses include metritis, coliform mastitis, grass tetany, acute indigestion, traumatic gastritis, coxofemoral luxations, obturator paralysis, lymphosarcoma, spinal compression, and fracture of the pelvis. Some of these diseases, in addition to aspiration pneumonia and degenerative myopathy, may also occur concurrently with parturient paresis or as complications. (*See also* THE DOWNER COW, p 555.)

Treatment: Treatment is directed toward restoring the serum calcium level to normal; this must be done as soon as possible to avoid muscular and nervous damage and recumbency. Cows that have calved in the preceding 72 hr should be watched closely. Calcium borogluconate is most commonly used (250-500 mL, 25% solution), preferably by IV injection, but the subcut. and IP routes also are used. Subcut. administration permits slow absorption of the calcium ion and may lessen the danger of cardiac arrest. Strict asepsis and limiting the volume injected at one site to ~50 mL reduce the chances of local reactions.

Animals that relapse or fail to get up after 8-12 hr should be treated again, although at the time of each repeated treatment, the diagnosis should be reconfirmed and complications ruled out. In the absence of blood analysis, it is often impossible to decide which element is low: in addition to calcium, other ions, eg, phosphorus or potassium, or most probably magnesium, may be indicated for nonresponsive cases. In cases complicated by ketosis (qv, p 446), 250-500 mL of 50% dextrose should be given IV.

In the few cases that do not respond to any other treatment, the udder may be inflated. Each quarter is inflated through a sterile teat tube until firm and, if necessary, the teats are gently tied with gauze to prevent escape of the air. The gauze is removed after 2-3 hr, and the udder is partially milked out. If necessary, inflation may be repeated 6-8 hr later.

Prophylaxis: Feeding normal-to-high phosphorus/low-calcium diets during late pregnancy helps to prevent parturient paresis, but such rations are difficult to devise in a practical form and, if continued for long periods in heavy-milking cows, may result in dangerous depletion of skeletal mineral reserves. Delayed or incomplete milking after calving, by maintaining pressure within the udder, is of doubtful value in reducing the number of attacks and may aggravate a latent infection into acute mastitis. Massive doses of vitamin D (20-30 million u daily), given in the feed for 5-7 days before parturition, reduces the incidence, but if administration is stopped >4 days before calving, the cow is more susceptible. This contingency can be avoided by the simultaneous injection of a corticosteroid to induce parturition. Dosing for periods longer than those recommended should be avoided because of the danger of toxicity. A single IV or subcut. injection of 10 million u of crystalline vitamin D given 8 days before calving is an effective preventive. The dose is repeated if the cow does not calve on the due date. Newer compounds used (where approved and available) in lieu of vitamin D and less likely to cause hypervitaminosis D are 25-hydroxycholecalciferol, 1,25-dihydroxycholecalciferol, and 1α-hydroxycholecalciferol. After calving, a diet high in calcium is required. Administering large doses of calcium in gel form (PO) following calving to ensure a high intake of calcium is commonly practiced. Doses of 150 g of calcium are given 1 day before, at, and 1 day after calving.

PARTURIENT PARESIS IN EWES

A disturbance of metabolism in pregnant and lactating ewes characterized by acute hypocalcemia and rapid development of hyperexcitability, ataxia, paresis, coma, and death.

Etiology: The exact cause is unknown, but the conditions under which field outbreaks occur are fairly well defined. Deficiency of calcium and/or magnesium may be contributing factors. The disease occurs at any time from 6 wk before lambing to 10 wk after, principally in highly conditioned older ewes at pasture. The onset is sudden and almost invariably follows—within 24 hr—an abrupt change of feed, a sudden change in weather, or short periods of fasting imposed by circumstances such as shearing, crutching, or transportation (see also TRANSPORT TETANY IN RUMINANTS, p 458).

Clinical Findings and Diagnosis: Characteristically, the disease occurs in outbreaks. The incidence is usually <5%, but in severe outbreaks, 30% of the flock may be affected at one time. The earliest signs are slight hyperexcitability, muscle tremors, and a stilted gait. These are soon followed by dullness, sternal decubitus, often with the hindlegs extended backward, mild ruminal tympany and regurgitation of food through the nostrils, staring eyes, shallow respiration, coma, and death within 6-36 hr.

Diagnosis is based on the history and clinical signs. In outbreaks occurring before lambing, pregnancy toxemia is the main differential diagnosis. A tentative diagnosis of acute hypocalcemia can be confirmed readily by a dramatic and usually lasting response to calcium therapy.

Prophylaxis and Treatment: Treatment consists of IV or subcut. calcium (eg, 100 mL of 25% w/v calcium borogluconate), preferably with some added magnesium. Affected sheep should be handled with care, lest sudden deaths occur from heart failure. Prevention is largely a matter of avoiding the predisposing causes.

PHYSICAL EXHAUSTION

A condition due to a complex series of metabolic events that occur when an individual is extended beyond its normal capacity for endurance. (It is different from fatigue, which can be considered as extreme tiredness within the individual's normal capacity.) It is most apt to occur in animals subjected to prolonged physical exercise, often under severe environmental conditions. Horses engaged in endurance and marathon events are the animals most commonly affected.

Pathophysiology: At the onset of exercise, the body responds to increased metabolic demands by increasing the supply of oxygen to the locomotor muscles, which synthesize ATP for the production of energy. If the exercise intensity is maintained at aerobic levels, it can be sustained for considerable periods. When exercise intensity increases above what can be sustained aerobically, energy is produced anaerobically, and fatigue ensues rapidly. Whether the energy is produced aerobically or anaerobically, heat is always produced. In the normal horse, this heat is dissipated by the evaporation of sweat. If the elements lost in the sweat during prolonged exercise are not replaced, particularly under conditions of high environmental temperature and humidity, metabolic disorders associated with exhaustion occur.

It is difficult to measure fluid losses accurately; however, changes in body weight provide a good quantitative index under the prevailing circumstances. Clinical signs of dehydration become apparent when loss of body weight is 4-5%, and signs are severe at ~10% loss. The concentrations of potassium and chloride are greater in sweat than in plasma; therefore they are lost more rapidly than sodium. Chloride is more important since its sustained loss results in alkalosis as the body adjusts to the anion loss by conserving bicarbonate ions.

The changes in plasma composition that occur during endurance rides vary with duration of the ride, environmental temperature and humidity, vigor of the ride, and the access to water (with or without electrolytes added) during the course of the ride. The general tendency is for electrolytes to change little or decrease somewhat during rides of 60 miles (100 km) provided the conditions are not too hot. When conditions are warm or hot, and sweating is profuse, plasma electrolyte concentrations may decline significantly. However, as concentrations of calcium and magnesium fall, that of phosphorus may rise significantly.

Also, plasma protein and albumin increase, a reflection of dehydration. This effect is also seen in the PCV and RBC, both during and after the ride. Rising concentrations of creatinine, urea, and bilirubin in plasma also reflect the effects of dehydration, while those of CPK and AST (SGOT) indicate increased leakage from the muscle fibers. In normal horses, these all return to normal after the endurance ride; failure to do so may indicate exhaustion. Persistent elevations of CPK or AST can indicate overt muscle damage, as occurs in exertional rhabdomyolysis (qv, p 553), which may be part of the exhaustion complex.

Accompanying these changes, a rise in blood pH, bicarbonate, and base excess, particularly during the middle stages of the ride, indicate development of metabolic alkalosis. Marked falls in blood glucose and rises in free fatty acids and glycerol concentrations, particularly toward the end of long rides, reflect the increasing contribution of lipid metabolism to energy production as carbohydrate sources in the liver gradually decline.

Within the fibers of the locomotor muscles, energy production depends on either aerobic or anaerobic pathways. At submaximal levels of work under aerobic conditions, the duration of work is limited by factors that govern the supply of glucose (from IM and hepatic glycogen) and/or non-esterified fatty acids (from body lipid stores). When the capacity for aerobic energy production is exceeded, either by the failure to supply sufficient oxygen or by a work load that exceeds the animals aerobic capacity, the gap in energy requirements is met by anaerobic pathways. As a result, lactic acid is produced, which is accompanied by the onset of fatigue. The fatigue process has 2 stages: 1) the failure of calcium release from the sarcoplasmic reticulum, and its binding by troponin; and 2) the turnover of the actin-myosin cross bridges. Both of these require energy from ATPase reactions, and are inhibited when ATP content is low, when reaction products that inhibit ATPase action reach sufficient levels, or when the muscle pH declines to an inhibitory low level. Low pH also decreases the release of calcium and its affinity for troponin. During prolonged exercise under aerobic conditions without lactic acid accumulation, fatigue occurs when glycogen stores are depleted.

However, fatigue also may occur when energy substrate reserves are adequate, and without the accumulation of lactic acid and the resulting fall in pH. The accumulation of potassium ions or depletion of sodium in the extracellular space or sarcotubular system can result in fatigue by affecting, or even preventing, the propagation of action potentials. An uneven inward spread of tubular excitation and, therefore, myofibrillar activation may also occur.

Additionally, the role of accumulating inorganic phosphorus during exercise, and its role in fatigue, particularly in the absence of high hydrogen ion concentration, needs further clarification.

Clinical Findings: Typically, an exhausted horse is lethargic and shows little interest in its surroundings. The corneas are glazed, ears expressionless, and the face may have an anxious, grimacing appearance reflecting colic or muscular spasms. Animals are usually anorectic and often, despite being dehydrated, will not drink. Hyperthermia is usually present, although rectal temperatures may be misleading if air has dilated the rectum because of a decrease in anal sphincter tone. The anal sphincter reflex may be absent.

Persistent tachycardia and tachypnea are evident. A shallow respiration at a faster rate than that of the heart can cause inefficient gas exchange. Synchronous diaphragmatic flutter, arrhythmias, murmurs, and obvious jugular pulse may be further signs of failure of the cardiovascular and pulmonary systems to reestablish normal function.

The most consistent clinical finding is dehydration, reflected as loss of skin elasticity, sunken eyeballs, and dry mucous membranes. These changes indicate a fluid loss of 7-10% of body wt, which can amount to 8-10 gal. (30-40 L) of water. This loss is complicated by the accompanying severe electrolyte imbalance. Fatigue, weakness, trembling, stiffness, pain, and possibly tying-up are the usual muscular signs.

Postexhaustion renal shutdown, hepatic dysfunction, rhabdomyolysis, and even laminitis result if the appropriate supportive fluid and electrolyte therapy is not administered. The development of these problems is indicated by high plasma concentrations of creatinine, urea, CPK, and AST (SGOT) for several days after the ride. A reduced flow of normally concentrated urine occurs during the course of a ride, which then returns to normal with the restoration of hydration afterwards. There is virtually no change in the composition of the urine between normal and exhausted horses, except for a positive test for blood in the urine in those with myoglobinuria.

Synchronous Diaphragmatic Flutter (SDF, "thumps"): Often related to athletic stress and not infrequently seen in endurance rides, this has also occurred with other conditions, including traumatic pressure on the phrenic nerve, persistent vomiting, electrolyte imbalance, and hypocalcemic states such as parturient paresis. The 3 common pathophysiological changes that occur are alkalosis (usually metabolic), hypocalcemia, and electrolyte imbalance. Horses may be withdrawn during an endurance ride due to SDF when they are likely to be somewhat alkalotic, normocalcemic, and variably dehydrated. They are almost certainly tired, but not necessarily exhausted. Whatever the specific cause, the mechanism of SDF is probably stimulation of the phrenic nerve by cardiac electrical discharge. The diaphragm then contracts simultaneously with the heartbeat.

Treatment and Prevention: Horses will maintain their hydration, within reasonable limits, if adequate water is provided at frequent intervals throughout a ride. Small drinks at regular intervals are of more value than occasional large ones. Supplementing water with salt or electrolytes is also advantageous. Should dehydration and exhaustion occur, the immediate need is restoration of body water and electrolyte balance. Horses that are willing to drink can be treated PO with a balanced electrolyte solution, and then allowed access to water as required. As a result of the electrolyte losses and the resulting plasma concentrations (eg, low sodium), there may be no thirst drive and the horse will have to be treated by gavage until the desire to drink returns. In severely affected horses, it may be necessary to provide the initial treatment IV to restore hydration rapidly; maintenance therapy is then continued PO as required. When complicated by SDF and if hypocalcemia is part of the metabolic imbalance, the provision of calcium borogluconate is often of value in stopping the "thumps". Simply correcting the alkalosis usually stops the "thumps". Evidence of myoglobinuria necessitates rigorous fluid therapy to ensure a substantial diuresis to reduce the degree of renal tubular damage that occurs from the filtered myoglobin. If there are clinical signs of pain, analgesics can be provided. In general terms, a horse that finishes a 50-100 mile (80-160 km) ride and is moderately dehydrated needs oral fluids (5-13 gal. [20-50 L]), containing 13-30 g sodium chloride and 8-20 g potassium chloride per liter, to restore hydration. If severely dehydrated, 2.5-5 gal. (10-20 L) of balanced electrolyte solution (eg, lactated Ringer's solution) IV is also needed. Proper conditioning and training of horses, careful pacing of events by the rider, and providing water during the ride, especially if >30 miles (50 km), contribute substantially to the prevention of exhaustion and its complications.

POSTPARTURIENT HEMOGLOBINURIA

Primarily a disease of high-producing dairy cows that occurs 2-4 wk after parturition. It is characterized by intravascular hemolysis, hemoglobinuria, and anemia.

The cause is unknown. The disease is rare in beef animals or animals <3 yr old, and is uncommon >4 wk after parturition. The incidence is generally low, but up to 50% of affected animals may die. Diets high in cruciferous plants (such as rape or kale) or beet pulp, and prolonged feeding on phosphorus-deficient diets are predisposing factors. In North America, the disease may occur after prolonged stabling. The hemoglobinuria is believed to be associated with hypophosphatemia since serum phosphorus levels are always subnormal (0.8-1.4 mg/dL) in acutely ill cows. In New Zealand, a nutritional deficiency of copper is the most common cause, although selenium deficiency may be responsible for some. The widely held hypothesis based on these field observations is that hemolytic agents occur in pasture plants as well as rape, turnips, and other cruciferous plants, and that hypophosphatemia or hypocuprosis renders the RBC more susceptible to the hemolysins.

Rapid IV hemolysis leads to hemoglobinuria, extreme pallor, and a rapid pulse. Dehydration, weakness, and a marked drop in milk yield are prominent signs. The temperature may be elevated to 103°F (39.5°C). Some respiratory distress may be seen. Hemolysis continues for 3-5 days, and in cows that recover, the return to normal is slow. Jaundice may occur in the late stages. Without treatment, death is usual.

Transfusion of large quantities of whole blood may be the only effective treatment of severely affected animals. In less severe cases, 2 oz (60 g) of sodium acid phosphate in 300 mL of distilled water may be administered IV followed by subcut. injections at 12-hr intervals or by daily oral doses of the same amount of phosphate. If injected subcut., sodium acid phosphate should be well distributed to avoid tissue necrosis. Bone meal should be added to the ration. It is important to avoid copper or phosphorus deficiency in the diet and prevent access to plants known to contain hemolysins.

PREGNANCY TOXEMIA IN COWS

A sporadic disease that is most common in beef cows that have become fat because of heavy feeding in early pregnancy, but which suffer a severe nutritional stress during the 2 mo before calving. (*See also* FAT COW SYNDROME, p 444.) Morbidity is low, and is highest when pastured cattle deplete the natural feed and are not supplemented. When the disease is clinically apparent, it is usually far advanced and treatment is unrewarding; mortality is virtually 100%.

Affected cows are often fat, completely anorectic, in the last stages of pregnancy, and often carry twins. There is a transitory period of restlessness and incoordination, the pulse is weak and fast, and feces are scant and firm. Sternal recumbency follows. There is a greater than normal amount of clear nasal discharge, the skin on the muzzle is dry, cracked, and may peel; respirations are rapid and grunting. The cow's condition remains unchanged for 7-10 days. Terminally, the feces become soft and smelly, tend to be orange, and remain scant; the cow becomes comatose and dies quietly.

Laboratory findings show marked ketonemia and ketonuria, hypoglycemia, and proteinuria. The hepatic enzyme levels in serum are raised and, terminally, the blood glucose is often raised to high levels. At necropsy, the liver is grossly enlarged, and obviously fatty. Ostertagiasis is often a significant concurrent disease, and the abomasal mucosa may be obviously abnormal.

Treatment is generally ineffective, especially if the cow is recumbent. Anabolic steroids are useful, and supportive therapy with glucose, fluids and electrolytes (IV and PO), and propylene glycol (PO) is recommended. Although it is likely at the cost of the calf, the cow may be saved by inducing parturition with corticosteroids or by cesarean section.

Adequate supplemental feeding of concentrates during the last trimester of pregnancy is preventive.

PREGNANCY TOXEMIA IN EWES
(Ovine ketosis)

A disease of preparturient ewes, characterized primarily by impaired nervous function.

Etiology: The primary predisposing cause is undernutrition in late pregnancy. Overfed ewes carrying twins or triplets are more susceptible than ewes in poor condition and those carrying single lambs. Anything that interrupts feed intake (eg, storms, transport, other disease conditions) may induce the disease. The primary lesion is hypoglycemic encephalopathy, the result of inability of the ewe to supply sufficient glucose (from products of digestion or catabolized tissues) to meet the carbohydrate demands of large multiple fetuses and herself. The defect appears to be in maintaining the blood glucose level, since utilization of available glucose is unimpaired. As the disease progresses, severe ketosis and acidosis may develop, together with hepatic, renal, and possibly endocrine disorders. The blood glucose may rise without alleviating the signs of encephalopathy. At this stage, the ewe is refractory to treatment.

Clinical Findings and Diagnosis: Early clinical signs may be erratic and difficult to detect. The usual course, lasting 2-5 days, includes listlessness, inappetence, aimless walking, "propping" against any kind of obstruction, muscle twitching (of the ears, around the eyes, and perhaps of other parts), unusual postures, grinding of the teeth, progressive loss of reflexes, blindness, ataxia, and finally sternal decubitus, coma, and death.

Laboratory tests usually reveal hypoglycemia early, with normoglycemia or hyperglycemia later, and hyperketonemia. Acidosis and high blood nonprotein nitrogen are variable concomitant findings. Necropsy findings include fatty livers, indistinguishable from those found sometimes in apparently healthy ewes underfed near term. The adrenal glands may be swollen, hyperemic, or grayish. Pulmonary changes are associated with recumbency.

Acute hypocalcemia before lambing is the main differential diagnosis. In this, the course is shorter (deaths occur within 24 hr), and usually there is a marked, immediate, and persistent response to IV calcium therapy.

Treatment: Once signs are advanced, no treatment is highly effective. Mortality of untreated cases is ~80%. With early diagnosis, such as may be made by gentle driving of the flock, particularly when the disease has been induced by relatively sudden fasting, glycerol or propylene glycol (PO, 4 oz [120 mL] b.i.d.) decreases mortality. Best results are obtained by the combination of one of these with an anabolic steroid and fluid therapy to counter acidosis, but the mortality is still likely to be ~50%. Cesarean section or induced abortion early in the course of the disease usually leads to recovery and, if near term, the offspring may be saved. Palatable feed and water and protection from extremes of weather should be provided. Force-feeding b.i.d. with soaked alfalfa pellets given by stomach tube may be a worthwhile practice with especially valuable animals; treatment should be continued until the appetite returns.

Prophylaxis: Obesity should be avoided in early pregnancy, and adequate good feed supplied during the last 6 wk of pregnancy. Feed supplementation depends on the condition of the pastures and weight of the ewes. When the pastures become poor, heavy feeding may be necessary. If adequate and suitable feed is not available for the whole flock during late pregnancy, early cases can be identified by gentle driving. These can be separated from the flock and given special care and nourishment, but any interruption of feed intake should be avoided.

When the disease occurs in fat ewes on good pastures, perhaps associated with mild foot conditions, gentle driving for 30 min may prevent incipient cases from developing by elevating the blood glucose for a period. When supplementary feeding can be provided as prophylaxis, it is important to prevent overeating, which may cause lactic acidosis and laminitis. Both diseases are probable if grain is made available *ad lib.*

PUERPERAL TETANY
(Eclampsia)

A disease most frequently encountered in small, excitable breeds of dogs such as Chihuahuas, Toy Poodles, and small terriers, particularly 1-3 wk after parturition. It also occurs sporadically in larger dogs and in cats.

Etiology and Pathogenesis: Considerably less is known about the pathogenesis of postparturient hypocalcemic syndromes in dogs and cats than in cattle (qv, p 451). There is little evidence to suggest that puerperal tetany in lactating bitches is the result of an interference in parathyroid hormone (PTH) secretion; in fact, PTH levels appear to be increased in response to the hypocalcemia. The severe hypocalcemia and hypophosphatemia that develop near the time of peak lactation (1-3 wk postpartum) most likely result from an imbalance between the rates of inflow and outflow from the extracellular calcium pool.

The functional disturbances associated with hypocalcemia in the bitch primarily are the result of increased neuromuscular tetany, in contrast to those in the cow in which the clinical signs are dominated by muscular paresis. The occurrence of either tetany or paresis in response to hypocalcemia appears to result from basic physiological differences between the bitch and cow in the function of the neuromuscular junction. The release of acetylcholine and transmission of nerve impulses across neuromuscular junctions are blocked by the severe hypocalcemia in cows, which leads to muscle paresis. Dogs appear to have a higher margin of safety in neuromuscular transmission, in that the degree to which end-plate potential exceeds the firing threshold is greater than in cows. Excitation-secretion coupling is maintained at the neuromuscular junction in the bitch with hypocalcemia. Tetany occurs as a result of spontaneous repetitive firing of motor nerve fibers. As a result of the loss of stabilizing membrane-bound calcium, nerve membranes become more permeable to ions and require a stimulus of lesser magnitude to depolarize.

Clinical Findings and Diagnosis: The clinical course in canine parturient hypocalcemia is rapid, with only an 8- to 12-hr interval between the onset of signs and development of tetany. Premonitory signs include restlessness, excess panting, and excitable behavior. Within a few hours, ataxia, trembling, muscular tetany, and convulsions may develop. Hyperthermia frequently is associated with the increased muscular activity; body temperatures of 107°F (42°C) are not uncommon.

In most cases, diagnosis is based on history, clinical signs of increased neuromuscular excitability, and response to therapy. Demonstration of hypocalcemia with serum calcium (Ca) levels of <7 mg/dL is confirmatory. Serum phosphorus (P) often is lowered to a comparable degree. Blood glucose is in the low-normal range or decreased as a result of the intense muscular activity associated with tetany.

Treatment: Slow IV administration of an organic Ca solution such as calcium gluconate should result in rapid clinical improvement and cessation of tetanic spasms within 15 min. In most bitches weighing 5-10 kg, 5-10 mL of 10% calcium gluconate provides sufficient Ca. Administration should be slow to avoid inducing ventricular fibrillation and cardiac arrest.

Puppies should be removed from the bitch for 24 hr to reduce the lactational drain of Ca. During this period, they should be fed a milk substitute or other appropriate diet; if mature enough, they should be weaned. Supplemental dietary Ca and vitamin D have been useful in preventing relapses in certain bitches.

Although some advocate the use of corticosteroids in addition to Ca and vitamin D to prevent relapses after the original therapy, their value is questionable; they may interfere with intestinal Ca transport and increase urinary loss of Ca.

Prevention: During gestation, a good-quality balanced diet with a Ca:P ratio of ≤1:1 that provides the required (but not excess) amount of Ca may provide a more responsive Ca homeostatic mechanism to meet the markedly increased demands of lactation. Clinical experience in cows suggests that increased control of Ca homeostasis by PTH secretion occurs with the approach of parturition and initiation of the lactational drain in animals fed balanced or relatively low-calcium diets during gestation.

TRANSPORT TETANY IN RUMINANTS
(Railroad disease, Railroad sickness, Staggers)

A condition that affects well-fed cows and ewes in advanced pregnancy, during or immediately after extended transportation and stress. It is also reported in lambs during transport to feedlots. The specific cause is unknown, but the condition in sheep may be a form of acute hypocalcemia brought on by adverse conditions during shipping. In cattle, hypomagnesemia may be the precipitating cause. Crowded, hot, poorly ventilated railroad cars or trucks with no provision for feed or water seem to be predisposing factors. Evidence of the condition is more commonly observed at destination, but may develop while in transit. Early signs of restlessness and uncoordinated movements are followed by a partial paralysis of the hindlegs and a staggering gait. Later, the animal is unable to rise and assumes an attitude similar to that observed in parturient paresis in cows. A pulse rate of 100-120 may be noted, and respiration is rapid and labored. The temperature may be elevated slightly, and congestion of the mucous membranes is common. Extreme thirst may develop, while anorexia is regularly observed; peristaltic and rumen activity may be reduced or completely absent. Abortion may occur as a complication. Progressive paralysis, gradual loss of consciousness, and death result within a few days, unless suitable treatment is undertaken soon after onset.

Animals in advanced pregnancy should be given only dry feed that contains adequate calcium and magnesium for 1-2 days preceding shipment. Loading should be accomplished with a minimum of excitement, and overcrowded, poorly ventilated vehicles should be avoided. If the in-transit time will be long, arrangements should be made to have the animals fed, watered, and rested. Promazine hydrochloride or other suitable ataractics (unless transport is to slaughter) given IM 30 min before loading are effective in alleviating the stress of transportation and may help to prevent the disease. For treatment, IV injections of calcium borogluconate (25% solution, 400-800 mL/cow, ~100 mL/ewe), or calcium borogluconate with magnesium sulfate (5% solution, same volumes) given very slowly, preferably with 250-500 mL of 50% dextrose solution, have been recommended, but results are poor. In affected cows, repeated IV injections of electrolyte solutions should be administered and the cow moved onto soft bedding with sure footing underneath. Induction of parturition is a logical treatment but is ineffective in most cases. Sedation is indicated if the animals are hyperexcitable.

MUSCULOSKELETAL SYSTEM

MUSCULOSKELETAL SYSTEM, INTRODUCTION

The musculoskeletal system is composed of the bones and striated muscles of the body, along with the articulations, tendons, and ligaments connecting the components. Its primary functions are to support the body, provide a means of motion, and in some instances, to provide protection to certain vital structures, eg, the brain, eyes, and viscera. It also provides the principal storage system for calcium and phosphorus and contains a major portion of the hematopoietic tissue. Disorders of interrelated systems, eg, nervous, blood-vascular, enzyme, and integumentary systems, may influence the function of the musculoskeletal system.

Diseases of the musculoskeletal system are most often manifest by impairment of motion or function; the degree of impairment depends on the specific cause and severity of changes. Most are due to skeletal disorders and articular changes, though some are due to muscular diseases, neurological disorders, toxins, endocrine imbalances, metabolic disorders, infectious diseases, blood-vascular diseases, nutritional deficiencies or imbalances, and occasionally, congenital defects.

Diseases of the musculoskeletal system also may affect other body systems, the primary complaint often being dysfunction. Ocular motion and control, respiration, bladder function, penile retraction, mastication, and deglutition all are partially a function of the musculoskeletal system. Complete or partial paralysis may be due to primary muscular dysfunction (infectious, toxic, or congenital), though in most instances the nervous system is the primary problem and the muscular dysfunction is secondary (eg, tetanus, rhinopneumonitis, canine distemper, hydrocephalus).

The structural and functional unit of skeletal muscle is the motor unit. It consists of the ventral motor neuron with its cell body in the central horn of the spinal cord and its peripheral axon, the neuromuscular junction, and the muscle fibers innervated by the neuron. Each component must be intact for the muscle to function normally. The ventral motor neuron is the final common pathway, which conducts neural impulses from the CNS to the muscle.

The first step in the transmission process is the propagation of the nerve action potential into the axon terminal. This results in depolarization of the axon terminal membrane because of the increased permeability of the membrane to sodium ions. Calcium ions, which enter the axon terminal as a result of depolarization, are necessary for release of the neurotransmitter acetylcholine from the synaptic vesicles in the axon terminal into the synaptic cleft of the neuromuscular junction. If calcium ions are absent or inhibited by magnesium ions, no acetylcholine will be released.

When acetylcholine unites with its receptors, permeability of the muscle membrane to sodium and potassium ions increases, which changes the muscle membrane potential. Passage of the action potential along the membrane initiates the contraction-coupling mechanism of muscle. The hydrolysis of acetylcholine into choline and acetate by cholinesterase concludes the transmission process.

Normal muscle and its associated motor units can be considered as a multifaceted dynamic organ. Many diseases can alter its structure and function. Disorders of the neuromuscular junction result in muscle fatigue, weakness, and paralysis. Conditions that interfere with function of the neuromuscular junction include myasthenia gravis, drugs (eg, curare, succinylcholine, certain antibiotics), toxins (eg, botulism, tetanus, snake bite, tick paralysis), hypocalcemia, and hypermagnesemia.

Diseases of muscle tissue are called myopathies; these include disorders of the membrane and contents of the muscle fiber. Myopathies primarily involving the muscle fiber membrane may be hereditary (eg, myotonia congenita in goats) or acquired (eg, vitamin E and selenium deficiencies, hypothyroidism, hypokalemia). Myopathies involving the muscle fiber contents include muscular dystrophy, polymyositis, eosinophilic myositis, malignant hyperthermia, glycogen and lipid storage diseases, vitamin E and selenium deficiencies (white muscle disease, azoturia), and exertional rhabdomyolysis. Differential diagnosis of these diseases is greatly facilitated by laboratory aids, eg, muscle biopsies, serum enzyme levels, electromyographic studies, thermography, and nerve conduction velocity studies.

Most bone diseases are congenital, nutritional, or traumatic. Congenital disorders include distortion of bones in utero as well as genetic defects. Examples of the latter include some cases of equine ataxia (wobbles) and hip dysplasia in certain breeds of dogs, and abnormal bone formation or growth such as due to parathyroid hypoplasia.

Nutritional causes are due primarily to imbalances or deficiencies of minerals, particularly calcium and phosphorus, although other trace minerals may be involved. Other nutritional causes include excessive protein in the ration of growing animals. Either a deficiency or an excess of certain vitamins, particularly A and D, may influence growth and integrity of bone. Osteomalacia is a classic example of calcium and phosphorus imbalance or deficiency. Epiphysitis may be due to imbalances or deficiencies of minerals or protein in the ration.

Traumatic causes include fractures, both complete and incomplete; periostitis; sequestra formation; and exostoses due to acute or chronic trauma, particularly at the insertion of tendons or ligaments. Limited motion, pain, heat, and swelling usually accompany any of these disorders.

Articulations are divided basically into 2 classifications: synarthroses, in which the segments are united by fibrous tissue or cartilage and are essentially immovable; and diarthroses, which are mobile joints characterized by the presence of a joint cavity with a synovial membrane. Synarthroses rarely are involved in diseases of the musculoskeletal system other than from trauma such as fractures. Diarthroses frequently are involved, and various portions of the joint may be affected: the fibrous capsule, the ligaments, the cavity itself (including menisci), the synovial membrane, synovial fluid, the subchondral bone, and the articular cartilages.

Diseases affecting the diarthroses may be due to acute trauma, chronic inflammation, developmental defects, or to bacterial or fungal infections. Acute trauma may result in luxations, subluxations, or fractures of the joints. Direct trauma may also partially or completely rupture the ligaments of the joint or the fibrous capsule.

Developmental defects include osteochondritis dissecans, equine ataxia, lumbar disk syndrome (as found in certain breeds of dogs due to conformational defects as a result of selective breeding), extension of epiphysitis into the joint, and damage due to abnormal angulation of a joint. Bacterial and fungal infections within the joint or involving the ligaments, fibrous capsule, or tendons of insertion near the joint are generally quite evident.

Chronic inflammation of the joints and surrounding structures is most common in those joints involved in locomotion, although others such as the temporomandibular may be affected. Synovial fluid acts as a lubricant for the joint surfaces and nourishes the articular cartilage. In any joint injury, the synovial fluid is altered in volume and composition: there is an effusion of fluid, an increase in protein content, and decreased resorption. Production of enzymes that often are destructive to the articular cartilage also occurs. Focal ulceration of the articular cartilage and proliferation of the synovial membrane and bone along the joint margin results. In some instances, the process continues until the bone underlying the articular cartilage erodes, which leads to irreparable degenerative joint disease.

Many diseases of the musculoskeletal system are relatively simple to diagnose, although interrelation with other body systems, particularly the nervous system, can complicate the diagnosis. Diagnostic procedures to determine the exact cause or localize the particular joint may include visual and manual examination, radiography, local or regional anesthesia, arthroscopy, scintigraphy, thermography, ultrasonography, and other laboratory examination of the synovial membrane and synovial fluid.

ARTHRITIS AND RELATED DISORDERS, LG AN
(Degenerative joint disease, Osteochondrosis, Septic arthritis, Traumatic arthritis)

Joint inflammation is a nonspecific condition that represents a spectrum of various diseases with varied pathogeneses. While common in all large animals, arthritis is best known in horses because of the significant effect on locomotion in that species. (*See also* LAMENESS IN CATTLE, p 494; IN GOATS, p 503; IN HORSES, p 507; IN PIGS, p 532; and IN SHEEP, p 540.)

SPECIFIC TYPES OF ARTHRITIS

Traumatic synovitis and capsulitis, intra-articular chip fractures, sprains and ruptures of intra-articular ligaments, and other traumatically induced articular cartilage lesions are all forms of **traumatic arthritis**. In all these diseases, the joint capsule (synovial membrane and fibrous capsule) is inflamed, which results in hyperemia, edema, and varying levels of pain and lameness. The amount of articular cartilage damage depends on severity of the trauma.

Degenerative joint disease (osteoarthritis) is a group of disorders characterized by a common end-stage: progressive deterioration of the articular cartilage accompanied by changes in the bone and soft tissues of the joint. Ringbone and bone spavin are examples. The disease may be due to repeated trauma, or wear and tear with undue stress and faulty conformation as contributing factors or, alternatively, any other arthritic entity may lead to this permanent stage of degeneration of the articular cartilage. The degree of loss of articular cartilage as well as the degree of osteophytosis and enthesopathy varies. In cattle, the condition commonly develops secondary to injuries to the cruciate ligaments, menisci, or joint capsule.

Septic or infectious arthritis (sometimes called purulent arthritis) results from sequestration of bacterial infection in a joint. An infected joint develops in 3 main situations: 1) hematogenous infection (navel ill), common in foals, calves, and lambs; 2) traumatic injury with local introduction of infection; and 3) iatrogenic infection associated with joint aspiration, infection, or surgery (usually in horses). Septic arthritis is characterized by extreme pain and distention of the joint with cloudy, turbid synovial fluid that contains many neutrophils. The articular cartilage, subchondral bone, and synovial membrane sustain permanent damage if effective treatment is not instituted quickly. The rate of damage depends on the causative organism. In foals, primary osteomyelitis also is caused by infection with a *Salmonella* sp, commonly as a polyarthritis in a hematogenous syndrome. In young lambs, *Actinobacillus seminis* causes polyarthritis, as do *Chlamydia psittaci* and *Erysipelothrix insidiosa*. The latter follows docking, castration, or navel infection. Viruses and mycoplasma may also be etiologic agents in food-producing animals. In mature goats, the caprine arthritis and encephalitis virus (qv, p 393) is an important cause of arthritis. In young goats, *Chlamydia psittaci* and *Mycoplasma mycoides* are frequent causes.

Infectious swine arthritis is a common term for a group of bacterial (including mycoplasmal) arthritides in younger pigs. In newborn pigs, septic arthritis usually is due to intrauterine or navel infection with *Escherichia coli*, or *Corynebacterium, Streptococcus*, or *Staphylococcus* spp; control is best directed toward reducing the possibility of infection from the environment. Older pigs sometimes develop arthritis as a sequela of infection with *Haemophilus, Erysipelothrix*, or *Mycoplasma* spp; although diagnosis in the early stages is not difficult, the more chronic stages can be confused with articular lesions produced by dietary hypervitaminosis A.

Osteochondritis dissecans is an important arthritic entity in horses. It is due to the more generalized condition of osteochondrosis (qv, p 558). Osteochondrosis is also an important disease in pigs and is seen in cattle. Osteochondritis dissecans is probably the most important orthopedic disease of young horses, and the stifle, hock, fetlock, and shoulder are frequently affected.

Clinical Findings: Arthritis produces pain and altered function of the joint. If the process is active or acute, the joint capsule is usually distended, and the surrounding tissues are swollen and warm. Manipulation of the joint causes pain in more severe cases. In more subtle cases, flexion tests are required to elicit lameness in horses. In more chronic cases, the range of motion is reduced, and there is decreased flexion and fibrous thickening in the area of the joint. Radiographic evaluation is necessary for positive confirmation of a number of disease entities. Arthroscopy is used to accurately assess the amount of damage to the articular cartilage and establish a prognosis.

Treatment: Treatment of acute traumatic synovitis and capsulitis includes rest and physical therapy regimens such as cold-water treatment, ice, passive flexion, and swimming. Nonsteroidal anti-inflammatory drugs are usually used. Lavage of the joint is used for removal of inflammatory products produced by the synovial membrane, as well as articular cartilage debris that exacerbates the synovitis. Joint drainage has been recommended for relief of capsular distention but is of minimal benefit on its own. Various intra-articular medications have been used. Corticosteroids are the most potent anti-inflammatory agent and are effective in acute traumatic synovitis. However, they do have some deleterious effects on cartilage metabolism and should be used carefully. Sodium hyaluronate is effective for synovitis and capsulitis, but has minimal effect when articular cartilage damage or intra-articular fractures are present. Polysulfated glycosaminoglycan has chondroprotective properties and is indicated to prevent ongoing degeneration of articular cartilage. Direct traumatic damage to the articular cartilage or intra-articular chip fractures are best treated with arthroscopic surgery to minimize the ongoing development of degenerative joint disease. Osteochondritis dissecans lesions also are treated this way.

Septic arthritis requires prompt treatment to avoid irreparable damage. Systemic broad-spectrum antibiotics are indicated; the initial choice is based on the most likely pathogen, but is subject to change based on culture and sensitivity tests. Systemic antibiotic treatment is combined with local therapy, which variously consists of joint lavage and arthrotomy to provide drainage. Arthrotomy or arthroscopy is needed to remove fibrin deposits. Adjunctive anti-inflammatory treatment (eg, phenylbutazone) is also used.

For degenerative joint disease, treatment is largely palliative. The permanence of degenerative joint disease emphasizes the need for prompt diagnosis and correct management of traumatic synovitis and capsulitis, intra-articular fractures or cartilage damage, osteochondritis dissecans, or septic arthritis. When degenerative joint disease is advanced, surgical fusion may be performed on selected joints. While treatment is usually unsuccessful in chronic cases, eg, chronic degenerative joint disease of bulls and cows, restricted exercise and good feeding may prolong the life of and be worthwhile for valuable breeding animals. In bulls that are unable to mount, semen for artificial insemination can be collected by electroejaculation, but the humane aspects of this treatment should also be considered.

BURSITIS

An inflammatory reaction within a bursa that can range from mild inflammation to sepsis. It is more common and important in horses. It can also be classified as true or acquired. True bursitis is inflammation in a congenital or natural bursa (deeper than the deep fascia), eg, trochanteric bursitis and supraspinous bursitis (fistulous withers). Acquired bursitis is development of a subcut. bursa where one was not previously present and/or inflammation of that bursa, eg, capped elbow over the olecranon process, shoe boil over the point of the elbow, and capped hock over the tuber calcaneus.

Synovitis may manifest as an acute or chronic inflammation. Examples of acute bursitis include bicipital bursitis and trochanteric bursitis in the early stages. It is generally characterized by swelling, local heat, and pain. Chronic bursitis usually develops in association with repeated trauma, with fibrosis and other chronic changes, eg, capped elbow, capped hock, and carpal hygroma. Excess bursal fluid accumulates, and the wall of the bursa is thickened by fibrous tissue. Fibrous bands or a septum may form within the bursal cavity, and generalized subcut. thickening usually develops. These bursal enlargements develop as cold, painless swellings, and unless greatly enlarged, do not severely interfere with function. Septic bursitis is more serious, and is associated with pain and lameness. Infection of a bursa may be hematogenous or follow direct penetration.

The pain in acute bursitis may be relieved by application of cold packs, aspiration of the contents, and intrabursal medication. Repeated injections may result in infection. Treatment of chronic bursitis is surgical. Cases of infected bursitis require treatment with systemic antibiotics as well as local drainage.

CAPPED ELBOW AND HOCK

Inflammatory swelling of the subcut. bursa located over the olecranon process and tuber calcaneus, respectively, of horses. Trauma from lying on poorly bedded hard floors, kicks, falls, riding the tailgate of trailers, iron shoes projecting beyond the heels, and prolonged recumbency are frequent causes.

Circumscribed edematous swelling occurs over and around the affected bursa. Lameness is rare in either case. The affected bursa may be fluctuating and soft at first, but in a short time, a firm fibrous capsule forms, especially if there is a recurrence of an old injury. Initial bursal swellings may be hardly noticeable or quite sizable. Chronic cases may progress to abscessation.

Acute early cases may respond well to cold-water applications, followed in a few days by aseptic aspiration and injection of a corticosteroid. The bursa may also be reduced in size by application of a counterirritant or by ultrasonic or radiation therapy. Older encapsulated bursae are more refractory. Surgical treatment (usually curettage and drainage) is recommended for advanced chronic cases or those that have become infected. A shoe-boil roll should be used to prevent recurrence of a capped elbow if the condition has been caused by the heel or the shoe.

FISTULOUS WITHERS—POLL EVIL

Two inflammatory disorders of horses that differ from one another essentially only in their location in the respective supraspinous and supra-atlantal bursae. This discussion is of fistulous withers but, except for anatomic details, applies in general also to poll evil. In the early stage of the disease, a fistula is not present. When the bursal sac ruptures or when it is opened for surgical drainage, and secondary infection with pyogenic bacteria occurs, it usually assumes a true fistulous character. It is rarely seen today.

Etiology: Evidence suggests that the condition is primarily infectious in origin, and agglutination titers support the theory. *Brucella abortus*, and occasionally *B suis*, can be isolated from the fluid aspirated from the unopened bursa, and outbreaks of brucellosis in cattle have followed contact with horses with open bursitis. A *Brucella* titer should always be evaluated in these cases, and if significant, the owners should be made aware of the public health significance.

Clinical Findings: The inflammation leads to considerable thickening of the wall of the bursa. The bursal sacs are distended and may rupture when the sac has little covering support. In more chronic, advanced cases, the ligament and the dorsal vertebral spines are affected, and occasionally these structures necrose.

In the early stage, the supraspinous bursa distends with a clear, straw-colored, viscid exudate. The swelling may be dorsal, unilateral, or bilateral, depending on the arrangement of the bursal sacs between the tissue layers. It is an exudative process from the beginning, but no true suppuration or secondary infection occurs until the bursa ruptures or is opened.

Treatment and Prevention: The earlier treatment is instituted, the better the prognosis. The most successful treatment is complete dissection and removal of the infected bursa. The expense of the protracted treatment required in chronic cases often exceeds the value of the animal. *Brucella* vaccines have not proved helpful. Sodium iodide therapy is of very limited value. It is reasonable to keep horses separate from *Brucella*-infected cattle, and horses with discharging fistulous withers from cattle.

CHLAMYDIAL POLYARTHRITIS-SEROSITIS
(Transmissible serositis)

An infectious disease affecting sheep, calves, goats, and pigs. Chlamydial polyarthritis of sheep was first described in Wisconsin, and has since been recognized in western USA, Australia, and New Zealand. The disease was identified in calves from the USA, Australia, and Austria; and in pigs from Austria, Bulgaria, and the USA.

Etiology and Epidemiology: Strains of the causal agent, *Chlamydia psittaci*, isolated from affected joints of sheep and calves are identical, but strain-specific antigens in their cell walls distinguish them from those that cause abortions in sheep and cattle (qv, p 651).

The GI tract is of prime importance in the pathogenesis of chlamydial polyarthritis. The disease has been reproduced experimentally by oral inoculation. Since chlamydiae can be recovered from the feces of clinically normal calves and lambs, it is most likely the GI tract wherein the host and parasite stay frequently in balance. If there is a shift in favor of the chlamydiae, then a systemic infection and chlamydemia ensues; the ultimate site of replication is the synovial membrane. The GI tract also has been infected after experimental intra-articular inoculations. Chlamydiae are excreted in the feces and urine, and transmitted via ingestion or, in some cases, inhalation.

Clinical Findings: Chlamydial polyarthritis is observed in lambs on range, on farms, and in feedlots. Morbidity may be 5-75%. Rectal temperatures are 102-107°F (39-41.5°C). Varying degrees of stiffness, lameness, anorexia, and a concurrent conjunctivitis (qv, p 294) may occur. Affected sheep are depressed, reluctant to move, and often hesitate to stand and bear weight on one or more limbs, but they may "warm out" of stiffness and lameness following forced exercise. The highest incidence of the disease in sheep on range occurs between late summer and early winter.

The disease affects cattle of all ages but 4- to 30-day-old calves are affected more severely. Calves may have fever, are moderately alert, and usually nurse if carried to the dam and supported while sucking. They invariably also have diarrhea, which can be severe. Affected calves assume a hunched position while standing; their joints usually are swollen, and palpation causes pain. Navel involvement and nervous signs are not observed.

Chlamydial polyarthritis has been recognized in older pigs as well as in young piglets. The affected piglets become febrile and anorectic, and may develop nasal catarrh, difficulties in breathing, and conjunctivitis. This condition has not been clearly differentiated from other infections that lead to polyserositis and arthritis in pigs.

Lesions: The most striking tissue changes are in the joints. In lambs, enlargement of the joints is not often noticed, but in chronic advanced cases, the stifle, hock, and elbow may be slightly enlarged. In calves, periarticular subcut. edema along tendon sheaths, and fluid-filled, fluctuating synovial sacs contribute to enlargement of the joints. Most affected joints of lambs or calves contain excessive, grayish yellow, turbid synovial fluid. Fibrin flakes and plaques in the recesses of the affected joints may adhere firmly to the synovial membranes. Joint capsules are thickened. Articular cartilage is smooth, and erosions or evidence of marginal compensatory changes is not present. Tendon sheaths of severely affected lambs and calves may be distended and contain creamy, grayish yellow exudate. Surrounding muscles are hyperemic and edematous, with petechiae in their associated fascial planes.

Diagnosis: The history and careful examination of the pathological changes in the joints and other organs can be of diagnostic value. Cytological examination of synovial fluids or tissues may reveal chlamydial elementary bodies or cytoplasmic inclusions. Isolation and identification of the causative agent from affected joints confirms the diagnosis. Bacteriological cultures of affected joints are usually negative, but *Escherichia coli* or streptococci occasionally may be isolated. If the joints of young calves are arthritic, and navel lesions are absent, chlamydial polyarthritis should be considered.

Clinical and pathological features distinguish chlamydial polyarthritis from most other conditions that cause stiffness and lameness in lambs. Lambs with mineral deficiency or osteomalacia usually are not febrile. The abnormal osteogenesis in these 2 conditions and the distinct lesions of white muscle disease are virtually pathognomonic. In arthritis caused by *Erysipelothrix rhusiopathiae*, there are deposits on and pitting of articular surfaces, periarticular fibrosis, and osteophyte formation. Laminitis due to bluetongue virus infection can be differentiated clinically and etiologically. Detailed microbiological investigations are required to differentiate chlamydial arthritis from mycoplasmal arthritis.

Treatment and Prevention: If begun early, therapy with long-acting penicillin, tetracyclines, or tylosin appears to be beneficial. More advanced lesions do not respond satisfactorily. Daily feeding of 150-200 mg of chlortetracycline to affected lambs in feedlots reduces the incidence of chlamydial polyarthritis. No approved vaccines are available.

TENDINITIS
(Bowed tendon)

Acute or chronic inflammation of a tendon with varying degrees of tendon fibril disruption. Tendinitis is most common in horses used at fast work, particularly racehorses. The problem occurs in the flexor tendons and is more common in the forelimb than the hindlimb. In racehorses, the superficial flexor is involved most frequently. The primary lesion is a rupture of tendon fibers with associated hemorrhage and edema.

Etiology: Tendinitis usually appears following fast exercise, and is associated with overextension and poor conditioning, fatigue, poor racetrack conditions, and persistent training when inflammatory problems in the tendon are already present. Improper shoeing may also predispose to tendonitis. Poor conformation and poor training also have been implicated.

Clinical Findings: During the acute stage, the horse is severely lame and the structures involved are hot, painful, and swollen. In chronic cases, there is fibrosis with thickening and adhesions in the peritendinous area. The horse with chronic tendinitis may go sound while walking or trotting but suffer recurrence under hard work. Ultrasonography has vastly improved definition of the problem and delineates many defects and injuries that are undetectable, or at least ill-defined, by palpation.

Treatment: Tendinitis is best treated in the early, acute stage. The horse should be stall-rested, and the swelling and inflammation treated aggressively with cold packs and systemic anti-inflammatory agents. Some degree of support or immobilization should be used, depending on the amount of damage to the tendon. Intratendinous corticosteroid injections are contraindicated. The horse should be brought back slowly into an exercise regimen to try to reduce the amount of adhesion formation. Superior check ligament desmotomy has been used more recently as an adjunctive treatment to minimize recurrence of the problem when the horse is put back into training.

Other treatments for chronic tendonitis have included superficial point firing (benefits of this are questionable), percutaneous tendon splitting, and carbon fiber implantation. Localized opening of the tendon, based on ultrasonographic identification of a hypoechoic area, has also been used, the rationale for which is to decrease intratendinous pressure due to serum or hemorrhage. The prognosis for a racehorse to return to racing following a bowed tendon is guarded, regardless of treatment. Annular ligament desmotomy is also used when tendonitis involves this area.

TENOSYNOVITIS

Inflammation of the synovial membrane and usually the fibrous layer of the tendon sheath. The condition is characterized by distention of the tendon sheath due to synovial effusion, and has different causes and clinical manifestations. The various types of tenosynovitis include idiopathic, acute, chronic, and septic (infectious).

Idiopathic synovitis refers to synovial distention of tendon sheaths in young animals, in which the cause is uncertain. Acute and chronic tenosynovitis are due to trauma. Septic tenosynovitis may be associated with penetrating wounds, local extension of infection, or a hematogenous infection.

There are varying degrees of synovial distention of the tendon sheath and lameness, depending on the severity. Horses are markedly lame in septic tenosynovitis. Chronic tenosynovitis is common in horses in the tarsal sheath of the hock (thoroughpin) and the digital sheath (tendinous windpuffs). These 2 entities must be differentiated from bog spavin and synovial effusion of the fetlock.

Acute cases may be treated symptomatically with cold packs, nonsteroidal anti-inflammatory drugs, and rest. Application of counterirritants and bandaging has been used in more chronic cases. Radiation therapy is helpful. Septic tenosynovitis requires systemic antibiotics and drainage. If adhesions develop between the tendon sheath and the tendon, persistent effusion and lameness is the rule.

ARTHRITIS AND RELATED DISORDERS, SM AN

See also LYME DISEASE, p 359, and LAMENESS IN SM AN, p 545.

BURSITIS

The bursae over joints may become inflamed, especially in larger breeds of dogs. Bursal cavities are connective tissue sacs lined with synovial membrane located between tendons and bone. Inflammation frequently resolves with rest, application of crushed ice compresses, or aspiration of fluid. The site should be protected from further injury. It is necessary to ascertain if the fluid of the inflamed bursa is sterile before administering corticosteroids. If septic, antibiotics can be injected directly into the bursa.

HIP DYSPLASIA (HD)

A developmental disease of dogs in which joint instability due to disconformity of the head of the femur and the acetabulum allows excessive movement of the femoral head.

Etiology: The cause is unknown. HD is common in large breeds, but also occurs in smaller ones. Males and females are affected with equal frequency. The pattern of inheritance suggests that it is polygenic. HD is a complex disease also influenced by environmental stresses, which results in abnormal articular modelling, the end point of which is secondary osteoarthritis (OA). Development does not depend on the degree of inclination of the femoral head with reference to the shaft of the femur, or the degree of femoral head rotation about the femur. However, abnormalities in these angles often coexist with HD and may play a role in progression of clinical signs. Parents with "normal" hips may have dysplastic offspring. However, sound dogs are more likely to be born to parents with normal hips. Breeding dogs for desirable traits, eg, good temperament or large size, may result in selection of animals that are susceptible to HD. Many offspring of dogs with HD also become dysplastic.

Clinical Findings: Decreased activity and evidence of joint pain are often observed between 4 mo and 1 yr of age. Young dogs have a swaying and unsteady gait; the hindlegs are drawn forward with the hocks displaced laterally, placing more weight on the forelimbs and attempting to force the femoral heads into the acetabula. Dogs often run with both hindlegs moving together (bunny hopping) and have difficulty rising from a sitting or lying position. Stairs are difficult to climb, and the dog may whimper or snap when the affected joint is manipulated. The disease is progressive and often crippling, but some dogs experience little discomfort despite abnormal changes in their joints. Intense activity can aggravate the condition and reveal signs of disease in an animal previously thought to be unaffected.

The hip joint becomes damaged, inflamed, and weakened, which ultimately results in severe secondary OA. The amount of synovial fluid is increased, and the round ligament becomes swollen, stretched, and eventually ruptures. The normally smooth articular cartilage covering the ends of the opposing bones is abraded, and the joint capsule becomes chronically inflamed and thickened. Muscles of the hip joint are weakened and atrophy.

Diagnosis: This can be established by radiography under general anesthesia or deep sedation. The animal is placed on its back, with both hindlegs fully extended and the stifles rotated inward. In the "normal" joint, the head of the femur conforms to the acetabulum; in the dysplastic joint, more space is evident between the bones. Displacement of the femoral head is the hallmark of the disease. In most dogs, if a radiograph reveals that the dorsal region of the acetabulum shadows <50% of the femoral head, the joint is subluxated. If the center of the femoral head is directly below the acetabular rim, the severity of HD is "moderate"; if displaced further, it is "severe". Femoral head displacement (ie, joint laxity) also can be revealed by taking a pelvic radiograph with a solid object between the femurs and squeezing the stifles medially; femurs should be perpendicular to the table. Often, the acetabulum appears shallow and osteophytes are evident. Characteristic changes may not be detected until animals are 2 yr old.

Treatment and Prevention: Walking, swimming, or slow running is beneficial, but jumping and prolonged running should be avoided. Buffered aspirin can relieve the pain, but aspirin and other medications do not arrest the destructive changes in the joint. Nutritional supplements have not been proved to be beneficial. Surgical procedures have been devised to treat dogs with pain and lameness; however, normal joint function is not fully restored.

Occurrence of HD can be reduced by selecting (radiographically) for breeding only those animals that have disease-free hips. A better method is to select breeding dogs based on family performance and progeny testing.

Development of HD is delayed and its severity diminished when the growth rate of puppies is restricted. The reverse is also true, ie, dysplasia can be accelerated by increasing the rate of growth during the first 4 mo of life. Dogs carrying the undesired genes can be identified by this procedure. The strategy is to "force" expression of HD in dogs being considered as breeding stock through diet and possibly other management practices. The procedure also can reveal the potential for disease in apparently healthy parents. By excluding dysplastic and potentially dysplastic animals from the breeding population, the frequency of dysplasia-free offspring should be increased.

IMMUNE-MEDIATED ARTHROPATHIES

In dogs, there are 2 types of systemic immune-mediated arthropathies, both of which are inflammatory, purulent, and noninfectious. In rheumatoid arthritis (RA)—erosive type—there is destruction of the articular cartilage and, in severe cases, even the subchondral bone. In systemic lupus erythematosus (SLE)—nonerosive type—destruction of the articular cartilage is not a main feature. The initiating cause is unknown for either type. SLE affects principally medium and large breeds, while RA is more common in small and toy breeds. Comparison of clinical pathological tests and radiological findings help differentiate the 2 conditions. There are no known cures; the best that can be done for these lifelong diseases is to keep them in remission with a combination of therapies, exercise, diet, and weight control.

OSTEOARTHRITIS
(OA, Degenerative joint disease)

OA is a common joint disease that, depending on its etiology, can afflict animals of all ages. It can be classified as primary, being synonymous with the "wear and tear" arthritis of old age; or secondary, implying that the OA is secondary to an infectious agent (septic arthritis), a mobile intra-articular bone piece, an ununited anconeal process, a malaligned fracture, or a developmental disease such as hip dysplasia. OA is distinct from rheumatoid arthritis (RA), which is a chronic, systemic, inflammatory disease that results in progressive destruction of the synovial joints. In OA, the articular cartilage is affected initially. The usual smooth, glistening, resilient hyaline cartilage begins to crack and fibrillate.

The lesion is usually chondromalacic due to chondrocytic necrosis and release of the degradative enzymes of the cell, which results in matrical destruction. The product released stimulates the synovial membrane, resulting in a synovitis that assists in enhanced degradation of the articular cartilage and causes a dull, constant joint pain. Due to the pain, the joint is protected, the surrounding muscles atrophy, the joint capsule thickens, and effusion can occur initially. With loss of the articular cartilage, the bony components of the joint articulate on each other (eburnation), and peripheral shelves of bone (osteophytes) result from the abnormal locomotor pattern of the articulation. OA can affect one or many joints; in quadrupeds, the weight-bearing joints (eg, hip, stifle, shoulder, and elbow) are involved most frequently.

Clinical Findings and Diagnosis: Affected animals are reluctant to jump, perform tricks, walk, run, or hunt; they bear less weight on the affected limb. They may limp, appear stiff, have difficulty rising from a lying or sitting position, and whine or snap when the affected joint is manipulated. Pain is worsened by cold or a sudden change in weather and by heavy exercise.

Evidence of OA includes joint capsule thickening, mineral deposits in soft tissues surrounding the joint, osteophytes at the edge of the joint, narrowing of the joint space (due to loss of articular cartilage), and changes in the thickness and density of the bones. Synovial fluid from disease-free joints contains only a small amount of clear, viscous fluid; discoloration of the fluid, or an increase in tissue cells or WBC are indicative of disease. Confirmation should include radiographic examination.

Treatment: Walking and swimming keep muscles and joint capsules limber, and promote lubrication and nutrition of the articular cartilage of the joints. Rest and weight loss (if obese) are important. Excessive use of a diseased joint aggravates pain and causes further damage. Anti-inflammatory drugs (eg, buffered aspirin) relieve the pain; corticosteroids can be used sparingly in advanced cases and only after a definitive diagnosis has been made. However, when pain is relieved, the animal becomes more active, and the condition may be aggravated. Medications make arthritic dogs more comfortable, but do not arrest the degenerative process. Vitamins and dietary supplements neither arrest the process nor restore joint function. Affected dogs should be kept warm and dry. Pain of a recent injury can be eased by local application of crushed ice compresses. When OA is secondary to osteochondritis dissecans of the shoulder and hock, patellar displacement, or elbow dysplasias, surgical correction of the primary condition is effective, but the OA continues to progress. When pain cannot be controlled by medication, the last resort is surgical implantation of an endoprosthesis.

SPONDYLOSIS DEFORMANS

Degenerative osteoarthritis of the spine, particularly of the lumbar area, characterized by development of osteophytes at the ends and near the ventral border of the vertebrae. A similar condition affects the lumbosacral region. A degenerative arthropathy of the articular processes accompanies the pathological lesions of the anterior column. The disease usually occurs as a chronic, progressive disease of older dogs, particularly in larger breeds. Degenerative change in the annulus fibrosus is one of the known causes; the nucleus pulposus plays a lesser role in the pathogenesis. Most affected dogs exhibit no clinical signs unless the osteophytes exert pressure on nerve roots (after which pain becomes evident and affected dogs are reluctant to move normally).

Radiographically, the osteophytes have sloping, smooth ventral or lateral surfaces that blend with the cortex of the vertebral body. The disk spaces may be of normal width. One or several pairs of vertebral bodies may be involved. Treatment is indicated only to allay pain. Aspirin alone or in conjunction with steroids is beneficial (*see also* pp 585 and 1399).

SUPPURATIVE ARTHRITIS
(Septic arthritis)

Usually caused by the introduction of infection into a joint by trauma; the affected joint is swollen, hot, and painful, and body temperature is elevated. Lameness is marked. Examination may disclose a wound leading into the joint, or a mucoid discharge from the joint composed of pus and synovial fluid. Suppuration in the joint cavity may have a lytic effect on the articular cartilage, followed by subchondral bone destruction.

If aspiration of the synovial fluid is unsuccessful, surgical drainage of the joint may be necessary. The fluid should be cultured and antibiotic sensitivity determined. Appropriate antibiotics should be used locally and systemically for several weeks. Intrasynovial injection of antibiotics often aids in shortening the acute inflammatory phase.

CONGENITAL AND INHERITED ANOMALIES OF THE MUSCULOSKELETAL SYSTEM

The inability of an animal to walk normally often is evident at birth. Some of these abnormalities are inherited; others result from ingestion of toxic plants or other toxic agents by the dam during early pregnancy, or from viral infections that invade the fetus. *See also* PATELLAR LUXATION, p 560. Conditions affecting the nervous system also may impair gait (eg, *see* DEFECTS OF CEREBELLUM AND BRAIN STEM, p 578).

ANGULAR LIMB DEFORMITIES OF FOALS
(Carpal or tarsal valgus, Knock-knees)

Congenital or acquired skeletal defects that allow the distal portion of a limb to deviate laterally (or medially) in early neonatal life. *In utero* malposition, hypothyroidism, trauma, poor conformation, excessive joint laxity, and defective endochondral ossification of the carpal or tarsal and long bones have been implicated. Both fore- and hindlimbs may be affected, often concurrently.

Clinical Findings: The carpus is affected most frequently, but the tarsus and fetlocks are occasionally involved. The deviation is obvious, but varies in severity. A lateral deviation (valgus) of up to 4° of the distal portion of a limb may be regarded as normal, yet may be the basis for an owner's complaint. Most foals are asymptomatic, but lameness and soft-tissue swelling can accompany severe deviation. Outward rotation at the fetlocks invariably accompanies carpal valgus. Foals in which there is defective ossification of the carpal cuboidal bones or excessive joint laxity frequently are painfully lame, and the legs become progressively deviated. Affected limbs must be palpated carefully to detect ligamentous laxity and specific areas that may be painful.

Diagnosis must include a precise determination of the site (level) and the cause for the deviation. The distal radial metaphysis, physis, or epiphysis, or the cuboidal bones may be the site of deviation. Radiography is indispensable. Films should include lengths of radius and metacarpus (or tibia and metatarsus) to augment tracings and measurement of the angle of deviation. Straight lines drawn through the longitudinal axes of the radius and cannon intersect at the site of deviation, aiding diagnosis and the selection of treatment. Physeal flaring, epiphyseal wedging, and deformation of carpal bones are frequent findings in addition to the deviation. Mild cases frequently improve spontaneously without treatment. Sequential examinations and radiographs, days or weeks apart, are necessary to follow spontaneous improvement or to establish a need for surgery.

Without treatment, the prognosis for carpal valgus is poor. The conformational anomaly leads to early degenerative joint disease. Likewise, deformity of the cuboidal carpal bones contributes to a poor prognosis. However, with early detection, careful evaluation, and proper surgical treatment, most cases respond favorably.

Treatment: Surgery is the primary treatment. Excessive joint laxity, with or without cuboidal carpal bone involvement, requires tube casts or padded gutter splints and carefully monitored exercise. To aid development of tendon and ligament tone, the fetlock and phalangeal region should be unrestricted by the casts. The casts protect the lax joint from trauma while allowing exercise to improve tissue tone. Such limb support may be required for up to 6 wk.

Physeal and epiphyseal defects are also amenable to surgical improvement. The success of these surgeries depends on continued growth and development of the bones, and they must be performed before physeal growth plates close, preferably as early as 2-4 mo of age.

ARACHNOMELIA AND ARTHROGRYPOSIS

A syndrome (SAA) that occurs in Brown Swiss calves, with the major lesions in the musculoskeletal system. Most calves with SAA are dead at birth or die within hours. The limbs appear slender and long and are curved. The muscles are atrophic. Carpal, hock, and fetlock joints usually have contractures. Additional malformations are brachygnathia, a short skull, kyphoscoliosis, and aneurysms of vessels. The defect is inherited as a simple autosomal recessive.

CONGENITAL MYOPATHIES

ASYMMETRICAL HINDQUARTER SYNDROME OF PIGS

A disorder, described in several European countries, that becomes apparent when pigs reach ~60 lb (30 kg) live wt, and is manifest by atrophy of either the right or left posterior thigh muscles. Some evidence suggests a complex inheritance for the disease.

BROWN ATROPHY
(Xanthosis, Lipofuscinosis)

The skeletal muscles and myocardium are yellow-brown to bronze in dairy cattle with this condition. The masseter muscles and the diaphragm are affected most frequently. No clinical disease is produced. Microscopically, brown pigment granules accumulate under the sarcolemma, or centrally in the muscle fibers. There is presumption of genetic cause, since certain breeds (eg, Ayrshire) are more predisposed than others.

DOUBLE MUSCLING IN CATTLE
(Myofibrillar hyperplasia, Doppellendigkëit, Muscular hypertrophy)

A disorder described in many cattle breeds and that also may affect lambs. An autosomal recessive mode of inheritance is involved in cattle. Affected calves have bulging muscles and only small amounts of subcut. fat. Microscopically, increased numbers of small muscle fibers with tapered ends and hypertrophied type II fibers are present. Affected calves may cause dystocia. Attempts to exploit this condition in the production of meatier carcasses generally have been unsuccessful because of inferior meat quality, reproductive efficiency, and skeletal structure.

MUSCULAR STEATOSIS

A condition in which fat replaces muscle fibers, observed occasionally in cattle and pigs at slaughter; no clinical disease is produced, and the cause is unknown. The gross lesions are symmetrical pale areas in affected muscles, especially of the back, neck, and upper limbs. Microscopically, many muscle fibers are replaced by fat cells.

MYOPATHY ASSOCIATED WITH CONGENITAL ARTICULAR RIGIDITY
(CAR, Arthrogryposis)

This syndrome, one of the more common congenital defects of calves, is characterized by rigid fixation of the limbs in abnormal postures, and often produces dystocia. Affected animals may have other anomalies including hydrocephalus, palatoschisis, and spinal dysraphism. The condition may be lethal, but some mildly affected animals recover completely. The muscle lesions may be primary in some types of the disease, but generally, neural lesions are primary and the muscular alterations represent denervation atrophy. CAR occurs in cattle, sheep, horses, and pigs. Numerous etiological factors have been recognized; these include viral (Akabane virus [qv, p 333]) and plant (*Lupinus* sp [qv, p 1689]) teratogens and a heritable recessive trait in cattle (*see* below). In sheep, plant (locoweed) and viral (Akabane, Wesselsbron [qv, p 408], and Rift Valley fever [qv, p 403]) teratogens, parbendazole exposure, and inherited autosomal recessive primary myopathies of Merino and Welsh Mountain lambs may cause CAR. In pigs, CAR may be inherited as an autosomal recessive, or result from vitamin A or manganese deficiency, or exposure of pregnant sows to plant toxins (tobacco, thorn apple, hemlock, and black cherry).

MYOPATHY ASSOCIATED WITH CONGENITAL HYDROCEPHALUS

Inherited in Hereford cattle as an autosomal recessive, affected calves may be blind and are unable to stand. The skeletal muscles are pale and soft and have various microscopic changes. Although details are unclear, the muscle lesions probably are secondary to the underlying neurological lesions.

SPLAYLEGS IN PIGLETS
(Spraddled legs, Myofibrillar hypoplasia)

A condition of neonates in which the hindlegs are spread apart or extended forward. Appropriately treated pigs usually recover within a few days, although few recover if the front legs are also affected. The immediate cause is weakness of the adductor muscles relative to the abductors. Affected pigs are susceptible to overlaying, starvation, and chilling because of poor mobility.

Etiology: Genetic influence has been demonstrated. There are significant differences in the incidence among the litters of different sires and breeds. It occurs more frequently in males than females and in lower-birthweight pigs. The incidence may be increased if glucocorticoids are administered during pregnancy, and it appears possible that stress-sensitivity of the heavily muscled parent(s) may be a contributing factor. However, any cause of stretching of the adductor muscles increases the incidence. Stretching can result from slippery floors, struggling while legs are caught in cracks in the floor, and as the result of damage to nerve pathways from intrauterine viral infections. Mycotoxins have been implicated in some cases. The general nutrition of the sow (choline, methionine, and vitamin E levels) may influence the incidence.

Diagnosis: The clinical signs are distinctive. *In utero* infections with hemagglutinating encephalitis virus, enteroviruses, other viruses, and postpartum bacterial meningeal infection and trauma should be considered. The affected muscles are generally hypoplastic, and the small muscle fibers contain few myofibrils, as would be found in muscles of normal fetuses nearing parturition.

Prophylaxis and Treatment: Dry, nonslippery floors should be provided, with no cracks in which the legs can become trapped, especially for the first 2 days. Pigs should be protected from injury by the sow, and adequate suckling should be ensured. In affected piglets, the hindlegs should be secured together above the hocks with a loose "figure 8" of adhesive tape for 2-4 days. Nutritional deficiencies in the sow ration should be corrected. Glucocorticoids should not be administered late in gestation. Highly susceptible blood lines should be eliminated.

CONTRACTED FLEXOR TENDONS

Probably the most prevalent abnormality of the locomotor system of newborn calves of almost all breeds, this is caused by an autosomal recessive gene; position *in utero* may affect degree of disability. Newborn foals also may be affected (qv, p 530).

At birth, the pastern and fetlocks of the forelegs, and sometimes the carpal joints, are flexed to varying degrees due to shortening of the deep and superficial digital flexors and associated muscles. A cleft palate may accompany this condition in some breeds. Slightly affected animals bear weight on the soles of the feet and walk on their toes. More severely affected animals walk on the dorsal surface of the pastern and fetlock joints; if not treated, the dorsal surfaces of these joints become damaged and suppurative arthritis develops.

Signs are very suggestive, but this condition must be differentiated from arthrogryposis (qv, p 477).

Mild cases recover without treatment. In moderate cases, a splint should be applied to force the animal to bear weight on its toes; however, the pressure of the splint must not compromise the circulation, or the foot may undergo ischemic necrosis. Frequent manual extension of the joints, attempting to stretch the ligaments, tendons, and muscles, aids in treating these intermediate cases. Severe cases require tenotomy of one or both flexor tendons. A plaster-of-Paris cast may also be indicated in some cases. Extreme cases may not respond to any treatment.

DEFECTS OF THE SPINE OF FOALS
(Swayback, Roachback)

Defects of the spine are uncommon in foals, but of these, congenital scoliosis is encountered most frequently and is present at birth. On clinical examination, it is often difficult to assess its severity, and a better appreciation can be obtained by radiographic examination. In mild cases, improvement is spontaneous and may be complete. Even in the more severe cases, there is rarely any obvious abnormality in gait or maneuverability. However, these foals frequently are not raised since they appear unlikely to be able to withstand being ridden or worked.

Another occasional congenital deformity is that of synostosis (fusion of vertebrae), which may be associated with a secondary scoliosis. Radiography is necessary for confirmation.

The condition of congenital lordosis (swayback) is associated with hypoplasia of the intervertebral articular processes. In adult horses, degrees of acquired lordosis and kyphosis (roachback) are occasionally seen, which contribute to back weakness. Diagnosis is based on the clinical appearance and can be confirmed by radiography, which reveals an undue curvature of the vertebral column, usually in the cranial thoracic region (T_{5-10}) in lordosis, and in the cranial lumbar region (L_{1-3}) in kyphosis.

DYSCHONDROPLASIA

Bovine: Dyschondroplasia of genetic origin occurs in most breeds of cattle. The forms range from the so-called Dexter "Bulldog" lethal, which is invariably stillborn, to those animals that are so mildly affected that diagnosis by visual inspection alone is unreliable.

The **brachycephalic dwarfs** that were common in Hereford cattle in the 1950's largely have been eliminated through genetic selection. They are characterized by short faces, bulging foreheads, prognathism, large abdomens, and short legs. They are approximately half normal size. The **dolichocephalic dwarf**, most commonly seen in Angus cattle, is of the same general body conformation as the brachycephalic dwarf, except that it has a long head and does not have either a bulging forehead or prognathism. The short-faced calves are frequently referred to as "snorter" dwarfs because of their labored, audible breathing. Both types are of low viability, and susceptible to bloat. Their carcasses are undesirable, and they are rarely saved except for research purposes.

Various mating studies indicate that brachycephalic and dolichocephalic dwarfs, and various types of "compressed" animals are all part of the same genetic complex that also may include the Dexter lethal. Analogous "dwarf types" also occur in other breeds. Few of these animals are now being used in breeding. Originally, it was believed that a single, autosomal recessive gene, with complete penetrance, would account for the brachycephalic dwarfs, and this still appears to be the case when matings are confined to compacts. However, when matings are confined to nondyschondroplastic carriers, the ratio of nondwarfs to dwarfs is ~15:1, thereby implicating recessive genes at 2 loci. However, there is no single genetic hypothesis that accounts for all the various dyschondroplastic types.

Canine: Dyschondroplasias of the appendicular and axial skeletons occur in dogs. The former is reported in Poodles and Scottish Terriers; the latter in Alaskan Malamutes, Basset Hounds, Dachshunds, Poodles, and Scottish Terriers. In some breeds (Bassets, Dachshunds, Pekingese), the appendicular dyschondroplastic characters are an important feature of breed type. In Malamutes, the condition is accompanied by anemia.

FEMORAL NERVE PARALYSIS

Unilateral hindlimb lameness that follows a difficult birth. The condition, identified in many breeds of cattle, is most often found in the offspring of first-calf heifers. The cause is overstretching of the femoral nerve with contusion and partial or total rupture. Affected calves are large or delivered through a small pelvis in anterior presentation with a "hip-lock" or "stifle-lock" dystocia. Occasionally, affected calves are born without assistance, but usually much traction is required for delivery.

The affected limb is unable to support weight, and spontaneous or induced patellar luxation, flexion of the hock and stifle when walking, diminished tone and atrophy of the quadriceps femoris, and hypometria are evident. Other findings compatible with severe dystocia and forced traction, such as fractured bones and contusions, also may be present. A history of forced traction, a large calf, a partially or completely paralyzed hindlimb, and muscle atrophy after several days are usually adequate to make a diagnosis.

There is no satisfactory treatment for severely affected calves, but those affected only slightly often recover after several weeks or months.

LIMBER LEG

A hereditary condition of Jersey cattle, apparently controlled by a simple recessive gene. Some affected calves are born dead. Living calves appear normal at birth, but are unable to stand; they may struggle to stand, but cannot because of incompletely formed muscles, ligaments, tendons, and joints. The shoulder and hip joints can be rotated in any direction without apparent discomfort. Diagnosis is based on signs, necropsy findings, and identification of carrier animals.

There is no treatment, but the sire and dam of every affected animal should be reported to the breed association and semen supplier so that carrier animals can be identified.

OSTEOGENESIS IMPERFECTA

A generalized, inherited bone defect in cattle, dogs, and cats, characterized by extreme fragility of bones and joint laxity. The long bones are slender and have thin cortices. Calluses and recent fractures may be present. The sclera of the eyes may be bluish.

OSTEOPETROSIS

A rare disease that appears to be inherited as a simple autosomal recessive in Angus and Hereford cattle, and is also seen in dogs, foals, and Simmental calves. On the average, affected Angus calves are aborted dead at 263 days of gestation. Affected calves have a short lower jaw that is nearly immobile. The molar teeth are impacted. The long bones are fragile. There is no differential density between cortical areas and bone marrow areas of long bones. Diagnosis is confirmed by longitudinal bisection of long bones. There are no bone marrow cavities; the diaphyses of the long bones are filled with a plug of bone. Thus, osteopetrosis is characterized by solid bone that is not resorbed or remodeled.

POLYDACTYLY

A genetic defect of cattle, sheep, pigs, and occasionally horses. In its most common and genetic form, it affects both forefeet symmetrically. The second digit is developed, but the medial dewclaws are missing. Toes may be fused to give rise to polysyndactyly. Sometimes only one leg is involved; still less common is occurrence of polydactyly on all 4. Polydactyly in cattle appears to be polygenic with a dominant gene at one locus and a homozygous recessive at another.

SYNDACTYLY
(Mule foot)

The partial or complete fusion of digits of one or more feet. Reported in numerous cattle breeds, it is most prevalent in Holsteins. It is inherited as a simple autosomal recessive. The forefeet are affected most often, but one or all 4 feet may be completely or partially syndactylous. Affected animals walk slowly with a high-stepping gait, and with difficulty if all 4 feet are affected. Syndactyly may be associated with susceptibility to hyperthermia.

There is no treatment. The sire and dam of affected animals should be reported to the breed association and semen suppliers so that carrier animals can be identified.

DYSTROPHIES ASSOCIATED WITH CALCIUM, PHOSPHORUS, AND VITAMIN D·

The principal causes of osteodystrophies are deficiencies or imbalances of dietary calcium (Ca), phosphorus (P), and vitamin D. Their interrelationships are not easily defined, and deficiencies of any of the 3 may be absolute or relative. Deficiencies must be assessed in relation to availability and growth rate.

In all species, an absolute or relative deficiency of Ca causes hyperparathyroidism (qv, p 483) and development of osteoporosis or fibrous osteodystrophy, or both. Calcium deficiency does not cause rickets or osteomalacia in mammals. Absolute deficiency is less common than relative deficiency conditioned by excess P.

Phosphorus deficiency causes rickets or osteoporosis in growing animals and osteomalacia or osteoporosis in adults. It occurs mainly in grazing ruminants, rarely in animals consuming grain or meat. Poor appetite and growth rate, pica, and abnormalities of gait occur. Decreased milk yield, infertility and, occasionally, anemia (*see* POSTPARTURIENT HEMOGLOBINURIA, p 455) are seen in cows.

Vitamin D deficiency is the classic cause of rickets (growing animals) and osteomalacia (adults). It usually results from insufficient exposure of animals or their feed to sunlight. It is influenced by deficiencies or imbalances of Ca and P; high levels of carotene in green feed also may produce signs of vitamin D deficiency.

Hypervitaminosis D may be iatrogenic or result from accidental dietary supplementation, or ingestion of rat poison. Single, massive overdosage causes hemorrhagic gastritis and interstitial pneumonia. Persistent moderate overdosage results in hypercalcemia, wasting, and mineralization of soft tissues, especially kidney, stomach, lung, and blood vessels. Histologically, accumulation of basophilic osteoid on bone surfaces is characteristic. Pseudohyperparathyroidism occurs in some dogs with nonparathyroid neoplasms, particularly anal sac adenocarcinoma and lymphosarcoma, and also results in severe hypercalcemia (*see also* HUMORAL HYPERCALCEMIA OF MALIGNANCY, p 285). Renal, less often gastric and endocardial, mineralization occurs. Animals grazing plants with vitamin D activity also may show signs of hypercalcemia and soft-tissue mineralization (*see* ENZOOTIC CALCINOSIS, p 488).

More than one disease due to deficiencies and imbalances of Ca, P, and vitamin D may coincide in an animal or group of animals, and descriptions of such cases as pure deficiencies have confused interpretation of naturally occurring osteodystrophies. Diagnosis of these osteodystrophies is based on histological criteria. Bone ash analyses generally can differentiate between the various diseases. Often, P deficiency is accompanied by hypophosphatemia, vitamin D deficiency by hypocalcemia, and Ca deficiency by normocalcemia. (*See also* DEGENERATIVE ARTHROPATHY OF CATTLE, p 496.)

PRIMARY HYPERPARATHYROIDISM

Excess production of parathyroid hormone (PTH) by an autonomous functional lesion in the parathyroid gland. This disease is encountered infrequently in older dogs, and it does not appear to be a sequela of chronic secondary hyperparathyroidism (*see* below). In primary hyperparathyroidism, the normal control mechanisms for PTH secretion by the concentration of blood calcium (Ca) are lost, and the parathyroid produces excess PTH despite increased levels of blood Ca.

PTH acts on cells of the renal tubules initially to promote the excretion of phosphorus (P) and retention of Ca. A prolonged increased secretion of PTH results in accelerated osteocytic and osteoclastic bone resorption. Mineral is removed from the skeleton and replaced by immature fibrous connective tissue. Fibrous osteodystrophy is generalized throughout the skeleton but is accentuated in local areas such as the cancellous bone of the skull. The elevated PTH levels also inhibit the renal tubular resorption of P.

The lesion in the parathyroid gland in dogs is usually an adenoma, occasionally a carcinoma, composed of active chief cells. Adenomas usually are single, light brown-red, and located in the cervical region near (but sharply demarcated from) the thyroid gland. Rarely, they are in the anterior mediastinum near the base of the heart.

Clinical Findings: Lameness follows severe osteoclastic bone resorption, and fractures of long bones occur after minor physical trauma. Compression fractures of weakened vertebral bodies may exert pressure on the spinal cord and nerves, resulting in motor and sensory dysfunction.

Facial hyperostosis with partial obliteration of the nasal cavity by poorly mineralized woven bone and highly vascular fibrous connective tissue, and with loss or loosening of teeth has been observed in dogs. This may result in an inability to close the mouth properly and development of gingival ulcers. The maxillae and rami of the mandibles often are coarsely thickened by the excess woven bone. Bones of the skull are markedly thinned by the increased resorption and have a characteristic "moth-eaten" appearance radiographically.

Lesions: Histological demonstration of a rim of normal tissue and a partial to complete fibrous capsule in an enlarged parathyroid suggests an adenoma rather than focal hyperplasia. Chief cell carcinomas tend to be larger than adenomas and fixed to the underlying tissues due to local infiltration of neoplastic cells.

Diagnosis: Although other laboratory findings may be variable, hypercalcemia is consistent and results from accelerated release of Ca from bone. The blood Ca in normal dogs is ~10 ± 1 mg/dL depending on age and diet (and assay method). Serum Ca values consistently >12 mg/dL should be considered to be hypercalcemic. Dogs with primary hyperparathyroidism usually have a serum Ca of ≥12-20 mg/dL. The blood P is low or in the low-normal range (≤4 mg/dL). The urinary excretion of P, and often of Ca, is increased and may result in nephrocalcinosis and urolithiasis. Accelerated bone matrix metabolism is reflected by increased urinary excretion of hydroxyproline. Serum alkaline phosphatase activity may be elevated in animals with overt bone disease. Demonstration of elevated levels of PTH by a species-specific assay in an adult to aged dog with hypercalcemia, hypophosphatemia, and evidence of generalized bone disease provides conclusive evidence of primary hyperparathyroidism. PTH can be measured by sensitive radioimmunoassays or immunoradiometric assays.

The intact N-terminal PTH assay can be run on either serum (preferred) or plasma that has been separated and frozen (-70°C in either glass or plastic tubes) as soon as possible after collection. Using this method, circulating levels of PTH in most animals are near 20 pg/mL (eg, dog, 20 ± 5 pg/mL; cat, 17 ± 2 pg/mL), with levels in nonhuman primates being slightly lower. PTH assays that utilize antibody generated against the carboxy terminal end of the human molecule usually give less consistent results in animals other than man.

Differential diagnoses include other causes of hypercalcemia, such as vitamin D intoxication (overdosage), enzootic calcinosis (qv, p 488), malignant neoplasms with osseous metastasis, and humoral hypercalcemia of malignancy (qv, p 285). The hypercalcemia of hypervitaminosis D may be as high as that in primary hyperparathyroidism but is accompanied by varying degrees of hyperphosphatemia and normal serum alkaline phosphatase activity. Skeletal disease usually is absent, since the increased concentrations of blood Ca and P are derived principally from augmented intestinal absorption rather than bone resorption.

Malignant neoplasms with osseous metastases may cause moderate hypercalcemia and hypercalciuria, but the alkaline phosphatase activity and serum P level usually are normal or only slightly elevated. These changes are believed to be due to the release of Ca and P into the blood from areas of bone destruction at rates greater than can be cleared by the kidneys and intestine. Bone involvement is more sharply demarcated and localized to the area of metastasis. Osteolysis associated with tumor metastases results not only from a physical disruption of bone by proliferating neoplastic cells, but also from local production of humoral substances that stimulate bone resorption, such as prostaglandins and interleukin-1.

Primary parathyroid hyperplasia has been described in German Shepherd pups associated with hypercalcemia, hypophosphatemia, increased immunoreactive PTH, and increased fractional clearance of inorganic P in the urine. Clinical signs include stunted growth, weakness, polyuria, polydipsia, and a diffuse reduction in bone density. IV infusion of Ca fails to suppress the autonomous secretion of PTH by the diffuse hyperplasia of chief cells in all parathyroids. Lesions include nodular hyperplasia of thyroid C-cells and widespread mineralization of the lungs, kidneys, and gastric mucosa. The disease is inherited as an autosomal recessive.

Hypercalcemia also may be associated with multifocal osteolytic lesions associated with septic emboli, complete immobilization, osteosarcoma, hypoadrenocorticism (Addison's-like disease), hypocalcitoninism due to a destructive thyroid lesion, chronic renal disease, hemoconcentration, or hyperproteinemia. Hypercalcemia is detected occasionally in dehydrated animals but usually is mild. It is attributed to fluid volume contraction that results in hyperproteinemia and increased concentrations of ionized and nonionized Ca; it resolves rapidly following fluid therapy.

Treatment: The objective is to eliminate the source of excessive PTH production. An attempt should be made to identify all 4 parathyroid glands before excising any tissue. Single or multiple adenomas should be removed *in toto*. If all identifiable parathyroids in the cervical region appear to be of normal or smaller size, and the diagnosis is reasonably certain, surgical exploration of the thorax near the base of the heart may be necessary to localize the parathyroid neoplasm.

Removal of the functional parathyroid lesion results in a rapid decrease in circulating PTH levels because the half-life of PTH in plasma is <15 min. Since plasma Ca levels in animals with overt bone disease may decrease rapidly and be subnormal within 12-24 hr after surgery, they should be monitored frequently. Postoperative hypocalcemia ($\leq$5 mg/dL) can result from: 1) depressed secretory activity of chief cells due to suppression by the chronic hypercalcemia or injury to the remaining parathyroid tissue during surgery, 2) abruptly decreased bone resorption due to lowered PTH levels, and 3) accelerated mineralization of osteoid matrix formed by the hyperplastic osteoblasts, which was previously prevented from undergoing mineralization by the elevated PTH levels. Infusions of calcium gluconate to maintain the serum Ca between 7.5 and 9 mg/dL, plus feeding high-calcium diets and supplemental vitamin D therapy will correct this serious postoperative complication. If hypercalcemia persists for $\geq$1 wk after surgery, or recurs after initial improvement, a second adenoma or metastases from a carcinoma should be suspected.

SECONDARY HYPERPARATHYROIDISM

NUTRITIONAL HYPERPARATHYROIDISM
(Fibrous osteodystrophy)

Increased secretion of parathyroid hormone (PTH) as a compensatory mechanism induced by nutritional imbalances. In general, growing animals are affected most severely because their requirement for calcium (Ca) is high. A large portion of the skeletal dystrophies diagnosed as rickets and osteogenesis imperfecta in kittens and puppies are manifestations of nutritional hyperparathyroidism.

Etiology and Pathogenesis: Dietary mineral imbalances of etiological importance are: 1) low Ca content (most grains) or unavailable Ca (plants high in oxalates, such as *Setaria sphacelata, Cenchrus ciliaris*, and *Panicum maximum*), 2) excess phosphorus (P) with normal or low Ca (muscle and organ meats), and 3) inadequate amounts of cholecalciferol (vitamin D_3) in New World primates. The significant end result is hypocalcemia that results in parathyroid stimulation.

A diet low in Ca fails to supply the daily requirement even though a greater portion of ingested Ca is absorbed, and hypocalcemia develops. Ingestion of excess P results in increased absorption and elevation of blood P. Hyperphosphatemia does not stimulate the parathyroid gland directly but does so by lowering blood Ca.

The disease develops frequently in puppies and kittens fed an unsupplemented, predominantly meat diet. (*See also* NUTRITION: DOGS and CATS, pp 1201 and 1160.)

Clinical Findings: Kittens that are fed beef heart exclusively develop locomotor disturbances within 4 wk, even though the high content of digestible protein (>50% on a weight basis) and fat promotes rapid growth, the animals appear well nourished, and their coat maintains a good luster. The predominant clinical signs are reluctance to move, posterior lameness, and ataxia. The kittens often stand with characteristic deviation of the paws. The skeletal disease becomes progressively more severe after 5-14 wk. The kittens become quiet and reluctant to play, and assume a sitting position or sternal recumbency with the hindlegs abducted. Normal activities may result in the sudden onset of severe lameness due to incomplete or folding fractures of one or more bones.

Lameness is the initial functional disturbance in growing dogs and may vary from a slight limp to inability to walk. The bones are painful on palpation, and folding fractures of long bones and vertebrae are common. In adult dogs, clinical signs usually are related to resorption of jaw bone. PTH-stimulated resorption of alveolar bone results in loosening and subsequent loss of teeth, with recession of gingiva and partial root exposure in advanced cases.

In horses, nutritional hyperparathyroidism is known as **bran disease, miller's disease**, and **"big head"**. The diet of "pampered" horses is often too high in grains and low in forage, which provides a high-phosphorus/low-calcium intake. Many of the obscure lamenesses of horses have been attributed to nutritional hyperparathyroidism. The pathological changes are similar to those in other species, with the provisos that the bones of the head are particularly affected in severe cases and that gross or microscopic fractures of subchondral bone, with consequent degeneration of articular cartilage and tearing of ligaments from periosteal attachments, are a dominant influence on the clinical signs.

Nutritional hyperparathyroidism is uncommon in cattle and sheep, but is seen occasionally in feedlots. Marrow fibroplasia is not a feature of the condition in these species. Osteoporosis is the dominant lesion, but "big head" may occur in goats. Bone deformities in recovered animals can cause obstipation or dystocia.

Diagnosis: To establish a definite diagnosis, the diet should be evaluated for Ca, P, and vitamin D content. There is radiographic evidence of generalized skeletal demineralization, loss of lamina dura dentes, subperiosteal cortical bone resorption, bowing deformities, and multiple folding fractures of long bones due to intense localized osteoclast proliferation. Laboratory values used to assess renal function should be within normal limits in animals with nutritional hyperparathyroidism.

Only one measurement of serum Ca, P, and alkaline phosphatase may be of limited diagnostic value. Since the homeostatic mechanisms are functioning and kidney function is normal, serum Ca and P levels usually are in the low-normal range. Alkaline phosphatase activity often is elevated in animals with overt bone disease. The increased PTH secretion acts on the normal kidneys to increase P and decrease Ca excretion into the urine.

Treatment: The objective is to decrease PTH secretion by correcting the dietary mineral imbalance or deficiency. Pups and kittens with the disease should be fed a diet that fulfills their daily requirements for protein, Ca, and P. Calcium gluconate, lactate, or carbonate should be used as dietary supplements to achieve a Ca:P ratio of 2:1 during the healing phase in young animals with severe bone disease. Additional vitamin D usually is not necessary; however, it may be indicated in primates with a vitamin D_3 deficiency. Calcium gluconate should be given parenterally if the appetite is depressed. Excess dietary Ca should be avoided because it may retard growth and alter remodeling of bone in young animals. Even animals with advanced disease respond favorably to dietary supplementation. Good nursing care is essential to prevent complications such as decubital ulcers, constipation, and additional fractures.

Affected animals should be confined for several weeks after initiation of the supplemental diet. Response to therapy is rapid, and within 1 wk the animals become more active and their attitude improves. Jumping or climbing must be prevented because the skeleton is still susceptible to fractures. Restrictions can be lessened after 3 wk, but confinement with limited movement is indicated until the skeleton returns to normal (response to treatment should be monitored radiographically). In young animals, recovery usually is complete in 8-9 wk.

RENAL SECONDARY HYPERPARATHYROIDISM

A complication of chronic renal failure characterized by an excess, but not autonomous, rate of parathyroid hormone (PTH) secretion. It occurs frequently in dogs and occasionally in cats and other animals. The secretion of hormone by the hyperplastic parathyroid glands usually remains responsive to fluctuations in blood calcium (Ca).

Etiology and Pathogenesis: The primary etiologic mechanism is chronic, progressive renal disease with impaired function. Chronic renal insufficiency in older dogs results from interstitial nephritis, glomerulonephritis, nephrosclerosis, or amyloidosis. Conditions such as renal dysplasia, familial renal diseases, polycystic kidneys, and congenital bilateral hydronephrosis may be responsible in younger dogs.

When renal disease significantly reduces the glomerular filtration rate, phosphorus (P) is retained and progressive hyperphosphatemia develops. Although the concentration of blood P has no direct regulatory influence on the synthesis and secretion of PTH, it may do so indirectly by lowering blood Ca, which stimulates the parathyroid. In chronic renal failure, hypocalcemia also results from an acquired defect in vitamin D metabolism, in which the diseased kidney is unable to convert inactive precursor forms into the active form of vitamin D (1,25-dihydroxycholecalciferol).

Clinical Findings: The predominant signs of vomiting, dehydration, polydipsia, polyuria, depression, and ammoniacal breath odor are related to progressive renal insufficiency and uremia. A spectrum of skeletal lesions of secondary hyperparathyroidism may be present, ranging from minor changes with early (or mild) renal disease to severe fibrous osteodystrophy of advanced renal failure. The volume of affected bones usually is normal (isostotic), particularly in older dogs because of the slow onset of renal failure and lower metabolic activity of bones. Hyperostotic bone lesions, such as facial swelling, may be seen in younger dogs in which deposition of unmineralized osteoid by hyperplastic osteoblasts and production of fibrous connective tissue exceed the rate of bone resorption.

Although skeletal involvement is generalized, all parts are not affected uniformly. Lesions become apparent earlier and reach a more advanced stage in certain areas, such as cancellous bones of the skull. Resorption of alveolar bone occurs early and results in loose teeth, which may be dislodged easily and interfere with mastication. As a result of accelerated resorption of cancellous bone of the maxilla and mandible, bones become softened and pliable ("rubber jaw disease"), and the jaws fail to close properly. This often results in drooling and protrusion of the tongue. Severely demineralized mandibles are predisposed to fractures and displacement of teeth from alveoli. Long bones are less dramatically affected. Lameness, stiff gait, and fractures after minor trauma may result from increased bone resorption.

Lesions: All parathyroid glands are enlarged, initially due to hypertrophy of chief cells, and subsequently by compensatory hyperplasia. Although the parathyroids are not autonomous, the concentration of PTH in the peripheral blood often exceeds that of primary hyperparathyroidism.

Diagnosis: Serum should be analyzed for Ca, P, and alkaline phosphatase. Multiple determinations are more reliable because of the considerable variation that exists, depending on the stage of the disease and the body's compensatory mechanism. Blood Ca usually is in the low-normal range because of mobilization of skeletal reserves. Blood P is increased because the progressive glomerular and tubular dysfunction with loss of target cells interferes with the phosphaturic response to the increased levels of PTH. Phosphorus is retained, and the blood concentration continues to rise despite the secondary hyperparathyroidism.

Alkaline phosphatase activity may be elevated in animals with overt bone disease. Of dogs with chronic renal failure, ~10% have a moderately elevated serum Ca ($\geq$12 mg/dL).

Treatment: Treatment usually is directed toward reducing the excretory load and providing substances (such as sodium [as chloride or bicarbonate] and water) that the failing kidney is unable to conserve. A special diet with supplemental Ca (gluconate or lactate) and vitamin D may diminish the severity of hyperparathyroidism and accompanying bone lesions. Small doses (0.003 μg/kg body wt/day) of 1,25-dihydroxycholecalciferol appear to reduce the degree of hyperparathyroidism.

HYPOPARATHYROIDISM

A metabolic disorder in which either subnormal amounts of parathyroid hormone (PTH) are secreted, or the hormone secreted is unable to interact normally with target cells. It has been recognized primarily in dogs, particularly in smaller breeds such as Miniature Schnauzers, but other breeds may be affected.

Etiology and Pathogenesis: Various pathogenic mechanisms can result in inadequate secretion of PTH. Parathyroid glands may be damaged or inadvertently removed during thyroid surgery. Following damage to the glands or their vascular supply, adequate functional parenchyma often regenerates and clinical signs subsequently disappear.

Idiopathic hypoparathyroidism in adult dogs usually is the result of diffuse lymphocytic parathyroiditis that causes extensive degeneration of chief cells and replacement by fibrous connective tissue. Other possible causes of hypoparathyroidism include destruction of parathyroids by primary or metastatic neoplasms in the anterior cervical area, and atrophy of parathyroids associated with chronic hypercalcemia. The presence of numerous distemper virus particles in chief cells of the parathyroid gland may contribute to the low blood Ca in certain dogs with this disease. Agenesis of the parathyroids is a rare cause of congenital hypoparathyroidism in pups. Certain cases of idiopathic hypoparathyroidism with histologically normal parathyroids in animals (including man) may be due to lack of the specific enzyme in chief cells that converts the pro-PTH molecule to the biologically active PTH secreted by the gland. Other cases may develop by means of an immune-mediated mechanism, since a similar destruction of secretory parenchyma and lymphocytic infiltration has been produced experimentally in dogs by repeated injections of parathyroid tissue emulsions.

Pseudohypoparathyroidism is a variant that occurs in man, but it is uncertain whether it occurs in other animals. Target cells in kidney and bone are unable to respond to normal or elevated amounts of PTH, and severe hypocalcemia develops even though parathyroid glands are hyperplastic.

Clinical Findings and Lesions: The functional disturbances and clinical manifestations of hypoparathyroidism primarily are the result of increased neuromuscular excitability and tetany. Bone resorption is decreased because of the lack of PTH, and blood Ca levels diminish progressively (4-6 mg/dL). Affected dogs are restless, nervous, and ataxic, with weakness and intermittent tremors of individual muscle groups that progress to generalized tetany and convulsions. Blood P levels are elevated substantially, owing to increased renal tubular reabsorption.

In the early stages of immune-mediated lymphocytic parathyroiditis in dogs, there is infiltration of the gland with lymphocytes and plasma cells, and nodular regenerative hyperplasia of remaining chief cells. Later, the parathyroid gland is replaced by lymphocytes, fibroblasts, and capillaries, with only an occasional viable chief cell.

Diagnosis: This is based on clinical signs of increased neuromuscular excitability, severe hypocalcemia, and often moderate hyperphosphatemia in a nonparturient animal, and the response to therapy. Some of the signs (eg, tetany) and laboratory data (eg, hypocalcemia) are similar to those of puerperal tetany (qv, p 457). However, puerperal tetany usually is accompanied by hypophosphatemia and a low-normal or subnormal blood glucose concentration as a result of the associated intense muscular activity.

Treatment: The neuromuscular tetany should be treated initially by restoring blood Ca levels to near normal by IV administration of organic Ca solutions. Long-term maintenance of blood Ca levels in the absence of normal PTH secretion should be attempted by feeding diets that are high in Ca and low in P, and that are supplemented with Ca (gluconate or lactate) and vitamin D_3.

Large doses of vitamin D_3 ($\geq$25,000-50,000 u/day, depending on the size of the dog) may be required initially to elevate the blood Ca level in hypoparathyroid animals, since the lack of PTH diminishes the rate of formation of the biologically active vitamin D metabolite in the kidney. To prevent hypercalcemia and extensive soft-tissue mineralization, the dosage of vitamin D should be carefully adjusted following frequent determination of the serum Ca level. After adjusting the dose of vitamin D, a 4- to 5-day interval should precede the next blood Ca determination. Once the blood Ca has returned to normal, substantially lower doses of vitamin D are indicated for long-term maintenance; in some dogs, only dietary Ca supplementation is required for long-term stabilization.

RICKETS

A disease of growing animals characterized by interference with mineralization, and consequently with normal resorption of growth-plate cartilage and interference with mineralization of bone matrix. Rapidly growing plates in rapidly growing bones are most severely affected.

Etiology: Deficient intake or absorption, or both, of vitamin D or phosphorus, or both, are most often causative. In housed animals, vitamin D deficiency is important; pastured animals are more likely to be deficient in phosphorus. Abnormal metabolism of vitamin D (as occurs, eg, in uremia or inherited biochemical defects) should be considered in rachitic animals on apparently normal diets, as should improper compounding of the diet. Failure to absorb vitamin D may be caused by steatorrhea. Endogenous vitamin D is produced in the epidermis from the action of ultraviolet light on a precursor. Exogenous vitamin D is absorbed from the diet or an injection site.

Clinical Findings and Diagnosis: In severe cases, there is lameness associated with enlargement of the ends of fast-growing bones, and deformities of the weight-bearing long bones. Lameness and enlargement of the joints more commonly is due to chronic polyarthritis and, in young large dogs, to hypertrophic osteodystrophy. Radiographs of rachitic bones show wide growth plates and demineralization. Demineralization in nutritional hyperparathyroidism is accompanied by normal growth plates.

Widening of the growth plate due to failure to resorb cartilage is not pathognomonic of rickets. It occurs in certain inherited chondrodysplasias, and any factor that interferes with normal metaphyseal vascularization or sinusoidal invasion of cartilage, or both, may cause widening of the plate. This should be considered when interpreting radiographs of single joints. In rachitic animals, the blood Ca times the blood P (in mg/dL) is usually <30. This is a useful aid to diagnosis if serum is collected before therapy or dietary correction. Confirmation of the diagnosis in mild cases requires histological examination of active growth plates. Since rachitic animals may be hypocalcemic, histological changes of hyperparathyroidism may be present.

Treatment: Accurate diagnosis is imperative since vitamin D without calcium exacerbates those conditions associated with nutritional hyperparathyroidism. Rickets caused by simple deficiencies of vitamin D or phosphorus should be treated according to standard nutritional recommendations after detailed consideration and, if possible, analysis of the existing diet. Secondary deficiencies require correction of the underlying cause.

ENZOOTIC CALCINOSIS
(Enteque seco, Enteque ossificans, Espichamento, Espichacao, Manchester wasting disease, Naalehu disease, Weidektankheit)

A disease complex of ruminants and horses, caused by plant poisoning or mineral imbalances and characterized by extensive calcification of soft tissues. The prevalence of the disease in cattle varies widely, from 10% to as high as 50%, in areas of Argentina, Brazil, Papua-New Guinea, Jamaica, Hawaii, and Bavaria. It is said to cause up to 60% mortality and affect 17% of the sheep in southern Brazil and Mattewara (India), respectively. Incidence elsewhere (Australia, Israel, South Africa, and southern USA) is less well documented, and in many areas it is rare or nonexistent.

Etiology and Pathogenesis: Known causes fall into 2 categories: plant poisonings and mineral imbalances in the soil, the first probably being the more important. *Cestrum diurnum* (wild jasmine, day-blooming jessamine, king-of-the-day), *Trisetum flavescens* (golden oats or yellow oat grass), *Nierembergia veitehii, Solanum esuriale, S torvum*, and *S malacoxylon (glaucophyllum)* contain $1\alpha,25$-dihydroxycholecalciferol (calcitriol) glycoside or a substance that mimics its calcinogenic action. Studies indicate that *S malacoxylon* has the required enzyme systems for the synthesis of calcitriol from vitamin D_3. No concrete evidence incriminating other plants is available.

The imbalance of minerals in certain soils in Hawaii, India, Austria, and possibly elsewhere has been thought to be the main etiological factor; dietary mineral imbalance may contribute to the calcification chiefly associated with plant poisoning. Excessive phosphate or calcium, absolute or conditioned magnesium deficiency, and deficiency of potassium and nitrogen have all been incriminated or suspected.

Osteodystrophy of bulls following prolonged excessive calcium intake is a similar condition; calcification of the cardiovascular system associated with aging and such cachectic diseases as tuberculosis is not identical. Excessive vitamin D_3 and normal or excessive calcium intake induces aortic calcification and atherosclerosis in ruminants.

Normally, the conversion of 25-hydroxycholecalciferol (calcifediol) to calcitriol in the kidney is controlled by a feedback mechanism. The calcitriol-like factor in the leaves of plants bypasses this mechanism and more calcium is absorbed than can be accommodated physiologically. Hypercalcemia promotes calcitonin production, calcinosis, and osteoporosis.

Changes in plasma calcium, phosphorus, and magnesium are different in different species. Horses develop hyperphosphatemia; plasma calcium remains normal, but does rise with excess doses of calcitriol. Frequently, both serum calcium and inorganic phosphorus are elevated in cattle. Hypomagnesemia also may be present.

Clinical Findings: The disease is progressive and chronic, extending over weeks or months. The earliest signs are stiffened and painful gait, which is most pronounced when the animal gets up after prolonged rest. Forelimbs are particularly affected, and some animals even walk or graze on their knees. When standing, the forelimbs bow forward since the joints cannot be extended completely. The animal shifts weight to the forepart of the hooves, or alternatively to each forelimb to ease stress on the carpus, which is thickened and painful. The distal joints become abnormally straight. When affected animals are forced to walk, their gait is awkward, stiff, and slow, the steps short, and after only short distances breathing becomes shallow and diaphragmatic, the nostrils are flared, and the head and neck are extended. Varying degrees of heart murmur are detectable, usually as a double or blurred second sound; these are exaggerated after exercise. Pulse rate is increased after slight exercise. Jugular pulse is prominent in some cases.

As the disease progresses, the animal loses weight and becomes weak and listless. The coat becomes shaggy, dull, and faded, particularly in cattle. There is wasting of muscles, a prominent skeleton, tucked up abdomen, kyphosis, and raised tailhead. Ovarian function is impaired. Appetite is usually unimpaired but sometimes becomes depraved. Calcification of vessels is palpable on rectal examination.

Osteodystrophy is observed in calcinosis due to *Trisetum flavescens* and *Cestrum diurnum* toxicities in Bavarian cattle and Florida horses, respectively. Severely affected horses stand with forelimbs somewhat abducted and luxated caudally at the shoulder joints. The flexor tendons, particularly the suspensory ligaments, are painful. Fetlock joints are overextended to varying degrees.

Lesions: Degeneration and calcification of soft tissues occur, with emaciation and varying amounts of excess fluid in the thoracic and abdominal cavities and pericardial sac. The cardiovascular system is the first to be involved, followed by lung, kidney, and tendons. The heart and aorta show the most marked effects. The left side of the heart is more affected than the right. In extreme cases, calcified foci are seen on valves and chordae tendinae. White, elevated plaques of irregular size and shape are seen on the luminal surface; in advanced cases, these occur throughout the length of the aorta and its main branches. Mineral deposits occur on the pleura, the surface and edges of the diaphragmatic and apical lobes of lungs, in the renal artery and pelvis of the kidney, and the ligaments and tendons (particularly of the forelimbs). Capsular thickening and irregular erosions of articular surface of cartilage and joints occur, especially of the carpus and hock.

The basic histological evidence is necrosis and calcification of connective tissue followed by cellular proliferation in the affected area.

Diagnosis: This is usually based on the history, signs, and lesions but may be difficult at early stages. Radiography and electrocardiography may be helpful.

Control: Removal of the causal factor(s) is essential, but when the disease is associated with the mineral content of the soil, control may be difficult. Change of pasture, forage, and environment may effect clinical improvement and even diminish the soft-tissue mineral deposits. Experimentally, daily administration of 15 g of aluminum hydroxide, PO, prevented the development of calcinosis in sheep fed *Trisetum flavescens.*

HYPERTROPHIC OSTEOPATHY
(Marie's disease)

A condition in which osseous changes of the limbs are associated with intrathoracic lesions. It has occurred in conjunction with tuberculosis, bronchopneumonia, and pulmonary abscesses. More commonly it is associated with primary or metastatic pulmonary neoplasms. It also has been associated with granulomatous processes in the thoracic cavity. The disease is more common in dogs but has been reported in horses, cattle, sheep, and other animals.

The cause is unknown. There is a rapid initial increase in the peripheral blood flow to the lower portion of the limbs, possibly from vagal stimulation. This is followed by connective tissue proliferation in the phalangeal region of the legs, which progresses proximally. The next change is a bony proliferation involving the phalanges and long bones.

Clinical Findings: Dogs usually are affected later in life; other species may be affected at any age. The usual history is that legs have become progressively thicker during the past few months, most often with accompanying lameness. Sometimes the history also includes chronic cough with some dyspnea, especially after mild exercise. Appetite and bowel function usually are normal. In advanced cases, there may be a stilted gait or even an inability to stand. Movement or palpation of the affected bones causes pain, and the thickened limbs are warm.

Lesions: The long bones of the limbs are involved most frequently. The affected bones are either partially or completely covered with uneven and irregular new-bone deposits on the cortex. The joint surfaces are not involved, but the soft tissue around the joints may swell and the joint capsules thicken.

Diagnosis: This is based on physical examination and characteristic radiographic findings. Radiographs reveal extensive proliferation of new bone, almost always bilateral, along the shafts of the long bones and phalanges. This bilateral distribution of new bone, together with the absence of cortical erosion, helps to distinguish the condition from bone neoplasia. Radiographs of the chest often disclose primary or metastatic neoplasia in the lungs.

Treatment: There is no specific treatment, although treatment of the intrathoracic lesion by surgery or chemotherapy may lead to a temporary regression of the bone changes. Vagal neurectomy also has been reported to be of value.

LAMENESS, GENERAL PRINCIPLES

Lameness is a departure from the normal stance or gait resulting from a structural or functional disorder of one or more limbs or the trunk. In most cases, there is associated pain, but occasionally there is none, and a mechanical type of lameness is observed. It is not a disease, but an indication of pain, weakness, deformity, or other impediment in the musculoskeletal system. *See also* the section (MUS) table of contents, pp 460-465, for related topics, EVALUATION OF GAIT, p 572, and DISEASES OF THE SPINAL COLUMN AND CORD, p 584.

Lameness can be classified into weight-bearing (supporting-leg) and nonweight-bearing (swinging-leg) disorders. A supporting-leg lameness is seen when the animal reduces the extent and duration of weight bearing by taking a shorter step and elevating the body during the support phase of the stride; it occurs with injuries to the feet, bones, tendons, ligaments, and motor nerves. A swinging-leg lameness is seen during the swing phase of the stride cycle when the limb is being brought forward. A mixed swinging and supporting lameness can occur. Furthermore, it is frequent for a lesion in one limb to cause secondary soreness or lameness in another area in the same limb or in any of the other 3 limbs from the effort to protect the original injury. Biomechanical laminitis in the opposite foot is a common complication of severe orthopedic problems in horses. Racehorses develop secondary soreness or even tendinitis and/or suspensory desmitis in the forelimbs following hindlimb lameness or vice versa. This situation is referred to as a complementary lameness.

ETIOLOGY AND PREDISPOSING FACTORS

The causes of lameness may be classified as 1) predisposing, which involve immaturity or poor condition, faulty conformation, systemic disease, lack of attention to the feet, or in horses, bad shoeing, or 2) exciting, due to direct or indirect trauma; incoordination of muscle action, as may occur in tired animals; and bacterial infection, especially of the feet, tendon sheaths, and joints.

Terms such as shoulder lameness, hip lameness, and tarsal lameness are often used to describe so-called regional lameness. However, these terms do not specifically indicate the structure involved, eg, shoulder lameness does not indicate whether the causal lesion is in the scapulohumeral joint, tendon of origin of the biceps, the bicipital bursa, or any of the muscles in that region. Shoulder lameness may be secondary to foot disease. The action or alteration in stride characteristics does not denote the precise region involved, although it may indicate the possible problem.

In large animals, except for Standardbred horses, most lamenesses affect the fore-limbs, usually from the carpus distally. Age is often a predisposing factor. The intensity of racing competition in Greyhounds and young, immature horses (ie, 2-yr-olds) means a high incidence of sore shins, stress fractures, splints, and tendon injuries. The type of surface on which the animal performs may aggravate any conformational abnormalities. Fatigue or improper fitness is another predisposing factor, particularly in tendon and ligament injuries. In small animals, trauma is probably the single most important factor in causing lameness, although conformation, growth, environment, and even neoplasia also must be considered. In farm animals, nutrition and the environment (ie, climate, housing, herd size, hygiene) are all important.

Breed may be a significant predisposing factor, eg, elbow osteochondrosis in Rottweilers, laminitis in ponies, and spastic paresis in Friesian calves.

DIAGNOSIS

A careful and systematic investigation is required to accurately define the location and cause. Lameness may be evident during rest, during progression, or by manual examination including passive movement (ie, in horses by testing with hoof testers or hammer). There are many sophisticated aids to diagnosis, but there is no substitute for clinical acumen, experience, palpation, and a good working knowledge of anatomy. Even with all of these, obscure lameness (eg, musculoligamentous injuries and back problems) may defy a definitive diagnosis.

Signalment and History: A complete and objective history should always be obtained before the physical examination. The type and age of the animal and amount of exercise provide important diagnostic clues. For example, young Thoroughbreds on a high-grain ration are prone to low-grade exertional myopathy or rhabdomyolysis (tying up). Older jumping horses are more predisposed to navicular disease and ringbone). Laminitis is most common in fat ponies on lush pastures. In cattle, a rich diet is linked not only to high production, but also to laminitis and other disorders of the digits. Historically, most cases of forelimb lameness in horses involved the foot, while the hock was the frequently affected region of the hindlimb; in today's light horses, most cases of forelimb lameness arise from the fetlock distally. However, in the Thoroughbred and Standardbred in training, the carpus frequently is involved. Developmental orthopedic diseases, eg, osteochondritis dissecans, may be generalized, and affect any joint or bone in the body; they are common in both companion and farm animals.

The onset and duration of the lameness, the existence of an inciting cause (eg, pricked foot, kick, or fall), when the horse was last shod (eg, nail prick), and the effects of any previous treatments are all helpful in defining the particular lameness. The type of rest (ie, stall or pasture) as well as any change in the lameness when the animal is exercised (ie, warming into or out of the lameness) must be determined. In horses, stumbling may be a feature of a specific lameness (eg, navicular disease) or be due to a neurological problem.

Examination at Rest: The examination should begin with a visual inspection. Conformational defects (eg, calf knees, sickle hocks) should be observed and recorded as possible predispositions. Faults in conformation must be considered, but as with many chronic swellings (eg, splints), they may not be the primary cause of lameness. Similarly, old wounds, scars, or swellings may or may not be relevant. The general demeanor of the animal may indicate pain (eg, sweating, pawing the ground, pointing, or favoring a limb). An abnormal stance may suggest a particular problem (eg, the typical posture of laminitis, locking of the patella, or radial paralysis). Abnormal mobility or position of a part of a limb may indicate a ruptured tendon or fractured bone. Adduction or abduction of a limb may also be noted in hip or stifle lamenesses, respectively.

Examination During Exercise: After visual inspection at rest, the animal should be viewed in motion. Lameness usually is demonstrated best at a slow trot on a hard, even surface. The animal should be trotted in a straight line both toward and away from the examiner. For the horse, the handler should keep a slack rein to allow unrestricted head movement. Initially, the examiner should look "up" at the backline of the horse to determine if there is a head nod or hip hike. Attention also should be directed to the body axis to determine whether the axis is in the same line as the direction of movement. Subsequently, it should be noted whether the legs are carried in a straight line or are adducted, abducted, or circumducted while in motion. Finally, the action should be viewed from the side to identify variations in stride length and restricted joint flexion.

Forelimb Lameness: The head is raised when the lame limb bears weight and is dropped when the unaffected limb is in support. In the horse, the sound made by each hoof as it strikes the ground may also indicate the lame limb. The head nod may not be apparent in bilateral lameness of near-equal severity, but the action in front is stilted, and the stride length is reduced. If the lameness is of unequal severity, the head nod is present as in unilateral lameness. In such a case, the less lame limb is likely to be overlooked. If the limb with obvious lameness is subjected to anesthetic blocking to desensitize the painful area, the apparent soundness of that limb and the head movement indicate that the other limb also is lame.

Hindlimb Lameness: The croup on the affected side is generally raised when the lame limb is in support; the degree of elevation of the croup varies with the source and severity of lameness. When both hindlimbs are lame, the gait is stiff and restricted, similar to that seen with back problems. When the lame leg has been identified, the following should be assessed: degree of flexion of the joints, length of stride, adduction or abduction of the limb, placement of the foot, and height to which the hocks are carried.

The animal should be turned in a tight circle in both directions. Difficulty turning on a lame or painful limb often can be seen as well as stiffness in the neck, back, or hindquarters. Forcing the animal to "back up" a few steps may also highlight some types of lameness (eg, vertebral damage, stringhalt).

In horses, mild lameness (eg, spavin) often can be demonstrated by trotting in a 4-5 yard (meter) circle on a lunge rein. Usually, the lameness is aggravated when the affected limb is on the inside of the circle. The effect that forced flexion or, in some instances, extension has on the degree of lameness (eg, spavin test) should be evaluated systematically, by attempting to maximally flex individual joints or regions of the limb for ~60 sec and then trotting the horse off for assessment of lameness. Flexion tests are particularly helpful in horses with mild lamenesses. All flexion tests should be compared with the effect on the opposite limb.

If the degree or site of lameness still is not clear, the horse should be lunged, ridden, or driven for ~20 min. The additional weight of the rider sometimes accentuates the lameness, and some horses must be examined at fast or maximal pace for the lameness to be seen effectively. After this sort of exercise, the horse should be rested for ~30 min and reexamined.

Physical examination of the lame limb should begin with the foot, and abnormalities of the hooves (eg, laminitic rings, sandcracks, contracted heels) and the state of the shoeing noted. Detectable heat in the foot or coronary band can be evaluated by comparison with the opposite limb. All identifiable structures should be gently, but thoroughly palpated, both with the foot on the ground and raised. The shoe should be removed and the hoof thoroughly cleaned and inspected for cracks, uneven wear, or discharge. Frequently, the hoof must be trimmed to aid examination. The hoof can be tested for pain by percussion of both wall and sole, using a light hammer, and then by compression, using hoof testers.

All anatomical landmarks from the pastern to the shoulder should be palpated systematically while the leg bears weight. The flexor tendons and suspensory ligament should be palpated individually with the limb semiflexed. Any heat, pain, joint distention, or other suspicious finding should be noted and compared with the opposite limb. The range of flexion and extension of the pastern, fetlock, carpus, elbow, and shoulder joints should be checked.

The hindlimb should be examined similarly with particular attention to the hock for palpable signs of tibiotarsal joint distention or spavin. If an upper hindlimb or low back condition is suspected in large animals, a rectal examination should be done.

A detailed examination of the back of the horse is best performed with the animal restrained in stocks. The dorsal midline of the back should be straight and show no lateral curvature suggestive of unilateral muscle spasm (spastic scoliosis). Any asymmetry of the pelvis or muscle wastage over the quarters should be noted, particularly if the history suggests sacroiliac damage. It is difficult to palpate more than the tips of the dorsal spinous processes, although in most normal horses the interspinous spaces can be identified. It should be possible to detect protrusion of the summits of the dorsal spinous processes and spasm of the longissimus dorsi muscles. Thin-skinned or hypersensitive horses cringe away when the dorsal midline is palpated deeply, but unless the response is dramatic (eg, kicking, rearing, grunting), it should not be considered clinically significant. The sacral spinous processes (S_{2-5}) should be palpated, particularly in horses used for harness racing, since pain may be detected over the tendinous insertion of the longissimus dorsi muscle onto the spines of S_2 and S_3.

By alternate pinching of the midline in the caudal thoracic and sacral region, the animal should flex (ventroflex or arch) and extend (dorsiflex or dip) its spine, respectively. Reluctance to perform this maneuver suggests some underlying pain due to soft-tissue or bony lesion of the thoracolumbar spine. Significant discomfort produced by this test is usually accompanied by spasm of the longissimus dorsi muscles. Skin sensitivity over the back and loins is an unreliable test because of its variability among individuals. However, firm stroking of the longissimus dorsi muscles with a pencil to produce muscular contraction and lateral flexion of the thoracic and lumbar spine is a useful technique. Normally, there should be no marked resentment to this test unless there is some painful muscle involvement. If some chronic bony or muscular problem is present in the midback, then a reluctance or difficulty in lateral flexion in one or both directions is often seen.

Aids to Diagnosis: While a thorough knowledge of musculoskeletal anatomy and physiology is essential for the diagnosis of lameness, it frequently is insufficient in itself. Additional techniques may be required; some require expensive equipment and experienced personnel, and are available only in large or institutional practices.

Local Anesthesia: Selective nerve blocks and intra-articular anesthesia are of primary assistance in confirming the site or region causing lameness in large animals. Experience and an accurate knowledge of topographical anatomy is essential, and the site should always be disinfected thoroughly. The procedure should be done systematically, beginning with the palmar digital nerves to desensitize the caudal part of the foot and sole, then gradually working up the limb proximally.

Radiology: In small animals, radiography is usually done after a careful clinical examination. In horses, radiography should not be done until the site of lameness has been confirmed by local anesthesia. A number of radiographic views help ensure accurate evaluation; the extent of any changes help establish the prognosis. (*See also* p 953.)

Ultrasonography: This is well established for assessment of soft tissues, and complements radiography. Proper interpretation requires complete knowledge of anatomy, and experience. It has become particularly valuable in horses for diagnosis and prognosis of tendinitis (bowed tendons) and desmitis (suspensory ligament strain). (*See also* p 957.)

Bone Scintigraphy: A means of detecting bone turnover and new bone formation that involves IV administration of radioactive material. Areas of increased radioactivity indicate bone growth, active bone damage, or fracture healing. The technique has become established in the diagnosis of obscure lameness and in monitoring the progress of lameness.

Arthroscopy: Endoscopy of joints enables accurate evaluation of the synovial membrane, articular cartilage, intra-articular ligaments, and menisci. It is a valuable tool in both diagnosis and treatment of orthopedic conditions in horses. The technique is being used increasingly in small animals.

Synovial Fluid Analysis: Collection and analysis of synovia for cytology, viscosity, protein, hyaluronic acid, cartilage degradation products, and certain enzymes can provide useful information about joint effusion, synovitis, and septic arthritis. It is the most reliable way of distinguishing between traumatic and/or septic processes in a joint.

Clinical Pathology: Measurement of the muscle-derived enzymes (CPK [also called creatine kinase], lactic dehydrogenase, and AST [SGOT]) can assist in the diagnosis of lameness or other musculoskeletal problems due to muscular disease or trauma.

Faradism: Rhythmically surged faradic current to induce contractions of specific muscle groups has been used in both diagnosis and treatment of muscle damage. However, the value of the method appears to vary directly with the ability of the operator.

Electromyography (EMG): This technique greatly facilitates the investigation of peripheral nerves, their insertions into muscles, and the muscles themselves. Needle electrodes inserted into the muscle are used to localize a lesion or to aid in identifying primary muscular disease. Changes in the electromyograph result from denervation and myopathies. By nerve stimulation, the severity and prognosis of a neuropathy can be assessed.

Muscle Biopsy: In horses, muscle biopsy samples can be taken by a simple percutaneous technique. Histological examination is being used for diagnosis, as well as for the evaluation of fitness and performance potential. Special histochemical techniques are used to determine fiber types as well as glycogen and various enzyme concentrations that are altered by exercise and training.

Thermography: Graphic imaging of temperature gradients of the skin is valuable for early detection of pathological changes, often before clinical signs become apparent. Thermograms of both limbs must always be obtained for comparison.

Gait Analysis: High-speed cinematography can be used to record and study the movements of horses at different speeds and gaits (kinesiology). Computerized film and video analyses now permit a much more complete and rapid assessment of gait and performance. Associated techniques in gait analysis include: 1) electrogoniometry, which provides the continuous recording of joint motion to determine patterns of joint movement, the range and amplitude of motion, angular velocities and accelerations, and swing support and total stride times; and 2) dynamography, which involves the use of force plates to directly measure the locomotive forces exerted by the foot on the ground or by specially designed shoes. The high-speed treadmill is augmenting the clinical application of gait analysis technology, and may become a standard method of analyzing and diagnosing gait abnormalities and lamenesses in racehorses and sporting animals of all kinds.

LAMENESS IN CATTLE

Lameness reduces performance in both beef and dairy cattle; it has a negative influence on feed intake and conversion, body weight, milk production, sexual activity, fertility and, in some instances, longevity.

Recent developments in breeding, feeding, and management practices have contributed to an increased incidence of lameness. Selection based on conformational characteristics can be counterproductive to functional efficiency. Prominent among these is lack of angulation of the limbs, which does not permit the tendons, ligaments, and muscles to assist in absorbing concussion and stress in the limbs.

Feeding high-energy rations deficient in adequate quality fiber is believed to cause softer-than-normal hoof horn, which wears, erodes, disintegrates, and is more easily traumatized than normal horn. Rapid growth in animals <18 mo old, inadequate exercise, and psychosomatic stress may exacerbate the predisposing causes of lameness. Certain types of flooring, both slatted and solid concrete, and cubicle and stanchion design can contribute to the managemental stress. Regular hoof trimming and use of "foot baths" are positive aspects of management. Lameness in cattle should be studied from an epidemiological perspective; a complete history of the herd should be considered.

As with most diseases, successful treatment, prevention, and control depend on accurate diagnosis. Observation from a distance while an animal is standing and moving yields valuable information. Abnormal posture and gait should not be confused with conformational defects. The diagnostician should be familiar with acquired physical changes in the musculoskeletal system, eg, swelling of the limbs, inflammatory reactions around the digital region, and distortions or defects of the hooves. Palpation or auscultation of a joint may be helpful. Rectal palpation is appropriate if pelvic abnormality is suspected. (*See also* DISEASES OF THE SPINAL COLUMN AND CORD, p 584.)

Since ~90% of lesions that cause lameness occur in the digital region, this area should be given special attention, even if the cause appears to be located elsewhere in the limb. The interdigital space, the coronary band, and the sole should be examined in every case. Every discoloration or break in the sole, white line, and wall must be investigated thoroughly. Using appropriate techniques, the limbs can be lifted in dairy cattle and some tranquilized beef cattle. A tipping table may be required. Xylazine hydrochloride is used extensively to sedate animals that are difficult to control, although it is not officially approved for use in cattle. Radiography, arthrocentesis, and regional nerve blocks may be required to confirm a diagnosis. (*See also* the section [MUS] table of contents, pp 460-465, for related topics, eg, MYOPATHIES; ARTHRITIS AND RELATED DISORDERS, LG AN; CONGENITAL ANOMALIES; and RUPTURE OF THE ACHILLES TENDON.)

Lameness may be secondary to or accompany numerous diseases such as bovine viral diarrhea; foot-and-mouth disease; mastitis; avitaminosis A, E, or D; ketosis; deficiency of calcium, phosphorus, or copper; photosensitization; intoxication with fescue, fluoride, or ergot; mycotic stomatitis; malignant catarrhal fever; and lymphocytoma. Recovery follows successful treatment of the primary disease. (*See also* THE DOWNER COW, p 555.)

CALVING PARALYSIS
("Obturator paralysis")

Paresis or paralysis of the adductor and caudal thigh muscles of the hindlimbs. The condition is a result of intrapelvic damage, primarily to the ventral branch of the L_6 spinal nerve, a major contributor to the obturator and sciatic nerves; direct obturator nerve damage may also occur. These lesions are most frequently associated with dystocia.

The signs are paralysis, paresis, or ataxia of one or both hindlimbs. The condition is most common in cows, but other species also may be affected. Nerve injury occurs when the fetus lies in the pelvic canal for an extended period, or a large fetus is forced through the pelvic canal. There is nearly always some degree of hindlimb paresis, ataxia, or paralysis in cows when a "hip lock" exists for >1 hr; severity ranges from slight difficulty in rising for a few days to permanent paralysis.

Paresis or paralysis of the muscles of the hindlimbs results in ataxia or inability to stand; flexion of the fetlock may be noted. The cow may lie on her sternum with the hindlegs in extreme abduction or held parallel with the body. Usually, after a few days, she is able to "creep", and then rise and walk with short choppy strides, only to fall frequently, with fetlock joints flexed and limbs abducted. Paralyzed cows are bright and alert in contrast to those with other postparturient diseases such as milk fever, acute mastitis, or metritis. The condition should be differentiated from fractures, muscle trauma, tumors, and abscesses involving the pelvic nerves and posterior spinal cord. Paralyzed animals may develop pressure ischemic myopathy, found in the thigh muscles of many "downer cows" within 6 hr of recumbency. The danger of ischemic myopathy can be reduced by turning the cow from side to side q2hr and using soft bedding.

Usually, history and signs allow a diagnosis. If the cow is not fully alert, cautious administration of calcium gluconate can rule out milk fever (qv, p 451). *See also* THE DOWNER COW, p 555, for other diagnostic possibilities and for treatment.

Calving paralysis can be prevented by early cesarian section or fetotomy, before prolonged or brutal fetal passage through the pelvic canal has occurred.

CORNS
(Hyperplasia interdigitalis)

Interdigital growths occur in both beef and dairy cattle, but the incidence is much higher in beef cattle. Hereditary predisposition and overfinishing appear to be the basic causes. Stretching of the distal interphalangeal (cruciate) ligament occurs with exostosis formation on the axial surface of the intermediate phalanx.

Corns begin with a ventral out-pouching of the interdigital fat, followed by thickening of the skin. As the mass projects downward, it is compressed between the claws and irritated by contact with the ground and foreign objects. This continual irritation stimulates further enlargement, and walking becomes extremely painful as the mass increases in size. Eventually, it may become one-fourth the size of a claw. Usually, ≥2 feet are affected.

The mass of connective tissue projecting downward between the claws usually is not difficult to diagnose, but it must be differentiated from a primary wound infection, and from dermatitis verrucosa (*see* below).

Surgical excision, combined with immobilization of the digits is usually successful for treatment. Cryosurgery also has been effective.

DEGENERATIVE ARTHROPATHY
(Degenerative joint disease, Osteoarthritis)

A nonspecific condition affecting mainly the hip and stifle, and characterized by degeneration of articular cartilage and eburnation of subchondral bone, joint effusion, fibrosis with calcification of the joint capsule, and osteophytes.

Many causes and predisposing factors probably influence the development, age of onset, and severity. Inherited predisposition to degenerative arthropathy occurs. Certain conformations, eg, straight hocks in beef bulls, are incriminated. Joint instability following trauma is a common cause. Nutritional factors involved in some cases are high-phosphorus and low-calcium rations, which probably influence the strength of subchondral bone. Copper deficiency or fluoride poisoning also may act similarly. Forced traction of a calf in breech presentation can embarrass the blood supply to the hip joint and arthritis may result. The role of infection is unclear. Infectious arthritis in calves usually produces severe changes in the hock, but degenerative arthropathy rarely involves this joint.

Bulls fed for show on high-grain diets may become lame when as young as 6-12 mo, but most cases are first noticed at 1-2 yr. Onset is gradual and usually affects both hip joints; stifle involvement is rare. Signs progress concomitantly with degeneration of cartilage and development of osteophytes. Lameness to the point of incapacitation, with crepitation of degenerate joints, may develop in a few months; however, correlation between pathological changes and clinical signs is poor. The earliest changes occur in the acetabulum and on the dorsomedial surface of the femoral head.

In cows, the stifle is affected most often, and the medial condyle of the femur shows the earliest changes. Onset of signs is later than in bulls, usually occurring in adults. Since degenerative arthropathy may result from any of several initiating factors, a specific diagnosis may be difficult. Radiographic, cytologic, and microbiologic evaluation of the synovial fluid are useful diagnostic aids. Arthroscopy of articular surfaces and ligaments may help attain a definitive diagnosis and prognosis.

Changes in the joints are usually irreversible by the time the diagnosis is made. Palliative treatment in valuable breeding animals should be undertaken with the knowledge that the condition or predisposing factors may be inherited. The diet should be carefully inspected, analyzed and, if necessary, corrected. This is especially important in fast-growing animals, in which adequate exercise is indicated and overfinishing should be avoided.

DERMATITIS VERRUCOSA
(Verrucosa granulosa)

A proliferative lesion of the skin just anterior and posterior to the interdigital space, nearly always of the hindfeet. Usually only one animal is affected, but on rare occasions, it may become a herd problem, usually if the lot is filthy. Numerous bacteria have been cultured from the lesions; if it becomes a herd problem, a viral etiology should be considered.

Initially, there is chronic irritation of the skin due to poor lot conditions, followed by proliferation of the epidermal cells and underlying fibrous connective tissues. Histological lesions include dermatitis, hyperkeratosis, and papilloma. A cauliflower-like mass appears, which eventually may invade the interdigital space. The mass gradually increases in size and becomes roughened on the surface, with cilia- or finger-like projections. Similar lesions also may appear just beneath the dewclaws. Lameness is only slight until after several months, when the lesions have become large and abraded. The location and rough cilia-like surface help to differentiate this condition from corns (*see* above).

Surgical removal and cauterization of the underlying tissue with antimony trichloride or copper sulfate is the preferred treatment. Cryosurgery of the lesion is also effective. When numerous animals in a herd are affected, commercial or autogenous wart vaccines may be indicated.

DISLOCATIONS

Coxofemoral dislocation and stifle injuries are often the result of allowing cows in estrus to remain with a herd that is confined on a slippery surface. Bulls serving cows in such an environment, and cows riding each other are likely to damage these joints. Resolution of an upward luxation of the coxofemoral joint is possible, provided that the head of the femur or the rim of the acetabulum has not been fractured; correction of stifle injuries has had limited success in both cows and bulls.

Dislocation of the fetlock occurs frequently in young cattle when they cross cattle guards (grillwork laid over a pit as a gate substitute). Tranquilization or light anesthesia facilitates replacement of dislocated structures. A padded fiberglass cast maintained in place for 3 wk usually promotes a satisfactory recovery.

Traumatic dislocation of the tibiotarsal joint has a good prognosis if the small tarsal bones are not fractured or prolapsed. General anesthesia is necessary to permit sufficient muscle relaxation to allow manual reduction. (*See also* PATELLAR LUXATION, p 560.)

ERGOTISM

A disease of cattle and other farm animals due to continued ingestion of sclerotia of the parasitic fungus *Claviceps purpurea*. Lameness is the first sign. (*See also* p 1684.)

FESCUE LAMENESS
(Fescue foot)

A dry gangrene of the extremities caused by consumption of toxic tall fescue, *Festuca arundinacea*. (*See also* FESCUE POISONING, p 1687.) Reliable reports of fescue lameness have come from many states in the USA, as well as New Zealand, Australia, and Italy.

The first signs develop within 10-14 days of grazing on tall fescue grass. There is local heat, swelling, severe pain, and lameness of one or more feet. Usually, a hindfoot is affected first. With continued feeding on fescue, an indented line appears at some point, usually between the hock and the claws. Dry gangrene affects the distal part, which eventually may slough. Low environmental temperature is thought to contribute to the severity of the lesions. Affected animals usually have a fever, seek shade in warm weather, and stand in water if it is available. At necropsy, there are few (if any) lesions other than those associated with the swelling or dry gangrene, although abdominal fat necrosis has been reported.

Lameness; poor condition; dry gangrene of distal extremities of the ears, tail, and feet; and a history of grazing tall fescue are diagnostic.

There is no satisfactory treatment, but it may be helpful to supplement fescue forage with grain. Application of high-nitrogen fertilizer to established stands of fescue should be avoided. Supplying other feed results in recovery if the lesions have not progressed to dry gangrene, and the animals are kept warm. Risk of fescue lameness is reduced by maintaining legumes in the sward since the tall fescue will not be consumed in large amounts when other forage is available. Endophyte-free seed should be used when establishing new pastures. Tall fescue varieties with reduced endophytic fungus infestations have been developed.

FOREIGN BODY PENETRATION OF THE SOLE

This most common foot injury in cattle occurs when a sharp object, eg, nail, wire, or glass, penetrates the sole. Lameness occurs immediately if the foreign body remains in place and continues to press on the nerve endings of the corium of the hoof. If an infection of the corium occurs before the foreign body is dislodged, an abscess forms at the point of penetration. If the abscess is located in the anterior region of the sole, onset of lameness is rapid, and pain is severe. When the infection is in the posterior aspect of the sole, the onset is slower and less severe; natural release of pus at the coronary band may occur.

An abscess may be detected by exerting pressure on the sole with pincers. More often, the sole must be pared to reveal either the foreign body or the track to the abscess. For treatment, the foreign body is removed and the tract probed to determine its extent. Exploration should continue until adequate drainage is provided, but destruction of healthy tissue must be minimized. The injury should be cleansed and dressed with an antibiotic, preferably in powder form. The affected digit may be enclosed in a small plastic bag that is retained in position and protected by a strong adhesive bandage. If the opening on the sole is located within 2 cm of the abaxial wall, a portion of the wall may be removed to permit drainage laterally; this creates a self-draining surface. Parenteral administration of penicillin is appropriate for 2-3 days at 10,000 u/lb (22,000 u/kg) body wt.

FRACTURES

Although bone fractures occur in cattle of all ages, they are most common in those <1 yr old. Appropriate procedures may be justified economically in this age group, provided that joints are not involved. External fixation techniques and/or a Thomas splint may be used successfully. In selected cases, percutaneous transfixation or internal fixation may be attempted.

Fractures of major long bones in adult cattle usually are not treated. Fracture of the tuber coxae may occur when cattle are hurried through narrow doorways. In these cases, spicules of bone may penetrate the skin or unsightly distortions of the flank can result. Fractures of the proximal and intermediate phalanges may be considered for treatment in tractable, young adult cattle.

Fracture of the distal phalanx is a relatively common fracture of adult cattle. Onset of lameness is rapid and the pain usually are severe. If the medial digit is involved, the animal may seek relief from the pain by crossing its legs. Natural recovery is prolonged, and because most such fractures occur into the distal interphalangeal joint, a debilitating arthritis may initiate at the fracture site. If this lesion is treated, the sound digit should be elevated on a wooden block, and the affected digit immobilized in a flexed position to the block using methyl methacrylate adhesive.

The risk of fractures is minimized if the most common causes are avoided. Slippery surfaces are hazardous, particularly to animals in estrus. Narrow doorways should be avoided for the passage of several animals at any one time.

FROSTBITE
(Hypothermia)

A calf born into an environment with a windchill factor of <0°F (-18°C) is at risk. A weak calf, born to an exhausted cow after a long labor in a cold and windy environment (eg, a temperature of 20°F [-7°C] and a wind of 30 mph [50 km/hr] making a wind chill factor of -20°F [-29°C]), can suffer frostbite of the feet and other extremities.

After several days, the calf becomes reluctant to follow its dam and to stand, but has a normal appetite. Inspection of a severely affected calf reveals a crusted muzzle, devitalized ear tips and tail end, and cold hindfeet. The hindfeet are usually affected, because they are placed away from the body when the calf lies down, while the front feet are placed under the body and protected from the cold by body heat. Several days to weeks later, the devitalized tissue (including the hooves) begins to slough, and the calf refuses to stand. (*See also* p 627). The major diagnostic problem is differentiation from fescue toxicity (qv, p 1687). Age of the animal, and temperature and windchill on the day of birth verify the diagnosis. Once signs are apparent, there is no treatment.

HOOF WALL FISSURES

The incidence of both vertical and horizontal fissures (fractures, cracks) of the hoof wall is increasing. Although it may not be identifiable, there is nearly always some predisposing impairment of the hoof wall, such as a conformational defect, perhaps due to faulty feeding; the one exception is a laceration. When a fissure is found in one claw, the corresponding claw on the opposite foot should be examined as well.

VERTICAL FISSURES
(Fissura ungulae longitudinalis, Sandcrack)

These occur on the dorsal and dorsoabaxial surface of the hoof wall. The brittleness of the hoof that precedes appearance of this condition is caused by water loss from the hoof horn, which occurs when the periople is absent. The periople is the waterproof stratum externum of the hoof, which diminishes with age, and is lost due to mechanical abrasion on sandy soils. Some believe that inappropriate nutrition (zinc deficiency) is implicated in the etiology.

Large sandcracks can occur on all 8 digits without any sign of lameness. Very small sandcracks that involve only the coronary band can be much more of a problem. The horn of the band is soft and flexible. As the animal moves, the pressures created can open the fissure sufficiently to permit infection to reach the structures beneath. The most serious sequela is an infected distal interphalangeal joint. Because a small sandcrack can be obscured easily, especially by mud, palpation of the coronary band should be a routine procedure.

Large sandcracks rarely need attention, but occasionally cosmetic care is requested. In these instances, the broken horn should be removed, and the crack filled with methyl methacrylate. Embedding staples is also useful. The proximal end of the fissure can be sealed with a hot iron. The loss of water from the hoof horn may be slowed down by applying thick oil or a varnish to the hoof wall.

For a small septic sandcrack of the coronary band, a small portion of the horn overlying the abscess should be removed, and antibiotic powder applied to the wound beneath. A small gauze dressing should be placed over the wound and held tightly in place with a 1 in. (2.5 cm) adhesive bandage around the coronary band.

HORIZONTAL FISSURES
(Fissura ungulae horizontalis, Thimbling)

These fissures occur primarily in mature dairy cattle following laminitis. Continuity of the hoof wall is lost in a plane parallel to the coronet. Usually all 8 claws are affected. The condition frequently follows a severe systemic illness that is accompanied by a marked fever. Nutritional and metabolic disturbances also may be basic causes. During active disease, a poor quality of hoof develops at the coronary band.

Initially, there may be some inflammation at the coronary band and slight lameness or stiffness. Despite apparent recovery, a depression in the hoof wall, encircling it except at the heel, soon becomes evident. Several months to ~1 yr later, when the grooved area has grown to within several centimeters of the sole, the hoof distal to the groove separates due to weight bearing and leverage on the toe. The separated portion appears as a thimble placed on the hoof, and movement of this portion causes a horizontal fissure to develop and penetrate the underlying sensitive tissues. The signs are pathognomonic.

Treatment consists of removing as much of the distal portion of hoof as possible without entering the sensitive tissue. After several weeks or months, new hoof extends and recovery occurs.

LAMINITIS
(Founder, Pododermatitis aseptica diffusa, PAD)

Many lesions of the hoof are associated with laminitis, which compromises the quality of the horn of the hoof and renders it susceptible to damage and erosion. The chronic form of laminitis is referred to as slipper foot. The major cause of laminitis is either a sudden massive ingestion of high-energy feed (acute) or the sustained intake of high levels of carbohydrate (subacute or subclinical). (See also GRAIN OVERLOAD, p 175.)

Dairy cows usually show the first signs of subclinical laminitis immediately after calving. The deterioration in quality of hoof horn predisposes to lesions such as white line disease, sole ulcers, and heel erosions. The sole also wears more rapidly, which makes it more susceptible to trauma.

Feedlot steers also may be affected with acute or subclinical laminitis. The latter form is of little economic importance.

Beef bulls on feeding trials and replacement dairy heifers are highly susceptible to subclinical laminitis. This condition is not clinically evident immediately, but causes pathological changes in the hoof that are seriously counterproductive. The condition is considered to result from lactic acidosis, which causes vasoactive endotoxins to be released from gram-negative organisms. The pathological changes in the microcirculation of the corium cause irreversible damage. Alternative etiologies are being investigated, eg, the role of epidermal growth factor. It is clear that subclinical laminitis has a more complex etiology than was originally believed. Managemental stresses as well as restricted exercise have been implicated.

In acute laminitis, usually there is a history of overconsumption of grain. The animals are reluctant to move and have diarrhea. The posture may be characteristic: all 4 limbs under the body, or fore- and hindlimbs extended forward. The animal may try to walk on its knees. Leg crossing or walking narrow is an indication that only the medial claws are affected. In chronic laminitis, the hooves are long, and turned up at the toes; heavy ridging is present. In subacute laminitis, there are no aberrations of gait or posture. The horn is soft, blood-stained, and has a yellow waxy appearance. The high incidence of mid-lactation lameness and the presence of white line lesions and sole ulcers confirm the diagnosis on a herd basis.

For treatment of acute cases, see GRAIN OVERLOAD, p 175. Trimming the slipper foot of the chronic case of laminitis is palliative at best (see HOOF TRIMMING, p 1111). Subclinical laminitis is extremely common in high-production dairy herds. These cases require special investigations aimed at identifying the relative importance of the epidemiologic factors involved.

Corkscrew claw and slipper foot are 2 deformities that are believed to be hereditary. Resolution of either of these deformities is not possible.

PERONEAL NERVE PARALYSIS

This usually appears shortly after parturition, but may not be related to it; nor is it restricted to adult cows. The cause is trauma or pressure on the peroneal nerve. Injuries at parturition, abscesses, tumors, and vertebral exostoses have been incriminated.

This condition is marked by flexion of the fetlocks and pasterns, and may affect one or both hindlegs. The flexion may be so severe that the animal bears weight on the dorsal surface of these joints; after several days, erosions may appear on these surfaces and suppurative arthritis results. A lameness with fetlocks and pasterns flexed is usually sufficient evidence for diagnosis.

A light plaster-of-paris cast to keep the fetlock and pastern joints extended is effective treatment in most cases, particularly if parturition injuries were the cause.

Tension to keep these joints in extension can be applied by anchoring the toes to webbing or a leather strap, which is placed around the limb just proximal to the hock.

PODODERMATITIS

FOOT ROT
(Interdigital necrobacillosis, Interdigital phlegmon)

The major cause of lameness in beef and dairy cattle of all ages.

Etiology: *Fusobacterium necrophorum* has long been considered the bacterium responsible for this disease, although conclusive evidence is hard to produce. More recently, *Bacteroides nodosus and B melaninogenicus* also have been incriminated. The disease occurs during all seasons, but tends to be most prevalent during wet seasons. However, it has occurred during dry weather when the ground is firm, and also when cattle have access to muddy areas, or have been forced to traverse newly broken land. Probably the hard, dry ground predisposes the interdigital tissue and heels to bruises. Once the skin is broken, the organisms in soil readily infect the wound. One or more feet may be affected at any given time.

Clinical Findings and Diagnosis: Symmetrical edema and erythema of the interdigital region with no evidence of foreign bodies is indicative of this condition. Lameness is severe, body temperature is elevated, and lactation may cease. Eventually, necrosis occurs and longitudinal fissures appear, which reveals a purulent, foul-smelling discharge and central mass of necrotic tissue. When this necrotic tissue is removed or sloughs, healing usually progresses rapidly. In some cases, the infection invades deeper structures and suppurative arthritis develops.

Treatment: Systemic and local treatment with antibiotics and sulfonamides appears to shorten the course of disease. Other procedures that may speed recovery are cleaning the foot, applying a protective dressing, wiring the claws together, and removing the necrotic interdigital mass. Zinc methionine has been recommended for both treatment and prevention. Walking cattle through a 3% formalin foot bath, a 5% copper sulfate foot bath, or mixed powdered copper sulfate and lime b.i.d. decreases the incidence. Oral iodides and zinc compounds have been beneficial as preventives in some cases.

Suppurative arthritis or tenosynovitis is an occasional sequela of foot rot. Surgical removal of an affected claw produces rapid relief, but >80% of cattle that have had a digit removed are culled within 1 yr. Surgical drainage and arthrodesis of the distal interphalangeal joint is worthwhile in valuable breeding cattle if more conservative methods are not successful.

STABLE FOOT ROT
(Interdigital dermatitis, Chronic necrotic pododermatitis)

This is most common under unhygienic conditions and is caused by *Bacteroides nodosus*. It starts as a moist interdigital dermatitis. Secretions ooze to the dorsal commissures of the cleft, where they dry and form a crust. At this point lameness is not present; there is no digital swelling, but the animal paddles from side to side. Up to 60% of the herd can be affected. In a few cases, the infection progresses to cause erosion of the heel. First seen as an ulcer between the cheeks of the bulbs, the condition can progress until the entire bulb is lost. At this stage the animal becomes lame, and complications may result.

Walking the herd through a formalin foot bath (3%) daily for 1 wk reduces the incidence. Improved hygiene is extremely important. The condition usually resolves spontaneously when the animals are turned out on pasture. Individual cases that have progressed to the stage of showing lameness should be isolated on clean bedding, and the affected region treated topically with a 50% mixture of anhydrous copper sulfate and sulfamethazine.

ULCERATION OF THE SOLE
(Pododermatitis circumscripta)

One of the most common causes of lameness in cattle, a sole ulcer is caused by mechanical pressure on the center of the sole at the sole-heel junction. At this point, the proximal process of the distal phalanx is close to the inner aspect of the sole. Therefore, any process that permits the sole to bend under pressure leads to pressure necrosis in the area. When damaged, the corium ceases to produce horn and granulation tissue forms; excessive wear of the sole and/or subclinical laminitis decreases the strength of the sole. Hoof trimming that removes too much abaxial wall leads to weight bearing being transferred from the wall to the center of the sole. If the heels have been eroded completely, weight bearing is transferred forward, and an ulcer can result. An excessive buildup of horn in the central sole, or permitting an animal to walk on a rocky surface, leads to trauma in the area.

Ulceration is seen at the junction of the posterior and middle thirds of the sole, ~0.5 in. (1.25 cm) from the axial border. Most lesions are found in the lateral hind claws, with a tendency for the lesion to be bilateral. The animal frequently stands with the affected legs extended backward. Medial front claws are sometimes affected. In some cases, the ulcer may not be encountered until the overlying sole has been pared away. The typical granulating lesion is usually 0.5 in. (1.25 cm) in diameter.

Corrective hoof trimming is an appropriate first step; rotten horn should be removed carefully from the circumference of the lesion without destroying any normal sole. A wooden block or rubber shoe should be applied to the sound digit. Granulation tissue need not be removed nor any dressing applied; a bandage is contraindicated.

RUPTURE OF THE GASTROCNEMIUS MUSCLE

Rupture of this muscle is relatively rare, but occurs often enough to be of significance. It is most likely to be associated with deficiencies of calcium, phosphorus, and vitamin D. Prolonged recumbency with resulting myositis and struggling to rise occasionally precipitates rupture of one or both of these muscles. Occasionally, the condition has been associated with pyelonephritis, which presumably caused a myositis, and weakened the muscle enough to permit rupture. Injections of irritating medicaments into the gastrocnemius muscle may cause necrosis and rupture.

The hock remains flexed; when completely ruptured, the standing animal rests the hock and distal portion of the limb on the ground or walking surface, which is diagnostic, although rupture of the Achilles tendon (qv, p 561) may produce an identical gait.

Successful treatment is extremely unlikely in heavy adult animals. A leg cast or splint that maintains the hock in extension, supplying adequate vitamins and minerals, and proper nursing may be successful, but a long recovery period is required.

SPASTIC PARESIS
(Elso heel)

A hereditary spastic condition seen in many breeds, most commonly Holstein and Angus. It appears first in one or both hindlimbs at 3 mo to 2 yr. Eventually, both hindlimbs become affected, even though only one initially exhibited signs. The cause is not known. Recent findings provide good evidence that the disease is not transmitted as a simple recessive. CSF contains a reduced amount of phosphorus, calcium, and homovanillic acid, the major metabolite of the neurotransmitter dopamine. AST (SGOT) is lowered and alkaline phosphatase is raised.

Taut gastrocnemius and superficial flexor muscles are characteristic. The hock and stifle are maintained in full extension, and the calcaneus is pulled into close apposition to the distal tibia. This anatomical relationship results in an excessively straight lower limb and a small, weak-appearing hock. Tremulous muscle contractions are evident in the affected limb when the animal is forced to move. The affected limb appears to be shorter and may not touch the ground; it swings as a pendulum when the animal walks or runs. An arched back and elevated tailhead also are often noted. Differential diagnoses include spastic syndrome, gonitis, dorsal luxation of the patella, and progressive posterior paralysis. The age at which first signs appear, the initial unilateral involvement, and the dorsal displacement of the tuber calcaneus are aids in the diagnosis.

Muscle relaxants may give slight temporary relief. Tenotomy of the gastrocnemius tendon and partial or complete tenotomy of the superficial flexor tendon 3-4½ in. (8-12 cm) dorsal to the tuber calcaneous may be beneficial. Tibial neurectomy has produced better results, but there is no real justification for any treatment of breeding animals, since this condition is apparently inherited. Treatment of nonbreeding animals may be justified for humane reasons, while they are being finished for market.

SPASTIC SYNDROME
(Crampy, Krampfigkeit, Stretches)

Intermittent, bilateral, tonic spasms of skeletal muscle groups in standing, older animals, primarily affecting dairy cattle. (*See also* p 593.) Although the cause frequently is listed as a simple autosomal recessive with incomplete penetrance, it is more likely inherited through a multiple gene mechanism. Onset of the syndrome appears to be dependent on and modified by factors such as pain, standing position, fear, and excitement.

Signs first appear when animals are ≥3 yr old. Initially very mild, the signs become progressively more severe over a period of years. They begin with slight muscle spasms that occur in conjunction with sudden movement, walking on a slippery surface, or excitement. Signs are absent in the recumbent animal. In time, spasms of one or both hindlimbs last for several minutes. Severely affected animals raise their head and turn it to the side, which appears to relieve acute attacks. They may elevate a forelimb and extend the hindlegs posteriorly. Occasionally, the hindlegs may be flexed one at a time. Eventually, spastic contraction of muscles extends to the entire body. These severe attacks may come intermittently at weekly or monthly intervals; as they become more frequent and persist for longer periods, slaughter or euthanasia is required.

It is most likely to be confused with tetanus (qv, p 330) and spastic paresis (*see* above). Absence of signs while the animal is recumbent differentiates it from tetanus. History of a gradual onset beginning at ~3 yr of age or more, and the signs, are usually sufficient to differentiate it from spastic paresis.

There is no permanent treatment. Muscle relaxants and CNS depressants provide only minimal, temporary relief.

LAMENESS IN GOATS

Abnormality of gait is a sign common to many diseases and conditions. A complete history is important for diagnosis; it should include incidence and duration in the herd, nutrition, feed changes, method of rearing, and recent introductions to the herd. (*See also* DISEASE-MANAGEMENT INTERACTION: GOATS, p 1114.)

The hoof of the affected leg(s) should be examined, and excess horn material removed to leave a level weight-bearing surface. If the feet have not been trimmed for a long period, or the goats have been on soft ground or bedding, excess horn commonly overgrows from the walls, toes, and heels, and folds over the sole. With severe neglect, "turkish slipper"-type hooves (elongated toes) may cause the goat to walk on its heels. During foot paring, any portion of the horn that is abnormally thickened, any underrunning of the heel or sole, any abnormal wear of one claw, or any abnormal or necrotic smell should be noted.

After paring, the feet should be scrubbed clean and inspected for puncture wounds, foreign bodies (eg, stones or clover burrs caught in the interdigital area), or pus from a discharging abscess—especially about the coronet.

The rest of the leg should be palpated carefully, including the bones, tendons, and muscles. Any muscle atrophy or restriction of movement should be noted. The joints also should be checked for heat, swelling, or pain.

If the clinical examination fails to identify a definite diagnosis, it may be necessary to aseptically collect some joint fluid from an affected joint (usually the carpus) for Gram stain and culture and sensitivity tests.

If the joint fluid contains pus alone, or gram-positive bacteria, this indicates joint-ill; fibrin alone suggests joint-ill or *Chlamydia* sp; fibrin and pus combined suggest *Mycoplasma* spp; clear or cloudy joint fluid with many mononuclear cells suggests CAE virus (qv, p 393) or *Erysipelothrix* sp. A blood sample may also be useful. In joint-ill or erysipelas, the WBC count is high, with neutrophilia. In laminitis, the eosinophil count may be normal or high. Blood calcium, phosphorus, and vitamin D levels may help diagnose bent leg, although these often return to normal before the affected goat is examined. If CAE is suspected, titers may be taken; however, false negatives may occur during severe stress, and positive titers may be coincidental to another cause of lameness if serological incidence is high in the herd of origin.

Radiography may be helpful. In "bent leg", the growth plates should be checked; there is also lateral deviation of the radii and occasionally thinness of the bone. In CAE virus infection, the initial swelling of the soft tissue surrounding the affected joint is followed by calcium deposits in the swollen periarticular tissue, joint capsule, ligaments, tendons, tendon sheaths, and finally the muscle bellies. Later changes consist of mild periarticular oesteophyte production, joint mice, and rough extensions of the periarticular bone proximally and distally.

Some of the more important conditions that cause lameness in goats are discussed below. *See also* THE TABLE OF CONTENTS, p 460.

BENT LEG
(Epiphysitis)

A calcium:phosphorus imbalance of young, rapidly growing kids, more often in males than in females; and in young does in the later stages of their first pregnancy or in the early stages of their first lactation. These does are either young (eg, 12 mo), extremely heavy milkers, or carrying twins or triplets. Bent leg is sometimes compounded by rickets (qv, p 487).

Clinical Findings and Diagnosis: Bent leg starts with lateral or medial bowing of one or both radii. Later changes may consist of lateral deviation of the fore or hind digits; lameness and reluctance to walk; an arched back; and soft swelling and pain in the carpal, metacarpophalangeal, tarsal, and metatarsophalangeal joints. Diagnosis can be confirmed with radiography.

Conditions that have been implicated in the cause include: an excess of dietary calcium with a ratio of calcium:phosphorus of >1.4:1 (generally >1.8:1), excess protein intake (has caused epiphysitis in other species), excess dietary iron (has reduced serum phosphorus levels in lambs by decreasing vitamin D metabolite formation), and housing of kids or lack of vitamin D caused by prolonged overcast weather and low vitamin D levels in the feed. Lush green feed, seed, and seed by-products have low vitamin D levels. Carotene has an antivitamin D effect. Vitamin D has poor stability in prepared feed, especially when mixed with minerals. Alfalfa is high in calcium (1.4% calcium to 0.2% phosphorus) and protein. Owners frequently keep kids on fresh milk for prolonged periods since they often have no commercial outlet for the milk.

Treatment and Control: Once the probable cause(s) is identified, the diet should be corrected and the appropriate supplement given. This is usually injectable vitamin D and phosphorus and/or oral balanced calcium/phosphorus supplements.

Predisposing factors must be corrected also. The diet of growing kids should be changed to slow their growth rates. The mating of very young does should be discouraged. Buck kids should be separated from doe kids when 3-4 mo old. Young does in milk with limb deformities should be managed so that full lactation is discouraged, eg, by not milking out fully and drying off as early as possible.

Treatment stops any worsening of limb deformities and should improve them to a great extent; however, a return to completely normal limbs is rare.

CONTRACTED TENDONS IN KIDS

A usually bilateral, congenital condition that is a genetic defect in Angoras in Australasia. It is due to a recessive autosomal allele that must reach a certain level before affected animals appear; the time between purchase of a carrier buck and appearance of affected kids may be 5-6 generations. Either the fore- or hindlimbs are affected. In rare cases, only one foreleg is twisted. In severe cases the kid is unable to stand, or walks on its fetlocks. In less severe cases, it may move relatively easily with permanently partly flexed fetlocks. In mild cases, the limbs may be splinted gradually straighter and straighter until the kid is able to bear weight on its feet.

In Anglo-Nubians in the USA, Canada, Australia, and New Zealand, there is a similar genetic condition called β-mannosidosis. At birth, these kids have varying degrees of fixed flexion of the forelimbs and fixed extension of the hindlimbs. They can see and bleat, and suckle if held up to the teat. Their withdrawal reflexes are normal or depressed, and there is intention tremor, especially of the head. There may be nystagmus, deafness, and facial abnormalities.

There are no gross abnormalities at necropsy, although cutting the tendons allows free movement of the limbs. Histology reveals a typical storage disease. Affected kids have no plasma levels of β-mannosidase, and both parents have half of the normal range.

COPPER DEFICIENCY

This can cause problems similar to those in cattle (*see* pp 1197 and 596).

FOOT ROT/FOOT SCALD

Both conditions are serious problems of goats and other species (*see* pp 501 and 541).

JOINT-ILL

A nonspecific bacterial infection of several joints of kids. Bacteria that have been incriminated are mainly gram positive, and include staphylococci, streptococci, *Corynebacterium* spp, and coliforms. *Erysipelothrix rhusiopathiae* also causes joint-ill although it is uncommon in goats, and when it does occur, it is mainly in 3- to 4-mo-old kids.

Environmental bacteria gain entry to the neonate's circulation, usually via the umbilical cord. Other methods of entry include contamination of breaks in the skin, or via the GI or respiratory tract. Predisposing factors include lack of routine dipping of the umbilical cord, poor sanitation in the kidding pens, or does kidding in overcrowded dirty conditions. *Erysipelothrix rhusiopathiae* are soil-living bacteria that may persist on farms or in pens used by sheep or pigs. Mycoplasma infection is also a differential diagnosis.

Clinical Findings: More than one joint is hot, swollen, and painful. Often, the affected limb(s) will not bear weight. Kids with >1 leg affected may be unable to stand. The more commonly affected joints are the carpus, shoulder, hock, and stifle. Generally, there is a fever but no reduction in appetite. Sometimes the navel area is inflamed, but often there is no visible abnormality. An abscess may form on the navel long after the kid has recovered. There is an increased WBC count with a left shift.

If the condition becomes chronic, the limbs are stiff, some joints may be ankylosed, and overall growth is poor. At this stage the temperature is normal.

Treatment: To be successful, treatment must be given as early as possible. Frequent injections of high doses of antibiotics given for ~1 wk often effect a cure if combined with careful nursing. Penicillin and its derivatives are the drugs of choice for erysipelas. Complications should be prevented by providing soft bedding, frequently turning any kid unable to stand, and massaging the affected joints. If ankylosis starts to develop, the kid should be supported in a sling for short periods as frequently as possible.

In large commercial herds, treating severely affected kids may not be economically justified; many that do recover remain unthrifty for the rest of their lives.

Control: Hygiene at parturition is essential. A deep bed of clean sawdust, wood shavings, or straw should be provided; it is often better to allow the doe to kid on fresh pasture if the weather is warm.

The umbilical cords of newborn kids should be dipped several times in a strong antiseptic, eg, Lugol's solution or iodophor teat dip. Cords should be dipped each time the kid is handled in the first 24-48 hr. Does frequently lick and bite the umbilical cord for several hours after the birth. Owners should clean their footwear before entering kidding pens.

LAMINITIS
(Founder)

A worldwide problem, the incidence in goats is lower than in dairy cattle and horses. Predisposing causes include overeating or sudden access to concentrates, high-grain and low-roughage diets, and/or high-protein diets. Laminitis can also occur as a complication of acute infections such as mastitis, metritis, or pneumonia, especially after kidding.

When severe, the affected goat is lame, reluctant to move, has a fever, and all 4 feet are hot to the touch. Touching the coronet elicits a severe pain reaction. In slightly less severe cases, only the forefeet are affected. Laminitis can become chronic if the initial phase is not diagnosed or treated successfully. The onset is insidious, but eventually the goat is observed walking on its knees, with "sled-runner" deformities of its hooves.

In acute laminitis, the primary condition, if any, must be treated promptly. The laminitis is treated with antihistamines, IV, t.i.d. After the first 12 hr, corticosteroids are useful; however, their use is contraindicated in pregnant does. Analgesics (eg, phenylbutazone 2-4 mg/kg, flunixin meglumine 1.1 mg/kg, or aspirin 30-100 mg/kg) daily, and hosing or soaking the affected feet is useful. Chronic laminitis with deformed hooves is treated by routine vigorous foot trimming.

MYCOPLASMOSIS

See also pp 658 and 754. Kids infected with *Mycoplasma mycoides* subsp *mycoides* (large colony variant [LC]) may show severe lameness with multiple hot swollen joints, weight loss, pyrexia, and poor coats. Some have diarrhea, and some have increased lung sounds and respiratory rates. Affected kids are generally 2-4 wk old. Morbidity and mortality rates of 90 and 30%, respectively, have been recorded.

TRAUMA/PAIN

Goats, in general, are very agile creatures, but if frightened they may attempt impossible jumps, with resultant fractures or other injuries. Yards designed for goats that are infrequently handled should have a visual as well as physical barrier. Fortunately, most fractures of the lower limbs heal rapidly with normal casting. Shearing of Angoras is a source of potential problems, eg, when the shearer's comb cuts into or through the Achilles tendon. Orthopedic procedures suitable for large dogs can be used.

Some IM injections can cause problems; eg, mixed clostridial vaccines can cause severe soft-tissue swelling and lameness for ≥48 hr, and irritant drugs can damage nearby nerves and cause lameness. In some cases of severe mastitis, especially gangrenous, there is a hindlimb lameness on the affected side. The doe changes her gait due to the swelling and pain in the udder. Aspirin, phenylbutazone, or flunixine meglumine are suggested as analgesics.

WHITE MUSCLE DISEASE

See also p 548. Most affected kids have been in good condition and 2-3 mo old (range 1 wk to 4 mo). Commonly, sudden death is associated with cardiac muscle damage. Other kids are depressed, reluctant to move, and appear stiff with a "saw-horse" stance. Muscles, especially of the hindlimbs, are firm and painful to the touch.

LAMENESS IN HORSES

See also LAMENESS, GENERAL PRINCIPLES, p 490.

CONDITIONS OF THE FOOT

BONE CYST IN PEDAL BONE

A large cyst in the pedal bone produces a chronic lameness that may be severe and is unresponsive to anti-inflammatory medication. This uncommon condition may be seen in any foot, but is more often in a hindfoot. There is no apparent age, breed, or sex predisposition. It is assumed to be traumatic in origin and not part of the osteochondrosis syndrome. Cystic demineralization can accompany prolonged subsolar abscesses. The cyst may communicate with the distal phalangeal joint. Multiple cysts are sometimes present; they may enlarge and eventually involve a large part of the pedal bone. Diagnosis is confirmed by volar nerve block and radiography. Differential diagnoses include keratoma, navicular disease, pedal osteitis, and pedal bone abscess. Surgical treatment is not always successful because of the site and size of the lesion. Secondary fracture of the pedal bone can occur due to progressive weakening of the bone. Some horses do return to performance status, and others are salvaged for alternative uses such as breeding.

BRUISED SOLE AND CORNS

Bruising on the volar surface of the foot usually is caused by direct injury from stones, irregular ground, or other trauma. Poor shoeing, especially in animals with flat feet or dropped soles, predisposes to bruising, usually around the periphery of the sole. Bruising may or may not be associated with lameness, but if it becomes chronic, the affected area can become infected. Persistent, nonresponsive bruised sole suggests pedal osteitis.

A "corn" is a specific type of bruising that occurs in the sole at the buttress (ie, the angle between the wall and the bar). It is most common in the forefeet on the inner buttress and is usually associated with the heel of a shoe that was improperly placed or left on too long and caused pressure on the sole. Shoes that have been fitted too closely at the quarters can also cause corns. Faulty foot conformation, straight walls that tend to turn in at the quarters, or contracted feet may predispose to corns. Other causes include excess trimming of the sole (which exposes the sensitive tissue to contusion) or neglect of the feet to the extent that they become long and irregular.

Corns are described as "dry" when only mild inflammatory changes exist, as "moist" when there is excess inflammatory exudate, and as "suppurative" once they become secondarily infected.

When the foot is raised and the solar surface freed of dirt and loose horn, a discoloration, either red or reddish yellow, is noted. Supporting-leg lameness is an early sign, but lameness is not always seen. Tapping with a light hammer over the area or applying pressure with a hoof tester usually causes discomfort. If infection is present, pain is pronounced when pressure is applied with hoof testers; if not promptly treated, a tract may extend through to the coronet to produce a suppurating sinus.

The prognosis is favorable. In uncomplicated dry corns, relief from pressure on the affected area is the first consideration. This can be achieved by shortening the toe if it is too long, and by applying a bar shoe to promote frog pressure. A three-quarter-bar shoe may be of value in relieving pressure.

If the corn is suppurating, it should be drained at once by a surgical opening directly through the sole. Following drainage, the foot should be dressed to permit drainage. Hot foot baths and poultices may be helpful. The horse should be kept in a dry, clean box stall. After infection is controlled, the cavity can be packed with sterile gauze and topical antibiotic ointment, and a metal, rubber, or leather sole placed between the shoe and the foot. Parenteral antibacterial therapy is of questionable value unless systemic illness is present.

CANKER

A chronic hypertrophy and apparent suppuration of the horn-producing tissues of the foot, involving the frog and the sole. The cause is unknown. Primarily a disease of the heavy draft horse, it is seldom seen today, although certain stables of light horses in the southern USA have had frequent occurrences. It is most often found in the hindfeet and is frequently well advanced before detection. The frog may appear to be intact but has a ragged, oiled appearance. The horn tissue of the frog loosens easily, and reveals a swollen, foul-smelling corium covered with a caseous exudate. The surface of the corium is irregular with a characteristic vegetative growth. The disease process may extend to the sole and even to the wall, showing no tendency to heal.

The prognosis is guarded. Treatment must be radical and intensive. All loose horn and affected tissue should be removed, and an antiseptic or antibiotic dressing applied daily. A clean, dry wound environment must be maintained to allow healing, which may take weeks or months. Waterproof materials and plastic boots are used for such purposes. If the horse is not lame, it can be returned to work during the period of healing by use of a special shoe with a removable sole plate to maintain the dressing.

CONTRACTED HEELS

Seen principally in the front feet of light horses, this may be caused by improper shoeing that draws in the quarters, which prevents hoof expansion and adequate frog pressure. Dry hooves, excess rasping of the wall, and trimming of the bars are pedisposing factors. It may follow the use of a hoof-immobilizing shoe, as used for fracture of the third phalanx.

The frog is narrow and shrunken, the bars may be curved or almost parallel to each other, and the quarters and heels are markedly contracted and drawn in. The hoof horn is dry and hard. Lameness is evident when the horse is worked at speed. The length of stride is shortened, and heat may be noticed around the heels and quarters.

The prognosis is guarded; recovery in advanced cases takes 6-12 mo. The most important factors in treatment are to moisturize the hooves and promote expansion. This can be achieved by soaking the feet in water daily for 10-14 days followed by corrective shoeing. Hoof-moisturizing products that contain oils or waxy substances should be used with caution because they can seal the water out of the hoof. Slipper shoes with no more than 3 nails in each branch promote hoof expansion. Quarter clips and the fourth nail must be avoided.

Thinning the wall of the quarters just below the coronary band with a rasp, or grooving the walls parallel to the coronet, 3/4 in. (2 cm) below the hairline from the heel halfway to the toe, aids in expanding the heels; second and third grooves should be 1/2 in. (1.2 cm) apart, and parallel to the first. As the quarters grow out, the procedure may need to be repeated until the heels and quarters are expanded normally.

FRACTURE OF NAVICULAR BONE

This may occur as a result of trauma or concussion to the foot, or be a sequela of navicular disease (qv, p 512). It is much less common than pedal bone fracture but may be seen in fore- or hindfeet. Although pain is variable, hoof testers will usually indicate the general site. Lameness is persistent and can be eliminated by palmar digital nerve block. Radiography will confirm the diagnosis; however, care should be taken with interpretation since congenital bipartite navicular bones can be confused with fractures.

Treatment is prolonged rest and corrective trimming to alleviate tendon adhesions, but a satisfactory bony union at the fracture site seldom occurs. Surgical repair by lag screw has been described. Prognosis is guarded to poor. Although this is the type of malunion fracture that might respond to low-intensity magnetic field therapy, supportive evidence is lacking.

FRACTURE OF PEDAL BONE
(Fracture of third phalanx, os pedis, or distal phalanx)

Not an uncommon injury, which occurs due to concussion, this produces a sudden onset of lameness during exercise or a race. Most fractures occur through the lateral wing and often extend into the distal phalangeal joint.

Acute weight-bearing lameness occurs, and usually there is pain on compression of the foot with hoof testers. Lightly tapping the hoof with a hammer also may elicit pain. Lameness is exacerbated by turning the horse or making it pivot on the affected leg. If the fracture does not extend into the joint, the lameness may improve considerably after only 48 hr stall rest.

The clinical signs may be suggestive, but the diagnosis is confirmed by distal palmar nerve block and radiography. Often, >2 views are required before the fracture line is evident. Radiographic confirmation may be difficult immediately after the injury because the fracture is only a hairline at this stage. Repeating the radiography 48-72 hr later and using oblique views may be necessary to confirm the presence and exact site of the fracture. It is important to establish whether the fracture extends into the distal phalangeal joint.

Conservative treatment of 6-9 mo rest is usually all that is required for fractures that do not involve the joint. Fractures often heal with a fibrous union, so that even though the animal returns to soundness, radiographic evidence of the fracture remains. It is usual to fit a plain bar shoe with a clip well back on each quarter to limit expansion and contraction of the heels. In young horses (<3 yr), fractures into the joint usually heal satisfactorily, provided a 12-mo rest period is given. Older horses (>3 yr) have a much less favorable prognosis, and insertion of a cortical bone screw using interfragmentary compression across the fracture site is indicated. However, infection is a frequent complication. Many fractures heal in the presence of infection, but the screw must be removed at a second surgery to restore the horse to complete working soundness. Palmar digital neurectomy of racehorses with wing fractures has been used to allow return to competition without the delay for complete healing.

KERATOMA
(Keraphyllocele)

Hypertrophy of horn on the inner aspect of the wall, usually at the toe. It is believed to follow a chronic inflammatory process of the laminar matrix caused by "nail bind", mechanical injury to the wall or coronet, or following hoof-grooving. The disease often is not obvious until the growth is well advanced. Examination of the palmar surface shows that the growth, commonly cylindrical, has pushed the white line in toward the center of the sole. Pressure atrophy of the pedal bone commonly follows in severe cases. Surgical removal of the mass is indicated. In mild cases, corrective shoeing may give some temporary relief. The prognosis is guarded.

LAMINITIS
(Founder, Fever in the feet)

Traditionally defined as inflammation or edema of the sensitive laminae of the hoof, laminitis is now thought to be a transient ischemia associated with coagulopathy that leads to breakdown and degeneration of the union between the horny and sensitive laminae. In refractory cases, rotation of the pedal bone is a common sequela that may progress to perforation of the sole. The disease is a local manifestation of a more generalized metabolic disturbance, and the hoof problems are classified as acute, subacute, or chronic. It can occur in the fore, all 4, or occasionally, only in the hindfeet. Biomechanical laminitis can occur in a single foot, usually as a complication of a severe lameness or orthopedic disease in the contralateral limb.

Etiology: The most common causes of laminitis are ingestion of excess carbohydrate ("grain overload"); grazing of lush pastures, especially in ponies; and excess exercise and concussion in an unfit horse. It also may occur secondary to postparturient metritis, endotoxemia, colic and enteritis, or administration of an excess of corticosteroid or some other medicament. The risk is higher in ponies and in horses that are overweight and unfit. There is a higher incidence of the acute and subacute forms whenever there is a flush of new grass.

The initial change in acute laminitis is ischemia of the lamellar arterioles and venules. The arterial blood is then "shunted" to the venous return via the many anastomotic blood vessels in the foot (especially at the coronary band) and bypasses the corium, which causes stagnation of blood, and functional congestion and thromboembolism of the capillary beds. Laminar necrosis contributes to rotation.

These disturbances in the circulation to the foot, which initially are reversible, probably cause the exhibited pain. However, if the condition becomes protracted and there is chronic hypoxia and a lack of essential sulfur-containing amino acids for the corium, then slowing or cessation of keratinization occurs between the stratum germinativum and keratogenous zone. The end result, in mild cases, is production of "laminitic rings"; pedal rotation or complete separation of the hoof from the underlying tissues occurs in severe cases. The separation of the horny and sensitive laminae is due to ischemia, faulty keratinization, and the constant pull of the deep flexor tendon on the pedal bone, along with the upward push of the toe as the horse stands. There is some support at the back of the pedal bone from the deep digital flexor tendon and the digital cushion; however, these supportive structures may serve as a fulcrum, resulting in pedal bone rotation. If the separation occurs rapidly, a "sinking" of the pedal bone within the hoof may occur. In chronic cases, the corona of the pedal bone may penetrate the sole just in front of the frog. The prognosis in severe cases is poor because the changes become irreversible and secondary infection is common. In subacute and chronic cases, the rotation of the pedal bone occurs relatively slowly. The sole tends to become convex and thicken, and the hoof alters shape to accommodate the new position.

Clinical Findings: In acute laminitis, the animal is depressed, anorectic, and stands reluctantly. Resistance to any exercise is marked, and the normal stance is altered in attempts to relieve the weight borne by the affected feet. If forced to walk, the animal shows a slow, crouching, short-striding gait. Each foot, once lifted, is replaced as quickly as possible.

Usually, heat is apparent in the whole hoof, especially near the coronary band. An exaggerated and bounding pulse can be palpated and may be visible in the digital arteries. Pain can cause muscular trembling, and a fairly uniform tenderness can be detected when pressure is applied to the feet. The pedal bone may rotate during or after the acute stage if efficacious treatment is not given rapidly. Radiographic evidence of rotation can be present as early as the third day. The visible mucosae are often injected, with increased body temperature (104-106°F [40-41°C]), pulse rate (80-120/min), and respiratory rate (80-100/min). In exceptionally severe cases, for which the prognosis is unfavorable, a blood-stained exudate may seep from the coronary bands.

The subacute case may exhibit any or all of the above clinical signs, but to a lesser degree. Often, there is only a mild change in stance, with reluctance to walk and some increased sensitivity to concussion on the soles of the affected feet. There may be no demonstrable heat in the coronary band or increase in digital pulse. The acute and subacute forms of laminitis tend to recur at varying intervals and may develop into the chronic form.

Chronic laminitis is characterized by changes in the shape of the hoof and usually follows one or more attacks of the acute form. Bands of irregular horn growth (laminitic rings) may be seen in the hoof, close at the toe and diverging at the heel. The hoof itself becomes narrow and elongated, with the wall almost vertical at the heel and horizontal at the toe.

As the condition progresses, the sole becomes thickened and either flattened or somewhat convex in outline. The gait is similar to that already described, and when standing, the body weight is continually shifted from one foot to the other. Radiography reveals rotation and some osteoporosis of the pedal bone. The corona of the bone is forced downward and presses on the horny sole. In severe cases, it may penetrate the sole just in front of the point of the frog.

Diagnosis: In acute and severe laminitis, diagnosis is based on the history (eg, grain overload) and posture of the animal, increased temperature of the hooves, a hard pulse in the digital arteries, and reluctance to move. Mild cases with no visible hoof deformity can be identified via radiography of the affected feet, which show a lack of parallelism on the lateral projection between the hoof wall and cranial face of the third phalanx. Divergence of $\geq 11°$ indicates a guarded to unfavorable prognosis for return to performance.

Treatment: Acute laminitis constitutes a medical emergency because pedal rotation can occur rapidly. Despite prompt therapy, the prognosis is guarded until recovery is complete and it is evident that the hoof architecture is not altered. In acute laminitis, especially in cases of grain overload, mineral oil is indicated; 1 gal. (4 L) PO acts as a laxative and tends to prevent absorption of toxic material from the GI tract. Purgation should not be employed in the acute phase because most horses tend to be dehydrated.

Traditionally, cold packs or ice packs applied to the affected feet have been advocated, but recent evidence suggests that hot packs used early in the course of the disease may be more beneficial. Antihistamines are of doubtful value during acute lameness, but isoxsuprine hydrochloride paste, a peripheral vasodilating agent, may be of value. Some are using heparin (40 u/kg, t.i.d. for 3 days) because of the suspected accompanying coagulopathy and thromboembolism; however, heparin therapy in the horse has been associated with RBC clumping which, in a dehydrated animal, could aggravate local blood flow dynamics in the feet.

Flunixin meglumine and phenylbutazone are the preferred anti-inflammatory agents, and meclofenamic acid also has been of value; however, all 3 may be toxic. These agents are nonsteroidal anti-inflammatory agents; each should be used according to label instructions and, if used in combination, the dosage of each should be reduced accordingly.

Phenoxybenzamine hydrochloride (0.66 mg/kg, IV in 500 mL saline), which is an α-adrenergic blocker that causes vasodilation for up to 24 hr, has been used in severe and acute cases of laminitis. However, it may cause depression and should be avoided in animals in shock.

Heart-bar shoes have been used in acute cases in an attempt to diffuse sole pressure and avoid pedal rotation. Because an improperly fitted heart-bar shoe aggravates the pain, correct fitting is essential.

Administration of corticosteroids is contraindicated because serious cellular catabolism and inhibition of the immune responses often result in muscular wasting and worsening of the laminitis. Because gram-negative endotoxins due to carbohydrate overload have been implicated in laminitis, it is especially important to preserve the normal immune responses during treatment.

Experimentally, a combination vaccine consisting of a killed *Salmonella* mutant bacterin, an endotoxoid, and an aluminum hydroxide adjuvant has been effective in reducing the endotoxin-related complications of laminitis.

Digital nerve blocks in the early stages of the disease permit the animal to be walked, which increases the arterial blood flow through the terminal arch. However, nerve blocking and walking are contraindicated once pedal rotation has commenced. Because of its value in hoof keratinization, methionine has been used at doses of 10 mg/lb (22 mg/kg), daily for 1 wk followed by 5 mg/lb for the second week and 2.5 mg/lb for the third.

Treatment of chronic laminitis has consisted of attempting to restore the normal alignment of the rotated coffin bone and encouraging frog pressure by lowering the heels, removing excess toe, and protecting the dropped sole. This requires corrective hoof trimming and the use of full leather pads or a heart-bar shoe. Acrylic compounds are useful in conjunction with proper trimming to build up the toe and to protect the sole. The hoof should be trimmed and the shoe reset at 4- to 6-wk intervals. This approach can be successful in selected cases but is expensive, labor intensive, and prolonged.

Resection of the separated hoof wall may also be indicated and has been used in acute and chronic cases, particularly those with seedy toe and/or infection. This surgical procedure carries risk and should follow consultation between the veterinarian and farrier.

NAVICULAR DISEASE
(Podotrochlosis, Podotrochlitis)

Essentially, a chronic degenerative condition of the navicular bursa and navicular bone that involves damage to the flexor surface of the bone and the overlying deep digital flexor tendon with osteophyte formation on the lateral and proximal borders of the bone. Thus, it is a syndrome with a complex pathogenesis rather than a specific disease entity. It is primarily a disease of the forefeet and is essentially unknown in ponies and donkeys.

Etiology: The exact cause is unknown; however, it is suggested that arterial thrombosis and ischemic necrosis within the navicular bone are involved. It is considered to be a disease of the more mature riding horse, but radiographic signs have been seen in 3-yr-olds. It may be partially hereditary; certainly it is associated with upright conformation of the forefoot. The conformation of the foot in chronic cases becomes abnormal; it is upright and narrow and has a small frog. Defective shoeing that inhibits the action of the frog and the quarters may be contributory. Concussion between the flexor tendon and the navicular bone can cause a local bursitis that leads to hyperemia and rarefaction of the bone with resultant alteration of the flexor surface of the bone.

Clinical Findings and Diagnosis: Usually, the disease is insidious in onset. Attention is first directed to the affected foot or feet by the attitude of the animal when at rest. The horse relieves the pressure of the deep flexor tendon on the painful area by pointing or advancing the affected foot with the heel off the ground. If both forefeet are affected, they are pointed alternately. An intermittent lameness is manifest early in the course of the disease. The stride is shortened, and there may be a tendency to stumble. A flexion test involving the distal forelimb usually produces a transient exacerbation of lameness. There may be soreness in the brachiocephalic muscles secondary to the changes in posture and gait, thus the frequent complaint of "shoulder lameness".

Clinical diagnosis is reasonably straightforward, and is based on a complete history (pointing) and careful physical examination. The lameness can be eliminated by palmar digital nerve block. Radiographs usually reveal degenerative lesions in the bone with a change in shape of the so-called vascular channels from the normal hair-line appearance to a triangular or inverted flask shape. These lesions may result from navicular disease or natural aging, and must be interpreted in light of the history and clinical findings.

Treatment: Since the condition is both chronic and degenerative, it can be managed in some horses but not cured. With severe lameness, rest is indicated. Foot care is directed to trimming and shoeing that restores normal phalangeal alignment and balance. Thinning the quarters with a rasp and proper hoof moisturization may relieve hoof contraction. Slippered branches and a wedge pad assist hoof expansion, but the normal angle must be maintained and only 3 nails used in each branch; a fourth nail in the heel will nullify the slipper effect. Toes should be rounded to facilitate the "break-over". Nonsteroidal anti-inflammatory drugs such as phenylbutazone, along with proper foot management, extend servicable soundness in some horses. Intrabursal injection of corticosteroid also is more palliative than curative. Another therapy is isoxsuprine hydrochloride (0.27 mg/lb [0.6 mg/kg], PO, b.i.d. for 6-14 wk) in a paste form, which acts as a peripheral vasodilator, but recurrences follow cessation of therapy.

Palmar digital neurectomy may render relief from pain and prolong the usefulness of the animal, but no neurectomy should be considered curative. Digital neurectomy can be accompanied by severe complications such as painful neuroma formation. Volar and higher neurectomy should never be done.

Recently, a technique of desmotomy of the collateral sesamoidean ligament has been described. By cutting this ligament, the concussive forces between the navicular bone and the deep digital flexor tendon are thought to be reduced. The results are preliminary and unsubstantiated.

Although the prognosis is guarded to poor, a carefully designed therapeutic regimen can prolong the usefulness in most cases, and the competitive status in many. Over months or years, all affected horses reach a point of nonresponsiveness to treatment.

PEDAL OSTEITIS

An inflammation of the sensitive structures of the volar aspect of the forefeet, associated with osteitis and demineralization of the coffin bone. Repeated concussion, laminitis, persistent corns, and chronic bruised sole have been implicated as causes. It is common in performance horses and usually is associated with work on hard tracks. Lameness may not be obvious because usually both forelimbs are affected. There may be a stilted or shuffling action in front with signs of discomfort in the hoof region. Percussion and pressure from hoof testers usually reveal tenderness over the whole of the sole. Radiography is helpful in diagnosis and in differentiating the possibility of navicular disease.

Treatment involves prolonged rest, anti-inflammatory medication, and careful shoeing to relieve sole pressure. Prognosis is guarded, but the servicable soundness of many horses can be extended by proper management.

PUNCTURE WOUNDS OF THE FOOT
(Pricked foot, Nail prick or bind, Subsolar abscess)

Puncture wounds are usually the result of poor farriery technique, but can occur when a horse steps on a penetrating foreign body. "Nail bind" implies that a nail has been driven close to the sensitive structures of the foot, causing acute pain. "Nail prick" means the corium has been penetrated.

Puncture of the sole by a foreign body is associated with introduction of pathogenic microorganisms. Lameness is usually severe, especially when bearing weight; the degree may be similar to that of a fracture. The horse may stand pointing the affected foot. There is increased heat and pain in the foot, which progress to the coronary band as abscess formation proceeds. Subsequently, there is edematous swelling of the pastern and fetlock areas. Neglected cases drain at the coronary band after 2-3 wk. Diagnosis is made by confirming the site of pain by pulling the shoe, using hoof testers, and paring the suspect area to locate the foreign body or its track.

Prompt treatment with disinfectants and poultices is important for nail bind and nail prick. Ensuring adequate drainage from the site helps prevent abscess formation. In pricked foot, the prognosis is good, provided diagnosis is made and therapy begun early. If a chronic subsolar abscess has developed, treatment may be prolonged and the prognosis guarded. If infection spreads to the distal interphalangeal joint, the prognosis is unfavorable. If present, foreign bodies must be found and removed, and the infected area pared with a hoof knife to establish adequate drainage. The foot should then be kept in a rubber or plastic boot for 3-5 days with a cotton pad soaked in saturated magnesium sulfate solution or other suitable poultice. All horses with puncture wounds should be immunized against tetanus. If pain is severe, a palmar nerve block provides temporary relief. Local and systemic antibiotic therapy are not necessary, provided the infection is localized and good drainage has been achieved. Deep punctures of the foot that involve the deep digital flexor tendon, navicular bursa, navicular bone, or third phalanx are surgical emergencies.

PYRAMIDAL DISEASE
(Extensor process disease, Buttress foot)

Once classified as a type of low ringbone (qv, p 517), this arises from a traumatically induced periostitis or an avulsion fracture of the extensor process of the third phalanx caused by excess tension at the tendon insertion. The close association of the extensor process with the distal phalangeal joint means secondary arthritis is a likely complication. In the early case, heat and pain on pressure may be manifest. An enlargement of the toe region just above the coronet is usually present, which results in the "buttress foot" appearance. Systemic anti-inflammatory medication may be beneficial. Surgery has been successful for avulsion fractures.

QUITTOR
(Coronary sinus)

A chronic, purulent inflammation of the alar cartilage of the third phalanx characterized by necrosis of the cartilage and one or more sinus tracts extending from the diseased cartilage through the skin in the coronary region. It is seldom encountered today, but used to be common in working draft horses. Quittor follows injury to the coronet or pastern over the region of the alar cartilage, by means of which infection is introduced into the deep tissues to form a subcoronary abscess, or it may follow a penetrating wound through the sole. The first sign is an inflammatory swelling over the region of the alar cartilage, which is followed by abscessation and sinus formation. During the acute stage, lameness occurs.

Surgery to remove the diseased tissue and cartilage is usually successful. Local and/or parenteral therapy without surgery is likely to fail. In the absence of any therapy, poor drainage, cartilage necrosis, and recurrent abscessation lead to chronic lameness and extension to deep structures. If damage is extensive and the coffin joint has been invaded, the prognosis is unfavorable.

SANDCRACK
(Toe crack, Quarter crack)

Cracks in the wall of the hoof that begin at the coronet and run parallel to the horn tubules. Quarter cracks are most common in race horses. While excess drying of the hoof is predisposing, trauma or conformational factors are cited as the most likely causes. Extensive injury to the coronet may give rise to a crack in the wall characterized by buildup and overlapping of the hoof wall at the site of injury. This latter condition is referred to as false quarter.

A crack in the horn emanating from the coronet is the most obvious sign. Lameness is usually not a problem. If infection is established, there may be a bloody or purulent discharge and signs of inflammation and lameness. Therapy involves surgery and corrective shoeing to change the distribution of weight on the hoof. Growth of new horn may be encouraged by application of a counterirritant (eg, tincture of iodine) to the coronet over the crack. Iodine should be used with caution on light colored or white skin. If the crack has become infected, an antiseptic pack is indicated. Patching techniques using acrylics or fiberglass are useful if properly and judiciously applied. Complete stripping of the wall caudal to the crack, being careful not to damage the coronet, is often the treatment of choice in early and severe quarter cracks, or when a hoof spur has formed. The hoof is then bandaged until new horn formation is evident. The animal is then shod with a three-quarter or three-quarter-bar shoe to relieve any pressure over the stripped portion of the wall.

SCRATCHES
(Greasy heel, Dermatitis verrucosa)

A chronic, seborrheic dermatitis characterized by hypertrophy and exudation on the caudal surface of the pastern and fetlock. It often is associated with poor stable hygiene, but no specific cause is known. Heavy horses are particularly susceptible, and the hindlimbs are more commonly affected. Standardbreds frequently are affected in the spring when tracks are wet. The common use of limestone on racetracks has been associated with the condition.

The disease may go unnoticed for some time because it is masked by the "feather" at the back of the pastern. The skin is itchy, sensitive, and swollen during the acute stages; later, it becomes thickened and most of the hair is lost. Only the shorter hairs remain, and these stand erect. The surface of the skin is soft, and the grayish exudate has a fetid odor. The condition can become chronic, with vegetative granulomas. Lameness may or may not be present; it can be severe and associated with generalized cellulitis of the limb. As the condition progresses, there is thickening and hardening of the skin of the affected regions, with rapid hypertrophy of subcut. fibrous tissue.

Persistent and aggressive treatment is usually successful. This consists of removing the hair, regular washing and cleansing with warm water and soap to remove all soft exudate, drying, and applying an astringent dressing. If granulomas appear, they should be cauterized. Cellulitis requires systemic antibiotic therapy and tetanus prophylaxis.

SEEDY TOE
(Hollow wall, Dystrophia ungulae)

A condition of the hoof wall in the toe region, characterized by loss of substance and change in character of the horn. It is most often a sequela of mild chronic laminitis. The outer surface of the wall appears sound, but on dressing the palmar surface of the hoof, the inner surface of the wall is seen to be mealy, and there actually may be a cavity due to loss of horn substance. Tapping on the outside of the wall at the toe elicits a hollow sound over the affected portion. The disease may involve only a small area or nearly the entire width of the wall at the toe. Lameness is infrequent, but accompanies the occasional infection and abscessation.

The prognosis is usually good. The diseased portion should be cleaned and packed with juniper tar and oakum. In the absence of lameness, shoeing and work can continue. If the condition is extensive, the outer wall may need to be removed over the affected area.

SHEARED HEELS

Severe acquired imbalance of the foot with asymmetry of the heels. The imbalance results in one side of the heel contacting the ground before its mate, which creates a shearing force at the bulbs of the heel, asymmetrical growth of the toe, and severe overriding contraction of the heels. There is chronic heel soreness indistinguishable from that of navicular disease. The asymmetrical foot must be viewed carefully from all angles, and the gait observed at a slow walk to detect the abnormal weight-bearing and shearing stresses in the central sulcus region. Hoof cracks, deep fissuring between the bulbs of the heel, and thrush frequently accompany the problem. Navicular disease may be a concomitant diagnosis.

Corrective trimming and shoeing to restore proper heel alignment and foot balance are required. A full bar shoe with a reinforcing diagonal bar to support the affected quarter and heel is used. Several shoe resettings are required before improvement is evident. The prognosis is good in uncomplicated cases if the corrective measures are consistently applied until new hoof growth occurs.

SIDEBONE

Ossification of the alar cartilages of the third phalanx. The disease is most common in the forefeet of heavy horses working on hard surfaces. It also is frequent in hunters and jumpers, but rare in racing Thoroughbreds. Repeated concussion to the quarters of the feet is probably the essential cause, but there may be an inherited predisposition. The condition also is promoted by improper shoeing that inhibits normal physiological movement of the quarters. Some cases arise from direct trauma.

Loss of flexibility on digital palpation of either one or both alar cartilages is indicative of sidebone. Since the rigidity of the cartilages is accompanied by ossification, the cartilages may protrude prominently above the coronet. Lameness may be a sign, depending on the stage of ossification, the amount of concussion sustained by the feet, and the character of the terrain. Lameness is most likely when sidebone is associated with a narrow or contracted foot or an accompanying condition such as navicular disease. The stride may be shortened, and walking the horse across a slope may exaggerate the soreness. Mules often have prominent sidebones, yet seldom show any lameness.

Sidebone may be suspected following palpation and observation, but radiographic examination is essential for confirmation. (Ossification of the alar cartilages commonly occurs without signs of lameness.) When lameness is present, corrective shoeing to promote expansion of the quarters and to protect the foot from concussion is often of value. Grooving the hooves, along with a counterirritant (eg, tincture of iodine) to the coronary region to promote hoof growth, also may promote expansion of the wall.

THRUSH

A degeneration of the frog with secondary bacterial infection that commences in the central and collateral sulci. It results from poor management and hygiene that permit horses to stand in wet conditions for prolonged periods, and failure to clean the hooves regularly. It is more common in the hindfeet. The affected sulcus is moist and contains a black, thick discharge with a characteristic foul odor. These signs alone are sufficient to make the diagnosis.

Treatment should begin by providing dry, clean standings, and cleaning out the hoof with removal of all macerated horn. An astringent lotion, used with daily hoof cleaning, aids recovery following removal of the diseased tissue. Use of a bar shoe after the disease process has been arrested may help in the regeneration of the frog. The prognosis is usually favorable, but if the corium of the frog has been damaged, all diseased frog tissue must be removed.

CONDITIONS OF THE FETLOCK AND PASTERN

FRACTURE OF FIRST AND SECOND PHALANGES AND PROXIMAL SESAMOIDS

Fractures of the first phalanx are not uncommon in racehorses. They may be small "chip" fractures along the dorsal margin of the proximal joint surface, longitudinal fractures (split pastern), or comminuted. Another category, seen exclusively in Standardbreds, involves chip or avulsion-type fractures of the palmar or plantar proximal aspect of the first phalanx (Birkeland fractures).

Signs of longitudinal fractures involve acute weight-bearing lameness following work or a race. There may be little or no swelling initially, but there is intense pain on palpation or flexion of the fetlock. Lameness may be less pronounced with chip or avulsion fractures, but flexion of the joint exacerbates the problem.

Diagnosis is confirmed by radiography, although a number of oblique views may be necessary to ensure visibility of the fracture line, which may be seen initially as a fine fissure extending from the fetlock joint out into the distal cortex.

Chip and avulsion fractures can be removed by arthroscopic surgery. Longitudinal fractures can be repaired by internal fixation using ≥2 cortical bone screws by the technique of interfragmentary compression. Conservative treatment of severely comminuted fractures involves plaster/fiberglass cast immobilization for up to 12 wk. However, complications include poor alignment at the fracture site and secondary arthritis.

Fractures of the second phalanx are similar to those of the first phalanx, but less common. Treatment and prognosis are similar.

Fractures of the proximal sesamoid bones are relatively common. They are caused by overextension and often are associated with suspensory ligament damage, as in the forelimb of the Thoroughbred. The lateral proximal sesamoid in the hindlimb of the Standardbred may be fractured as a result of torque forces induced by shoeing with a trailer-type shoe. The fractures may be apical, middle, basal, or multiple, and involve one or both sesamoids. Clinical signs include heat, pain, and acute lameness, which is worsened by flexion of the fetlock. There is hemarthrosis and synovial effusion of the fetlock joint. Diagnosis is confirmed radiographically. Prompt surgical removal of small fragments carries a fairly good prognosis. Standardbreds respond more favorably than Thoroughbreds because of their 2-beat gait. The prognosis in large basilar fractures is poor, regardless of surgical approach. Complete disruption of the suspensory apparatus, including fractures of both sesamoid bones, is a catastrophic injury accompanied by vascular compromise of the foot; however, some horses can be salvaged for breeding by surgical arthrodesis of the fetlock joint.

OSSELETS
(Osslets, Periostitis and serous arthritis of the fetlock joint)

An inflammation, usually bilateral, of the periosteum on the dorsal distal epiphyseal surface of the large metacarpal bone and the associated capsule of the fetlock joint. The proximal end of the first phalanx may also be involved. Hence, this condition constitutes a form of periostitis and serous arthritis that may progress to degenerative joint disease. The exciting cause is the strain and repeated trauma of hard training in young animals. It has come to be recognized as an occupational hazard of the young Thoroughbred.

The gait is short and choppy. Palpation and flexion of the fetlock joint produce pain, and examination reveals a soft, warm, sensitive swelling over the front and sometimes the side of the joint. Radiography in the initial stages may show no evidence of new bone formation, in which case the condition is called "green osselets". Later, enthesopathy may be seen in the area of attachment of the fetlock joint capsule to the large metacarpal bone and first phalanx. New bone or spur formation may break off and appear as "joint mice".

Rest is very important and can be curative for early cases. The inflammation may be relieved by the application of cold packs for several days. Systemic anti-inflammatory agents such as phenylbutazone may also be employed. Some prefer the intra-articular injection of a corticosteroid; however, this and other forms of anti-inflammatory medication, if used along with continued training or racing, inevitably lead to destruction of the joint surfaces. Intra-articular sodium hyaluronate is a useful means of treatment aimed at reestablishing normal synovial viscosity. This can also be done by synovial fluid transfer by removing ~5 mL synovia from a normal joint (eg, tibiotarsal) and injecting it into the affected fetlock.

RINGBONE

A periostitis or osteoarthritis of the phalanges that leads to exostoses. Faulty conformation, improper shoeing, or repeated concussion through working on hard ground are causative; trauma and infection, especially wire-cut wounds, are also incriminated. In light horses, the strain of ligaments and tendinous insertions in the pastern region are frequent causal factors. It may be a part of the osteochondrosis syndrome (qv, p 558) in young, rapidly growing horses.

There is a characteristic bell-shaped appearance to the pastern region. Lameness due to periostitis is seen initially. Once bone proliferation has occurred, lameness may not be present, particularly if there is no involvement of the articular surfaces.

However, lameness usually persists if the joint surfaces are involved, and this may progress to ankylosis.

Clinical diagnosis is based on visualization and palpation of soft-tissue thickness and new bone proliferation in the pastern region. Usually, the range of joint movement is restricted, and there is pain on forced flexion of the involved articular surfaces. Regional nerve blocks identify the pastern region as the site of pain. Radiography confirms the diagnosis.

Complete rest is the most important requirement for treatment. Cold and astringent applications, and radiation therapy in the early stages may be beneficial. Anti-inflammatory medication may relieve the signs of lameness. Surgical arthrodesis of the pastern joint is curative and is used successfully to restore the performance future of young horses with osteochondrosis.

SESAMOIDITIS

The sesamoid bones are maintained in position by the suspensory ligament proximally, and a number of sesamoidean ligaments distally. Due to the great stress placed on the fetlock during fast exercise, the insertion of some of these ligaments can tear, which results in sesamoiditis.

The clinical signs are similar to, but less severe than, those resulting from sesamoid fracture. Depending on the extent of the damage, there are varying degrees of lameness and swelling. Reduced speed may be the only manifestation of lameness. Pain and heat are evident on palpation and flexion of the fetlock joint. The radiographic features include periosteal new bone proliferation and/or osteolytic lesions, particularly on the abaxial surface of the affected sesamoid, and radiolucent lines, which look similar to fracture lines except there is no fragment distraction, running obliquely across the bone. These lines are prominent vascular channels. Oblique radiographic views are essential for accurate diagnosis and evaluation.

Despite various treatments, the prognosis is guarded or poor. Even after 9-12 mo rest, many horses become lame 6-8 wk after recommencing training. The recommended treatment is a 2-to 3-wk course of phenylbutazone. For mild sesamoiditis, ≥6 mo rest is required; for severe cases, 9-12 mo.

VILLONODULAR SYNOVITIS

An inflammation of the synovial membrane of the dorsoproximal aspect of the forelimb fetlock joints. The cause is unknown. Affected animals are 2-18 yr old. Incidence is slightly higher in males. Bilateral involvement has been reported. The intra-articular nodules are usually attached by a broad stalk to the dorsal portion of the dorsal proximal pouch of the fetlock joint, are firm and grayish white, and may be circumscribed or lobulated. Erosive bone lesions are typically associated with the mass and, in some cases, may extend to erosion of the articular surface. Microscopically, the lesions consist of dense, well-collagenized stroma lined by synovial cells. Vascularization is prominent, and hyaline change in the stroma and osseous metaplasia are occasionally seen.

Diagnosis can be suspected by palpation and confirmed radiographically. Treatment is by surgical excision of the lesion. Smaller masses are amenable to arthroscopic surgery. Radiation therapy appears to help prevent recurrences after surgical excision.

WINDGALLS
(Windpuffs)

Puffy, fluid-filled swellings around the fetlock joints (of either or both fore- and hindlimbs) that usually are not accompanied by heat, pain, or lameness. They are said to be associated with trauma and hard exercise, but the exact pathogenesis is uncertain. Although usually benign, they should be regarded with suspicion in the presence of lameness. Some horses, particularly heavy ones, seem to be more susceptible. Treatment is problematical; in the absence of lameness it is unwarranted. Windgalls may disappear spontaneously or respond to periods of rest, bandaging, and exercise. Recurrence is common.

CONDITIONS OF THE CARPUS

BUCKED SHINS
(Sore shins, Saucer fractures)

A periostitis on the cranial surface of the large metacarpal or metatarsal bone, most often seen in the forelimbs of young Thoroughbreds (2-yr-olds) in training and racing. It is much less common in Standardbreds.

This injury is generally brought about by concussion in young horses in which the bones are not fully conditioned. Microfractures (ie, stress fractures) are believed to be involved. It may progress to a cortical saucer fracture or even incomplete longitudinal fracture. In mild cases, subperiosteal hematoma formation and thickening of the superficial face of the cortex may be all that is clinically apparent. There is a warm, painful swelling on the cranial surface of the affected bone. The horse is usually lame initially, the stride is short, and the severity of the lameness increases with exercise.

Rest from training is important until the soreness and inflammation have disappeared. The acute inflammation may be relieved by application of cold packs. If the condition is associated with a stress fracture, counterirritation and local corticosteroid injections are contraindicated. Screw fixation of fissure fractures may be indicated in selected cases.

CARPAL HYGROMA

A prominent, fluid-filled swelling on the dorsal aspect of the carpus when repeated trauma causes a local bursitis (*see* CAPPED ELBOW AND HOCK, p 469). In some cases, tenosynovitis of the extensor carpi radialis or common digital extensor, or occasionally, synovitis of the radiocarpal or intercarpal joint develops and is visually indistinguishable. The animal usually is not lame, but in severe cases, the range of joint flexion may be restricted. Conservative treatment of simply withdrawing the fluid and injecting corticosteroid is rarely effective; the swelling rapidly recurs. It is necessary to open the lesion surgically, insert a drain for up to 3 wk, and keep a pressure bandage on the limb. In some instances, the bursal lining must be dissected out to prevent repeated recurrence.

CARPITIS
(Sore knee, Popped knee)

An acute or chronic inflammation of the joint capsules and associated structures of the carpus. Exostoses (enthesophytes) may develop in chronic cases. The acute form is common in Thoroughbreds in training. The condition is usually attributed to concussion from hard training, especially in immature and unfit horses. Injury to the dorsal aspect of the carpus is a common cause, especially in hunters and jumpers. Some cases are the result of undetected chip or slab fractures, or osteitis/sclerosis of one of the carpal bones. If conformation is poor, the condition may appear without any obvious history of trauma or injury.

The initial lameness and swelling of the carpus may consist of distention of a joint capsule and related synovial structures, or be a true soft-tissue swelling. The chronic case may show well-developed exostoses on the distal radius or on the dorsal surfaces of any of the carpal bones, usually the radial or third carpal. The diagnosis usually is simple; however, there may be an underlying carpal bone fracture. Radiography, with all views, should be a routine part of the evaluation. The tangential ("sunrise") view is important for detecting osteitis/sclerosis, particularly the third carpal bone. Arthroscopy is useful for evaluating articular cartilage in the absence of bony changes.

Rest is the best treatment; if adequate time is given, the prognosis for acute cases is good. Pain may be relieved by aspiration of excess fluid from the joint and the intra-articular injection of a corticosteroid, but adequate rest is still mandatory. This procedure may be repeated after 4 or 5 days if necessary. Intra-articular hyaluronic acid or the polysulfated glycosaminoglycans have received widespread acceptance for this condition. The presence of chip fractures or degenerative bony changes is an indication for arthroscopy and surgery. Anti-inflammatory treatment combined with continued training and racing accelerates the degenerative process within the joint. The prognosis is based on the efficacy of treatment and the degree of bony changes.

FRACTURE OF THE CARPAL BONES

Most of these are caused by "shear-type" stresses; they usually occur toward the end of a race when the possibility of maximal overextension of the joint is greatest. Most fractures occur on the dorsal aspect of the carpal joint and particularly involve the radial and third carpal bones. Both chip and slab fractures occur, although chip fractures of the distal radius and radial carpal bones predominate, and slab fractures of the third carpal bone are usually seen. Another carpal fracture is a longitudinal fracture of the accessory carpal bone.

Chip fractures may not produce obvious signs until the animal is cooling down after fast work, when swelling of the carpus and accompanying lameness may be noticed. Slab or compression fractures of the carpal bones usually result in immediate swelling and severe supporting-leg lameness. If the fracture is incomplete, or if the fragment is small, the animal may walk relatively soundly in 7-10 days following simple anti-inflammatory measures, such as rest and local applications of cold packs. Intra-articular injection of steroids and administration of phenylbutazone also relieve the inflammation. However, lameness recurs with any strenuous work.

A diagnostic set of radiographs entails 6 exposures to ensure that a fracture line is not missed. Dorsopalmar, lateromedial, obliques of both the medial and lateral aspects, and lateromedial flexed views are necessary. A "skyline" projection is valuable to delineate the extent of a slab fracture.

The combination of intra-articular or systemic anti-inflammatory treatment and continued work may be used for economic reasons, but usually leads to degenerative changes within the joint; therefore, arthroscopic surgery is the treatment of choice. Slab fractures require screw fixation using interfragmentary compression.

Fractures of the accessory carpal bone may be treated conservatively by allowing stall rest for 8-12 mo to permit a fibrous union at the fracture site; however, return to full athletic activity is unlikely. The prognosis for carpal fractures is directly related to the severity of the injury and the efficacy of surgery or other treatment(s).

FRACTURES OF THE SMALL METACARPAL AND METATARSAL (SPLINT) BONES

Fractures of the second and fourth metacarpal and metatarsal (splint) bones are not uncommon. The cause may be from direct trauma, such as interference by the contralateral leg, but splint fractures more often follow a suspensory desmitis and the resulting fibrous tissue buildup and encapsulation of the distal, free end of the bone. The usual site of these fractures is through the distal end, ~2 in. (5 cm) from the tip. Immediately after the fracture occurs, acute inflammation is present, usually involving the suspensory ligament. A supporting-leg lameness is noted, which may recede after several days rest and recur only after work.

Chronic, long-standing fractures cause a supporting-leg lameness at speed. Thickening of the suspensory ligament at and above the fracture site results. The fracture may show a considerable buildup of callus at the fracture site, but little tendency to heal.

Diagnosis is confirmed by an oblique radiograph. Surgical removal of the fractured tip and of the callus is the treatment of choice. The prognosis is based on severity of the associated suspensory desmitis, which has a greater bearing on future performance than the splint fracture itself.

FRACTURE OF THE THIRD METACARPAL (CANNON) BONE

A transverse fracture in the midmetacarpal region can occur from direct trauma, usually from a kick. The stress of racing on a hard surface may result in a longitudinally oblique (ie, condylar) fracture that progresses up the metacarpal shaft from the fetlock and sometimes also involves the proximal sesamoids. Small saucers or incomplete fractures of the dorsal cortex of the midmetacarpal region can occur as stress-type fractures. Diagnosis is confirmed by radiography; the fissure fractures can be difficult to demonstrate, and a range of oblique views may be necessary. Midmetacarpal fractures may heal with just a cast, although prolonged immobilization may be necessary since delayed union often occurs. Malunion and the encroachment of callus on surrounding tendons and ligaments cause further problems. Internal fixation with compression plates and screws is the treatment of choice. Condylar fractures can be treated conservatively by casting, but such articular injuries are best managed by screw fixation using interfragmentary compression if osteoarthritis is to be minimized or avoided. Fissure fractures also may show delayed union unless a cortical bone screw is applied. (*See also* BUCKED SHINS, p 519.)

SPLINTS
(Interosseous desmitis)

This condition primarily involves the interosseous ligament between the large (third) and small (second) metacarpal (less frequently the metatarsal) bones. The reaction is a periostitis with production of new bone (exostoses) along the involved splint bone. Trauma from concussion or injury, strain from excess training (especially in the immature horse), faulty conformation, or improper shoeing may contribute to their development.

Splints most commonly involve the medial rudimentary metacarpal bones. Lameness is observed only when splints are forming and is seen most frequently in young horses. Lameness is more pronounced after the animal has been worked. In the early stages, there is no visible enlargement, but deep palpation may reveal local painful subperiosteal swelling. In the later stages, a calcified growth appears. Following ossification, lameness disappears, except in rare cases in which the growth encroaches on the suspensory ligament or carpometacarpal articulation. Radiography is necessary to differentiate splints from fractured splint bones.

Complete rest is indicated. Local use of steroids delays the consolidation process and is contraindicated. In Thoroughbred practice, it has been traditional to point-fire a splint, the aim being to accelerate the ossification of the interosseous ligament. However, in most cases irritant treatments are contraindicated. If the exostoses impinge against the suspensory ligament, then surgical removal may be necessary.

CONDITIONS OF THE SHOULDER AND ELBOW

ARTHRITIS OF THE SHOULDER JOINT

Inflammation of the structures of the shoulder joint is uncommon. It is secondary to changes in the joint capsule, or more frequently, bony changes of the articular surfaces of the humerus or scapula, such as might be caused by osteochondritis dissecans. Occasionally, fractures involving the articular surfaces are present. Trauma to the point of the shoulder is a frequent cause. Bacterial infection of the joint from puncture wounds or of hematogenous origin (pyosepticemia) in foals results in a purulent arthritis.

A swinging- and supporting-leg lameness is present in severe cases. In milder cases, only the swinging-leg lameness may be noted. The forward phase is shortened, the toe may be worn, and the leg is often circumducted to avoid flexion of the joint. Forced extension of the leg, which pulls the shoulder forward, often causes pain. Radiographs of the shoulder joint, preferably taken with the horse in lateral recumbency, may demonstrate the arthritic changes.

Often, treatment is ineffective because of severe arthritic changes. Intra-articular injections of a steroid may be of some benefit. Systemic steroids or phenylbutazone may relieve signs of pain. Hyaluronic acid, because of its apparent benefit in cases of degenerative disease in other joints, may be worthy of consideration.

BICIPITAL BURSITIS

An inflammation of the bursa between the tendon of the biceps and the bicipital groove of the humerus. The usual cause is direct trauma to the point of the shoulder. Essentially, the condition produces a swinging-leg lameness with the forward phase being shortened. The animal may stumble because the toe is not being lifted sufficiently to clear the ground. In severe cases, a supporting-leg lameness is also present; the animal rests the limb in a characteristic semiflexed position. Forced extension of the leg usually causes a pain reaction, as may deep digital pressure over the bursa and the tendon of the biceps. Ultrasonography can demonstrate the excess fluid and associated lesions of the biceps tendon. Radiographs may be of aid in chronic cases in which calcification of the bursa is a common sequela.

Prolonged rest is indicated (>6 mo), particularly in acute cases. Intrabursal injection of hyaluronic acid or steroids may be successful. Phenylbutazone and oral steroids may also be helpful. The prognosis is guarded.

FRACTURES OF THE ELBOW

Fractures of the elbow are not uncommon orthopedic injuries in horses, the most frequent being fracture of the ulna. They occur at any age as a result of a kick or fall. In foals (<12 mo), they involve the physeal plate of the olecranon. Onset of lameness is sudden, and there is pain and swelling of the elbow. The fracture is usually transverse, extending through the semilunar notch, and is frequently articular. The olecranon is distracted by the pull of the triceps tendon of insertion; the elbow is dropped and cannot be extended, which produces signs similar to those of radial nerve paralysis. The carpus and fetlock are flexed, with the toe resting on the ground. Diagnosis must be confirmed radiographically.

Treatment may be conservative or surgical. In nonarticular and nondisplaced fractures, full-leg splinting and stall rest are successful. Otherwise, open reduction and internal fixation using a tension band plate is the method of choice. The prognosis is favorable with proper treatment.

FRACTURES OF THE SHOULDER

Fractures of the distal scapula (tuber scapulae) and proximal humerus (lateral tuberosity) are the most common shoulder fractures. They usually result from falls or kicks. Lameness is severe and sudden in onset. Often, there is much local soft-tissue swelling and hematoma formation. Diagnosis is confirmed radiographically. Conservative treatment by prolonged stall rest often results in improvement. Surgical treatment can be successful in selected cases. Unless treated surgically, both types of fractures heal with fibrous union. The prognosis is poor if the articular surfaces are involved.

SWEENEY
(Shoulder atrophy, Slipped shoulder)

Disuse or neurogenic atrophy of the supraspinatus and infraspinatus muscles. Disuse atrophy, sometimes involving the triceps also, follows any lesion of the limb or foot that leads to prolonged diminished use of the limb. Neurogenic atrophy is due to damage to the suprascapular nerve, which supplies the supraspinatus and infraspinatus muscles. Polo ponies are occasionally affected because of collision during competition.

Clinical Findings and Diagnosis: If trauma is not evident, pain may be absent, and lameness may be difficult to detect until atrophy occurs. If injury is evident, there is usually some difficulty in extending the shoulder. As atrophy proceeds, there is a noticeable hollowing on each side of the spine of the scapula, especially in the infraspinous area, resulting in prominence of the spine. Since the tendons of insertion of the 2 affected muscles act as lateral collateral ligaments to the humeroscapular joint, atrophy of the muscles leads to a looseness in the shoulder joint. Abduction of the shoulder follows and, in severe cases, is sometimes erroneously diagnosed as a dislocation. The affected limb, when advanced, takes a semicircular course and, as weight is borne by the limb, the shoulder joint moves laterally (shoulder slip). At rest, along with abduction of the shoulder, there is an apparent abduction of the lower part of the limb.

Treatment and Prognosis: Treatment for disuse atrophy consists of removing the cause of the failure to use the limb. For neurogenic atrophy, massage with stimulating liniments or by an electrical vibrator may be of benefit. Rhythmic muscular contractions by faradism have "kept the affected muscles alive" until nerve regeneration has occurred. Based on success with a limited number of cases, surgical release of the suprascapular nerve from scar tissue impingement, by "notching out" the rostral border of the scapula, has been recommended. For best results, the surgery should be performed before looseness and slipping of the shoulder joint are advanced.

The prognosis for cases with disuse atrophy depends on removal of the primary cause. In neurogenic atrophy, the prognosis is guarded; in mild cases, recovery should occur in 6-8 wk. When damage to the nerve has been severe, spontaneous recovery may take many months if it occurs at all. Such cases are candidates for surgical release. If the nerve has been severed, recovery is unlikely.

CONDITIONS OF THE TARSUS

See also FRACTURE OF THE SMALL METACARPAL AND METATARSAL (SPLINT) BONES, p 520.

BOG SPAVIN
(Tarsal hydrarthrosis)

A chronic synovitis of the tibiotarsal joint characterized by distention of the joint capsule. Faulty conformation may lead to weakness of the hock joint and increased production of synovia. In such cases, both limbs are affected. The unilateral case is more likely to be a sequela of a sprain or some underlying problem within the joint, such as osteochondrosis.

The horse usually is not lame unless the condition is complicated by bone involvement. The primary distention of the joint capsule is on the dorsal medial surface of the hock, while smaller swellings occur on each side of the proximal caudal aspect. Uncomplicated bog spavin rarely interferes with the usefulness of the animal, but is an unsightly blemish and signals the need for radiographic evaluation. Spontaneous appearance and disappearance of the distention may occur in weanlings and yearlings.

The excess fluid within the joint capsule may be aspirated. Intra-articular corticosteroids provide variable and transient relief. The procedure may be repeated 3 wk later if necessary. Arthroscopy should be done when osteochondral involvement is suspected. The condition tends to recur, especially if poor conformation is a factor.

BONE SPAVIN

Osteoarthritis or osteitis of the hock joint, usually the distal intertarsal and tarsometatarsal articulations and, occasionally, the proximal intertarsal joint. Lesions involve degenerative joint disease, particularly on the craniomedial aspect of the hock with periarticular new bone proliferation, which eventually leads to ankylosis. Although the condition usually causes lameness, this may be obscured if the lesions are bilateral. Theories advanced to explain this condition include faulty hock conformation, excessive concussion, and mineral imbalance. All breeds can be affected, but it is most prevalent in Standardbreds and Quarter Horses.

The lame horse tends to drag the toe. The forward flight of the hoof is shortened, and hock action is decreased. The lameness sometimes is continuous since the bone lesions involve the articular surfaces. The heel may become elongated. Standardbreds develop soreness in the gluteal musculature (so-called trochanteric bursitis) secondary to spavin. In advanced cases, the bony proliferation may be visible on the distal craniomedial aspect of the hock (seat of spavin). When standing, the horse may rest the toe on the ground with the heel slightly raised. The lameness often disappears with exercise and returns after rest. The spavin test (moving at a trot after flexing the affected joint for 1-2 min) may be a useful aid to diagnosis, but is not specific for this condition or even this joint. In so-called occult spavin, there are no visible or radiographic exostoses. Local anesthesia of the individual tarsal joints is necessary to localize the exact site of pain responsible for the lameness.

The disease is self-limiting, ending with spontaneous ankylosis of the affected joint(s) and a return to soundness. In the early stages, intra-articular corticosteroids and/or sodium hyaluronate injection may be beneficial. Nonsteroidal anti-inflammatory drugs (eg, phenylbutazone) eliminate or reduce the clinical signs. Working the horse following this treatment is aimed at promoting ankylosis and resolution of lameness. Surgical arthrodesis is another means of accelerating ankylosis of the affected joint. Cunean tenotomy is commonly used, but of questionable value by itself. Deep point firing used to be advocated for hastening ankylosis, but it is very doubtful that it has any beneficial effect beyond encouraging rest. Corrective shoeing by raising the heels and rolling the toe may help, but is unlikely to eliminate lameness on its own.

CURB

A thickening or bowing of the plantar tarsal ligament due to strain. Inflammation and thickening of this ligament may occur after falling, slipping, jumping, or pulling. It is most common in Standardbreds in which poor conformation of the hock is a predisposing factor. There is an enlargement over the caudal surface of the fibular tarsal bone ~4 in. (10 cm) below the point of the hock. It is easily seen when observing the animal from the side. A recently formed curb is associated with acute inflammation and lameness. The horse stands and favors the limb with the heel elevated. In chronic cases, there is rarely any lameness or pain.

If the condition is due to acute inflammation, cold packs and rest are indicated. Little can be done to overcome the curb that is secondary to poor conformation. Fortunately, the problem seems to be self-limiting, without lasting effects on performance.

DISPLACEMENT OF SUPERFICIAL FLEXOR TENDON FROM THE POINT OF THE HOCK

Damage to the medial attachment of the superficial flexor tendon as it passes over the tuber calcaneus can cause a lateral luxation of the tendon. The injury occurs due to sudden flexion of the hock, and the tendon can occasionally slip to the medial aspect of the hock. Initially, there is lameness in the limb, with local heat and swelling. Treatment involves rest for ≥3 mo, possibly with application of a cast. The lameness improves, but the animal may be left with a permanently displaced flexor tendon and a rather jerky hock action. There is usually no difficulty during fast exercise or jumping, but dressage movements may be affected. Surgical treatment has been reported in a limited number of cases. The results have not been very successful, particularly in larger horses.

FRACTURE OF THE TARSUS

Fractures of the hock occur as a result of trauma or as a secondary complication of degenerative joint disease. The hock is a complex joint that comprises 8 bones. As in the carpus, a wide range of locations and types of fractures can occur. Specific diagnosis depends on careful radiographic examination.

Some of the more common fractures involve chips of the tibiotarsal bone and the medial or lateral malleolus of the tibia. Slab fractures of the central and third tarsal bones are also encountered, particularly in Standardbreds. Since these often are quite small and may not cause lameness, it is important to use local anesthesia to positively identify the site of lameness. In many instances, a rest period (3-6 mo) is all that is required for full recovery, although with large chip fragments, surgical removal may be better. The tibiotarsal joint is amenable to arthroscopy and surgery, with most involved areas being accessible. Slab fractures are amenable to lag screw fixation.

HINDLIMB TENDON RUPTURES

Laceration of the entire Achilles tendon (*see also* p 561) involving both the gastrocnemius and superficial flexor tendons is rare. The hock drops to the ground, and is unable to bear weight. The prognosis is grave.

Gastrocnemius muscle rupture is more common and can result from excess stress applied to the hock (eg, sudden stopping). It can be bilateral and weight can be borne, but there is excess flexion of the hock, which makes walking difficult. There is no satisfactory treatment. Splinting the limb and slinging the animal have been attempted, but are usually unsuccessful.

Injuries to the extensor tendons, the long and lateral digital extensors, frequently accompany hindlimb lacerations. If one tendon is involved, the prognosis is usually good. If both extensor tendons are severed, the horse may be left with a gait deficit for performance, but be useful for slow speeds or for breeding. Conservative treatment leads to wound healing, but surgical repair and casting should be considered if both tendons are severed and/or performance status is desired.

Rupture of the superficial and deep flexor tendons sometimes occurs as a racing injury or accompanies lacerations. These are serious injuries with marked lameness and varying degrees of overextension of the fetlock and pastern. Treatment involves surgical repair with splinting and casting the limb, but the prognosis is poor for future performance.

PERONEUS TERTIUS RUPTURE

Injury to the peroneus tertius muscle affects the stay apparatus of the hindlimb and disrupts the reciprocal action of the stifle and hock joints. The most characteristic diagnostic feature is the ability to extend the hock and flex the stifle simultaneously. The horse is lame, but usually able to bear weight on the limb. The affected hindleg exhibits a jerking motion as it is brought forward. Conservative treatment consisting of prolonged rest (usually 4 mo) is indicated; the prognosis is favorable.

STRINGHALT
(Springhalt)

A myoclonic affliction of one or both hindlimbs seen as spasmodic overflexion of the joints. The etiology is unknown, but lesions of a peripheral neuropathy have been identified in the sciatic, peroneal, and tibial nerves. Severe forms of the condition have been attributed to lathyrism (sweet pea poisoning) in the USA and possibly to flat weed intoxication in Australia. Horses of any breed may be affected, but it is rare in foals.

All degrees of hyperflexion are seen, from the mild, spasmodic lifting and grounding of the foot, to the extreme case in which the foot is drawn sharply up until it touches the belly and then struck violently on the ground. In severe cases, there is atrophy of the lateral thigh muscles. In Australian stringhalt and lathyrism, the condition may be progressive and the gait abnormality become so severe that euthanasia is necessary.

Mild stringhalt may be intermittent. The signs are most obvious when the horse is sharply turned or backed. In some cases, the condition is seen only on the first few steps after moving the horse out of its stall. The signs are often less intense or even absent during warmer weather. Although it is regarded as unsoundness, stringhalt may not materially hinder the horse's capacity for work, except in severe cases when the constant concussion gives rise to secondary complications. The condition may also make the horse unsuitable for equestrian sports (eg, dressage).

Diagnosis is based on clinical signs, but can be confirmed by electromyography. If in doubt, the animal should be observed as it is backed out of the stall after hard work for 1 or 2 days. False stringhalt sometimes appears as a result of some temporary irritation to the lower pastern area or even a painful lesion in the foot. The occasional case of momentary upward fixation of the patella may exhibit a stringhalt-like gait.

When intoxication is suspected, removal to another paddock may be all that is required. Many of these cases apparently recover spontaneously. In chronic cases, tenectomy of the lateral extensor of the digit, including removal of a portion of the muscle, has given best results. Improvement may not be evident until 2-3 wk after surgery. Prognosis following surgery is guarded—not all cases respond. This is not surprising since the condition is a distal axonopathy. Other methods of treatment include large doses of thiamine and phenytoin.

THOROUGHPIN

A distention of the tarsal sheath of the deep digital flexor tendon just above the hock. It is characterized by plantar fluid-filled swellings visible on both medial and lateral sides proximal to the tibiotarsal joint, which distinguish it from bog spavin. It is usually unilateral and varies in size. The lesion is referred to as a tenosynovitis of traumatic origin, but it may not be associated with any detectable inflammation, pain, or lameness. It essentially constitutes a blemish and so is of major clinical importance in show horses. Treatment is by withdrawal of the fluid and injection of hyaluronic acid or a long-acting corticosteroid, which may need to be repeated until the swelling does not recur. Radiation therapy also helps reduce the secretory property of the tendon sheath.

CONDITIONS OF THE STIFLE

FRACTURE OF THE STIFLE

Severe fractures of the stifle involving either the distal femur or proximal tibia are uncommon. The associated damage to the femorotibial joint, ligaments, and menisci, and marked soft-tissue swelling make treatment in adult horses difficult or impossible.

Fractures of the patella usually cause much less severe lameness and swelling, and radiography is necessary to confirm the diagnosis. Patellar fractures may respond to conservative treatment or, if a large bone fragment is involved, require surgical repair. Fracture of the tibial crest also occurs occasionally and requires surgical repair.

GONITIS

An inflammation of the stifle leading to degenerative joint disease. The joint is complex and the condition may be precipitated by multiple causes: osteochondrosis, persistent upward fixation of the patella, injuries to the medial or lateral collateral ligaments, injuries to the cruciate ligaments or the menisci, erosions of the articular cartilage, or bacterial infection of the joint from puncture wounds or of hematogenous origin (eg, pyosepticemia).

Signs vary with the cause and extent of the pathological changes. The distended femoropatellar capsule is seen just below the patella.

A swinging-leg lameness is noted as a shortening of the forward phase. At rest, the fetlock is flexed with only the toe touching the ground. In moderately severe cases, both a supporting- and a swinging-leg lameness are noted. In severe cases, the leg may be carried in a flexed position. Crepitation may be noted if the menisci, cruciate ligaments, or the collateral ligaments of the joint have been ruptured. Radiographs are of value in confirming osteochondral involvement, whereas ultrasonography is of value for evaluating ligaments, menisci, and soft tissue.

Prolonged rest is indicated. Repeated intra-articular injections of steroids or hyaluronic acid may be useful. Phenylbutazone and systemic steroids may relieve the lameness in less severe cases. Those cases due to rupture of ligaments or damage to the menisci rarely respond satisfactorily, and rapidly progress to secondary arthritis. The prognosis is poor if the condition is chronic or if severe injuries to the articular surface, ligaments, or the menisci have occurred.

PATELLAR LUXATION

True dislocation of the patella is uncommon in horses (*see also* p 560). When it does occur it is usually a serious injury, and the lateral luxation is readily apparent. In some breeds, a congenital form of lateral luxation occurs similar to that seen in small dogs. The most frequent problem involving the patella is upward fixation or locking of the medial patellar liagment over the proximal part of the medial femoral trochlear ridge. Some pony breeds may have a hereditary predisposition, but the condition is also seen in immature animals with poorly developed thigh muscles. It may be uni- or bilateral. The classical signs are of an intermittent locking of the limb in extension followed by a sudden jerk or hyperflexion as the patellar ligament becomes freed from the medial trochlear ridge. The signs are most frequently seen after standing still for any period (eg, overnight in the stable, or after travelling in a trailer). However, the clinical signs are often much less dramatic, which makes diagnosis difficult. There may simply be a lack of hindlimb impulsion associated with a rather jerky patellar action.

In many cases, a general improvement in fitness and muscle tone of the hindquarters effects a cure. In the more severe and persistent cases, desmotomy of the medial patellar ligament is indicated. Desmotomy has been commonly employed in the past, but currently is in disfavor. A fragmentation of the distal extremity of the patella and osteochondrosis are believed to follow the surgery, particularly if postoperative exercise is initiated early. When surgery is done, rest should be sufficient (eg, 4-6 wk) to permit complete healing before training is resumed.

SUBCHONDRAL BONE CYST
(Osseous cyst-like lesion)

Large, radiolucent, cyst-like structures that may occur in various sites in the body, but particularly in the stifle. Their pathogenesis is not completely understood, but they may arise following trauma to the articular cartilage or as a result of an osteochondritic lesion. They seem to appear at a point of load-bearing; the common sites are the medial condyle of the femur, the third phalanx, the shoulder, the fetlock, and the carpus.

In the stifle, cysts are most frequently seen in young Thoroughbreds (1-2 yr olds); usually, lameness is first noticed when breaking-in or training begins. Although femoropatellar joint distention is characteristic, these cystic lesions can cause quite severe lameness without joint distention or pain on palpation. They are readily diagnosed radiographically. Some horses respond to rest for 4-6 mo and improve with phenylbutazone medication. When this conservative treatment fails, particularly in more mature animals, surgery is indicated. This involves drilling and curetting the cyst lining and packing the space with an autogenous bone graft. Because of the favorable results, some are recommending surgery before more conservative treatment. Both arthroscopy and arthrotomy are being used.

CONDITIONS OF THE HIP

COXITIS
(Osteoarthritis of the hip)

Inflammation of the hip that leads to osteoarthritis of the coxofemoral joint. Most cases are traumatic in origin, secondary to falls or being stall-cast in recumbency; however, tears of the rim of the acetabulum or fractures through the acetabulum, and localization of a systemic infection, particularly pyosepticemia in young animals, have occurred.

Both a supporting- and a swinging-leg lameness are noted. In severe cases, the leg may be carried. In less severe cases, the gait is rolling, ie, the affected quarter is elevated as weight is borne on the leg. The limb is advanced in a semicircular manner with the forward phase of the stride shortened. The toe may be worn from dragging. The animal often stands with the limb partially flexed, the stifle turned out, and the point of the hock turned inward. Atrophy of the muscles of the quarter occurs in chronic cases. Rectal palpation may reveal an enlargement over the acetabulum, particularly if a fracture through it has occurred. Radiography of the joint confirms the diagnosis.

The prognosis is poor. Rest is indicated, and intra-articular steroids may relieve the lameness temporarily in milder cases. Phenylbutazone is useful, but many cases are too painful for the drug to have a beneficial effect.

DISLOCATION OF THE HIP

Dislocation of the hip can occur in association with rupture of the teres (round) ligament, accessory ligament, or joint capsule. This type of injury occurs secondary to trauma, but is quite uncommon. Fracture of the dorsal acetabular rim frequently accompanies the dislocation. Dislocation with dorsal displacement of the femoral head is accompanied by upward fixation of the patella.

Rupture of the round ligament of the hip joint is associated with a typical appearance of the hindlimb, in which the stifle and toe rotate outward and the hock rotates inward. Complete dislocation of the hip joint does not always occur; when it does, there is a marked effect on gait, with a reluctance to bear weight. The femur is rotated outward, and the greater trochanter is more prominent than usual.

Relocation of the hip joint may be attempted under general anesthesia, but the long-term results are usually poor.

PELVIC FRACTURE

This can occur at any age, but is most prevalent in horses 6 mo to 2 yr old. Almost any part of the pelvic girdle may be involved. The site and extent of soft-tissue damage affect the ultimate prognosis. There is sudden onset of hindlimb lameness with considerable pain. Crepitus may be difficult to appreciate initially. It is usually possible to confirm a pelvic fracture by rectal examination, especially if the fragments are displaced. If the lameness is not too severe, but a fracture is suspected, it is better to rest the animal for 4-6 wk before giving a general anesthetic for radiographic examination.

In more chronic cases, the lameness is associated with atrophy of the gluteal muscles. Radiography can demonstrate the site and assist with the prognosis. Fractures of the tuber coxae, wing of the ilium, tuber ischii, and ischial shaft carry a hopeful prognosis, particularly in young animals. Rest (9-12 mo) is usually the only treatment necessary. Fractures of the acetabulum, shaft of the ilium, and pubis have a much more guarded prognosis.

TROCHANTERIC BURSITIS
("Whirlbone" lameness)

An inflammation of the tendon of the middle gluteal muscle, of the bursa between this tendon and the trochanter major, or of the cartilage of the trochanter major. It is most common in Standardbreds, in which bursitis and gluteal myositis are secondary to hock problems.

The weight is placed on the medial wall of the foot so that it is worn more than the lateral wall. The stride of the affected leg is shorter, and the leg is rotated inward. The horse tends to carry the hindquarters toward the sound side. In chronic cases, the muscles between the external and internal angles of the ilium are atrophied, giving the croup a flat appearance. Pressure over the greater trochanter gives evidence of pain.

If the inflammation is acute, the animal should be rested and hot packs applied over the affected area. Injection of corticosteroid into the bursa temporarily relieves the inflammation. In chronic cases, the injection of 1 mL of 5% Lugol's solution diluted with equal parts of distilled water into or around the bursa as a counterirritant has been recommended.

CONDITIONS OF THE BACK

FRACTURES

Multiple fractures of the summits of the dorsal spinous processes of $T_{4\text{-}10}$ are sometimes seen in young horses that have reared up and fallen over backwards. The tips of the summits and centers of ossification are fractured and displaced laterally. After the initial pain and local reaction have subsided, recovery is satisfactory. Usually, there is no permanent effect on performance, but a persistent swelling over the withers may require use of a special saddle. Occasionally, other fractures of individual spinous processes occur, and their presence can be confirmed by radiography. The clinical signs in these cases are variable.

Fractures of the vertebral bodies are more serious. There is often a history of a bad fall entailing a somersault, and complete or partial paraplegia results from damage to the spinal cord. The prognosis is grave.

MUSCLE AND LIGAMENT STRAIN

See also MYOPATHIES, p 547.

Damage to the soft tissues is undoubtedly the most common cause of back soreness in the horse. This mostly involves the longissimus dorsi complex of muscles, which act to extend (dorsiflex) and laterally flex the spine. Strain of all or part of the longissimus muscles usually occurs during ridden exercise, and clinical signs are associated with altered performance and back pain of acute onset. The principal sites of damage are the caudal withers and cranial lumbar regions (just in front of and behind the saddle area). Most of these injuries respond to rest and physiotherapy, although several weeks may be needed for full recovery.

Another fairly common site of soft-tissue damage is the so-called supraspinous ligament, which runs down the middle of the back and is adherent to the summits of the thoracic and lumbar dorsal spinous processes. It is made up of the multiple tendinous insertions of the various parts of the longissimus dorsi complex and, therefore, is subject to the same strains as the muscles. The clinical signs usually persist longer, and the chances of complete recovery are not as good as for the uncomplicated muscle strains.

There is considerable controversy over the diagnosis and treatment of back problems in horses. Much credit is given to the value of physiotherapy, particularly chiropractic and osteopathic manipulation, but there are no substantiated reports of their efficacy.

OSSIFYING SPONDYLOSIS

Spondylitic lesions of the vertebral bodies of the mid-to caudal thoracic region are uncommon in working horses. However, when they do occur, they have serious effects, and little can be done in the way of permanent treatment to keep the animal in work.

Osteoarthritic lesions of the transverse and articular processes of the lumbar vertebrae are much more common, especially in older horses. However, they appear to cause little inconvenience to the animal because this part of the spine is kept particularly rigid even when the horse is jumping.

OVERRIDING OF THE DORSAL SPINOUS PROCESSES
(Kissing spines syndrome)

Impingement of the summits of the dorsal spines beneath the saddle area predisposes to back pain in some horses. Pressure points between adjacent overriding spines are shown by local periosteal reaction, small bone cysts, and false joint formation. Radiographic lesions of this type are sometimes seen in animals that do not suffer from back trouble, although incidence is lower and lesions are less severe. Diagnosis can be aided by injection of local anesthetic into the affected interspinous spaces. Many cases respond to rest and physiotherapy, but treatment in persistent cases is by resection of one or more of the summits to relieve the crowding of the spines.

SACROILIAC INJURY
(Sacroiliac subluxation, Sacroiliac strain, Sacroiliac arthrosis, Hunter's bumps)

Acute and severe strain of the sacroiliac ligaments is associated with a history of injury and of severe pain in the pelvic or sacroiliac region, often with marked hind-limb lameness. Subacute or chronic sacroiliac strain is low-grade damage that causes typical back soreness. It represents incomplete healing or reinjury of an acute strain. There may be a history of poor performance with an intermittent, often shifting, hindlimb lameness. This may be associated with some restriction in hindlimb action and dragging of the toe of one or both hooves. There usually is prominence or asymmetry of the sacral tuber. Rectal palpation aids the identification of crepitation or shifting in the sacroiliac region.

This syndrome is common in Standardbreds and hunt-jump horses, and has been confused with chronic stifle problems. Usually, there is rather poor muscling of the gluteal masses and, when viewed from behind, some asymmetry of the croup. This may be due to some tilting or rotation of the pelvis or muscle wastage of one quarter, or both. The tail may be held slightly to the side. Pain in the early stages may be evinced when pressure is applied to the midline in front of the tuber coxae, and usually there is a reluctance to ventroflex the back. If these cases are diagnosed early and the animal rested sufficiently for complete healing of the damaged ligaments (6-9 mo), they can recover. However, Standardbreds usually do not then compete well. Chronic cases continue to show poor performance, despite rest and anti-inflammatory medication.

MISCELLANEOUS CONDITIONS

FLEXION DEFORMITIES
(Contracted tendons, Club foot, Knuckling)

A syndrome of flexor tendon disorders associated with postural and foot changes, lameness, and debility. There are congenital and acquired causes. Uterine malposition, teratogenic insults (arthrogryposis, qv, p 477), and genetic defects have been either implicated or proved to cause contracted limbs in newborn foals. Chronic pain is the most common cause of acquired tendon contracture. Pain can arise from physitis, osteochondrosis, degenerative joint disease, or soft-tissue wounds and infection. Pain induces the withdrawal reflex with shortening of the musculotendinous units. Flexors are stronger than extensors, so the animal walks on its toes or knuckles in the fetlocks. Nutritional errors referable to problems associated with bone growth (ie, osteochondrosis and physitis, see [both] below) are intimately associated with the syndrome and must be addressed as a part of the treatment. (*See also* p 478.)

Clinical Findings: Signs vary widely in newborn foals. Some cannot stand; some attempt to walk on the dorsum of their fetlocks; and others can stand, but knuckle in the fetlocks or carpi. One foal may improve spontaneously yet another, seemingly normal at birth, may become progressively worse. Sucklings and weanlings 3-12 mo old may exhibit a rapid onset and walk around on their toes with their heels off the ground. A slower onset is characterized by a "boxy" hoof with an elongated heel and concave toe. Physitis frequently is evident in these animals. Involvement of both forelimbs is the rule, with a tendency to be worse in one leg. Toe abscesses are a frequent complication of the hoof and locomotion changes, and add to the pain and deformity.

Older animals (1-2 yr) commonly knuckle in the metacarpophalangeal joints, which are swollen and enlarged. These animals are upright and straight-legged in both fore- and hindlimbs with flexor tendon and suspensory ligament involvement. Yearlings usually are more severely affected and more difficult to treat than younger animals. The specific diagnosis of tendon involvement is not difficult if a complete examination and careful judgement is rendered. The associated or underlying bone or joint disease and nutritional mismanagement must be identified and corrected.

Treatment: Various types of splints and casts are used for foals with contracted tendons. Forced extension of the limbs induces the inverse myotatic reflex with relaxation of the flexor muscles. Early cases in sucklings and weanlings can be managed conservatively with nutritional correction, proper hoof trimming, and analgesia. Surgical treatment can be simple or complex, depending on the degree of involvement. Desmotomy of the accessory ligament of the deep digital flexor tendon (inferior check desmotomy) is the most successful and commonly used procedure, and does not interfere with future performance. Other types of surgery, including tenotomy and tendon lengthening, tend to be less successful. Joint capsule contracture, collateral ligament malformation, and bone involvement are complications in chronic cases that preclude a successful outcome. Nutritional correction, proper foot trimming, and analgesia are integral to recovery, even when surgery is indicated. The prognosis is fair to good for those that are detected early and managed properly.

OSSIFYING MYOPATHY
(Fibrotic myopathy)

An uncommon condition seen chiefly in working Quarter Horses as a result of trauma to the semimembranosis, semitendinosis, and biceps femoris muscles. Usually, it is unilateral and involves a progressive fibrosis with local adhesions of the affected muscles, which eventually ossify. The gait is fairly characteristic; the forward phase of the stride is jerky, and the foot is jerked back a short distance before being placed on the ground. The action is appreciably different from those of stringhalt and upward patellar fixation. The hardening of the muscles can be palpated in some cases. Radiography and ultrasonography help to establish the degree of involvement. Treatment involves surgery to incise the medial ligament of the semitendinosis at the stifle. Results from a limited number of cases are encouraging. Otherwise, the prognosis is poor.

OSTEOCHONDROSIS
(Osteochondritis dissecans, OCD, Dyschondroplasia)

A metabolic disease of cartilage maturation and defective endochondral ossification that results in a syndrome of bone and joint defects (*see also* p 558). Causes include rapid growth, trauma to cartilage, malnutrition, and mineral imbalances, including trace mineral deficiencies and heavy metal toxicities in isolated circumstances. Genetic factors are unproved, but a familial tendency among fast-growing bloodlines seems to exist. Trauma to the growing cartilage damages budding capillaries, which arrests endochondral ossification and leads to physical deformity of the cartilage model. If the physeal-metaphyseal cartilage is affected, bone contours and longitudinal growth are disturbed (*see* PHYSITIS, below). Involvement of articular cartilage at the periphery of joint surfaces leads to regressive changes at the joint margins, dissecting lesions, and the formation of flaps (osteochondritis dissecans). Central articular lesions, because of weight-bearing effects, involve focal retention of cartilage within the subchondral bone (*see* SUBCHONDRAL CYSTS, p 527). Axial skeletal involvement includes vertebral articular facets, spinal instability, spinal cord damage, and ultimately, ataxia and proprioception deficits.

Clinical Findings: The syndrome varies depending on the cartilage structure(s) affected. Many horses have multiple lesions. Young, growing horses are affected, but the occasional subchondral cyst may not be evident until 2-3 yr of age. Pain and deformity are the initial signs. Angular limb or flexion deformities suggest inclusion of osteochondrosis in the differential diagnosis. Likewise, synovial joint effusions associated with variable degrees of lameness are indicative of articular cartilage defects. Any bone or joint can be affected, but the tibiotarsal, femoropatellar, femorotibial, elbow, and shoulder joints are sites of predilection; the meta-carpophalangeal and proximal interphalangeal joints also are frequently affected. Involvement of the pastern joint results in ringbone (qv, p 517), although in a younger than expected animal. Radiography is essential. Because lesions are frequently bilateral, the contralateral part should be radiographed for comparison. Because articular cartilage lesions are commonly missed with radiography, arthroscopy is becoming increasingly important in diagnosis and evaluation.

Treatment: Treatment is primarily surgical. Both flexion limb and angular limb deformities are amenable to surgery with predictably favorable results in properly selected cases. Surgical treatment of OCD of the tibiotarsal, metacarpophalangeal, femoropatellar, and shoulder joints has been successful. Arthroscopic techniques are used. Subchondral cysts of the femorotibial joint have been successfully managed by curettage, with and without cancellous bone grafts. Pastern disease can be managed by surgical arthrodesis.

In addition to the surgical considerations, nutritional imbalances must be corrected, and toxic elements eliminated. Overfeeding of high-energy feeds is a common error. Exercise must be regulated according to the site(s) and severity of involvement. The prognosis is guarded but depends on the age of the animal, the nature and location of lesion(s), the detection and correction of predisposing factors, and the response to treatment.

PHYSITIS
(Epiphysitis, Physeal dysplasia, Dysplasia of the growth plate)

Physitis involves swelling around the growth plates of certain long bones in young horses. It can be a component of osteochondrosis. Suggested causes include malnutrition, conformational defects, faulty hoof growth, compression of the growth plate, and toxicosis. The most acceptable hypothesis at this time appears to be the compression theory. However, the changes observed in physitis also occur in clinically normal animals; the condition is seen frequently in well-grown, fast-growing, heavy-topped foals during the summer when the ground is dry and hard, and on stud farms where the calcium:phosphorus ratio in the diet is imbalanced.

The condition occurs in young horses and most commonly involves the distal extremities of the radius, tibia, third metacarpal/metatarsal bone, and the proximal aspect of the first phalanx. It is characterized by swelling at the level of the growth plate, giving a typical "boxy" appearance to the affected joints. Radiographs aid the clinical assessment. Microscopically, the physeal cartilage appears crushed and thinned, and new bone is formed.

Treatment consists of reducing food intake to reduce body weight or at least growth rate; confining exercise to a yard or a large, well-ventilated loose box with a soft surface (peat moss, deep straw, shavings, or sand); ensuring that the feet are carefully and frequently trimmed; and correcting the diet if necessary. The calcium:phosphorus ratio should be adjusted to 1.6:1, and protein content limited to <10% of dry matter. In general terms, bran should not be fed, and dicalcium phosphate or bone flour (10-30 g daily) should be added to the diet. Vitamin D supplements (PO or parenteral) are indicated, but the dosage must be monitored closely to avoid hypervitaminosis D.

As a preventive measure, the older foal or yearling that is over-fat or heavy-topped should be watched carefully for clinical signs, especially when the ground is hard and dry. When these conditions prevail, food rations and exercise should be restricted.

LAMENESS IN PIGS

Locomotor disturbances are becoming more common in pigs, probably because of trends toward increased production and intensive housing, particularly when slotted/perforated floors are in use. Lameness may result in failure to reach marketable weight, reduced performance, and partial or total condemnation at slaughter. Heavy losses in breeding stock can occur, and boar/gilt selection rates may be compromised. Locomotor disturbances in sows may be a major reason for culling; additional losses arise from 1) replacement costs, 2) increased numbers of sows needed to maintain production, 3) increased preweaning mortality resulting from clumsy sows, and 4) poorer reproductive performance due to a reduction in the average parity of the sow herd. Since lame boars are unable to breed, losses include 1) additional replacement costs (otherwise the physically fit boars are overworked), 2) reduced litter size and conception rates, and 3) more boars have to be maintained.

The locomotor system involves muscles, bones, joints, tendons, ligaments, and claws, all regulated by the central and peripheral nervous systems. Dysfunction in any area may result in lameness. Only the common abnormalities affecting the skeletal system and feet are discussed here, and these need to be differentiated from lamenesses resulting from neuromuscular abnormalities.

Whenever a problem is encountered, a full history should be taken, and include the morbidity, ages affected, type of onset and progression of lameness, and other clinical signs. Animal flow, management practices, and vaccination programs also need to be evaluated.

CONDITIONS OF THE FOOT

FOOT LESIONS AND FOOT ROT

Foot rot is a septic laminitis that follows cracks in the hoof wall (quarter cracks). These lesions are seen primarily on the lateral claw of fore- and hindlimbs, particularly the latter. The cracks originate on the volar aspect of the wall, and generally occur in the distal two-thirds of the hoof. Foot rot may also occur in pigs of all ages as a result of infection following penetration of the sole or heel. On the "average" farm, ~15-20% of pigs may be affected during a year, and up to 50% in problem herds. In pigs of market weight, up to 85% may have evidence of hoof lesions, although most are not severe. Heel erosions, separation along the white line, erosion of the sole, and hoof-wall cracks are the more common lesions.

Breeding stock may have a high incidence of foot lesions. "False sand cracks" (wall cracks originating on the volar surface), "bush foot" (deformity of the foot resulting from septic laminitis), bruising of the sole or heel, and hyperkeratinization of the heel seem to be the lesions most frequently associated with lameness.

Pathogenesis: Mixed populations of gram-negative cocci, gram-negative filamentous organisms, and spirochetes have been recovered; cultures have yielded *Fusobacterium necrophorum* and *Corynebacterium pyogenes*. Development of necrotic sinuses in the corium, and microbial invasion of underlying structures may result in tenosynovitis, osteomyelitis, or suppurative arthritis. These tracts may migrate dorsally within the corium, and cellulitis with fistulas above the coronary band commonly develops. Severely affected claws become enlarged and deformed due to a proliferation of fibrous connective tissue, but most infections are confined to the hoof or the area of the fetlock joint. Occasionally, probably when osteomyelitis of the pedal bone is present, foot lesions are the route of entry for systemic infection and resultant localized infection in other body regions. Pigs fed on the floor can develop septic laminitis from cracked corn (maize) penetrating the sole and migrating dorsally. Traumatic laminitis may follow trauma to the hoof wall with or without superficial changes in the hoof. Not all hoof lesions result in septic or traumatic laminitis, so care should be taken to determine whether a hoof lesion is the cause of lameness. The following factors influence the development of foot lesions.

Hoof Size and Consistency of the Horn: In neonates, the medial claws, particularly of the hindlimb, are most commonly affected because of lateral thrusting while nursing. In other age groups, the lateral claws, particularly the hind, are most commonly affected for several reasons: the medial digit is shorter in both fore- and hindlimbs; the volar surface of the medial digit is also shorter and narrower than the lateral; and the area of the volar surface of the hoof, along with the length and angle of the toe, can be influenced by the floor surface on which the animal is housed. The composition of the hoof horn may influence the incidence of foot lesions: more calcium is present in damaged horn, and the horn produced by inflamed corium is more porous and less resistant to damage. Pigmented horn has been found to contain more mineral than nonpigmented horn, and the incidence of foot lesions is higher in the latter, possibly because they are softer.

Floor Surfaces: Animals housed on artificial floors develop more foot lesions. The ideal floor should provide adequate traction, and be nonabrasive and comfortable to lie on, self-cleaning or easily cleaned, durable, and inexpensive. Many floors, while satisfying some of the above criteria, have a major deficiency; it is difficult to produce a nonabrasive, yet nonslip surface. Concrete has been used extensively in all phases of production, and solid, partially slatted, or fully slatted floors have been used. Unfortunately, concrete surfaces vary tremendously because of differences in composition, laying conditions, and finishing, and also because of factors that precipitate excessive wear of floor and foot.

Freshly poured or "green" concrete can produce a higher incidence of lesions than a seasoned surface. Rough finishes and worn solid concrete floors with exposed sharp aggregates increase the risk of foot and leg lesions. Concrete slats with sharp or chipped edges are traumatic to hooves and legs, while "pencil-edged" slats tend to be less so. Partially slatted floors cause fewer hoof lesions than those fully slatted. Slat width is of importance for growing and finishing pigs: 8 in. (20 cm) concrete slats produce fewer foot lesions than 5 in. (13 cm) ones.

Efforts to determine the optimal layout, design, and composition of slats for piggery floors have given equivocal results. Wooden surfaces may produce fewer lesions than concrete, but are less durable. Plastic and aluminum slats seem to predispose to more severe heel and sole lesions, whereas concrete floors or steel slats favor cracks in the wall of the foot. Plastic-coated metal panels are less abrasive, especially to knees of neonates. Many of the above criticisms apply to the various forms of punched or woven metal floors, and care must be taken with the finish, void-size, and laying of such floors. Consideration also must be given to cleaning and disinfecting flooring materials.

Nutrition: Nutrition plays a part in the incidence of foot rot. Pigs fed whey or skim milk may have a high incidence, while offal- or garbage-fed pigs may be less likely to have foot rot. Supplemental biotin, 200 μg/kg in noncorn-based diets, may reduce the incidence of foot lesions in sows and help to prevent their development. Diets having corn (maize) as the base may be adequate in available biotin, but supplementation could still prove beneficial.

Clinical Findings and Diagnosis: A unilateral, nonweight-bearing lameness may result from a hoof lesion with subsequent laminitis, or from traumatic laminitis with no evidence of a hoof lesion. The hoof should be cleaned and palpated. Digital pressure may aid in localizing the area of pain.

Treatment and Control: Therapy usually involves treatment of the secondary infection. Topical chemotherapeutic agents, such as antibiotic ointment, formalin solution, and copper sulfate have been used in outbreaks of foot rot. Large IM doses (6 million IU) of procaine penicillin are claimed to be effective. It may be of benefit to place animals in a bedded pen or outside on dirt. Foot lesions may improve if animals are housed in individual crates. Chronically affected claws can be amputated, but conservative treatment with astringents is as effective, if not more so.

The most important control measures are to provide a floor surface that is clean, dry, and nonabrasive. Bedding should be kept clean and dry and of adequate depth. Rough concrete floors should be resurfaced; a variety of bitumen and epoxy resin-based paints have been used, but the former may not be sufficiently durable, and the latter can make floors too slippery. The slipperiness may be partially overcome by incorporating sand or sawdust in the resin, but the floor can then be too abrasive. If the edges of concrete slats are sharp or chipped, they may need to be replaced.

Formalin or copper sulfate foot baths can aid in prevention. Animals with equal-sized digits should be selected for the breeding herd and their diet supplemented with biotin.

LAMINITIS

Inflammation of the corium of the foot, whether infectious or noninfectious, may result in lameness. Systemic diseases such as postparturient fever and mercury toxicity can occasionally result in laminitis, as can overfeeding. Since laminitis is not the main clinical sign of a systemic disease, the frequency with which the 2 are associated is unknown. Perhaps the most common form of laminitis is observed in sows with postparturient fever or mastitis. Lameness is usually observed in the forelimbs, although all 4 limbs are affected. Heat and pain may be evident in the hoof, and a digital pulse may be detected if the fetlock is palpated. Hyperemia, hemorrhage, and dilation of the lymphatics are observed in histological sections. Thrombosis and suppurative inflammation are seen at the base of the laminae. Treatment is usually directed toward the primary systemic illness, but corticosteroids or antihistamines may be used to reduce inflammation of the corium.

Laminitis, with or without infection, is a common problem in animals raised on artificial floors. Trauma to the hoof, which produces hemorrhage and inflammation in the corium, is a common noninfectious cause; hemorrhage is particularly obvious in animals with nonpigmented horn.

LOSS OF ACCESSORY DIGITS

Loss of, or damage to, the medial accessory digit of the hindlimb in neonatal pigs or sows in farrowing crates with certain types of punched or expanded metal floors has been reported. The digits may be infected during the suckling period and shed after weaning.

OVERGROWN HOOVES

Changes in the structure of the hoof do not necessarily indicate a problem in the foot. Overgrown hooves are common in animals housed on nonabrasive floor surfaces or allowed only limited exercise, eg, boars and sows in stalls in soft dirt lots. Changes in the shape of the hoof may occur when any cause leads to altered gait, and thus to an altered wear pattern. Elongated toes may result from exostosis and fracture of the distal end of the third phalanx. Painful lesions in the heel, or a lesion on the anterior aspect of the articular surface of the distal humerus that causes an animal to bear weight mainly on the sole and toe of the hoof, cause shortening of the toe and proliferation of the heel. Treatment of uncomplicated overgrowth of the heel or toe usually involves trimming the excess horn. Breed type may also predispose to some conformational changes of the foot.

INFECTIOUS ARTHRITIDES

MYCOPLASMAL ARTHRITIS

Mycoplasma hyosynoviae is a common early inhabitant of the nasopharynx. It can produce acute synovitis and subsequent lameness in pigs 10-30 wk old, more commonly at the upper end of this range.

Clinical Findings: Clinical signs may be preceded by changes in management, such as transport, mixing, and sorting. Walking in dirt lots following heavy rain may also precipitate an outbreak. Synovitis due to *M hyosynoviae* can be secondary to degenerative joint disease. Affected pigs are usually afebrile and reluctant to rise. Joints commonly affected include the carpus, elbow, stifle, and tarsus, but hindlimb lameness is most common. When the forelimbs are affected, animals shift weight to the hindlimbs, flex the carpus, and extend the elbow. Hindlimb involvement is characterized by attempts to shift weight to the forelimbs. The animal stands uneasily with a stiff-legged posture, repeatedly shifts weight from one hindleg to the other, and frequently flexes the affected leg. Immediately after standing, such animals may walk with a stiff gait, but often walk more normally following forced exercise. Kyphosis may be observed. Joint distention is visible and palpable when the carpus and tarsus are involved, but distention of other joints is difficult to detect.

Lameness normally decreases ~1 wk after onset, and clinical signs continue to diminish until recovery is complete. Morbidity is variable (1-50%), and mortality is low.

Mycoplasma hyosynoviae has recently been isolated from the lesions of adventitious bursitis of the hocks, but whether it is involved with development of these bursae is not clear.

Diagnosis and Lesions: The synovial membranes are hyperplastic, edematous, and hyperemic. There is excessive serosanguineous joint fluid, but the articular and periarticular surfaces are unaffected. Diagnosis is based on history, signs, and lesions; an acute, nonfebrile, nonsuppurative synovitis in a 12- to 24-wk-old pig is highly suggestive. Diagnosis is confirmed by isolation of the organism and serology.

Treatment and Control: *Mycoplasma hyosynoviae* is sensitive to parenteral tylosin, lincomycin, and tiamulin. A corticosteroid injection at the first signs of illness reduces the severity of lameness. Identification and correction of predisposing factors are the best means of prevention; experimentally, vaccination has proved effective.

MYCOPLASMAL POLYSEROSITIS

Mycoplasma hyorhinis is a common commensal in the nasal secretions of growing pigs. If the animal is stressed, septicemia may result, with subsequent colonization of the serous and synovial membranes. Although *M hyorhinis* is commonly isolated from pneumonic lesions, it is not known whether it is a contaminant or a secondary pathogen (*see also* p 748).

The lameness is usually acute and accompanied by other signs of systemic infection such as moderate fever (104-105°F [40-41°C]), anorexia, and depression. Pigs show dyspnea, and stand with an arched back. The tarsal and carpal joints may be swollen. The stifle, shoulder, and atlanto-occipital joints may also be involved. Two weeks later, the predominant sign is lameness with distended joints, which occasionally persists for up to 6 mo. Polyarthritis usually occurs in animals 3-10 wk old, and there may be a history of concurrent pneumonia or enteritis. The mortality is usually low, although morbidity occasionally reaches 25%.

Culture and histopathology may differentiate the gross lesions of *M hyorhinis* polyserositis and arthritis from those due to *Haemophilus parasuis*. The chances of isolating the organism are better when animals are in the acute stages of the disease. Serology also may aid diagnosis.

Mycoplasma hyorhinis is sensitive to tylosin or lincomycin, but often, treatment is not very effective unless given at the first signs of illness. Preventing concurrent diseases, avoiding stresses, eg, extreme temperature fluctuations, mixing, movement, and overcrowding, aid in prevention.

NEONATAL SEPTIC POLYARTHRITIS
(Joint-ill)

Septic polyarthritis is an important cause of preweaning mortality: up to 30% or more of litters may be affected, and the average herd incidence is >17%. Average morbidity is ~3.3% and the mortality 1.5%, but >50% of the neonates that develop septic arthritis survive and contribute to the lameness problems observed in the growing and finishing stages.

The main routes of entry of bacteria in young pigs are thought to be the tonsils and small intestine, but the navel may also be important. In fact, any surgical break in the integument (eg, tail docking, ear notching, teeth clipping) may provide a portal of entry for infection that localizes in the joint(s), as may foot lesions, generalized skin infections, and knee abrasions resulting from rough floor surfaces.

Colostral immunity is important in the prevention of septic arthritis. The incidence is higher in the progeny of gilts and young sows, and in herds that have been recently repopulated or that purchase large numbers of replacement gilts.

Clinical Findings: Lameness may be observed as early as 3-4 days (usually ~10), and joint distention by 7-15 days after farrowing, but mortality peaks between 2 and 5 wk. Any joint may be affected, but there is a predilection for the carpus, elbow, hip, and tarsus.

Diagnosis and Lesions: Most cases are suppurative in nature. The most common isolates are streptococci (~55%), particularly serogroups C, L, and D; staphylococci (~6%); *Escherichia coli* (~4%); and *Corynebacterium pyogenes* (~3%). *Pasteurella* and *Moraxella* spp, *Erysipelothrix rhusiopathiae* (nonsuppurative), *Actinobacillus (Haemophilus) pleuropneumoniae*, and *H parasuis* are involved occasionally.

In subacute cases, group C streptococci, *E coli*, and staphylococci are the common isolates. Joint capsules are filled with necrotic material, fibrin, or flecks of purulent material. The synovial membranes are hyperemic and show a degree of proliferation, but cartilage erosion is rare. Group L streptococci usually cause chronic infections with large amounts of purulent material in the joint capsule.

Corynebacterium pyogenes is most commonly isolated from joints with chronic lesions, severe periarticular fibrosis, necrosis, and fibrosis of surrounding muscles. Copious pale-green, purulent material is present in the joint capsules, and extensive ulceration of the articular surfaces may occur.

Demonstration of the infectious agent in stained smears and cultures of the joints and spleen or brain confirm the diagnosis.

Treatment and Control: If given as soon as signs of lameness appear, treatment is more effective than when joint distention is visible. Choice of antibiotic should be based on the infectious agent involved. When given in adequate dosage, penicillin is usually effective against streptococci.

Polyarthritis can be prevented by 1) ensuring an adequate intake of colostrum during the first few hours of life; 2) performing tail docking, teeth clipping, ear notching, castration, etc, hygienically; and 3) providing nonabrasive floors. Since the problem is most severe in gilt litters, the average age of the sow herd should be allowed to increase, and gilts should be introduced from one source only.

Vaccination of sows to prevent polyarthritis in neonates has not been evaluated thoroughly, but it may be effective for groups C and L streptococci. Passive protection of neonates can be obtained by vaccination of sows against erysipelas, but there are no effective vaccines against *C pyogenes* or staphylococci. Vaccines for *E coli*, *A pleuropneumoniae*, *H parasuis*, and *Pasteurella* spp are available, but their efficacy in preventing neonatal polyarthritis is unknown.

Dipping navels in iodine is a commonly practiced preventive measure but must be performed soon after birth. Ligation/clamping of navels is time-consuming, but benefits are claimed. An antibiotic injected into the piglet shortly after birth is helpful in some cases. The use of antibiotics in sow feed is not effective.

SUPPURATIVE ARTHRITIS AND OSTEOMYELITIS IN OLDER ANIMALS

Suppurative arthritis also occurs in older animals, although some cases originate in suckling pigs. The etiological agents involved are somewhat different from those causing arthritis in neonates: *Corynebacterium pyogenes* is more common, and streptococci and staphylococci also occur. Occasionally, *Brucella suis* causes suppurative arthritis.

Streptococci invade the palatine tonsil, but damage to mucosal surfaces and skin may also provide entry for streptococci, staphylococci, and *C pyogenes*. Routes of entry in older animals include injection sites, wounds from tail and vulval biting, foot lesions, dystocias, udder lacerations, and unsanitary surgical procedures.

Signs depend on the region of the body involved, but the problem is usually chronic and progressive. When the pyemia is intra-articular, joint distention is marked. Periarticular areas may also be abscessed. Spondylitis and osteomyelitis of the lumbar vertebrae, as well as epidural abscesses, may result in hypersensitivity over the spine, and kyphosis or paraplegia may occur. Traumatic or pathological fractures, degenerative joint disease, and other abnormalities of the skeletal system are often complicated by pyemia. Such animals should be culled.

Arthrocentesis reveals a large amount of purulent material—creamy in the case of streptococci or staphylococci, or yellowish green if *C pyogenes* is the cause. *Corynebacterium pyogenes* tends to be more chronic and associated with extensive articular damage and periarticular fibrosis.

Treatment with an appropriate antibiotic is effective only in the early stages. The same is true for osteomyelitis or epidural abscesses. Joint lavage and instillation of antibiotics may be effective, but are time-consuming and costly.

Prevention should aim at eliminating the route of entry of the organism. There is no effective vaccine against staphylococci or *C pyogenes*, but streptococcal vaccines may be useful in the neonatal disease. If suppurative arthritis in weaned animals is considered a residual problem from the farrowing house, preventive measures should be instituted there.

NONINFECTIOUS SKELETAL ABNORMALITIES

APOPHYSIOLYSIS OF THE ISCHIATIC TUBEROSITY

An apophysis is a growth plate that is associated with a projection of bone, such as the ischiatic tuberosity. Bilateral separation of the ischiatic tuberosity usually occurs in young sows, typically in those heavily pregnant or that have just farrowed. A "dog-sitting" posture is often adopted; the animal may stand with assistance, but usually only for a brief period. Palpation over the ischiatic tuberosity may demonstrate crepitus or swelling. The cause of this condition is unknown, but as with epiphysiolysis (*see* below), separation is thought to follow an abnormal endochondral ossification that results in a thick and weakened physis. Thickening of the physis associated with the ischiatic tuberosity has been seen in osteochondrosis. Unilateral separation with evidence of repair also has been observed, which suggests that animals suffering from a mild, unilateral apophysiolysis may not need to be slaughtered.

DEGENERATIVE JOINT DISEASE AND OSTEOCHONDROSIS

Degenerative joint disease—also termed arthropathy, arthrosis, polyarthrosis, osteoarthritis, and osteoarthrosis—is a cause of lameness in young adult and older pigs.

Pathogenesis: Microbiological examination has failed to reveal infectious agents. The histological changes in the articular cartilage, subchondral bone, and synovial membrane support that finding.

Degenerative joint disease in pigs is usually secondary to osteochondrosis (*see also* p 558). Osteochondrosis in pigs usually refers to a focal failure in endochondral ossification both in epiphyseal and physeal cartilage. This is probably a misnomer, since osteochondrosis implies degeneration and necrosis of both bone and cartilage of an ossification center. Osteonecrosis is not observed in early lesions, but sclerosis and bone marrow fibrosis may be observed during the later stages. Chondronecrosis is most commonly observed in the articular-epiphyseal complex and only occasionally observed in the physeal cartilage. The incidence and severity of osteochondrosis cannot be related to locomotor abnormalities in pigs under market weight. Lameness develops when an area of the articular-epiphyseal cartilage complex, weakened by osteochondrosis, separates from the underlying subchondral bone.

Degenerative joint disease and osteochondrosis have been reported in many of the synovial joints of the limbs and axial skeleton. There is a predilection for certain joints and sites in the articular surface of these joints. The surfaces most commonly affected are the axial aspect of the medial condyle of the femur, the anterior of the trochlea of the humerus, the lumbar intervertebral synovial joints, and the lateral aspect of the head of the humerus. Osteochondrosis is also observed in several physeal areas. The physes most commonly involved are those of the distal ulna and the proximal and distal femur. It also has been seen in nonweight-bearing physes such as the trochlear physis of the proximal ulna and apophysis of the ischiatic tuberosity. Osteochondrosis has been observed in the area of endochondral ossification of the ribs. There is some doubt as to whether osteochondrosis of certain physeal areas leads to lameness by producing abnormalities in the angulation of the long bones, or whether these abnormalities are the reason for the development of osteochondrosis. Without a serial study of the progression of the disease, it is impossible to say what is cause and what is effect.

The cause of osteochondrosis and degenerative joint disease has not been determined. Growing pigs develop more serious lesions as their weight increases, but it is not known whether the lesions are related to the rate of gain or actual body weight. Litter and breed differences are also recognized, but there is still some question as to whether osteochondrosis can be eliminated through selection without sacrificing desirable production traits, especially when the prevalence of osteochondrosis of the ulna, humerus, and femur in slaughter-weight animals approaches 100%.

Clinical Findings, Lesions, and Diagnosis: Degenerative joint disease usually is a chronic, progressive, bilateral lameness, and although signs may be observed as early as 4 mo of age, >6 mo is more typical. The elbow, stifle, and lumbar intervertebral joints are involved most commonly. Animals with involvement of the elbows initially exhibit slight flexion of the carpal, metacarpal, and interdigital joints, with extension of the elbow during the weight-bearing phase of the stride and while standing. The stride length is shortened slightly. Lameness progresses from this straight-legged appearance to one of walking on the toes with visible flexion of the carpus. Severely affected animals may walk on the carpus.

When the stifles are affected, the animal bears weight with the stifle and tarsus extended. As the lameness progresses, the stride is shortened, and the animal may bear weight on the toe only. When observing the gait from the rear, there is a noticeable lateral swaying of the hindquarters. Kyphosis may be observed with quadrilateral lameness due to involvement of both the elbow and stifle. Kyphosis is also observed with spondylosis secondary to osteochondrosis in the growth areas of the centrum of the lumbar vertebrae.

Necropsy usually reveals bilateral lesions of similar or differing severities in the joints most often involved. In the stifle, lesions are located mainly on the axial aspect of the medial condyle of the femur. Lesions in the elbow may be observed on the medial condyle or the capitulum humeri. Involvement of the articular surfaces of ulna and radius occurs only late in the disease.

Articular lesions first appear as corrugations of the cartilage, with no involvement of the superficial articular cartilage. Progression of the lesion may result in the formation of a cartilage flap (osteochondritis dissecans), with ulceration of the articular cartilage and exposure of subchondral bone in severe cases. Chronic lesions have evidence of fibrocartilaginous repair. Synovial fluid may be slightly increased and serosanguineous in appearance. Ankylosis and formation of osteophytes may occur in chronic, severely affected joints. Radiography of valuable breeding stock may aid in diagnosis, but detects only lesions involving subchondral bone.

Treatment and Control: Prognosis is poor. Early surgical intervention to remove cartilage and curette the affected area is seldom economical. Because the etiology is uncertain, recommendations for prevention tend to be general and vague. Providing adequate nutrition, limiting energy intake of animals selected for breeding stock to slow their growth, basing selection on certain conformations or on the severity of lesions in performance-tested progeny, increasing exercise, and providing better floor surface have been recommended.

FRACTURES

Fracture of a bone can occur in a pig of any age. Most fractures in neonates are caused by the sow. Fractures in adults may be associated with severe, direct trauma on the farm or in transport. As a result of osteomalacia, sows and gilts not uncommonly develop fractures of the proximal femur or vertebrae following weaning of large litters. They are most common in sows that have suckled piglets in crates and then been mixed with other sows at weaning. Affected pigs should be slaughtered.

NUTRITIONALLY INDUCED SKELETAL ABNORMALITIES

Deficiencies or excesses of various nutrients have been associated with skeletal abnormalities in pigs. (*See* DYSTROPHIES ASSOCIATED WITH CALCIUM, PHOSPHORUS, AND VITAMIN D, pp 481 and 1252.) Alterations in bone growth and remodeling are seen as nutritional problems in young, growing animals. Bone deformation may result. In older animals, nutritional imbalances predominantly affect the remodeling process, usually resulting in changes in the strength of cortical and trabecular bone. Osteomalacia is most common in adult sows nursing large litters for ≥4 wk.

Skeletal lesions have been reported in pigs with hyper- or hypovitaminosis A; deficiencies in manganese, magnesium, and copper; and zinc and fluoride toxicosis. However, most trials on nutritional imbalances affecting the skeletal system have been concerned with levels of calcium, phosphorus, and vitamin D.

PROXIMAL FEMORAL EPIPHYSIOLYSIS

A fracture through the physis or growth plate of the proximal femur, in which the head of the femur separates from its neck. This is usually observed in pigs between 5 mo and 3 yr old. Closure of the proximal femoral physis occurs when pigs are 3-3½ yr old. Pathogenesis is uncertain, but it is thought that the condition is due to a weakened physeal region associated with alteration in endochondral ossification in growing animals. Osteochondrosis has been incriminated as an alteration in endochondral ossification that may weaken the physeal growth plate.

The condition may be unilateral or bilateral; onset is usually acute and extremely painful; occasionally, the lameness is more insidious and then abruptly becomes severe 5-10 days after onset. If bilateral, the animal is usually unable to rise, but may accept food and water; with unilateral lameness, weight is not borne on the affected limb. Manipulation of the affected limb is resented, and crepitus may be heard or felt over the hip.

Unilateral epiphysiolysis should be differentiated from unilateral fracture of the femur associated with trauma or osteomalacia. Bilateral epiphysiolysis should be differentiated from bilateral fractures and from paraplegia due to lumbosacral fractures, spondylosis, or spinal abscessation. There is no treatment.

LAMENESS IN SHEEP

A number of systemic diseases may cause lameness in sheep. The more common conditions, listed by age group usually affected, are: **lambs**—joint-ill, tetanus, white muscle disease, enzootic ataxia (copper deficiency), polyarthritis (chlamydial), rickets, poisonous plant intoxication (eg, sneezeweed), contagious ecthyma (orf); **adults**—mastitis, epididymitis, mineral and trace element imbalances; **any age**—erysipelas (one of the more important, qv, p 335), laminitis, bluetongue, ulcerative dermatosis, foot-and-mouth disease, dermatophilosis. Additional information on differential diagnosis, treatment, and prevention can be found under the specific topics. (*See also* ARTHRITIS AND RELATED DISORDERS, LG AN, p 467; DISEASES OF THE SPINAL COLUMN AND CORD, p 584; CONGENITAL ANOMALIES, p 475; and MYOPATHIES, p 547.)

Many lamenesses are due to injuries. The general principles of treatment and prevention of these are the same for sheep as for other species.

In addition to the diseases that also affect other parts of the body, there is a group of infections specific to the feet. They are due to mixed infections with combinations of bacteria including *Fusobacterium necrophorum*. The skin between the claws is the primary site of invasion, but this usually does not occur when the stratum corneum is dry and intact. Predisposing causes are damage by water, maceration, frostbite, or mechanical trauma. Epidermal penetration by *F necrophorum*

and *Corynebacterium pyogenes* induces a transient condition, ovine interdigital dermatitis; when there is concurrent invasion by *Bacteroides (Fusiformis) nodosus*,
foot rot results. This may be benign or virulent, depending on the strain of *B
nodosus*. When the dermal and subdermal invasion by *F necrophorum* and *C pyogenes* involves the distal interphalangeal joint, foot abscess develops. Infection of
the hoof matrix with these organisms results in septic laminitis. Descriptions of
these 5 distinct but related conditions follow:

FOOT ABSCESS
(Infective bulbar necrosis, Heel abscess, Bumblefoot)

A necrotizing or purulent infection involving the distal interphalangeal joint.
The incidence is usually sporadic, but up to 15% of rams or ewes in late pregnancy
may be affected.

The 2 organisms most consistently recovered from foot abscess are *Fusobacterium necrophorum* and *Corynebacterium pyogenes*. Most commonly, foot abscess
develops as a complication of ovine interdigital dermatitis (OID, qv, p 544) by
extension of the necrotic process into the subcutis, and thence into the distal interphalangeal joint. This joint is vulnerable to infection on the interdigital aspect
where the joint capsule protrudes above the coronary border as the dorsal and volar
pouches. At these 2 sites, the joint capsule is protected only by the interdigital skin
and a minimal amount of subcut. tissue.

Sporadic cases may also arise following penetration by sharp objects or careless
paring of the hoof.

Foot abscess develops most often when the soil and pastures are wet. Rams,
particularly in their first winter, and ewes during late pregnancy are affected most
commonly. The disease causes an acute lameness, usually restricted to one foot. In
the early stages, it may be possible to express necrotic material through an opening
in the interdigital skin via the channel caused by the bacterial invasion. Later, the
sinuses may extend to break out at one or more points above the coronet. In ~50%
of the cases, movement of the affected digit is exaggerated, which indicates that the
ligaments about the distal interphalangeal joint have ruptured; it is likely that there
will be displacement of the digit during locomotion, and permanent deformity.

Acute lameness, swelling of one digit, and discharging sinuses distinguish foot
abscess from foot rot. Radiographs can help determine the extent of joint damage.

Once the infection becomes established in the joint, treatment is of limited
value. Therapy should be aimed at maintaining the integrity of the joint ligaments
by draining the abscess, bandaging to reduce stress on the ligaments, and countering
the bacterial infection with antibiotics or sulfonamides.

Although the prognosis for complete recovery is poor, in most cases the foot
heals sufficiently to allow adequate locomotion after ~2 mo.

Control depends on early treatment and avoiding the conditions that lead to
OID. Although *F necrophorum* vaccines are available, they have not proved to be
entirely satisfactory.

FOOT ROT

BENIGN FOOT ROT (BFR)

A form of foot rot in which the infection is confined largely to the interdigital
skin, with minimal underrunning of the adjacent horn. Clinically, it is similar to
OID (qv, p 544), but *Bacteroides nodosus* is involved. Lameness is common but
less severe than in virulent foot rot (VFR, *see* below). The etiology and pathogenesis are the same as in VFR, but the causal strains of *B nodosus* are less virulent.
Bacteroides nodosus isolated from cattle usually causes only the benign form of
foot rot in sheep. The economic effect of BFR is much less than is that of VFR.
Foot baths with 5% formaldehyde solution are usually adequate for control.

VIRULENT FOOT ROT
(VFR, Malignant foot rot, Contagious foot rot)

A specific, chronic, necrotizing disease of the epidermis of the interdigital skin and hoof matrix. It commences as an interdigital dermatitis and extends to involve large areas of the hoof matrix. Because the infected tissue is destroyed, the hoof loses its anchorage and becomes detached. Foot rot is contagious and, under suitable conditions, morbidity may approach 100%. The infection is also found in goats and deer, but rarely in cattle.

Etiology: Foot rot is due to a mixed infection in which synergism between 2 gramnegative, anaerobic bacteria is essential. *Fusobacterium necrophorum* is a normal resident of the sheep's environment, but infection depends on the presence of *Bacteroides nodosus*, a strict parasite that does not survive for more than a few days in the soil or pastures. Because the prolonged availability of *B nodusus* depends on the presence of infected animals, it is regarded as the transmissible and specific causal agent of foot rot, although its contribution to the disease process is not necessarily greater than that of *F necrophorum*.

The transmission of foot rot to healthy animals requires a warm, moist environment. Under these conditions, the interdigital stratum corneum becomes macerated; filaments of *F necrophorum* invade the superficial epidermis and induce OID (qv, p 544). If *B nodosus* is in contact with the skin at this stage, foot rot results. Injuries to the feet enhance the transmission of foot rot, although it usually does not occur when the soil temperature is <40°F (4.5°C).

Clinical Findings: The most obvious sign is lameness, which may be severe. Some animals remain recumbent or on their brisket and knees, which tend to become depilated and ulcerated. Affected animals lose body condition. Rams infected in the hindfeet may be unable to serve, and similarly, ewes with hindfeet lesions may be unable to bear the weight of a ram at service. Wool production is reduced. In early cases, examination of the feet may reveal nothing more than dermatitis similar to OID. In slightly more advanced cases, in which the infection has begun to extend into the hoof matrix, there is slight detachment of areas of the hoof. As the disease progresses, the epidermal necrosis and separation of the horn spread further under the heel and sole, and finally the outer wall, so that the hoof may eventually be attached only at the coronet. The necrotic tissue has a characteristic odor. Myiasis is a common sequela and may extend to the sides of the sheep at sites where the infected feet are placed when the sheep lie down. The disease persists for years in some sheep. In others, the infection may be hidden in small pockets within the foot where it is detectable only on extensive paring; sheep so affected act as subclinical carriers. These small pockets may become active within the foot or open up and contaminate the soil when favored by a moist external environment. Recovery from foot rot occurs but is not followed by appreciable immunity.

Diagnosis: Early cases confined to the interdigital space may be confused with OID or BFR, advanced ones with foot abscess (*see* above). In flocks affected with VFR, underrunning and separation of the hard horn of the hoof, usually of more than one foot, are characteristic. In foot abscess, there is a deeper invasion and discharge of necrotic and purulent material; usually, only one foot is affected. *Bacteroides nodosus* usually can be identified in smears of stained necrotic material from foot rot, although other bacteria predominate.

Treatment: Treatment efforts may be directed toward temporary control of the disease or to eradicating it from the flock. At certain times, eg, during a wet season, temporary control may be the only realistic goal.

Treatment may be topical or parenteral. Topical treatment requires careful hoof paring to remove all underrun horn and expose necrotic tissue. Bactericidal solutions are then applied by aerosol spray, footbathing, or footsoaking. Common footbathing solutions are 10% zinc sulfate, 10% copper sulfate, or 5% formaldehyde.

The solutions used as aerosol sprays include those used for footbathing as well as 20% cetrimide and 1.3% oxytetracycline in water/alcohol.

For footsoaking, the sheep are kept standing for 1 hr in a solution of 10% zinc sulfate and 0.2% v/v of laundry detergent containing nonionic surfactants or the surfactant sodium lauryl sulfate. In moist conditions, it is not necessary to pare the feet previously, but if the feet are dry and hard, paring improves the recovery rate. Usually the footsoaking should be repeated in 5-10 days.

Parenteral treatment consists of injections of penicillin and dihydrostreptomycin at 22,500-31,750 u/lb (50,000-70,000 u/kg) and 22.5-31.75 mg/lb (50-70 mg/kg), respectively (this dose exceeds by 2-3 times the approved dose in most countries); oxytetracycline; or benzathine penicillin G (not an approved use in all countries).

The success rate for either method of treatment is substantially improved if the treated sheep are kept in a dry environment after treatment (even for 24 hr). The feet of treated sheep should be examined q1-2wk to identify those not responding to treatment or those needing further paring.

Reports from several countries indicate an improved response from the use of oral zinc sulfate along with vitamin A. The dosages used and time of treatment have varied widely, but it appears that an extended treatment period (1 tablet containing 210 mg zinc sulfate and 50,000 IU of vitamin A, given every 10 days for 7 doses) is beneficial. Laser therapy has been used experimentally with success.

Combining both topical and parenteral methods of treatment will not result in immediate eradication of foot rot. Time is necessary to identify the subclinical or relapsing cases.

Prevention and Control: Flocks that are free of foot rot may be kept free by preventing the introduction of *B nodosus*. Any sheep to be added to the flock should be examined, isolated for 1 mo, and then reexamined. Any vehicles or facilities in which unknown or infected sheep have been held must be cleaned and disinfected before placing clean sheep in them.

During periods of the year that favor transmission of foot rot, some control may be achieved by footbathing the affected flock and individual treatment (either topical or parenteral) of severely affected sheep.

Bacteroides nodosus vaccines accelerate healing in affected animals and aid in protecting unaffected ones. Alum-precipitated vaccines require 2 doses 4-6 wk apart to establish effective immunity, which persists for ~2 mo. Lesions heal within 4-6 wk if immunity is established. Oil-emulsion vaccines induce immunity within 3 wk of the initial dose and may persist for 3-4 mo. In endemic areas, revaccination is recommended at intervals of 3-6 mo. Vaccination alone usually does not provide complete control or eradication.

Eradication: Eradication may be achieved only by eliminating all cases of virulent *B nodosus* infection and preventing its reintroduction. This can be done by replacing the affected flock with disease-free sheep, or disposing of affected animals that do not respond readily to treatment, and rigorously treating all new infections. Affected animals are identified by clinical examination; no other diagnostic tests are practical under such circumstances. Subclinical cases constitute a major problem since they may relapse during the next 2-3 mo and transmit infection. Other ruminants (goats, deer, cattle) are potential sources of *B nodosus* and should be considered in eradication programs.

Eradication should be undertaken only when the environment is dry; at other times, treatments should be directed toward control within the flock. A successful eradication program requires planning, commitment, and an investment of time and money; however, it is usually well worth the effort and expense when compared with trying to manage a permanently infected flock.

Before eradication is attempted, prevalence should be reduced to <15% by use of chemotherapy and/or vaccination. Once this is achieved, or if the prevalence is already low, the feet of all sheep in the flock should be examined, and the flock divided into affected and unaffected groups. Those with no visible VFR lesions are isolated, footbathed, and placed on clean, dry ground. This group should be footbathed weekly during the next 2-3 mo, and any lame sheep should be removed immediately. The sheep with VFR lesions are either disposed of or, following careful and extensive foot paring, medicated topically (and parenterally also if desired), and then kept separate from the group with no lesions. The affected group should be footbathed or medicated topically every 3-4 days, and their feet examined and pared q1-2wk. Eventually, a "potentially clean" group can be formed from those appearing to respond to treatment in the affected group. This potentially clean group must be monitored for 1-3 mo or through a period conducive to the spread of foot rot to detect and re-isolate any subclinical cases that relapse. Eventually, this group may be placed with the clean flock.

Most affected sheep recover from foot rot with adequate treatment and time. Placing just one active or subclinical case in the clean flock, however, may lead to failure of the eradication program.

IMPACTED OR INFECTED OIL GLAND

Sheep have a sebaceous (oil) gland in the skin of the digit. An oily, glandular secretion is stored in a small pouch lying between the phalanges. A duct in the skin allows discharge of the secretion to the skin surface. Occasionally, the duct may be occluded and cause impaction and distention of the oil pouch. This may cause lameness as well as distortion in the appearance of the interdigital tissues. The oil sac also may become infected and result in a local cellulitis or abscess. Expression of the contents by manual pressure relieves impaction. Infected glands also can be expressed and then treated with local or systemic antibiotics or both, depending on the extent and severity of the infectious process.

INTERDIGITAL FIBROMA

A mass of fibrous tissue between the toes; it may resemble a papilloma and, if not removed, grows upward between the first phalanges and may cause severe lameness. If detected early, surgical removal (cryosurgery and electrocautery) is successful.

OVINE INTERDIGITAL DERMATITIS
(OID, Foot scald)

A necrotizing condition of the interdigital skin due to a mixed infection with *Fusobacterium necrophorum* and *Corynebacterium pyogenes*. Cold weather and damp pastures are considered to be predisposing factors. A similar condition has been attributed to mechanical damage inflicted by short, stiff stubble. Similar injuries to the interdigital epithelium frequently result from "clay balling", a condition in which balls of clay, molded into the shape of the interdigital space, harden and become difficult to dislodge and cause constant irritation and enhance bacterial invasion.

Lameness may be seen in 90% of sheep, and all 4 feet may be affected. In milder cases, the interdigital skin is red and swollen, and covered by a moist film of whitish necrotic material. However, in severely affected cases, the interdigital skin is necrotic and eroded, and subcut. tissues are exposed. Suppuration and swelling of the deeper interdigital tissues may develop. The wall of the hoof does not separate from the underlying tissue, and the characteristic odor associated with *Bacteroides nodosus* infections is not present. Under dry conditions, the disease often is transient but may persist or recur while pastures remain wet.

The clinical appearance is characteristic, but similar conditions involving other organisms must be excluded. In foot rot (*see* above), microscopical examination of stained smears reveals *B nodosus*. Dermatophilosis (strawberry foot rot, qv, p 787) affects the hairy skin of the coronet and pastern. Viral diseases such as ulcerative dermatitis, contagious ecthyma, and foot-and-mouth disease may be excluded by flock history, clinical signs, and serology. *Fusobacterium necrophorum* may also infect the lesions caused by these diseases.

Treatment and Control: Most lesions heal rapidly with the advent of dry conditions or removal to drier pastures. When the disease is associated with stubble, improvement usually follows removal to ordinary pastures. External application of disinfectants such as 5% formaldehyde or 10% zinc sulfate may help. In severe cases, housing in dry conditions may be appropriate.

SEPTIC LAMINITIS
(Lamellar suppuration, Toe abscess)

An acute bacterial infection of the laminar matrix of the hoof, usually restricted to the toe and abaxial wall. The disease is sporadic and the etiology variable, but cases due to *Fusobacterium necrophorum* and *Corynebacterium pyogenes* usually are more severe and extensive than those involving streptococci or other organisms. Infection probably enters through fissures between the wall and sole and through vertical and horizontal fractures of horn. Sometimes, it is enhanced by impaction with mud and feces, by overgrowth of the hoof, or by separation of the wall following laminitis.

Front feet are affected more commonly. Lameness is severe, and the affected digit hot and tender. There may be a sinus above the lesion at the coronet. Affected sheep usually recover rapidly after paring of the horn to provide dependent drainage.

LAMENESS IN SMALL ANIMALS

A deviation from the normal gait, usually because of injury or defect in the limb, especially of the foot or leg. Spinal pathology may be involved (*see* DISEASES OF THE SPINAL COLUMN AND CORD, p 584). Lameness may be acquired or inherited. The origin of a lameness may be skeletal, from the joint or surrounding soft tissues, or from a defect in a nerve pathway. To assess the course of a lameness, the degree of lameness must be recorded. One method to rate a lameness is on a 1-10 scale, 1 being sound and 10 being nonweight-bearing.

Before examination, the dog should be observed at both a walk and a trot on a surface that is not slippery. The leash should be slack to avoid altering the gait pattern. The examiner should observe the dog walking toward, past, and away (to allow viewing from one side and then from the rear), and then toward and past from the other side. The procedure is repeated with the dog trotting; mild lamenesses not seen at a walk may become apparent at a slow trot. The trot should not be accentuated, and the dog should not be allowed to lope. It is normal for some dogs to pace instead of trot. A useful technique is to develop the ability to imagine a replay, in slow motion, of what was seen during the examination. The examination should be repeated until the affected leg and, if possible, site of the lameness can be determined. (*See also* LAMENESS, GENERAL PRINCIPLES, p 490.)

During the excitement of a visit to a clinic, a lameness may "disappear"; it may be necessary to have the dog remain for 1-2 days to see whether it recurs.

The following should be observed: the length of the swing phase, the duration of the stance phase, the position of the contact point and the lift point, and whether the limb is swung forward and carried backward normally or abducted or adducted. Any alteration in normal joint angles during the stride should be noted. A decrease in movement in a joint indicates pain in that area; the area of the foot that first contacts the ground should be noted in particular. The dog's head goes down when the sound leg is on the ground and up when the lame leg contacts the surface. The head is usually carried lower than normal in hindlimb lamenesses and sometimes higher than normal in forelimb lamenesses.

Most cats will carry a painful limb, but if allowed to roam around indoors, sometimes the site of the lameness can be determined by using the same techniques as for the dog.

Forelimb Lameness: An animal lame in the forelimb has a shortened step, reaches forward with the sound limb and lurches over the arc of the step when using the lame limb, while lifting the head up at the same time. With severe lameness, the spine may arch excessively.

Shoulder Lameness: "Freezing" (lack of movement) of the shoulder joint occurs, and movement occurs between the scapula and the thorax. A short, choppy stride is observed at slower gaits.

Elbow Lameness: Posterior positioning of the stance phase is decreased; the limb unloads abruptly at the point of maximum load. When standing, the elbow tends to be adducted.

Carpus and Foot Lameness: There is good movement in the swing phase but a marked limitation of loading in the stance phase.

Hindlimb Lameness: Weight is shifted to the forequarters, the neck is extended, and the head is carried lower. The forelimbs tend to be positioned more posteriorly.

Hip Lameness: The hindlimbs are spread abnormally far apart to make use of lateral bending of the lumbar spine; the swing phase is reduced, and the head may be thrown up on the lame side. Young, dysplastic pups tend to have a weak, wobbly gait and usually "bunny hop" when running. Subluxating hips usually can be palpated (positive Ortolani sign) or may be audible.

Stifle Lameness: Movement of the joint is decreased, the sound leg collapses in the stance phase, the swing phase is taken up by the hip movement, and tarsal movement is minimal. This latter phenomenon occurs because the hock and the stifle move concomitantly.

Hock and Foot Lameness: The joint angle may be fixed. With tarsal osteochondritis dissecans, dogs frequently stand with their hocks hyperextended.

SPECIFIC CAUSES OF LAMENESS IN YOUNG ANIMALS

Forelimb: 1) nutritional imbalance (pathologic fractures); 2) shoulder—congenital luxation, osteochondritis dissecans, physeal fracture; 3) elbow—fragmented coronoid process, ununited anconeal process, elbow subluxation, physeal fracture, osteochondritis dissecans (distal-medial humeral condyle); 4) carpus—angular limb deformity (secondary to physeal injury), retained cartilage core, hyperextension with ligamentous injury; 5) lameness originating from long bones—fractures, panosteitis, bone cysts, osteomyelitis, hypertrophic osteodystrophy, neoplasia.

Hindlimb: 1) nutritional imbalance (pathologic fractures); 2) hip—hip dysplasia, avascular necrosis, growth plate injury, slipped capital femoral physeal fracture; 3) stifle—osteochondritis dissecans, medial patellar luxation, distal femoral and proximal tibial physeal fractures; 4) tarsus—osteochondritis dissecans; 5) lameness originating from long bones—fractures, panosteitis, hypertrophic osteodystrophy, osteomyelitis, neoplasia.

SPECIFIC CAUSES OF LAMENESS IN ADULTS

Forelimb: 1) general degenerative joint disease—arthritis, infectious arthritis, immune-mediated arthritis, osteochondritis dissecans, cervical spine disease; 2) shoulder—bicipital bursitis, traumatic luxation, scapular fracture, humeral fracture, osteomyelitis, neoplasia, neuromuscular pathology, chronic degenerative joint disease secondary to developmental abnormalities; 3) elbow—distal humeral fracture, rupture of the tendon of insertion of the triceps, biceps tendon avulsion, chronic degenerative joint disease secondary to developmental abnormalities, acute or chronic luxation, subluxation secondary to asynchronous growth; 4) antebrachium—fracture, Monteggia fracture, osteomyelitis, neoplasia; 5) carpus—luxation, subluxation, osteomyelitis, avulsion of flexor tendons, metacarpal fracture, sesamoid fracture, nail bed infection, neoplasia.

Hindlimb: 1) hip—spinal disk disease (Type I or II), diskospondylitis, sacroiliac subluxation, pulled or ruptured muscles, inguinal hernia, lumbosacral syndrome, thromboembolism, traumatic hip luxation, fracture, hip dysplasia, neoplasia; 2) femoral shaft—fracture, osteomyelitis, neoplasia; 3) stifle—local fracture (femur, patella, or tibia), cranial or caudal cruciate rupture, rupture of collateral ligaments, meniscal injury, long digital extensor avulsion, chronic osteochondritis dissecans, patellar luxation; 4) tibial shaft—fracture, osteomyelitis, neoplasia; 5) tarsus and metatarsus—fractures (all bones), luxation, subluxation, degenerative joint disease, hyperextension, plantar ligament rupture, superficial digital flexor tendon luxation.

MYOPATHIES

Diseases that produce primary damage to the skeletal muscle fiber, excluding those of inflammatory origin and those secondary to neural lesions. Many examples of myopathy occur in animals; some, such as the nutritional myopathies, have great economic importance. Other myopathies in animals are important models of human diseases. (*See also* CONGENITAL MYOPATHIES, p 476.)

DYSTROPHY-LIKE MYOPATHIES

Numerous examples of progressive myopathies have been described in animals; many are heritable, and many resemble various types of muscular dystrophy in man. Affected muscles have a variety of degenerative and atrophic changes. In Meuse-Rhine-Yssel cattle of Holland, a progressive fatal myopathy of the diaphragm and intercostal muscles has been described. Another dystrophy in cattle is weaver syndrome in Brown Swiss. Hyperplasia, commonly called "double muscling" (qv, p 477), is a congenital myopathy found in some European breeds of cattle. Progressive myopathies have been reported in Merino sheep (an inherited autosomal recessive), in Pietrain pigs (Pietrain creeper syndrome), and in dogs, cats, chickens, turkeys, and mink. Inherited muscular dystrophy of mice and hamsters has been studied extensively; the hamsters have severe myocardial lesions and serve as a model for studies of cardiomyopathy.

NUTRITIONAL MYOPATHIES

The most common and economically important myopathies of domestic animals are those due to deficiency of selenium or vitamin E, or both. Characteristically, these are acute diseases and most often, but not exclusively, affect young animals of suckling age. The clinical signs vary widely, depending on the distribution and severity of muscle damage. Frequently, they include stiffness or inability to stand as a result of symmetrical damage to the girdle muscles or the large muscles of the limbs. Complications, such as bronchopneumonia or inability to nurse, may lead to prostration and death within a few days to ~1 wk after onset. Acute cardiac failure is often the precipitating cause of death, especially in calves.

The lesions in heart or skeletal musculature vary from diffuse, light-colored areas to well-defined, white streaks or patches, and almost always are bilaterally symmetrical. Most muscles can be involved, but macroscopic lesions are most common in the heart or in the large muscles of the shoulder girdle, back, and thighs; those of the diaphragm and tongue also may be affected. Examples have been described under various names in most domestic and laboratory animals, including muscular dystrophy, white muscle disease, nutritional muscular dystrophy, stiff-lamb disease, equine degenerative myeloencephalopathy, late-lactation paralysis, white flesh, fish flesh, waxy degeneration, paralytic myoglobinuria, and selenium-responsive myopathy.

Pathological changes in other tissues often occur in association with some of the myopathies. These include liver necrosis, subcut. and pulmonary edema with exudation into the body cavities, steatitis, gastric ulceration, pancreatic necrosis, gizzard myopathy, anemia, intestinal lipofuscinosis, testicular degeneration, embryonic death and resorption, and encephalomalacia and other nervous system lesions. In some cases, the lesions in other tissues predominate or appear to constitute the sole pathology: eg, exudative diathesis (qv, pp 1271 and 1273) and encephalomalacia in the chick (qv, p 1273); necrosis of heart, liver, muscle, and kidney in the mouse; dietary liver necrosis in the rat; and perhaps, massive liver necrosis in the sheep. Some, but not all, reports have attributed a causative role to selenium and vitamin E deficiency in the occurrence of these myopathies and of mastitis, metritis, placental retention, cystic ovaries and impaired reproductive performance in dairy cattle, and of immunosuppression in calves.

In addition to structural changes in the various myopathies, chemical changes may be detected in muscle tissue, blood, and urine. Lowered concentrations of muscle creatine are generally observed, with increased calcium and sodium and decreased potassium. Selenium levels in serum from myopathic animals are decreased, as is the activity of glutathione peroxidase, while activities of lactic dehydrogenase, AST (SGOT), and CPK are increased. The urine frequently has an increased creatine:creatinine ratio as a result of increased creatine excretion, and may contain myoglobin.

NUTRITIONAL MYOPATHY OF CALVES AND LAMBS
(White muscle disease [WMD], Stiff lamb disease, Enzootic muscular dystrophy)

A myodegeneration frequently occurs in calves and lambs of dams that received selenium-deficient feed during or before gestation. Legume forages grown in certain areas where selenium is either deficient or unavailable in the soil seem to be particularly involved and appear to be less effective in taking up selenium from the soil than are grasses. When the diet is restricted to such feeds, as in range cattle or sheep production, the cows and ewes may receive inadequate selenium. This condition has been recorded in many countries, and has been produced experimentally in several species of animals by restricting their intake of selenium and vitamin E. A similar myopathy occurs naturally in yearling and young adult cattle, goats (see p 507), deer, foals, adult horses, dogs, rabbits, poultry, fish, and various laboratory and wild animals.

Etiology: Some myopathies (especially in herbivores) and some of the related conditions listed above have been attributed to a deficiency of vitamin E, which may be caused by large amounts of unsaturated fatty acids and other peroxide-forming substances in the diet, eg, continuous supplementation with cod liver oil has induced cases of vitamin E deficiency. WMD in pastured cattle following spring turn out has been attributed to absorption of the portion of polyunsaturated fatty acids in lush grasses that escapes ruminal hydrogenation. In many cases of nutritional myopathy, selenium deficiency is present. This may be a simple deficiency caused by animals eating forage grown on selenium-deficient soils, or it may be precipitated by antagonistic effects of various metals (silver, copper, cobalt, cadmium, mercury, tin). High dietary intake of phosphorus has enhanced the severity of WMD and resulted in decreased hepatic selenium content in sheep. Application of sulfur to pasture soils, as elemental sulfur or gypsum, may interfere with uptake of selenium by forage plants and precipitate the disease in grazing ruminants.

Some myopathies and related conditions respond only to selenium, some only to vitamin E, others to either. While vitamin E cannot completely satisfy the need for selenium, it can reduce the amount required to protect against exudative diathesis. The converse is also true. A vitamin E deficiency in chicks (qv, p 1273) apparently leads to development of encephalomalacia and muscular dystrophy even in the presence of selenium sufficient to protect against exudative diathesis (on a low-methionine, low-cystine diet). Similarly, selenium cannot replace vitamin E to prevent the sterility and myopathy in some experimental animals (rabbits) or encephalomalacia in chicks produced by vitamin-E-deficient diets. Conversely, a naturally occurring infertility in ewes, apparently relating to fetal deaths, and sometimes associated with a high incidence of WMD in lambs receiving adequate vitamin E, responds remarkably to minute supplements of selenium, as does alopecia in rats and primates. The hepatic necrosis observed in rats and pigs appears to respond to either nutrient.

Clinical Findings: The congenital type of myopathy may result in sudden death within 2-3 days of birth, usually with involvement of the myocardium. The delayed type of WMD is associated with cardiac or skeletal muscle involvement, or both, and may be precipitated by vigorous exercise. Affected animals may move stiffly with an arched back and frequently become recumbent. If the condition is severe enough to prevent nursing, either from dysfunction of the muscles of the legs or the tongue, death may result from starvation. Sometimes there is profuse diarrhea. In chronic cases, there may be relaxation of the shoulder girdle and splaying of the toes. In progressive cardiac failure, dyspnea results. Signs vary with dietary selenium status and, in some areas, general unthriftiness may be the only sign associated with selenium deficiency.

Lesions: Generally, skeletal muscle lesions are bilaterally symmetrical and may affect one or more muscle groups. Grossly, the affected muscle is pale and dry, and usually shows distinct longitudinal striations or a pronounced chalky whiteness due to abnormal calcium deposition, but sometimes the involvement may be diffuse. Cardiac lesions occur as well-defined subendocardial plaques that often are more pronounced in the right ventricle in lambs, and in the left ventricle in calves. Microscopically, evidence has been established for sequential changes in damaged muscle progressing from mitochondrial swelling and myofibrillar lysis to either hyaline or granular necrosis. When the heart is involved, Purkinje fibers may be damaged; pleural, pericardial, and peritoneal effusions with pulmonary congestion and edema are not uncommon.

Diagnosis: In lambs, outbreaks of infectious, nonsuppurative arthritis produce a clinical syndrome similar to that of WMD, and sudden deaths from heart failure might be confused with enterotoxemia. The history and necropsy findings, however, are usually characteristic. In mild cases and in very young lambs, laboratory studies such as histological examination, and glutathione peroxidase, AST (SGOT), and CPK levels may be necessary.

In calves, the typical syndrome and lesions are reasonably definitive. In mild cases—and particularly in older animals—diagnosis can be difficult, and laboratory studies (as with lambs) may be necessary.

Prevention: To prevent WMD within 4 wk after birth, ewes are given 5 mg and cows 15 mg of selenium, PO or subcut., usually as sodium selenite 4 wk before expected parturition. For prevention of delayed WMD, lambs are given 0.5 mg and calves 5 mg selenium at 2-4 wk of age and 2 more times at monthly intervals. A selenium and vitamin E mixture is advocated in some areas. Other procedures for selenium supplementation include administration of intraruminal selenium pellets, use of selenium-fortified salt or mineral mixtures, subcut. implantation of selenium pellets, or soil application of selenium at 4 g/acre (10 g/hectare) in fertilizer.

Adding selenium to feed for breeding animals or their young is useful in areas of known deficiency or unavailability of selenium. The recommended supplemental level is 0.3 ppm selenium, calculated on the basis of total dry-matter intake. It is added as sodium selenite, which contains 45.65% selenium; because of the minute quantities involved and the toxicity of excess intake, premixing and thorough subsequent mixing is necessary. In some countries, including the USA, addition of selenium to feeds is controlled by law, and appropriate authorities should be consulted; in all areas, caution in its use is indicated.

Treatment: Lambs and calves may be given sodium selenite and vitamin E in sterile emulsion, subcut. or IM, at 1 mg selenium and 50 mg (68 IU) of vitamin E per 40 lb (18 kg) body wt. This may be repeated after 2 wk, but not to exceed 4 doses. Larger doses are sometimes advocated, but caution is advised since they approach the toxic level. In practice, several products are available for use with designated animal species. When simple vitamin E deficiency is apparent, dietary supplementation with α-tocopherol or substances rich in vitamin E should be instituted. Minimum dosages have not been established; however, cures have been reported following daily doses with 5 mg of α-tocopherol to rabbits; 500 mg initially, followed by 100 mg on alternate days to lambs; and 600 mg initially, followed by daily doses of 200 mg to calves. When the causative diet contains substances antagonistic to vitamin E, such as unprotected, polyunsaturated fats, these must be removed or stabilized by addition of an appropriate antioxidant. Dry concentrates of vitamins A and D may substitute for cod-liver oil, thus removing a potential source of oxidative damage.

NUTRITIONAL, SKELETAL, AND CARDIAC MYOPATHIES IN PIGS
(Hepatosis dietetica [HD], Mulberry heart disease [MHD])

There are several specific diseases of pigs in which muscle degeneration may be extensive, such as MHD; and others in which the degeneration is frequently less conspicuous, such as HD.

Etiology: MHD and HD are associated with diets low in selenium or vitamin E. Administration of iron dextran to piglets having low vitamin E may precipitate a severe myopathy (qv, p 1673) with lesions identical to selenium/vitamin E deficiency. Other factors that may increase the selenium requirement include diets with low protein and especially low sulfur-containing amino acid concentrations, feeding an excess of selenium antagonistic compounds, and possibly genetic influences on selenium metabolism. Vitamin E may be less available in diets with high concentrations of polyunsaturated fatty acids, vitamin A, or mycotoxins. There is evidence that MHD is not always caused by deficiencies of vitamin E/selenium. It appears to be related to rapid growth in quite young pigs.

Clinical Findings: These conditions have certain characteristics in common. Losses tend to occur sporadically, and rapidly growing pigs 2-16 wk old are affected. Death almost invariably occurs suddenly, and is often precipitated by exercise.

Lesions: In MHD, the characteristic lesion is a pericardial sac grossly distended with straw-colored fluid that contains fibrin strands, and extensive hemorrhage throughout the epicardium and myocardium. Microscopically, hearts show both vascular and myocyte lesions; in addition to interstitial hemorrhage, there is usually extensive myocardial necrosis together with fibrin thrombi in capillaries. If animals survive for a few days, nervous signs may be seen as a result of focal encephalomalacia.

In HD there is often subcut. edema and varying amounts of transudate in serous cavities. Fibrin strands adhere to the liver, which has a characteristic mottled appearance caused by irregular foci of parenchymal necrosis and hemorrhage. Focal lesions of myocardial necrosis and, less frequently, skeletal myonecrosis may be apparent. Acute lesions may appear as scattered, red, swollen lobules and edema of the gallbladder wall.

Many pigs that die with selenium/vitamin E deficiency have esophagogastric ulceration or pre-ulcerative changes.

Diagnosis: The history and gross necropsy findings may be distinctive, but histology to demonstrate specific cardiac and skeletal muscle lesions may be necessary. Differential diagnoses for MHD include acute septicemic diseases (eg, salmonellosis, erysipelas, and streptococcosis), pericarditis, polyserositis, and edema disease. For HD, pitch poisoning and gossypol toxicosis also should be considered, and for pigs with prominent skeletal muscle lesions, porcine stress syndrome might also be considered. As in other species with selenium/vitamin E deficiency, cases may be identified by decreased selenium, vitamin E, and glutathione peroxidase levels in the serum and tissues; and increased levels of CPK and AST (SGOT) in the serum.

Prevention and Treatment: Rations may be supplemented with selenium or vitamin E or both, as for ruminants. Affected pigs and their herdmates may be given injections of selenium/vitamin E to increase tissue levels rapidly; injection of sows in late gestation increases tissue levels in newborn piglets.

NUTRITIONAL MYOPATHY OF EQUIDAE

Myodegeneration, associated with selenium/vitamin E deficiency, may occur in adult horses, donkeys, and mules. The disease in adult equids may manifest in the acute form with sudden unexpected death, or in the subacute form by staggering gait, myoglobinuria, dysphagia with swelling of the masseter and lingual muscles, and dyspnea and tachycardia. Lesions involve the skeletal muscles and myocardium. Diagnosis and treatment are as for ruminants and pigs (*see* above). In foals, a myopathy that appears similar to the vitamin-E/selenium-responsive disorders of other species may occur at birth or shortly thereafter, and may be accompanied by steatitis or "yellow fat" (*see* below). Stiffness and pain on palpation of subcut. fat masses is noticeable, and severely affected foals may be unable to suckle. Selenium and glutathione peroxidase levels in affected foals may be no lower than in normal ones. Treatment with vitamin E appears more effective than with selenium.

"YELLOW FAT" DISEASE
(Nutritional steatitis, Nutritional panniculitis)

A disease characterized by a marked inflammation of adipose tissue and deposition of "ceroid" pigment in fat cells. It may occur alone in cats, or with accompanying myopathy in affected rats, mink, foals, and pigs.

It is believed that an overabundance of unsaturated fatty acids in the ration, together with a deficiency of vitamin E or other antioxidants, results in lipid peroxidation and deposition of "ceroid" pigment in the adipose tissue. Most naturally occurring and experimentally produced cases have occurred in animals that have had fish or fish by-products as all or part of the diet. The specific cause is believed to be related jointly to the high unsaturation of the fish oil fatty acids and their lack of protection with vitamin E or other antioxidants.

Affected cats are frequently obese, usually young, and of either sex. They lose agility, are unwilling to move, and resent palpation of the back or abdomen. In advanced cases, even a light touch causes pain. Fever is a constant finding and anorexia may be present.

In mink, kits may be affected with steatitis shortly after weaning and, if untreated, losses may continue to pelting time. Signs appear suddenly; the kits may refuse a night feeding and be dead by morning. Affected animals may refuse their feed and show a peculiar, unsteady hop, followed by complete impairment of locomotion, and coma. At pelting, survivors show yellow fat deposits and hemoglobinuria.

The typical laboratory finding is an elevated WBC count, with neutrophilia and sometimes eosinophilia. Biopsy of the subcut. fat shows it to be yellowish brown and firm. Microscopical examination reveals severe inflammatory changes and associated ceroid pigment.

A somewhat similar syndrome, caused by infection with fungi or bacteria (eg, *Mycobacterium*) occurs in the same animals, and others, including dogs.

The offending excessive fat source must be removed from the diet. The administration of vitamin E, in the form of α-tocopherol, at least 30 mg daily for cats, or 15 mg daily for mink, is necessary. Antibiotics are of doubtful value, in spite of the fever and leukocytosis. Parenteral use of fluids is not advisable unless dehydration exists. Because of associated pain, affected animals should be handled as little as possible.

HYPOKALEMIC POLYMYOPATHY IN CATS

Affected cats have acute onset of generalized muscular weakness, persistent ventroflexion of the neck, apparent muscular pain on palpation, stiff stilted gait, and reluctance to walk. Administration of potassium PO or parenterally reverses the syndrome. Affected cats have elevated serum CPK activity and low serum potassium concentrations. Muscle biopsies reveal either no alterations or, occasionally, mild myonecrosis. Affected cats require long-term dietary potassium supplementation to prevent recurrence.

TOXIC MYOPATHIES

See also IRON DEXTRAN TOXICITY, p 1673.

IONOPHORE TOXICITY

Monensin, lasalocid, salinomycin, and narasin may cause myopathy. Horses are highly susceptible, and reports of toxicity also exist for cattle, sheep, pigs, dogs, chickens, turkeys, and guinea fowl. Toxicity has generally resulted from exposure to undiluted premixes or from mixing errors. Toxicosis may be potentiated by various antibiotics and sulfonamides incorporated into feeds in combination with ionophores. Affected horses and cattle may develop anorexia, cardiac failure with tachycardia, dyspnea, diarrhea, stiffness, muscular weakness, and myoglobinuria. At necropsy, pale areas of myocardial necrosis and pulmonary congestion are usually prominent in horses and cattle. Pigs and sheep tend to have mainly skeletal muscle lesions that appear quite similar grossly and histologically to those of nutritional myopathy. Diagnosis requires history of exposure with development of characteristic clinical and pathological alterations.

PLANT INTOXICATION

Degeneration of skeletal and cardiac muscles results when cattle and some other animals, notably goats, consume the fruit or beans of certain plants. *Karwinskia humboldtiana* (coyotillo) and *Cassia* spp (sennas) have been incriminated, but other species also may cause similar damage. Affected animals show weakness and gait abnormalities, and there is pallor of severely degenerated muscles. Microscopic lesions consist of hyaline necrosis and granular degeneration. Some blood enzymes are elevated, and myoglobinuria may occur. Treatment consists of removal of animals from offending range, and supplemental feeding.

EXERTIONAL MYOPATHIES

AZOTURIA AND "TYING-UP" OR "CORDING-UP" SYNDROME OF HORSES
(Paralytic myoglobinuria, Exertional rhabdomyolysis)

Tying-up or cording-up is thought to be a mild form of azoturia and therefore to have a similar etiology. The terms are applied mainly to light horses and to heavier breeds, respectively; both are associated with skeletal myopathy. (*See also* PHYSICAL EXHAUSTION, p 453.)

Etiology: The cause is unknown. Both entities are usually associated directly with forced exercise after a period of rest during which feed has not been restricted, but the disease has been observed in horses on pasture. The cause seems to relate more to excess total feed energy consumption than specifically to the carbohydrate content of the diet as once believed.

Clinical Findings: In both tying-up and azoturia, the first signs are profuse sweating, trembling, and rapid pulse followed by weakness of the hindlimbs, which results in a stiff gait and reluctance to move, and in severe cases, myoglobinuria. In azoturia, the disease quickly progresses to recumbency, often with nervous signs. Elevated serum activities of AST (SGOT) and CPK are useful indicators of the extent of muscle damage. Prognosis depends on the extent of muscle damage; it is good for those animals that remain standing. It is also fairly good for those animals that go down due to loss of use of their hindquarters, providing that they remain quiet and contented, and the pulse returns to normal within 24 hr. However, survivors sometimes suffer from lameness and prolonged, or occasionally permanent, muscle atrophy.

The prognosis is poor for nervous, restless, recumbent animals that continue to struggle and are not quieted by sedatives or tranquilizers; for those that are forced to continue moving after the signs become apparent; and for those that after 24 hr show progressive inability to roll up on the sternum and retain that position. A weak or irregular pulse is most unfavorable.

Lesions: Extensive pale areas of myonecrosis are present, especially in the thigh, pelvic, and loin muscles. Muscles are generally moist and dark, but pale areas of myocardial necrosis may occur, and swollen kidneys with a brown cortex and brown-red streaks in the medulla may be seen. Brown urine reflects myoglobinuria. Microscopical study reveals hyaline degeneration, myonecrosis, and myoglobinuric nephrosis. Calcification usually is not a component.

Treatment: Good management is important. The animal should be kept as quiet as possible, and attempts should be made to keep it standing. Close attention should be given to its comfort, and precautions taken against the development of decubital ulcers. Nervous, restless animals, or those showing evidence of pain, should be given sedatives such as chloral hydrate or tranquilizers. If conditions indicate a period of recumbency, an oily laxative should be given. Quick-acting purgatives, such as arecoline and physostigmine, should not be used.

When signs are slight, there is no history of previous occurrence, and serum enzyme activities are not significantly elevated, moderate tranquilization may be sufficient. More severely affected horses should not be moved, but provided with on-the-spot shelter. They should be rubbed dry and blanketed according to the weather. Selenium and vitamin E injections appear to give favorable results in many cases; however, no evidence of underlying selenium/vitamin E deficiency has been found in affected horses.

EXERTIONAL RHABDOMYOLYSIS IN DOGS

An azoturia-like syndrome occasionally occurs in dogs following strenuous exercise. The condition usually is reported in racing Greyhounds or coursing dogs, but may follow fighting in aggressive dogs. The typical signs include stiffness of the lumbar muscles, polyuria, polydipsia, and myoglobinuria. Serum enzymes are elevated and, in severe cases, there is complete renal failure. The presumptive diagnosis is based on the clinical signs and history, and is confirmed by renal biopsy. Mild cases may benefit from IV fluids to combat shock and aid renal excretion of myoglobin, and from 20 mL/kg of 4.2% bicarbonate solution given IV and continued (at 1.4%) for 2-3 days. Mortality reportedly is ~25%.

CAPTURE MYOPATHY OF WILD ANIMALS

This syndrome often occurs following restraint of wild animals. Affected animals may die acutely from lactic acidosis or may live several days and show muscular stiffness or become recumbent. Severe skeletal muscle lesions with myocardial necrosis and myoglobinuric nephrosis may be present. Careful handling and reduction of stress are useful; IV fluids and sodium bicarbonate may help. If the animals are from areas considered to be deficient in selenium, the condition may be an exercise-induced myopathy that is responsive to selenium or vitamin E. (*See also* MALIGNANT HYPERTHERMIA, p 448.)

MISCELLANEOUS MYOPATHIES

ISCHEMIC MYOPATHY

Thrombosis of the iliac artery in horses results in extensive ischemic necrosis of the musculature of the hindlimb. In cattle, massive necrosis of the thigh muscle may be present in "downer cows" (qv, p 555), and probably is due to the effects of both ischemia and physical trauma associated with prolonged recumbency and abortive attempts to rise.

POSTANESTHETIC MYOPATHY IN HORSES

Complications of general anesthesia in horses may cause muscle lesions due to regional ischemia from anesthetic-induced arterial hypotension. This syndrome may occur as a localized form in muscle groups in contact with the surgery table or as a generalized form with features similar to azoturia.

FIBROTIC AND OSSIFYING MYOPATHY IN QUARTER HORSES

Physical tearing of muscles, especially in the posterior thigh, during intensive exertion results in healing with extensive fibrosis and ossification. Lesions have also been associated with IM injections. (*See also* p 531.)

MYOSITIS OF UNDETERMINED ETIOLOGY

EOSINOPHILIC MYOSITIS IN DOGS
(Atrophic myositis)

An acute, relapsing inflammation of the muscles; it is common in German Shepherd Dogs and most frequently affects the muscles of mastication. The initiating cause is unknown, but recent evidence strongly supports the role of an immune-mediated selective injury directed against specific proteins of masticatory type 2M muscle fibers.

The onset is usually abrupt. During an attack, the jaws become fixed, and the muscles of mastication swell symmetrically and interfere with drainage from the retrobulbar tissues, which produces edema of the conjunctiva, prolapse of the nictitating membrane, and exophthalmos. The mouth is held partially open; the animal has recurrent attacks of pain and eats with difficulty. The attacks last 1-3 wk and in eosinophilic myositis are accompanied by a marked eosinophilia. In atrophic myositis, which occurs in other, long-nosed breeds, eosinophilia is mild or absent. Periods between attacks vary from 3 wk to 6 mo. After each attack, the affected muscles become more atrophied; with each succeeding attack, the severity decreases and the interval between attacks tends to shorten. In late stages, involvement of the esophagus makes swallowing difficult.

During acute attacks, the affected muscles are enlarged and doughy in consistency, darkened, and hemorrhagic with focal pale areas. The regional nodes are enlarged and firm. During early attacks, the lesions are confined to the muscles of mastication; as the attacks continue, additional muscles may become involved. The histological lesion is an acute eosinophilic myositis. Although the eosinophilic infiltration is usually quite diffuse, actual muscle involvement is patchy. Frequently, necrotic muscle fibers appear to be the focus of the reaction. In late lesions, extensive atrophy and fibrosis, and infiltrations of plasma cells and lymphocytes are present in the affected masticatory muscles.

The periodic nature of the disease and its unusual selectivity for site and breed usually make the diagnosis obvious. Eosinophilia is generally supportive and if any doubt remains, histological examination of a muscle biopsy can be used to confirm the diagnosis.

The disease is progressive, and no therapy has yet been able to alter its recurrent nature and course; however, corticosteroids and adrenocorticotropic hormone markedly minimize the discomfort and muscle swelling during an attack.

EOSINOPHILIC MYOSITIS IN CATTLE AND SHEEP

A focal myonecrosis associated with large numbers of eosinophilic granulocytes. Sudden deaths in cattle and sheep may involve myocarditis. The cause is unknown in most instances, but the presence of degenerate *Sarcocystis* spp (qv, p 562) in the center of some of the necrotic lesions suggests that they may be implicated. Alternatively, the cause may be an allergic reaction focused on muscle. This condition is seen at slaughter as focal, greenish gray discolorations in skeletal and occasionally cardiac musculature, which fade when exposed to air.

POLYMYOSITIS IN DOGS

Affected dogs may have stiff painful muscles and muscular atrophy, be exercise intolerant, and have dysphagia from involvement of eosphageal and laryngeal muscles. The disease, which occurs in mature large breeds, may develop acutely or have a slow and progressive course; it is suspected to be immune-mediated. Diagnosis is confirmed by muscle biopsy that shows focal infiltrations of lymphocytes and plasma cells with accompanying muscle fiber necrosis. Most cases respond to corticosteroid therapy.

NEUROMUSCULAR OR SKELETAL PARESIS IN COWS FOLLOWING PROLONGED RECUMBENCY
(Downer cow)

Recumbent cows that have failed to respond to treatment of their primary or initially diagnosed disease may be referred to as downer cows. Such cows are generally alert with no forelimb problems, but have hindlimb paresis or paralysis. This syndrome develops most commonly following parturient paresis (qv, p 451), but can be a sequela of any disease that causes recumbency for a few hours, eg, metritis, mastitis, calving paralysis (qv, p 495), ketosis, arthritis, exhaustion, grass tetany, toxicity, anesthesia, and trauma. See also PROTEIN, NUTRITION: CATTLE, p 1187.

Experimental evidence has shown that, in <6 hr, the pressure on the sciatic nerve and muscles in the caudal thigh of a downer cow can cause hindlimb paresis or paralysis. The pressure causes severe ischemic myonecrosis and neuropathy (the "compartmental" or "crush" syndrome). Paretic cows recumbent on concrete floors are especially at risk, and even more so if the cow cannot turn herself from side to side. Thus, this syndrome has a final common pathway of pathogenesis, but many possible initiating factors; causes of these factors must be diagnosed so that specific therapeutic, prognostic, and preventive measures can be instituted.

Clinical Findings: Affected cows usually are seen 6-24 hr after treatment for parturient paresis when they are still recumbent, although they have usually responded well to calcium therapy in all other respects. Vital signs are normal; they are bright, alert, and will eat and ruminate, although their appetite is usually diminished. There are no other clinical abnormalities, but when urged to rise they either will not try, or make an unsuccessful attempt. In some cases, this unsuccessful attempt is associated with an inability to extend the fetlocks and flex the hocks. This is an indication of probable damage to the sciatic nerve, or its peroneal branch, suffered during recumbency associated with parturient paresis. Clinical examination will not reveal the severe nerve and muscle necrosis in the thigh. Nerve conduction velocity between the sciatic notch (ischium) and the lateral aspect of the stifle can be measured to confirm the lesion. A normal conduction velocity in the fibular-sciatic nerve is 80-110 m/sec. A damaged sciatic has a slowed conduction (<50 m/sec).

Serum calcium, magnesium, and inorganic phosphorus levels are usually low normal after adequate treatment for the initial hypocalcemia. Serum enzymes (AST [SGOT], CPK) are markedly elevated within 12-36 hr as a result of the ischemic muscle necrosis.

Treatment: There is little experimental support for any of the treatments that have been suggested. These include administration of phosphorus, potassium, adrenocorticotropic hormone, corticosteroids, and antihistamines. Additional calcium should be given only with caution to recumbent cows if they do not have other signs of hypocalcemia. Good nursing is the best treatment; the recumbent cow should be moved promptly (and with care) to an area with deep, soft bedding and good footing (either outside, or on a solid manure pack). Most cows will then move from side to side; those that do not should be turned q2-4 hr. Their hindlimbs should be flexed, extended, and massaged. Adequate nursing and feeding care are essential for good recovery. Most affected cows will try to get up within 1 wk; those that are recumbent for 2 wk without improvement are unlikely to ever get up, although if given sufficient attention some apparently hopeless cases do recover. In paretic or ataxic cows, a temporary fetlock knuckling may be noted from the sciatic injury in the thigh or peroneal nerve damage lateral to the stifle.

Great care must be taken if "hip-lifters" are used on large cows; they may do more harm than good by adding to the muscle damage. Slings are less likely to cause additional injury, although they are more difficult to use. Slings (or "hip-lifters") may be helpful if used with care once daily. If these are not used, the cow should be stimulated to rise daily—some apparently fail to realize they have recovered. Good footing should be maintained to minimize slippage. If a slippery surface is unavoidable, tying burlap bags over the feet, or tying the hindfeet together with a yard long (1 m) rope or strap may be helpful.

For humane reasons, slaughter should be considered if the environment and care are unsuitable.

Control: Prevention and prompt treatment of parturient paresis are the best ways to avoid this condition. Dairymen should learn to recognize the earliest clinical signs of milk fever so cows can be treated before they become recumbent. Cows that are candidates for parturient paresis should calve outside, or in a box stall with a dirt floor and straw, or a well-bedded manure pack. They should be in one of these areas at least 4 days before and 4 days after calving.

OSTEITIS

Inflammation of bone marrow (osteomyelitis), cortical bone, and periosteum (periostitis), usually caused by bacteria, occasionally by fungi, and rarely by migrating foreign bodies or electrolytic reaction to metallic implants.

Etiology and Pathogenesis: Necrosis of tissue and an infectious agent are necessary to produce infectious osteitis. Most cases are secondary to trauma (with or without fracture) or orthopedic surgery. Staphylococci, streptococci, and coliforms usually are responsible. Organisms may arrive hematogenously or by direct extension, but the former is rare, especially in adult and small animals. Involvement of metaphyses and epiphyses follows bacteremia in foals (*Salmonella* spp, *Escherichia coli*) and calves (*Corynebacterium (Actinomyces) pyogenes*). Metaphyseal and epiphyseal localization is favored by the sinusoidal circulation of the spongiosa. Vertebral body lesions occur in pigs (*Brucella suis*) and calves (*C pyogenes*). Vertebral localization is permitted by connections between vertebral medullary venous sinuses and the major veins of the abdomen and thorax. *Nocardia* spp occasionally cause thoracolumbar vertebral osteitis in dogs with intrathoracic infections.

In endemic areas, the systemic mycoses, coccidioidomycosis (South and Central America, Arizona, California, Texas) and blastomycosis (Africa, central Atlantic states, Mississippi-Ohio River basins, northern border of Ontario and Manitoba) often cause hematogenous osteitis in dogs.

Osteitis from direct extension may follow bite wounds in dogs and cats (*Pasteurella* spp, oral anaerobes); penetrating foreign bodies, chronic arthritis, and decubitus ulcers in large animals; and dental diseases in all species (*see also* ACTINOMYCOSIS, p 318). The latter is due to periodontal lymphatic drainage into adjacent bone.

Clinical Findings and Diagnosis: Pain, soft-tissue swelling, fever, and often depression and anorexia characterize early osteomyelitis. Leukocytosis with a left shift and an increased sedimentation rate may be noted. The animal may be reluctant to use the limb.

If infection spreads to a joint, it may become swollen and painful. In chronic osteitis, fluctuant swellings or draining fistulas may develop. Samples should be collected for culture and sensitivity testing, microscopy of exudates, and histological examination. They must be obtained from deep within the lesion, using surgical exposure if necessary. Biopsy samples should be chosen to avoid nonspecific periosteal reaction.

Radiography is essential to define the extent of disease and response to treatment. Radiographic changes may be absent in early osteomyelitis. Bone lesions may be visible first at ~2 wk, with onset of increased medullary density and irregular thickening at the periosteal surface. Later, extensive periosteal new bone may develop in reaction to circulatory disruption and inflammatory exudate in the marrow. Rarely, large volumes of dead bone (sequestra) are visible as they become isolated in pus by living involucra.

In dogs, acute osteomyelitis must be distinguished radiographically from other causes of bone pain, eg, hypertrophic osteopathy and panosteitis. Chronic osteomyelitis with periosteal reaction should be confirmed by biopsy. Squamous cell carcinoma of the digit is often complicated by osteitis in small animals, and in all species, periosteal proliferation is a nonspecific response to many insults, including neoplasms and trauma.

Treatment: Effective treatment of acute or early osteomyelitis depends on identification of the organism and its antibiogram. Systemic antibiotics, preferably bactericidal, are recommended. These include ampicillin, cephaloridine, chloramphenicol, gentamicin, and kanamycin. Treatment for 1-2 mo is advisable. Drainage of the infected site may be necessary.

Success with chronic osteomyelitis requires long-term therapy, often including surgery. An appropriate antibiotic should be started before surgery. All sequestra should be removed, and fibrous and necrotic tissue debrided. Fistulas should be explored, and the bone curetted until bleeding occurs. Internal fixation should be left if it is providing rigid support; if it is not, it should be removed and replaced with something that will. The surgical wound can be left open to drain and heal by granulation, or closed meticulously taking care to eliminate all dead space provided that drainage tubing has been installed. Fenestrated tubing can allow flushing with large volumes of sterile saline, antibacterials, and enzyme preparations. Tyloxapol can be flushed into the site to help break up mucoid material and maintain drain patency.

At 2- to 3-wk intervals during treatment, culture and sensitivity tests should be done and the animal's progress followed clinically and radiographically. Large surgical defects may be repaired with bone grafts once infection is overcome. Inadequate antibacterial therapy of acute osteitis may eliminate clinical signs but allow infection to persist, which may lead to chronic osteitis months or years later. Amputation may be the best initial treatment in osteitis of the digit, and must be considered in other cases if long-term intensive therapy fails.

CANINE PANOSTEITIS
(Eosinophilic panosteitis, Panostosis, Enostosis, Juvenile osteomyelitis)

A disease characterized by intermittent shifting lameness and spontaneous remission, which affects mainly young (5-12 mo old) male dogs of large and giant breeds, but smaller and older dogs may be affected.

The etiology is unknown. Suggested causes include allergens, hyperestrogenism, stress, and infectious agents. About 75% of cases involve German Shepherd Dogs and ~66% are males; thus, genetic and hormonal factors may be predisposing.

The disease develops as a localized area of granular degeneration of the adipose bone marrow, followed by edema and medullary fibrovascular proliferation usually near the nutrient artery of a long bone. Later the fibrovascular tissue ossifies. The proliferating tissue may occupy most of the diaphyseal medullary cavity, and if it involves the endosteum, secondary periosteal proliferation occurs. With remission, the medullary and periosteal bone is resorbed but, in chronic cases, the affected long bones become cubical from repeated remodeling.

Mild to severe lameness with bone pain that tends to be intermittent and shifting is typical. Firm palpation of long bones in the affected limb may elicit pain. Some dogs may be febrile and anorectic in early stages. Rarely, tonsillitis may be present. Long bones, especially of the foreleg, are most often affected. Multiple bone involvement occurs in ~50% of dogs. Spontaneous remission and exacerbation of signs occur, and usually the disease within a bone resolves within 3 mo. In older dogs, the disease becomes more protracted.

Radiographic findings are diagnostic, but lesions may not be visible until 10-14 days following onset of signs, and then may be subtle enough to escape detection.

Areas of medullary blurring or soft-tissue density may be seen in the marrow cavity, especially in the region of the nutrient artery. Sometimes, only endosteal roughening may be apparent. Later, the areas of radiodensity may coalesce and expand to fill most of the marrow space. A mild periosteal reaction may be visible, and ossification of the soft tissue will render the lesions more prominent.

There is no specific treatment. Usually, symptomatic treatment with analgesics, and rest or restricted exercise as necessary, are sufficient. Panosteitis tends to run a course of remission and exacerbation over one to several months. The osseous lesions regress gradually after the clinical signs disappear.

OSTEOCHONDROSIS

A disturbance in endochondral ossification sometimes classified as chondrodysplasia. It may involve the separation of the immature articular cartilage from the underlying epiphyseal bone (sometimes dissecting completely free and floating loose in the synovial cavity—osteochondritis dissecans), or may result in the retention of pyramidal cores of physeal cartilage projecting into the metaphysis (eg, osteochondritis in pigs). Often these 2 lesions occur simultaneously in the same bone. The disease occurs during maximal growth when the biomechanical stresses are greatest in the immature skeleton (4-8 mo in dogs, 80-120 lb [36-54 kg] in pigs). It is most common in large and giant breeds of dogs, and rapidly growing pigs, horses, turkeys, and chickens.

OSTEOCHONDRITIS DISSECANS (OCD)

A focal area of the immature articular cartilage becomes thickened and contains a decreased number of chondrocytes, which are disorganized. The matrix in the basal area of this region becomes chondromalacic and acellular. There is separation of the immature articular cartilage from the underlying trabecular bone. The chondral fracture extends horizontally and vertically until a flap is formed. Synovial fluid gains entrance to the underlying medullary space and subchondral cysts may form (usually only in larger animals). The flap of immature articular cartilage may break away completely (joint mice), or may reattach by endochondral ossification to the underlying bone, especially in pigs, and result in a wrinkled articular surface. The latter occurs only if the joint is rested or protected, which permits reestablishment of the circulation necessary for endochondral ossification. If the flap is torn free by joint motion, it may be ground into smaller pieces during locomotion and disappear, while the larger plaques may become attached to the synovial membrane, become vascularized, and ossify. The resultant articular defect, in time, fills with fibrocartilage.

Etiology: The exact cause is unknown. Trauma due to excessive biomechanical stresses in focal areas has been implicated. In pigs, complementary lesions in the immature articular cartilage and the adjacent physeal cartilage are not uncommon. The inheritance of predisposing characteristics (rate of growth, excitability, size of skeleton, muscle mass, etc) is not known. The joint most commonly affected varies among species, eg, shoulder in dogs, elbow in pigs. The stifle (medial or lateral condyle) and hock (caudal aspect of medial trochlea of the talus) also may be involved.

Clinical Findings: OCD causes an insidious and usually persistent lameness beginning, in dogs, at 4-8 mo of age. Lameness is often unilateral, even though the lesions can be bilateral. Occasionally, several joints are affected. The animal may be stiff after resting, and lameness is aggravated by exercise. Depending on which joint is affected, pain can be elicited by hyperextension or hyperflexion, eg, shoulder joints are most painful on hyperextension. Untreated, the lameness persists and becomes permanent due to secondary osteoarthritis. The joint is crepitant, and muscular atrophy is observed in the chronic condition. When the articular cartilage does not fracture, the condition may go undetected; however, the silent lesions may be demonstrated radiographically.

Diagnosis: The history, age, breed, sex, and clinical signs provide useful information; however, radiographs are required to substantiate the diagnosis. The shoulder lesion is observed on a lateral radiograph as a flattened irregularity of the central caudal half of the humeral articular surface. OCD of the femoral condyles in the dog is observed best from a lateral radiograph in which the condyles are not superimposed. Anteroposterior radiographs of the hock in full extension reveal the characteristic depression of the affected surface. The specific lesions in the elbow and hock are not visible on radiographs until after proliferative osteoarthrosis develops.

Treatment: A few animals recover spontaneously with 4-6 wk of rest and restricted exercise. Anti-inflammatory drugs are not indicated since they promote physical activity, and thus aggravate the condition. If surgery of affected shoulder joints is performed soon after diagnosis, the prognosis is good. Joint bodies should be removed and the lesion in the subchondral bone curetted. Lesions involving the stifle, elbow, and hock also should be treated surgically; however, the prognosis for these joints is guarded.

ELBOW DYSPLASIA

Three conditions that affect the canine elbow have been classified under the general term elbow dysplasia: ununited anconeal process, ununited medial coronoid process, and ununited medial humeral epicondyle; all result in secondary osteoarthritis (OA, qv, p 474).

Ununited Anconeal Process: UAP, which occurs principally in the same breeds as OCD (*see* above), is separation of the ossification center of the anconeal process from the proximal ulnar metaphysis. Fusion should be completed by 5-6 mo of age. The fracture is postulated to result from a biomechanical imbalance of force and movement in the rapidly growing elbow. Initially, the anconeal process is connected to the ulna by a bridge of fibrous tissue, which fragments to form a pseudoarthrosis, and the elbow becomes unstable. This joint laxity continues to damage the articular cartilage, and secondary OA results. A hereditary basis has been implicated, but not proved.

Lameness develops insidiously between 4 and 8 mo of age; however, some bilateral cases may not be diagnosed until the dogs are >1 yr old. Affected elbows may deviate laterally, and the range of motion is restricted. Advanced cases have OA, joint effusion, and crepitus. Clinical signs are suggestive, and the diagnosis is confirmed by radiography. A lateral radiograph of the elbow in the flexed position allows visualization of the ununited process. Both elbows should be examined because the condition can be bilateral.

Surgical removal of the UAP soon after diagnosis is the treatment of choice. OA will occur, but to a lesser degree, and the activity of the animal is markedly improved with surgery.

Ununited Medial Coronoid Process: UMCP is a condition of the medial compartment of the canine elbow, in which the coronoid process fails to unite, either partially or totally, with the ulnar diaphysis, and thus does not become a part of the articular surface of the trochlear notch. Joint laxity, irritation, and finally OA result. This condition and osteochondrosis of the medial humeral condyle are considered to be the 2 most common causes of OA of the canine elbow. Before the onset of OA of this condition, the fragments can be demonstrated radiographically. Diagnosis is confirmed by arthrotomy and removal of the fragments, which is followed by an improvement of the clinical signs. However, the secondary OA will continue to cause intermittent lameness.

Ununited Medial Humeral Epicondyle: UMHE results from a disturbed endochondral fusion of the epiphysis of the medial epicondyle with the distal end of the humerus. The exact cause is unknown, but since the carpal and digital flexors originate from the ventral aspect of this structure, it may represent an epiphyseal avulsion. It occurs in young dogs (6-8 mo) of large breeds, results in pain on flexion of the elbow or deep digital palpation, and is accompanied by soft-tissue swelling. Radiographically, radiodense structures have been observed caudal and distal to the area of the medial epicondyle. Reported treatment has been surgical excision; however, if it is an epiphyseal avulsion, reattachment would seem more appropriate. OA is the usual accompaniment; severity and time of onset of this condition depend on the expediency of diagnosis and amount of tissue damage at the time of surgery.

PATELLAR LUXATION

In large animals, patellar luxation occurs as 3 clinical syndromes: 1) Congenital hypoplasia or malformation of the trochlear ridges seen in neonatal calves, lambs, and foals. An inherited basis for this condition has not been proved, although patellar luxation has been observed in mares and their foals. 2) Progressive destruction of the lateral trochlear ridge resulting from osteochondritis dessicans, seen in young, fast-growing animals. 3) Luxation at any age due to trauma and rupture of the patellar ligaments.

In small animals, patellar luxation usually is seen in toy and miniature breeds of dogs, in which it should be considered heritable. Usually it is termed congenital since the predisposing conditions are present at birth. It is characterized by coxa vara and a decrease in femoral neck anteversion. Signs may be intermittent. In older animals, the condition may appear acutely as a result of minor trauma, worsening of degenerative joint disease pain, or breakdown in soft tissue. Luxation in large and giant breeds, also called genu valgum, is seen in the same breeds that are affected by hip dysplasia. In these cases, it usually is bilateral and is apparent by 5-6 mo of age.

Clinical Findings—Large Animals: *See also* p 527. Bilaterally afflicted neonates have difficulty in rising; the stifle and hock are markedly flexed, and the affected limb(s) will not bear weight. The patella can be palpated as a hard mass lateral to the stifle, and can be replaced within the trochlear groove if the limb is extended. Unilateral lateral luxation produces similiar signs, although the animal may be able to rise and ambulate with partial weight bearing on the affected limb. An important condition to rule out in neonatal calves is femoral nerve paralysis subsequent to dystocia. Juvenile animals with osteochondritis may have uni- or bilateral lameness and moderate to profound femoropatellar effusion. A crescent-shaped, calcified osteochondral body, the remains of the lateral trochlear ridge, is often palpable laterally within the joint space (*see also* OSTEOCHONDROSIS, p 558). Traumatic patellar luxation is usually unilateral and accompanied by profound periarticular swelling and joint effusion. Otherwise, clinical signs are similar to those of the congenital form.

Small Animals: In small breeds, luxation is medial in 75-80% of the cases, and nearly all traumatic cases are medial; lateral luxations are seen, but usually later in life (5-8 yr). The condition in large breeds, described above, usually results in lateral luxation.

In all cases, the gait is affected; medial luxations usually cause a bow-legged appearance, and lateral luxations cause a knock-kneed stance. The stifle is flexed to varying degrees, and the degree of weight bearing also varies. Especially in the congenitally affected small breeds, luxation may be intermittent; even when luxated, the effect on gait may not be apparent at every stride. In 15-20% of middle-aged and older dogs with chronic luxation, the cranial cruciate ligament is ruptured.

Diagnosis: Clinical signs are strongly suggestive, and palpation or radiographic visualization of the displaced patella is diagnostic. This condition may resemble femoral nerve paralysis, rupture of the cranial cruciate ligament, or gonitis of any form. Radiography and arthroscopy are helpful in evaluating osteochondritic lesions and deformities of the trochlear groove or ridges, especially when surgical treatment is contemplated.

Treatment: Animals with profound congenital deformities of the trochlear ridges have a poor prognosis, especially if the patella does not stay within the trochlear groove for some time after manual replacement. Surgical techniques to deepen the trochlear groove and reconstruct the periarticular ligaments or the joint capsule may be successful in selected cases.

RUPTURE OF THE ACHILLES TENDON

A partial or complete disruption in the continuity of the gastrocnemius and superficial flexor tendons. It may be the result of trauma from automobile accidents, laceration from mowing machinery or wire, extreme stress during a race or hunt, or occasionally, a severe local infection. Lacerations may occur anywhere along the course of the tendon; however, ruptures are usually at the point of insertion on the calcaneus, in connection with an avulsive fracture of the tuber calcaneus, or at the juncture of the muscle and tendon.

Rupture of the gastrocnemius muscle (qv, p 502) produces a gait similar to that of rupture of the Achilles tendon. Careful examination, both radiographic and by palpation, should be done to determine the exact nature of the lesion and the possibility of bone involvement. Ultrasonography is useful to identify tendon or muscletendon junction defects when the limb is diffusely swollen and palpation is unrevealing.

There is a characteristic alteration of the stance and gait. The animal is no longer able to stand or walk on the toes of the affected limb. The degree of flexion of the hock is increased without concurrent flexion of the stifle. The plantar surface of the metatarsus may touch the ground. On palpation, the tendon is flaccid and sometimes swollen. Pain is not an outstanding sign.

Treatment is surgical, and musculotendinous ruptures require immediate attention. Ruptures with sharp division of the tendon are easier to repair than indistinct lacerations. After surgical repair, the leg should be immobilized in a slightly flexed position for 5-6 wk. Fixation of the tuber calcaneus to the tibia with a bone screw has been recommended as a method of immobilization.

RUPTURE OF THE CRUCIATE LIGAMENTS

The cranial and caudal cruciate ligaments are responsible for maintaining the craniocaudal stability of the stifle in flexion and extension; rupture of either results in marked joint instability, which may predispose to degenerative joint disease.

Injury to the cruciate ligaments can be related directly to their function as constraints of joint motion. Excessive forces during extremes of these constraints result in damage to the ligaments. Because of its position in the joint and because it is the primary constraint against cranial instability, internal rotation, and hyperextension of the stifle, the cranial cruciate ligament is injured most often.

Injury to the cranial cruciate ligament is usually associated with a sudden rotation or hyperextension of the stifle; injury to the caudal cruciate ligament is usually a result of a direct force on the tibia driving it caudally. Acute cruciate ligament injury can be isolated, or associated with other stifle pathology. Depending on the mechanism of injury, the collateral ligaments, menisci, and/or other cruciate ligaments may be involved. Because of the associated joint instability, chronic injury usually results in degenerative joint changes that include periarticular osteophyte formation, capsular thickening, and medial meniscal degeneration.

Rupture of either or both ligaments usually causes an acute hindleg lameness and is diagnosed by demonstrating abnormal cranial or caudal excursion of the tibia on the femur, the so-called drawer sign. The cruciate ligaments are best evaluated for integrity with the limb in a functional position. A small animal is placed in lateral recumbency, and the examiner grasps the distal femur with one hand and the proximal tibia with the other. With the limb in a functional position, attempts are made to subluxate the tibia cranially or caudally; abnormal excursion in either direction indicates cruciate ligament insufficiency. Large animals are examined while standing. The palms of the hand are then used to quickly and forcefully push and pull the proximal tibia in an effort to demonstrate an abnormal cranial or caudal excursion.

Because of the joint instability and subsequent progression of degenerative joint changes, surgical stabilization of the stifle is indicated. Prognosis is based on the amount of surgical stabilization and the extent of degenerative changes already present.

SARCOCYSTOSIS
(Sarcosporidiosis)

An invasion of the endothelium and muscles by protozoans of the genus *Sarcocystis*. As the name implies, *Sarcocystis* spp form cysts in the muscles of the various intermediate hosts—man, horses, cattle, sheep, goats, pigs, birds, rodents, and reptiles—which vary in size from a few micrometers to several centimeters, depending on the host and species.

Etiology: *Sarcocystis* spp develop in 2-host cycles consisting of an intermediate host (prey) and the final host (predator). Prey-predator life cycles have been demonstrated for cattle-dog (*S cruzi*), cattle-cat (*S hirsuta*), cattle-man (*S hominis*), sheepdog (*S tenella, S arieticanis*), sheep-cat (*S gigantea, S medusiformis*), goat-dog (*S capracanis, S hircicanis*), goat-cat (*S moulei*), pig-dog (*S meischeriana*), pig-man (*S suihominis*), pig-cat (*S porcifelis*), and others. About 1 wk after ingesting musculature containing *Sarcocystis* cysts (sarcocysts), the final hosts begin to shed infective sporocysts in their feces; shedding continues for several months. Following ingestion of sporocysts by a suitable intermediate host, sporozoites are liberated and initiate development of schizonts in vascular endothelia. Merozoites are liberated from the mature schizonts and produce a second generation of endothelial schizonts. Merozoites from this second generation subsequently invade the muscle fibers and develop into the typical sarcocysts. Initially, sarcocysts contain only a few metrocytes—round, noninfective parasites that give rise to the banana-shaped infective zoites found in mature cysts beginning 2-3 mo after infection. Sarcocysts of some species grow so large that they are easily visible with the unaided eye. The presence of such sarcocysts can cause condemnation of the carcass during meat inspection. Sarcocysts of other species remain microscopic even though tremendous numbers of cysts may be present in the muscles.

Pathogenicity: *Sarcocystis* spp were considered of doubtful pathogenicity, until induced infection with *S cruzi* sporocysts from canine feces caused acute disease in calves, and abortions, stillbirths, and deaths in pregnant cows. Similar pathogenicity has been demonstrated for *S tenella* in lambs and ewes. The clinical signs were similar to those reported from natural outbreaks of sarcocystosis in cattle in Australia, Canada, England, Ireland, Norway, and the USA. Man also may serve as the intermediate host and suffer myositis and vasculitis, but the source of such human infection has never been determined, and only ~40 such cases are known worldwide. Human illness has followed ingestion of sarcocysts of *S suihominis* in uncooked pork, and *S hominis* in uncooked beef; clinical signs of nausea, abdominal pain, and diarrhea lasted up to 48 hr. The extent of human illness from ingestion of infected meat has not been documented.

Clinical Findings: Most animals are asymptomatic, and the parasite is discovered only at slaughter. In cattle severely affected by *S cruzi*, the signs include fever, anorexia, cachexia, decreased milk yield, diarrhea, muscle spasms, anemia, hyperexcitability, weakness, prostration, and death. Cows infected in the last trimester of pregnancy aborted. After recovery from acute illness, some calves failed to grow well and eventually died in a cachectic state. Sheep, goats, and pigs have similar clinical signs. After recovery from acute illness, some sheep lost their wool. At necropsy, acutely affected animals have hemorrhage of the serous membranes of the viscera and myocardium.

Control: The livestock become infected by sporocysts from the feces of carnivores. Because most adult cattle and sheep, and many pigs, harbor cysts in their muscles, dogs and other carnivores should not be allowed to eat raw meat, offal, or dead animals. Supplies of grain and feed should be kept covered; dogs and cats should not be allowed in buildings used to store feed or house animals. Amprolium (100 mg/kg body wt, daily for 30 days), fed prophylactically, reduced illness in cattle inoculated with *S cruzi*. Prophylactic administration of amprolium or salinomycin also protected experimentally infected sheep. Therapeutic treatment of cattle and sheep has been ineffective. Vaccines are not available.

NERVOUS SYSTEM

NERVOUS SYSTEM, INTRODUCTION

The nervous system, by generation, propagation, and integration of electrical activity, detects changes in the external or internal environment of the body, interprets the sensory information, directs coordinated muscular responses, and releases hormones.

ORGANIZATION

The nervous system has evolved with simple reflexes involving 2 or 3 neurons as its basic mechanism, eg, the knee jerk and withdrawal reflexes. These reflexes are modified with increasing degrees of variation and integration as the sensory (afferent) information passes from the limbs, eyes, tongue, nose, ears, or vestibular system through the spinal cord and/or the primitive brain stem, cerebellum, thalamus, and cerebral hemispheres. The connections between areas of the nervous system are called tracts.

The motor (efferent) commands are modified in a similar hierarchy: cerebral hemispheres, basal nuclei, brain stem, and spinal cord. More highly evolved species have the greatest ability to vary and learn their responses to a stimulus. In animals, this usually is thought of as intelligence. Human characteristics of intelligence (abstract problem solving and appreciation of the future) are handled by "association" areas of the cerebral hemispheres, which among nonhuman species are well developed only in the higher apes. The alert state and sleep are interactions of the brain stem with the cerebrum. Consciousness (what we know we feel) is cerebral, largely in "association" areas. Fortunately, most sensory data and motor control do not or need not involve consciousness, eg, gut movements, sphincter control, and regulation of heart rate.

The cerebellum is the highest motor coordination center of the nervous system, and the hypothalamus the highest control of the visceral nervous system (sympathetic, parasympathetic) and hormones. A combination of brain structures, which include evolutionarily older parts of the cerebrum and hypothalamus, is involved in emotions and behavior.

Thus, sensory, motor, coordination, visceral, intelligence, emotional, and behavioral activities are, to a considerable extent, independent of each other. A disease may severely damage one function, yet have little effect on the others.

FUNCTION

The **central nervous system** (CNS) comprises the brain and spinal cord; the **peripheral nervous system** (PNS), the cranial and spinal nerves. Spinal and cranial nerves contain axons of lower motor neurons (LMN) of various sizes that drive skeletal and smooth muscle. Loss of LMN leads to flaccid paralysis, loss of reflexes, and rapid atrophy of skeletal muscles. All other motor neurons in the CNS are called upper motor neurons (UMN), and can affect muscles only via LMN, the final common pathway to muscles. Loss of UMN leads to a spastic (tonic) paralysis, exaggerated reflexes, and a slow disuse atrophy of skeletal muscles supplied by the affected LMN. Partial and complete loss of voluntary motor function are termed paresis and paralysis, respectively.

Separate sensory fibers in spinal nerves mediate conscious sense of position (conscious proprioception [CP]) and touch via the cerebrum; and subconscious proprioception via the cerebellum; as well as pain, heat, and cold sensation. Thus, there can be analgesia (loss of pain) without complete loss of all sensation (anesthesia), loss of CP without cerebellar input loss, and vice versa. Cranial nerves mediate the specialized sensory functions of smell, taste, vision, hearing, and balance, as well as various amounts of motor and visceral activities and skin sensation.

Ascending and descending spinal tracts associated with motor and sensory function traditionally have been termed long tracts. Injury to these tracts typically causes UMN paralysis and loss of CP or pain sensation in the limbs and trunk caudal to the lesion. In contrast, injury to similar fibers in the peripheral nerves produces segmental sensory signs (focal loss of pain sensation or reflex function) and LMN paralysis in only some muscles of a limb.

Units of the nervous system generally function by modifying the existing or inherent electrical activity of other units; eg, LMN have a natural electrical firing rate in response to a tap on their muscle or its tendon, which is suppressed by many UMN (eg, cerebral) but increased by some UMN (eg, vestibular).

Time of arrival and sequencing of sensory data are important, especially in coordination of movements. The cerebellum is informed of most UMN commands to LMN and achieves coordination by comparing the original command to the proprioception data that result from the muscle movements. Any lesion, whether inflammatory or compressive, may delay arrival of data in the cerebellum. The resulting ataxia, hypermetria, or tremor may be as severe as if the cerebellum or its tracts were physically destroyed. Balance is further coordinated by the vestibular system with information initially sensed by receptors in the labyrinth of the inner ear (peripheral) and then relayed to vestibular nuclei in the brain stem (central). Peripheral and central lesions can be distinguished because other evidence of brain-stem disease (depression, cranial nerve deficits, CP loss, weakness) accompanies the latter.

Neurotransmitters are chemicals that relay electrical impulses (data) across a synaptic gap to the next neuron. Chemical synapses offer several evolutionary advantages over simple electrical synapses in data processing and complexity of possible responses. Neurotransmitters are excitatory (eg, glutamate) or inhibitory (eg, γ-aminobutyric acid [GABA]) and may evolve into circulating hormones (eg, noradrenaline) or also be used in other body functions (eg, serotonin in local inflammation). Chemicals, toxins, antibodies, or enzymes that destroy, mimic, enhance, or block the effects of these neurotransmitters may produce widespread or local nervous system changes (eg, atropine, organophosphates, strychnine, tetanus toxin).

Thus, disease processes may affect the timing, excitation, inhibition, and transmission of electrical data in the nervous system, as well as physically damage the organ. Physiological changes may not be detectable by light or even electron microscopy.

INTERACTION WITH OTHER ORGANS

Nervous system function requires that blood electrolytes, glucose, oxygen, temperature, pH, osmolarity, pressure, and other variables be maintained within narrow limits. Only oxygen, carbon dioxide, and glucose readily cross the blood-brain barrier. Oxidative metabolism of glucose provides most of the brain's energy requirements. Supply of both oxygen and glucose to the brain depends on cerebral blood flow (CBF). Normal CBF depends on cerebral perfusion pressure, which equals mean arterial pressure minus intracranial pressure. Therefore, either reduced mean arterial pressure or increased intracranial pressure could reduce CBF. Fortunately, however, CBF is maintained at a relatively constant rate at mean arterial pressures of 50-160 mm Hg by appropriate dilation or constriction of cerebral blood vessels (pressure autoregulation), and also when intracranial pressure is high by increasing mean arterial pressure (Cushing response). Cerebral blood vessels also are sensitive to the chemical content of blood; systemic hypoxia and hypercapnia both cause vascular dilation to prevent cerebral hypoxia and acidosis, respectively (chemical regulation). Despite these safeguards, neurons can become deprived of oxygen (hypoxic hypoxia), and a characteristic lesion of ischemic neuronal cell change occurs. Other potential causes of cerebral hypoxia include anemia (anemic hypoxia), selective impairment of CBF (ischemic hypoxia), and reduced cardiac output (stagnant hypoxia). Ischemic neuronal cell change also occurs due to hypoglycemia, as occurs with insulin-producing tumors of the pancreas, and certain other metabolic insults, eg, thiamine deficiency of ruminants and salt poisoning of pigs. Many other organ system diseases can thus affect the nervous system, usually producing seizures, depression, or coma.

Conversely, nervous system changes can produce surprising changes in other organ functions; eg, increased vagal tone, caused by brain-stem inflammation or a rise in CSF pressure, can produce severe bradycardia, heart block, and sinoatrial arrest. Emotional shock or brain damage can cause neurogenic shock. Emotional stress affects pyloric emptying and can also cause colitis. Fainting is a vasovagal phenomenon. Brain trauma can cause fatal neurogenic pulmonary edema.

CLINICAL RESPONSES TO DISEASE

Despite the many mechanisms by which disease or injury can affect the nervous system, only 4 basic types of clinical responses are seen: deficiency, shock, release, and discharge.

Deficiency is the most likely response to be seen, eg, a nerve is injected accidentally, a vertebral fracture damages spinal cord tracts, infection damages a reflex, a tumor presses on the optic nerves causing blindness, or otitis interna causes loss of vestibular function.

CNS shock is mostly limited to concussion; spinal shock occurs only transiently following spinal injury in animals. Concussion is a temporary "shake up" of neurons, not bruising or hemorrhage as occurs with contusion.

Release phenomena include hyperreflexia after UMN loss to LMN has occurred, and perhaps some instances of loss of learned self-control leading to vicious attacks.

Discharge refers to electrical bursts in the brain seen as seizures (convulsions), sensory nerve irritation (pain), and LMN irritation (muscle fasciculations).

Thus, clinical signs reflect not only the disease process, but the part of the nervous system affected.

The nervous system responds to disease in a limited number of ways. The principal forms of brain edema are vasogenic (fluid passes into the extracellular spaces because of vascular injury), cytotoxic (fluid accumulates intracellularly due to failure of the sodium pump), and interstitial (fluid passes from the ventricles into the interstitium due to hydrocephalus). Most brain diseases cause a certain degree of necrosis, which may be concentrated in either gray matter (polioencephalomalacia) or white matter (leukoencephalomalacia). Demyelination is frequent and may occur independent of axonal or neuronal cell-body injury (primary demyelination) or because of it (secondary demyelination). Degeneration of the axon and its myelin sheath distal to the point of axonal or neuronal injury is called wallerian degeneration. This is typical of chronic, compressive spinal cord disease. Acute spinal cord injuries, in contrast, often cause central hemorrhagic necrosis.

PRINCIPLES OF DIAGNOSIS

The classical steps in diagnosis are localization of the lesion and determination of its character (irritative or obliterative) and cause. This fits in well with the problem-oriented medical record system but emphasizes neurologic localization. Detailed knowledge of neuroanatomy is not needed to make a diagnosis and select a treatment, but is needed to explain all the signs.

Efficiency in neurological diagnosis usually depends on collection and interpretation of the history and neurological and physical examinations. Important factors in differential diagnosis are: species, breed, age, speed of onset of signs, improvement, deterioration, cyclic or episodic signs, evidence of focal pain, possibility of trauma, recent vaccination, and access to poisons or infected animals.

The Neurological Examination: The examination has 3 objectives: characterize the presenting sign, find any other nervous system changes, and localize the lesion(s) as well as possible. Even in obscure cases, the lesion usually can be localized to the spine, brain, or peripheral nervous system. Within the brain, lesions may be localized to 1 of 4 main areas based on signs: cerebrum-thalamus (change in attitude, compulsive walking, circling, seizures), cerebellum (ataxia, dysmetria, tremors), brain stem (depression, paresis, cranial nerve deficits), or vestibular system (ataxia, head tilt, nystagmus). Spinal cord lesions should be localized to either C_{1-5} (UMN paralysis in all 4 limbs, hindlimbs perhaps worse), C_6-T_2 (LMN paralysis in forelimbs, UMN paralysis in hindlimbs, forelimbs worse), T_3-L_3 (normal forelimbs, UMN paralysis in hindlimbs), or L_4-S_3 (normal forelimbs, LMN paralysis in hindlimbs). Lesions may be localized to specific peripheral and cranial nerves based on changes in reflex function and the pattern of loss of sensation and muscle mass. The severity and left-right symmetry also can be estimated (the crossover of functions in the brain should be remembered). Left limb functions are mediated by the right midbrain and right cerebrum. Therefore, lesions at or rostral to the midbrain cause contralateral clinical deficits, and lesions caudal to the midbrain usually cause ipsilateral deficits. Left side cranial nerve reflexes are mediated by the ipsilateral brain stem, but left side conscious vision by the contralateral cerebrum. Tract functions generally are used to estimate severity; reflexes are used more for localization. (*See* CLINICAL EXAMINATION OF THE NERVOUS SYSTEM, below.)

Neurological localization helps diagnosis in general ways. For example, multifocal lesions suggest infectious disease, while focal lesions are more suggestive of neoplasia or infarction. Other tests usually are necessary for specific disease identification (radiology, hematology, blood chemistries, serology, CSF tap). Knowledge of the severity of a lesion aids selection and urgency of treatment, prognosis, and owner education. In general, spinal cord lesions that cause LMN paralysis or loss of pain sensation have a poorer prognosis.

Differential diagnosis is facilitated by having a list of diseases that can cause every presenting sign, preferably subdivided by species. A perspective of the combination and rate of development of clinical signs possible with each disease is also needed. Traumatic and vascular diseases usually cause acute, nonprogressive signs; infectious, metabolic, neoplastic, and degenerative diseases cause chronic, progressive signs.

Laboratory Tests: Electrical testing of the neuromuscular systems is now done in most species. Electroencephalography (EEG) is of some help in seizure diagnosis and may provide indirect evidence of other disease. Electromyography (EMG) identifies spontaneous muscle activity (fibrillation potentials, positive sharp waves) associated with nerve injuries and also may help to identify myogenic disorders (bizarre muscle potentials). Sensory and motor nerve conduction velocities (NCV) are most helpful in diseases such as coonhound paralysis, in which the NCV is reduced. Repetitive nerve stimulation is used to diagnose myasthenia gravis, in which there is a characteristic decrement of the evoked muscle potential. Spinal- and brain-evoked potentials give information regarding the integrity of brain (vision, hearing) and spinal cord (pain, proprioception) pathways.

CSF pressure measurement, cell counting, culture, and chemical analysis are all possible. In general, bacterial diseases cause the WBC to increase dramatically ($>1000/\mu L$) in CSF with most being neutrophils, and viral diseases cause mild or moderate increases ($<100/\mu L$) with most being lymphocytes or macrophages. Other inflammatory or neoplastic diseases cause variable changes, often intermediate between those seen with bacterial and viral diseases.

Muscle biopsies can reflect changes typical of both primary muscle (variation in fiber size, increased internal nuclei, hyalin fibers) or nerve (angular fibers, small group atrophy) disease. Biopsies of sensory nerve branches or partial biopsies of motor nerves may identify demyelination or inflammation typical of certain diseases. Serological and urine tests for many nervous system metabolites are available.

Diagnostic imaging techniques often have an important role (*see* p 952 *et seq*). Plain and contrast radiographs aid in identifying spinal lesions. More recently, use of computed tomography and magnetic resonance scans have allowed clearer identification of intracranial neoplasia. In a herd or flock situation, necropsy of an affected individual should be considered.

CLINICAL EXAMINATION OF THE NERVOUS SYSTEM

An accurate history and thorough physical and neurological examinations are necessary to evaluate a problem involving the nervous system. An understanding of neuroanatomy, neurophysiological concepts, and neuropathological processes is a requisite for accurate interpretation of clinical findings. From the initial clinical assessment, the problem may be defined as diffuse, multifocal, or focal; symmetrical or asymmetrical; mild, moderate, or severe; and the anatomical locations determined. Consideration of the potential mechanisms of disease as congenital and familial, inflammatory, metabolic, toxic, nutritional, traumatic, vascular, degenerative, neoplastic, or idiopathic is necessary to formulate an accurate differential diagnosis list. Further clinicopathological tests may be needed to obtain a final diagnosis, including CSF analysis, plain and contrast radiography, and other special diagnostic tests.

HISTORY

Neurological diseases tend to have a species, age, breed, and occasionally, a sexual predilection. The primary complaints for neurological problems often include behavioral changes, seizures, tremors, cranial nerve deficits, ataxia, and paresis or paralysis of one or more limbs. Information about the onset, course, and duration of the primary complaint can be used to determine the most probable disease mechanisms. Congenital and familial disorders most commonly are seen at birth or within the first 1½ yr of life and may be static or progressive. Inflammatory, metabolic, toxic, and nutritional disorders tend to have an acute or subacute onset and usually are progressive. Vascular and traumatic disorders have an acute onset and rarely are progressive. Degenerative and neoplastic disorders tend to occur most frequently in older animals, and to have a chronic onset and progressive course. Many idiopathic disorders begin acutely and improve over a short time. Information about similar familial problems, concurrent or recent systemic disease, vaccination status, other affected animals, diet, possible exposure to toxins or trauma, and past neoplastic disorders may be useful to further support certain mechanisms of disease.

PHYSICAL AND NEUROLOGIC EXAMINATIONS

Evidence of disease in other body systems may be associated with inflammatory, metabolic, toxic, or metastatic neoplastic disorders of the nervous system. External signs of traumatic or toxic exposure may support these mechanisms of disease.

Neurologic examination may be divided into 4 sections: evaluation of the head; the gait; the neck and forelimbs; and the trunk, hindlimbs, anus, and tail. Initially, an attempt should be made to relate all deficits to a focal anatomical lesion.

If abnormalities are found on evaluation of the head, then an initial attempt should be made to explain hindlimb abnormalities due to a lesion above the foramen magnum. If no abnormalities are found in the head, but forelimb abnormalities are present, then an attempt should be made to explain hindlimb abnormalities due to a cervical lesion. Paralysis or paresis of all 4 limbs with loss of all spinal reflexes (with or without cranial nerve deficits) is often associated with diffuse peripheral nerve or neuromuscular junction disease.

Knowledge of specific diseases within a certain mechanism for a given species, age, breed, and sex of animal enables an accurate differential diagnosis and diagnostic plan to be formulated after the history and physical and neurologic examinations are completed. Toxic, metabolic, and nutritional mechanisms rarely produce asymmetrical neurologic deficits. The other mechanisms may be symmetrical or asymmetrical.

EVALUATION OF THE HEAD

The mentation, head posture, coordination, and cranial nerve functions are observed during evaluation of the head. Abnormal findings are due to lesions above the level of the foramen magnum in the cerebrum, the brain stem (diencephalon, midbrain, pons, or medulla oblongata), or the cerebellum. Dementia, compulsive pacing, or other behavioral abnormalities are frequently due to lesions in the cerebrum or diencephalon. Depression, semicoma, or coma may be due to lesions of the cerebrum, diencephalon, or midbrain. Seizures are due to involvement of the cerebrum or diencephalon. A head tilt or compulsive circling without a head tilt is also associated with a cerebral or diencephalic lesion on the side toward which the animal turns. A true head tilt is due to vestibular system disease. Abnormal head coordination, bobbing, and tremors result from cerebellar dysfunction.

The **cranial nerves** are located at specific sites along the brain stem and are simple to test. Abnormal findings are produced by peripheral cranial nerve or brain-stem lesions. If a brain-stem lesion is present, abnormalities are seen in the gait, forelimbs, or hindlimbs. If only a peripheral cranial nerve is affected, the other 3 parts of the examination are normal.

I. Olfactory: The olfactory nerve is used for smelling.

Tests: Observe the animal's ability to find food or the reaction to chemicals such as cloves, benzene, and xylol (do not use substances that irritate the nasal mucosa and the trigeminal nerve endings, such as camphor or phenol).

Signs of Dysfunction: An abnormal response is an inability to find food or respond to nonirritating chemicals, and is found with disease of the cribriform plate, olfactory bulbs, and diencephalon.

II. Optic: The optic nerves are necessary for vision and also carry the afferent fibers of the pupillary light reflex center to the midbrain.

Visual Tests: Perform the menace test by making a threatening gesture toward each eye, taking care to avoid excessive air currents or touching the hair. Obstacle testing may be necessary when visual acuity is in doubt. It is useful to blindfold one eye at a time to detect asymmetrical blindness.

Pupillary Light Reflex: A bright focal light is directed into each pupil toward the temporal retina and the pupil observed for immediate constriction. The opposite pupil should constrict consensually.

Ophthalmoscopic Examination: This detects local eye diseases. Chorioretinitis or papilledema may be associated with central or peripheral nervous system diseases.

Signs of Dysfunction: Optic nerve dysfunction results in a decrease or loss of vision and pupillary light reflexes on the affected side. Consensual pupillary constriction should still occur when the opposite eye is stimulated. Optic tract, optic radiation, thalamic (lateral geniculate nucleus), or occipital cortex lesions usually produce a contralateral blindness with normal pupillary light reflexes, eg, a lesion of the left cerebral hemisphere causes a right-sided blindness with normal pupil reactions.

III. Oculomotor: This nerve carries efferent parasympathetic fibers from the pupillary light reflex center to the fibers of the ciliary ganglion, which innervate the constrictor muscle of the pupil. It is also efferent to the levator palpebrae muscle; the dorsal, medial, and ventral rectus muscles; and the ventral oblique muscle of the eye.

Tests: 1) Perform the pupillary light reflex test as for the optic nerve. 2) Observe for presence or absence of ptosis of the upper eyelid, and ventrolateral strabismus.

Signs of Dysfunction: Oculomotor nerve or midbrain lesions result in a dilated pupil unresponsive to light, but the eye is visual. The animal may or may not have ventrolateral strabismus and ptosis. With unilateral lesions, ipsilateral (direct) pupillary constriction does not occur, but contralateral (consensual) constriction does.

IV. Trochlear: This is the motor nerve to the dorsal oblique muscle of the eye.

Test: Observe the eyeball for dorsomedial strabismus (easiest to see in cats because of the vertical pupil).

Signs of Dysfunction: Trochlear nerve or midbrain lesions may result in dorsomedial strabismus.

V. Trigeminal: This nerve has 3 branches. The mandibular branch is the motor nerve to the muscles of mastication and sensory to the floor of the oral cavity, ventral arcade, and the skin of the ventrolateral head. The ophthalmic and maxillary branches are sensory to the skin of the dorsolateral head; mucous membranes of the roof of the oral cavity, the dorsal arcade, and the nasal cavity; and the eyeball, including the cornea (pain).

Tests: 1) Evaluate jaw tone and masticatory movements and palpate masseter and temporalis muscles to evaluate the motor component of the trigeminal nerve. 2) The sensory function can be evaluated by stimulation of the medial and lateral canthi of the eyes, which elicits the **palpebral reflex** (closure of the eyelids), and stimulation of the cornea, which results in globe retraction. In stoic dogs, a pinprick to the nasal mucosa may be necessary, and an avoidance response will be observed.

Signs of Dysfunction: A lesion of the trigeminal nerve or pons produces temporal and masseter muscle atrophy and/or loss of sensation to the face, cornea, and nasal mucosa. A bilateral trigeminal motor nerve lesion produces a dropped jaw.

VI. Abducens: This is the motor nerve to the lateral rectus and retractor bulbi muscles of the eye.

Tests: 1) Observe the eyeball for medial strabismus. 2) Elicit the corneal reflex with the eyelids held open, and observe for retraction of the eyeball and prolapse of the third eyelid.

Signs of Dysfunction: Abducens nerve or rostral medulla oblongata lesions result in medial strabismus and lack of globe retraction.

VII. Facial: This is the motor nerve to the muscles of facial expression (ear, eyelids, nose, and mouth).

Tests: 1) Elicit the palpebral, menace, and corneal reflex for orbicularis oculi muscle function. 2) Observe the nose for deviation (with unilateral lesions). 3) Pinch the lip to see if it retracts. 4) Tickle the ear to see if it moves.

Signs of Dysfunction: A facial nerve lesion (middle or inner ear or rostral medulla oblongata) results in an inability to blink the eyelid or move the lips or nose, and usually produces a droopy face, drooling, and accumulation of food in the affected cheek.

VIII. Vestibulocochlear: There are 2 main divisions of this nerve; the first, the **cochlear nerve**, functions to provide the sense of hearing. The second branch, the **vestibular nerve**, allows maintenance of normal posture, muscle tone, and equilibrium.

Tests: Total deafness (qv, p 306) is easily detected by creating loud noises near the sleeping animal. Observe for head tilt, disequilibrium, and tendency to fall, roll, or circle with unilateral or asymmetrical lesions. Check for the presence of abnormal nystagmus with the head in normal position (resting spontaneous nystagmus) and with the head held in a deviated position (positional nystagmus).

Signs of Dysfunction: Unilateral vestibulocochlear nerve (inner ear) or rostral medulla oblongata lesions produce disequilibrium with head tilt toward the side of the lesion. A spontaneous or positional horizontal and rotary nystagmus is often present. A bilateral lesion results in disequilibrium on both sides, wide excursion movements of the head, and deafness. A unilateral cerebellar lesion may result in a head tilt away from the side of the lesion.

IX. Glossopharyngeal and **X. Vagus:** These provide sensory and motor control of the pharynx, larnyx, and of the viscera.

Tests: 1) Pinch the hyoid bones to elicit a **gag reflex.** 2) Observe for normal phonation and respiratory sounds.

Signs of Dysfunction: Glossopharyngeal and vagus nerves or caudal medulla oblongata lesions result in dysphagia, megaesophagus, laryngeal paresis or paralysis, and a change in phonation.

XI. Spinal Accessory: Innervates the trapezius, sternocephalic, and brachycephalic muscles.

Tests: Palpate the innervated muscles.

Signs of Dysfunction: Cranial cervical spinal cord or caudal medulla oblongata lesions may result in atrophy of the sternocephalicus muscle.

XII. Hypoglossal: This is the motor nerve to the tongue and geniohyoid muscles.

Test: Observe for muscular control of the tongue during licking and lapping of water.

Signs of Dysfunction: Hypoglossal nerve or caudal medulla oblongata lesions may result in deviation or atrophy of the tongue.

EVALUATION OF GAIT

Gait is observed while the animal walks, trots, gallops, turns, sidesteps, and backs. In large animals, ambulation up and down a grade and while blindfolded may accentuate subtle gait deficits. Evaluation of the gait is especially important in ambulatory large animals since postural reactions are difficult to obtain because of size, and spinal reflexes usually are not tested unless the animals are recumbent. In small animals, subtle deficits may be detected by postural reaction testing of the limbs (in the next 2 parts of the examination, *see* below). Hemistanding and hemiwalking (standing or walking on one side) are also observed in small animals. Animals with lesions in the cerebral cortex and diencephalon usually have a relatively normal gait, but may circle compulsively. Animals with lesions of the midbrain, pons, and medulla oblongata have paresis or paralysis of the limbs, with deficits often more severe on the side of the lesion. Cerebellar lesions produce ataxia and dysmetria. Vestibular dysfunction causes ipsilateral falling, rolling, or circling. If no abnormalities are found on evaluation of the head, but the gait is abnormal, a lesion most likely is located in the spinal cord, peripheral nerves, or muscles.

EVALUATION OF THE NECK AND FORELIMBS

The neck is examined for pain and, in large animals, atrophy and desensitization to pinprick, which indicate a cervical spinal cord lesion.

Wheelbarrow: The hindlimbs of small animals are lifted off the ground, and the animal is evaluated while walking on the forelimbs alone. This test is used to detect subtle deficits of the forelimbs. Normal animals should not stumble or knuckle over on the toes as they walk.

Tonic Neck and Eye: With the animal (dog or cat) standing, its nose is elevated and the eyes observed to see if they coordinately adjust to the center of the palpebral fissures. Simultaneously, the forelimbs should extend with no tendency to knuckle or collapse. If neck pain is present, a lesion in this area should be considered.

Proprioceptive Positioning: Each foot is displaced by turning it onto its dorsum or by abducting or adducting the limb widely. The animal should immediately replace the leg to a normal position. Conscious proprioception is often the first modality to be affected by subtle lesions of the nervous system.

Placing: Small animals may be carried toward a table top; on seeing the table, a normal animal anticipates placing its forepaws on the surface. If blindfolded, the animal should place the forepaws on the table only when the limbs contact the edge of the table. A loss of placing response may be present in subtle dysfunction when the gait is normal.

Hopping: This can be tested only in small animals. While holding the other 3 limbs off the ground, the animal is forced to move or hop on the fourth limb; motor and proprioceptive loss, cerebellar incoordination, and cerebrocortical deficiency may be detected. This procedure also is useful to detect subtle dysfunction.

Righting: The animal is observed to see if it can right itself from lateral recumbency. A small animal suspended upside down by the hips attempts to hold its head up when the trunk is rotated from side to side and extends its forelimbs to support weight when lowered to the ground. With vestibular dysfunction, the animal twists toward the side of the lesion or curls its head under.

Spinal Reflexes: The spinal reflexes are tested with the animal in lateral recumbency with the limbs relaxed. When the toes or skin of the distal limb are pinched, that limb should withdraw and the opposite limb usually does not move. This is the **flexor** or **withdrawal reflex**; it is present if spinal cord segments C_6-T_2 and nerves of the brachial plexus are intact. Intramedullary spinal cord lesions at C_6-T_2 usually depress or abolish the reflex, but mild extramedullary lesions may produce no change. With lesions cranial to C_6, a simultaneous extension of the opposite limb (the **crossed extensor reflex**) may occur when the tested limb flexes.

Other tendons (biceps and triceps) and muscle (extensor carpi radialis) may be tapped with a percussion hammer and the response evaluated to test C_{6-7} or the musculocutaneous nerve, and C_7-T_2 or the radial nerve, respectively. These reflexes can be difficult to obtain in normal animals, so changes should be interpreted with caution. All reflexes may be normal or exaggerated with lesions above C_6.

Muscle Atrophy: Severe localized muscle atrophy of the limbs or neck indicates damage to the particular nerve (cell body, root, or peripheral portion) that innervates that muscle and can be helpful in localizing a lesion to that site.

Sensation: Conscious perception of superficial (skin) or deep (osseous) pain is tested by applying forceps to the skin or bone and observing a behavioral response. Such a response indicates that the peripheral sensory nerve and spinal cord, as well as the pathways through the brain stem to the cortex, are intact.

If the animal has abnormal findings on the evaluation of the head, any forelimb abnormalities should be initially related to the lesion above the foramen magnum. If the forelimb abnormalities cannot be explained by the lesion in the head, then a multifocal or diffuse disease process such as an inflammatory, toxic, metabolic, nutritional, or metastatic neoplastic disorder must be present.

If there are no abnormalities on evaluation of the head, and the forelimbs are abnormal, then a cervical spinal cord and brachial plexus lesion is present. In cervical spinal cord lesions, the forelimbs are abnormal and hindlimb spinal reflexes are normal or exaggerated.

If no abnormalities are found on evaluation of the head and forelimbs, then a lesion, if it exists, must be below T_2 spinal cord segments.

EVALUATION OF THE TRUNK, HINDLIMBS, ANUS, AND TAIL

The trunk of the animal is observed for abnormal posture or deviation of the vertebral column, pain, desensitization or hyperesthesia to light pinpricking, and focal muscle atrophy.

Cutaneous Trunci and Panniculus Reflex: Pinpricks applied to the skin of the thorax and abdomen result in contraction of the cutaneous trunci muscle. This reflex arc uses the cutaneous branches of the lumbar and thoracic spinal nerves as afferent pathways and the lateral thoracic nerve of the brachial plexus as the efferent pathway. The reflex is used to localize spinal cord lesions between the site of afferent stimulation and caudal brachial plexus levels.

Attitudinal and Postural Reactions: Wheelbarrowing, proprioceptive positioning, placing, and hopping are evaluated on the hindlimbs in a manner similar to that used for the forelimbs. As with the forelimbs, these tests require complete integrity of the brain, spinal cord, and peripheral nerves; thus, they are not useful for localizing lesions, but are useful in detecting subtle deficits that support the presence of a neurologic lesion.

Spinal Reflexes: The hindlimb spinal reflexes are more reliable for localizing thoracolumbar lesions than are the forelimb reflexes. Spinal reflexes may be normal or exaggerated with lesions above the reflex arc level, or depressed or abolished with lesions at the reflex site. Percussion of the patellar tendon should produce extension of the stifle if L_{4-5} spinal cord segments and the femoral nerve are intact. Percussion of the gastrocnemius and cranial tibial muscles causes extension or flexion of the hock, respectively, and tests the tibial and peroneal nerves and L_6-S_2 spinal segments and the lumbosacral plexus. A **crossed extensor reflex** may be associated with lesions above L_6. When the anus is pinched or pricked with a pin, the sphincter tightens and the tail pulls down if S_{1-3} (anus) and caudal (tail) segments and nerves are intact. An atonic (flaccid) bladder, anus, and tail are seen with lesions affecting S_1-Cd_5 or the cauda equina.

Muscle Atrophy: Focal muscle atrophy of the trunk or hindlimb localizes a lesion to the nerve that innervates that muscle.

Sensation: In moderate to severe spinal cord lesions, superficial sensation may be absent from the cranial aspect of the lesion caudally. In severe spinal cord lesions, deep sensation is absent from bones of all toes and the tail.

Schiff-Sherrington Phenomenon: In some animals with acute, severe spinal cord lesions between T_2-L_3, the hindlimb paralysis is accompanied by an extensor rigidity of the forelimbs when the animal is in lateral recumbency. Although a severe lesion produces this syndrome, the prognosis is probably not hopeless if deep pain can be elicited.

CEREBROSPINAL FLUID (CSF)

The pressure and composition of CSF may further aid in the determination of the mechanism of CNS disorders. The technique of collection is simple and safe with practice. Analysis of CSF requires minimal special equipment, but cell counts and identification must be performed within 30 min after collection. Analysis of CSF is usually necessary to detect CNS infections. Collection can be done by puncture of the cerebellomedullary cistern in small animals, or of the subarachnoid space at the lumbosacral junction in large animals. Elevations of pressure to >170 mm H_2O in small animals indicate a space-occupying lesion or a defect in drainage of CSF into the venous system. Elevation of protein is often associated with encephalitis, meningitis, neoplasia, or spinal cord compression. Increased cellular content suggests inflammation of the CNS. Neutrophils are indicative of bacterial infections, subarachnoid hemorrhage (RBC are also present), brain abscess or a steroid-responsive suppurative meningoencephalitis, or in some cases, necrosis within a tumor. Increased numbers of lymphocytes, monocytes, and neutrophils are most common in granulomatous meningoencephalitis, fungal infections, or toxoplasmosis. Cultures of CSF may demonstrate the causative agent in bacterial and fungal infections. Serology can identify antibodies to other agents, particularly viruses.

CLINICAL PATHOLOGY

Metabolic causes of behavioral abnormalities and seizures include hypoglycemia, hepatic encephalopathy, uremic encephalopathy, hypocalcemia, hypomagnesemia, and hyperosmolar and hyposmolar syndromes. Serum glucose, liver enzymes, BUN, bile acids, serum ammonia, and electrolytes should be evaluated to detect most metabolic dysfunctions. Serum cholinesterase and lead determinations are invaluable for the diagnosis of acute organophosphate and lead toxicity, respectively.

RADIOGRAPHY

Plain radiographs of the skull and vertebral column are useful to detect fracture, subluxation, infection, or neoplasia of osseous structures. In most cases, brain and spinal cord infections or neoplasia have normal plain radiographs. Myelography is used to detect compressive spinal lesions, including herniated or protruded intervertebral disks and spinal cord tumors. Cerebral angiography, pneumoventriculography, computed tomography, and magnetic resonance imaging are other diagnostic techniques used to evaluate animals with neurological disease.

OTHER DIAGNOSTIC EVALUATIONS

Electroencephalography, electromyography, and other special electrodiagnostic procedures are available at most neurology referral practices.

PRINCIPLES OF THERAPY

See also NERVOUS SYSTEM, PHM, p 1397.
The aim of surgical therapy is to reduce compression of the spinal cord, brain, or nerves. This is best accomplished as soon as possible after injury, since prolonged compression may cause irreversible damage.

Brain swelling due to edema is medically decompressed with combinations of metabolic diuretics (eg, furosemide, 1 mg/kg, b.i.d.), osmotic diuretics (eg, mannitol, 0.25-1 g/kg, t.i.d.), large "membrane-stabilizing" doses of glucocorticoids (eg, prednisolone 30-50 mg/kg, or dexamethasone 2-4 mg/kg, q.i.d.), dimethylsulfoxide (DMSO), and adequate oxygenation. Deep anesthesia and hyperbaric oxygen have not been effective experimentally, but various specific antiprostaglandins may become available to block arterial vasospasm in the brain.

Glucocorticoids, phenylbutazone, DMSO, and various other anti-inflammatories can be used when there is noninfectious inflammation (eg, demyelination, edema, peri-infarct hypoxia). Cage or stall confinement may be used if trauma or an intervertebral disk lesion is suspected. Reduction of pain (eg, with glucocorticoids) in an animal with a spinal lesion should be done with strict confinement, lest freedom from pain allow the animal to move excessively and worsen the lesion. Animals with severe neurological dysfunction or chronic pain may require surgery. Immune-mediated demyelination or inflammation may need glucocorticoid therapy on alternate days for 3-12 mo.

Care in drug selection is necessary if active infection is suspected. Cage confinement and perhaps aspirin are preferable to glucocorticoids, which may suppress immune function. Sedation can be used for relaxation. Diazepam is not only a tranquilizer but a specific muscle relaxant. Relaxants (eg, methocarbamol) help relieve muscle spasm associated with spinal pain or even tetanus. Morphine derivatives should be avoided in animals with CNS lesions since they may increase edema.

Infections: Few antiviral agents are available, and antifungals are of limited use in the CNS. Most antibacterial agents do not cross the intact (noninflamed) blood-brain or blood-CSF barrier, and many do not cross adequately even when inflammation is present. Chloramphenicol, trimethoprim, and sulfas do cross the intact blood-CSF barrier; ampicillin and penicillin cross it adequately when it is inflamed. The aminoglycoside antibiotics (gentamicin, neomycin, etc) do not cross the blood-CSF barrier well, even when it is inflamed. If intrathecal (inside the subarachnoid space or ventricular system) instillation is necessary, the agent should be administered into a lateral ventricle. An injection into the cerebellomedullary cistern is acceptable for spinal lesions. The CSF drains from the ventricles over the brain surface and down the spinal cord.

When the animal is recumbent, special attention is required to prevent or treat decubital ulcers. Slings, pads, straw, and sawdust can help distribute the animal's weight. Water beds also may be helpful but must be fashioned from sturdy material to avoid puncture. Preventing urine scald, keeping the animal dry, and turning the animal q2hr are helpful. Effective treatment of a decubital ulcer is difficult until the animal begins to regain motor function.

Cystitis may be a sequela of paralysis or incontinence; acidifiers, antiseptics, and antibiotics may be necessary once infection is detected. Manual expression of the bladder t.i.d. helps prevent and treat cystitis. Catheterization should be avoided if possible.

Metabolic and Toxic Diseases: The brain is especially sensitive to electrolyte changes or reductions in blood glucose and vitamins necessary for its metabolism (eg, thiamine). Rises in ammonia and other compounds in the blood due to a failing liver or kidneys may have dramatic effects on the brain. Toxic compounds usually cause coma or seizures, change electrolyte ratios, block metabolic pathways, or affect neurotransmitters or the liver. Specific treatment depends on disease or agent identification and a knowledge of the metabolic pathway affected.

Physiotherapy and Rehabilitation: Manual extension and flexion of paralyzed limbs (eg, for 15 min, t.i.d) help retain muscle bulk and limit fibrotic contracture of muscles, but only for a few months. Percutaneous electrical stimulation is more effective. Swimming and sling support can be used once some motor function returns. Ultrasonic therapy may help muscles maintain and improve function, but it is not therapeutic for CNS lesions.

Devices that allow movement, eg, carts, are effective for dogs and cats with posterior paresis but do not solve the problem of incontinence. Little other rehabilitation has been tried in animals.

Specific therapy for seizures depends on their cause, eg, antibiotics for infectious meningitis, calcium EDTA for lead poisoning, calcium gluconate for hypocalcemia, and glucose for hypoglycemia. Anticonvulsants can help treat such diseases, but their primary use is to control epilepsy. Phenobarbital, primidone, diazepam, valproate, paramethadione, phenytoin, and progesterone-like compounds can raise the brain cells' threshold to seizures and slow the spread of abnormal electrical activity between cells. Of these drugs, phenobarbital appears to be most effective for long-term control of seizures in dogs and cats. Diazepam is most useful in status epilepticus. Estrogen lowers the seizure threshold as does any excitement, stress, or irritation; hence, neutering of epileptics is advised. Anticonvulsant dose rates vary tremendously among species and may be metabolized differently (especially phenytoin). Because of this, measurement of serum levels is advisable.

Behavioral Therapy: Training and owner education are the most needed treatments for many problem animals, but hormones, neutering, anticonvulsants, and tranquilizers can help. Specific drugs aimed at neurotransmitter metabolism may become better understood and new ones made available. Surgical treatments, eg, prefrontal lobotomy and focal lesioning in the brain, have rarely been effective.

Oral choline loading seems to have a temporary (weeks) effect in most "senile" animals.

Episodic Weakness: Many systemic and neurological diseases may cause weakness or exercise intolerance. One such disease, myasthenia gravis, may be treated specifically with acetylcholine potentiators or parasympathomimetics such as edrophonium (IV—short acting), physostigmine, and neostigmine (IM or PO). These agents help maintain neuromuscular synaptic transmission (nicotinic effects), but some also stimulate muscarinic synapses (excess salivation). Atropine, an acetylcholine blocker, prevents unwanted muscarinic effects but does not affect nicotinic synapses.

BOVINE SPONGIFORM ENCEPHALOPATHY
(BSE)

A progressive, fatal, nervous disease of adult domestic cattle, which closely resembles scrapie of sheep and goats (qv, p 622); it was first diagnosed in Britain in 1986.

Etiology, Epidemiology, and Pathogenesis: The causal agent has not been identified, but similarities between BSE and scrapie suggest that it belongs to a group of incompletely characterized microorganisms called unconventional viruses or prions. These agents, in addition to scrapie, cause transmissible mink encephalopathy (qv, p 1054), chronic wasting disease of mule deer, and kuru and Creutzfeldt-Jakob disease of man. Infectivity of such agents is detected only by biological assay in experimental host species, notably mice and hamsters. Transmissibility of BSE has been established in mice and cattle. There is no evidence that the transmissible spongiform encephalopathies of man are acquired from animals.

Initial studies in Britain showed an extended common source epidemic, consisting solely of index cases with no evidence of transmission between cattle. The incidence of affected herds increased with herd size. Nevertheless, national- and within-herd incidence was generally low. The peak incidence was in 4-yr-old cattle. There was no sex or breed predisposition. Available evidence supports a food-borne exposure to a scrapie-like agent by contamination of concentrate rations.

The pathogenetic mechanisms are as yet unknown, but data indicate an oral route of infection and a minimum incubation period of 22 mo.

Clinical Findings and Lesions: The clinical signs are principally neurological, insidious in onset, progress variably over weeks to months, and end in death. Clinical onset is independent of season or stage of lactation; signs include apprehensive behavior that may progress to aggression and frenzy, hyperesthesia with kicking during milking, gait ataxia, and reduced milk yield or live weight loss. Incoordination, hypermetria, falling, and generalized paresis are concurrent with behavioral changes, and later become the dominant signs. Tremors and muscle fasciculations also occur. Intense pruritus, as seen in scrapie, is not a feature, but some affected cattle do rub and scratch. Welfare considerations, unmanageable behavior, recumbency, or emaciation necessitate slaughter.

Significant necropsy findings are confined to histological changes in the CNS. These comprise bilateral, usually symmetrical, vacuolation of gray matter neuropil (spongiosis) and neurons, similar to the lesions seen in scrapie.

Diagnosis: Initial clinical signs may be subtle or resemble those of hypomagnesemia or nervous ketosis. Metabolic disorders can be ruled out on serum biochemistry and failure to respond to therapy. Clinical evaluation must be based on repeated examinations at intervals sufficient to detect progress of the signs. Subsequent histological examination of the brain is essential to confirm the diagnosis. Behavioral changes of BSE could be confused with those of the furious form of rabies (qv, p

619), but the usually protracted clinical course of BSE contrasts with that of rabies. Differential diagnoses also include encephalic listeriosis (qv, p 356), lead poisoning (qv, p 1674), and downer cow syndrome (qv, p 555).

Control: Treatment is ineffective. Interim statutory control measures have been initiated in Britain, which assume that exposure of cattle to scrapie-contaminated tissue in meat and bone meal is the source of the problem. These comprise notification of suspected clinical cases to regulatory authorities, compulsory slaughter, histopathology of the brain, destruction of the carcass, and payment of compensation. The use of ruminant-derived protein in ruminant rations was prohibited in July 1988.

CONGENITAL AND INHERITED DISEASES OF THE CNS

Congenital defects of the CNS are common, and most can be recognized by structural change, which may involve both the CNS and the skeletal structures, or only the former. Some congenital defects are known to be inherited, others are caused by environmental factors (toxic plants, nutritional deficiencies, viral infections); for many, the cause is still unknown. In animals born with a well-developed nervous system (foals, calves, lambs, pigs), inherited neurological disorders may be recognized at birth. In kittens and puppies, which are born less well developed, neurological disorders may not be noticeable until they would normally begin to walk. (*See also* DISEASES OF THE SPINAL COLUMN AND CORD, p 584.)

CEREBELLAR AND BRAIN-STEM DEFECTS

Arnold-Chiari malformation consists of herniation of tongue-like processes of cerebellar tissue through the foramen magnum into the anterior cervical spinal canal and caudal displacement and elongation of the medulla oblongata, pons, and the fourth ventricle. Often it is associated with spina bifida, hydrocephalus, and meningomyelocele. It is rare in domestic animals, and the cause is unknown.

Cerebellar aplasia, hypoplasia, and **degeneration** have been described in many species. Their pathogenesis and causes must be reevaluated since prenatal and neonatal infection (feline panleukopenia virus and bovine viral diarrhea) may be causative. The main signs are ataxia at birth or shortly after, violent muscular movements, coarse tremors, and opisthotonos. The pathological features include atrophy of all or parts of the layers of the cerebellar cortex, but particularly, loss of the Purkinje cell layer. Cerebellar hypoplasia in puppies and kittens often is accompanied by hypoplasia of the pons, the inferior olivae, and sometimes the optic tracts. Clinical signs consist of tumbling, circling, and ataxia, and often a head tremor. Another type of cerebellar disorder, in which the cerebellar white matter is predominantly affected, has been seen in Jersey and other calves in North America. Lesions also occur in other parts of the brain, the most notable being a lack of myelin formation. In Britain, a somewhat similar condition, **hypomyelinogenesis congenita**, has been described in newborn paralytic lambs. Throughout their entire nervous system, axis cylinders develop, but myelination is deficient. Myoclonia congenita in pigs (qv, p 583) may represent a variation of hypomyelinogenesis congenita.

Cerebellar cortical atrophy has been described in Holstein calves with clinical and morphological features comparable to those of the defect in lambs (**daft lambs**) and dogs. A similar condition has been described in Angus calves as **familial convulsions and ataxia**; almost identical pathological changes have been described in Holstein calves and in a Charolais. The clinical signs usually appeared during the first few hours of life and were characterized by single or multiple, sudden tetaniform seizures of variable intensity, lasting 3-12 hr or longer. Inheritance appeared to be dominant with incomplete penetrance (20-30%).

Hereditary neuraxial edema and congenital brain edema were first reported in neonatal polled Herefords. The calves were unable to rise, and lay quietly without struggling. There was incoordination and coarse muscular tonic contraction. Sudden touch or clapping of hands elicited vigorous extension of the legs and neck. Brains were grossly normal, but microscopical examination revealed spongy vacuolar appearance of the CNS tissue along the long axis of myelinated fibers in white and gray matters.

Progressive ataxia is a clinical and pathological entity, most likely of genetic etiology, in Charolais cattle. Clinical signs were first noticed in cattle 8-24 mo old, and progressed in 1-2 yr from slight ataxia involving all 4 limbs, to recumbency. Histological lesions consisted of eosinophilic plaques in the white matter of the internal capsule, cerebellar white matter, and spinal cord. There was myelin breakdown but no phagocytic response.

CEREBRAL DEFECTS

Agenesis of the corpus callosum, absence of all or part of the corpus callosum, has been described rarely in domestic animals and its cause is unknown.

Anencephaly, nonclosure of the cranial portion of the neural tube and subsequent failure of the cranium to develop, has been described in cattle. Its cause is unknown. The pituitary may be absent, and its absence probably is responsible for the prolonged gestation of some calves affected with anencephaly. Associated defects include cleft palate, no tail, atresia ani, and patent fontanelle.

Arhinencephaly (absence of the rhinencephalon) is a rare deformity in cattle characterized by unilateral or bilateral absence of olfactory bulbs, tract, or nerves. Prolonged pregnancy may accompany the condition. Breeds involved are Simmental, Guernsey, and Angus. Cause of the deformity is unknown, although it was once assumed to be a dominant lethal mutation.

Cranioschisis, a cleft in the cranial skeleton, is usually associated with herniation of the meninges and parts of the brain.

Cyclopia and **cebocephalia** are severe defects involving the cranium as well as the facial skeleton. The cause in lambs is ingestion of the range plant *Veratrum californicum* (qv, p 1705).

Exencephaly is a brain entirely exposed or extruding from a large defective skull (acrania). The defect is rare and its cause unknown.

Hydranencephaly is complete or almost complete absence of the cerebral hemispheres in a cranium of normal conformation. The space is filled with CSF encased by thin membranous cerebral tissue and meninges. The congenital syndrome of hydranencephaly, with or without arthrogryposis, occurs sporadically or as epidemics in calves. The chief clinical signs are blindness, incoordination, and arthropathy. Other pathological changes observed are cerebellar hypoplasia, muscular atrophy, cleft palate, scoliosis, and spina bifida. Abortion, stillbirth, or premature birth may occur. Several causes, including hyperthermia and the viruses of ephemeral fever, Japanese encephalitis, bluetongue, and Akabane disease, have been identified.

Hydrocephalus, an excess accumulation of fluid within the ventricular system, is common in cattle and other domestic animals. Calves with internal hydrocephalus (*see also* p 477) may be dead at birth or within a few days. In many breeds of cattle, it appears to be inherited as a simple autosomal recessive. In Hereford and Shorthorn calves, it is accompanied by a stenotic aqueduct, cerebellar hypoplasia, myopathy, multiple ocular anomalies, retinal detachment and dysplasia, cataracts, microphthalmia, and persistent pupillary membranes. Hydrocephalus varies considerably; one or both lateral ventricles may be involved, the third ventricle and anterior portion of the aqueduct may be dilated, and the fourth ventricle may be normal. In Hereford calves, there may be dorsal kinking and lateral compression of the midbrain with stenosis of the middle part of the mesencephalic aqueduct. Doming of the skull is not consistent in domestic animals. Dyschondroplastic calves (*see also* p 479) usually are affected with internal hydrocephalus.

Meningocele and **meningoencephalocele** are characterized by protrusion of meninges and brain tissue through a cranial cleft (cranioschisis). The herniated portion sometimes forms a large liquid-filled sac. Meningoencephalocele usually occurs in the frontal region (proencephaly) but may be midfrontal, parietal, or occipital. In most domestic animals, it is not known if the defect is inherited; in piglets, it is a simple autosomal recessive. (Meningoceles occur in the spinal column also, as a type of spina bifida.)

Micrencephaly is rare and has been described as a normal-sized cranial cavity only partly filled by brain. In the reported cases, there was a decrease in number of gyri, and the corpus callosum and fornix were absent; all were stillborn or died soon after birth. Associated defects were micrognathia, multiple ear and eye defects, vesicular cerebral hemisphere, and absent septum pellucidum.

SPASTIC AND PARALYTIC DISEASES

A group of diseases, some of which are hereditary, with clinical evidence of CNS involvement; however, pathogenesis and neurological lesions have not been well defined.

Citrullinemia, a hereditary metabolic defect in Holstein-Friesian calves, was first described in Australia. It is due to an elevation of citrulline in plasma caused by deficiency of the urea cycle enzyme arginosuccinate synthetase. Affected calves appear normal at birth but die of acute fatal neurologic disease in 1-4 days. Signs are sudden in onset and consist of depression, aimless wandering, blindness, seizures, opisthotonus, and recumbency. There are no gross lesions in the brain; the GI mucosa may reveal congestion and edema, and the liver is pale and yellow. There is diffuse cerebrocortical edema, congestion, some neuronal degeneration, and astroglial swelling. Similar changes are present in the midbrain, cerebellum, and brain stem but are less severe.

Epilepsy is a functional disease of the brain characterized by recurrent periodic tonic-clonic convulsions, usually of short duration, and apparently similar to epilepsy in man. "Idiopathic" epilepsy has been described in many species but probably is seen most often in dogs (*see* below); it has been recorded in Swedish Red cattle as an autosomal recessive, and in Brown Swiss cattle as an autosomal dominant. (*See also* CONVULSIVE SEIZURES [DOGS], below.)

The typical history is that of recurrent seizures with few or no other physical signs. Convulsions may begin in the first year of life, but more frequently begin in the second year. The typical seizure lasts for 1-2 min and consists of a staring expression, falling on the side, and running movements of the extremities. Evacuation of the bladder and bowel is common during seizures. After the convulsion, the animal may quickly regain its normal state, or act dazed and uncoordinated for a few minutes.

GM_1 gangliosidosis occurs in inbred Friesian calves in Ireland, and involves a reduction (70-80%) in β-galactosidase activity. Clinical signs become evident during the first few weeks of life, and include swaying of the hindquarters, reluctance to move, and stiffness. Microscopic lesions are primarily vacuolation of neurons.

Lethal spasm (lethal neonatal spasticity) has been reported in Jersey and Hereford cattle as a simple autosomal recessive.

Mannosidosis (originally reported as **pseudolipidosis**) in Angus, Murray Grey, Galloway, and possibly a few other breeds is due to deficiency of the enzyme mannosidase and is a simple autosomal recessive. Clinically, there is ataxia, head tremor, aggression, and failure to thrive. There also may be abortions and neonatal death. Most affected calves die within the first year, sometimes shortly after birth. Vacuolation of neurons, macrophages and reticuloendothelial cells of lymph nodes, and exocrine pancreas cells are typical. Affected (homozygous) calves have an absolute deficiency of α-mannosidase, and heterozygotes are partially deficient. Thus, mannosidosis can be controlled by identifying and eliminating heterozygotes on the basis of biochemical testing.

Maple syrup urine disease is a genetic aminoaciduria in polled and possibly horned Hereford calves. Affected calves have severe neurologic disease in the first week of life. They are dull, become recumbent in 2-4 days, and finally have opisthotonus. The severe histologic lesions consist of status spongiosus.

Spastic paresis occurs in many breeds of cattle, and is characterized by spastic contracture of the muscles and extension of the stifle and tarsus of one or both hindlegs. It has been referred to as "contraction of the Achilles tendon", "straight hock", and "Elso heel". (*See also* LAMENESS IN CATTLE, p 494.) Spasticity affects the gastrocnemius and superficial flexor muscles and tendons and, in some cases, also the biceps femoris, semitendinosus, semimembranosus, quadriceps, and abductor muscles. It is a progressive disease and varies in severity and time of onset; it is usually noted first in 3- to 6-mo old calves.

Radiographs of affected hocks are characterized by increased joint angle, osteoporosis, exostosis of the distal epiphyseal line of the tibia, curvature and exostosjs of the dorsal aspect of the calcaneus, and widening of the epiphyseal line of the calcaneus. Genetic influence(s) as well as environmental factors interact to express spastic paresis. Affected bulls should not be used for breeding.

A **spastic syndrome** (remittent or periodic spastic syndrome, crampy neuromuscular spasticity, progressive posterior paralysis, stretches, or barn cramps) is observed in cattle >3 yr old and is characterized by sudden, spastic, muscular contractions of one or both hindlegs. (*See also* pp 502 and 503.)

SPINAL MUSCULAR ATROPHY

A disease of Brown Swiss calves, suspected to be inherited. The first clinical sign is weakness of the hindlegs at 3-4 wk of age; calves have difficulty getting up and become recumbent. Terminal stages are characterized by severe muscular atrophy. Histopathologic examination reveals degeneration and loss of motor neurons in the ventral horns of the spinal cord. Neurogenic atrophy of muscles is a consistent lesion.

BOVINE PROGRESSIVE DEGENERATIVE MYELOENCEPHALOPATHY (BPDME) OF BROWN SWISS CATTLE

BPDME may be a congenital metabolic defect of axon transport that is familial and appears to be inherited. Four basic criteria are required to establish the clinical diagnosis: 1) onset of bilateral hindleg weakness and ataxia between 5 and 8 mo of age; 2) deficient proprioceptive reflexes, with no other clinically detectable neurological abnormality; 3) absence of clinically significant musculoskeletal abnormality; and 4) adherence to familial relationship. Initially described as "weaver" because of the peculiar weaving gait, the disease is frequently associated with back injury or joint disease.

Clinical signs of BPDME reflect the 4 diagnostic criteria. Affected animals eventually become recumbent and die or must be slaughtered because of ruminal tympany. There are no typical gross lesions. Primary microscopic lesions are confined to the CNS. Spinal cord lesions consist of axonal degeneration, including spheroid formation; loss of axons and myelin; and vacuolation of white matter due to large, empty intercellular spaces. Lesions are qualitatively similar at all levels of the spinal cord but quantitatively dissimilar at different levels in the same funiculi. Ascending and descending fibers are involved, and involvement is most severe in the thoracic area. Electron microscopy demonstrates axonal and myelin changes and reactive changes in glial cells. Little or no glial response, no inflammatory response, and no involvement of gray matter are observed in the spinal cord. Cerebellar lesions are limited to selective degeneration and loss of Purkinje cells and occasional swelling of Purkinje cell axons in the granular layer of the cerebellar cortex.

DISORDERS OF DOGS

Convulsive seizures appear to be hereditary in certain breeds of dogs. Spastic attacks in Labrador Retrievers resembled epilepsy (in EEG readings). "Fits" in Belgian Tervurens probably have a genetic basis.

Epilepsy (*see* p 580) in Beagles has a genetic basis. The higher rate in males than in females suggests a genetic hypothesis involving 2 loci, one an autosomal recessive, the other, a sex-linked suppressor gene. Epilepsy in German Shepherd Dogs also appears to be inherited as an autosomal recessive. A high incidence of epilepsy has been noted in Cocker Spaniels. Electroencephalograms may be used to detect at an early age neurological disorders that are likely to manifest as convulsions when the dog is older.

Convulsions in dogs also have been associated with deficiencies of vitamins A and B, hypocalcemia, intestinal parasitism, intestinal obstructions, and hyperthermia; they may precede tick paralysis. Since the cause is unknown, treatment must be aimed at alleviating the clinical signs. Drugs commonly used to control epileptic seizures in dogs include phenobarbital, primidone, and phenytoin, given singly or in combination.

Familial amaurotic idiocy, possibly inherited as a simple autosomal recessive, has occurred in German Shorthaired Pointers; clinical signs at 6 mo of age were nervousness and decreased ability for training. Progressive ataxia and impaired vision developed later. Neurons with soluble and insoluble granules and an increase of GM_2 gangliosides in the cerebral cortex were seen histologically.

Globoid cell leukodystrophy (Krabbe's disease), reported in Cairn Terriers, West Highland White Terriers, and Miniature Poodles, is inherited as a simple autosomal recessive that causes deficiency of a β-galactosidase. Clinically, 2 major syndromes are seen: at 3-6 mo little pelvic stiffness is seen in some dogs, while in others, a cerebellar disturbance is the main clinical sign. Death occurs 2-3 mo after the onset of signs. Total protein content of 80 mg/dL in the CSF compares with the normal 27.5 mg. Large globoid cells are distributed throughout the white matter of the spinal cord and brain.

Hallucinatory behavior in the King Charles Spaniel is characterized by persistent "fly-catching" in the absence of stimuli (flying insects).

Hereditary ataxia, a simple autosomal recessive trait, appears in 2- to 4-mo-old Fox Terriers. Progression is rapid, then slows, but the general ataxia progresses until the dog is unable to walk. Histological lesions are bilateral demyelination of the dorsolateral and ventromedial columns of the spinal cord. Ataxia in Jack Russell Terriers is clinically similar.

Heritable cerebellar hypoplasia and degeneration, reported in 12-wk-old Airedales, was manifest by signs of ataxia and hypermetria. There was absence and degeneration of Purkinje cells as well as chromatolysis of the neurons of the central cerebellar nuclei.

Juvenile amaurotic idiocy in the English Setter, most likely inherited as a recessive, was characterized by reduced vision and dullness, manifest when the dog was 12-15 mo old. By 18 mo, muscle spasms appeared and, eventually, seizures progressed to severe, tonic-clonic spasms. Gross pathological findings were enlarged lymph nodes and brain atrophy. Histologically, lipid granules were observed in neurons, heart, lungs, liver, and GI tract.

Neuronal abiotrophy in Swedish Laplands, inherited as a simple autosomal recessive, is characterized by a sudden onset of weakness in either fore- or hindlimbs when dogs are 5-7 wk old. It progresses to tetraplegia, atrophy of the limbs, and joint flexion. Central peripheral chromatolysis, cell-body shrinkage, neurophagia, and axonal and myelin degeneration is seen histologically.

A **neurotropic osteopathy** in 3- to 9-mo-old Pointers, considered to be hereditary, was characterized by toe-gnawing, self-mutilation, and low sensitivity in distal parts of the limbs. Spinal cord sections revealed demyelination and vacuolar degeneration of the white matter.

Paralysis of the hindlimbs of the first cross of St. Bernard × Great Dane and Great Dane × Bloodhound developed when the dogs were 3 mo old. Death of motor and preganglion sympathetic neurons in the spinal cord was thought to be inherited.

Recurrent tetany in Scottish Terriers, referred to as **Scotch cramp** and usually first seen at ~1 yr of age, is characterized initially by an arching back followed by a stiff-legged gait due to overflexed hindlimbs and abducted forelimbs. Signs, which may result from abnormal serotonin metabolism, are seen when the dogs are excited or strenuously exercised and abate with rest. It is a simple autosomal recessive.

Spinal dysraphism in Weimaraner dogs is an inherited disorder, although the mode of inheritance is not clear. Major clinical signs are hopping gait, crouching stance, abduction of one limb, and abnormal proprioception in the hindlegs when the dogs are 4-6 wk old. The disease is not progressive. Spinal cords have duplication, absence, and malformation of the central canal; thinning and absence of central gray matter; and areas of ectopic gray matter in the ventral median sulcus. **Syringomyelia** (cavitation of the spinal cord) may develop in older dogs.

A permanent **trembling condition** in the hindquarters and tail occurs in Airedale Terriers, usually after the dogs are ≥6 mo old.

PORCINE CONGENITAL TREMOR SYNDROME
(Myoclonia congenita, Shaker pigs, Dancing pigs, Congenital trembles)

A distinctive neurological syndrome of newborn piglets characterized clinically by trembling. Congenital tremor is indicative of a diffuse CNS disorder, and generally is associated with abnormalities of central myelin formation. It sometimes also involves cerebellar hypoplasia. Pathological and neurochemical studies have established 5 etiological entities within the syndrome.

Etiology and Epidemiology: Transplacental viral infections of fetuses during the first half of gestation cause most incidents of the syndrome. Hog cholera (qv, p 381) virus is the only identified infectious etiology. Another transmissible agent, presumably viral, is probably responsible for most outbreaks of congenital trembling in countries free of hog cholera. Inherited causes have also been recognized, but only rarely reported, in male Landrace and Landrace-cross pigs as a sex-linked recessive, and in British Saddleback and Chester White pigs as an autosomal recessive. The organophosphate trichlorfon has produced the syndrome in piglets when used in sows in mid-gestation. Probably there are other etiological entities.

Infectious causes give rise to epidemics that usually affect many litters and up to 100% of the pigs within litters. In the most common infectious form, mortality is usually low, especially under conditions of good management, but in outbreaks resulting from infection with hog cholera virus, it can be high. Outbreaks persist for 2-3 mo. Subsequent litters from parents of an affected litter are likely to be normal. Subclinical infection is spread by adults with the common infectious form. Trichlorfon, when used therapeutically as an acaricide, can produce incidents in which many affected litters with high morbidity and mortality are born over a short period. The epidemiology of genetically determined congenital tremor conforms to simple Mendelian inheritance; ~25% of the piglets in each litter are affected, and mortality is high. Breed and sex predispositions help to identify these uncommon forms.

Clinical Findings: The principal manifestation is a diffuse rhythmic tremor or repetitive myoclonus present at or developing within a few hours of birth. When piglets rest, the tremors diminish or cease, only to resume following external stimulation. During voluntary motor activity they are constant. When the tremors are so severe as to preclude nursing, the piglets soon die of starvation. In most survivors the tremor disappears within 3 wk, but occasionally it persists for months, even to maturity. Mild ataxia and sometimes dysmetria may accompany the tremors, especially when they are severe. Occasionally, in an outbreak of infectious congenital tremor, some of the affected piglets are concurrently splaylegged (*see also* p 477). There is, however, no known pathogenetic association between the 2 syndromes.

Lesions: Pathological alterations are limited to the CNS and have been characterized morphologically and neurochemically for the defined entities. Spinal hypo- or dysmyelinogenesis occurs in all of the congenital tremor entities described, but is variable in nature and extent between different etiological forms and variable in severity among cases of a single form. Alterations in oligodendrocytes probably underlie the myelin deficits. The spinal cord generally is reduced in size in all forms except the most commonly occurring infectious form. In this, morphological changes are minimal, and myelin deficits are virtually confined to the spinal cord. In some other etiological entities, the brain myelin is also affected. The correlation between the degree of myelin abnormality and severity of clinical signs is not always close. Although the tremor is considered to originate in the spinal cord, the mechanism is unknown. Cerebellar hypoplasia and dysplasia are present in forms that result from transplacental infection with hog cholera virus or fetal exposure to trichlorfon.

Diagnosis: The distinctive clinical sign in live, affected piglets readily allows diagnosis of the syndrome. Etiological diagnosis requires knowledge of the epidemiological and pathological findings. The hereditary types generally involve specific breeds and have a low incidence even in affected herds. The infectious types tend to occur in outbreaks with initial high morbidity and, if due to hog cholera, may give rise to other forms of reproductive loss. Demonstration of antibodies to hog cholera in the sera of sows with affected litters confirms exposure of the sow to the virus.

Demonstration of spinal myelin deficits requires careful comparison of stained histological sections of spinal cord from affected and normal piglets of the same age. Although neurochemical methods are more exact, the laboratory techniques are not routinely available. The objective assessment of cerebellar hypoplasia depends on the weight of the cerebellum relative to the weight of the whole brain, and comparison with appropriate control data. If cerebellar hypoplasia is found in affected piglets, hog cholera should be suspected initially, especially in countries where this disease remains endemic.

Treatment and Control: Specific prophylactic biologicals or treatments have not been developed. However, since death is caused by inability to nurse, individual pigs may be saved by helping them nurse, or by providing them with sustenance until, with age, the intensity of the tremors diminishes. If they survive the first 5 days, their chances of survival without help are good.

Herd control measures depend on etiological diagnosis. Infectious causes (often hog cholera) produce economically more important disease than do hereditary causes. Transplacental infection by an unidentified virus, which is most common, can be controlled by deliberate exposure of unbred sows to affected piglets; this should result in protection of piglets from subsequent pregnancies. In unaffected herds, use of boars from infected herds may introduce the disease.

Hereditary causes can be eliminated by culling carriers identified by statistical analysis of breeding data. Piglets that survive congenital tremor, whatever the cause, should not be retained for breeding.

DISEASES OF THE SPINAL COLUMN AND CORD

Diseases of the spinal column and cord of dogs and cats include congenital diseases, degenerative diseases, inflammatory and infectious diseases, neoplasia, nutritional diseases, trauma, and storage diseases. Several of these diseases also affect other animals. General discussions, with emphasis on the diseases in small animals, appear below; discussions of more specific diseases in cattle, horses, pigs, and sheep and goats are presented separately, p 592 *et seq.*

DOGS AND CATS

CONGENITAL DISORDERS

Atlantoaxial subluxation is an instability of the atlantoaxial articulation that results from separation, absence, or malformation of the odontoid process (dens). It may produce acute, severe neurological deficits because of excessive flexion of the joint. It is most common in dogs <1 yr old, but can occur in older animals as a result of trauma. It also has been reported in cats. Clinical signs range from cervical rigidity and pain, through spastic tetraparesis, to tetraplegia. Signs may occur acutely or develop slowly over several months. Diagnosis is based on radiographic findings. The prognosis is guarded. Surgical decompression with stabilization of the luxation is mandatory.

Cervical malformation-malarticulation (wobbler syndrome) represents a malformation of the lower cervical vertebrae that results in varying degrees of spinal cord compression. The disease is characterized radiographically by displacement of the craniodorsal aspect of the vertebra into the vertebral canal, stenosis of the cranial orifice of the vertebral foramen, and sometimes, by malformation of the craniodorsal or cranioventral aspects of the vertebral body. It occurs in horses (*see* EQUINE WOBBLER SYNDROME, p 593) and several breeds of dogs, but most commonly in younger (<1 yr) Great Danes and older (>5 yr) Doberman Pinschers. There have been isolated reports in other breeds, including Borzoi, Rhodesian Ridgeback, Old English Sheepdog, Irish Setter, Fox Terrier, Boxer, Chow Chow, Weimaraner, Golden Retriever, and Pyrenian Mountain Dog. The cause is unknown, although rapid growth rates and nutrition, mechanical factors, and genetics may be implicated. Signs tend to be progressive and range from mild paraparesis to tetraplegia. The hindquarters sway awkwardly while walking. This disorder needs to be differentiated from skeletal diseases such as coxofemoral dysplasia, osteochondrosis dissecans, hypertrophic osteodystrophy, and from genu valgum, cervical spinal cord neoplasms, and intervertebral disk protrusions in older dogs. Spinal cord changes consist of variable degrees of necrosis and demyelination at the level of injury. Diagnosis is based on clinical signs, breed, and radiography. Spinal contrast studies are essential to establish an accurate diagnosis. Prognosis depends on the severity of the defect and age of the dog. Young dogs occasionally recover spontaneously. In others, corticosteroid therapy may help. In severe cases, the prognosis is poor, even with decompressive and stabilizing surgery. A possible hereditary malformation of C_{2-3} vertebrae occurs in Basset Hounds <6 mo old, in which spinal cord compression can be successfully relieved by surgery.

Dermoid sinuses are neural tube defects that result from incomplete separation of skin and neural tube during embryonic development. The condition is more common in Rhodesian Ridgeback dogs, but other breeds may be affected. Clinical signs can occur when the sinus communicates with the dura mater and becomes infected. Clinical signs reflect the location of the lesion and may range from weakness to paralysis of one or more limbs. Surgical excision is the treatment of choice.

Hemivertebra is a congenital malformation characterized by the presence of one or more wedge-shaped vertebral bodies, which results in dorsal deviation (kyphosis) of the thoracic vertebral column (usually between T_7 and T_9). It is most common in English Bulldogs, French Bulldogs, and Boston Terriers, usually <1 yr old. Signs of paraparesis or paraplegia and urinary incontinence result from progressive kyphosis that produces spinal cord compression, or may follow vertebral luxation or fracture at the site of the hemivertebra secondary to a sudden jump, fall, or trauma. Diagnosis is by radiography and/or myelography. Prognosis for clinically affected animals is guarded. Spinal cord compression requires surgical decompression and stabilization. **Block vertebra** and **butterfly vertebra** are vertebral malformations that rarely are clinically significant.

Hereditary canine spinal muscular atrophy is a dominantly inherited disease of Brittanys that is characterized by degeneration of selected brain-stem and ventral horn neurons of the spinal cord. The disease has been clinically defined as: 1) early onset—progressive tetraparesis from 1-4 mo of age; 2) intermediate onset—signs of paresis begin at 4-6 mo of age, and progressive tetraparesis occurs over the next 2 yr; and 3) late onset—a slowly progressive disease with animals surviving well into adulthood. Animals walk in a waddling fashion, and muscle atrophy becomes prominent in the proximal muscles of the hindlimbs and paraspinal muscles. Severely affected animals remain in lateral recumbency and are unable to raise their heads. Diagnosis is based on clinical signs and breed. There is no treatment.

Hereditary myelopathy of Afghan Hounds is an autosomal recessive disease that is characterized by cavitation and necrosis of the spinal cord from the low-cervical to mid-lumbar segments. Clinical signs occur between 3 and 8 mo of age. Hindlimb paresis progresses over several weeks to paraplegia and forelimb paresis. Spinal reflexes may be depressed and breathing may be abdominal. Death frequently results from respiratory failure. Hindlimbs may be analgesic. Radiography is normal. Diagnosis is based on age, breed, and clinical signs. There is no treatment and prognosis is poor.

Lumbosacral stenosis can be congenital or acquired in dogs. Synonyms are "cauda equina syndrome" and "spondylolisthesis". It is characterized by shortening of the pedicles, thickening and sclerotic apposition of the lamina and articular processes, infolding and hypertrophy of the ligamentum flavum, and sclerotic articular facets that bulge into the vertebral canal. The congenital form is common in small breeds, whereas the acquired form is more common in large breeds, particularly German Shepherd Dogs. In both forms, signs are usually noted in mature to middle-aged dogs. Clinical signs include pain on palpation of the lumbosacral area, difficulty in rising, paraparesis, fecal and urinary incontinence, and hypotonia of the anal sphincter. Diagnosis is by radiography. Prognosis is usually favorable with surgical decompression.

Multiple cartilaginous exostosis is a benign proliferative disease of cartilage and bone that may involve vertebrae. It occurs infrequently in dogs and cats. There is no breed or sex predisposition, although a familial tendency is probable. The condition is related to abnormal differentiation of cartilage cells, which gives rise to exostoses. Neurological signs relate to spinal cord compression secondary to vertebral exostoses, which are most common in thoracic and lumbar regions. Signs, which appear before 1 yr of age, progress from hindlimb paresis to paralysis. Diagnosis is based on radiography and myelography. Surgical excision is necessary if there is evidence of spinal cord compression. Prognosis is guarded.

Occipital dysplasia refers to an abnormally large foramen magnum, the result of a developmental defect of the occipital bone. It is common in small or toy breeds of dogs, usually seen as an incidental finding on skull radiographs. It is not believed to cause clinical signs.

Sacrococcygeal dysgenesis (caudal dysgenesis) is an inherited malformation of the lower spine and spinal cord in tailless Manx cats, in which sacral and coccygeal vertebrae may be absent. Sometimes, it is associated with spina bifida, meningomyelocele, syringomyelia, spinal cord dysplasia, and absence of the cauda equina. Affected cats have a plantigrade posture, hopping gait, hindlimb paresis or paraplegia, fecal and urinary incontinence, and perineal analgesia. Diagnosis is based on age, breed, and radiographic findings. Prognosis is guarded. Animals may steadily deteriorate after birth, or a partial disability may not progress. Mildly affected cats may attain longevity if fecal and urinary incontinence are managed. There is no treatment.

Spina bifida is a congenital malformation that results from failure of fusion of the halves of the dorsal spinous processes, with or without protrusion of the spinal cord (myelocele) or its membranes (meningocele), or both (myelomeningocele). The condition has been reported commonly in dogs and cats. The incidence is high in young English Bulldogs. It occurs most commonly in the lumbar region. Clinical signs, which may be seen as soon as the animal begins to walk, include hindlimb weakness, fecal and urinary incontinence, perineal analgesia, and flaccid anal sphincter. The site of the bony defect may be marked by dimpling of the overlying skin, streaming of coat, or palpable cavitation in the dorsal spinous process. Diagnosis is confirmed by radiography or myelography. Prognosis is guarded to poor, and treatment usually is not attempted.

Spinal dysplasia is an inherited disorder of the spinal cord of dogs that often is characterized by hydromyelia, duplication of the central canal, syringomyelia, and gray matter ectopias. It is most common in Weimaraners, in which it is inherited. Clinical signs usually appear by 4-6 wk of age and include symmetrical "bunny-hopping" hindlimb gait, wide-based stance and overextension of hindlimbs, and depressed proprioception. Less constant signs include scoliosis, abnormal hair streams on the dorsal neck region, and koilosternia. Clinical signs neither progress nor retrogress. Animals may lead a normal life. There is no treatment.

DEGENERATIVE DISEASES

Arachnoid cysts are reported sporadically in dogs 1-10 yr old. They are characterized as dorsal midline cavitational lesions that result in spinal cord compression. To date, cervical and thoracolumbar clinical syndromes have been observed. Diagnosis is by myelography. Surgical excision is the treatment of choice.

Degenerative myelopathy is a disease that occurs most frequently in German Shepherd Dogs, and occasionally in other large breed dogs, usually >5 yr old. An inherited basis is suspected. A similar disease also occurs in cats. The cause and pathogenesis are unknown, but it is unrelated to disk disease, spondylosis deformans, or dural ossification. Pathologically, the most severe changes are found in the thoracic spinal cord and are characterized by degeneration of white matter. Onset of the disease is insidious. Clinical signs include progressive weakness and knuckling of the paws of the hindlimbs, and truncal ataxia. Some dogs have a depressed patellar reflex. Diagnosis is based on age, breed, and clinical syndrome. Ancillary tests, including radiography and myelography, are normal. Prognosis is poor. There is no treatment.

Dural ossification is a degenerative disorder of dogs that is characterized by formation of bone plaques on the inner surface of the dura mater. These plaques occur in >60% of dogs >2 yr old and are most common in cervical and lumbar areas. Usually, it is a subclinical condition detected radiographically as an incidental finding. It is characterized by thin, radiopaque, linear shadows within the vertebral canal, especially at the site of the intervertebral foramina.

Fibrocartilaginous emboli, believed to arise from intervertebral disks, result in ischemic necrosis of the spinal cord. This disorder occurs in immature and adult dogs, especially in larger breeds, and in cats. Infarction at the level of the cervicothoracic or lumbosacral spinal cord results in necrosis of ventral horn cells. Onset of clinical signs is typically hyperacute (within seconds) with paralysis of one or more limbs, depending on the level of spinal cord infarction. The most common sites are lumbar and cervical cord segments. Affected animals typically do not manifest pain. Diagnosis is based on the rapidity of onset and normal radiographic/myelographic findings. CSF may have increased protein and an elevated neutrophil count within a few hours of clinical onset. Prognosis is guarded. Any improvement should be apparent in 1-2 wk. Corticosteroids (1 mg/kg, b.i.d.) may be beneficial in reducing cord edema during the first 24 hr. In large animals, fibrocartilaginous emboli have been reported in low cervical segments of horses, and in low lumbar segments of a sow.

Intervertebral disk disease is one of the most common neurological disorders; it results from extrusion of disk material into the vertebral canal with subsequent compression of the spinal cord or spinal nerve roots, or both. It occurs in all breeds of dogs, but is most common in Dachshunds, Beagles, Pekingese, Poodles, Cocker Spaniels, Shih Tzus, and Welsh Corgis, 3-7 yr old. The risk of occurrence in Dachshunds is said to be 10-12 times greater than for all other breeds combined. It is rare in cats. The most common sites are the thoracolumbar (85%) and cervical (15%) regions. Clinical signs of cervical disk disease are characterized by cervical pain and spasms, and tetraparesis. Tetraplegia is unusual. Dogs may assume a posture with the nose held close to the ground and the back arched. With thoracolumbar disease, they may be paretic or paraplegic. Forelimb function is normal. Digital pressure on the spine at the level of disk extrusion usually elicits pain. Animals are usually incontinent. As a result of an acute, explosive extrusion of material from a thoracolumbar disk, progressive diffuse myelomalacia may develop in a small percentage of dogs, and cause ascending and descending paralysis. As this condition progresses, hind- and forelimbs may become flaccid. Affected animals die from respiratory paralysis as the condition spreads to involve the cervical cord. Definitive diagnosis of disk disease is based on radiographic, and sometimes myelographic, studies. Prognosis depends on the acuteness of disk extrusion, degree of cord injury, and duration of cord compression. In general: 1) Animals that are paretic or paralyzed, but still maintain bladder control and have normal pain sensation, have a favorable prognosis following medical or surgical treatment. 2) Animals that are paralyzed, incontinent, and show reduced pain sensation have a guarded prognosis following surgical decompression. 3) Animals that are paralyzed, incontinent, and have loss of pain sensation have an extremely poor prognosis regardless of treatment.

Treatment may be conservative (cage rest, restricted activity, analgesics and corticosteroids [eg, prednisolone, 0.5 mg/kg, b.i.d. for 72 hr and then discontinued] for severe pain) for animals manifesting their first episodes of pain, or pain with mild weakness. Following conservative management, >50% of dogs have recurrences. Surgical treatment is indicated by recurrent or progressive clinical signs, signs unresponsive to medical management, paresis or paralysis with deep pain, and paralysis and absence of deep pain of <24 hr duration. In such animals, prompt surgical decompression and removal of extruded material are required. Rehabilitation includes bladder management (manual emptying, catheterization), prevention of decubital ulcers, swimming exercises, and standing/walking exercises. Potential complications of high dosage and/or long-term glucocorticoid therapy are GI hemorrhage and ulceration, colonic perforation, and pancreatitis. These complications can be averted by minimizing use of steroids and by prophylactic use of GI protectants, antacids, and H_2 antagonists.

Spondylosis deformans is a degenerative disorder of the spinal column characterized by vertebral osteophytes at intervertebral spaces, which result in the formation of spurs or complete bony bridges; in dogs, this occurs most often at T_{9-10} and L_7-S_1 sites. Flat-coated Retrievers, Irish Setters, Bloodhounds, and Rhodesian Ridgebacks may have a high risk of spondylosis deformans. The incidence in dogs and cats increases with age. It is usually a subclinical disorder; however, localized pain may occur in association with fracture of bony spurs or bridges. Osteophytic projections into the spinal canal with compression of the spinal cord are rare. Diagnosis is based on radiographic findings. Treatment is symptomatic and prognosis is good.

INFLAMMATORY AND INFECTIOUS DISEASES

Distemper (qv, p 408) remains one of the most common CNS disorders in dogs. Spinal cord signs range from weakness to paralysis in one or more limbs. Rhythmic flexor spasms are often present in limb flexor muscles, abdominal muscles, and the cervical musculature. These contractions are not necessarily associated with limb paresis or paralysis and usually persist during sleep. Multifocal encephalomyelitis occurs in mature dogs (4-8 yr old) and is characterized by a chronic course (eg, 6-12 mo). The incidence of this disease is low and it is not preceded by, nor coincident with, the systemic signs that are seen in younger dogs. Initial signs include weakness of the hindlimbs, generalized incoordination, and occasional falling, which frequently progress to tetraplegia. Generalized seizures or personality changes are not features of this disease. Some animals have facial paralysis, head tilt, and nystagmus, and head tremors may be seen.

Rabies (qv, p 619) is caused by a rhabdovirus that reaches the CNS via the peripheral nerves. The virus has high tropism for neurons, and Negri bodies may be seen in large neurons such as the pyramidal cells in the hippocampus. It produces multifocal polioencephalomyelitis with mononuclear perivascular infiltrates. There is a predilection for localization in the brain stem and spinal cord. Spinal cord signs may be characterized by ascending spinal paresis or flaccid paralysis. Spinal reflexes are often depressed. Differential diagnosis of flaccid paralysis includes tick paralysis, botulism, and coonhound paralysis. A paralytic syndrome (similar to that seen in rabies itself) may occur in dogs and cats after vaccination with modified live vaccine, but clinical recovery may occur within 1-2 mo.

Among farm animals, cattle are affected most commonly. Spinal cord signs include knuckling of the hind fetlocks, sagging and swaying of the hindquarters while walking, decreased sensation (most evident over the hindquarters), tail flaccidity, paralysis of the anus, tenesmus, recumbency, and death usually within 48 hr. Similar signs are seen in sheep. Horses and pigs usually show excitement and mania. Terminal paralysis and death ensue as in cattle.

Bacterial meningitis is uncommon in dogs and cats. Bacterial invasion of the CNS usually results in both encephalomyelitis and meningitis. *See* MENINGITIS AND ENCEPHALITIS, p 608.

Epidural abscessation may result from blood-borne septic emboli. Clinical signs usually reflect a focal space-occupying lesion. An epidural abscess rarely invades the dura and breaks into the spinal cord. Accordingly, CSF is usually normal. Diagnosis may require contrast radiography. Prognosis is poor, especially if the mass is large and encapsulated, which makes it refractory to antibiotic therapy.

Feline infectious peritonitis (FIP, qv, p 415) is an immunopathological disease caused by a coronavirus. It is characterized by granulomatous lesions, principally of the ependymal surfaces, choroid plexuses, and leptomeninges, although spinal cord lesions are not infrequent. The clinical and neurological vagaries of FIP include hindlimb paresis, generalized ataxia, dorsal thoracolumbar hyperesthesia, nystagmus, anisocoria, seizures, tetraparesis, and intention tremors. Prognosis for clinically affected cats is poor since most animals die within a few weeks or months. There is no satisfactory treatment.

Feline polioencephalomyelitis is a chronic, slowly progressive disease. Pathological findings consist of perivascular cuffing and severe neuronal degeneration and loss, especially in the thoracic spinal cord, together with diffuse degeneration (demyelination and axonal necrosis) of spinal cord white matter. The cause is unknown, although pathological changes suggest a viral infection. It may be associated with panleukopenia or feline leukemia virus. Clinical signs include paraparesis, ataxia, and sometimes hypermetria. An intention tremor of the head may be seen. Affected cats are usually mentally alert. Cranial nerve function is normal except for depressed direct and consensual pupillary reflexes in some animals. Postural reactions and segmental spinal reflexes may be depressed in affected limbs. Occasionally, a localized area of apparent hyperesthesia is evident. Some cats have leukopenia, myeloid hyperplasia, and nonregenerative anemia. Prognosis is guarded to poor. There is no definitive treatment.

Granulomatous meningoencephalomyelitis (GME) is a worldwide, sporadic, nonsuppurative, inflammatory disease of dogs, most commonly young and middle-aged small breeds, especially Poodles. Lesions may be disseminated or focal. The disseminated form has been previously described as "inflammatory reticulosis", the focal form as "neoplastic reticulosis". Lesions are confined to the CNS and are characterized by dense aggregations of mesenchymal cells arranged in a whorling perivascular pattern. Perivascular cuffs are usually composed of histiocytic elements and lymphoplasmic cell infiltrates.

Neutrophils and multinucleate giant cells are sometimes present in small numbers. In the disseminated form, lesions are distributed widely throughout the CNS, especially in the white matter of the cerebrum, lower brain stem, cerebellum, and cervical spinal cord. Coalescence of granulomatous lesions from many adjacent blood vessels can produce a true mass, which represents the focal form of GME. In some dogs, an ocular form occurs in which granulomatous cuffs initially involve the optic nerves, optic disk, or retina. The cause is unknown; however, it is possible that GME represents an altered host response to an infectious agent.

Disseminated and focal forms of GME are more common than the ocular form. The onset of disseminated GME usually is acute with a progressive course over 1-8 wk. In ~25% of affected dogs, deterioration is rapid, and leads to death within 1 wk. In >50% of cases, the clinical course is 2-6 wk. The focal form of GME has a more insidious onset and can progress slowly over 3-6 mo. The ocular form tends to have a sudden onset and may remain static or be progressive.

Clinical signs are variable and reflect lesion localization. Signs of focal GME usually are suggestive of a single, space-occupying lesion, eg, cerebral, pontomedullary, vestibular syndromes, etc. Signs of disseminated GME usually reflect a multifocal syndrome. Common signs include incoordination, ataxia and falling, cervical pain, head tilt, nystagmus, facial/trigeminal paralysis, circling, seizures, and depression. Occasionally, fever accompanies the clinical signs. Cervical cord signs (cervical pain and rigidity) need to be differentiated from cervical disk disease and meningitis. CSF is abnormal, with increased protein levels (100-1000+ mg/dL) and mononuclear pleocytosis (50-800 WBC/mL).

Although temporary remission may follow corticosteroid therapy, the prognosis is poor. Cessation of corticosteroid therapy is followed by rapid and dramatic deterioration.

Mycotic diseases sporadically produce a granulomatous meningoencephalomyelitis in dogs and cats. Mycotic infectious agents, including *Cryptococcus neoformans, Blastomyces dermatitidis, Histoplasma capsulatum,* and *Coccidioides immitis,* may reach the CNS hematogenously (eg, from primary infection in the respiratory tract) or by direct spread from an adjacent infection, eg, from the nasal chambers, tooth alveoli and sinuses, outer ear, eustachian tube, middle or inner ear, petrous temporal bone, or basilar bone. While the incidence of CNS involvement in mycotic diseases is low, *C neoformans* may be more likely to be incriminated than the other organisms, and especially in immunosuppressed animals. Cats contract the disease more frequently than dogs. A striking feature of mycotic lesions, particularly in the CNS, is the relative lack of a tissue response by the host. Neurological signs vary according to location and severity of the lesion, and may reflect either a focal mass or a diffuse multifocal disease process; they may include seizures, depression, disorientation, circling, ataxia, falling, hindlimb paresis, paraplegia, anisocoria, pupillary dilatation, and blindness. Organisms may be demonstrated in CSF, which is pleocytic (mononuclear and polymorphonuclear) and has an elevated protein level. Eosinophils may be present with cryptococcosis. Prognosis for animals with CNS involvement is poor, even when treated with amphotericin B.

Other mycotic agents have been reported to produce CNS infection sporadically. These include *Cladosporium trichoides, Paecilomyces* sp, *Flavobacterium meningosepticum, Geotrichum candidum,* and *Aspergillus* sp. *(See also* FUNGAL INFECTIONS, p 340 *et seq.*)

Osteomyelitis-diskospondylitis is an inflammatory disorder of the vertebral bodies and associated intervertebral disks. It is common in young to middle-aged adult dogs, usually of the larger breeds. Affected male dogs outnumber females by ~2:1. It also has been reported in cats. The condition may occur following iatrogenic trauma of the vertebral column (eg, disk curettage), foreign body migration, or more commonly, blood-borne septic emboli. The source of infection is not established in most cases. Possible sites include the urinary tract, skin, gingiva, and heart valves. Organisms identified include *Staphylococcus aureus, Brucella canis, Nocardia* sp, *Streptococcus canis,* and *Corynebacterium diphtheroides.* Clinical signs, which reflect the degree of bone proliferation and compression of spinal cord, range from subtle spinal hyperesthesia to severe paresis/paralysis. Affected animals may be depressed, anorectic, and febrile. Diagnosis is based on radiographic findings that may include bone lysis (especially in vertebral areas adjacent to the disk), proliferation, vertebral sclerosis, shortening of vertebral bodies, and narrowed intervertebral disk spaces. Common sites of diskospondylitis are thoracic and lumbar vertebrae and the lumbosacral joint. Prognosis is usually favorable with long-term antibiotic therapy. Cephalosporins have been effective in most instances in small animals. Vertebral curettage may expedite clinical resolution. In animals with spinal cord compression, decompression and vertebral immobilization are required.

Polyradiculoneuritis (coonhound paralysis) is a common neurological disease of dogs, occurring especially in raccoon-hunting breeds. However, a similar condition can occur in dogs with no possible exposure to raccoons. The pathogenesis is unclear. A raccoon bite has been a consistent antecedent, and an immunological basis is suspected.

Clinical signs frequently appear 7-11 days after an encounter with a raccoon. Onset is marked by weakness and hindlimb hyporeflexia. Paralysis progresses rapidly, and results in a flaccid symmetrical tetraplegia. In severely affected animals, there may be facial weakness and dyspnea. The paralysis lasts for several weeks to 2-3 mo. Prognosis is usually favorable with symptomatic treatment and supportive nursing care; however, protection from future attacks is short-lived or nonexistent. Death may occur from respiratory paralysis.

Tetanus (qv, p 330) is caused by *Clostridium tetani* toxin. Susceptibility varies markedly among species. Clinical signs usually are observed within 5-10 days of infection. These include stiffness of gait with extensor rigidity in all limbs, dyspnea, spasms of the masticatory and pharyngeal muscles (which result in trismus and dysphagia), elevation of the tail, and contracted facial muscles (which give a sneering expression). Animals are hypersensitive to external stimuli. In severe disease, the animal may be recumbent and opisthotonic, and death may result from respiratory failure. Diagnosis is usually based on the characteristic clinical signs. Prognosis is usually favorable with treatment.

Toxoplasmosis (qv, p 365) in the CNS may cause perivascular cuffing; meningeal infiltration by lymphocytes, plasma cells, and histiocytes; necrosis; and neuronal degeneration. Signs in dogs and cats may include hyperexcitability, depression, tremors, paresis, paralysis, and seizures. In dogs <3-4 mo old, rigid hyperextension and gross atrophy of the hindlimb muscles may be present. Recently, *Toxoplasma* polymyositis/polyneuropathy has been reported in adult dogs with rapidly progressive tetraplegia. CSF is usually abnormal (elevated protein and a mixed monocytic-polymorphonuclear pleocytosis). Diagnosis is confirmed by serology and histopathology. Prognosis is poor in animals with CNS involvement; however, some dogs may respond favorably to clindamycin.

Vertebral osteomyelitis, diskospondylitis, or **epidural abscessation** also occurs commonly in large animals following foreign body migration, or more commonly, from blood-borne septic emboli secondary to navel ill in foals and calves; metritis, mastitis, and traumatic peritonitis in cattle; tail docking in lambs; and tail biting in pigs. Clinical signs are referable to the site of the lesion. Bacteria often involved include *Corynebacterium pyogenes* and *Fusobacterium necrophorum* in cattle; *C pseudotuberculosis* in sheep and goats; *Salmonella* spp, *Actinobacillus equuli*, or *Rhodococcus equi* in foals; *Mycobacterium tuberculosis* or *Brucella abortus* in adult horses; and *B suis* in boars.

NEOPLASIA

Neoplasia of the spinal cord in dogs and cats occurs less frequently than neoplasia of the brain (*see* p 610).

NUTRITIONAL DISORDERS

Nutritional disorders that affect the spinal column or cord are unusual in dogs and cats, except for hypervitaminosis A and hound ataxia. **Hypervitaminosis A** occurs in cats fed predominantly a liver diet. The excess vitamin A results in bone hypertrophy and ankylosing spondylosis of cervical vertebrae. Clinical signs include "kangaroo-sitting", inability to move head or neck, pain, and forelimb lameness. Diagnosis is by radiography. Prognosis is guarded to poor. Alterations in diet may stop further progression but do not significantly reduce the spondylosis that is present. **Hound ataxia** has been seen in Foxhounds, Harriers, and Beagles in the UK. Affected animals are usually 2-6 yr old. Severe wallerian degeneration occurs in the spinal cord. Clinical signs are hindlimb weakness, ataxia, and hypermetria. The clinical course may be 6-18 mo. Forelimb function remains normal. A dietary factor is implicated, since the disorder is associated with feeding paunch (the forestomachs of cattle and sheep).

SPINAL TRAUMA

This is common in dogs and cats, and is most often caused by automobiles, falls, fighting, or gunshot wounds. Spinal fractures and luxations may occur at any level but are most frequent at the thoracolumbar junction, an area that comprises movable and stable spinal segments. Resulting spinal cord injuries are characterized pathologically by variable degrees of ischemia, edema, hemorrhagic necrosis, neuronal degeneration, demyelination, and focal malacia. Localized edema may result in pronounced cord swelling. Clinical signs usually occur immediately, and generally are nonprogressive. Severe thoracolumbar spinal cord injury in dogs results in paraplegia and forelimb hyperextension (**Schiff-Sherrington syndrome**). Radiography usually demonstrates obvious fractures and luxations of the vertebral column. Prompt surgical decompression, vertebral reduction, and stabilization are indicated, often combined with corticosteroid therapy (dexamethasone 2-4 mg/kg, IV, repeated at 6- to 8-hr intervals). Prognosis is guarded. Animals that have lost pain sensation have a poor prognosis.

Horses are prone to sacral fractures following falls while backing off transportation carriers, and to cervical trauma associated with violent jerks to the halter. Cattle are susceptible to lumbosacral fractures from breeding accidents. Vertebrae of calves, foals, or pigs with calcium deficiency may be more susceptible to fracture.

STORAGE DISEASES

See also CONGENITAL AND INHERITED DISEASES OF THE CNS, p 578.

These are rare diseases that result from genetically determined enzyme defects with subsequent accumulation and storage of substrates within the nervous system.

Progressive paraparesis may be seen in animals 3-4 mo old. Signs of cerebral disease also are frequent. Storage diseases that produce spinal cord signs in dogs and cats include gangliosidosis, sphingomyelinosis, globoid cell leukodystrophy, and mucopolysaccharidosis. These diseases usually are fatal. There is no treatment.

CATTLE

Vertebral osteomyelitis, rabies, axonal degeneration in Brown Swiss cattle, and spinal trauma are mentioned in the discussion centered on dogs and cats (*see* above). Additional diseases of the spinal column and cord in cattle are discussed below.

Bovine atlantoaxial subluxation and secondary cervical cord compression occur in Holstein and crossbred cattle between birth and 1 yr old. The dens is small or absent, and the axis is displaced ventral to the atlas. The atlas and occipital bones may be fused. Clinical signs range from paresis to tetraplegia.

Focal symmetrical poliomyelomalacia has been reported in a purebred herd of Ayrshire cattle. Affected animals are normal at birth but become weak in the hindquarters and paraplegic by 10 days; forelimbs also can be involved. There is muscle atrophy, and spinal reflexes are reduced or absent. Lesions appear to be restricted to the spinal cord and are characterized by necrosis (malacia) of ventral horns with accumulation of lipid-laden phagocytes. Areas of the cord that appear to be susceptible are the cervical and lumbar enlargements. The cause of the condition is unknown, but genetic factors may play a role. There is no treatment.

Infectious bovine rhinotracheitis meningoencephalomyelitis is caused by a herpesvirus that infrequently causes CNS disease in cattle. Signs include depression, ataxia, blindness, seizures, and death (*see also* p 730.) Sometimes only ataxia and paralysis of the hindlimbs may be seen. There is no treatment.

Myelin disorder of Charolais cattle is a progressive neurological disorder characterized by multiple plaques of abnormal myelin throughout the white matter of the CNS. It has been recognized in the UK, France, and Canada. It is believed to be familial, and the pathological process suggests a basic derangement of the oligodendrocyte—the myelin-forming cell. Clinical signs are first recognized at 8-24 mo of age, and progress from slight hindlimb ataxia to recumbency over 1-2 yr.

Myelodysplasia is a congenital malformation due to defective development of any part of the spinal cord before complete differentiation of gray and white matter. It may occur sporadically in calves born with moderate to severe hindlimb ataxia and nonprogressive spastic paresis. Some animals manifest a "bunny-hopping" hindlimb gait. Vertebral column malformation may accompany the spinal cord anomaly.

Neoplasia of the spinal column and cord in cattle usually is restricted to the epidural space. Lymphosarcoma (qv, p 391) often may develop in the epidural space at any spinal level and produce clinical signs referable to the compressed area of the spinal cord. An elevated antibody titer to bovine leukemia virus may suggest this disease, which may involve other body systems. Neurofibroma of spinal nerves occasionally may extend into the vertebral canal and compress the spinal cord.

Organophosphate toxicity in cattle may cause paraparesis. (*See* HALOXON INTOXICATION IN SHEEP, below, and the discussion in the TOX section, p 1669.)

Parasitic migration: (*See also* p 603.) Larvae of *Hypoderma bovis*, the cattle grub (qv, p 781), migrate through the epidural space of cattle, usually during July through October; they have been implicated in the development of paraparesis and hindlimb ataxia in cattle treated for the grub infestations. Other parasitic disorders that may cause similar clinical signs in cattle include *Coenurus cerebralis* and *Parelaphostrongylus tenuis*.

Progressive degenerative myeloencephalopathy (weaver syndrome, qv, p 581) is inherited in Brown Swiss cattle.

Spastic paresis (bovine spastic paralysis, Elso heel) is common in young dairy and beef calves (1-9 mo old), especially among those nursing. (*See also* p 502.) The cause is not clear; however, a neurotransmitter imbalance is suspected. Signs are characterized by progressive, tremulous spasms of the gastrocnemius and digital flexor muscles. Signs are usually asymmetric, initially with the affected limb swinging as a pendulum when the animal moves. Tenotomy of the gastrocnemius tendon, and tibial neurectomy have proved beneficial in some cases.

Spastic syndrome (qv, p 503), also known as periodic spasticity, crampy, or stretches, is most common in Holstein and Guernsey cattle, usually 3-7 yr old. The syndrome is believed to be inherited. Signs are characterized by episodes of hindlimb extension that last from a few seconds to several minutes; they usually occur when the animal is rising to stand, or on sudden movement after a period of relaxation. There are extensor muscle spasms of the back and hindquarters with caudal extension of the hindlimbs and difficulty in moving. Signs are usually permanent and may progress to the point that an animal cannot stand. Lesions are inconsistent and there is no treatment. The prognosis is guarded.

Tremors may occur in cattle feeding on various grasses, including paspalum, canary grass, and rye grass. Animals often manifest a spastic hindlimb gait, accompanied by falling and trembling. In cases of paspalum staggers (qv, p 1689), a mycotoxin produced by the fungus *Claviceps paspali* has been identified as the tremorgenic agent.

HORSES

Spinal trauma, rabies, tetanus, vertebral osteomyelitis, and fibrocartilaginous emboli are mentioned in the discussions centered on dogs and cats (*see* above). Additional diseases of the spinal column and cord in horses are discussed below.

Acute hematomyelia has been reported in some horses following anesthesia in dorsal recumbency. There is widespread hemorrhage in the gray matter of the spinal cord. Affected animals remain paralyzed.

Atlanto-occipital malformation is believed to be a recessively inherited disorder in Arabian foals of both sexes. Usually, the atlas is fused with the occipital bone, and the axis is displaced ventrally. The foramen of the atlas may be markedly reduced. Signs of cranial cervical cord compression may be present at birth and cause severe paresis and ataxia or tetraparesis and an inability to stand. An audible click at the site of malformation may occur when the head is moved. Diagnosis is confirmed by radiography. Prognosis is guarded to poor. A similar disorder has been described in Holstein cattle.

Cervical malformation-malarticulation or **cervical stenotic myelopathy** (also known as **wobbler syndrome** and **equine sensory ataxia**) is a vertebral disorder affecting horses, usually within the first 1-2 yr of life. The incidence is highest in Thoroughbreds; signs are frequently noted in weanlings or yearlings. Stenosis of the vertebral canal, most frequently involving C_{5-7}, results in a focal compressive myelopathy. Demyelination is the main pathological change. Pronounced hindlimb ataxia and paresis are manifest. Forelimbs may be spastic. Diagnosis is by radiography and/or myelography. Prognosis is guarded. Surgical arthrodesis may be successful.

Degenerative encephalomyelopathy is a slowly progressive neurological disorder of young horses and zebras (from birth to 3 yr). The cause is unknown; however, it is possible that genetic predisposition and nutritional factors (eg, vitamin E) both contribute to the disease. Lesions consist of bilaterally symmetrical areas of diffuse myelin degeneration, extending from cervical to lumbar cord segments, especially in lateral and ventral funiculi. Neuroaxonal dystrophy, nerve cell loss and pigment accumulation may also be seen in the spinal cord. Clinical signs usually begin in the hindlimbs and progress to involve the forelimbs. Signs are characterized by symmetrical ataxia, spasticity, and paresis. Clinically, it may not be possible to differentiate this disease from cervical stenotic myelopathy. All ancillary tests are normal. A similar syndrome has been described in Morgan horses and in captive Mongolian Przewalski wild horses.

Equine herpesvirus 1 myeloencephalopathy is a disease of horses (adults and foals) that occasionally accompanies outbreaks of abortion and respiratory disease (*see also* p 734). The neurological syndrome may occur as the only illness on the farm. All ages of animals may be affected, but mares 3-9 mo pregnant are particularly susceptible. Lesions in the spinal cord are characterized by multiple necrotic foci in both gray and white matter that result from vasculitis accompanied by thombosis. The vasculitis may have an immunological basis. Neurological signs are of sudden onset, usually symmetrical, and vary in severity from mild ataxia to paralysis. Paresis may progress to tetraplegia, but usually there is little change in signs after 2-3 days.

Equine infectious anemia (qv, p 27) occasionally produces neurologic disease in horses. Neuropathologic changes include nonsuppurative granulomatous ependymitis, choroid plexitis, meningitis, and encephalomyelitis. Clinical signs include hindlimb ataxia. Signs may begin acutely or insidiously. Diagnosis is by positive agar gel immunodiffusion test. Affected animals should be euthanized because the disease is contagious.

Lathyrism is a chronic, progressive neurological disorder that occurs in horses that ingest sorghums or Sudan grass. (*See also* p 1730.) The disease is believed to be associated with hydrocyanic acid found in these plants. Degenerative changes occur in nerve roots of lumbar, sacral, and coccygeal segments. Clinical signs include dribbling of urine, urine scalds over the buttocks and thighs, flaccid anal sphincter, and paraparesis. Cystitis and hematuria develop secondary to neurogenic urine retention. Horses should not be permitted to graze sorghum pastures while the plants are rapidly growing or are stunted by drought. There is no definitive treatment. Prognosis is guarded to poor.

Neoplasia of the spinal column and cord is rare in horses.

Neuritis of the cauda equina is a slowly progressive idiopathic polyradiculoneuritis that affects adult horses of either sex and of any breed. Pathological findings include granulomatous inflammation and axonal degeneration in nerves of the cauda equina. The cause has not been determined; however, allergic and immune-mediated factors are thought to play a role. Clinical signs are characterized by fecal and urinary incontinence, flaccid anal sphincter, inability to retract the penis, perineal analgesia, tail paralysis, and gluteal muscle atrophy. Mild ataxia and paresis may be observed. Some animals show signs of cranial nerve involvement (eg, facial paralysis and vestibular disease). The CSF is abnormal, with increased protein levels (100-300 mg/dL) and mononuclear/polymorphonuclear pleocytosis (>100 cells/mL). Differential diagnoses include sacral trauma, herpesvirus 1 myeloencephalopathy, rabies, lathyrism, protozoal myelitis, and spinal nematodiasis. Prognosis is poor. There is no treatment.

Parasitic migration through the spinal cord of horses (qv, p 603) may occur with several organisms, including *Micronema deletrix, Strongylus vulgaris, Setaria* sp, and *Hypoderma lineatum*. Clinical signs usually are sudden in onset, and depend on the location of the lesion. Examination of the CSF may reveal increased numbers of eosinophils and RBC. Prognosis is guarded. There is no definitive therapy.

Protozoal myelitis is a common sporadic disease of young adults (it has not been observed in foals) that produces a necrotizing, nonsuppurative encephalomyelitis. The disease was once thought to be restricted to horses living east of the Rocky Mountains in the USA; however, reports have come from Canada and California. In a few horses, protozoa are abundant, mostly contained within macrophages. The identity and life cycle of the parasite have not been determined (it closely resembles *Sarcocystis* sp). The disease most frequently affects young adult Thoroughbred and Standardbred horses. It does not appear to be contagious. Clinical signs are variable and depend on the location of the lesion; they range from paraparesis to tetraparesis. The neurological signs often are asymmetric. Involvement of cervical or lumbar intumescence results in muscle atrophy, hypotonia, and hyporeflexia. The clinical course may be moderately progressive. CSF may be abnormal, with increased protein levels and pleocytosis. The prognosis is guarded to poor, even with anti-folic-acid drugs (trimethoprim-sulfadiazine at 15 mg/kg, PO b.i.d., and pyrimethamine at 0.25 mg/kg, PO once daily, for up to 2 mo). Diagnosis is based on age and clinical and historical data. It is not unusual for only a single animal on a farm to be affected.

Synovial cysts associated with articular facets of lower cervical vertebrae may cause spinal cord compression in horses, 1-6 yr old. The cause is unknown. Diagnosis is by radiography and myelography.

PIGS

Vertebral osteomyelitis, rabies, and fibrocartilaginous emboli are mentioned in the discussions centered on dogs and cats (*see* above). Additional diseases of the spinal column and cord in pigs are discussed below.

Arsanilic acid poisoning (qv, p 1640) is due to overdosing feed rations with organic arsenical growth promoters. Clinical signs may progress from hindlimb ataxia and paresis to tetraparesis. Affected animals may assume a "dog-sitting" position. Early withdrawal of the arsenical may result in complete spontaneous recovery. Lesions in the nervous system are characterized by myelin and axonal degeneration in peripheral nerves, optic nerves, and optic tracts.

Nutritional myelopathy is a rapidly progressive spinal cord disorder of young pigs 3½-6 mo old. Clinical signs progress from hindlimb paresis to paraplegia. The spinal cord lesion consists of bilaterally symmetrical demyelination. The cause is copper deficiency. Similar clinical signs may occur in 3-mo-old pigs fed only milk, as a result of vitamin A deficiency. (*See also* pp 19 and 1252.)

Parasitic migration through the spinal cord by the kidney worm of pigs, *Stephanurus dentatus* (qv, p 876), can produce hindlimb ataxia and paresis. Onset of clinical signs is acute. Individual pigs are usually affected. The condition occurs especially in the southeastern USA. No effective treatment is known. Similar signs can be caused by *Ascaris suum*.

Poliomyelomalacia, which occurs in pigs 6 wk to 5 mo old, may occur as an outbreak in several pigs. Clinical signs occur suddenly and include ataxia, paresis and loss of reflexes of all 4 limbs, and inability to stand. Degenerative lesions are present in spinal cord gray matter, especially in cervical and lumbar segments. The disease may be related to nicotinamide deficiency.

Porcine enteroviral encephalomyelitis (qv, p 616), also termed Teschen disease, Talfan disease, porcine poliomyelitis, and benign enzootic paresis, is most common in suckling, weaned, or early grower pigs. This enterovirus has a predilection for spinal cord gray matter, in which it causes neuronal degeneration, glial cell proliferation, and vascular congestion and cuffing. Clinical signs include ascending, progressive hindlimb ataxia and weakness, with generalized muscle tremors. In severe cases, nystagmus, convulsions, opisthotonus, and coma may be seen. There is no treatment, but some animals may survive, often with permanent neurological deficits.

Porcine hemagglutinating encephalomyelitis (qv, p 388) is caused by a neurotropic coronavirus that sporadically affects young pigs. Clinical signs may include muscle tremors, ataxia, hyperesthesia, and coma. Morbidity and mortality can approach 100%.

SHEEP AND GOATS

Rabies and vertebral osteomyelitis are mentioned in the discussions centered on dogs and cats (*see* above). Additional diseases of the spinal column and cord in sheep and goats are discussed below.

Acute necrotizing myelopathy has recently been described in lambs 8-12 wk old. Clinical signs ranged from hindlimb ataxia to paralysis. Changes in the cord included focal necrosis in the white matter and axonal swelling. The cause of the lesion was believed to be fibrocartilaginous emboli.

Haloxon intoxication may occur following exposure to the organophosphate anthelmintic haloxon. Clinical signs usually occur 3-5 wk following exposure, and are characterized by symmetrical spastic paraparesis and ataxia. The hindlimbs are partially flexed, often with the dorsal surface of the hoof on the ground. Signs usually remain static. Swollen axons may be present in the lumbar spinal cord and sciatic nerve. Prognosis is guarded. (*See also* ORGANOPHOSPHATE TOXICITY, p 1669.)

Parasitic migration through the spinal cord of sheep is often associated with the meningeal worm of white-tailed deer, *Parelaphostrongylus tenuis* (qv, p 605). Signs are abrupt in onset and may range from hindlimb paresis and ataxia to tetraparesis. Affected animals have a history of grazing on pastures that have been exposed to white-tailed deer. The clinical course is variable, often related to the migratory route of the parasite. Signs may progress, remain static, or improve. CSF is often abnormal, with increased protein levels and a mononuclear and eosinophilic pleocytosis. Treatment with diethylcarbamazine, levamisole, or thiabendazole is recommended. The prognosis is guarded. Similar signs can be caused by larvae of *Setaria digitata* and *Coenurus cerebralis* (gid larvae) that localize in the spinal cord.

Swayback, also known as enzootic ataxia (qv, p 1197), is a neurological disease in sheep and goats that is associated with copper deficiency of the dam and offspring. Lesions in the spinal cord and brain stem are characterized by myelin deficiency and neuronal degeneration. Initial signs, seen from birth to 3-4 mo of age, include hindlimb ataxia and paresis that usually progresses to tetraparesis. Treatment with copper sulfate may result in marked improvement.

Viral leukoencephalomyelitis of goats is a highly infectious disease caused by a nononcogenic retrovirus of the lentivirus group. Lesions are characterized by diffuse demyelination and disseminated inflammatory granulomatous changes that often involve gray matter. This virus may also produce an interstitial pneumonitis and arthritis (qv, p 393). It is shed in colostrum and milk of infected does. Signs are usually seen in kids <5 mo old. The incidence of subclinical infection is high. Signs range from paraparesis to tetraparesis and progress rapidly over a 2-wk period. The CSF is abnormal with elevated protein levels and usually mononuclear pleocytosis. Prognosis is poor; there is no treatment.

DYSAUTONOMIA

CANINE DYSAUTONOMIA

Five cases have been documented from the UK and Norway. In addition, 3 cases have occurred in dogs of North American origin. Dysuria and loss of the anal reflex were seen in each dog along with other signs typical of feline dysautonomia. Histopathologic features were similar to those seen in the equine and feline disorders (*see* below).

EQUINE GRASS SICKNESS

A fatal dysautonomia of unknown etiology that causes marked reduction in GI motility due to widespread degeneration in the autonomic nervous system. It is seen throughout the UK and northern Europe and has been reported once in Australia. Outbreaks of disease in Colombia are disputed. Japanese literature contains reports of possibly related conditions.

Grass sickness occurs at any age after weaning and at any time of the year, but the peak incidence is in spring in 2- to 7-yr-old horses. All Equidae appear susceptible. Although associated with recently acquired horses kept solely at grass, the condition has been seen in housed stock. Peracute, acute, subacute, and chronic forms are recognized. Death occurs within 24 hr, 4 days, and 21 days, respectively, for the first 3 forms. Horses with the chronic form may live for weeks or months; some survive. Experimental evidence suggests the presence of a neurotoxic factor in the plasma of affected horses.

Clinical Findings: The condition is afebrile and characterized by profound depression, restlessness, elevated pulse rate, ileus, and colic. Patchy sweating and fine muscular fasciculations occur over the shoulders and flanks. In contrast to feline dysautonomia, pupillary light reflexes and tear production are normal, and plasma catecholamines are elevated. Affected horses may show dysphagia and esophageal dysfunction. This causes drooling of saliva, nasal reflux of stomach contents, and difficulty passing a stomach tube. On rectal palpation, the mucosa is dry and tacky, and feces are scant and hard. Distended loops of small intestine and an impacted large colon are features of acute cases. In more chronic cases, cachexia occurs, and penile prolapse may be seen in geldings. Secondary ileal impaction and large colon displacement may be confusing features.

Lesions: In acute cases, fluid distention of the stomach and small intestine is marked, and the large intestine is impacted. Gastric rupture may occur. The GI tract is usually empty in chronic cases. All forms may show splenomegaly, linear ulceration of the esophagus, and hard, dry, dark fecal balls. The pathognomonic lesion is a chromatolytic-type neuronal degeneration throughout the entire autonomic nervous system, and, to a lesser degree, in certain nonautonomic neurons.

Diagnosis: No reliable *in vivo* diagnostic test is available, but demonstration of esophageal dysfunction or elevated plasma catecholamine levels may be helpful. Confirmation of the diagnosis depends on histopathological examination of autonomic ganglia. Obstruction of the small intestine must be ruled out in the more acute forms. In the chronic form, other possible causes of emaciation should be considered.

Treatment: Symptomatic fluid therapy with gastric decompression may provide temporary relief, but the prognosis is bleak. Early euthanasia is desirable on humane grounds. Stabling of at-risk stock for part of the day is recommended.

FELINE DYSAUTONOMIA
(Key-Gaskell syndrome)

A newly recognized condition of domestic cats, characterized by dysfunction of the autonomic nervous system. All breeds and ages appear susceptible. The first cases were reported in early 1982 in the UK. The condition became widespread, but later declined in incidence and severity. Cases have also been recorded in other European countries, New Zealand, Dubai, and Venezuela. In the last few years, 5 cases have been reported in the USA, and 2 of these did not originate in the UK. The disorder appears to affect neuronal protein biosynthesis, but the etiology is unknown. Equine grass sickness and canine dysautonomia (*see* above) appear to be similar to the feline syndrome.

Clinical Findings and Lesions: Affected cats initially exhibit depression and anorexia, often with signs of upper respiratory tract infection or transient diarrhea. More definite features appear over several days, although in some cats the onset may be peracute, while others may show vague malaise for a few weeks. The most common signs are dilated nonresponsive pupils, a dry rhinarium, reduced lacrimal secretion, esophageal dysfunction with regurgitation, and constipation. Other features include dry oral mucosa, prolapse of the membrana nictitans, bradycardia, anisocoria, and urinary or fecal incontinence. These signs reflect both sympathetic and parasympathetic dysfunction. Nonautonomic signs include occasional hindleg proprioceptive deficits and anal areflexia. When measured, plasma catecholamines or their urinary metabolites have been decreased.

Necropsy may show megaesophagus, dry mucous membranes, an atonic bladder, and accumulation of feces in the rectum. In recently ill cats, a chromatolytic-type degeneration is seen in neurons throughout the autonomic nervous system, and to a lesser degree in certain nonautonomic neurons. Chronic cases show a marked depletion of neurons in autonomic ganglia.

Diagnosis: Definitive diagnosis depends on histopathological examination of autonomic ganglia. Clinical confirmation may be aided by contrast radiography of the esophagus and demonstration of reduced lacrimal secretion (<5 mm/min when measured by the Schirmer tear test). Pilocarpine (0.1%) applied to the cornea of an affected cat causes profound miosis within 10-15 min, but has no effect on a normal cat. Feline leukemia virus (FeLV) infection (qv, p 39) can cause both anisocoria and urinary incontinence, but cats with feline dysautonomia usually show other distinct clinical signs and are FeLV-negative.

Treatment: The aim of therapy is to stabilize the cat and to maintain adequate fluid balance. Total parenteral nutrition can be useful in the initial stages, but should be followed by nasogastric or gastrostomy tube feeding. When regurgitation resolves, maintaining an upright position after oral intake is helpful. Multivitamin preparations, warmth, manual evacuation of the bladder, and attention to grooming and cleanliness are beneficial. Artificial tears and intermittent steam vaporization may help relieve the dryness of the eyes and mucous membranes. Liquid paraffin is helpful for constipation but may increase the risk of aspiration. Danthron (5-15 mg, PO, daily) is a safer alternative. Parasympathomimetics such as bethancol (2.5 mg, b.i.d. or t.i.d.) may be of use; however, their effect is crude, and overdosage may require treatment with atropine. Metoclopramide (0.1 mg/kg, IV, or 0.3 mg/kg, t.i.d., subcut.) has been used to improve gastric emptying. A small portion of cats has recovered, while others may be able to cope with residual autonomic deficits. However, such improvements often require up to 1 yr, and the prognosis remains poor.

EDEMA DISEASE
(*Escherichia coli* enterotoxemia)

An acute, highly fatal, neurological disorder of pigs that usually occurs 5 days to 2 wk (commonly 10 days) after weaning. It is found worldwide. Early weaning seems to have reduced the frequency but may have shortened the incubation period.

Etiology and Pathogenesis: The disease depends on colonization of the small intestine by toxigenic strains of *E coli* that produce the edema disease principle (EDP). The EDP-producing strains of *E coli* are few, the most important being 0138:k81, 0139:k82, and 0141:k85. Most, if not all, produce hemolysin. Absorbed EDP causes arterial degeneration and increased vascular permeability, which result in edema formation at various locations, and focal malacia in the brain stem.

Clinical Findings and Lesions: Sudden death of well-fleshed, rapidly growing pigs may be the first sign. Characteristic neurological signs include apparent blindness, ataxia, and circling, which progress to lateral recumbency with opisthotonos and paddling. Edema of the eyelids or forehead may be evident, and edema of the larnyx may cause a characteristic squeaky voice. Death usually follows in several hours to 2 days. Some pigs that recover have persistent neurological signs of varying severity. Morbidity in an affected group may be ~15%. Neither diarrhea nor constipation are consistent findings.

Although some pigs show no gross lesions, others, particularly those recently dead, have obvious subcut. edema, notably of the head region. The submucosa of the greater curvature of the stomach and the mesentery of the spiral colon may show gelatinous edema. The serous cavities may contain excessive clear amber fluid.

Diagnosis: Carcasses are usually in good condition, and the clinical signs and necropsy findings in recently dead animals are distinctive. Isolation of nearly pure cultures of specific hemolytic *E coli* serotypes from the small intestine of acute cases is helpful. Confirmation is based on histological demonstration of focal malacia in the brain stem, or typical degenerative vascular lesions at various locations. Differential diagnoses include *Streptococcus suis* meningitis, pseudorabies, *Salmonella* septicemia, and salt and organic arsenical poisoning.

Treatment and Control: Affected pigs rarely recover. Preventive measures should aim at reducing the buildup of heavy *E coli* populations in the gut. Minimizing dietary change at weaning and increasing the amount of fiber in the diet may be helpful. Prophylactic feeding of, or in-water medication with, antibiotics to inhibit *E coli* multiplication over the risk period is beneficial in some cases. Some growth promoters (qv, p 1532) may also help. Stimulation of local intestinal immunity to *E coli* colonizing factors before weaning may reduce the severity of the outbreak.

Because there is evidence of a hereditary predisposition, genetic selection may be the future means of prevention.

EQUINE ENCEPHALOMYELITIS
(Equine encephalitis)

The equine encephalitides are clinically similar syndromes characterized by signs of CNS dysfunction and moderate to high mortality. Various arboviruses classically have been regarded as the causal agents, but toxoplasma-like protozoal agents also have been incriminated (*see also* pp 365 and 594). The causal arboviruses are transmitted by mosquitoes or ticks and infect a variety of other vertebrate hosts, including man, in which they occasionally cause serious infections. In general, these arboviruses utilize a rodent- or bird-mosquito cycle.

Etiology and Epidemiology: Horses may be infected by alphaviruses, family Togaviridae, or flaviviruses, family Flaviviridae. The alphaviruses most closely associated with equine encephalitis include Eastern (EEE), Western (WEE), and Venezuelan (VEE) equine encephalomyelitis viruses. Other alphaviruses associated virologically or serologically with clinical encephalitis in Equidae are Aura, Ross River, Semliki Forest, and Una viruses, but these agents appear to be only infrequently or incidentally associated with disease, and do not occur in North America. Recent evidence suggests that the Snow Shoe Hare virus of the California antigenic group of the Bunyaviridae family also is capable of causing clinical disease. EEE virus occurs in the eastern USA and Canada, where disease in horse and man has been associated with outbreaks in domestic fowl, especially in the Atlantic and Gulf coastal states. Virus activity also occurs in Mexico, Panama, Central and South America, and the Caribbean islands. While the geographic distribution of WEE virus appears to encompass virtually all of the Americas, clinical WEE has been reported only in the western USA and Canada, Mexico, and South America. VEE variants that are nonpathogenic for horses occur in sylvatic cycles in the Florida Everglades, western USA, Mexico, Panama, Central and South America, and some Caribbean islands. Periodic outbreaks of VEE have occurred naturally in equids and man in northern South America for ≥60 yr. VEE virus pathogenic for horses has been isolated only during equine epidemics, and its origin has no known association with sylvatic VEE virus.

EEE and WEE have been associated with naturally occurring and experimentally induced neurological diseases in calves. EEE also has been associated with clinical and experimental disease in pigs.

In terms of public health, Japanese encephalitis virus is the most important flavivirus that causes equine encephalitis; it is recognized throughout the Far East. Mortality in horses is low (<5%), and it causes abortion in pigs without other clinical signs. In addition, other flaviviruses isolated from encephalitic Equidae are those of louping ill, and Murray Valley and West Nile encephalitides. Other flaviviruses, eg, the cause of St. Louis encephalitis, can produce serological evidence of infection in horses without clinical disease.

Maindrain virus, a *Culicoides*-transmitted bunyavirus found in the western USA has been isolated from encephalitic horses. **Borna disease**, a meningoencephalitis of horses, is not of arbovirus etiology nor is it known to be a zoonosis. It is caused by an unclassified RNA virus that is isolated in Europe during the spring and early summer. Clinically, the disease resembles the alphavirus encephalitides.

EEE, WEE, and sylvatic VEE viruses are transmitted to mammalian hosts by biting insects, principally mosquitoes of the genera *Aedes, Anopheles, Culex* (including the subgenus *Melanoconion*), and *Culiseta*. The sylvatic VEE virus of the western USA can be isolated from swallowbugs (*Oeciacus vicarius*). Equine-virulent VEE virus has been isolated from many genera of mosquitoes and other hematophagous insects, but only during epidemics. Mosquitoes are biologic vectors, ie, the viruses replicate in the body and persist in the salivary glands. Transmission by arthropods other than mosquitoes probably is unimportant. Wild birds serve as principal reservoirs of EEE and WEE viruses. Forest rodents and wild birds are the most probable reservoirs of sylvatic VEE virus; the reservoir or origin of epidemic VEE virus is unknown. Reservoir hosts tend to develop viremia with blood titers adequate to infect mosquitoes, and actively contribute to the cycle of virus survival. Horses are considered dead-end hosts for WEE and sylvatic VEE viruses; horses with EEE infections may develop viremia adequate to infect vectors, but probably do not contribute significantly to viral transmission or persistence. Horses are the most important amplifiers of epidemic VEE virus and produce a viremia adequate to infect mosquitoes. Unlike EEE and WEE viruses, epidemic VEE virus may, on occasion, also spread between horses and to man by contact or aerosol. These diseases occur more frequently in pastured than in stabled horses and are concentrated in areas having the appropriate combination of susceptible reservoir hosts and mosquitoes. Epidemics of EEE and WEE tend to occur in mid to late summer.

Clinical Findings and Lesions: The sequential clinical and serological events following infection with EEE, WEE, or VEE viruses are similar. Clinical signs of an encephalomyelitis occur ~5 days after infection, and most deaths occur 2-3 days later. Signs include fever, impaired vision, irregular gait, wandering, reduced reflexes, circling, incoordination, yawning, grinding of teeth, drowsiness, pendulous lower lip, inability to swallow, photophobia, head-pressing, inability to rise, paralysis, occasional convulsions, and death. Mildly affected animals may slowly recover in a few weeks but may have residual brain damage (dullness, dementia), and have been referred to as "dummies". Mortality in horses is 20-50% from WEE, 50-90% from EEE, and 50-75% from VEE.

No characteristic gross lesions are observed. Microscopically, hemorrhage and degeneration of neurons occur in the cerebral cortex, thalamus, hypothalamus, and other parts of the CNS. Gliosis, perivascular cuffing with polymorphonuclear (especially in EEE and VEE) and mononuclear (especially in WEE) cells, microglial proliferation, and meningitis may be present. Inclusion bodies are present only in Borna disease.

Diagnosis: A presumptive diagnosis can be based on clinical signs, history, and seasonal occurrence and is aided by knowledge of endemic areas or known epidemic activity of a virus type. Demonstration of typical histological lesions of a viral encephalitis strengthens the diagnosis. Diagnostic specificity results from virus neutralization, hemagglutination inhibition, or complement fixation tests during acute and convalescent phases. Because of the high mortality and rapid death of affected horses, it is difficult to obtain paired sera. Neutralizing antibody is detectable about the time signs of CNS dysfunction occur, and viremia terminates 4-5 days after infection. A 4-fold rise in titer between acute and convalescent sera or a very high titer (particularly of IgM) in an unvaccinated animal is considered positive. Diagnosis is confirmed by isolation and identification of virus from brain or blood. With VEE and EEE viruses, isolation is difficult after CNS signs are seen; blood should be collected for virus isolation from clinically normal, febrile horses in the same or an adjacent pasture.

Differential diagnoses include hepatoencephalopathy, rabies, protozoal myeloencephalitis, verminous encephalitis, and leukoencephalomalacia.

Prophylaxis and Treatment: No specific antiviral agents are available. Supportive treatment (anti-inflammatory drugs, control of seizures) and intensive nursing care aid in the recovery of mild cases. Since the encephalitides are spread primarily by mosquitoes, control measures should be directed against them; these include drainage and insecticide treatment of mosquito-breeding areas, and application of insect repellent to horses. Removing horses from pasture and stabling them is advisable during outbreaks.

Inactivated chick embryo or cell-culture origin vaccines are now used almost exclusively and generally are considered effective. Monovalent, bivalent (EEE and WEE), and trivalent (EEE, WEE, VEE) vaccines are available. Monovalent VEE vaccine is an attenuated virus of cell-culture origin and should not be used in pregnant mares or young foals. The attenuated VEE vaccine has been largely replaced by a formalinized product incorporated into a trivalent vaccine with EEE and WEE antigens. Vaccine should be given ~1 mo before the mosquito season and, where the mosquito season is long, should be repeated within the year. In areas where mosquito activity is year round, foals should be vaccinated when 3, 4, and 6 mo old, and annually thereafter.

FACIAL PARALYSIS

Facial paralysis is common in dogs, especially Cocker Spaniels. The facial nerve is particularly vulnerable to damage in its course through the middle ear, and where its branches divide more superficially into the auriculopalpebral and dorsal and ventral buccal nerves that innervate the muscles of facial expression (ears, eyelids, cheeks, lips, nose). Most facial palsies in dogs occur as an idiopathic syndrome that can be transient or permanent. The second most common cause is inflammatory damage from chronic otitis media/interna. The nerve is also susceptible to surgical trauma during external ear canal ablation and bulla osteotomy procedures. Neoplasms and inflammatory processes in the cerebellomedullary angle, or within the rostral medulla where the facial nucleus is located, can cause facial paralysis. Cats are predisposed to squamous cell carcinomas and adenocarcinomas of the ear canal, which often spread to affect the facial nerve. Facial paralysis in dogs is occasionally associated with hypothyroidism, pituitary tumors, myasthenia gravis, and polyneuritis due to coonhound paralysis or idiopathic syndromes. Horses commonly suffer facial paralysis from pressure trauma to the superficial branches of the facial nerve as it crosses the mandible. Protozoal encephalomyelitis and cauda equina neuritis are central and peripheral nerve diseases, respectively, in which unilateral or bilateral facial paralysis may be seen (*see* [both] p 594). Acute head trauma that causes fractures and hemorrhage into the petrous temporal bone, otitis media/interna, guttural pouch infections, and osteoproliferative lesions at the articulation of the stylohyoid bone with the temporal bone are other causes of facial paralysis in horses. Listeriosis in ruminants is a classical cause of facial paralysis. Brain abscesses, basilar fibrinous meningitis, and suppurative otitis/media are also common causes in pigs, cattle, sheep, and goats.

Clinical Findings: Total unilateral facial paralysis is characterized by absence of the palpebral reflex, immobility of the ear, and flaccidity of the muscles of facial expression with subsequent deviation of the nose toward the normal side. In dogs and cats, the palpebral fissure is opened widely, and in response to the menace test, the animal may retract the globe and flick the third eyelid instead of blinking. Signs of exposure keratitis may occur in conjunction with facial paralysis because of inability to blink or flick the third eyelid to lubricate the cornea. Keratitis sicca also may occur if there is a loss of tear production because of damage to the parasympathetic fibers in the facial nerve. In cattle and horses, the upper eyelid may droop slightly because of atony of the frontalis muscle. Injury to the auriculopalpebral branch as it crosses the zygomatic arch causes paralysis of only the ear and eyelid.

Depending on the site and degree of injury to the nerve, facial paralysis may be total or partial. For instance, in horses, damage to the buccal branches may result only in slight deviation of the nose and flaccidity of the lips, but drooling liquids and impaction of food in the buccal area of the mouth on the affected side is common. Also, the nostril may fail to dilate actively on inspiration. The site of underlying nerve damage frequently can be localized to the inner ear by the concomitant vestibular disturbance manifest by head tilt, nystagmus, and incoordination in the acute stages. Lesions of the brain stem near the facial nucleus may cause bilateral signs. In addition, limb weakness and other cranial nerve deficits can help differentiate a central disease from peripheral lesions.

Treatment: Depending on severity of the lesion, traumatic and idiopathic neuritis of the facial nerve often resolve spontaneously within a few weeks. Corticosteroids are useful to control acute edema and inflammation, particularly if used within 24 hr of injury. Infections must be treated vigorously with the appropriate drug. Protective ophthalmic ointments or surgical closure are necessary to prevent keratitis when the eyelids are paralyzed. With impairment of the prehensile lips of horses, wet bulky mashes and deep water containers are needed for supportive care. In performance horses, surgery and prostheses have been used to prevent total collapse of the nostril during vigorous exercise.

HAEMOPHILOSIS
(Thromboembolic meningoencephalitis, TEME)

An acute, septicemic disease primarily of the CNS and eye, characterized by fever, severe depression, weakness, ataxia, blindness, coma, and death within 1 hr to several days. It is most common in feedlot cattle but occurs in calves, dairy cattle, and pastured animals. Although found worldwide, most reports are from North America.

Etiology: The causal organism, *Haemophilus somnus*, is a small, gram-negative, nonmotile, nonsporeforming, pleomorphic coccobacillus that grows best in an atmosphere that contains carbon dioxide and on media that contains calf's blood and yeast extract (thiamine pyrophosphate). It appears to be identical to *Histophilus ovis*, an etiologic agent of ovine septicemia, mastitis, and epididymitis. Different strains are recognized, and there appears to be some relationship between strain and disease.

Transmission, Epidemiology, and Pathogenesis: The mechanisms by which *H somnus* is spread are unknown. The organism is often found in the respiratory tract, which suggests an aerosol route. It is also excreted with urine and in discharges from the vagina and prepuce of infected animals. It can survive for >70 days in blood or nasal mucus, but only for brief periods in urine. Infection from contaminated pasture has been suggested. The infection rate in healthy cattle is high, but morbidity in infected groups generally is 2-5%, occasionally approaching 30%. Mortality in untreated clinically affected animals often is 100%. In addition to the CNS, the GI, auditory, musculoskeletal, ocular, renal, reproductive, and respiratory systems may be affected. *Haemophilus somnus* also causes pneumonia (resembling shipping fever), vaginitis, mastitis, and rarely abortion.

The pathogenesis is poorly understood, although the organism circulates in the bloodstream and causes disseminated intravascular coagulation, severe vasculitis, hemorrhage, thrombosis, and infarction in many organs.

Clinical Findings: A temperature as high as 108°F (42°C) is often the first sign of disease, but this falls rapidly to normal or subnormal. Other characteristic signs are stiffness, knuckling at the fetlocks, severe depression, ataxia, paralysis, and opisthotonos, followed by coma and death within 1-48 hr. Affected animals may be blind, and retinal hemorrhages with gray foci of retinal necrosis are sometimes observed. Other signs, such as hypersensitivity, convulsions, excitement, nystagmus, and circling, occur inconsistently. Occasionally, animals are found dead without signs of illness.

Other manifestations of *H somnus* infection have also been reported: vaginitis, endometritis, infertility, abortion, possibly repeat breeding, laryngitis, tracheitis, suppurative pneumonia, myocarditis, otitis, mastitis, and arthritis.

A marked change in the total and differential WBC count is common; leukopenia and neutropenia occur in severe cases, and neutrophilia in less severe cases. In the CSF, the total cell count is markedly elevated and neutrophils predominate. In acute stages of the disease, the organism can be cultured from blood, synovial fluid, CSF, and brain.

Lesions: Red to brown foci of necrosis with hemorrhage are frequently present on the surface and cut sections of the brain and spinal cord. A fibrinous meningitis may extend over the brain and spinal cord in some animals, and the CSF may be cloudy. Necrosis and ulceration are often present in the larynx and trachea. An interstitial pneumonia may accompany the septicemic form, or an acute fibrinous bronchopneumonia may occur separately. Serofibrinous polyarthritis is common. Hemorrhagic necrosis may be observed in the myocardium, skeletal muscle, serosa of esophagus and intestine, bladder, and renal cortex. Fibrinous pericarditis, and peritonitis are sometimes observed. Retinal hemorrhage and thrombosis are common in the septicemic form. Corneal opacity may be present occasionally but probably is associated with trauma.

Diagnosis: Presumptive diagnosis is based on clinical signs, examination of CSF, and gross necropsy findings, and confirmed by histopathology and isolation of the bacterium. Differential diagnoses include polioencephalomalacia, hypovitaminosis A, lead poisoning, rabies, pseudorabies, and listerial meningoencephalitis.

Treatment and Control: Clinically affected animals should be segregated and treated immediately with penicillin and streptomycin, or oxytetracycline. Treatment is most effective in the early stages of the disease. Once the animal becomes recumbent, the prognosis is poor. Cattle in feedlots in which the disease has been confirmed should be checked every few hours; constant surveillance and immediate treatment of new cases is recommended. Tetracyclines (eg, oxytetracycline or chlortetracycline) in the feed or water may reduce the incidence of new cases. Most outbreaks run their course in 2-3 wk. The organism usually is resistant to lincomycin, neomycin, and sulfonamides. Mortality may be controlled by management practices that emphasize growth rather than finishing.

Bacterins may reduce morbidity and mortality and decrease the number of animals requiring treatment. Susceptibility to the development of clinical disease does not appear to be related to serum antibody titers.

CNS DISEASES CAUSED BY HELMINTHS AND INSECT LARVAE

A number of parasites are associated with the CNS of vertebrates and may be categorized as follows:

1) **Immature stages of parasites of carnivorous animals:** These parasites may induce behavioral changes in the intermediate host that are likely to enhance transmission to the final host by means of predation, eg, *Taenia multiceps*.

2) **Neurotropic species:** These require conditions provided by the CNS for their growth and development, eg, *Parelaphostrongylus (Pneumostrongylus) tenuis*. In the normal host, these parasites usually do not cause neurological signs; in others, they may be highly pathogenic.

3) **Anomalous or accidental parasites:** A number of parasites that migrate in host tissues may reach the CNS, although it is not a requirement for their development and transmission; in some instances, the biological significance of the association with the CNS is unclear, eg, certain ascaridoid nematodes.

Pathogenicity in the CNS usually can be attributed to trauma caused by activities of the parasites; the role of excretory and secretory products is unknown. Also, the parasites may transport pathogenic microorganisms to the CNS. Clinical signs are related to the location of the parasite and the lesions produced by it. Signs include motor weakness, ataxia, head deviation, circling, depression, blindness, drooping of the ear or eyelid, loss of fear or herding instinct, paresis, and paralysis.

Successful chemotherapeutic treatment for cerebrospinal nematodiasis has been reported with diethylcarbamazine at 100 mg/kg (45 mg/lb). Ivermectin and organophosphates kill bots and at least some nematodes, but killing parasites in the CNS may provoke additional tissue damage. Surgery may be useful as for coenurosis (*see* below).

CESTODES

Coenurosis: *Taenia (Multiceps) multiceps* is an intestinal parasite of canids (especially dogs, foxes, and jackals) and man. Intermediate hosts are sheep, goats, deer, antelope, chamois, rabbits, hares, horses, and less commonly, cattle, which acquire the eggs while grazing. Some oncospheres reach the brain and develop by endogenous budding of scolices into coenuri (once known as *Coenurus cerebralis*). Initial invasion and development of the oncospheres may be responsible for acute suppurative meningoencephalitis. The fully developed coenurus may be 5-6 cm in diameter and cause increased intracranial pressure resulting in ataxia, hypermetria, blindness, head deviation, stumbling, and paralysis. The clinical condition is commonly known as **gid, staggers,** or **sturdy.** In sheep, palpation of the skull caudal to the horn buds may reveal rarefaction; surgery to remove the cyst, including its wall, has a reasonable chance of success and is justified in valuable animals. Dogs associated with livestock should not be fed the heads of infected animals and should be dewormed regularly (especially if associated with sheep).

Cysticercosis: *Taenia solium* is an intestinal parasite of man. Cysticerci (once regarded as a separate parasite, *Cysticercus cellulosae*) occur in the flesh of pigs, but may also develop in man and dogs that have ingested the eggs. They commonly localize on the meninges and in the neuropil, and may cause convulsions and locomotor disturbances.

Hydatid Disease: *Echinococcus granulosus* is a parasite of dogs and wolves. Eggs are ingested by wild and domestic herbivores, eg, sheep, cattle, and moose. After hatching, the oncospheres invade the circulatory system and lodge in various parts of the body (especially the liver and lungs). They develop into large cysts (hydatids) that bud scolices endogenously. Hydatids have been reported rarely in the CNS of animals, including man, in which they produce signs and symptoms similar to those of brain tumors.

A related species, a parasite of foxes, *E multilocularis*, utilizes the vole as an intermediate host. It has rarely been found in the brain of man, in which the hydatid does not produce scolices. As mentioned above (coenurosis), surgery may be useful.

INSECT LARVAE

Myiasis involving the CNS is rather uncommon except for *Hypoderma bovis*, the larvae of which develop normally in burrows between the periosteum and dura mater before migrating to the subcut. tissue of the back. Neurological signs, varying from a transient, stiff, unsteady gait to paralysis, may occur in cattle given systemic insecticides when the larvae are present in the spinal canal (qv, p 781).

The larvae of *Oestrus ovis*, the nasal fly of sheep (qv, p 758), are reported rarely to penetrate the ethmoid bone and reach the forebrain. However, it is possible that other factors facilitate entry of larvae into the brain.

Bots and warbles may move rapidly after death of the host and migrate into tissues far from the site of origin.

NEMATODES

ASCARIDOIDEA

Ascaridosis: The larvae of some ascaridoid roundworms, including *Baylisascaris* spp of mustelids and *Toxocara canis* of dogs and cats, may invade the CNS as well as other tissues of groundhogs, rabbits, mice, beavers, dogs, and man. These larvae apparently are transported to various tissues by the arterial system. Larvae are active in the neuropil, and those of some species, eg, *B columnaris*, grow markedly and may cause considerable tissue trauma; such infections generally result in neurological disturbances that can lead to death of the host.

FILARIOIDEA

Elaeophorosis: *Elaeophora schneideri*, a filarioid of the carotid arteries and its branches, is common in mule deer, mainly in western North America. Microfilariae accumulate in the skin of the cephalic region; vectors are species of Tabanidae. Larvae develop in arteries of the leptomeninges before migrating to the carotids. The infection is usually silent in the normal host.

In wapiti, moose, white-tailed deer, sheep, and goats, worms in the arteries cause degeneration and loss of the endothelium and accumulation of plasma proteins and platelets on and within the intima. Thrombosis, infiltration of the intima, and fibroblastic proliferation may eventually result in occlusion and ischemic necrosis in associated tissues. Necrotic lesions associated with occlusion of leptomeningeal arteries are commonly found in the brain. Neurological signs include blindness, head deviation, circling, ataxia, and paralysis (*see also* p 807).

Setariosis: *Setaria digitata* is a common parasite of the peritoneal cavity of cattle in Asia. Microfilariae occur in the blood; mosquitoes are vectors. The infection appears to be silent in cattle. Details of development in the normal host are unknown. In horses, goats, and sheep, the developing worms invade the CNS and cause motor weakness, ataxia, lameness, drooping eyelids or ears, and lumbar paralysis. Lesions include focal malacia and degeneration of axis cylinders and myelin sheaths in all regions of the CNS.

Setaria cervi (Elaphostrongylus altaica) has been reported on the leptomeninges of deer in Europe and the USSR, often in association with *E cervi. Setaria* sp has also been found in the CNS of horses. The significance of these findings is unclear.

METASTRONGYLOIDEA

Angiostrongylosis: *Angiostrongylus cantonensis* is a common parasite of the pulmonary arteries of rats in southeast Asia and the south Pacific. Terrestrial gastropods are intermediate hosts. Larvae invade the cerebrum and develop in the neural parenchyma for ~2 wk, then enter the subarachnoid space and migrate, ~1 mo after infection, to the pulmonary arteries via the venous system. Neurological signs are rare in rats with light to moderate infections, but circling, cannibalism, and paraplegia may occur in heavy infections. The infection is frequently acquired by people in endemic regions.

Elaphostrongylosis: *Elaphostrongylus cervi (rangiferi)* is a common parasite of the skeletal musculature of *Rangifer* and *Cervus* spp (reindeer and elk) in the holarctic region, especially in Eurasia. It is transmitted through terrestrial gastropods and apparently develops for a time in the CNS before migrating to the muscles. Infection is associated with lumbar weakness, paresis, and paralysis in cervids in Sweden and the USSR.

Parelaphostrongylosis: *Parelaphostrongylus (Pneumostrongylus) tenuis* occurs normally in the subdural space and venous sinuses of the cranium of white-tailed deer in eastern North America. Eggs reach the lungs in the venous blood and develop into larvae, which pass up the bronchial tree and out with the feces. Infective larvae, acquired from terrestrial snails and slugs as the deer feeds, invade the spinal cord and develop for several weeks in the dorsal horns of the gray matter; then, they invade and mature in the subdural space. The infection is usually silent in white-tailed deer.

Parelaphostrongylus tenuis invades the CNS of various wild cervids (moose, caribou, wapiti), antelope, sheep, and goats. In these hosts, the parasite produces considerable trauma in the CNS. In addition, eggs deposited in the neural tissue provoke marked inflammatory reactions. Clinical signs consist of lumbar weakness, ataxia, lameness, stiffness, circling, abnormal positions of the head, and paralysis. Signs vary in onset and character in individual animals. Temporary remissions are typical.

Skrjabingylosis: *Skrjabingylus nasicola* and *S chitwoodorum* are found in the frontal sinuses of mustelids, especially mink, weasels, and skunks. Larvae acquired from terrestrial gastropods develop for a time in the gut wall, then migrate to the spinal cord. They move on the leptomeninges to the brain and along the olfactory tracts to the cribriform plate, which they penetrate to reach the frontal sinuses. Their presence on the leptomeninges elicits hemorrhage and leptomeningitis. In heavy infections, some subadult worms may invade the brain and cause neurological signs, including paralysis.

RHABDITOIDEA

Micronemosis: *Micronema deletrix* is a free-living cephalobid nematode that has been reported in the CNS of horses and man. It may reach the CNS through wounds contaminated by soil that contains the worms or through abscesses in the oral and nasal cavities. The nematode multiplies in the CNS and is highly destructive of neural tissues, which causes death of the host.

MISCELLANEOUS NEMATODES

Migrating larvae of strongyles (perhaps *Strongylus vulgaris*) have been reported in the CNS of horses; the phenomenon appears to be rare. Larvae of *Stephanurus dentatus* rarely invade the CNS of pigs; larvae of *Trichinella spiralis* have been found in the brain in fatal human cases of trichinosis and in experimentally infected mice. Larvae of *Baylisascaris procyonis*, a roundworm of the small intestine of raccoons, infect many intermediate hosts (including man), and not uncommonly migrate through the CNS, with serious consequences. Larvae of *Strongyloides stercoralis* may invade the brain of experimentally infected animals. *Splendidofilaria quiscali* is found in the cerebral hemispheres of grackles (*Quiscalus quiscula*) and other birds in North America. *Paronchocerca helicina* occurs in the cranial leptomeninges of the snake bird (*Anhinga anhinga*) in the USA. *Gnathostoma spinigerum* has been found rarely in the CNS of man. *Eustrongylides ignotus* implanted subcut. in rats and chickens migrated to the CNS and caused death of the host. (*See also* p 203.)

TREMATODES

Paragonimiasis: Adults and eggs of *Paragonimus westermani* have been reported rarely in the CNS of man, dogs, cats, and rats (the latter 3 were experimentally induced).

Schistosomiasis: Schistosomes normally deposit their eggs in small vessels of the gut and urinary bladder, from which they pass into the feces or urine. Some eggs, however, get into the general circulation and may reach the CNS where they become encapsulated. This condition has been noted in man and a few other animals.

Troglotremiasis: *Troglotrema acutum* inhabits the frontal and ethmoidal sinuses of foxes and mustelids in Europe. Rarefying osteitis may result and allow microorganisms to reach the cranial cavity, leading to fatal purulent meningitis.

LOUPING ILL
(Ovine encephalomyelitis)

An acute, tick-transmitted viral disease of the CNS, ranging from inapparent to fatal. It primarily affects sheep, but cattle, goats, horses, dogs, pigs, red deer, roe deer, red grouse, and man also can be infected; man can be infected by tick bites or exposure to infected tissues or instruments. The disease occurs throughout the rough hill grazings of the British Isles wherever the vector tick, *Ixodes ricinus*, is prevalent. Diseases of sheep indistinguishable from louping ill and caused by viruses that have not been differentiated from louping-ill virus have occurred recently in Norway, Spain, Turkey, and Bulgaria, which suggests that the condition may not be restricted to the British Isles.

Etiology and Transmission: The virus belongs to the Flaviviridae family and is part of an antigenically closely related complex of viruses distributed throughout the northern temperate regions known as the tick-borne encephalitides, which are primarily associated with disease in man. Infection is transmitted trans-stadially by the host tick; it appears that transovarial transmission does not occur. In sheep, mortality ranges from 60% in newly introduced stock to 5-10% in previously exposed animals. On farms where the disease is endemic, losses are mainly confined to animals <2 yr old; adults tend to be immune as a result of previous infection, and lambs are protected in their first season by colostral antibody. However, when the disease appears for the first time, or after a lapse of several years, all ages of sheep are susceptible. Mortality is variable in other species, but tends to be high in red grouse. Only sheep and grouse appear able to pass the infection to the vector tick. Infection also can be spread through contact with contaminated instruments or tissues. Infected lactating goats can excrete high titers of virus in their milk, which may cause fatal infection of their kids and be a potential health hazard to man.

Pathogenesis, Clinical Findings, and Lesions: The course of infection in all species is similar, and varies only in the intensity of viremia and frequency with which clinical signs develop. Following inoculation by an infected tick, virus initially replicates in lymphoid tissues, which gives rise to viremia that lasts 1-5 days. Only individuals that develop high titers can transfer the virus to ticks. During viremia, a febrile reaction may occur, but overt clinical signs are generally absent until the virus enters the CNS and begins replication, even though the immune response has eliminated the virus from the extra-neuronal tissues. The extent of neuronal damage consequent to viral replication determines the severity of signs, from none to apparent neurological dysfunction. Histological lesions may be present whether or not signs develop. Signs include fine muscular tremors, nervous nibbling, ataxia (particularly of the hindlimbs), weakness, and collapse; death may occur 1-3 days after onset of signs. Peracute deaths may also occur. In some recovered animals, residual paresis or torticollis may persist. All recovered individuals are solidly immune.

The severity of clinical disease in animals recently infected with *Cytoecetes phagocytophila* (the cause of tick-borne fever [qv, p 405]) is markedly increased, presumably due to the immunosuppressive effect of this organism. The accompanying pathology may be complex, and may account for the high mortality experienced when naive flocks are introduced to tick-infested pasture.

No specific gross lesions are present, although secondary pneumonia may develop. Histological examination of the CNS usually shows a nonsuppurative polioencephalomyelitis with lesions predominantly in the brain stem.

Diagnosis: The disease normally occurs only in animals that have had access to tick-infested pasture; however, the variable clinical picture necessitates differentiation from other conditions that cause locomotor or neurological dysfunction. Confirmation is by histological examination of the brain, virus isolation from CNS tissue, and serology. As much of the brain and brain stem as possible should be fixed in formaldehyde solution (10% in saline), and sections examined for the characteristic lesions, which can be useful in reaching a presumptive diagnosis; a definitive diagnosis requires virus isolation. Brain stem (1 cm^3) should be collected aseptically into 50% glycerol saline for isolation of the virus by mouse or tissue-culture inoculation, and subsequent identification by FA tests or neutralization with specific antibodies. Measurement of serum neutralizing and hemagglutination inhibiting (HI) antibodies also can be useful in reaching a diagnosis and for surveys. The presence of IgM antibody in cattle and sheep, detected by the HI test, provides good evidence that infection occurred within the preceding 10 days.

Treatment and Control: No specific treatment is available, but nursing, hand-feeding, and sedation may be helpful. An inactivated, tissue-culture-propagated vaccine is available and has successfully protected sheep, cattle, and goats. A single injection provokes an antibody response that persists for ≥2 yr. Colostrum from the vaccinated ewe prevents infection of lambs in their first months. Generally, all animals to be retained for breeding are vaccinated at 6 mo of age. Use of insecticidal dips to protect against exposure to ticks generally is inadequate, although the recently developed "pour-on" preparations may reduce exposure.

MENINGITIS AND ENCEPHALITIS

In most species, meningitis tends to occur in association with or secondary to encephalitis. However, signs of meningism may precede the encephalitic phase in certain infections. In dogs, several syndromes are recognized in which meningeal signs predominate throughout the course of the disease. Causes of meningitis and encephalitis other than bacteria include viruses, fungi, protozoa, parasitic migration, chemical agents, and immune-mediated disease.

Etiology and Pathogenesis: Bacterial meningoencephalitis often affects neonatal farm animals as a sequela of septicemia caused by *Escherichia coli* or streptococci; *Actinobacillus equuli* infection is an important cause in foals. Failure of passive transfer of immunoglobulins is the single most important factor predisposing neonates to omphalophlebitis and/or enteritis with subsequent hematogenous spread of the infection to the CNS. In older or adult animals, well-recognized disease entities such as thromboembolic meningoencephalitis (TEME [*Haemophilus somnus*]) of cattle, Glässer's disease of pigs (*H parasuis*), and *H agni* septicemia in feeder lambs also cause meningoencephalitis by the hematogenous route. Listeriosis (*Listeria monocytogenes*), which is common in cattle, sheep, and goats, is an example of a multifocal brain-stem meningoencephalitis that ascends to the CNS via cranial nerves. *Pasteurella haemolytica* and *P multocida*, which usually cause fibrinous pneumonia and hemorrhagic septicemia in ruminants, occasionally produce a localized fibrinopurulent leptomeningitis. Meningoencephalitis due to *P haemolytica* also has been reported in horses, donkeys, and mules. *Actinomyces, Cryptococcus,* and *Streptococcus* spp are sporadic causes of meningitis in adult horses.

In any species, direct extension of bacterial or mycotic infections to the CNS can occur from sinusitis, otitis media or interna, vertebral osteomyelitis, diskospondylitis, or deep bite or traumatic wounds adjacent to the head or spine. Iatrogenic infections are possible from contaminated spinal needles or surgical instruments. Brain abscesses also can arise from direct infection or by septic embolism of cerebral vessels. Pituitary abscesses in ruminants are thought to originate from bacterial invasion of the rete mirabile surrounding the pituitary gland. In chronic brain abscesses, an adjacent or occasionally diffuse fibrinous leptomeningitis may develop. Although less commonly than in farm animals, dogs can develop a spontaneous bacterial meningitis or meningoencephalitis from which various bacteria (*P multocida, Staphylococcus aureus, S epidermidis, S albus, Actinomyces* spp, and *Nocardia* spp) have been isolated. Bacterial endocarditis is also an important source of CNS infection in dogs.

Pathological changes characteristic of bacterial meningoencephalitis include diffuse infiltration of both neutrophils and mononuclear cells into the leptomeninges. Frequently, the entire subarachnoid space of the brain and spinal cord is inflamed. Vasculitis is often pronounced. Bacteria may also invade the CNS parenchyma, which results in mononuclear and polymorphonuclear infiltration and large areas of perivascular cuffing. Necrosis of gray and white matter may be observed, with infiltrations of macrophages, neutrophils, and plasma cells. Listeriosis uniquely causes microabscesses consisting of accumulations of neutrophils and microglial cell reaction with central liquefaction necrosis.

Other agents that can cause meningoencephalitis, especially in dogs and occasionally cats and other species, include *Toxoplasma* and *Toxoplasma*-like protozoa, *Neospora caninum, Acanthamoeba castellani, Cryptococcus neoformans, Blastomyces dermatitidis, Histoplasma capsulatum, Aspergillus* sp, *Coccidioides immitis,* and *Rickettsia* spp (Rocky Mountain spotted fever, salmon poisoning, and ehrlichiosis). Rarely, other fungi such as *Cladosporium trichoides, Paecilomyces variotii, Flavobacterium meningosepticum,* and *Geotrichum candidum* cause meningoencephalomyelitis. Aseptic suppurative encephalitis associated with aberrant migration of parasites into the CNS occurs with a number of species (*see* pp 603-

606). Viruses such as those of canine distemper, canine parvovirus, feline infectious peritonitis, malignant catarrhal fever in ruminants, and sporadic bovine encephalomyelitis also produce meningitis in addition to encephalitis. Eosinophilic meningoencephalitis is an unusual inflammatory response to salt poisoning in pigs. Unicellular plants, *Prototheca wickerhamii* and *P zopfii*, can also produce an eosinophilic meningoencephalomyelitis in dogs.

Several idiopathic meningoencephalitides are recognized in dogs. A **pyogranulomatous meningoencephalomyelitis** occurs in mature Pointer dogs. It has been reported as an acute, rapidly progressive disorder. The lesions consist of extensive mononuclear cells and neutrophils infiltrating the leptomeninges and parenchyma, especially in the cervical spinal cord and brain stem. An etiologic agent has not been identified. **Granulomatous meningoencephalomyelitis** (GME, qv, p 589) or **inflammatory reticulosis** is a more common nervous disease that affects dogs with a mean age of 5 yr (range 8 mo to 10 yr). Recently, a steroid-responsive suppurative meningitis affecting mainly large dogs <2 yr old, and a severe **necrotizing vasculitis** syndrome in Beagles, Bernese Mountain Dogs, and German Shorthaired Pointers, have been identified as possible immunologic disorders with a hereditary predisposition.

Clinical Findings: The usual signs of bacterial meningitis are pyrexia, hyperesthesia, neck rigidity, and painful paraspinal muscle spasms. Dogs and occasionally horses display this syndrome acutely and sometimes chronically without clinical signs of brain or spinal cord involvement. However, in diffuse meningoencephalitis due to any agent, depression, blindness, progressive paresis, cerebellar and/or vestibular ataxia, opisthotonus, cranial nerve deficits, seizures, delerium, and terminal coma can develop, depending on the severity and localization of the lesions. In neonatal infections, omphalophlebitis, polyarthritis, and ophthalmitis with hypopyon can accompany the CNS inflammation. Because of its unusual pathogenesis, *Listeria monocytogenes* often causes unilateral vestibular imbalance, and facial and pharyngeal paralysis. In TEME of cattle, the nervous signs tend to be peracute with the animal suddenly collapsing into a semicoma. Fever and limb stiffness may be the only signs detectable in the prodromal stages. Clinical signs of pyogranulomatous meningoencephalomyelitis include cervical rigidity, kyphosis, nose held close to the ground, reluctance to move, and an incoordinated hypermetric gait. Sometimes, bradycardia, vomiting, and atrophy of cervical muscles are observed. Cranial nerve signs may include Horner's syndrome and those of paralysis of trigeminal. and facial nerves. The signs of granulomatous meningoencephalomyelitis in dogs vary with distribution of the lesions. Neck pain, depression, behavioral disturbances, ataxia, paresis, and cranial nerve deficits may be seen. The disseminated form of GME has a shorter, more fulminating course of 1-8 wk in comparison to the focal form, which often has an insidious progression over many months.

Diagnosis: In addition to the history, environmental conditions, species or breed predispositions to certain diseases, and clinical signs, examination of CSF is the most accurate means of identifying an inflammatory process of the CNS. Unless a spinal tap has ruled out meningitis, the animal exhibiting pain with no neurologic deficits may be misdiagnosed as having disk disease, pleuritis, pancreatitis, polyarthritis, or malaise and discomfort from septicemia. Dogs with bacterial meningitis and encephalitis, steroid-responsive suppurative meningitis, and vasculitis typically have high numbers of neutrophils (100's-1000's/μL) in the CSF. The protein content of the CSF is usually significantly elevated (100-5000 mg/dL) as well. Occasionally, bacteria are seen on cytological examination of the CSF and identified with Gram's stain. Culture of bacteria from CSF is more likely in large animals than in dogs. In some cases, serial blood cultures are more successful for isolation of the causative organism. Viral infections and listeriosis typically produce a mononuclear pleocytosis in CSF; the total cell count and protein levels are mildly to moderately elevated. Granulomatous inflammations usually induce moderate to high cell numbers and elevated protein in the CSF. The cell population is predominantly mononuclear, and it can be difficult to distinguish between infections and idiopathic causes of GME. However, in pyogranulomatous meningoencephalomyelitis, CSF analysis usually reveals a neutrophilic pleocytosis (500-1000 WBC/mL). Cryptococci and occasionally protozoa have been identified in CSF, but usually serology is necessary to confirm mycotic and protozoan infections *in vivo*.

Treatment: The prognosis for bacterial meningoencephalomyelitis is guarded. Appropriate use of antibiotics, according to culture results, is basic to successful therapy. Relapses are frequent, and prolonged therapy is often necessary. Correction of the immunodeficiency is mandatory in neonatal large animals. Broad-spectrum antibacterials such as ampicillin, chloramphenicol, tetracyclines, trimethoprim-sulfas, and third-generation cephalosporins are used, but higher than normal dosages may be necessary to achieve adequate concentrations in the CNS.

Mycotic infections of the CNS in man have been successfully treated with amphotericin B; toxoplasmosis may respond to a sulfa/pyramethamine combination, or to clindamycin therapy. Glucocorticoids are usually contraindicated with bacterial, mycotic, or protozoal infections; however, a high-dose, short course of dexamethasone or methylprednisolone may control life-threatening complications such as acute cerebral edema and impending brain herniation. Immunosuppressive doses of corticosteroids are recommended for idiopathic inflammations in dogs. Supportive care consists of analgesics, anticonvulsants, fluids, a high-quality diet, and physiotherapy.

NEONATAL MALADJUSTMENT SYNDROME
(NMS, Barkers, Wanderers, Dummies, Convulsive foals)

A noninfectious condition of foals characterized by gross behavioral disturbances. Affected foals may appear normal at birth and delivery is uncomplicated. The first signs, which usually appear within 24 hr, are loss of affinity for the mare and of the sucking reflex. As the condition progresses, hyperexcitability, bruxism, apparent blindness, aimless wandering, and clonus appear. Foals often make "barking" noises during the wandering stage, and mildly affected foals may exhibit only those signs related to the wanderer stage. Opisthotonos and extensor rigidity, loss of righting reflex, recumbency, and finally, a comatose state ensue in that order. Hypoxia and acidosis accompany the behavioral changes.

The exact cause of NMS is unknown; possibilities include cerebral vascular disturbance that may result in edema and hemorrhage, cranial or thoracic trauma, or hypoxia and increased intracranial pressure during parturition. Differential diagnoses include prematurity, dysmaturity, acute cranial trauma, congenital hydrocephalus, and septic meningitis.

Treatment is supportive and symptomatic. It is essential to maintain normal body temperature, acid-base balance, optimal body fluid levels, and adequate nutrition, and to assist ventilation and prevent secondary infection. Chemical control of convulsions is often necessary (barbiturates, phenytoin, diazepam, or primidone).

The prognosis is good if uncomplicated by septicemia. Survival is >50% with appropriate treatment. If the foal recovers, neurological functions return in the reverse order in which they were lost.

NEOPLASIA OF THE NERVOUS SYSTEM

Primary tumors of the nervous system originate from neuroectodermal or mesodermal cells in or associated with brain, spinal cord, or peripheral nerves. Secondary tumors may originate from surrounding tissues or from hematogenous metastasis. Primary nervous system tumors rarely metastasize outside the cranium and vertebral canal, and in dogs and cats, they are more common in the brain than in the spinal cord or peripheral nerves. Age and breed (but not sex) are predisposing factors. In veterinary medicine, nervous system tumors have been classified according to criteria used to classify tumors in man, but 15-20% of neuroectodermal tumors remain unclassified.

Because secondary effects may mask the location of intracranial tumors, accurate clinicopathologic correlations are difficult. In addition to actual infiltration of brain tissue, a tumor within the cranium may lead to local necrosis, edema, and cerebral or cerebellar herniation. Herniation may cause an increase in intracranial pressure with subsequent development of hydrocephalus. Herniated tissue also may result in compression of the brain stem.

Primary tumors generally grow slowly; secondary, highly malignant, metastatic tumors and bone tumors frequently grow rapidly. Topography, growth patterns, and resulting changes within and around the tumor tend to be characteristic for the specific neoplasm. Primary glial tumors, eg, astrocytomas and oligodendrogliomas, tend to be deep-seated and to infiltrate the surrounding parenchyma. Neoplastic granulomatous meningoencephalomyelitis (primary reticulosis) also tends to infiltrate the CNS. They all have a predilection for the cerebral hemispheres.

Meningiomas in dogs and cats usually are benign tumors that tend to grow slowly under the dura mater and expand toward the brain or spinal cord; they produce pressure atrophy rather than infiltrate. They may adhere to the dura mater or lie within the leptomeningeal tissue. Spinal meningiomas tend to occupy an intradural-extramedullary position. Intracranial meningiomas may produce bone erosion. Hyperostosis (thickening of bone adjacent to meningiomas) has been reported in dogs and cats. In dogs with spinal meningiomas, radiography may depict scalloped-appearing, laminar changes in the affected vertebrae, indicative of pressure atrophy-like changes associated with the slow tumor growth.

Ependymomas arise from the ependymal cells lining the ventricular system. They tend to penetrate the brain parenchyma but can project into the lumen of the ventricle. Metastasis can occur via the CSF. Ependymomas of the fourth ventricle may extend out of the foramina and girdle the brain stem. Choroid plexus papillomas expand the ventricle locally, and rarely show invasive destructive growth or metastasis. Because of their location, particularly when they arise in the fourth ventricle, ependymomas and choroid plexus papillomas tend to interfere directly with the CSF flow in the ventricular system.

Incidence: Most data on the frequency of neoplasia of the nervous system in domestic animals relate to dogs, in which intracranial tumors are 1-3% of all tumors. In large animals, nervous system tumors are rare except for lymphosarcomas and neurofibromas in cattle.

Brain Tumors: In dogs, the most common brain tumors are meningiomas, gliomas (astrocytomas, oligodendrogliomas), and undifferentiated sarcomas. Primary reticulosis, pituitary adenomas, and choroid plexus papillomas are also common. Among domestic animals, Boxers, English Bulldogs, and Boston Terriers >5 yr old have the highest incidence of brain tumors, usually gliomas. Pituitary adenomas are also frequent in brachycephalic breeds.

Most meningiomas occur in dogs >7 yr old. They are intracranial, and frequently occur in the falx cerebri, convexities of the cerebral hemispheres, and ventral surface of the brain, especially in the middle cranial fossa. Some are found in the retrobulbar space arising from the sheath of the optic nerve.

Most ependymomas in dogs appear to be in the lateral and third ventricles. Of choroid plexus papillomas, ~50-60% occur in the fourth ventricle, the rest with equal incidence in the lateral and third ventricles.

In cats, meningiomas (often multiple) are the most commonly reported primary brain tumors; ~70-75% occur in cats >9 yr old.

Spinal Cord Tumors: The most common spinal cord tumors in dogs are extradural, primary, malignant bone tumors, and metastatic tumors in bone and soft tissues. Metastasis to the spinal cord is unusual in animals, although an incidence of 16% has been reported in dogs. Spinal cord blastomas are extramedullary tumors with a predilection for the T_{10}-L_3 cord segments. They are observed in young dogs, and more frequently in German Shepherd Dogs. Most spinal meningiomas in dogs are in the cervical region, whereas astrocytomas tend to locate in the lower cervical and upper thoracic segments. Epidural lymphosarcomas are the most common spinal tumors in cats, pigs, and cattle.

Peripheral Nerve Tumors: Peripheral nervous system (PNS) tumors are more frequent than CNS tumors in horses and cattle. Neurofibroma is the most frequently seen PNS tumor in cattle. Not common in dogs, nerve sheath tumors mainly involve the roots of cranial nerve V and brachial plexus. In dogs, cats, horses, and cattle, lymphosarcomas can occur in nerve roots or nerves.

Clinical Findings: Signs associated with various brain, spinal cord, and peripheral nerve syndromes are shown in TABLE 1. Clinical signs may be acute or insidious in onset, and progress rapidly or slowly. Dogs with intramedullary tumors usually do not seem to have the long history of obscure pain as do dogs with other types of spinal cord/peripheral nerve tumors. Perhaps this is due to lack of nerve root compression and/or lack of bony destruction. Signs, including onset of paresis/paralysis, tend to develop rapidly in intramedullary spinal tumors. Neurological signs that are asymmetrical initially may quickly become bilaterally symmetrical.

A paraneoplastic syndrome (reduced or absent spinal reflexes, muscle atrophy, reduced tone) may occur in animals with malignant neoplasms that may or may not have metastasized to the CNS.

Table 1. Clinical Signs Associated with Various Brain, Spinal Cord, and Peripheral Nerve Syndromes

Syndrome	Signs
Cerebral/diencephalic	1) Behavior/mental status change (apathy, disorientation, hyperexcitability, aggression) 2) Abnormal posture/movement (circling, pacing, head pressing, pleurothotonos) 3) +/− Visual impairment, seizures, papilledema, hypothalamo-hypophyseal syndrome (pituitary)
Cerebellar	1) Dysmetria (usually hypermetria) 2) Intention tremor (head, body) 3) Wide-based stance 4) Truncal ataxia 5) +/− Menace deficit, eye tremors
Vestibular	1) Head tilt 2) Circling/falling/rolling 3) Nystagmus 4) Vestibular strabismus
Cervical (C_{1-5})	1) Hemiparesis—tetraplegia 2) Upper motor neuron (UMN) signs* in fore- and hindlimbs 3) Cervical pain, +/− cervical rigidity
Cervicothoracic (C_6-T_2)	1) Hemiparesis—tetraplegia 2) Lower motor neuron (LMN) signs** in forelimbs 3) Upper motor neuron signs in hindlimbs 4) Absent panniculus reflex (C_8-T_1) 5) +/− Horner's syndrome (T_{1-3}) (miosis, ptosis, enophthalmos, prolapse of third eyelid)
Thoracolumbar (T_3-L_3)	1) Upper motor neuron signs in hindlimbs 2) Hypalgesia—analgesia caudal to lesion site
Lumbosacral (L_4-S_3 .. Cd)	1) Lower motor neuron signs in hindlimbs 2) Dilated anal sphincter, urine retention
Neuropathic	1) Lower motor neuron signs in all hindlimbs 2) Significant skeletal muscle atrophy (neurogenic atrophy) 3) +/− Hypalgesia

* spastic paresis/paralysis, hyperreflexia, hypertonia
** flaccid paresis/paralysis, hyporeflexia, hypotonia

Adapted from Braund, K.G., Neoplasia, In: *Veterinary Neurology*, Oliver, J.E., Hoerlein, B.F., Mayhew, I.G. (ed.), W.B. Saunders Co., Philadelphia, 1987.

Diagnosis: Diagnosis is based on age, breed, clinical signs, CSF analysis, and radiography. In deep-seated tumors, CSF analysis is often unremarkable. Occasionally, protein concentration may be mildly to moderately increased. When the meninges are involved, the CSF typically has a neutrophilic pleocytosis with increased protein concentration. Tumor cells are rarely seen in primary CNS neoplasia.

Usual radiologic studies include survey film radiography and myelography. For brain tumors, ventriculography, cerebral sinus venography, and cerebral angiography are being replaced by more accurate, safer imaging techniques such as scintigraphy, computerized tomography (CT), and magnetic resonance imaging. Survey film radiography may detect proliferation, lysis, or lucency of bone secondary to neoplasms. Because of calcification in the tumor, intracranial meningiomas may be radiodense; increased or decreased density of the skull may be seen at the site of the tumor in cats.

Loss of bone density of the vertebral canal (which appears as a widening of the canal) may be caused by tumors in the canal, and nerve root neurofibromas may cause enlargement of the intervertebral foramina. Myelography outlines spinal tumors and helps identify their location. CT may accurately localize brain tumors, and may also provide information pertaining to tumor malignancy. Meningiomas, choroid plexus tumors, and pituitary tumors are readily distinguished via contrast agent enhancement.

Electrophysiology is occasionally used when brain neoplasms are suspected. Electroencephalography may identify an area of abnormal electrical activity associated with a space-occupying lesion. Electromyography, performed frequently in peripheral nervous sytem disorders, is helpful in differentiating root from spinal or peripheral nerve tumors.

Histopathology of tissue obtained by surgical biopsy or tumor removal is the final step toward a definitive diagnosis.

Prognosis and Treatment: Prognosis is guarded to poor. Although early accurate localization of a brain tumor mass is seldom possible, removal of intracranial tumors is becoming more frequent. Spinal cord tumors can be better localized, but intramedullary masses are not surgically resectable, and extradural tumors are frequently primary bone or metastatic tumors.

Although some consider intradural-extramedullary tumors to be surgically correctable, others have reported that most are not completely resectable and that recurrence is high.

If they have not invaded the spinal cord, peripheral nerve or root tumors may be resected, but the affected nerve or root also must be removed. When more than one root or nerve is involved (as may occur with a tumor of the brachial plexus), amputation of the limb may be necessary. The use of radiotherapy and chemotherapy for tumors of the nervous system has been infrequent in veterinary medicine. Corticosteroids may reduce edema around tumors; for lymphoid and reticulohistiocytic tumors, they may induce temporary regression.

PARALYSIS OF THE FORELIMB

The innervation of the foreleg is commonly damaged by direct trauma, ischemia from restraint or prolonged anesthesia of heavy horses and cattle in lateral recumbency, and occasionally, by tumors involving the nerves or rootlets of the brachial plexus. Traction on the forelimb severe enough to cause excessive abduction of the shoulder can avulse or severely stretch the entire plexus. The resulting clinical signs reflect varying degrees of damage to intradural ventral and dorsal nerve roots. The radial nerve is most vulnerable to injury at the level of the first rib and at the humerus where it lies in the musculospiral groove.

Characteristically, any animal with complete brachial plexus paralysis stands with the elbow dropped, and the carpus and metacarpal joint in partial flexion. The limb is dragged, and weight-bearing causes collapse at the elbow and carpus. Of the

5 major nerves of the plexus (musculocutaneous, axillary, radial, ulnar, and median), injury to the radial nerve proximal to the elbow produces the greatest motor disability because the elbow, carpus, and digits cannot be extended to bear weight. A lesion of the nerve distal to the elbow results in knuckling of the digits and carpus only. With severe radial nerve lesions, desensitization occurs primarily over the dorsum of the forelimb and digits. Impaired flexion of the digits and carpus occurs with ulnar and median nerve paralysis. Axillary and musculocutaneous nerve damage affects shoulder movement and elbow flexion, respectively. When a neoplastic, traumatic, or inflammatory process affects the spinal cord segments from which the brachial plexus arises (C_6-T_2), bilateral paresis of fore- and hindlimbs may occur. Neurofibromas originating in a nerve of the brachial plexus often progress to the spinal cord and cause a discrete hemiplegia. Involvement of the first thoracic root often produces Horner's syndrome on the same side as the limb paralysis. Within 1-2 wk, severe neurogenic muscle atrophy develops in the denervated muscle groups.

In dogs, a form of brachial plexus neuritis has been reported that is characterized by shifting forelimb lameness. There are diffuse electromyographic abnormalities typical of denervation; CSF and spinal myelography are normal. These dogs improve with glucocorticoid therapy. Dietary beef and/or equine products have been implicated in this disorder.

An accurate history and careful neurological examination of the forelimb are essential and usually adequate for a diagnosis. Radiographic evidence of fractures may suggest the site of injury. The prognosis is guarded when sensory loss is complete, and 2-4 mo of convalescence may be necessary for nerve regeneration. Electromyographic analysis of the various muscle groups can determine the extent of injury. By sequential nerve conduction studies, signs of nerve regeneration can be detected sooner and a more definite prognosis given.

In cases of acute contusion of the nerves, edema and pressure should be relieved. When it is suspected that a nerve(s) has been severed, surgical exploration and repair is indicated. If the foot is dragged and prone to laceration, it can be protected with a leather boot. During a prolonged period of convalescence, physiotherapy (consisting of muscle massage), and flexion and extension of all joints of the affected limb may help prevent joint fixation due to muscle contracture. Prognosis for animals with brachial plexus avulsion is guarded to poor. Amputation of the limb in small animals may be necessary in irreversible cases.

POLIOENCEPHALOMALACIA
(PEM, Cerebrocortical necrosis)

A noninfectious neurological disease of ruminants characterized by amaurosis and strabismus, followed by recumbency, opisthotonos, and convulsions. Tissue thiamine and related enzymatic activity are depressed, and lead to necrosis and autofluorescence of affected brain tissue; the latter is useful in diagnosis. Young, intensively reared cattle and sheep are at greatest risk, but it also occurs in goats, antelope, deer, and in pastured cattle and sheep under special circumstances. It occurs worldwide, notably in North and South America, Europe, the Middle East, and Australia.

Etiology and Epidemiology: In all cases, tissue thiamine is deficient; however, the cause of this deficiency is varied and not completely clear. When the diet is abruptly changed to concentrates and corn (maize) silage, the amount of thiamine in the rumen falls rapidly, and the GI microflora changes demonstrably; gram-positive bacilli with thiaminase type I activity, gram-negative cocci, and coccobacilli become dominant. The type I thiaminase leads automatically to production of thiamine analogs, some of which have been demonstrated in brain tissue of affected animals; however, their etiological role is still uncertain. Ultimately, low tissue levels of thiamine-dependent enzymes impair energy metabolism, particularly in brain and heart, tissues that depend on glucose catabolism. This results in changes consistent with acute metabolic arrest in glial cells and neurons in brain areas of high vulnerability, and the less commonly recognized focal myocardial necrosis. PEM also occurs in poisoning by bracken fern (*Pteridium aquilinum*), nardoo (*Marsilea drummondii*), and rock fern (*Cheilanthes sieberi*) since these contain thiaminase type I. (*See also* p 1641.) Moldy feed also may be associated with PEM since some molds produce thiaminase type I, or they or their metabolites may act by interfering with the balance of GI microflora and the endogenous synthesis of thiamine. Ingestion of excessive amounts of sulfate fed to limit concentrate intake or as a contaminant in water also has been associated with outbreaks of PEM. The mechanism is not yet understood. Molasses toxicity in Caribbean nations produces similar signs and lesions, but its relationship to PEM is uncertain.

Virtually all cases relate to disturbances of the rumen and intestinal ecosystem by intensive farming practices and the feeding of large quantities of carbohydrate. In sheep, a rate of change of >280 g of water-soluble carbohydrate per head per feeding has been associated with the disease. Cases occurring at pasture in New Zealand and Europe relate to lush high-protein grass. In Australia, previously flooded pastures repopulated with the nardoo fern induce PEM, while in South America PEM has been observed in starving pastured cattle that have cannibalized rotting carcasses.

Pathogenesis: Thiamine pyrophosphate is a coenzyme required in the tricarboxylic acid cycle and the pentose shunt, both of which are vital to brain cell energy production. Lack of energy causes neuronal necrosis and swelling of astrocytes. Due to the distribution of terminal branches of cerebral arteries, variable neuronal metabolic requirements, and intrinsic neuronal biochemical differences, brain lesions in PEM are worst in the cortex (frontal, parietal, and occipital), thalamus, lateral geniculate bodies, and posterior collicular nuclei. Secondary ischemic lesions due to brain swelling include subtentorial herniation of parts of the cortex and herniation of the cerebellum into the foramen magnum. Focal myocardial necrosis occurs principally in the atria. More recently, disturbances of bone marrow activity in thiamine inadequacy have been noted, and may account for rare subserosal hemorrhages in the viscera of calves and the hemorrhagic nature of cortical lesions sometimes seen in lambs.

Clinical Findings and Lesions: Prodromal signs are isolation and anorexia. Sudden depression, ruminal hypoactivity, medial dorsal strabismus ("star gazing"), moderate opisthotonos, disturbed gait, cortical blindness, and preserved pupillary light reflex are the most common signs. Hyperesthesia, recumbency, severe opisthotonos, and tonic-clonic convulsions follow in untreated cases. Elevated CSF pressure, pleocytosis of monocytes and macrophages, and papilledema may be noted within 24-48 hr. Unless convulsions follow, the temperature remains normal. Bradycardia and arrhythmias occur occasionally, and a grunting expiration and transitory diarrhea may be noted. In untreated recumbent cattle, the mortality approaches 100% in 3-4 days. The morbidity in feedlot cattle is usually <5%, but in 3- to 5-mo-old calves it may be up to 50%. In sheep, the clinical course tends to be more rapid.

In animals affected <24 hr, gross lesions are subtle. Characteristic symmetrical cortical yellowing of the frontal, occipital, and parietal lobes is best seen in animals surviving for 2-3 days. Subtentorial occipital herniation and coning of the cerebellum into the foramen magnum create focal necrotic and hemorrhagic lesions. The brain lacks normal turgor. After 24 hr of clinical disease, under ultraviolet light, at 365 nm in darkness, the zones of necrosis in the cortex and deep brain structures fluoresce yellow-blue. Histological lesions include laminar cortical necrosis with shrunken, eosinophilic, "metabolic arrest" neurons; fine spongy vacuolation of the neuropil; and occasionally, small perivascular hemorrhages. Severity of capillary hypertrophy and macrophage activity in necrotic tissues is progressively time dependent.

Diagnosis: In live animals, assay of RBC transketolase and fecal or ruminal thiaminase, and response to thiamine therapy are helpful diagnostic procedures. Fecal thiaminase in neurologically normal animals having blood thiamine levels of <50 nmol/L may indicate a subclinical thiamine inadequacy associated with poor weight gain. Elevated blood pyruvate and lactate are suggestive, but prone to misleading elevation due to muscular exertion. In dead animals, the gross cortical fluorescence and characteristic histological brain lesions are confirmatory. Thiamine levels in brain, liver, and heart are low. Subacute lead poisoning, salt poisoning, and water intoxication are also capable of causing areas of cortical degeneration with a histological pattern that may be difficult to distinguish from that of PEM.

Differential diagnoses in cattle and sheep include acute lead poisoning, nitrofuran toxicity, hypomagnesemia, vitamin A deficiency, chlorinated hydrocarbon toxicity, infectious thromboembolic meningoencephalitis (TEME), brain abscess, and type D clostridial enterotoxemia.

Treatment: PEM is an emergency; since neurons are dying by millions, therapy should begin immediately after onset of signs. Thiamine hydrochloride, at 10-15 mg/kg, IV or IM, ensures rapid reactivation of the deficient enzyme complexes. Excess parenteral thiamine is lost rapidly in the urine. Continued antagonism and destruction of GI-derived thiamine may necessitate repeat treatments at lower dose rates (2-10 mg/kg, b.i.d. or q.i.d. for 3 days). In valuable animals, dexamethasone (1-2 mg/50 kg, IM for 3 days) and an IV mannitol drip may minimize brain swelling and facilitate recovery. Rapidity of recovery relates directly to the speed of diagnosis and therapy. Recovery of vision and restoration to normal function are often achieved but may require 2-3 wk convalescence. Since others in the flock or herd are at risk, dietary concentrate and corn (maize) silage should be decreased and additional quality roughage supplied for 5 days before a gradual return to higher-energy rations. Parenteral thiamine and dietary change is the preferred prophylaxis. Supplementary dietary thiamine is contraindicated as it may further stimulate thiaminolytic organisms in the gut. However, oral prophylaxis or supportive therapy may be achieved by administration of the less-soluble thiamine propyl disulfide or thiamine tetrafurfuryl disulfide. These are not destroyed by thiaminase type I and are readily absorbed from the GI tract.

PORCINE ENTEROVIRAL ENCEPHALOMYELITIS
(Teschen disease, Porcine polioencephalomyelitis, Talfan disease, Benign enzootic paresis)

An infectious disease of pigs, analogous to human poliomyelitis. Severe disease is now rare; it occurs in the USSR and Africa but was last reported in Europe from Austria in 1980. In other countries, sporadic mild disease is reported, or the disease is unrecognized.

Etiology, Epidemiology, and Pathogenesis: Enteroviruses (Picornaviridae) are ubiquitous in swine populations throughout the world. Many strains are nonpathogenic. Using the virus-neutralization test, 11 porcine enterovirus serogroups have been defined. Most neurotropic strains belong to one of the first 3 serogroups, and serogroup 1 contains not only the highly virulent but also many of the less virulent neurotropic strains. Although antigenic subtypes are recognized, they do not distinguish between more or less virulent strains of virus. Enteroviruses can survive in the environment for months.

Transmission is by direct or indirect contact with infected pigs. The virulent serogroup 1 strain of classical Teschen disease produces high morbidity and mortality in all ages of pigs but apparently has remained confined to certain geographic areas. Mild, sporadic disease occurs elsewhere. Conventional herds are usually endemically infected, and exclusion of enteroviruses from SPF herds is difficult to maintain. Infection is mainly inapparent and occurs usually at weaning with the decline of passive maternal immunity and mixing of pigs. Sporadic clinical cases of nervous disease occur mainly around this time, although disease is more common in unweaned piglets following introduction of a serotype to which the herd has not been exposed.

Ingested virus replicates in the GI tract and its associated lymphoid tissue. There is no destruction of gut epithelium, but virus is shed from multiplication sites into the feces for several weeks. In some pigs, especially those infected with virulent strains, viremia ensues and results in spread of infection to the CNS. (*See also* p 595.)

Clinical Findings and Lesions: In acute virulent infection, clinical signs appear 1-4 wk after exposure in pigs of all ages. Ataxia is often the first sign observed, followed by fever, lassitude, and anorexia. Seizures, nystagmus, opisthotonus, and coma may occur. Paralysis, initially evident as paraplegia but progressing to quadriplegia, is frequent in severe cases. Death is common within 3-4 days of onset of signs.

Mild disease signs are essentially ataxia and paresis, the latter more rarely progressing to paralysis. Only young pigs (unweaned or weaned) are susceptible, and recovery is frequent.

There are no gross lesions. Microscopic changes are most prominent in the gray matter of the brain stem, cerebellum, and spinal cord. The nonsuppurative encephalitis is characterized by neuronal necrosis, neuronophagia, glial foci, and perivascular lymphocytic cuffing. Meningitis is often present over the cerebellum.

Diagnosis: The clinical signs (especially those of locomotor disturbance), the epidemiology, and the absence of specific gross necropsy findings offer a presumptive diagnosis. The nature and distribution of histological lesions offer supportive evidence. Acute and convalescent serum samples, taken ≥2 wk apart, may demonstrate a rise in neutralizing or complement-fixing antibodies. Virus isolation from the CNS is required to confirm the diagnosis. Differentiation of severe and more mild forms of the disease can be based only on serological, clinical, and epidemiological evidence.

Differential diagnoses include the many other viral encephalitides of pigs, particularly hog cholera, African swine fever, pseudorabies, rabies, and the encephalopathies of edema disease and water deprivation/salt intoxication. The prominent locomotor signs in enteroviral encephalomyelitis also can be confused with several toxic and nutritional neuropathies.

Treatment and Control: There is no treatment. Live attenuated vaccine is used for control in areas experiencing severe endemic disease. In the past, eradication measures in central Europe have involved ring vaccination and slaughter, and restrictions on importation of pigs and pork products. In many countries, suspected classical Teschen disease must be reported to regulatory authorities. In herds with endemic mild clinical disease, introduction of new breeding stock ≥1 mo before breeding should enhance passive immunity in offspring.

PSEUDORABIES
(Aujeszky's disease, Mad itch)

A viral infection, primarily of pigs, that affects the CNS. The host range is broad, although the infection is fatal in virtually all animals that become infected except pigs. Man, apes, chimpanzees, poikilotherms, and insects are resistant to infection. The virus can survive on the body surface of domestic flies, which may serve as a source of virus. Pseudorabies has been reported in the USA, Central and South America, Europe, India, Southeast Asia, Taiwan, Japan, northern countries of Africa, and New Zealand. It has not been detected in Canada or Australia.

Etiology, Epidemiology, and Pathogenesis: The causal herpesvirus has a double strand of DNA and a lipoprotein envelope. There are at least 5 glycoproteins that project from the envelope. Virus persists in a latent state in ganglion neurons in a high percentage of infected pigs. Many strains of virus exist and vary from apparent avirulence for pigs to highly virulent.

The pig is the primary host and only known reservoir. Pigs excrete large quantities of virus in saliva and nasal secretions for up to 2 wk after primary infection, and small quantities only rarely in urine or feces. Pigs may be latently infected for life and may shed virus for up to 1 wk if sufficiently stressed. Although survival in the environment depends on the temperature, humidity, and medium, the virus generally does not survive >2 wk outside the live pig. Most animals become infected by direct contact with pigs that are shedding virus. Infection by ingesting contaminated tissue or inhaling contaminated aerosol is less common, although aerosol transmission over significant distances does appear to occur.

The pathogenesis and disease expression is similar in all susceptible species. The virus is taken into the oronasal passages and initiates infection in epithelial cells; it travels in the axoplasm of the cranial nerves to the brain, and simultaneously, infects the upper respiratory tract and may progress to the alveoli. Viremia is intermittent and of low titer, but does give the virus access to all parts of the body.

Clinical Findings: The incubation period in pigs is 30-48 hr. The first signs are sneezing and coughing, followed quickly by pyrexia, anorexia, and lassitude. Neurologic involvement may follow and is manifest by trembling, incoordination, convulsions, and coma. Vomiting and diarrhea occur in some young pigs. Death may occur 3-6 days after infection. Mortality may approach 100% in suckling pigs, but decreases with increasing age; few if any adults die. Incidence of abortion, mummification, and/or stillborn piglets may increase depending on the stage of gestation at infection. After the initial outbreak in a herd, passive immunity protects the pigs until 6-12 wk old, and signs may be observed only in the growing-finishing pigs. Although outbreaks can cause severe losses, it is not unusual for an infected herd to have no obvious clinical effects.

The disease in cattle, sheep, and goats most often follows a short clinical course of 36-48 hr. There is a brief excitement phase in which cattle occasionally are aggressive; trembling and apparent anxiety occur as respiration rate and salivation increase, and are accompanied by licking of the nares. As the neurologic involvement progresses, pruritus with savage efforts to relieve the itching may develop, and culminate in incoordination, recumbency, convulsion, exhaustion, coma, and death.

The disease in dogs and cats follows a course similar to that in ruminants with certain exceptions. Dogs have not been found to be aggressive, and the length of the syndrome is more variable. In cats, the excitement phase is preceded by a period of sluggishness; at the onset of salivation, mewing becomes persistent and the cat resists being caught. Pruritus may or may not be present in dogs and cats.

Lesions: Congestion of the vessels of the meninges is often grossly evident. Petechiation of the renal papillae and cortex, necrotic tonsillitis, and diffuse necrotic foci in the liver and spleen are seen less frequently. Vesicles are sometimes present on the skin of the nares and the buccal mucosa. Other signs of CNS involvement are the microscopic lesions of nonsuppurative meningoencephalomyelitis, encephalomyelitis, meningitis, and ganglioneuritis. Occasionally, eosinophilic intranuclear inclusions may be found in glial cells or neurons. There are necrotic foci of parenchymal cells in the tonsils, liver, spleen, and lungs.

Diagnosis: Tentative diagnosis may be based on history, prevalence of pseudorabies in the area, clinical signs, and postmortem lesions. When clinical signs are mild, differential diagnoses include: for suckling pigs—*Escherichia coli, Streptococcus suis*, transmissible gastroenteritis, hemagglutinating encephalomyelitis virus; for growing-finishing pigs—chlorinated hydrocarbon or arsenical toxicity, *S suis*, water deprivation; for adults—parvovirus, encephalomyocarditis virus, leptospirosis, or influenza virus. Virus isolation or FA technique may be used to detect virus in tissues. Tonsil and brain are best, but liver, spleen, and lung may be positive. Abnormal fetuses may also yield virus. Serological tests, including serum neutralization, ELISA, and latex agglutination, are commonly used to detect pigs that had been exposed ≥2 wk previously.

In other species, the usually dramatic clinical signs combined with a history of exposure to pigs are quite suggestive.

Control: There is no treatment. Attenuated and inactivated vaccines are effective in preventing disease, but do not prevent infection by field virus. Vaccinated pigs also shed virus after infection with field strain, although at lower concentrations and for shorter periods than do nonvaccinated infected pigs. Genetically altered vaccines are available; accompanying serological tests allow vaccinated pigs to be differentiated from those infected with field strain of virus. Each of these tests is designed to be used in conjunction with a specific vaccine.

To maintain a herd free of pseudorabies virus: 1) add only seronegative pigs to the herd; 2) avoid visiting infected premises and deny public access to the pigs' facility; 3) keep wildlife, particularly feral pigs and stray animals, away from the herd; and 4) avoid using equipment from other premises. In case of an outbreak, isolation of noninfected pigs may limit the spread within the herd.

RABIES

An acute, viral encephalomyelitis that affects all warm-blooded animals. The mortality rate is close to 100%. Although rabies occurs throughout the world, a few countries are free of the disease due to successful eradication programs, or by virtue of their island status or enforcing rigorous quarantine regulations.

Etiology and Epidemiology: Of the 4 lyssavirus serotypes currently recognized, serotype 1 is responsible for classical terrestrial animal rabies. Serotypes 2, 3, and 4 are rabies-related viruses that have antigenic and epidemiological differences from rabies proper. Rabies viruses recently identified in European bats are currently classified as serotype 4.

The predominant animal species in which rabies is maintained varies in different parts of the world. Dog rabies predominates in Africa, Asia, Latin America, and the Middle East. In North America and Europe, where dog rabies has been effectively controlled, the disease is maintained in wildlife species. In North America, skunk, raccoon, and fox rabies are each found in fairly distinct geographic regions, although some overlap in distribution occurs. These distribution differences can also be detected as differences in viral strains by monoclonal antibody typing, with a "skunk-associated" or "raccoon-associated" strain predominating in a given region. Bat rabies is distributed throughout the USA, and monoclonal antibody typing can differentiate rabies viruses of bat origin from those of terrestrial wildlife origin. In Europe, fox rabies predominates. In certain parts of northern Europe, rabies in the raccoon dog is of increasing concern, and it now appears that rabies in serotine bats may be widely distributed in Europe. The vampire bat is an important reservoir in Mexico, Central and South America, and parts of the Carribean, and is the source of outbreaks in cattle. Other wildlife species may play an important role in the maintenance of rabies in certain areas, including mongooses in the Carribean and southern Africa, jackals in certain parts of Africa, and wolves in parts of northern Europe.

Transmission and Pathogenesis: Transmission is usually by the bite of a rabid animal, via saliva rich in virus. Less commonly, virus may be introduced into existing cuts or wounds on skin, or through intact or abraded mucous membrane. Virus may be present in the saliva and be transmitted by an infected animal some days before onset of clinical signs. Rarely, transmission has been recorded by nonsalivary routes. These include aerosol transmission to man in the laboratory and in bat-infested caves.

The incubation period is prolonged and variable. Most cases in dogs occur within 21-80 days after exposure, but the incubation period may be shorter or considerably longer.

Most infections occur by the deposition of infected saliva into muscle or mucous membranes. Following replication at the site, the virus travels via the peripheral nerves to the spinal cord and ascends to the brain. The considerable interval during which the virus remains at the inoculation site justifies the local infiltration of hyper-immune serum as one of the treatment methods advocated for use in man. Having reached the brain, the virus usually travels from the CNS and reaches the salivary glands via their nerve supply. It is rare to find virus in the salivary gland and not in the brain. Hematogenous spread can occur but is rare. Although the disease usually is fatal once clinical signs appear, recovery has been recorded in several animals, including man.

Clinical Findings: Rabid animals of all species exhibit typical signs of CNS disturbance, with minor variations peculiar to carnivores, ruminants, bats, and man. (*See also* p 588.) The clinical course, particularly in dogs, can be divided into 3 phases: the prodromal, the excitative, and the paralytic. The term "furious rabies" refers to animals in which the excitative phase is predominant, and "dumb or paralytic rabies" to those in which the excitative phase is extremely short or absent and the disease progresses quickly to the paralytic phase. In any animal, the first sign is a change in behavior, which may be indistinguishable from a GI disorder, injury, foreign body in the mouth, poisoning, or an early infectious disease. Temperature change is not significant, and driveling may or may not be noted. Animals usually stop eating and drinking and may seek solitude. Frequently, the urogenital tract is irritated or stimulated as evidenced by frequent urination, erection in the male, and sexual desire. After the prodromal period of 1-3 days, animals either show signs of paralysis or become vicious. Carnivora, pigs, and occasionally, horses and mules bite other animals or people at the slightest provocation. Cattle butt any moving object. The disease progresses rapidly after the onset of paralysis, and death is virtually certain within 10 days of the first signs.

Paralytic Form: This is characterized by early paralysis of the throat and masseter muscles, usually with profuse salivation and inability to swallow. Dropping of the lower jaw is common in dogs. Owners frequently examine the mouth of dogs and cattle, searching for a foreign body, or administer medication with the bare hands, thereby exposing themselves to rabies. These animals are not vicious and rarely attempt to bite. The paralysis progresses rapidly to all parts of the body, and coma and death follow in a few hours.

Furious Form: This is the classical "mad-dog syndrome" in which the animal becomes irrational and viciously aggressive. The facial expression is one of alertness and anxiety, with pupils dilated; noise invites attack. Such animals lose all caution and fear of natural enemies. There is no evidence of paralysis during the excitatory stage. Dogs rarely live >10 days after the onset of signs. Dogs with this form of rabies frequently roam streets and highways, biting other animals, people, and any moving object. They commonly swallow foreign objects, eg, feces, straw, sticks, and stones. Rabid dogs chew the wire and frame of their cages, breaking their teeth, and will follow a hand moved in front of the cage, attempting to bite. Young pups apparently seek human companionship and are overly playful, but bite even when petted, usually becoming vicious in a few hours. As the disease progresses, muscular incoordination and seizures become common. Death is the result of progressive paralysis.

Rabid domestic cats and bobcats attack suddenly, biting and scratching viciously. Rabid foxes frequently invade yards or even houses, attacking dogs and people. The irrationality of behavior that can occur is demonstrated in the fox that attacks a porcupine; finding a fox with porcupine quills can, in most cases, support a diagnosis of rabies. Rabid foxes and skunks are responsible for most pasture cattle losses, and have attacked cattle in barns.

The rabid raccoon is characterized by its loss of fear of man, its frequent aggression and incoordination, and its activity during the day, being predominantly a nocturnal animal. In urban areas, they often attack domestic dogs.

Rabies in cattle follows the same general pattern, and those with the furious form are dangerous, attacking and pursuing man and other animals. Lactation ceases abruptly in dairy cattle. Instead of the usual placid expression, there is one of alertness. The eyes and ears follow sounds and movement. A most typical clinical sign in cattle is a characteristic bellowing. This may continue intermittently until shortly before death.

Horses and mules may show extreme agitation evidenced by rolling as with colic. As with other species, they may bite or strike viciously and, because of size and strength, become unmanageable in a few hours. Such animals frequently suffer self-inflicted wounds.

In general, rabies should be suspected in terrestrial wildlife acting abnormally. The same is true of bats that are observed flying in the daytime, resting on the ground, attacking people and animals, or fighting. Insectivorous bats, though small, can inflict a wound with their teeth and should never be caught or handled with bare hands.

Diagnosis: Clinical diagnosis is usually possible but may be difficult; in the prodromal stage, rabies may easily be confused with other diseases. In all species of animals, inability to swallow saliva is suggestive of an obstruction in the throat, a foreign body lodged between the teeth, or ingestion of irritating substances. Furthermore, many normal animals fight when injured, when provoked, or for possession of food or a mate; cats, particularly males, may make sudden unprovoked attacks on other animals or man. All of these behavior patterns may be present with rabies, but also can be unrelated.

The FA staining technique on fresh brain tissue combines the speed of histological techniques with the greater sensitivity of biological examination. The test is based on direct visual observation of a specific antigen-antibody reaction. Brain tissues examined must include hippocampus, medulla oblongata, and cerebellum (and should be preserved by refrigeration with wet ice or cold packs). When properly used, it can establish a highly specific diagnosis within a few hours, and it has become the test of choice in most laboratories. Although utilized by many laboratories as a back-up procedure, results of the mouse inoculation test rarely disagree with the FA test.

Control: Based on reduction or elimination of cases in domestic carnivores and the appropriate wildlife reservoir, control programs work best on a national or regional basis. Comprehensive guidelines for control in dogs have been prepared by the World Health Organization and include: 1) notification of suspected cases, and destruction of dogs with clinical signs and those bitten by a suspected rabid animal; 2) reduction of contact rates between susceptible dogs by leash laws, dog movement control, and quarantine; 3) mass immunization of dogs by campaigns and by continuing vaccination of young dogs; 4) stray dog control and destruction of unvaccinated dogs with low levels of dependency on, or restriction by, man; and 5) dog registration.

Many effective vaccines are available throughout the world; in the USA, there are currently 19 approved for use in dogs by the National Association of State Public Health Veterinarians (NASPHV), of which 18 are inactivated. Modified live virus (MLV) vaccines are still in widespread use for dogs in many other parts of the world. Recommended vaccination frequency is 1 or 3 years (manufacturer's recommendations should be followed). Several NASPHV-approved vaccines are also available for use in cats, and a few for use in horses and domestic livestock. No NASPHV-approved vaccine is available for use in wildlife kept as pets, and protective immunity from the commercially available vaccines in these species has not been demonstrated.

Until recently, the control of rabies in wildlife populations relied on the destruction of wildlife in an attempt to reduce the contact rate between susceptible animals. However, this proved ineffective and has led to the widespread (and effective) use of oral MLV vaccines distributed in baits to control fox rabies in Europe. The disease has now been eradicated from Switzerland. Further research is underway in an attempt to apply this method to the control of wildlife rabies in North America, and to assist in the control of dog rabies in developing countries.

Management of Suspected Rabies Cases—Exposure of Pets: It is important to ascertain whether exposure to rabies infection has occurred. It should be presumed that a domestic animal has been exposed if saliva or nervous tissue from a rabid or potentially rabid animal could have had direct contact with mucous membranes or a break in the skin, even though an actual bite was not witnessed or the potentially infective animal was not available for testing. Where terrestrial wildlife or bat rabies are known to occur, any domestic animal that is bitten or scratched by a wild carnivore or bat that is not available for testing should be regarded as having been exposed to a rabid animal. The NASPHV recommends that any unvaccinated dog or cat exposed to rabies infection be destroyed immediately. If the owner is unwilling to do this, the animal should be placed in strict isolation for 6 mo and vaccinated against rabies 1 mo before release. If vaccination of an exposed animal is current, it should be revaccinated immediately and confined for 90 days observation.

Exposure of Man: When a person is exposed to an animal suspected of having rabies, the circumstances should be evaluated carefully. This should include consideration of the species of animal involved, the rabies risk in the area, whether exposure sufficient to transmit rabies virus occurred, and the current disposition of the animal and its availability for diagnostic testing. Wild carnivores and bats present a considerable risk where the disease occurs, and abnormal behavior may not be present when the animals are rabid. Any wild carnivore or bat suspected of exposing a person to rabies should, if feasible, be tested. In some countries it is considered that any wildlife species in which rabies is known to occur and that has exposed man or a domestic animal is rabid unless proved otherwise. Exposure of people to rabies from their "pet" wildlife should be considered likewise. Any healthy dog or cat, whether vaccinated against rabies or not, that exposes a person should be confined for 10 days; if the animal develops any signs of rabies during that period, it should be destroyed humanely and its brain promptly submitted for rabies diagnosis. If the dog or cat responsible for the exposure is stray or unwanted, it should be destroyed immediately and submitted for rabies diagnosis.

Human Immunization: It is strongly recommended that all people in high-risk groups of the population, such as veterinary practitioners, animal control officers, rabies and diagnostic laboratory workers, and people travelling to countries in which dog rabies is endemic receive pre-exposure immunization. However, pre-exposure prophylaxis cannot be relied on in the event of subsequent rabies exposure and must be supplemented by a limited postexposure immunization regimen.

SCRAPIE
(Tremblante du mouton, Rida)

A degenerative neurologic disease of sheep, it is the prototype of the "slow virus" infections that produce subacute spongiform encephalopathies in animals and man. Each of transmissible mink encephalopathy (TME), chronic wasting disease of captive mule deer and elk, kuru, Creutzfeldt-Jakob disease, and bovine spongiform encephalopathy (BSE, qv, p 577) is defined by the clinicopathologic features in their natural hosts; all are transmissible to other species in which they are virtually indistinguishable.

Etiology, Transmission, and Pathogenesis: The causal neuropathogens have properties so unusual that they are called "unconventional viruses". Although viral or subviral in size, the lack of identification of any agent-specific nucleic acids or proteins has severely limited progress in their characterization and lead to speculation that they represent new forms of "infectious" entities capable of producing cell death and tissue degeneration.

Scrapie is naturally transmitted to susceptible sheep by contact with infected animals or pastures. There is no clear evidence that it is vertically transmitted in the genome or by embryo transfer, despite its common familial occurrence. During the first year after natural exposure, presumably orally, the agent slowly replicates in lymphoreticular tissues before spreading to the CNS, either by intermittent hematogenous seeding of the blood-brain barrier or by centripetal passage along nerve pathways. Once in the CNS, the scrapie agent replicates. Degeneration of targeted neurons after 2 yr of age results in onset of clinical signs.

Susceptibility to infection by natural exposure is controlled genetically. In the USA, it is almost exclusively a disease of purebred sheep, notably Suffolks.

Clinical Findings: The onset is insidious. Affected sheep become more excitable, and fine tremors of the head and neck may be observed. The most characteristic feature is intense pruritus, which often begins over the rump. In some cases, the pruritus makes it difficult for the animal to feed and rest normally. Nervous signs may be elicited from a quiet but affected sheep by sudden noise or movement. The wool is dry, separable, and brittle, which results in loss of fleece over large areas. Other areas may be rubbed raw. Occasionally, convulsions occur. When made to trot, there is often a peculiar hypermetria of the forelegs, sometimes with galloping movements of the hindlegs. After 2-6 mo of progressive neurologic deterioration characterized by emaciation, weakness, and ataxia, the affected sheep becomes totally debilitated and soon dies.

Lesions: Lesions are microscopic and confined to the CNS; they include microvacuolation of the gray matter and neuronal degeneration and astrocytic hypertrophy. There are no inflammatory cell infiltrates, and no agent-specific immune reactions have been demonstrated. Examinations of infected brain material for virus-like particles have been unsuccessful, but amyloid-like fibrils have been identified and found to be specific. These structures, called scrapie-associated fibrils (SAF), are composed of a single sialoglycoprotein (prion protein) which is coded for by a host gene. Regulation of this gene is thought to be important in determining the length of the incubation period in experimentally infected mice, and may also be important in sheep susceptibility.

Diagnosis: This is based on clinical signs, flock history, and microscopical examination of the CNS. Studies are in progress to determine if isolation of SAF and detection of prion protein by Western blot analysis can be used to supplement clinicopathologic findings.

Epidemiology and Control: There is no treatment. Sheep, goats, mink, mule deer, elk, and cattle are presently affected, but it is not known which are incidental hosts and which are potential sources of natural infection for other species. Goats seem to be incidental hosts; their rare infections are associated with commingling with scrapie-infected sheep or exposure to contaminated pastures. Captive mule deer and elk may become affected only after being housed in facilities previously used for sheep. Mink are dead-end hosts that were originally thought to become exposed only when scrapie-infected sheep tissues were fed to ranch-reared mink. However, recent epidemiological studies of TME suggest that cattle may also be a source of infection. Other studies on BSE in the UK indicate that this new explosive outbreak may have resulted from feeding contaminated processed animal protein supplements to dairy cattle.

One of the main concerns of infections that affect both man and other animals is whether they are zoonotic, eg, there is no evidence that the occurrence of Creutzfeldt-Jakob disease is influenced by contact with any animal species.

Following first appearance in the USA (in 1947), the Scrapie Eradication Program was established. This involved identification of affected animals and destruction of all sheep in the flock as well as other exposed flocks. This procedure was modified in 1983 to destroy mainly bloodline animals because of the strong familial occurrence of the disease.

SPORADIC BOVINE ENCEPHALOMYELITIS
(SBE, Chlamydial encephalomyelitis)

Outbreaks of SBE have occurred in various parts of the world. Reports indicate that chlamydiae can also cause infections of the brain in man, opossums, dogs, and several avian species.

Etiology and Epidemiology: SBE is caused by immunotype 2 strains of *Chlamydia psittaci*. Isolates of *C psittaci* from cattle and sheep fall into 5 immunotypes. Immunotype 2 strains have also been isolated from lambs and calves with polyarthritis (qv, p 470), conjunctivitis (qv, p 294), and enteritis (qv, p 137).

Subclinical intestinal infections in cattle as well as other animals are probably much more common than reported, and may well be the source of infection in chlamydial encephalomyelitis. It is not understood why in sporadic cases chlamydiae leave a balanced host-parasite relationship in the intestine, penetrate the intestinal barrier, establish a blood-infectious phase, and infect the brain as the target organ.

The disease is most often seen in cattle 3 mo to 3 yr old. Morbidity rates are usually low but can reach 50%; many of the sick calves die if not treated at an early stage.

Clinical Findings and Lesions: The incubation period in experimentally infected calves is 6-30 days. The first sign in natural and experimental cases is fever (104-107°F). The temperature remains elevated until shortly before death or recovery. Appetite remains good for the first 2-3 days despite the fever. Afterward, depression, excess salivation, diarrhea, anorexia, and weight loss occur. Calves are incoordinated and stagger or fall over objects. Head pressing and blindness are not observed. In the terminal stage, the calves are frequently recumbent and may develop opisthotonus. The course of the disease is usually 10-14 days.

Lesions are not limited to the brain; vascular damage can be seen in many different organs. Serofibrinous peritonitis, pleuritis, and pericarditis are common, and are especially pronounced in more chronic cases. Microscopic lesions in the brain consist of perivascular cuffs and inflammatory foci in the parenchyma composed primarily of mononuclear cells.

Diagnosis: A tentative diagnosis can be based on clinical signs and particularly on the presence of a serofibrinous peritonitis in the absence of causes of peritonitis such as intestinal volvolus, intussusceptions, traumatic perforations of the reticulum, perforated abomasal ulcers, or displaced organs. Differential diagnoses also include rabies, infectious bovine rhinotracheitis/encephalitis, listeriosis, thromboembolic encephalomalacia, polioencephalomyelitis, pseudorabies, and malignant catarrhal fever. A diagnosis of SBE is confirmed by isolation of the organism from brain tissue in either developing chicken embryos or cell cultures, by histological changes in brain sections, or by evaluation of tissue impression smears after Giemsa or immunofluorescent staining.

Treatment: The antibiotics of choice are tetracyclines, oxytetracyclines, and tylosin. For treatment to be effective, it must be given as early as possible in the disease course, in high doses (eg, oxytetracyclines at 20-50 mg/kg/day) and for ≥1 wk. If effective, the fever should drop significantly within 24 hr. Vaccines are not available.

TICK PARALYSIS

A toxin-induced, afebrile, ascending, symmetrical, flaccid tetraplegia with functional impediment to the reflexes of the superficial and deep tendons of the limbs and abdomen. This syndrome differs both clinically and etiologically from all viral encephalitides and other tick-borne diseases. The host range depends principally on the vertebrate preference of the tick species involved. Accordingly, man, especially children, and a wide variety of mammals as well as birds and marsupials may be affected. Dogs are affected most commonly but losses can occur in cats, lambs, calves, goats, and foals. Rapid modern transport may be responsible for spread of tick paralysis to other regions, not necessarily limited to the locale of the particular tick species.

Although the disease has an almost worldwide distribution, some responsible tick species are of particular relevance in certain regions. For human medicine these are, in Australia, *Ixodes holocyclus*, and in North America, *Dermacentor andersoni* and *D variabilis*. Of particular interest in veterinary medicine are the same species as well as *I rubicundus* (Karoo tick paralysis) in South Africa, *Rhipicephalus evertsi evertsi*, and *Argas (Persicargas) walkerae* in sub-Saharan Africa and, probably, *A (Persicargas) radiatus* in North America.

Etiology, Epidemiology, and Pathogenesis: The potential for inducing paralysis has been demonstrated, described, or suspected in 54 species of ticks belonging to 7 ixodid and 3 argasid genera. The substance responsible for tick paralysis is generally assumed to be a neurotoxin. Several hypotheses regarding the nature of the toxin describe it either as a product of the tick *per se*, as a toxic metabolite resulting from the interaction of tick saliva with host tissue, or as a product of a microbial organism or symbiont.

Toxicity is associated principally with female ixodid ticks and is limited, at least in *R evertsi evertsi*, to a brief sucking phase of a few hours between day 4 and 5 of infestation. The toxicity of female ticks is initiated, or at least partially activated, by copulation and successful transfer of spermatophores. In most argasid ticks, however, the larvae are the causative stage.

Host parameters that influence epidemiology include sensitivity to toxin, age, immunity, behavior, reactivity, and population density. Antitoxic immunity, starting at least 2 wk after primary tick exposure and lasting a few weeks, can be boosted by further infestations. Tick factors include the dynamics and virulence of paralysis-inducing capability, sexual activity, rate of infestation, and the sucking phase. Maximal incidence of tick paralysis is always associated with seasonal activity of female ticks, and occurs mainly in spring and early summer.

Tick paralysis is a motor polyneuropathy, and involvement of the afferent pathways is limited, although recent studies suggest that sensory and autonomic pathways are also affected. The neurotoxin circulates in the host animal and interferes with acetylcholine liberation at the neuromuscular junction. Functional impairment during paralysis also affects the efferent nerve fibers that serve the respiratory muscles; as a result, carbon dioxide levels increase, and the partial oxygen pressure and blood pH fall. Respiratory acidosis impairs the organs that influence hemodynamic functions.

Clinical Findings: The incubation period, which depends on the duration of tick feeding, is usually 5-7 days. Hindlimb paralysis is initially characterized by slight to pronounced incoordination and weakness. These signs intensify and extend within a few hours; the animal becomes unable to move fore- or hindlegs, or to stand or sit. Sensation usually is preserved. There are also nystagmus and difficulties in breathing, chewing, and swallowing. Death can occur in several hours from respiratory paralysis. Temperature is normal; blood and humoral values are unchanged. In the latter stages of tick paralysis, acute ventilatory failure, pulmonary congestion, moderate hypoxemia, and a mild nonrespiratory acidosis have been documented. Elevated serum levels of CPK also have been reported in canine tick paralysis caused by *D andersoni* and *I holocyclus*. Phosphate levels are reportedly elevated in the latter stages of paralysis caused by *I holocyclus*. There are no morphologically manifest lesions. Electrophysiological studies reveal diminution of maximal motor nerve conduction velocities; decrease in nerve compound action potentials, as well as in the compound potentials from the corresponding muscles; and impairment of impulse propagation of afferent fibers and the simultaneously required heightening of the stimulating current potentials necessary to elicit a response. The encephalogram is normal. Paralysis peaks within a few hours; recovery is rapid (1-3 days) and complete if the ticks are removed in time. In dogs with tick paralysis caused by *I holocyclus*, several stages of the disease have been outlined: 1) weakness, 2) inability to walk, 3) inability to right, 4) inability to right and loss of withdrawal reflexes, and 5) moribund state, with death following within 2 hr.

Diagnosis: This is based on the presence of ticks, sudden appearance of paralysis, rapid course, and quick clinical recovery after tick removal. As a rule, and unlike other tick-borne diseases of the peripheral nervous system, temperature is normal, and blood and fluid values are unchanged. Specific laboratory diagnostic techniques are not available.

Botulism and polyradiculoneuritis (in dogs, qv, p 590) are differential diagnoses.

Treatment and Control: Treatment of tick paralysis is limited to the timely removal of attached ticks, either manually or by using a suitable acaricide dip or sponge-on. A therapeutically effective immune serum is available only for *I holocyclus* paralysis. The prognosis for this form of tick paralysis is doubtful even with tick removal, acaricide treatment, and hyperimmune serum. Treatment is supportive.

Prophylactic biological or chemical control (or both) of ticks, and adherence to certain husbandry practices may greatly reduce the risk of paralysis. Active immunization by injection of crude and purified extracts of salivary glands of *I holocyclus* also may be considered.

PHYSICAL INFLUENCES

COLD

HYPOTHERMIA

A profound fall in body temperature resulting from exposure to external cold, effects of drugs, or failure of internal temperature-regulating mechanisms. In endotherms, hypothermia can be classified as mild, moderate, or profound when the body temperature is 86-89.5°F (30-32°C), 71.5-77°F (22-25°C), or 32-46.5°F (0-8°C), respectively. The prognosis varies accordingly.

Hypothermia in neonates (especially piglets and lambs) is an important cause of death. Susceptibility is greatest during their first 48 hr. Drafts and faulty or misplaced infrared lamps are the main causes in piglets; inclement weather and wet birth coats are the main ones in lambs. Chilled piglets may crowd close to the sow, which increases the risk of death by crushing. Shivering, lowered ability and instinct to nurse, and burning calories for heat rather than growth and energy lead to death through the hypothermia/starvation syndrome.

Rewarming and maintenance of normal body temperature can be accomplished externally or internally. In external or surface warming, the body surface is warmed by warm water immersion, blankets, warm room, hot water bottles, etc. Shock can be avoided during rewarming by warming slowly, if possible. In more critical cases when rewarming quickly is important, peritoneal dialysis with the dialysate preheated to 122-131°F (50-55°C) provides an excellent method of internal or core warming. Neonates require not only rewarming but careful attention to nutritional needs.

FROSTBITE

Destruction of superficial tissues as a result of exposure to cold with secondary structural and functional disturbances of the smaller surface blood vessels. Frostbite is not uncommon in young animals, especially poorly nourished calves and foals exposed to storms and extreme cold. (*See also* p 498.) Pigs farrowed in extreme cold may suffer from frostbite of exposed parts, especially the ears and tail. Sometimes the combs of chickens are affected. (*See also* HYPOTHERMIA, above.)

Slight frosting causes the skin to become pale and bloodless. This is soon followed by intense redness, heat, pain, and swelling. In such cases, the hair may fall out and the epidermis may peel. Usually, the inflammation subsides, the swelling disappears, and only an increased sensitivity to cold remains; irritation and itching may continue for some time.

If freezing is more severe, the affected part becomes swollen and painful, remains cold, and later begins to shrivel. In severe cases, patches of skin are devitalized, and a line of demarcation forms between the affected and normal parts. Finally, the destroyed portion sloughs and leaves a raw surface.

Small, simple lesions may be treated with mild antiseptics and thoroughly covered with healing ointment. Simple frostbite is treated by rapidly warming the affected part by water bath or pack (105-108°F [40.5-42°C]) for 15-20 min, and by applying antiseptic dressing. As sensation returns, self-trauma should be prevented. Severe freezing may be treated conservatively until a line of demarcation appears. The necrotic portion of severely affected tissue should then be removed surgically and the defect treated as an open wound.

ELECTRIC SHOCK

LIGHTNING STROKE AND ELECTROCUTION

Injury or death of an animal due to high-voltage electrical currents may be the result of lightning, fallen transmission wires, faulty electrical circuits, or chewing on an electrical cord (*see also* ELECTRIC SHOCK, SM AN, p 635). Lightning stroke is seasonal and tends to be geographically restricted.

Certain types of trees, especially those that are tall and have spreading root systems just beneath the ground surface, tend to be struck by lightning more often than others. Electrification of such roots charges a wide surface area, particularly when the ground is already damp; passage of charged roots beneath a shallow pool of water causes it to become electrified. A tile drain may spread an electric charge over an entire field. Fallen transmission wires also may electrify a pool of water. Differences exist in conductivity of soil; loam, sand, clay, marble, and chalk (in decreasing order) are good conductors, while rocky soil is not.

Accidental electrocution of farm animals usually occurs as a result of faulty wiring. Electrification of a water or milk line, or a metal creep or guard rail can result in widespread distribution of an electric current throughout the stable (*see also* STRAY VOLTAGE IN ANIMAL HOUSING, below).

Death from electric shock usually results from cardiac or respiratory arrest; passage of current through the heart usually produces ventricular fibrillation; involvement of the CNS may affect the respiratory or other vital centers.

Clinical Findings: Varying degrees of electric shock may occur. In most instances of lightning stroke, death is instantaneous, and the animal falls without a struggle. Occasionally, the animal becomes unconscious but may recover in a few minutes to several hours; residual nervous signs, eg, depression, paraplegia, cutaneous hyperesthesia, may persist for days or weeks, or be permanent. Singe marks on the carcass, damage to the immediate environment, or both, occur in ~90% of cases of lightning stroke, but are less likely to be found if the animal is electrocuted by standing on electrified earth. Singe marks tend to be linear and are more commonly found on the medial sides of the legs, although rarely much of the body may be affected. Beneath the singe marks, capillary congestion is common; the arboreal pattern characteristic of lightning stroke can be visualized best from the dermal side of the skin by subcut. extravasations of blood. Singe marks are difficult to find on the recovered animal. Smaller animals such as pigs that contact electrified water bowls or creeps may be killed instantly or be thrown across the pen from the strength of the shock.

Diagnosis: History of a recent storm may be confusing; finding a dead or injured animal under a tree or near a fence is significant only if one finds evidence of recent burning of bark, splitting of fence posts, welding of wire, etc. *Rigor mortis* develops and passes quickly. Postmortem distention of the rumen occurs rapidly and must be differentiated from antemortem ruminal tympany (qv, p 163); in both conditions, the blood tends to clot slowly or not at all. The mucosae of the upper respiratory tract, including the turbinates and sinuses are congested and hemorrhagic; linear tracheal hemorrhages are common, but the lungs are not compressed as in bloat. All other viscera are congested, and petechiae and ecchymoses may be found in many organs. Due to postmortem ruminal distention, the poorly clotted blood is passively moved to the periphery of the body, resulting in postmortem extravasation of blood in muscles and superficial lymph nodes of the head, neck, and thoracic limbs, and to a lesser extent, in the hindquarters. Probably the best indication of instantaneous death is the presence of hay or other feed in the animal's mouth; supportive evidence includes the presence of normal ingesta (especially in the rumen), lack of frothy ingesta (frothy bloat), absence of a distended gallbladder, and presence of normal feces in the lower tract and occasionally on the ground behind the animal. Bone fractures occur occasionally.

Treatment: Those animals that survive may require supportive and symptomatic therapy.

STRAY VOLTAGE IN ANIMAL HOUSING

The term "stray voltage" refers to small electric currents that flow through a barn; when of sufficient voltage, they can pass through an animal's body and adversely affect its behavior. The electrical resistance of the cow is usually lower than that of man; thus, she may be affected by voltages too low to be perceived by the dairyman. The pathway from mouth to hooves is the most sensitive. It is generally believed that for cows the threshold of behavioral modification is 0.5-1 volt of alternating current (AC); higher levels produce correspondingly greater alterations. At 2 volts AC, 90% of cows can be expected to respond. Intermittent exposure seems to be more disturbing than continuous exposure. Even when the threshold is exceeded, not all the animals respond all the time, nor with the same signs, but as the voltage increases, signs in the herd are more widespread and uniform.

A growing amount of evidence suggests there is no relationship between behavioral responses to stray voltage and physiological or hormonal responses. There is no apparent relationship between behavioral modifications and milk production.

Stray voltage problems can also affect beef cattle, pigs, and poultry, although less frequently, because the electrical demand in those operations is lower.

Clinical Findings: No one sign is pathognomonic: a wide variety of signs has been reported in cows exposed to different levels of stray voltage. Documented signs are behavioral changes, decreased drinks of water per day, and decreased length of time per drink. Amount of water consumed is not affected. Intermittent periods of poor performance, poor milk let-down and incomplete or uneven milk-out, abnormal behavior during milking, increased milking time, refusal of feed or water, increased somatic cell counts in milk, and increased mastitis are signs often attributed to stray voltage that may also be caused by other factors, such as abusive cow handling, faulty milking machine, poor milking techniques and hygiene, and nutritional deficiencies. Therefore, a thorough investigation should be conducted before stray voltage is blamed as the sole cause.

Signs in pigs are similar, although growing pigs are 2.5 times more resistant to stray voltage than dairy cows. Sows show aggressive behavior, reduced appetite, lowered water consumption, and uneven milking (increased starve-out in litters). Post-farrowing anorexia with some constipation is a major complaint.

The problem in poultry is not well defined, but a significant mortality rate has been reported in turkey poults.

Diagnosis: For confirmation, a potential of ≥1 volt AC must be measured between 2 points that a cow might contact, and some cows should exhibit signs of exposure. Voltage levels may need to be monitored at different times of the day and on different days since the threshold level may be exceeded intermittently. When exposure during milking is suspected, measurements should be made with all electrical milking equipment turned on (both 110 and 220 volt). Although levels of exposure between 0.5 and 1 volts AC are thought not to be detrimental, farms on which these levels have been detected should be monitored to ensure that higher levels do not occur intermittently. Since electrical usage is greater in the evening than in the morning, stray voltage may be more of a problem during evening milkings.

Stray voltage can be measured point-to-point or point-to-reference ground. Point-to-point refers to measurements made between 2 contact points that the cow might touch simultaneously. Point-to-reference ground measurements utilize, as one measuring point, a 4 ft (1.3 m) copper-clad rod driven into the ground ≥25 ft (8.5 m) from any grounding rods or electrical equipment, and a cow as the other contact point. Both methods have been used satisfactorily. Long, insulated meter leads (6-10 ft [2-3 m]) facilitate taking measurements on the farm. The voltmeter should have a full scale reading of 2-5 volts in 0.1 volt increments. It is advisable to have a qualified electrician evaluate the situation and devise corrective action. If ≥1 volts are detected, the source should be determined: an electrician can do so by measuring the voltage between an isolated reference ground rod representing true earth and a ground wire at the barn service entrance under different loads.

An on-farm problem needs immediate correction for the safety of people and livestock. If voltage varies >0.5 volts in the absence of any on-farm load or approaches 1 volt with typical on-farm loads included, the problem is off-farm, and the local power supplier should be contacted about possible solutions.

Prevention and Control: Most on-farm sources of stray voltage are due to wiring systems that do not meet the usual standards. Deficiencies may include actual ground faults (shorts), undersized wiring, loose or corroded connections, or wiring damaged by animals, accidents, or moisture. An electrician should examine the system and repair any defects. Elimination of off- or on-farm sources created by nonfaulty 240-volt service usually is the responsibility of the utility company.

The response of cows varies when stray voltage is eliminated, depending on the length, magnitude, and consistency of exposure. When exposure has been low (<2.5 volts), recovery from abnormal behavior may be almost immediate; when exposure has been to higher voltages, behavior may not change until cows have left the milking herd and gone through a dry period. When exposure has been through feeding or watering, response is usually prompt, but the response reflected by production and new cases of mastitis is variable. The reservoir of mastitis will remain until it is controlled by an udder health program.

Electrical systems should comply with the code standards at all times. Whenever suggestive signs cannot be attributed to other causes, measurements should be taken to determine if a voltage potential exists, and the results recorded for future comparisons. Monitors are available for continuous on-farm surveillance.

HEAT

BURNS

The destruction of epithelium or deeper tissues by direct heat, radiant heat, flames, friction, electricity, or corrosive chemicals.

Etiology: Thermal burns result from scalding with hot liquids, contact with hot objects, or exposure to flame or radiant heat. Pigs, dogs (especially the "hairless" breeds), and closely shorn sheep may suffer radiant heat burns (sunburn). Burns resulting from friction most commonly are caused by rubbing rough ropes against the skin during restraint of large animals, or by dragging or rubbing the skin along pavement in small animals hit by motor vehicles. In large animals, electrical burns most commonly are caused by lightning stroke (qv, p 628) in open pastures and less frequently by contact with live electric wires (as in small animals, qv, p 635). In small animals, electrical burns are most often the result of chewing an electrical cord or use of a defective hair dryer. Corrosive chemicals include acids, phenols, and strong alkalies. *See also* PHOTOSENSITIZATION, p 820.

Clinical Findings: Burns in animals are not strictly comparable to those of man. First-degree burns with reddening of the skin may occur, but formation of vesicles and blisters is uncommon except in pigs. The usual lesion of a moderately severe burn in animals is diffuse edema of the skin and subcut. tissues, with or without formation of small vesicles and sloughs. Charring of tissue occurs in severe burns, and the skin may be wholly devitalized and the injury may extend into the deeper structures. Sloughing of the skin may follow, leaving large denuded areas from which constant exudation or effusion of serum can lead to considerable loss of protein and fluid. Burns of small areas of the body cause only discomfort; animals with more severe burns are reluctant to move, resent handling, and may be indifferent to normal stimuli. Extensive burns with considerable loss of plasma may result in shock. Later complications include infection, impaired cardiac and liver function, and pneumonitis. The prognosis depends on the total area of the burn, depth of penetration (partial or full thickness), location, and age and condition of the animal.

Treatment: Shock, renal failure, anemia, and respiratory disorders should be treated as necessary. If burns are severe and involve more than 50% of the body, euthanasia should be considered. Less severe burns or those involving smaller areas usually can be treated successfully. Initially, the application of cold packs may reduce pain and edema. The burned area should be clipped since the extent of damage may not be readily visible through the hair, and sloughing of the necrotic tissue may not occur for several days. Cleansing of the wound is imperative to remove sloughing tissue and debris, and can be accomplished by hydrotherapy or local washing with saline or iodine solution. Local application of antibacterial creams such as silver sulfadiazine should follow the cleansing procedure. Occlusive dressings and ointments are contraindicated although light bandages may be necessary. Systemic antibiotics are seldom required.

Sunscreen creams may be used to protect hairless dogs.

HYPERTHERMIA
(Heat exhaustion, Heat cramps, Heatstroke, Sunstroke)

An increase in body temperature to or beyond the point of physiological regulation, generally secondary to high environmental temperature, high humidity, and inadequate ventilation. Exposure to direct rays of the sun may be contributory.

All domestic animals are susceptible to heatstroke. Dogs confined to close quarters in hot weather, and cattle, horses, or other stock being driven in large numbers or being transported in hot weather are affected most commonly. Predisposing factors include physical effort, obesity, and stagnation of the air.

Heat exhaustion occurs in draft horses, cattle, and pigs. It is unusual in dogs. Prolonged exposure to high environmental temperature causes the peripheral blood vessels to dilate. When dilation occurs without a compensatory increase in blood volume, circulatory collapse may ensue.

Heat cramps are most common in animals doing hard work in intense heat. Animals with the ability to sweat are most commonly affected, eg, draft horses. Heat cramps are rare in dogs other than those working or racing in a hot environment. Deranged electrolyte balance (acute salt loss) is the cause.

The outstanding signs of heat exhaustion are weakness, muscle tremors, and collapse. There may be hyperpnea and rapid pulse. Body temperature is not necessarily elevated, and onset of signs is not as sudden as in heatstroke. Heat cramps are characterized by severe muscle spasm, with cessation of sweating in horses and working animals other than dogs.

Clinical signs of heatstroke include hyperpnea and collapse. A staring expression, vomiting, and diarrhea are not uncommon. The oral mucosa may be bright red, and the rectal temperature is greatly elevated (up to 109.5°F [43°C]). Disseminated intravascular coagulation (qv, p 24) and cerebral edema may occur as complicating factors in dogs.

In heat exhaustion, cold water should be applied to the body, and the animal moved to a cool, shaded area. Isotonic saline solution may be given IV to animals suffering from heat cramps. (*See also* VENTILATION, p 1106.)

Heatstroke requires immediate therapy. Animals respond best to immersion in cold water. Cold water enemas are also useful. The rectal temperature should be checked q10min and treatment stopped as the temperature approaches normal. Rectal temperature may not be an accurate indicator if cold water enemas have been used.

HIGH-MOUNTAIN DISEASE
(Brisket disease, Pulmonary hypertensive heart disease)

A noninfectious disease of cattle characterized by the clinical signs and lesions of congestive heart failure (CHF). It affects cattle in high mountain areas of the western USA and South America (usually above 2200 m), and has been reported in certain other mountainous areas of the world. The syndrome may also occur in sheep and deer under extreme stress. A similar disease is of clinical importance in chickens in the Andes Mountains. The incidence in cattle at risk is 0.5-5% but usually is <2%. Occurrence depends on altitude, but not exclusively. Newly introduced cattle tend to be more susceptible than native cattle. In those areas in North America where cattle spend summer and fall grazing at high altitude and return to lower elevation later in the fall, the disease is usually manifest after being at high altitude for ≥2 mo. In areas where cattle live year-round at high altitude, the disease incidence is greater in winter or early spring, presumably due to stress of winter weather. It affects both sexes, all ages, and probably most breeds—but not necessarily equally. It is more common, for instance, in cattle <1 yr old and in steer calves.

Etiology: The disease is related to the chronic hypoxia of a high-altitude environment, which causes pulmonary vasoconstriction, hence pulmonary hypertension and ultimately CHF. The necessity of some other inciting or causative factor(s) is often indicated circumstantially. Absence of the disease on browse-type ranges in certain geographic areas at altitudes as high as 3400 m has been documented, as has high incidence on nearby nonbrowse-type ranges having similar cattle strains and management procedures. Altered chemoreceptor activity and myocardial metabolism have been implicated as possible contributory factors. Recent studies suggest that phenotypic alteration of smooth muscle cells following hypoxic or pressure-induced injury induces extracellular deposition of elastin and collagen in pulmonary vasculature, a contributing factor in the development of right heart failure. Marked variation occurs in individual susceptibility (ostensibly inheritable, at least in part). The pathway varies by which the pulmonary hypertension proceeds to CHF. In uncomplicated cases, it appears related to individual susceptibility and permanent pulmonary vascular damage. Other kinds of stress, such as pneumonia, plant poisoning, lungworm infection, subzero weather, chronic pulmonary lesions, or ruptured diaphragm, are often superimposed on the already partially compromised pulmonary circulation and may obscure the etiology.

Locoweed (certain species of the genera *Oxytropis* and *Astragalus*), when consumed by cattle, especially calves, at high elevation markedly increases the prevalence and severity of CHF. The condition develops within 1-2 wk, and the incidence may be as high as 100% if cattle are allowed to graze the locoweed for more than short periods. The toxin in locoweed, the indolizidine alkaloid swainsonine, is excreted in the milk, thus nursing calves develop CHF. These animals have the signs and lesions of high-mountain disease and lesions of locoweed poisoning. These observations suggest that other factors may enhance the incidence of high-mountain disease.

Clinical Findings: The disease usually develops slowly. Periods of severe cold or other environmental stress appear to precipitate onset of signs. The affected animals are first noted to be depressed. As the syndrome progresses, subcut. edema may develop in the brisket region and extend cranially to the intermandibular space and caudally to the ventral abdominal wall. Occasionally, the marked fluid imbalance and edema are not evident; instead, the animal is emaciated. Ascites and marked distention and pulsation of the jugular vein are usually present, and profuse fluid diarrhea may develop. Respiration is labored, and the animals may appear cyanotic. They are reluctant to move, may become recumbent, and on forced exertion, may collapse and die.

Lesions: Generalized edema is usually present, particularly of the ventral subcutis, skeletal musculature, perirenal tissues, mesentery, and GI tract wall. Ascites, hydrothorax, and hydropericardium are present. The liver lesions, due to chronic passive congestion, vary from an early "nutmeg" appearance to severe lobular fibrosis. The lungs may have varying degrees of atelectasis, interstitial emphysema, edema, and in some cases, pneumonia. Marked right ventricular hypertrophy and dilatation of the heart are present. Displacement of the cardiac apex to the left gives the heart an enlarged, rounded contour. Occasionally, pulmonary arteries contain thrombi. Microscopically, hypertrophy of the media of small arteries and arterioles in the lung is a consistent finding. This disease must be differentiated from other diseases that cause CHF in cattle, such as traumatic pericarditis, chronic pneumonia, congenital anomalies, and primary myocardial lesions.

Treatment and Control: Affected animals should be removed with minimal restraint, stress, and excitement to a lower altitude, where some will recover spontaneously. General supportive therapy, including antibiotics to combat pneumonia, should be administered. Large amounts of effusion can be removed by paracentesis. Digitalis and diuretic therapy has been beneficial. At high altitudes, use of oxygen to lower pulmonary arterial pressure may be considered for valuable animals. Because the disease may recur, recovered animals should not be returned to high altitudes, and since an inherited susceptibility is likely, affected cattle should not be retained for breeding. Long-term studies strongly suggest that measurement of pulmonary arterial pressure of new sires could be an important management tool to reduce the incidence of this disease.

MOTION SICKNESS

A condition characterized by nausea, manifest as excessive salivation and vomiting, and other signs generally referable to stimulation of the autonomic nervous system. It is usually seen during travel by land, sea, or air. Man and many domestic animals may be affected. The principal causative mechanism involves stimulation of the vestibular apparatus in the inner ear, which has connections to the emetic center in the brainstem. Fear of the vehicle may be a contributory factor in dogs and cats (typical signs may be seen in a stationary vehicle).

The outstanding signs are salivation and vomiting. Animals may yawn, whine, and show signs of uneasiness or apprehension; severely affected ones may also have diarrhea. Signs usually disappear when vehicular motion ceases.

Motion sickness at times may be overcome by conditioning the animal to travel. If not, some ataractic and antinausea drugs have been used in dogs with good results. Antihistamines such as diphenhydramine hydrochloride, dimenhydrinate, and promethazine hydrochloride prevent motion sickness, provide sedation, and inhibit drooling. The centrally acting phenothiazine derivatives, such as triethylperazine, chlorpromazine, prochlorperazine, and acepromazine maleate, have antiemetic as well as sedative effects. Phenobarbital also has been used to produce a general sedative effect. Oral administration of one of these drugs several hours before departure should reduce or eliminate the signs of motion sickness. (*See also* DRUGS AFFECTING GASTRIC FUNCTIONS, p 1376.)

TRAUMA, SM AN

Automobiles, other animals, sharp objects, gun shots, blunt impact, or falling may cause trauma to small animals. Trauma-induced injuries are often life-threatening, and require rapid evaluation. Vital signs are determined immediately: heart rate, pulse, mucous membrane color, capillary refill time, breathing rate and effort, limb movement, and motor and cranial nerve function (see CLINICAL EXAMINATION OF THE NERVOUS SYSTEM, p 569). The abdomen is palpated for evidence of a fluid wave and an intact urinary bladder. Initial laboratory data should include PCV, total protein, ECG, blood test strips for BUN and glucose, and eventually, radiographs of affected areas.

The most life-threatening problem should be addressed first. Active hemorrhage should be stopped with pressure bandages, and open chest wounds immediately covered with sterile bandages and pleural air aspirated. Dyspnea and shock (qv, p 1369) should be treated with oxygen, fluids, and steroids as indicated. Often, diagnostic and therapeutic procedures such as radiographs and wound management are delayed until the animal has stabilized. Appropriate monitoring procedures should be initiated for early detection of complications or decompensation. PCV, total protein, urine output, respiratory rate and effort, heart rate, blood pressure, core body and peripheral temperatures, central venous pressure, ECG, pulse intensity, and repeated neurological exams are commonly assessed for that purpose.

Fractures commonly occur with automobile accidents. The obvious treatment is surgical; however, cleansing of open wounds and temporary immobilization are indicated, and reduction and fixation should be delayed until the animal is stable.

DROWNING

Fatalities result from complex pathophysiological events that differ according to the composition of the liquid. Hypoxia is the most consistent finding, and is more severe when seawater is inhaled. Initial therapy uniformly involves clearing and suctioning the airways, judicious fluid and electrolyte replacement, and support of the cardiovascular system.

Evaluation and prognosis are based on physical examination, arterial blood gas analysis, radiographs, and response to therapy. Initial radiographs may be normal, and changes detected only on arterial blood gas analysis. Typical radiographic changes include ventrocaudal alveolar patterns with bronchial and interstitial components that progress with time.

Mechanical support of ventilation is often required in both freshwater and seawater "near drownings". Intermittent positive pressure ventilation and/or positive end expiratory pressure are often the modalities of choice. Response to mechanical ventilation is determined by blood gases. The prophylatic use of antibiotics is controversial; some advocate their use only when secondary infection has been documented.

Near drowning in freshwater results in large quantities of hypotonic fluid entering the lungs and being rapidly absorbed into the bloodstream. Hypervolemia and hemodilution occur and are associated with hemolysis of RBC. Ventricular fibrillation may result from dilution of electrolytes and Hgb, and associated with anoxia. Treatment is aimed toward supporting ventilation and oxygenation, stabilizing the cardiovascular system, promoting renal perfusion and eliminating excessive fluids, establishing normal electrolyte balance, and preventing pneumonia. Exchange transfusions provide a possible means of reestablishing the normal blood volume and electrolyte balance. Peritoneal dialysis can be done to remove excessive water.

Seawater is hypertonic. Rapid diffusion of salts into the blood occurs and water moves into the pulmonary alveoli. Marked hemoconcentration, hypernatremia, and pulmonary edema result. Oxygen, fluid, ventilation, and cardiovascular support are required. Colloid infusion (eg, plasma, dextrans, hetastarch) may be required to reestablish circulating volume and increase plasma oncotic pressure.

ELECTRIC SHOCK

See also p 628. In puppies and kittens, this usually results from chewing on electrical cords. The severity of the problem varies with the voltage and pathway of the current through the body. The most common signs are tissue damage (burns, necrosis), cardiac dysrhythmias, and acute pulmonary edema. As the electricity traverses the skin and mucosa, the energy is converted to heat; coagulation necrosis occurs at the sites of entry and exit, and within the striated muscle it passes through. Wounds of the palate, lips, and tongue are frequent, and may require debridement, antibiotic therapy, and temporary nasogastric tube feeding to bypass the oral cavity.

Cardiac dysrhythmias are secondary to electrophysiologic changes within the heart produced by the electric current. Any arrhythmia can occur, but the most common are ventricular tachycardia, ventricular fibrillation, and A-V conduction disturbances. Treatment is symptomatic, using antiarrhythmic drugs or defibrillation as indicated. Careful fluid administration is indicated to avoid circulatory collapse.

Pulmonary edema, with the resultant dyspnea and cyanosis, is a common sequela in small animals. Usually, it is severe, and the onset is within 12 hr of insult. Leakage of fluid from disrupted pulmonary capillaries, cardiac failure, or neurogenic mechanisms may contribute to the edema. Radiograhic abnormalities characteristically involve the dorsocaudal lung fields, which show a mixed interstitial and alveolar pattern. Oxygen therapy and judicious fluid administration are required. Furosemide, bronchodilators, and corticosteroids may be beneficial early in the course of treatment. If the animal decompensates, mechanical ventilation may be necessary. If needed, low doses of oxymorphone (0.025-0.05 mg/kg) or morphine may be used to decrease anxiety.

Stupor, coma, hypovolemic shock, convulsions, or death are possible complications. Focal necrosis may occur in nerves, spinal cord, and brain. Renal tubular necrosis is possible with acute renal failure.

THORACIC TRAUMA

Trauma to the chest may lead to life-threatening interference with oxygenation. Diagnosis must be made quickly and proper treatment instituted. Primary differentials to consider are chest wall injuries (eg, flail chest), pneumothorax, hemothorax, pulmonary contusions, and diaphragmatic hernia. Diagnosis of thoracic trauma is based on history and physical examination, including auscultation, percussion, and palpation. Radiography is done after initial stabilization.

Initial medical management includes oxygen by face mask or nasal catheter, fluids, and other appropriate medications for cardiopulmonary support and stabilization.

Penetrating chest wounds are cleaned quickly and covered with a sterile bandage. Pleural air is evacuated as quickly as possible. Fractured ribs or a flail chest is diagnosed by observation and palpation. In flail chest, paradoxical movement of the chest wall is seen with each respiration; the chest wall may be stabilized temporarily by placing the animal in lateral recumbency with the affected side down. External or internal fixation is required for permanant repair.

Pneumothorax, a common sequela of injury to the chest wall, lung parenchyma, or airways, may be open or closed to the environment. A pneumothorax is classified as simple when the intrapleural pressure is less than or equal to atmospheric pressure. When a piece of tissue or a foreign object acts as a one-way valve and allows airflow into the pleural space on inspiration but prevents escape of the air on expiration, tension pneumothorax occurs: the intrapleural pressure is greater than atmospheric, which causes impaired venous return and hypoxia. This is life-threatening.

Pneumothorax is diagnosed by history, observation, palpation, auscultation, and percussion. Severity of signs is directly related to rapidity of onset, severity of the damage, and type of pneumothorax. Tachypnea and anxiety are usually present. Pale mucous membranes, with or without cyanosis, and open-mouth breathing may be present. A barrel-shaped chest with poor chest-wall movement indicates tension pneumothorax. On auscultation, vesicular lung sounds are decreased or absent dorsally. Ventral lung sounds are normal, and heart sounds may be normal or muffled.

Percussion of a pneumothorax reveals hyperresonance, and the chest is tympanic if a tension pneumothorax is present.

Treatment depends on the severity and type of pneumothorax. All penetrating wounds should be covered with a sterile bandage. If the pneumothorax is mild and has minimal associated clinical signs, cage rest is frequently all that is required. If the pneumothorax is moderate to severe, the pleural space is evacuated by thoracocentesis or chest tube. A tension pneumothorax requires immediate drainage and equilibration of intrapleural and atmospheric pressures. High intrapleural pressures may be relieved quickly by placing a large gauge (14-18) needle or catheter into the pleural space. Chest tube placement is required if the pneumothorax is severe, if air accumulates quickly after thoracocentesis, or if tension pneumothorax is present.

In **hemothorax**, the dorsal lung sounds are normal and the ventral lung sounds are decreased or absent. Heart sounds are usually muffled. On percussion, the chest is dull ventrally. Treatment is based on severity of signs. Mild to moderate hemothorax may require cage rest only; severe or ongoing hemothorax may require thoracocentesis, blood transfusions, or chest tube placement. When the bleeding is continuous, surgical exploration and autotransfusion are required.

Pulmonary contusions, alone or with other thoracic injuries, usually occur soon after the traumatic insult, but may increase in severity during the first 72 hr. Diagnosis is by history, physical examination, auscultation, and radiography. Respiration is labored and may be fast and shallow. Bronchovesicular sounds or crackles may be increased over the contused areas. If injury is severe, lung sounds may be absent in the affected area. Radiographs show an increased interstitial and alveolar pattern.

Treatment for pulmonary contusions depends on the severity of insult and clinical signs. Alveolar ventilation and gas exchange decrease due to accumulation of blood and fluid in the lung parenchyma. Animals mildly affected respond to cage rest with or without oxygen supplementation. The animal may be in shock and restless. Fluids are given to improve perfusion, but overhydration must be avoided since it may worsen pulmonary edema and hemorrhage. Judicious use of diurectics and bronchodilators may be useful. Morphine at small dosages (0.1-0.5 mg/kg) may relieve anxiety and thereby improve alveolar ventilation. Corticosteroids may be beneficial when given early, although their use, as well as that of antibiotics, is controversial. Animals with severe pulmonary contusions are at an increased risk of respiratory failure.

If radiographs reveal a diaphragmatic hernia (qv, p 711), surgical repair is required once the animal has stabilized. Emergency surgery is indicated if the ventilatory space is significantly compromised by viscera in the thorax, the stomach is in the thorax, visceral blood supply is compromised, or shock cannot be stabilized.

WOUNDS

Wounds may result in loss of continuity and function, pain, and hemorrhage. Basic wound management incorporates procedures to prevent further contamination, remove debris, debride tissue, provide drainage, promote vascularization, and allow eventual closure of the wound.

Compression bandages are a first aid measure to control bleeding. Once bandages become soaked with blood, additional dressings are placed over these rather than removing and replacing them. Tourniquets should be used only when pressure bandages are ineffective. Later, bleeding vessels are ligated or coagulated.

Once bleeding is controlled, the wound is covered with sterile, water-soluble lubricant while the hair around it is clipped and the skin cleaned with germicidal soap. A sterile dressing with antibiotic ointment, 0.5% povidone iodine solution, or 0.5-1% chlorhexidine is then applied until the animal stabilizes. Small, clean wounds may be infiltrated with local anesthetics for debridement.

Narcotic sedation or general anesthesia may be required for more involved wound care. Debris should be flushed out thoroughly with warm sterile saline. Nonviable tissue and foreign materials that remain after lavage should be excised. If the wound is extensive or deep, debridement may be done in stages. Degloving injuries require wet-to-dry bandage changes at least daily until a healthy granulation bed is present. Contaminated wounds may be left open under sterile dressings, and drains are placed if dead space cannot be obliterated. Open abdominal wounds require careful bandaging. Wet abdominal bandages should be changed immediately to prevent contamination.

Final closure of wounds is by primary closure, delayed primary closure, secondary closure, or second intention healing. Primary closure is appropriate for a clean wound <6 hr old. If the wound is contaminated, primary closure is delayed. The wound is cleaned, debrided, lavaged, and left open under a bandage made of sterile wet gauze, absorbent cotton, and elastic tape. Sutures are placed on day 4 or 5 if the tissues appear vital and not infected. Infected wounds are left open under bandages for 5-10 days after cleansing and debridement. Secondary closure then can be accomplished by direct suture apposition of 2 granular surfaces, or by excision of the granulation tissue and primary closure. For old wounds or large infected skin defects, closure by second-intention healing through epithelialization and contraction is recommended. These wounds are left open under appropriate bandages after debridement and lavage. Skin flaps or grafting techniques provide an option for faster or more cosmetic healing.

Bacterial cultures may be obtained before wound flushing, and systemic antibiotic therapy initiated and maintained for at least 7-10 days. Complications of wound healing generally are associated with drying of tissues, bacterial or fungal infection, poor nutrition, self-mutilation, immunosuppression, or improper surgical technique.

Bite wounds usually appear as small puncture wounds of the skin, but massive subcut. and muscle contamination and maceration may be present under the surface; the formation of bite-wound abscesses is especially common in cats. Such wounds need exploration. Should the wound appear to penetrate the chest or abdominal cavity, signs of fever, pain, effusion, high WBC count, or depression can indicate a need for exploration of the appropriate cavity. A diagnostic peritoneal or pleural lavage with fluid analysis aids in the detection of subacute or acute contamination (ie, bacterial with WBC) before systemic signs.

REPRODUCTIVE SYSTEM

REP

REPRODUCTIVE SYSTEM, INTRODUCTION

All functions of the reproductive system must be considered when resolving reproductive problems. The differences of the reproductive system between the sexes and species are complex. In both sexes, there are primary sex organs and primary regulatory centers. Gonads and function-adapted, tubular, genital organs constitute primary sex organs in both sexes. The pituitary gland and the hypothalamus are the main primary regulatory centers; thus, the regulatory function is, in part, neuroendocrine in nature. In pregnant females, the fetoplacental unit has a significant role in maintaining and terminating pregnancy.

REPRODUCTIVE PHENOMENA

The temporal and physiological features of the reproductive cycle in several species are summarized in the following tables.

THE GONADS

Both sexes have a pair of gonads, the main functions of which are gametogenesis and steroidogenesis. Both functions are regulated primarily by gonadotropins released by the anterior pituitary gland under the influence of the hypothalamus. The latter is mediated by a peptide, gonadotropin-releasing hormone (Gn-RH); the secretion and release of Gn-RH are governed by CNS stimuli and, through a feedback mechanism, by hormones produced by other endocrine organs such as the gonads, pituitary, thyroid, and adrenal glands.

The Ovaries: The intra-abdominal female gonads vary in size and location depending on species. Only those of the cow and the mare can be directly examined by rectal palpation. Once puberty is reached (*see* TABLE 3) and an animal starts cycling, the size and form of the ovaries are altered by cyclic functional structures, namely corpora lutea (CL) and follicles. According to a simplified concept, follicle-stimulating hormone (FSH) is responsible for development of follicle(s) and synthesis of estrogens by the theca cells. Once a certain estrogen level is attained, luteinizing hormone (LH) is released in spontaneously ovulating species. This LH peak precedes ovulation, which is followed by development of CL. The increase of luteal cells parallels a rise of serum progesterone. In nonpregnant polyestrous and seasonally polyestrous females (*see* TABLE 3), the functional and morphological life of the CL is terminated by endogenous prostaglandin (PG) $F_{2\alpha}$ from the uterus. As the CL regresses, a new ovulatory follicle(s) develops, which completes the estrous cycle. The hormonal changes during the estrous cycle can be monitored by radioimmunoassay and ELISA of hormones in blood, milk, or other body fluids. Estrual cycling continues after puberty unless interrupted by pregnancy, and in some species, by season or lactation during the immediate postpartum period. Cycling is also blocked by pathological conditions of the ovaries (eg, nutritional and stress atrophy

Table 1. Gestation Periods*

Domestic Animals	Days	Wild Animals	Days
Cat	58-65	Barbary Ape	210
Cattle, Angus	281	Bear, black	210
Ayrshire	279	Bison	270
Brahman	292	Camel	~410
Brown Swiss	290	Coyote	60-64
Charolais	289	Deer, Virginia	197-220
Guernsey	283	Elephant	600-660
Hereford	285	Elk, Wapiti	240-250
Holstein	279	Giraffe	420-450
Jersey	279	Hare	38
Limousin	289	Hippopotamus	225-250
Shorthorn	282	Kangaroo, red	38**
Simmental	289	Leopard	92-95
Dog	58-70	Lion	108
Donkey	365	Marmoset	140-150
Goat	145-155	Monkey, macaque	150-180
Horse, heavy	330-340	Moose	240-250
light	340-342	Muskox	270
Llama	330	Opossum	12-13
Pig	112-115	Panther	90-93
Sheep, meat breeds	144-147	Porcupine	112
wool breeds	148-151	Pronghorn	230-240
Fur Animals	**Days**	Raccoon	63
		Reindeer	210-240
Chinchilla	110-120	Rhinoceros, African	530-550
Ferret	42	Seal	330
Fox	49-55	Shrew	20
Marten, European	236-274	Skunk	62-65
Mink	40-75	Squirrel, gray	30-40
Muskrat	28-30	Tapir	390-400
Nutria (coypu)	120-134	Tiger	105-113
Otter	270-300	Walrus	330-360
Rabbit	30-35	Whale, sperm	480-500
Wolf	60-68	Woodchuck	31-32

*See also SOME PHYSIOLOGICAL DATA OF LABORATORY ANIMALS, p 1031.
**Delayed development as long as a "joey" is in the pouch.

Table 2. Incubation Periods

Domestic Birds	Days	Caged and Game Birds	Days
Chicken	20-22	Budgerigar	17-18
Duck	26-28	Finch	11-14
Muscovy duck	35	Parrot	17-31
Goose	25-28	Pheasant	24
Guinea fowl	28	Pigeon	10-18
Turkey	28	Quail	21-23
		Swan	33-36

Table 3. Features of the Reproductive Cycle

Species	Age at Puberty	Cycle Type	Cycle Length	Duration of Estrus	Best Breeding Time	First Estrus After Parturition	Remarks
Cattle	4-18 (12) mo, usually first bred ~15 mo	Polyestrous, all year.	21 days (18-24)	18 hr (10-24)	Insemination from mid-estrus until 6 hr after end	Varies,* best to breed at 60-90 days	Ovulation 10-12 hr after end of estrus. Uterine bleeding ~24 hr after ovulation in most but may require vaginal examination for detection.
Horse	10-24 (18) mo	Seasonally polyestrous early spring on.	Very variable, ~21 days (19-26)	6 days (2-10)	Last few days; should be bred at 2-day intervals	4-14 days (9)	Double ovulation occurs in ~20% of estrous periods, but twins rarely progress to term.
Sheep	7-12 (9) mo	Seasonally polyestrous, early fall to winter. Prolonged seasons in Dorsets and Merinos.	16½ days (14-20)	24-48 hr	18-20 hr after onset of estrus	Next fall	Ovulation near end of estrus.
Pig	4-9 (7) mo	Polyestrous, all year.	21 days (16-24)	2-3 days	~24 hr after onset of estrus	4-10 days after weaning	Ovulation usually ~40 hr after beginning of estrus.
Goat	4-8 (5) mo	Seasonally polyestrous, early fall to late winter.	18-21 days (19)	2-3 days	Daily during estrus	Next fall	Many intersexes born in hornless strains.

Dog	5-24 mo; earlier in smaller breeds later in larger breeds	Unseasonally monestrous.	3½-13 mo	2-21 days (6-12 av)	From day 2 of estrus, and on alternate days thereafter until end of estrus	Few months (2- to 3½-mo period of metestrus, followed by a highly variable period of anestrus)	Proestrous bleeding 7-10 days. Ovulation usually 1-3 days after first acceptance. Ova shed before 1st polar body has been extruded. Pseudopregnancy usually ends between 60 and 70 days.
Cat	4-12 (10) mo; 12-18 mo in Persians	Provoked ovulation, seasonally polyestrous spring and early fall.	14-21 days	6-7 days	Daily from day 2 of estrus	4-6 wk	Ovulation 24-48 hr after coitus. Pseudopregnancy lasts 36 days. Infertile matings prolong onset of next cycle ~45 days.
Fox	10 mo	Monestrous December to March, but mostly late January to February.		2-4 days		Next winter	Ovulation usually on 1st or 2nd day of receptivity. Ova shed before 1st polar body has been extruded. No proestrous bleeding.
Mink	10 mo	Provoked ovulation, seasonally polyestrous mid-February to early April.	Waves of follicles at intervals of 7-10 days	2 days	Induced ovulator	Next spring	Ovulation begins 36-48 hr after coitus, which must last ≥30 min.

(continued)

Table 3. Features of the Reproductive Cycle (continued)

Species	Age at Puberty	Cycle Type	Cycle Length	Duration of Estrus	Best Breeding Time	First Estrus After Parturition	Remarks
Chinchilla	400-600 g (6-8½ mo)	Polyestrous, intense in November to May.	30-50 days (41)	Vagina perforated ½-6 days during estrus; mate at night	Mate on 2nd night, rarely on 3rd night	2-48 hr, ovulation on 2nd night	
Nutria	5-8 mo	Polyestrous.	24-29	2-4 days		48 hr	
Rabbit	5-9 mo; range 4-12 mo for most breeds	Provoked ovulation. Breed all year, more or less; may show seasonal anestrus.	No regular estrous cycles	To 1 mo	When vulva is enlarged and hyperemic	Immediately, but blastocysts die if doe suckles large litter	In USA do not breed well in summer. Ovulation 10½ hr after coitus. Pseudopregnancy lasts 14-16 days.
Rhesus monkey (*Macaca mulatta*)	3 yr	Polyestrous all year, tendency to anovulatory cycles in summer in USA.	27-28 days (23-33)	~3 days	Near ovulation, day 10-13 of cycle	After weaning of previous young	Menstruation lasts 4-6 days. Ovulation usually ~13 days after onset.
Rat	37-67 days, varies with strain; body length at puberty 148-150 mm	Polyestrous, all year.	4-5 days	~14 hr (12-18), usually begins ~7 pm	Near ovulation	Within 24 hr	Ovulation soon after midnight. Cervical stimulation causes pseudopregnancy lasting 12-14 days.

Mouse	35 days (28-49)	Polyestrous, all year.	Usually 4 or 5 days	A few hr from 10 pm on	Female most receptive during 1st 3 hr	Within 24 hr	Ovulation soon after midnight. Stimulation of cervix causes pseudopregnancy lasting 10-12 days.
Guinea pig	55-70 days	Polyestrous, all year.	16½ days	6-11 hr, usually begins in evening	Mid-estrus on	Usually immediately	Ovulation ~10 hr after onset of estrus.
Hamster	4-6 wk	Polyestrous, all year. Few pregnancies in winter.	4-5 days	12 hr, one night	Mid-estrus	After weaning	Ovulation 8-12 hr after onset of estrus. Pseudopregnancy lasts 7-13 days.
Gerbil, Mongolian	9-12 wk	Polyestrous.	4-6 days	12-15 hr	Mid-estrus	1-3 days	Ovulation spontaneous 6-10 hr after mating.

*Many normal cows ovulate as early as 8-12 days after parturition, with or without detectable signs of estrus.

and ovarian cysts) and by uterine disease (eg, pyometra and severe endometritis), which may result in persistent CL. Estrogens and progesterone, the principal gonadal hormones, act locally, affect target organs such as the tubular genital tract, and regulate gonadotropin release by feedback mechanism on both the hypothalamus and anterior pituitary. In addition to these sites of action, female sex hormones are responsible for sex characteristics, behavior, and lactation.

The Testes: Like the ovaries, the testes have a dual function: spermatogenesis and steroid hormone secretion. In simple terms, spermatogenesis is stimulated by FSH and augmented by androgens, primarily testosterone. Leydig cells, under the influence of LH, produce testosterone and, in some species (eg, equine), also estrogens. Testosterone is required for development and function of accessory glands, copulatory organs, male sex characteristics, and behavior. For optimal spermatogenesis, mammalian testes must descend into the scrotal cavity; however, intra-abdominal testicular steroidogenesis occurs, and the libido of cryptorchid stallions, boars, and dogs is not impaired. Photoperiod affects both sperm cell formation and steroidogenesis in males of species with a seasonal reproductive pattern. Semen quality, libido, and mating ability are reduced during the anestrous period of the females. Methods for evaluation of representative semen samples and hormone assays are available for assessment of testicular function. Palpation and measurement of the testicles may reveal pathological conditions.

THE FEMALE TUBULAR GENITAL TRACT

Except for the vestibulum, which develops from the urogenital sinus, the female genital tract is derived from the embryonic paramesonephric (müllerian) ducts. Each of the segments is adapted to fulfill its function. Thus, the oviduct, through its motility, acquires the egg(s) and propels the zygote(s) into the uterus, while its secretion provides a proper environment for survival of gametes, fertilization, and the first few critical days of embryonic life. Interference with motility or secretion leads to infertility. Species variation of the bicornual, Y-shaped uterus involves the size of the body and length of horns, which are adapted to accommodate species-specific number and form of fetus(es). The cervix provides a protective barrier, relatively effective against ascending infections except for species in which semen is deposited intrauterinally, eg, equine. Morphological and functional integrity of the uterus and cervix are required for establishing and maintaining pregnancy and for parturition. Infections, contracted at mating and during parturition and puerperium, and their sequelae are common causes of female infertility. They interfere with normal uterine function, including release of $PGF_{2\alpha}$. Applicability of diagnostic methods for detection of uterine and cervical abnormalities depends on species, size of the animal, and anatomy of the cervix. Clinically, cases are diagnosed by rectal and abdominal palpation, vaginoscopy and fiberoptic hysteroscopy, radiography, and transrectal ultrasonography. Laboratory diagnostic aids include microbiological and cytological examination of exudate or secretion, histological examination of biopsies, endometrial cytology, and hormone assays.

The posterior tract, consisting of vagina, vestibulum, and vulva, serves as the copulatory organ and as the last segment of the birth canal. It also provides a pathway for ascending infections, particularly when effectiveness of the sphincter of the vulva is lost or reduced due to trauma or relaxation. Puerperal infections commonly involve the entire tubular tract. In addition, vestibulovaginal infection perpetuated by urovagina and pneumovagina sustains chronic infection of the bovine and equine uterus. However, the vestibulum and vagina can be inflamed, even when the uterus is normal, or even pregnant. Conversely, in closed-cervix pyometras in cows and bitches, the vagina and vestibulum may be essentially normal.

THE MALE TUBULAR GENITAL TRACT

In males, the tubular tract provides a pathway for sperm cells and semen. It begins as the efferent ductules of the testes, includes the head, body, and tail of the epididymis, and continues on as the ductus deferens. The ductus deferens ascends into the abdominal cavity via the inguinal ring and passes over the dorsal aspect of the bladder to enter the pelvic urethra. The pelvic and penile urethras are shared as an outlet for semen and urine. Along this pathway, certain segments of the tract have evolved morphologically and functionally to perform additional specific functions. The epididymides are involved in sperm cell maturation, storage, and selective absorption of abnormal spermatozoa. Ampullae and accessory sex glands (ie, seminal vesicles, prostate, bulbourethral glands) contribute to the formation of seminal plasma. The size and form of the accessory sex glands vary among species. The seminal vesicles and the bulbourethral (Cowper's) glands are absent in dogs. In bulls, the epididymides and seminal vesicles are common sites of infection. Epididymitis is also common in rams. Prostate hypertrophy and malignancy are found primarily in dogs, and may be detected by rectal palpation. Pathological conditions of the epididymides, eg, various forms of inflammation, cystic dilatation (spermiostasis), and segmental aplasia, can be diagnosed by scrotal palpation in most animals. Other diseases or functional disturbances may require evaluation of one or several semen samples. The seminal vesicles can be assessed clinically only in animals that are large enough for rectal palpation.

INFERTILITY AND ITS MANIFESTATIONS

Interaction of the CNS, hypothalamus, pituitary gland, gonads, and their target organs results in finely coordinated chains of physiological events that lead to estrus and ovulation in the female, and ejaculation of fertile semen by the male. For optimal results, ovulation and deposition of semen into the female genital tract must be closely synchronized. Failure of any single functional event in either sex leads to infertility or sterility.

The ultimate manifestation of infertility is failure to produce offspring. In polyestrous animals, a subnormal number of offspring also constitutes infertility. In females, infertility may be due to failure to cycle, aberrations of the estrous cycle and period (based on dysfunction of the ovaries or the hypothalamus-pituitary axis), failure to conceive, or prenatal and perinatal death. Major infertility problems in males are disturbances of the production, transport, or storage of spermatozoa; aberration of libido; and partial or total inability to mate.

Most, if not all, major infertility problems have a complex etiology; several factors, singly or in combination, can cause reproductive failure. Pathogenesis may be equally complex.

DIAGNOSTIC APPROACH TO INFERTILITY PROBLEMS

Since the female bears the offspring, she reflects either success or failure of reproduction. However, especially in naturally mated animals but also with AI, the first diagnostic step, regardless of the complaint, is to establish the etiological role of the female and the male.

In recent years, man has assumed more and more responsibility for certain aspects of reproduction, such as observation of estrus, preservation of semen, and insemination; each point of interference is a potential source of error. Thus, human errors, which are detected or ruled out by assessment of performance with the main emphasis on techniques and procedures, and their adequacy and quality, must be considered.

Diagnostic methods have been developed to test the anatomical and functional soundness of both sexes. They range from clinical examination, supported by diagnostic aids such as endoscopy and ultrasonography, to laboratory tests including hormone assays, microbiology, cytology, serology, cytogenetic examination, semen evaluation, etc.

The choice of examination methods is determined by the species and size of the animal. Decisions with regard to type and extent of laboratory tests are based on history and information gained during the course of examination. The diagnostic plan should provide evidence for establishing the role of the female, the male, and the manager in each case of reproductive failure. Reproductive problems are seldom accompanied by alarming signs of disease. Furthermore, there is a time interval between when a failure occurs and when it becomes apparent. Examples are intervals between unsuccessful service and return to estrus or failure to give birth. This lag period may allow recovery, and examination may yield negative results. Interpretation of results also must account for species differences and, in species with a seasonal reproductive pattern, that infertility may be physiological during certain periods of the year.

PRINCIPLES OF THERAPY

(*See also* MANAGEMENT OF REPRODUCTION, p 1127 *et seq.*) The increasing demands for production efficiency, along with changing environments (eg, housing and management systems) and, in many instances, the successful eradication of specific infections (eg, brucellosis, tuberculosis, campylobacteriosis) have caused a shift in therapeutic strategies in several domestic species. Especially for food animals, and to some extent for horses, the therapeutic approach of choice often is a combination of pharmacological agents and correction of management problems. Treatments on a herd basis also have become more important, especially in light of the need for cost effectiveness, eg, the increased use of pharmacological agents in reproductive management such as synchronization of estrus, superovulation, induction of parturition, and treatment of anestrus and substestrus. Other therapeutic trends in food animals are the result of an increasing awareness of the possible hazards of antimicrobial and hormone residues in tissues and milk; alternatives to antibiotic therapy warrant increased attention.

In small animals, the change of the therapeutic strategy is not as evident as in large animals. The individual animal is still in focus, and the environment of these species has not undergone the same changes as for large animals. However, diagnostic techniques and treatments have become more sophisticated. More effective therapy may propagate hereditary predisposition for lowered fertility by curing diseases that previously were self-limiting; this should be considered whenever one deals with fertility problems.

Pharmacological Control of Reproduction: Control of the estrous cycle—most commonly synchronization of estrus—usually is based on agents that act directly on the ovaries (eg, FSH, LH, or preparations with similar effect, such as pregnant mare serum gonadotropin [PMSG], or human chorionic gonadotropin [HCG], and prostaglandins) or on agents acting mainly at the pituitary-hypothalamic level (Gn-RH, progesterone, progestins). Superovulation, which has become an essential part of embryo transfer, usually is achieved by hormonal treatment during a certain stage of the cycle with FSH or agents with FSH effect (eg, PMSG) combined with a drug with LH effect (eg, HCG). In ruminants, $PGF_{2\alpha}$ or its analogs are used to lyse the CL and induce estrus following FSH stimulation of multiple follicle development.

Pathological conditions of the ovaries (cystic ovaries, delayed ovulation) are often treated with preparations with LH effect (eg, HCG) or Gn-RH. For persistent CL, prostaglandins have become the treatment of choice. Postpartum ovarian inactivity (postpartum anestrus) has been experimentally treated with pulses of FSH or Gn-RH repeated over time. However, practical delivery systems for these products are currently unavailable, and conditions such as lactation anestrus remain difficult to treat. Delayed puberty in some species (eg, pigs) frequently responds to treatment with a drug with follicle-stimulating effect (FSH, PMSG, or a combination of PMSG and HCG).

Other areas in which exogenous hormones can play a role in the control of reproduction are pregnancy and parturition. Estrogens are used as abortifacients in some species (eg, bovine), but prostaglandins are usually more effective. Estrogens are also used for prevention of pregnancy following undesired mating (eg, dog). Progesterone or various progestogens can be used for suppression of estrus to prevent mating in all species. For induction of parturition, which has become an important management tool in some species (eg, pigs and cattle), corticosteroid treatment or $PGF_{2\alpha}$ or a combination thereof is used. Dams with a dead fetus usually do not respond well to corticosteroids. In pigs, it appears that either $PGF_{2\alpha}$ or a combination of $PGF_{2\alpha}$ and oxytocin is best. In mares, oxytocin is most effective. It is important in all species that the animal is prepared for parturition. The less prepared the reproductive tract (eg, cervix, fetoplacental unit, and mammary gland), the higher the risk of complications.

For conditions such as prolonged gestation, the same agents are used as for induction of parturition in normal animals. In uterine disorders (pyometra, retained placenta, and endometritis), the best nonantibiotic agents are those that can cause myometrial contractions, increase uterine blood flow, and mobilize defense mechanisms to the uterus. This can be achieved with estrogens and oxytocin. Prostaglandins have a strong stimulus on myometrial contractions in dogs and cycling cows, but not in postpartum cows. Pyometra in cows is best treated with $PGF_{2\alpha}$ since the condition is defined as including presence of a CL.

Antimicrobial Treatment: Antimicrobial agents, most commonly antibiotics, are used for treatment of infections of the reproductive tract in all species. Drug selection should be based on microbiological identification and sensitivity tests. The dose, route of administration, and the dosage interval vary among species and with microbiological status, blood and tissue distribution, etc. Most systemically administered antibiotics penetrate the reproductive tract tissues better than those administered locally, especially when severe endometritis or metritis is present. A recent trend is the use of higher doses or a shorter dosing interval to achieve effective blood levels, tissue distribution, and minimum inhibitory concentration of the drug. In general, this means that doses higher than those officially approved are used.

Nonantibiotic Alternatives: Unsatisfactory results with antibiotics and increased concern about bacterial resistance and tissue residues, at least for food animals, emphasize the need for nonantibiotic alternatives for treatment of reproductive infections. In general, there are 2 effects of nonantibiotics on the reproductive tract that are desirable: the contractile effect that causes the evacuation of the tubular tract, and the positive effect on the cellular and humoral local defense. Drugs of primary interest for evacuation of the uterus are oxytocin, ergonovine, estrogens, and in some species (eg, dogs), $PGF_{2\alpha}$. Of these drugs, estrogens and $PGF_{2\alpha}$ may have a dual beneficial effect, stimulating the contractions of the uterus (eg, in cases of retained lochia or placenta, or postpartum metritis) and stimulating the local cellular defense. In addition to its contractile effect on the myometrium, $PGF_{2\alpha}$ causes regression of the CL in several species. This induces estrus, which reinforces the effect on the myometrium and produces endogenous estrogen. In pyometra, these effects may work synergistically. Drugs with contractile effect on the tubular tract, or with stimulatory effect on the local defense, are used in combination with antibiotics or as the only treatment in cases of retained placenta, metritis, delayed uterine involution, lochial retention, metrorrhagia, uterine prolapse, pyometra, etc. Oxytocin is commonly used to stimulate milk ejection in mastitis in some species (cattle, horses, dogs, and pigs).

In the past, use of disinfectant douches (eg, Lugol's solution, chlorhexidine, hydrogen peroxide, various iodophors, etc) was rather common for certain infections. They are still used for that purpose, especially in large animals; however, some of these substances are irritating, and there are indications that the local use of disinfectants may disturb the local immune defense (eg, the phagocytic ability of the WBC). Since the beneficial effects have not been confirmed, this type of treatment is now less frequently recommended. For certain purposes, eg, to induce premature estrus in cows during a certain stage of the cycle, it might still have a place among possible treatments. However, the beneficial effect in such cases is associated more with the induction of endogenous $PGF_{2\alpha}$ and estrogen production than with the antimicrobial effect of the drug.

ABORTION, LG AN

Many abortions in cattle and sheep result from infection that reaches the fetus via the maternal circulation. The first step is to identify the cause of the abortion so that preventive measures can be taken. However, diagnosis of the cause is difficult, and a positive diagnosis is made in only ~25% of cases.

The important infections that may lead to abortion are discussed under their respective headings. *See* MANAGEMENT OF REPRODUCTION: CATTLE—CAUSES OF ABORTION, p 1133, and OF HORSES—ABORTION, p 1142.

In **sheep** in the USA, the most common cause of abortion is campylobacteriosis. Other agents associated with abortion in sheep include: *Toxoplasma gondii*, bluetongue virus, *Brucella ovis*, chlamydiae, leptospires, *Listeria monocytogenes*, and *Salmonella* spp. Similarly, the important infectious diseases causing abortion in **pigs** (*see* below) include brucellosis, leptospirosis, pseudorabies, and parvovirus.

Trauma, fatigue, surgical shock, poisons, and certain drugs and chemicals have been incriminated as causes of abortion, but specific proof usually is lacking. Certain genes (recessive or lethal) may be involved. Nitrate poisoning has been mentioned frequently as a cause of abortion; however, all controlled experiments and observations concerning the effects of nitrate on the fetus have failed to link this chemical with fetal disease or abortion. The factors listed above may affect pregnancy through stress or direct effect on the fetus. In all probability, most chemicals exert their effect by crossing the placenta and affecting the fetus or the placenta, or both. Such chemicals may cause fetal death, and/or anomalies of varying severity. Their effect on the fetus depends on the dosage and the specific time of gestation (decrease with the age of the fetus), eg, *Veratrum californicum* produces adenohypophyseal aplasia and skeletal malformations in fetal lambs when ingested by the ewe on day 14 of gestation (*see* p 579).

Most equine twin pregnancies end in abortion. Introduction of bacterial contaminants into the uterus, by an AI pipette or other means, may cause death of the fetus and abortion.

INDUCED ABORTION AND PARTURITION

Cattle can be aborted by IM injection of a luteolytic dose of prostaglandin (PG) $F_{2\alpha}$ or its analogs. This is nearly 100% effective through the fourth month but tends to be less effective as pregnancy progresses. Abortion can be induced (95%) during the months 5-8 by injecting a combination of a luteolytic dose of PG and 25 mg of dexamethasone. Either drug induces parturition; however, when both are given, calves tend to be born at a more predictable time following treatment (39 ± 1.5 hr). Parturition is induced in 85-100% of cows when the drugs are injected 0-14 days before term, but up to 75% of successful inductions have retained placentas; colostrum and milk production are not significantly affected. Calves born up to 14 days before term have normal viability and normal blood levels of γ globulins.

Mares can be aborted with PG. After the fourth month, a double dose or repeated treatment at 48-hr intervals (or both) is necessary. In late pregnancy, PG will induce parturition but not a live foal. Douching the uterus with dilute antiseptic, saline, or antibiotic solutions results in abortion in the mare at any stage of pregnancy. Depending on the stage of pregnancy, 200-500 mL of fluid is sufficient.

In mares, when the cervix has begun to relax, and colostrum is in the udder, parturition may be induced by administering 40 u of oxytocin IV. Parturition occurs in ~30 min. This is accompanied by premature release of the allantochorion, and assistance should be available to aid in delivery and to remove the membranes from the foal. A variation of this treatment is to give 3 doses of 5 u of oxytocin at 15-min intervals, and then increase the dosage to 10 u at 15-min intervals until parturition occurs.

ABORTION IN PIGS

Abortions are frequently dramatic but usually only as individual events. Early fetal resorption without obvious abortion may be more significant economically. Most abortions are the result of noninfectious causes. Despite a complete history and laboratory evaluation, often it is impossible to determine the specific cause. Reproductive failure is only rarely due to a single disease. Most problems are prevented by good management and husbandry, and good record-keeping. Careful collection of retrospective information is critical. *See* MANAGEMENT OF REPRODUCTION: PIGS, p 1143.

Some specific causes of abortion or other reproductive failure are listed below. General discussions of the specific diseases listed can be located via the INDEX.

Parvovirus: This virus is present in most swine populations. Maternal immunity persists in gilts until sexual maturity, and may prevent them from becoming naturally immune. They may then be exposed near breeding time and experience reproductive failure. Early fetal resorption and irregular return to estrus are most common. Reduced litter size, abortion, and increased numbers of mummies may be observed. Diagnosis is best based on records and submission of mummified fetuses to a diagnostic laboratory.

Pseudorabies: Reproductive problems may include abortions, stillbirths, mummies, and weak pigs. In a recently infected herd, other signs may include fever, and respiratory and nervous signs. A number of different laboratory tests may be used for confirmation depending on the type of specimens available. Evidence of reproductive failure in the chronically infected herd may be more subtle.

Other Viruses: Other viruses, eg, enterovirus and influenza virus, may contribute to reproductive failure. A complete diagnostic investigation is required for identification.

Brucellosis: An uncommon and closely monitored disease, this is transmissible to man and is the subject of regulations governing movement of breeding stock. Brucellosis is the only venereal disease of pigs. All producers of breeding stock should maintain certification of regular testing and freedom from this disease. It may cause abortions or other failures, and is diagnosed by laboratory testing, primarily serology of sows.

Leptospirosis: Epidemiology of this disease is complex, and it is one of the most common causes of reproductive failure. There are a number of potential sources of infectious serotypes, and any number of clinical manifestations including abortions may result. Complete evaluation may include serology, but specific diagnosis without a full investigation is difficult.

Other Bacterial Infections: Numerous bacterial pathogens can induce infertility and abortion: any organism that produces a febrile response may result in abortion. Resulting losses are usually sporadic and diagnosis may be difficult.

Mycotoxins: Molds may produce toxins, usually in feed grains, that can induce abortions. Sudden onset of feed refusal, diarrhea, or abortions may be cause to consider mycotoxins. Usually, they are an insidious cause of lowered reproductive efficiency. A complete epidemiologic study should be conducted as soon as possible. Laboratory support may be helpful, but affected feed is often not available for evaluation. This is one reason for the value of a regular program to sample and retain feed.

Carbon Monoxide: Various environmental influences such as severe ambient temperatures may have subtle effects on reproduction. In facilities with poor ventilation and some types of carbon-monoxide-generating heaters, accumulations of carbon monoxide may cause multiple abortions and danger to caretakers. Air sampling and diagnostic evaluation of aborted pigs may result in a relatively prompt diagnosis.

Physiological Accidents: Many abortions in pigs result from various physiological incidents in individual sows. These are often hormonal, and may not have any obvious relationship to disease. Attempts at diagnosis are almost always retrospective and fruitless. If autumn abortions or shortening daylight reproductive inefficiencies are recognized, artificial lighting and improved energy intake in late summer and early fall should be considered.

CHLAMYDIAL ABORTION

CATTLE

Chlamydiae have been identified as causes of abortion in cattle in North America, Europe, Africa, and Asia. In the USA, chlamydial abortions have been diagnosed in Colorado, Arizona, California, Utah, Wisconsin, Wyoming, Montana, and Texas.

Etiology and Epidemiology: Abortions are caused by immunotype 1 strains of *Chlamydia psittaci* (*see also* ENZOOTIC ABORTION IN SHEEP AND GOATS, below). Immunotype 1 strains represent the only immunotype recovered from aborted placentas and fetuses of cows, and they are also frequently isolated from cows with subclinical intestinal infections. A separate entity known as epizootic bovine abortion, or foothill abortion (*see* below), once thought to be caused by chlamydial infection, is now associated with a borrelial agent transmitted by the soft-shelled tick *Ornithodoros coriaceus*. Chlamydial agents have been isolated from bovine abortions in the California foothills where this tick is known to occur, as well as in areas where it is not. Transmission of the agent of chlamydia-induced abortion depends not on vectors, but on the fecal-oral route. Subclinical intestinal infections (qv, p 137) are common in cattle, and abortions have been induced experimentally with such intestinal isolates. Genital chlamydial infections of bulls cause a **seminal vesiculitis syndrome**, in which the semen contains chlamydiae. Heifers inseminated with such semen did not conceive because chlamydia-induced endometritis prevented embryo nidation and resulted in sterility. Infertility is a problem in herds with affected bulls, but abortions have not been reported in such herds.

Clinical Findings and Lesions: Abortions usually occur without prior signs. They are frequently sporadic in nature, but up to 20% of the cows have aborted in a given herd. Cows of all ages are susceptible; abortions can occur as early as month 5, although most occur during the last trimester. Stillborn and weak calves can also be born. Placentas may be retained, and endometritis can result in rebreeding difficulties.

A consistent and significant lesion is severe placentitis, which can be localized. The trophoblastic epithelium is necrotic, especially in the inter- and periplacentomal areas. Fibrinopurulent exudate may be present between the endometrium and chorion. The intercotyledonary chorion may be of a gelatinous (edematous) or leathery consistency.

Lesions in the fetus vary considerably depending on the stage of the infection. They may be minimal if the infection remains localized in the placenta and the abortion is simply a result of fetal hypoxia that occurs before fetal chlamydemia. If the fetus becomes infected with chlamydiae, then lesions such as focal necrosis, vasculitis, and other inflammatory reactions may be seen in various organs including the brain. There are petechiae in the subcutis, thymus, and various mucosal/serosal surfaces. The liver is swollen with a mottled surface, and there is ascites and enlarged lymph nodes.

Diagnosis: The fetal or placental lesions are not characteristic enough for a specific diagnosis without laboratory confirmation. Exfoliative cytology reveals intracytoplasmic chlamydial inclusions or elementary bodies abundant in the chorionic placental epithelial cells from affected placental parts. Chlamydiae can also be isolated in chicken embryos or tissue culture from the placenta or various fetal tissues, but infectivity in these samples can be low by the time of abortion.

Antibody responses of pregnant cows with placental and fetal chlamydial infections and abortions are detectable with the ELISA or the indirect inclusion FA test. The responses are diagnostically indicative. An initial mild rise of antibodies is observed. The titers decline to low levels before abortion or parturition, provided these events occur later than 4 wk after inoculation or exposure. Delivery of chlamydia-infected dead or live fetuses with infected placentas stimulates a rapid rise in antibody titer that reaches maximum levels 2-3 wk after termination of pregnancy. Accordingly, paired serum samples, taken at the time of abortion and 2-3 wk later, show a significant rise in titer if the abortion resulted from chlamydial infection. The major chlamydial antigens reactive in these tests are proteinaceous antigens specific to species, type, and strain. The previously employed standard complement fixation (CF) test was genus-specific and relatively insensitive. Fetuses may have elevated levels of immunoglobulins that are not reactive in the CF test, but they react with chlamydial antigens in the double immunodiffusion test or ELISA.

Treatment and Prevention: Since cows show no signs before abortion, it is difficult to prevent abortions by antibiotic treatment. Chlortetracycline, 2-5 g/cow/day, incorporated in pelleted alfalfa or protein-molasses blocks did reduce the abortion rate in a field trial. This, however, is an expensive prophylactic regimen and is not practical except in special circumstances in which a severe, confirmed, chlamydial abortion problem exists in a given herd. Effective chlamydial vaccines are not available for use in cattle.

ENZOOTIC ABORTION IN SHEEP AND GOATS

A worldwide, infectious disease manifest by abortion and, to a lesser extent, by stillbirth or premature parturition. Eye infections in laboratory workers, and abortions in women who had contact with aborting sheep have been reported.

Etiology and Epidemiology: The causative agent comprises immunotype 1 strains of *Chlamydia psittaci*, identical to the one associated with bovine chlamydial abortion (*see* above). Strains recovered from aborted fetuses of sheep or cattle cause abortion in either species. The organisms from ovine tissues can be propagated in the yolk sac of chicken embryos, in cultured cells, in mice by nasal instillation, and in guinea pigs by IP inoculation.

The natural mode of infection is oropharyngeal exposure, ingestion, or inhalation. The portals of entry and penetration are in the nasopharynx, possibly the tonsillar crypts, and intestinal sites. The disease can be produced experimentally by either parenteral or oral inoculation. There is no evidence of arthropod-mediated transmission. Rams can have infections in genital organs and shed chlamydiae in semen that contains abundant WBC. The conception rate of ewes bred by such rams is reduced. Open ewes may become infected, and the infection persists. After conception and placental and fetal development with associated immune responses, chlamydemic phases occur; the agent invades the placenta and fetus, and abortion ensues. Occasionally, only one lamb of a set of twins will be infected. Up to 30% of pregnant ewes may abort when the infection is newly introduced into a flock, while lower losses occur year after year among yearling and younger ewes in endemically infected flocks.

Clinical Findings: Abortion, stillbirth, or premature parturition in the last month of gestation are characteristic. The placenta is retained in a small portion of the abortions. Dead fetuses may be carried *in utero* and sometimes mummify before being expelled. Such ewes lose condition rapidly and may die. Apart from these cases, the disease has little effect on the dam.

Lesions: Aborted fetuses are well preserved and may be covered with clay-colored, flaky material. Petechiae may be detected in the subcutis on skinning, and lymph nodes are enlarged and edematous. Placentitis is the most consistent finding, with a variable portion of necrotic cotyledons and tough, granular thickening of the intercotyledonary chorion. The margins of the lesions are hyperemic. Other parts of the placenta may appear normal.

Diagnosis: Laboratory assistance is essential in differentiating chlamydial abortion from abortions due to other infectious causes. Chlamydial elementary bodies appear as single or aggregated, small, red dots in Gimenez-stained impression smears. Cryostat sections of affected cotyledons or intercotyledonary tissues contain red elementary bodies in cytoplasmic inclusions. FA reveals, with immunologic specificity, chlamydial antigens in placental samples. Isolation and identification of causative chlamydiae constitute a conclusive diagnosis, but are time consuming and of little value in an outbreak. Antibodies against chlamydial antigens rise significantly after abortion. Antibodies may be detected in fetal serum. The tests of choice are the ELISA or the indirect inclusion FA test, which principally detect antibodies against protein chlamydial antigens. The previously used complement fixation test detects antibodies against genus-specific antigens.

Abortion due to *Campylobacter* sp can be differentiated by examination of impression smears and bacterial culture. *Brucella ovis* and *Coxiella burnetii* cause similar syndromes and may be differentiated through exfoliative cytology or culture.

Treatment and Control: Abortions in susceptible ewes were significantly reduced by 2 injections (2 wk apart) of a long-acting preparation of oxytetracycline at midgestation. Tetracycline therapy is recommended for infected neonates and dams that aborted. However, effective doses have not yet been established.

A killed vaccine has given good protection when administered before breeding or early in gestation; it should be repeated at intervals of 3 yr or less. However, it is not fully effective, and shedding of the organism may still occur in a vaccinated flock. Isolation of aborting ewes for 2-3 wk, removal of all placentas, and sanitation of the area reduces hazard to the rest of the flock.

EPIZOOTIC BOVINE ABORTION
(EBA, Foothill abortion of cattle)

An infectious disease of cattle manifest by abortion or weak calves at birth. It is endemic in the foothills of California, Nevada, and southern Oregon.

Etiology and Transmission: The distribution of EBA is closely associated with that of the vector, the soft-shelled pajaroello tick, *Ornithodoros coriaceus*. This tick is usually found in the ground litter of deer bedding areas; under the foothill chaparral, scrub oak, and manzanita; as well as in the higher wooded elevations in the Sierra Nevada, Cascade, and Coastal ranges. The feeding of combinations of nymphal and adult ticks on susceptible pregnant cows produces abortion in the third trimester of pregnancy after an incubation period of 90-150 days. Because the tick is active during the warm dry months of the year and is relatively dormant during colder wet months, infection is most common from May through October.

Chlamydia and *Borrelia* spp and 3 viruses have been isolated from pajaroello ticks. Borrelial organisms were cultured from maternal and fetal tissues but did not induce EBA when pregnant cows were inoculated. The viral agents from ticks did not induce abortions in pregnant cows, but chlamydial inoculation reliably caused abortion. However, *Chlamydia*-induced abortion (qv, p 651) appears to be a separate entity from EBA. The infectious cause of EBA has not yet been definitely established.

Animals at risk are primarily those that are in the second trimester of pregnancy when taken into an endemic area for the first time. Heifer calves do not appear to develop immunity in endemic tick areas and remain susceptible to abortion as pregnant yearlings. The incidence of abortion and weak calves from potentially exposed cows is 10-90%, depending on degree of tick exposure, stage of gestation, and susceptibility of animals in the herd.

Clinical Findings, Lesions, and Diagnosis: Infected cows normally show no signs of disease; those that abort generally recover quickly with few sequelae and conceive at subsequent breedings. Cows that are stressed additionally or are undernourished are more likely to have a retained placenta. Infected calves that are born alive may be premature or smaller than normal. Palpable lymph node enlargement helps to identify affected calves. Survival may depend on weather and availability of protection and feed.

Diagnostic lesions do not develop in the fetus until >100 days after infection. The most characteristic lesion is an enlarged and nodular liver, the result of chronic congestion. Lymphoid tissue throughout the fetus is enlarged; the lymph nodes may be 3 times normal size. Other lesions in aborted fetuses include edema of the subcut. tissues and ascites; erythema may be present over the skin of the flank and abdomen. Petechial hemorrhages often are scattered throughout the subcut. tissues, over the ventral surface of the tongue, the mucosa of the trachea and oral cavity, and in the conjunctivae.

Histologically, acute necrotizing lesions are superimposed on chronic proliferative ones. The proliferative lesions involve the cells of the monocyte-macrophage system that infiltrate various organs, most obviously lymph nodes, spleen, and liver. Acute necrotizing foci frequently form pyogranulomas in several organs, particularly lymph nodes and spleen. Acute vasculitis may be present in any organ.

The unique changes that occur in the thymus include atrophy of the cortical mantle of thymocytes and infiltration by macrophages. The acute lesions appear similar to immune-mediated changes that result from deposition of toxic complexes in the tissue.

A tentative diagnosis can be made on history and gross lesions, and confirmed by typical histological changes. Although serology is unreliable in view of the uncertain cause, specific tests are helpful for differentiating other infectious causes of abortion.

Prophylaxis and Treatment: Immunizing agents and antibiotics have not proved useful in preventing or treating EBA. Management successfully minimizes the impact of EBA in known endemic areas. Keeping known susceptible pregnant heifers and cows out of endemic areas during the months of pajaroello tick activity or until after the cow is 6 mo pregnant has proved beneficial. Manipulation of cattle on the same ranch between known tick-exposure and non-tick-exposure pastures, based on gestational susceptibility and seasonal tick activity, has helped to reduce the incidence of EBA. Exposed cattle appear not to abort a second time, although the length of protection from natural exposure is unknown. Changing the calving season (eg, spring to fall or fall to late summer) has improved calf crops.

OVINE GENITAL CAMPYLOBACTERIOSIS

An infectious disease characterized by abortion and caused by *Campylobacter fetus* subsp *fetus* or *C jejuni*. It causes serious economic losses in sheep in the USA and other countries. Both species of *Campylobacter* cause sporadic abortion in cattle, and diarrhea, bacteremia, abortion, and perinatal sepsis in man. *Campylobacter jejuni* has also been associated with diarrhea in various other animals (*see* p 102).

Etiology and Transmission: Both organisms cause epidemics of ovine abortion. Ingestion with food or water is followed by a transient bacteremia and infection of the placenta and fetus. Experimental efforts to transmit the disease venereally have failed. Carrier sheep probably are the major source of infection—via organisms shed in the feces from GI and gallbladder infections, or in uterine discharges, or aborted fetuses and membranes. *Campylobacter jejuni* is widespread in nature and has been isolated from the feces of sheep, goats, cattle, chickens, turkeys, ducks, many other birds, cats, dogs, and zoo animals. In most instances the carriers were asymptomatic. *Campylobacter fetus* subsp *fetus* has been isolated from the blood, feces, aborted fetuses, and bile of cattle, sheep, and man.

The incubation period is 7-53 days after ingestion of the organism. Some outbreaks follow by a few weeks a single primary abortion. An outbreak produces immunity in the flock, possibly of lifetime duration, but there is no cross-protection between the 2 species and both may be involved. Outbreaks in susceptible replacement ewes are not uncommon.

Clinical Findings: Abortion during the last 8 wk of pregnancy or, in some instances, the delivery of weak lambs at term constitutes the typical syndrome. Fetal death usually occurs 1-2 days before abortion. Usually, there is no indication of the impending abortion, but a few ewes show a prior vaginal discharge. Usually, recovery is prompt and fertility in subsequent breeding seasons is good. Occasionally, abortion is complicated by metritis and subsequent death of the ewe. Ewe mortality is 0-5%. In recently affected flocks, abortion may be confined chiefly to unvaccinated replacement ewes. Usually, the incidence of abortion is not >10-20%, but it may be as high as 70%.

Lesions: In some aborted fetuses, most frequently those near term, the liver shows typical gray, necrotic foci 1-3 cm in diameter. Usually, the fetus is edematous, and the body cavities contain a reddish fluid. The fetal membranes are edematous and the cotyledons pale and necrotic, but the lesions are variable and not specific.

Diagnosis: Campylobacteriosis must be differentiated from chlamydial abortion (qv, p 651), since the latter produces nearly identical clinical findings and can occur concomitantly. An early diagnosis is necessary for early treatment and protection of the rest of the flock. A tentative diagnosis can be based on a history of abortion in the last 8 wk of pregnancy, or birth of living but weak lambs, and the observation of slender curved bacteria in stains of cotyledon impressions, vaginal discharges, or the fetal abomasal fluid. The organisms are gram negative, but can be stained with most simple stains to reveal their characteristic morphology. Necrotic foci in the liver are pathognomonic, but occur in <40% of fetuses.

Diagnosis is confirmed by isolation and identification of the organism, which can be accomplished readily from satisfactory specimens. The fetal abomasal fluid and liver are the most appropriate sources for isolation. If the abdominal organs are removed by scavengers, isolations can sometimes be made from the heart, lung, or brain.

Treatment and Control: Aborting ewes should be isolated, and strict hygienic practices adopted; these include removal of aborted fetuses and associated discharges. If possible, unaffected ewes should be moved to a clean area and provided with uncontaminated feed and water.

Vaccination in the face of an experimental outbreak has proved effective in reducing abortions, and should be considered when abortions occur appreciably before the lambing date.

Treatment with penicillin-streptomycin IM on 2 consecutive days has reduced abortion experimentally, but many strains of both species are resistant to these antibiotics. Because resistant strains occur, sensitivity testing should be done. Other antibiotics, usually effective, that could be considered are erythromycin, tylosin, gentamicin, neomycin, and some of the tetracyclines.

Feeding chlortetracycline daily from time of diagnosis until lambing has been used with some success but has disadvantages of expense, time lost in preparation of a custom mix, and palatability. Sanitation, treatment with parenteral antibiotics, and possibly vaccination should control most outbreaks.

Vaccination with bivalent vaccine is effective for prevention of abortion due to *C fetus* subsp *fetus*, but abortions due to *C jejuni* sometimes occur in vaccinated ewes. Ewes should be vaccinated shortly before or after breeding and given a booster vaccination shortly after the second month of gestation. Annual booster vaccinations should be given at that time.

AGALACTIA SYNDROME

SOWS

Agalactia is a total failure of production or letdown of milk. It is unusual in sows; however, hypogalactia or lactational insufficiency (*see* below) is not, and occurs in individual sows or herd outbreaks. A number of mammary gland conditions are so devastating to the piglets (because of agalactia or hypogalactia [*see* p 1093]) that prompt diagnosis and therapy or cross-fostering is essential.

Because the sow may have agalactia or hypogalactia in one or more glands, individual piglets that select and "fix" on to a single gland by 24 hr of age may suffer while their littermates are normal. This commonly occurs as a result of bacterial mastitis in a single gland with no obvious clinical signs in the sow but severe consequences for the piglet "affixed" to that gland.

In another condition, individual teats may be occluded or nonexistent; in either case, the most common cause is teat necrosis, which is a consequence of trauma to the teats on rough, usually concrete, floors within the first days of life. Varying numbers of glands in varying portions of the female piglets may be affected. The trauma and inflammation lead to teat ablation or duct occlusion, which can cause "blind teats" in later life. It may be prevented by changing the surface of farrowing crate floors from concrete to one of the available plastic materials.

A condition often referred to by farmers as "hard udders" is extremely common. Circumstantial evidence suggests that this is usually associated with increasing milk production and, for various reasons, a failure of the piglets to consume all the available milk, eg, when piglets are debilitated by diarrhea or chilling. The condition is self-limiting: the sow responds by producing less milk, with the potential loss of subsequent growth in the piglets. "Hard udders" should not be confused with lactational insufficiency. Apart from a reluctance to nurse, sows with "hard udders" show none of the other clinical signs of hypogalactia. Similarly, hypogalactia should not be confused with bacterial mastitis in which, in severe cases that involve many glands and *Klebsiella* or staphylococci infections, the sow may die. Diagnosis is largely through careful clinical examination.

LACTATIONAL INSUFFICIENCY IN PERIPARTURIENT SOWS
(Mastitis-metritis-agalactia complex [MMA], Periparturient hypogalactia)

A syndrome of complex etiology; the most frequently used name, MMA, is a misnomer. Although the mammary glands are swollen, tender, and frequently warmer than normal, grossly detectable mastitis is found in only slightly >50% of affected sows. Likewise, metritis is only an occasional finding and not a clinically important aspect of this problem. Finally, only rarely is there complete agalactia; most sows continue to produce milk, but at a greatly reduced rate. The consequence is piglet death from acute starvation, hypoglycemia-induced weakness and an increased incidence of crushing by the sow, and increased susceptibility to diarrhea and other problems.

Etiology and Pathogenesis: The etiology is multifactorial. Evidence suggests that lipopolysaccharide (LPS) endotoxins, a portion of the cell wall of all gram-negative bacteria, play a role in some cases. It has been hypothesized, and partially demonstrated, that such toxins are readily absorbed from the mammary glands. In addition to the isolation of numerous streptococci and staphylococci, field surveys of mastitis in pigs have reported a high incidence of *Escherichia coli* and *Klebsiella* spp, which further supports the proposed role of gram-negative bacteria. It has also been demonstrated that endotoxins may be absorbed from the uterus, but not from the vagina of the postpartum sow.

In addition to producing a wide range of cardiovascular and immunologic changes, LPS endotoxins also suppress prolactin production by the anterior pituitary, decrease circulating thyroid hormone, and increase cortisol concentrations. These changes adversely affect milk production. Systemic administration of purified *E coli* endotoxins has produced clinical, endocrine, and hematologic changes indistinguishable from those seen in field cases of lactation failure. The circumstantial evidence that LPS endotoxins may play a role in lactation failure is strong, but the extent of their involvement has not yet been determined.

Clinical observations have suggested that constipation and/or feeding finely ground feed to sows can result in bacterial overgrowth and subsequent absorption of endotoxins from the intestines, but this theory has been largely disproved.

Other causes of hypogalactia that should be considered include udder and teat abnormalities, udder edema, hypocalcemia, bacterial mastitis, active viral infection (eg, pseudorabies, transmissible gastroenteritis), and chronic ergotism. Ergot derivatives suppress prolactin release in other species, a mechanism of action presumably applicable in sows. Incidence of lactational insufficiency is ~3 times higher in multiparous than in nulliparous animals, and does not follow a discernible seasonal pattern. Incidence of inadequate milk production varies from only an occasional sow to >50% of those in a herd.

Clinical Findings and Lesions: The problem is observed almost exclusively within the first 3 days postpartum; >50% of affected sows show signs of decreased milk production within the first 24 hr. Clinical examination is best conducted while the piglets are nursing. Milk ejection in affected sows is either absent or of brief duration, which causes the piglets to continue to actively nurse for an extended time. As a result of vigorous nursing efforts, the teats may be traumatized. The mammary glands vary from grossly normal to swollen, firm, and warm to the touch, with blotched purple skin. Rectal temperature of the sow varies from normal to markedly elevated (>106°F [41°C]). Anorexia, constipation, and depression may also be manifest. Some vaginal discharge is normal during the first few days postpartum, and metritis is rarely present.

During the initial stages, the piglets repeatedly attempt to nurse at frequent intervals and do not "settle" following nursing. Face biting is frequent as the piglets jostle for position and more milk. As the piglets' energy reserves are depleted, attempts to nurse decrease, and they often migrate to the warmest portions of the farrowing crate. Crushing by the sow is common.

There are no consistent macroscopic lesions. Some sows may have a few small foci of inflammation in the mammary glands. One or more glands may have a severe necrotizing mastitis.

Diagnosis: Diagnosis is usually based on clinical signs. Weak emaciated piglets, a significant number of crushed piglets, and a failure of the litter to quiet down following nursing are signs of inadequate milk production. In sows, mild to moderate pyrexia, constipation, diarrhea, decreased appetite, and mammary tenderness, swelling, and teat damage are consistent with a diagnosis of lactational insufficiency. Pure bacterial cultures may be isolated from milk samples.

Treatment and Control: Several therapeutic or other means are available for treatment; by far the most effective is to cross-foster the piglets from affected to normal sows. A sow that has farrowed within 24 hr, or one that has had its litter weaned at 2-3 wk of age, makes a suitable foster mother. The latter should not have the piglets introduced until ~3 hr after her own litter has been removed. Oxytocin (5-10 u/ sow) is occasionally effective in reestablishing lactation if used 2-3 times at 3- to 4-hr intervals. In herds in which a substantial percentage of the sows and gilts are affected, prostaglandin-$F_{2\alpha}$-induced parturition has reduced the incidence of lactational insufficiency. Although the mechanism is unclear, it has been hypothesized that with a rapid induction of labor, the teats are dilated for a shorter period of time, and the potential for a coliform mastitis is reduced. Broad-spectrum antibiotics are appropriate if the sow shows signs of mastitis. Some reports have suggested that glucocorticoids are effective for treating udder edema. Some success has been reported using flunixin meglumine to counteract some of the effects of endotoxins. There is no clear evidence that vaccines offer a beneficial prophylactic effect. Good sanitation tends to decrease the incidence of mastitis in the sow and diarrhea in the piglets. Subsequent litters are not likely to be affected.

CONTAGIOUS AGALACTIA (CA) AND OTHER MYCOPLASMAL MASTITIDES OF SMALL RUMINANTS

Although CA is usually caused by *Mycoplasma agalactiae*, at least 3 other mycoplasmas, viz *M mycoides mycoides* (large colony type, *Mmm* LC), *M capricolum*, and *M putrefaciens*, can cause a transmissible mastitis in small ruminants, particularly goats. Although, occasionally, several other mycoplasma species can be isolated from the udder of sheep and goats, they probably do not cause disease at this site.

Mycoplasma agalactiae and *M putrefaciens* most frequently localize in the udder, and *M capricolum* in the joints, while *Mmm* LC is usually associated with a complex syndrome of signs. However, distinguishing between these organisms clinically can be difficult, and in those countries where 2 or more of them commonly occur (eg, Spain, Portugal, France), the term CA is applied to a syndrome of agalactia and polyarthritis, with or without other signs and regardless of the cause.

Etiology and Clinical Findings: *Mycoplasma agalactiae* causes subacute or chronic disease in both goats and sheep. It has been reported from many countries around the world, most often in the Mediterranean basin.

Disease appears at or shortly after parturition. The udder becomes hot and swollen; pyrexia and inappetence are followed by decreased milk production. The milk may become thick and yellow, and separates on standing. One or both glands of the udder may be affected; hardened nodules and, later, atrophy may develop. Milk production may completely cease. Polyarthritis is frequent; keratoconjunctivitis is less common. In serious outbreaks, most animals can be affected, and mortality may be 10-20%.

Mmm LC is serologically indistinguishable from the causal agent of contagious bovine pleuropneumonia, but differs from it in several biological characteristics, most notably in producing large colonies on agar media. It occurs almost entirely in goats, and rarely in sheep. It is a major cause of disease in goats in the USA, France, and Israel, but also occurs in many other countries. *Mmm* LC usually causes acute or subacute disease, more severe than that produced by *M agalactiae*. Mortality may reach 25% in does and be >90% in kids. Any or all of the signs of mastitis, polyarthritis, pleuropneumonia, keratonconjunctivitis, and peracute or acute death, sometimes with CNS signs, may be seen. Signs and severity can vary markedly between outbreaks and herds, and, with time, even within the same herd. In endemic situations, disease may be sporadic and of low prevalence, with reduced milk production the most apparent outcome. In acute outbreaks, the udder is usually firm and affected bilaterally, and the milk watery and greenish, with a flaky deposit. On endemically infected farms, often only one gland is affected, and milk, though reduced in volume, often appears normal despite containing large numbers of mycoplasmas. In both situations, the condition may resolve or progress to atrophy of the gland. In one outbreak in sheep, pleuropneumonia and polyarthritis caused 60% mortality.

Mycoplasma capricolum causes sporadic, acute disease in goats, rarely sheep. Most commonly reported from France, the USA, and Spain, although also from many other countries, this organism is one of the "*M mycoides* group (cluster)" and is particularly closely related to the agent of contagious caprine pleuropneumonia. It may cause agalactia, polyarthritis, and occasionally, abscesses in does after a septicemic stage. Pneumonia and arthritis are seen in kids; in sheep, the organism has been associated with arthritis and an ulcerative vulvovaginitis.

Mycoplasma putrefaciens causes subacute or chronic disease in goats only. It has been reported most frequently from the USA, occasionally France and Australia. It is the least pathogenic of the 4 species, and signs are normally limited to the udder, although agalactia may be followed by severe polyarthritis. Milk production falls abruptly, with or without gross changes in milk. A putrefactive odor may be detectable in the bulk milk tank.

Transmission and Epidemiology: Milk is a major source of infection, either directly in the suckled young, through contaminated milking equipment or milker's hands, or through contaminated bedding or water troughs. Infection appears to be principally by the oral route in young animals, though the respiratory route is also implicated in *Mmm* LC infection. Ascending infection of the teat canal is also important in the lactating adult, especially with *M agalactiae* and *M putrefaciens*.

Carriers are a major source of infection. Animals may excrete mycoplasmas, especially *M agalactiae*, through a lactation and into the succeeding one(s). All 4 mastitogenic mycoplasmas may be harbored in the external ear canal of goats and in mites occurring at this site. The importance of this in the epidemiology of mycoplasmoses of small ruminants is not yet known. Although mycoplasmas have been regarded as fragile and short-lived away from the host, there have been reports of long-term survival in soil, dung, or secretions, especially at low temperatures.

Diagnosis: New outbreaks should be investigated by culture of the agent(s) involved. *Mycoplasma agalactiae* and *M putrefaciens* are relatively easily identified, although identification of *M capricolum* and *Mmm* LC may require a specialized laboratory. Serology (usually the complement fixation and indirect hemagglutination tests) is less frequently applied and useful only on a herd basis, preferably after cultural demonstration that the specific mycoplasma examined for occurs in the herd or locale.

Differential diagnoses include infection with *Pasteurella haemolytica*, which can cause pneumonia, mastitis, and occasionally arthritis; mastitis due to staphylococci, streptococci, or other bacteria; and arthritis caused by caprine arthritis encephalitis virus or *Erysipelothrix rhusiopathiae*.

Treatment and Control: The most efficacious antibiotics are the tetracyclines, the macrolides (tylosin, erythromycin, josamycin), and tiamulin fumarate. If administered promptly and for sufficient duration (at least 3-5 days), signs generally ameliorate, although affected joints may be recalcitrant. Moreover, antibiotic therapy is expensive and rarely eliminates mycoplasma infection.

Improved hygiene and management can markedly reduce the prevalence and severity of mycoplasmal disease. Infected animals should be isolated, and milking adults kept apart from younger animals. If possible, newborn animals should be separated from their dams at birth and fed colostrum, then milk, both heat treated at 56°C for 30 min. Housing and milking utensils should be disinfected regularly, and hygienic principles strictly observed during milking.

Commercial vaccines are available only for *M agalactiae*. Both killed and attenuated forms have reduced disease; however, killed vaccines are expensive and of low efficacy, and live vaccines, though more effective, may cause disease and live organisms may be secreted in the milk. Furthermore, live vaccines used so far have not prevented infection with, and excretion of, virulent strains.

BOVINE GENITAL CAMPYLOBACTERIOSIS

A venereal disease of cattle characterized by infertility and early embryonic death. Abortion occurs in a small percentage of infected cows. Distribution is worldwide.

Etiology and Transmission: *Campylobacter fetus* subsp *venerealis*, the usual cause of this disease, is a gram-negative, curved or spiral-shaped rod, which is motile by means of a polar flagellum. This subspecies is not known to infect man. Exposure to heat, drying, and atmospheric levels of oxygen quickly destroys the organism. The 2 known biotypes do not differ in pathogenicity.

Sporadic abortions in cattle without evidence of infertility can be caused by *C fetus* subsp *fetus* or *C jejuni* following ingestion of the organisms. These species cause enzootic abortion in sheep and goats (qv, p 655), enteritis in various animals (qv, p 102), and bacteremia and enteritis in man.

Campylobacter fetus is transmitted under natural conditions by coitus, and may be spread by contaminated instruments or untreated semen in artificial insemination. Infection may spread between bulls by contact with contaminated semen-collecting equipment, or by lying on contaminated bedding. Some bulls are refractory to infection, but others become permanent carriers. Duration of the carrier state in cows is quite variable; in one trial, 37% remained infected 5-10 mo after exposure. The development of local immunity usually results in clearance from the fallopian tubes and uterus within 3 mo, but vaginal infection may persist after pregnancy is established.

Clinical Findings: The primary effect is temporary infertility; abortion is of secondary importance. Irregularity of the estrous cycle is a prominent sign: conception occurs and is interrupted by infection, the embryo is resorbed, and a new cycle begins. If the embryo is expelled, it is often so small that the abortion goes unrecognized. The variable degree of endometritis, and the slight vaginitis and cervicitis sometimes produced, also may be overlooked.

Under conditions of natural breeding, the first evidence of disease may be increased numbers of cows returning to estrus late in the breeding period and greater than normal loss in flesh of the breeding bulls due to overwork. In herds not under close observation, disease may be unsuspected until many open cows and greater than normal differences in stages of pregnancy are detected.

Conception rates of 40-50% or lower occur in newly infected herds. Where the disease is endemic, conception rates may be only moderately below normal, with severe infertility confined to replacement heifers or susceptible cows bred with the herd. Usually no more than 5% of a herd aborts; abortions may occur anytime during gestation, but are most common between months 4 and 6. In late abortions, the placenta may be retained. The placental and fetal lesions are not characteristic enough to be diagnostic.

Diagnosis: Bovine genital campylobacteriosis and trichomoniasis (qv, p 662) are clinically similar, and difficult or impossible to differentiate without laboratory procedures. On occasion, the 2 diseases are found concurrently in a herd. Campylobacteriosis can be diagnosed tentatively by the clinical history and observation of slender, curved bacteria in stains of cotyledon impressions or fetal abomasal fluid. The organisms are gram negative, but will stain with most simple stains, which reveals their characteristic morphology. They can often be seen in wet preparations of the abomasal fluid examined by darkfield or phase-contrast microscopy. Microscopical examination of preputial fluid or cervicovaginal mucus is not useful due to the frequent occurrence of commensals such as *C sputorum* in healthy animals. Suspected campylobacteriosis can be confirmed by:

1) Isolation of *C fetus* subsp *venerealis*. The most efficient and specific procedure is isolation of causative organisms from the herd bulls, which are the principal carriers, or from selected infertile, nonpregnant cows. Isolations can be made from aborted fetuses, usually without use of selective media, if the tissues are sent to the laboratory in good condition. Tissues should be held slightly above freezing for transportation. Abomasal fluid and liver are the best sources for isolation, but recoveries can sometimes be made from other organs, including the brain. A low-oxygen atmosphere is required for incubation of cultures.

Preputial fluid or cervicovaginal mucus can be collected for culture. Lavage of the preputial cavity or vagina with fluid can result in reduced isolations due to overgrowth of cultures by contaminating organisms and is not recommended. Because of the sensitivity of the organisms to atmospheric levels of oxygen, the samples should either be cultured on selective media soon after collection, or placed in vials of transport-enrichment medium for transport to the laboratory. Cervicovaginal mucus samples can be transported in pipettes on dry ice, but there is some reduction in number of viable organisms, which can result in false-negative results.

Bulls and cows are sometimes examined for campylobacteriosis before export or sale; a minimum of 3 negative cultures, from samples collected ≥5 days apart, is required for reasonable assurance of freedom from infection.

2) FA stains. FA examination of preputial and cervicovaginal mucus complements culture, and use of both procedures identifies a slightly higher number of infected animals than either alone. FA also has been used after incubation of transport-enrichment medium. A disadvantage of FA is the inability to distinguish between *C venerealis* and *C fetus*.

3) Serology. The vaginal mucus agglutination test has been used as a herd test but is of limited value in detecting infection in individual animals. Antibody may not appear until the animal has been infected for several months, and some animals become negative quickly. The ELISA test has not been used extensively, but preliminary results indicate it is more sensitive and detects antibodies earlier than the agglutination test.

The blood serum agglutination and complement-fixation tests are of limited value because most cows develop only low titers and some virgin disease-free heifers develop titers, presumably due to contact with organisms sharing antigens with *Campylobacter* spp.

Treatment and Control: Control measures are based on assumptions that transmission occurs only at coitus and that carriers are present in the herd. The infection is confined to the genital tracts of both sexes, and systemic immune responses do not develop naturally. Following infection, most cows develop local immunity that clears the bacteria from the fallopian tubes and uterus within 3 mo. Pregnancy can then occur, although the vagina may remain infected for several months or through one or more successful pregnancies. Persistence of infection is thought to be due to the ability of the bacteria to change the surface antigens exposed to the immune defenses of the host during the course of infection. Convalescent cows may develop vaginal infection again on exposure to infected bulls, but develop an anamnestic response that prevents infection of the uterus and permits conception. A natural immunity in bulls has not been identified; some bulls remain infected for life unless treated or vaccinated.

Control measures are usually made in preparation for the next breeding season. Culling open cows will not eliminate herd infection because of pregnant carriers, and their retention should be considered because developing immunity will result in reasonably good fertility. All animals should be vaccinated as soon after the diagnosis as is feasible, and again in 6-8 wk; a booster vaccination should be given ~1 mo before start of breeding. The interval between vaccinations should not be <4 wk.

Vaccination of infected cows hastens elimination of infection to some extent, but the effect may be minimal in well-established infection. However, vaccination dramatically improves the fertility of infected cows, although some remain vaginal carriers. Vaccination of bulls can cure infection and prevent permanent infection, but in one trial, 3 vaccinations were required to eliminate infection from all bulls. Vaccinated bulls can transmit infection for a few hours after breeding an infected cow. There is some indication that double the vaccine dosage used for cows may be best for bulls.

Artificial insemination can prevent spread of infection. Semen is preferably obtained from uninfected bulls, and diluted 1:25; 500 u of penicillin and 0.5 mg of dihydrostreptomycin are added per mL of diluted semen. The treated semen should be held at 40°F (4.4°C) for ≥6 hr before use. Procedures for heat detection and insemination should be designed to eliminate any possibility of transmission between cows.

Although antibiotic treatment of infected cows has given variable results and is seldom practiced, treatment of bulls is usually effective, and in some circumstances may be appropriate. Local or systemic treatment, or both, may be used. The bull is given a subcut. injection (25 mg/kg) and a preputial infusion (10 mL) of 50% aqueous dihydrostreptomycin; the preputial orifice is held closed, and the exterior of the sheath massaged for 1 min before the orifice is released. Two or 3 treatments at 48-hr intervals are advised. Ulceration of penile mucosa, of undetermined significance, has been observed in some bulls following local treatment.

Vaccination should be practiced in clean herds at risk due to potential of mixing of cattle during breeding, or when nonvirgin animals are added to the herd. Although recommendations of vaccine manufacturers vary, the following vaccine program is based on research results. Cows and bulls not previously vaccinated should be vaccinated twice at an interval of ≥4 wk, with the last vaccination given ≤1 mo before start of breeding. Annual booster vaccinations are required (because most vaccinated animals do not develop an anamnestic response on exposure to infection) and should be given before breeding. Booster vaccinations given a considerable period before breeding, eg, at time of pregnancy examination, are of some value, but not as effective as if given just before breeding.

BOVINE TRICHOMONIASIS

A venereal, protozoal disease of cattle characterized by early fetal death and infertility associated with greatly extended calving intervals. Distribution is worldwide.

Etiology and Epidemiology: The causative piriform protozoan, *Tritrichomonas (Trichomonas) foetus*, is ordinarily 10-15 × 5-10 μm, but there is considerable pleomorphism, and organisms cultivated in artificial media tend to become spherical. At the anterior end of the organism, there are 3 flagella about the same length as the parasite. An undulating membrane extends the length of the trichomonad and is bordered by a marginal filament that continues beyond the membrane as a posterior flagellum. A few organisms can survive the freezing procedures used for storing semen, but they do not survive drying or high temperatures.

The organism is found only in the genital tract of the cow and bull. Of cows serviced by a diseased bull, >90% may become infected. Transmission by artificial insemination (AI) can occur; therefore, only semen from bulls known to be uninfected should be used. It may be assumed that transmission occurs only during coitus and that most bulls remain permanently infected unless properly treated. The bull is usually the source of initial and continuous infection in a herd. Infected cows usually recover spontaneously after mean durations of 20 wk (primary exposure) and 10 wk (secondary exposure).

Cows can remain infected throughout pregnancy and discharge trichomonads from the genital tract following calving. However, most previously infected cows that undergo 3 mo of sexual rest after calving with normal uterine involution are free of infection.

Clinical Findings: The most common sign is infertility caused by death of the fetus, usually 2-4 mo after conception, and characterized by repeat breeding and greatly delayed calving. If pregnancy continues into the third and fourth months, abortion may occur. Cows that carry their calves beyond the fourth month usually deliver a live calf. A practical measure of the infertility in cows infected for the first time is an increase in the mean calving interval by 90-100 days.

Trichomoniasis is a cause of postcoital pyometra, which results from death and maceration of the developing fetus. In infected herds, this complication usually occurs in <5% of the cows. The corpus luteum and, in some instances, the cervical seal persist so that there is no discharge of pus. More frequently, however, the cervix opens and there is a slight nonodorous discharge. As in all pyometras, estrus does not occur, and the condition may persist for months.

Diagnosis: A tentative diagnosis may be based on the history and clinical signs, but confirmation depends on finding the organism in at least one animal in a herd. Organisms may be found in the placental fluid, the stomach contents of an aborted fetus, the uterus for several days after an abortion, and exuded pus. They also can be found in the vagina in large numbers 12-19 days after infection. Subsequently, the numbers regularly increase and decrease according to the phase of the estrous cycle, and are highest 3-7 days before each estrus.

In bulls, the organisms are in the prepuce, frequently in small numbers. Microscopical examination of preputial smegma for trichomonads is the most common method to confirm a herd diagnosis. While trichomonads may be found in all parts of the sheath and on the penis, they occur in the greatest numbers in the fornix and on the glans penis. An AI plastic pipette can be used to collect preputial fluid. The pipette is introduced into the fornix of the prepuce, and smegma is collected with a combination of scraping and aspirating via an attached rubber bulb or syringe. Samples of vaginal mucus are aspirated from the anterior vagina with a glass or plastic pipette and a long rubber tube. Diagnosis is simplified and efficiency improved by culturing samples for 4-7 days at 37°C before microscopical examination (high power).

A larger volume of fluid may be examined if no cover slip is used. The organisms may not be numerous, and careful systematic examination is often necessary. Identification can be made at low power and is based on the size and shape of the organisms as well as the characteristic aimless, jerky motion. Only living organisms are useful for diagnostic purposes.

Treatment and Control: Control measures are based on the assumption that transmission occurs only during coitus. Animals with pyometra or other genital abnormalities should be culled. Most of the remaining cows can recover if AI with semen free of *T foetus* is used. If AI is not possible, the herd can be divided into exposed and unexposed groups. In the unexposed group, service is resumed using uninfected bulls. The exposed group is treated for recognizable uterine disease and allowed 3 mo of sexual rest. For breeding, the exposed herd should be divided into as many groups as practical, with one young bull for each group. Bulls and cows should be examined for reinfection. Control may also be gained in large herds by eliminating all bulls >3 yr old and using only younger bulls for mating. This is based on the relative lack of susceptibility of young bulls to trichomonad infection.

Slaughter, rather than treatment, of bulls is generally recommended. Successful treatment has been reported with dimetridazole, ipronidazole, or metronidazole. However, such usage lacks official approval.

BOVINE UDDER DISEASES

See also MASTITIS, p 686, and COWPOX and PSEUDOCOWPOX, p 823.

BOVINE ULCERATIVE MAMMILLITIS

A severe ulcerative condition of the teats of dairy cows that can occur in outbreaks and result in marked loss of milk production and a high incidence of secondary mastitis. Initially reported in the UK, it also occurs in the USA and other countries. It is caused by bovine herpesvirus 2, which is the same as the Allerton strain of Group II lumpy-skin-disease viruses (qv, p 824).

The lesions begin as one or more thickened plaques of varying size on the skin of one or more teats. Vesiculation of these plaques occurs quickly, and the surface sloughs, leaving a raw ulcerated area that becomes covered with a black-brown scab. The scabs tend to crack and bleed, especially if milking is attempted. Much of the teat wall may be involved, and often the lesion includes the teat orifice, which predisposes to mastitis and obstruction of the streak canal. In the early stages, before vesiculation is marked, intranuclear inclusions may be detected in the cells of the epidermis. The disease is more severe in cows that have recently calved, especially those with udder edema. Severe lesions may take several weeks to heal.

Diagnosis is based on the signs and confirmed by histopathology or by virus isolation from early lesions. Virus neutralization titers rise quickly, and the first serum sample must be taken early in the course of disease.

Affected cows should be isolated and separate milking utensils used. Cannulas may be necessary to remove milk. Emollient antiseptic ointments used after milking may reduce further trauma, hemorrhage, and secondary bacterial infections. Prophylactic infusions for mastitis should be considered if the teat orifice is involved. Iodophor solutions (1:320 v/v) may be useful as teat and udder disinfectants to aid control in infected herds.

CONGENITAL AND PHYSIOLOGICAL DISEASES

Congenital aberrations include many structural defects, eg, fusion of the front and hind teats, large-base or funnel-shaped teats, small short teats, improperly placed teats, "cut-up" udders, predisposition to pendulous or swinging udders, hypoplasia of front- or hindquarters, and supernumerary teats. Except for the latter condition, there is no treatment. These defects should be eliminated by selective breeding.

Agalactia is observed occasionally in heifers and probably is a hereditary condition associated with an imbalance of the hormones that control udder growth and development, or lactation. Response to treatment is equivocal. Occasionally, this condition is due to a severe systemic disease in the recently fresh animal, or it may be associated with advanced chronic mastitis with extensive fibrosis of the mammary gland. Animals affected with the latter condition never produce a normal supply of milk.

Failure of milk letdown is observed occasionally after parturition in young dairy cattle. This may be caused by the pain and discomfort of a large and edematous udder, or by fear and stress during the initial milking procedure. If usual methods of massage, use of warm compresses, sucking, and frequent milking fail to result in proper letdown of milk, administration of posterior pituitary extract or oxytocin may be successful. This treatment may have to be repeated at each milking for several days. An exact milking and feeding routine is important in training heifers to develop a proper letdown habit.

Inversion of the teat orifice is congenital and may be hereditary. Although associated with ease of milking, it is undesirable because the teats frequently spray. This type of teat orifice favors udder infection.

Necrotic dermatitis (sometimes called seborrhea of the udder) is observed in cows or first-calf heifers with large edematous udders several weeks after calving. In heifers, the area usually involved is the lateral aspect of the udder and medial aspect of the thigh; the udder is pressed tightly against the leg and causes chafing, dermatitis, and finally, necrosis. In cows, it is usually observed at the anterior portion of the udder between the 2 forequarters. Possibly, poor circulation or ischemia due to the extensive edema causes the necrosis at this site. In heifers, treatment consists of reducing udder congestion as rapidly as possible with diuretics or diuretics and corticosteroids, limiting movement, daily cleansing with an antiseptic solution, and applying mild astringents. In cows, the swollen necrotic area should be washed daily to control the odor, and astringent and drying powders should be applied, along with fly repellents during the summer. There is no specific treatment to hasten the normal tissue sloughing and repair.

Physiological udder edema and congestion is common in high-producing dairy cattle before and after parturition. This problem cannot be controlled satisfactorily, but several practices may help. Some advise milking cows before parturition as a means of reducing the congestion and edema, but this may predispose older cows to parturient paresis. Frequent milkings may be helpful. Massage and hot compresses stimulate circulation and promote reduction of the edema. The massage should be repeated as often as possible. When milk letdown fails, udder edema and congestion appear to increase. In severely affected cows, the udder often "breaks down" and becomes pendulous. Diuretics, eg, chlorothiazide or similar preparations, have proved highly beneficial in reducing udder edema, especially in young cattle.

Rupture of the suspensory ligaments of the udder (mainly the medial ligaments) occurs gradually in some older cows over several lactations, leads to a dropping of the udder, and causes the teats to point somewhat laterally. Occasionally, acute rupture can occur at or just after parturition; this is characterized by a sudden dropping of the udder, hardness and swelling, and by marked edema with serous exudation at the base of the udder, especially anteriorly. There is no successful treatment; supportive trusses generally are not satisfactory.

Supernumerary teats may be located on the udder behind the posterior teats, between the front and hind teats, or attached to either the front or hind teats. They are easily removed surgically when the animal is from 1 wk to 1 yr old; it is best done at 3-8 mo of age. Removal just before or during lactation is undesirable since a teat fistula often forms that is difficult to correct. Removing supernumerary teats from dairy heifers is desirable to improve appearance of the udder, eliminate the possibility of mastitis in the gland above the extra teats, and facilitate milking.

Urticaria or allergic swelling of the udder and teats is observed in association with generalized urticaria (qv, p 867), and occasionally, it may be localized when cows are bedded on buckwheat straw or other allergenic plants.

TRAUMATIC DISEASES

Superficial wounds to the udder and teats may be cleaned with suitable antiseptic solutions and treated as open wounds with frequent application of antiseptic powders or sprays. If the teats are involved, adhesive tape may hasten healing. Those involving the teat orifice should be dressed with antiseptic creams and bound b.i.d. to prevent udder infections. Severe hemorrhage that requires prompt compression and ligation may result from wounds that sever a large milk vein.

Deeper wounds of the udder and teats should be promptly (within 6 hr) cleansed and sutured under local anesthesia, with physical or chemical restraint, to promote first-intention healing. When the wound involves the teat cistern, it may be necessary to insert a self-retaining teat cannula with removable cap into the teat for the first 24 hr to prevent milk seeping through the wound (which would delay or prevent healing) and to aid in milking. Aftercare includes infusion of the affected quarter with antibiotic preparations and maintenance of high blood levels of antibiotic by parenteral therapy.

Abscesses of the udder may be secondary to wounds, advanced mastitis, infected hematomas, or severe contusions. They should be incised and drained when they are chronic and near the surface of the udder. The wound should be packed for 2 days with gauze that contains a counterirritant (eg, a 2.5% alcoholic solution of iodine) and washed daily thereafter with an antiseptic solution.

"Black spot" and **teat "spider"** or **"black scab"** may cause necrosis, scab formation, and fibrous thickening of the teat orifice and sphincter, and may lead to teat stenosis (*see* below). They frequently respond to regular applications of antibiotic-corticosteroid ointment, in the early stages. Outbreaks may be due to faulty milking machine function, especially faulty pulsation, liners too short, or excessively high vacuum level and over-milking. Such faults may initially cause eversions and vegetative growths at the teat orifice, and residual milk in these lesions can favor bacterial growth and development of a local infection, which can lead to "black spot" and secondary mastitis.

"Blind" or nonfunctional quarters usually are the result of a severe infection, which may occur in the dry or lactating cow or in the heifer due to sucking by other heifers or calves. If treated, the infection may be overcome and the quarters will milk fairly satisfactorily during the next lactation if fibrosis is not extensive. Blind quarters that still contain a small amount of pus may be dried up permanently by infusion of 3% silver nitrate solution (30-50 mL). Rarely, blind or nonfunctional quarters may be congenital.

Bloody milk frequently is seen following calving when the udder usually is severely congested and edematous, as well as following udder trauma. This condition is most common at the first to third parturitions. It usually resolves without treatment in 4-14 days, providing the gland is milked out regularly.

Chapping and cracking can occur when teats are exposed to frequent washing and drying, irritant solutions, or cold wet winds. In some countries, teat chapping and pseudo-cowpox (qv, p 823) may occur simultaneously and lead to severe lesions. Both conditions can be treated with antiseptic udder ointments such as those that contain chlorhexidine or iodophors. Teat dips with the latter plus 5-10% glycerin, applied after milking, may help prevent teat chapping and aid in mastitis control.

Complete teat obstruction is caused by the same factors that cause stenosis, or by a congenital membranous obstruction. Treatment is similar to that for stenosis, but the prognosis usually is more guarded. Occasionally, if the injury is severe enough, milking of the quarter should be discontinued for the remainder of the lactation period or permanently. Corpora amylacea, firm blood clots, small pedunculated tumors of the teat lining, or foreign bodies (eg, teat dilators) may be present in the teat cistern and intermittently obstruct the internal teat orifice. These may be removed by massage, or by dilation or incision of the teat orifice and grasping and removing the object with a pair of fine forceps.

Contusions and hematomas of the udder and teats produce painful swellings and frequently result in bloody milk. Also, temporary stenosis of the teat canal or orifice may occur. Cold applications applied regularly at intervals over several days, and then warm applications or hot packs and gentle massage may hasten resolution of the swelling. In these conditions, machine milking should be replaced by gentle hand milking until recovery is complete. Rarely, large hematomas may interfere with circulation of blood in the skin of the udder, and necrosis and infection may occur. Hematomas should not be incised or drained unless they become infected.

"Leakers" are cows with teats that drip milk continuously or after the stimulus that causes milk letdown. These cows usually have sustained a severe teat injury or have a large streak canal. In general, little can be done to correct this condition satisfactorily. Injecting small amounts of Lugol's solution around the teat sphincter with an intradermal syringe, cauterizing the external teat orifice or teat end, and surgical correction have been tried with limited success.

Permanent fistulas into the teat or gland cisterns are best repaired surgically when the cow is dry.

Teat stenosis is characterized by a marked narrowing of the teat orifice or streak canal (or both), which makes milking difficult. Occasionally a congenital condition affecting all teats, more often it results from a contusion or wound that produces swelling or formation of a blood clot or scab. In acute cases, conservative treatment as outlined for wounds and contusions is indicated. Machine milking should be discontinued temporarily in favor of hand milking of the affected teat(s). In rare cases, a teat cannula taped in place may be used, with proper aseptic precautions, for withdrawing the milk. Many acute cases of stenosis progress to the more chronic form, characterized by a fibrous thickening of the canal lining and sphincter tissues, especially if a wound is present in or around the teat orifice. In chronic cases, surgery may sometimes correct the stenosis. All injuries to, or surgical procedures on, the teat should be handled carefully to prevent infection. Prophylactic antibiotic infusions of the quarter are indicated when the teat or teat orifice is involved.

UDDER ACNE

A disease of dairy cows characterized by pustules on the skin of the udder and teats, often near the teat base. It tends to spread in some herds. Staphylococci usually can be isolated from the pustules. A predisposing factor may be excessive teat-cup "crawl" at milking associated with a prolonged interval between cessation of milk flow and teat-cup removal. Hair should be clipped from the affected area, the skin thoroughly washed with chlorhexidine (5000 ppm) or iodophor (10,000 ppm), and an antibacterial ointment such as chlorhexidine or sulfathiazole applied b.i.d. after milking. Use of iodophor or chlorhexidine solutions as udder washes and postmilking teat dips helps prevent spread of the disease.

BRUCELLOSIS

A contagious disease primarily affecting cattle, pigs, sheep, goats, and dogs, caused by bacteria of the genus *Brucella* and characterized by abortion and, to a lesser extent, orchitis and infection of the accessory sex glands in males. The disease is prevalent in most of the world. Brucellosis occasionally affects horses. The disease in man, often referred to as undulant fever, is a serious public health problem.

BRUCELLOSIS IN CATTLE
(Contagious abortion, Bang's disease)

Etiology and Epidemiology: The disease in cattle is caused almost exclusively by *Brucella abortus*; however, *B suis* or *B melitensis* is occasionally implicated. Infection spreads rapidly and causes many abortions in unvaccinated herds. Typically, in a herd in which disease is endemic, an infected cow aborts only once after exposure; subsequent gestations and lactations appear normal. Following exposure, many cattle become bacteremic for a short period and develop agglutinins and other antibodies; most of the remainder resist infection, and a small percentage of infected cows recover. A positive serum agglutination test usually precedes abortion, but may be delayed in some animals. Organisms are shed in milk and uterine discharges, and the cow may become temporarily sterile. Bacteria may be found in the uterus during pregnancy, uterine involution, and infrequently, for a prolonged time in the nongravid uterus. Some infected cows that aborted previously shed brucellae from the uterus at subsequent normal parturitions. Secondary infections contribute to infertility and may prolong involution and the presence of *B abortus* in the uterus and its discharges. Organisms are shed in milk for a variable length of time—in some animals for life.

Natural transmission may occur by ingestion of organisms, which can be present in large numbers in aborted fetuses, fetal membranes, and uterine discharges. Cattle may ingest contaminated feed and water, or lick contaminated genitals of other animals. Venereal transmission by infected bulls to susceptible cows may occur but is rare. Transmission may occur by artificial insemination when *Brucella*-contaminated semen is deposited in the uterus but reportedly not when deposited in the mid-cervix. Brucellae may enter the body through mucous membranes, conjunctivae, wounds, or even intact skin.

Mechanical vectors (eg, other animals including man) may spread infection. Brucellae have been recovered from fetuses and from manure that has remained in a cool environment for >2 mo. Exposure to direct sunlight kills the organism in a few hours.

Clinical Findings: Abortion is the most obvious manifestation. Infections may also cause stillborn calves, retained placentas, and reduced milk yield. Usually, general health is not impaired in uncomplicated abortions.

Seminal vesicles, ampullae, testicles, and epididymides may be infected in bulls; therefore, organisms are in the semen. Agglutinins may be demonstrated in seminal plasma from infected bulls. Testicular abscesses may occur. The organism has been isolated from arthritic joints.

Diagnosis: Diagnosis is based on bacteriology or serology. *Brucella abortus* can be recovered from the placenta, but more conveniently in pure culture from the stomach and lungs of an aborted fetus. Most cows cease shedding organisms from the genital tract when uterine involution is complete. Foci of infection remain in the reticuloendothelial system and udder, and *B abortus* is frequently isolated from milk and secretions of the nonlactating udder.

Serum agglutination tests have been the standard diagnostic method. Agglutination tests may also detect antibodies in milk, whey, and plasma. More recently, an ELISA has been developed to detect antibodies in milk and serum, and *Brucella* antigens in vaginal discharges. A test utilizing vaginal mucus to detect *Brucella* agglutinins may also be of diagnostic value. When the standard plate or tube serum agglutination test is used, complete agglutination at dilutions of 1:100 or more for nonvaccinated animals, and of 1:200 for animals vaccinated between 3 and 9 mo of age are considered positive, and the animals are classified as reactors.

Screening test procedures: 1) *Brucella* milk ring test (BRT)—In the official control and eradication on an area basis, the BRT has been efficient and accurate for locating infected dairy herds. The brucellosis status of dairy herds in any area can be monitored by implementing the BRT at 3-to 4-mo intervals. Pooled milk samples from individual herds are collected at the farm, milk processing plant, or creamery, and tested. Herds with a positive BRT are individually blood tested, and reactors are slaughtered. The cost of a BRT program in an area is ~10% of serological testing. Efficacies of the 2 test programs in reducing infection rates are comparable.

2) Market cattle testing (MCT)—Nondairy herds in an area also may be screened for brucellosis by testing sera collected from cattle destined for slaughter through intermediate and terminal markets, or at abattoirs. Reactors are traced to the herd of origin, and entire herds are tested. The cost of identifying reactors by this method is minimal compared to the cost of testing all cattle in all herds. Additional screening tests, including the card test and plate test, may be used to identify presumptively infected animals, thus reducing the number of more expensive diagnostic tests.

Brucellosis-free areas can be achieved and maintained, effectively and economically, by using the BRT on dairy herds and MCT on nondairy herds.

Supplemental tests may be used in herds from which brucellosis has not been eradicated despite continued application of standard tests. Utilization of a battery of these tests improves the probability of detecting infected animals that have remained in these herds as reservoirs of infection. They are also used to clarify the results of plate or card tests, especially among sera from vaccinated cattle. These tests, which include complement fixation and rivanol precipitation, are designed to detect primarily the antibodies specifically associated with *Brucella* infection. Another supplementary diagnostic procedure is testing milk samples from individual udder quarters by serial dilution BRT; this is often an excellent method for detecting chronic infection in udders of cows that may have equivocal serum reactions.

Control: Since no practical treatment is known, efforts are directed at detection and prevention. Eventual eradication depends on testing and eliminating reactors. The disease has been eradicated from many individual herds and areas by this method. Herds must be tested at regular intervals until 2-3 successive tests are negative.

Noninfected herds must be protected. The greatest danger is from replacement animals. Additions should be vaccinated calves or nonpregnant heifers. If pregnant or fresh cows must be added, they should originate from brucellosis-free areas or herds and be seronegative. Replacements should be isolated for ≥30 days and retested before being added to the herd.

Vaccination of calves with *B abortus* Strain 19 increases resistance to infection. Resistance may not be complete, and some may become infected, depending on severity of exposure. A small percentage of vaccinated animals develop antibodies that may persist for years, and thus may confuse diagnostic test results. To minimize this problem, calves in the USA are vaccinated with a vaccine that contains 3-10 billion viable *B abortus* Strain 19 organisms per 2 mL dose.

Whole-herd adult cattle vaccination using from 300 million to 1 billion viable Strain 19 organisms per 2 mL dose has been practiced in certain high incidence areas in the USA; however, it is not recommended in areas where the disease has been eliminated.

Brucella abortus 45/20 bacterin in adjuvant is another vaccine that has been used in some countries. Most studies indicate that 45/20 vaccine, when used as recommended, may induce immunity comparable to that of Strain 19. Current recommendations are for 2 initial injections at specific intervals and an annual booster. An advantage is that a positive serum agglutination test seldom occurs. Disadvantages include multiple injections at specific intervals, cost of additional vaccine and labor, and local reactions at injection sites.

Vaccination as the sole means of disease control has been effective. Reduction in the number of reactors in a herd is directly related to the percentage of vaccinated animals. However, when proceeding from a control to an eradication program, a test and slaughter program is necessary.

BRUCELLOSIS IN DOGS

Although dogs occasionally become infected with *Brucella abortus, B suis,* or *B melitensis,* these sporadic occurrences are usually closely associated with infected domestic livestock. A cause of abortion in kenneled dogs is *B canis.* Dogs appear to be the definitive host of this organism. Infection has caused a reduction of 75% in the number of pups weaned in some breeding kennels. The disease disseminates rapidly among dogs closely kenneled, especially at time of breeding or when abortions occur. Transmission is congenital, venereal, or by ingestion of contaminated materials. All ages and both sexes appear to be equally susceptible. Transmission of brucellosis from dogs to man and occasionally to other animals has been reported.

Primary signs are abortion without premonitory signs during the last trimester of pregnancy, stillbirths, and conception failures. Prolonged vaginal discharge usually follows abortion. Abortions may occur during subsequent pregnancies. Infected dogs develop generalized lymphadenitis, and frequently epididymitis, periorchitis, and prostatitis. Bacteremia is frequent and persists for ~18 mo after exposure. Pyrexia is not characteristic.

Diagnosis is based on isolation and identification of the causative agent or by serology. The organism can usually be readily isolated from vaginal exudate, aborted pups, blood, milk, or semen of infected dogs. The most widely used serological test is the agglutination test. Nonspecific agglutination reactions occur in some dogs from which *Brucella* has not been isolated; to eliminate nonspecific antibodies, the serum is treated with 2-mercaptoethanol and retested (qv, p 952).

Attempts at immunization or treatment have not been uniformly successful. Control is based on elimination or isolation of infected dogs identified by positive cultural or serological tests. Incidence of infection is much lower in kennels where dogs are caged individually. Long-term therapy, eg, with a combination of streptomycin and tetracycline, has been successful in most cases.

BRUCELLOSIS IN GOATS

The signs of brucellosis in goats are similar to those in cattle. The disease is prevalent in most countries where goats are a significant part of the animal industry.

It is rare in the USA. The causal agent usually is *Brucella melitensis*, but *B abortus* has been implicated. Infection occurs primarily through ingestion of the organism, but conjunctival, vaginal, and subcut. inoculations will produce disease. The disease causes abortion about the fourth month of pregnancy. Rarely, arthritis and orchitis occur, and keratitis and chronic bronchitis may be caused by infection with *B melitensis*. Diagnosis is made by bacteriological examination of milk or an aborted fetus, or by serum agglutination tests. If any goat in a herd shows a titer of ≥1:100, all goats with titers of 1:50 or 1:25 should be considered positive. In the USA, the disease is controlled by slaughter of reactors; in other countries, vaccination is used.

BRUCELLOSIS IN HORSES

Horses can be infected with *Brucella abortus* or *B suis*. Suppurative bursitis, most commonly recognized as "fistula of the withers" or "poll evil" (qv, p 469) is the most frequent ailment associated with brucellosis in horses. Occasionally, abortion has been reported.

BRUCELLOSIS IN PIGS

Clinical manifestations of brucellosis in pigs vary considerably, but are similar in many respects to those seen in cattle and goats. Although the disease is often self-limiting, it has remained in some herds for years. Brucellosis caused by *B suis* also occurs in other domestic animals and man. Epidemics of human brucellosis have been reported among packing-house workers, and the usual source is infected pigs.

Etiology and Transmission: *Brucella suis* is spread mainly by close animal contact, usually by ingestion of infected tissues or wastes. Infected boars may transmit the disease during service; the organism can be recovered from semen.

Pigs raised for breeding purposes constitute an important source of infection. Although infrequent, natural transmission among infected weanling pigs has been reported. Suckling pigs may become infected from sows, but most reach weanling age without becoming infected. The disease is usually more severe in breeding pigs than in young pigs, but both age groups are susceptible.

Clinical Findings: Following exposure to *B suis*, pigs develop a bacteremia that may persist for up to 90 days. During and following the bacteremia, localization may occur in various tissues. Signs depend considerably on the site(s) of localization. Common manifestations are abortion, temporary or permanent sterility, orchitis, lameness, posterior paralysis, spondylitis, and occasionally, metritis and abscess formation in extremities or other areas of the body.

The incidence of abortion may be 0-80%. Abortions may also occur early in gestation and be unobserved. Usually, sows or gilts that abort early in gestation return to estrus soon afterward and are rebred.

Sterility in sows, gilts, and boars is common and may be the only manifestation. Before attempting treatment, it is logical to test for brucellosis in herds in which sterility is a problem. Sterility may be permanent in sows, but is more frequently temporary. In boars, orchitis, usually unilateral, may occur; fertility appears to be reduced, but complete sterility may not ensue.

Diagnosis: The principal means of diagnosis in pigs is the brucellosis card test. Various other serum agglutination tests or complement fixation tests have been used. It is generally accepted that the tests are effective in determining the presence of brucellosis in a herd, but have limitations in detecting it in individual animals. Thus, entire herds or units of herds, rather than individual animals, must be tested in any control program. Low agglutinin titers occur in almost any sizable herd, infected or not, and a few infected pigs may have no detectable titer. The card test is usually more accurate than conventional agglutination tests. Supplemental tests designed for cattle also can be used for pigs.

Prophylaxis and Control: Caution should be followed in the purchase of individual pigs that exhibit a low agglutinin titer, unless the status of the entire herd of origin is known. Pigs should be isolated on return from fairs or shows before entering the herd. Replacements should be purchased from herds known to be free of brucellosis, or should be tested and isolated for 3 mo and retested before being added to the herd. Vaccination is unreliable, and no practical recommendations can be made for treatment. Control is based on test and segregation, and slaughter of infected breeding stock. The following plans can be used to eliminate brucellosis from a herd.

1) Sale of entire herd for slaughter: This plan is usually the most rapid, reliable, and economical. Replacements should be from herds free of infection and made after premises and equipment are cleaned and disinfected. The replacement herd should be placed on ground that has been free of pigs for ≥60 days.

2) Test, segregation, and delayed slaughter of infected herd: This plan is recommended for use only in purebred herds when it is desired to retain valuable bloodlines. Weanling pigs ≤6 wk old should be isolated (on uncontaminated ground); the remainder of the herd should be marketed as soon as practicable. Pigs should be tested ~30 days before breeding, and only gilts that test negative should be saved. Breeding should be only to boars known to be negative. Gilts should be retested after farrowing. If infection is found, the entire plan should be repeated, or abandoned in favor of plan 1.

3) Slaughter of reactors only: This is not generally recommended except in herds in which only a very few reactors are found, no clinical signs of brucellosis have been noted, or there is doubt that reactor titers were caused by *Brucella*. A herd retest at 30-day intervals is recommended, with removal of reactors until the herd is negative.

Swine breeders in the USA should be encouraged to validate their herds as brucellosis-free. Details of validation procedures are available from state regulatory veterinarians.

BRUCELLOSIS IN SHEEP

Brucella melitensis infection in sheep causes clinical disease similar to that in goats (*see above*). However, *B ovis* produces a disease unique to sheep: epididymitis and orchitis impair fertility, which is the principal economic effect. Occasionally, placentitis and abortion are observed and there may be perinatal mortality. The disease was first described in New Zealand and Australia, and has since been reported from most sheep-raising areas of the world.

Rams as young as 8 wk have been infected experimentally by various nonvenereal routes. The disease can be transmitted among rams by direct contact. Active infection in ewes is unusual but has developed after mating with naturally infected rams. Contaminated pastures do not appear to be important in spread of the disease. Infection frequently persists in rams, and a high percentage shed *B ovis* intermittently for ≥4 yr.

Primary manifestations are lesions of the epididymis, tunica, and testis in rams; placentitis and abortion in ewes; and occasionally, perinatal death in lambs. Lesions may develop rapidly: in rams, the first detectable abnormality may be a marked deterioration in semen quality associated with the presence of inflammatory cells and organisms. An acute systemic phase is rarely observed in naturally occurring infections. Following regression of the acute phase—which may be so mild as to go unobserved—lesions may be palpated in the epididymis and scrotal tunics. Epididymal enlargement may be unilateral or bilateral. The tail of the epididymis is involved more frequently than the head or body, and the most prominent lesion is spermatoceles of variable size containing partially inspissated spermatic fluid. The tunics frequently become thickened and fibrous, and extensive adhesions develop between them. The testes may show fibrous atrophy; these lesions are usually permanent. In a few cases, palpable lesions are transient, while in others, organisms may be present in semen over long periods without clinically detectable lesions.

Since not all infected rams show palpable abnormalities of scrotal tissues (nor are all cases of epididymitis due to brucellosis), the remaining rams must be examined further. Rams shedding organisms, but having no lesions, must be identified by culture of semen. Repeated examinations may be necessary to identify intermittent shedders. Microscopical examination of stained semen smears may also be helpful; FA examination is a highly specific diagnostic aid. Serological tests used for eradication of disease and certification of animals have included ELISA, complement fixation, hemagglutination inhibition, indirect agglutination, and gel diffusion. Delayed hypersensitivity skin tests have also been utilized, particularly in Romania, the USSR, and South America.

Incidence and spread of the disease may be reduced by regular examination of rams before the breeding season, and culling of those with obvious genital abnormalities. Since suseptibility in rams increases markedly with age, it is advantageous to keep a young ram flock and isolate noninfected rams from older, possibly infected rams.

Immunization of rams has been practiced extensively in New Zealand using 2 doses of killed *B ovis* cells in adjuvant. Immunization of weaner rams with attenuated *B melitensis* has been recommended in South Africa. Since infection in ewes apparently originates almost exclusively from service by infected rams, lamb losses through infection of ewes may be controlled economically by restricting vaccination to rams.

Chlortetracycline and streptomycin used concomitantly have effected bacteriologic cures. However, treatment is not economical except in especially valuable rams, and even if infection is eliminated, fertility may remain impaired.

CONGENITAL AND INHERITED ANOMALIES OF THE REPRODUCTIVE SYSTEM

Cryptorchidism is failure of one or both testicles to descend into the scrotum. It is most common in pigs and horses, and is hereditary in these species. It is suspected to be hereditary in dogs and cats. Bilateral retention results in sterility due to thermal suppression of spermatogenesis. The normal temperature of the scrotum necessary for mammalian spermatogenesis is 1-8°F (0.5-4.5°C) below the normal body temperature. Unilateral cryptorchids have normal spermatogenesis in the scrotal testicle, are fertile, and may pass the trait on to their offspring. Abdominal testicles produce male hormones, and cryptorchids have normal secondary sex characteristics and mating behavior. Because cryptorchid testicles may become neoplastic, affected animals should be castrated. Gonadotropic hormones administered to prepubertal animals may sometimes cause the testicles to descend.

Monorchidism, anorchidism, and **gonadal hypoplasia** occur. The hereditary gonadal hypoplasia of Swedish Highland cattle has largely been eliminated by a controlled breeding program. A similar gonadal hypoplasia has not been observed in the USA. Idiopathic hypoplasia is common. Other anomalies of the testis and epididymis are rare. Ovarian agenesis or supernumerary ovaries are extremely rare, and hypoplasia is infrequent.

Prolapse of the prepuce in bulls occurs as a breed characteristic or may result from edema following trauma. Prolapse predisposes to further injury and if untreated results in abscessation, scarring, adhesions, and phimosis. Prolapse of the prepuce can be corrected by surgical removal of redundant tissue. Secondary infection following surgery may result in adhesions and stenosis.

Deviations of the penis in bulls may result from injury, but in most cases the etiology is obscure; a heritable factor has been suggested. Deviations are lateral, downward, or upward, and if severe, prevent copulation. Surgical correction by removing 1-2 pieces of tunica albuginea on the convex side has been done. Such operations are difficult because of the chance of infection and the difficulty in removing exactly the right amount of tissue, and should not be done if inheritance seems to be involved.

Corkscrew penis is a result of extreme erection in which the dorsal and lateral tunica albuginea of the penis stretches more than does the thicker and stronger tunic around the urethral groove. Most affected bulls eventually overcome this difficulty without treatment. They learn to insert the penis before the corkscrew occurs, or libido may decrease so that there is a less vigorous erection. Corkscrew penis is sometimes seen when using high voltages for electroejaculation.

The penile urethra may open on the ventral surface of the penis (**hypospadias**) or on its dorsal surface (**epispadias**) and interfere with natural insemination.

Persistent frenulum in young bulls can be cut with scissors. **Congenitally short penis** may occur in bulls. **Diphallus** is rare in bulls.

Hermaphroditism or intersexuality may occur in all species of domestic animals. The true hermaphrodite has both ovarian and testicular tissue. Such a condition is usually bilateral and may result in anomalies of the external genitalia. The most common hermaphrodite is in fact a pseudohermaphrodite in which there are present either ovaries or testes, and there is an anomaly of the external genitalia, which resemble, to some degree, those of the opposite sex. Pseudohermaphroditism is most common in goats (qv, p 1114) and pigs.

The most frequent congenital disorder of the uterus is **segmental uterine aplasia**, which occurs in inbred cattle. Although often referred to as **white heifer disease**, this is a misnomer since it has no connection with coat color. The portion of the uterus without outside opening may fill with fluid, which results in a distended, cyst-like structure. Aplasia may occur at various levels, including the cervix, so that the description of the condition is quite variable between animals. The vagina may be involved and may fill with mucus. These animals are sterile. There is no treatment.

Cattle frequently have a **double cervix**. Usually, this is not a complete double cervix, but rather a double external os with 2 cervical canals that join before reaching the internal os. This condition is inherited. It has no effect on fertility, and in most cases is found only incidentally during a genital examination. **Cystic Gartner's ducts** on the floor of the vagina are of no clinical importance. Rarely, cows may have an **imperforate hymen**, which causes accumulation of fluid in the vagina.

One of the most frequent congenital anomalies of cattle is the **freemartin**, a female born as a twin of a normal male. Over 90% of such females have such extreme hypoplasia of the genital tract that the uterus and ovaries may be observed only histologically. The anterior portion of the vagina is hypoplastic, while the vulva and the posterior portion of the vagina are usually normal. Diagnosis of freemartinism based on vaginal hypoplasia usually can be determined by a vaginal examination of the calf with either the finger or a suitably small speculum. The fusion of the placental circulation of the twins allows interchange of embryonic cells and possibly also hormones. The interchange of cells results in a dual genetic pattern in the twins, which can be detected by the combination of 2 different blood types in a single animal. This specific blood-typing test is available through the purebred cattle associations and elsewhere.

Rectovaginal constriction of Jersey cattle is a congenital defect resulting from homozygosity of a simple autosomal recessive gene. In females, the defect is characterized by inelastic constrictions at the junction of the anus, rectum, vestibule, and vulva. The male has anal stenosis. Affected cows develop severe dystocia. Rectal examinations are difficult to perform on affected cattle. In addition, affected cows are prone to develop udder edema at calving, frequently followed by severe mastitis. Mammary blood flow is significantly lower at parturition. However, there is a significant increase of blood pressure in the cranial superficial epigastric vein at parturition.

Mares may be sterile as a result of **chromosome abnormalities**; such mares are usually smaller than the breed average. There is no cyclic pattern of estrous behavior, and although there may be reaction to the teaser, they are usually passive to the stallion's advances. External genitalia are slightly smaller than usual. The striking abnormalities are confined to the internal genitalia. The ovaries are very small, smooth, firm, and have no follicles or corpora lutea. Histological examination reveals that these ovaries consist of undifferentiated stroma. The uterus is small and flaccid, and the cervix is flaccid with the os remaining open. The usual chromosome abnormality in these mares is an absence of one of the sex chromosomes, and they are designated XO. Autosomes appear to be normal. Sometimes there is a mosaic involving a mixture of XO and XX, or XY. There is no treatment.

CYSTIC OVARY DISEASE

Among domestic animals, cystic ovary disease is most common in cattle, particularly the dairy breeds, but it occurs sporadically in dogs (qv, p 678), cats, and pigs. Multiple large follicles are occasionally found in one or both ovaries of the mare, primarily during the spring or fall transition phases of the reproductive cycle. Their appearance, however, is not accompanied by the clinical picture and behavioral aberrations typical of the disease in cattle. Ovarian cysts in cattle can be of 3 types: follicular, luteal, or cystic corpus luteum (CL). In contrast to the others, the cystic CL arises following ovulation. A cystic CL is considered a normal stage or variation of CL development since they are found in normally cycling and pregnant cows without concurrent signs of infertility. Cystic CL have a softer, more mushy core area, due to presence of fluid or a degenerating blood clot, than a typical CL, and are most often detected ~ 1 wk after estrus when the structure is nearing the end of the corpus hemorrhagicum, ie, developmental, phase. Cystic as well as typical CL may or may not possess an ovulation crown or papilla at the apex of the structure. Absence should not be considered diagnostic of the cystic condition since 10-20% of functional, normal CL fail to develop this feature. The discussion below is limited to the 2 pathologic forms of bovine cystic ovary disease, follicular cysts and luteal cysts. Although etiologically and pathogenetically related, their clinical differences justify separate description.

FOLLICULAR CYSTIC OVARY DISEASE
(Follicular cysts, Cystic follicles, Nymphomania, "Bulling")

Behavioral and conformational manifestations of the disease vary considerably, as does the overall clinical picture. However, all the signs relate to the focal primary lesions, viz, thin-walled cysts in the ovary.

Cystic ovary disease primarily affects dairy cattle, although it has been reported occasionally in beef cattle. This difference is due to the more intensive management and treatment methods used on individual dairy cows. The disease is more common among certain family lines within breeds, which implicates hereditary factors in the etiology.

The cystic ovary syndrome is commonly thought to be caused by high production. The observation is biased, however, since higher-producing cows are more likely to be examined, more likely to be treated if found to have cystic ovary disease, and more likely to be allowed to stay in the herd despite some reduction in reproductive performance. Evidence indicates that cystic ovary disease causes cows to produce more milk rather than that high production causes cows to develop the disease. Incidence increases with age. Within age groups, most cases occur within 3-8 wk of lactation at the first attempted postpartum ovulation, coincidental with peak daily milk production. The reported herd incidence is 5-25%, or higher in some problem herds, and can be influenced by herd-health programs in which examination and detection are emphasized.

Etiology and Pathogenesis: Hereditary predisposition has been implicated in dairy cattle, eg, daughters of previously cystic cows had a higher incidence of cystic ovary disease than did daughters of unaffected cows. Preparturient stress apparently serves as a trigger. The mechanism by which stress elicits the hypothalamic and pituitary defects in genetically predisposed animals is most commonly thought to be a relative deficiency in the release of luteinizing hormone (LH) at estrus. This may be a reflection of failure of hypothalmic release of gonadotropin-releasing hormone (Gn-RH). Another mechanism known to exist in some cows with cysts is a deficiency of LH and follicle-stimulating hormone (FSH) receptors in developing follicles.

During normal proestrus, regression of the CL coincides with development of a selected follicle, while the growth of any additional follicles is inhibited. In animals developing cystic ovary disease, ovulation fails to occur. Moreover, in the absence of the inhibitory effect of adequate LH, several follicles (including the one failing to ovulate) may grow and form multiple cysts either bi- or unilaterally. Grossly, the cysts resemble enlarged follicles, varying in size from normal to 5-6 cm in diameter. The size and form of an affected ovary depend on the number and size of cysts present. The cystic ovary is at least initially capable of steroidogenesis, and its products vary from estrogens to progesterone to androgens. The action of the various hormones produced is responsible for the observed changes of the genital tract as well as for body conformation and general behavior.

Clinical Findings: Behavioral aberrations range from frequent, intermittent estrus with exaggerated monosexual drive to bull-like behavior, including mounting, pawing the ground, and bellowing. This behavior often is accompanied by masculinization of the head and neck. Relaxation of the vulva, perineum, and the large pelvic ligaments, which causes the tail head to be elevated, is common in chronic cases. Most affected animals show these signs, but others may be sexually quiescent. This variation is due to the duration of the disease and the nature of the hormone secreted by the diseased ovary. The affected ovaries generally are enlarged and rounded, but their size varies, depending on the number and size of cysts. Their surface is smooth, elevated, and blister-like, particularly when cysts exceed 2.5-3 cm in diameter. Frequently, the cysts are multiple and may exceed 2.5 cm in diameter. Under the influence of hormones produced by the cystic ovary and/or the lack of hormones normally present during estrous cycles, the uterus undergoes palpable changes, which in turn vary with the duration of the cystic condition. Thus, during the first week, the uterine wall is thickened and edematous as an extension of the normal postestrual edema. Toward the end of the week, the uterine wall attains a sponge-like texture. In chronic cases, atony and atrophy of the uterine wall are common. Less commonly, the uterine horns are markedly shortened but otherwise feel normal. Some degree of mucoid to mucopurulent vaginal discharge is common. Hydrometra, a fluid-filled, extremely thin-walled uterus, occurs rarely.

Diagnosis: The larger, multiple cysts are easily identified by rectal palpation. History, conformation, and uterine changes, when present, provide supplemental diagnostic evidence. Palpation characteristics of the uterus are helpful for differentiation between a single follicular cyst and a mature graafian follicle. Only the estrous cow has a coiled, extremely turgid uterus.

Prognosis: From one viewpoint, the disease responds readily to treatment, be it mechanical (manual rupture) or hormonal. The success rate of manual rupture, when measured in terms of conceptions within 24 days, is ~50%; hormone therapy (*see* below) appears to be slightly more successful. Aberrant behavior ceases within 3-4 days after successful therapy. This is followed by normal conformation of the ovary; a normal, fertile estrus can be expected within 4-7 days after manual rupture and 10-30 days following hormonal therapy. With Gn-RH, 25% of cases required a second treatment, and 5% required a third. One-third of the cases treated for the third time failed to respond. Self-recovery is possible and common in cases arising during the first 50 days following calving. That, and the observation that self-recovery involves the same sequence of events as recovery in response to hormonal therapy, suggests caution in evaluating therapeutic efficiency. Owners should be made aware that each successfully treated cow is more likely to require treatment after the next parturition than are previously unaffected cows. Likewise, successful treatment encourages perpetuation of the disease in the herd if the offspring are used for breeding. While the cystic ovary condition in cattle clearly has a genetic component, it is unlikely that a single farm using AI can have significant influence on its incidence. Sweden has made progress in reducing the condition through culling and selection procedures for bulls used in AI, but affected cows are still treated.

Treatment: The oldest treatment is manual rupture—the ovary is grasped and moderate pressure applied with finger pads, not tips, against the palm until the cyst(s) bursts. Following successful rupture, the ovary may be compressed briefly to minimize hemorrhage; however, hemorrhage is rarely a sequela of rupture of correctly diagnosed follicular cysts. This complication probably occurs most often when a misdiagnosis is made and rupture of a CL or corpus hemorrhagicum is attempted. The potential danger of traumatizing the ovary and causing hemorrhage with subsequent local peritonitis should not be overlooked. It should be weighed against the cost of hormone therapy.

Of several hormone preparations recommended and used in the past, human chorionic gonadotropin (HCG) remains the only one still available and used. It is most efficacious at 10,000 USP units IM, although some have reported success with lower doses given IM or IV. Newer hormone therapy includes a Gn-RH product known as LH-RH, which is efficacious at 100 µg IM. It is equally effective but less antigenic than HCG. Use of the 2 products may be alternated, particularly in refractory cases. To hasten the onset of the first estrus following treatment, prostaglandins can be administered 9-10 days after HCG or Gn-RH. The claim that breeding on the first estrus is prone to produce twins has not been substantiated. In fact, breeding on the first estrus appears to reduce the danger of recurrence.

Progesterone (or its analogs) has been given parenterally and PO to cows failing to respond to HCG and Gn-RH therapy. Progesterone treatment has been continued at least 10-12 days, if not 20, in expectation of a normal estrus on withdrawal; however, results have been less than encouraging.

CYSTIC OVARY DISEASE AS A HERD PROBLEM

Occasionally, individual herds experience exceptionally high rates (~50%) of cystic ovary disease over a period of months. Determining the cause of these episodes is not easy, but the following questions should be addressed: 1) Is the diagnosis accurate, eg, are the structures being identified as cysts really cysts? This can be established via second opinion diagnoses, milk or plasma progesterone determination, and/or honing of diagnostic skills by continuing education. 2) Has the palpation examination schedule for the herd changed? Initiating routine postpartum examinations for all cows, and increasing frequency of herd visits can result in an increased apparent incidence. 3) Has the herd's incidence of periparturient complications and stress increased? Cows having problems around calving are much more likely to develop cysts. Attempts to reduce these complications are indicated. 4) Has the herd's nutritional program been evaluated? Nutritional aberrations are frequently implicated as causing cows to develop cysts, but rarely have these concerns been confirmed in controlled experiments. Inadequacies or imbalances involving calcium and phosphorus, vitamin E and selenium, and energy have been implicated most often. Moldy feed or roughages that contain high concentrations of estrogenic substances are also frequently suspected, but better testing methods are needed.

LUTEAL CYSTIC OVARY DISEASE
(Luteal cysts)

This type of cystic ovary disease is characterized by enlarged ovaries with one or more cysts—the walls of which are thicker than those of follicular cysts because of a lining of luteal tissue. Incidence ratios of follicular versus luteal cysts vary greatly among veterinarians, depending on their individual diagnostic tendencies. The incidence pattern is similar to that of follicular cysts.

Etiology and Pathogenesis: The basic causes of luteal cysts are the same as for follicular cysts. Superimposed is release of LH sufficient to initiate luteinization of follicles, but inadequate to cause ovulation. Luteal cysts are an extension of follicular cysts such that the nonovulatory follicle is partially luteinized spontaneously or in response to hormonal therapy.

Clinical Findings: Luteal cysts are accompanied by normal conformation and anestrous behavior. Rectal palpation reveals a quiescent uterus characteristic for the luteal phase of the estrous cycle. Luteal cysts are recognized as smooth, fluctuant domes protruding above the surface of the ovary. Usually, they are single, but may be multiple or appear concurrently with follicular cysts unilaterally or bilaterally. Luteal cysts are differentiated from follicular cysts on the basis of palpable characteristics of the structure and the uterus, and to some extent, on body conformation and behavior. Progesterone assay and ultrasonography can help differentiate between follicular and luteal cysts. On attempts to manually rupture the cystic structure, follicular cysts explode under minimal pressure while luteal cysts cannot be ruptured without applying considerable pressure, often in excess of that considered safe. Both types of cysts respond to LH or Gn-RH therapy, but prostaglandin (PG) $F_{2\alpha}$ will lyse some luteal cysts and, when applicable, this treatment is preferable due to its much shorter time from administration to estrus and its lower cost than HCG or Gn-RH.

Treatment and Control: The treatment of choice is luteolytic doses of $PGF_{2\alpha}$. Luteal cysts also respond to HCG and Gn-RH therapy effective in the treatment of follicular cysts. Manual rupture of luteal cysts is not recommended.

Preventive measures are common to both cyst types (*see* above).

DISEASES OF THE REPRODUCTIVE SYSTEM, SM AN

See also MANAGEMENT OF REPRODUCTION: SM AN, p 1154.

DISORDERS OF THE FEMALE

ACUTE METRITIS

Acute infection of the uterus is usually a postpartum disorder that may be associated with abortion, fetal infection, retained placentas, obstetrical manipulation, or ascending infection following apparently normal parturition. Uncommonly, metritis occurs following breeding. *Escherichia coli* is the most common bacterium isolated from the infected uterus; streptococci, staphylococci, and others are isolated less frequently.

Animals with metritis are usually quite ill with fever, lethargy, and inappetence. A purulent, foul-smelling vaginal discharge is usually found. The dam may neglect the young. Acute metritis should be considered in any postpartum animal with signs of systemic illness or an abnormal vaginal discharge. A large, flaccid uterus may be palpable. Radiographs should be taken to determine if fetuses are retained. The hemogram may show a leukocytosis with a left shift.

Therapy includes supportive care, IV fluids, and broad-spectrum bactericidal antibiotics, preferably those effective against *E coli*. Prostaglandin $F_{2\alpha}$ (0.1-0.25 mg/kg body wt, subcut. for 2-3 days) or oxytocin (5-20 u bitches, 2-5 u queens, IM) may help evacuate the uterine contents. Ovariohysterectomy is indicated following initial stabilization if the animal is extremely ill or if future reproduction is unimportant. Otherwise, it should be considered an elective procedure to be performed when lactation has ceased.

DYSTOCIA

Difficult birth may result from myometrial defects, metabolic abnormalities such as hypocalcemia, inadequate pelvic diameter, insufficient dilation of the birth canal, fetal hormone deficiency (fetal corticosteroid deficiency), fetal oversize, fetal death, or abnormal fetal presentation.

Dystocia should be considered in any of the following situations: an animal with a history of previous dystocia or reproductive tract obstruction; no parturition within 24 hr of the drop in rectal temperature (to <100°F [37.7°C]); 1-2 hr of strong abdominal contractions without passage of a puppy or kitten; 1-2 hr of active labor without delivery of subsequent puppies/kittens; the resting period during active labor exceeds 4-6 hr; the bitch or queen is in obvious pain (crying, licking, or biting the vulva); there is a black, purulent, or hemorrhagic vaginal discharge; there are signs of systemic illness; or gestation is prolonged.

To enable a rational therapy, the cause of the dystocia (obstructive versus non-obstructive) must be determined and the condition of the animal assessed. A thorough history regarding previous parturitions, pelvic trauma, and breeding dates is desirable. The animal should be examined for signs of systemic illness which, if present, may necessitate immediate cesarean section. The normal vaginal discharge at parturition is a dark green color; abnormal color or character requires immediate attention. A sterile vaginal examination should be performed to evaluate the degree of cervical dilation, the patency of the birth canal, and the position and presentation of the fetus(es). Radiography or ultrasonography can be used to determine the presence of fetuses, their size, number, position, and viability.

Medical management may be considered when the condition of the dam and fetuses are stable, when there is proper fetal position and presentation, and when there is no obstruction. Oxytocin IM (3-20 u in bitches, 2-5 u in queens) up to 3 times at 30-min intervals, with or without 10% calcium gluconate (3-5 mL, IV slowly, once) may be given in an attempt to promote uterine contractions. If no response follows, a cesarean section should be performed.

Forceps may be used (carefully) to remove dead fetuses or to facilitate delivery of malpresented or partially delivered fetuses. Gentle manipulation and adequate lubrication must be used to prevent damage or death to living fetuses. Episiotomy may be helpful.

Surgery is indicated for obstructive dystocia, if dystocia is accompanied by shock or systemic illness, for primary uterine inertia, when active labor is prolonged, and/or if medical management has failed.

FALSE PREGNANCY IN BITCHES
(Pseudopregnancy, Pseudocyesis)

False pregnancy is common in bitches, uncommon in queens. It occurs at the end of diestrus and is characterized by hyperplasia of the mammary glands, lactation, and behavioral changes. Some bitches behave as if parturition has occurred, "mothering" by nesting inanimate objects, and refusing to eat. The history, abdominal palpation, and abdominal radiographs/ultrasonography exclude the possibility of true pregnancy.

The falling progesterone and increasing prolactin concentrations associated with late diestrus are believed to be responsible for the clinical signs. No treatment is recommended because the condition resolves spontaneously in 1-3 wk. Tranquilizers may be considered for bitches with significant behavioral changes, although some may increase prolactin release. Estrogens should not be used because of the potential for bone marrow suppression. Progestins usually stop lactation, but when they are discontinued, prolactin again increases and lactation may recur. Androgens could be considered to stop lactation. If owners are distressed by repeated bouts of pseudopregnancy, the bitch should either be bred or undergo ovariohysterectomy. Ovariohysterectomy prevents recurrence.

FOLLICULAR CYSTS: NYMPHOMANIA

Follicular cysts are rare, and result in prolonged estrogen secretion and continued signs of proestrus or estrus, and attractiveness to males. Ovulation may not occur during this abnormal estrous cycle. Follicular cysts should be suspected in any bitch showing clinical manifestations of estrus for >21 days, or when proestrus plus estrus have lasted for >40 days. Cystic follicles may be difficult to differentiate from normal, frequent cycles in queens. An estrogen-secreting ovarian tumor is the other diagnostic consideration.

Ovariohysterectomy is curative. If the animal is to be bred, ovulation may be induced by using gonadotropin-releasing hormone (Gn-RH, 25 μg total in bitches ≤11 kg, and 2.2 μg/kg in bitches >11 kg; 25 μg, IM, total in queens for 2 days). Breeding should probably continue throughout the prolonged estrus since the time of ovulation is unknown. Gn-RH is not an effective treatment for ovarian tumors.

MASTITIS

A septic or nonseptic inflammatory process involving one or more mammary glands, which usually occurs during lactation. Septic mastitis may occur via an ascending infection from the nipples, penetrating wounds, or hematogenous spread. Staphylococci and streptococci are the most common bacteria isolated from the milk. The source of infection usually is not found. Affected mammary glands are usually swollen, warm, and painful. Milk from affected glands may be hemorrhagic or purulent, may have an alkaline pH, and often is more viscous than normal milk. The bitch/queen may or may not show signs of illness such as fever, listlessness, inappetence, and neglect of the young.

Diagnosis is made easily from the history and physical examination. Milk from each gland should be evaluated in any postpartum bitch or queen with signs of systemic illness. Before beginning therapy, a milk sample should be collected for bacterial culture and sensitivity. Fluid for culture also can be obtained by fine needle aspiration. Broad-spectrum, bactericidal antibiotics should be chosen based on sensitivity tests, and with the realization that they will be passed in the milk to the young. Antibiotics such as tetracycline, chloramphenicol, or aminoglycosides should be avoided during lactation unless the neonates are weaned. Hot-packing the affected glands encourages drainage and seems to relieve discomfort. An abscessed mammary gland should be lanced, drained, flushed, and treated as an open wound.

Nonseptic mastitis occurs most commonly at weaning. The affected gland(s) are warm, swollen, and painful to the touch, but the animal is alert and healthy. The nursing dam with nonseptic mastitis should have warm compresses applied locally 4-6 times daily, and the young should be encouraged to nurse from these glands. When galactostasis occurs at weaning, lactation can be diminished by reducing food and water intake of the dam. The mammary glands should not be stimulated during this time. Appropriate food and water must be provided for the young.

PYOMETRA

A diestrual disorder characterized by an abnormal uterine endometrium with secondary bacterial infection. In the normal bitch, the corpora lutea produce progesterone for 9-12 wk following ovulation in each estrous cycle. If pregnancy does not occur after a cat is induced to ovulate, the corpora luteal life span is ~45 days.

Etiology: Progesterone promotes endometrial growth while decreasing myometrial activity. Cystic endometrial hyperplasia and accumulation of uterine secretions ultimately develop. Progesterone may also inhibit the WBC response to bacterial infection. Bacteria from the normal vaginal flora are the most likely source of uterine contamination. *Escherichia coli* is the most common bacterium isolated in cases of pyometra, although *Staphylococcus, Streptococcus, Pseudomonas,* and *Proteus* spp, and other bacteria also have been recovered. Since queens require copulatory stimulation to ovulate, form corpora lutea, and produce progesterone, pyometra is less common in queens than in bitches. Administration of medroxyprogesterone has been associated with development of pyometra in bitches and queens. Pyometra can develop in uterine tissue left after ovariohysterectomy (stump pyometra).

Estrogen, by itself, does not contribute to the development of cystic endometrial hyperplasia or pyometra. However, it does increase the stimulatory effects of progesterone on the uterus. Administration of exogenous estrogens (eg, "mismate shots") during diestrus greatly increases the risk of developing pyometra; estrogen injections to prevent pregnancy should be discouraged.

Clinical and Laboratory Findings: Clinical signs are seen during diestrus, usually 4-8 wk after estrus, or following administration of exogenous progestins. The signs are variable and include lethargy, anorexia, polyuria, polydipsia, and vomiting. When the cervix is open, a purulent vulvar discharge, often containing blood, is present. When the cervix is closed, there is no discharge and the large uterus may cause abdominal distention. Signs can progress rapidly to shock and death.

Physical examination reveals lethargy, dehydration, uterine enlargement, and if the cervix is patent, a sanguineous to mucopurulent vaginal discharge. Fever is found in only 20% of affected animals. Shock may be present.

The leukogram of animals with pyometra is variable, and may be normal. Leukocytosis characterized by a neutrophilia with a left shift is usual. Leukopenia may be found in animals with sepsis. A mild, normocytic, normochromic, nonregenerative anemia (PCV of 28-35%) may also develop. Hyperproteinemia due to hyperglobulinemia may be found. Results of urinalysis are variable. With *E coli* uterine infection, isosthenuria due to endotoxin-induced impairment of renal tubular function and/or insensitivity to antidiuretic hormone may develop. A glomerulonephropathy caused by immune complex deposition may result in proteinuria. These renal lesions are potentially reversible once the pyometra is resolved.

Diagnosis: Pyometra should be suspected in any ill, diestrual bitch or queen, especially if polydipsia, polyuria, or vomiting is present. The diagnosis can be established from the history and physical examination, and abdominal radiography/ultrasonography. Vaginal cytology is often helpful in determining the nature of the vulvar discharge. The complete blood count, biochemical profile, and urinalysis help exclude other causes of polydipsia/polyuria and vomiting, and evaluate renal function, acid-base status, and septicemia. A culture and sensitivity should be performed on the uterine exudate. Differential diagnoses include pregnancy and other causes of vulvar discharge, polyuria and polydipsia, and vomiting.

Treatment: Ovariohysterectomy is the treatment of choice, but medical management could be considered if it is desired to salvage the reproductive potential of the bitch or queen. IV fluids and broad-spectrum, bactericidal antibiotics should be administered. Fluid, electrolyte, and acid-base imbalances should be corrected as quickly as possible, before ovariohysterectomy is performed. The bacterial infection is responsible for the illness and will not resolve until the uterine exudate is removed. Oral antibiotics (based on the results of the culture and sensitivity) should be continued for 7-10 days after surgery.

Medical therapy with prostaglandin (PG) $F_{2\alpha}$ can be used for animals to be bred in the future, although PG are not approved in the USA for use in cats or dogs. PG cause contraction of the myometrium, relaxation of the cervix, and expulsion of the uterine exudate, and at therapeutic doses, do not cause luteolysis in dogs or cats. Probably, PG should not be used in animals >8 yr old or those not intended for breeding. The delay before clinical improvement and the many side effects of $PGF_{2\alpha}$ preclude its use in a severely ill animal. It also should be used with caution in the bitch or queen with a closed-cervix pyometra because the risk of uterine rupture is increased. Pregnancy must be ruled out since PG can induce abortion.

Only naturally occurring $PGF_{2\alpha}$ (0.25 mg/kg body wt, subcut. once daily for 5 days) should be used in the bitch and queen. Synthetic analogs, eg, cloprostenol, fluprostenol, and prostalene, are much more potent than natural $PGF_{2\alpha}$, but have not been evaluated for use in dogs or cats. Broad-spectrum, bactericidal antibiotics, chosen on the basis of culture and sensitivity tests should be given for ≥2 wk. Other effects of $PGF_{2\alpha}$ include restlessness, panting, hypersalivation, pacing, abdominal pain, tachycardia, vomiting, and defecation. In cats, vocalization and intense grooming behavior also may be seen. These reactions disappear within 2 hr of the injection. The LD_{50} of $PGF_{2\alpha}$ in dogs is 5.13 mg/kg body wt. Severe ataxia, respiratory distress, and muscle tremors may be seen in queens given 5 mg/kg. If severe side effects occur, IV fluids at rates appropriate for treatment of shock are indicated. Uterine evacuation after an injection is variable.

The animal should be reexamined 2 wk after completion of medical therapy. If a sanguineous or mucopurulent vulvar discharge, or uterine enlargement is still present, $PGF_{2\alpha}$ therapy, using the same protocol, may be repeated; however the prognosis for recovery is much worse.

Prognosis: Usually, the prognosis for an animal undergoing ovariohysterectomy is good. Following medical therapy, the prognosis for initial resolution of the pyometra is good if the cervix is open, but guarded to poor if closed. Of those animals that respond, as many as 90% of the bitches and 70% of the queens with open-cervix pyometra may be fertile. Only 50% of bitches with closed-cervix pyometra are reported to return to fertility. Recurrence is likely: of bitches treated medically for pyometra, 70% had recurrence within 2 yr. It is recommended that the animal be bred on the next and each subsequent cycle until the desired number of puppies or kittens has been obtained, and then spayed.

VAGINAL HYPERPLASIA

A proliferation of the vaginal mucosa, usually originating from the floor of the vagina anterior to the urethral orifice. It occurs during proestrus and estrus, as a result of estrogenic stimulation. The most common sign is a mass protruding from the vulva, initially smooth and glistening; with prolonged exposure the surface becomes dry and fissures develop, so the mass has a tongue-like appearance. A slight vaginal discharge may be present. Although the hyperplastic tissue originates near the urethral orifice, dysuria is uncommon. Vaginal hyperplasia interferes with copulation. Reluctance to breed may be the only clinical sign if the hyperplastic tissue is contained within the vaginal vault. Vaginal hyperplasia resolves spontaneously as soon as estrogen declines. The diagnosis is made by the history (stage of the estrous cycle) and examination of the vagina. Estrogenic stimulation could be confirmed by vaginal cytology if the history is questionable. The 2 differential diagnoses are vaginal prolapse and neoplasia. The former can be excluded by the historical and physical findings, the latter by biopsy.

If the mass is not causing problems, therapy is not indicated. However, if the hyperplastic tissue protrudes from the vulva, it should be kept clean and moist, and an antibiotic ointment applied. An Elizabethan collar may be necessary to prevent self-trauma. These animals may be bred by artificial insemination. The hyperplasia regresses as soon as the follicular phase of the estrous cycle has passed. Rarely there is a recurrence at parturition, presumably associated with a burst of estrogen. Submucosal resection may be necessary if the mass is extremely large or mucosal damage is extensive. Recurrence is common even after surgical resection. Vaginal hyperplasia resolves within days of removal of estrogen. Ovariohysterectomy hastens resolution and prevents recurrence, and is the treatment of choice.

VAGINITIS

Inflammation of the vagina may occur in prepuberal or mature, intact or spayed bitches. It is rare in queens. Vaginitis usually is due to bacterial infection, which may be secondary to conformational abnormalities such as vestibulovaginal strictures. Viral infection (herpes), vaginal foreign bodies, neoplasia, hyperplasia of the vagina, androgenic steroids (eg, mibolerone), or intersex conditions also may cause vaginitis.

The most common clinical sign is a vulvar discharge. Licking of the vulva, attraction of males, and frequent micturition also may be seen. Signs of systemic illness are not present, nor are there abnormalities in the hemogram or biochemical profile. Absence of these alterations helps differentiate vaginitis from open-cervix pyometra, the most important differential diagnosis. The diagnostic evaluation should include a digital examination of the vagina, vaginoscopy, cytology and culture of the exudate and, if necessary, abdominal radiographs or ultrasonography to evaluate the uterus. An anterior vaginal culture may be obtained utilizing a guarded sterile culture swab. The vagina contains normal bacterial flora; therefore, culture results must be interpreted cautiously. A heavy growth, especially of one organism, is probably more significant than a light growth of several organisms.

Predisposing factors such as foreign material or anatomic abnormalities should be corrected. Bacterial infection may respond to local treatment (vaginal douches). Systemic, broad-spectrum, bactericidal antibiotics may be needed for persistent infections. Prepuberal animals often do not require treatment because the vaginitis nearly always resolves with the first estrus. For this reason it may be wise to delay elective ovariohysterectomy in affected animals until after their first estrous cycle.

DISORDERS OF THE MALE

For a discussion of prostatic disorders, *see* p 695.

ACUTE ORCHITIS/EPIDIDYMITIS

Acute inflammation or infection of the testis and/or epididymis may be caused by trauma, infection (fungal, bacterial, or viral), or testicular torsion. Clinical signs are pain and swelling of the testes, epididymides, and/or scrotum. There may be wounds or draining tracts in the scrotal skin.

The scrotal contents, including the vas deferens and pampiniform vessels, should be carefully palpated for evidence of torsions, foreign material, or focal lesions of the testes or epididymis. Semen should be collected for cytology, and bacterial and mycoplasmal culture. Collection of semen may be difficult in an animal with acute orchiepididymitis. A fine needle aspirate of the involved testis or epididymis provides material for cytology and culture. A rapid slide agglutination test for *Brucella canis* should be performed.

If maintaining the dog's fertility is not important, castration and broad-spectrum, bactericidal antibiotics for 7-10 days is the treatment of choice. Lesions of the scrotal skin are treated appropriately. If fertility is important, therapy for bacterial orchitis is broad-spectrum bactericidal antibiotics. Antifungal agents are indicated for fungal infections. In addition, anti-inflammatory agents (eg, prednisone [0.5 mg/kg, daily] or aspirin [10 mg/kg, b.i.d.]) and local hypothermia (eg, cool water packs) may decrease testicular damage caused by local swelling and hyperthermia.

The prognosis for maintaining fertility is guarded despite aggressive therapy because of the potential for irreversible damage to the germinal epithelium, tubular degeneration, development of immune-mediated orchitis, or blockage of the duct system with necrotic debris and fibrous tissue. These sequelae may take months to occur. There is no successful treatment for *B canis* infection. All the antifungal agents interfere with spermatogenesis, directly or indirectly. The ischemic damage caused by testicular torsion becomes irreversible within hours.

CHRONIC ORCHITIS/EPIDIDYMITIS

Chronic orchiepididymitis may develop as a sequela of the acute syndrome, or may arise with no previous history of testicular inflammation. Possible causes include those of acute orchiepididymitis, immune-mediated orchitis/epididymitis, neoplasia, and spermatocele or granuloma formation. The usual clinical presentation is infertility; most animals are otherwise asymptomatic. Physical examination may reveal testicular atrophy and fibrosis. Palpation of the epididymis may reveal induration or enlargement. Tumors may be palpable.

Diagnostic tests should include cytological examination of semen with bacterial and mycoplasmal culture, and a rapid slide agglutination test for *Brucella canis*. Fine needle aspiration, especially of focal lesions, is often helpful. A testicular biopsy for histopathology and bacterial culture may be performed when less invasive diagnostic tests have been exhausted.

Treatment is difficult because often the underlying cause is unknown. If bacterial cultures are positive, appropriate systemic antibiotics should be administered for ≥3 wk. If histopathology is suggestive of an immune-mediated process (lymphocytic, plasmacytic infiltration), treatment with immunosuppressive drugs (eg, prednisone, 1 mg/kg body wt, b.i.d.) may be indicated. However, as a result of inhibitory effects on the hypothalamic-pituitary-gonadal axis, glucocorticoids can cause testicular atrophy and infertility. The prognosis for return of fertility is grave. The treatment for testicular neoplasia is castration.

BALANOPOSTHITIS

Inflammation of the preputial cavity is common in dogs. Mild balanoposthitis, resulting in a slight mucopurulent preputial discharge, is present in many mature dogs and is of little clinical significance. Trauma, lacerations, neoplasia, foreign bodies, or phimosis may result in development of severe balanoposthitis. Balanoposthitis is rare in cats.

Signs include mucopurulent preputial discharge, swelling of the prepuce, and possibly pain. The penis and prepuce should be examined thoroughly for underlying predisposing factors. Bacterial cultures of the preputial cavity, although sometimes difficult to interpret because of the normal flora, are helpful in identifying unusual organisms or antibiotic sensitivities for refractory cases.

Treatment includes correcting any predisposing factors, cleaning and thorough flushing of the preputial cavity with a mild antiseptic (eg, povidone-iodine douche) or sterile saline solution, and infusing an antibiotic ointment into the preputial cavity for 7-10 days. This should be combined with 7-10 days of broad-spectrum systemic antibiotics if systemic illness is present. Recurrence of mild balanoposthitis is common despite therapy. Castration may be helpful.

PARAPHIMOSIS

Inability to completely retract the penis into the preputial cavity usually occurs following erection and development of a functional phimosis. It is seen most often after semen collection or coitus. The skin at the preputial orifice becomes inverted and impairs venous drainage from the penis. Other causes include mild phimosis, foreign objects around the penis, trauma, or chronic balanoposthitis. Paraphimosis must be differentiated from priapism, congenitally shortened prepuce, congenital deformity of the os penis, or paralysis of the retractor penis muscles.

Paraphimosis is a medical emergency. The exposed penis becomes edematous, dessicated, and painful. If untreated, ulceration, ischemic necrosis, and/or gangrene may develop. If recognized early, before severe edema and pain develop, paraphimosis is easily treated. The prepuce is slid gently in a posterior direction, extruding the penis further—this everts the skin at the preputial orifice; then the prepuce usually slides easily over the penis. With paraphimosis due to other causes, or of longer duration, sedation or general anesthesia is required. It may be necessary to incise the preputial skin to thoroughly examine the preputial cavity, remove restricting material, and relieve venous obstruction. After circulation has been reestablished, bathing the exposed penis in cold or hypertonic solutions may also help reduce swelling. The penis is then replaced in the preputial cavity, and the incision is closed. If the urethra has been damaged, an indwelling urinary catheter may be needed to prevent stricture formation. If necrosis or gangrene is severe, amputation of the penis and prepuce, and castration may be necessary.

PHIMOSIS

A congenital or acquired inability to extrude the penis through an abnormally small preputial orifice. It may develop because of inflammation, neoplasia, edema, or fibrosis following trauma, irritation, or infection. Clinical signs are variable. Usually, the problem is unnoticed until the dog attempts to mate and is unable to copulate. Diagnosis is established by physical examination of the prepuce and penis. Treatment depends on severity of the stenosis and intended use of the dog. If the dog is not used for breeding, therapy probably is not needed, although castration should be considered to prevent unexpected arousal. Surgical enlargement of the preputial orifice is indicated if the animal is to be used for breeding, if the phimosis contributes to balanoposthitis, or in the unlikely event that phimosis interferes with normal micturition.

TRANSMISSIBLE CANINE VENEREAL TUMOR

A cauliflower-like, pedunculated, nodular, papillary, or multilobulated tumor, it ranges from a small nodule (5 μm) to a large mass (>10 cm), and is firm, though friable. The surface is often ulcerated and inflamed, and may be hemorrhagic and infected. The tumor may be solitary or multiple, and is almost always located on the external genitalia, although it may occur in adjacent skin and oral, nasal, and conjunctival mucosae.

Incidence varies from relatively high in some areas to rare in others. The tumor may arise deep in the prepuce or vagina and be difficult to see. This may lead to misdiagnosis if bleeding is incorrectly assumed to be hematuria. The tumor is spread from site to site and dog to dog by implantation. Initially it grows rapidly. Metastasis is uncommon (5%); when it occurs, it is usually to the regional lymph nodes. Metastases are also seen in the kidney, spleen, eye, brain, pituitary, skin and subcutis, mesenteric lymph nodes, and peritoneum. Usually, it is easy to diagnose by cytology of fine needle aspirates of the mass. In contrast to the cytological appearance, the histological appearance of transmissible venereal tumor may be difficult to distinguish from other round cell tumors such as histiocytoma, lymphosarcoma, or mast cell tumors. This is especially true when tumors occur in extragenital locations.

Because transmissible venereal tumors may not spontaneously regress, they should be considered progressive, and treated accordingly. Although surgical excision, radiation therapy, and immunotherapy have been used, chemotherapy is considered the treatment of choice. Vincristine sulfate (0.5 mg/m^2, IV, once weekly for 3-6 wk) is reported to be effective, except when the tumor is in the eye or brain. Usually, total remission can be expected by the sixth treatment. Adriamycin (30 mg/m^2, IV, once q3wk) also has been effective; however, because of the greater incidence of adverse reactions, it should be reserved for those animals that do not respond to vincristine. The prognosis for total remission is good, unless metastatic involvement of the CNS or eye is present.

EQUINE COITAL EXANTHEMA

A benign venereal disease of horses.

Etiology and Epidemiology: The disease occurs worldwide. It affects both sexes and is primarily spread at coitus; although rare in unmated horses, transfer by gynecological manipulations is possible. Abortion under natural conditions has not been substantiated. Immunity is short-lived. The causal equine herpesvirus 3 (EHV-3) is of one antigenic type, but a mixed population of small and large plaque variants can be isolated from clinical specimens.

Clinical Findings: In mares, multiple, circular, red nodules up to 2 mm in diameter develop on vaginal and vulval mucosae and skin (especially on the perineum) 4-8 days after mating; the vaginal mucosa appears inflamed. Lesions progress to vesicles and pustules that rupture and form shallow, coalescing ulcers. Healing, which usually occurs within 3 wk, leaves unpigmented areas (white scars) that permit identification of potential carriers. Lesions of the clitoris and vagina heal more slowly. No accompanying systemic disturbance occurs unless complicated by bacterial infection. Similar lesions occur on the penis and prepuce of stallions; those acutely affected may be reluctant to serve. Recurrence is common when matings are frequent. Fertility of either sex is not affected. Extragenital lesions on the teats, lips, and nasal mucosa are rare.

Diagnosis: The typical appearance and distribution of lesions afford ready recognition of the disease, but are easily overlooked. Herpesviruses can be seen in electron microscope preparations of epithelial cells from the margin of ulcers, and if required, virus can be isolated and identified. Serological tests for serum neutralizing antibodies are useful only for epidemiological studies. EHV-1 and EHV-4 infections (qv, p 734) can produce similar lesions on the genital mucosae.

Prophylaxis and Treatment: Treatment of stallions for 3 days with topical antibiotics to combat secondary infection, and sexual rest provide sufficient control to permit mating in 1-2 wk. Mares can be treated with chlorhexidine and cortisone-antibiotic creams.

MAMMARY TUMORS

The frequency of mammary neoplasia in different species varies to an astonishing degree. The dog is by far the most frequently affected domestic species. The prevalence in dogs is ~3 times that in women; ~50% of all tumors in the bitch are mammary tumors. In cats, the prevalence of lymphoid and skin tumors is higher. Mammary tumors are rare in cows, mares, goats, ewes, and sows. There are differences in both biological behavior and histology of mammary tumors in cats and dogs. Although both are house pets and have a similar diet, environment, and life span, the prevalence is higher in dogs; however, only ~45% are malignant in dogs, whereas ~90% are malignant in cats. Dogs have a much higher number of complex and mixed tumors than cats.

Etiology: The cause of mammary tumors is unknown in any species except mice, in which an oncornavirus is causative in certain inbred lines. Hormones play an important role in the hyperplasia and neoplasia of mammary tissue, but the exact mechanism is unknown. Recent work in animals has demonstrated estrogen and/or progesterone receptors on mammary tumor cells, which may influence the pathogenesis of hormone-induced mammary neoplasia as well as response to hormone therapy.

Genetic and nutritional effects on mammary neoplasia have been identified in mice and in some people, but not in dogs or cats. From a practical view, all mammary tumors should be regarded as potentially malignant regardless of the size or number of glands involved. Spread of mammary carcinomas in both dogs and cats is primarily to regional lymph nodes and lungs. In dogs, 5-10% of mammary carcinomas may produce skeletal metastases, primarily in the axial skeleton, but also in long bones.

Canine Mammary Tumors: These occur most frequently in intact bitches; they are extremely rare in male dogs. Ovariectomy before the first estrus reduces the risk of mammary neoplasia to 0.5% of the risk in intact bitches; ovariectomy after one estrus reduces the risk to 8% of that in intact bitches. Those neutered after maturity have the same risk as intact bitches. The 2 caudal mammary glands are involved more often than the 3 anterior glands. Grossly, the tumors appear as single or multiple nodules in one or more glands, ranging in size from 1 to 25 cm. The cut surface is usually lobulated, gray-tan, and firm, often with fluid-filled cysts. Mixed mammary tumors may contain grossly recognizable bone or cartilage on the cut surface.

Of canine mammary tumors, >50% are benign mixed tumors; a smaller portion is malignant mixed tumors. In the latter, epithelial or mesenchymal components, either singly or in combination, may produce metastases. Histologically, canine mammary gland tumors have been classified by the World Health Organization (WHO) as carcinomas (with 6 types and additional subtypes), sarcomas (with 4 types), carcinosarcomas (mixed mammary tumors), or benign adenomas. This classification scheme is based on the extent of the tumor, involvement of lymph nodes, and the presence of metastatic lesions (TNM system), and includes unclassified tumors and apparently benign dysplasias.

Feline Mammary Tumors: These occur mostly in older (av 11 yr) intact female cats. Spaying at an early age, especially before the first estrus, has a sparing effect and reduces the risk, but the degree of protection is less precisely documented than for dogs. The 2 anterior or thoracic mammae are more frequently involved than the posterior glands.

Histologically, most feline mammary tumors are adenocarcinomas, with tubular or papillary types more common than solid or mucoid types. Mixed mammary tumors and sarcomas are less commonly diagnosed than carcinomas. Benign tumors of the feline mammary gland are relatively infrequent and account for only ~10% of these tumors. The WHO TNM clinical staging system (*see* above) also applies to feline mammary tumors.

A distinct entity called fibroadenomatous hyperplasia has been noted in cats. Other names for this are feline mammary hypertrophy, benign mammary hypertrophy, and fibroglandular mammary hypertrophy. It affects primarily young, actively cycling, or pregnant cats. It also has been seen in neutered cats, including older males given exogenous progestational drugs (megestrol acetate). The disorder is marked clinically by the rapid growth of one or more mammary glands.

Diagnostic Methods (Dogs and Cats): A mammary tumor is usually suspected on detection of a mass on physical examination. The duration is unclear, but the rate of growth may be helpful in determining prognosis. Palpation of the regional lymph nodes helps to determine the extent of spread. Thoracic radiographs should be taken to detect pulmonary metastases. Fine needle aspirates may differentiate between inflammatory and neoplastic lesions, but may lead to erroneous conclusions and delay of surgery.

Treatment and Prognosis: Mammary tumors are best treated by surgery, although there is no consensus as to the best procedure. Removal of the tumor alone (lumpectomy), simple mastectomy (removal of the affected gland only), modified radical mastectomy (removal of the affected gland and those that share lymphatic drainage and associated lymph nodes), and radical mastectomy (removal of the entire mammary chain and associated lymph nodes) all have their proponents. The more involved procedures have not been shown to prolong survival compared to the others, and the advantages of the simpler procedures are obvious. In cats, radical mastectomy has increased the disease-free interval but not survival time.

Chemotherapy has not been an effective treatment in canine mammary tumors; a combination of doxorubicin and cyclophosphamide has been used with limited efficacy in feline mammary tumors. Radiation therapy has not been effective.

The prognosis is based on multiple factors. Most canine mammary gland tumors that are going to cause death do so within 1 yr. Sarcomas are associated with shorter survival times than carcinomas. Other factors, including size, lymph node involvement, and nuclear differentiation also affect the prognosis. In cats, tumor volume is important; cats with large tumors (>3 cm diameter) have a median survival time of 6 mo, but those with tumors <2 cm in diameter have a median survival of >4 yr.

MASTITIS, LG AN

Inflammation of the mammary gland, almost always due to the effects of infection by bacterial or mycotic pathogens. Although of greatest economic importance in dairy cows, it may affect other species and is handled in much the same way in each of them. Brief notes on mastitis in ewes, goats, sows, and mares are given separately below. (*See also* the discussions on DISEASE-MANAGEMENT INTERACTIONS in the MHN section.)

Factors that predispose to infection within the gland are poor milking hygiene, milking machine faults, faulty milking management, teat injuries, teat sores, and environmental populations of pathogens. Infection is diagnosed by culture and identification of the pathogen from a sample of milk collected aseptically. Mastitis is detected by clinical signs or results of tests designed to detect increases in the number of WBC in the milk (in subclinical cases). In clinical cases, a provisional diagnosis usually is based on signs and knowledge of the predominant pathogens in the herd, but it should be confirmed by culture. Sensitivity tests on isolates are used to determine or confirm suitability of antibiotics used in therapy.

The 4 clinical types of mastitis are: 1) peracute—swelling, heat, pain, and abnormal secretion in the gland are accompanied by fever and other signs of a systemic disturbance such as marked depression, rapid weak pulse, sunken eyes, weakness, and complete anorexia; 2) acute—changes in the gland are similar to those above, but fever, anorexia, and depression are slight to moderate; 3) subacute—there are no systemic changes, and the changes in the gland and its secretion are less marked; and 4) subclinical—the inflammatory reaction is detectable only by tests, such as the California Mastitis Test (*see* below), the Wisconsin Mastitis Test, the Nagase test, or other tests and the electronic cell count, which are used at intervals to detect a persistently high WBC content in the milk.

Changes in the secretion can vary from a slight wateriness with a few flecks (eg, subacute staphylococcal mastitis), through watery or serous with large yellow clots (eg, acute and peracute streptococcal, staphylococcal, or mycoplasmal mastitis), to watery and brownish with fine mealy flakes (eg, coliform or mycoplasmal mastitis). With severe chronic mastitis, the affected gland gradually loses its productive capacity and may either atrophy or slowly develop firm nodular abscesses or granuloma-like masses within the parenchyma.

The most common bacterial pathogens (in approximate order of decreasing frequency) are: *Staphylococcus aureus, Streptococcus uberis, Str agalactiae, Str dysgalactiae*, other streptococci, and coliforms. Mastitis may be associated with infection with many other organisms, including *Corynebacterium pyogenes, Pseudomonas aeruginosa, Nocardia asteroides, Clostridium perfringens, Mycobacterium* spp, *Mycoplasma* spp, *Pasteurella* spp, yeasts, and *Prototheca* spp.

Treatment of Mastitis: Treatment almost always is recommended when clinical mastitis occurs. Penicillin is the drug of choice for streptococcal mastitis and nonresistant staphylococci. However, most staphylococcal isolates in some herds are resistant, so that semisynthetic penicillins, such as cloxacillin, which is not affected by staphylococcal penicillinase, are more effective. Although treatment usually hastens return of production, a high percentage of staphylococcal infections may not be eliminated during lactation. A somewhat better cure rate results from dry-cow therapy. Coliforms vary widely in their antibiotic sensitivity.

Certain antibiotics, such as penethamate hydriodide and erythromycin, reach much higher levels in the milk than in plasma after systemic administration, and may be useful in acute and peracute cases due to susceptible organisms.

Milk samples for culture should be taken before treatment, which is then initiated immediately. Culture and antibiotic sensitivity testing permit accumulation of data on the common infectious agents in each herd, which serve to guide future recommendations for treatment and control.

Depending on which antibiotic and base is infused into the udder, and what repository form is injected, the milk collected for several milkings following treatment must not be used for human consumption. Recommended withdrawal times should be observed. In case of doubt, milk should be tested before marketing.

CALIFORNIA MASTITIS TEST (CMT)

A kit consisting of a plastic paddle plus all the necessary reagents is available commercially. Equal quantities (2 mL) of reagents and milk are mixed in the cups of the plastic paddle by a swirling motion. Negative samples are free from gel formation, positive samples show various degrees of gelling, which is a reflection of the degree of udder inflammation. There is a high degree of correlation between the CMT and the somatic cell count. The CMT may be used to estimate the somatic cell count of bulk herd milk, bucket milk, or quarter milk.

MASTITIS IN COWS

Streptococcal Mastitis: The mammary gland is required for perpetuation of *Streptococcus agalactiae* in nature. All other streptococci, whether saprophytes or potential pathogens, enter the mammary gland by chance and do not depend on it for survival. Therefore, *S agalactiae* mastitis is a specific infectious disease that can be eradicated from dairy herds. The organism enters the gland through the teat opening and resides in the milk and on the surface of the milk channels. It does not penetrate the tissue. Initially, it multiplies rapidly and causes an outpouring of neutrophils into the ducts and damages the ductal and acinar epithelium, which leads to ductal obstruction with cells and cellular debris. Fibrosis of interalveolar tissue and involution of acini in affected lobules quickly follow and lead to a loss of secretory function.

Because *Streptococcus agalactiae* spreads from cow to cow during milking, shedder cows should be milked last. Some believe that calves fed on milk containing the pathogen may transmit it to the immature glands of penmates if they are permitted to suckle each other. For this reason, milk-fed calves are housed separately.

The other streptococci that may cause mastitis are *S dysgalactiae*, *S uberis*, *S zooepidemicus*, and Lancefield groups D, G, L, and N streptococci. Both *S dysgalactiae* and *S uberis* are common to the environment of dairy farms; *S agalactiae* is most likely to contribute substantially to unacceptable bacterial counts in milk, and may be totally responsible.

Mastitis caused by *S agalactiae* responds well to penicillin, but some of the other streptococci appear to be more resistant; the antibiotic is infused into the infected gland through the teat canal after thorough disinfection of the teat orifice. Chlortetracycline, oxytetracycline, cephalosporin, or sodium cloxacillin also may be used. Variable results have been reported for neomycin. Benzathine cloxacillin, penicillin-novobiocin, cephalosporin, or long-acting penicillin preparations may be used in dry-cow treatment.

Staphylococcal Mastitis: *Staphylococcus aureus* is the most important cause of mastitis in most dairy areas today because it causes both acute and chronic mastitis, the infections respond poorly to treatment, and it is easily transmitted at milking time. But, contrary to prior opinion, it does not colonize the skin, and is found there only with udder infection.

In herds in which staphylococcal mastitis is a problem, ≥50% of the cows may have chronic subclinical infections. *Staphylococcus aureus* may cause peracute mastitis; peracute gangrenous mastitis (in which the skin of the quarter and teat becomes cold and bluish and eventually sloughs); as well as the acute, subacute, and chronic subclinical types. Infections lasting more than a few months often are refractory to treatment because of the development of a tissue barrier between the antibiotic and the organism.

Treatment of cows with subclinical infections during lactation is not as successful as dry-cow treatment; hence, these should be treated at drying off with an appropriate long-acting infusion, eg, penicillin-streptomycin preparations, cephalosporin, novobiocin, or benzathine cloxacillin. The latter drug is preferred if sensitivity tests have not been done.

Peracute and acute staphylococcal mastitis may be treated systemically with an appropriate antibiotic, eg, erythromycin, streptomycin, oxytetracycline, or chlortetracycline. For intramammary therapy, cloxacillin is recommended, but sensitivity tests may reveal that other infusions, such as erythromycin, lincomycin, penicillin-streptomycin, chlortetracycline, or neomycin, may be more effective in some instances. Staphylococcal vaccines have been recommended, but their value in the control of the disease appears to be limited.

Coliform Mastitis: The most frequently encountered coliforms are *Escherichia coli*, *Enterobacter aerogenes*, and *Klebsiella* spp. In quarters with low cell counts, coliforms multiply rapidly. The inflammatory reaction that follows destroys the coliform population, thereby releasing their endotoxin. The resulting toxemia produces the local and systemic signs of acute or peracute mastitis (including gangrene in occasional cases), and death may occur. The temperature in acute or peracute mastitis is 103-108°F (39-42°C), milk secretion ceases even though usually only one gland is infected, and anorexia, depression, dehydration, and rapid weight loss are prominent. The secretion of the clinically affected quarter(s) is usually brownish and watery. Diarrhea also may occur. A unique feature is that, on recovery, the udder tissue generally returns to normal so that, in a subsequent lactation, no fibrosis is found and the gland is capable of producing to capacity. Cows producing milk with low WBC counts (<100,000 cells/mL) are more subject to episodes of acute coliform mastitis, and older cows may be even more so because of increased patency of the streak canal.

In peracute coliform mastitis, systemic treatment with sulfamethazine or antibiotics, such as penicillin-streptomycin combinations, oxytetracycline, or ampicillin, is indicated together with a mastitis infusion of the same antibiotic into the affected quarter q24hr for 3-4 treatments. The affected quarter is infused after the evening milking and repeatedly stripped out during the day to remove bacteria and toxins. Oxytocin may be used to remove more secretion before treatment. Single or repeated injections of flunixin meglumine, antihistamine, or IV administration of a corticosteroid with isotonic, balanced electrolyte solutions may be of use as supportive therapy in severe cases. Calcium borogluconate or isotonic bicarbonate solutions may be needed if levels are low.

In acute mastitis, intramammary antibiotic infusions with or without systemic antibiotics initially (depending on the severity) are usually sufficient if the organism is sensitive to the antibiotic in use. Dihydrostreptomycin sulfate, ampicillin, chlortetracycline, oxytetracycline, and neomycin have been used with variable results. Frequent stripping is also recommended. Fortunately, most coliform udder infections are eliminated by the cow, often before treatment can be instituted; therefore, cultures of clinical cases may often be negative.

Pseudomonas aeruginosa Mastitis: Generally, a persistent infection occurs, which may be characterized by intermittent acute or subacute exacerbations. The organism is found in soil-water environments common to dairy farms. Herd-wide infections have been reported following extensive exposure to contaminated wash water, teat cup liners, or intramammary treatments administered by milkers. Failure to employ aseptic techniques for udder therapy or use of contaminated milking equipment may lead to establishment of *P aeruginosa* infections within the mammary glands. Severe peracute mastitis with toxemia and high mortality may follow immediately in some, while subclinical infections may occur in others. The pathogen has persisted in a gland for as long as 5 lactations, but spontaneous recovery may occur.

The pathogen often is sensitive to streptomycin, neomycin, and carbenicillin *in vitro*, but results have been variable when these drugs have been infused into the udder. Carbenicillin appears to be the drug of choice, but a satisfactory treatment for *P aeruginosa* mastitis has not been developed.

Corynebacterium pyogenes Mastitis: This pathogen is common in suppurative processes of cattle and pigs, and it produces a characteristic mastitis in heifers and dry cows; occasionally, it is observed in mastitis in the lactating udder, and it may be a secondary invader. The inflammation is typified by the formation of profuse, foul-smelling, purulent exudate. The foul smell is not caused by *C pyogenes*, but by an anaerobic micrococcus, *Peptococcus indolicus*, that commonly is found in association with the former; in the rare instances of *C pyogenes* mastitis in which *P indolicus* is not present, the exudate is odorless.

Mastitis due to *C pyogenes* occurs in epidemic form among dry cows, heifers, and calves pastured during the summer months in northern European countries when the vector *Hydrotaea irritans* is present. In other countries, where the fly is absent, cases are sporadic. Epidemics may be controlled by fly control or removal of animals from fly-infested areas. Prophylactic treatment of heifers and dry cows in endemic areas with long-acting penicillin preparations has been effective in reducing infections. Cows are treated at drying off and again in 4-6 wk. Therapy is rarely successful, and the infected quarter is usually lost to production. Infected animals may be systemically ill, and animals with abscesses usually should be slaughtered.

Unusual Forms of Mastitis: *Mycoplasma* spp can cause a severe form of mastitis that may spread rapidly through a herd with serious consequences. *Mycoplasma bovis* is the most common cause. Other significant species include *M californicum, M canadense,* and *M bovigenitalium.* Typically, onset is rapid. Some or all quarters become involved. Loss of production is often dramatic, and the secretion is soon replaced by a serous or purulent exudate. Initially, a characteristic fine granular or flaky sediment may be seen in the material removed from infected glands. Despite the severe local effects on udder tissue, cows usually do not manifest signs of systemic involvement. The infection may persist through the dry period. Since there is no satisfactory treatment, affected cows should be segregated at least for that lactation or for their lifetimes, or slaughtered and sanitary measures strictly enforced, especially at milking or during treatment.

Nocardia asteroides causes a destructive mastitis characterized by acute onset, high temperature, anorexia, rapid wasting, and marked swelling of the udder. Response in the udder is typical of a granulomatous inflammation and leads to extensive fibrosis and formation of palpable nodules. Herd histories suggest that infection of the udder may be associated with failure to ensure asepsis in intramammary treatment of the common forms of mastitis. Slaughter is recommended for obvious clinical cases, but intramammary infusions of a furaltadone-penicillin preparation may successfully remove latent and subclinical infections.

Mastitis due to various yeasts has appeared in dairy herds, especially following the use of penicillin in an attempt to eradicate *S agalactiae*, or in association with prolonged repetitive use of antibiotic infusions in individual cows. Yeasts grow well in the presence of penicillin and some other antibiotics, and if accidentally introduced during udder infusions of antibiotics, they may be able to multiply and cause mastitis. Signs may be severe with a high temperature, followed by spontaneous recovery in ~2 wk or by a chronic destructive mastitis. Other yeast infections cause minimal inflammation and are self-limiting. If mastitis due to yeast is suspected, antibiotic therapy should be stopped immediately.

A chronic indurative mastitis similar to that caused by the tubercle bacillus has been reported to be caused by acid-fast bacilli derived from the soil, such as *Mycobacterium fortuitum, M smegmatis, M vaccae, and M phlei*, when such organisms are introduced into the gland along with antibiotics, especially penicillin, in oil or ointment vehicles. The oil apparently enhances the invasiveness of these organisms, and such therapy is contraindicated.

These organisms otherwise tend to be saprophytic and to disappear from infected quarters, at least by the next lactation. In the meantime, mastitis is usually moderate. Distinct outbreaks do occur and several have been reported, especially with *M fortuitum* and *M smegmatis*.

CONTROL OF BOVINE MASTITIS

Control and eradication of the contagious forms of mastitis due to *Str agalactiae* and *S aureus* are accomplished by adherence to the 8 points listed below, plus a specific program for each pathogen.

Since 90-95% of *Str agalactiae* infections can be cured by penicillin therapy during lactation, infected dry and lactating cows should be identified by culture and treated at once. Treatment of late lactation cows may be postponed until drying off. Dry-cow therapy should cure most remaining infected cows. The herd should be monitored to detect reintroduction of infection.

A much smaller percentage of cows infected with *S aureus* are cured by either lactation or dry-cow therapy. Therefore, all infected cows should be maintained in a segregated group until culled from the herd. This group is always milked last (unless there is also a group infected with *Mycoplasma*) to stop transfer of infection at milking. Dry-cow therapy is administered to this group and clinical cases are treated, but they are never regarded as cured, even if a negative culture is obtained. Any other cows with new *S aureus* infections should be transferred to this group. The herd should be monitored by culture of clinical mastitis and bulk tank milk samples to detect reintroduction of infection.

There are 8 related points to consider: 1) Check (and correct when necessary) milking machine function and milking procedures. The following factors have been associated with higher incidences of mastitis: a) Excessive irregular vacuum fluctuation in the teat cup and in the vacuum or milk line. This sometimes occurs due to inadequate vacuum reserve or faulty handling of teat cups ("liner slips" toward the end of milking, letting excess air into the system, is particularly harmful). b) Vacuum levels of ≥2 in. (5 cm) of mercury above or below the recommended 13 in. (33 cm) at the teat cup. c) Blocked air-admission holes in the claw pieces. d) Narrow-bore milk liners (<1 in. [2.5 cm] internal diameter are preferred to wide-bore liners). e) Gross abnormalities in pulsation rate (normal 40-60/min) and ratio (40-50 rest:50-60 vacuum). f) Effective liner length too short (minimum of 5 ½ in. [14 cm] recommended from top of liner to lowest point of collapse). Short liners prevent adequate massage and allow congestion of the end of the teat. g) Incorrect cluster removal. The vacuum should be released first and the cups removed soon after the cow has milked out, to avoid overmilking. h) Inadequate stimulation before applying teat clusters.

2) Observe and correct milking hygiene. A recommended hygiene system is: a) Initially milk out 1-2 streams of milk. b) Wash teats in clean or sanitized running water and dry with disposable paper towels. c) Dip teats at end of milking in a hypochlorite solution (4% available chlorine), a chlorhexidine solution (0.5%), an iodophor solution (5000-10,000 ppm iodine), or other effective dip. d) Milkers should wear rubber gloves and disinfect their hands when going from cow to cow, especially in outbreak situations. e) To control coliform mastitis, dip teats before milking in 2500-5000 ppm iodophore and wipe teats dry with a towel. Continue post-milking teat-dipping, but use a hypochlorite dip to prevent bulk milk iodine levels exceeding acceptable limits.

3) Detect infected cows by repeat CMT (qv, p 687) or cell counts and cultures. Culture all clinical cases. Isolate infected cows and milk them last. Milk clean heifers first, then clean cows, then recently treated cows, and finally, infected cows.

4) Treat clinical infections as they occur and subclinical infections at drying off (especially *S aureus* and streptococcal infections). Cows carrying *Str agalactiae* infections can be treated during lactation with a reasonable degree of success. Treat all quarters at drying off with an appropriate long-acting antibiotic infusion.

5) Cull any cows that have had 3-5 or more clinical attacks of mastitis during the lactation, have failed to respond to repeated therapy (including dry-cow therapy), or have persistently high somatic cell counts.

6) Examine all introductions to the herd by udder palpation, culture, and CMT of secretion from all quarters.

7) Control teat cracks, chapping, and pseudo-cowpox by appropriate measures, since they may predipose to a high incidence of mastitis.

8) Maintain owner interest and awareness of the mastitis problem by regular discussions of cell count (or CMT) and culture results on monthly bulk-tank samples, pretreatment samples saved from all clinical cases, and monthly analyses of somatic cell counts from processor and herd records.

MASTITIS IN GOATS

The organisms infecting the udder of goats are similar to those in cows. Coagulase-negative staphylococci have a high prevalence and appear to cause persistent infections that result in elevated cell counts and low-grade mastitis with some recurring clinical episodes. The level of infection and incidence of mastitis due to *Staphylococcus aureus* and *Streptococcus agalactiae* and other streptococci tend to be low, but major differences between herds may occur.

Mycoplasma infections, primarily *Mycoplasma mycoides mycoides* (large colony type) and *M putrefaciens*, sometimes cause serious outbreaks of mastitis in goats (*see also* p 658). The latter also causes septicemia, polyarthritis, pneumonia and encephalitis, together with serious disease and mortality in suckling kids. *Mycoplasma capricolum* has also been reported to cause severe mastitis in goats and infection in kids. Does usually recover in ~4 wk.

As with cows, gram-negative organisms cause intermittent infections that may be severe, but are usually self-limiting. *Corynebacterium pyogenes* sometimes produces multiple nodular abscesses.

Programs for diagnosis, control, and treatment of bacterial mastitis in goats are similar to those in cows. Milking and environmental sanitation need to be good to reduce the prevalence and spread of infection. Chronically infected goats should be culled, as should goats with *M mycoides mycoides* infections and those not recovering from *M putrefaciens* or *M capricolum* infections.

MASTITIS IN MARES

Acute mastitis occurs occasionally in lactating mares, most commonly in the drying-off period, in one or both glands. *Streptococcus zooepidemicus* is the most frequent pathogen. *Streptococcus equi, S equisimilis, S agalactiae*, and *S viridans* are also found. A variety of gram-negative bacteria has also been reported. Marked painful swelling of the affected gland and adjacent tissues occurs, and the secretion is often seroflocculent. Fever and depression may be present. The mare may walk stiffly or stand with hindlegs apart due to the discomfort.

Treatment is similar to that in cows, but when intramammary infusions are used, they should be inserted separately into both orifices of the teat. Culture and antibacterial sensitivity testing aid selection of appropriate local and systemic antimicrobial therapy. Without prompt treatment, abscessation or induration of the gland can occur. Little is known about the frequency and persistence of subclinical intramammary infections in mares.

MASTITIS IN SHEEP

This can be quite an important disease, with an incidence of ≥2%. Apart from deaths from peracute infections, the disease can be a cause of lamb mortality from starvation, or of depressed weaning weights of lambs. Peracute, gangrenous (usually due to *Staphylococcus aureus*), acute, subacute, and probably subclinical types occur. The organisms most commonly involved are *S aureus*, coagulase-negative staphylococci, streptococci, *Escherichia coli, Pasteurella haemolytica*, and *Corynebacterium pyogenes*.

The principles of diagnosis and treatment used in bovine mastitis can be applied to ewes. Little is known about the control of ovine mastitis, but careful inspection of the mammary glands of ewes before mating to detect and eliminate those with acute, subacute, and chronic mastitis should be beneficial.

MASTITIS IN SOWS

Mastitis can be important in swine-raising units. Peracute mastitis can affect sows and gilts and is most commonly associated with coliform (*Escherichia coli, Enterobacter aerogenes*, and *Klebsiella*) infections. It is most common at or just following parturition, and affected sows have a moderate to severe toxemia. The sow's temperature may be elevated to 107°F (42°C) or may be subnormal. The affected glands are swollen, purple, and have a watery secretion. Sow mortality is high, and the litter will die unless fostered or fed artificially. Recovered sows may have impaired milk production in the next lactation. The treatment of peracute coliform mastitis in sows is similar to that in cows (*see* above). Ampicillin, dihydrostreptomycin, or oxytetracycline administered systemically has been used.

Subacute mastitis may occur in older sows and lead to induration of one or more glands and impair the sow's ability to nurse a large litter. This form of mastitis is more likely to be associated with infection by streptococci or staphylococci. Granulomatous lesions in the mammae of sows have been associated with *Actinobacillus lignieresii, Actinomyces bovis*, and *Staphylococcus aureus* infections. *Fusobacterium necrophorum* and *Corynebacterium pyogenes* also have been incriminated in sow mastitis. A thorough examination and culture of the mammary glands of the sow is important to diagnose any of the above peracute and subacute types of mastitis. (*See* AGALACTIA SYNDROME, p 656.)

The control of porcine mastitis has not been extensively investigated, but isolating sows in adequately disinfected pens before, during, and for an adequate period after farrowing should help prevent the severe losses associated with coliform mastitis.

METRITIS, LG AN

Inflammation of the muscular and endometrial layers of the uterus. Acute metritis almost always occurs after abnormal parturition or gross uterine contamination. Delayed uterine involution is a major predisposing factor. It is often accompanied by retention of the fetal membranes (qv, p 698). Contaminants enter the uterus during parturition and establish infection, especially in association with stress caused by dystocia, abortion, concurrent systemic disease, or malnutrition. Commonly, there is a fetid discharge from the uterus. In severely affected animals, the uterus is atonic, and in cows and mares several gallons of fluid may accumulate. Systemic signs include fever, anorexia, depression, and in mares, toxemia and laminitis. The uterus may be swollen and fragile so that caution should be used in examination. Manipulation of the uterus by rectal palpation may cause perimetritis.

Treatment should be both systemic and local with broad-spectrum antimicrobials. Systemic treatments, indicated when systemic signs are present, include trimethoprim with sulfadoxine, tetracyclines, ampicillin (especially when urinary tract infection also is present), and penicillin. Evacuation of the uterine contents is essential before treating locally. Oxytocin usually is effective within 48 hr of parturition. Siphoning must be used if there is a poor response.

For local treatment of the postpartum uterus of cows, some medications in concentrations likely to be achieved in the uterus are ineffective against common bacteria (eg, *Corynebacterium pyogenes*). Some drugs or their vehicles elicit severe inflammatory responses in the endometrium. The anaerobic environment of the postpartum uterus may be unsatisfactory for some drugs (eg, aminoglycosides). The uterine contents may also contain substances such as penicillinase that inhibit particular drugs. Oxytetracycline in a povidone base infused into the uterus every second day, with systemic penicillin therapy when fever is present, has been suggested as a treatment regimen. Selection of antibiotics for treatment of lactating dairy cows must consider milk withholding times.

The antibiotic selected for local treatment of mares with metritis should be one known not to be irritating to the endometrium, eg, the tetracyclines. Uterine lavage, used in conjunction with local antibiotics is useful in removing fluids and toxic by-products of inflammation; in mares with severe septic metritis, the physical removal of uterine contents may be critical to survival. Repeated large-volume (10-12 L) lavages with warm saline or water cause uterine contraction as well as enhance removal of the offending material.

When the cow has not been systemically ill, spontaneous recovery from metritis is common. If the disease becomes chronic, the uterus may become thick-walled and fibrotic. Chronically affected cows may lose condition, and fertility potential may be impaired. Chronic cases may be treated with antibiotic infusions, or with disinfectants such as Lugol's solution. The latter agent causes necrosis of the superficial endometrium, which subsequently regenerates and may possess improved potential.

If mares survive the acute phase of metritis, there is generally no negative aftereffect. Careful inspection for damage to the endometrium and cervix caused by parturition, metritis, or treatment should provide data that correlate well with future fertility.

(*See also* CONTAGIOUS EQUINE METRITIS, below, and MMA, p 657.)

CONTAGIOUS EQUINE METRITIS (CEM)

A highly contagious venereal disease of horses and, experimentally, donkeys. In most areas, the disease must be reported to regulatory authorities.

Etiology, Epidemiology, and Clinical Findings: The causal agent is a gram-negative coccobacillus, once arguably classified in the genus *Haemophilus*, now designated *Taylorella equigenitalis*. It is fastidious and best cultivated on chocolate Eugon agar at 37°C in a microaerophilic atmosphere.

In infected stallions, *T equigenitalis* resides in the smegma of the prepuce and on the surface of the penis, especially in the urethral fossa, without producing clinical disease. Infection is transmitted at coitus, but potential transfer between mares and between stallions, and by attendants and instruments is a serious hazard. Severely affected mares develop endometritis manifest by a profuse, sticky, mucopurulent, vulval discharge 2-6 days after service; signs are less severe or insignificant in others. Conception rate is low, presumably due to salpingitis, but after infection subsides, fertility is regained. Diestrus may be shortened. Abortion is uncommon, but foals may be exposed at birth and retain infection until breeding age.

Diagnosis: In mares, this is based on recovery of *T equigenitalis* from the endometrium, cervix, clitoral fossa, and sinuses at various stages after exposure, and subsequent development of specific complement fixation (CF) and hemagglutination (HA) antibody 1-2 wk after clinical signs appear (8-14 days after mating). Indirect immunofluorescence may also be of value. Specimens for bacteriology should be taken with care to prevent lateral spread of infection. In acute infections, *T equigenitalis* can best be isolated from guarded endometrial swabs; in chronic infections, from a combined swab of clitoral fossa and sinuses. For stallions, swabs of prepuce, penis, and urethral fossa are required. Use of transport media held at 4°C (Amies medium is preferable, but Stuart's medium is satisfactory when delay between collection and processing of swabs is short) enhances survival of *T equigenitalis*. Overgrowth by saprophytic microbes may interfere with isolation. Adding trimethoprim, clindamycin, and antifungal agents (amphotericin) to Eugon chocolate agar supplemented with 5% lysed horse blood aids isolation of both streptomycin-resistant and streptomycin-sensitive strains, but should be used in parallel with nonselective media. FA is of limited value for identification of the causal agent in clinical material although useful in identifying suspicious colonies. Serology can be used to monitor mares mated with stallions of uncertain disease status, and to assess mares that have recently contracted infection but for which bacteriology results are inconclusive. CF titers persist for 4-6 wk, HA titers longer. Serological tests are not useful in infected stallions.

Treatment and Control: The stallion should be teased, and the extended penis and sheath washed thoroughly with chlorhexidine (smegma must be removed from the urethral fossa); after 2 min, the antiseptic is washed off; the penis, fossa, and sheath are dried and smeared liberally with nitrofurazone cream. This is repeated daily for 5 days. After ≥1 wk, it is advisable to test mate the stallion before resuming breeding. Prolonged prophylactic use of chlorhexidine on stallions before and after service to minimize the possibility of their acquiring *T equigenitalis* is not recommended; it can inhibit the normal flora and allow *Pseudomonas* to build up on the skin of the penis, which can be transferred to mares. Acute CEM infection of most mares resolves without treatment in 3 wk, but many retain infection in the clitoral fossa and sinuses. Cleaning the fossa of smegma and local application of chlorhexidine and antibiotic creams to the fossa and sinuses (variable in number and location) often overcome residual infection; in others, ablation of the clitoral sinuses is necessary.

PROLONGED GESTATION IN CATTLE AND SHEEP

Gestation is prolonged when a lesion in the pituitary-adrenocortical axis of the fetus interferes with release of cortisol necessary for initiation of parturition. Two forms of prolonged gestation seen in cattle are inherited via a homozygous autosomal recessive gene. One form, seen in Holstein and Ayrshire cattle, is due to hypoplasia of fetal adrenals and lack of an adrenal enzyme necessary for the synthesis of glucocorticoids. These fetuses continue to grow 20-90 days beyond term and may exceed 200 lb (90 kg). At the end of normal pregnancy, affected cows show some mammary hypertrophy with no other signs of parturition. Spontaneous initiation of parturition, which occurs only after the fetus dies, results in dystocia, and cesarean section is indicated. Live calves delivered by cesarean section are hypoglycemic and have a hypoadrenocorticism-like syndrome. Continuous corticosteroid and supportive therapy may keep these calves alive but is impractical.

A second form of prolonged gestation, which occurs in Guernsey and Swedish Red and White cattle, is due to aplasia of the pituitary and lack of sufficient adrenocorticotropic hormone (ACTH) to stimulate glucocorticoid release. Characteristics of these fetuses include arrested growth at ~7 mo of gestation, deformed limbs, hairlessness, and hydrocephalus, anencephaly, or cyclopia. The adrenals also may be hypoplastic or absent. These fetuses may live *in utero* for long periods, and gestations of up to 18 mo have been reported. Parturition occurs following death of the fetus.

Another form of prolonged gestation in Holstein cattle has been associated with cerebral herniation (Catlin mark) in the fetus. Such a fetus continues to grow *in utero* and parturition may be initiated 20-60 days late, resulting in dystocia due to a larger than normal fetus. The characteristics of these fetuses include cerebral herniation, a sloping forehead, and reduced cranial cavity. Hypoplasia of the adrenals or aplasia of the pituitary also has been reported.

Veratrum californicum ingested by the ewe between days 14 and 30 of gestation interferes with development of the CNS (qv, p 579) and results in severe deformities of the head and face, cyclopia, hypoplasia or aplasia of the pituitary, and prolonged gestation. These fetuses continue to grow *in utero* up to 230 days and may result in death of the ewe if not removed by cesarean section. *Veratrum album*, found in Europe, may cause a similar condition of the fetus when ingested by cattle.

Prolonged gestation associated with giant fetuses has been described in Karakul sheep. It is believed that the sheep consume a shrub (*Salsola tuberculata*) that inhibits fetal hypothalamic-releasing factors. The affected ewes fail to develop normal preparturient udder enlargement. Fetuses have small pituitaries and hypoplastic adrenals.

Parturition may be induced by IM injection of glucocorticoids in cases of prolonged gestation. Prostaglandin analogs or combinations of prostaglandin and glucocorticoids also may be used. (*See also* FAILURE OF FETAL ENDOCRINE FUNCTION, p 259.)

PROSTATIC DISEASES

Uncommon to rare in other species, diseases of the prostate are common in dogs. They include benign prostatic hyperplasia, bacterial prostatitis, prostatic abscesses, prostatic and paraprostatic cysts, and prostatic neoplasia; all have similar clinical signs because they all cause prostatic enlargement or inflammation. The most common signs include tenesmus, blood dripping from the penis, hematuria, and recurrent urinary tract infections. Additional nonspecific signs such as fever, malaise, and caudal abdominal pain are often present with bacterial infections and neoplasia. Prostatic adenocarcinoma with pelvic and lumbar vertebral metastases may cause gait abnormalities. Prostatic enlargement may mechanically interfere with other abdominal organs. Less commonly, prostatic diseases may cause infertility, urinary incontinence, or urethral obstruction.

The prostate is examined physically by abdominal and rectal palpation. Rarely is the enlarged prostate located completely within the pelvic canal. Size, shape, symmetry, consistency, mobility, and the presence or absence of discomfort are assessed by palpation. The clinical signs and physical findings are usually sufficient to localize a disease process to the prostate gland, but not to differentiate between the various conditions.

Abdominal radiographs may further define the size, shape, and position of the prostate. The sublumbar lymph nodes, lumbar vertebrae, and bony pelvis should be evaluated radiographically for evidence of metastases. A positive contrast cystourethrogram can be performed when an abnormal prostate is difficult to differentiate from the bladder. Ultrasonography provides additional information about the homogeneity of the prostatic parenchyma, urethral diameter, and the diffuse or focal nature of the disease. Urethral invasion or destruction, as identified by contrast radiology or ultrasonography, is highly suggestive of prostatic neoplasia. Other radiographic/ultrasonographic findings do not differentiate between cysts and abscesses, or hyperplasia, diffuse neoplasia, and prostatitis.

Material for cytologic and microbiologic examination can be obtained by prostatic massage followed by aspiration via a urinary catheter, collection of the prostatic fraction of the ejaculate, fine needle aspiration, and/or biopsy. Prostatic massage is easily performed; however, samples are always contaminated by material from the bladder. Since prostatic fluid normally refluxes into the bladder, urinary tract infection is usually present with bacterial prostatitis. Microbiologic examination of the prostatic portion (third fraction) of the ejaculate is more accurate than is examination of prostatic massage specimens when urinary tract infection is present. Neoplastic cells are often not recovered in specimens obtained by ejaculation or prostatic massage. Fine needle aspiration can be performed transrectally or percutaneously, with or without ultrasonographic guiding; while generally safe and simple, this is not without some risk of penetration of surrounding structures. Biopsy is the most definitive, but also the most invasive, diagnostic procedure for differentiating prostatic diseases. Prostatic biopsy is probably best performed via celiotomy.

BENIGN PROSTATIC HYPERPLASIA

The most common prostatic disorder, this is found in most intact male dogs >6 yr old. It is a result of androgenic stimulation, but why some males are affected and others are not is unknown. There may be no clinical signs, or tenesmus, hematuria, and bleeding may occur. The diagnosis is suggested by physical and historical findings. Radiology can confirm prostatomegaly. Ultrasonography should show diffuse, relatively symmetrical involvement. Multiple, diffuse, cystic structures are fairly common. Cytologic examination of massage or ejaculate specimens reveals hemorrhage with mild inflammation without evidence of sepsis or neoplasia. Castration is the treatment of choice; prostatic involution is usually evident within a few weeks and is often complete in several months.

For males intended for use in breeding, other therapy may be feasible. However, treatment with antiandrogens is not nearly as effective as is castration. The drugs that either inhibit androgen synthesis or "counteract" the effects of androgens have the potential of inhibiting spermatogenesis, and their long-term use may not have a more desirable outcome than castration. The use of estrogens to reduce prostatic hyperplasia cannot be recommended. Squamous metaplasia of the prostate can occur whenever estrogenic stimulation is present (exogenous administration or endogenous production by Sertoli cell tumor). Squamous metaplasia can cause prostatic enlargement and worsen the clinical signs. It may also enhance the risk of cystic changes and infection within the prostate. Estrogens can cause negative feedback to the hypothalamus and pituitary, thereby diminishing spermatogenesis. Also, estrogens are potentially toxic to the bone marrow.

Long-term studies with other antiandrogens such as ketoconazole, flutamide, or megestrol acetate are currently lacking. Megestrol acetate (0.25 mg/lb [0.55 mg/kg], PO, daily for 10 days) has been recommended for the treatment of benign hyperplasia in valuable studs. Limited experience suggests that any beneficial effects may be temporary. Castration remains the treatment of choice.

CALCULI

When prostatic calculi occur (rarely), there is usually some other prostatic disease as well. Rarely, radiopaque prostatic calculi are incidental findings on abdominal radiographs.

NEOPLASMS

Adenocarcinoma is the most common neoplasm of the prostate. Transitional cell carcinoma arising from the bladder occasionally invades the prostate. Castration is not protective against future development of prostatic neoplasia in dogs.

The clinical signs of prostatic neoplasia parallel those of other prostatic diseases. Pain and fever may be present. If the neoplasm infiltrates the urethra, dysuria or urethral obstruction is likely. Prostatic adenocarcinoma metastasizes to the regional lymph nodes, lumbar vertebrae, and bony pelvis. Spread to distant sites such as lungs is uncommon until late in the course of disease. Metastasis often has occurred before the diagnosis is made. Whenever prostatic disease causes urethral obstruction in dogs, neoplasia should receive highest consideration. Likewise, prostatomegaly in a previously castrated dog is highly suggestive of neoplasia. Diagnosis is made by biopsy.

There is no effective treatment. Consultation with a veterinary oncologist is recommended.

PROSTATIC AND PARAPROSTATIC CYSTS

Large cysts are occasionally encountered within or associated with the prostate gland. The signs are similar to those encountered with other types of prostatic enlargement, and usually become apparent only when the cyst reaches a size sufficient to cause pressure on adjacent organs. Large cysts may result in abdominal distention and must be differentiated from the bladder and prostatic abscesses.

Medical treatment is ineffective, and estrogen therapy is contraindicated. Castration alone is unlikely to be of benefit but may be indicated following removal of the cyst. Total excision of the cyst is the only satisfactory treatment. Surgical excision is preferable to marsupialization because chronic management of the fistula is often problematic.

PROSTATITIS

Inflammation of the prostate gland usually is suppurative, and may result in abscesses. It may be associated with prostatic hyperplasia (*see* above). Various organisms have been incriminated. Infection may be hematogenous or ascending from the urethra. Because prostatic fluid normally refluxes into the bladder, urinary tract infection often accompanies prostatic infection.

The signs resemble those of prostatic hyperplasia. In addition, malaise, pain, and fever are common. Dehydration, septicemia, and shock may occur in severe cases of acute bacterial prostatitis or prostatic abscess.

The historical, physical, and radiographic findings are suggestive of acute bacterial prostatitis and abscesses. Neutrophilia with a left shift, monocytosis, and/or toxic WBC may be seen. Ultrasonography shows hypoechoic areas consistent with pockets of fluid. Ideally prostatic material is obtained by ejaculation, prostatic massage, or fine needle aspiration for cytologic examination and for culture and sensitivity testing. Massage of an acutely infected prostate may liberate organisms into the blood and cause bacteremia/septicemia. For this reason, other methods are preferred. Fine needle aspiration may liberate organisms into the peritoneal cavity. Dogs with acute bacterial prostatitis or abscesses may be reluctant to ejaculate. Urinalysis shows hematuria, pyuria, and bacteriuria. The urine should be submitted for culture and sensitivity testing. Often the urine and prostatic material yield the same organisms.

Chronic bacterial prostatitis may cause no clinical signs except recurrent urinary tract infection. Physical abnormalities may be limited to the urinary tract. Prostatic size and shape may be normal. Dogs with chronic bacterial prostatitis are usually willing to ejaculate. Prostatic fluid and urine should be submitted for cytologic and microbiologic examination. Prostatic massage or fine needle aspiration could also be used to obtain specimens.

Fluid therapy is indicated for dehydration or shock. Antibiotics should be selected on the basis of sensitivity testing and given for 1-2 wk. Large prostatic abscesses are best treated by surgical drainage. After the infection is controlled, castration could be considered. Urine and/or prostatic fluid should be cultured again after antibiotic therapy and 2-4 wk later, to be certain that infection is resolved.

Chronic bacterial prostatitis may be difficult to resolve. Antibiotic therapy should continue for ≥4 wk. Cultures should be repeated during, and for several months after, antibiotic therapy to ascertain whether resistance or persistent infection has developed. The benefits of castration for treatment of chronic bacterial prostatitis are uncertain; however, it seems reasonable that the prostatic involution following castration would at least help prevent recurrence of infection.

RETAINED PLACENTA, LG AN

COWS

The fetal membranes are normally expelled within 12 hr of parturition; expulsion occurring 12-24 hr after calving is considered to be delayed, and if not expelled within 24 hr, membranes are considered to be retained. The incidence of retained placenta following normal parturition is 3-12%. Following abnormal births, or when the reproductive tract is infected, 20-50% of the cows may be affected.

In normal placental expulsion, the placentomes begin to loosen during late pregnancy. Collagenization of the maternal and fetal connective tissues in the placentome is the major change. During parturition, changes in uterine pressure, alteration of blood flow, and flattening of the placentome contribute to prompt expulsion. Retention may be related to immature placentomes, as in premature delivery or abortion; placentitis or cotyledonary inflammation, as in bacterial or mycotic infections; edema of the chorionic villi due to any cause; and uterine atony or delayed involution. Specific diseases associated with abortion, eg, brucellosis, are important causes of retained placenta. Various nutritional and metabolic etiologies are also recognized.

Usually, degenerating, discolored membranes are seen hanging from the vulva after 24 hr. Occasionally, they may persist within the tract and cause a foul-smelling discharge. Often, there is no systemic illness, but appetite and milk yield may be decreased. Systemic involvement may occur when the uterus is atonic or traumatized. Closure of the cervix before expulsion of the membranes may precipitate severe metritis with systemic signs.

The traditional manual removal of retained placenta has been replaced with a more conservative approach, which is less traumatic and generally less complicated. In cows not showing signs of systemic disease, gentle daily traction on the membranes is usually sufficient to cause expulsion in a few days. Excess tissue should be removed to prevent further gross contamination of the tract. Examinations and local treatments should be done with scrupulous cleanliness.

When signs of systemic illness are noted, intrauterine therapy is indicated. The tetracyclines are the best choice because penicillinase production is characteristic of the typical flora associated with metritis in cows (which makes penicillin ineffective), the involvement of anaerobic bacteria limits the effectiveness of aminoglycosides, and tissue debris in the uterus of affected cows inactivates sulfonamides. Antiseptic therapy of the uterus has not proved to be beneficial. Systemic antibiotics should be given when there is a fever, or trauma or necrosis of the tract.

A follow-up examination in 10-20 days to determine whether residual metritis is present is advised in an attempt to reduce the calving interval.

MARES

The placenta normally is expelled within 3 hr of foaling but may be delayed until 8-12 hr without untoward sequelae. Retention beyond this is uncommon and tends to be associated with infection, dystocia, or an atonic uterus. Uncomplicated cases may be managed by administering oxytocin, either as repeated small doses (20-30 u) IM, or by slow IV drip of 50-100 u over 1-2 hr. Discomfort associated with uterine contraction may be noted.

Since bacteria multiply logarithmically after 8 hr, it is prudent to initiate local and systemic antibiotic therapy when retention exceeds this time. Whenever the uterus is medicated or explored manually, cleanliness and gentleness is imperative. Exploration may be combined with local administration of medication to reduce the number of times the uterus is invaded. Careful manipulation of the membranes may result in separating them, but in no case is forceful extraction justified.

The most serious complications of retained placenta in mares are metritis, septicemia, and laminitis. To minimize these, uterine lavage with large volumes of warm water or saline is helpful.

OTHER SPECIES

In ewes and does, local and systemic treatment to guard against infection, and gentle traction on the membranes are usually used. The retained placenta usually is expelled within 2-10 days.

In sows, signs of systemic illness and a purulent discharge containing shreds of membrane indicate the uncommon case of retained placenta. If seen early, oxytocin may assist. Intensive treatment to combat infection is indicated.

ULCERATIVE POSTHITIS AND VULVITIS
(Sheath rot, Pizzle rot, Enzootic balanoposthitis, Caprine herpesvirus vulvovaginitis)

Ulcerative posthitis (or vulvitis), a moderately contagious disease of sheep and goats and occasionally of cattle, is characterized by ulcerative lesions with scab formation on the prepuce, and less frequently on the lips of the vulva. It is prevalent in castrated male sheep and goats and in rams, and less frequent in ewes; the incidence in does is unknown. The highest incidence occurs in Merino and Angora wethers. Posthitis is also seen in steers and sometimes in bulls.

Etiology and Epidemiology: A combination of high levels of urinary urea and the causative organism, *Corynebacterium renale*, is necessary to establish ulcerations. Animals on high-protein diets (16-18%) produce alkaline urine, which is high in urea (up to 4%), and *C renale*, a normal inhabitant of the skin, can hydrolize urea to ammonia. A caprine herpesvirus has been isolated from goats with vulvovaginitis.

The higher incidence in Merino and Angora wethers is correlated with the long, heavy wool and mohair surrounding the prepuce, which allows the area to become contaminated with urine. Seasonal severity fluctuates with the availability of protein-rich forages, time of shearing, and possibly other influences unrelated to protein intake. The condition in the USA usually is limited to Angora wethers and rams retained for breeding, since castrated sheep are not retained beyond the market lamb stage. The condition can be transmitted to wethers, rams, and ewes by infective material from an external preputial or vulval ulcer. Intact male lambs (2-3 wk) usually are resistant. Ewe lambs (1 mo) may show blister-like lesions under the tail.

Clinical Findings: Ulcers develop around the preputial orifice (external ulcerative posthitis), and a brownish crust develops over the lesion. Removal of this crust rarely produces hemorrhage. If untreated, the condition may progress and partially or totally occlude the preputial orifice. Further progression to the internal preputial mucosa causes a serious and debilitating condition, internal ulcerative posthitis.

Ulcerative vulvitis begins with vulval inflammation and a yellowish encrustation of the labia. The condition may resolve or progress to swelling, ulceration, and scab formation at the ventral commissure, clitoris, and posterior vagina.

In advanced cases of internal ulcerative posthitis, there are typical external lesions, plus enlargement and elongation of the prepuce due to partial or complete occlusion of the preputial orifice. These cases are accompanied by a thickened preputial wall and the accumulation of a foul-smelling mixture of urine and necrotic exudate.

Diagnosis: Ulcerative lesions of the prepuce or vagina, covered by brownish crusty scabs that on removal produce minimal hemorrhage, are characteristic of ulcerative posthitis. Ulcerative dermatosis (UD, qv, p 866), a viral disease, must be considered and can be differentiated on the basis that UD forms a rigid, firmly attached scab that on removal reveals a granular and hemorrhagic surface. UD may also involve the glans penis and cause phimosis or paraphimosis. Ulcerative lesions at other locations, such as the face and legs, suggest a diagnosis of UD.

Enlargement and elongation of the prepuce due to ulcerative posthitis must be differentiated from urinary calculi (qv, p 885).

Treatment and Control: Effective treatments are difficult and often unsuccessful in wether sheep and goats kept for fleece production in extensive range operations. Reducing the protein intake, removing wool or hair from the preputial area, and implanting 100 mg of testosterone q3mo (where available) reduces incidence and severity. Zeranol in the ration has given limited success.

Treatment consists of debriding affected tissue and weekly applications of an ointment containing penicillin, bacitracin, or 5-10% copper sulfate. Animals should be isolated until remission of clinical signs. Early treatment (and isolation) is necessary to prevent the more serious and debilitating internal ulcerative posthitis, which may require surgery.

UTERINE PROLAPSE AND EVERSION

Prolapse of the uterus may occur in any species; however, it is most common in dairy cows and sows, less frequent in ewes, and rare in mares, bitches, and queens. Etiology is unclear and occurrence is sporadic. Recumbency with the hindquarters lower than the forequarters, invagination of the uterus, excessive traction to relieve dystocia, and hypocalcemia all have been incriminated as contributory causes. Prolapse of the uterus usually occurs within a few hours after parturition, when the cervix is open and the uterus lacks tone. Prolapse usually is complete, and the mass of uterus usually hangs below the hocks of the affected animal. An exception occurs in sows, in which one horn may become everted while unborn piglets in the other prevent further prolapse.

In cows, treatment involves removing the placenta (if still attached) and thorough cleaning of the endometrial surface. The uterus is then returned to its normal position by one of several methods. First, an epidural anesthetic should be administered. If the cow is standing, the uterus should be cleaned, elevated to the level of the vulva on a tray (or by means of a hammock held by 2 assistants), and then replaced by applying steady anterior pressure beginning at the cervical portion and gradually working toward the apex. Once the uterus is replaced, the hand should be inserted to the tip of both uterine horns to be sure that there is no remaining invagination. If recumbent, the cow should be positioned with the hindquarters elevated by moving her onto a sloping area or placing her in sternal recumbency with hindlegs extended backwards.

An alternative method involves elevating the hindquarters with some type of lift attached to the hindlegs, thus placing the cow in dorsal recumbency. The uterus is replaced as indicated above. In sows and small animals, reposition may be achieved by simultaneously manipulating the uterus from outside with one hand and through an abdominal incision with the other. Resection of the prolapsed uterus is indicated in long-standing cases in which tissue necrosis has occurred. Once the uterus is in its normal position, antibiotics are placed in the uterus, oxytocin is administered, and a Caslick suture is placed in the vulva. Infusions of warm sterile saline may help prevent recurrence.

The prognosis depends on the amount of injury and contamination of the uterus. Prompt replacement of a clean, minimally traumatized uterus allows a favorable prognosis. There is no tendency for the condition to recur at subsequent parturitions. Complications tend to develop when laceration, necrosis, and infection occur, or when treatment is delayed. Shock, hemorrhage, and thromboembolism are common sequelae of a prolonged prolapse and require aggressive supportive therapy. In some instances, the bladder and intestines may prolapse into the everted uterus. These require careful replacement before replacement of the uterus. The bladder may be drained with a catheter or needle passed through the uterine wall. Elevation of the hindquarters and pressure on the uterus aid in replacement of bladder and intestines. It may be necessary to incise the uterus to replace these organs.

In the cow, amputation of a severely traumatized or necrotic uterus may be the only means of saving the animal. Supportive treatment and antibiotic therapy are indicated.

VAGINAL AND CERVICAL PROLAPSE

Eversion and prolapse of the vagina, with or without prolapse of the cervix, occurs in all species, but is most frequent in cattle and sheep. It is referred to as casting of wethers in sheep. Occasionally, the bladder may be contained within the prolapsed vagina.

The condition usually occurs in mature females in late pregnancy. Predisposing factors include relaxation and increased mobility of the soft-tissue structures in the pelvic canal and perineum as parturition approaches and increased intra-abdominal pressure due to increasing fetal size, intra-abdominal fat, or rumen distention. The condition may also have a genetic component since it is reported to occur frequently in some families and may occur in young nonpregnant animals. However, most prolapses occur in multiparous cows, which suggests that multiple calvings predispose to eversion. Relaxation of the vulva, vagina, and soft tissue surrounding the vagina in late pregnancy allows for increased mobility of the caudal reproductive tract. When the animal is down, gravity and increased intra-abdominal pressure temporarily evert the vagina through the vulva. Irritation and swelling of the exposed mucosa follows repeated eversion; this results in straining and a prolapse occurs.

In sheep, predisposing factors include genetics, increased intra-abdominal pressure due to multiple lambs or rumen distention, estrogens in the feed, and grazing in areas that have estrogenic plants (*Trifolium subterraneum*). Use of stilbestrol or estradiol to fatten lambs may predispose to vaginal prolapse.

The floor of the vagina prolapses first, and repeated eversions may result in a diverticulum of one or both sides of the vagina. The cervix occasionally prolapses through the vulva. The external cervical os may be enlarged and erythematous; however, pregnancy usually is not interrupted. The urethra may be occluded and prevent urination, which may lead to rupture of the bladder. If untreated, it results in uremia, vascular stasis, necrosis and infection of the vagina, and eventually, death.

Families predisposed to the condition and those animals that have been affected previously should not be bred. Feeding practices should be evaluated to ensure that animals are gaining weight in the last trimester but are not overconditioned, and that estrogenic sources are eliminated. Animals should be kept on level ground during late pregnancy. Methods to prevent intermittent prolapse in late pregnancy include various suturing techniques or use of a retention device (Johnson prolapse retainer). For sheep that are pastured on estrogenic feed and chronically affected, a commercially available vaginal retention device (a bearing retainer) may be useful. Resection of some of the mucosa of the vaginal wall, cervical or vaginal wall fixation, and epidural anesthesia using alcohol to prevent straining are other long-term solutions for recurrent prolapse. After administering an epidural anesthetic, the organ is washed with soap and water, and rinsed thoroughly; the bladder is emptied if necessary; congestion and edema are reduced by applying gentle pressure; the vagina is replaced, and topical antibiotic applied. The vagina must then be retained in position. Only the last procedure presents serious difficulty. The irritation of the vaginal mucosa results in extreme tenesmus, and retention devices must be strong to prevent recurrence. Temporary or permanent retention is accomplished through various methods of suturing the vulva. Metal prolapse pins with heavy buttons or similar devices also have been used. These devices are removed during stage 1 of parturition.

VAGINITIS AND VULVITIS, LG AN

Bruising or laceration of the vagina and vulva frequently result from parturition. Infrequently, **traumatic vaginitis** may result from malicious injury, service from a large and vigorous bull, or prolapse of the vagina (*see* above). The inflamed vagina is painful and edematous, and often there is a fetid exudate, which indicates bacterial infection. Usually, vaginal lacerations are limited to the retroperitoneal area, and cellulitis with accompanying edema, necrosis, and fetid discharge are common, often with an accompanying acute metritis. There may be tenesmus, and swelling of the vulva. The degree of depression, anorexia, and fever depends on severity of the infection. Malignant edema (qv, p 327) occasionally establishes itself in the injured tissue.

Examination and treatment must be done with a clean, well-lubricated, gloved hand to minimize pain and straining. If the fetal membranes are retained, they should be removed if this can be done easily and quickly. Since metritis (qv, p 692) is usually present, it should be treated. Antibiotics placed in the uterus escape through the vagina and assist in treating the infection there. Oily antibiotic preparations may be placed in the vagina with a catheter. Animals with severe vaginitis should be treated by parenteral antibiotics or sulfonamides. Tenesmus in traumatic vaginitis usually is transitory or caused by examination; it should be controlled by epidural anesthesia. Inflammatory changes usually prevent prolapse in these cases.

Granular vaginitis is characterized by spherical nodules, ~1 mm in diameter, on the vulval mucosa of cattle. Similar hyperplasia may occur in the lymphatic follicles of the bull's penis. It is a nonspecific hyperplastic response of the lymphatic tissue of these areas to an irritant or an antigen. Infectious pustular vulvovaginitis (IPV, qv, p 730) is one disease in which hyperplasia occurs after recovery from the acute infection. In other cases, the stimulus for hyperplasia frequently is unknown. Treatment of females is not indicated, and the condition subsides spontaneously in several weeks to several months. Young animals are affected most frequently since they experience the most exposure to new antigens. In females, the condition is not related to fertility, although the predisposing agent may influence fertility.

Mucopurulent vaginitis, sometimes with cervicitis, endometritis, and associated balanoposthitis in bulls, is difficult to define etiologically. Viruses, including the herpesvirus of IPV and the virus of "Epivag" in South Africa, are at times clearly involved. Bacteria, such as streptococci, coliforms, corynebacteria, and mycoplasmas, are often present. Outbreaks occur in some herds after service; often, there are no associated deeper infections and fertility is not impaired. A viral etiology has been postulated. *Haemophilus somnus* (qv, p 602) may play a role since it has been isolated frequently from affected herds. Spontaneous recovery is usual. When there is infertility, treatment with antibiotics often is unrewarding. Suspension of natural mating and use of artificial insemination is indicated.

RESPIRATORY SYSTEM

RESPIRATORY SYSTEM, INTRODUCTION

Nature and Function of the Respiratory Tract: The respiratory system performs several functions. Most importantly it delivers oxygen to the cardiovascular system for distribution to the body, and removes carbon dioxide. Gas transfer occurs in the alveoli of the lungs, where the air-blood barrier is a thin, permeable membrane.

Failure or major dysfunction of gas transfer due to disease processes that compromise this membrane or its air or blood supply have serious effects. In addition to gas exchange, the respiratory system performs numerous other functions, including maintaining acid-base balance, acting as a blood reservoir, filtering and probably destroying emboli, metabolizing some bioactive substances (such as serotonin, prostaglandins, corticosteroids, and leukotrienes), and activating some substances (such as angiotensin). The system must also protect its own delicate airways, and does so by warming and humidifying inhaled air, and filtering out particulate material. The upper airways also provide for the sense of smell (olfaction) and play a role in temperature regulation in panting animals.

Large airborne particles are usually deposited on the mucous lining of the nasal passages, trachea, and bronchi, after which they are carried by the mucociliary "blanket" to the pharynx to be swallowed or expectorated. Small particles may be deposited as deep as the alveoli, where they are phagocytized by macrophages. Defense against invasion by microorganisms and other foreign particles is provided by anatomical structures, and by both nonspecific and immunological mechanisms (both cellular and humoral). These are the factors that determine species and individual susceptibility to disease, and which may be manipulated by using husbandry, vaccines, antimicrobials, and new biotechnological products such as interferon and lymphokines. Other factors include the tortuosity of nasal passages; presence of hairs, cilia, and mucus; the cough reflex; and bronchoconstriction. Cellular defenses include the macrophage, which phagocytizes invaders and presents them, or at least their important antigens, to lymphocytes for stimulation of an immune response, and the neutrophil, which dies in its fight against invaders and must be removed along with its potentially damaging enzymes. Secretory defenses include interferon for antiviral defense, complement for lysis of invaders, surfactant lining the alveoli to prevent their collapse and facilitate macrophage function, fibronectin to block bacterial attachment, and antibodies and mucus.

The respiratory system must perform many functions, preferably while expending minimal energy. The required effort is increased by processes that oppose expansion of the lung (eg, fibrosis, or hydro-, chylo-, pneumo-, or hemothorax), impede the flow of air (eg, nasal tumors, bronchiolitis, bronchoconstriction, or pulmonary edema), or thicken the air-blood interface (eg, interstitial pneumonia due to viruses or toxins, pulmonary edema).

The anatomy of the respiratory tract differs markedly among species in: shape of both the upper and lower respiratory tract; extent, shape, and pattern of the turbinate bones; branching patterns of bronchi; anatomy of terminal bronchioles, including collateral ventilation; lobation and lobulation; thickness of pleura; completeness of the mediastinum; relationship of pulmonary arteries to bronchial arteries and bronchioles; presence of vascular shunts; distribution of mast cells; and blood supply to the pleura. Each variation in anatomical structure implies variation in function, each of which can influence the pathogenesis of respiratory disease in a particular species. The 3 main groups of species that have anatomically similar respiratory tracts are: 1) cattle, sheep, and pig; 2) dog, cat, monkey, rat, rabbit, and guinea pig; and 3) horse and man.

Marked physiological variations also exist between different species; eg, cattle are prone to retrograde drainage from the pharynx, are predisposed to pulmonary hypertension and reduced ventilation in a cold environment, have relatively small lungs with low tidal volume and functional residual capacity, and are more sensitive to changes in environmental temperatures than are most other species. These anatomical and physiological differences largely determine why some pathogens affect only some species (eg, *Pasteurella haemolytica* affects cattle but not pigs), and why pneumonia is very important in some species (cattle, pigs) but less so in others (dogs, cats).

Hypoxia (lowered oxygenation, often termed anoxia) causes clinical signs of respiratory disease. It can result from: 1) reduced oxygen-carrying capacity of the blood (anemic anoxia, such as in carbon monoxide or nitrite poisoning, or true anemia due to various causes), 2) reduced blood flow (stagnant anoxia, such as in congestive heart failure or shock), 3) insufficient alveolar ventilation or diffusion impairment (anoxic anoxia, such as in pneumonia, pulmonary edema, chronic congestion, pneumothorax, or paralysis of respiratory muscles), or 4) inability of tissues to use available oxygen (histotoxic anoxia as in cyanide poisoning).

Compensatory mechanisms for hypoxia include increased depth and rate of breathing, which is mediated by chemoreceptors located in the carotid and aortic bodies; contraction of the spleen, which forces more RBC into the circulation; and increased cardiac stroke volume and heart rate. If cerebral hypoxia develops, respiratory function may be reduced even further due to depression of neuronal activity. Stimulation of erythropoiesis also occurs with hypoxia, although the degree of polycythemia is species dependent. In addition, myocardial, renal, and hepatic functions may be reduced, as may motility and secretions of the intestine. If compensatory mechanisms are inadequate, a vicious cycle may begin in which all body tissues function less efficiently.

Clinical Signs of Respiratory Malfunction: Nasal discharge may be serous, catarrhal, purulent, or hemorrhagic, depending on the degree of mucosal damage. It indicates increased production of normal secretions, sometimes supplemented by neutrophils (purulent) or blood (hemorrhage). It probably also indicates decreased ''grooming'' of the nostrils with the tongue when animals are ill. **Epistaxis,** the presence of blood in the upper airways or nose, is often caused by vascular rupture, such as in mycotic infection of the guttural pouch or exercise-induced pulmonary hemorrhage in horses. **Hemoptysis,** the coughing up of blood, occurs following rupture of pulmonary aneurysms in the lungs of cattle with chronic lung abscesses. Bleeding may also result from polyps, neoplasms, granulomas, trauma, thrombocytopenia, and bracken fern or sweet clover toxicity.

Hyperpnea, an increase in rate and depth of pulmonary ventilation, becomes **dyspnea** when the breathing appears labored and to be causing distress. Infectious processes that cause toxemia further compromise the host, eg, bovine pneumonia due to *Pasteurella haemolytica.* Dyspnea can be caused by disease of the respiratory tract itself, eg, airway obstruction, pneumonia, or hydrothorax, or by other problems, eg, heart failure, acid-base imbalances, abnormal oxygen-carrying capacity of the blood, or even disorders of nervous function. Labored inhalation, as seen with obstruction by tumors or exudates, is termed inspiratory dyspnea, whereas labored expiration, such as with emphysema, is termed expiratory dyspnea. Other responses include coughing to clear exudates, and shallow breathing with grunting, often associated with the pain of pleuritis.

Causes of Malfunction: Anomalies of the respiratory tract are rare, but do occur. Examples include cysts in the sinuses and turbinates, tracheal hypoplasia, and accessory lungs. The most common cause of upper respiratory tract malfunction is rhinitis (which results in exudation of neutrophils, macrophages, and fluids), or erosion and ulceration, or both, of the nasal mucosa. It may be caused by viral, bacterial, fungal, or parasitic agents, as well as by hypersensitivity reactions, such as localized allergies and anaphylaxis (*see* THE IMMUNE SYSTEM, p 421 *et seq*). Atrophy of the turbinates, eg, in atrophic rhinitis of pigs, removes a major filtration function and exposes the lungs to much heavier loads of dust and microorganisms. Obstruction of the nasal cavity may be caused by tumors, granulomas, abscesses, or foreign bodies. Sinusitis can be a complication of upper respiratory infections or dehorning.

Laryngitis, tracheitis, and bronchitis result in coughing, inspiratory and expiratory dyspnea, and prolonged inspiration. Coughing may be dry if the irritation is caused by mucosal erosion, or moist if due to copious exudate in the major airways. Severe pulmonary edema causes extreme respiratory insufficiency, as does emphysema.

The most common respiratory disease is **pneumonia,** which is defined as inflammation of the lungs. There are many systems for classifying the various types of pneumonia. One useful method is to classify according to the distribution of lesions in the lungs, as follows: **Focal pneumonia** has one or more discrete foci in a random pattern, eg, abscessation due to emboli from other sites, tuberculosis, or actinomycosis. **Lobular pneumonia** accentuates the anatomical pattern of lobules, as in bronchopneumonia caused by *Pasteurella multocida*. **Lobar pneumonia** covers large areas of lobes and is often severe, such as in fibrinous pneumonic pasteurellosis of cattle. **Diffuse** or **interstitial pneumonia** often involves the entire lung, as in maedi of sheep, or hypersensitivity reactions. The appearance or etiology of a particular pneumonia can be described further, eg, gangrenous, parasitic (verminous), aspiration, etc. The initial problem in many pneumonias is thought to be a sudden alteration in the normal nasal bacterial flora, which results in a sudden dramatic increase in one or more species of bacteria. These bacteria are breathed into the lung in large numbers and may overwhelm the normal defense mechanisms, localize, multiply, and initiate inflammation. In addition, often as a precursor, a viral respiratory infection probably occurs, particularly in groups of animals that have recently been congregated and stressed by travel, handling, and mixing. Some respiratory viral infections can cause temporary dysfunction of phagocytic mechanisms of the alveolar macrophages. This usually occurs several days following viral exposure. Inhaled bacteria proliferate and pneumonia ensues, often with an overwhelming infection and massive exudation into the alveoli.

Pneumonia also can be caused by direct infection with viruses, bacteria, and fungi, as well as by toxins arriving hematogenously or by inhalation.

Through natural processes, possibly aided by appropriate therapy, the exudate may be removed from the lungs, and the mucosal lesions of the air passages may heal. However, serious sequelae may persist. **Bronchiectasis** is a chronic lesion of the bronchi and parenchyma characterized by irreversible cylindrical or saccular dilatation, secondary infection, and atelectasis. Ulceration of bronchioles caused by viral agents may lead to organized plugs of connective tissue in small bronchioles, a lesion called "**bronchiolitis obliterans**", which may cause permanent obstruction, atelectasis, and severe respiratory insufficiency. Constriction of bronchioles in chronic allergic bronchitis and bronchiolitis results in similar clinical signs. Some chronic pneumonias, eg, maedi in sheep, are characterized by firm diffuse lesions, due to hyperplasia of lymphoid follicles, hyperplasia of smooth muscle around bronchioles, diffuse fibrosis, and diffuse lymphocytic infiltration. Aspiration pneumonia often leads to gangrene with severe toxemia accompanying the acute inflammatory reaction.

Most infectious pneumonias occur in the anteroventral portions of the lungs. However, infectious agents, as well as neoplasms, can invade the lungs via the blood, which may extensively impair pulmonary function, as can pulmonary edema from chronic heart failure. Pleuritis, empyema, hydrothorax, chylothorax, atelectasis, diaphragmatic hernia, or pneumothorax can also seriously impair respiratory function. Pulmonary thrombosis can lead to pulmonary edema. Infarction of the lung can reduce respiratory function but is rare because of the dual blood supply of the organ. Toxic injury, such as in 3-methylindole toxicity in cattle, causes edema, emphysema, and necrosis of alveolar epithelium followed by compensatory hyperplasia of these cells; the effects on gas exchange result in severe hypoxia and dyspnea.

Although pneumonia is most important, several other conditions that occur in the thorax can cause respiratory dysfunction. **Pulmonary edema**, the abnormal accumulation of fluid in the interstitial tissue, airways, or alveoli of the lungs, may occur in conjunction with circulatory disorders, particularly left ventricular failure or increased capillary permeability, occasionally in anaphylactic and allergic reactions, and in some infectious diseases. Head trauma can cause pulmonary edema in dogs. Dyspnea and open-mouth breathing may occur. Animals stand in preference to lying down or lie only in sternal recumbency, or may assume a sitting position. Auscultation of the chest may reveal wheezing and fluid sounds.

Pleuritis or pleurisy may be caused by any pathogen that gains entrance to the pleural cavity, but is often an extension of pneumonia. Rapid shallow breathing, elevated temperature, and thoracic pain are suggestive of pleuritis. Auscultation of the chest may reveal friction sounds.

Empyema, purulent exudate in the pleural cavity, is caused by pyogenic bacteria or fungi reaching the thoracic cavity via the blood, or by extension of a pneumonia, traumatic reticulitis, or penetrating wounds of the chest. Cough, fever, pain, and dyspnea may be present.

Hemothorax, the accumulation of blood in the pleural cavity, is usually caused by trauma to the thorax. **Hydrothorax,** the accumulation of transudate in the pleural cavity, is usually due to interference with blood flow or lymph drainage. **Chylothorax,** the accumulation of chyle in the pleural cavity, is relatively rare, and is seen most often in cats. It may be caused by rupture of the thoracic duct, but often is idiopathic. The signs of all 3 conditions include respiratory embarrassment and weakness.

Pneumothorax, air in the pleural cavity, may be of traumatic or spontaneous origin. Air can enter the pleural cavity through penetrating wounds of the thoracic wall or by extension from pulmonary emphysema. The lung collapses if a large volume of air enters the pleural cavity. Bilateral pneumothorax may develop if the mediastinum is weak or incomplete. Dyspnea is evident.

Control of Respiratory Disease: Sudden dietary changes, weaning, cold, drafts, dampness, dust, high levels of ammonia, poor ventilation in general, and the mixing of widely divergent age groups are major influences in respiratory disease in groups of animals. Stress and mixing of animals from several sources should be avoided or minimized. Establishing individual animal identification, making accurate clinical and postmortem diagnoses, and maintaining a record system of diagnosis and treatment are important to minimize or control outbreaks of pneumonia.

Immunization can help control respiratory infection. However, control may be compromised by improper timing, use of ineffective or inappropriate vaccines, or overwhelmingly negative management practices. In most cases, severe insults to the natural defenses cannot be reversed later by therapeutic agents and biologicals.

The mucosal surfaces of the respiratory tract contain lymphoid follicles that exchange cells with other parts of the body. However, most of the lymphocytes in the respiratory lining produce only IgA, whereas the cells in the lymph nodes of the respiratory tract produce IgM and IgG. Depending on the agent involved, various cell- and antibody-mediated immune responses occur in the respiratory tract and include: opsonization, agglutination, immobilization, neutralization of toxin and virus, blockage of adherence to cells, lysis, and chemotaxis. Variation in the type of immune response occurs because of age, species, and the means to respond to specific virulence mechanisms of the pathogens involved. Species vary in the type of immune response available at different sites in the respiratory tract. Large droplets of antigen may immunize the upper tract with IgA, but small replicating particles may be necessary to immunize the lower tract. To develop adequate levels of antibody to protect the lungs, repeated doses of antigen plus adjuvant, or a replicating antigen are often necessary. These results are seldom achieved under field conditions, eg, many field trials using respiratory vaccines in cattle have not demonstrated statistically significant efficacy.

PRINCIPLES OF THERAPY

(*See also* p 1402.) Respiratory disease is often characterized by abnormal production of secretions and exudates, and by a reduced ability to remove them. The primary goal is to reduce the volume and viscosity of the secretions, and facilitate their removal. This can be accomplished by controlling infection, modifying the secretions, and when possible, improving postural drainage and mechanically removing the material. Therapeutic methods include altering the inspired air and administration of expectorants, antitussives, bronchodilators, antimicrobials, diuretics, and other drugs.

Hydration should be maintained. Inhalation of humidified air may facilitate removal of airway secretions. Expectorants are sometimes used with the intention of liquefying these secretions. However, they should be used in conjunction with ancillary respiratory therapy such as improved postural drainage, mild exercise, and thoracic percussion, which (in addition to coughing) encourages expectoration and removal of secretions. The value of expectorants at traditional dosages is questioned. Mechanical removal of tenacious and viscid secretions by aspiration may be necessary in severe airway obstruction.

Antitussive agents are indicated to relieve the discomfort associated with unproductive coughing, but contraindicated when airway mucous secretion is excessive. Products that contain atropine also are contraindicated, at least in theory, because atropine increases the viscosity of airway secretions.

Increased airway resistance caused by bronchial smooth muscle contraction can be alleviated with bronchodilators, which may be indicated in animals with asthmalike conditions and chronic respiratory disease. Methylxanthines, such as theophylline and aminophylline, are effective bronchodilators in species other than cattle. Isoproterenol, clenbuterol, and epinephrine are also generally effective, and sodium cromoglycate is used in horses for treating small airway disease (eg, heaves). The use of corticosteroids is justified in allergic conditions. Antihistamines can be used to alleviate the bronchoconstriction caused by histamine release. Bronchospasm also can be reduced significantly by removing irritating factors, using mild sedatives, or reducing periods of excitement.

In bacterial infection, antimicrobial therapy should be instituted. The basic goal is to select the most effective agent against a specific organism, or the least toxic agent of several alternatives. Culture and sensitivity testing of airway secretions provide a worthwhile, though not infallible, guide to determining the appropriate antibiotic. Knowledge of tissue penetration and pharmacokinetic characteristics of the antimicrobial agents is important as well. The following agents have proved effective in the listed species: cattle—oxytetracycline, erythromycin, penicillins, and sulfonamides; sheep and goats—oxytetracycline, penicillins, and sulfonamides; pigs—lincomycin, spectinomycin, penicillins, and sulfonamides; dogs and cats—cephalosporins, chloramphenicol, erythromycin, lincomycin, clindamycin, penicillins, sulfonamides, and tetracyclines; horses—penicillins, sulfonamides, and tetracyclines, the latter with caution due to an occasional side effect of severe diarrhea. Aminoglycosides are useful but can be nephrotoxic. Trimethoprim, usually in combination with a sulfonamide, is useful for respiratory therapy in most species but is not licensed for food-producing animals in the USA. New drugs such as enrofloxacin (approved in small but not large animals in the USA) and ceftiofur may prove to be efficacious. Broad-spectrum antibiotics should be used if specific bacteria cannot be identified, and once begun, a full course of therapy should be completed. Multiple antimicrobial agents should be used only with full knowledge of the potential drug interactions. Because of residues in food-producing animals, veterinarians must use these products appropriately and provide sound advice to producers.

The hypoxemia caused by most lung disorders usually can be corrected by administering oxygen. However, continuous administration of high concentrations increases the tendency for regional resorption atelectasis, thus worsening the hypoxemia, and can cause pneumonitis on its own. Hypoxemia is often accompanied by variable degrees of hypercapnia and acidemia. Endotracheal intubation and mechanical ventilation may be necessary in animals with acute respiratory failure or in animals that are comatose or apneic. Arterial blood gas and pH determinations, when practicable, are extremely valuable in monitoring treatment.

Diuretics may be indicated in pulmonary edema. The osmotic diuretics have a minimal action on diuresis. A profound diuretic effect can be produced with carbonic anhydrase inhibitors (eg, acetazolamide) and with loop-active diuretics (eg, furosemide).

ASPIRATION PNEUMONIA
(Foreign-body pneumonia, Inhalation pneumonia, Gangrenous pneumonia)

A form of pneumonia characterized by pulmonary necrosis and caused by foreign material in the lungs.

Etiology: Faulty administration of medicines is the most common cause. Liquids administered by drench or dose syringe must not be given faster than the animal can swallow, and drenching is particularly dangerous when the animal's tongue is drawn out, when the head is held high, or when the animal is coughing or bellowing. Administration of liquids by nasal intubation is not without risk, and careful technique is especially necessary in debilitated animals. Animals (especially cats) are particularly susceptible to pneumonia caused by aspiration of tasteless products such as mineral oil. Inhalation of food sometimes occurs in calves and pigs. Attempts by animals to eat or drink while partially choked, or aspiration of vomitus may result in aspiration pneumonia. Disturbances of deglutition, as in anesthetized or comatose animals (eg, mature cattle under general anesthesia and cows in lateral recumbency with milk fever), or in those suffering from vagal paralysis, acute pharyngitis, abscesses or tumors of the pharyngeal region, esophageal diverticula, cleft palate, or encephalitis, are frequent predisposing causes. In sheep, poor dipping technique may cause aspiration of fluid. Inhalation of irritant gases or smoke is an infrequent cause.

Some anesthetics, eg, thiobarbiturates, stimulate salivation. Atropine sulfate helps to control salivation, while use of an endotracheal catheter with an inflatable cuff prevents fluid aspiration during surgery.

Clinical Findings: A history that discloses an event within the previous 1-3 days when foreign-body aspiration could have occurred is of great diagnostic value. In horses, the temperature usually rises to 104-105°F (40-40.5°C) during the first few days and then becomes remittent. Pyrexia is also observed in cats, dogs, and cattle, but sometimes cattle develop little or no fever. The pulse is accelerated, and respiration rapid and labored. A sweetish, fetid breath characteristic of gangrene may be detected, the intensity of which increases as the disease progresses. This is often associated with a purulent nasal discharge that sometimes is reddish brown or green. Occasionally, evidence of the aspirated material can be seen in the nasal discharge or in expectorated material, eg, oil droplets. On auscultation, fluid sounds over one or both sides of the chest are heard early in the condition, followed by wheezing sounds, pleuritic friction rubs, and sometimes, the crackling sounds of subcut. emphysema. In cows that aspirate ruminal contents, toxemia is usually fatal within 1-2 days. Cattle and pigs recover more frequently than horses, but in all species, mortality is high. Recovered animals often develop pulmonary abscesses. In outbreaks following dipping of sheep, losses rise from day 2 to about day 7, and then decrease gradually.

Lesions: The pneumonia is usually in the anteroventral parts of the lungs and may be unilateral or bilateral. In the early stages, the lungs are markedly congested, with areas of interlobular edema. The bronchi are hyperemic and full of froth. The pneumonic areas tend to be cone-shaped with the base toward the pleura. Suppuration and necrosis follow, the foci becoming soft or liquefied, reddish brown, and foul smelling. There usually is an acute fibrinous pleuritis, often with pleural exudate.

Treatment: The animal should be kept quiet. A productive cough should not be suppressed. Broad-spectrum antibiotics should be used in animals known to have inhaled a foreign substance, whether it be a liquid or an irritant vapor, without waiting for signs of pneumonia to appear. Care and supportive treatment are the same as for infectious pneumonias. In small animals, oxygen therapy may be beneficial. Despite all treatments, prognosis is poor and efforts must be directed at prevention.

CHLAMYDIAL PNEUMONIA

Chlamydiae have been identified in various parts of the world as one of the causes of enzootic pneumonia in calves (qv, p 727). These organisms also cause pneumonia in mice, sheep, and goats. In cats, it may occur as a rare sequela of the much more common chlamydial conjunctivitis and rhinitis. Chlamydiae have also been isolated on rare occasions from pneumonic samples from piglets and foals. The main clinical sign of zoonotic chlamydiosis in man is pneumonia, which is generally contracted from birds (*see also* p 1568).

Etiology and Epidemiology: The causative agent is *Chlamydia psittaci*. Some of the respiratory isolates from calves have properties of immunotypes 1 and 6, and are similar to strains recovered from intestinal infections or abortions of cattle and sheep. Immunotype 6 was recovered from pneumonic lungs of calves and pigs. Thus, the GI tract must be considered as an important site in the pathogenesis of chlamydial infections (*see also* p 137), and as a natural reservoir and source of the organisms. Chlamydial pneumonia has affected calves under range conditions as well as on dairy farms. The disease in sheep is most frequently seen in feeder lambs assembled from different sources in feedlots or irrigated pastures. Stressed lambs under these husbandry conditions are frequently subjected to various secondary bacterial infections, which can result in much higher mortality and morbidity rates than is seen in uncomplicated chlamydial respiratory infections.

Clinical Findings and Lesions: Calves with chlamydial pneumonia are usually febrile, lethargic, have a serous and later mucopurulent nasal discharge, and have a dry hacking cough and dyspnea. Weanling-age calves are affected most frequently, but older cattle may also show signs. Lambs and goats show similar signs.

The acute pulmonary lesion is a lobular, interstitial pneumonia. The anteroventral parts of the lungs are consolidated but, in severe cases, entire lobes can be involved. The dry cough is attributed to tracheitis. Microscopic changes in the lungs are typical of an exudative bronchopneumonia with an exudative and proliferative bronchiolitis.

Diagnosis: Neither the clinical signs nor the lesions allow even a presumptive diagnosis of chlamydial pneumonia; they are not sufficiently different from those seen in the bovine/ovine respiratory disease complex with its multiple etiologies. Diagnosis requires isolation of chlamydiae from affected tissues in a tissue culture or chick embryo. A rise in antibody titers using ELISA in sera collected during the acute and convalescent stages of the disease can be an aid in diagnosis. Predominant IgG_2 antibodies are induced by chlamydial infections in cattle. Subclinical chlamydial infections are not uncommon.

Prophylaxis and Treatment: Vaccines are not available. Several antimicrobials such as penicillin, erythromycin, tylosin, and tetracyclines can interfere with chlamydial multiplication, but tetracyclines are generally the drug of choice. Treatment must start as early as possible. Injections of oxytetracycline at 25-50 mg/kg, daily for 5-7 days, are recommended.

DIAPHRAGMATIC HERNIA

A break in the continuity of the diaphragm with protrusion of abdominal viscera into the thorax.

Etiology: Trauma is the usual cause, although congenital defects of the diaphragm may result in herniation as seen in peritoneopericardial hernia. In small animals, automobile-related trauma is a common cause, whereas in large animals, falling and parturition must also be considered. Its prevalence in water buffalo suggests a hereditary basis in this species. In cattle, adhesions to the diaphragm adjacent to the reticulum must be differentiated from those resulting from traumatic reticuloperitonitis with subsequent diaphragmatic herniation.

Clinical Findings: The signs vary, depending on the species affected. Dogs characteristically show dyspnea, and frequently assume a sitting position to lessen the pressure of the abdominal viscera on the lungs. Incarceration of the stomach or intestine may mimic or actually result in obstruction, and obstructive signs may occur, especially in chronic cases. Congenital peritoneopericardial hernia is most frequently an incidental finding, although findings may be related to the respiratory or GI systems, or due to compromised venous return to the heart. Horses may have a history of recurrent colic. Subsequent acute obstruction may necessitate surgery, and the hernia is diagnosed on exploration of the diaphragm. Cattle and water buffalo ingest foreign bodies and suffer GI disturbances related to traumatic reticuloperitonitis. Weakening of the diaphragm and subsequent herniation may be difficult or impossible to differentiate from congenital diaphragmatic defects.

A considerable volume of abdominal viscera may gradually pass through a relatively small tear because of the negative pressure in the thoracic cavity. Radiographs usually show the herniated viscus and the irregularity or disruption of the diaphragmatic line.

Diagnosis and Treatment: Evidence of previous trauma and clinical signs of dyspnea or GI disturbance are suggestive. Radiographs (contrast if necessary) can confirm the diaphragmatic abnormality. In large animals, exploratory celiotomy may be necessary to substantiate clinical findings suggestive of diaphragmatic herniation. Differential diagnosis in small animals must include other causes of dyspnea, and in large animals, other causes of GI problems.

Surgical repair is the only treatment.

DISEASES OF THE LARYNX

Laryngitis, an inflammation of the mucosa or cartilages of the larynx, may be secondary to an upper respiratory tract infection. It may also arise by direct irritation due to inhalation of dust, smoke, or irritating gas; foreign bodies; or the trauma of intubation or excess vocalization. Laryngitis may accompany infectious tracheobronchitis and distemper in dogs; infectious rhinotracheitis and calicivirus infection in cats; infectious rhinotracheitis and calf diphtheria in cattle; strangles, herpesvirus 1 infection, viral arteritis, and infectious bronchitis in horses; *Fusobacterium necrophorum* or *Corynebacterium pyogenes* infections in sheep; and influenza in pigs.

Edema of the mucosa and submucosa is frequently an integral part of laryngitis, and if severe, the rima glottidis may be significantly obstructed. However, edema may also result from allergy, inhalation of irritants, or surgery in the area. Intubation for anesthesia, especially when attempted with inadequate induction or poor technique, is likely to provoke laryngeal edema. Brachycephalic and obese dogs, and dogs with laryngeal paralysis (*see* below) develop laryngeal edema and laryngitis through severe panting or respiratory effort during excitement or hyperthermia. In cattle, laryngeal edema has been observed in blackleg, urticaria, and serum sickness. In pigs, it may occur as a part of edema disease. In horses, cattle, and sheep, laryngeal edema may lead to arytenoid chondropathy.

Laryngeal chondropathy is a suppurative condition of the cartilage matrix that can afflict horses, sheep, and cattle, most often young males. There is a distinct breed predisposition in Thoroughbred horses, Texel and Southdown sheep, and Belgian Blue cattle.

Clinical Findings: A cough is the principal sign of laryngitis when edema is slight and the deeper tissues of the larynx are not involved. It is harsh, dry, and short at first, but becomes soft and moist later and may be very painful. It can be induced by pressure on the larynx, exposure to cold or dusty air, swallowing coarse food or cold water, and attempts to administer medicines. Vocal changes may be evident in small animals. Stridor may result from swelling and reduced motility of the arytenoid cartilages in laryngeal chondropathy. Halitosis and difficult, noisy breathing may be evident, and the animal may stand with its head lowered and mouth open. Swallowing is difficult and painful. Systemic signs are usually attributable to the primary disease, as in calf diphtheria, in which temperatures of 105°F (40.5°C) may occur. Death due to asphyxiation may occur, especially if the animal is exerted.

Edema of the larynx may develop within hours. It is characterized by increased inspiratory effort and stridor arising from the larynx. Respiratory rate may slow as the effort of breathing becomes exaggerated. Visible mucous membranes are cyanotic, the pulse rate is increased, body temperature rises, and horses may sweat profusely. Dogs with obstructions of the conducting airways may show extreme disturbance of thermoregulation in hot weather; marked hyperthermia is not uncommon.

Diagnosis: A tentative diagnosis is based on the clinical signs. Definitive diagnosis requires laryngoscopy. In conscious horses and cattle, this can be achieved with a flexible endoscope passed per nasum; in dogs and cats, usually anesthesia or analgesia is required. The history and signs usually permit rapid identification of the primary disease and the associated laryngeal involvement.

Treatment: In laryngeal obstruction, a tracheotomy tube should be placed immediately. Corticosteroids should be administered to reduce the obstructive effect of the inflammatory swellings—hydrocortisone IV is appropriate initially. Concurrent systemic antibiotic therapy is also necessary. Identification and treatment of the primary disease is essential. Palliative procedures to speed recovery and give comfort to the animal include inhalation of humidified air, confinement to a warm clean environment, feeding soft or liquid foods, and avoiding dust. The cough may be suppressed with antitussive preparations, and bacterial infections controlled with antibiotics or sulfonamides. Control of pain with judicious use of an analgesic, especially in cats, allows the animal to eat, and thus speeds recovery. Subtotal arytenoidectomy is an effective remedy for laryngeal chondropathy of horses, sheep, and cattle, although a return to full athletic capacity in competitive horses is uncertain.

LARYNGEAL PARALYSIS

A disease of the upper airway, common in dogs and rare in cats. Signs include a dry cough, voice changes, noisy breathing that progresses to marked dyspnea with stress and exertion, stridor, and collapse. Regurgitation and vomiting may occur. It is a common acquired problem in middle-aged to older, large and giant breeds of dogs, eg, Labrador Retrievers, Irish Setters, and Great Danes. It is seen less often as a hereditary, congenital disease in Bouvier des Flandres, Leonbergers, Siberian Huskies, and racing sled dogs.

Diagnosis is based on clinical signs. Laryngoscopy under light anesthesia is needed for confirmation. Laryngeal movements are absent or paradoxical with respiration. Electromyography shows positive sharp waves, denervation potentials, and sometimes myotonia. Radiographs are not diagnostic. Denervation atrophy is seen on histologic sections of laryngeal muscles.

Differential diagnoses include myositis, recurrent laryngeal or vagal nerve tumor, inflammation, myasthenia gravis, severe hypothyroidism, trauma, and more widespread generalized neurologic degeneration. Therapy is directed at relieving signs of airway obstruction. Tranquilization and corticosteroids are effective temporarily in mild cases. Severe obstruction may require tracheotomy. Definitive therapy is surgical and is directed at enlarging the glottic opening.

HYPOSTATIC PNEUMONIA

A condition arising from failure of the blood to pass readily through the vascular structures of the lungs, which may lead to a shift in fluid from the vascular to the pulmonary spaces. It is due to passive congestion of the lungs and is seen most commonly in old or debilitated animals. It is usually secondary to some other disease process, eg, congestive heart failure. Animals recovering from anesthesia or that are otherwise recumbent sometimes develop hypostatic pneumonia if they are not moved regularly.

Any primary disease must be diagnosed and treated. Coughing is not always a prominent sign, but as the condition progresses, dyspnea and cyanosis become apparent. Secondary bacterial infection is common. Radiographs reveal increased density of the lungs, and the mediastinal space may be shifted to the atalectic side.

The animal's position must be changed hourly. Exercise must be encouraged insofar as it is compatible with the animal's condition. If a primary cause can be determined, specific therapy, eg, digitalis for congestive heart failure or chlorothiazide for edema, should be instituted.

Use of narcotics and sedatives should be minimal to encourage movement and to avoid depression of the cough reflex. Maintenance of proper hydration is important, but overhydration may increase congestion and should be avoided.

LUNGWORM INFECTION
(Verminous bronchitis, Verminous pneumonia)

An infection of the lower respiratory tract, resulting in bronchitis or pneumonia, or both, by any of several parasitic nematodes, including: *Dictyocaulus viviparus* in cattle and deer; *D arnfieldi* in donkeys and horses; *D filaria, Protostrongylus rufescens*, and *Muellerius capillaris* in sheep and goats; *Metastrongylus apri* in pigs; *Filaroides (Oslerus) osleri* in dogs; and *Aelurostrongylus abstrusus* in cats. Other lungworm infections occur but are less common. Lungworms are found in many countries, particularly in those with a temperate climate.

The first 3 lungworms listed above belong to the superfamily Trichostrongyloidea and have direct life cycles; the others belong to the Metastrongyloidea and, except for *F osleri*, have indirect life cycles.

Some nematodes that inhabit the right ventricle and pulmonary circulation, eg, *Angiostrongylus vasorum* (qv, p 75) and *Dirofilaria immitis* (qv, p 73), both found in dogs in certain areas of the world, may be associated with pulmonary disease. Clinical signs relating to a cardiac or a pulmonary syndrome, or a combination of both, may occur.

The cattle lungworm, *D viviparus*, is common in northwest Europe. It causes "husk" or "hoose", an economically important disease in the British Isles. The lungworm of goats and sheep, *D filaria*, is recognized as a pathogen in Australia, Europe, and North America but is thought to be more important in the Mediterranean countries, the Middle East, and India. *Muellerius capillaris* is prevalent worldwide, but it is usually not considered to cause obvious clinical signs in infected sheep. Other lungworm infections of horses, pigs, dogs, and cats are recognized in many countries, and sporadically, they may cause serious clinical disease.

Epidemiology: Adult females in the bronchi lay larvated eggs that may hatch in the bronchi (eg, *D viviparus*) or in the host's feces (eg, *D arnfieldi*) after having been coughed up and swallowed. The first-stage larvae in feces develop to infective third-stage larvae in a minimum of 1 wk, but may take longer depending on ambient temperature and humidity. Viability of infective larvae is enhanced by moderate temperatures and high humidity. Larvae may be disseminated on a pasture by fluid feces, the wheels of vehicles, and in the case of *D viviparus*, by being projected from dung pats by the sporangia of the fungus *Pilobulus*.

Following ingestion, the infective larvae undergo 2 further molts while migrating to the lungs from the intestines via the lymphatic system and the pulmonary arterial blood supply. Larvae emerge into the alveoli and migrate to the bronchioles and bronchi where they mature. The prepatent period is ~4 wk for *D viviparus*, 5 wk for *D filaria*, and 8-16 wk for *D arnfieldi*. Of the latter, patent infections occur only in donkeys or foals, not older horses.

Pastures become a source of infection early in the year as a result of larvae surviving on the herbage or in the soil during the previous winter (which they can do even at low temperatures), or by being grazed by apparently normal animals that carry light infections from the previous year. Donkeys are considered to be the prime source of pasture contamination with *D arnfieldi* for horses.

Most of the metastrongyloidean lungworms have indirect life cycles. Adult *M apri* are found in small bronchi in the caudal lung lobes of pigs. After the larvated eggs are passed in the feces, they are ingested by earthworms in which infective third-stage larvae develop in 3 wk; an earthworm may contain ≥1000 infective larvae. Pigs become infected by eating the earthworms, and the infection becomes patent in 4 wk.

Muellerius capillaris, P rufescens, and *A abstrusus* require slugs or snails as intermediate hosts; sheep and goats become infected by eating the hosts, but cats probably become infected with *A abstrusus* by eating a paratenic host such as a bird or a rodent that had previously eaten the slugs or snails. For these infections to become patent, at least 4-6 wk is required; for *M capillaris,* 10 wk may be required.

Filaroides osleri lays larvated eggs in the dog's trachea, where they hatch. Pups become infected by ingesting first-stage larvae in either the feces or the saliva of an infected dog, probably in the latter case while being licked by their dams. The first-stage larvae molt in the duodenum, and eventually the adults are found within nodules that develop in the mucous membrane of the trachea and the origins of the lobar bronchi; 10-18 wk are required for the infection to become patent. (*See also* RESPIRATORY DISEASES OF SM AN, p 758.)

In general, the epidemiology of lungworm infections is reflected by the problems caused in cattle by *D viviparus.* Clinical disease is usually observed in the young when they are first exposed to infective larvae; in calves, this is during their first season at pasture. Adults are generally immune, although they may have light subclinical infections and serve as a source of larvae for the contamination of pasture or other environments. Patent parasitic bronchitis may occur when individuals or groups are first exposed as adults with no age-immunity (eg, following a move to a new area), or reinfection may occur when adult animals with waning immunity encounter an overwhelming challenge of infective larvae.

Although young cattle are exposed at pasture early in spring, severe clinical disease usually does not occur until fall. The reasons for this are not completely understood, but may include the behavior of infective larvae in soil and recycling of the infection in the population at risk. The epidemiology of many lungworm infections is not known in detail.

Pathogenesis: The pathogenic effect of lungworms depends on their location within the respiratory tract, the number of infective larvae ingested, and the animal's immune state. During the prepatent phase of *D viviparus* infection, the main lesion is blockage of bronchioles by an infiltrate of eosinophils in response to the developing larvae; this results in obstruction of the airways and collapse of alveoli distal to the block. The clinical signs are moderate unless large numbers of larvae are present, in which case the animal may die in the prepatent phase with severe interstitial emphysema. In the patent phase, the adults in the segmental and lobar bronchi cause a bronchitis, with eosinophils, plasma cells, and lymphocytes in the bronchial wall; a cellular exudate, frothy mucus, and adult nematodes are found in the lumen. The bronchial irritation causes marked coughing, and the entire reaction leads to increased airway resistance. A major component of the patent stage is development of a chronic, nonsuppurative, eosinophilic, granulomatous pneumonia in response to eggs and first-stage larvae aspirated into alveoli and bronchioles. This is usually in the caudal lobes of the lungs, and is severe when widespread; in combination with the bronchitis, death may result. Interstitial emphysema, pulmonary edema, and secondary infection are complications that increase the likelihood of death. Survivors may suffer considerable weight loss. If the animal survives until the end of patency (~2-3 mo for *D viviparus*), most or even all of the adult worms are expelled, and the cellular exudate resolves over the ensuing 4 wk. Most recover unless secondary infection occurs in the damaged lungs during the postpatent phase. In a few animals, clinical signs are exacerbated in the postpatent phase. This is due to development of a diffuse, proliferative alveolitis characterized by hyperplasia of the type II alveolar epithelial cells; the cause is unknown.

Dictyocaulus filaria is similar to *D viviparus,* but interstitial emphysema is not a common complication. Bronchial lesions predominate in *D arnfieldi* infections, and when an alveolar reaction occurs, as in donkeys or foals, there are lobular areas of overinflation due to intermittent obstruction of small bronchi.

The pathogenic effect of the other lungworms has a similar basis, but frequently such severe clinical signs are not produced, perhaps due to a more restricted localization in the lungs. The patent phase and the associated lesions last ≥4 mo for some lungworms (*M apri* and *A abstrusus*) but can be >2 yr (*M capillaris*). The lesions in pigs with *M apri* are a combination of localized bronchitis and bronchiolitis with overinflation of related alveoli, usually at the edges of the caudal lobes. In pigs, hypertrophy and hyperplasia of bronchiolar and alveolar duct smooth muscle with marked mucous cell hyperplasia are striking features. Near the end of the patent period (as the adult worms are killed), gray lymphoid nodules (2-4 mm) are formed; fragments of dead worms may be found microscopically in these nodules.

In *M capillaris* and *P rufescens* infections, chronic, eosinophilic, granulomatous pneumonia seems to predominate; the reaction is in the bronchioles and alveoli that contain the parasites, their eggs, and larvae. They are surrounded by macrophages, giant cells, eosinophils, and other immuno-inflammatory cells, which produce gray or beige plaques (1-2 cm) subpleurally in the dorsal border of the caudal lung lobes. Small (1-2 mm), greenish, nodular lesions may also occur. The effect of these lesions in sheep is minor, perhaps because of the predominately subpleural location. This infection represents the lower end of the pathogenic spectrum for lungworms.

In cats, *A abstrusus* produces nodular areas of granulomatous pneumonia in the caudal lobes that, if sufficiently generalized, can be clinically significant and occasionally fatal; a notable feature is the hypertrophy and hyperplasia of the smooth muscle in the media of pulmonary arteries and arterioles. The nodules of *F osleri*, found in the mucous membrane of the trachea and large bronchi, can produce extreme airway irritation and persistent coughing.

In adult animals not previously exposed to infection, the lesions and pathogenesis are the same as in young animals. However, in adults with some degree of immunity, reexposure to the parasite (eg, husk in adult cattle) can result in different lesions. Since the immune response is imperfect, many larvae are able to reach the lungs before they are killed in the terminal bronchioles and alveoli. The gray-green, subpleural nodules (2-4 mm) that form around the dead parasite are composed of lymphocytes and plasma cells surrounding a central zone of eosinophils. Eventually, the parasite and the eosinophils disappear to leave a residual lymphoid nodule that also regresses with time. Larvae that are not killed in the terminal bronchioles may reach the bronchi and cause a bronchitis characterized by marked eosinophilic infiltration of the bronchial walls and greenish yellow exudate in the lumen comprising eosinophils, other inflammatory cells, and parasitic debris. The reaction associated with this process can lead to severe clinical signs if the nodules are numerous and the eosinophilic bronchitis extensive; this is responsible for the reinfection phenomenon.

Clinical Findings: Signs of lungworm infection range from moderate coughing with slightly increased respiratory rates to severe persistent coughing, and respiratory distress and even failure. Reduced weight gains, reduced milk yields, and weight loss accompany many infections in cattle, sheep, and goats. Patent subclinical infections can occur in all species.

The most consistent signs in cattle are tachypnea and coughing. Initially, rapid shallow breathing is accompanied by a cough that is exacerbated by exercise. Respiratory difficulty may ensue, and heavily infected animals stand with their heads stretched forward and mouths open, and drool saliva. The animals become anorectic and rapidly lose condition. Lung sounds are particularly prominent at the bronchial bifurcation. In adult dairy cattle, milk yield drops severely and abnormal lung sounds are heard over the caudal lobes. The reinfection phenomenon in adult dairy cattle is usually seen in the fall; although less severe than in initial infections, the signs are widespread coughing and tachypnea with a marked drop in milk yield.

The signs in sheep and goats infected with *D filaria* are similar to those in cattle. Pulmonary signs usually are not associated with *M capillaris* or *P rufescens* in sheep or goats. *Dictyocaulus arnfieldi* is associated with coughing, tachypnea, and unthriftiness in older horses, but few if any signs in foals or donkeys.

The main clinical sign of *M apri* in pigs is a persistent cough that may become paroxysmal. Coughing and dyspnea occur in cats and dogs with *A abstrusus* and *F osleri* infections, respectively. Fatalities are relatively uncommon with these lungworms, although they do occur in kittens.

Diagnosis: Diagnosis is based on the clinical signs, epidemiology, presence of first-stage larvae in feces, and necropsy of animals in the same herd or flock. Bronchoscopy and radiography may be helpful. Larvae are not found in the feces of animals in the prepatent or postpatent phases and usually not in the reinfection phenomenon. In the early stages of an outbreak, larvae may be few in number. First-stage larvae or larvated eggs can be recovered using most fecal flotation techniques with the appropriate salt solutions. A convenient method for recovering larvae is a modification of the Baermann technique in which feces (25 g) are wrapped in tissue paper or cheese cloth and suspended or placed in water contained in a beaker. The water at the bottom of the beaker is examined for larvae after 4 hr; in heavy infections, larvae may be present within 30 min.

Necropsy should include examination of the trachea, particularly at the bifurcation, for *F osleri* and the lesions they induce. Adults of *Dictyocaulus* spp and *M apri* are readily visible in the bronchi during the patent phases of infection. However, examination of smears from bronchial mucus or histological sections from lesions may be necessary to confirm a diagnosis during other stages of lungworm infection, and also for some of the other lungworms.

Bronchoscopy can be used to detect nodules of *F osleri* or to collect tracheal washings (dogs and horses) to examine for eggs, larvae, and eosinophils.

Treatment: Several drugs are useful. Levamisole, the benzimidazoles (fenbendazole, oxfendazole, and albendazole), and ivermectin are frequently used in cattle, and are effective against all stages of *D viviparus*. These drugs are also effective against lungworms in sheep, horses, and pigs. Fenbendazole has been used successfully in cats for *A abstrusus*. *Filaroides osleri* in dogs is a problem, but there is evidence that fenbendazole and albendazole are effective if treatment is prolonged.

Animals at pasture should be moved inside for treatment, and supportive therapy may be needed for complications that can arise in all species.

Control: Control of lungworm infections by pasture management alone is unreliable. To minimize the hazard for cattle, calves should not be allowed to graze with other animals or on pastures with a recent history of lungworm infection. Avoiding paddocks grazed by donkeys may be useful for lungworm control in horses. Combining a grazing routine with strategic anthelmintic dosing also has been unreliable. However, the availability of anthelmintics with prolonged activity (eg, ivermectin, which is effective for up to 2 wk against *D viviparus*) or a sustained-release bolus (eg, morantel tartrate) now make this a more reliable approach. In first-season grazing cattle, 2 treatments with ivermectin 3 and 8 wk after turn out, provide effective control of parasitic bronchitis unless pasture challenge is heavy and the grazing season prolonged; in this case, an additional treatment at 13 wk may be necessary. To avoid environmental contamination, dosing animals that may be carriers is a sensible precaution. Lungworms that require an intermediate host may be controlled by eliminating contact with this host, eg, by housing pigs indoors.

Vaccination against the cattle lungworm is practiced widely in northwest Europe and is effective in controlling husk. The vaccine comprises attenuated (X-irradiated), infective larvae administered PO in 2 doses 4 wk apart. The animals should be housed during the vaccination period and for 2 wk after the second dose to allow time for adequate resistance to develop before release to pasture. A similar vaccine is used against *D filaria* in southeast Europe.

MYCOTIC PNEUMONIA

A chronic inflammation of the lungs caused by fungi or yeasts. (It has been customary to include the lung infections caused by *Actinomyces* and *Actinobacillus* spp.)

Etiology: *Cryptococcus, Histoplasma, Coccidioides, Blastomyces,* and *Aspergillus* spp, and other fungi and yeasts, have been incriminated as causative agents of this condition in domestic animals (*see* FUNGAL INFECTIONS, p 340). The tissues and secretions of the respiratory passages are an excellent environment for these organisms. Fungal infections are often concurrent with bacterial infections. The source of most infections is believed to be soil-related and not horizontal transfer from other animals. Considering the high rate of exposure to these pathogens in certain circumstances, there are unresolved questions on the epidemiology of the condition, including individual susceptibility, toxigenicity of the organisms, the role of immunity, and concurrent disease.

Clinical Findings and Lesions: A short, moist cough is characteristic, but the disease is more one of general debilitation. As in other pneumonias, a thick mucoid nasal discharge may be present. As the disease progresses, dyspnea, emaciation, and generalized weakness become increasingly evident. Respiration becomes abdominal, resembling that seen in diaphragmatic hernia. On auscultation, harsh respiratory sounds are heard. In advanced cases, the normal sounds of breathing are decreased or almost inaudible. Leukocytosis and periodic fever occur, probably concurrent with bacterial infections. Dissemination often occurs with blastomycosis. Changes in the eyes, eg, corneal ulcers, blindness, and purulent discharge, are not uncommon, and lesions may be evident in the skin, lymph nodes, bones, and joints.

Focal lesions of chronic inflammation are present in the lungs. Abscess formation and cavitation may be seen in conjunction with yellow or gray areas of necrosis. Some animals show numerous miliary nodules that can be seen on radiographs.

Diagnosis: A tentative diagnosis of mycotic pneumonia may be made if an animal with chronic pneumonia exhibits the signs described and does not respond to antibiotics. However, a definitive diagnosis requires laboratory assistance, and radiography may be useful. Some antigens, eg, histoplasmin and blastomycin, have been developed and are an aid in diagnosis. Culture of the sputum that is expelled in spasms of coughing may reveal the infective organism. The clinical diagnosis can be confirmed at necropsy by appropriate cultural and histopathological techniques.

Treatment: There is no entirely satisfactory method of treating systemic mycotic infections; amphotericin may be helpful but is undesirably toxic. Ketoconazole has activity against several fungal pathogens in man; it may be effective in dogs and other animals.

NECROBACILLOSIS

The term necrobacillosis is used to describe any disease or lesion with which *Fusobacterium necrophorum (Sphaerophorus necrophorus)* is associated. It includes calf diphtheria (*see* below), necrotic rhinitis of pigs (qv, p 750), foot rot of cattle (qv, p 501), foot abscess of sheep (qv, p 541), postparturient necrosis of the vagina and uterus, focal necrosis of the liver of cattle and sheep, quittor of horses (qv, p 514), and numerous other necrotic lesions in ruminants and, less commonly, pigs, horses, fowl, and rabbits. The organism is probably a secondary invader rather than a primary cause and is usually part of a mixed infection. However, its necrotizing exotoxin undoubtedly plays a role in the production of characteristic lesions. It is part of the normal flora of the mouth, intestine, and genital tract of many herbivores and omnivores, and is widespread in the environment. It is thought to gain entry to the body through wounds in the skin or mucous membranes.

CALF DIPHTHERIA

An infectious disease of calves affecting the larynx (necrotic laryngitis), oral cavity (necrotic stomatitis), or pharynx, characterized by fever, ulceration, and swelling of the affected structures.

Etiology: *Fusobacterium necrophorum* has long been considered to be the cause of this disease. However, traumatic injury to the mucous membranes of the oral cavity by coarse feed or feed containing an excessive quantity of thistles or tough stems is predisposing. Similarly, erupting teeth or other infections, eg, mucosal disease, may cause preliminary damage to the mucous membranes. Contributing factors include dirty barns and feedlots.

Clinical Findings and Lesions: Calf diphtheria usually occurs as necrotic stomatitis in calves <3 mo old and as necrotic laryngitis in older calves. The calf with necrotic stomatitis has difficulty in nursing, is depressed and anorectic, and has a temperature of up to 104°F (40°C). The cheeks may be swollen, saliva may drip from the mouth, and the breath has a foul odor. In calves with necrotic laryngitis, the most prominent sign in severe cases is loud wheezing. The early signs may include a fever as high as 106°F (41°C), tachypnea, and salivation. Later, protrusion of the tongue and a nasal discharge may be noted. Calves may develop both necrotic stomatitis and necrotic laryngitis; an acute, necrotizing pneumonia due to aspiration of infected tissue debris may be a sequela. Untreated calves may succumb to toxemia and pneumonia within 2-7 days.

The chief lesions are necrotic ulcers of varying depth on the oral, pharyngeal, or laryngeal mucous membranes, most often on the tongue (particularly its borders), the inner surface of the cheeks, and the lining of the pharynx. In severe cases, lesions extend into the nasal cavity, larynx, trachea, and even the lungs.

Diagnosis: The signs are usually sufficient to establish a diagnosis. Difficulties may be encountered in outbreaks when an older calf is the first to become ill, or in herds in which the disease affects only 1 or 2 calves. The filamentous, beaded, gram-negative bacteria may be demonstrated in smears from the deeper parts of the lesions or by culture on blood agar under anaerobic conditions; the colonies are β-hemolytic.

Treatment and Control: Affected animals must be isolated from healthy ones. Cleaning and disinfecting the feeding and drinking areas and sheds are important steps in preventing spread of the disease. All young calves should be examined daily for early recognition of new cases. The sulfonamides of choice are sulfamerazine and sulfamethazine. Penicillin or tetracyclines are usually beneficial, and also chloramphenicol where its use is permitted. Supplemental feeding with milk, eggs, and nutritious gruel is advisable.

PHARYNGITIS

Inflammation of the walls of the nasopharynx or oropharynx.

Etiology: Pharyngitis may accompany infections of the upper respiratory tract; arise from direct physical, chemical, or traumatic insult; or develop through extension of inflammatory disease of adjacent structures. The pharyngeal submucosa of all species contains generous deposits of lymphoid tissue, which in the immature animal tend to become hyperplastic. In the young racehorse, generalized pharyngeal lymphoid hyperplasia (PLH) is a universal finding on endoscopy, but it tends to be aggravated by viral infections or particulate air pollutants, especially when the horse is in full training. PLH is regarded by some as a cause of upper airway obstruction, but recent evidence suggests that it has little impact on racing performance. It often becomes chronic, and then is characterized by nodules on the walls of the pharynx and pharyngeal recess that contain masses of lymphocytes. It improves with rest but often recurs when training is resumed. PLH usually disappears spontaneously during the 3-yr-old stage. Trauma to the pharynx may result from foreign bodies or unskilled use of instruments, eg, balling guns. Oropharyngeal foreign bodies are common in dogs and less so in cats. They fall into 2 groups, those that become wedged and are too firmly lodged to be displaced by the animal and those that penetrate mucosa. Penetrating foreign bodies range from pins and needles to sticks, which may impale the pharyngeal wall when being swallowed and cause severe local cellulitis and esophageal rupture or, if broken off, act as a focus for suppuration. Inhalation or ingestion of drugs and chemicals may cause intense irritation. Regardless of etiology, dysphagia of any kind is likely to be accompanied by pharyngitis. Horses with pharyngeal paralysis from guttural pouch mycosis (qv, p 739), dysautonomia (qv, p 596), or strangles (qv, p 744) all show secondary pharyngitis. Similarly, dogs with palatal defects, megaesophagus, or esophagitis develop inflammation of the tonsils and pharynx. Thermal irritation of the pharynx occurs in dogs as a result of ingesting hot food or liquids. Elongation of the soft palate or eversion of the lateral ventricles of the larynx in brachycephalic dogs can cause respiratory distress and dysphagia, with resulting pharyngitis and tonsillitis.

Clinical Findings and Diagnosis: In general, animals with pharyngitis have a normal desire to eat and drink but decline to do so because of the pain of ingestion and deglutition. Palpation of the pharynx reveals increased sensitivity. The submaxillary, retropharyngeal, and pharyngeal lymph nodes may be swollen, and the tonsils often are enlarged and inflamed. If there is accompanying laryngitis, a suppressed cough can be elicited by pressure on the pharynx. If pain causes resistance to opening the mouth, general anesthesia can facilitate examination. Inability to swallow may cause drooling; retching and coughing are common, and the possibility of aspiration pneumonia should be considered.

Pharyngeal paralysis (qv, p 148) may be a sign of rabies (qv, p 619). Severe PLH increases turbulence of airflow through the pharynx and may cause respiratory noise during exercise. It is also thought to trigger dorsal displacement of the soft palate. On endoscopy, PLH is visible in the pharyngeal walls, pharyngeal recess, guttural pouch mucosa, and on the dorsal surfaces of the soft palate and epiglottis.

The causes of pharyngitis are variable, and no single prognosis is applicable. The outcome depends on the nature of the precipitating factors.

Treatment: The primary objectives are to identify and control the predisposing factors. If the condition has been caused by foreign bodies, removal of the offending object and local application of an expectorant-antiseptic solution (eg, Mandl's solution [iodine 0.6 g, potassium iodide 1.2 g, peppermint oil 0.25 g, glycerin *qs ad* 30 mL]) is usually effective. The affected animal should receive soft or liquid foods that can be swallowed easily. Supplemental IV feeding may be necessary during the acute stage.

Large animals should be given sulfonamides or antibiotics parenterally. In horses, PLH is a disease of adolescence that tends to resolve spontaneously as the animal matures. When the hyperplasia is severe, the horse should be rested in a clean stable environment and treated with topical pharyngeal sprays and systemic antibiotics. In horses with infectious pharyngitis (ie, strangles), in which swelling and exudates may cause distressing dyspnea, steam vapors with cresol are helpful and may avoid the need for tracheotomy; abscessed lymph nodes are common and should be encouraged to drain, by lancing if necessary. The cough may be relieved by applying syrupy expectorants on the tongue. It is unwise to restrain and attempt to force oral medication because of the danger of causing fatal asphyxiation.

Similarly, management of pharyngitis in small animals aims to control or eliminate the causes. Calicivirus infection in cats may cause marked ulceration of the oropharyngeal mucosa. Treatment is essentially supportive to control secondary bacterial infections and to maintain normal hydration while providing adequate nutrition. This may include IV fluid therapy and/or a pharyngostomy or gastrostomy tube.

Elongated soft palate, glosso-epiglottic entrapment, and everted laryngeal ventricles should all be treated surgically in dogs.

PULMONARY EMPHYSEMA

Two major forms of emphysema occur in the lungs. **Alveolar emphysema** (in horses, called "heaves" or chronic obstructive pulmonary disease, qv, p 733) is permanent enlargement of alveolar spaces accompanied by rupture of alveolar septa. **Interstitial emphysema** is the presence of air within interlobular, subpleural, and interstitial areas of the lungs. Emphysema must be distinguished from simple hyperinflation of alveoli, which is a common postmortem finding that occurs temporarily secondary to obstruction of outflow of air.

Emphysema is an important disease in man; in other animals it is almost always secondary to another pulmonary disease process. The pathogenesis is not fully understood, but at least 2 possibilities have been suggested: 1) there may be degradation and weakening of the interstitium by proteolytic enzymes, particularly elastase, released by inflammatory cells; 2) more commonly, the condition develops secondary to either chronic bronchitis or bronchiolitis, which cause obstruction of airways on expiration but still allow air to enter alveoli on inspiration or through communicating pores in alveolar walls.

Interstitial emphysema is most common in cattle and pigs due to the well-developed interlobular septae of their lungs. In cattle, severe interstitial emphysema can be accompanied by subcut. emphysema over the back when air dissects along fascial planes from the lungs through the mediastinum and thoracic inlet to the subcutis of the back. Interstitial emphysema frequently follows severe expiratory distress in cattle, particularly acute (atypical) interstitial pneumonia (*see* ABPE, p 724). Minor degrees of emphysema may precede death if there was a prolonged struggle and exaggerated respiration. These agonal changes must be differentiated from antemortem lesions.

RESPIRATORY DISEASES OF CATTLE

BOVINE RESPIRATORY DISEASE COMPLEX

INTRODUCTION

Bovine respiratory disease (BRD) can be caused by a variety of factors that interact to allow microbial colonization of the lungs, which results in severe respiratory distress and possibly death. The host's immune system, various viruses and bacteria, including chlamydiae and mycoplasmas, and even helminths and fungi play a role in determining the severity of disease. Management, by altering the environment of the animal, affects all these factors and, consequently, directly influences the possible economic losses. Thus, if animals are stressed as a result of weaning, transportation, alteration or deprivation of diet, etc, which may adversely affect the animal's defense mechanisms, and then mixed with animals that are shedding various pathogens, disease is likely to ensue. If the animals are crowded or if ventilation is inadequate, transmission is enhanced. In many cases, the pathogens themselves cause immunomodulation; thus, viral infections not only induce anatomical alterations of the respiratory tract, which improve the cultural conditions for bacteria, but they also alter the host's clearance mechanisms. This synergism is seen often between viruses and bacteria in BRD.

VIRUS-INDUCED BOVINE PNEUMONIA

PARAINFLUENZA-3 VIRUS (PI-3)

Historically, PI-3 has been linked with bovine respiratory disease (BRD), although opinions have varied as to what role it plays in the disease. It can infect many species, including man, cattle, dogs, horses, monkeys, and sheep. It is found worldwide.

PI-3 virus is capable of causing disease by itself, but is probably much more often involved as a primary infection followed by *Pasteurella haemolytica* as a secondary invader. Clinical signs include fever, anorexia, serous nasal discharge, lacrimation, and coughing.

Uncomplicated, fatal PI-3 viral pneumonia, although probably rare, can be seen as severe consolidation of anteroventral lobes of the lungs. Histological lesions include bronchiolitis, and alveolitis with marked congestion and hemorrhage. The pathological picture is usually seen as *Pasteurella*-induced, fibrinopurulent pneumonia.

PI-3 virus infection with or without secondary bacterial infection is difficult to separate from other virus-induced pneumonia in cattle. Adenoviruses, enteroviruses, rhinoviruses, reoviruses, caliciviruses, coronaviruses, and possibly others probably play a major role in some BRD outbreaks, and disease caused by them is not easily differentiated from that induced by PI-3 virus. *See also* BRSV INFECTION, below.

Treatment includes antibiotic therapy for bacterial invaders. Good management practices such as appropriate feed, and ready access to fresh water and shelter help to reduce losses.

Several vaccines are available for PI-3 that provide protection if used as a rational part of a disease prevention and management program.

BOVINE RESPIRATORY SYNCYTIAL VIRUS (BRSV)

Infection occurs worldwide with some antigenic variation among virus isolates. The host range of BRSV includes all bovine species and may include sheep, goats and other animals, including man. BRSV, a pneumovirus, family Paramyxoviridae, apparently is indigenous in cattle populations, in which it causes cyclic inapparent infection, and results in substantial serum antibody titers in most cattle. These antibodies may protect the animal from developing clinical disease, but do not prevent infection. As with other respiratory viruses, BRSV is spread by aerosol droplets. There is evidence that BRSV is a major agent involved in the initiation of bovine respiratory disease, and that bacteria and stress factors contribute to precipitate clinical disease. (*See also* PI-3 INFECTION, above.)

Clinical Findings: BRSV is capable of producing acute viral pneumonia, and is implicated in some cases of feedlot emphysema. However, more often, it probably is a prelude to pneumonic pasteurellosis. Fever ($>108°F$ [$42°C$]) can be found in the early stages of infection and peaks at 5-7 days, thereafter dropping to 104-106°F (40-$41°C$), accompanied by secondary bacterial infection and pneumonia. Initially, these animals may appear alert and feed normally and then become anorectic and depressed, and often have mucopurulent nasal discharge, coughing, and dyspnea.

Lesions: Uncomplicated pneumonia caused by BRSV is not common. However, the virus can cause a severe bronchopneumonia that is diffuse, usually with some degree of emphysema and edema. Froth in the bronchi and trachea is common. Pneumonia as a result of BRSV infection is usually reflective of secondary infection by *Pasteurella haemolytica* (*see* below). This pneumonia is fibrinopurulent, and there is severe consolidation of the cranioventral lobes. Edema and emphysema of the diaphragmatic lung lobes may vary in severity.

On histopathological examination, necrotizing bronchiolitis with syncytia (multinucleated cells) may be present in the epithelial lining and alveolar walls. Interstitial edema and emphysema with alveolar epithelialization and hyaline membrane formation also have been noted.

Diagnosis: There are no cardinal features that make a diagnosis of BRSV-induced respiratory disease easy. In some studies, >50% of feedlot respiratory disease involved BRSV. In addition, the virus is common in beef and dairy herds, and is involved in many, if not most, respiratory disease problems. Usually, it can be just as certain that the viral infection is complicated by secondary bacteria. Some also think that BVD (qv, p 166) may play a prominent tandem role with BRSV to produce disease.

Virus isolation from nasal swabs is usually futile, as is recovery of the virus from necropsy specimens. The virus is fragile and probably is "tied up" early by antibodies.

Serology appears to be the definitive method of diagnosis; however, this is always retrospective. Paired serum samples are imperative. However, the antibody titer of animals with well-developed clinical disease may be higher in the acute sample than in the sample taken 2-3 wk later. This is because the antibody response often develops rapidly, and clinical signs follow virus infection by up to 10-12 days. Single serum samples showing high antibody titers from a number of animals in a respiratory outbreak may be useful in making a diagnosis if coupled with clinical signs.

Treatment and Prophylaxis: Treatment focuses on secondary bacterial invaders. Use of antibiotics with supportive therapy usually reduces losses. In pure virus-induced severe disease with emphysema, treatment must be early and vigorous. Death loss may be substantial. Antihistamines and corticosteroids appear to be beneficial.

Field experience indicates that vaccines, both inactivated and modified live, reduce losses due to BRSV-induced respiratory disease.

PNEUMONIC PASTEURELLOSIS
(Shipping fever, Transit fever)

All ages are susceptible, but severe respiratory disease associated with *Pasteurella* spp generally occurs in younger animals following shipping; thus, it is often called shipping fever. (*See also* HEMORRHAGIC SEPTICEMIA, below.) However, other forms of stress combined with simultaneous exposure to one or more of numerous viruses and bacteria may also result in pneumonia.

Etiology: *Pasteurella haemolytica* is the agent most frequently isolated from the lungs of infected animals. However, *P multocida*, as well as various other bacteria, also can cause pneumonia. In most cases, both of these *Pasteurella* spp are inhabitants of the upper respiratory tract of healthy animals; under normal conditions they remain confined to the upper respiratory tract, especially in the tonsillar crypts. Following stress or viral infection (*see* above), the replication rate of the bacteria appears to increase rapidly, which results in bacterial colonization of the lungs. The increased bacterial growth rate and colonization of the lungs may be due to anatomical and environmental alterations of the respiratory tract as well as to a suppression of the host's defense mechanism. The disease is most common in feedlot cattle within the first few weeks of entry into the feedlot. In some cases, up to 50% of the animals may require treatment, and 1-10% mortality is common.

Clinical Findings: Affected cattle are depressed, anorectic, and have a fever (104-106°F [40-41°C]) and a serous to mucopurulent nasal discharge with rapid shallow breathing. They often cough if they move. In severe cases, there is pleurisy; breathing is irregular and animals may grunt on exhalation. Eventually, they may refuse to get up. Lung auscultation may reveal moist rales, pleuritic friction rubs, and crackling. As lung consolidation progresses, lung sounds may be decreased. The course of the disease can be shortened if treatment is initiated early, but may become chronic if delayed; animals may become unthrifty and die a few weeks or months later.

Lesions: On necropsy, the anteroventral portions of the lungs are dark red, swollen, and hard, and often covered with fibrin. Adhesions between adjacent surfaces are common. In addition, a serofibrinous pleural exudate is present. On the cut surface, fibrin is evident between lobules, and areas of necrosis are scattered throughout the lobe. As the disease progresses, these necrotic areas become demarcated by a white outline. Pure cultures of *P haemolytica* can be isolated from most cases; these are associated with fibrinous pleuropneumonia with extensive thrombosis of interstitial lymphatics, marked involvement of macrophages, and foci of lung necrosis, but few signs of airway inflammation. In contrast, *P multocida* infections are associated with suppurative bronchitis and bronchopneumonia, minimal exudation with fibrin, and less thrombosis of the lymphatics. These findings may help differentiate the infections. Although it is believed that viruses predispose to bacterial superinfection, the virus and its lesions generally have disappeared before fatalities occur.

Treatment: Affected cattle must be treated early for best results. Animals should be identified, isolated, and treated with broad-spectrum antibacterials. Unless long-acting drugs are used, treatment should be repeated for at least 3-4 days. Treatment failures may occur if treatment is initiated late, or if the organisms are resistant to the selected antibiotic. Mass medication in feed or water generally is of limited value since sick animals do not eat or drink enough to achieve inhibitory blood levels of the antibiotic.

Control: Management is the key to control of bovine respiratory disease. Calves should be immunized against the major viral pathogens before weaning and transport (*see* ENZOOTIC PNEUMONIA OF CALVES, below). The value of *Pasteurella* bacterins has yet to be determined; some reports indicate that they may even exacerbate the disease. However, field tests of newer, live culture, modified culture, and subunit (leukotoxin, etc) vaccines have shown considerable efficacy when used as part of a disease prevention and control program. Vaccination should be undertaken ≥3 wk before shipment and movement to a feedlot. Immunizations may be repeated on entry into the feedlot. Processing procedures should be reduced and spread out as much as possible to reduce stress. Animals could be creep-fed before weaning to allow time for them to adjust to dietary alterations. Ventilation (qv, p 1106) is an important management tool; frequent air changes remove infected airborne droplets from the environment, which temper the insult to the animal's respiratory system. (*See also* DISEASE-MANAGEMENT INTERACTION: CATTLE, p 1108.)

ACUTE BOVINE PULMONARY EMPHYSEMA AND EDEMA
(ABPE, Fog fever, Bovine atypical interstitial pneumonia)

One of the more common causes of acute respiratory distress in cattle, particularly adult beef cattle, characterized by sudden onset, minimal coughing, and a course that terminates fatally or goes on to dramatic improvement within a few days. It is a disease of groups; morbidity ranges to >50%, although usually only a small minority develops severe respiratory distress. Typically, it occurs in autumn, 5-10 days after a change to a better, often lush, pasture. The term fog fever derives from its association with "fog" pastures, ie, foggage or aftermath.

Etiology: Metabolites of the naturally occurring amino acid L-tryptophan probably are responsible for many outbreaks. In the rumen, L-tryptophan is degraded to indoleacetic acid, which can be converted to 3-methylindole (3-MI) by some ruminal microorganisms. 3-MI is absorbed into the bloodstream and is the source of the pneumotoxicity after metabolism by the mixed-function oxidase system, which is very active in the lungs. Apparently, the L-tryptophan level of crops is most likely to be high in lush, rapidly growing pastures, particularly (but not exclusively) in the fall. Indistinguishable clinicopathological syndromes occur on rape pasture and following the ingestion of either moldy sweet potatoes infested with *Fusarium solani*, or the wild mint, *Perilla frutescens*. Wild mint contains perilla ketone, which is pneumotoxic; sweet potatoes infested with *F solani* contain several pneumotoxic substances, especially 4-ipomeanal.

Clinical Findings: ABPE is most common in heavy beef cows, but may occur in either sex and in dairy or beef cattle under similar management conditions. Outbreaks usually develop within 5-10 days of a change to better grazing, and rarely occur in animals that have been on a field >3 wk. Morbidity ranges up to 50% or even to 100%, but usually only a few are severely affected.

Mild cases may go unnoticed: cattle are subdued but still alert; there is tachypnea and hyperpnea, but auscultation is usually unrewarding. Such cattle usually recover spontaneously within days. Severely affected cattle show extensive respiratory distress with mouth breathing, extension of the tongue, and drooling of saliva. A loud expiratory grunt is common, but coughing is unusual. In the early stages, auscultation reveals surprisingly soft respiratory sounds; rales are rare. If death does not occur (up to 1 in 3 die), the animals improve dramatically and resume eating by the third day. At this stage, auscultation reveals harsh respiratory sounds and, in some animals, dorsal (emphysematous) crackles. Some cattle have subcut. emphysema extending along the back from the withers. Full clinical recovery may require 3 wk.

Lesions: Significant lesions are limited to the respiratory tract. In affected cattle that have died or have been slaughtered *in extremis*, the lungs are heavy and do not collapse normally. They are widely affected with various degrees of rubbery firmness; there is extensive edema and emphysema, often with the formation of large air-filled bullae in interlobular and subpleural regions. Submucosal hemorrhages are often present on the larynx and in the trachea and larger bronchi. Histologically, the lesion is characterized by congestion, alveolar edema, hyaline membrane formation, and areas of early alveolar epithelial hyperplasia of type II pneumonocytes; occasionally, areas of bronchiolar necrosis may be found. The emphysema is often dramatic and is limited to interstitial fascia where it is accompanied by edema.

In animals that are slaughtered after 3 days of illness, the lungs are still heavy and do not collapse normally; they are a pinkish gray and of increased firmness; edema and emphysema are inconspicuous or absent. Histologically, widespread alveolar epithelial hyperplasia characteristic of a diffuse, acute, proliferative alveolitis is seen.

Diagnosis: Diagnosis is based on history, signs, and lesions. Since the syndrome is not specific with regard to cause, clues must be obtained from management factors such as change in pasture, or exposure to perilla mint or moldy sweet potatoes.

Treatment and Prophylaxis: Severely affected animals have so little reserve that any driving or handling must be done with caution to prevent immediate deaths. No drug has proved effective in controlled trials, but epinephrine, aminophylline, and corticosteroids are used widely. Even severely affected animals can recover if removed from the offending pasture and handled quietly. After 1 wk, the cattle may be gradually reintroduced to the pasture.

ATYPICAL INTERSTITIAL PNEUMONIA
(Farmer's lung disease)

A condition that appears to be similar to farmer's lung disease in man occurs in both acute and chronic forms in adult cattle. The human and bovine forms of the disease may coexist on problem farms due to common exposure to dust from moldy hay.

Etiology: The disease occurs when sensitized individuals inhale antigens from thermophilic actinomycetes, commonly the spores of *Micropolyspora faeni*. The actinomycetes proliferate in vast numbers in hay, grain, or other vegetable material that has overheated to ~150°F (65°C) following damp storage (30-40% moisture content). Dust that contains large numbers of spores is released when this moldy hay is shaken. The small size (1 μm) of the spores allows them to reach the smallest airways and alveoli to provoke a reaction that has been termed a "hypersensitivity pneumonitis"; this is considered to be predominantly a type III hypersensitivity reaction (Arthus), although a type IV hypersensitivity component is suspected (*see* IMMUNOPATHOLOGICAL DISEASES, p 433 *et seq*).

Affected herds exist in areas where significant rainfall usually occurs during the haymaking season, suggesting that a clinical problem may arise only after repeated sensitization and challenge from the spores. Clinical disease tends to arise during the latter half of the winter feeding period and usually only when moldy hay is fed indoors. Under such circumstances, serum antibodies (usually detected by immunodiffusion) to *M faeni* are widespread among the adult cattle by the end of each winter feeding period, and many apparently normal cattle are seropositive. By contrast, few adult cattle are seropositive on other farms where "good" hay is the norm or where grass silage is fed.

Clinical Findings: Individuals may succumb to the **acute** form of the disease over a period of weeks. Usually, only severe acute cases are noticed: there is respiratory distress, anorexia, and agalactia in animals ≥5 yr old; coughing and pyrexia also occur and adventitious sounds are occasionally heard on auscultation; death is rare.

The **chronic** disease usually has a higher morbidity; in most instances, the signs are weight loss, poor production, and persistent coughing. Affected individuals are fairly bright and eat reasonably well, but tachypnea, hyperpnea, and coughing are widespread in the group. Auscultation may reveal anteroventral crackles and sometimes, in more severe cases, scattered rhonchi. Exercise intolerance may be seen, and congestive cardiac failure can develop if pulmonary fibrosis is widespread.

Lesions: The macroscopic lesions are often unremarkable; usually, there is mild peripheral lobular overinflation with diffusely scattered, small, gray, subpleural spots. Although transient pulmonary edema may be a feature of severe acute cases, the histological lesions that are consistently found are interalveolar cellular infiltration, epithelioid granulomata, and bronchiolitis obliterans. In some chronic cases, small foci of alveolar epithelial hyperplasia and metaplasia with interstitial fibrosis may be found. These areas may extend to include most, if not all, of the lung substance to produce cases clinically indistinguishable from diffuse fibrosing alveolitis (DFA). Circumstantial evidence suggests that some cases of DFA are end-stage chronic farmer's lung disease.

Treatment and Control: Since it is often impossible to completely shield cattle from further challenge, most recover only partially following dexamethasone treatment (1 mg/5-10 kg body wt). However, improvement is usually marked when they are turned out in the spring. Prevention is difficult in areas where hay is likely to be wet during the curing process and it is not possible to alter the feeding regimen.

CONTAGIOUS BOVINE PLEUROPNEUMONIA

A highly contagious pneumonia generally accompanied by pleurisy. It is present in Africa, the Iberian peninsula, and parts of India and China; minor outbreaks occur in the Middle East. The USA has been free of the disease since 1892, the UK since 1898, and Australia since 1973.

Etiology: The causal organism is *Mycoplasma mycoides mycoides*. (*See also* CONTAGIOUS CAPRINE PLEUROPNEUMONIA, p 754.) Susceptible cattle become infected by inhaling droplets coughed out by affected cattle. Goats and sheep are not important in the epidemiology. Septicemia produces lesions in the kidneys and placenta, which can be sources of infection. Transplacental infection of the fetus can occur. Viability of the organism in the environment is poor. The incubation period of the disease varies, but most cases occur 3-8 wk after exposure. In some localities, susceptible herds may show up to 100% morbidity, but much lower infection rates (~10%) associated with clinical signs are more common. Mortality is likely to be ~50%. Of recovered animals, 25% may become carriers with chronic lung lesions in the form of sequestra of variable size. Since carriers may not be detectable clinically or serologically, they constitute a serious problem in control programs. Breed susceptibility, management systems, and general health of the animal are important factors that influence the infection.

Clinical Findings: In acute cases, signs include fever up to 107°F (41.5°C), anorexia, and painful difficult breathing. In hot climates, the animal often stands by itself in the shade, its head lowered and extended, its back slightly arched, and its elbows turned out. Percussion of the chest is painful; respiration is rapid, shallow, and abdominal. If the animal is forced to move quickly, the breathing becomes more distressed and a soft, moist cough may result. The disease progresses rapidly, animals lose condition, and breathing becomes very labored, with a grunt at expiration. The animal becomes recumbent and dies after 1-3 wk. Chronically affected cattle usually exhibit signs of varying intensity for 3-4 wk, after which the lesions gradually resolve, and the animals appear to recover. Subclinical cases occur and may be important as carriers.

Lesions: The thoracic cavity may contain up to 10 L of clear yellow or turbid fluid mixed with fibrin flakes, and the organs in the thorax are often covered by thick deposits of fibrin. Varying amounts of one or both lungs may be involved, the affected portion being enlarged and solid. On section, the typical marbled appearance of pleuropneumonia is evident due to the widened interlobular septa and subpleural tissue that encloses gray, yellow, or red consolidated lung lobules. Microscopically, this is a severe, acute, fibrinous pneumonia with fibrinous pleurisy, thrombosis of pulmonary blood vessels, and areas of necrosis of lung tissue; the interstitial tissue is markedly thickened by edema fluid containing much fibrin. In chronic cases, the lesion has a necrotic center sequestered in a thick, fibrous capsule, and there may be fibrous pleural adhesions. Organisms may survive in these sequestra and the animals become carriers.

Diagnosis: This is based on clinical signs, the complement fixation test, and necropsy, and is confirmed by histopathology, detection of organisms in pleural fluid using darkfield microscopy, isolation of the organism from lung or pleural fluid, or demonstration of specific antigens in lung tissue by immunodiffusion or immunofluorescence and hyperimmune antigalactan serum. Subclinical disease is detected by use of the complement fixation test. As soon as an outbreak is suspected, slaughter and necropsy of a suspect animal is advisable.

Control: The disease is reportable by law in many countries from which it has been eradicated by slaughter of all infected and exposed animals. In countries where cattle movement can readily be restricted, the disease can be eradicated by quarantine, blood testing, and immunization with attenuated vaccine (eg, T1/44 strain). Where cattle cannot be confined, the spread of infection can be limited by vaccination. Tracing the source of infected cattle detected at abattoirs, blood testing, and imposition of strict rules for cattle movement also can contribute to the control of the disease in such areas.

Treatment is recommended only in endemic areas because the organisms may not be eliminated and carriers may develop. Tylosin (10 mg/kg, IM, b.i.d. for 6 injections) is said to be effective.

ENZOOTIC PNEUMONIA OF CALVES

A name commonly used for infectious respiratory disease of calves maintained in groups confined in a communal pen, either in a building or outdoors. It is primarily a problem in calves <6 mo old but may occur in those up to 1 yr old, and is more common in dairy than beef calves. Morbidity rates may approach 100%; mortality rates are extremely variable but frequently are >20%.

Etiology: The causes are those of bovine respiratory disease (*see* above) in general: the triad of stress plus a primary respiratory viral infection followed by a bacterial superinfection. Stress results from poor husbandry, eg, failure of transfer of passive immunity, inadequate ventilation, continually adding calves to a group, poor-quality milk replacers, or inadequate space. Any of several viruses may be involved. Similarly, a variety of bacteria may be recovered from chronically affected calves. Antimicrobial susceptibility tests of the isolates should be done to determine the most effective treatment. Isolation of viruses from nasal swabs or transtracheal washing is difficult, as the acute viral infection may be over by the time clinical signs are observed. The viral entities could be identified serologically with paired serum samples, the first taken when a calf enters an infected group and the second following clinical respiratory disease. However, this may be of limited value since calves often seroconvert to multiple viruses under these conditions.

Clinical Findings: During acute outbreaks, body temperature is 103-107°F (39.5-41.5°C). Initially, breathing is rapid and shallow with soft coughing, accompanied by a serous nasal discharge. The condition may resolve slowly or become more severe, characterized by harsh coughing, marked dyspnea, tenacious nasal discharge, anorexia, dehydration, and weakness. The disease may be insidious in onset with vague clinical signs. Such calves develop chronic respiratory disease, cough sporadically, have rough coats, fail to gain weight, and are often culled as "poor doers" following one or more regimens of treatment.

    Lesions: These are bilateral and confined to the apical and anterior portions of the cardiac lobes of the lungs. A fibrinopurulent bronchopneumonia with pleural adhesions are typical lesions when death is due to *Pasteurella* pneumonia. The consolidated areas are red and gray. Fibrin is present on the surface of the lungs. Numerous abscesses may be found that are the result of infection with *Actinobacillus* (*Corynebacterium*) *pyogenes*.

Treatment: Although antimicrobials should be chosen based on susceptibility tests, it is often necessary to initiate treatment before laboratory results are available. In such cases, the medicament of choice is a broad-spectrum antibiotic that has been effective in treating similar cases on the same premises or in the area. Treatment should be continued ≥48 hr after clinical signs are markedly improved, with a body temperature of <103°F (39.5°C).

Control and Prevention: When calves are placed in communal pens that contain calves of varying ages, control of enzootic pneumonia is extremely difficult. Severity of the pneumonia may be modified by improved husbandry, proper housing, adequate ventilation, and good nursing care. Prevention begins with vaccinating the cows against specific respiratory viruses and bacteria 3-4 wk prepartum, to improve the quality of colostral antibodies. Calves should receive colostrum at 8-10% of body wt in the first 12 hr after birth. Newborn dairy calves should be housed individually in hutches or stalls and fed whole milk or a high-quality milk replacer with a fiber content of <0.5% until 8-12 wk old. Calves should be vaccinated against respiratory viruses 3-4 wk before the first grouping. When establishing groups, calves should be of similar age, and the group should be limited to ≤10. As calves mature, groups can become larger as the size of the herd, facilities, and available labor dictate. An "all-in/all-out" policy should be practiced when establishing and terminating a group. Newborn beef calves and their dams should be moved from concentrated calving areas as soon as the calf is nursing well and strong enough to travel.

HEMORRHAGIC SEPTICEMIA (HS)

An acute pasteurellosis, principally of cattle and water buffalo, that frequently reaches epidemic proportions. The only true outbreaks in North America have occurred in bison in Yellowstone National Park. Occurrence in Central and South America has not been confirmed. HS is a major disease of cattle and water buffalo in southern and eastern Asia, Africa, and some countries of southern Europe and the Middle East. Although it may occur at any time of year, the worst epidemics occur during the rainy season. It is most common in the river valleys and deltas of southeast Asia among buffaloes used in rice cultivation. Water buffalo are thought to be more susceptible than cattle. There have been reports of HS in horses, pigs, deer, bison, camels, elephants, and yaks. It is likely that wild cattle and buffalo are also susceptible. As few as 20,000 bacteria given subcut. can kill a susceptible buffalo. Laboratory rabbits and mice are highly susceptible to experimental infection.

Etiology: HS is caused by 1 of 2 serotypes of *Pasteurella multocida*, designated B:2 and E:2. Serotype E:2 has been recovered only in Africa; B:2 causes the disease elsewhere, and also has been recovered from cases in Egypt and the Sudan. *Pasteurella multocida* is an extracellular parasite and immunity is primarily humoral. HS is essentially an endotoxemia.

As many as 5% of cattle or water buffalo may carry the potentially pathogenic serotype in the nasopharynx. It is hypothesized that under various stresses, carriers may become clinical cases and shed virulent organisms (via saliva and nasal discharges) that are spread by direct and indirect contact to susceptible animals. The outbreaks that ensue may result in enormous losses in some regions. The heaviest losses occur during the monsoon rains in southeast Asia, and it is thought that the organisms, which can survive for hours and probably days in the moist soil and water, are transmitted widely at this time.

Clinical Findings: Most cases are acute or peracute, resulting in death within 8-24 hr after onset. Because the course is so short, clinical signs may not be seen. Animals first evince dullness, then reluctance to move, fever, salivation, and serous nasal discharge. Edematous swelling is frequently seen, beginning in the throat region and spreading to the parotid region, neck, and brisket. Mucous membranes are congested; there is respiratory distress, and usually the animal goes down and dies within hours. Occasional cases linger for several days. Recovery is rare. There appears to be no chronic form.

Lesions: The most obvious changes in affected animals are the edema, widely distributed hemorrhages, and general hyperemia. Most cases have an edematous swelling of the head, neck, and brisket region. Incision of the swellings reveals a clear or straw-colored serous fluid. The edema is also found in the musculature, and the subserous petechial hemorrhages, which are found throughout the animal, are particularly characteristic. Blood-tinged fluid is often found in the pericardial sac and in the thoracic and abdominal cavities. Petechial hemorrhages are particularly prominent in the pharyngeal and cervical lymph nodes. Gastroenteritis is seen only occasionally, and unlike pneumonic pasteurellosis, pneumonia usually is not extensive.

Diagnosis: Outbreaks can be readily identified, particularly if there is a history of earlier outbreaks and a recent failure to vaccinate. Sporadic cases are more difficult to diagnose clinically. The season of the year, rapid course, and high herd incidence, with fever and edematous swellings indicate typical HS. Characteristic necropsy lesions support the clinical diagnosis. Although typical outbreaks are not difficult to recognize clinically, acute salmonellosis, anthrax, pneumonic pasteurellosis (other serotypes), and rinderpest should be considered.

A presumptive diagnosis is based on the isolation of *P multocida* from the blood and vital organs of an animal with typical signs; definitive diagnosis depends on identifying the serotype as B:2 or E:2. Other serotypes cause various infections in cattle and buffalo but not typical HS. The passive mouse protection test employing specific B:2 and E:2 immune rabbit sera is used in Asia and Africa to identify these serotypes. More precise tests such as indirect hemagglutination, coagglutination, and counterimmunoelectrophoresis and immunodiffusion tests are available in some laboratories.

If there is postmortem decomposition, the causative agent may be overgrown and obscured by extraneous bacteria. In such cases, the subcut. inoculation of mice or rabbits with small amounts of blood and tissue suspensions facilitates the recovery of the pasteurellae in pure or nearly pure culture.

Serology is of no value in diagnosis. However, the indirect hemagglutination procedure and passive mouse protection test are of value in determining the immune status of animals.

Treatment and Control: Various sulfonamides, tetracyclines, penicillin, and chloramphenicol (where its use is permitted) are effective if administered early. Because of the rapid course of the disease and the frequent difficulty of access to animals, antimicrobial therapy often is not practicable. Although multiple antibiotic resistance has been reported for some strains of *P multocida*, it has not been described for the HS serotypes. The principal means of control is by vaccination. Three kinds of vaccine are widely used: plain bacterin, alum-type precipitated bacterins, and an oil-adjuvant bacterin. The most effective bacterin is the oil-adjuvant—one dose provides protection for 9-12 mo; it should be administered to all animals annually. The alum-precipitated-type bacterin is given at 6-mo intervals. Maternal antibody interferes with vaccine efficacy in calves. The oil-adjuvant vaccine has not been popular because of difficulty in syringing, and occasional adverse tissue reactions.

INFECTIOUS BOVINE RHINOTRACHEITIS (IBR), INFECTIOUS PUSTULAR VULVOVAGINITIS (IPV), AND ASSOCIATED SYNDROMES

Bovine herpesvirus 1 (BHV-1) can cause mild to severe syndromes in cattle of all ages and breeds. Furthermore, it can affect many body systems and thereby manifest itself in several forms, including respiratory disease, abortions, encephalitis, a systemic disease, conjunctivitis, or genital infection. In feedlot cattle, the respiratory form is most common; in breeding cattle, abortions or genital infections are more common. Following recovery from infection, the virus usually is maintained in a latent state that can be reactivated periodically following transport, concurrent disease, other stress, or corticosteroid treatment. Animals with latent infections generally show no clinical signs when the virus is reactivated, but they do serve as a source of infection for other susceptible animals and thus perpetuate the disease.

Etiology and Epidemiology: Although there are strain differences within the BHV-1 group, there is little association with particular syndromes; all forms of the disease can be caused by the same isolate under appropriate conditions. The virus can be isolated from nasal, ocular, and vaginal secretions, and semen and preputial washings.

The **respiratory form** is most prevalent in feedlot situations in which large numbers of animals are crowded or transported. This allows rapid spread of the virus to susceptible animals from a few carrier animals. Virus infection alone often is not life-threatening, but concurrent infection with bacteria (most commonly *Pasteurella* spp) increases the severity of respiratory disease with subsequent development of pneumonia and possibly death.

Genital infections occur in bulls (infectious pustular balanoposthitis) and cows (IPV) within 1-3 days of mating or close contact with an infected animal. Transmission can occur in the absence of visible lesions and through artificial insemination with semen from subclinically infected bulls.

Clinical Findings: The incubation period for the respiratory and genital forms generally is 2-6 days. In the respiratory form, the animal may be depressed, anorectic, and have a fever of 104-108°F (40-42°C) and a nasal discharge and highly inflamed nares ("red nose"). Close examination demonstrates numerous papules or ulcers in the nasal mucosa. At this time, the animal may exhibit dyspnea, mouth breathing, and excess salivation. Many animals also exhibit conjunctivitis, and in mild cases, this may be the only evidence of BHV-1 infection. If concurrent bacterial infection does not occur, animals generally recover without treatment 4-5 days after peak temperature and respiratory signs occur.

Abortions occur regardless of the severity or form of the disease. Abortions can occur as late as 90 days after infection; thus, it may be difficult to relate them to BHV-1 infection, especially if the disease was mild or subclinical. Abortions generally occur in the second half of pregnancy. Early embryonic mortality and return to service also may occur.

In genital infections of cows, the first signs are frequent urination, elevation of the tailhead, and a mild vaginal discharge. The vulva is swollen, and small papules, then erosions and ulcers, are present on the mucosal surface. If secondary bacterial infections do not occur, animals recover in 10-14 days. If bacterial infection occurs, there may be inflammation of the uterus and transient infertility with purulent vaginal discharge for several weeks. In bulls, similar lesions occur on the penis and prepuce.

BHV-1 infection can be severe in young calves. Pyrexia, ocular and nasal discharges, respiratory distress, diarrhea, incoordination, and eventually convulsions and death may occur in a short period following generalized viral infection. A strain of BHV-1 has been isolated that can cause encephalitis in adults as well as in the young.

Lesions: The extent of lesions depends on the time at which an animal is examined following the primary infection as well as on the extent of secondary bacterial complications. In uncomplicated IBR infections, most lesions are restricted to the upper respiratory tract and trachea. Petechial to ecchymotic hemorrhages may be found in the mucous membranes of the nasal cavity and the paranasal sinuses. Focal areas of necrosis develop in the nose, pharynx, larynx, and trachea. The lesions may coalesce to form plaques.

The sinuses are often filled with a serous or serofibrinous exudate. As the disease progresses, the pharynx becomes covered with a serofibrinous exudate, and blood-tinged fluid may be found in the trachea. The pharyngeal and pulmonary lymph nodes may be acutely swollen and hemorrhagic. The tracheitis may extend into the bronchi and bronchioles and terminate in bronchopneumonia. When this occurs, epithelium is sloughed in the airways. The viral lesions are often camouflaged by secondary bacterial infections (*see* BOVINE RESPIRATORY DISEASE COMPLEX, above). In young animals with generalized BHV-1 infection, erosions and ulcers overlaid with debris may be found in the nose, esophagus, and forestomachs; and white foci may be found in the liver, kidney, spleen, and lymph nodes. In young calves suffering from encephalitis, the meninges are hyperemic only. Aborted fetuses may have pale, focal, necrotic lesions in all tissues. They are especially visible in the liver.

Diagnosis: Uncomplicated BHV-1 infections can be diagnosed on the characteristic signs and lesions. However, since the severity of disease can vary, it is best to differentiate BHV-1 from other viral infections by viral isolation. Samples should be taken early in the disease, and a diagnosis should be possible in 2-3 days. A rise in antibody titer also can be used to confirm a diagnosis, although a single sample, even if it has a high titer, is of little value. It is not possible to detect a rising antibody titer in abortions, since infection occurs a considerable time before abortion and titers are already maximal. BHV-1 abortion can be diagnosed by identifying characteristic lesions and demonstrating the virus in fetal tissues by FA and culture. Gross and microscopic lesions from animals shortly after death may help.

Treatment and Control: Immunization with modified live or killed virus vaccines generally provides adequate protection by reducing the severity of disease. Use of live vaccines is not without risk due to persistence of the virus and its potential for reactivation. Both IM and intranasal modified live vaccines are available, but the IM types may cause abortion. The intranasal vaccines are more highly attenuated and therefore recommended for use in breeding herds, including pregnant cows. The IM vaccines are easier to use and often are the vaccines of choice in feedlots. Breeding and replacement heifers and bulls should be immunized when 6-8 mo old, before breeding, and q1-2yr thereafter. Some recommend not vaccinating young bulls because they may be discriminated against when sold for breeding if they have titers. Feedlot cattle should be immunized 2-3 wk before entry into the feedlot. Antibiotics are of no value against the viral infection but may reduce secondary bacterial infections. Eradication of the virus is possible by serological testing and either culling reactors or running a strict 2-herd system.

TRACHEAL EDEMA SYNDROME OF FEEDER CATTLE
(Honker syndrome)

Extensive edema of the mucosa-submucosa in the dorsal membrane of the lower trachea, with attendant diarrhea and often obstructive asphyxiation. The syndrome occurs in feedlot cattle throughout the plains of the USA, during the last two-thirds of their feeding period.

The cause is unknown. To date, no infectious agents have been incriminated. While it occurs year-round, it is more common in the summer. There may be a relationship between dust in the air and rate/depth of breathing and incidence, but seldom are more than 1 or 2 animals involved on a given day or in one pen. There appears to be a subclinical state that can be triggered by movement and exercise.

Usually, the first sign is a loud guttural inspiratory sound even before any visual sign of distress. With time, and especially if the animal is moved, respiratory distress worsens, and the animal may become excited or belligerent. If the lesion is deep in the tracheal tree, little sound is produced and signs are largely visual. The animal becomes cyanotic, and typically collapses and dies in <24 hr.

Most often, the lesion extends from the midcervical region to the thoracic inlet; it may reach the tracheal bifurcation. Slight to moderate lesions have been seen in animals that appear normal at slaughter time. In fatal cases, the lesion is completely obstructive, and often accompanied by hemorrhage.

Differential diagnoses include tracheal abscesses, necrotic laryngitis, and other causes of thickening of the dorsal tracheal membrane—which are usually less obstructive.

Corticosteroids, if given early—before body temperature reaches 104°F (40°C)—and with a minimum of handling stress, can be lifesaving. Keeping the animal calm and cool is important. Penicillin at 10,000 u/lb (22,000 u/kg) body wt has been effective when given in time, but should not be used if salvage slaughter is anticipated within 1 mo. Response to diuretics has been poor, and that to antiprostaglandins not yet well evaluated.

RESPIRATORY DISEASES OF HORSES

INTRODUCTION

A number of viruses affect the equine respiratory tract, notably the influenza, herpes, rhino, and arteritis viruses. Adenovirus pneumonia has been reported in association with combined immunodeficiency in Arabian foals. The significance of parainfluenza and reoviruses is obscure. Equine herpesvirus type 1 (rhinopneumonitis) and influenza are commonly involved in clinical infections; however, frequent vaccination (q2-3mo) of many horses against the latter virus has dramatically reduced its incidence.

Viral respiratory infections usually produce pyrexia, nasal discharge, and frequently, a cough. Secondary bacterial infections, which produce a mucopurulent nasal discharge and exacerbate the cough, are not uncommon. Affected horses usually look "sick" and don't eat. Other signs include lymphadenitis, and sometimes, hematological or blood biochemical changes. Although culture of respiratory viruses from nasopharyngeal swabs or blood in acutely viremic horses is possible, viral infections are usually confirmed by serology.

Viral respiratory infections may affect all parts of the airway, including the paranasal sinuses and guttural pouches. Occasionally, lung abscessation, pneumonia, or pleurisy may develop; such complications are usually associated with stress, eg, travel or hard exercise.

Many bacteria and fungi can be isolated from the respiratory tract of normal horses. However, they may become opportunistic pathogens in certain situations, eg, following viral infection. *Streptococcus zooepidemicus* is probably the most common, although *Actinobacillus equuli, Bordetella bronchiseptica, Escherichia coli, Pasteurella* spp, and *Pseudomonas aeruginosa* have also been isolated. Isolation of *S equi* indicates strangles infection (*see* p 744). Recently *S pneumoniae* has been identified from racehorses with bronchiolitis.

Streptococcus spp are probably the most common organisms isolated from foals with pneumonia or pulmonary abscesses. However *Rhodococcus (Corynebacterium) equi* (*see* below) infection produces a severe pneumonia, and may be endemic on some stud farms. Mycoplasmas are of uncertain significance but were incriminated in one outbreak of pleurisy.

Bacterial pathogens may be identified by culture from a nasal swab but more satisfactorily from a nasopharyngeal swab or a tracheobronchial wash. The cause of respiratory infections is usually determined by a combination of history and clinical, endoscopic, radiological, and in some cases, ultrasonographic examinations. Hematological and blood biochemical investigations are also helpful in most respiratory infections.

Respiratory infections may predispose to irritant/allergic bronchiolitis if affected horses are exposed to pollution by stable dusts (eg, fungal spores—*see* COPD [HEAVES], below).

Vaccines of variable effectiveness are available for equine influenza, viral rhinopneumonitis, and strangles. General recommendations are impossible because of the various views of different national regulatory agencies and the rapid development of new vaccines. The cost and hazards of each vaccination must be weighed against the probability of exposure and potential losses in economic and sentimental value. The strength of arguments supporting vaccination increases with the probability of exposure.

In acute viral respiratory disease, affected horses are rested under dust-free stable conditions. Broad-spectrum antibacterials (eg, potentiated sulfonamides) may prevent secondary bacterial infection. If affected horses are exercised, more serious complications, eg, pleurisy, may develop. Antipyretic drugs can be used if pyrexia is severe.

If clinical signs persist, antibacterials (eg, penicillin, potentiated sulfonamide), perhaps combined with bronchodilators, may be given. A tracheal wash for culture and sensitivity testing should be collected in unresponsive cases or in a few selected individuals after a respiratory outbreak has occurred on a stud farm. Transtracheal washes should not be performed in animals undergoing treatment at the time. Biochemical analysis of blood may indicate a severe inflammatory problem such as bronchopneumonia, lung abscessation, or pleurisy. Radiography of the chest may help confirm the diagnosis and monitor progress following treatment. Ultrasonography may also be useful. In horses with pleural effusion, thoracocentesis and pleural drainage should be done from both sides of the chest. Dust- and ammonia-free stable management and rest for horses with severe lower respiratory diseases such as pneumonia, lung abscessation, or pleurisy are of great importance.

CHRONIC OBSTRUCTIVE PULMONARY DISEASE
(COPD, Heaves, Chronic alveolar emphysema)

A chronic, noninfectious respiratory disease of Equidae characterized by dyspnea, chronic coughing, nasal discharge, and lack of stamina.

Etiology: Although there is debate about the primary cause, the most commonly recognized cause is exposure to dust, molds, or other air pollutants. However, triggering factors may include respiratory tract infections or a hereditary predisposition. The condition is uncommon in horses <6 yr old.

Clinical Findings and Lesions: The disease usually is insidious in onset and progressive in nature. Many horses may be affected mildly or only during certain seasons. However, acute 'asthmatic" episodes are not uncommon. In most cases, respiratory distress occurs when the horse is stabled, particularly when it is exposed to dusty surroundings. The signs may be aggravated by exercise and feeding of certain roughages, particularly dusty or moldy hay. Expiration is labored. Contraction of the abdominal muscles over a long period may result in muscular hypertrophy and the formation of a ridge ("heave line") along the costal arch. In advanced cases, the nostrils are flared, and the anus may protrude if dyspnea is severe. Persistent, occasionally paroxysmal, coughing is usually a feature. This cough may be productive, and often occurs during feeding or exercise. A nasal discharge is common. High-pitched, end-expiratory rhonchi and rales are heard on thoracic auscultation in severe cases, but such sounds may be heard only after using a rebreathing bag.

Horses stabled on straw and fed dry hay frequently have subclinical bronchiolitis. In such cases, tracheal endoscopy reveals a mucopurulent exudate. However, many horses with a chronic cough and nasal discharge do not have adventitious lung sounds on thoracic auscultation.

The most consistent lesion is generalized bronchiolitis, but in severe chronic cases there may be emphysema with permanent structural changes in the alveolar walls and interstitial tissues.

Diagnosis: Differentiation from other causes of a chronic cough or nasal discharge (eg, parasitic bronchiolitis) is based on the history and other diagnostic procedures such as endoscopy, evaluation of a tracheobronchial exudate, and chest radiography. In its most subtle form, the only clinical sign may be hyperpnea at rest.

Treatment: Most horses improve dramatically if the respiratory environment is improved, eg, the horse is turned permanently out of doors, or all straw and hay is removed from the stable environment. Dust-free stable management involves the use of paper or wood chips for bedding, and feeding complete cubes, vacuum-packed grass, or even thoroughly soaked hay. Occasionally, affected horses may show clinical signs at grass, probably because of exposure to tree or grass pollens.

Awareness of the owner to the initiating cause is vital to successful management. Judicious use of bronchodilator and mucolytic drugs may speed recovery. Corticosteroids may also be useful in poorly responsive cases. In the small percentage of horses that improve only slightly, chronic pulmonary changes are probably irreversible. Affected horses should be kept dust-free for the rest of their lives.

EQUINE HERPESVIRUS 1 INFECTION
(Equine viral rhinopneumonitis, Equine abortion virus)

Etiology and Epidemiology: Equine herpesvirus 1 (EHV-1) comprises 2 genetically and antigenically distinct groups of viruses now commonly referred to as subtypes 1 and 2 of EHV-1, but until recently considered separate herpesviruses designated EHV-1 and EHV-4. EHV-1 is ubiquitous in horse populations throughout the world. Both subtypes produce acute febrile respiratory disease on primary infection, characterized by rhinopharyngitis and tracheobronchitis. Outbreaks of respiratory disease occur annually among foals in areas with concentrated horse populations; elsewhere episodes are sporadic. Most of these outbreaks in weanlings are caused by subtype 2 strains. The age, seasonal, and geographic distributions vary, and probably are determined by immune status and concentration of horses. In individuals, the outcome of exposure is determined by viral strain involved, immune status, pregnancy status, and possibly age. Infection of pregnant mares with subtype 2 strains rarely results in abortion.

Mares may abort several weeks to months after clinical disease or, in most instances, after subclinical infection with subtype 1 strains of EHV-1. A further infrequent clinical sequela of EHV-1 infection, which is caused solely by certain subtype 1 strains of the virus, is development of neurologic disease. The natural reservoir of

EHV-1 is the horse; there is increasing evidence of latent carriers of both virus subtypes. Transmission occurs by direct or indirect contact with infective nasal discharges, aborted fetuses, placentas, or placental fluids. Enzyme restriction analysis of EHV-1 has confirmed the existence of multiple, genetically distinct strains within both virus subtypes; these strains or electropherotypes co-circulate and may be the cause of outbreaks of respiratory disease, abortion, and in some instances, associated neurologic disease.

Clinical Findings: After an incubation period of 2-10 days, susceptible horses may develop any of the following signs: fever of 102-107°F (39-42°C) persisting for 1-7 days, neutropenia and lymphopenia, congestion and serous discharge from nasal mucosa and conjunctiva, malaise, pharyngitis, cough, inappetence, and sometimes edematous mandibular and/or retropharyngeal lymph nodes, or constipation followed by diarrhea. Horses infected with subtype 1 strains often develop a diphasic fever, with the viremia coinciding with the second temperature peak. Secondary bacterial infections are common, with resultant mucopurulent nasal exudate and coughing. The infection is mild or inapparent in horses previously exposed and immunologically sensitized to the virus.

Mares that abort after infection with EHV-1 seldom display any premonitory signs. Abortions occur 2-12 wk after infection, usually between months 7 and 11 of gestation. Aborted fetuses are fresh or minimally autolyzed, and the placenta is expelled shortly after abortion. There is no evidence of damage to the mare's reproductive tract, and subsequent conception is unimpaired.

Mares exposed late in gestation may not abort, but give birth to live foals with a fulminating viral pneumonitis; these are very susceptible to secondary bacterial infections and usually die within hours or days. Infrequently, EHV-1 has been associated with development of herpetic lesions on the external genitalia of mares.

Some animals in certain outbreaks of EHV-1 infection develop neurologic disease of varying clinical severity (*see also* p 593). Depending on the location and extent of the lesions, signs vary from mild incoordination and posterior paresis to severe posterior paralysis with recumbency, loss of bladder and tail function, and loss of sensation to the skin in the perineal and inguinal areas, and even the hindlimbs. In exceptional cases, the paralysis may be progressive and culminate in quadriplegia and death. Prognosis depends on severity of signs and the period of recumbency. Although EHV-1-associated neurologic disease is seen most frequently in mares shortly after foaling during outbreaks of abortion, it can also occur in barren mares, stallions, geldings, and foals after an outbreak of EHV-1 respiratory infection. Myeloencephalitis with recovery of the virus has been reported in certain cases. It has not been established whether neuritis of the cauda equina is a sequela of EHV-1 infection.

Lesions: There are significant differences in pathogenetic mechanisms between the 2 subtypes of EHV-1: subtype 2 infections are restricted to respiratory tract epithelium and associated lymph nodes; subtype 1 strains also have a predilection for vascular endothelium, especially in the nasal mucosa, lungs, adrenal, thyroid, and CNS. Of additional significance is the leukocyte-associated viremia that occurs in subtype 1 infections, which may result in abortion or neurologic disease.

Gross lesions of viral rhinopneumonitis are hyperemia and ulceration or necrosis of the respiratory epithelium, and multiple, tiny, plum-colored foci in the lungs. Histologically, there is evidence of inflammation, necrosis, and intranuclear inclusions in the respiratory tract epithelium and in the germinal centers of the associated lymph nodes. Lung lesions are characterized by neutrophilic infiltration of the terminal bronchioles, peribronchiolar and perivascular mononuclear cell infiltration, and serofibrinous exudate in the alveoli.

Typical lesions in EHV-1 abortions include interlobular lung edema with excessive fluid in the thoracic cavity; multifocal areas of necrosis in the liver; petechiation in the myocardium, the adrenal, and beneath the splenic capsule; lymphoid hyperplasia of the spleen; and thymic necrosis. Intranuclear inclusions are found in lung, liver, adrenal, and lymphoreticular tissues.

Horses with EHV-1-associated neurologic disease may have no gross lesions, or only minimal evidence of hemorrhage in the meninges, brain, and spinal cord parenchyma. Histologically, lesions are discrete and comprise vasculitis with endothelial cell damage and perivascular cuffing, thrombus formation and hemorrhage, and in advanced cases, areas of malacia. Lesions may be at any level of the brain or spinal cord.

Diagnosis: Equine viral rhinopneumonitis cannot be differentiated from equine influenza (*see* below), equine viral arteritis (qv, p 376), or certain other equine respiratory infections solely on the basis of clinical signs. Confirmation can be achieved by virus isolation, preferably from nasopharyngeal swabs and citrated blood samples taken very early in the course of the infection and by serological testing of acute and convalescent sera.

In cases of suspect EHV-1 abortion, a diagnosis is based on characteristic gross and microscopic lesions in the aborted fetus, virus isolation, and demonstration of viral antigen in fetal tissues. Lung, liver, adrenal, and lymphoreticular tissues are productive sources of virus. Serological testing of aborting mares has little diagnostic value (*see also* abortion in horses, p 1142).

Although subtype 1 strains of virus have been isolated from certain cases of EHV-1-associated neurologic disease, and homologous neutralizing antibody on occasion has been found in CSF of affected animals, this is uncommon, and diagnosis depends on demonstration of the characteristic vascular lesions in sections of CNS tissue.

Treatment: There is no specific treatment. Rest during the acute febrile phase of respiratory disease caused by EHV-1, and several days thereafter, is indicated to minimize secondary bacterial complications. Antipyretics are recommended for horses with a fever of ≥105°F (40.5°C). Antibiotic therapy should be instituted at the first sign of purulent nasal discharges or pulmonary involvement. Most foals infected prenatally with EHV-1 succumb shortly after birth despite intensive nursing and antimicrobial medication. If animals with EHV-1-associated neurologic disease are nonrecumbent, or recumbent for only 2-3 days, the prognosis is usually favorable. Intensive nursing care is necessary to avoid pulmonary congestion, pneumonia, ruptured bladder, or bowel atony. Recovery may be complete, but a small percentage of cases have neurological sequelae.

Control: Immunity following natural infection with either subtype of EHV-1 appears to involve a combination of both humoral and cellular immune factors. While little cross-immunity occurs between the 2 subtypes after primary infection of the respiratory tract of immunologically naive foals, significant cross-protection develops in horses after repeated infections with a particular virus subtype. Immunity to reinfection of the respiratory tract may persist for up to 3 mo, but multiple infections result in a level of immunity that prevents clinical signs of respiratory disease. Immunity to infection that leads to abortion seems to be related to the level of resistance at the pharyngeal lymphatic ring. Diminished resistance may lead to development of a leukocyte-associated viremia, which in turn may result in transplacental infection of the fetus.

Recommended management practices for the prevention and control of EHV-1-related diseases include: 1) Avoid introducing the virus into a susceptible group of horses from an exogenous source. Horses arriving on a farm from other farms or sales or returning from the racetrack should be isolated for 3-4 wk before commingling with resident horses, especially with pregnant mares. 2) Reduce management-related stress-producing circumstances, and the possibility of stress-induced reactivation of latent EHV-1 in carrier animals. 3) Segregate horses on breeding farms or at racetracks into small separate groups. This is especially relevant with respect to pregnant mares, which if possible should be maintained in a group away from weanlings, yearlings, and horses out-of-training. In an outbreak of respiratory disease or abortion, affected animals should be isolated, appropriate sanitary measures taken, and no horse should leave the premises for 3 wk after recovery of the last clinical case. On small farms where close contact has already occurred, attempted isolation of affected animals may be considered pointless.

Parenterally administered modified live vaccines are licensed in some countries but banned in others. An inactivated vaccine is the only product currently recommended by the manufacturer as an aid in prevention of EHV-1 abortion. It should be administered during months 5, 7, and 9 of pregnancy. Immunity produced by available vaccines persists for only 2-4 mo. To maximize its effectiveness against respiratory disease, vaccination should commence when foals are 3-4 mo old, and depending on the vaccine used, a second dose given 4-8 wk later. Booster vaccinations may be indicated as often as q2-3mo through maturity. Vaccination programs against EHV-1 should not be limited to pregnant mares, but include all horses on a premises. Such programs should not engender a false sense of security; vaccination against this infection is not a substitute for sound management practices.

INFECTION BY OTHER HERPESVIRUSES

Equine herpesvirus 2 (EHV-2) is ubiquitous on the respiratory mucosa, conjunctivae, and in the WBC of normal horses as well as those affected with a diversity of diseases. It is present in horses of all ages. Its pathogenic significance remains obscure. It has been suggested that EHV-2 is the cause of herpetic keratoconjunctivitis. Equine herpesvirus 3 (EHV-3) is the cause of the equine coital exanthema (qv, p 684), a benign, progenital exanthematous disease.

EQUINE INFLUENZA

An acute, highly contagious, febrile respiratory disease.

Etiology and Epidemiology: Two immunologically distinct influenza viruses have been found in horse populations worldwide except in Australia and New Zealand. Orthomyxovirus A/Equi-1, although probably present for decades, has not been isolated anywhere since 1980; orthomyxovirus A/Equi-2 was first recognized in 1963 as a cause of widespread epidemics, following which the virus has become endemic in many countries. Endemicity is maintained by sporadic clinical cases, and by mild or inapparent infection in susceptible horses that are constantly introduced into the population by birth, through waning immunity, or after movement from other areas or countries. It is not known if a carrier state exists. The clinical outcome following viral exposure largely depends on immunological conditioning; in susceptible animals this may vary from a mild, inapparent infection to severe disease that is rarely fatal except in young, old, or otherwise debilitated horses and in donkeys. Transmission occurs by the respiratory route through contact with infective respiratory secretions. Epidemics arise when one or more acutely infected horses are introduced into a susceptible group assembled for show, sale, training, or racing. The epidemiologic outcome depends on the antigenic characteristics of the circulating virus and the immune status of a given population of horses at time of exposure to, and possible infection with, that virus. Frequent natural exposure or regular vaccinations may have contributed to the degree of antigenic drift that has occurred with certain strains of A/Equi-2 virus in some parts of the world. Should new mutants of the virus arise with antigenicity that differs significantly from strains in current circulation, then widespread outbreaks of disease can be expected.

Clinical Findings and Lesions: The incubation period is usually 1-3 days, but ranges from 18 hr to 5 or, rarely, 7 days. Onset is abrupt, with fever up to 107.5°F (42°C), usually lasting <3 days in uncomplicated infections. Coughing, usually dry, harsh, and nonproductive, is a significant feature; it is observed early in the course of the disease and may persist for several weeks, especially if bacterial infection supervenes. Nasal discharge, though scant and serous initially, usually becomes profuse and mucopurulent later in the presence of a superimposed streptococcal infection. Depression, anorexia, and weakness are frequent. Lacrimal discharge, enlargement of the lymph nodes in the head, limb edema, stiffness, laminitis, expiratory dyspnea, and pneumonia are sometimes present. Mildly affected horses recover uneventfully in 2-3 wk; severely affected animals may convalesce for up to 6 mo. Recovery from the cough and incapacitating sequelae of the disease are hastened by complete restriction of strenuous physical activity.

The risk of complications caused by secondary bacterial infections, eg, pneumonia, pleurisy, chronic bronchitis, and COPD (heaves), are minimized by restricting exercise, controlling dust, providing superior ventilation, and practicing good stable hygiene.

Lesions usually are not observed, but interstitial pneumonia, pleurisy, bronchitis, peribronchitis, perivasculitis, and interstitial myocarditis may be seen in fatal cases.

Diagnosis: Laboratory assistance is often required to differentiate influenza from equine viral rhinopneumonitis, equine viral arteritis, and other respiratory infections. However, occurrence of a rapidly spreading respiratory infection in a group of horses, characterized by rapid onset, high fever, depression, weakness, and widespread coughing is usually sufficient to make a presumptive diagnosis of equine influenza. Confirmation is based on virus isolation and/or serology of acute and convalescent sera. Nasopharyngeal swabs are the clinical specimens of choice for attempted virus isolation; they should be taken as soon as possible after the onset of illness.

Treatment and Control: Horses without complications require only rest and good nursing. Antipyretics are recommended for horses with a fever of ≥105°F (40.5°C). Antibiotics are indicated when fever persists beyond 3-4 days, or when purulent nasal discharges or pulmonary involvement are present. Rest should be complete and for a sufficient time after cessation of clinical signs to prevent long-term lung or myocardial damage.

Control requires sound management and use of an inactivated adjuvanted vaccine that contains both A/Equi-1 and A/Equi-2 viruses. The likelihood of exposure to infection can be reduced by isolation of any horses newly introduced into a stable or other group of horses, and by minimizing contact with other horses. Racing and other equine authorities require that horses be given 2 vaccinations, not <3 wk or >3 mo apart, followed by an initial booster 6 mo later, and annually thereafter. In view of the limited duration of protection provided by current vaccines, booster injections probably should be administered more often, eg, q3-6mo. Available vaccines need to be monitored continuously for strain content to reflect as closely as possible the antigenicity of current field virus strains.

EXERCISE-INDUCED PULMONARY HEMORRHAGE
(EIPH, Epistaxis, "Bleeder")

Blood in the tracheobronchial airways during or after exercise. Hemorrhage is believed to occur from the bronchial arterial circulation. The lungs have extensive bronchiolitis in the dorsal regions of the caudal lobe with concurrent bronchial arterial neovascularization, interstitial fibrosis, and sequestration of macrophages containing hemosiderin (hemosiderophages).

Etiology: Although several mechanisms have been proposed, the definitive cause is not known. One theory is that small airway disease, probably a consequence of inhaled particulate matter and previous respiratory disease, predisposes lung regions to abnormal mechanical stresses, especially during severe exertion. These abnormal stresses are believed to occur because the equine lung has poor collateral ventilation, and lung segments with diseased small airways do not inflate uniformly. Shear stresses at the interface between slow and normally expanding lung segments result in disruption of lung tissue with subsequent hemorrhage. Bronchial arterial neovascularization of the diseased segments occurs as part of the repair response, and it is thought that subsequent bleeding probably occurs from these vessels. It is likely that this process occurs each time the horse is exercised strenuously.

There are no apparent geographic differences in the prevalence of EIPH, and ~30% of Standardbreds and >75% of racing Thoroughbreds, Quarter Horses, and

Appaloosas have evidence of EIPH after strenuous exertion. It also has been reported in horses used for jumping, barrel racing, roping, and polo, but does not occur often in horses used for endurance riding. Although EIPH has been recognized after trotting, it is associated more commonly with speeds >14 m/sec, or short periods of strenuous exercise. The absence of EIPH in horses undergoing prolonged low-intensity exercise, and its occurrence in horses after vigorous exercise, supports the premise that the hemorrhage is a consequence of the increased pressures applied to the pulmonary vascular circulation.

Diagnosis: Endoscopic observation of blood in the airways after exercise provides definitive evidence of EIPH. Other sources of hemorrhage in the upper airway, particularly guttural pouch mycosis (*see* below) and ethmoidal hematoma, must be excluded during endoscopy, which is usually recommended within 60-90 min after exercise. If EIPH is suspected and the horse cannot be examined after exercise, cytological examination of a tracheobronchial aspirate for hemosiderophages is considered diagnostic. Stains that highlight iron-containing pigments facilitate recognition of these cells. Abnormalities in the hemogram or in hemostasis have not been noted.

Treatment and Control: Treatment of horses with severe pulmonary hemorrhage is generally ineffective, while those with mild hemorrhage may not require therapy. Efforts should be directed toward symptomatic treatment of any recognized respiratory disease, improvements in stable ventilation, appropriate training and fitness, and adequate convalescence after viral or bacterial respiratory infection. The drug used most in control attempts is furosemide. Other medications used for prevention include conjugated estrogens, vitamin K, and vitamin C. Oral products that have been used (also with variable results) include the bioflavinoid product hesperidan, as well as oral vitamins C and K.

GUTTURAL POUCH DISEASE

EMPYEMA

An accumulation of pus that may develop secondary to upper respiratory tract infections in horses, especially those caused by streptococci, or as a complication of other guttural pouch diseases. Bacterial infection in one or both pouches produces an intermittent nasal discharge, painful swelling in the parotid area, and in severe cases, stiff head carriage and stertorous breathing. Body temperature is elevated, and depression and anorexia occur often. Diagnosis can be made by endoscopy of the pharynx and affected guttural pouch, and radiographs can demonstrate partial obliteration of the normal guttural pouch contour by accumulated fluid.

Treatment with antibiotics alone is frequently unsuccessful, although a course of penicillin therapy combined with daily lavage of the guttural pouches with a nonirritating solution usually is effective. Refractory cases require surgical drainage, and surgery is the treatment of choice in those rare cases in which the purulent material becomes inspissated and forms "chondroids". Congenital tympany of the guttural pouch may develop empyema. Surgery is the only treatment.

GUTTURAL POUCH MYCOSIS

A localized or diffuse fungal invasion on the roof of the guttural pouch, usually by *Aspergillus* spp (*see also* p 341). Other fungal organisms and bacteria also can be isolated; however, the true cause of this disease and the role of fungi remain unknown. A variety of clinical signs arises from damage to the cranial nerves and the arteries contained within the mucosal lining of the guttural pouch. The most common sign is epistaxis, due to fungal erosion of the wall of either the internal carotid artery or branches of the external carotid artery. Hemorrhage is usually spontaneous and severe, and repeated bouts may precede a fatal episode. Dysphagia, Horner's syndrome, laryngeal hemiplegia, and dorsal displacement of the soft palate may develop in response to fungal damage to the cranial and sympathetic nerves in the affected guttural pouch. If dysphagia develops, the prognosis is poor. Diagnosis can be made by endoscopy. Solutions containing an antifungal agent should be delivered directly to the affected tissues by infusion through the biopsy channel of an endoscope. Surgical removal of the lesion is effective but not recommended unless the affected arteries are occluded. Hemorrhage can be prevented by occluding the affected arteries along their course through the guttural pouch by means of balloon-tipped catheters. Oral and systemic antifungal agents generally are not recommended because of the expense and potential toxic effects.

GUTTURAL POUCH TYMPANY

Tympany develops shortly after birth, more commonly in fillies than in colts, but also may be evident in horses up to 1 yr old. The affected pouch becomes distended with air and forms a characteristic nonpainful, elastic swelling in the parotid region. Breathing may become stertorous in severe cases; however, most affected foals appear normal. The cause is unknown, although a defect in the pharyngeal orifice of the eustachian tube may allow air to enter the affected guttural pouch but prevent its return into the pharynx. Diagnosis is usually based on the clinical signs and age of the affected animal. Severe cases may develop a secondary empyema, which can complicate the clinical manifestation. The condition is usually unilateral, but bilateral cases have been reported. The treatment of choice is fenestration of the membrane that separates the affected guttural pouch from the normal one; this provides a route for air in the abnormal guttural pouch to pass to the normal side and be expelled into the pharynx. The prognosis following surgery is good.

LARYNGEAL HEMIPLEGIA
(Roaring, Recurrent laryngeal neuropathy)

A permanent paresis or paralysis of the left arytenoid cartilage and vocal fold, manifest clinically by exercise intolerance and abnormal respiratory noise, primarily inspiratory stridor (whistling or roaring), during exercise. Right-sided and bilateral involvement (laryngeal paraplegia) are uncommon.

Etiology and Pathogenesis: This is a distal axonopathy, usually congenital (and likely heritable), that affects the recurrent laryngeal nerves, and possibly the peroneal nerves and long fibers of the CNS. The cause of the axonal degeneration is unknown. Progressive loss of the large myelinated fibers in the distal portion of the recurrent laryngeal nerves results in neurogenic atrophy of the intrinsic laryngeal muscles, except for the cricothyroid muscle, which is innervated by the cranial laryngeal nerve. Initially, the adductor muscles, notably the lateral cricoarytenoid muscle, are affected, and clinical signs become evident with involvement of the principal abductor, the dorsal cricoarytenoid muscle. The left recurrent nerve is thought to be involved more commonly because of its longer length, and the initial involvement of the lateral cricoarytenoid muscle because of the larger fibers distributed to this muscle. Less common causes include direct trauma to the vagus or recurrent laryngeal nerve, accidental perivascular injection of irritating substances, and plant (*Cicer arietinum* [chick peas] and *Lathyrus* spp) and chemical (lead, organophosphate) intoxications.

Although all breeds can be affected, there appears to be a higher prevalence in larger breeds, and in males and larger horses within a breed. Estimates of the prevalence in Thoroughbreds are 2-95% depending on the diagnostic criteria.

Loss of neuromuscular control of the abductor muscle results in collapse of the associated arytenoid cartilage and vocal fold, which reduces the glottal cross-sectional area. The increased impedance to flow necessitates greater effort by the accessory muscles of respiration to maintain the airflow necessary for gas exchange. Because of the pliable nature of the glottis, the exaggerated collapsing forces result in further collapse of the arytenoid cartilage and exacerbation of the impedance to airflow. During strenuous exercise, the affected side collapses completely so that the left arytenoid cartilage is drawn across the midline until it abuts the abducted normal arytenoid, effectively occluding the airway (dynamic collapse). The characteristic inspiratory whistle results from resonance within the open ventricle on the affected side. The harsher stridor, or roar, is produced by vortex shedding from the edges of the arytenoid cartilage and vocal fold.

Clinical Findings and Diagnosis: Affected horses are usually asymptomatic at rest. Abnormal respiratory noise during exercise, and exercise intolerance are the principal clinical signs. Diagnosis is confirmed by endoscopic observation of abnormal motion of the arytenoid cartilage and vocal fold. With laryngeal hemiplegia, the arytenoid cartilage and vocal fold are located in a median position within the laryngeal lumen and are immobile. Incomplete abduction, or early adduction after complete abduction are considered diagnostic of laryngeal hemiparesis. Asynchronous movements of the laryngeal cartilages occur commonly; their relationship to recurrent laryngeal neuropathy remains controversial. Horses with laryngeal asynchrony, exercise intolerance, and abnormal respiratory noise during exercise should have their laryngeal function examined immediately after strenuous exercise, or preferably during treadmill exercise, in an effort to confirm laryngeal dysfunction.

Other physical tests, such as laryngeal palpation, the arytenoid depression test, the laryngeal adductory reflex (slap test), and observation of arytenoid movement during swallowing and nasal occlusion, are useful aids but do not provide definitive evidence of laryngeal hemiplegia.

Differential diagnoses include other causes of upper airway obstruction and exercise intolerance. Arytenoid chondropathy (chondritis) is the only other disorder of the arytenoid cartilages that may be confused with laryngeal hemiplegia on endoscopy. Misdiagnosis can be avoided by careful observation of the shape and size of the arytenoid cartilages—in arytenoid chondropathy, they thicken transversely and lose their characteristic "bean" shape. Abduction and adduction are usually limited, and often the margin of the palatopharyngeal arch is evident on the affected side. With progression, the axial (medial) surface of the arytenoid cartilage may be distorted with granulation tissue protruding through the mucosa, and a contact lesion may be present on the contralateral arytenoid cartilage. Differentiating between the conditions is usually difficult only when thickening of the arytenoid cartilage is minimal, or if both arytenoid cartilages are affected similarly. Arytenoid chondropathy should always be considered if motility of the right arytenoid is reduced. Radiographs usually show small foci of mineralization within the arytenoid in cases of chondropathy.

Treatment: Recurrent laryngeal neuropathy is incurable; current "treatments" are intended to stabilize the affected side of the larynx during inspiration, and thus prevent dynamic collapse of the airway during exercise. Laryngeal ventriculectomy is helpful in affected horses not normally used for strenuous exercise. Prosthetic laryngoplasty is commonly used in racing horses, and is the only technique that satisfactorily reduces the impedance to inspiratory flow. Although complications such as coughing or nasal reflux of ingesta occasionally develop, the risks of prosthetic laryngoplasty are justified in horses that cannot otherwise be effective athletes. Subtotal arytenoidectomy is of limited value.

PLEURISY
(Pleuritis, Pleuropneumonia)

Acute or chronic inflammation of the pleural membranes, characterized by signs related to pleural pain and pleural effusion.

Etiology and Pathogenesis: Pleural effusion can be idiopathic but usually is associated with pneumonia, lung abscess, penetrating thoracic wounds, esophageal rupture, neoplasia, or peritonitis. In North America, pleuropneumonia is the most common cause of pleural effusion, especially in racing horses. Stress associated with transportation, exercise, surgery and anesthesia, and recent viral respiratory infection are considered to be important predisposing factors.

Microbes can be isolated in ~2 of 3 horses with parapneumonic pleural effusion. Typical organisms include *Streptococcus zooepidemicus, Escherichia coli, Pasteurella* spp, *Klebsiella* spp, *Rhodococcus (Corynebacterium) equi*, and anaerobes such as *Bacteroides* and *Clostridium* spp. *Mycoplasma felis* and other *Mycoplasma* spp also have been isolated. In certain dry dusty regions, lung infections with *Coccidioides immitis* and *Nocardia* spp have been associated with pleural effusion.

Clinical Findings and Diagnosis: Early signs include fever, inappetence, depression, dyspnea, standing with abducted elbows and reluctance to move, and subcut. edema of the ventral thorax and limbs. A flinching response to thoracic percussion indicates pleural pain. Often, horses with pleurisy appear to have colic. In chronic cases, there is often anorexia, weight loss, intermittent fever, abnormal respiratory effort, and in horses with sterile or neoplastic effusion, reduced exercise tolerance.

Definitive diagnosis requires detection of pleural effusion and collection of pleural fluid samples for gross and cytological evaluation, Gram's stain, and culture. Cytologic examination allows differentiation of infectious from neoplastic and other noninfectious causes of pleural effusion. If fluid is present in both pleural cavities, samples should be evaluated from both sites as it is not uncommon for the fluid character and microorganisms to be different. Since about one-third of horses with pleuropneumonia have sterile pleural effusion, concurrent collection of a transtracheal aspirate for cytology and culture for anaerobic organisms (including *Mycoplasma* spp) in addition to aerobic organisms is recommended. A foul odor to the breath or pleural fluid is strongly suggestive of anaerobic infection.

Ultrasonography is useful to estimate the quantity of pleural fluid and to ascertain the degree of loculation. Gas bubbles within the fluid are indicative of anaerobic infection. Radiography is of limited value until the pleural cavity is drained. Radiographs often confirm coexisting pulmonary pathology, and are useful for monitoring the resolution of pneumonic lesions after the effusion has resolved.

Hematologic findings are relatively nonspecific and usually indicate inflammation or infection. Anticipated changes include hyperfibrinogenemia, mild anemia, neutrophilic leukocytosis, hyperproteinemia, hypoalbuminemia, and hyperglobulinemia.

Auscultation and percussion of the thorax are useful for monitoring resolution of the effusion and changes in lung aeration. With lung consolidation and pleural effusion, cardiac sounds usually can be detected over a larger region of the thorax, particularly dorsally and caudally. Abnormal lung sounds include complete absence of air movement, inspiratory wheezes and crackles, friction rubs, and musical sounds. Careful auscultation with and without the aid of a rebreathing bag, combined with outlining regions of abnormal sound and fluid levels on the chest wall, are important for monitoring progression of the disease.

Treatment: Drainage of the pleural cavities combined with antibiotics, anti-inflammatories, analgesics, and supportive nursing care are important. Broad-spectrum antimicrobial therapy (penicillin and gentamicin) should be used initially, and changed if culture results indicate more appropriate antibiotics. Tetracycline is indicated for *Mycoplasma* spp infection, and metronidazole may be required for some anaerobic infections. The pleural space can be drained by intermittent thoracentesis as fluid reaccumulates, or by continuous drainage with tube thoracostomy and a one-way Heimlich chest drain valve or an underwater seal. Open chest drainage is indicated when the fluid is too viscous to drain through a tube or if it is contained within a well-demarcated abscess cavity. Ultrasonographic guidance may be necessary for drainage of multiloculated regions.

Pleural effusion secondary to peritonitis requires identification and appropriate treatment of the cause of the peritonitis. Malignant pleural effusions are often refractory to treatment because the neoplastic process is usually advanced by the time signs become evident. Effusion secondary to esophageal perforation and rupture requires recognition and repair of the site of the esophageal defect. Extensive contamination of the mediastinal space with feed material often precludes successful repair. Penetrating thoracic wounds should be debrided vigorously and repaired.

Lavage of the affected hemithorax, aspiration of the pneumothorax, and broad-spectrum antimicrobial therapy are important to minimize empyema.

With early recognition and appropriate treatment, recovery can be expected in ≥50% of horses with parapneumonic pleural effusion; return to comparable levels of activity occurs in ~50% of the survivors. Prognosis is guarded to poor for those with pleural effusion secondary to neoplasia or esophageal rupture.

RHODOCOCCUS EQUI LUNG ABSCESSATION IN FOALS
(Granulomatous pneumonia)

A worldwide, infectious disease of foals, acquired by inhalation of dust from soil contaminated with the causative organism, and characterized by bronchopneumonia and lung abscessation.

Etiology and Pathogenesis: The causal bacterium, *Rhodococcus (Corynebacterium) equi*, is a gram-positive, pleomorphic, aerobic, nonsporeforming, encapsulated rod. It affects primarily 2- to 6-mo-old foals; horses >6 mo old are resistant unless immunocompromised. It has been associated with diarrhea and abortion in horses, and with various suppurative lesions in several other hosts, including cattle, sheep, goats, cats, and man.

The bacterium is a soil saprophyte; its growth is considerably enhanced by constituents of herbivore manure, such as acetic acid, and high temperatures. Under ideal conditions, eg, high summer heat, it may multiply thousands of times in soil. In addition, the organism will grow to large numbers in the intestine of foals <12 wk old, but its presence in the feces of older horses represents pasture acquisition. It resists sunlight and dessication, and is relatively resistant to most disinfectants. Thus, over the years, infection may progressively build up on breeding farms that have large numbers of foals or allow manure to accumulate in the immediate environment.

Inhalation of contaminated dust results in a cranioventral distribution of lung abscesses, which may be more extensive in the right lung than in the left. Granulomatous enteritis and lymphadenitis may follow swallowing of infected sputum. In rare cases, enteritis without pneumonic change may occur.

Rhodococcus equi is an opportunistic pathogen; it affects foals when maternal antibody levels decline and their own immune system is immature. Animals with a compromised immune system (ie, combined immunodeficiency, qv, p 435) are at high risk of infection. There may also be a genetic predisposition to disease, particularly in Arabians. The mechanism of pathogenicity remains unknown but relates to the ability of the organism to survive within and eventually destroy alveolar macrophages of young foals. The severity of the disease process appears to be related to the number of organisms inhaled into the lungs. Most foals appear to encounter and successfully resist small numbers of *R equi* early in life.

Clinical Findings: The disease process begins with increased diffuse bronchial sounds, often accompanied by a cough. This develops into wheezes, which may be localized to a small area of the lungs (most often the anteroventral area), in some cases unilaterally. Pyrexia (>102°F [39°C]) follows over the next few days, with an increased respiratory rate (>40/min) and abdominal "tucking" on inspiration. Bronchovesicular sounds are increased over the large airways, and wheezing occurs over the small airways. Untreated foals develop progressive crackles that can be heard over the entire lung field, often accompanied by stridor. Coughing becomes more severe and intense. Foals commonly remain bright, alert, and vigorous, despite severe lung involvement, often until in the late stages of the disease. Neutrophilic leukocytosis, monocytosis, and marked fibrinogenemia occur. Mucopurulent nasal discharge is common, but lymphadenopathy of the throat region is absent. Eventually, the untreated foal may become cyanotic and collapse. There may be severe respiratory embarrassment and fever up to 106°F (41°C) when the lungs are extensively abscessed and consolidated. On farms where the infection is endemic, morbidity may be 90% and mortality in untreated animals as high. Where the disease is not endemic, foals probably often experience subclinical pneumonia, with perhaps development of a solitary small abscess in the lungs as the only manifestation of disease. In some cases, *R equi* causes severe diarrhea, due to granulomatous colitis and mesenteric lymphadenitis from swallowing infected sputum. Terminally, foals may become bacteremic and develop osteomyelitis or hypopyon.

Lesions: Typical gross lesions include bronchopneumonia with generalized irregular distribution of abscesses that are 0.3-6 cm in diameter and may be caseous. The pulmonary parenchyma is often consolidated, and there is mucopurulent exudate in some airways. Abscessation of regional lymph nodes is common. Histologically, the lesions are pyogranulomatous and contain thick, caseous material and a core of necrotic debris that is surrounded by numerous macrophages and neutrophils containing intact bacteria.

Diagnosis: The optimal method is by positive culture of transtracheal bronchoalveolar aspirates, but false negative results may occur. Thoracic auscultation may be of limited value early in the course of the disease since airway involvement may not be fully evident. Radiographic lesions of a prominent alveolar pattern characterized by ill-defined regional consolidation is typical; such consolidated lesions are often nodular or cavitary. Mediastinal lymphadenopathy is evident radiographically in advanced cases. In suspected cases, initiation of therapy should be based on radiographic evidence of granulomatous pulmonary disease and clinical signs. Diagnostic serological tests have been described but are not readily available. Quantitative fecal culture, demonstrating $>10^6$ *R equi*/g of feces, using selective media may be useful.

Treatment and Control: Systemic antimicrobial therapy should be instituted at once and maintained for 4-10 wk. The antibiotic combination of choice is erythromycin estolate or ethylsuccinate at 25 mg/kg body wt, PO, t.i.d. with rifampin at 10 mg/kg, PO, once daily. This synergistic combination has had excellent clinical results, probably because both drugs are lipid soluble and penetrate phagocytes well. Most foals recover with early treatment. Alternative drugs include trimethoprim (6.6 mg/kg, PO, t.i.d.) in fixed combination with sulfamethoxazole, and sodium ampicillin (11-15 mg/kg, IM, q.i.d.) in combination with gentamicin (2.2 mg/kg, IM, t.i.d.). The latter drug should not be used for >7 days without monitoring for nephrotoxicosis. Response to treatment is evaluated on radiographic evidence of resolution and the return of plasma fibrinogen concentration to normal levels.

Dehydrated animals should be given a balanced polyionic solution (eg, lactated Ringer's) IV. Fever may be controlled with dipyrone, 22 mg/kg; phenylbutazone, 0.5-1 mg/kg; or flunixin meglumine, 0.5-1 mg/kg. Optimal ventilation should be provided and exercise restricted.

To prevent buildup of *R equi* in the environment of young foals, manure should be removed. Loafing paddocks for young foals and their dams should be grassed and rotated. Dusty conditions within stables should be prevented, eg, by concreting walkways and damping them down. Foals should be moved away from heavily infected environments as soon as possible; on endemically affected farms, foals should be examined (temperature, respiratory rate, auscultation of lung fields) every 2-3 days during their first 4 mo, and all with suspected disease treated. By this means, mortality can be prevented, but only good husbandry will reduce the level of infection.

No commercial vaccines are available. Antibody appears to have a protective effect and, in severe cases, administration of serum (500 mL to 1 L) obtained from the mare may be beneficial. Vaccination against debilitating viral agents (eg, equine herpesvirus 1 and equine influenza virus) and routine parasite control programs should be instituted.

STRANGLES
(Distemper)

An infectious, transmissible, worldwide disease of Equidae, characterized by inflammation of the upper respiratory tract and most often by abscessation of the adjacent lymph nodes.

Etiology and Pathogenesis: The causal agent, *Streptococcus equi*, is a gram-positive, capsulated, β-hemolytic, Lancefield group C coccus that forms chains. A single antigenic type has been recognized, but more than one strain may exist. It is transmitted through the purulent discharges of infected animals. It is susceptible to desiccation, sunlight, and disinfectants. Affected animals are infectious for ≥4 wk after onset. An atypical and endemic, but milder form of the classical disease is caused by a capsule-deficient variant of the bacterium. A chronic, convalescent carrier state exists. While primarily a disease of the young, animals of any age without previous infection or immunization may be affected.

Infection is by inhalation or ingestion, followed by invasion of upper respiratory and pharyngeal mucosa in which enzymes and toxins released by the organism induce inflammation. The organism then spreads to local lymph nodes, where it causes lymphadenitis and abscessation. Bacteremia may occur, which disseminates the organism to lymphoid tissues throughout the body. Local spread may cause guttural pouch inflammation and sinusitis. Production of specific antibodies (secretory IgA and IgG) by the nasopharyngeal mucosa, and maturation and drainage of the abscesses effect recovery. Immunity following recovery is not long lasting.

Clinical Findings: The incubation period is 3-6 days. Inappetence and fever up to 106°F (41°C) are the first signs. Inflammation of the upper respiratory mucosa and lymphoid tissue of the pharynx occurs within 1-2 days, which makes swallowing painful. A serous or mucopurulent bilateral nasal discharge and, sometimes, ocular discharge follow. Lymphadenopathy is the major clinical finding. The infection spreads to the intermandibular and parapharyngeal lymph nodes, and often to the anterior cervical nodes. Abscessation of the nodes then occurs. The hemogram of infected horses is nonspecific, and shows neutrophilia with or without a left shift and hyperfibrinogenemia. The normal course of the disease is 10-14 days when the abscesses mature and drain.

Morbidity may approach 100% in a previously unexposed population, although mortality is <2%. Death may result from a CNS infection, pneumonia, abscessation of viscera, or asphyxiation due to compression of the pharynx or larynx. Myocarditis and pericarditis may occur. Equine purpura (qv, p 58) may accompany or follow the disease. Empyema of the guttural pouch (*see* above) occurs in a few animals either through primary diverticulitis or drainage of local lymph node abscesses into the pouch.

"Bastard strangles" is characterized by abscessation in other areas of the body, particularly of the lymph nodes in the abdomen and less frequently the thorax. Rupture of mesenteric or mediastinal abscesses causes purulent peritonitis and pleuritis. It occurs in animals that apparently fail to develop an immune response, or in those that have been treated with inadequate doses of penicillin during the course of the disease, thus modifying the bacterial cell wall antigens.

Diagnosis: When strangles occurs in epidemic form, its clinical features—high fever and the formation of abscesses in the lymph nodes of the head and pharyngeal region—are almost pathognomonic. Infection of the upper respiratory mucosa and lymph nodes by *S zooepidemicus* secondary to viral disease may mimic strangles, but the fever and characteristic rapid development of abscesses can differentiate the disease clinically. Definitive diagnosis depends on identification of *S equi*, preferably from pus obtained by surgical drainage of mature abscesses. Abscesses that drain naturally are rapidly invaded by *S zooepidemicus*, which may confuse bacteriological diagnosis. Identification of *S equi* from one horse (with or without typical signs of strangles) is reliable warning of the imminence of this disease in the herd.

Treatment: Complete rest and nursing care should be provided. Hot packs over the abscesses may speed their maturation; when mature, they should be incised and drained. Dysphagic animals should be provided with soft, moist, palatable feeds. Horses showing marked dyspnea and/or dysphagia may require a tracheostomy, feeding by stomach tube, and IV fluid therapy. The use of antimicrobials is controversial, although *S equi* is sensitive to penicillin, sulfamerazine, sulfamethazine, and trimethoprim-sulfadiazine. Penicillin or the sulfonamides are indicated in nursing foals, severe acute cases, and animals that require a tracheostomy. If antibiotic therapy is used, high doses of penicillin (25,000-100,000 IU/kg, IV, q.i.d.) for 7-10 days is recommended.

Prophylaxis: Animals to be added to a band of horses should be isolated for several weeks before mingling. Any nasal discharge that develops should be cultured for *S equi*. If positive, these animals should be isolated until free of infection. Stalls, water troughs, and tack and grooming utensils should be disinfected and left unused for ≥4 wk.

In the USA, 3 vaccines are currently available, although vaccination is of some benefit only in herds in which the disease is endemic. Vaccination frequently leads to an abscess at the injection site, and does not prevent infection but does result in milder disease in infected animals.

Because of the generally unsatisfactory results following vaccination with killed bacteria or their products, the current focus is on development of a stable avirulent strain of *S equi* that when administered intranasally will stimulate local mucosal immunity.

RESPIRATORY DISEASES OF PIGS

INTRODUCTION

Respiratory diseases of pigs can be classified into 2 broad categories based on the extent and duration of overt disease: those that affect large numbers of pigs and may be serious but of limited duration; and those that persist in a large portion of the pigs for indefinite periods. Those in category 1 can be very costly, but the losses are limited rather than ongoing. They include swine influenza (*see* below), hog cholera (qv, p 381), and pneumonic forms of pseudorabies (qv, p 617). The causal viruses may persist in a herd, but outbreaks of overt disease tend to be self-limiting. The most important syndromes in category 2 are atrophic rhinitis, mycoplasmal pneumonia, and pleuropneumonia (*see* below for all 3). Moderate levels of atrophic rhinitis, in which crooked snouts are not evident, are not too damaging. Enzootic pneumonia, when caused by mycoplasma alone, is of little consequence but when combined with secondary infections, eg, *Pasteurella multocida,* the resulting conditions may be severe. *Actinobacillus pleuropneumoniae* may be associated with considerable losses in some herds. Migrating worm larvae or the infections listed in group 1 often lead to severe problems when they occur with the infections in group 2.

The severity and economic importance of diseases in category 2 also are related to population density and to the type and size of herd. They may be of little importance in herds producing weaners for sale, but become of major importance in high-density feeder-pig units. Mortality from these diseases usually, though not always, is low. Economic damage results from an adverse and uneven effect on growth rate, an adverse effect on feed efficiency, and additional cost of drugs, particularly of feed medication. Although these costs are variable, they are serious because they are continuous. However, when stress can be avoided by proper management, these diseases may be present but cause only minimal losses.

It is possible to set up herds free of diseases in category 2 by techniques such as SPF repopulation or medicated early weaning, or by buying pigs from a pneumonia-free herd. The latter method is the least expensive, but since the etiology of diseases in category 2 is complex, all the pigs should be purchased from one source. (This is also true when purchasing weaners for feeder-pig units.)

It is difficult to keep herds free of respiratory diseases since most are transmitted by aerosol; they can be windborne over distances ≥2 miles, depending on climate, terrain, and density of pigs in the locality.

Closed herds, ie, buying in no living animals (using artifical insemination or embryo transfer to bring in new genetic material), help establish immunity to the present organisms and avoid introduction of new infections, strains, or serotypes. An "all-in/all-out" policy, in which the entire barn or air space is emptied before refilling, is a powerful tool in minimizing the potential effect of chronic pneumonia.

Respiratory disease is endemic in most herds. The main factors in control are stress management, stocking density, ventilation, temperature control, and freedom from mixing and moving. These, together with the "all-in/all-out" and closed-herd management practices greatly lessen or avoid the need for prophylactic and therapeutic medication.

ATROPHIC RHINITIS

A disease of pigs characterized by sneezing, followed by atrophy of the turbinate bones, which may be accompanied by distortion of the nasal septum, and shortening or twisting of the upper jaw.

Etiology: The etiology is complex and involves at least 2 organisms. Various infections, eg, inclusion body rhinitis and pseudorabies, and noninfectious agents may cause sneezing and tear-staining, usually without leading to atrophic rhinitis. *Bordetella bronchiseptica* has long been implicated as a major cause. This bacterium is not host-specific, although strains that cause atrophic rhinitis are generally isolated only from pigs. Dogs, cats, rodents, and other species may harbor *B bronchiseptica* for long periods, but their role in the spread of atrophic rhinitis in pigs is uncertain. Certain toxigenic strains of *Pasteurella multocida*, often acting with *B bronchiseptica*, cause permanent turbinate atrophy and nasal distortion. Because both organisms can cause clinical atrophic rhinitis, the disease has now been divided into 2 forms: **regressive** atrophic rhinitis, due to *B bronchiseptica*, is mild and transient and probably does not affect the animal's growth and performance; **progressive** atrophic rhinitis, caused by toxigenic *P multocida*, is severe and permanent and usually results in poor growth.

Outbreaks of disease usually follow the introduction of pigs, or mixing of pigs from different sources. Piglets may become affected at any age, especially with *P multocida*, which may infect mature animals. Crowding, inadequate ventilation, mixing and moving, and other concurrent diseases are important contributory factors in intensification of the disease.

Clinical Findings: Acute signs usually appear between 3 and 8 wk of age and, in severe cases, nasal hemorrhage may occur. The lacrimal ducts may become occluded, and tear stains then appear below the medial canthi of the eyes. As the disease progresses, some affected pigs may develop lateral deviation or shortening of the upper jaw; others may suffer some degree of atrophy of the turbinates with no apparent outward distortion. The degree of distortion can be judged from the relationship of the upper and lower incisors if breed variations are considered.

The severity of atrophic rhinitis in a herd depends largely on the presence of toxigenic strains of *P multocida*, the level of management, and the immune status of the herd. The latter is related to both vaccination status and the parity distribution of the sow herd, since younger sows tend to be infected more and have less lactogenic immunity than older ones.

Lesions: The degree of atrophy and distortion is best assessed by examining a transverse section at the level of the second premolar tooth (the first cheek tooth, up to 7-9 mo of age); some recommend additional parallel sections. In the active stages of inflammation, the mucosa has a blanched appearance, and purulent material may be present on the surface. In later stages the nasal cavities may be clear, but there may be variable degrees of softening, atrophy, or grooving of the turbinates; deviation of the nasal septum; and asymmetric distortion of the surrounding bone structure.

Diagnosis: The signs and lesions are commonly the basis for diagnosis; however, bacteria should be identified by culture. Routine monitoring is done in some breeding herds, with the degree of atrophy in slaughter pigs measured and the herd given a score. Atrophic rhinitis must be differentiated from necrotic rhinitis (*see* below).

Control: It is rarely possible to keep herds entirely free from mild outbreaks of sneezing, and a low level of aberrant turbinates and nasal bones at necropsy is common, even in herds that show no clinical signs of rhinitis. When atrophic rhinitis rises to an unacceptable level in a herd, the control measures adopted are usually strategic: chemoprophylaxis, vaccination, temporary closure of the herd to introductions of new pigs, and improvements in husbandry (eg, better ventilation and hygiene, and less dusty feed). Chemoprophylaxis usually includes administration of antibacterial drugs to all sows, particularly prefarrowing, as well as the newborn piglets, and sometimes the newly weaned pigs. Medication of weaner and grower rations, and sometimes sow rations, is often helpful. Drugs commonly used are sulfonamides, trimethoprim, tylosin, and tetracyclines.

Bacterins against toxigenic *P multocida*, *B bronchiseptica*, or both, have been developed. Both toxoid vaccines and bacterin-toxoid mixtures are available against *P multocida*; while both give satisfactory results in most herds, infection can be best prevented with bacterin-toxoid mixtures. The sows are vaccinated 4 and 2 wk before farrowing, and the young pigs at 1 and 4 wk of age. A high level of colostral immunity develops in piglets nursing vaccinated sows.

INCLUSION BODY RHINITIS (IBR)

A rhinitis caused by cytomegalovirus, which produces inclusion bodies in the nasal mucosa. Infection of pregnant sows rarely may lead to mummified fetuses, stillbirths, and neonatal deaths; inclusion bodies are demonstrable in the fetal viscera. Infection of young pigs (<2 wk) may be fatal in the absence of lactogenic immunity; if circulating antibody is present, infection results in a moderately severe rhinitis and conjunctivitis, often with copious discharge, from which recovery is uneventful. Infection of older pigs normally leads to no clinical signs, although large basophilic inclusions are present in the nasal mucosa. It is suggested, but not proved, that IBR predisposes to bacterial infections that lead to atrophic rhinitis (*see* above). The virus is widespread; serological surveys suggest it is ubiquitous in North America, although clinical signs are unusual.

MYCOPLASMAL PNEUMONIA
(Enzootic pneumonia, EP)

A chronic, clinically mild, infectious pneumonia of pigs, characterized by its ability to become endemic in a herd and to produce a persistent dry cough, retarded growth rate, sporadic "flare-ups" of overt respiratory distress, and a high incidence of lung lesions in slaughter pigs. It occurs worldwide.

Clinical outbreaks of mycoplasmal pneumonia may impair growth rate and feed conversion. This effect is enhanced when large numbers of pigs are closely confined in poorly ventilated buildings under poor husbandry conditions. The effects of the disease are uneven and unpredictable, and place limits on the efficiency and flexibility of large production units. However, in modern units with good disease control, mycoplasmal pneumonia remains largely subclinical and is of little economic importance.

Etiology and Epidemiology: The terms "virus pneumonia" and "enzootic pneumonia" are frequently used to describe a characteristic disease syndrome now known to be caused primarily by *Mycoplasma hyopneumoniae*. The pleomorphic organism is fastidious, smaller than most bacteria, and difficult to see clearly under ordinary light microscopes. It can be cultured in specially prepared media, but isolation from field cases is difficult. It is rapidly inactivated in the environment and by disinfectants, but it may survive longer in cold weather. It appears to be host specific. Field investigations suggest that different strains vary in pathogenicity.

In addition, mycoplasmal pneumonia is frequently complicated by other mycoplasmas, bacteria, and viruses, which affect the severity of the disease. Certain strains of *M hyorhinis*, and perhaps some viruses, may themselves act as primary agents to produce a syndrome resembling the pneumonia caused by *M hyopneumoniae*.

In most countries that use modern pig-farming methods, the lungs of 30-80% of the pigs slaughtered show pneumonic lesions of the type associated with mycoplasmal infection. Pigs of all ages are susceptible, but within a herd, pigs become infected in the first few weeks of life either by their dam or by other young pigs after mixing. The incidence of lung lesions is highest in 2- to 4-mo-old pigs. Immunity develops slowly, the lung lesions regress, and older growing and mature pigs may recover completely.

Clinical Findings and Lesions: In herds in which the disease is endemic, morbidity is high, but clinical signs may be minimal and mortality is low. Coughing is the most common sign and is most obvious when pigs are roused. Sporadically, individual pigs or groups develop severe pneumonia. A common predisposing factor is a change of weather, but other stresses, eg, transient viral infections and mixing pigs, may also cause flare-ups. The disease is usually more severe when it first enters a herd.

The lesions in the lungs are gray or purple, and most common in the apical and cardiac lobes. Old lesions become clearly demarcated. The associated lymph nodes may be enlarged. Histologically, inflammatory cells are present in the bronchioles; there is perivascular and peribronchiolar cuffing and extensive lymphoid hyperplasia.

Diagnosis: Clinical, pathological, and epidemiological findings are usually adequate for diagnosis. *Mycoplasma hyopneumoniae* can be demonstrated in impression smears of the cut surface of the affected lung, identified by FA technique, and sometimes isolated and identified in culture. Serological tests, principally the complement fixation test, are occasionally used on a herd basis, but results are difficult to interpret because of false positive and false negative results.

Mycoplasmal pneumonia must be differentiated from swine influenza, pasteurellosis, *Bordetella* pneumonia, severe ascariasis, lungworm, and other pneumonias.

Control: When the disease first enters a herd, mass treatment with antibiotics, eg, tylosin, spiramycin, tiamulin, or a tetracycline, helps to control the severity of signs. When it flares up in herds in which it is endemic, treatment of individual pigs with antibiotics usually results in remission, presumably by controlling secondary bacteria.

Inactivated mycoplasmal cultures have been developed as vaccines, but are of doubtful value. The economic effects of the disease can be reduced, and sometimes eliminated, by improvements in housing and husbandry, particularly ventilation and overcrowding.

In large intensive units, starting with foundation stock free of mycoplasmal pneumonia and adopting strict precautions against direct and indirect contact with pigs from other herds is advisable. Unfortunately, many herds set up in this way do not remain free of mycoplasmas for very long, particularly in pig-dense areas. Field observations suggest that infection can be windborne for at least a mile between large herds in cold, wet weather.

In the USA and parts of Europe, most of the mycoplasmal-pneumonia-free herds were established by the pig repopulation technique. More recently, some have been established by medicated early weaning. The biggest problems with these herd programs are the breakdown rate and the difficulty of monitoring the herds that claim to be free of mycoplasmal pneumonia. Early detection of a herd breakdown may also be extremely difficult.

NECROTIC RHINITIS
(Bull-nose)

An uncommon and sporadic disease of young pigs characterized by suppuration and necrosis of the snout, arising from wounds of the oral or nasal mucosa. Confusion exists in the literature because of the use of the misnomer "bull-nose" to also describe atrophic rhinitis (*see* above).

Etiology: *Fusobacterium necrophorum* is commonly isolated from the lesion and undoubtedly contributes to the disease, but many other types of organisms are frequently present. They gain entry through damage to the roof of the mouth, often as a result of clipping the needle teeth too short or using blunt clippers.

Clinical Findings and Lesions: Signs include swelling and deformity of the face, occasionally hemorrhage, snuffling, sneezing, foul-smelling nasal discharge, sometimes involvement of the eyes with lacrimation and purulent discharge, loss of appetite, and emaciation. Generally, only 1 or 2 pigs in the herd are affected.

The facial swelling usually is hard, but incision reveals a mass of pinkish gray, foul-smelling, necrotic tissue, or greenish gray tissue debris, depending on the age of the lesion. The nasal and facial bones become involved; as a consequence, facial deformity may be marked.

Diagnosis: Necrotic rhinitis is readily differentiated from atrophic rhinitis by the bulging type of facial distortion observed in the former. Atrophic rhinitis causes no swelling other than that due to the upward or lateral deviation of the snout. The character of the exudate and its location within the tissue of the snout or face are distinctive of bull-nose.

Prophylaxis and Treatment: Prevention is directed toward avoiding injuries to the mouth and snout, and improved sanitation. When the disease occurs repeatedly, needle teeth should be clipped carefully.

If the condition is advanced, it is doubtful that treatment is advisable. Early surgical intervention and packing the cavity with sulfonamide or tincture of iodine may be useful. In young pigs, sulfamethazine given PO is of value.

PASTEURELLOSIS

Pasteurellosis is most commonly seen in pigs as a complication of mycoplasmal pneumonia (*see* above), although swine influenza, Aujeszky's disease, *Bordetella bronchiseptica*, or *Actinobacillus (Haemophilus) pleuropneumoniae* may also cause changes in the lungs that lead to disease caused by *Pasteurella* spp. The causative organism usually is *Pasteurella multocida*. It produces an exudative bronchopneumonia, sometimes with pericarditis and pleuritis. Primary, sporadic, fibrinous pneumonia due to pasteurellae, with no epidemiological connection with mycoplasmal or other pneumonia, may also occur in pigs. In both primary and secondary forms, chronic thoracic lesions and polyarthritis tend to develop. Diagnosis is based on necropsy findings and recovery of pasteurellae from the lesions. Nontoxigenic strains of capsular type A are the predominant isolates from cases of pneumonia. Toxigenic strains of *P multocida*, in the presence of *Bordetella bronchiseptica*, are now associated with atrophic rhinitis (*see* above).

Septicemic pasteurellosis and meningitis occasionally occur in piglets. *Pasteurella haemolytica* has been recovered from aborted fetuses, and septicemia may also occur in adult pigs. There are no distinctive lesions, and the pathogenesis is obscure. Porcine strains of *P haemolytica* are often untypeable and do not belong to the common ovine and bovine serotypes. However, some outbreaks in the UK have been associated with close contact with sheep.

Control of the secondary, pneumonic form of the disease is generally based on prevention or control of mycoplasmal pneumonia. Early and vigorous therapy with antibiotics, or antibiotics combined with sulfonamides, for all forms of the disease is indicated to prevent chronic sequelae. An increasing resistance to some antibiotics has been noted among the pasteurellae.

PLEUROPNEUMONIA

A severe and contagious respiratory disease, primarily of young pigs (up to 6 mo), although in an initial outbreak, adults may be affected. It has a sudden onset, short course, and high morbidity and mortality. It occurs worldwide and appears to be increasing in incidence, although some reports suggest that severity is declining in countries where it has been long established.

Etiology: The causal organism is *Actinobacillus (Haemophilus) pleuropneumoniae.* Transmission is by aerosol, and many recovered pigs are carriers. Clinical signs develop within 4-12 hr in experimental infections.

Clinical Findings: Onset is sudden, and in herds that have not been infected previously, spread is rapid. Some pigs may be found dead without having shown clinical signs. Respiratory distress is severe; there are "thumps", and sometimes a blood-stained frothy nasal and oral discharge. Fever up to 107°F (41.5°C), anorexia, and reluctance to move are typical signs.

Although primarily a disease of growing pigs, adults may suffer abortions or fatal infections. The course is typically 1-2 days. Morbidity may reach 50%, and in untreated cases, mortality is high. Survivors generally show reduced growth rates and persistent cough.

Once established in a herd, the disease may be evident only as a cause of reduced growth rate and pleurisy at the abattoir, although acute flare-ups may occur. However, severe lesions may not always be accompanied by equally severe clinical signs, and deaths in transit or carcass condemnation may result. Concurrent infection with mycoplasma, pasteurellae, or swine influenza virus is common.

Lesions: Fibrinous pleurisy and pericarditis may be severe. In acute cases, the lungs are dark and swollen and ooze blood and fluid from the cut surface; hemorrhagic, even necrotic bullae of various sizes may be present. The trachea may contain much blood-stained froth. In chronic cases, the lesions are more organized and localized. Extrathoracic lesions are uncommon, although there are reports of associated osteomyelitis.

Diagnosis: An explosive onset is suggestive, and when combined with clinical signs and gross lesions often justifies a tentative diagnosis. Concurrent infections, eg, with pasteurellae, may complicate diagnosis. In herds that have been exposed and developed at least a degree of immunity, the pattern may be less distinctive. Many serological tests have been used to help confirm a herd diagnosis or detect carriers, but results are not always clear-cut. A definitive diagnosis depends on isolation and identification of *A pleuropneumoniae.*

Treatment and Control: Rapidity of onset and persistence in infected herds makes treatment difficult. Kanamycin, spiromycin, tetracyclines, trimethoprim, synthetic penicillins, tylosin, and sulfonamides have been used. The first treatment should be parenteral, followed by in-water or in-feed medication, which also may protect in-contact pigs.

Because survivors frequently remain carriers, control is difficult, although good results are being claimed for some vaccines. "All-in/all-out" management, reduced stocking rates when possible, and improved ventilation are recommended. Herds free of the disease should try to purchase replacements from *A-pleuropneumonia*-free herds; if the disease proves difficult to control, herd repopulation should be considered.

SWINE INFLUENZA
(Hog flu, Pig flu)

Experimentally, an acute, highly contagious, respiratory disease may result from infection with type A influenza virus. However, in the field, isolates of variable virulence exist, and clinical manifestation may be determined by secondary organisms. Pigs are the principal hosts of classical swine influenza virus (SIV). (Human infections have been reported, but porcine strains of influenza A do not appear to spread in the human population.) The disease occurs commonly in the midwestern USA, occasionally in other states; in Mexico, Canada, and South America; in Europe, from the UK to the USSR, and from Sweden to Italy; in Kenya; and in Japan, Taiwan, and other parts of eastern Asia. It appears to be absent from Australia.

Etiology: SIV is an RNA orthomyxovirus of the influenza A group with hemagglutinating antigen H1 and neuraminidase antigen N1 (ie, H1N1) and also H3N2 and their recombinants. Influenza B and C viruses have been isolated from pigs but may not cause the classical disease. The classical type A infection with isolates of mild virulence may favor replication of pseudorabies virus (qv, p 617), *Haemophilus parasuis* (*see* p 381), and *Actinobacillus (H) pleuropneumoniae* (*see* above) or *Mycoplasma hyopneumoniae* (*see* above), any of which may complicate outbreaks. The mixing of carrier and nonimmune pigs is an important predisposing factor. The virus is unlikely to survive outside living cells for >2 wk except in cold conditions. It is readily inactivated by disinfectants.

Within an infected area, outbreaks are most common in fall or winter, often at the onset of particularly cold weather in North America. In warmer areas of the world, infection may occur at any time. Usually, an outbreak is preceded by 1 or 2 individual cases and then spreads rapidly within a herd, mainly by airborne and pig-to-pig transmission. The virus survives in carrier pigs for up to 3 mo and can be demonstrated in unaffected animals between outbreaks. In antibody-positive herds, outbreaks of infection recur as immunity wanes. Up to 40% of herds may contain antibody-positive pigs. Carrier pigs are usually responsible for the introduction of swine influenza into previously uninfected herds and countries.

Pathogenesis: There is a spectrum of virulence from mild to acute, but in the classical acute form, the virus multiplies in bronchial epithelium within 16 hr of infection and causes focal necrosis of the bronchial epithelium, focal atelectasis, and gross hyperemia of the lungs. Bronchial exudates and widespread atelectasis, seen grossly as plum-colored lesions affecting individual lobules of apical and intermediate lobes, occur after 24 hr. The lesions continue to develop until 72 hr after infection, after which the virus becomes more difficult to demonstrate. Bronchial epithelial hyperplasia, neutrophils in the exudate, and coagulative necrosis of some alveoli occur and are accompanied by lesions in the diaphragmatic lobes. Interstitial pneumonia, mononuclear cells in exudates, and bronchial hyperplasia all occur in the healing lesion and most virus disappears by day 9. Losses in reproduction associated with primary outbreaks appear to be secondary as virus has not been recovered.

Clinical Findings: A classical acute outbreak is characterized by sudden onset and rapid spread through the entire herd, often within 1-3 days. The main signs are depression, fever (to 108°F [42.2°C]), anorexia, coughing, dyspnea, weakness, prostration, and a mucous discharge from the eyes and nose. Mortality is generally ~1-4%. The overt course of the disease is usually 3-7 days in uncomplicated infections, with clinical recovery of the herd almost as sudden as the onset. However, virus may continue to recycle with clinical signs being suppressed by immune responses; some pigs may become chronically affected. In herds that are in good condition, the principal economic loss is from stunting and delay in reaching market weight. Some increase in piglet mortality has been reported, and effects on herd fertility, including abortions in late pregnancy, may follow outbreaks in nonimmune herds.

Lesions: In uncomplicated infections, the lesions usually are confined to the chest cavity. The pneumonic areas are clearly demarcated, collapsed, and purplish red. They may be distributed throughout the lungs but tend to be more extensive and confluent ventrally. Nonpneumonic areas are pale and emphysematous. The airways contain a copious mucopurulent exudate, and the bronchial and mediastinal lymph nodes are edematous, but rarely congested. There may be severe pulmonary edema, especially of interlobular septae, or a serous or serofibrinous pleuritis. Histologically, the lesions are primarily those of an exudative bronchiolitis with some interstitial pneumonia when fully developed.

Diagnosis: In typical outbreaks, a presumptive diagnosis can be made on clinical and pathological findings, but confirmation depends on isolation of the virus or demonstration of specific antibody. Virus can be isolated from nasal secretions in the febrile phase or from affected lung tissue in the early acute stage by inoculating embryonated hens' eggs, harvesting the amniotic fluid after 72-96 hr, and examining for specific hemagglutinating activity. It may be necessary to passage material at least twice before considering it negative. A retrospective diagnosis can be made by demonstrating a rise in specific antibodies in acute and convalescent serum samples, using the hemagglutination-inhibition test. H3 and H1 subtype antigens must be included. This test is also used for herd surveys. To diagnose uncomplicated influenza infection, conditions such as pasteurellosis; pseudorabies; and chlamydial, *Haemophilus*, and *Actinobacillus* infections must be eliminated.

Treatment and Control: There is no effective treatment, although antimicrobials may reduce secondary bacterial infections. Vaccination and import controls are the only specific preventive measures; H1N1 and H3N2 strains are often included together with oil or alum adjuvants. Good husbandry and freedom from stress, particularly due to crowding and dust, help to reduce losses.

RESPIRATORY DISEASES OF SHEEP AND GOATS

INTRODUCTION

Some, but not all, of the discussions in this chapter are of diseases common to sheep and goats. Emphasis in the introduction is on diseases of sheep but, in general terms, it applies to both species. The importance of respiratory diseases depends on their prevalence (which tends to fluctuate seasonally), their effects on productivity, and with some diseases, their international spread.

Diseases of the upper respiratory tract of sheep and goats include sinusitis caused by larvae of *Oestrus ovis* (*see* below), nasal polyps in older sheep, and endemic nasal adenocarcinomas in several sheep breeds. Retrovirus-like particles have been demonstrated on histologic sections of endemic nasal adenocarcinomas.

Many viruses and bacteria, including mycoplasmas and chlamydiae, have been recovered from the respiratory tract of sheep and goats, but not all have been shown to cause disease. The importance of bacteria such as *Pasteurella haemolytica* has been established in pneumonia of sheep, but no clear etiological role has been identified for certain mycoplasmas (eg, *Mycoplasma arginini*), some viruses (eg, reovirus), and chlamydiae. Many sheep carry *P haemolytica* in their upper respiratory tract and tonsils. Infection with parainfluenza-3 (PI-3) virus is common, whereas adenovirus (of which at least 6 serotypes are known in sheep) and respiratory syncytial virus infections generally are less frequent.

Respiratory disease syndromes may be divided broadly into short-duration (acute) exudative pneumonias and prolonged (chronic) proliferative diseases. Not all factors predisposing to acute respiratory diseases are known, but acute viral infections in a susceptible population of sheep can alter the protective mechanisms in the respiratory tract so that certain commensal bacteria may invade, multiply, and cause serious disease. One confirmed synergism is an initial infection with PI-3 virus followed by invasions of biotype A *P haemolytica*. The result is often severe pneumonia in one or several sheep in a flock. Introduction of new stock, high-density stocking, or reduced ventilation can act as associated predisposing factors. In such outbreaks, red consolidated anterior lobes of the lungs are common at necropsy.

Chronic, progressive, proliferative changes in the lungs are usually associated with so-called slow virus infections. The prevalence of such infections, of which 2 specific entities have been described in sheep, varies throughout the world, but may be high in some regions. In progressive pneumonia (maedi, qv, p 756), the entire lung can change in a gradual process of cellular proliferation (type I pneumocytes and lymphocytes) which, through time, results in dyspnea and marked wasting. The other slow virus disease is pulmonary adenomatosis (see below), in which the type II pneumocytes and related bronchiolar cells proliferate so that tumor masses form in the lung tissue.

Chronic bronchitis and pneumonia that affect principally the diaphragmatic lobes can also result from lungworm infection (Dictyocaulus filaria, Muellerius capillaris, or Protostrongylus rufescens. A further chronic but nonprogressive pneumonia, which can resolve over months, is called "atypical pneumonia" (see below). This proliferative exudative pneumonia, which primarily affects the anterior lobes of the lungs, is associated with Mycoplasma ovipneumoniae and P haemolytica (type A serotypes). PI-3 virus also may be involved in outbreaks of this disease. Caseous lymphadenitis (qv, p 64) caused by Corynebacterium pseudotuberculosis may result in abscessation of the lungs and associated lymph nodes, and cause progressive debilitation of sheep and goats. A herpesvirus recovered from the lungs of sheep with pulmonary adenomatosis has been shown experimentally to cause a mild chronic interstitial pneumonia.

For the control of respiratory disease, predisposing management conditions should be avoided. Vaccination using bacterins that contain P haemolytica has given equivocal or disappointing results. Vaccination with intranasal or other PI-3 vaccines may be useful. The control of slow virus diseases, atypical pneumonia, and caseous lymphadenitis are considered below.

In all respiratory disease outbreaks, laboratory assistance with necropsies, serology, or microbiology can aid the diagnosis and result in more effective control.

CONTAGIOUS CAPRINE PLEUROPNEUMONIA

A contagious pneumonia with pleurisy; it occurs commonly in goats in many parts of the Middle East, Africa, and Asia, less commonly in the Mediterranean countries and Central and North America.

Etiology: Acute pneumonias in goats are caused by Mycoplasma strain F38, M mycoides mycoides (large colony type, Mmm LC), and M mycoides capri. (See also CONTAGIOUS BOVINE PLEUROPNEUMONIA, p 726.) Strain F38 causes a highly contagious lethal disease most resembling the earlier descriptions of classical contagious caprine pleuropneumonia, and appears to be transmitted by infective aerosol. Morbidity can be 100% and mortality 60-100%. Gathering or housing animals together facilitates spread of the disease.

The disease caused by the other mycoplasmas is not particularly contagious. Both Mmm LC and M mycoides capri have been isolated in Australia, the former in North America.

Clinical Findings and Lesions: Weakness, anorexia, cough, hyperpnea, and nasal discharge accompanied by fever (106°F [41°C]) are often found. Exercise intolerance and, eventually, respiratory distress develop. A septicemic form of the disease without specific respiratory tract involvement has been described.

Typically, the thorax contains an excess of straw-colored fluid, and there is acute fibrinous pneumonia with overlying fibrinous pleurisy. Consolidation is sometimes confined to one lung. The degree of distention of interlobular septa by serofibrinous fluid varies, and is said to be less conspicuous with strain F38 infection than with the other mycoplasmas. The tendency to form necrotic sequestra is less than in contagious bovine pleuropneumonia, and lesions may resolve slowly in surviving animals. Fibrinous pericarditis, fibrinopurulent arthritis, and meningitis also occur with some infections.

Diagnosis: The clinical signs, epidemiology, and postmortem findings are used to establish a diagnosis. The causative organism should be isolated and identified, but isolation may be difficult in some cases: Pasteurella spp are often associated with pneumonias in goats and may complicate the identification of the main etiological agents. The filamentous forms of the mycoplasma can often be detected on darkfield microscopical examination of the pleural fluid from acute cases. There are no serological tests in general use, but complement fixation tests may be useful.

Control: Quarantine of affected flocks is desirable. Vaccines, both killed and live, have been used, but their efficacy has not been established. Treatment with tylosin at 10 mg/kg, IM, daily for 3 days, has been effective.

NONPROGRESSIVE (ATYPICAL) PNEUMONIA

A chronic, infectious, infrequently fatal disease that generally affects sheep up to 1 yr old, and occasionally adults.

Etiology: *Mycoplasma ovipneumoniae, Pasteurella haemolytica* biotype A, and perhaps parainfluenza-3 (PI-3) virus have been implicated. *Pasteurella multocida* may constitute the bacterial component of the disease in some countries and cases, but *Mycoplasma arginini* and *Chlamydia psittaci*, which are also isolated from a small portion of cases, appear to play no role in the disease.

Transmission is probably exclusively by the respiratory route, and ewes are the main source of infection for lambs. Microorganisms may colonize the upper respiratory tract as early as 1-2 days after birth. The endemic form occurs when the number of respiratory agents increases as the lambing period progresses and increasing numbers of infected animals excrete the organisms. Decline of colostral antibodies permits the development of chronic, nonprogressive pneumonia as early as 2-3 wk, but more usually at 2-3 mo of age. Many factors, primarily stocking density and management before and after lambing, influence the incidence and severity in a flock. In housed flocks, ≥40% lambs may be affected. Outbreaks may occur in older lambs and even ewes following stresses, eg, movement or mixing of animals from different sources.

Pathogenesis: *Mycoplasma ovipneumoniae* produces only mild changes in the lungs, but these permit secondary invasion by *P haemolytica*, with concomitant exacerbation of lesions and clinical signs. The mycoplasma may persist in the lungs for ≥7 mo after initial infection, but pasteurellae are generally eliminated within 3 mo, and lesions start to resolve after this time. Although nonprogressive pneumonia is experimentally reproducible only with these 2 organisms, PI-3 virus infection may be a necessary precursor to the field disease.

Clinical Findings: The disease is often mild enough to be overlooked. Signs include coughing, mucopurulent nasal discharge, depression, hyperpnea, and occasionally dyspnea; they are particularly evident after exercise. Sporadic deaths may occur. Pyrexia may be observed in the early stages. Inappetence and poor growth may be seen in housed lambs.

Lesions: The clearly demarcated lung lesions, which range from red-brown (in the early stages) to gray, are generally found in the apical, cardiac, and anterior portions of the diaphragmatic lobes. Pleurisy may be present. Histological changes include nodular lymphoid hyperplasia, often with peribronchiolar and perivascular lymphoid cell cuffing, bronchiolar epithelial hyperplasia, and hyaline-like "scars" within or close to bronchiolar walls. Cellular exudate in alveolar lumina consists principally of macrophages and, in the early stages when pasteurellae are present, of neutrophils.

Diagnosis: Signs of respiratory disease concurrently in several sheep <1 yr old is suggestive, but confirmation depends on gross and microscopical examination of lung lesions. Microbiology and serology assist in identifying the disease, but are not diagnostic since both organisms occur widely in normal sheep populations (and goats, in the case of the mycoplasma) and readily invade lung tissue diseased by other causes.

Differential diagnoses include pulmonary adenomatosis, maedi, pasteurellosis, and lungworm infection. Absolute differentiation relies on pathologic examination of the lungs. Pulmonary adenomatosis and maedi generally affect animals >1 yr old and involve single animals, while pasteurellosis causes more acute signs and deaths and affects animals of all ages.

Treatment and Control: *Pasteurella* vaccines have been ineffective experimentally; mycoplasma vaccines have not been assessed. Treatment should incorporate either injectable tiamulin, shown experimentally to prevent lesion development, or tylosin; both are administered at 10 mg/kg, preferably over 3 consecutive days. Oxytetracycline is less effective. Tiamulin or tylosin on a prophylactic basis would seem to be the most promising means for combating endemic atypical pneumonia.

Control requires good management to maximize ability to resist infection and minimize transmission of respiratory organisms. Stocking densities and, in housed systems, good ventilation are important. Lambs should be exposed as little as possible to older animals. Purchased animals should be isolated until they have recovered from transport stress.

PROGRESSIVE PNEUMONIA
(Maedi-Visna, Zwoegersiekte)

A chronic, progressive, viral disease of sheep and goats. In sheep, the virus affects principally the lungs and udder, but the CNS and joints also may be affected. The disease has been reported from North and South America, Europe, Africa, and Asia. The disease in sheep has never been encountered in Australia and New Zealand, although the disease in goats is prevalent in these countries.

Etiology: The causal RNA virus (a lentivirus), which persists in the WBC of infected sheep in the presence of a humoral and cell-mediated immune response, is detectable by several serological tests. Neutralizing antibodies appear more slowly than other antibodies, generally several months after infection. Seropositive sheep must be considered infected and capable of transmitting the virus. Transmission is considered to occur usually by ingestion of colostrum or milk that contains virus, or by inhalation of aerosol droplets. Intrauterine infection is thought to occur infrequently. All breeds of sheep appear susceptible, although Border Leicester sheep seem more susceptible than down-breed sheep. Management practices can influence morbidity rates.

A similar disease of goats, caprine arthritis-encephalitis (qv, p 393), is caused by a closely related retrovirus.

Clinical Findings: Signs rarely occur in sheep <2 yr, and are most common in sheep >4 yr old. The disease progresses slowly, with wasting and increasing respiratory distress (maedi or zwoegersiekte) as the main signs. Coughing and bronchial exudate are seldom evident. Affected sheep may die from secondary *Pasteurella* pneumonia. A noninflammatory, indurative mastitis is common. Other, but rarer, forms of disease produced by this virus are encephalitis and arthritis. All are low-grade, progressive infections. In the encephalitic form (visna), ataxia, muscle tremors, or circling progresses to paresis and eventually to complete paralysis.

Acute neurological disease is a frequent occurrence in 1- to 6-mo old kids on farms where there is a high incidence of arthritis in lactating does. Unlike the slowly progressive arthritic disease in adults, infected kids show signs of ataxia within 1 mo of birth, and this may progress to paralysis within the following 2 mo.

Lesions: Macroscopic lesions of progressive pneumonia are confined to the lungs and associated lymph nodes. The lungs do not collapse when the thorax is opened and are abnormally firm and heavy (2-4 times normal weight). Early lung changes may be difficult to detect, but later in the disease, lungs are mottled by gray and brown areas of consolidation. The mediastinal and tracheobronchial lymph nodes are enlarged and edematous. Interstitial pneumonia, perivascular and peribronchial lymphoid hyperplasia, and hypertrophy of smooth muscle are seen throughout the entire lung. CNS lesions, when they occur, are those of meningoleukoencephalitis with secondary demyelination. All lesions are progressive and result from the cellular immune response of the host, and not directly from viral damage.

Diagnosis: Clinical diagnosis of progressive pneumonia cannot be made with certainty. Pulmonary adenomatosis, verminous pneumonia, and pulmonary caseous lymphadenitis are differential diagnoses. Necropsy can rule out both of the latter and, in most cases, pulmonary adenomatosis also. Listeriosis, scrapie, louping ill, rabies, and space-occupying lesions should be considered when neurological signs are observed. In flocks experiencing progressive pneumonia for the first time, the diagnosis should be confirmed by histopathology, serology, or isolation of the virus.

Control: There is no effective treatment. Methods of control include slaughter of all seropositive sheep (sometimes including their lambs) and retesting at intervals of ~6 mo until ≥3 negative tests are obtained. Alternatively, lambs may be isolated at birth, denied access to colostrum and milk from positive ewes, and reared artificially.

PULMONARY ADENOMATOSIS
(Jaagsiekte)

A contagious, viral, neoplastic disease of the lungs of sheep and more rarely of goats. It has been reported from Europe, Asia, Africa, and South and North America.

Etiology: Respiratory exudates from affected sheep are infectious. The causal agent has not been established, although a retrovirus has been identified in the tumor and fluids. A herpesvirus also has been recovered from the tumor, but does not appear to have an etiological role. Natural transmission seems to occur generally by the respiratory route. Close contact, eg, at feeding troughs, may assist spread of the virus.

Clinical Findings: The period of incubation following natural infection extends over months so that clinical signs generally become evident when sheep are 3-4 yr old. The tumors produce clinical signs when they become sufficiently large or numerous to interfere with respiration. Affected sheep lose weight and show increasing respiratory embarrassment. Moist rales may be heard even without a stethoscope. Coughing is not prominent. Forced lowering of the head often causes frothy mucus to run from the nostrils. Clinical disease ends fatally after days or weeks, sometimes due to secondary pasteurellosis.

Lesions: Tumors are confined to the lungs and rarely the associated lymph nodes. They vary from small nodules to extensive solid areas involving the ventral parts of ≥1 lobe(s). These are firm, gray, and flat, and sharply demarcated. Copious amounts of white, frothy fluid are present in the air passages. Histological changes are caused by uncontrolled proliferation of columnar-shaped type II pneumonocytes and similar cells in the bronchioles.

Diagnosis: No available serological or biochemical tests can positively identify affected sheep before clinical signs develop. Although several sheep in a flock may be affected, usually a single sheep is noticed at any one time. Age of the sheep, moist rales, and evidence of abnormal volumes of respiratory fluid in an afebrile sheep aid the diagnosis. However, such cases may be complicated by a terminal *Pasteurella* pneumonia, and histological examination is often essential to confirm the presence of tumor tissue.

Control: Treatment is not practical, and control in flocks in which the disease is known to occur must be based on reducing crowding and early elimination of any sheep that is thin, losing weight, or showing respiratory signs.

SHEEP NOSE BOT

The sheep nose bot fly, *Oestrus ovis*, is a cosmopolitan parasite that, in its larval stages, inhabits the nasal passages and sinuses of sheep and goats. It also has been seen in bighorn sheep (*Ovis canadensis*) and European ibex (*Capra ibex*) and in uncharacteristic hosts such as man and dogs. While its incidence in some northern European countries has decreased in recent years, it continues to be one of the most widely distributed sheep parasites in South Africa, Brazil, and countries in the Mediterranean basin.

The adult fly is grayish brown and ~12 mm long. The female deposits larvae in and about the nostrils of sheep without alighting. These small, clear white larvae (initially <2 mm long) migrate into the nasal cavity, many of them spending at least some time in the paranasal sinuses. As the larvae (bots) mature, they become cream-colored, then darken, and finally show a dark or black band on the dorsal surface of each segment. The larval period, which is usually shortest in young animals, is said to vary from 1-10 mo. When mature, the larvae leave the nasal passages, drop to the ground, burrow down a few inches, and pupate. The pupal period lasts 3-9 wk, depending on the environmental conditions, after which the fly emerges from the pupal case and pushes its way to the surface. Mating soon occurs and the female begins to deposit larvae.

Clinical Findings: Once the larvae begin to move about in the nasal passages, a profuse discharge occurs, at first clear and mucoid, but later mucopurulent and frequently tinged with fine streaks of blood emanating from minute hemorrhages produced by the hooks and spines of the larvae. Continuing activity of the larvae, particularly if they are numerous, causes a thickening of the nasal mucosa that, together with the mucopurulent discharge, leads to impairment of respiration. Paroxysms of sneezing accompany migrations of the larger larvae. Larvae present in the sinuses are sometimes unable to escape; they die and may gradually become calcified or lead to a septic sinusitis. The purulent inflammation produced in the sinuses occasionally may spread to the brain with fatal results. However, the principal effects of the nose bot are annoyance, with a resulting reduction in grazing time, and loss of condition. Infestations may consist of ≥80 larvae, but usually only 4-15 are found.

To avoid the fly's attempts at larval deposition, a sheep may run from place to place, keeping its nose close to the ground, and may sneeze and stamp its feet or shake its head. Commonly, especially during the warmer hours of the day when the flies are most active, small groups of sheep gather and face the center of a circle, heads down and close together.

Treatment: Ruelene given PO at 50 mg/lb (110 mg/kg) as a drench should afford good control. Rafoxanide, given PO at 7.5 mg/kg as a drench or bolus, trichlorfon administered PO at 75 mg/kg as a drench or IM, and nitroxynil given subcut. at 20 mg/kg have been reported to be effective. Ivermectin administered at 200 μg/kg, PO or subcut., is effective.

RESPIRATORY DISEASES OF SMALL ANIMALS

INTRODUCTION

Respiratory diseases occur frequently in dogs and cats. Although clinical signs such as coughing and dyspnea are commonly referable to primary problems of the respiratory tract, they may also occur secondary to disorders of other organ systems, eg, congestive heart failure.

Both young and aged animals are at increased risk of developing respiratory disease. At birth, the respiratory and immune systems are incompletely developed; this facilitates the introduction and spread of pathogens within the lungs, and alveolar flooding may occur. In aged animals, chronic degenerative changes that disrupt normal mucociliary clearance and immunologic anergy may render the lungs more vulnerable to airborne pathogens and toxic particulates.

A varying flora of indigenous commensal organisms (*Pasteurella multocida, Bordetella bronchiseptica*, streptococci, and coliform bacteria) normally reside in the canine and feline nasal passages, nasopharynx, and upper trachea, and at least intermittently in the lungs without causing clinical signs. Opportunistic infections by these bacteria may occur when respiratory defense mechanisms are compromised by: 1) infection with a primary pathogen such as distemper, parainfluenza virus, or canine type 2 adenovirus in dogs, and rhinotracheitis virus or calicivirus in cats; 2) other insults such as inhalation of smoke or noxious gases; or 3) diseases such as congestive heart failure and pulmonary neoplasia. Secondary bacterial infections complicate the management of viral respiratory infections of both dogs and cats. Pathogens may continue to reside in the respiratory tract of convalescent animals. When stressed, these animals may relapse; they can also act as a source of infection for others. Poor husbandry practices, eg, overcrowding, are often associated with poor hygienic and environmental conditions, and the resultant stress increases both the incidence and severity of infections. Conditions that favor the spread of infections often occur in catteries, kennels, pet shops, boarding facilities, humane shelters, etc.

Congenital abnormalities, such as stenotic nares, elongation of the soft palate, and tracheal stenosis, can cause respiratory dysfunction. Neoplastic masses and degenerative changes of the airways, eg, laryngeal paralysis (qv, p 713) and tracheal collapse, can result in dyspnea and other clinical manifestations of respiratory disease.

Tracheal collapse is most common in toy and miniature breed dogs, and rare in cats. The etiology is unknown. Affected animals have a chronic cough and inspiratory or expiratory dyspnea. Frequently, they are obese and have concurrent cardiovascular or other pulmonary disease. Weight loss (if obese) is an important part of management. Other measures include exercise restriction, reduction of excitement and stress, and medical therapy, eg, antitussives, antibiotics, and bronchodilators.

ALLERGIC PNEUMONITIS

Acute or chronic hypersensitivity reaction of the lungs and small airways.

Etiology: An underlying etiology is rarely determined in pulmonary hypersensitivity reactions in dogs and cats. Type I or immediate hypersensitivity is probably the most common mechanism, although Type III and IV mechanisms may also be involved (*see also* p 424 *et seq*). The cellular infiltrate is typically eosinophilic; however, mixed inflammatory infiltrates consisting of mononuclear cells, eosinophils, and neutrophils, or predominantly lymphocytic infiltrates can be observed. Pulmonary infiltration with eosinophilia (PIE, qv, p 426) is a group of diseases associated with both pulmonary-associated and peripheral eosinophilia. Not all types of allergic pneumonitis, however, are associated with PIE. Causes of PIE include migrating parasites, reaction to microfilariae of heartworms, lungworms, chronic bacterial or fungal infections (histoplasmosis, aspergillosis), viruses, external antigens, and unknown precipitating factors. Canine heartworm (qv, p 73) pneumonitis occurs when dogs become sensitized to microfilariae. A similar reaction may be seen in cats with heartworms. Migrating intestinal parasites and primary lung parasites may induce either subclinical or mild signs of allergic pneumonitis. Pulmonary hypersensitivity also may be caused by drugs and reactions to inhaled allergens; however, this is poorly documented in small animals.

Clinical Findings: Chronic cough is the most common sign. It may be mild or severe, productive or nonproductive, and progressive or nonprogressive. Weight loss, tachypnea, dyspnea, wheezing, exercise intolerance, and occasionally, hemoptysis may be observed. Severely affected animals may exhibit moderate to severe dyspnea and cyanosis at rest. Auscultation varies from unremarkable to increased breath sounds, crackles, or wheezes. Fever is usually absent. The degree of dyspnea and coughing is related to the severity of inflammation within the airways and alveoli.

Diagnosis: This is based largely on history, and radiographic and clinicopathological findings. Thoracic radiographs frequently show irregular patchy alveolar infiltrates, and increased bronchial and interstitial markings. Radiographic evidence of heartworm disease or parasitic pulmonary disease may suggest an underlying etiology. Typical hematological changes are mild leukocytosis, variable peripheral eosinophilia (4-50%), and occasionally basophilia. Fecal analysis and Knotts' test or an occult heartworm test are indicated when lung parasitism or heartworm disease is suspected. A tracheal wash for cytological analysis, culture, and detection of larval forms is often helpful. In allergic pneumonitis, tracheal wash cytology generally reveals a predominance of eosinophils. Bacterial cultures of aseptically collected tracheal washes are commonly negative.

Treatment: When an underlying cause can be found, elimination of the offending agent and a short-term course of glucocorticoids resolves the problem. Prednisolone beginning at 1-2 mg/kg body wt, PO and tapered over 10-14 days is often sufficient. When PIE is secondary to heartworm disease or pulmonary parasites, treatment with prednisolone before or during treatment for the parasite controls the pulmonary signs. When an underlying etiology cannot be determined, prolonged therapy with prednisolone for 3 wk to 3 mo is often required. When severe bronchoconstriction is suspected, bronchodilators may be helpful. Severely dyspneic animals may require short-term oxygen therapy.

FELINE RESPIRATORY DISEASE COMPLEX

A complex that includes those illnesses typified by rhinitis, conjunctivitis, lacrimation, salivation, and oral ulcerations. The principal diseases, feline viral rhinotracheitis (FVR) and feline calicivirus infections (FCV), affect exotic as well as domestic species. Feline pneumonitis (*Chlamydia psittaci*) and mycoplasmal infections appear to be of lesser importance. Feline infectious peritonitis and pleuritis (qv, p 415) typically causes a more generalized condition but may cause signs of mild upper respiratory tract infection.

FVR and caliciviruses are host-specific and pose no known human risk. Human conjunctivitis caused by the feline chlamydial agent has been reported.

Etiology: Probably 40-45% of feline upper respiratory infections are caused by FVR virus, a herpesvirus; FCV has a similar incidence. Dual infections with these viruses are common. Other organisms such as *Chlamydia psittaci, Mycoplasma* spp, and reoviruses are believed to account for most of the remaining infections.

Natural transmission of these agents occurs via aerosol droplets and fomites, which can be carried to a susceptible cat by a handler. Convalescent animals may continue to harbor virus for many months. Calicivirus is shed continuously, while infectious FVR virus is released intermittently. Stress may precipitate a secondary course of illness. The incubation period is 2-6 days for FVR and FCV, and 5-10 days for pneumonitis.

Clinical Findings: The onset of FVR is marked by fever, frequent sneezing, conjunctivitis, rhinitis, and often salivation. Excitement or movement may induce sneezing. The fever may reach 105°F (40.5°C), but subsides and tends to fluctuate from normal to 103°F (39°C). Initially, a serous nasal and ocular discharge occurs; it soon becomes mucopurulent and copious, at which time depression and anorexia are evident. Severely debilitated cats may develop ulcerative stomatitis, and ulcerative keratitis occurs in some. Signs may persist 5-10 days in milder cases, and up to 6 wk in severe cases. Generally, the mortality is low and prognosis good except for young kittens and aged cats. The illness often is prolonged and a marked weight loss may occur. FVR often is complicated by secondary bacterial infections; abortions and generalized infections have been associated with it.

There are many serologically related strains of feline caliciviruses. They appear to have predilection for the epithelium of the oral cavity and the deep tissues of the lungs. Some caliciviruses are nonpathogenic. Some induce little more than salivation and ulceration of the tongue, hard palate, or nostrils; others produce pulmonary edema and interstitial pneumonia. Two strains may produce a transient "limping syndrome" without signs of oral ulceration or pneumonia. These latter 2 strains produce a transient fever, alternating leg lameness, and pain on palpation of affected joints. These signs occur most often in 8- to 12-wk-old kittens, and usually resolve without treatment. The syndrome may occur in kittens vaccinated against FCV, as no vaccine protects against both strains of the caliciviruses that produce the "limping syndrome".

Calicivirus has also been found in cats with lymphocytic-plasmacytic gingivitis and stomatitis. The superficial lesions heal rapidly, and the infected cat regains appetite 2-3 days after onset. The clinical course usually is 7-10 days. An acute febrile response, inappetence, and depression are common signs. Serous rhinitis and conjunctivitis also can occur.

Chlamydia psittaci infections characteristically produce conjunctivitis; infected cats sneeze occasionally. Fever may occur as the disease progresses beyond serous lacrimal discharge to mucopurulent conjunctivitis, lymphoid infiltration, and epithelial hyperplasia. Convalescent animals may undergo relapses.

Mycoplasma may infect the eyes and upper respiratory passages, characteristically producing severe edema of the conjunctiva and a less severe rhinitis.

The occurrence of severe viral upper respiratory disease is rare in adult, properly vaccinated cats. These cats should be tested for concurrent immunodeficiency diseases including feline leukemia virus and feline immunodeficiency virus.

Lesions: Lesions generally are confined to the respiratory tract, conjunctivae, and oral cavity. In FVR, the conjunctivae and nasal mucous membranes are reddened, swollen, and covered with a serous to purulent exudate. In severe cases, focal necrosis of these membranes may occur. The larynx and trachea may be mildly inflamed. The lungs may be congested, with small areas of consolidation; however, pulmonary changes are rarely remarkable in FVR except possibly in stressed, young kittens. The characteristic histological lesion of FVR is the acidophilic intranuclear inclusion body. During the early stage of the illness, inclusions may be present in sites of epithelial necrosis on the tongue, nasal membranes, tonsils, epiglottis, trachea, and nictitating membranes. Inclusion bodies are transitory. Inclusions do not occur in calicivirus infections.

The characteristic lesion caused by FCV is ulceration of the oral mucosa. Lesions on the tongue or hard palate initially may appear as vesicles, which subsequently rupture. Ulcerations occasionally occur on the epithelium covering the median nasal septum. The more virulent caliciviruses destroy epithelial cells of the bronchioles and alveoli, which causes acute pulmonary edema that progresses through seropurulent bronchiolar hyperplasia and interstitial pneumonia.

Early in the clinical course of feline pneumonitis, the causative organism may be identified in Giemsa-stained conjunctival smears or scrapings. The elementary bodies are intracytoplasmic. Mycoplasmas occur as extracellular coccoid bodies often seen on the surface of conjunctival epithelial cells.

Diagnosis: The presumptive diagnosis is based on such typical signs as sneezing, conjunctivitis, rhinitis, lacrimation, salivation, oral ulcers, and dyspnea. FVR tends to affect the conjunctivae and nasal passages, caliciviruses the oral mucosa and lower respiratory tract. Chlamydial infections result in chronic, low-grade conjunctivitis. These characteristics may be obscured in mixed infections. Cytological examination of Giemsa-stained conjunctival scrapings is of value for the identification of chlamydiae and mycoplasmas. A definitive diagnosis is based on isolation and identification of the agent. The oropharyngeal mucosa, external nares, and conjunctival sacs are the preferred sampling sites.

Treatment: Treatment is largely symptomatic and supportive, but the broad-spectrum antibiotics are useful against secondary invaders as well as directly against *C psittaci*. Tetracyclines are the most effective against *C psittaci*. Nasal and ocular discharges should be removed frequently for the comfort of the animal. Nebulization may aid in the removal of tenaceous secretions. Nose drops containing a vasoconstrictor (eg, 2 drops of ephedrine sulfate, 0.25% solution, in each nostril b.i.d.) and antibiotics may be helpful in reducing the amount of nasal exudate. A bland ophthalmic ointment containing antibiotics (tetracyclines in *C psittaci* infections) is indicated 5-6 times daily to prevent corneal irritation produced by dried exudate. If corneal ulcers occur in FVR infections (herpetic keratitis), ophthalmic preparations containing idoxuridine or acyclovir are indicated in addition to other antibiotic ophthalmic preparations. If dyspnea is severe, the cat may be placed in an oxygen tent. Fluids may be indicated to correct dehydration, and force-feeding may be necessary. Esophagostomy and gavage may be appropriate for alimentation of severely debilitated cats. Antihistamines (eg, chlorpheniramine maleate, PO, b.i.d. [8 mg for adults, 4 mg for kittens]) may be beneficial early in the course of the disease.

Prophylaxis: Two types of modified live virus FVR-FCV vaccines are available. The first type is intended for parenteral administration; cats >9 wk old should be vaccinated twice, with a 3-wk interval. Kittens should be vaccinated at intervals of 3-4 wk until they are ≥12 wk old. Annual revaccination with a single dose is indicated.

The second type of vaccine is administered to healthy cats by instillation into the conjunctival cul-de-sacs and nasal passages. (Owners should be advised that cats inoculated oronasally may sneeze 4-7 days after vaccination.) Kittens vaccinated when <12 wk old should be revaccinated on reaching this age. Annual revaccination with a single dose is recommended.

Modified live virus FVR-FCV vaccines intended for parenteral administration are available in combination with either chemically inactivated or modified live virus feline panleukopenia vaccines. A parenterally administered vaccine composed entirely of inactivated viruses also is available.

Vaccines containing either chick-embryo- or cell-line-origin *C psittaci* are administered parenterally. A single dose is recommended for cats >12 wk old; younger kittens should be revaccinated when they reach 16 wk; all should be revaccinated annually. These vaccines are indicated in catteries or on premises where *C psittaci* infection has been confirmed. The chlamydial vaccines are available in combination with FVR-FCV and panleukopenia vaccines. Systematic vaccination and control of environmental factors (exposure to sick cats, overcrowding, and stress) provide excellent protection against upper respiratory disease.

LUNG FLUKES
(*Paragonimus kellicotti, P westermani*)

These parasites usually are found in cysts, primarily in the lungs of dogs, cats, and several other domestic and wild animals. They also have been encountered rarely in other viscera or the brain. Infection is most common in China, southeast Asia, and North America. *Paragonimus westermani* is a parasite of man and other animals in China and other countries in the Far East.

The adults are fleshy, reddish brown, oval, and measure ~14 × 7 mm. The eggs are golden brown, oval, distinctly operculated, and measure ~100 × 60 μm. The eggs pass through the cyst wall, are coughed up, swallowed, and passed in the feces. The life cycle includes several snails as the first intermediate host, and crayfish or crabs as the second. Dogs and cats become infected by eating raw crayfish or crabs that contain the encysted cercariae. After penetration of the intestinal wall and wandering in the peritoneal cavity, the young flukes pass through the diaphragm to the lungs where they become established.

Infected animals may have a chronic, deep, intermittent cough, and eventually become weak and lethargic, although many infections pass unnoticed. Finding the characteristic eggs in feces or sputum is diagnostic. The location in the lungs is ascertained by radiography. Aberrant infections can be determined serologically.

Daily administration of bithional for 1 wk or every other day for 1 mo is an effective treatment. Fenbendazole or albendazole given daily for 2 and 3 wk, respectively, also are valuable treatments for reducing the number of eggs deposited and eventually killing the parasites.

LUNG NEMATODES

See *also* LUNGWORM INFECTION, p 714.

AELUROSTRONGYLUS ABSTRUSUS

This nematode, the most common lungworm of cats, is found in many parts of the world, including the USA, Europe, and Australia. They are small parasites (males 7 mm, females 10 mm), deeply embedded in the lung tissues. The eggs are forced into alveolar ducts and adjacent alveoli where they form small nodules. The eggs hatch within these nodules. Once the larvae escape, they are coughed up, swallowed, and passed in the feces. The larvae observed in the feces of infected animals are tightly coiled, have an undulating tail with a spine, and measure <400 μm long. The life cycle includes snails or slugs as first intermediate hosts, and frogs, lizards, birds, or rodents as vectors of encysted larvae. When one of these transport hosts is eaten, the larvae migrate from the stomach to the lungs via the peritoneal and thoracic cavities. They reach the lungs within 24 hr, and larvae are seen in the feces in ~1 mo.

Although prevalence of this infection can be high, clinical and diagnostic signs are often lacking. Chronic wasting, cough, dyspnea, and pulmonary rales may be observed. The lungs usually have solidified, gray, raised nodules 1-10 mm in diameter; generalized alveolar disease has been observed in chronic cases. Treatment is difficult and not often necessary, but levamisole and other newer anthelmintics may be effective.

CAPILLARIA AEROPHILA

Although usually parasites of the frontal sinuses, trachea, bronchi, and rarely nasal cavities of foxes, *C aerophila* are found in dogs and other carnivores. They are 25-35 mm long. The females produce eggs with bipolar plugs that resemble those of whipworms; however, their shells are colorless-to-greenish and pitted. The eggs are laid in the lungs, coughed up and swallowed, and passed in the feces. The eggs can be identified either from tracheal washes or fecal flotation. The life cycle is direct; dogs become infected through consumption of feed or water contaminated with larvated eggs. After hatching in the intestine, the larvae reach the lungs and bronchi via the circulatory system. They mature ~40 days after infection. Clinical signs include coughing, sneezing, and nasal discharge. Treatment may be attempted through extended administration of levamisole or fenbendazole.

FILAROIDES SPP

Filaroides osleri are tracheal worms of dogs, usually found in thin-walled nodules around the bronchial bifurcation. They have been found in the USA, South Africa, New Zealand, India, Great Britain, France, and Australia. The males are ~5 mm long, and the females 10-15 mm. The life cycle is direct, and an infected bitch can transfer larvae in her saliva to her pups while licking and cleaning them. On ingestion, the larvae pass to the blood and are carried to the lungs and bronchi.

A persistent, dry cough is the most common clinical sign. Coughing may later become severe with respiratory distress. Finding the larvae in the feces is diagnostic, but since these larvae are lethargic and few in number, bronchoscopy is a better method. Surgical excision of the nodules, combined with administration of fenbendazole, levamisole, or thiabendazole has been effective in treating infected animals. Chemotherapy alone can be successful but does not always give a complete cure.

Filaroides hirthi is similar to *F osleri* but is found in the lung parenchyma. The females are oviparous. The adults occur in nests in the lung parenchyma, where a focal granulomatous reaction occurs. Diagnosis of low-grade infections can be difficult. Zinc sulfate flotation is usually more successful than using a Baermann apparatus. Treatment with thiabendazole or levamisole has been reported to be effective.

NEOPLASIA OF THE RESPIRATORY SYSTEM

TUMORS OF THE NOSE AND PARANASAL SINUSES

These account for 1-2% of all canine or feline tumors. The incidence in dogs is twice that in cats; males of both species have a higher incidence than females. The mean age at time of diagnosis is 10 ½ yr for dogs and 12 yr for cats. In dogs, 80% of these tumors are malignant and 60-70% are adenocarcinomas and squamous cell carcinomas. In dogs, the ethmoturbinates tend to be the site of predilection. Dolicocephalic and mesocephalic breeds appear to be at higher risk than brachycephalic breeds. Of nasal tumors in cats, 90% are malignant, the most common being carcinomas and lymphomas. Tumors of the nose and paranasal sinuses typically are very invasive locally and metastasize infrequently; metastasis is more likely in carcinomas, and usually occurs late in the disease. Common sites of metastasis are regional lymph nodes, lungs, and brain. Invasion of the paranasal sinuses tends to be greater in dogs than in cats. In general, if untreated, survival is 3-5 mo after diagnosis.

Chronic nasal discharge is the most common clinical finding; it may be mucoid, mucopurulent, or serosanguineous. Initially the discharge is unilateral but often becomes bilateral. Periodic sneezing, epistaxis, and respiratory stertor may occur. Facial and oral deformities result from destruction of bony or soft tissue sinonasal structures. Retrobulbar extension of these tumors results in exophthalmos and exposure keratitis. Secondary epiphora may occur if the nasolacrimal duct is blocked. Late in the disease, CNS signs, eg, disorientation, blindness, seizures, stupor, and coma, may result if the tumor extends into the cranial vault.

Diagnosis is made from the history and clinical findings, and by eliminating other causes of nasal discharge, sneezing, or facial deformation. Cranial radiographs typically show increased density of the nasal cavity and frontal sinuses, and evidence of bone destruction. Definitive diagnosis is based on biopsy of tumor tissue.

Treatment is largely palliative since permanent cure is rare. Aggressive surgical excision, chemotherapy, radiation therapy, or combinations afford a more favorable prognosis when diagnosis is made early.

TUMORS OF THE LARYNX AND TRACHEA

Both these are rare in dogs and cats. Tumors of the larynx most frequently reported in dogs are oncocytoma, squamous cell carcinoma, mast cell tumor, melanoma, and osteosarcoma; and in cats, squamous cell carcinoma, lymphosarcoma, and adenocarcinoma. Benign inflammatory polyps of the larynx also occur in dogs and cats. Tumors of the trachea are particularly rare. Osteochondral dysplasia of the trachea (osteochondroma) is a benign tumor of the trachea primarily seen in dogs <1 yr old. Other benign mesenchymal tumors, carcinomas, and sarcomas are occasionally seen.

The most common signs of tumors of the larynx include inspiratory dyspnea, stridor, voice change (hoarse bark or loss of voice), coughing, and exertional dyspnea. Findings typically associated with tumors of the trachea are coughing, dyspnea, stridor, and rarely, hemoptysis. Both laryngeal and tracheal tumors may be associated with signs of fixed upper airway obstruction (inspiratory and expiratory dyspnea). The degree of dyspnea often relates to the degree of luminal obstruction.

Diagnosis is made from the history and clinical findings, and by eliminating other causes of upper airway obstruction or coughing. Laryngoscopy or tracheoscopy affords visualization of the tumor mass. Definitive diagnosis is made on biopsy.

Surgical excision and resection is the treatment of choice. Radiation therapy may be palliative for radiosensitive tumors such as squamous cell carcinoma, mast cell tumor, and lymphoma. Surgical resection of tracheal osteochondral dysplasia in dogs is curative.

PRIMARY LUNG TUMORS

These are rare in dogs and cats; however, the reported incidence of lung carcinomas has increased at least 100% during the last 20 yr. This is attributed to an increased average life span and better detection and awareness. Most primary lung tumors occur in dogs at a mean age of 10 yr, and in cats at a mean age of 12 yr. There is no consistent breed or sex predilection in either. Primary lung tumors usually originate from the terminal bronchioles and alveoli; occasionally they occur as a second coincidental tumor, which may make the differentiation between primary and metastatic disease difficult. Of the primary lung tumors in dogs and cats, ≥80% are malignant. Adenocarcinoma and anaplastic carcinoma are the most common types in dogs and cats. Squamous cell carcinoma is observed more frequently in cats than in dogs. Primary lung sarcomas and adenomas are rare in both species. Metastatic spread of primary lung tumors is generally to other areas of the lungs, tracheobronchial lymph nodes, bone, and brain. Intrapulmonary spread via the airways occurs in ~50% of dogs with adenocarcinoma. Metastatic spread to the pleurae, pericardium, heart, and diaphragm may occur; miscellaneous extrathoracic sites include liver, spleen, and kidney. Dogs with adenocarcinoma have a better prognosis than those with squamous cell carcinoma (mean survival time, 19 mo and 8 mo, respectively). Both recurrence and metastasis tend to occur earlier and with greater frequency in dogs with primary pulmonary squamous cell carcinoma.

Clinical Findings: Primary lung tumors have variable manifestations, which depend on the location of tumor, rapidity of tumor growth, presence of previous or concurrent pulmonary disease, and awareness of the owner. Common signs include cough, inappetence, weight loss, reduced exercise tolerance, lethargy, tachypnea, dyspnea, wheezing, vomiting or regurgitation, pyrexia, and lameness. The most common clinical finding in dogs is a chronic, nonproductive cough. Coughing is uncommon in cats, and nonspecific signs such as inappetence, weight loss, and tachypnea and dyspnea are more common. In either species, tachypnea or dyspnea indicates massive tumor burden or pleural effusion. Pleural effusion is particularly common in cats with primary lung tumors. Lameness may be due to hypertrophic osteopathy (unusual in cats, [qv, p 489]), or metastasis to bone or skeletal muscle. Thoracic auscultation may be normal, reflect increased breath sounds compatible with pulmonary congestion, or be muffled due to pulmonary consolidation or pleural effusion.

Diagnosis: One-third or more of the primary lung tumors are recognized incidentally during radiography for other problems, or at necropsy. Thoracic radiographs are essential for a tentative diagnosis in those animals exhibiting compatible clinical signs. Primary lung tumors in dogs may occur as single or multiple circumscribed mass lesions, as a diffuse lung pattern, or as a lobar consolidation. In cats, single circumscribed mass lesions are less common, whereas a diffuse lung pattern and lobar consolidation are more frequent. Pleural fluid accumulation is common in cats and less frequent in dogs. In either species, chest wall involvement and hilar lymphadenopathy may occur. Tentative diagnosis can be made by ruling out other causes of pulmonary disease with similar radiographic lung patterns. Definitive diagnosis requires biopsy.

Treatment: Surgical resection of tumor via lobectomy of diseased lung lobes is the treatment of choice. Inoperable lesions or metastatic disease may be controlled with chemotherapy. Mean survival time for operable primary lung tumors in dogs is 10-13 mo; if the lymph nodes are involved at the time of diagnosis, survival time is shortened. Recurrence or metastasis of tumor is a common cause of death.

METASTATIC TUMORS, LUNGS

A localized tumor may extend to the lungs by dissemination through hematogenous or lymphatic routes, or by direct extension of tumor cells. Certain primary tumors, such as mammary adenocarcinoma, osteosarcoma, and oral melanoma, most commonly metastasize to the lungs. The lungs may be the only site of metastasis or there may be concurrent metastasis in other organs; in the former, the diagnostic approach is to identify an occult primary tumor or to carefully review the medical history for disclosure of previous tumor removal. Because pulmonary metastasis occurs late in the clinical course of a malignant tumor, prognosis is poor.

The signs of metastatic pulmonary disease are similar to those of primary lung tumors except that coughing is less common. Severity of signs depends on the anatomic location of the tumor and whether the lesions are solitary or multiple.

The diagnosis is similar to that for primary lung tumors. Because of limitations in the resolution of small lesions ($\leq$3 mm in diameter) on routine radiography, $\geq$40% of cases with pulmonary metastasis may not be visualized.

Radiography of the chest should precede removal of tumors with a known high incidence of metastatic spread to the lungs. The major goal of cancer therapy is prevention of metastasis rather than its eradication. Slow-growing or solitary metastatic lesions are best treated by surgical excision. Chemotherapy or radiation therapy may be useful with certain tumor types not amenable to surgical resection. Overall, pulmonary metastasis has a poor prognosis.

PNEUMONIA

Acute or chronic inflammation of the lungs and bronchi, characterized by disturbance in respiration and hypoxemia and complicated by the systemic effects of associated toxins. The usual cause is primary viral infection of the lower respiratory tract.

Canine distemper virus, adenovirus types 1 and 2, parainfluenza virus, and feline calicivirus cause lesions in the distal airways and predispose to secondary bacterial invasion of the lungs. Parasitic invasion of the bronchi, as by *Filaroides, Aelurostrongylus*, or *Paragonimus* spp may result in pneumonia. Protozoan involvement, eg, by *Toxoplasma gondii* (qv, p 365), is rarely seen. Tuberculous pneumonia, although uncommon, is seen more often in dogs than cats. Mycotic granulomatous pneumonias (*see* FUNGAL INFECTIONS, p 340) also have a greater incidence in dogs. Cryptococcal pneumonia has been described in cats. Injury to the bronchial mucosa and inhalation or aspiration of irritants may cause pneumonia directly and predispose to secondary bacterial invasion. Aspiration pneumonia may result from persistent vomiting, abnormal esophageal motility, improperly administered medications (eg, oil) or food (forced feeding), or may follow suckling in a neonate with a cleft palate.

Clinical Findings: The initial signs are usually those of the primary disease. Lethargy and anorexia are common. A deep cough of low amplitude is noted. Progressive dyspnea, "blowing" of the lips, and cyanosis may be evident, especially on exercise. Body temperature is increased moderately, and there may be leukocytosis. Auscultation usually reveals consolidation, which may be patchy but more commonly is diffuse. In the later stages of pneumonia, the increased lung density and peribronchial consolidation caused by the inflammatory process can be visualized radiographically. Complications such as pleurisy, mediastinitis, or invasion by opportunistic organisms may occur.

Diagnosis: Analysis of tracheal wash fluid is valuable for the diagnosis of bacterial infections. Cytologic examination will indicate the animal's immune response and intracellular or extracellular location of bacteria. Bacterial culture and sensitivity testing is required and may include anaerobe and mycoplasma culture, especially in refractory animals. A viral etiology generally results in an initial body temperature of 104-106°F (40-41°C). Leukopenia, often expected, may not occur in many viral respiratory infections (eg, canine infectious tracheobronchitis, feline calicivirus pneumonia, feline infectious peritonitis pneumonia). A history of recent anesthesia or severe vomiting indicates the possibility of aspiration pneumonia. Acutely affected animals may die within 24-48 hours of onset. Mycotic pneumonias are usually chronic in nature. Miliary nodules seen at necropsy may suggest protozoal pneumonia.

Treatment: The animal should be placed in a warm, dry environment. Anemia, if present, should be corrected. Oxygen therapy may be used if cyanosis is severe and is best applied by means of an oxygen cage, with a concentration of 30-50%. Empirical antimicrobial chemotherapy should be initiated and altered based on results of transtracheal wash fluid analysis. Supportive therapy should be instituted as needed and may include oxygen supplementation, pulmonary physiotherapy (nebulization and coupage), and bronchodilators. A negative response after 48-72 hr of therapy warrants reassessment of the treatment plan. Antimicrobial chemotherapy should be continued 1 wk beyond resolution of clinical and radiographic signs.

Animals should be reexamined frequently. Chest radiographs should be repeated at regular intervals to monitor recurrence or note a primary underlying disease process, and to detect complications such as lung consolidation, atelectasis, or abscessation.

RHINITIS AND SINUSITIS

Acute or chronic inflammation of the mucous membranes of the nose and sinuses.

Etiology: Viral infection is the most common cause of acute rhinitis/sinusitis in dogs and cats. Feline viral rhinotracheitis (FVR), feline calicivirus (FCV), canine distemper, canine adenovirus types 1 and 2, and canine parainfluenza are most frequently incriminated. Chronic states exist for FVR and FCV, with intermittent shedding associated with stress. Bacterial rhinitis/sinusitis frequently is a secondary complication. Primary bacterial rhinitis in dogs may be from infection with *Bordetella bronchiseptica* or *Pasteurella multocida*. Allergic rhinitis/sinusitis is a poorly defined atopy that occurs seasonally in association with pollen production, and perennially, probably in association with housedusts and molds. Smoke aspiration, inhalation of irritant gases, or foreign bodies lodged in the nasal passages also may cause acute rhinitis.

Chronic rhinitis most commonly is due to bacterial infection following inflammation or trauma, foreign bodies, neoplasia, or mycotic infection. In cats, chronic rhinosinusitis is a frequent sequela of acute viral infections of the nasal and sinus mucosa that result in hyperplastic glandular and epithelial changes. Rhinitis or sinusitis or both may result when an apical tooth root abscess extends into the maxillary recess. Mycotic rhinosinusitis may be caused by *Cryptococcus neoformans*, *Aspergillus* spp, and *Penicillium* spp. Cats more often are affected with *Cryptococcus* sp than dogs, whereas aspergillosis is frequent in dogs but rare in cats.

Clinical Findings and Diagnosis: Acute rhinitis is characterized by one or more of nasal discharge, sneezing, pawing at the face, respiratory stertor, open-mouth breathing, or inspiratory dyspnea. Lacrimation and conjunctivitis often accompany inflammation of the upper respiratory passages. Affected tissues are often hyperemic and edematous. The nasal discharge is serous, but becomes mucoid as a result of secondary bacterial infection. If inflammatory cells infiltrate the mucosa, the discharge may become mucopurulent. Sneezing, in an attempt to clear the upper airways of discharge or exudate, is observed most frequently in acute rhinitis and tends to be intermittent in chronic rhinitis. Aspiration reflex ("reverse sneeze"), a short paroxysmal episode of inspiratory effort in an attempt to clear the nasopharynx of obstructing material, may also be seen. Respiratory stertor, open-mouth beathing, and inspiratory dyspnea occur when the nasal passages are narrowed from inflamed mucosa, glandular elements, and secretions. An acute unilateral nasal discharge, possibly accompanied by pawing at the face, suggests a foreign body. Neoplastic or mycotic disease is suggested by a chronic nasal discharge that was initially unilateral but becomes bilateral, or changes in character from mucopurulent to serosanguineous or hemorrhagic.

Diagnosis is based on history, physical examination, radiographic findings, and elimination of other causes of nasal discharge and sneezing.

Treatment: In mild or acute cases, supportive treatment may be effective. Severe cases of rhinosinusitis in kittens or adult cats may require parenteral fluids to prevent dehydration, and nutritional support via a nasogastric tube to maintain weight. Chronic secondary bacterial rhinosinusitis may be treated with antimicrobial chemotherapy for 3-6 wk based on sensitivity of the predominant organism(s) cultured. Intermittent use of vasoconstrictive nasal decongestants usually provides only temporary relief of congestion of the nasal mucosa. Mycotic rhinosinusitis requires antifungal therapy based on identification of a fungal etiologic agent. (*See also* ANTIFUNGAL AGENTS, p 1464.) Cases unresponsive to medical therapy may require surgery consisting of sinusotomy and/or rhinotomy, lavage, and antimicrobial chemotherapy. Radiation therapy following debulking turbinectomy is the most viable treatment for intranasal neoplasia.

TONSILLITIS

Etiology: Tonsillitis is common in dogs, but rare in cats. In dogs, it may occur as a primary disease, frequently in small breeds. It also may be secondary to nasal, oral, or pharyngeal disorders (eg, cleft palate); chronic vomiting or regurgitation (eg, from megaesophagus); or chronic coughing (eg, with bronchitis). Chronic tonsillitis may occur in brachycephalic dogs in association with pharyngitis accompanying soft palate elongation and redundant pharyngeal mucosa. Chronic tonsillitis in young dogs is thought to represent maturation of pharyngeal defense mechanisms.

Escherichia coli, Staphylococcus aureus, and hemolytic streptococci are the pathogenic bacteria most often cultured from diseased tonsils. Plant fibers or other foreign bodies that lodge in the tonsillar fossa may produce a localized unilateral inflammation or a peritonsillar abscess. Other physical and chemical agents may cause irritation of the oropharynx and one or both tonsils. Tonsillitis may also accompany neoplastic tonsillar masses because of physical trauma or secondary bacterial infection.

Clinical Findings and Diagnosis: Tonsillitis is not always accompanied by obvious clinical signs. Fever and malaise are uncommon unless consequent to systemic infection. Gagging, followed by retching or a short, soft cough may result in expulsion of small amounts of mucus. Inappetence, listlessness, salivation, and dysphagia are seen in severe tonsillitis.

Tonsillar enlargement may range from protrusion just out of the crypts, to a mass of sufficient size to cause dysphagia or inspiratory stridor. A septic, suppurative exudate may surround the tonsil, which may be reddened with small necrotic foci or plaques. Tonsillitis may be a sign of generalized or regional inflammatory disease; therefore, primary tonsillitis should be diagnosed only after underlying diseases have been ruled out. Squamous cell carcinoma, malignant melanoma, and lymphosarcoma commonly occur in canine tonsils and should be distinguished from tonsillitis. Tonsillar lymphosarcoma generally results in bilateral symmetrical enlargement, whereas nonlymphoid neoplasia is usually unilateral.

Treatment: Prompt systemic administration of antibiotics is indicated for bacterial tonsillitis. Penicillins are often effective, but in refractory cases, culture and sensitivity testing may be needed. Mild analgesics are appropriate for severe pharyngeal irritation, and a soft palatable diet is recommended for a few days until the dysphagia resolves. Parenteral administration of fluids is required for those animals that are unable to take food by mouth.

Tonsillectomy is rarely required for chronic primary tonsillitis, but provides permanent relief. Other indications for tonsillectomy include tonsillar enlargement that interferes with airflow (eg, in brachycephalic breeds) and tonsillar neoplasia.

TRACHEOBRONCHITIS

Acute or chronic inflammation of the trachea and bronchial airways. Bronchitis may extend from the bronchioles to the lung parenchyma. Tracheobronchitis may be primary or secondary depending on the etiologic agent.

Etiology: Canine infectious tracheobronchitis (kennel cough, *see* below) is often secondary to viral infection of the respiratory system. Other causes of tracheobronchitis include parasites, eg, *Aelurostrongylus abstrusus* (cats and dogs), *Capillaria aerophila* (dogs), *Crenosoma vulpis* (dogs), and *Filaroides osleri* (dogs). Tracheitis may be secondary to diseases of the oropharynx, or to chronic coughing related to heart disease or noncardiac pulmonary disease. Other causes include smoke aspiration and exposure to noxious chemical fumes. Exacerbation of a chronic bronchitis affecting middle-aged and older dogs may follow sudden changes in the weather or other environmental stresses. Bronchial asthma has been diagnosed in cats, but is rare. Foreign bodies in the airway, and developmental abnormalities such as laryngeal deformities may predispose to bronchitis. Bronchiectasis may occur as the end stage of chronic bronchitis in dogs. Recognition of tracheobronchitis as an often secondary disease syndrome underlies the importance of diagnosis and control of an associated primary disease.

Clinical Findings: Spasms of coughing are the outstanding sign. These are most severe after rest or a change of environment, or at the beginning of exercise. On auscultation, the respiratory sounds may be essentially normal. In advanced cases, sonorous rales are heard. The temperature is slightly elevated. The acute stage of bronchitis passes in 2-3 days; the cough, however, may persist for 2-3 wk. Severe bronchitis and pneumonia are difficult to differentiate; the former often extends into the lung parenchyma resulting in pneumonia. Feline bronchial asthma may result in cyanosis and dyspnea, and is accompanied by eosinophilia.

Lesions: During the acute and subacute inflammatory stages, the air passages are filled with frothy, serous, or mucopurulent exudate. In chronic bronchitis, they contain excessive viscid mucus. The epithelial linings are roughened and opaque, a result of diffuse fibrosis, edema, and mononuclear cell infiltration. There also is hypertrophy and hyperplasia of the tracheobronchial mucous glands and goblet cells. The act of coughing is an attempt to remove the accumulations of mucus and exudate from the respiratory passages.

Diagnosis: The diagnosis is made from the history and clinical signs, and by elimination of other causes of coughing. In chronic bronchitis, chest radiographs may show an increase in linear and peribronchial markings. Bronchoscopy reveals inflamed epithelium and tacky, often mucopurulent mucus in the bronchi. In addition, the procedure allows collection of biopsy and swab samples for *in vitro* assay. Bronchial washing is an additional diagnostic aid that may demonstrate causative agents or significant cellular responses, eg, eosinophils.

Treatment: In mild or acute cases, supportive therapy may be effective; however, treatment of concurrent disease is indicated. Rest, warmth, and proper hygiene are important. Broad-spectrum antimicrobial chemotherapy is indicated for treatment of cough. Persistent, productive coughing is best controlled by codeine-containing expectorants or similar antitussives. Animals refractory to conservative medical management should have radiographs taken of the thorax and cervical trachea, and a laboratory data base evaluated to rule-out other differential diagnoses. Transtracheal wash for cytology and culture sensitivity may be indicated to identify an etiologic agent and to determine appropriate antimicrobial chemotherapy. Pulmonary physiotherapy consisting of sodium chloride nebulization and gentle coupage may loosen secretions and stimulate expectoration. A bathroom environment with steam from a hot shower may be substituted for nebulization.

INFECTIOUS TRACHEOBRONCHITIS OF DOGS
(Kennel cough)

Generally, a mild, self-limiting disease that affects dogs of all ages, and results from inflammation of the upper airways. It may progress to fatal bronchopneumonia in puppies, or to chronic bronchitis in debilitated adult or aged dogs. The illness spreads rapidly among susceptible animals housed in close confinement, eg, veterinary hospitals or kennels.

Etiology: Canine parainfluenza virus, canine adenovirus 2 (CAV-2), or canine distemper virus can be the primary or sole pathogen involved. Canine reoviruses (types 1, 2, and 3), canine herpesvirus, and canine adenovirus 1 (CAV-1) are of questionable significance in this syndrome. *Bordetella bronchiseptica* may act as a primary pathogen, especially in dogs <6 mo old; however, it and other bacteria (usually gram-negative organisms such as *Pseudomonas* sp, *Escherichia coli*, and *Klebsiella pneumoniae*) may cause secondary infections following viral injury to the respiratory tract. Concurrent infections with several of these agents are common. The role of *Mycoplasma* sp has not been clearly established. Stress and extremes of ventilation, temperature, and humidity apparently increase susceptibility to, and severity of, the disease.

Clinical Findings and Diagnosis: The prominent clinical sign is paroxysms of a harsh, dry cough, which may be followed by retching and gagging. The cough is easily induced by gentle palpation of the larynx or trachea. Affected dogs demonstrate few if any additional clinical signs except for partial anorexia. Body temperature and WBC counts usually remain normal. Development of more severe signs including fever, purulent nasal discharge, depression, anorexia, and a productive cough, especially in puppies, indicates a complicating systemic infection such as distemper or bronchopneumonia. Stress, particularly due to adverse environmental conditions and improper nutrition, may contribute to a relapse during convalescence.

Tracheobronchitis should be suspected whenever the characteristic cough suddenly develops 5-10 days following exposure to other susceptible or affected dogs. Usually severity diminishes during the first 5 days, but the disease persists for 10-20 days. Tracheal trauma secondary to intubation may produce a similar but generally less severe syndrome.

Treatment: Preferably, affected animals should not be hospitalized, because the disease is usually highly contagious, and also is self-limiting. Appropriate husbandry practices including good nutrition, hygiene, and nursing care, as well as correction of predisposing environmental factors, hasten recovery. Cough suppressants containing codeine derivatives, such as hydrocodone (0.25 mg/kg body wt, q6-12hr, PO) or butorphanol (0.05-0.1 mg/kg, q6-12hr, PO or subcut.), should be used only as needed to control persistent nonproductive coughing. Antibiotics are usually not needed except in severe chronic cases; cephalosporins, chloramphenicol, and tetracycline are preferable because they reach effective concentrations in the tracheobronchial mucosa. When needed, the antibiotic should be selected by culture and sensitivity tests of specimens collected by transtracheal aspiration or bronchoscopy. Antibiotics given PO or IM may not significantly reduce the numbers of *B bronchiseptica* in the distal trachea or major bronchi. Thus, in severe cases not responsive to parenteral antibiotics, kanamycin sulfate (250 mg) or gentamicin sulfate (50 mg) diluted in 3 mL of saline may be administered by aerosolization b.i.d. for 3 days. Dogs to be aerosolized should be pretreated with bronchodilators. Endotracheal injection of antibiotics (eg, gentamicin) is a possible alternative to aerosolization. Corticosteroids may help alleviate clinical signs, but should be used concurrently with an antibacterial agent; they are contraindicated in severely ill, coughing dogs.

Prophylaxis: Dogs should be immunized with modified live virus vaccines against distemper, parainfluenza, and CAV-2, which also provides protection against CAV-1. Commercial products frequently combine these agents and often include modified live parvovirus and leptospiral antigen vaccines. An initial vaccination should be given at 6-8 wk and repeated twice at 3- to 4-wk intervals until the animal is 14-16 wk old. Revaccination should be performed annually. When the risk of *B bronchiseptica* infection is considered to be significant, use of a live, avirulent, intranasal vaccine is preferable to parenteral products containing inactivated bacteria or bacterial extracts. A combination of an avirulent *B bronchiseptica* and a modified live parainfluenza vaccine is available for intranasal use. One inoculation is administered (intranasally) to puppies >3 wk old.

SKIN

SKIN, INTRODUCTION

The skin represents the anatomical boundary and principal organ of communication between the animal and its environment. It is the largest body organ, constituting 12-24% of the animal's body weight, depending on age. An extremely heterogeneous organ, it consists of various cellular and tissue components: an epidermis, an appendageal system, dermis, arrector pili muscle, panniculus carnosus (twitch muscle), and panniculus adiposus (a fatty subcut. layer).

The main activity of the **epidermis** is to produce keratin and melanin. The former is a product of the keratinocyte, the latter of the melanocyte. Another cell type in the epidermis is the Langerhans' cell, a dendritic but non-neural cell that is active in immunological processes and possibly in regulation of keratin formation.

The rate of mitosis in the epidermis and the normal processes of keratinization are under complex chemical control. Chemicals, eg, adrenalin, may interact with growth factors, and result in a decrease in mitotic activity and keratinization. Other factors that affect epidermal mitosis and keratinization include steroids, vitamin A, chalones, and possibly the estrous cycle and ambient conditions of light. The epidermis is intimately related to and dependent on the underlying dermis; there is evidence that the dermis contains factors that affect the activity of the epidermis.

The most important part of the epidermis is its superficial layer, the stratum corneum, since much of the functional activity of the skin resides in this layer (*see* below). The integrity of this layer depends on the proper structural arrangement of the keratin it contains and probably on its lipid content. The latter has an effect on adhesion of the keratinocyte, waterproofing of the skin, and absorption or penetration of agents into the body. The stratum corneum is continuously shed or desquamated. In man, ~2 g of stratum corneum is shed daily. Little is known about the desquamative process and its control mechanisms.

The **appendageal system** is an outgrowth of (and continuous with) the epidermis, and consists of hair follicles and sebaceous and apocrine glands. The hair follicles in dogs, cats, sheep, and goats are compound, often consisting of a primary follicle (coarse and long hair) surrounded by varying numbers (3-12) of secondary follicles (fine, short undercoat hairs), all usually exiting through a single pore. In cattle and horses, the follicles are simple with only a single hair emerging from each pore. The hair follicle is not a static organ but rather goes through periods of growth (anagen) and inactivity (telogen). There is normally also a transitional stage of involution (catagen) between anagen and telogen. Shedding is a seasonal event and usually represents loss of telogen hair as new anagen hair grows. It occurs during the early spring and fall and is related primarily to photoperiodicity, ie, changes in the duration and intensity of light. It follows one of 3 patterns: synchronous, wave, or mosaic.

Hormonal, neural, and vascular control factors may influence hair growth. The endocrine control mechanisms are the most important; they are complex and probably depend on a balance of various hormones. In general, hair growth is increased by thyroxine, adrenalectomy, and gonadectomy. Glucocorticoids and estrogens tend to retard hair growth. Nutritional factors, particularly proteins, fats, and vitamins (and to a lesser degree, caloric intake), also may affect hair growth. The size, shape, and length of hair in animals is genetically controlled, although these may be influenced by environmental factors.

The remainder of the appendageal system consists of sebaceous glands and apocrine and eccrine sweat glands. Sebaceous glands are simple alveolar, holocrine glands that secrete sebum into the follicles and thus to the epidermal surface. Sebum is a complex lipid material containing cholesterol, cholesterol esters, triglycerides, diester waxes, and fatty acids. Sebaceous glands become fully functional at puberty and are under the primary influence of androgenic hormones. Diet also has an effect; decreases in fat intake may lead to an initial reduction in sebum production followed by a compensatory increase.

The apocrine sweat glands are present wherever hair follicles exist (*see also* CUTANEOUS APOCRINE GLAND TUMORS, p 851). Their ducts enter the follicle just above the entrance of the sebaceous ducts. The product of the sweat gland is a white, proteinaceous, lipid material. The glands do not become functional until puberty and are under both humoral and nervous control.

Eccrine sweat glands are present in limited areas (usually on the foot pad and planum nasale) in many animals. They empty directly onto the skin surface. In primates, these are the organs most responsible for sweating.

The **dermis** is a mesenchymal structure that supports, nourishes, and to some degree, regulates the epidermis and appendages. It consists of fibers (collagen, reticular, and elastic), ground substance (a mucopolysaccharide gel), cells (fibroblasts, mast cells, and histiocytes), and vast nervous and vascular plexuses. Both myelinated and nonmyelinated nerves are present in the dermis. Motor nerves are predominantly adrenergic in type, and innervate blood vessels and arrector pili muscles. Except in horses, apocrine glands appear to be non-innervated. Sensory nerves are distributed in 3 networks: dermal, follicular, and specialized end organs. Touch, pressure, pain, itch, heat, and cold are cutaneous sensations perceived by the brain.

The major function of the skin is protection. The pelage provides mechanical protection and also serves as an important filtering system and insulator. Additionally, it may serve to conceal or camouflage an animal. The stratum corneum, a highly developed, tough, durable, flexible membrane, serves as a chemical and waterproofing structure; if it is removed, the skin acts much like a mucous membrane and is freely permeable to almost all agents. Cutaneous temperature, hyperemia, hydration of the stratum corneum, and mechanical or chemical injury to the membrane itself affect it and alter its protective function. Increased cutaneous temperature and hydration of the epidermis, hyperemia, and mechanical or chemical injury to the surface increase the dermal penetration of noxious materials. The pelage also helps protect against the penetration of toxic or allergenic agents through the skin surface by mechanical filtration and by the adsorption of positively charged molecules to the negatively charged keratin of the hair.

The third type of protection afforded by the skin is that against actinic irradiation. Ultraviolet light is filtered by the coat, and absorbed by melanin granules in the epidermis and hair.

The skin is important for thermal regulation in man and some domestic animals, particularly in horses and to a lesser degree in pigs, sheep, and goats. In those animals that have apocrine sweat glands, their function normally is not thermal regulation; other adaptive mechanisms, such as panting in dogs, and slobbering and smearing saliva on the pelage in cats and mice are used for dissipating heat. Conservation of heat is accomplished through vasoconstriction, shivering, and the insulation provided by subcut. fat and erection of hair. The secondary hairs, rather than the primary, insulate the animal through dead air spaces contained within the hair coat, particularly when erected. For this to function properly, the hair must be dry and waterproof.

The epidermis also serves as an immunologic messenger. For example, antigenic and allergenic material may be processed by Langerhan's cells and transported by them to local and nodal T cells to induce hypersensitivity reactions. Epidermal protein may conjugate with exogenous haptens rendering them antigenic.

Also, 7-dehydrocholesterol, the precursor of vitamin D, is formed in the epidermis.

The functions of the sweat and sebaceous glands of the skin and their products are not well understood. Mutant hairless animals without apocrine or sebaceous glands function quite normally without them. Although in horses, sheep, and goats, apocrine sweat glands play a part in heat regulation, it is quite uncertain what function they serve in other domestic animals. Apocrine sweat may affect the hydration of the stratum corneum and viscosity of the lipid film. The sebaceous glands provide the epidermal surface with a lipid film that has antibacterial and antifungal activity; they may affect epidermal hydration, and possibly desquamation. The sebaceous lipids are important in providing a gloss or sheen to the coat.

Reaction Patterns: Although the skin is a complex organ and heterogeneous in structure, it reacts only in a limited number of patterns. These basic patterns are expressed clinically as primary and secondary lesions. Primary lesions include: 1) macules (≤10 mm) and patches (>10 mm)—nonelevated discolored areas of the skin; 2) papules, nodules, and tumors—solid, elevated lesions (in order of increasing size); 3) wheals—flat-topped, steep-walled, solid elevations of the skin resulting from release of histamine from mast cells; 4) vesicles (≤10 mm) and bullae (>10 mm)—elevated, fluid-filled lesions; and 5) pustules—elevated lesions containing pus. Secondary lesions include: 1) scales—desquamated stratum corneum; 2) crusts—the dried remains of exudative lesions; 3) lichenification—bark-like, usually pigmented skin in which normal skin markings are exaggerated; and 4) alterations in pigmentation resulting from inflammatory or neoplastic processes.

Many agents may produce identical reactions or lesions in the skin. For example, a pustule may be a reaction to an irritant, an infection, a ruptured apocrine cyst, or associated with an autoimmune disease (eg, pemphigus). Conversely, any one agent may produce a variety of reactions. A dermatophytic infection may be asymptomatic, or produce alopecia with or without inflammation, or a papule, pustule, or granulomatous nodule (kerion). Actinic irradiation may result in erythema and inflammatory changes or induce neoplastic changes. Therefore, it is often difficult (and sometimes impossible) to make an etiologic diagnosis based on the primary eruption alone. Rather, a complete history, definition of the topographical distribution, cultures, smears, scrapings, and histopathology are essential to a definitive diagnosis. Additionally, as primary lesions may be obliterated by self-trauma and/or secondary bacterial infections, the history and topographical distribution of lesions often become increasingly important in diagnosis.

When the skin is insulted, it reacts in a limited (genetically conditioned) manner to eliminate or neutralize the injury through a number of inflammatory or proliferative events: 1) the influx of inflammatory cells, edema, chemotactic factors, etc in the dermis—usually producing solid elevated lesions in the skin as papules or nodules; 2) inflammation sweeping through the epidermis—producing vesicles, pustules, or exudation; 3) acceleration of the turnover time of the epidermis—producing scales; 4) increased mitotic activity—leading to thickening of the epidermis; or 5) increased melanocyte activity—producing pigmentation. Some of these events may actually be detrimental to the healing process, eg, crusting in the skin tends to trap and maintain an infection. The response to pruritus (scratching, licking, biting) may intensify inflammation. Disruption of the epidermis may predispose to secondary infection or entry of harmful substances, and surface exudation may favor proliferation of bacteria. Thus, in treating any condition, the correct balance of anti-inflammatory agents and the disease process must be considered.

History: Information should be obtained and interpreted as follows:
1) When and where did disease start and how did it progress?
2) If pruritus is present, the owner should be asked to grade its intensity on a scale of 1 to 10. (However, people's perception of the intensity of pruritus is extremely variable—eg, animal has no excoriations and yet owner reports grade 10 pruritus.) a) Slight to moderate—occurs in most diseases and is not diagnostic. b) Severe—scratching in the examination room, eg, scabies, flea allergy dermatitis, food allergy dermatitis. c) Continuous—acral pruritic nodule and "hot spot". d) Minimal—localized demodectic mange, ringworm, most endocrine alopecias, seborrhea, and impetigo in young animals.
3) Responsiveness to previous treatment? a) Steroids—many dermatoses are controlled by steroids. Exceptions include autoimmune disease treated with anti-inflammatory doses, and variable responses in food allergy dermatitis, sex hormone aberrations, scabies, and lick granulomas. b) Antibiotics—responsiveness is expected in treatment of pyodermas but not in vesiculopustular, crusty diseases

that resemble bacterial infections, eg, ringworm, contact dermatitis, autoimmune diseases, seborrhea.

4) Involvement of family members?—Most bacterial infections are not contagious. When other animals or household members are involved, ectoparasites or changes in diet or environmental conditions should be considered.

5) Age of animal?—Many dermatoses have a distinct age pattern, eg, first year of life—juvenile pyoderma, demodectic mange, zinc-responsive dermatosis, congenital dermatoses, ringworm; between years 1 and 3—atopy (inhalant dermatitis); middle and late years—endocrine dermatoses, tumors.

6) Breed predispostion—eg, Boxers: Cushing's disease, atopy, demodectic mange, "hot spots", lick granulomas, nasal solar dermatitis, lupus; Irish Setters: seborrhea, atopy, neurotic self-inflicted trauma; Cocker and Springer Spaniels: seborrhea; German Shepherd Dogs: pyoderma, food allergy dermatitis or idiosyncracies, demodectic mange, perianal fistulas.

7) Did lesions precede or follow any self-trauma?—Primary lesions should precede self-trauma.

8) Does the disease have any relationship to the estrous cycle?—Certain dermatoses worsen or improve during estrus or begin 4-6 wk after estrus ('blown coat" syndrome). Castrated males have a variety of dermatologic problems, often seen 2-4 yr after castration, that are responsive to testosterone replacement therapy.

9) Has there been a change in the animal's environment or diet that might relate to the onset of disease?

10) Does the disease have a seasonal pattern? Is it constant throughout the year or does it wax and wane? Atopy, sex hormone aberration, flea allergy dermatitis, seborrhea, and pyoderma may have definite seasonal patterns.

A number of dermatologic diseases have distinct topographical patterns. 1) Atopy (inhalant allergy)—face (including ears), axillae, and feet; 2) Food allergy dermatitis—as above, and/or lower back and perineum; 3) Endocrine disorders (in general)—trunk, sparing head and extremities; 4) Sex-hormone related dermatoses—lower back, perineum, groin, folds of flank, axillae, digits, and face; 5) Seborrhea—pinnae, periocular, perilabial, median trunk, preen area on tail, perianal, groin, umbilical and nipples, interdigital; 6) Contact dermatitis—feet, scrotum, groin, axillae, pinnae, and lips.

Conversely, specific areas of the body are more commonly affected by certain conditions. 1) Face—autoimmune disease, pyoderma, demodectic mange, contact dermatitis, ringworm, scabies, seborrhea; 2) Feet—neurotic dermatoses, pyodermas, demodectic mange, atopy, hookworm infection, vasculitis; 3) Carpi and tarsi—lick granulomas; 4) Lateral elbows—scabies, calluses, pressure point pyoderma; 5) Trunk—pyoderma, seborrhea, demodectic mange, *Cheyletiella*, endocrine disorders; 6) Pinnae—scabies, seborrhea, autoimmune disease, hives, pyoderma, vasculitis; 7) Lower back—flea allergy dermatitis, food allergy dermatitis, anal sac impaction or infection, hyperesthesia syndrome (cats); 8) Groin—pyoderma, autoimmune disease, contact dermatitis, atopy, seborrhea.

PRINCIPLES OF THERAPY

There are particular difficulties related to the practice and understanding of dermatotherapy. The mode of action of many drugs used in dermatology is unknown (eg, tars and sulfur are used extensively with remarkable success but without knowledge of the molecular mechanisms involved); there have been few in-depth studies.

The influence of other systems on the integument often demands that treatment be internal as well as topical, eg, it is irrational to treat a dermatosis due to hypothyroidism by external application of medicaments rather than with thyroid hormone. Properly selected topical measures may be the best form of treatment if the cause is unknown or uncertain. The choice of topical measures is determined largely by the morphological characteristics, and by the stage and site of the eruption. A dermatosis should be classified as acute or chronic, dry or exudative, infected or uninfected, superficial or deep, and treated accordingly.

Topical remedies are chosen to produce specific effects according to the character of the lesions. It is better to use a few well-understood remedies rather than be confused by the abundance of available dermatological drugs. A remedy may harm rather than help; when in doubt, the mildest and most indifferent agent should be used. When using a new medicament, the effect should be observed on a small area before proceeding to a larger area; a new remedy should not be tried as long as the dermatosis is improving satisfactorily with the older one. When a remedy disagrees with the animal, it should be discontinued at once and the cause of the disagreement found (if possible). The action of topical remedies often depends on the mode of application and removal. Owners must be given adequate instructions and often a demonstration for correct use, including application and removal. Whether or not the diagnosis is certain, topical therapy in many dermatoses is important in therapeutic management.

Topical therapy is of value or most suitable when: 1) a definitive diagnosis cannot be made, or has not yet been made; 2) it will hasten the recovery as an adjunct to systemic treatment; or 3) experience indicates that it will be as successful as systemic treatment. *See also* ANTISEPTICS AND DISINFECTANTS, p 1527.

ACANTHOSIS NIGRICANS

A descriptive term for a clinical syndrome with multiple potential underlying etiologies. It occurs in dogs, particularly Dachshunds. Potential causes are many, and more than one may be found in the same animal. Underlying causes to consider include mechanical trauma from friction (especially in obese animals), inhalant allergy, food allergy, contact allergy, pyoderma, hypothyroidism, hyperadrenocorticism, and sex-hormone-related dermatoses. Some cases are idiopathic, and may be hereditary.

Lesions consist of varying degrees of symmetrical axillary erythema, alopecia, hyperpigmentation, and thickening and lichenification of the skin. Signs may progress to involve the medial forelimbs, ventral neck, thorax, and abdomen. The surface of affected skin frequently has a greasy or waxy texture. Pruritus may be present.

Underlying and contributing causes should be identified. A complete evaluation includes skin biopsy, allergy testing, a hypoallergenic diet trial, thyroid and adrenal evaluation, and other tests as appropriate for the individual animal. A diagnosis of idiopathic acanthosis nigricans is made by excluding all known causes.

Many therapies have been advocated, and the variable benefit obtained with each probably reflects the multiple underlying etiologies. Treatment should be specific when possible. Melatonin (1 u/dog, subcut. once daily for 3 days, then as needed) has been advocated for idiopathic cases, but is rarely effective and is difficult to obtain. Vitamin E (dl-α-tocopherol acetate) at 200 IU, PO, b.i.d. for 1-2 mo is beneficial for some idiopathic cases. Topical therapy with antiseborrheic shampoos and weight reduction in obese animals are helpful.

ALLERGY TESTING

Tests for diagnosis of allergic skin disease in animals include intradermal skin testing and *in vitro* serum-based tests such as radioallergosorbent test or ELISA. They are used primarily to detect allergy to airborne substances; their use in food allergy is controversial.

Intradermal Skin Testing: IDST is the most commonly used and best characterized test. It is used in dogs and cats for diagnosis of allergic inhalant dermatitis (atopy or atopic dermatitis) and flea allergy, and in horses for diagnosis of inhalant-allergy-related urticaria and insect hypersensitivity. IDST relies on the presence of sensitized mast cells in the skin. When an offending allergen is injected intradermally, these cells degranulate and release inflammatory chemical mediators. The result is a wheal and erythema at the injection site if the animal is allergic.

IDST requires experience and an investment in materials, so it is often done by specialists on a referral basis.

IDST reactions can vary by season; the optimal time for testing most animals is shortly after the worst of the allergy season. Thus, the ideal time to test in the Northern Hemisphere is September-November. Corticosteroid drugs (oral, injectable, and topical forms) interfere with IDST, and must be withdrawn at least 2-4 wk before testing. Antihistamines and tranquilizers can be administered up to 1 wk before testing. During drug withdrawal, concurrent problems such as seborrhea or pyoderma should be treated.

Specific allergens that should be used for testing vary geographically. Individual specific extracts (eg, birch pollen) are preferred to mixed extracts (eg, mixed tree pollens). Allergen extracts are purchased in concentrated form without glycerine preservative and must be diluted before use. Depending on manufacturer, allergen concentration is expressed either as protein nitrogen units/mL (PNU/mL) or weight:volume (w:v). Usual testing dilutions are 250-1000 PNU/mL or 1:5000 to 1:1000 w:v. Potency of testing dilutions deteriorates with time; fresh dilutions should be made q6wk. A positive control (1:100,000 histamine phosphate) and a negative control (allergen diluent solution) are always used.

Sedation may be necessary for testing. Drugs that do not interfere with IDST include xylazine hydrochloride for dogs or horses and ketamine hydrochloride for cats. Small animals are restrained in lateral recumbency and the lateral thoracic region clipped of hair; ~0.05 mL of each test allergen and both controls are injected intradermally at appropriately marked sites. In horses, the lateral cervical skin is used and a volume of 0.1 mL injected.

Immediate reactions are observed 15-30 min after injection. Wheal diameter, and degree of induration and erythema should be noted. The negative control should produce no wheal. The positive control should produce a large (>12 mm), erythematous, indurated wheal; failure to observe a strong positive control reaction indicates a problem with the test, usually drug interference. Reactions are most commonly recorded as 0, 1 +, 2 +, 3 +, or 4 +, with the negative control receiving a score of 0 and the positive control a 4 +. Positive reactions are much more subtle in cats, which makes interpretation difficult.

Transient pruritus at injection sites may occur in ~10% of animals. Severe adverse reactions such as anaphylaxis can occur, but are rare.

In Vitro Testing: These tests, performed in commercial laboratories, detect presence of allergen-specific reaginic antibody (IgE) in the serum. They are available only for dogs. Their usefulness in diagnosis and management of canine allergic disease has not been fully documented. Advantages include ease of use, lack of requirement for special reagents, and lack of necessity to withdraw drugs such as corticosteroids. Sample requirements, test scoring, and interpretation vary according to the laboratory performing the test.

ALOPECIA
(Atrichia, Baldness)

Local or general loss of hair, fur, or wool. Alopecia can be primary, or secondary to many inflammatory skin disorders.

Etiology: Congenital alopecia has been described in cows, horses, dogs, cats, and pigs. Hairless strains of mice and rats have been selected, and are commercially available. Hairlessness invariably accompanies congenital goiter in pigs farrowed by iodine-deficient sows. Acquired alopecia is due to a variety of diseases and intoxications, eg, dietary deficiencies; infectious diseases, particularly those causing febrile reactions or epithelial destruction; and poisoning as by mercury, thallium, iodine, or formaldehyde. Endocrine disorders (hypothyroidism, hyperadrenocorticism, growth-hormone-responsive alopecias, and sex hormone imbalances) are common causes of noninflammatory alopecia, especially in dogs. Temporary alopecia in horses, sheep, and dogs can occur during pregnancy, lactation, or several weeks after a severe illness or fever. Localized hair loss may result from repeated local friction; the continued application of chemicals, irritants, or radiation; ectoparasites; and bacterial and dermatophyte infections.

Clinical Findings and Diagnosis: Alopecia is a frequent sign of a specific skin disease, eg, dermatophytosis or endocrine abnormalities. In acquired alopecia, hair loss usually starts as a focal patch that may enlarge and coalesce with adjacent lesions, or remain static. Pruritus is variable, depending on the primary cause. In endocrine alopecia, the lesions develop in a symmetrical pattern, and pruritus is absent unless there is a secondary bacterial infection. The course of alopecia is chronic and the prognosis unfavorable unless the primary cause is identified and treated.

Skin scrapings for ectoparasites (especially, in dogs, for *Demodex*) should be performed. Bacterial and fungal cultures also may be indicated, especially if the hair loss pattern is patchy and multifocal. The best diagnostic tool is a skin biopsy of representative lesions. Serum concentrations of thyroid hormones, growth hormone, cortisol, estrogens, and androgens should be determined if a bilateral symmetrical alopecia is present. Severe inflammatory diseases can result in permanent scarring and nonresponsive alopecia.

Treatment: Successful therapy depends on the underlying cause and specific diagnosis. The degree of recovery depends on the duration of the disease and amount of damage to the hair follicles. Bacterial infections should be treated for ≥3 wk with an appropriate drug (eg, in dogs, lincomycin 20 mg/kg, b.i.d.; erythromycin 20 mg/kg, t.i.d.; cephalosporin 20 mg/kg, t.i.d.; trimethoprim-sulfa 15 mg/kg, b.i.d.). Dermatophyte infections should be treated as recommended (*see* RINGWORM, p 789). In dogs, if imbalances of the gonadal hormones are the cause of alopecia, neutering is indicated. In hypothyroidism (qv, p 280), therapy with L-thyroxine (0.5 mg/m^2, b.i.d.) is usually effective (for formula to calculate body surface area, *see* p 48.) Gonadal hormone replacement therapy may be given when indicated by examination and serology; however, estrogen (and possibly androgen) therapy may have serious side effects.

For male dogs, methyltestosterone, 1 mg/kg (maximum 30 mg) may be given every other day. For female dogs, 0.1 mg of diethylstilbestrol may be given every day for 3 wk, then discontinued for 1 wk; this cycle is repeated for 3 mo. Care should be taken to avoid bone marrow depression. If successful, sex hormone therapy should be tapered to the lowest possible effective dosage.

CATTLE GRUBS
(*Dermatobia hominis* and *Hypoderma* spp)

Hypodermosis of cattle in the Northern Hemisphere is caused by the larvae (cattle grubs or ox warbles) of flies of the genus *Hypoderma* (order Diptera, family Oestridae). *Hypoderma (Oedemagena) tarandi* parasitizes native Cervidae and reindeer in Arctic regions. In Central and South America, larvae (tropical warbles) of *Dermatobia hominis* (Diptera, Cuterebridae) are important pests of cattle.

DERMATOBIA HOMINIS

The tropical warble fly or torsalo, one of the most important parasites of cattle in Latin America, is distributed between southern Mexico and northern Argentina. Larval stages are found in many hosts: cattle, sheep, goats, pigs, buffaloes, dogs, cats, rabbits, and man. Cattle and dogs are infected most commonly.

Life Cycle: The adult fly is 12-15 mm long; its life span is short (av 4 days). The adult fly fastens its eggs to different types of insects (49 [mostly mosquitoes and flies] have been described as vectors of *D hominis* in Latin America) that then transport them to the mammalian hosts where they hatch as the insects feed. The larvae migrate under the skin of the animal within a few minutes of hatching and remain in the subcut. tissue for 39-50 days. During this period, the larvae grow and produce warbles with a breathing hole. When mature, the larvae leave the host and drop to the ground, burrow, and pupate. The pupal period lasts 32-43 days; the flies then emerge as adults. The complete life cycle takes 78-117 days.

Larval penetration of the skin is accompanied by severe pain and local inflammation, and pus gradually forms. Hides are condemned at slaughter, and production of milk and meat is reduced.

Treatment and Control: Different systemic insecticides in various formulations are available for treatment. Organophosphorus insecticides such as dichlorvos and fenthion are used in Latin America as spray or spot-on products; trichlorfon is available as an oral, spray, or injectable product; ivermectin may be given subcut. or as a pour-on.

HYPODERMA SPP

Two species of *Hypoderma*, *H bovis* and *H lineatum*, are important pests of cattle. They occur between 25° and 60° latitude in the Northern Hemisphere, in more than 50 countries of North America, Europe, Africa, and Asia. In North America, *H lineatum*, the common cattle grub, is found in Canada, the USA, and northern Mexico; *H bovis*, the northern cattle grub, is found generally north of the 35th parallel. Occurrence in cattle and American bison is common. Larvae of *Hypoderma* spp also have been reported in horses, sheep, goats, and man.

Life Cycle: Adult *Hypoderma* (heel flies) are hairy and ~15 mm long. In late spring or early summer, they attach their eggs on the hair of cattle, particularly on the lower legs. The eggs hatch in 3-7 days, and first-stage larvae emerge, travel down the hair, and penetrate the skin. Larvae appear to travel almost exclusively through connective tissue. They secrete proteolytic enzymes that dissolve tissue and facilitate their movement. During autumn-winter, larvae migrate toward 2 different regions, depending on the species. *Hypoderma lineatum* migrates to the connective tissue of the esophageal wall where they congregate for 2-4 mo. *Hypoderma bovis* larvae migrate to the region of the spinal canal; some are found in the epidural fat of the canal where they congregate for a similar period.

Beginning in early winter, the larvae begin their final migration, again through connective tissue, and arrive in the subdermal tissue of the back of the host where they make a breathing hole through the skin. Cysts or "warbles" are formed around the larvae, and they undergo 2 molts (second and third stage). This warble stage lasts 4-6 wk. Finally, the third-stage larvae emerge through the breathing holes, drop to the ground, and pupate. The flies emerge from the pupae in 1-3 mo, depending on weather conditions. The adult flies, which do not feed, live <1 wk. The life cycle is complete in 1 yr.

For the 2 species, seasonal events are similar except that those for *H lineatum* occur ~6-8 wk earlier than those of *H bovis*. These events vary from year to year, but are fairly well correlated with local and regional climatic conditions. In southern USA, larvae first appear in backs of cattle about mid-September, whereas at northern latitudes appearance is delayed until late January or later. Grubs first emerge from the back during the last half of November in Texas and during the first half of March in Montana. When both species are present, grubs may appear in the back for ~5-6 mo; when only *H lineatum* is present, for ~3-4 mo. In southern USA, the activity of ovipositing female flies is at its height January-March and in the northern states, May-July.

Clinical Findings and Pathogenesis: During periods of sunshine on warm days, cattle may run with their tails high in the air when chased by female heel flies, particularly *H bovis*. Not all stampeding or "gadding" of this kind is the result of heel fly attacks; this activity has been observed in absence of heel flies.

In otherwise normal cattle, *H bovis* larvae and their secretions in the epidural fat of the spinal canal are associated with dissolved connective tissue, fat necrosis, and inflammation. Sometimes, the inflammation extends to the periosteum and bone, producing a localized area of periostitis and osteomyelitis. Occasionally, the epineurium and perineurium may become involved. In rare severe cases, paralysis or other nervous disorders may occur. Similarly, *H lineatum* in the submucosa of the esophagus may cause sufficient inflammation and edema in the surrounding tissues to hinder swallowing or eructation. It is unusual, however, for clinical signs of parasitism to be evident during the migratory phase.

Penetration of the skin by newly hatched larvae produces a hypodermal rash. The points of penetration are painful and inflamed, and usually exude a yellowish serum. Grubs may occur in the back from tailhead to shoulders, and from topline to about one-third the distance down the sides. The cysts or warbles are firm and usually raised considerably above the normal contour of the skin; in each there is a breathing hole, ranging in size from a small slit to a round hole, 3-4 mm in diameter, for mature larvae. Secondary infection of cysts may result in large suppurating abscesses. The emergence of the grub, its forced expulsion, or its death within the cyst usually results in healing of the lesion without complications. Carcasses and hides of cattle infested with cattle grubs show marked evidence of the infestation and are reduced in value.

The number of warbles in an infested animal is 1 to ≥300; infested herds may have animals with no grubs. Younger animals are more heavily infested.

As *Hypoderma* larvae migrate through connective tissue toward their predilected sites, if they die in either site, especially near the spinal cord, they can cause severe reactions that are sometimes fatal; these reactions appear to be related to grub abundance, but are rare in any case.

Death of first-stage larvae of *H bovis* in the spinal canal of cattle following systemic insecticide treatment has produced stiffness, ataxia, muscular weakness, and paralysis of hindlimbs. Recovery is usually rapid and complete, but occasionally paralysis may be permanent.

Death of the first-stage larvae of *H lineatum* causes inflammation of the esophageal wall, dysphagia, drooling of saliva, and bloat. Again, recovery is usually rapid and complete (48-72 hr after treatment), but in severe cases the bloat may be fatal. Rupture of the esophagus may be caused by attempted passage of a stomach tube.

Diagnosis: Third-stage larvae can be easily differentiated: *H bovis* is generally larger, has no spines on the tenth segment, and the spiracular plate is funnel shaped; *H lineatum* is smaller, has spines on the tenth segment, and the spiracular plate is generally flat. In cases of bloat or paralysis, presence of disintegrating grubs and the associated hemorrhage and tissue damage distinguishes between parasitized and "clean" animals.

Treatment and Control: Six different systemic insecticides, in various formulations, are available for treatment. Pour-on treatments of coumaphos, famphur, fenthion, phosmet, trichlorfon, or ivermectin should be poured evenly along the midline of the back. Fenthion in a 20% formulation should be applied to a single spot on the animal's midline.

Sprays containing coumaphos or phosmet also control cattle grubs; sufficient volume and pressure are needed to thoroughly wet the entire surface of the skin for maximal absorption. Coumaphos and phosmet also may be used as a dip. Ivermectin is systemically active against cattle grub larvae when administered subcut., PO, or as a pour-on.

No organophosphate systemic agent should be used in conjunction with another since their actions may be synergistic. Cattle stressed by castration, overheating, vaccination, or shipping should not be treated. Use of these organophosphates and of ivermectin is prohibited in lactating dairy animals. Because residues are present in cattle for varying periods after treatment, withdrawal times should be observed strictly.

Cattle, especially calves, in areas where grub numbers are high, should be treated as soon as possible after the end of the heel fly season. They should not be treated later than 8-12 wk before the anticipated first appearance of grubs in the backs, since adverse reactions may occur when migratory larvae are killed.

Where systemic insecticides cannot be used and rotenone is approved, cattle grubs can be controlled by applying rotenone to the warbles in the back. Since new grubs continue to appear in the back, and since rotenone kills only those with which it comes in contact through the breathing holes, treatment must be repeated every 30-45 days during the warble season. A wash or dust with crude rotenone should be applied to the animal's back and worked into the grub holes. This treatment, if properly applied, kills >90% of the grubs in the back.

On small groups of tractable animals, extraction by instrument or hand expulsion (by squeezing) of the individual grubs is effective. Rarely, when this procedure is carelessly performed, the grub is crushed in its cyst and an anaphylactic reaction may result.

CONGENITAL AND INHERITED ANOMALIES OF THE SKIN

Congenital defects involving the skin and its adnexa are not uncommon, and most are genetic.

Albinism is classified as partial, incomplete, or complete. Partial albinism is characterized by an iris that is blue and white centrally and brown peripherally, and a coat color that is usually characteristic of the breed or more dilute. Animals with incomplete albinism, which is inherited as an autosomal dominant, may have colobomas of the nontapetal fundus and tapetal fibrosum hypoplasia.

Chédiak-Higashi syndrome (qv, p 63), characterized by partial albinism, is inherited recessively; affected animals have abnormally large, membrane-bound organelles in various cell types, and increased susceptibility to infection. Complete albinos have pure white coats and white to pink irises, but a normal tapetum lucidum. Complete albinism is inherited as a simple autosomal recessive.

An albinotic color deficiency in Angus cattle, oculocutaneous hypopigmentation, is inherited as a simple autosomal recessive. Brown hair is seen over the entire body, and the muzzle, hooves, and scrotum also are brown. Skin surface is brown to gray, and this is particularly obvious on the glabrous skin around eyelids, ears, muzzle, anus, and vulva. The most distinguishing feature involves iris color: the black iris is replaced by a light, usually dual-colored iris giving a double-ringed appearance. The pupils always appear constricted in daylight, and from a distance, the eyes appear white. The ocular fundus is albinotic.

Skin fragility, similar to Ehlers-Danlos syndrome in man, is characterized by extreme skin fragility, joint laxity, cutaneous fragility, and delayed healing of skin wounds. Collagenous tissues of the body reveal fragmentation and disorganization of fibers and lack of maturity. Skin from affected calves contains 12% less protein and 36% less glycine than normal skin. The defect has been identified in the Middle and High Belgian, Hereford, Simmental, Charolais, and German Black Pied breeds of cattle.

Epitheliogenesis imperfecta is inherited as a simple autosomal recessive and occurs in Holstein, Ayrshire, Jersey, Shorthorn, and Angus calves. Holstein calves have large epithelial defects distal to the carpal and tarsal joints, and one or more defective claws. Muzzle, nostril, tongue, hard palate, and cheeks also have epithelial defects. The ears are deformed by rolled margins and adhesions on the contacted surfaces. Ayrshire calves have similar but less extensive lesions and are without horn or claw defects. Jersey calves have extensive epithelial defects in the oral cavity and on the body and legs. They also have gross defects such as brachygnathia inferior and atresia ani. Shorthorn and Angus calves have large epithelial defects distal to carpal and tarsal joints and have one or more defective claws and dewclaws. There are also epithelial defects in the oral cavity and esophagus. Calves affected with epitheliogenesis imperfecta either are born prematurely or die shortly after birth from septicemia.

Imperfect keratogenesis (inherited parakeratosis, adema disease) is inherited as a simple autosomal recessive in Black Pied cattle and British Friesians. The disease possibly is present in Holsteins in the USA. Affected calves appear normal at birth but after 1 mo, exanthema of the legs develops with symmetrical hair loss. Some calves develop diarrhea; others, CNS signs, conjunctivitis, rhinitis, and bronchopneumonia. Calves develop scaly, thickened, and folded skin over the neck and shoulders; they are alopecic and the horns fail to grow. Lesions of exudative dermatitis develop on the legs, and erosions of the mucosa of the oral cavity, esophagus, and forestomachs are seen. Skin lesions are followed by deterioration of body condition. The pathogenesis of imperfect keratogenesis involves deficient uptake of zinc in the intestine (chromosomal defects are common in these calves but are considered a sequela rather than the cause of this defect).

Congenital ichthyosis, due to homozygosity of a simple autosomal recessive gene, has been described in Pinzgauer, Canadian Holsteins, and Chianina calves. The defect is characterized by absence of hair, and the entire body is covered by horn plaques measuring up to 1 in. in diameter. The horn plaques are separated by deep fissures, from which hair sprouts. The defect is lethal. Associated defects include microtia, cataracts, and thyroid dysplasia.

Six different kinds of **hypotrichoses** may be distinguished in cattle, all sensitive to environmental influences. All 6 types are inherited and severity varies; some are lethal. Lethal hairless, semihairless, and viable hypotrichosis are simple autosomal recessive characters; hypotrichosis with anodontia is considered to be a sex-linked recessive trait; hypotrichosis with missing incisor teeth is possibly a dominant trait; and streaked hairlessness is a dominant sex-linked gene. A patterned hairlessness with anodontia is seen in Chinese Crested dogs.

The single most common trait is viable hypotrichosis in horned and polled Hereford calves. The defect ranges from slight to severe. Huxley's cells of the hair follicles contain spheroidal microdroplets of semitranslucent, pleomorphic material, abundant in the region of differentiation and transformation of papillary cells into inner and outer hair sheaths. These microdroplets are electron-dense trichohyaline granules and lack the micro- and macrofilaments usually seen in normal cattle.

Dermatosis vegetans is a relatively rare hereditary condition of pigs caused by a semilethal, autosomal recessive factor thought to have originated in the Danish Landrace breed. Erythematous plaques, progressing to wart-like lesions, on the feet, belly, and inner thighs can be seen at birth or developing during the first 3 wk of life. Growth is retarded and death usually occurs from an associated giant-cell pneumonitis within 6 mo, although some appear to recover completely.

Congenital erythropoietic protoporphyria is an uncommon hereditary photosensitizing disease recognized only in Limousin cattle and man. Decreased activity of the mitochondrial enzyme ferrochelatase throughout the body allows accumulation of free protoporphyrin in developing RBC, which by diffusion, enters the plasma and intercellular fluids, and ultimately the feces. Protoporphyrin in the plasma and extracellular fluid is associated with cutaneous photosensitivity.

Affected animals are photosensitive in areas of skin exposed to near ultraviolet light. Calves may also suffer seizures. Affected animals sheltered from light grow well. The defect is inherited as a simple autosomal recessive and has been identified in the USA and Canada. Diagnosis is based on clinical signs and analysis of porphyrin levels in the RBC and feces. There should be no protoporphyrin in the urine. Clinically normal heterozygous animals have a distinct but moderately elevated concentration of free protoporphyrin in the RBC. A similar disease, congenital erythropoietic porphyria (qv, p 444), occurs in cattle and other species and is characterized by additional problems and signs. (*See also* PHOTOSENSITIZATION, p 820.)

CONTAGIOUS ECTHYMA
(Contagious pustular dermatitis, Sore mouth, Orf)

An infectious dermatitis of sheep and goats, affecting primarily the lips of young animals. Encountered in all parts of the world, it is most common in late summer, fall, and winter on pasture, and in winter in feedlots. The condition may occur in young lambs in early spring and occasionally in mature sheep that do not have immunity from natural exposure. Man is occasionally affected, and the disease has been reported in dogs that have eaten infected carcasses.

The causal poxvirus (a parapoxvirus) is related to those of pseudo-cowpox and bovine papular stomatitis. Infection occurs by contact. The virus is highly resistant to desiccation, having been recovered from dried crusts after 12 yr. It is also resistant to glycerol and to ether.

Clinical Findings and Diagnosis: The primary lesion develops on the skin of the lips, with frequent extension to the mucosa of the mouth. Occasionally, lesions are found on the feet, usually in the interdigital region and around the coronet. Ewes nursing infected lambs may develop lesions on the udder. In young lambs, the initial lesion may develop on the gum below the incisor teeth. The lesions develop as papules and progress through vesicular and pustular stages before encrusting. Coalescence of numerous discrete lesions often leads to the formation of large scabs, and the proliferation of dermal tissue produces a verrucose mass under them. When the lesion extends to the oral mucosa, secondary necrobacillosis (qv, p 718) frequently develops.

During the course of the disease (1-4 wk), the scabs drop off and the tissues heal without scarring. During active stages of the infection, the more severely affected lambs fail to eat normally and lose condition. Extensive lesions on the feet lead to lameness. Mastitis may result in ewes with lesions on the udder.

The lesion is characteristic. The disease must be differentiated from ulcerative dermatosis (qv, p 866), the virus of which produces a different kind of reaction leading to tissue destruction and formation of crateriform ulcers. Ecthyma usually affects younger animals than does ulcerative dermatosis, although this criterion can only be used presumptively. A positive differentiation may be obtained by inoculating susceptible and ecthyma-immunized sheep.

Treatment and Control: Antibacterials may help combat secondary infection. In endemic areas, appropriate repellents and larvicides should be applied to the lesions. The virus is transmissible to man, and the lesions, usually confined to the hands and face, are more proliferative, and occasionally very distressing. Veterinarians and sheep handlers should exercise reasonable protective precautions. Diagnosis in man is established by transmitting the virus to sheep; a complement-fixation test may be of value.

Sheep recovered from a natural attack are highly resistant to reinfection. Despite a multiplicity of immunogenic virus strains, with an occasional exception, the presently employed commercial single-strain vaccines have produced fair immunity in all parts of the USA. Vaccine "breaks" appear to be due to the virulence of the infecting strain rather than differences in antigenicity of the vaccine. Sheep immunized against contagious ecthyma remain susceptible to ulcerative dermatosis.

Vaccines should be used cautiously to avoid contaminating uninfected premises, and vaccinated animals should be segregated from unprotected stock until the scabs have fallen off. A small amount of the vaccine is brushed over light scarifications of the skin, usually on the inside of the thigh. Lambs should be vaccinated when ~1 mo old. For best results, a second vaccination ~2-3 mo later is suggested. Nonimmunized lambs should be vaccinated before going into infected feedlots. Experimental work suggests that parenteral administration of virulent vaccine induces better immunity than does the current procedure.

CUTEREBRA INFESTATION, SM AN

The presence of the larva of a rodent or rabbit bot fly, *Cuterebra* spp (order Diptera, family Cuterebridae), in the subcutis. Adult *Cuterebra* are nonparasitic and seldom observed. Females deposit eggs in or near nests, or along runways of the normal hosts. Infective larvae, which develop inside the eggs, hatch in response to heat from a nearby host. Although larvae usually enter the host via the mouth and nares, other body openings as well as skin lacerations may be used. Following penetration, they migrate to various subcut. locations in different hosts. The route of migration is variable. The larva may reach 25 mm in length and 10 mm in diameter. Black cuticular spines give fully developed larvae a dark color. The larva takes ~1 mo to develop, after which it exits to pupate in the soil. The duration of pupation varies considerably, depending on environmental factors and winter diapause. Adult flies, which deposit 5-15 eggs per site, may deposit >2000 eggs.

A thick-walled, subcut. abscess of variable size forms around the developing larva. Pus may exude from the breathing hole made through the skin by the parasite. Aberrant larval migration may occur, including invasion of the brain with fatal CNS disturbances.

Cuterebra are incidental parasites of those aberrant hosts likely to make contact with eggs. Dogs and cats may become infested, presumably from investigating rodent burrows or other egg sites. Lesions are found most often under the skin of the neck and chest during late summer and early fall. Constant licking of the chest area is frequently the most obvious clinical sign in cats.

On rare occasions, dogs and cats may be infested with *Hypoderma* spp, or more commonly, with *Dermatobia hominis* in areas where it is present.

The lesion should not be squeezed since rupture of the parasite may result in anaphylaxis. The breathing hole through the skin should be enlarged surgically to permit careful removal of the larva. The lesion is then treated as any abscess with flushing and instillation of antibiotic preparations.

DERMATITIS

Inflammation of the skin can be produced by myriad agents, including external irritants, burns, allergens, trauma, and bacterial, viral, parasitic, or fungal infections. It can be associated with concurrent internal or systemic disease, and hereditary factors also may be involved. Allergies (qv, p 425 *et seq*) form an important group of etiological factors, especially in small animals.

The most common sign is scratching, followed by skin lesions that progress from edema and erythema to papules, vesicles, oozing, and crusting or scaling. Secondary infection may occur. As the disease becomes chronic, the erythema decreases and there are fewer papules, but the lesions are drier and the skin may develop fissures. Findings may vary considerably with the species affected and the cause.

Since palliative measures rarely effect a cure, it is important to determine the underlying cause. A thorough history should be taken, noting the progression (pruritic? seasonal?), the environment, food, exposure to and involvement of other animals or persons, and any prior treatment. Physical examination should define the areas affected: generalized, trunk, face, mucous membranes, etc. Diagnostic tests such as skin scrapings for ectoparasites, skin culture for bacteria and fungi, skin biopsy, endocrine evaluation, hypoallergenic diet, or intradermal skin testing should be employed when indicated.

Until the underlying cause is diagnosed, or in idiopathic dermatitis, both topical and systemic palliative therapy may be used. The hair should be clipped from the affected and surrounding areas. Acute moist dermatitis may be treated with astringent soaks (eg, Burow's solution) or a minimally occlusive corticosteroid lotion or cream. Chronic dry dermatitis is usually helped by application of a corticosteroid ointment. To remove scales or crusts, a sulfur and salicylic acid or tar and sulfur shampoo may be used. Tar products are contraindicated for cats.

Unfortunately, topical medicaments often are licked or rubbed off; systemic therapy with anti-inflammatory doses of corticosteroids is usually the best alternative. A short-acting, oral drug should be used (prednisone, prednisolone). Initial dosage is 1 mg/kg, PO once daily; this should be gradually reduced to the lowest possible every-other-day dose that provides symptomatic relief. Before using either systemic or topical costicosteroids, infectious etiologies must be eliminated.

Restraining devices (hobbles, Elizabethan collars) and sedatives should be used only as last resorts in the therapy of pruritus. They contribute little to the comfort of the animal or diagnosis of the disease.

DERMATOPHILOSIS

(Dermatophilus infection, Cutaneous streptotrichosis, Lumpy wool, Strawberry foot rot)

An infection of the epidermis, seen worldwide, but more prevalent in the tropics, also called, erroneously, mycotic dermatitis. The lesions are characterized by exudative dermatitis with scab formation. *Dermatophilus congolensis* has a wide host range. In domestic animals, the condition most frequently affects cattle, sheep, and goats; it occasionally affects horses, but is rare in pigs, dogs, and cats. It is commonly called cutaneous streptotrichosis in cattle, goats, and horses; in sheep, it is termed lumpy wool when the wooled areas of the body are affected, and strawberry foot rot when the distal portions of the limbs are affected. The few human cases reported usually have been associated with handling diseased animals.

The natural habitat of *D congolensis* is unknown. Although probably a saprophyte in the soil, attempts to isolate it from soil have been unsuccessful; it has been isolated only from the integument of various animals, and is restricted to the living layers of the epidermis. Asymptomatic chronically infected animals are considered the primary reservoir.

Etiology, Transmission, and Epidemiology: *Dermatophilus congolensis*, the only species in the genus, is a gram-positive, non-acid-fast, facultative anaerobic actinomycete. It has 2 characteristic morphologic forms: filamentous hyphae and motile zoospores. The hyphae are characterized by branching filaments (1-5 μm in diameter) that ultimately fragment by both transverse and longitudinal septation into packets of coccoid cells. The coccoid cells mature into flagellated ovoid zoospores (0.6-1 μm in diameter).

Factors such as prolonged wetting by rain, high humidity, high temperature, and various ectoparasites that reduce or permeate the natural barriers of the integument influence the development, prevalence, seasonal incidence, and transmission of dermatophilosis. The organism can exist in a quiescent form within the epidermis of lesions until exacerbated by climatic conditions. Epidemics usually occur during the rainy season. Moisture facilitates release of zoospores from pre-existing lesions and their subsequent penetration of the epidermis and establishment of new foci of infection. High humidity also contributes indirectly to the spread of lesions by allowing increases in the number of biting insects, particularly flies and ticks, which act as mechanical vectors. Infection can be spread by shearing, dipping, or introducing an infected animal into a herd or flock.

Dermatophilosis is contagious only in that any reduction in systemic or local skin resistance favors establishment of infection and subsequent disease.

Pathogenesis: To establish infection, the infective zoospores must reach a skin site where the normal protective barriers are reduced or deficient. The respiratory efflux of low concentrations of carbon dioxide from the skin attracts the motile zoospores to susceptible areas on the skin surface. Zoospores germinate to produce hyphae, which penetrate into the living epidermis and subsequently spread in all directions from the initial focus. Hyphal penetration causes an acute inflammatory reaction. Natural resistance to the acute infection is due to phagocytosis of the infective zoospores, but once infection is established, there is little or no immunity. In most acute infections, the filamentous invasion of the epidermis ceases in 2-3 wk, and the lesions heal spontaneously. In chronic infections, the affected hair follicles and scabs are sites from which intermittent invasions of noninfected hair follicles and epidermis occur. The invaded epithelium cornifies and separates in the form of a scab. In wet scabs, moisture enhances the proliferation and release of zoospores from hyphae. The high carbon dioxide concentration produced by the dense population of zoospores accelerates their escape to the skin surface, thus completing the unique life cycle.

Clinical Findings: Dermatophilosis occurs in all ages, but is most prevalent in the young. Lesions are not at the same stage of progression, and in an individual animal can vary from acute to chronic. Variation also occurs because of age, sex, and breed. Few animals exhibit pruritus, and most recover spontaneously within 3 wk of the initial infection or during dry weather. Uncomplicated skin lesions heal without scar formation. These infections usually have little effect on general health. Animals with severe generalized infections often lose condition, and movement and prehension are difficult if the feet, lips, and muzzle are severely affected; these are often sent to slaughter as incurable. Deaths occasionally occur, particularly in calves and lambs, because of generalized disease with or without secondary bacterial infection and secondary fly or screwworm infestation. The primary economic consequences are damaged hides in cattle and wool loss in sheep.

Lesions: Distribution of the gross lesions on cattle and sheep usually correlate with the predisposing factors that reduce or permeate the natural barriers of the integument. In cattle, the lesions can be observed in 3 stages: 1) hairs matted together as "paintbrush" lesions, 2) crust or scab formation as the initial lesions coalesce, and 3) accumulations of cutaneous keratinized material forming "wartlike" lesions that are 0.5-2 cm in diameter. Typical lesions consist of circular dome-shaped scabs 2-8 mm in diameter. Most lesions associated with prolonged wetting of the skin are distributed over the head, dorsal surfaces of the neck and body, and upper lateral surfaces of the neck and chest. Cattle that stand for long periods in deep water and mud develop lesions in areas such as skin folds of the flexor surfaces of the joints. Lesions initiated by biting flies (mechanical vectors) are found primarily on the back, whereas lesions induced by ticks are primarily on the head, ears, axillae, groin, and scrotum.

Chronic lumpy wool infections are characterized by pyramid-shaped masses of scab material bound to wool fibers. The crusts are primarily on the dorsal areas of the body and prevent the shearing of sheep. Spiny plants often predispose to lesions on the lips, legs, and feet. Strawberry foot rot is a proliferative dermatitis affecting the skin from the coronet to the carpus or hock.

Histopathological examination of the lesions reveals the characteristic branching hyphae with multidimensional septations, coccoidal cells, and zoospores in the epidermis. The organisms are usually abundant in active lesions, but can be sparse or absent in chronic lesions.

Diagnosis: Presumptive diagnosis depends largely on the appearance of lesions in clinically diseased animals and demonstration of *D congolensis* in stained smears or histological sections from scabs. A definitive diagnosis is made by culture and identification. Differential diagnoses include the dermatomycoses in most species, warts and lumpy skin disease in cattle, and contagious ecthyma and ulcerative dermatosis in sheep.

Treatment and Control: Since acutely infected animals usually heal rapidly and spontaneously, treatment is indicated only for cosmetic reasons. Usually, chronic infections can be rapidly and effectively cured with a single IM injection of procaine penicillin (22,000 IU/kg) and streptomycin (22 mg/kg). If this fails, the penicillin-streptomycin combination can be administered for 5 days, or a single injection of long-acting oxytetracycline (20 mg/kg) can be substituted.

Isolating clinically affected animals, culling affected animals, and controlling ectoparasites are methods used to break the infective cycle. External treatment with disinfectants that contain a cresol or copper salt base can decrease the spread of infection if applied at times when transmission is likely. Insecticides applied externally are frequently used to control biting insects.

DERMATOPHYTOSIS
(Ringworm)

An infection of keratinized tissue (skin, hair, and nails) by one of several genera of fungi collectively called dermatophytes. (*See also* FUNGAL INFECTIONS, p 340). All domestic animals are susceptible. Pathogenic fungi are found worldwide. A few dermatophytes (eg, *Microsporum gypseum*) normally inhabit soil (geophilic) but can cause disease in animals, including man. Other dermatophytes (eg, *M audouinii*) are adapted to man and infect animals rarely (anthropophilic); still others are primarily animal pathogens (eg, *M canis, Trichophyton equinum,* and *T verrucosum*) but can cause disease in man (zoophilic). Transmission occurs primarily by contact with infected individuals, contaminated fomites such as furniture, grooming tools or tack, or with soil that contains a geophilic species. Occasionally, spread of thallic conidia (arthrospores) through the air may occur. Zoonotic transmission sometimes occurs, and is especially common with *M canis*. Contact with a dermatophyte does not always result in infection. Whether infection is established depends on the fungal species and host factors, such as age, immunocompetence, fungistatic activity of skin secretions, concurrent disease, and nutritional and hormonal status. The most susceptible hosts are young, debilitated, or immunocompromised. Recovery from infection is accompanied by development of cell-mediated immunity against dermatophyte antigens, and usually results in immunity to further infection.

Under most circumstances, dermatophytes grow only in dead keratinized tissue, and advancing infection halts on reaching live cells or inflamed tissue. Zoophilic fungi are host-species adapted, and rarely cause severe inflammatory reactions in animals; in man, they often cause acute inflammatory reactions that limit their progress. Infection begins in a growing hair or in the stratum corneum, where thread-like hyphae develop from conidia. The hyphae penetrate and invade the hair shaft, thus weakening it, and grow downward as the hair grows upward. Fungi do not penetrate the living, mitotic region of the hair; when hair growth terminates, fungal growth terminates. The important species of animal dermatophytes produce clusters of arthrospores primarily along the outer surface of the hair (ectothrix type) rather than within the hair shaft (endothrix type).

Dermatophytoses are extremely variable in their clinical appearance. Diagnosis is accomplished by culture, examination with a 366 nm wavelength ultraviolet lamp (Wood's lamp), or direct microscopical examination of hairs or scrapings.

Fungal culture is the most effective and specific means of diagnosis. It frequently shows infections missed by the other procedures, and permits fungal species identification. Dermatophyte Test Medium (DTM) may be used. Following mild cleansing of the affected area with water or 70% alcohol to reduce saprophytic contamination, hairs and scales are removed and placed on the agar plate, which is then covered or sealed to reduce evaporation. Incubation at room temperature is sufficient. Dermatophyte growth usually is apparent within 3-7 days, but may require up to 3 wk. Dermatophytes cultured on DTM produce a color change in the medium from yellow to red at the time the colony is first visible; the colonies themselves are white to off-white. Saprophytic fungal colonies are white or pigmented, but almost never produce an initial color change. Saprophytes turn DTM red with prolonged incubation, so it is crucial to examine cultures daily for color change. Definitive diagnosis and species identification require removal of hyphae and macroconidia from the surface of the colony with acetate tape, and microscopical examination with lactophenol cotton blue stain.

The Wood's lamp is useful in screening examinations for *M canis* infections in animals (and *M audouinii* infections in man). Infected hairs fluoresce yellowish green; infected scales do not fluoresce. This procedure has limited application, since only ~50% of *M canis* infections fluoresce, and other animal dermatophyte species are nonfluorescent. False-positive fluorescence may occur, especially with the scaling and crusting seen in canine seborrheic disease. Also, certain topical medications (soap, petrolatum, tetracyclines) and keratin may fluoresce. Iodine or other medications that contain halogens may block fluorescence in infected hairs. Fluorescing hairs should always be cultured to confirm presence of a dermatophyte.

Direct microscopical examination of hairs or skin scrapings sometimes permit definitive diagnosis by demonstrating characteristic hyphae and/or arthrospores. Hairs or scrapings from the periphery of a suspicious area are examined for fungal elements in a wet preparation (20% potassium hydroxide [KOH] in water) that has been gently warmed and squashed out under a coverslip.

Addition of a stain specific for chitin in the fungal cell wall (chlorazole black E, 100 mg/100 mL KOH solution) facilitates identification of arthrospores and hyphae.

DERMATOPHYTOSIS IN CATTLE

Trichophyton verrucosum is the usual cause of ringworm in cattle, but other *Trichophyton* spp are isolated occasionally. The disease is most common in calves. After an incubation period of 2-4 wk, the hair in the infected area breaks off or falls out, and by 2-3 mo, thick, round, raised, sharply circumscribed, gray-white, crusting plaques are seen. Lesions expand at the periphery and can reach 5-10 cm in diameter. Sites of predilection include the head, neck, and perineum. If untreated, lesions can generalize, especially in calves. Pruritus is usually absent, and secondary pyoderma is unusual. Ringworm is more common during the winter in stabled animals, but may occur at any time. A presumptive diagnosis can be based on typical clinical signs, and confirmed by culture.

For treatment, many topical medications are apparently successful. Since spontaneous recovery is common, the main virtue of topical therapy probably is to prevent progression of existing lesions and limit spread of infective material to other animals. Thick crusts should be removed gently with a brush and mild soap, and the contaminated material burned. Effective topical therapy includes washes or sprays of 0.5% lime-sulfur, 0.5% sodium hypochlorite (1:10 chlorine bleach), 0.5% chlorhexidine solution, 1% povidone-iodine, or 1:300 Captan. These medications are applied to the entire body surface of affected animals daily for 5 days, then weekly until the infection is controlled. Individual lesions also can be soaked regularly in a 5% suspension of thiabendazole in dimethyl sulfoxide. An attenuated fungal vaccine is in use in Europe, and provides effective prophylaxis; it is not available in the USA or Canada.

DERMATOPHYTOSIS IN DOGS AND CATS

In dogs, ~70% of cases are caused by *Microsporum canis*, 20% by *M gypseum*, and 10% by *Trichophyton mentagrophytes*. In cats, ~98% are caused by *M canis*, with *M gypseum* and *T mentagrophytes* accounting for the remainder. Because of the high prevalence of *M canis* infections, the Wood's light is a useful screening tool for these species. However, since *M gypseum*, *T mentagrophytes*, and half of the *M canis* strains do not fluoresce, a negative Wood's lamp examination does not rule out dermatophytosis. Diagnosis should always be confirmed by culture. Detection of infection in asymptomatic carrier animals is facilitated by brushing the coat with a new toothbrush or nylon scalp massager, then inoculating a culture plate by pressing the bristles to the surface of the medium.

The clinical appearance of feline ringworm is quite variable. Kittens are affected most commonly. Lesions often consist of focal alopecia, scaling, and crusting, are minimally erythematous, and most often occur around the ears, face, and extremities. There may be no clinically apparent lesions, or there may be only a few broken hairs around the face and ears. Such animals often serve as carriers and create a particular problem in catteries or multiple-animal households. Up to 90% of "infected" cats may appear normal. Occasionally, dermatophytosis in cats occurs as a "miliary dermatitis"-like condition. Pruritus may or may not be present.

Lesions in dogs usually consist of alopecic, scaly patches with broken hairs. Atypical forms of canine dermatophytosis may be seen. In one form, lesions consist of papules and pustules without alopecia or scaling. Sharply demarcated, raised, erythematous, alopecic plaques or nodules are termed kerion ringworm, and may be associated with a local hypersensitivity reaction. *Trichophyton mentagrophytes* can cause localized, somewhat symmetrical infection on the bridge of the nose that is easily confused with many other diseases. Generalized ringworm is rare in the dog unless accompanied by immunodeficiency (including that due to corticosteroid or other immunosuppressive therapy and hyperadrenocorticism) or a metabolic disease such as diabetes mellitus. Differential diagnoses in dogs include demodectic mange, bacterial folliculitis, and circular seborrheic lesions.

Dermatophytosis in small animals is usually self-limiting. The primary objective of therapy is to prevent spread of infection to other animals and owners. Topical therapy almost always suffices. Whole-body treatment is preferred over spot treatment of lesions, since the latter may miss grossly inapparent areas of infection. Lime-sulfur (0.5%), chlorhexidine (0.5%), or 1:300 Captan solution can be used as a rinse twice weekly. For chronic or severe cases, systemic therapy with griseofulvin is warranted. The dose for dogs is 40-120 mg/kg body wt of the microcrystalline form administered once daily or in divided doses, with a high-fat meal. Cats should not receive >20-50 mg/kg/day, due to potential bone marrow toxicity. Griseofulvin-resistant strains are seen occasionally in man, but have not been reported in animals. Dermatophytes may be sensitive to ketoconazole (10-30 mg/kg, daily), although this drug is not approved for use in animals. All treatments for dermatophytosis are continued for 2-4 wk past clinical cure or negative fungal culture. Treatment for 1-3 mo is usually necessary.

DERMATOPHYTOSIS IN HORSES

Trichophyton equinum is the primary cause of ringworm in horses, although *Microsporum equinum* (often confused with *M canis*) is important in some localities; *T mentagrophytes, M canis,* and *M gypseum* are found occasionally. Clinical signs consist of one or more patches of alopecia; erythema, scaling, and crusting are often present but vary in severity. Early lesions may resemble urticaria, then progress to alopecia and crusting in a few days. Diagnosis is confirmed by culture. Differential diagnoses include dermatophilosis and bacterial folliculitis. Transmission by contaminated grooming equipment, saddle blankets, and harnesses is especially common.

Successful treatment requires medication of the animal and decontamination of the environment. Ideally, affected animals should be isolated. Topical treatment consists of whole-body rinsing in an antifungal agent (*see* above [cattle] for recommendations) daily for 5-7 days, then weekly until cure results. The rinse may be preceded by a povidone-iodine shampoo if desired. Grooming tools and tack should be disinfected frequently and not transferred from affected to unaffected animals.

DERMATOPHYTOSIS IN OTHER SPECIES

Dermatophytosis in pigs usually is caused by *Microsporum nanum*. Lesions consist of centrifugally spreading rings of inflammation with central alopecia and reddish brown crusts. Typically, lesions are 4-6 cm in diameter. Affected pigs should be isolated until lesions heal. Pens and rubbing posts should be cleaned and disinfected. For treatment, *see* DERMATOPHYTOSIS IN CATTLE, above.

Ringworm is uncommon in sheep and goats. The primary infecting species is *Trichophyton verrucosum*. Lesions are most often found on the head, neck, and shoulders. Treatment is the same as in cattle.

MISCELLANEOUS DERMATOSES

A number of systemic diseases produce various lesions in the skin. Usually the lesions are noninflammatory, and alopecia is common. In some instances, the cutaneous changes are characteristic of the particular disease. Often, however, the dermatosis is not obviously associated with the underlying condition, and must be carefully differentiated from primary skin disorders. Some of these secondary dermatoses are mentioned briefly below, and also are described in the chapters on the specific disorders.

Dermatosis may be associated with nutritional deficiency, especially of proteins, fats, minerals, some vitamins, and trace elements. However, this is uncommon in dogs and cats fed modern diets because of improvements in pet food nutrition. Siberian Huskies, and occasionally other breeds, may develop a disease similar to parakeratosis in pigs and require additional zinc in their diet (220 mg zinc sulfate, q12-24hr). Zinc-responsive dermatoses have also been reported in cattle, sheep, and goats, and are associated with a higher individual requirement, not a dietary deficiency.

Dermatitis is sometimes observed in the course of chronic disorders of internal organs, such as nephritis, hepatitis, or pyometra, and with diseased anal sacs. Poisoning by thallium sulfate (rat poisons), ergot, mercury, and iodides may cause various skin changes. Hyperkeratosis in cattle can be caused by chlorinated naphthalene toxicity.

In dogs, dermatosis can develop as a result of endocrine dysfunction. In males with Sertoli cell tumors, bilateral alopecia and occasional pruritus with a papular eruption may be seen. Intact female dogs with hormonal imbalances are usually pruritic and have a papular eruption, mammary tissue enlargement, and frequent estrous cycles. The skin lesions of both disorders may begin in the inguinal or flank region and progress cranially. Dermatosis following neutering is not common in dogs and cats; when it does occur, it is generally nonpruritic, with mild alopecia in the perineal or inguinal areas. However, feline endocrine alopecia is seen mainly in neutered male cats. It is characterized by a bilaterally symmetrical diffuse thinning of the hair, which begins in the genital and perineal regions. The etiology is unknown, but it usually responds to sex-hormone therapy.

Dermatoses have been observed in hypothyroidism. The skin lesions are characterized by diminished hair growth and bilaterally symmetrical alopecia. The skin is dry, scaly, thickened, and folded. Acanthosis and seborrheic disorders also may occur. In rare cases, cutaneous myxedema develops.

Faulty production of hypophyseal hormones may rarely cause dermatoses. Hypopituitarism is characterized by alopecia, especially in the axillary regions and on the lateral thorax and abdomen. Hyperadrenocorticism also is manifest by skin changes such as hyperpigmentation, alopecia, seborrhea, calcinosis cutis, and secondary pyoderma. In diabetes mellitus, pruritus and secondary infection may occur.

Treatment of all these conditions depends on a specific etiological diagnosis. Once this is established and managed, the skin lesions usually need only symptomatic care (eg, control of scratching) until they disappear with resolution of the primary disease. (*See also* THE ENDOCRINE SYSTEM, p 254 *et seq.*)

ECZEMA NASI OF DOGS
(Collie nose, Nasal solar dermatitis)

Nasal dermatitis of dogs should be considered as a clinical sign of many diseases. Lesions may affect the bridge of the nose, the planum nasale, or both. In pyoderma, dermatophytosis, and demodicosis, the haired portions of the nose are affected. In lupus or pemphigus, the whole muzzle is often crusted with occasional oozing of serum or ulceration. In systemic and discoid lupus, and occasionally in pemphigus and cutaneous lymphoma, the planum nasale is depigmented, erythematous, and eventually may ulcerate. Eczema nasi due to solar radiation probably is a rare disease, often a misdiagnosis for the lupus variants. In nasal solar dermatitis, the nonpigmented areas of the nasal planum are affected first, and occasionally the bridge of the nose may become inflamed and sometimes ulcerated. The lesions are worse in the summer, although lupus and pemphigus may also show this seasonal variation. Any of the above diseases may affect the periocular areas. (*See also*, SYSTEMIC LUPUS ERYTHEMATOSUS, p 430, and PEMPHIGUS, p 429.)

Treatment depends on etiology. Diagnostics should include skin scrapings, bacterial and fungal cultures, and biopsies for both histopathology and immune testing.

If the diagnosis is nasal solar dermatitis, a topical corticosteroid lotion (betamethasone valerate, 0.1%) is helpful in relieving inflammation. Exposure to sunlight must be severely curtailed. Topical sunscreens may be effective, but need to be applied at least b.i.d.

EOSINOPHILIC GRANULOMA COMPLEX

A group of diseases that affects cats, dogs, and horses. The etiology is unknown, although in cats an underlying hypersensitivity reaction may be present.

Clinical Findings: In cats, 3 disease entities have been grouped in the complex.

Eosinophilic ulcer: A well-circumscribed, erythematous, ulcerative lesion, usually not painful or pruritic, and usually found on the upper lip (*see also* p 126). These lesions occasionally progress to squamous cell carcinoma, which is the major differential diagnosis. Histology shows an ulcerative dermatitis, with a cellular infiltrate of neutrophils, plasma cells, and mononuclear cells predominating. Tissue or peripheral eosinophilia is uncommon.

Eosinophilic plaque: A well-circumscribed, erythematous, raised lesion that occurs most commonly in the medial thigh region and is extremely pruritic. Histology shows a diffuse eosinophilic dermatitis, with marked inter- and intracellular edema and vesicles containing eosinophils in the epidermis. Mast cells are often present in large numbers, and this condition must be distinguished from mast cell tumor. Peripheral eosinophilia is common.

Linear granuloma: This is usually raised, well circumscribed, yellowish to pink, with a distinctly linear configuration, although this pattern may be less noticeable when the lesions occur in the mouth. Usually they occur on the caudal aspect of the rear legs. Histologically, a granulomatous inflammatory response surrounds degenerative collagen. Tissue and peripheral eosinophilia are marked when the lesions are in the mouth, but vary when lesions are on the skin.

In **dogs**, the lesions reported as eosinophilic granulomas histologically resemble the linear granuloma of cats, with marked collagen degeneration surrounded by a granulomatous and eosinophilic infiltrate. These lesions may occur as ulcerated or vegetative masses in the oral cavity or, less commonly, as plaques, nodules, or papules on the lips and other areas of the body. Any breed may be affected, but Siberian Huskies may be at greater risk.

In **horses**, the disease has been termed equine eosinophilic granuloma with collagen degeneration. Other names are nodular necrobiosis of collagen, collagenolytic granuloma, and axillary nodular necrosis. The lesions are nodular, nonulcerative and nonpruritic, often occur in the saddle area, and may have a gray-white central core. Older lesions may become mineralized. Both insect bites and trauma have been suggested as etiologies, although the occasional onset during winter in cold climates and in noncontact saddle or tack areas suggest multifactorial causes. Histology reveals multifocal areas of collagen degeneration surrounded by granulomatous inflammation containing eosinophils. Thus, histologically this lesion is similar to linear granuloma of cats and eosinophilic granuloma of dogs.

A rare disease of horses, characterized grossly by a progressive exfoliative dermatitis and histologically by an eosinophil-rich perivascular infiltrate with occasional spongiosis and eosinophilic pustules, has been termed equine exfoliative eosinophilic dermatitis and stomatitis. Eosinophilic granulomas in internal organs and the oral cavity have been noted in severe cases. A similar hypereosinophilic syndrome has been identified in cats.

Treatment: In cats, hypersensitivity disorders (allergy to fleas, food, or inhalants) should be investigated. If no underlying cause can be determined and the condition is causing discomfort, corticosteroids such as methylprednisolone acetate (4 mg/kg), given IM once q2wk for 2-3 injections, or triamcinolone tablets (4 mg/5 kg body wt) every 1-3 days may be used. In cases of relapse, one injection of methylprednisolone acetate q6wk is often effective. In dogs, the lesions seem much more responsive to corticosteroids, and therapy is oral prednisone or prednisolone (0.5 to 2 mg/kg/day initially, and tapering the dosage over 20-30 days). Lesions recur in some dogs, in which case low-dose, every-other-day corticosteroid therapy is indicated. In horses with solitary lesions of equine eosinophilic granuloma with collagen degeneration, the lesions may be treated by surgical excision or sublesional corticosteroid injections. Mineralized lesions require excision. Triamcinolone acetonide (3-5 mg/lesion) or methylprednisolone acetate (5-10 mg/lesion) is effective. No more than 20 mg triamcinolone acetonide should be administered sublesionally because of the potential to induce laminitis. Horses with multiple lesions may be treated with oral prednisone or prednisolone at 1.1 mg/kg, q24hr for 2-3 wk. In equine exfoliative eosinophilic dermatitis and stomatitis and feline hypereosinophilic syndrome, corticosteroids, even at high doses, have been ineffective. The prognosis for this disease is grave, and affected animals are usually euthanized.

EXUDATIVE EPIDERMITIS
(Greasy pig disease)

An acute, generalized dermatitis that occurs in 5- to 60-day-old pigs, characterized by sudden onset, with morbidity of 10-90% and mortality of 5-90%. It has been reported from most swine-producing areas of the world and occurs frequently in the corn-belt area of the USA.

Lesions are caused by *Staphylococcus hyicus (hyos)*, but the bacteria seem unable to penetrate intact skin. Abrasions on the feet and legs or lacerations on the body frequently precede infection. A vesicular-type virus may be a predisposing factor.

Pigs develop resistance with age, but the organism may be recovered from the skin of older pigs, the vagina of sows, and the preputial diverticulum of boars. Suckling pigs are usually infected by their dams, but cross-infection occurs after mixing at weaning.

Clinical Findings and Lesions: The first signs are listlessness and reddening of the skin in one or more piglets in the litter. Affected pigs rapidly become depressed and refuse to eat. Body temperature may be elevated early in the disease but thereafter is near normal. The skin thickens, reddish brown spots appear from which serum exudes, and pain is evident in acutely affected pigs. Often, there is suppurative inflammation of the external ear and catarrhal inflammation of the eyes.

Vesicles, possibly caused by a virus, develop on the skin, burst, and become infected. The body is rapidly covered with a moist, greasy exudate of sebum and serum, which becomes crusty. Vesicles and ulcers also occur on the nasal disk and tongue. The feet are nearly always involved with erosions at the coronary band and heel; the hoof may be shed in rare cases. In the acute disease, death occurs within 3-5 days. Otherwise, particularly in older animals, the disease is milder; circumscribed lesions develop slowly and do not coalesce. Mortality is low except in those affected while very young, but recovery can be slow and growth retarded.

Necropsy of severely affected pigs reveals marked dehydration, congestion of the lungs, and inflammation of the peripheral lymph nodes. Distention of the kidneys and ureters with mucus, cellular casts, and debris is common in peracute and acute forms of the disease.

Treatment: The causative organism is inhibited by most antibiotics, and penicillin in heavy dosage can be successful if started early. Treatment may be less effective in young pigs and in advanced cases. Infected litters should be isolated and a broad-spectrum antibiotic administered. In severe outbreaks, pigs in contact may also be given antibiotics for several days. Thorough washing of severely affected pigs with soap and a warm, mild disinfectant solution can aid recovery. Sows due to farrow, and their housing, should be disinfected thoroughly to halt an outbreak. Other control measures include raising the zinc and biotin levels of the diet, and vaccination.

Recently, bacterial interference by nonpathogenic strains of *S hyicus* has been demonstrated.

FLEAS

Ubiquitous bloodsucking ectoparasites, principally of dogs and cats, that can cause pruritus and subsequent severe dermatological problems. The 2 species commonly found infesting household premises, *Ctenocephalides felis* and the less prevalent *C canis*, readily feed on dogs, cats, and man. *Pulex irritans*, considered a flea of man, also feeds on dogs and cats. Fleas require warmth and moisture to complete their life cycle; in temperate climates they may be only a seasonal summer problem, but in more tropical zones or warm indoor areas, serious perennial infestations are common. Fleas also act as intermediate hosts for the common tapeworm *Dipylidium caninum*, and can transmit the filarial parasite *Dipetalonema reconditum*. Transmission of other diseases by the common cat or dog flea is not currently recognized.

Dog and cat fleas are not known to transmit disease to man, but their ability to feed on human blood indicates that they are undesirable from a human health perspective. Additionally, dogs and cats may serve as transient carriers of other species of fleas that may transmit other diseases (*see* PLAGUE, p 363). Papular urticaria and multiple pruritic skin lesions caused by flea bites are quite common in both children and adults, and may be the first noticeable signs of flea infestation of the pets of the household.

Etiology and Epidemiology: Adult fleas can jump long distances and readily attach themselves to animals moving through infested environments. Minor irritation may be caused by their crawling on the skin surface and piercing the epidermis. The major problem is frequent induction of allergic hypersensitivity by salivary secretions of the flea.

In a humid environment, fleas can survive off the host for up to 7 mo without a blood meal. When attached to a host, they feed voraciously but digest only a small percentage of ingested blood, the remainder being excreted as small, black, fecal "flea dirts". Feeding stimulates egg laying while on the host, and adult female fleas lay several hundred eggs during their lifetimes. The small white eggs do not adhere to skin or hair but fall freely off the host to contaminate bedding, floors, carpets, and the environment. The legless larvae that emerge from the eggs are virtually invisible to the unaided eye. They actively feed on local proteinaceous debris, particularly the dried blood feces of adult fleas. The larvae pupate, and adult fleas later emerge from the tiny cocoons. The entire flea life cycle is completed in ~3 wk under favorable environmental conditions.

Fleas can rapidly reproduce into epidemic populations during a few warm months. Severe infestations in pet-owning households can result in a massive number of adult fleas, which readily bite human skin and can make premises almost uninhabitable.

Pathogenesis: Fleas feed quickly by biting through the epidermis and sucking blood from damaged skin capillaries. Multiple feeding bites may be made at a site within a few minutes, and several fleas can cause hundreds of individual skin penetrations over a brief period. Hosts that have not become hypersensitive to flea salivary antigens may experience little or no skin reaction to flea bites; however, many individuals eventually develop allergic hypersensitivity to fleas (**flea allergy dermatitis** [FAD]) and may exhibit both immediate urticarial skin wheals and delayed inflammatory lesions that are intensely pruritic. Much of the resulting skin damage is then caused by self-inflicted scratching, chewing, biting, and rubbing. Severity of clinical signs is related more to the degree of hypersensitivity than to the number of fleas present. In a highly sensitive individual, very few fleas can cause severe disease, and the duration of clinical signs may be for many days past the time of the actual bite. Individual animals vary in their sensitivity to flea allergens; in dogs, this depends in part on their prior exposure pattern to flea bites—intermittent exposure leads to greater hypersensitivity than continuous exposure. Allergic skin reactions to flea bites are less well documented in cats.

Clinical Findings: Pruritus is usually the first sign of flea infestation in dogs and cats, often in the absence of any obvious dermatological lesions. Lesions are most common on the dorsal lumbosacral area, dorsum of the tail, medial and caudal aspects of the hindlimbs, and abdominal and inguinal areas. Repeated scratching may not cause much significant skin damage but often annoys owners of household pets. Occasionally, a cat (or a dog) may be infested but asymptomatic. Because massive numbers of fleas can remove significant amounts of blood from small animals, anemia is not uncommon in heavy infestations.

Lesions: A wide variety of skin lesions can develop in hypersensitive animals. Classical evidence is dorsal alopecia with inflamed exudative dermatitis, particularly near the base of the tail. Chronically affected dogs may develop marked hair loss and hyperkeratosis or "elephant hide". Patches of acute moist dermatitis or "hot spots" may arise in dogs when skin is damaged by self-inflicted scratching or chewing, although fleas are not always the cause of this condition. Cats with chronic flea infestations may have no lesions or pruritus, or develop miliary dermatitis ("scabby cat disease"), with multiple, small, raised papules and crusts found mainly on the skin of the back. However, these lesions are not always flea-related, and the degree of pruritis may vary. In addition, fleas may be responsible for excess grooming behavior and have been implicated as contributing to the eosinophilic granuloma complex.

Diagnosis: Adult fleas are visible, particularly if an illuminated magnifying lens is used, although not always found on the animal. A diagnostic aid is the "wet paper test": a sheet of plain, white paper is thoroughly moistened and held under the animal while the dorsal hair coat is briskly combed with the fingers. Any dislodged "flea dirts" produce visible reddish brown blood stains on the paper. It is not easy to prove that pruritus or exudative dermatitis is being caused by fleas; however, they are the most common cause, and it is reasonable to initiate insecticidal treatment.

The severity of a household flea infestation cannot be fully assessed by examination of resident animals; the owners must also be questioned to learn if human skin is being bitten and which areas or rooms are most used by the animals and therefore most likely to be infested.

Differential diagnoses of FAD include atopy, food allergy, seborrheic disorders, pyoderma, dermatophytosis, and canine scabies. A positive intradermal test with commercial flea antigen lends support to the diagnosis and aids in owner education, but not all dogs with FAD have a positive intradermal test. Any pruritic dermatitis with a primarily caudodorsal distribution, presence of fleas or flea feces, or inadequate flea control measures appropriate for the geographic region should be treated initially as FAD. If the animal fails to respond to vigorous flea control measures within 4 wk, coexisting disease or other differential diagnoses should be considered.

Diagnosis in cats is based on history, clinical signs, and response to therapy. Differential diagnoses include food hypersensitivity, cheyletiellosis, trombiculidiasis, dermatophytosis, atopy, bacterial folliculitis, and idiopathic miliary dermatitis.

Treatment and Control: There are no "easy" effective flea controls; the infestation must be persistently controlled on several fronts. The elements of a successful program are: 1) All animals in a household should receive regular insecticidal treatment appropriate to seasonal needs. A direct skin application is required in the form of a spray, aerosol, bath, rinse, dust, or foam application. A flea collar may be used for additional protection but should not be regarded as the sole means of control. Oral dosing of dogs with cythioate or topical administration of fenthion may be tried, but efficacy is variable, and toxicity must be avoided. 2) Animal sleeping quarters should be primary targets for insecticidal application because flea feces, eggs, larvae, and pupae accumulate there. Bedding should also be regularly washed, and the entire area kept clean by rigorous vacuuming and sanitizing as often as necessary. 3) Rooms frequented by animals may benefit from occasional use of flea control foggers or hand sprayers. Frequent use of a vacuum cleaner reduces accumulation of flea eggs and debris. 4) Outdoor areas where animals play, rest, or sleep should be sprayed with insecticide, especially during warmer weather. 5) For a controlled household, all visiting animals should be treated on arrival unless their flea-free status is certain. Animals returning from boarding kennels should be treated immediately. 6) An ideal program probably should include prophylactic treatment early in the season before any fleas are seen. The appearance of adult fleas on animals usually indicates that infestation of the entire premises has already occurred, and the parasite population is rapidly escalating.

The choice of chemicals is critical for the success of a control program. Synergized pyrethrins, synthetic pyrethroids, carbamates, and organophosphates (OP) all have their place, and new formulation technology promises to extend residual effects. Methoprene is an insect growth regulator approved for flea control; it inhibits maturation of larvae into adults. It is also available in a spray formulation, in which it has ovacidal effects. Its use in combination with insecticides appears to offer better overall sustained premises control. (*See also* EXTERNAL PARASITICIDES, p 1497.)

OP toxicity (qv, p 1669) can occur in animals if they are exposed to simultaneous multiple use of this class of compounds in flea collars, sprays, rinses, oral cythioate, fenthion, or dichlorvos anthelmintic treatment. Cats are particularly susceptible; if an OP is used, it should be with caution. Similar advice may apply to Greyhounds. Concentrated OP preparations should be handled with caution as spillage on unprotected skin can cause serious systemic toxicity in man.

Resistance of fleas to certain chemicals has been reported but is often used as an excuse for inadequate epidemiological control.

Effective treatment of FAD hinges on eradication of fleas, along with other appropriate measures to control secondary pyoderma, seborrhea, or pyotraumatic dermatitis. As a temporary measure to provide relief from pruritus while flea control is underway, short-acting corticosteroids may be used (eg, prednisolone, 0.5-1 mg/kg, once daily for 4-7 days, then every other morning [in dogs—in cats, every other evening] for an additional 10 days). There is no justification for repeated use of injectable long-term corticosteroids to control FAD in dogs, since this may lead to iatrogenic hyperadrenocorticism. Attempts to hyposensitize animals with commercial flea antigen preparations are rarely successful.

FLIES AND MOSQUITOES

FLIES

BLACK FLIES AND BITING GNATS

Black flies, also known as buffalo gnats, are members of the family Simuliidae, order Diptera. They are characterized by a strongly humped thorax, a marked enlargement of the anterior wing veins, and the absence of simple eyes. Few species are >5 mm long. They range in color through gray, olive, and black. Only the females feed on blood, and their mouthparts include blade-like piercing stylets. The antennae consist of 9-12 segments. Eyes of the female are distinctly separated; those of the male, with rare exceptions, are contiguous above the antennae. The palpi have 5 segments. Although there are >1000 species of Simuliidae, only a few are considered important as pests. Black flies feed on all classes of livestock, wildlife, birds, and man.

Simuliidae are distributed throughout the world in areas where conditions permit development of the immature forms. Black flies often occur in swarms where strong or swiftly flowing streams provide well-aerated water for larval development. Larvae nearly always are found in running water; shallow mountain torrents are favored breeding places. Some species, including some notable pests, breed in larger rivers; others live in temporary or semipermanent streams. Black flies are particularly abundant in the north temperate and subarctic zones, but many species occur in the subtropics and tropics where factors other than seasonal temperatures affect their developmental and abundance patterns.

Larvae attach to rocks or other solid objects (eg, the sides and concrete drop structures in irrigation canals, concrete dams) in the stream, sometimes clinging to aquatic or emergent vegetation.

Black flies have 1-6 generations per year, depending on the species and climatic conditions. Adult female activity may last from 2-3 wk up to 3 mo. Nectar from flowers provides carbohydrates for flight energy for both females and males, but females usually require blood for ovarian development.

Adults may fly 8-11 miles (12-18 km) from their breeding places, but migrating wind-borne swarms may go much farther. *Simulium arcticum* may travel ≥90 miles (150 km) in this way in western Canada, and other species are reported to travel ≥250 km. *Simulium colombaschense* may travel 200-450 km with wind currents in the Danube Valley.

Another group of biting gnats belongs to the family Ceratopogonidae. These small, bloodsucking flies are often referred to as midges, sandflies, punkies, or "no-see-ums". *Culicoides* spp are the most common. They are associated with wet or semiaquatic habitats, such as in mud or moist soil around streams, ponds, and marshes. They are vicious biters and can cause irritation to both people and livestock. (*See also* SWEET ITCH IN HORSES, p 804.)

In addition to local reactions (reddened, itching wheals) at the bite site, there may be general conditions that vary in intensity with the sensitivity of the individual and the number of bites. Attacks by large numbers of black flies can cause heavy damage and high mortality in livestock, and man may be viciously attacked.

Death from black-fly attack apparently results from a toxin in the saliva, which increases the permeability of the capillaries and permits the fluid from the circulatory system to ooze out into the body cavity and tissue spaces. The animal rapidly succumbs to a mass attack, but can recover quickly if protected from further onslaughts. Reductions in meat, milk, and egg production may result from less extensive attacks. Certain species of black flies sometimes cause losses in poultry either by direct attack or through the transmission of *Leucocytozoon* spp. In Africa, members of the complexes grouped around *S damnosum* and *S neavei* are important as vectors of *Onchocerca* spp. In Central America, *S ochraceum, S metallicum, S callidum,* and *S exiguum* are important vectors of *Onchocerca. Simulium ochraceum* and *S metallicum* also can be vicious biters. The African species, *S neavei,* an important vector of *O volvulus,* and several other species have an obligate relationship with river crabs of the genus *Potamonautes.*

Culicoides spp also are vicious biters and can cause intense irritation and annoyance. In large numbers, they can cause livestock to be very nervous and interrupt their feeding pattern. *Culicoides* midges are also capable of transmitting diseases, including onchocerciasis in horses and bluetongue in sheep and cattle.

Treatment and Control: Since area-wide control of black flies is difficult and expensive, livestock raisers frequently resort to the daily use of repellents for the protection of their animals. Extension entomology personnel should be contacted for the latest approved recommendations. If public funds and trained supervisory personnel are available, large-scale control of black flies is possible by treating breeding streams with an approved larvicide. Pesticide treatments involving water surfaces or large land areas are subject to governmental regulation and must be done with due regard for possible deleterious environmental effects and residues in food products. (*See also* ECTOPARASITICIDES, p 1497.)

BLOWFLY STRIKE
(Cutaneous myiasis, Fleece worms, Fly strike, Wool maggots)

Several species of blowflies cause myiasis in sheep. Primary flies in USA and Canada are the black blowflies, *Phormia regina* and *Protophormia terraenovae,* and the green bottle fly, *Lucilia sericata. Lucilia illustris, Cochliomyia (Callitroga) macellaria* (secondary screwworm), and some others are usually secondary invaders. *Lucilia cuprina* is the most important primary fly in Australia and South Africa; *L sericata* in Great Britain; and *L cuprina*, *L sericata*, and *Calliphora stygia* in New Zealand.

Eggs, usually laid below the tip of the fleece, hatch within 24 hr if conditions are moist. Moisture and nutrients from serum, feces, etc, are necessary for survival of the first-stage maggot. The second-stage larva can abrade the skin with its mouth hooks to obtain food. Once established, strikes can spread rapidly and attract more blowflies, secondary as well as primary. Bad strikes can be fatal, but even mild strikes can cause rapid loss of condition. Strikes should be diagnosed early; behavior of the sheep is a good indicator of myiasis. Screwworm (qv, p 830) may be suspected if the larvae are associated with wounds.

A common site of strike is the breech, where flies are attracted to wool soaked with urine or contaminated with feces. The body of the sheep also may be struck. This is usually associated with soaking rains that cause development of fleece-rot, often characterized by discoloration due to *Pseudomonas* sp, or dermatophilosis (qv, p 787). Other sites are heads of horned rams, wool around the prepuce, sides where feet with foot rot come in contact with the fleece, and wounds.

Blowfly infestation of the breech can be effectively controlled for ~6-8 wk by "tagging" or "crutching" (wool is shorn between the legs and around the tail). Complete shearing controls outbreaks involving other parts of the body. Wool removed from around the head and the prepuce can prevent strike in these areas. Urine staining of the crutch of Merino ewes can be virtually eliminated by removal of breech wrinkles (Australian Mules operation), and fecal contamination can be greatly reduced by docking tails correctly at the third joint. Scouring should be controlled. Odors and associated moisture attract flies and stimulate oviposition, particularly during hot, humid weather.

Chemoprophylaxis consists of wetting to complete saturation of susceptible areas with suitable insecticidal and larvicidal preparations such as the organophosphorous insecticides, or cryomazine, a specific larvicide in dips or sprays. The most efficient procedure is to force insecticide into the fleece (usually locally—to the breech, along the back, head) under high pressure ("jetting"). Protection can last 6-8 wk, but where the primary fly is resistant, eg, *L cuprina* in Australia, it may last only 2-3 wk. Weekly application of agents such as ronnel (2.5%) under pressure to wounds until healed can be highly beneficial, particularly for screwworm. Individual treatment should begin with removal of all the wool from the struck area and around it, before applying suitable agents. Burning, or deep burying of the carcass may be a valuable general hygienic measure, but may have little effect on primary strikes. The main source of primary flies is the struck sheep.

BUFFALO FLIES

Haematobia irritans exigua is similar to the horn fly, *H irritans*, in size and appearance, and in feeding and breeding habits. The buffalo fly is a primary pest of cattle and water buffalo but occasionally feeds on horses, sheep, or wildlife. It is distributed throughout northern Australia and New Guinea, and is found in parts of southern, southeastern, and eastern Asia, and Oceania but does not extend into New Zealand. Its development is similar to that of the horn fly; the adult leaves the host animal only long enough to oviposit on the fresh manure, where development occurs. The life cycle may take as little as 7-10 days, depending on weather conditions.

Of primary concern with buffalo flies is their irritation and annoyance to animals. Bite wounds usually occur about the shoulders and withers, and may provide a site for screwworm infestation. During hot weather, the flies move to shaded parts of the body. Affected animals suffer blood loss and are irritated by the flies; feed efficiency and production may be affected adversely.

These flies are easily controlled because they are very susceptible to insecticides. In areas where resistance is not a problem, the pyrethroid ear tag can be used;

however, resistance to pyrethroids has developed in parts of Australia. (*See also* ECTOPARASITICIDES, p 1497.)

FACE FLIES

Musca autumnalis is similar in appearance to the common house fly, and occurs on rangeland cattle throughout southern Canada and most of the USA. Its mouthparts consist of sponging labellae, and there are 4 longitudinal stripes on the abdomen. It can be differentiated from the house fly by the closeness and angles of the interior margins of the eyes and by the distinctive coloration of the face and abdomen.

Cattle are the principal host of the face fly in the USA, but it also will feed on horses and possibly sheep and goats. The face fly is a pest of range cattle, and breeds only in fresh cattle feces in rangeland situations. It does not develop in feedlot situations, and thus is not a pest of confined cattle. The eggs are laid on fresh manure and hatch in ~1 day. The yellowish larvae develop in 2-4 days, and when mature, leave the manure to pupate in the surrounding soil. The complete life cycle from egg to adult requires 12-20 days, depending on climatic conditions. The diapausing adult overwinters within buildings and other protective places.

Face flies often occur in large numbers around the eyes and on the muzzle of livestock. Females feed on facial secretions such as tear fluid, nasal mucus, and saliva to obtain protein for egg development. They also feed on other sources, such as blood from wounds and milk on calves' faces. Because face flies possess small, rough spines (prestomal teeth) on their sponging mouthparts, only a few flies can cause irritation and mechanical damage to the eye tissue of their host. The feeding activity of face flies enhances transmission of *Moraxella bovis*, the principal etiological agent of infectious bovine keratoconjunctivitis. Face flies can also serve as vectors of the nematode eyeworms, *Thelazia* spp, and are a natural vector of the cattle nematode *Parafilaria bovicola*.

Control of face flies is difficult. Much effort has been made using various insecticides and application techniques, such as dust bags, mist sprays, and wipe-on formulations. Also, insecticides and insect growth regulators are used as feed additives. Usually these efforts are less than satisfactory; the introduction of insecticide-impregnated ear tags has provided somewhat better control. However, with most of these devices, seasonal face fly reductions of only up to 70-80% have been achieved, even with 2 tags (one in each ear) per animal.

HEAD FLIES
(Plantation flies)

Hydrotaea irritans is a nonbiting muscid found in large numbers in northern European countries, especially Denmark and Britain, where it is a pest of cattle, sheep, and other livestock. It is a nuisance to domestic stock and man because it is attracted to the mouth, nose, ears, eyes, and wounds to feed on secretions. Unlike other *Hydrotaea* spp, *H irritans* produces one generation each year, with 3 larval instar stages. Eggs deposited in late summer hatch out larvae within a few days. This saprophagous stage is brief, before development to the stage that is predatory on other insect larvae. Overwintering occurs as late-stage larvae. Adults are most active from early June until late September, and are common in the vicinity of thickets or woodland in which they shelter between periods of feeding.

In Britain, sheep are mainly affected. Large swarms of flies, attracted by the movement of animals, congregate to feed on the secretions from the eyes and nose, and the cellular debris at the growing horn base. To alleviate the persistent irritation, the sheep scratch and rub their heads, which results in formation of raw wounds or "broken heads", especially on the poll. Flies, attracted by the blood, settle on these self-inflicted lesions and extend the margins by their feeding activity. Sheep of all ages are involved, but breeds with horns and without wool on the head are most severely affected.

Head flies also attack man, deer, horses, cattle, and rabbits. Although no corresponding "broken head" lesions develop in cattle, the association between the occurrence of summer mastitis (due to *Corynebacterium pyogenes*) and the seasonal activity of head flies is closely linked, especially in Denmark. Head flies may also be involved in the spread of myxomatosis in rabbits.

The development, emergence, and congregation of head flies, which occur away from farm areas, preclude the traditional methods of insecticide spraying of generalized breeding sites and resting habitats. Control at the point of contact between the feeding adult insects and the mammalian hosts is also limited in value. With sheep, the retention of organophosphorous compounds or pyrethrin derivatives on the susceptible head areas is of short duration, which necessitates impractical reapplications in free-ranging animals. Use of insecticide-impregnated ear tags in cattle decreases the incidence of summer mastitis, presumably by reducing transmission by the head fly.

Removal of livestock from infested locations during the fly season is the only completely effective way to prevent damage. Once "broken heads" have occurred, the housing of sheep is the only successful method of stopping further fly damage.

HORN FLIES

Haematobia irritans is a major cattle pest found in most cattle-producing regions of the world. Populations are common in Europe, North Africa, Asia Minor, and the Americas. In North America, the horn fly is found wherever cattle occur. However, it occurs in much larger numbers and for longer periods in the southern and southwestern USA.

Horn flies have the general color and appearance of stable flies, but are only about half the size and more slender. Their bayonet-type, piercing/sucking mouthparts are also similar in appearance and position. Horn flies are almost exclusively pests of cattle and reproduce only in bovine feces, but will also feed on horses, sheep, goats, and wildlife.

Adult horn flies spend their entire life on their host, and females leave only to oviposit eggs on fresh feces, where larval development occurs. In the southern USA, the life cycle can be as short as 1 wk, but in cooler climates and in the spring or fall, development can take 2-3 wk. In some warmer areas (south Florida and southernmost Texas), horn flies continue to reproduce actively throughout the entire year.

Newly emerged flies seeking their host may travel 7-10 miles (11-15 km), but usually find a host in much shorter distances, and migration seldom occurs over any great distance. In the southern USA, fly populations on individual animals may reach into the thousands, especially on bulls not receiving chemical treatment; in the north, they may not exceed 100, although the damage inflicted is similar.

Clinical Findings: Adults of both female and male horn flies pierce the skin to suck blood, which causes pain, annoyance, and blood loss in cattle. Since they feed up to 20 times per day, considerable quantities of blood must be replenished. Also, the irritated animals lose weight because of their less efficient use of feed. Heavy infestations cause lesions along the ventral midline of the animal. Horn flies cause great economic losses annually in the USA; 14% reductions in weight gains on range cattle and losses of 12-14 lb (5-6 kg)/head in weaned calves are common. In dairy cattle, milk production may be reduced 10-20%. In addition, the horn fly serves as the intermediate host of the cattle nematode *Stephanofilaria stilesi* (qv, p 811).

Treatment and Control: Horn flies are relatively easy to control with whole-animal chemical sprays and with self-treating devices, such as dust bags or back rubbers in a forced-use situation. Certain insecticides are also available as feed additives that pass through the animal to kill larval horn flies breeding in the feces. Another method of control is the use of insecticide-impregnated ear tags (pyrethroid or organophosphate). Unfortunately, horn fly resistance to pyrethroids, especially in ear tags, has developed across the south from Florida to Texas, north to Kentucky and Nebraska, and west to California and Hawaii. Consequently, certain guidelines should be followed in controlling horn flies in these areas and other areas where pyrethroid resistance might occur. Animals should be tagged according to label directions. Also, animals should be tagged at or near the beginning of fly season, the tags removed at or near the end of fly season, and alternate treatment methods with non-pyrethroid insecticides used near the end of fly season. If resistance is suspected, retreatment should not be with other brands of pyrethroid ear tags since cross-resistance is likely; use of alternative control methods with non-pyrethroids is indicated.

HORSE FLIES AND DEER FLIES

Flies of this family (Tabanidae) range in size from 6-10 mm up to 25 mm long. Within the family, the most important pests in North America are in the genera *Chrysops* (deer flies), and *Hybomitra* and *Tabanus* (horse flies). The latter 2 generally are larger than the former and are the more serious pests. The host range includes all livestock, wildlife, pet animals, and man. In the USA, the more serious problems are in the southeast, where conditions are moist and more favorable. However, even in upland or dryland areas during certain times of the year, large outbreaks can occur.

The larvae of horse flies are primarily aquatic or semiaquatic, but they can be found in upland areas where little moisture is associated with the soil. The life cycle of many of the species is unknown; it can last 1-2 yr, depending on the species and the location in which they are found. Most horse flies studied have a single brood each year and overwinter in the larval stage. The adult females require a blood meal for ovipositing, while the males feed on flowers and vegetable juices.

Horse flies can transmit the causal agents of anthrax, anaplasmosis, tularemia, and equine infectious anemia. In the Philippines and in Africa, tabanids can transmit several trypanosomes that are pathogenic to livestock. Transmission usually is mechanical, but the flies may also serve as an intermediate host for some agents, eg, *Trypanosoma theileri, Haemoproteus metchnikovi*, and at least 4 nematodes.

The blade-like mouthparts of the female cause a painful wound and a considerable flow of blood, which is then lapped up. A few individuals of the larger species can prevent cattle from feeding normally and add to the loss by the overactivity they stimulate. Blood loss becomes a significant factor when dozens of flies feed on an animal for several hours each day during the summer. Once feeding has ceased, blood may continue to flow from the feeding site and attract other flies, of which the screwworm *Cochliomyia hominivorax* is of the greatest concern in southern Mexico and Central America.

Treatment and Control: Horse flies are the most difficult to control of any of the bloodsucking flies. Many of the compounds used for other flies will kill tabanids; however, they may not be exposed long enough to be affected since they are intermittent feeders that stay on the host for only a short time, and so require larger doses of the compounds. Commercial repellents are protective for only short periods and need to be applied repeatedly to maintain effectiveness. Specific controls should be used only after checking with local regulatory officials.

HOUSE FLIES AND OTHER FILTH-BREEDING FLIES

The house fly, *Musca domestica*, is commonly found around livestock and poultry operations, where it readily breeds in accumulating manure sources. It is grayish with 4 dark thoracic stripes, and equipped with sponging, nonbiting mouthparts. Under favorable climatic conditions, the life cycle can be completed in as few as 10-14 days.

Even though house flies do not feed on blood, annoyance is caused by their movement on and off animals. This can lead to reduced performance. In addition, they have been implicated in the transmission of numerous pathogenic agents of medical and veterinary importance. Also, large house-fly populations may occur near poorly managed livestock or poultry facilities, and be a public annoyance.

Several other species of filth-breeding flies may occur around livestock and poultry facilities; these include little house flies (*Fannia* spp), dump or garbage flies (*Ophyra* sp), false stable flies (*Muscina* spp), black soldier flies (*Hermetia illucens*), various blow flies (family Calliphoridae), and moth flies (family Psychodidae).

A thorough sanitation program is necessary to control fly-populations in and around livestock and poultry facilities. All manure accumulations should be removed at least twice a week or handled properly, if stored on the premises, to minimize fly breeding. If solid manure management practices are applied, efforts should be made to reduce manure moisture. If a liquid manure pit is utilized, manure should not be allowed to accumulate above the waterline, either floating or sticking to the sides, since this is an ideal site for fly production. Insecticides should be considered as supplementary to sanitation and management measures aimed at preventing fly breeding. Residual sprays providing up to 2-4 wk of control with one treatment may be applied to fly-resting surfaces. Space sprays, mists, or fogs with quick "knockdown" but no residual action can be used for immediate reduction of high numbers of adult flies. Other measures for control of adult flies, such as the use of insecticide resin strips or various fly baits, can be taken. These measures are most useful as supplements to other fly-control practices. Larvicides also can be applied directly to fly-breeding sources; however, this should be considered only for fly-breeding spots that cannot be eliminated by normal sanitation practices.

STABLE FLIES

Stomoxys calcitrans has about the same size and general appearance as the house fly. It is brownish gray, the outer of 4 thoracic stripes is broken, and the abdomen has a checkered appearance. It has a needle-sharp proboscis that when at rest points forward from beneath the fly's face. The wings, when at rest, are widely spread at the tips. It is cosmopolitan throughout much of the world.

The stable fly feeds on most warm-blooded animals. Generally, it is found around barns or cattle-loafing areas; however, it also can be found feeding on animals in confined situations. The immature forms develop in decaying organic matter including grass clippings and seaweed along beaches. In the midwestern USA, larvae can be found in wet areas around the edges of hay stacks and silage pits. Where cattle are fed hay, breeding can occur at the edge of the feeding area where hay has become mixed with urine and feces. The life cycle in the field can be completed in 2-3 wk and adults may live 3-4 wk or longer.

Stable flies can be a problem in most areas of the USA but are predominant in midwestern feedlots. The damage inflicted to cattle is caused by the painful bite and blood loss, and the irritation causes animals to be less efficient in converting feed to meat or milk. The stable fly may also be a mechanical vector of anthrax or surra and is an intermediate host of *Habronema microstoma*, a nematode parasite of horses.

Stable flies are difficult to control by treatment of animals since they usually feed only once or twice daily, for short periods. Various approved insecticides can be sprayed where flies may be resting in barns or on fence rows. The main consideration in stable fly control is sanitation, which can effect up to 90% control. Areas along fence rows, under feed bunks, or wherever manure and straw or decaying matter can accumulate should be kept clean since this provides the development medium in which the flies are produced. If good sanitation procedures are practiced, then chemical control is less likely to be needed; without sanitation, chemical control measures are likely to fail.

SHEEP KED
(Sheep tick)

Melophagus ovinus is one of the most widely distributed and important external parasites of sheep. It is a true insect, a wingless fly, and not an acarine. The adult is ~7 mm long, a brown or reddish color, and covered with short, bristly hairs. The female gives birth to a single, fully developed larva, which is cemented to the wool and pupates within 12 hr. A young ked emerges after ~22 days; females live 100-120 days, males ~80 days. During this time, each female produces ~10 larvae.

The entire life is spent on the host. Keds that fall off the host usually survive <1 wk and present little danger of infestation to a flock. Ked numbers increase during the winter and early spring when they spread rapidly through a flock, particularly when sheep are assembled in close quarters for feeding or shelter.

To feed, keds pierce the skin with their mouthparts and suck blood. They usually feed on the neck, breast, shoulder, flanks, and rump, but not on the back where dust and other debris collect in the wool. They cause a defect in hides called cockle. The lesions create a blemish that affects the grade and value of the sheep skin.

The skin irritation causes sheep to rub and bite, and the fleece becomes thin, ragged, and dirty. The excrement of the keds causes permanent discoloration, which is likely to reduce the value of the wool. Infested sheep, particularly lambs and pregnant ewes, may lose vitality and be unthrifty. Keds also transmit *Trypanosoma melophagium*, which is believed to be nonpathogenic for sheep.

Control: Shearing removes many pupae and adults. Thus, shearing before lambing and the subsequent treatment of the ewes with insecticides to control the remaining keds can greatly reduce the possibility of lambs becoming heavily infested. Sheep are usually treated after shearing, and best results are obtained if an insecticide that has a residue that remains at least 3-4 wk is used. By this means, the keds that emerge from the pupae are also killed. Modern treatments to control lice also control the keds.

When vats are available, dipping is regarded as an effective method of treatment. Completely submerging the sheep ensures the destruction of all keds present, but in most instances does not kill the pupated larvae; a long-acting insecticide is required to kill the newly emerging keds. Large flocks of range sheep should be treated in a permanently constructed dipping vat. Smaller flocks and farm flocks may be successfully treated in portable, galvanized-iron dipping vats or in smaller tanks, tubs, or canvas dipping bags.

Spraying may be as effective as dipping, and is more convenient in some areas. Pressures of 100-200 lb/sq in. (7-14 kg/cm^2) for short wool and 300-350 lb/sq in. (21-28 kg/cm^2) for long wool are commonly used.

Shower dipping is also sometimes used; the sheep are held in a special pen and showered from above and below until the fleece is saturated. The run-off is returned for recirculation, and the concentration of insecticide used is the same as for dipping. The concentration of the insecticide can drop rapidly and become ineffective if the instructions for replenishment are not followed explicitly.

Jetting involves the forceful application of the insecticide by means of a hand-held, multiple-jet comb drawn through the short fleece. Although a little slower, and less effective than dips or sprays, it may be advantageous for smaller flocks, since it is economical and does not require a permanent installation.

Spot-on or pour-on formulations of the newer pyrethroids are easy to apply and very effective.

Power dusting is a method that fits well into management practices at shearing time. It is rapid and economical, and avoids wetting the animals. Various types of equipment for dusting are available commercially. (*See also* EXTERNAL PARASITICIDES, p 1497.)

SWEET ITCH IN HORSES

An annually recurring, seasonal, pruritic dermatosis of the horse, affecting the mane, tail, and belly regions, caused by an allergic reaction to *Culicoides* spp, family Ceratopogonidae. Sweet itch occurs worldwide and is known as "*Culicoides* hypersensitivity" in Canada, "Queensland itch" in Australia, and "Kasen" in Japan. *Culicoides* spp, often called midges, sandflies, punkies, or "no-see-ums" (*see also* p 798), are very small, blood-sucking insects. They fly only in the warm months of the year and are most active before and during dusk, feeding often at the mane, tail, and belly. The disease is a result of a type I hypersensitivity reaction.

Usually only a small percentage of horses in a group are affected, the number depending on the exposure to midges. Furthermore, immature horses are rarely affected, and clinical signs often worsen as a horse ages. Ponies may be more frequently affected. A familial predisposition has been observed.

Severe pruritus, alopecia, serous effusion, and crusting caused by excoriation and inflammation are common. In severe, chronic cases, lichenification is also present. The poll, mane, and tail areas are commonly affected, while the belly is rarely involved.

An intensely pruritic, crusting alopecia of the mane and tail regions, associated with exposure to midges, is very suggestive of the diagnosis. Clinical signs are evident only during the warmer months in most cases, but are seen throughout the year in severe cases. Differential diagnoses include onchocerciasis (qv, p 808), and reaction to *Haematobia irritans* (horn fly) and *Stomoxys calcitrans* (stable fly). Onchocerciasis is a nonseasonal dermatosis that is similar to sweet itch but usually is less pruritic and affects the head, neck, and belly. Onchocerciasis and *Culicoides* hypersensitivity are not mutually exclusive, and clinical signs may be similar. Often a definitive diagnosis is not reached until a positive response to treatment has been seen. The horn fly and stable fly both cause a pruritic seasonal dermatosis; the stable fly on the back, chest, neck, and legs; the horn fly on the ventral midline.

Treatment and Control: Prednisolone (400 mg, PO, b.i.d.) or, in severe cases, dexamethasone (10 mg, PO, b.i.d.) is effective in resolving clinical signs. The dose should be decreased gradually after 5 days, to the lowest dosage that controls pruritus. Alternate-day therapy is advised if corticosteroids are to be administered for a prolonged period. Topical cortisone and antibiotics are effective as adjunctive therapy only; the cream base is useful in preventing exposure of the skin to the midges. Antihistamines are ineffective in treating most cutaneous hypersensitivity diseases in horses.

Preventive measures to reduce exposure to midges are preferable to long-term corticosteroid therapy. Stabling affected horses before and during dusk is usually effective because midges rarely enter barns. The use of a fan in a stable to create air movement around the horse is beneficial as *Culicoides* are generally poor flyers. If this is not feasible, fly repellents used before dusk are occasionally effective. Fly-repellent ear tags attached to the horse's mane and tail (not approved in the USA); pyrethrum, synergized with piperonyl butoxide, applied weekly; butoxy-polypropylene glycol 800, applied daily; stable blankets; and fine screens on stable doors and windows have been used with mixed success.

MOSQUITOES

About 3000 species of mosquitoes have been described worldwide, with ~150 in temperate North America. Mosquitoes are the most prominent of the numerous kinds of bloodsucking arthropods. They are found from the salt marshes of the coastal plains to the snow pools above 14,000 ft (4300 m), and to 3600 ft (1100 m) below sea level in the gold mines of India. All classes of livestock, dogs, wildlife, and man are subject to attack.

Important genera include *Aedes, Anopheles, Culex, Culiseta,* and *Psorophora.* Mosquitoes lay their eggs either directly on the surface of standing water or, in the case of most *Aedes* and *Psorophora* spp, on a substrate such as damp soil where they hatch following flooding due to irrigation, rainfall, snow melt, etc. Larvae and pupae, also known as "wigglers" and "tumblers", respectively, are aquatic and occur in a wide variety of habitats from permanent ponds and marshes to flooded pastures and tree holes to an assortment of artificial containers (including old tires) that contain water. Some species have several generations per year, and alternate dry and wet periods due to rainfall or irrigation bring them out in enormous numbers. The flight habits of adults vary with species; some *Aedes* spp are reported to migrate many miles from their aquatic, larval habitat. *Aedes* and *Psorophora* spp usually overwinter in the egg stage, while *Anopheles, Culex,* and *Culiseta* spp generally overwinter in the adult stage.

Psorophora columbiae is a severe pest of both livestock and people in the rice-growing areas of Arkansas and Louisiana. *Culex tarsalis*, an important vector of western equine encephalitis, is found in the western, central, and southern states of the USA. *Aedes vexans* is an important nuisance species found in the Midwest, and certain species of the genus *Mansonia* are severe pests of livestock in Florida. *Aedes albopictus* is a recently introduced Asian species that could become an important disease vector.

The injuries that mosquitoes inflict on livestock consist mainly of severe annoyance, blood loss, and transmission of several diseases. Also, the toxins injected at the time of biting may cause systemic effects. Several diseases, including equine encephalomyelitis and canine dirofilariasis, are transmitted. In Central and South America, the adult of the bot fly *Dermatobia hominis* (qv, p 780) fastens its eggs to a species of *Psorophora* mosquito, which then transmits them to the mammalian host as the mosquito feeds. Apparent transmission of fowlpox by mosquitoes has also been reported.

Treatment and Control: The individual stockman should attempt to eliminate or reduce areas on his land that harbor mosquito larvae. Area control of mosquitoes usually involves the cooperation of many individuals and can be done successfully only by experienced personnel with proper equipment. In addition to eliminating aquatic breeding sites, area programs generally include extensive use of larvicides. In large outbreaks of adult mosquitoes, particularly when disease transmission is a concern, application of an insecticide active against the adults may be necessary.

Caution is advised with area treatment programs since many nontarget organisms, eg, fish, shrimp, bees, may be exposed to insecticides. A local extension entomologist should be consulted regarding appropriate materials for use on animals or premises. These large-scale programs usually are conducted by mosquito abatement districts or other government agencies.

It is difficult for the individual stockman to protect his animals; residual sprays on the animals do not prevent attack, and currently available repellents do not confer adequate protection during heavy outbreaks. Protection from adult mosquitoes may be provided by ground and, in some cases, aerial application of an insecticide at the time of maximum infestation. Depending on local conditions, this protection may be short-lived. Valuable animals should be housed in closed or screened buildings, and the mosquitoes inside killed with a fog or aerosol formulation of an approved insecticide. Temporary relief may be afforded by a spray or "wipe on" of materials commercially available.

HELMINTHS OF THE SKIN

CUTANEOUS HABRONEMIASIS
(Summer sores, Jack sores, Bursatti)

A skin disease of Equidae caused in part by the larvae of stomach worms (qv, p 201). When the larvae emerge from flies feeding on preexisting wounds or on moisture of the genitalia or eye, they migrate into and irritate the tissue, which causes a granulomatous reaction. The lesion becomes chronic, and healing is protracted. Diagnosis is based on finding nonhealing, reddish brown, greasy skin granulomas that contain rice-grain-sized, yellow, calcified material. Larvae, recognized by spiny knobs on their tails, can sometimes be demonstrated in scrapings of the lesions. Many different treatments have been used, most with poor results. Symptomatic treatment, including use of insect repellents, may be of benefit, and organophosphates applied topically to the abraded surface may kill the larvae. Surgical removal or cauterization of the excessive granulation tissue may be necessary. Treatment with ivermectin (200 µg/kg) has been effective, and although there may be temporary exacerbation of the lesions (presumably in reaction to the dying larvae), spontaneous healing may be expected. Control of the fly hosts and the regular collection and stacking of manure, together with regular anthelmintic therapy may help to reduce the incidence.

DRACUNCULUS INFECTIONS

Dracunculus insignis occurs mainly in the subcut. connective tissues of the legs of raccoons, mink, and other animals, including dogs, in North America and possibly other parts of the world. The females ($\geq$300 cm long) are much longer than the males ($\sim$20 mm). They produce ulcers in the skin of their host, through which their anterior end is protruded on contact with water. They lay characteristic long, thin-tailed larvae. Water fleas (*Cyclops* sp) are the intermediate host in which infective larvae develop. Dogs become infected through ingestion of contaminated water or a paratenic host (frogs).

Subcut., serpentine, inflammatory tracts and nonhealing, crater-like, edematous skin ulcers are observed. Although rare, infections are occasionally encountered around small lakes and bodies of shallow, stagnant water. Treatment is by careful, slow extraction of the parasite. Administration of miridazole or benzimidazole compounds may be useful.

Dracunculus medinensis, the "guinea worm" of parts of Africa, Asia, and the Middle East, although primarily a parasite of man, also occurs in dogs and other animals.

ELAEOPHOROSIS
(Filarial dermatosis, "Clear-eyed" blindness, Sorehead)

Elaeophora schneideri is a parasite of mule deer and black-tailed deer found in the mountains of western and southwestern USA; it also has been found in white-tailed deer in the southern and southeastern regions. Adult parasites are 60-120 mm long and usually are found in the common carotid or internal maxillary arteries. The microfilariae, $\sim$275 μm long and 15-17 μm thick, normally occur in capillaries of skin on the forehead and face. Development in the intermediate hosts, horse flies of the genera *Tabanus* and *Hybomitra*, requires $\sim$2 wk. Infective larvae invade the host as the horse fly feeds, migrate to the leptomeningeal arteries and develop to immature adults in $\sim$3 wk. These young adults migrate against the blood flow and establish in the common carotid arteries, where they continue to grow. The parasites reach sexual maturity $\sim$6 mo later and begin producing microfilariae. The life span of the adults is 3-4 yr.

Clinical Findings: Clinical disease has not been reported in mule deer and black-tailed deer; therefore, they are considered to be the normal definitive hosts. When horse flies transmit the infective larvae to elk, moose, domestic sheep, domestic goats, sika deer, and possibly white-tailed deer, they develop in the leptomeningeal arteries and cause ischemic necrosis of brain tissue, resulting in blindness, brain damage, and sudden death. Blindness in these animals is characterized by absence of opacities in the refractive media of the eye ("clear-eyed" blindness).

Domestic sheep and goats, especially lambs, kids, and yearlings, may die suddenly 3-5 wk after infection. Death is usually preceded by incoordination and circling, and often by convulsions and opisthotonos. Numerous thrombi occur in the cerebral and leptomeningeal arteries. One or more young adult *E schneideri* accompany each thrombus. If sheep or goats survive the early infection, a raw bloody dermatitis on the poll, forehead, or face ("sorehead") develops 6-10 mo later. Lesions occasionally occur on the legs, abdomen, and feet. These lesions are an allergic dermatitis in response to the microfilariae lodged in capillaries. Lesions persist, with periods of intermittent and incomplete healing for $\sim$3 yr, followed by spontaneous recovery. Hyperplasia and hyperkeratosis occur in the epidermis of the parasitized area.

Diagnosis: Differential diagnoses include coenurosis (*Taenia*, qv, p 604), cerebrocortical necrosis (qv, p 614), and enterotoxemia (qv, p 325). Elaeophorosis should not be considered unless sheep have been in endemic areas during the summer. Diagnosis in lambs, kids, or yearling and calf elk usually is made at necropsy; numerous thrombi and parasites are found in the common carotid, internal maxillary, cerebral, and leptomeningeal arteries. Presumptive diagnosis in mature sheep is based on history and location and type of lesion. The skin lesion must be differentiated from ulcerative dermatosis (qv, p 866). Confirmation is by recovery of microfilariae from the lesion, or postmortem recovery of the adult parasites. A skin biopsy of the lesion is macerated in isotonic saline solution, and allowed to stand ≥6 hr at room temperature. The skin is strained off and the fluid examined for the typical microfilariae.

Prophylaxis and Treatment: Piperazine salts are effective at 100 mg/lb (220 mg/kg) body wt, PO. Complete recovery occurs in 18-20 days. No treatment is available for the cerebral form of the disease.

ONCHOCERCIASIS

The taxonomic status of the 3 species of *Onchocerca* currently recognized in the USA, and other previously recognized species, is under debate. *Onchocerca cervicalis* occurs in the ligamentum nuchae and possibly other sites in Equidae. In cattle, *O gutturosa* locates in the ligamentum nuchae, and *O lienalis* in the gastrosplenic ligament. Adults are associated with connective tissues, are very thin, and are 3-60 cm long. Microfilariae are found in the dermis and on rare occasions circulating in peripheral blood. The microfilariae lack a sheath and are 200-250 μm long with a short, sharply pointed tail. *Culicoides* spp are the intermediate hosts for *O cervicalis*, and *Simulium* spp for *O gutturosa* and *O lienalis*.

Clinical Findings: *Onchocerca cervicalis* has been associated with fistulous withers, poll evil, dermatitis, and uveitis in horses (*see also* EYEWORMS OF HORSES AND CATTLE, p 304). However, because of the common presence of large numbers of the parasite in horses without these diseases, there is some debate about its role in the pathogenesis of these conditions.

Adults in the ligamentum nuchae induce inflammatory reactions ranging from acute edematous necrosis to chronic granulomatous changes, resulting in marked fibrosis and mineralization. Mineralized nodules are more common in older horses. Although lesions occur in these areas, presumably associated with dead parasites, it is generally agreed that fistulous withers and poll evil are not associated with *O cervicalis* infections.

Microfilariae concentrate in skin of the ventral midline. Large numbers can be found in horses without dermatitis as well as in horses with dermatitis of the face, neck, chest, withers, forelegs, and abdomen. These lesions often include areas of scale, crusts, ulceration, alopecia, and depigmentation, and may be pruritic. The dermatitis may be associated with an immunological reaction to dead and dying microfilariae. Although the pathogenesis of these lesions is unclear, treatment with microfilaricidal drugs may dramatically improve the conditions. Allergic reactions to the bites of small flies may produce similar lesions or exacerbate microfilaria-associated dermatitis. Thus, diagnosis of *Onchocerca*-associated dermatitis may be based on responsiveness to microfilaricidal treatment.

Microfilariae also accumulate in the eyes of horses, but not all agree that a clear association between equine uveitis (qv, p 302) or other ocular lesions in horses has been made.

Diagnosis: The most effective method is by skin biopsy; a full-thickness biopsy ≥6 mm is preferable. The tissue is minced and macerated in isotonic saline for several hours. Microfilariae are concentrated and stained with New Methylene Blue after removal of skin pieces. The microfilariae can be differentiated microscopically from *Setaria* spp, which occur in the blood of cattle and Equidae, by the presence of a sheath around *Setaria*. (*See also* SWEET ITCH IN HORSES, p 804.)

Treatment: No treatment is effective against the adults. Ivermectin (200 µg/kg) is efficacious (>99%) against microfilariae, and produces marked clinical improvement in horses with onchocercal dermatitis. A small portion of horses infected with *O cervicalis* react to the treatment with a marked, edematous ventral midline swelling 1-3 days following treatment. Ocular lesions have also been reported. These reactions usually resolve spontaneously, but symptomatic treatment may be necessary.

PARAFILARIA INFECTION

PARAFILARIA BOVICOLA

A filarial parasite of cattle that causes subcut. lesions that resemble bruising. It also has been reported from water buffalo (*Bubalus bubalis*). The worm is whitish; adult females are 50-65 mm long, and males 30-35 mm long. It occurs in Asia (Philippines, Japan, Russia, Pakistan, India), Europe (Bulgaria, Romania, France, Sweden), and Africa (Morocco, Tunisia, Rwanda, Burundi, South Africa, Namibia, Botswana, Zimbabwe). A specimen was recovered in Canada from a bull imported from France, but *P bovicola* does not appear to have established itself on the American continents, and has not been reported from Australia.

Parafilaria infection has been identified as a source of considerable economic loss to the beef industries of South Africa and Sweden, despite their climatic differences. The disease occurs primarily in range cattle in the savanna areas of southern Africa, whereas in Sweden, it has emerged as a problem in cattle in spring following turn out to pasture after winter housing.

The only external signs of infection in cattle are focal cutaneous hemorrhages ("bleeding spots") that may ooze for some hours before clotting and drying in the matted hair of the coat. Bleeding spots are induced by the female worm, which causes the formation of a small nodule, perforates the skin, and oviposits in the blood dripping from the central wound. The tiny eggs contain the first larval stage (microfilariae) of the parasite. In both the Northern and Southern Hemispheres, bleeding spots are markedly seasonal, being most common in spring and early summer. Most bleeding spots occur along the dorsum of the animal, particularly in the forequarters.

The invertebrate hosts are face flies of the genus *Musca* (subgenus *Eumusca*), which ingest the eggs when feeding at the bleeding points. *Musca autumnalis* has been identified as a host in Sweden, *M lusoria* and *M xanthomelas* in South Africa, and *M vitripennis* in Asia. Development to infective third-stage larvae in the fly takes 10-12 days. Transmission to cattle probably occurs when the flies feed on wounds, *Parafilaria* bleeding points, or on ocular secretions.

Because of seasonal bleeding and the cutaneous nodules, severe infections of *P bovicola* have been reported to impair the productivity of working bullocks in India; however, the major importance of *Parafilaria* is in beef-producing countries, and centers on the damage to the subcut. tissues. Carcasses of infected animals display irregular, edematous, greenish yellow lesions that resemble bruising. These are usually superficial, but occasionally underlying muscles are extensively involved. Lesions are most severe during the spring and summer.

The trimming of lesions from affected carcasses leads to considerable loss of saleable meat. Trimmed carcasses are often seriously disfigured and consequently downgraded. In severe cases, the carcass may be condemned. Lesions are more common and severe in bulls than in steers, which in turn are less severely affected than female animals.

The seasonal bleeding points are sometimes confused with those from injury by thorns, wire, ticks, or biting insects. For differentiation, either fresh or dried blood should be mixed with water in a test tube and centrifuged. The characteristic eggs are found on microscopical examination of the sediment.

Carcass lesions can be differentiated from bruising by the presence of numerous eosinophils in Giemsa-stained impression smears made from the lesions. In addition, affected tissue has a characteristic, disagreeable, metallic smell.

Usually, only small numbers of worms are present in affected carcasses, and are often difficult to find because of their color and the accompanying inflammatory reaction. Affected tissues can be incubated in warm saline to facilitate the recovery of parasites. An ELISA for the detection of antibodies against *P bovicola* has recently been developed.

Ivermectin (200 μg/kg) or nitroxynil (20 mg/kg) given by subcut. injection is effective in reducing the number and surface area of *Parafilaria* lesions. To provide sufficient time for resolution of lesions, animals should be treated at least 70-90 days before slaughter. The treatment-to-slaughter interval should not be >120 days because unaffected larval forms of the parasite may induce fresh lesions as they mature.

In trials in Sweden, use of pyrethroid-impregnated ear tags gave good control of flies and reduced parafilarial lesions at slaughter by 75%. Ear tagging all cattle in an area resulted in total control of the parasite. The use of residually active, synthetic pyrethroid dips has also been effective in reducing transmission.

It may be possible to screen imported animals with the ELISA to prevent spread of the disease to presently unaffected countries, or to use this test in conjunction with residual insecticides and effective anthelmintics to eradicate new foci of infection.

PARAFILARIA MULTIPAPILLOSA

Parafilaria multipapillosa occurs in the subcut. tissues of horses in various parts of the world; it is especially common in the Russian steppes and eastern Europe. It is similar in size, appearance, life cycle, and development to *P bovicola*. It is thought that blooksucking *Haematobia* spp are the invertebrate hosts.

In spring and summer, the parasite causes skin nodules, particularly on the head and upper forequarters. These bleed transiently but often profusely (''summer bleeding''), and then resolve; other hemorrhaging nodules develop as the parasite moves to a different site. Occasionally, the nodules suppurate. The nodules and bleeding are unsightly and interfere with the harness of working horses, but generally are of little consequence. The clinical signs are pathognomonic.

No satisfactory treatment is available, but fly control may help to reduce the incidence.

PELODERA DERMATITIS
(Rhabditic dermatitis)

A rare, nonseasonal, acute dermatosis that results from invasion of the skin by larvae of the free-living saprophytic nematode *Pelodera (Rhabditis) strongyloides*. The larvae are ubiquitous in decaying organic matter and on or near the surface of moist soil, but are only occasionally parasitic. Exposure to the larvae occurs through direct contact with infested material such as damp, filthy bedding. The larvae may not be able to invade healthy skin; preexisting dermatoses or environmental conditions favoring maceration of the skin, eg, constant exposure to mud or damp bedding, may facilitate invasion. *Pelodera* dermatitis has been reported in dogs, cows, horses, sheep, guinea pigs, and man.

Typically, lesions are confined to body areas in contact with the infested material, such as the extremities, ventral abdomen and thorax, and perineum. Affected skin is erythematous and partially to completely alopecic, with papules, pustules, crusts, erosions, or ulcerations. Pruritus usually is intense, but can be moderate or even absent. Differential diagnoses include demodicosis, canine scabies, dermatophytosis, pyoderma, and other rare cutaneous larval infestations such as hookworm dermatitis, dirofilariasis, dipetalonemiasis, and strongyloidiasis.

Diagnosis is confirmed easily by finding live, motile *P strongyloides* larvae in skin scrapings of affected areas. The larvae are cylindrical and ~600 μm x 38 μm. Histological examination of skin biopsy specimens reveals larvae in the hair follicles and superficial dermis, and usually an inflammatory dermal infiltrate. The larvae are easily cultivated on blood agar plates at 77°F (25°C).

Effective treatment consists primarily of removing and destroying moist, infested bedding material, and moving the animal to a clean, dry environment. Usually, spontaneous recovery ensues. It may be desirable to dip or spray the affected animals with an insecticidal preparation at least twice at weekly intervals. Short-term use of corticosteroids may be indicated if pruritus is severe.

STEPHANOFILARIASIS
(Filarial dermatitis of cattle)

Stephanofilaria stilesi is a small filarial parasite responsible for a circumscribed dermatitis along the ventral midline of cattle. It has been reported throughout the USA, but is more common in the west and southwest. The adult worms are 3-6 mm long and usually are found in the dermis, just beneath the epidermal layer. Microfilariae are 50 μm long and are enclosed in a spherical, semirigid vitelline membrane. The intermediate host for *S stilesi* is the female horn fly, *Haematobia irritans* (qv, p 801). Horn flies feeding on the lesion ingest microfilariae that develop to the third-stage infective larvae in 2-3 wk. The infective larvae are introduced into the skin as the horn fly feeds.

The dermatitis develops along the ventral midline, usually between the brisket and navel. With repeated exposure, the lesion spreads and often involves the skin posterior to the navel. Active lesions are covered with blood or serous exudate, while chronic lesions are smooth, dry, and devoid of hair. Hyperkeratosis and parakeratosis occur in the epidermis of the parasitized area.

Deep skin scrapings are macerated in isotonic saline solution and examined microscopically for adults or microfilariae. The microfilariae must be differentiated from microfilariae of *Onchocerca lienalis*, *O gutturosa*, and *Setaria* spp, which are much larger (200-250 μm), and *Pelodera strongyloides* (*see* above), a small free-living nematode that is occasionally responsible for a moist, superficial dermatitis. The rhabditiform esophagus of *P strongyloides* does not occur in filarial nematodes.

No approved treatment is available for *S stilesi*, but topically applied organophosphates (trichlorfon 6-10%, daily or on alternate days for 7 days) have proved effective against other species of *Stephanofilaria*.

HYGROMA

A false bursa occurring over bony prominences and pressure points, especially in large breeds of dogs. Repeated trauma due to the dog lying on hard surfaces produces an inflammatory response, which results in a dense-walled, fluid-filled cavity. A soft, fluctuant, painless swelling develops over pressure points, especially the olecranon. If long-standing, severe inflammation may develop, and ulceration, infection, and fistulas may be present. The bursa contains a clear, yellow to red fluid.

If diagnosed early and if still small, hygromas can be managed medically via aseptic needle aspiration, and prevention of trauma. Soft bedding or padding over pressure points is imperative to prevent further trauma. If chronic, surgical drainage, flushing, and placement of Penrose drains are indicated. Areas with severe ulceration may require complete excision and reconstructive surgery. Use of intrahygromal corticosteriods is highly controversial.

INTERDIGITAL "CYSTS"

Inflamed, multiform nodules (not true cysts) involving the interdigital webs of dogs. Histologically, they represent areas of furunculosis. Opinions differ as to etiology. The most probable causes are foreign bodies, eg, ingrown hairs, awns, and grains of sand (granulomatous reactions); and bacterial infections, mainly

staphylococcal (suppurative reactions). Hypersensitivity to contact or bacterial allergens also may play a role. *Demodex* mites often can be recovered from the interdigital area and may be an etiological factor. Cysts are common in dogs confined to
areas with wire flooring. It appears that the constant irritation and trauma, alone or
in combination with the above agents, are significant factors.

In its early stage, the interdigital lesion appears as a small papule, but later it
progresses to a nodule. The latter usually is 1-2 cm in diameter, reddish purple,
shiny, and fluctuant, and may rupture when palpated and exude a bloody material.
There may be single or multiple nodules on one or more feet. Those caused by
foreign bodies are usually solitary and often occur on a front foot; recurrence is not
common in these cases. If caused by bacteria, there may be several nodules with
new lesions developing as others resolve. Pain may not be apparent, but is common
in nodules that are about to rupture or that contain foreign bodies.

Foreign-body granulomas may respond to application of moist heat for 15-20
min 3-4 times a day, and removal of the foreign object. Resolution of the lesion
requires 1-2 wk. If hot foot baths are not effective, surgical excision is the most
practical approach.

Bacterial lesions are treated systemically with antibiotics selected according to
culture and sensitivity results. High doses and prolonged treatment for up to 6-8 wk
may be required. Lesions may need to be surgically incised and debrided. Antibiotic
dressings may then be applied for several days followed by daily soaking or washing with antiseptic solutions, eg, chlorhexidine. Therapy with staphylococcal bacterins also has been used successfully.

Lesions in confined dogs are likely to recur unless the dog is removed from the
wire surface.

MANGE

A contagious skin disease caused by one of several species of mites that may be
transmitted when larvae, nymphs, or fertilized females are transferred to a susceptible host directly by contact with diseased animals, or indirectly by fomites or contaminated quarters. Infested animals suffer alopecia and pruritus with intense
irritation and hypersensitivity, which can lead to debilitation and possibly death.
The incubation period is 2-6 wk and depends on the number of mites transferred,
the site of transfer, and host susceptibility. The developmental stages include egg,
larva (3 pairs of legs), nymph (1 or 2 pairs), and adult (4 pairs). Nymphs and adults
are sexually dimorphic. Two to 3 wk may be required to complete the life cycle,
which is spent entirely on the host. Although they are host-specific, some mange
mites are considered biological races rather than distinct species, and infestation—at least temporary—may result on other host species, including man, in contact with infested hosts.

MANGE IN CATTLE
(Barn itch)

Identification of the type of mange present and its differentiation from other
dermatoses are made by recovery of the mite in skin scrapings. Mange and ringworm may occur concurrently in herds and individual animals.

Scabies (*Sarcoptes scabiei* var *bovis*) lesions first appear on the head and neck
and then spread to other parts. Sometimes, the lesions appear in the perineal region
and between the thighs. The skin irritation and eruptions are similar to those in
horses (*see* below). They are characterized by a squamous, crusted appearance; the
skin thickens and forms large folds. The lesions may heal spontaneously during the
summer, particularly when the animals are kept on pasture.

Common scabies or **psoroptic mange** of cattle (*Psoroptes ovis*) is a notifiable
and quarantinable disease, and when suspected must be reported immediately to
regulatory officials. Owners in the USA should not attempt to treat cattle infested
with psoroptic mange; this must be done by government officials. The disease is

seen in range and feedlot beef cattle from the central and western states, with the largest numbers of outbreaks reported from Texas, New Mexico, Oklahoma, Kansas, Colorado, and Nebraska. It appears first on the withers and soon spreads along the neck and back, and over the shoulders and brisket to the belly and flanks. Larger mite populations develop when self-grooming is restricted, as may occur with cattle in stanchions. In severe cases, lesions may cover almost the entire body; deaths in untreated calves and yearlings are not uncommon. The course is usually chronic, but may be acute in younger animals, especially during winter. Prognosis following treatment is favorable. Infested cattle should be dipped, not sprayed.

Four dips are approved in the USA: toxaphene, 0.5-0.6% (28-day withdrawal time); coumaphos, 0.3% (no withdrawal time); phosmet, 0.2-0.25% (21-day withdrawal time); and hot lime-sulfur (2% calcium polysulfides heated to 95-105°F [35-40.5°C]) (no withdrawal time). Depending on the product used (label instructions should be checked), regulations may call for repeat dippings of infested animals at intervals of 7-14 days. Only hot lime-sulfur is registered for use on lactating dairy cows (one dip, no withdrawal time).

Ivermectin given subcut. at 200 μg/kg body wt is approved for control of psoroptic and sarcoptic mange (not in lactating dairy cattle). Although one treatment is effective, treated cattle should be isolated from other cattle for 2 wk.

Chorioptic mange (*Chorioptes bovis*) is the most common type of mange in cattle in the USA. The pastern areas of the legs are predilection sites for this mite. A high proportion of cattle may be infested without exhibiting clinical signs. Lesions usually start on the legs, and the disease is called "leg mange". The root of the tail frequently becomes affected and, if untreated, the condition may spread to other parts of the body. Cattle may be treated with crotoxyphos applied as a 0.25% spray at high pressure so as to completely wet the animal, including the legs and escutcheon. Dips and sprays containing 0.06% lindane are also effective where use of this drug is permitted. The dips permitted for bovine psoroptic scabies are effective against *Chorioptes*. Lime-sulfur dips are effective if 6 treatments are given at 7- to 10-day intervals. Ivermectin applied topically at 500 μg/kg body wt is effective against chorioptic mange (not for use in lactating dairy cattle).

Demodectic mange (*Demodex bovis*) is transferred from cow to calf while nursing and may cause considerable damage to hides. The lesions may be apparent on the neck, brisket, shoulder, and face of young dairy cattle, but are rarely visible or palpable on beef cattle. Rarely, lesions may appear over the entire body. Of hides dehaired before tanning, ~90% have been found to contain blemishes due to demodectic mites. First, small papules and nodules develop; sometimes they are red, and a thick, white, waxy material can be expressed from them. This material contains numerous mites. In rare cases, the nodules are filled with pus and may coalesce, forming abscesses covered with small scales. In some cases, cutaneous lesions consist of thick crusts, and the skin thickens and forms heavy folds. The course of bovine demodectic mange generally is mild, but may extend over many months. Recovery is usually spontaneous. There is no satisfactory treatment.

Itch mite infestations (*Psorergates bos*) of cattle have been reported in the USA and Canada. Alopecia and desquamation may occur, but lesions lack the scab formation associated with mange mite infestations. The mites are minuscule and difficult to collect. The acaricide of choice is a lime-sulfur spray or dip applied twice, with a 2-wk interval.

MANGE IN DOGS AND CATS

Cutaneous Acariasis: Skin disease caused by parasitic mites; sarcoptic mange is highly contagious, demodectic mange much less so.

Sarcoptic mange of dogs (*Sarcoptes scabiei* var *canis*) is found worldwide. The eggs are oval, and the body of the mite is almost circular with short legs. The nymphal and adult stages have 4 pairs of legs, the larval stage has 3. In the adult, the third and fourth pairs do not extend beyond the margin of the body. The entire life cycle is spent on the host and requires 17-21 days for completion. Eggs are laid in tunnels formed by the female burrowing in the skin. The **sarcoptic mange mite of cats**, *Notoedres cati*, is smaller and more circular than the mite that attacks dogs.

Canine demodectic mange (*Demodex canis*) typically infests the hair follicles and sometimes the sebaceous and apocrine sweat glands; healthy dogs also may harbor the mite. The developmental stages are egg, larva, protonymph, nymph, and adult. The life cycle requires 20-35 days to complete. Eggs are spindle-shaped and the mites are vermiform. The elongated abdomen is marked with transverse striations. *Demodex cati* is occasionally found on cats and may cause lesions similar to those in dogs.

Sarcoptic mange is readily transmitted by direct contact. Visible lesions may appear in 2-8 wk, depending on the number of mites transmitted, site of infestation, and susceptibility of the host.

Demodectic mange is transmitted when mites wandering on the skin are transferred from an infested to a susceptible host. Initial exposure usually occurs during the first few days of life, while puppies nurse an infested bitch. Susceptible young dogs may also contract mange from close contact with heavily infested dogs. Demodectic mites lose their capacity to invade hair follicles when off a host only briefly.

The sarcoptic mite causes intense itching; vigorous scratching, chewing, and rubbing leads to inflammation and secondary infection. Preferred regions for the mites are the head (around the eyes, ears, and muzzle), ventral thorax, and root of the tail. The skin becomes dry, thickened, and wrinkled. Crusts form in involved areas. In untreated animals, emaciation, debilitation, and even death may occur. Other animals may harbor mites for extensive periods with only localized involvement. In cats, mange usually starts at the tips of the ears, spreads to the face and then to the entire head. It also may extend to involve the rest of the body and legs.

Dogs with demodectic mange may have various lesions, from small patches of hairlessness around the eyes or over the body to extensive bloody or purulent lesions completely covering the body. In the localized form, small isolated areas of alopecia are seen on the face or forelegs, or both. The localized condition is mild, does not normally develop secondary pyoderma, and is not considered serious. In the pustular type (generalized), the skin is highly reddened, with blood and serum oozing from affected areas, along with purulent material resulting from bacterial invasion (usually *Staphylococcus aureus*, occasionally *Pseudomonas* spp).

The pathogenicity of sarcoptic mange depends on the interactions of parasite and host, complicated by secondary infections. The burrowing of mites in the epidermis causes mechanical damage, and irritation is produced by salivary secretions. Afflicted hosts typically develop hypersensitivity to allergens associated with the mites and their excretions and secretions, and a concomitant intense pruritus.

Demodectic mites feed primarily on the cells of the hair follicle, surrounding cells, and to a lesser extent, on sebum. In localized demodectic mange, the damage is restricted to isolated, nonpruritic areas accompanied by erythema and scales; there is no immune component. Conditions that favor mite proliferation and the development of generalized mange are not completely understood. In dogs with generalized demodecosis, blastogenesis of lymphocytes is severely depressed by a suppressive factor in the sera, but the suppression is seen only in cases complicated by bacterial infection.

Skin scrapings of several different sites may be required to find mites and confirm the diagnosis of sarcoptic mange. Regions with erythematous papules and crusting should be scraped vigorously to recover sarcoptic mites from their burrows. Demodectic mites may be squeezed from the hair follicles and collected by scraping with a scalpel blade those areas immediately adjacent to sites with alopecia, erythema, crusting, or folliculitis. Coating the scalpel blade lightly with mineral oil facilitates collection of skin debris and mites onto the blade. Mites are transferred from the blade to a drop of mineral oil on a microscope slide for examination under low power (40 ×). Examination is facilitated by clearing the sample with 10% NaOH or KOH. Even if mites are not demonstrable in skin scrapings, when typical signs are present, trial therapy with an approved miticide should be considered.

The affected animal should be prepared by clipping the hair and washing the skin with a keratolytic and antiseborrheic shampoo before treatment with an approved acaricide. Two or more treatments over several weeks may be necessary for a complete cure. (*See* EXTERNAL PARASITICIDES, SM AN, p 1500.)

Several acaricides are toxic to cats. Lime-sulfur washes or rotenone compounds may be used successfully; good results can be obtained by applying an ointment of sulfur to affected areas.

Canine demodectic mange, particularly the generalized form, may be persistent and often responds poorly to treatment. The squamous or localized form often heals spontaneously in 4-8 wk, but ~10% of dogs with localized mange develop the generalized form. Ronnel in a propylene-glycol mixture and amitraz are the 2 most efficacious acaricides for treating demodectic mange. The ronnel solution should be applied daily to no more than one-third of the body on a rotating basis. Topical application (by complete wetting of the dog) of amitraz q2wk is recommended, and should continue until no live mites are recovered after 2 successive applications. In cases with secondary infection, antibiotics should be administered since deaths may occur due to septicemia and abscesses.

Nasal acariasis (Nasal mites): An infestation of the nasal cavity and paranasal sinuses of dogs by the mite, *Pneumonyssus (Pneumonyssoides) caninum*, is usually without, or with only mild, signs. The adult mite has a pale-yellow body. The gravid female contains a fully developed embryo that nearly fills the abdomen. The method of transmission of the parasite is unknown.

Except for an accumulation of mucus and mild hyperemia of the mucous membranes, no signs or lesions are usually attributed to the infestation. A severe rhinitis may occasionally occur. Most infestations are found at necropsy. A few cases have been reported in which the mite was found on the nose of sleeping dogs. Treatment has not been attempted.

Otoacariasis (Otodectic mange, Ear mange, Parasitic otitis externa): An infestation of the ears with parasitic mites (*see* OTITIS EXTERNA, p 309).

Cheyletiella Infestations: Mite infestations of *Cheyletiella blakei* on cats, and *C yasguri* on dogs have occasionally been reported to extend to people who are closely associated with infested animals. A related species, *C parasitivorax* (the fur mite), occurs on rabbits and perhaps other animals. Most human infestations occur when infested cats are allowed to sleep on beds. The disease is highly contagious. *Cheyletiella* spp inhabit the pelage and skin surface of animals but also can live free in nature. They are large ($388 \times 266 \ \mu$m) and are easily identified microscopically by the large palpal claws, numerous feathered bristles, and cones on the tarsi.

Two clinical forms, exfoliative and crustose, have been recognized in dogs. In the first, a scaling process (mimicking dandruff) occurs primarily on the dorsal trunk, and is most evident on the skin, with a few scales in the pelage. Alopecia and inflammatory changes are usually present only secondary to scratching. Pruritus is moderate to intense. In the crustose form, multiple, discrete, circular, alopecic crusts (2-5 cm in diameter) are on the dorsal and lateral trunk. The lesions may expand or enlarge and appear similar to ringworm; however, no inflammatory border is evident and no dermatophytes can be demonstrated. The lesion also resembles the crustose form of seborrhea that commonly occurs in Cocker Spaniels. The crustose form of the disease is most common in cats; the lesions strongly resemble those of ringworm except that most occur on the neck and trunk.

Diagnosis depends on identification of the mites in skin brushings; scrapings are unnecessary. Material removed for examination should be placed in 10% potassium hydroxide and viewed under $25 \times$ magnification. Because cats groom themselves regularly, infestation can frequently be diagnosed by demonstrating mites or eggs during a routine fecal flotation. (This [grooming] is an additional reason to be careful in selection of ectoparasiticides for cats.)

Successful treatment (*see also* p 1500) may be achieved with derris washes or dusts, or the topical application of various insecticides including 0.02% lindane, organophosphorous compounds, benzyl benzoate-lindane solution, or potassium tetrathionate shampoo with lindane. Topical applications should be repeated until clinical cure is achieved and neither the mite nor its eggs can be demonstrated by microscopical examination.

MANGE IN HORSES

Sarcoptic mange (*Sarcoptes scabiei* var *equi*) is the most severe type. Early lesions appear on the head, neck, and shoulders. Regions protected by long hair, and lower parts of the extremities usually are not involved. The first sign is intense itching. Small papules and vesicles develop into an acute dermatitis; scaling increases rapidly, followed by crusting. The bald and encrusted patches enlarge and the skin thickens, forming folds, particularly in the neck region. In advanced cases, the lesions may extend over the entire body, leading to emaciation, general weakness, and anorexia. The course is chronic, and the prognosis is the most unfavorable of all types of mange in horses, particularly when the infestations are severe and the animals are in poor condition.

For treatment, acaricidal preparations are applied by spraying, rubbing, or dipping. For groups of animals, dipping is the most convenient and effective method. Lime-sulfur can be used if the dip is heated and the animals are dipped 4-6 times at intervals of 10-12 days. Toxaphene dip (0.5%) usually gives control with one application. Lindane (0.06%) can be used as a spray or dip where its use is permitted.

Psoroptic scabies (*Psoroptes ovis [equi]*) is a notifiable and quarantinable disease in the countries in which it is found. It produces lesions on sheltered parts of the body, such as under the forelock and mane, at the root of the tail, under the chin, between the hindlegs, and in the axillae. Mites are sometimes found in the ears and may cause head shaking. The lesions are similar to the sarcoptic type, but the crusts are larger and thicker, the skin is less folded, and the itching is less severe. The course is chronic and the prognosis favorable. Treatment corresponds to that for the sarcoptic type (*see* above), or to the dips used for psoroptic scabies of cattle (*see* above).

Chorioptic mange (*Chorioptes bovis*) is also known as "leg mange". Cutaneous lesions are found chiefly on the lower parts of the hindlegs. In severe cases, skin lesions may spread to the flanks, shoulders, and neck. The disease is characterized by intense itching, scales, crusts, thickening of the skin, and in neglected cases, a moist dermatitis in the fetlock region. The signs subside in summer, but recur with the return of cold weather. The course usually is chronic, the prognosis favorable. Treatments recommended for other mange mites are effective against chorioptic mange.

Demodectic mange (*Demodex equi*) is seldom diagnosed in horses. The mites live in the hair follicles and in the sebaceous glands and produce papules and ulcers, particularly around the eyes and on the forehead. Subsequently, the lesions spread to the shoulders and finally over the entire body. The affected skin is covered with scales. Pruritus is absent. There is no satisfactory treatment.

MANGE AND SCABIES IN SHEEP AND GOATS

In sheep, these diseases are caused by *Sarcoptes scabiei* var *ovis*, *Chorioptes bovis*, *Psoroptes ovis*, *P cuniculi*, *Demodex* sp, and *Psorergates (Psorobia) ovis*. **Sarcoptic mange** in sheep occurs only on the nonwooly skin, starting, as a rule, on the head and face; it is rare. **Chorioptic mange**, the most frequent type in sheep, is most often found on the hindlegs and between the toes, or on the scrotum of rams; it is commonly called "leg" or "foot mange". **Psoroptic scabies (sheep scab)** is a notifiable disease, and affected flocks are subject to quarantine and dipping regulations. No psoroptic scabies of sheep has been reported from the USA since 1970. Countries where sheep scabies (scab) is still a problem include the UK, Eire, France, Germany, Lebanon, Israel, Egypt, South Africa, Kenya, Argentina, Brazil, and Mexico. It occurs almost exclusively on the woolly parts of the body where it produces large, scaly, crusted lesions. Biting and scratching brought on by intense itching are generally the first signs. When large areas are involved, animals gradually become emaciated and suffer from anemia and cachectic hydremia. Psoroptic mites are sometimes found in the ears of sheep.

Injectable ivermectin is effective against psoroptic mange in sheep, although 2 injections with a 7-day interval are required to eliminate mites; one injection is effective against *Sarcoptes* and *Psorergates*. A single dipping in 0.5-0.6% toxaphene eliminates all mites that attack sheep except *Psorergates ovis*. Other dips approved for use against *Psoroptes*, viz, coumaphos (0.3%) and phosmet (0.2-0.25%), control chorioptic mites, but their efficacy against *Sarcoptes* has not been tested. In the UK, a single dipping for 1 min in currently approved dips containing diazinon, propetamphos, or flumethrin are fully effective; diazinon and fenvalerate are also used in South Africa.

Psoroptic mange (*P cuniculi*) of goats usually infests the ears but sometimes spreads to the head, neck, and body and causes severe irritation. This occurs particularly in Angora goats, in which the mohair is considerably damaged. The disease in Angora goats is notifiable in Texas. The course is chronic but the prognosis is good. Any of the acaricides approved for use as sheep dips will eliminate ear mange from goats. Lactating dairy goats should be treated only with lime-sulfur solution. *Psoroptes cuniculi* also infests the ears and sometimes the body of domestic rabbits.

Demodectic mange has been reported in sheep and goats, in which it causes skin lesions similar to those in other large animals. In goats, it is similar to that of dairy cattle. The lesions are found on the skin of the neck, shoulder, thorax, and flank. The nodules, ranging in size from pinhead to hazelnut, contain a thick, waxy, grayish material that can be easily expressed. Numerous demodectic mites are found in this material. The nodules in goats appear as cysts with mild inflammation in the surrounding tissue. In some countries, this infection in goats may be persistent, causing great damage to the hides. There is no satisfactory treatment. In valuable goats, incision of the nodules and painting with tincture of iodine gives the best therapeutic results.

"Itch mite" infestation: An infestation of sheep by *Psorergates ovis* in which the pruritus induced by the mite causes the host to bite and rub the affected areas and to damage the fleece. The disease has been reported from Australia, New Zealand, South Africa, the USA, Argentina, and Chile, but is not regarded as being of major economic importance. The life cycle (egg, larva, 3 nymphal stages, and adult) is completed in 4-5 wk. All stages undergo development in the epidermis, where the mites are believed to feed on cell fluids.

The first signs often occur ~2-3 yr after arsenical dips are abandoned in favor of the newer insecticides. The incidence increases slowly in the flock until, after 3-4 yr, 10% of the older sheep may be actively biting or rubbing. A damaged fleece, alopecia, crusting, or chronic dermatitis resulting mainly from self-inflicted trauma (in the absence of *Psoroptes*, lice, keds, dermatophilosis, fleece rot, or grass seeds) are suggestive of itch mite infestation. The withers and sides of the trunk are usual sites of involvement. Demonstration of the mites in skin scrapings (several may be necessary) is required for confirmation.

Dipping in 1% lime-sulfur or 0.2% arsenic is a satisfactory treatment. This need not be done annually, but only as the incidence in the flock warrants. In some countries, ivermectin is approved for itch mite in sheep.

MANGE IN PIGS

Sarcoptic mange (*Sarcoptes scabiei* var *suis*) is the only form of any importance in pigs. The lesions usually start on the head, especially the ears, then spread over the body, tail, and legs. Itching is usually intense and associated with a hypersensitivity reaction to the mites. As the hypersensitivity subsides, usually after several months, the thickened, rough, dry skin is covered with grayish crusts and thrown into large folds. Skin scrapings should be examined since pigs also suffer from other skin diseases, including ringworm. Pruritus is frequently a better indicator of infestation than mite recovery, especially in sows and nursing piglets. Spraying with lindane (0.05-0.1%) or malathion (0.05%) is effective; chlordane solution (0.25%) also has been used. (Use of some or all of these on food-producing animals is prohibited in some countries.) Ivermectin at 300 µg/kg body wt, subcut. is also effective.

Demodectic mange also occurs in pigs, causing skin lesions similar to those seen in other large animals. There is no reliable treatment.

PARAKERATOSIS

A nutritional deficiency disease of 6- to 16-wk-old pigs, characterized by lesions of the superficial layers of the epidermis. It is a metabolic disturbance resulting from a relative deficiency of zinc (*see also* p 1252) and an excess of calcium in the diet.

Signs are limited to the skin, although mild lethargy, anorexia, and growth depression may be seen in severe cases; there is little if any pruritus. The outstanding lesions are symmetrically distributed areas of excessive and abnormal keratinization of the epidermis with the formation of horny scale and fissures. Brown spots or papules are first seen on the ventrolateral areas of the abdomen and inner thigh, pastern, fetlock, hock, and tail regions, which coalesce to involve larger areas until the entire body may be covered. The scale is horny, dry, and usually easily removed. Occasionally, secondary infection of the cracks and fissures causes them to fill with dark, sticky exudate and debris, which may resemble exudative epidermitis (qv, p 794); however, this usually occurs in younger piglets.

Highly satisfactory results can be obtained by adjusting the intake of calcium and zinc. The calcium level in the diet of feeder pigs should be maintained at 0.65-0.75%, and supplemental zinc added at 50 ppm (equivalent to an addition of 0.4 lb of zinc sulfate or carbonate per ton [200 mg/kg] of feed). Correction of the deficiency results in rapid recovery.

PEDICULOSIS
(Louse infestation, Lousiness)

Various species of biting lice (order Mallophaga) and sucking lice (order Anoplura [Siphunculata]) infest domestic animals. Sucking lice infest mammals, but biting lice infest both mammals and birds (*see* ECTOPARASITISM OF POULTRY, p 1621).

Etiology: Lice of domestic animals are largely host specific. **Cattle** are most commonly infested with the cattle biting louse, *Damalinia (Bovicola) bovis*, and with 3 species of Anoplura: the shortnosed cattle louse, *Haematopinus eurysternus*; the long-nosed cattle louse, *Linognathus vituli*; and the little blue cattle louse, *Solenopotes capillatus*. In the tropics, the tail switch louse, *H quadripertusus*, is not uncommon (Florida and Gulf Coast in the USA). The louse of the domestic water buffalo, *H tuberculatus*, may infest cattle temporarily.

Horses may harbor 2 species of lice, the horse biting louse, *Damalinia (Bovicola) equi*, and the horse sucking louse, *Haematopinus asini*. **Pigs** are commonly infested with the hog louse, *Haematopinus suis*, which is very large (~5-6 mm).

Sheep may become infested with the sheep biting louse, *Damalinia (Bovicola) ovis*, and 3 sucking lice: the sheep foot louse, *Linognathus pedalis*; the body louse, *L ovillus*; and the African sheep louse, *L africanus*. **Goats** harbor many species of lice, the most common being the goat biting louse, *Damalinia (Bovicola) caprae*, and the goat sucking louse, *Linognathus stenopsis*. Two other Mallophaga, *D limbata* and *D crassipes*, also are frequently found.

Dogs may be infested with *Linognathus setosus* (Anoplura) and *Trichodectes canis* and occasionally *Heterodoxus spiniger*. *Felicola subrostrata* (Mallophaga) parasitizes **cats**.

Lice are wingless, flattened insects, usually 1-2 mm long. The legs are adapted for clinging to hairs and feathers. Anoplura are bloodsuckers. The mouthpart stylets are retracted within the head when not in use. Mallophaga have obvious ventral chewing mandibles and live on epidermal products; some species feed on blood and exudates when available.

Louse eggs are glued onto hairs and are pale, translucent, and suboval. Nymphal lice (3 stages) are smaller than adults, but otherwise resemble them in habits and appearance. About 3-4 wk are required to complete one generation, but this varies with species.

Clinical Findings and Diagnosis: Pediculosis is manifest by pruritus and dermal irritation with resultant scratching, rubbing, and biting of infested areas. A generally unthrifty appearance, rough coat, and lowered production in farm animals are common. In severe infestations, there may be loss of hair and local scarification. Extreme infestation with sucking lice can cause anemia. In sheep and goats, the rubbing and scratching often results in broken fibers, which gives the fleece a "pulled" appearance. In dogs, the coat becomes rough and dry and, if the lice are numerous, the hair may be matted. Sucking lice cause small wounds that may become infected. The constant crawling and either piercing or biting of the skin causes nervousness in hosts.

Diagnosis should be based on the presence of lice. The hair should be parted and an examination made of the skin and proximal portion of the coat under strong light. The hair of large animals should be parted on the face, neck, ears, topline, dewlap, escutcheon, tail base, and tail switch. The head, legs, feet, and scrotum should not be overlooked, particularly in sheep. On small animals, the ova (nits) are readily seen. Occasionally, when the coat is matted, the lice can be seen when the mass is broken apart. Biting lice are active and can be seen moving through the hair, while sucking lice usually move more slowly and are often found with mouthparts embedded in the skin.

Pediculosis of livestock is most prevalent during the winter; severity is greatly reduced with the approach of summer. Infestations, particularly of sucking lice, may become severe. In dairy herds, the young stock, dry cows, and bulls may escape early diagnosis and suffer more severely. Young calves may die. Effective treatment results in prompt improvement.

Transmission usually occurs by host contact. Lice dropped or pulled from the host die in a few days, but disengaged ova may continue to hatch over 2-3 wk in warm weather. Therefore, premises recently vacated by infested stock should be disinfected before being used for clean stock.

Treatment: Louse control usually requires application of effective insecticides (*see* EXTERNAL PARASITICIDES, p 1497) but products available are greatly influenced by local regulations. In many parts of the world, organochlorine insecticides are not available for use on livestock, and in the USA, some insecticides are approved only in certain states.

When livestock are dipped or sprayed, the manufacturer's instructions should be followed carefully, in part to avoid "stripping" of the dips, particularly by sheep, in which the fleece acts as a sieve and retains droplets of emulsions and particles of suspensions. Dipping is being replaced by delivery systems such as the "pour-on" and "low-volume spray" for application of pyrethroid insecticides.

Zero to very low tolerances for pesticides in milk limit the insecticides that may be used on dairy cattle and dairy goats. Effective compounds include crotoxyphos, crotoxyphos plus dichlorvos, and permethrin. Additionally, dairy cattle may be treated with coumaphos, fenvalerate, and stirofos. Nonlactating goats may also be treated with coumaphos, dioxathion, or fenvalerate. Beef cattle, sheep, and pigs may be treated with 0.06% coumaphos, 0.15% dioxathion, 0.5% malathion, methoxychlor, fenvalerate, permethrin, crotoxyphos, crotoxyphos plus dichlorvos, or ivermectin (for sucking lice). Phosmet, stirofos, stirofos plus dichlorvos, lindane, and amitraz may be used on beef cattle; 0.03% diazinon spray is effective against lice on sheep. Although rotenone should not be used on pigs, it is safe for use on other animals when regulations permit.

Dipping or thorough spraying provides excellent coverage, and usually 2 treatments 2 wk apart will effectively control lice. Effective spraying requires soaking the hair to the skin: as much as 3 gal. (12 L) may be required on large, long-haired cattle. Dipping consistently provides the most thorough coverage, but the number of formulations that can be applied by this method is limited.

Methods other than dipping or spraying, eg, the pour-on, may be desirable because stress to the animal is reduced as well as to the individual who makes the application. Several systemic insecticides approved for cattle grub control provide louse control as well; however, precautions should be taken to avoid host-parasite reactions (*see* CATTLE GRUBS, p 780). Pour-on formulations of fenthion control louse infestations on beef and nonlactating dairy cattle and pigs. Chlorpyrifos, applied to a single spot on the back of an animal, provides season-long control of lice on beef cattle, nonlactating dairy cattle, and sheep. A 1% permethrin pour-on is now available for lice control on beef and dairy cattle. Cattle that can be restrained, eg, dairy cattle in stanchions, can be treated with a low-volume mist application of 1% crotoxyphos plus 0.25% dichlorvos.

Lice on beef cattle can be controlled by wintertime use of backrubber devices or dust bags (coumaphos, crotoxyphos, dioxathion, malathion, phosmet, and stirofos) similar to those used against flies in the summer. Effectiveness depends on frequent use by all cattle in the herd. Crotoxyphos, dichlorvos, coumaphos, or 3% stirofos may be used on dairy cattle. Louse populations also can be reduced by hand-dusting with 5% malathion, 10% methoxychlor, or 1% phosmet on beef cattle; or 1% rotenone, 3% stirofos, or 1% coumaphos on dairy or beef cattle.

Injectable ivermectin is highly effective against sucking lice (less so against biting lice) in cattle, sheep, and pigs, but is not to be used in lactating animals when the milk is to be used for human consumption. Doses high enough to be effective for lice are not recommended in dogs.

Dogs can be treated with dips, washes, sprays, or dusts. Effective compounds include permethrin, pyrethrins, dioxathion, rotenone, methoxychlor, lindane, diazinon, malathion, or coumaphos. On cats, only carbaryl, rotenone, or pyrethrins should be used.

Lice on pigs can be controlled with dips and sprays of amitraz, 0.03% lindane, 0.15% dioxathion, and 0.5% methoxychlor, and sprays of 0.5% malathion, 0.06% coumaphos, crotoxyphos plus dichlorvos, crotoxyphos, ronnel, and 0.5% stirofos. Dust formulations of 3% stirofos, 1% coumaphos, or 1% phosmet also are effective. Dust formulations of 3% stirofos and 1% coumaphos may be used to treat bedding. Injectable ivermectin at 300 μg/kg is effective.

In most countries, regulatory agencies specify tissue residue limits of insecticides and carefully regulate their use on livestock. All such regulations are subject to change; pertinent current local laws and requirements should be determined. The treatment of meat and dairy animals must be restricted to uses specified on the labels and all label precautions carefully observed.

PHOTOSENSITIZATION

A condition in which lightly pigmented skin is hyperreactive to sunlight due to a photodynamic agent in the skin. Molecules of photosensitizing agents are energized by light. When the molecule returns to the less energized state, the released energy is transferred to receptor molecules that quickly initiate chemical reactions in components of the skin. Tissue injury probably results from the production of reactive oxygen intermediates or alterations in cell membrane permeability. Photosensitization differs from sunburn, in which lightly pigmented skin slowly becomes inflamed following exposure to ultraviolet rays.

Photosensitization occurs worldwide and may affect any species but is most common in cattle and sheep.

Etiology: Photosensitization can be classified as primary, secondary (hepatogenous), or as defective or aberrant pigment formation. *See also* CONGENITAL ERYTHROPOIETIC PORPHYRIA, p 444, and CONGENITAL ERYTHROPOIETIC PROTOPORPHYRIA, p

784. A wide range of chemicals may be photosensitizing agents, although most are from plant material.

Primary Photosensitization: The photodynamic agent is absorbed through the skin, or from the GI tract unchanged and reaches the skin in its "native" form. Examples of these are hypericin (from *Hypericum* [St. John's-wort]) and fagopyrin (from *Fagopyrum esculentum* [buckwheat]). Plants in the families Umbelliferae and Rutaceae contain photoactive furocoumarins (psoralens), which cause photosensitization in livestock and poultry. *Ammi majus* (bishop's weed) and *Cymopterus watsonii* (spring parsley) have produced photosensitization in cattle and sheep, respectively. Ingestion of *A majus* and *A visnaga* seeds has produced severe photosensitization in poultry. Species of *Trifolium, Medicago* (clovers and alfalfa), *Erodium*, and *Brassica* have been incriminated, eg, in "trefoil dermatitis" and "rape scald". Many other plants have been suspected, but the phototoxins have not been identified. Additionally, some coal tar derivatives, phenothiazine, sulfonamides, and tetracyclines have induced primary photosensitivity.

Secondary (Hepatogenous) Photosensitivity: This is by far the most frequent type in livestock. The photosensitizing agent, phylloerythrin (a porphyrin), accumulates in the plasma due to impaired hepatobiliary excretion. Phylloerythrin is derived from the anaerobic breakdown of chlorophyll by microorganisms in the forestomachs of ruminants. Phylloerythrin, but not chlorophyll, is normally absorbed into the circulation and is effectively excreted by the liver into the bile. Failure to excrete phylloerythrin due to hepatic dysfunction or bile duct lesions increases the amount in the circulation. Thus, it reaches the skin where it absorbs and releases light energy, which initiates a phototoxic reaction.

Phylloerythrin has been incriminated as the phototoxic agent in the following conditions: common bile duct occlusion; facial eczema (qv, p 1686); lupinosis (qv, p 1689); congenital photosensitivity of Southdown and Corriedale sheep (*see* below); and poisoning by *Tribulis terrestris* (puncture vine), *Lippia rehmanni, Lantana camara*, several *Panicum* spp (kleingrass, broomcorn millet, witch grass), *Myoporum laetum* (ngaio), and *Narthecium ossifragum* (bog asphodel).

Photosensitization also has been reported with liver damage associated with various poisonings: ragwort and other *Senecio* spp; blue-green algae; *Nolina texana* (bunch grass); *Agave lecheguilla* (lechuguilla); *Holocalyx glaziovii, Kochia scoparia*, or *Tetradymia* (horse brush or rabbit brush); *Brachiaria brizantha;* phosphorus; and carbon tetrachloride. It is likely that phylloerythrin is the phototoxic agent in many of these.

Aberrant Pigment Metabolism: The photosensitizing porphyrin agents are endogenous pigments that are normally absent or present in the circulation only in minute amounts.

Clinical Findings and Lesions: The syndrome has similar clinical signs regardless of the cause. Photosensitive animals are photophobic immediately when exposed to sunlight. They squirm in apparent discomfort and scratch or rub lightly pigmented, exposed areas of skin, eg, ears, eyelids, and muzzle. Severe phylloerythrinemia and bright sunlight can induce typical skin lesions, even in black-coated cattle and sheep. Erythema develops rapidly and is soon followed by edema. If exposure to light ceases at this stage, the lesions soon resolve; if prolonged, there is marked serum exudation, scab formation, and skin necrosis. In cattle and especially in deer, exposure of the tongue while licking may result in glossitis with ulceration and deep necrosis.

Depending on the initial cause of accumulation of the photosensitizing agent, other clinical signs may be seen, eg, if the photosensitivity is hepatogenous, icterus may be present.

Diagnosis: Marked photosensitivity presents well-recognized clinical signs, but early or mild cases are similar to the primary actinic effects of sunburn. Reference to the specific diseases in which photosensitization is an objective sign may assist in diagnosis of the underlying disease. Serum analysis and liver biopsy for indication of hepatic disease; and examination of blood, feces, and urine for porphyrins should be considered.

Treatment and Control: While photosensitivity continues, animals should be shaded fully or, preferably, housed and allowed out to graze only during darkness. The severe stress of photosensitization and extensive skin necrosis can prove highly debilitating and increase mortality. Corticosteroids, given parenterally in the early stages, may be helpful. Secondary skin infections and suppurations should be treated and fly strike prevented. The skin lesions heal remarkably well, even after extensive necrosis. The prognosis and eventual productivity of an animal is related to the site and severity of the primary lesion and to the degree of resolution.

CONGENITAL PHOTOSENSITIZATION IN SHEEP

Southdown and Corriedale sheep may inherit a hepatobiliary incompetence that results in photosensitization. In mutant Southdown sheep, the inherited defect is in hepatic uptake of unconjugated bilirubin and organic anions. Plasma levels of unconjugated bilirubin are consistently elevated and, since partial bilirubin excretion is maintained, icterus is not a clinical feature. Phylloerythrin is less effectively excreted, and affected lambs become photosensitized when they first commence grazing green plant material. Unless chlorophyll is excluded from the diet, or exposure to sunlight is prevented, the lesions and stress of photosensitization result in death within weeks. Mutant sheep so protected develop progressive renal lesions in which radial fibrous bands are formed in the medulla, along with increasing numbers of cystic tubules. The changes ultimately result in renal insufficiency and death. The liver is small, with pericanalicular deposits of lipofuscin.

This semilethal trait appears to be inherited as a simple recessive. Elimination of carriers is the only feasible control.

In mutant Corriedale sheep, the hepatocellular incompetence is in the excretion of conjugated bilirubin and other conjugated metabolites. There is no obvious icterus, but phylloerythrin excretion is sufficiently impaired to produce photosensitization. Hepatic pigmentation is an obvious gross feature. Brown-black, melanin-like pigment is confined to centrilobular parenchymal cells. The trait is transmitted as an autosomal recessive. Control is by detection and removal of carriers.

PITYRIASIS ROSEA IN PIGS

A sporadic disease of uncertain etiology of the skin of pigs, usually 8-12 wk old, but occasionally as young as 2 wk, and very rarely in pigs up to 10 mo. One pig or more, or the whole litter, may be affected. The disease is mild, but transient anorexia and diarrhea have been reported. The lesions are characterized by erythematous, ring-like patches with distinct raised and reddened borders. The lesions enlarge at their periphery, and adjacent lesions may coalesce. The center of the lesion is flat and covered with a bran-like scale that usually dries off and leaves normal skin. The lesions occur predominantly on the abdomen, but may be seen over the back, neck, and down the legs. Characteristically, there is no pruritus, and spontaneous recovery occurs in 6-8 wk. Treatment is generally considered unnecessary. Diagnosis is straightforward in most cases, but laboratory tests may be used.

The disease is considered to be partially hereditary, pigs of the Landrace breed being commonly affected, but the mode of inheritance is uncertain. Viral etiology is a possibility, since a similar disease in man is considered to be due to a virus.

POX DISEASES

Acute viral diseases of man, animals, and birds, excluding dogs. Typically, widespread lesions of the skin and mucosae occur and progress from macules to papules, vesicles, and pustules before encrusting and healing. Most lesions contain multiple intracytoplasmic inclusions, which represent sites of virus replication in infected cells. In some poxvirus infections, vesiculation is not clinically evident, but microvesicles can be seen on histological examination and, in some, proliferative lesions are characteristic.

Infection is acquired either by inhalation or through the skin (eg, sheeppox). In certain instances (eg, fowlpox, swinepox), the virus is transmitted mechanically by biting arthropods. Infection may be followed by generalized lesions (eg, sheeppox) or remain localized (eg, pseudocowpox). Strains of poxvirus with reduced virulence are used to immunize against some infections, the classical example being the global eradication of smallpox in man by immunization with strains of live vaccinia virus. The origin of this virus is obscure.

Poxviruses can be classified according to their physicochemical and biological properties. Immunologically, the viruses of smallpox, cowpox, monkeypox, etc, are closely related to vaccinia virus. The avian poxviruses, the myxoma viruses, and some of the other poxviruses (eg, swinepox) are species specific. The viruses of orf, pseudocowpox, and bovine papular stomatitis are parapoxviruses.

In Europe, localized skin infections, but in some cases fatal generalized disease, have been reported in cheetahs, lions, and domestic cats (*see* below).

COWPOX

A mild, eruptive disease of dairy cows with lesions occurring on the udder and teats. Once considered common, it is now extremely rare and is reported only in Western Europe (*see also* POXVIRUS INFECTION IN CATS, below).

The virus of cowpox is closely related antigenically to vaccinia and smallpox viruses. Indeed, the first 2 can be differentiated only by sophisticated laboratory techniques. Before vaccination against smallpox was discontinued, some outbreaks in cows were due to infection with vaccinia from recently vaccinated persons.

The disease spreads by contact during milking. After an incubation period of 3-7 days, during which cows may be mildly febrile, papules appear on the teats and udder. Vesicles may not be evident or may rupture readily, leaving raw, ulcerated areas that form scabs. Lesions heal within 1 mo. Most cows in a milking herd may become affected. If milkers have not been vaccinated against smallpox, they may develop fever and have lesions on the hands, arms, or face.

Cowpox or vaccinia infection may be confused with bovine herpes mammillitis (qv, p 664); because the lesions are similar, laboratory confirmation is required. Pseudocowpox is a milder disease.

Measures to prevent spread within a herd must be based on segregation and hygiene.

PSEUDOCOWPOX
(Milkers' nodes, Paravaccinia)

A common, mild infection of the udder and teats of cows, caused by a parapoxvirus, which is widespread worldwide. The virus of pseudocowpox is related to those of orf (qv, p 784) and bovine papular stomatitis (qv, p 125). These parapoxviruses differ morphologically from vaccinia virus and other poxviruses. They have a limited host range and have not been propagated in fertile eggs. They will grow in some cell cultures, though relatively poorly.

Lesions begin as small, red papules on the teats or udder. These may be followed rapidly by scabbing, or small vesicles or pustules may develop before scabs form. Scabs may be abundant but can be removed without causing pain. Granulation occurs beneath the scabs, resulting in a raised lesion that heals from the center and leaves a characteristic horseshoe or circular ring of small scabs. This stage is reached in ~7-12 days. Some lesions persist for several months, giving the affected teats a rough feel and appearance, and more scabs may form. The infection spreads slowly throughout milking herds, and a variable percentage of cows shows lesions at any time. Cattle may become reinfected in subsequent lactations.

The scabbed lesions may be confused with warts or mild traumatic injuries to the teats and udder. Scabs examined with the electron microscope frequently show characteristic virus particles.

Control of infection within the herd is difficult and depends essentially on hygienic measures, such as teat dipping, to destroy the virus and prevent transmission. Little immunity appears to develop.

Man may become infected with painless but itchy, purplish red nodules that are generally present on the fingers or hands. These lesions cause little disturbance and disappear after several weeks.

LUMPY SKIN DISEASE

An infectious, eruptive, occasionally fatal disease of cattle characterized by nodules on the skin and other parts of the body. Secondary infection often aggravates the condition. Traditionally, it occurs in southern and eastern Africa, but in recent years has extended northwest through the continent into sub-Saharan West Africa.

Etiology and Epidemiology: The causal virus is related to that of sheeppox. The prototype strain is known as the Neethling poxvirus. Lumpy skin disease appears epidemically or sporadically. Frequently, new foci of infection appear in areas far removed from the initial outbreak. Its incidence is highest in wet summer weather, but it may occur in winter. It is most prevalent along water courses and on low ground. Since quarantine restrictions designed to limit the spread of infection have failed, biting insects have been suspected as vectors, but outbreaks have occurred under conditions in which insects practically could be excluded. Because the disease can be transmitted by infected saliva, contact infection must be accepted as a method of spread. African buffalo are suspected of being carriers in Kenya.

Artificial infection can be produced by inoculation of cutaneous nodule suspensions or blood taken during the early febrile stage, or by feed or water contaminated with saliva from infected animals.

Clinical Findings: A subcut. injection of infected material produces a painful swelling and then fever, lacrimation, nasal discharge, and hypersalivation, followed by the characteristic eruptions on the skin and other parts of the body in ~50% of susceptible cattle. The incubation period is 4-14 days.

The nodules are well circumscribed, round, slightly raised, firm, and painful and involve the entire cutis and the mucosa of the GI, respiratory, and genital tracts. Nodules may occur on the muzzle and within the nasal and buccal mucous membranes. The skin nodules contain a firm, creamy-gray or yellow mass of tissue. Regional lymph nodes are swollen, and edema develops in the udder, brisket, and legs. Secondary infection sometimes occurs, and causes extensive suppuration and sloughing; as a result, the animal may become extremely emaciated and euthanasia may be warranted. The nodules either regress in time, or necrosis of the skin results in hard, raised areas ("sit-fasts") clearly separated from the surrounding skin. These slough off to leave ulcers, which heal and scar.

Morbidity is 5-50%; mortality is usually low. The greatest loss is due to decreased milk yield, loss of condition, and rejection or reduced value of the hide.

Diagnosis: The disease may be confused with **pseudo-lumpy skin disease** caused by a herpesvirus (bovine herpesvirus 2). These diseases can be similar clinically, though in some parts of the world, the herpesvirus lesions seem confined to the teats and udder of cows, and the disease is called herpes mammillitis (qv, p 664).

Pseudo-lumpy skin disease is said to be a milder disease than true lumpy skin disease, but differentiation depends essentially on isolation and identification of the virus. Histological and ultrastructural examination of nodules may be helpful. Poxlike intracytoplasmic inclusion bodies or eosinophilic intranuclear herpesvirus inclusions may be seen in the nodules, depending on the cause.

Dermatophilus congolensis also causes skin nodules in cattle (*see* DERMATOPHILOSIS, p 787).

Prophylaxis and Treatment: Quarantine restrictions are useless. Vaccination with attenuated virus offers the most promising method of control. Goat poxvirus and sheep poxvirus passed in tissue culture also have been used.

Administration of sulfonamides to control secondary infection, and good nursing are recommended.

POXVIRUS INFECTION IN CATS

A sporadic disease in domestic cats, recorded in the UK and possibly Western Europe. Affected cats usually have multiple skin lesions, although respiratory and other signs also may be seen.

Etiology and Epidemiology: To date, all isolates examined from domestic cats have been indistinguishable from cowpox virus. Cowpox or infection with other closely related viruses also has been recorded in captive Felidae and in other species, eg, elephants, rhinoceroses, and anteaters, in various European zoos. However, the relationship of some of these viruses to established species within the genus (*see* above) is not clear. Cowpox apparently does not occur in the USA, although another orthopoxvirus has been isolated from raccoons. It is possible that this virus may also infect other hosts. Cowpox virus is also infectious to man and cat-to-man transmission has been recorded. Owners should be advised accordingly.

Although traditionally described as a disease of cattle, cowpox virus is, in fact, rare, and it is generally accepted that its reservoir hosts are small wild mammals. Cats, which are now the most commonly recognized host of cowpox virus, are believed to become infected when hunting; most affected cats come from rural environments and are known to hunt rodents, and the initial lesion is often described as having originated as a small bite-like wound. Cat-to-cat transmission can also occur, but usually results in only subclinical infection. Rare bovine cases presumably result from direct or indirect contact with the reservoir host, as do some human cases. However, cat-to-man and cow-to-man transmission are also possible. Infection in cats has a marked seasonal incidence, with most cases occurring between September and November.

The significance of the disease and its relatively recent recognition in the cat is unknown. It may have always been present in the cat population but not recognized. Alternatively, the disease may be increasing in importance, either as a result of a change in the epidemiology of the disease in the reservoir host, or (perhaps less likely) in the nature of the dominant biotype of the virus itself.

Pathogenesis: The most common route of entry appears to be through the skin, but oronasal infection is also possible. After local replication and development of a primary skin lesion, the virus spreads to local lymph nodes and a leukocyte-associated viremia develops. The viremic phase may be associated with pyrexia and depression, and during this period, virus can be isolated from various tissues, including the skin, turbinates (and sometimes lungs), and lymphoid organs. Widespread secondary skin lesions appear a few days after the onset of viremia, and fresh lesions continue to appear for 2-3 days, at which time the viremia subsides.

Clinical Findings: Most affected cats have a history of a single primary skin lesion, usually on the head, neck, or a forelimb. The primary lesion can vary in character from a small, scabbed wound to a large abscess. About 7-10 days after the primary lesion appears, widespread secondary skin lesions begin to appear. Over 2-4 days, these develop into discrete, circular, ulcerated papules ~0.5-1 cm in diameter. The ulcers soon become covered by scabs, and healing is usually complete by ~6 wk. Many cats show no signs other than skin lesions, but ~20% may develop mild coryza and/or conjunctivitis. Some cats may also be pyrexic, depressed, and inappetent during the viremic phase just before and during the early development of secondary lesions. Concurrent bacterial infection, particularly of the primary lesions, may give rise to systemic signs. Most domestic cats, however, recover uneventfully. More severe pulmonary disease is uncommon in domestic cats, but frequently occurs in cheetahs, and is often fatal in both species. More severe disease in domestic cats is often associated with immunosuppression either following treatment with corticosteroids or associated with infection with feline leukemia virus or feline immunodeficiency virus.

Lesions: Because most cats survive, skin biopsies generally are the only tissue available for pathological examination. Histologically, early lesions consist of areas of epidermal hyperplasia and hypertrophy with vesiculation of the prickle cell layer. Many of the epidermal cells bordering such vesicles contain characteristic eosinophilic cytoplasmic inclusions. Later, there is ulceration and necrosis of the epidermis and replacement by an eosinophilic coagulum of necrotic cells and fibrin. A heavy, mixed inflammatory cell exudate is present in the dermis surrounding the lesion. As healing ensues, a thin layer of epidermis covers the skin beneath the scabs, early scar tissue is present, and there is a moderate, mainly mononuclear, cell infiltrate.

In rarer cases, in which the disease has generalized, lesions may also be present in the liver, lungs, trachea, bronchi, oral mucosa, and small intestine.

Diagnosis: If multiple, well-circumscribed skin lesions are present, and especially if there is a history of hunting or exposure to a rural environment, a presumptive diagnosis may be based on clinical signs. Cowpox virus infection also should be suspected when skin lesions do not respond to antibiotics. Differential diagnoses include miliary dermatitis, feline herpesvirus or calicivirus infection, eosinophilic granuloma, bite wounds, ringworm, and other chronic bacterial or fungal conditions.

Presumptive and rapid diagnosis can be made in most cases from unfixed scab, exudate, or biopsy material examined for characteristic brick-shaped orthopox virions by electron microscopy. A more accurate and sensitive method of diagnosis is isolation of virus in cell culture or on the chick chorioallantois. Fixed biopsy material for histological examination, and serum for antibody determination also can be sent to the laboratory, if no virus is isolated.

Treatment and Control: In both domestic cats and cheetahs, it is important that cowpox be diagnosed promptly because steroid treatment, which is often used in the therapy of other skin conditions in cats, is contraindicated. Although in cheetahs the disease is often severe, in domestic cats, if the condition is recognized, supportive treatment (broad-spectrum antibiotics, fluid therapy) is generally successful and mortality low.

At present, because it seems that infection in domestic cats is mainly sporadic and acquired from chance contact with an infected wildlife reservoir, control measures probably are not indicated. In wildlife parks, where big cats are at risk from contact with small wild rodents, and especially where the disease has already occurred, vaccination may be helpful. Vaccinia virus appears to be of low pathogenicity in domestic cats, and cheetahs appear to be refractive; no trials have yet been done with other orthopoxvirus vaccines. Thus, at present, management of outbreaks among large cats depends on prompt diagnosis and segregation of affected animals to reduce the possibility of cat-to-cat spread. As far as is known, γ globulin has little or no value, but may be worth using if available. Premises may be disinfected by hypochlorite bleach or detergents. At ambient temperatures, poxviruses are relatively resistant, and may remain infective in dried crusts for months.

SHEEPPOX AND GOATPOX

Serious, often fatal, diseases characterized by widespread skin eruption. Both diseases are confined to parts of southeastern Europe, Africa, and Asia. The poxviruses of sheep and goats (capripoxviruses) are closely related, both antigenically and physicochemically. They are also related to the virus of lumpy skin disease (*see above*). Reports on the natural susceptibility of sheep to goat poxvirus and *vice versa* are conflicting; at least some strains seem capable of infecting both species.

The incubation period of sheeppox is 4-8 days, and of goatpox 5-14 days. The clinical picture is similar in the 2 diseases, but is generally less severe in goats. Fever and a variable degree of systemic disturbance occur. Eyelids become swollen, and mucopurulent discharge crusts the nostrils. Widespread skin lesions develop that are most readily seen on the muzzle, ears, and areas free of wool or long hair. Palpation can detect lesions not readily seen. Lesions start as erythematous areas on the skin, and progress rapidly to raised, circular plaques with congested borders caused by local inflammation, edema, and epithelial hyperplasia. Although microvesicles are present histologically, vesicles and pustules are not evident clinically. Virus is abundant in skin lesions at this stage. As lesions start to regress, necrosis of the dermis occurs, and dark, hard scabs form, which are sharply separated from the surrounding skin. Regeneration of the epithelium beneath the scabs takes several weeks. When scabs are removed, a star-shaped scar, free of hair or wool, remains. In severe cases, lesions can occur in the lungs. In some sheep and in certain breeds, the disease may be mild or the infection inapparent.

It has been suggested that transmission may be airborne, or occur by direct contact with lesions, or mechanically by biting insects.

The disease in either species must be differentiated from the milder infection, orf (qv, p 784), which mainly causes crusty, proliferative lesions around the mouth.

Infection results in solid and enduring immunity. Live, attenuated virus vaccines give longer immunity than inactivated virus vaccines. Live, attenuated, lumpy skin disease virus also can be used as a vaccine against sheeppox and goatpox.

SWINEPOX

An acute, often mild, infectious disease characterized by skin eruptions, that affects only pigs. It is present in the USA, particularly in the Midwest, and has been reported from all continents, although the incidence is generally low.

Historically, in some outbreaks vaccinia virus was involved, but currently, swinepox virus appears to be the only cause. The disease described here is that caused by the latter. Swinepox virus is distinct from other poxviruses and does not protect against infection with vaccinia virus. It will grow on pig cell cultures, but not embryonating eggs. It is relatively heat stable and survives for ~10 days at 37°C.

The disease is most frequently seen in young pigs, 3-6 wk old, but all ages may be affected. Following an incubation period of ~1 wk, small red areas may be seen most frequently on the face, ears, inside the legs, and abdomen; these develop into papules and, within a few days, pustules develop or small vesicles may be seen. The centers of the pustules become dry and scabbed, and are surrounded by a raised, inflamed zone so that the lesions appear umbilicated. Later, dark scabs (1-2 cm in diameter) form, giving affected piglets a spotted appearance. These eventually drop or are rubbed off without leaving a scar. Successive crops of lesions can occur so that all are not at the same stage. The early stage of the disease may be accompanied by mild fever, inappetence, and dullness. Few pigs die of uncomplicated swinepox.

Virus is abundant in the lesions and can be transferred from pig to pig by the biting louse (*Haematopinus suis*). The disease also may be transmitted, possibly between farms, by other insects acting as mechanical carriers.

Recovered pigs are immune. There is no specific treatment. Eradication of lice is important.

PRURITUS
(Itching)

An unpleasant sensation that provokes the desire to scratch or, alternatively, an uneasy sensation of irritation within the skin. Many believe it can be elicited only from the epidermis and palpebral conjunctiva. There are no specialized itch receptors. The itch sensation is carried from the nerve ending to the spinal cord, and ascends the ventrolateral spinothalamic tract via the thalamus to the cortex.

The nature of the mediators of pruritus is controversial. It is now believed to include both histamines (released from mast cell degranulation) and proteolytic enzymes (proteases). Proteases are released by fungi, bacteria, and mast cell degranulation, and during antigen-antibody reactions. Leukotrienes, prostaglandins, and thromboxane A_2, which are broken down from arachidonic acid, are pro-inflammatory. Essential fatty acids, particularly γ-linolenic acid, have been used to counter the inflammation mediated by leukotrienes and thromboxane A_2.

A sign and not a disease, pruritus is commonly elicited in domestic animals by allergic diseases, ectoparasites, bacterial infections, and idiopathic conditions (eg, seborrhea). However, certain conditions can be designated as pruritic or nonpruritic only in general terms, since diseases vary among and within species as to their ability to produce pruritus; eg, while endocrinopathies generally cause nonpruritic dermatoses, concurrent secondary seborrhea or pyoderma can elicit pruritus and potentially cause a misdiagnosis or the underlying hormonal imbalance to be overlooked.

A thorough dermatologic history should be taken, and the type of lesions and their location(s) noted. Diagnostic techniques include skin scrapings, Wood's lamp examination, fungal culture, allergy investigations (dietary tests, patch testing, and intradermal testing), and biopsy. If pyoderma is noted, it must be determined whether it is the sole cause of the pruritus or whether it is secondary to an underlying allergy. This is best determined by treating the animal with an antibiotic effective against staphylococci (the most common bacterial pathogens in pyodermas in small and possibly also in large animals), and then reevaluating the pruritus in 7-10 days. A complete or near-complete resolution of the pruritus indicates that the pyoderma is the primary instigator; partial reduction of the pruritus indicates a concurrent allergic or ectoparasitic etiology.

Unfortunately, some animals have pruritus that must be classified as idiopathic after all diagnostic tests have been utilized. In these, therapy with corticosteroids or nonsteroidal antipruritic drugs (antihistamines, aspirin, or essential fatty acids) should be attempted. While the corticosteroids are more commonly effective in all species, the pruritic animal that may need a lifelong course of corticosteroids to control pruritus deserves a month of trial therapy on various nonsteroidal antipruritics. If such drugs are effective, the potential side effects of long-term corticosteriod therapy may be avoided.

PYODERMA
(Pyogenic dermatitis, Acne, Secondary pyoderma)

A pyogenic infection of skin, which can be primary or secondary, superficial or deep. Microorganisms commonly isolated include *Staphylococcus aureus, S epidermidis*, streptococci (both hemolytic and nonhemolytic), *Corynebacterium* spp, *Pseudomonas* spp, and *Proteus vulgaris*. Most causative staphylococci are now identified as *S intermedius*. Metabolic disorders, immune deficiencies, endocrine imbalances, or various allergies may predispose to development of pyoderma.

Clinical Findings: Dogs are the species most often affected. Superficial pyodermas are characterized by pustules, follicular papules, and epidermal collarettes. The latter are circular lesions with scaling margins, often mistaken for ringworm. While found in other skin diseases, epidermal collarettes are most common in superficial pyodermas. Deep pyodermas may be localized to the face, limbs, or interdigital areas (interdigital "cysts", qv, p 811), or may be generalized. Lesions are draining, purulent tracts. German Shepherd Dogs appear to be more susceptible.

Juvenile cellulitis (juvenile pyoderma, puppy strangles) usually occurs in dogs ≤12 wk old, most commonly in Labrador and Golden Retrievers, Dachshunds, Brittanys, and Springer Spaniels. It is characterized by enlarged lymph nodes; periaural, perioral, and periocular swelling; pustules; and alopecia. Affected dogs are usually febrile, anorectic, and lethargic. In dogs with any type of pyoderma, demodicosis must be the first differential diagnosis. Cats rarely get pyodermas, but when they do, clinical signs resemble those seen in dogs. Cats may get mycobacterial infections, such as feline leprosy.

In horses, folliculitis often develops in the saddle and lumbar regions (*see also* SADDLE SORES, below), particularly in summer. Staphylococci, *Dermatophilus* spp, or *Corynebacterium pseudotuberculosis* are isolated most commonly. Initially, the affected area may be swollen and sensitive; then, follicular papules and pustules develop. These may become confluent or rupture, and form plaques and crusts. Deep folliculitis followed by ulceration may develop over large areas of the body, especially on the neck, lateral thorax, inner surface of the thighs, or prepuce. Deep pyodermas in horses are usually caused by *C pseudotuberculosis*.

In cattle, folliculitis, which may progress to necrosis, develops mostly on the abdomen, groin, and medial thighs. Other primary pyodermas frequently occur on thin-skinned or frictional areas. Animals suffering from extensive deep pyoderma may have fever, anemia, leukocytosis, and enlargement of regional lymph nodes.

Treatment and Prognosis: Irritation of affected areas should be avoided. In the early stage, bathing in warm antiseptic solutions such as hexachlorophene or povidone-iodine is useful. Therapy of superficial or skin-fold pyodermas often is helped by benzoyl peroxide (2.5%) shampoos. In general, both superficial and deep pyodermas are best treated with antibiotics based on culture and sensitivity. When empiric antibiotic therapy is used (before results of culture and sensitivity are known), it should be remembered that most staphylococci that cause pyoderma are penicillinase producers. In persistent or recurring pyodermas, immunostimulants such as bacterins may be used.

Therapy of juvenile cellulitis (not a true bacterial infection) should include high doses of corticosteroids (prednisone or prednisolone) starting at 1 mg/kg, b.i.d. with gradual tapering over a 1-mo period. Antibiotics may be used concurrently.

The prognosis for superficial pyoderma may be more favorable in horses than in other animals. The prognosis for superficial pyoderma in other species, particularly dogs, and for deep pyoderma in any species may be unfavorable unless the predisposing factor(s) can be determined and corrected, or unless long-term, even lifelong, antibiotic therapy is used.

SADDLE SORES
(Collar galls)

The area of riding horses that is under saddle, or the shoulder area of those driven in harness, frequently is the site of injuries to the skin and deeper soft and bony tissues. Clinical signs vary according to the depth of injury and the complications caused by secondary infection. Sores affecting only the skin are characterized by inflammatory changes that range from erythematous through papular, vesicular, pustular, and finally, necrotic. Frequently, the condition starts as an acute inflammation of the hair follicles and progresses to a purulent folliculitis. Affected areas show hair loss and are swollen, hot, and painful. The serous or purulent exudate dries and forms crusts. Advanced lesions are termed "galls". In cases of more serious damage of the skin and underlying tissues, abscesses may develop. They are characterized by hot, fluctuating, painful swellings from which purulent and serosanguineous fluid can be aspirated. Severe damage to the skin and subcutis or deeper tissues results in dry or moist necrosis. Chronic saddle sores are characterized by a deep folliculitis (hard nodules) or a localized indurative and proliferative dermatitis. Lesions are usually caused by poorly fitting tack.

Excoriations and inflammations of the skin of the saddle and harness regions are treated as any other dermatosis. Absolute rest of the affected parts is necessary. During the early or acute stages, astringent packs (Burow's solution or 2% lead acetate) are indicated. Chronic lesions and those superficially infected may be treated by warm applications and massage with stimulating ointments (iodine), or systemic antibiotics. Hematomas should be aspirated or incised. Necrotic tissue should be removed surgically. A skin astringent and antiseptic consisting of 500 mL of 0.1% alcoholic sublimate, 30 g tannic acid, and 1 g gentian violet may be of value. In severe folliculitis/furunculosis, antibiotics are indicated. Identification and elimination of the offending portion of tack is more important than any other treatment.

SCREWWORMS

Screwworms are larvae of the blowfly, *Cochliomyia (Callitroga) hominivorax* (order Diptera, family Calliphoridae), which is an obligate myiasis-causing parasite. The female screwworm fly lays eggs on wounds, cuts, bites, navels of newborns, and other sites in the skin of all warm-blooded animals. *Cochliomyia hominivorax* is distributed throughout the neoarctic and neotropical regions of the Western Hemisphere. As a result of massive state, federal, and international eradication programs, extant populations of *C hominivorax* are no longer found in the USA or Mexico; the isolated reports of infestations are often traced to importation of infested animals from locations where the screwworm is still prevalent. Extant populations are found in Central and South America, and certain Caribbean islands. Another species of screwworm, the "old world" screwworm, *Chrysomyia bezziana*, is found in Africa and southern Asia, including Papua New Guinea.

Etiology, Epidemiology, and Pathogenesis: The screwworm fly, similar in appearance to other blowflies, deposits 200-400 eggs in rows that overlap like shingles in a mass on the edge of a wound. After 12-21 hr, larvae hatch, crawl into the wound, and burrow into the flesh. The larvae feed on wound fluids and live tissue and complete their growth in 5-7 days. Grown larvae then exit from the wound, fall to the ground, and burrow into the soil to pupate. The pupal period varies from 7 days to 2 mo, depending on temperature. Freezing or sustained soil temperatures (<46°F [8°C]) kill the pupae. The adults mate when 3-4 days old, and gravid females are ready to oviposit when ~6 days old. In warm weather, the life cycle may be completed in 21 days. Only female flies feed and oviposit on wounds; males and younger, virgin females gather to mate in vegetation, especially flowering vegetation.

Screwworm myiasis is spread by the movement of infested animals and by migration of the screwworm fly. The larvae have sharp, pointed mouth hooks that tear living flesh.

Clinical Findings and Diagnosis: Newly infested wounds contain screwworm larvae of a single age; older, larger wounds may contain larvae of various ages and often of different species of flies. The malodorous, reddish brown fluid produced in the wound usually drains and may stain the hair or wool around or below the wound. As the annoyance increases, the infested animal seeks protection by retreating to the densest available shade. Even a small and relatively inconspicuous wound infested with screwworm larvae attracts not only screwworm flies, but also house flies and blow flies; later, necrotic tissue attracts more flies. The wounds can become greatly enlarged due to multiple infestation and, unless treated, usually result in death of the animal.

Screwworm flies are bluish to bluish green, slightly larger than a house fly, and difficult to distinguish from other blowflies in the family Calliphoridae. The larvae are tapered, and have mouth hooks at the narrow end and breathing spiracles at the wide end. Body segments are ringed with spines. Because of their shape and appearance, they resemble woodscrews, hence the common name of screwworm. Screwworm larvae can be distinguished from larvae of other closely related species, especially *Cochliomyia (Callitroga) macellaria* (the secondary screwworm) by the tracheal trunks, which in true screwworm larvae are darkly pigmented and can be seen through the larval cuticle.

Control: Screwworms in wounds can be killed by direct application of a wound dressing, called a "smear". Such smears, which contain lindane or ronnel, may be difficult to find in the USA because of the eradication program. Smears are best applied with a 1-in. (2.5-cm) paint brush and should reach all the many pockets formed by the burrowing larvae in deep wounds. A thin layer should also be applied to the skin surrounding the wound to protect from reinfestation. Wounds may also be treated with aerosol, dust, or foam formulations of coumaphos, lindane, or ronnel. As a prophylactic measure to protect animals from infestation and also to kill larvae in small, difficult-to-detect wounds, animals can be sprayed thoroughly with ronnel or sprayed with or dipped in coumaphos. In cattle, subcut. injection of ivermectin has been shown to clear wounds of *C bezziana* larvae within 3 days and to prevent reinfestation for 14 days following injection.

Eradication Program: In 1958, the USA Department of Agriculture initiated a program in the southeastern states to eliminate the screwworm by the sterile insect technique. When reared artificially and exposed to γ irradiation shortly before they emerge from the pupae, male flies are sterile but able to mate. The female mates only once, and when mated with a sterile male, lays eggs that do not hatch. Release of sufficient numbers of sterile males in an area over a period of time leads to elimination. By 1959, the screwworm had been eliminated from Florida. The program had cost ~$11 million, whereas the fly (and its treatments) had been estimated to cost $20 million annually.

The program was expanded to cover the rest of the area involved in the USA and then, via a joint Mexico-USA agreement, to include most of Mexico. This, plus the use of a screwworm attractant and an insecticide system that attracted and killed adults, led to eradication of screwworms from Mexico. There is interest in expanding the area throughout Central America and the Caribbean. However, until this has been achieved, constant vigilance by all who deal with animals in the southern USA and Mexico is necessary to detect an infestation quickly and eradicate it before flies reproduce and spread. If a wound is found infested with larvae, appropriate samples should be collected and sent to eradication officials at P.O. Box 969, Mission, TX 78572 USA.

TICK INFESTATION

Ticks are obligatory bloodsucking ectoparasites of most types of terrestrial vertebrates virtually wherever these animals occur. Ticks transmit a large number and variety of infectious agents, eg, *see* TICK-BORNE FEVER, p 405, and TICK PYEMIA, p 407. Some of these are only slightly pathogenic to livestock but may cause disease in man (*see* ZOONOSES, p 1736); others cause diseases in livestock that are of tremendous economic importance. In addition, tick feeding activity produces host reactions such as toxicosis (eg, sweating sickness, qv, p 364; tick paralysis, qv, p 624) caused by salivary fluids and toxins, skin wounds susceptible to secondary bacterial infections and screwworm infestations, anemia, and death. The total effect—reduced production and performance—is incalculable, although research to quantify the various effects has been undertaken.

Economically developed nations spend huge sums to prevent and reduce losses from tick-borne diseases. In less developed nations with fewer resources for prevention and control, and a relatively greater need for animal protein to sustain the poorly nourished human population, losses from tick-borne diseases are especially harsh. International movement of animals infected with tick-transmitted *Theileria*, *Babesia*, *Anaplasma*, and *Cowdria* spp are widely restricted.

Primary factors in the extensive distribution and prevalence of many tick species and tick-borne disease agents are movement of tick-infested livestock over great distances, and introduction of livestock to tick species and tick-borne agents that they have not previously experienced and against which they have no immunity or innate resistance. A number of introduced tick species thrive in the vast grazing and browsing environments established during recent centuries as a result of human and livestock population explosions.

Two of the 3 families of ticks parasitize livestock: the Argasidae (argasids, "leathery" or "soft ticks") and the Ixodidae (ixodids, "hard ticks"). Although they share certain basic properties, argasids and ixodids differ in many structural, behavioral, physiological, feeding, and reproductive patterns. Tropical and subtropical species may undergo 1, 2, or rarely 3 complete life cycles annually. In temperate zones there is often one annual cycle; in northern regions, 2-4 yr are required by most species. There are 4 developmental stages: egg, larva, nymph, and adult. All larvae have 3 pairs of legs; all nymphs and adults, 4. Adults have a distinctive genital and anal area on the ventral body surface. The foreleg tarsi of all ticks bear a unique sensory apparatus—the Haller's organ—for sensing chemical stimuli (odor), temperature, humidity, etc. Pheromones stimulate group assembly, species recognition, mating, and host selection in ticks.

Certain tick species that parasitize livestock can survive several months, and occasionally a few years without food, if environmental conditions permit. Tick host preferences are usually limited to a certain genus, family, or order of vertebrates; however, certain ticks are exceptionally adaptable to a variety of hosts, so each species must be evaluated separately. The larvae and nymphs of most ixodids that parasitize livestock feed on small wildlife such as birds, rodents, small carnivores, or even lizards.

In the Argasidae, the leathery dorsal surface lacks a hard plate (scutum). Male and female argasids appear to be much alike, except for the larger size of the female and differences in external genitalia. The argasid capitulum (mouthparts) in larvae arises from the anterior of the body, but from the ventral body surface in nymphs and adults.

In the Ixodidae, the male dorsal surface is covered by a scutum. The scutum of the ixodid female, nymph, and larva covers only the anterior half of the dorsal surface. The ixodid capitulum arises from the anterior end of the body in each developmental stage.

Argasid Parasitism: The Argasidae are highly specialized for sheltering in protected niches or crevices in wood or rocks, or in ground-level or subterranean vertebrates' nests or resting places. Most of these leathery parasites inhabit tropical or warm temperate environments with long dry seasons. Hosts are those that either rest in large numbers near the argasid microhabitat, or return from time to time to rest there or seasonally to breed there.

Most of the 55 *Argas* spp parasitize birds that breed in colonies in trees or against rock ledges, others parasitize cave-dwelling bats. Few feed on reptiles or wild mammals, and none on livestock. Several species have become important pests of man's domestic fowl and pigeons; among these are the vectors of *Borrelia anserina* (avian spirochetosis) and *Aegyptianella pullorum* (aegyptianellosis). *Argas* spp also cause tick paralysis, and many are vectors of a variety of arboviruses, some of which also infect man.

The nearly 100 species of *Ornithodoros* shelter in caves, burrows, or dens; under the shade of trees; in the substrate or under stones or debris in ground-level bird breeding colonies; in bird nests in tree holes; or under large stones together with lizards or tenrecs. Different groups of the species parasitize reptiles, birds, or mammals. A few species have adapted to different environments where livestock are confined, and also are pests of man. Certain species are vectors of relapsing fever spirochetes (*Borrelia* spp) and the virus causing African swine fever; some species also cause toxicosis. Numerous *Ornithodoros*-transmitted salivary toxins or arboviruses cause irritation or febrile illnesses in man.

An argasid population normally parasitizes only a single kind of vertebrate and inhabits its shelter area, and they use multiple hosts, ie, the larvae feed on one host and drop to the substrate to molt; the several nymphal instars each feed separately, drop, and molt; adults feed several times (but do not molt). Argasid nymphs and adults feed rapidly (usually 30-60 min). Larvae of some argasids also feed rapidly; others require several days to engorge fully. Adult argasids mate off the host several times; afterward, females deposit a few hundred eggs in several batches and feed between ovipositions.

The unique argasid genus *Otobius* is discussed on p 844.

Ixodid Parasitism: The Ixodidae number over 650 species (vs about 155 argasid species), occupy many more habitats and niches than argasids, and parasitize a greater number of vertebrates in a wider variety of environments. More than 600 ixodid species have a 3-host life cycle; others have a 2-host cycle, and a few have a 1-host cycle. Each ixodid postembryonic development stage (larva, nymph, adult) feeds only once but for a period of several days. Males and females of most species that parasitize livestock mate while on the host, although some mate off the host on the ground or in burrows. Males take less food than females, but remain longer on the host and may mate with several females. During inactive seasons, few or no females are found feeding, even though males are still attached to the hosts. Larval and nymphal population activity generally peaks during the "off-seasons" of adults, although in some species there is more or less of an overlap in the seasonal dynamics of immatures and adults.

The ixodid male becomes sexually mature only after beginning to feed, after which he mates with a feeding female. Only after mating does the female become replete and fully sexually mature. She then detaches, drops from the host, and over a period of a few days, deposits a single batch of numerous eggs on or near the ground, usually in crevices or under stones or debris. Depending on species and quantity of female nourishment, the egg batch usually numbers 1000-4000, but may be >12,000. The female dies after ovipositing. Notably, ixodids (except 1-host species) spend ≥90% of their lifetime off the host, a fact of utmost significance in planning control measures. The several-day feeding process progresses slowly; the balloon shape characteristic of engorged larvae, nymphs, and females develops only during the final half day of feeding and is followed by detaching. The dropping time at certain hours of the day or night is governed by a circadian rhythm closely associated with the activity cycle of the chief host.

It is also vital to know whether immatures of an ixodid species feed on the same host species as do the adults, or on smaller vertebrates. Where acceptable smaller-sized hosts are scarce, immatures of some ixodid species can feed on the same livestock hosts as adults; immatures of other species seldom or never do so.

The proximity of acceptable hosts, air temperature gradients, and atmospheric humidity during "resting" and questing periods are among the numerous factors that regulate the development of each stage and, in the case of females, oviposition.

Three-host Ixodids: Most ixodids have a 3-host cycle. The recently hatched larvae quest for a suitable host, usually from vegetation, feed for several days, drop, and molt to nymphs, which repeat these activities and molt to adults. Of the 3-host species that parasitize livestock, a few have immatures and adults that parasitize the same kind of host; these often develop tremendous population densities. The success of ixodid species that require smaller-size hosts for immatures depends on the availability of those hosts in the livestock browsing and grazing grounds. The numerous natural hazards inherent in the 3-host cycle have been compensated for by the numerous benefits afforded adaptable tick species by animal husbandry practices. Only certain ixodids specific for herbivores have adapted to coexistence with livestock, and therein lies the answer to numerous livestock tick problems in Africa, where hosts for adults and immatures are abundant.

Two-host Ixodids: Some ixodids, especially those that parasitize wandering mammals (and also birds in certain cases) in inclement environments of the Old World, have developed a 2-host cycle in which larvae and nymphs feed on one host, and adults on another. As in 3-host species, both hosts may be different or may be the same species. Two-host parasites of livestock thrive in both inclement and clement environments and are difficult to control. This is especially true of 2-host species that feed in the ears and anal areas of livestock.

One-host Ixodids: Among the most economically important ticks are several 1-host species. These parasites co-evolved with herbivores that wandered in extensive ranges in the tropics (*Boophilus* spp, *Dermacentor nitens*, etc) or in temperate zones (*D albipictus*, *Hyalomma scupense*). Larvae, nymphs, and adults feed on a single animal until the mated, replete females drop to the ground to oviposit.

Feeding Sites: Each species has one or more favored feeding sites on the host, although in dense infestations, other areas of the host may be utilized. Some feed chiefly on the head, neck, shoulders, and escutcheon; others in the ears; others around the anus and under the tail. Other common feeding sites are the axillae, udder, male genitalia, and tail brush. Immatures and adults often have different preferred feeding sites. Attachment of the large, irritating *Amblyomma* spp is regulated by a male-produced aggregation-attachment pheromone, which ensures that the ticks attach at sites least vulnerable to grooming.

IMPORTANT IXODIDAE

AMBLYOMMA SPP

Amblyomma ticks are large, 3-host parasites. They have eyes, long and strong mouthparts, are more or less brightly ornamented, and generally are confined to the tropics and subtropics. Adults and immatures of 37 of the 102 known species in this genus parasitize reptiles, which together with ground-feeding birds, are often hosts of immature *Amblyomma* ticks that have adapted, in the adult stage, to parasitizing mammals. Their long mouthparts make *Amblyomma* ticks especially difficult to remove manually and frequently cause serious wounds that may become secondarily infected by bacteria or screwworms.

Most, if not all, African *Amblyomma* ticks that parasitize livestock are reservoirs and vectors of *Cowdria ruminantium*, the rickettsial agent of heartwater (qv, p 396). Certain American *Amblyomma* ticks that parasitize livestock are proved or potential vectors of this agent.

Amblyomma americanum, the lone-star tick, is abundant in southern USA from Texas and Missouri to the Atlantic Coast and ranges northward into New Jersey. It is also a notorious pest in Mexico, and Central and South America.

The scutum is distinctive because of pale ornamentation in the male and a conspicuous, silvery spot ("star") near the posterior margin in the female. Larvae, nymphs, and adults are indiscriminate in host choice and parasitize a variety of livestock and wildlife as well as man. Activity in the USA continues from early spring to late fall. Feeding sites on domestic and wild mammals are usually areas with sparse hair; wounds at these sites predispose livestock to attack by the screwworm fly, *Cochliomyia hominivorax*. The lone-star tick transmits the agents that cause tularemia, Rocky Mountain spotted fever, Q-fever, and Lyme disease, and may cause tick paralysis in man and dogs. Lone-star virus (Bunyaviridae) has been isolated from *A americanum* in Kentucky.

Amblyomma cajennense, the Cayenne tick, ranges from South America into southern Texas. As with *A americanum*, each active stage is indiscriminate in host choice: livestock and a large variety of avian and mammalian wildlife serve as hosts. People are severely irritated by clusters of *A cajennense* larvae ("seed ticks") in wooded and high-grass areas. Most adults attach on the lower body surface, especially between the legs, some feed elsewhere on the body. Activity continues throughout the year. *Amblyomma cajennense* is apparently a vector of the rickettsial agent of Rocky Mountain spotted fever. Wad Medani virus (an orbivirus, Reoviridae), an African virus transported to Caribbean islands by *A variegatum*-infested cattle from Senegal, has been isolated from *A cajennense* in Jamaica.

Amblyomma maculatum, the Gulf Coast tick, is an important pest of livestock, particularly cattle, from South America to southern USA. Optimal habitats are warm areas with high rainfall, close to seacoasts. Immatures usually parasitize birds and small mammals; adults parasitize deer, cattle, horses, sheep, pigs, and dogs. Adult feeding activity is chiefly in late summer and early fall but may begin later after a dry summer. Most adults infest the ears, where the feeding wounds are initial sites of screwworm infestations. Clustered feeding adults also cause much irritation to the upper parts of the neck of cattle and to the humps of Brahman cattle.

Amblyomma imitator parasitizes livestock from Central America to southern Texas. Occasional pests of livestock in tropical America are *A neumanni* (Argentina), *A ovale* and *A parvum* (Argentina to Mexico), *A tigrinum* (much of South America), and *A tapirellum* (Colombia to Mexico).

Amblyomma testudinarium inhabits Asian tropical wooded environments from Sri Lanka and India to Malaysia and Vietnam, Indonesia, Borneo, Philippines, Taiwan, and southern Japan. Adults are particularly abundant on wild and domestic pigs and also infest deer, cattle and other livestock, and man. Immatures parasitize birds and small mammals as well as man. In India and Sri Lanka, adult *A integrum* and *A mudlairi* also parasitize livestock, wild ungulates, and man.

Amblyomma hebraeum, the southern Africa bont tick, inhabits warm, moderately humid savannas of the Republic of South Africa, Namibia, Botswana, Zimbabwe, Malawi, Mozambique, and Angola. Immatures feed on various small mammals, ground-feeding birds, and reptiles. Adults infest livestock, antelopes, and other wildlife. Adults, attached chiefly to body areas with relatively little hair, cause serious wounds that become secondarily infected by bacteria and screwworm (*Chrysomyia bezziana*). Like other African *Amblyomma* ticks (bont ticks) that parasitize livestock, *A hebraeum* is an important vector of *Cowdria ruminantium*, and the larvae transmit *Rickettsia conori* (tick typhus) to man.

Amblyomma variegatum, the tropical African bont tick is an easily visible, brightly colored parasite found throughout sub-Saharan savannas southward to the range of *A hebraeum*, and also in southern Arabia and several islands in the Indian and Atlantic Oceans and the Caribbean. Host preferences are similar to those of *A hebraeum* but also include camels. Adults feed chiefly during rainy seasons, immatures during dry seasons. Most adults attach to the underside of the host body, on the genitalia, and under the tail. *Amblyomma variegatum* injuries to hosts and transmittal of *C ruminantium* are similar to those of *A hebraeum*. This tick is not considered to be an effective vector of Nairobi sheep disease virus but is a secondary vector of Crimean-Congo hemorrhagic fever (CCHF) virus. Dugbe virus has been isolated from *A variegatum* in 6 nations north of the equator; the Thogoto and Bhanja viruses are also associated with this tick in various areas north of the equator. Notably, yellow fever virus has been isolated from *A variegatum* collected from cattle in the Central African Republic and has been demonstrated to be transovarially transmitted to the progeny of infected females. Jos virus infects *A variegatum* from Ethiopia to Senegal and has been transported in this tick to Jamaica.

Amblyomma lepidum, the East African bont tick, inhabits xeric savanna environments from northern Tanzania to central Sudan. *Amblyomma gemma*, the gem-like bont tick, occurs in similar environments of Tanzania, Somalia, Kenya, and Ethiopia. A small variety of the buffalo bont tick, *A cohaerens*, is abundant on cattle in Ethiopian highlands, but from Zaire to Tanzania the larger variety of *A cohaerens* parasitizes chiefly the Cape buffalo. Other African *Amblyomma* ticks of the Cape buffalo and different large mammals and livestock are *A pomposum*, of humid highland forests in Angola, Zaire, Uganda, southern Sudan, Kenya, and Zimbabwe; and *A astrion*, of West Africa and Zaire.

BOOPHILUS SPP

Each of the 5 *Boophilus* spp has a 1-host life cycle that may be completed in 3-4 wk and results in a heavy tick burden. Under these conditions, acaricide resistance becomes a major problem in control efforts. Zebu cattle, which have served for centuries as hosts of *B microplus* in the region of India, have developed resistance to feeding by large numbers of *Boophilus* and are used purebred, or crossbred in integrated control programs. *Boophilus microplus*, considered the world's most important tick parasite of livestock, has been introduced from the bovid- and cervid-inhabited forests of the Indian region to many areas of tropical and subtropical Asia, northeastern Australia, Madagascar, coastal lowlands of southeastern Africa to the equator, and much of South and Central America, Mexico, and the Caribbean. *Boophilus microplus* and *B annulatus* were eradicated from the USA after a long, costly control program. Constant surveillance is maintained to prevent their reintroduction. *Boophilus annulatus* of southern USSR, the Near and Middle East, and the Mediterranean area, was introduced with livestock of the early Spanish colonialists into northeastern Mexico but has not spread into Central America. In Africa, south of the Sahara and north of the equator, cattle movements probably account for the many *B annulatus* populations. *Boophilus decoloratus*, which ranges from southern Africa to the Sahara, is being replaced in the southeastern part of this area by *B microplus*. In more humid West African zones, *B annulatus* mixes with or is totally replaced by *B geigyi*. Scattered *B geigyi* populations occur as far east as southern and central Sudan. In Sri Lanka, an unnamed species infests domestic cattle and buffalo and wild deer. The only boophilid restricted to sheep and goats (and occasionally horses) is *B kohlsi* of Syria, Iraq, Israel, Jordan, western Saudi Arabia, and the Yemen. *Boophilus microplus* and *B annulatus* are major vectors of *Babesia bigemina*, *B bovis*, and *Anaplasma marginale*. *Boophilus decoloratus* is an efficient vector of *Babesia bigemina* and *A marginale* but does not transmit *B bovis*.

DERMACENTOR SPP

Of the 30 *Dermacentor* spp, 19 inhabit temperate zones. Of the 11 tropical species, only *D nitens* is of major importance in veterinary medicine; the others may transmit zoonotic infections, and adults may be common on wildlife such as pigs, deer, and antelopes. Immatures infest chiefly rodents and also lagomorphs. *Dermacentor* spp in cold areas (and *D nitens* in tropical America) have specialized life cycles and seasonal dynamics of activity, each of which must be considered separately. Otherwise, the *Dermacentor* life cycle is of the typical 3-host pattern.

Dermacentor (Anocentor) nitens, the 1-host tropical horse tick, originally parasitized deer (*Mazama*) in the forests of northern South America. With the introduction of Equidae and other livestock into its habitat, it adapted to these animals. Spending its entire parasitic life deep in the hosts' ears, this parasite was easily spread by human activities to other areas of the Americas, including Florida and Texas. In addition to ear cavities, each active stage may infest nasal passages and the mane, ventral abdomen, and perianal area. *Dermacentor nitens* transmits *Babesia caballi* transovarially to successive generations and is important in the horse racing industry.

Another American 1-host species, *D albipictus*, the winter or moose tick, ranges from Canada and northern USA into western USA and Mexico. A brownish "form", sometimes called *D nigrolineatus*, is distributed from New Mexico to southern and eastern USA and probably merits subspecies if not full-species rank. The larval-nymphal-adult feeding period on a single host (moose, deer, elk, or domestic cattle or horses) extends from fall to spring. Heavily infested hosts may die. *Dermacentor albipictus* causes the often fatal "phantom moose disease" of Canada and is a secondary vector of Colorado tick fever virus.

The 6 other American *Dermacentor* spp have 3-host life cycles. The Rocky Mountain wood tick, *D andersoni*, occurs from Nebraska westward to the western mountains (Cascades and Sierra Nevadas), in northern New Mexico and Arizona, and in western Canada. The American dog tick, *D variabilis* occurs west of the Cascades and Sierra Nevadas, in Mexico, from Nebraska to the Atlantic, and in eastern Canada. Both species produce tick paralysis in livestock, wildlife, and man. They are the chief vectors of *Rickettsia rickettsii*, the agent of Rocky Mountain spotted fever. *Dermacentor andersoni* is also the chief vector of Colorado tick fever virus, and transmits Powassan virus, *Anaplasma marginale*, and the agents of tularemia and Q-fever. *Dermacentor variabilis* transmits Sawgrass virus and *A marginale*. Adults of both species parasitize livestock and wildlife such as deer, bison, and elk, but those of *D variabilis* prefer skunk, raccoon, puma, etc, and domestic dogs. Immatures feed on rodents and other small wild mammals. A related, biologically similar species, *D occidentalis*, is restricted to the Pacific lowlands from Oregon to Baja California.

In western USA and Mexico, *D parumapterus*, *D hunteri*, and *D halli* parasitize various hares and rabbits, mountain sheep, and peccaries, respectively. These ticks seldom make contact with livestock. In Mexico and Guatemala, *D dissimilis* parasitizes a variety of hosts; in Costa Rica and Panama, *D latus* infests tapirs.

In Eurasian steppes, forests, and mountains, *D marginatus*, *D reticulatus*, and *D silvarum*, collectively, are vectors of numerous viruses and *Babesia bovis*, *B caballi*, *B equi*, *B canis*, *Theileria ovis*, *Anaplasma ovis*, and the agents of tularemia and Q-fever. *Dermacentor marginatus* is found in forests, marshes, semideserts, and alpine zones from France to southwestern Siberia, Kazakh SSR, Xinjiang Uygur Autonomous Region of China, Iran, and northern Afghanistan. *Dermacentor reticulatus* ranges from Ireland and Britain to northwestern Siberia and Xinjiang, China, in meadows, floodplains, and deciduous and deciduous-conifer forests. *Dermacentor silvarum* ranges from central Siberia and northeastern China to Japan in marshes, meadows, shrubby and secondary forests, and farmlands in taiga forest areas. Some males in populations of each of these 3 species remain attached to the host during winter. Adults and immatures may overwinter on the ground. Greatest adult activity is from early spring to summer with a lower peak in fall. Larvae and nymphs are active from spring through fall. The life cycle may be completed in 1 yr or extended by one or more summer or winter diapauses, or both, to 2-4 yr.

About 12 other *Dermacentor* spp inhabit certain lowland and mountain steppe and semidesert areas of temperate Asia. Their adults are commonly taken from camels, cattle, horses, sheep, and goats. In tropical Asia, the several species of the *Dermacentor* subgenus *Indocentor* are parasites of wild pigs; they also infest larger wildlife but seldom if ever feed on livestock.

HAEMAPHYSALIS SPP

Few of the 155 species of *Haemaphysalis* parasitize livestock, but those that do are economically important in Eurasia, Africa, Australia, and New Zealand. Some haemaphysaline parasites of wild deer, antelopes, and cattle have adapted to domestic cattle and to a lesser extent to sheep and goats. Others, originally specific for various wild sheep and goats, have adapted chiefly to the domestic breeds of these animals. A few African species that co-evolved with carnivores now parasitize domestic dogs. Immatures of species that parasitize livestock generally feed on small vertebrates, but there are a few notable exceptions. All *Haemaphysalis* spp have a 3-host life cycle, and are small (unfed adults <4.5 mm long), brownish or reddish, and eyeless. Most have very short mouthparts. Different species produce tick paralysis and are vectors of the agents that cause Q-fever, tularemia, and brucellosis, and of *Theileria orientalis, T ovis, Babesia major, B motasi, B canis, Anaplasma masaeterum,* etc.

Haemaphysalis punctata is widely distributed where sheep, goats, and cattle feed in certain open forests and shrubby pastures from southwestern Asia (Iran and USSR) to much of Europe, including southern Scandinavia and Britain. Immatures infest birds, hedgehogs, rodents, and reptiles. In addition to transmitting *Anaplasma* and *Babesia* spp, different *H punctata* populations are infected by tick-borne encephalitis virus, Tribec virus, Bhanja virus, and CCHF virus.

Haemaphysalis sulcata adults parasitize livestock (chiefly sheep and goats) from northwestern India and southern USSR to Arabia, Sinai, and southern Europe. *Haemaphysalis parva (otophila)* adults parasitize these hosts from southwestern USSR and the Near East to the Mediterranean area (but not Egypt). Immature *H sulcata* are especially common on lizards, but the range of hosts of larvae and nymphs of both species is similar to that of *H punctata.*

Haemaphysalis longicornis is a parasite of deer and livestock in Japan and northeast Asia; there is a bisexual form (race) in southern areas and a parthenogenetic race in northern areas. The latter has been introduced into Australia, New Zealand, and the Pacific islands, where it preserves this unusual reproductive capacity. Immatures usually parasitize small mammals and birds but may also feed on livestock; heavy population densities may become a serious pest of deer and livestock. This tick is the chief vector of *Theileria orientalis,* and also transmits *Babesia ovata, B gibsoni,* and the agents of Q-fever, Powassan encephalitis, and Russian spring-summer encephalitis. Larval feeding causes acute dermatitis in man.

Other Eurasian haemaphysalines of livestock are *H inermis* (lowlands from northern Iran and southwestern USSR to central and southeastern Europe to Italy), *H pospelovashtromae* (mountains of southern USSR and Mongolia), *H kopetdaghicus* (Caspian Sea area, mountains of USSR, and Iran), and *H tibetensis, H xinjiangensis,* and *H moschisuga* (China).

Of the several haemaphysaline species of livestock parasites that occur chiefly in India, 3 are especially noteworthy: *H bispinosa* ranges to Pakistan, Bangladesh, Nepal, Bhutan, Sri Lanka, and Malaysia, and transmits *Babesia* spp to cattle, sheep, and dogs; *H spinigera* is the chief vector of Kyasanur Forest disease virus in man in Karnataka state, India; and *H anomala* ranges from the Nepal lowlands to Sri Lanka and the mountains of northwestern Thailand.

In temperate Asia, 18 other haemaphysalines parasitize livestock: 9 high in the Himalayas and outlying mountains, and 9 in northeastern USSR, Korea, and Japan. The yak and yak-cattle hybrid are among the livestock hosts of Himalayan haemaphysalines. Several Himalayan species appear to prefer sheep and goats.

In sub-Saharan Africa, 4 haemaphysalines infest livestock in highland forests or lowland, humid, secondary or riparian forests. These are *H parmata* (Ethiopia and Kenya, Central and West Africa, to Angola), *H aciculifer* (Ethiopia to Cameroon and Zimbabwe, introduced into South Africa), *H rugosa* (southern Sudan and Uganda to Ghana and Senegal), and *H silacea* (Zululand and eastern south Africa).

HYALOMMA SPP

Hyalomma ticks are often the most abundant tick parasites of livestock, including camels, in warm, arid, and semiarid, generally harsh lowland and middle altitude biotopes, and those with long dry seasons, from central and southwest Asia to southern Europe and southern Africa. Of the 30 known *Hyalomma* spp, ≥15 are important vectors of infectious agents to livestock and man. The 3-host life cycle predominates in this genus, but some species have either a 1- or 2-host cycle. Some 3-host species can develop in 1- or 2-host cycles, a capacity unique to this ixodid genus. Hyalommines are mostly moderately large to large ticks with long mouthparts.

In the subgenus *Hyalommasta*, immatures of the single species, *H aegyptium*, parasitize tortoises and small wildlife and livestock from Pakistan to both sides of the Mediterranean basin. Adults are specific for tortoises.

The subgenus *Hyalommina* centers in the Indian subcontinent and ranges to Somalia. Each of the 6 species has a 3-host cycle. Immatures parasitize small mammals, especially rodents. Adult host preferences among livestock reflect the wild gazelle, bovine, caprine, or ovine group with which each species co-evolved. Two species now infest chiefly cattle and the domestic buffalo: *H brevipunctata* (India and Pakistan) and *H kumari* (India, Pakistan, Afghanistan, northwestern Iran, and Tadzhik SSR). Three usually parasitize sheep and goats: *H hussaini* (India, Pakistan, Burma), *H rhipicephaloides* (Dead Sea and Red Sea areas), and *H arabica* (Yemen and Saudi Arabia). *Hyalommina punt* (Somalia and Ethiopia) feeds on antelopes, camels, cattle, sheep, and goats.

The subgenus *Hyalomma* contains 15 species of veterinary and public health importance. Three of the 15 species have 2, 3, and 4 subspecies, respectively. Chief among these is the 2-host *H anatolicum anatolicum*, which ranks high among the world's most damaging ticks and has been widely distributed by camels, cattle, and horses in steppe and semidesert environments from central Asia to Bangladesh, the Middle and Near East, Arabia, southeastern Europe, and Africa north of the equator. Immatures and adults generally infest the same kinds of hosts. Nymphs and unfed adults spend the dry and winter season in crevices in stone walls, stables, and weedy or fallow fields. When immatures infest smaller mammals, birds, or reptiles, the life cycle type is 3-host. *Hyalomma anatolicum anatolicum* transmits *Theileria annulata*, *Babesia equi*, *B caballi*, *Anaplasma marginale*, *Trypanosoma theileri*, and at least 5 arboviruses; it is a significant vector of CCHF virus to man. The numerous *H anatolicum anatolicum* immatures and adults that often parasitize livestock cause unthriftiness. Immatures of the subspecies *H anatolicum excavatum* (a 3-host parasite) infest chiefly burrowing rodents in somewhat different biotopes in the same environments as *H anatolicum anatolicum*. Adults of both subspecies may infest the same animal. Distribution of *H anatolicum excavatum* is somewhat more limited than that of *H anatolicum anatolicum*, but its winter season population densities are often greater than those of the latter. A closely related species, *H lusitanicum*, replaces *H anatolicum anatolicum* from central Italy to Portugal, Morocco, and the Canary Islands, and is associated with equine and bovine babesiosis. In addition to livestock, deer and rabbits serve as hosts.

The *Hyalomma marginatum* complex consists of 4 subspecies, each apparently invariably 2-host. Adults parasitize livestock and wild herbivores; immatures' primary hosts are birds; hares and hedgehogs are secondary hosts; and rodents are rarely, if ever, parasitized. The subspecies are: *H marginatum marginatum* (Caspian area of Iran and USSR to Portugal and northwestern Africa), *H marginatum rufipes* (south of the Sahara to South Africa, also Nile Valley and southern Arabia), *H marginatum turanicum* (Pakistan, Iran, southern USSR, Arabia, parts of northeastern Africa — introduced with sheep from Iran to Karoo), and *H marginatum isaaci* (Sri Lanka to southern Nepal, Pakistan, northern Afghanistan). *Hyalomma marginatum* subspecies are important vectors of CCHF virus and also transmit agents of livestock diseases and other viruses that infect wildlife, livestock, and man.

The *Hyalomma asiaticum* complex consists of 3 subspecies with 3-host life cycles and inhabits deserts, semideserts, and steppes from southwestern China, Mongolia, and southern USSR into the Middle East as far as Iraq. Rodents are the chief hosts of immatures; hares also may be infested. Adults parasitize livestock, particularly camels. The subspecies from east to west, *H asiaticum kozlovi*, *H asiaticum asiaticum*, and *H asiaticum caucasicum*, are of considerable veterinary and medical importance.

Three additional 3-host *Hyalomma* spp that parasitize camels (and other livestock) are *H dromedarii* (India to Africa north of the equator), *H schulzei* (eastern Iran to Arabia and northern Egypt), and *H franchinii* (Syria to Tunisia). Immatures parasitize rodents and other small mammals, birds, and reptiles; those of *H dromedarii* also infest livestock. *Hyalomma dromedarii* is of considerable veterinary and medical importance. The other 2 species have been little investigated in this respect.

Hyalomma detritum, an important vector of *Theileria annulata*, is a 3-host species; both adults and immatures parasitize livestock. Its biotopes are humid areas in steppes, deserts, and semideserts from southern China, Mongolia, and Nepal lowlands to southern Europe and northern Africa. *Hyalomma impeltatum* ranges from Iran and Arabia to northern Tanzania and Chad. Adults parasitize livestock; immatures feed on rodents and other small mammals, birds, and reptiles.

Hyalomma scupense, a 1-host parasite of cattle and horses in southwestern USSR and southeastern Europe, is unusual in that it overwinters on the host, which often suffers greatly from the long feeding period of numerous larvae (late autumn), nymphs (winter), and adults (spring). It is a vector of *Theileria annulata* and *Babesia equi*.

In addition to the several species already mentioned, the African savannas harbor 5 other *Hyalomma* spp of livestock and wildlife: *H truncatum* (southeastern Egypt to southern Africa), *H albiparmatum* (southern Kenya, northern Tanzania), *H erythraeum* (eastern Somalia and Ethiopia, and Yemen), *H impressum* (western Sudan and West Africa), and *H nitidum* (Central African Republic and West Africa). Immatures of these 3-host species generally infest small mammals, less often birds and reptiles. Each species is economically important. For instance, *H truncatum*, which causes bovine sweating sickness and lameness and also human and ovine tick paralysis, is a vector of CCHF virus, *Coxiella burnetii* (Q-fever), and *Rickettsia conori* (tick typhus).

IXODES SPP

This, the largest genus of the family Ixodidae, contains ~220 species and is highly specialized both structurally and biologically. So far as is known, all *Ixodes* spp have a 3-host life cycle. Almost all inhabit temperate or tropical forest zones or wooded or shrubby grasslands; fewer are adapted to humid areas in semideserts or to arctic or subantarctic nesting colonies of marine birds. Hosts are a wide variety of birds and mammals and a few reptiles. Most species parasitize burrowing hosts or those that return regularly to caves, dens, or terrestrial or arboreal nesting colonies. The few *Ixodes* spp that parasitize wandering artiodactyls or perissodactyls are exceptionally adaptable; they also parasitize livestock and are important pests or vectors of agents that infect livestock and man.

The *I ricinus* group of Eurasia, northwestern Africa, and North and South America is especially important. *Ixodes ricinus*, the so-called sheep tick and prototype of this group, inhabits relatively humid, cool, shrubby and wooded pastures, gardens, windbreaks, floodplains, and forest through much of Europe to the Caspian Sea and northern Iran, and also northwestern Africa. Its life cycle is 2-4 yr, depending on environmental temperature. (In drier, warmer, eastern Mediterranean biotopes, *I ricinus* is replaced by *I gibbosus*, which completes its life cycle in 1 yr.) *Ixodes ricinus* larvae feed on small reptiles, birds, and mammals; nymphs feed on small and medium-sized vertebrates; and adults feed chiefly on herbivores and livestock. All stages, especially nymphs and adults, parasitize man. Male *I ricinus* take little or no food but mate on the host while the female feeds. Adult activity peaks in spring; in some populations, there is a lower peak of adult activity in the fall. Chief among the numerous arboviral diseases transmitted by *I ricinus* are louping ill, tick-borne encephalitis, and CCHF. Other agents transmitted to livestock are *Coxiella burnetii, Anaplasma marginale, Babesia divergens*, and *Ehrlichia phagocytophila*.

Ixodes persulcatus, the taiga tick, is closely related to *I ricinus* and has similar host preferences; it ranges from the central and eastern mountains of Europe through the lowland forests from the Baltic Sea and Karelia eastward through the Siberian taiga to the Seas of Japan and Okhotsk and the northern islands of Japan. The life cycle is completed in 2-4 yr. It is the chief vector of Russian spring-summer encephalitis virus, and transmits *Babesia* spp and the agents of ovine anaplasmosis, plague, and tularemia.

Other Asian representatives of the *I ricinus* group are *I sinensis* of China; *I kashmiricus* of mountainous northern India, Pakistan, and Kirghiz SSR; *I pavlovskyi* of southern RSFSR; and *I kazakstani* of mountain taiga and deciduous forest in Kazakh SSR, Kirghiz SSR, and Turkmen SSR.

Ixodes dammini (also a member of the *I ricinus* group) is a vector of *Borrelia burgdorferi*, the agent of Lyme disease in northeastern and north central USA and southern Canada; it is also a vector of *Babesia microti*, the agent of human babesiosis in coastal areas from New York to Massachusetts. The chief hosts of adult *I dammini* are deer; livestock seldom graze in the wooded zones inhabited by this tick. Adults of the closely related *I scapularis* sometimes parasitize livestock in southern USA; those of *I pacificus* do so from Baja California to British Columbia and in inland pockets of Idaho, Nevada, and Oregon. *Ixodes pacificus* transmits the agents of Lyme disease, tularemia, and a rickettsia of the Rocky Mountain spotted fever group; its bite causes slowly healing ulcers. A related species, *I affinis*, ranges from South Carolina and Florida to Argentina. It is recorded chiefly from wildlife and has not been investigated for vectorial capacity.

In Africa, only 4 *Ixodes* spp have adapted to livestock. Chief among these is the South African paralysis tick, *I rubicundus*, of humid hill and mountain karoo vegetation in South Africa. Its salivary toxins cause a flaccid tetraplegia in livestock, man, dogs, and jackals. Immatures parasitize the rock hare, other hares, and elephant shrews. Other parasites of livestock in African highlands are *I drakenbergensis* (Natal), *I lewisi* (Kenya), and *I cavipalpus* (southern Sudan to Zimbabwe and Angola).

MARGAROPUS SPP

Closely related to *Boophilus*, the 3 highly specialized beady-legged, 1-host *Margaropus* spp are restricted to limited areas of Africa. *Margaropus reidi* and *M wileyi* are recorded from giraffe in the Sudan and in Kenya and Tanzania, respectively. *Margaropus wileyi* is also known to parasitize the zebra and gnu. *Margaropus winthemi*, a winter-feeding parasite of the zebra, horse, and less often other livestock and antelopes, is confined to mountains of South Africa and may contribute to loss of condition during winter.

NOSOMMA SP

Adults of the single species in this genus, *N monstrosum*, particularly parasitize wild and domestic buffalo, also man, livestock, and wildlife, through much of India, Nepal lowlands, Bangladesh, Thailand, and Laos. Immatures parasitize chiefly murid rodents.

RHIPICEPHALUS SPP

Rhipicephalid species occur in Eurasia and northern Africa (15 species) and in sub-Saharan Africa (~55 species). Adults of most species parasitize wild and domestic artiodactyls, perissodactyls, or carnivores. Immatures feed mostly on smaller mammals; however, of those that parasitize rodents or hyraxes, and of those that parasitize artiodactyls, a few feed on the same host as the adults. The rhipicephalid life cycle is typically 3-host, but in the Mediterranean climatic zone (long, warm summer with low rainfall), *R bursa* has a 2-host cycle. In sub-Saharan Africa with long dry seasons, *R evertsi* and *R glabroscutatum* also have 2-host cycles.

A number of abundant, economically important African *Rhipicephalus* spp have long been particularly difficult to identify or incorrectly identified. The taxonomy of these groups is presently being revised. When this revision is completed, numerous familiar species concepts will change. "Problem areas" are indicated below.

Tropical Asia is the home of 5 *Rhipicephalus* spp; adults of 2 species parasitize domestic animals. *Rhipicephalus haemaphysaloides* infests all types of livestock, and wild antelopes, deer, carnivores, and hares in continental southeast Asia (and Taiwan and the Philippines) westward to India, Sri Lanka, Nepal, Pakistan, and western Afghanistan. *Rhipicephalus pilans* infests livestock and wildlife in Indonesia and Borneo. Immatures of both species feed chiefly on rodents, also on shrews, hares, and smaller carnivores.

From central Europe to Kazakh SSR, *R rossicus*, *R schulzei*, and *R pumilio* are of medical and veterinary importance. In southwestern Europe, *R pusillus* infests dogs as well as the European rabbit, fox, and wild pig. *Rhipicephalus turanicus*, as presently recognized, ranges from China, southern USSR, and India into southern Europe, and Africa as far south as South Africa. A member of the taxonomically difficult *R sanguineus* group, "*R turanicus*" and its various populations, which may represent separate species, requires further studies of its capabilities as a vector.

An easily recognized, 2-host species, *R bursa*, ranges from the western Mediterranean area of Europe to Iran and Kazakh SSR. Adults and immatures both parasitize livestock, hares, deer, wild sheep and goats, and man. It causes ovine paralysis and transmits CCHF and other viruses to man, and *Babesia*, *Theileria*, and *Anaplasma* spp to livestock.

The best known African rhipicephalid, *R sanguineus*, the kennel tick or brown dog tick, has traveled worldwide with domestic dogs. It is now established in buildings as far north as Canada and Scandinavia and as far south as Australia. In Africa, the Near East, and parts of southern Europe, adults parasitize wild and domestic carnivores, sheep, goats, camels, other livestock, and various wild mammals, especially hares and hedgehogs. Immatures in nature in this area feed on small mammals. However, in urban situations everywhere, dogs are virtually the only hosts of immatures and adults. Man is rarely attacked. Strains of adult *R sanguineus* that feed on cattle are recorded in parts of Mexico and in Tahiti. This tick is active throughout the year in the tropics and subtropics but only from spring to fall in temperate zones. Newly active adults and nymphs are frequently observed climbing walls from floor-level cracks. *Rhipicephalus sanguineus* is a vector of *Babesia canis*, *Ehrlichia canis*, *Rickettsia rhipicephali*, *R conori*, CCHF, and Thogoto virus. In southcentral USA, *R sanguineus* is associated with scattered foci of *Leishmania mexicana*. Implications of this tick as a vector of other infectious agents require confirmation. Certain American populations have become resistant to insecticides. The hymenopteran (chalcid) parasite of ticks, *Hunterellus hookeri*, frequently infests nymphal *R sanguineus* in East Africa.

Rhipicephalus appendiculatus, the brown ear tick, is a major pest in cool, shaded, woody and shrubby savannas with ≥24 in. (600 mm) annual rainfall from sea level to 7400 ft (2300 m) from southern Sudan and eastern Zaire to Kenya and South Africa. Adults and immatures feed in the ears of cattle, other livestock, and antelopes, but also on other areas when the infestation is massive. Immatures may infest small antelopes and carnivores, and occasionally rodents. Seasonal activity is closely associated with temperature and rain periods. *Rhipicephalus appendiculatus* is the major vector of the *Theileria parva* group of diseases (East Coast fever, Corridor disease, Zimbabwe malignant theileriosis) and Nairobi sheep disease virus, and is also a vector of *Theileria taurotragi, Ehrlichia bovis, Rickettsia conori*, and Thogoto virus. Heavy infestations on susceptible *Bos taurus* cattle cause a sometimes fatal toxemia, loss of resistance to various infections, and severe damage to the host's ears.

The closely related *R zambeziensis*, with similar host preferences, occurs in drier lowland savannas in Tanzania, Zimbabwe, Zambia, Botswana, and Transvaal; it also is a vector of East Coast fever. Other species closely related to *R appendiculatus* include *R nitens* in the Cape Province of South Africa and *R duttoni* in Angola and Zaire.

The ivory-ornamented *R pulchellus*, a parasite of the zebra, also infests livestock and game animals east of the Rift Valley from southern Ethiopia to Somalia and northeastern Tanzania. Its habitats are savannas with grass, bushes, and scattered trees between 1000 and 4200 ft (300 and 1300 m) altitude where the annual rainfall is 10-24 in. (250-600 mm). Adults and immatures generally infest the same host; however, immatures also feed on hares, and larvae ("seed ticks") are notoriously annoying pests of man. *Rhipicephalus pulchellus* feeds in hosts' ears and on the lower abdomen, chiefly during wet seasons. This tick is a vector of *Babesia equi* (among zebra), *Theileria* spp, *Trypanosoma theileri, Rickettsia conori*, several Bunyaviridae (CCHF, Nairobi sheep disease, Kajiado, Kismayo, and Dugbe viruses), and Barur virus.

The 2-host African rhipicephalids are *R evertsi* subspecies and *R glabroscutatum*. *Rhipicephalus evertsi evertsi*, a large, beady-eyed, red-legged tick, a parasite of the East African zebra, parasitizes all types of herbivorous wildlife and livestock (but seldom pigs). Immatures and adults infest the same hosts; immatures are also recorded from hares. It ranges from South Africa through eastern Africa east of the Nile to southern Sudan, and is established in the mountains of Yemen. Scattered foci, introduced by domestic animals, occur west of the Nile. Immatures feed in the ear canal; adults mostly around the anus and under the tail, also in the axillae and groin and on the sternum. Large numbers on a single host are common on Equidae and are difficult to control because of their concentrations in difficult-to-reach feeding sites. The life cycle continues through the year but slackens in cooler seasons. *Rhipicephalus evertsi evertsi* transmit *Babesia equi, Theileria parva* (secondary vector), *Borrelia theileri, Rickettsia conori*, and Kerai, Wad Medani, and Thogoto viruses. The banded-legged (*Hyalomma*-like) western subspecies, *Rhipicephalus evertsi mimeticus*, found from western Botswana to Namibia, Angola, and Zaire, is like the nominate subspecies in host preferences, feeding sites, and life cycle.

The tiny *R glabroscutatum* has become a common pest of sheep, goats, and other livestock in the arid, small-shrub savanna of southeastern Cape Province, South Africa. The kudu and other small antelopes are also infested. The few records of immatures are from rodents.

The *R pravus* group, presently under taxonomic study, consists of ≥4 species of which the adults feed on livestock and herbivorous wildlife (including hares); immatures feed on elephant shrews (insectivores), hares, and other small mammals. *Rhipicephalus pravus*, a brown, convex-eyed tick, occurs in shrubby and wooded savannas in east Africa. It is infected by Kadam virus. The closely related *R occulatus*, a parasite of hares, and another related yet unnamed parasite of livestock occur in southern Africa.

The difficult-to-classify *R punctatus* group of parasites of livestock and wild artiodactyls consists of *R punctatus* (Angola, Mozambique, Tanzania), *R kochi* (*neavi*) (Botswana to Kenya and Zaire), and an as yet unnamed species from Zimbabwe and South Africa.

The *R capensis* group is also under study. Originally parasites of the Cape buffalo, these species now parasitize livestock and wildlife in Namibia and South Africa (*R capensis*, including the possibly synonymous *R gertrudae*), East Africa (*R compositus* and *R longus*), and West Africa to southwestern Sudan (*R cliffordi*).

Above 5900 ft (1800 m) altitude in East African forest and shrub zones, *R hurti* and *R jeanelli* infest livestock, and Cape buffalo and other large game animals.

Rhipicephalus hurti also inhabits mountains in Zaire. Both species feed chiefly in the hosts' ears; *R jeanelli* also feeds in the tail brush.

Rhipicephalus simus, the prototype of the *R simus* group and long considered to be a well-established species, is now divided into several species. In the new classification, *R simus sensu stricto* occurs through central and southern Africa, roughly south of latitude 8°S. In eastern and northern Africa, *R simus* is replaced by a less punctate species, *R praetextatus*, which ranges from central Tanzania to Egypt. Adults of both species parasitize livestock, dogs, wild carnivores, large and medium-sized game animals, and man. Occurrence and densities on livestock are inexplicably erratic. Immature stages feed on the common burrowing rodents in savannas. Both species cause tick paralysis of man and transmit *Rickettsia conori* and *Coxiella burnetii*. In Kenya, *R praetextatus* is a vector of Thogoto virus and may be a secondary vector of Nairobi sheep disease virus. West of the Nile, these species are replaced by *R senegalensis* and *R muhsamae*.

Much literature regarding *R tricuspis* (Tanzania to South Africa) and *R lunulatus* (West Africa to Ethiopia and Tanzania) has been incorrect. The chief feeding site of both on livestock and wildlife is the tailbrush, but other parts of the host are also feeding sites.

Rhipicephalus sanguineus and *R turanicus* of the *R sanguineus* group have been mentioned above. Related species are *R camicasi* and *R bergeoni* of northeastern Africa, *R guilhoni* and *R moucheti* of West Africa, and 2 widely distributed "forms" of *R sulcatus*, which are under study.

Two quite distinctive species often confused with *R appendiculatus* are *R supertritus* (Natal to southern Sudan) and *R muhlensi* (Kenya and southern Sudan to Central Africa). Adults of both species parasitize cattle, the Cape buffalo, antelopes, and big game animals; *R supertritus* also is found on carnivores.

IMPORTANT ARGASIDAE

ARGAS SPP

Most of the 56 known *Argas* spp are specific for birds or bats; a few parasitize wild terrestrial mammals or the Galapagos giant tortoise. The species of importance in transmitting *Aegyptianella pullorum* and *Borrelia anserina* to poultry are *A persicus* (many tropical and subtropical areas of the world), *A arboreus* (much of Africa, including Egypt), *A africolumbae* (tropical Africa), *A walkerae* (southern Africa), and *A miniatus* (South and Central America). Other species that infest poultry appear to transmit both *A pullorum* and *B anserina*. Tick paralysis is caused by feeding *A persicus*, *A arboreus*, *A walkerae*, *A miniatus*, *A radiatus*, and *A sanchezi* (USA). These and other *Argas* spp can cause great irritation when feeding on man.

ORNITHODOROS SPP

Few of the ~100 *Ornithodoros* spp have contact with livestock. Most inhabit protected niches in burrows, caves, dens, cliffsides, and bird colonies. Among those that parasitize livestock, *O savignyi* and *O coriaceus* are exceptional because they have eyes, and because they rest just below or above ground level under the shade of trees where livestock and game animals rest and sleep. *Ornithodoros savignyi*, the sand tampan, lives in semiarid areas from Namibia to India and Sri Lanka and is often tremendously abundant. Man and tethered livestock suffer severe irritation and toxicosis from sand tampan bites, and paralysis and death of animals are recorded. *Ornithodoros coriaceus*, the "pajaroello" of hillside scrub oak habitats from northern California to Chiapias, Mexico, occupies deer beds under trees and is famous for irritating deer, cattle, and man. Epizootic bovine abortion appears to be transmitted only by *O coriaceus*. *Ornithodoros guerneyi* shelters in tree-shaded soil in arid zones of Australia where kangaroos and man rest; livestock are rare or absent in these habitats.

Among the numerous *Ornithodoros* that inhabit burrows, several species are either naturally infected with African swine fever (ASF) virus in Africa, or have the laboratory-confirmed capacity to harbor and transmit the agent in Europe and the

Americas. The natural reservoir and vector of ASF virus is *O porcinus porcinus (O moubata porcinus)*, which is abundant in burrows of tropical African pigs and also of antbears and porcupines. Domestic pig populations in the vicinity of infected wild pigs often have been decimated by ASF. Wild and domestic pigs are not involved in the epidemiology of *Borrelia duttoni*, the agent of human African relapsing fever, which is transmitted by *O moubata*. ASF virus has been transported in infected meat to Spain where *O marocanus (erraticus)*, an inhabitant of rodent burrows and pig sties, is an efficient vector. *Ornithodoros marocanus* is also a reservoir and vector of *Borrelia hispanica*, the agent of Spanish-northwest African human relapsing fever. ASF has likewise been introduced in Brazil, Haiti, the Dominican Republic, and Cuba. The American *O puertoricensis, O turicata, O talaje, O dugesi*, and *O coriaceus* are potential vectors of ASF virus.

Ornithodoros tholozani (papillipes, also *crossi*) infests burrows, caves, stables, stone and clay fences, and human habitations in ancient and newly developed towns and cities in semidesert, steppe, and long-dry-season environments from China, southern USSR, northwestern India, and Afghanistan to Greece, northeastern Libya, and eastern Mediterranean islands. Numerous rodents, hedgehogs, porcupines, and domestic animals support *O tholozani* populations. Man suffers from severe, sometimes fatal, Persian relapsing fever when bitten by *O tholozani* infected with *Borrelia persicus*.

Ornithodoros lahorensis, originally a parasite of wild sheep resting in the lee of cliffsides, is an important pest of stabled livestock in lowlands and mountains of Tibet, Kashmir, and southern USSR to Saudi Arabia and Turkey, Greece, Bulgaria, and Yugoslavia. The 2-host life cycle and long wintertime attachment of *O lahorensis* is biologically remarkable. It is deleterious to livestock held for much of the winter in heavily infested stables; it may cause paralysis, anemia, and toxicosis, and it transmits the agents of piroplasmosis, brucellosis, Q-fever, and tularemia. In Iran and Turkmen SSR, the seldom studied *O canestrini* also parasitizes livestock in caves and stables.

Ornithodoros turicata parasitizes burrow-, crevice-, and cave-dwelling rodents, owls, snakes, and tortoises, and also domestic pigs and other livestock, in southern USA and Mexico. Contrary to most *Ornithodoros* feeding patterns, immature *O turicata* engorge in ≤30 min, but adults may attach for up to 2 days. *Ornithodoros turicata* has been associated with diseases of pigs, and serious toxic reactions and secondary infections can result when man is bitten.

Ornithodoros furucosus parasitizes man and livestock in houses and stables in northwestern South America. Other South American pests of livestock and man, probably originally parasites of the peccary, are *O braziliensis* and *O rostratus*.

OTOBIUS SPP

Otobius megnini, which is exceedingly specialized biologically and structurally, infests the ear canals of the pronghorn antelope, mountain sheep, and Virginia and mule deer in low rainfall biotopes of western USA and in Mexico and western Canada. Cattle, horses, goats, sheep, dogs, and man are similarly infested. This well-concealed parasite has been transported with livestock to western South America, Galapagos, Cuba, Hawaii, India, Madagascar, and southeastern Africa. Notably, adults have nonfunctional mouthparts and remain nonfeeding on the ground but may survive for almost 2 yr. Females deposit up to 1500 eggs in a 2-wk period. Larvae and 2 nymphal instars feed for 2-4 mo, mostly in winter and spring. There can be ≥2 generations annually. Man and other animals may suffer severe irritation from ear canal infestations, and heavily infested livestock lose condition during winter. Tick paralysis of hosts and secondary infections by larval screwworms are reported. *Otobius megnini* is infected by the agents of Q-fever, tularemia, Colorado tick fever, and Rocky Mountain spotted fever. The second *Otobius* sp, *O lagophilus*, feeds on the heads of jack rabbits (hares) and rabbits in western USA.

TICK CONTROL

Tick control is practiced in a wide variety of circumstances involving different tick and host species. The main reasons for tick control are to protect hosts from irritation and production losses, formation of lesions that can become secondarily infested, damage to hides and udders, toxicosis, paralysis, and of greatest importance, infection with a wide variety of disease agents. Control also prevents the spread of tick species and the diseases they transmit to unaffected areas, regions, or continents.

Cultural and Biological Control: These measures can be directed against both the free-living and parasitic stages of ticks. The free-living stages of most tick species, both ixodid and argasid, have specific requirements in terms of microclimate and are restricted to particular microhabitats within the ecosystems inhabited by their hosts. Destruction of these microhabitats reduces the abundance of ticks. Alteration of the environment by removal of certain types of vegetation has been used in the control of *Amblyomma americanum* in recreational areas in southeastern USA and in the control of *Ixodes rubicundus* in South Africa. Control of argasid ticks such as *Argas persicus* and *A walkerae* in poultry can be achieved by eliminating cracks in walls and perches, which provide shelter to the free-living stages.

The abundance of tick species may also be reduced by removal of alternate hosts or hosts of a particular stage of the life cycle. This approach has occasionally been advocated for the control of 3-host ixodid ticks such as *Rhipicephalus appendiculatus, Amblyomma hebraeum* and *Ixodes rubicundus* in Africa, and *Hyalomma* spp in southeastern Europe and Asia.

Rotation of pastures or pasture spelling has been used in the control of the 1-host ixodid tick *Boophilus microplus* in Australia. The method could also be applied to other 1-host ticks, in which the duration of the spelling period is determined by the relatively short life span of the free-living larvae. However, it has minimal application to multihost ixodid ticks or argasid ticks because of the long survival periods of the unfed nymphs and adults.

Predators, including birds, rodents, shrews, ants, and spiders, in some areas, play a role in reducing the numbers of free-living ticks. In the New World, fire ants (*Pheidole megacephala*) are noteworthy tick predators. Engorged ticks may also become parasitized by the larvae of some wasps (Hymenoptera), but these have not significantly reduced tick populations.

It is well established that Zebu (*Bos indicus*) and Sanga (a *Bos taurus, B indicus* crossbreed) cattle, the indigenous breeds of Asia and Africa, usually become very resistant to ixodid ticks following initial exposure. In contrast, European (*B taurus*) breeds usually remain fairly susceptible. The tick resistance of Zebu breeds and their crosses is being increasingly exploited as a means of control of the parasitic stages. The introduction of Zebu cattle to Australia has revolutionized the control of *B microplus* on that continent. Use of resistant cattle as a means of tick control is also becoming important in Africa and the Americas. In Africa, infestations of ixodid ticks on livestock and wild ungulates may also be reduced by oxpeckers (*Buphagus* spp), which are birds that feed on attached ticks.

Chemical Control: (*See also* EXTERNAL PARASITICIDES, p 1497.) Control of ticks with acaricides may be directed against the free-living stages in the environment or against the parasitic stages on hosts. Control of ixodid ticks by acaricide treatment of vegetation has been done in specific sites (eg, along trails) in recreational areas in the USA and elsewhere, to reduce the risk of tick attachment to people. This method has not been recommended for wider use, because of environmental pollution and the cost of treatment of large areas. Dog kennels, barns, and human dwellings may also require periodic treatment with acaricides to control the free-living stages of ixodid ticks such as the kennel tick, *Rhipicephalus sanguineus*.

The free-living stages of argasid ticks, which infest specific foci such as fowl runs, pigeon lofts, pig sties, and human dwellings, are more frequently and more effectively treated with acaricides.

Treatment of hosts with acaricides to kill attached larvae, nymphs, and adults of ixodid ticks and larvae of argasid ticks has been the most widely used control method. In the first half of the century, the main acaricide was arsenic trioxide. Subsequently, organochlorines, organophosphates, carbamates, amidines, and pyrethroids have been used in different parts of the world. The introduction of new compounds has been necessary because of the development of resistance in tick populations.

Acaricides are most commonly applied to livestock by use of dips or sprays, with dips being considered the more effective. In recent years, several other means of acaricide application have been developed, including slow release of systemics from implants and boluses, slow release of conventional acaricides from impregnated ear tags, "pour-ons" which are applied on the back and spread rapidly over the entire body surface, and "spot-ons" which are similar but have less capacity to spread. On fowl, acaricides are usually applied as dusts; on cats as dusts or washes; and on dogs as dusts, washes, or dips.

Vaccines: A recent advance of potentially great importance has been the production, using biotechnology, of an effective vaccine against *B microplus*. The immunizing agent is a "concealed" tick antigen, not normally encountered by the host. The immune mechanism that it stimulates is different from that stimulated by exposure to ticks (ie, tick feeding). The antigen was derived from a crude extract of partially engorged adult female ticks. It stimulates the production of an antibody that damages tick gut cells and kills the ticks or drastically reduces their reproductive potential. It is likely that similar vaccines will be developed in the future against other ixodid ticks of major economic importance. These could render most other forms of tick control obsolete and alter our approaches to the control of ticks and tick-borne diseases.

Control Strategies: Initially the main uses of acaricides were tick eradication, prevention of spread of ticks and tick-borne diseases (quarantine), and eradication and control of tick-borne diseases. The eradication programs were successful in some ecologically marginal subtropical areas, such as southern USA and central Argentina where *Boophilus* spp and babesiosis were eradicated, and southern Africa where East Coast fever (caused by *Theileria parva parva*) was eradicated. The programs were less successful in the ecologically more favorable tropical areas of northeastern Australia, Central America, the Caribbean Islands, and East Africa.

In the areas where eradication was not achieved, the costs of maintaining intensive tick control programs have become prohibitive. For this reason, integrated biological and chemical control strategies are being adopted. The design of these more cost-effective strategies has been facilitated by our increasing knowledge of the ecology and host-relationships of ticks, the effects of ticks *per se* on the productivity of livestock, the epidemiology of tick-borne diseases, and the control of these diseases by immunological methods. Tick population models and models of the epidemiology of tick-borne diseases are being used to simulate control strategies as a means of identifying the best strategies for use in different ecological and socioeconomic situations.

Strict quarantine measures to prevent reintroductions are enforced in countries from which ticks and tick-borne diseases have been eradicated. Climate-matching models, geographic information systems, and expert systems (models based on expert knowledge and artificial intelligence) are being used to identify unaffected areas in which tick pests could become established if introduced.

TUMORS OF THE SKIN AND SOFT TISSUES

INTRODUCTION

Cutaneous tumors are the most frequently diagnosed neoplastic disorders in domestic animals, in part because they can be identified easily and in part due to the constant exposure of the skin to the external environment. Chemical carcinogens, ionizing radiation, and viruses all have been implicated, but hormonal and genetic factors may also play a role in development of cutaneous neoplasms.

The skin is a complex structure composed of various epithelial (epidermis, adnexa), mesenchymal (fibrous connective tissues, blood vessels, adipose tissue), and neural and neuroectodermal tissues (peripheral nerve, Merkel cells, melanocytes), all with the potential of developing distinctive tumors. Because of the diversity of cutaneous tumors, their classification is difficult and, for many, there is controversy as to the cell of origin. There is also controversy as to what criteria should be used to establish whether a lesion that arises in the skin or soft tissues is or is not a neoplasm, and if so, whether it is benign or malignant. To avoid confusion, the following terms are used in this discussion: 1) A **nevus** (hamartoma) is a localized developmental defect in the skin that may or may not be apparent at birth. Nevi may arise from one or more cutaneous structures, eg, a sebaceous nevus refers to a localized developmental defect in skin, which involves the sebaceous glands. The term nevus is not applied to benign melanocytic lesions in veterinary medicine, although it is used to define such lesions in man. 2) A **benign neoplasm** is localized, noninfiltrative, and easily excisable. 3) A **neoplasm of intermediate malignancy** is locally infiltrative and often requires radical surgery. These recur frequently but seldom, if ever, metastasize. (Such a category is essential because many are neither obviously benign nor obviously malignant.) 4) A **malignant neoplasm** is infiltrative and has considerable metastatic potential.

Although cutaneous neoplasms characteristically are nodular or papular, they also can occur as localized or generalized alopecic plaques, erythematous and pigmented patches and plaques, wheals, or nonhealing ulcers. Because of this, distinguishing an inflammatory from a neoplastic disease is difficult based solely on clinical features; distinguishing a benign from a malignant tumor is even more subjective, as malignancies (especially early in their development) may palpate as discrete, encapsulated masses.

To establish a definitive diagnosis, histopathology is generally required. Cytologic evaluation can also be useful and, for some types (eg, mast cell tumors), can rival or even surpass the value of histopathologic examination.

Therapy depends largely on the type of tumor, its location and size, and signalment of the animal. For benign neoplasms that are associated with neither ulceration nor clinical dysfunction, no therapy may be the most prudent option, especially in aged dogs. For more aggressive neoplastic diseases or benign tumors that are cosmetically unpleasant or inhibit normal function, there are several therapeutic options. For most, surgery provides the best chance of cure at least cost, and often with the fewest side effects. Complete excision is best. Although a lumpectomy is adequate for benign lesions, if a malignancy is suspected, the lesion should be removed with wide surgical margins. For tumors that cannot be completely excised, partial removal or debulking may be done. Debulking may prolong the life of the animal as well as increase the effectiveness of radiation or chemotherapy. Cryosurgery is also an option; although most effective for benign, superficial lesions, malignant cutaneous neoplasms can be so treated. Radiation therapy is of most value for infiltrative neoplasms that are not surgically resectable, or when surgical intervention would cause unacceptable physical impairment. Chemotherapy may be used either as a primary method for malignant neoplasms or as an adjunct to surgical or radiotherapy. In the skin, it is most commonly used to treat round cell tumors (lymphosarcomas, mast cell tumors, transmissible venereal tumors, etc) or solid tumors that cannot be excised completely. Although generally palliative, long remissions may sometimes be obtained. Other forms of therapy include hyperthermia, laser therapy, and phototherapy.

EPIDERMAL AND HAIR FOLLICLE TUMORS

BENIGN, NON-VIRUS-ASSOCIATED PAPILLOMATOUS LESIONS

For viral warts, the most common lesions of the skin, *see* PAPILLOMATOSIS, p 854. However, benign, proliferative lesions not associated with papillomavirus infection can display the same morphology.

Epidermal nevi are rare proliferations that have been identified only in dogs, most often in the young. Grossly, they generally appear as pigmented, hyperkeratotic papules, plaques, or patches, often in a vague linear pattern. Although benign, their appearance is unpleasant, and the extensive hyperkeratosis is prone to secondary bacterial infection. Localized lesions can be excised; larger ones may be inoperable and controllable only by use of topical keratolytic shampoos and emollients.

Congenital papillomas of foals are rare, and probably a developmental defect rather than a result of papillomavirus infection. They occur anywhere on the body but most commonly on the head. Thoroughbreds may be predisposed. Present at birth, the lesions (often several centimeters in diameter) are hairless, pedunculated, and exophytic with a papillated surface reminiscent of a cauliflower. They are benign and excision is curative.

Warty dyskeratomas are rare, benign neoplasms of dogs with features that suggest hair follicle derivation. They appear grossly as verrucous papules with a keratotic umbilicated center. Excision is curative.

BASAL CELL TUMORS
(Basal cell epitheliomas, Basaliomas, Basal cell carcinomas)

Generally benign cutaneous tumors that are common in dogs and cats, less so in horses. It is not known if they arise from the epidermis, the hair matrix region, or both. In dogs and cats, some basal tumors are continuous with the epidermis; however, most are devoid of epidermal attachments. In dogs, a pattern reminiscent of a trichoblastoma (a hair matrix tumor in man) is common. Solar injury has not been proved as a cause of basal cell tumors in domestic animals. However, actinic damage to the skin of dogs may produce focal zones of basal cell proliferation originating in the epidermis.

Basal cell tumors are most common in middle-aged and older animals. In dogs, they are most common on the head, neck, and shoulders. Cocker Spaniels and Poodles appear to be predisposed. In cats, there is no site predilection, and the breeds most at risk appear to be domestic long hair, Angora, Siamese, and Himalayan. The tumors generally appear as firm, solitary, encapsulated, often hairless or ulcerated nodules that may be pedunculated, and vary in size from <1 cm to >10 cm in diameter. In cats, they are often cystic and variants may be multicentric. In cats and dogs, these lesions may often be pigmented. They also may have defined evidence of differentiation into sebaceous glands, apocrine glands, or hair follicles. They are benign, slowly expansive neoplasms, and may be associated with extensive ulceration and secondary inflammation. Complete excision is curative. Multicentric basal cell tumors of cats occasionally recur.

INTRACUTANEOUS CORNIFYING EPITHELIOMAS
(Keratoacanthoma or, incorrectly, Squamous papilloma)

Benign neoplasms of the dog and possibly the cat. As with human keratoacanthomas, these lesions most likely arise from the hair follicle and not from the interfollicular epidermis. They are most common on the back, neck, thorax, and shoulders in middle-aged to older dogs, more often in males than females. Norwegian Elkhound and Keeshond dogs are most predisposed; however, German Shepherd Dogs, Old English Sheepdogs, and Collies appear at risk for developing a generalized form of the disease. The lesions may be solitary or multiple, sometimes of a large number. Most commonly, these are umbilicated, exophytic and endophytic papules or nodules with vaguely papillated margins surrounding a central keratin plug, and can also involve the deeper dermis with no palpable epidermal involvement. This latter variant is clinically indistinguishable from a keratinized cyst. As they are benign, treatment is optional provided a definitive diagnosis has been established and there is no self trauma, ulceration, or secondary infection. Excision is curative; however, dogs that develop one may develop others over time. There is no evidence that chemotherapy or immunotherapy is of value in treating fully developed lesions or in preventing their recurrence.

SQUAMOUS CELL CARCINOMAS
(Epidermoid carcinomas)

Thought to arise from either the epidermis or the epithelium of the outer root sheath of the hair follicle, these have been recognized in all domestic animals but are uncommon in pigs. Forms have been associated with prolonged exposure to sunlight. Although widely recognized in man, the role of papillomaviruses in inducing squamous cell carcinomas in domestic animals remains poorly understood. Only squamous cell carcinomas of non-mucous membranes are addressed below.

In dogs, these are the most frequent carcinoma of the cutis, usually found on the distal extremities, the head, neck, shoulder regions, or the ventral abdomen. They are most common in Scottish Terriers, Pekingese, Boxers, Poodles, and Norwegian Elkhounds. In addition, some black-coated breeds such as Labrador Retrievers, Standard Poodles, and Schnauzers may infrequently develop subungual squamous cell carcinomas on multiple extremities. Incidence tends to increase with age. In dogs, the etiology of most remains undefined; some, which develop on the ventral abdominal, preputial, scrotal, and inguinal skin in white-skinned, short-coated breeds such as Dalmatians, Pit Bull Terriers, and Beagles, are induced by prolonged solar injury. These develop in a ventral location because: 1) the poorly haired skin offers minimal shielding from ultraviolet radiation, 2) many animals sun themselves lying on their backs, and perhaps, 3) solar radiation may reflect from the ground upward. Before a carcinoma develops, animals acquire focal zones of lichenification, hyperkeratosis, and erythema known as solar keratosis (solar dermatosis, actinic keratosis, senile keratosis).

In cats, cutaneous squamous cell carcinomas most commonly develop in conjunction with chronic solar injury, generally on the pinnae and/or eyelids, areas in which the coat and skin are white. As in dogs, a solar keratosis often precedes development of a malignant tumor. Those not caused by sun exposure most commonly develop on the digits.

In horses, most of these occur in the genital and ocular regions; they are rare in skin that is not adjacent to mucous membranes. Genital squamous cell carcinomas are more common in males than in females. Those that arise in the eyelids are most common in horses with white periocular regions and are assumed to be induced by solar injury.

In cattle, they are most common in breeds with white hair and poorly pigmented skin around the mucous membranes, usually at the mucocutaneous junctions, particularly the periocular and vulvar regions. In India, squamous cell carcinomas of the horn core are often found in aged bullocks. The most common cause is actinic injury. Solar keratoses often precede development of an invasive tumor; genetic factors, immunodeficiency, and viruses also have been suggested as playing a role.

In sheep, squamous cell carcinomas are of economic significance in some parts of the world; in a study in Australia, they were responsible for more than one-third of all condemnations before slaughter. The Merino breed is most at risk, and females more so than males. The most common sites are the poorly haired skin of the ears, lips, muzzle, and the vulvar lips after they have been externalized by Mule's operation to prevent fly strike. Tumors at all these sites occur in conjunction with solar injury, which is heightened when animals ingest photosensitizing plants. Tumors of the ears also occur more frequently after a procedure such as ear tagging. Squamous cell carcinomas can develop from follicular cysts on sites not commonly exposed to sunlight.

In goats, these occur most frequently in females, in which tumors develop on the perineal and vulvar regions as well as the skin of the teats and udders; both males and females can develop sun-induced tumors on the ears. Although Angora is the breed most at risk, Saanan goats occasionally develop squamous cell carcinomas on the udder in association with papillomas. The role papillomaviruses play in tumor progression is undefined.

Most squamous cell carcinomas are solitary lesions; however, multiple tumors may develop in conjunction with solar injury. They appear as endophytic or exo-endophytic lesions, the former as raised, irregular, dermal masses with an ulcerated surface; the latter as raised, irregular, dermal masses covered by a papillated epidermis. In cattle with involvement of the horn, the first sign is that of distorted growth.

Usually, they are highly infiltrative into adjacent soft and bony tissues, but tend to metastasize slowly. Infrequently, in cattle, they regress spontaneously. The most common modes of therapy are complete excision or cryosurgery. In cats, radiation has been reported to elicit a 2-yr control rate of 87%. Some success has been obtained using immunotherapy for treating bovine ocular or horn core squamous cell carcinomas, with either an autogenous vaccine made from the tumor tissue suspended in Freund's adjuvant, or nonspecific immunomodulation using *Corynebacterium parvum*. If the tumors are large, debulking is recommended before instituting immunotherapy. In dogs with multiple ventral actinic keratoses or squamous cell carcinomas not amenable to surgery, topical dinitrochlorbenzene or 5-fluorouracil (5%) have been suggested treatments.

KERATINIZED CUTANEOUS CYSTS

Most of these are malformations of the hair follicle. They are common in dogs; occasionally identified in cats, horses, goats, and sheep; and rare in cattle and pigs. Excision is the treatment of choice. Vigorous squeezing of these lesions is contraindicated, as it often incites a severe foreign body inflammatory response.

Epidermal inclusion cysts (epidermoid cysts, follicular cysts, infundibular type, often erroneously called sebaceous cysts) actually represent a cystic dilation of the hair follicle infundibulum (the upper region of the hair follicle that is indistinguishable from the epidermis). They vary in size from 2 mm to >5 cm (lesions <5 mm in diameter are often called milia). Despite their name, there is little evidence that epidermal inclusion cysts actually originate from an invagination of the epidermis. The only identified domestic animal at risk is the Merino sheep, in which these cysts are often multiple and may progress to squamous cell carcinomas. As with all follicular cysts, these are usually a solitary, papular to nodular lesion that is freely movable. They are generally partially compressible on palpation, and occasionally have a small opening through the epidermis from which the cystic contents drain. They are filled with a gray, brown, or yellowish, granular, "cheesy" material.

The term **tricholemmal** or **pilar cyst** is applied to follicular cysts that demonstrate the keratinization pattern of the lower portion of the outer root sheath. They have been definitively identified only in dogs and cats.

Matrix cysts, follicular cysts in which the wall resembles the epithelium of the hair bulb (the matrix portion of the hair follicle) and the inner root sheath, occur predominately in dogs and cats. Many progress to pilomatricomas (*see* below).

Hybrid cysts, follicular cysts that have a combination of the characteristics of epidermal inclusion, tricholemmal, and matrix cysts, occur predominately in dogs and cats. They may progress to trichoepitheliomas (*see* below).

Dermoid cysts, congenital malformations found most commonly on the dorsal midline of the head or along the vertebral column, are most commonly identified in Boxers, Kerry Blue Terriers, and Rhodesian Ridgeback dogs, Thoroughbred horses, and possibly, Suffolk sheep. Typically multiple, they differ from other follicular cysts in that on cut surface they contain fully formed hair shafts.

Keratomas, cystic lesions in the hoof wall of the toe or, less frequently, the quarter or heel in simple or cloven-hoofed animals, are often secondary to a traumatic injury; as such, they may actually represent true epidermal inclusion cysts. Lameness and deformity of the hoof wall or sole are seen. These lesions are seldom >5 cm in diameter, and contain white to brown laminated keratin, often with a necrotic center. They often become secondarily inflamed.

TUMORS OF THE HAIR FOLLICLE

The hair follicle is a complex structure composed of 8 different epithelial layers. Hair-follicle tumors display a similar complexity, and much work needs to be done to further characterize them. (*See also* INTRACUTANEOUS CORNIFYING EPITHELIOMAS, SQUAMOUS CELL CARCINOMAS, and KERATINIZED CUTANEOUS CYSTS, above.) They are most common in dogs, less frequent in cats, and rare in other domestic animals.

Tricholemmomas, rare, benign, hair-follicle neoplasms of dogs, are derived from the outer root sheath, with vague similarities to a tumor of the same name in man. They are most common in older dogs and most frequently identified on the head. Poodles may be predisposed. They appear as firm, ovoid masses, 1-7 cm in diameter. They are encapsulated but expand over time. Excision is curative.

Dilated pores of Winer, rare hair-follicle neoplasms that have been recognized only in aged cats, most often in males, are benign, solitary lesions with the appearance of a giant comedo. Excision is curative.

Trichoepitheliomas, benign, hair-follicle neoplasms in which all elements of the hair follicle (infundibulum, isthmus, and inferior portions of the follicle) are represented, with the infundibular and isthmic regions predominating, are most common on the trunk in dogs and the head in cats, usually in animals >5 yr old. They appear as palpably encapsulated nodules (1-5 cm in diameter) in the dermis and subcut. fat. They tend to ulcerate, and often a condensed, yellow, granular, "cheesy" material can be extruded. They consist of multiple cystic structures filled with keratin. Excision is curative. Animals that develop one often develop others over time.

Pilomatricomas (hair matrix tumors, calcifying epitheliomas [of Malherbe]) are benign hair-follicle neoplasms composed of all elements of the hair follicle; however, unlike the trichoepithelioma, the matrix component predominates. They are most common on the trunk of mature dogs, usually Kerry Blue Terriers, Poodles, Bedlington Terriers, and Schnauzers, and rare in cats. Grossly, they are indistinguishable from trichoepitheliomas except their cystic contents often are gritty due to mineralization. Excision is the treatment of choice. As with trichoepitheliomas, dogs that develop one such lesion often develop others over time.

Malignant pilomatricomas (malignant epithelial neoplasms with hair-follicle differentiation) are rare and have been identified almost exclusively in dogs, usually old ones. Grossly, they are characterized as solitary or multinodular tumors that have the appearance of pilomatricomas and recur following attempts at complete excision. They often metastasize to draining lymph nodes and internal organs, especially the lungs. Aggressive surgery is recommended. It is unknown if these are responsive to radiation or chemotherapy.

CUTANEOUS APOCRINE GLAND TUMORS

There are 2 types of sweat glands: apocrine and eccrine. Apocrine glands are tubular glands with a coiled secretory portion and a long straight duct that empties into the follicular infundibulum. In domestic animals, all hair follicles have apocrine glands. Apocrine glands in dogs and cats are also present in association with the anal sac, and modified apocrine glands, known as ceruminous glands, are present in the external auditory meatus. In most animals, apocrine glands produce an odiferous, oily compound that is a sexual attractant, a territorial marker, and a warning signal. In horses and cattle, these glands play a role in thermoregulation by producing sweat.

Apocrine gland tumors are most common in dogs and cats, usually in middle-aged or older animals, and rare in other domestic animals. Three diseases of haired skin can be characterized under this heading.

Cystic apocrine gland dilation (apocrine gland cyst, cystic apocrine gland hyperplasia) is best characterized as a nevus. It is common in the dog, and found most frequently on the head and neck. It is characterized by a focal region of dilated apocrine glands in non-traumatized skin, usually not grossly apparent until one or more of the glands become dilated until it can be palpated. They appear as fluctuant papules or nodules that are filled with a clear to brownish fluid. Complete excision is curative.

Apocrine gland adenomas are rare in all domestic animals but have been identified most frequently in dogs, cats, and horses. In dogs and cats, these are most common on the head and neck; in horses, on the pinnae and vulva. Grossly, they appear as firm to fluctuant, discrete, nodular masses seldom >4 cm in diameter. Ulceration is uncommon. They are benign, and complete excision is curative.

Apocrine gland adenocarcinomas of haired skin are rare in all domestic animals but most frequently identified in dogs and cats. In dogs, they most commonly develop in the axillary regions, and must be differentiated from mammary gland adenocarcinomas. They are frequently ulcerated, often are larger than apocrine gland adenomas, and have irregular margins. Occasionally, variants have been identified with extensive cytoplasmic vacuolations (clear cell hidradenocarcinomas). All are locally infiltrative but generally metastasize late. Complete excision is the treatment of choice.

APOCRINE GLAND TUMORS OF ANAL SAC ORIGIN

These have been identified only in dogs, most commonly in older females (intact or ovariohysterectomized). Most are malignant. (*See also* p 285.) They most commonly appear as deep, firm, nodular masses in the area of the anal sac. Many are associated with a paraneoplastic syndrome, which is characterized by hypercalcemia and results in anorexia, weight loss, polyuria, and polydipsia. They tend to be highly infiltrative into the pelvic canal. They commonly (90%) metastasize to the sublumbar lymph nodes and to distant internal organs (40%). Wide surgical excision including involved lymph nodes is the treatment of choice. Even if the tumor cannot be totally resected, surgery may be palliative as hypercalcemia appears to be related to the total tumor mass. Adjunct chemotherapy may also be of benefit, but all have a poor prognosis; few dogs live >1 yr after the tumor has been recognized.

CERUMINOUS GLAND TUMORS

Rare neoplasms that develop from the modified apocrine glands in the external auditory meatus, these are most common in cats but also occur in dogs, usually in middle-aged or older animals. They appear as firm, nodular, often pedunculated nodules that may completely obstruct the external ear canal, and are often associated with a secondary otitis externa. In cats, they need to be distinguished from inflammatory polyps that arise from the inner ear. In dogs, they can be confused with severe adnexal hyperplasia due to a primary otitis externa. These are benign in all respects, and excision is curative.

Ceruminous gland adenocarcinomas are rare, but most common in cats and also seen in dogs. Tumors of middle-aged or older animals, these are usually nodular or plaque-like with ill-defined borders. They tend to remain confined to the ear canal until late in the course of the disease when they extend into surrounding soft tissue, bone, and draining lymph nodes; distant systemic metastasis has been identified. Wide surgical excision, which may require ablation of the external ear, is the treatment of choice. The prognosis is good if the tumor is confined to the ear canal. For invasive tumors, external beam irradiation has been recommended; however, it is not known whether this combination therapy significantly prolongs survival.

ECCRINE GLAND TUMORS

Eccrine glands, coiled, tubular, sweat glands, are present on the foot pads of carnivores, the frog of ungulates, the carpus of pigs, and the nasolabial region of ruminants. Only anecdotal reports of these tumors exist. In dogs and cats, they develop exclusively on the foot pads. Most are malignant. Too few have been identified to characterize gross, microscopic, or behavioral features.

SEBACEOUS GLAND TUMORS

Tumors and tumor-like conditions of sebaceous glands are common in dogs, infrequent in cats, and rare in other domestic animals. Although 5 different categories have been described, all may represent variants of the same disease process.

Sebaceous gland nevi are solitary lesions that have been reported only in dogs. The only gross features that distinguish them from sebaceous gland hyperplasia and adenomas are that they tend to be linear or circumscribed and several centimeters in length or diameter.

Sebaceous gland hyperplasias represent a senile change, most common in dogs and cats. They appear on the eyelids, head, and trunk, as multiple papillated masses generally <1 cm in diameter with a shiny, keratotic surface.

Sebaceous gland adenomas may occur in all domestic animals but usually in mature dogs, most commonly Fox Terriers, Cocker Spaniels, Poodles, Beagles, and Dachshunds, although Kerry Blue Terriers, Boston Terriers, Norwegian Elkhounds, and Basset Hounds also may be predisposed. Often multiple, they most commonly develop on the abdomen and the thorax, and may be grossly indistinguishable from sebaceous gland hyperplasia.

Sebaceous gland epitheliomas (sebaceomas) are infrequently recognized and poorly defined benign tumors of dogs, and rarely cats, that appear as nodular, often ulcerated cutaneous masses that may be several centimeters in diameter. A papillated epidermal surface and pigmentation are variable findings.

Sebaceous gland adenocarcinomas are rare in domestic animals, recognized almost exclusively in dogs and cats, generally in middle-aged or older animals, and seldom >2 cm in diameter. They are often ulcerated and may appear indistinguishable from sebaceous epitheliomas. They tend to be locally infiltrative and may metastasize to regional lymph nodes late in the disease.

Treatment is optional for benign sebaceous gland tumors unless they are secondarily inflamed and infected. Excision is the treatment of choice for sebaceous gland adenocarcinoma, but this can be difficult due to its infiltrative nature, and adjunct radiotherapy may be required. Even benign sebaceous gland growths recur if remnants are left at the surgical site; this is common in adenomas of the eyelid. In addition, sebaceous gland hyperplasia and sebaceous gland adenomas often recur at other cutaneous sites even after complete excision. There is no established protocol of chemotherapy for any of these lesions, although oral retinoids have been reported to be effective in controlling recurrent hyperplasias and adenomas in man.

HEPATOID GLAND TUMORS
(Perianal gland tumors, Circumanal gland tumors)

Common canine neoplasms that arise from modified sebaceous glands. These glands are most common in the cutaneous tissues around the anus but may also be present along the ventral midline from the perineum to the base of the skull, the dorsal and ventral tail, and in the skin of the lumbar and sacral regions. Androgens stimulate the development of the hepatoid glands, resulting in benign pathologic changes, usually in older, intact, male dogs.

Benign hepatoid gland tumors are divided into hepatoid gland hyperplasias and perianal gland adenomas; however, criteria have not been established to distinguish between them, and they will be considered as a single entity. Hepatoid gland adenomas are most common in aged, male dogs and are uncommon in females. Cocker Spaniels, German Shepherd Dogs, Dachshunds, Beagles, English Bulldogs, and Samoyeds are affected most commonly. Tumors may develop at any site where hepatoid glands are present, but 90% occur in the perianal region. Grossly, they appear as one or (more commonly) multiple intradermal nodules 0.5-10 cm in diameter. They commonly ulcerate, and hemorrhagic, keratinaceous material can often be extruded with local pressure. Large tumors can compress the anal canal making defecation difficult. Up to 95% of male dogs respond completely to castration; in those that do not, adrenocortical function should be evaluated, and if no abnormality is detected, the dog should be reevaluated for the presence of a low-grade hepatoid gland adenocarcinoma. Excision may be used concurrently to remove extremely large or ulcerated tumors that have become secondarily infected. Surgery is the treatment of choice for females with hepatoid gland tumors, but may need to be repeated because recurrence is common. Radiation therapy is also an option and has been effective in eliciting a 2-yr cure rate of 69% in benign tumors. Diethylstilbestrol may serve as an alternative to castration, but because of the side effects, which include aplastic anemia and cystic prostatic hyperplasia, its use should be severely restricted.

Hepatoid gland adenocarcinomas are uncommon canine neoplasms, of which <1% are malignant. They do not appear to be influenced by hormones, and occur in aged dogs with equal frequency in males and females. They are generally ulcerated with palpable evidence of invasion into deep perianal tissues. They have marked metastatic potential and often spread to regional lymph nodes. Treatment consists of wide surgical excision including involved lymph nodes, and possibly subsequent radiation. These tumors are generally not responsive to castration or estrogen therapy, and it is unknown if chemotherapy is of benefit for metastatic disease. The prognosis is guarded.

PRIMARY CUTANEOUS NEUROENDOCRINE TUMORS
(Merkel cell tumors, Atypical histiocytomas, Trabecular carcinomas, Extramedullary plasmacytomas)

In veterinary medicine, whether tumors develop from Merkel cells (tactile, neurosecretory cells of uncertain derivation, present in the basal cell layer of the epidermis) remains controversial. There are descriptions of neoplasms in the skin and oral cavity of dogs with membrane-bound, intracytoplasmic granules characteristic of neuroendocrine tumors. However, these are often indistinguishable from cutaneous extramedullary plasmacytomas; most likely they are the same tumor.

PAPILLOMATOSIS
(Warts)

Multiple papillomas of skin or mucosal surfaces generally are seen in younger animals, and are caused by viruses; single papillomas are more frequent in older animals, but their cause is unknown. The term papillomatosis is sometimes used to describe the multicentric form that occurs most often on skin, and upper GI, genital, and bladder mucosae in a variety of mammals, including man. Warts have also been reported in some species of fish, and in birds. No virus-induced warts have been recognized in Felidae. The papillomavirus-induced warts are quite species-specific under natural conditions, and frequently site-specific. Papillomatosis is most common in horses, dogs, and cattle.

Wart viruses are small (av 55 nm), double-stranded DNA viruses of the Papovaviridae family. Some mammals have several distinct papilloma viruses, eg, man has >20; cattle, 5; dogs, 2; and rabbits, 2. The virus is transmitted by direct contact, fomites, and possibly by insects.

Clinical Findings—Cattle: Warts commonly occur on the head, neck, and shoulders, and occasionally on the back and abdomen. The extent and duration of the lesions depend on type of virus, area affected, and degree of susceptibility. Warts appear ~2 mo after exposure, and may last ≥1 yr. Papillomatosis becomes a herd problem when the infection occurs in a large group of young susceptible cattle. Immunity to re-exposure usually develops 3-4 wk after initial infection, but recurrences occasionally occur, probably due to loss of immunity.

The bovine wart contains a fibromatous element. This is particularly prominent in the venereal form of the disease, in which fibropapillomas may be a serious problem on the penis of young bulls, and can cause dystocia when the vaginal mucosa of heifers is affected.

A form of persistent cutaneous papillomatosis with small warts may occur in herds of older cattle. Bovine papillomavirus has been demonstrated in bladder tumors associated with bracken fern ingestion (qv, p 1641) in several parts of the world, and in upper GI tract papillomas of cattle in Scotland. It is believed that the papillomavirus acts as a co-carcinogen. When bovine papillomavirus is injected into the skin of horses, a fibrosarcoma-like tumor similar to sarcoid develops.

Horses: Small, scattered warts occur on the nose and lips, presumably at the sites of abrasions when colts nuzzle each other. It is common when young horses are kept together, but regresses in a few months, due to complete immunity. So-called aural plaques are also thought to be a form of papilloma. These occur on the inner surface of the pinnae, and occasionally around the anus, mammary glands, and vulva.

Equine papillomas must be differentiated from sarcoid, which has a similar appearance. Equine sarcoid (qv, p 857) is a more common tumor of horses that may resemble ulcerated warts.

Dogs: Two forms of canine papillomas occur, both primarily in young dogs. Oral papillomas are multiple, gray or white, cauliflower or piliform growths that in extreme cases may cover a large portion of the palate, tongue, and esophagus, and interfere with mastication. Necrosis and secondary infection may occur and cause a putrid odor. Viral inclusions are present in the granular layer. The cutaneous form appears like its counterpart in cattle, with multiple warts on face, neck, and limbs. Oral papillomavirus does not cause cutaneous papillomas when injected into the skin.

Other Species: Warts affecting various areas of the skin have been described in goats; some on the teats and udder become carcinomas. Warts are rare in sheep; they can be transmitted to other sheep, but not to other species. Papillomas are rare in pigs, and viral etiology is suspected but not proved. Lesions may be solitary or multiple, and occur on the face or genitalia. For papillomas in rabbits, *see* p 1066. Transmissible, cutaneous papillomatosis has been reported in monkeys, but the species specificity was not established.

A cutaneous fibroma occurs in white-tail, black-tail, and mule deer, and in antelope, moose, and caribou. It is caused by a papillomavirus found only in the epithelium that covers the tumors, and resembles bovine papillomavirus.

Treatment and Control: Infectious papillomatosis is a self-limiting disease, although the duration of warts varies considerably. A variety of treatments has been advocated without agreement on efficacy. Surgical removal is recommended if the warts are sufficiently objectionable. However, because surgery in the early growing stage of warts may lead to recurrence and stimulation of growth, they should be removed when near their maximum size or when regressing. Affected animals may be isolated from susceptible ones, but with the long incubation period, many are likely to have been exposed before the problem is recognized.

Most vaccines have had limited success as a preventive in cattle, but not for treatment. Since wart viruses are mostly species-specific, there is no merit in using a vaccine derived from one species on another.

When the disease is a herd problem, it can be controlled by vaccination with a suspension of ground wart tissue in which the virus has been killed with formalin. Autogenous vaccines may be more effective than those commercially available. It may be necessary to begin vaccination as early as 4-6 wk of age in calves with a dose of ~0.4 mL intradermally at each of 2 sites. The vaccination is repeated in 4-6 wk and at 1 yr of age. Immunity develops in a few weeks, but is unrelated to whatever mechanism is involved in spontaneous regression. If exposure to the virus occurred before vaccination, immunity may develop too late to prevent warts. A vaccination program must be in effect for ~3-6 mo before its preventive value will be evident. Vaccination should be continued for ≥1 yr after the last wart disappears since the premises may still be contaminated. Stalls, stanchions, and other inert materials can be disinfected by fumigating with formaldehyde.

CONNECTIVE TISSUE TUMORS

BENIGN FIBROBLASTIC TUMORS

Collagenous nevi, benign, focal, developmental defects associated with increased deposition of dermal collagen, are relatively common in dogs, uncommon in cats, and rare in large animals. They generally occur in middle-aged or older animals, and are most frequently on the proximal and distal extremities, head, and neck. They are sessile to raised, dermal nodules, often with a papillated surface; occasionally, coarse hairs exit from them. Infrequently, they may occur in the subcut. fat. Excision is curative.

Generalized nodular dermatofibrosis, recognized in German Shepherd Dogs, is a syndrome in which multiple collagenous nevi are associated with renal cystadenocarcinomas and, in females, multiple uterine leiomyomas. Believed to be inherited as an autosomal dominant, it is first recognized when the animal is 3-5 yr old. It is characterized by development of multiple collagenous nevi varying from barely palpable to large and nodular, generally on the limbs, feet, head, and trunk, and may have a symmetrical distribution. Renal disease develops ~3-5 yr after the skin lesions are recognized. No known therapy can prevent development of the renal and uterine neoplasms.

Fibromas, discrete, generally cellular proliferations of dermal fibroblasts, rare in all domestic species but most common in aged dogs and cats, are solitary, firm to fluctuant, often hairless papules or nodules. As these lesions are benign, treatment is optional; however, complete excision is recommended for histopathologic confirmation.

Acrochordons (cutaneous tags, soft fibromas, fibrovascular papillomas) are distinctive, benign, cutaneous lesions of older dogs. These lesions are common, may be single or multiple, and can occur in any breed, but large breeds may be at increased risk. Most commonly, they appear as pedunculated exophytic growths, often covered by a verrucous epidermal surface. Treatment is optional, but biopsy is recommended to confirm the diagnosis. They are amenable to excision, electrosurgery, and cryosurgery, but dogs that develop one acrochordon are prone to develop others over time.

MALIGNANT FIBROBLASTIC TUMORS

One of a group of malignant neoplasms known as spindle cell sarcomas, which includes equine sarcoids, fibromatoses, fibrosarcomas, malignant fibrous histiocytomas, neurofibrosarcomas, leiomyosarcomas, rhabdomyosarcomas, and variants of liposarcomas, angiosarcomas, synovial cell sarcomas, mesotheliomas, and meningiomas. As a group, these are perhaps the most widely recognized yet least defined neoplasms. The confusion stems in part from the fact that all spindle cell sarcomas have a common cell of origin: a primitive mesenchymal cell. Thus, the characterization of spindle cell sarcomas is based not on its cell of origin, but on the cell line toward which it is differentiating. Because this primitive mesenchymal cell is apparently more capable of dedifferentiation and differentiation than the basal cell (the cell of origin of most epithelial tumors), generally there is considerably greater morphologic overlap in sarcomas than carcinomas. This makes it difficult to define histopathologic criteria necessary for making an unequivocal diagnosis of specific spindle cell sarcomas.

A second cause for the confusion stems from the difficulty in determining whether these are benign or malignant. Most spindle cell sarcomas of domestic animals are locally infiltrative, difficult to excise, and yet seldom metastasize. Logically, these tumors should be considered benign because by definition, only malignant tumors have metastatic potential; however, equal logic counters that these tumors should be considered malignant because by definition, benign neoplasms are not infiltrative. In human pathology, infiltrative but nonmetastasizing mesenchymal spindle cell tumors have been defined as "sarcomas of intermediate malignancy", a concept utilized below.

Because spindle cell sarcomas are usually considered as a group, some general comments can be made. Clinically, 4 general principles relate to spindle cell sarcomas and soft-tissue sarcomas: 1) the more superficial the location, the more likely the tumor is to be benign (deep tumors tend to be malignant); 2) the larger the tumor, the more likely it is to be malignant; 3) a rapidly growing tumor is more likely to be malignant than one that develops slowly; 4) benign tumors are relatively avascular, whereas most malignancies are hypervascular.

Excision is the treatment of choice; wide excision or amputation should be performed when anatomically feasible because spindle cell sarcomas often infiltrate along fascial planes, making it difficult to determine from gross examination the peripheral margins of the tumor. The best, if not only, opportunity to completely remove a spindle cell sarcoma is during the first surgical attempt; those that recur have a greater potential for metastasis, and the time between recurrence tends to shorten with each subsequent attempt at excision. In addition, many soft tissue tumors have a "pseudocapsule", which on gross examination gives the impression of complete encapsulation; these tumors should not be "shelled out" because neoplastic cells are almost always present in the pericapsular connective tissues. Except for equine sarcoids, cryosurgery is usually not used for these tumors as some types, most notably fibrosarcomas, have thick cell membranes, making them resistant to freezing. Spindle sarcomas generally do not respond well to conventional doses of radiation, however, higher doses have been reported to control ~50% of them for 1 yr. Surgical debulking followed by radiation is also an option for local control. Although chemotherapy has been effective in treating similar tumors in man, no chemotherapeutic protocol is known to be of value in treating these in other animals.

Equine sarcoids are the most frequently recognized neoplasm in horses. Their etiology is undefined, but most likely they are caused by a papillomavirus distinct from those in cattle. There is evidence of a familial predisposition, and they may be transmissible through direct contact, via arthropod vectors, or via fomites, eg, contaminated brushes and needles. They develop in horses, donkeys, or mules, most commonly in those <4 yr old. Sarcoids may occur anywhere on the body, and up to 84% of affected animals have multiple lesions. The most common site varies with geographic area: in the UK, the penis appears to be the most common site, while in the northwest USA, the limbs are affected most frequently. Sarcoids are highly variable in appearance, and 4 manifestations are recognized: 1) verrucous, which may be confused with squamous papillomas or squamous cell carcinomas; 2) fibroblastic, which may be confused with granulation tissue or fribromas; 3) sessile or flat, which may be confused with flat warts (verruca plana); and 4) mixed verrucous and fibroblastic, which may be confused with fibropapillomas. They should be considered as sarcomas of intermediate malignancy; they do not metastasize but commonly recur. Cryosurgery (after surgical debulking of larger lesions) is the treatment of choice. A 1-yr remission rate of ~90% has been reported. Also, nontreated lesions may regress spontaneously, although ≥50% of equine sarcoids recur following surgery alone. Radiation therapy using iridium may be of value when lesions are present in locations not amenable to cryosurgery or excision. Immunotherapy with inoculations of Bacillus Calmette-Guerin (BCG) remains controversial; both good results and fatal anaphylaxis have been reported. Treatment with flunixin meglumine and prednisolone 30 min before BCG inoculation is recommended. Sarcoids inoculated with BCG may take several months to regress entirely. Lastly, this form of therapy should not be utilized when treated animals could be exposed to cattle, as BCG can induce a positive tuberculin reaction in cattle.

Fibromatosis (aggressive fibromatosis, extra-abdominal desmoids, desmoid tumors, low-grade fibrosarcomas, nodular fasciitis) is a sclerosing and infiltrative proliferation of well-differentiated fibroblasts derived from aponeuroses and tendon sheaths. They may occur in other locations, but are generally observed on the head of dogs, where they are commonly diagnosed as nodular fasciitis. (In veterinary medicine, the term nodular fasciitis is applied to 2 different diseases: one that behaves as a fibromatosis and one that commonly affects the periocular tissues [known as canine fibrous histiocytoma—*see* below]). Fibromatoses are infrequent in cats and horses. Grossly, fibromatoses are generally indistinguishable from infiltrative fibrosarcomas; however, they can be differentiated on histological examination. Focal lymphoid nodules are scattered throughout the tissues. The fibromatoses are locally infiltrative with essentially no metastatic potential. If feasible, excision is the treatment of choice. Recurrence is common, and radiation therapy may be of value for local control.

Fibrosarcomas, aggressive mesenchymal tumors in which fibroblasts are the predominant cell type, are most common in cats, in which they are the most common soft-tissue tumor. They are also common in dogs, but rare in other domestic animals. Two forms are recognized in cats: a multicentric form in the young (generally <4 yr old) caused by the feline sarcoma virus (FSV), and a solitary form in the young or old, in which FSV has not been implicated. In all other species, fibrosarcomas tend to be solitary. In dogs, these tumors are most common on the trunk and extremities, and females and Cocker Spaniels may be predisposed.

Fibrosarcomas vary markedly in size. They appear as firm, fleshy lesions involving the dermis and subcut. fat, and may invade the underlying musculature along fascial planes. When tumors are multiple, they are usually located within the same anatomic region. Fibrosarcomas with abundant interstitial proteoglycans (connective tissue mucins) are called myxosarcomas or myxofibrosarcomas. Myxosarcomas remain poorly defined in veterinary medicine, and many of them might be better characterized as variants of liposarcomas or malignant fibrous histiocytomas. Fibrosarcomas should be considered invasive tumors; ~10% metastasize. The ability to successfully excise fibrosarcomas depends on the degree of cellular atypia (as defined by the mitotic index), the infiltrative nature of the tumor, and its size and anatomical location. Cats with tumors on the pinna or flank have relatively long postoperative survival times; if on the head, back, or limbs, 70% recur <1 yr after the initial surgery.

FIBROHISTIOCYTIC TUMORS

Pleomorphic, mesenchymal tumors composed of fibroblasts and histiocytic cells (often present as multinucleated giant cells), these benign lesions remain poorly defined in veterinary medicine. A lesion called **canine fibrous histiocytoma** (nodular granulomatous episclerokeratitis, nodular fasciitis, proliferative keratoconjunctivitis, conjunctival granuloma, Collie granuloma) is recognized at the episcleral junction and cornea in young to middle-aged (2- to 4-yr old) Collies, but the histologic features are more suggestive of a granulomatous inflammatory response than a neoplasm. As might be expected for a noninfectious inflammatory process, these are generally responsive to sublesional injections of 10-40 mg of methylprednisolone.

Malignant fibrous histiocytomas (extraskeletal giant cell tumors, giant cell tumors of soft parts, dermatofibrosarsomas) are uncommon in the skin and soft tissues of cats, horses, and mules. They have been described but remain poorly defined in dogs. In cats, malignant fibrous histiocytomas are most common on the distal extremities or ventral cervical regions of the aged. In horses and mules, these have been described as giant cell tumors of soft parts. They appear to occur in horses 3-12 yr old. They are firm, nodular to diffuse swellings that are white on cut surface, with variable hemorrhage. Malignant fibrous histiocytomas are sarcomas of intermediate malignancy. They are locally invasive and tend to recur after attempts at complete excision but seldom metastasize. Radical excision is recommended.

PERIPHERAL NERVE SHEATH TUMORS

Amputation neuromas (traumatic neuromas) are non-neoplastic, disorganized proliferations of peripheral nerve parenchyma and stroma in response to amputation or traumatic injury. They are most commonly identified in conjunction with tail docking in dogs or neurectomy in the distal extremities of horses. In dogs, amputation neuromas are generally recognized in the young, and are associated with extreme self-trauma to the tail tip. In horses, such a lesion appears as a firm, often painful swelling at the surgery site. Excision is curative.

Neurofibromas and **neurofibrosarcomas** (perineuromas, neurilemmomas, nerve sheath tumors, hemangiopericytomas, neurothekomas, schwannomas) are spindle cell tumors that arise from the connective tissue components of the peripheral nerve. They are believed to arise from Schwann cells, but they could also arise from mesenchymal cells, which manufacture the non-myelinated connective tissues that surround the myelinated nerve fiber. In dogs, forms of this tumor can be virtually indistinguishable from hemangiopericytomas, and may be the same tumor.

In dogs and cats, peripheral nerve sheath tumors of the skin occur in older animals. In cattle, they have a suspected genetic basis, may be multiple, can occur in both the young and old, and are most commonly an incidental finding at slaughter, appearing as one or more nodose swellings of deep nerves of the thoracic wall and viscera. Cutaneous involvement is rare. They appear as white, firm, nodular lesions that may be identified in association with peripheral nerves. Both benign and intermediate-grade malignant variants are recognized. Benign ones are most common in cattle in which, due to their indolent nature, treatment is optional; also additional tumors tend to develop spontaneously at other sites over time. In dogs, cats, and horses, most are locally infiltrative but do not metastasize. Complete excision is the treatment of choice.

ADIPOSE TISSUE TUMORS

Lipomas represent benign tumors of adipose tissue, perhaps more accurately characterized as nevi. They are common in dogs, occasionally occur in cats and horses, and are rare in other domestic species. In dogs, they generally occur in older, obese females, most commonly on the trunk and proximal limbs. The breeds most at risk are Cocker Spaniels, Dachshunds, Weimeraners, Labrador Retrievers, and small terrier breeds. Most affected cats are spayed or neutered, and 6-12 yr old. Obesity does not appear to be a factor in their development. Affected horses are generally <2 yr old. Lipomas typically appear as soft, occasionally pedunculated, discrete nodular masses, and most are freely movable. In dogs and cats, they are frequently multiple. A rare variant of this tumor, diffuse lipomatosis, has been identified in Dachshunds, in which virtually the entire skin is affected, resulting in prominent folds on the neck and truncal skin. Many lipomas merge imperceptibly with the adjacent non-neoplastic adipose tissue, making it difficult to determine when the entire lesion is excised. Lipomas with an abundant connective tissue stroma (fibrolipomas) or a prominent vascular component (angiolipomas) are also recognized. Despite their benign nature, lipomas should not be ignored due to their tendency to enlarge over time, and their gross presentation, which may be indistinguishable from infiltrating lipomas or liposarcomas (see below). Excision is curative. In dogs, dietary restriction several weeks before surgery may allow for better definition of the surgical margins of the tumor. About one-third of dogs and cats that develop one such tumor develop others over time.

Infiltrative lipomas (intramuscular and intermuscular lipomas) are rare in dogs, cats, and horses. In dogs, they are most common in middle-aged females, usually on the neck and limbs. They are poorly confined, soft, nodular to diffuse swellings that typically involve the subcut. fat and underlying muscle and connective tissue stroma. Infiltrative lipomas, which dissect along fascial planes and between skeletal muscle bundles, are considered sarcomas of intermediate malignancy. Rarely, they metastasize. Aggressive excision is recommended, and amputation may be necessary.

Liposarcomas are uncommon in all domestic animals. In cats, feline leukemia virus infection has been infrequently associated with their development; whether this is a coincidence or such infections play a causative role remains undefined. These tumors generally occur in older animals. They are nodular, soft to firm, and may exude myxoid fluid when sectioned. Many have palpable, partially encapsulated areas, but these zones should not be construed as evidence of a benign tumor. Liposarcomas are malignant neoplasms that have a low metastatic potential but are extremely infiltrative. Wide excision is recommended even for those that appear to be partially encapsulated. Recurrence is common, especially for anaplastic variants.

VASCULAR TUMORS

Hemangiomas of the skin and soft tissues are benign proliferations that closely resemble blood vessels. Whether these actually are neoplasms, nevi, or vascular malformations remains undefined, and no clear criteria allow for their separation. They are most commonly identified in dogs, occasionally in cats and horses, rarely in cattle and pigs, and exceptionally in other animals. Boxers, Scottish Terriers, Airedales, and Kerry Blue Terriers have been suggested as the canine breeds most at risk. In horses, they are most common on the distal extremities of those <1 yr old. In cattle, they occur in older animals or as congenital lesions. Dairy cattle are predisposed to developing disseminated hemangiomas (angiomatosis) in the skin and internal organs. In pigs, these lesions generally occur in the scrotal or perineal skin of Yorkshire, Berkshire, and less commonly, Chester White boars. In the first 2 breeds, the disease is believed to be genetically transmitted. Hemangiomas are single to multiple, circumscribed, often compressible, red to black nodules. The lining epidermis may be unaffected or, especially in horses and cattle, ulcerated or papillated.

When RBC are sparse or absent, the term lymphangioma is applied. Hemangiomas present solely in the superficial dermis and that have induced epidermal hyperplasia are known as angiokeratomas.

Hemangiomas are benign but their tendency to ulcerate, as well as the importance of confirming the diagnosis to make a prognosis, indicates removal. Excision is the treatment of choice; however, in large animals, in which the lesions may occur on the distal extremities, this may be difficult. In these cases, cryosurgery or radiation therapy may be necessary. Except for dairy cattle with angiomatosis, development of additional tumors at new sites after complete excision is uncommon.

Hemangiopericytomas (canine spindle cell sarcoma, canine malignant fibrous histiocytoma, canine neurofibrosarcoma, canine perineuroma) are common in dogs, and rare (if they occur) in cats. They are most common on the distal extremities of older dogs. Females appear to be predisposed and Boxer, German Shepherd Dogs, Cocker and Springer Spaniels, Fox Terriers, Airedales, and Doberman Pinschers are the breeds most at risk. They are firm, multilobulated but solitary lesions with irregular borders, most commonly in the subcut. fat but sometimes in the dermis. Hemangiopericytomas are of intermediate malignancy and have limited metastatic potential. Complete excision is the treatment of choice, but due to their infiltrative nature, ~30% recur.

Angiosarcomas are malignant neoplasms, the cells of which have many functional and morphological features of normal endothelium. Although these tumors are often divided into hemangiosarcomas (of purported blood vessel origin) and lymphangiosarcomas (of lymphatic vessel origin), such a distinction is arbitrary. The term angioendothelioma is also used. Their cause is unknown, but in dogs with a short white coat, eg, Pit Bull Terriers, chronic solar injury has induced a change in the superficial vascular plexus, which initially appears as a hemangioma and then progresses to a malignant vascular tumor.

Angiosarcomas of the skin and soft tissues occur in all domestic animals but are most common in dogs, generally in adult or aged animals. In dogs, they most frequently develop on the trunk, hip, thigh, and distal extremities. Males are more frequently affected than females, and German Shepherd Dogs, Boxers, and Bernese Mountain Dogs are most at risk. Most commonly they are solitary, poorly confined, erythematous nodules present anywhere in the skin or underlying soft tissues. Less frequently, they appear as a poorly defined bruise. All grow rapidly, often associated with large zones of necrosis and thrombosis, and typically are red to black on cut section. Characteristically, they create their own vascular space by dissecting through soft tissues. In dogs, angiosarcomas are the most aggressive of all soft-tissue sarcomas. Distant metastasis, especially to the lung and liver is common. In other domestic animals, these tumors do not appear to behave as aggressively, and postexcisional recurrence rather than metastasis is more common. For all species, wide excision is the treatment of choice. Recently, adjuvant chemotherapy consisting of vincristine, doxorubicin, and cyclophosphamide have been reported to shrink angiosarcomas; however, effects of this therapy on long-term survival remain to be defined.

CUTANEOUS SMOOTH MUSCLE TUMORS

Either because they are not recognized or because they do not occur with any regularity in domestic animals, cutaneous smooth muscle tumors (leiomyomas or leiomyosarcomas) are diagnosed rarely. Those reported generally have been malignant and limited to dogs and cats. Usually they are firm cutaneous masses. Leimyomas are smaller and tend to be limited to the dermis, whereas leiomyosarcomas are larger and most arise from (or extend into) the subcut. fat. The behavior of malignant smooth muscle tumors remains poorly defined. Complete excision is the treatment of choice for both leiomyomas and leiomyosarcomas.

UNDIFFERENTIATED AND ANAPLASTIC SARCOMAS

These are malignant mesenchymal tumors that are difficult to characterize microscopically. Undifferentiated sarcomas lack distinctive features (architectural patterns, cytoplasmic and nuclear features, cell products). Anaplastic sarcomas have most of the following features: variations in size and shape of nuclei, nuclear hyperchromasia, striking irregularity of chromatin pattern, abnormal mitotic figures, and large numbers of mitotic figures. As such, anaplastic sarcomas are generally undifferentiated, but undifferentiated sarcomas do not have to be anaplastic. Both should be treated with wide excision; however, the prognosis for anaplastic sarcomas is generally poorer than for undifferentiated sarcomas.

LYMPHOCYTIC, HISTIOCYTIC, AND RELATED CUTANEOUS NEOPLASMS

LYMPHOID NEOPLASMS OF THE SKIN

Canine extramedullary plasmacytomas (atypical histiocytomas, cutaneous neuroendocrine tumors [qv, p 854]) are recently recognized but relatively common cutaneous tumors, believed to be of plasma cell origin. Most of these tumors were previously diagnosed as reticulum cell sarcomas.

This neoplasm is most common on the digits, lips, external aural pinnae, and in the oral cavity in mature to aged dogs. They are seldom >5 cm in diameter. Cocker Spaniels, and possibly Golden Retrievers, are the breeds most at risk. These tumors are red, occasionally pedunculated, and frequently ulcerated. Although generally solitary, the lesions are multiple in ~10% of animals. Extracutaneous plasmacytomas may be locally invasive, especially when in the oral cavity; complete but conservative excision is usually curative. Treatment for recurrent or multiple tumors remains poorly defined. Radiation therapy appears to be the best secondary treatment. For radioresistant tumors, chemotherapeutic agents including melphalan, cyclophosphamide, and glucocorticoids have been recommended.

Cutaneous lymphosarcomas may occur as a disease in which the skin is the initial and primary site of involvement, or occur secondary to systemic, internal disease. *See also* LYMPHOSARCOMA, pp 32, 39, and 391. Cutaneous lymphosarcoma is uncommon but has been identified in all domestic species. In general, 2 distinct forms are recognized: an epitheliotropic form (assumed to be of T-lymphocyte origin) in which there is infiltration by malignant lymphocytes into the epidermis, and a nodular, nonepitheliotropic form (assumed to be of B-lymphocyte origin).

Epitheliotropic lymphosarcomas (mycosis fungoides), the most common form of cutaneous lymphosarcoma in dogs, is uncommon in cats, and rare in others. In both dogs and cats, it occurs in middle-aged or older animals. It has numerous gross manifestations, and initially may be difficult to diagnose based on clinical features. Early, it can appear as irregular erythematous patches, excess scaling, a primary alopecic disease, an erosive and ulcerative gingivitis, plaques and nodules, or a combination of one or more of the above. As it progresses, plaques and nodules generally become a major feature. In veterinary medicine, the term pagetoid reticulosis is used when epitheliotropic lymphosarcoma is devoid of significant dermal involvement. A progressive and incurable disease, lymph node involvement generally occurs late in the tumor's progression. In most cases, the skin becomes so severely involved that euthanasia is necessary. In the rare cases in which there is evidence of malignant cells within the peripheral blood, the term Sezary syndrome is applied. No effective therapy for this neoplasm has been established.

Nonepitheliotropic cutaneous lymphosarcomas (NECL) are the most commonly recognized form of cutaneous lymphosarcoma in all domestic animals but the dog, but are rare to uncommon in all species. In dogs, NECL are most common in middle-aged or older animals. Lesions are nodules or plaques, most commonly on the trunk. Lesions may be single or multiple, and frequently ulcerate. In many cases, NECL are grossly indistinguishable from epitheliotropic lymphosarcoma, and histologic evaluation may be necessary to distinguish them. Canine NECL are aggressive, and secondary systemic involvement is frequent. Various modes of therapy including excision, chemotherapy and, less frequently, radiotherapy have been utilized both singly and in combination. Excision is the choice when the disease is limited to a solitary tumor, and complete cures have occasionally been obtained. Excision or cryosurgery in more diffuse forms infrequently elicit long-term remissions. Chemotherapy or chemoimmunologic protocols utilized for other forms of canine lymphosarcoma should be considered as palliative. The average remission time is ~8 mo.

In horses, NECL (nodular lymphosarcoma, subcut. lymphosarcoma, lymphohistiocytic lymphosarcoma) may be recognized at any age, but is most common in middle-aged animals. Firm, nonulcerated nodules are most common in the subcut. fat of the ventral body surface. Microscopically, 2 types of equine nodular lymphosarcoma are recognized: the most common consists of a mixture of histiocytes and small, well-differentiated lymphocytes, occasionally with plasmacytoid features; the second consists of a monomorphic population of large atypical lymphocytes, with only occasional histiocytic cells. Differentiation of these is important as most cases of equine cutaneous lymphosarcoma, which have a monomorphic pattern of cells, have internal involvement and progress rapidly. In contrast, the lymphohistiocytic form seldom tends to be associated with internal involvement, and affected horses may live for months or years. As the lymphohistiocytic form progresses, the nodules tend to become more frequent on the ventral cervical regions. In many cases, euthanasia may be warranted when pharyngeal involvement induces dyspnea. There is no known therapy for either form.

In cattle, cutaneous lymphosarcoma is a disease of young animals (generally <4 yr old). It is not associated with bovine leukemia virus infection. The lesions are typically nodular, involve the dermis and/or subcut. fat, and are often ulcerated. There is no known therapy.

In cats, NECL is a disease of middle-aged or older animals. The role of feline leukemia virus remains undefined. The lesions are plaques or nodules that may be solitary or multiple, alopecic or haired, and ulcerated or lined by an intact epidermis. Feline NECL is aggressive; even when complete excision of a solitary nodule is attempted, recurrence is common. To date, no therapy is known; it is unknown if chemotherapeutic protocols used in treating other forms of feline lymphosarcoma are of value for NECL.

CUTANEOUS MAST CELL TUMORS

These (also called mastocytomas, mast cell sarcomas) are the most frequently recognized malignant or potentially malignant neoplasms of dogs. In addition, leukemic and visceral forms can occur. A viral etiology has been speculated but remains controversial. These may occur in dogs of any age (av 8-10 yr). They may occur anywhere on the body surface as well as in internal organs, but the upper posterior limbs, perineal, and preputial regions are the most common sites; ~10% of them are multicentric. They vary markedly in size, and clinical appearance alone cannot establish a diagnosis. Most commonly, they appear as soft to solid, raised, nodular masses. Although they often appear to be encapsulated, they are not; they are a dense aggregate of mast cells surrounded peripherally by a "halo" of smaller numbers of mast cells that palpate as normal skin. Dogs may also develop clinical signs associated with the release of vasoactive products from the malignant mast cells. Most common is gastroduodenal ulceration that may be present in up to 25% of cases. Cytological evaluation of Wright's-stained, fine needle aspirates or impression smears can be used to establish the diagnosis of canine mast cell tumors. However, cytology is no substitute for histopathology, as only the latter has been correlated with prognosis. Two systems of histopathologic grading have been defined, and to avoid confusion, it is essential to know which of the 2 systems is being used.

Although there is believed to be a benign variant of canine mast cell tumor, there is no clinical or microscopical means of identifying it. In addition, small mast cell tumors may remain quiescent for long periods before becoming aggressive.

Thus, all should be treated as malignancies. Treatment depends on clinical stage of disease.

The preferred treatment of Stage I tumors is complete excision, with a liberal margin: a minimum of 3 cm of healthy tissue surrounding all palpable borders should be removed in an attempt to excise both the nodule and its surrounding "halo" of neoplastic cells. If histological evaluation suggests that the tumor extends beyond the surgical margins, additional surgery or, alternatively, radiation therapy should be initiated.

At present, there is no agreed upon mode of therapy for Stage II-IV mast cell tumors. For Stage II tumors, several options are available including excision (including the affected regional node, if feasible), prednisolone, and radiotherapy used either singly or in combination. Treatment of Stage III and IV tumors is generally palliative. One recommended therapy is prednisolone (2 mg/kg body wt, PO, for the first 5 days, followed by a maintenance dose of 0.5 mg/kg, daily) or intralesional injections of triamcinolone (1 mg/cm diameter of tumor, q2wk). Cimetidine (4 mg/kg, PO, q.i.d.) should be administered concurrently to inhibit the formation of gastroduedenal ulcers. In addition, cimetidine may have some antitumor activity.

Feline cutaneous mast cell tumors are common. In addition to cutaneous tumors, systemic, leukemic, and GI forms have been recognized. Two distinct variants of the form are recognized: 1) a mast-cell type analogous to, but not identical with, cutaneous mast cell tumors in dogs, and 2) a histiocytic-type unique to cats.

The mast-cell type is most common. It occurs chiefly in cats >4 yr old, and may develop anywhere on the body, but most commonly on the head and neck. They are single, alopecic nodules, generally 2-3 cm in diameter, occasionally with extension into the subcut. fat. Lymphoid nodules are common, eosinophils are rare. As with canine cutaneous mast cell tumors, there is a correlation with cellular atypia and clinical behavior; however, no histopathologic grading system has been established. Complete excision is the treatment of choice; <20% recur following surgery and of those that do, considerably fewer metastasize.

The histiocytic type of feline cutaneous mast cell tumor is recognized primarily in Siamese cats <4 yr old. Lesions may develop anywhere on the body and appear as multiple, small (generally 0.5-1 cm in diameter), firm, subcut. papulonodules. Usually, the older the cat, the less numerous the lesions. This variant may be difficult to distinguish morphologically from a granulomatous inflammatory response. As they tend to resolve spontaneously, no treatment is necessary.

Equine mast cell tumors are uncommon, benign tumors. There is debate as to whether they actually represent a neoplastic process or an unusual inflammatory response. Lesions may develop anywhere on the body but are most common on the head and legs. Typically there is a single, solitary mass in the dermis and/or subcut. fat, which may expand to involve the underlying musculature. Alopecia and ulceration are variable features. Excision is the treatment of choice. These lesions do not metastasize. A variant of cutaneous equine mast cell tumor occurs in newborn foals, in which the lesions may become generalized but regress over time, suggesting an equine equivalent of urticaria pigmentosa in man.

Mast cell tumors in pigs and cattle are rare. In pigs, most appear as discrete, solitary, cutaneous nodules. Most are benign, but disseminated and leukemic variants do occur. In cattle, most are malignant, and characterized by multiple cutaneous nodules often accompanied by systemic involvement; purely cutaneous forms have been recognized occasionally.

TUMORS WITH HISTIOCYTIC DIFFERENTIATION

These comprise a group of poorly defined skin diseases all characterized by a proliferation of histiocytes (tissue macrophages) in the absence of any known stimulus.

Cutaneous histiocytomas are common in dogs and rare in cats, goats, and cattle. The lesions may arise from modified cutaneous macrophages known as Langerhan's cells; however, the exact cell of origin is unknown. There is evidence of a viral etiology for canine histiocytoma, but a causative agent has not been identified. In dogs, these are most common on the head, pinnae, and limbs, where they appear as solitary, raised, generally ulcerated nodules that are freely movable. Although typically seen in dogs <2 yr old, they can occur in those of any age. Boxers, Dachshunds, Cocker Spaniels, Great Danes, and Shetland Sheepdogs are the breeds most at risk. Although a common neoplasm, histiocytomas are not always easy to diagnose histologically, and can be confused with granulomatous inflammation, mast cell tumors, plasmacytomas, and cutaneous lymphosarcomas. Canine histiocytomas should be considered benign, and most resolve spontaneously without treatment within 2-3 mo. However, complete but conservative excision is the standard treatment; cryosurgery or electrosurgery may be equally effective.

Similar tumors have been reported in young cats. Whether these truly represent a feline variant of the canine disease or whether they are a variant of the histiocytic form of feline mast cell tumor remains undefined.

In goats and cattle, histiocytomas are extremely rare and behave similarly to the canine tumors.

Cutaneous histiocytosis is rare in dogs, associated with development of numerous plaques and nodules involving the dermis and/or the subcut. fat. It can occur at any age but is most common in young adult animals. German Shepherd Dogs appear to be predisposed. The nodules and plaques tend to wax and wane, with multiple lesions often occurring at the same time. The face, neck, back, and trunk are involved most commonly. Most lesions are nonpruritic, but they may ulcerate. Cutaneous histiocytosis does not progress to involve internal organs, but its diffuse nature and the unsightly appearance of the lesions often force the owner to consider euthanasia. Various forms of therapy have been tried, including systemic glucocorticoids, and a combination of glucocorticoids and chemotherapy. In some cases, glucocorticoids appear to induce remissions.

The **histiocytoses of Bernese Mountain Dogs** are systemic, familial disorders of unknown etiology with 2 manifestations: a more indolent and generally cutaneous form known as systemic histiocytosis; and a more aggressive form in which skin lesions are extremely rare, known as malignant histiocytosis. Malignant histiocytosis has been infrequently identified in other canine breeds. In systemic histiocytosis, males (mean age at onset 4 yr) are more often affected than females. There are multiple cutaneous nodules, papules, and plaques involving the skin (especially of the scrotum), nasal mucosa, and eyelids. The lesions are poorly circumscribed, variably alopecic, and may be ulcerated. The lesions develop in waves and slowly regress, only to recur several months later. The clinical disease tends to become more severe with each new wave of eruptions. Although the skin is the primary target organ, lesions may also develop in other organs including lymph nodes, spleen, and bone marrow. The disease may be episodic in its clinical presentation, but it is progressive and eventually fatal.

Malignant histiocytosis occurs in male Bernese Mountain Dogs (mean age at onset 7 yr) and, less frequently, in other canine breeds. The lungs, lymph nodes, and liver are the most common organs affected, and the disease tends to spare the skin. Grossly, the lesions appear as large, solitary, firm masses that may efface large portions of affected internal organs. It is rapidly progressive and does not wax and wane as does systemic histiocytosis. Few dogs survive >6 mo.

Various chemotherapeutic regimens have been used to treat both forms: bovine thymosin fraction 5 may be of benefit in inducing remissions, especially in the systemic form; however, both forms of the disease are ultimately fatal.

TRANSMISSIBLE VENEREAL TUMORS

See TRANSMISSIBLE CANINE VENEREAL TUMOR, p 683. These can also develop initially on haired skin due to inoculation via cutaneous injuries.

NEOPLASMS OF MELANOCYTIC ORIGIN

Melanocytic neoplasms are most common in dogs, gray horses, and miniature pigs, uncommon in goats and cattle, and rare in cats and sheep. Because of the importance of melanocytic lesions in human dermatology, 2 points need to be made: 1) The terminology used to describe melanocytic lesions in animals is markedly different from that used in human dermatology. In animals, the term "benign melanoma" and "malignant melanoma" are utilized to distinguish innocuous and aggressive neoplasms, respectively. In man, the term "nevus" is applied to all benign melanocytic lesions, and the term "melanoma" refers to all malignant melanocytic neoplasms. 2) Although solar injury is a common cause of melanocytic tumors in man, there is no evidence to suggest actinic damage can stimulate the development of these lesions in domestic animals.

In dogs, **benign melanomas** of the skin (considerably more common than malignant melanomas) most commonly develop on the head and forelimbs in middle-aged or older dogs; Scottish Terriers, Schnauzers, Doberman Pinschers, and Irish Setters are most at risk. They can appear as macules or patches, as papules or plaques, or as elevated, occasionally pedunculated masses. Most have a pigmented surface. Although generally solitary, multiple lesions may be present in the breeds at risk. These tumors are benign, and complete excision is curative.

Canine malignant melanomas most commonly develop at the mucocutaneous junctions of the lips, in the oral cavity (*see also* p 130), and in the nail beds. Malignant melanomas of haired skin are rare, and most arise on the ventral abdomen and the scrotum. Scottish Terriers and Golden Retrievers are the breeds most at risk for malignant melanomas that do not arise in the oral cavity. Males are affected more commonly than females. Most malignant melanomas appear as raised, generally ulcerated nodules that are variably pigmented. When present on the mucocutaneous regions of the lip, some tumors may be pedunculated with a papillated surface; when present in the nail bed, they appear as swellings of the digit, often with loss of the nail and destruction of underlying bone. Canine malignant melanomas are aggressive, and have considerable metastatic potential. Treatment generally consists of complete excision; however, the infiltrative nature of the tumor may make this difficult. Melanomas are generally considered insensitive to radiation therapy, and there is no established chemotherapeutic protocol.

Feline cutaneous melanocytic neoplasms are most commonly identified on the head and distal extremities, generally in middle-aged or older cats. Most are benign. Excision is the treatment of choice.

Most **melanocytic lesions in horses** occur in dark-skinned horses, in which the coat turns gray (or white) with age. They are especially common in Lippizaners, Arabians, and Percherons. They are generally recognized in older animals, but usually begin their development when animals are 3-4 yr old. They most commonly arise in the perineum and on the base of the tail, but may occur in any location including the parotid area. The tumors are often multiple and may appear as coalescent, frequently pedunculated nodules that may extend in a linear arrangement up the tail base. They are usually black on cut section.

Melanomas of gray horses increase in size and number over time and most are slowly infiltrative. Some are more aggressive, with wide cutaneous dissemination. Many gray horses have evidence of lymph node involvement; however, there is debate as to whether this represents metastasis or whether the intranodal melanocytes and melanophages represent a stimulation of extracutaneous melanocytes that are normally present in the lymph node. Treatment consists of surgical or cryosurgical removal; however, animals that develop one such tumor are predisposed to develop others over time.

Melanomas of non-gray horses are rare, considered to be a disease of older horses, and generally solitary on initial presentation. In general, they are highly infiltrative and have true metastatic potential. Excision or cryosurgery is the treatment of choice. The long-term prognosis is guarded.

Melanomas of pigs are rare except for congenital lesions in Sinclair (Hormel) miniature pigs and Duroc breeds. Selective breeding in these strains has increased the prevalence of tumors. These tumors develop both pre- and postnatally, and can occur anywhere on the body. Generally multiple, they can appear as pigmented macules or patches with smooth borders; as raised, often ulcerated pigmented lesions; or as deeper, slightly raised, blue masses. Deeply invasive melanomas are often associated with metastatic disease. The lymph nodes and lungs are the most common sites of metastasis. Not all become invasive; many undergo spontaneous regression associated with an intense lymphocytic infiltrate. Melanocytic lesions in pigs are not treated; because of the heritable nature of the disease, prevention by selective breeding is recommended if it is frequently recognized in a herd.

Melanomas in cattle develop infrequently anywhere on the body. They can occur at any age but are most commonly recognized in young animals; congenital forms have been recognized. Angus cattle appear to be predisposed. Most commonly they are large nodular masses, densely pigmented on cut surface. Excision is curative for most; however, rare malignant variants have been recognized with distant metastasis.

Melanomas in sheep occur most frequently in middle-aged or older animals but have been recognized in neonates. They are most common in Suffolks and Angoras. Most occur as multiple, densely pigmented dermal and/or subcut. masses. They should be considered malignant; metastasis is common.

Melanocytic tumors in goats are rare. They are most common in middle-aged or older animals, and possibly in Angoras. There may be a site predilection for the coronary band and udder. Lesions occur as solitary or multiple masses with variable pigmentation on cut surface. Most tend to grow rapidly and metastasis is common.

METASTATIC TUMORS, SKIN

The spread of a primary neoplasm to the skin is unusual in domestic animals. It is occasionally identified in dogs, less commonly in cats and rarely in horses, cows, sheep, goats, and pigs. Although all malignant neoplasms are capable of secondary cutaneous involvement, mammary gland adenocarcinomas, squamous cell carcinomas, transitional cell carcinomas, transmissible venereal tumors, and hemangiosarcomas are those with the greatest metastatic potential. Although appearance is variable, the lesions most commonly are multiple, ulcerated papulonodules. Early cutaneous metastasis is characterized by aggregates of neoplastic cells within superficial and deep dermal vessels. As these lesions evolve, they extend into the dermis and are associated with effacement of adnexa. Generally, it is difficult to distinguish the primary neoplasm based on the morphologic features of a metastatic site. This is because only a small population of cells in the primary tumor have the potential for metastasis, and these cells may have different microscopic features. Cutaneous metastasis has a guarded prognosis.

ULCERATIVE DERMATOSIS OF SHEEP
(Lip and leg ulceration, Venereal balanoposthitis and vulvitis)

An infectious, ulcerative, viral disease of sheep manifesting itself in 2 somewhat distinct forms, one characterized by formation of ulcers around the mouth and nose or on the legs (lip and leg ulceration), and the other as venereally transmitted ulceration of the prepuce and penis or vulva.

Clinical Findings: The lesion, regardless of location, is an ulcer with a raw, easily bleeding crater that varies in depth and extent, and contains an odorless, creamy pus; it is covered from the beginning with a scab.

Face lesions occur on the upper lip, between the border of the lip and the nasal orifice, on the chin, and on the nose. The ulcerative process may, in severe cases, perforate the lip. Foot lesions occur anywhere between the coronet and the carpus or tarsus.

Venereal lesions partially or completely surround the preputial orifice and may become so severe as to produce phimosis. Rarely, the ulcerative process may extend to the glans penis so that the ram becomes unfit for natural breeding. In ewes, edema, ulceration, and scabbing of the lips of the vulva have less serious consequences.

There are no noticeable early systemic reactions. Often, the disease remains unrecognized until the lesions are so advanced that signs of lameness or disturbed urination become apparent.

Diagnosis: This depends entirely on recognition of the characteristic ulcerative lesion. Differentiation between this lesion and that of orf (qv, p 784), which is essentially proliferative in character, is fundamental. The question of the similarity of the agents of ulcerative dermatosis and orf is not clearly defined, but inoculation of sheep previously immunized against orf helps in making a diagnosis. It is also difficult and, in some instances, impossible, without resorting to sheep inoculation, to differentiate between ulcerative posthitis and vulvitis (qv, p 699) and ulcerative dermatosis.

Prophylaxis and Treatment: Infected animals should be isolated, and those with genital lesions should not be bred. Recovery takes 2-8 wk and is not greatly influenced by treatment, which therefore, is usually not attempted unless the animals are to be bred soon, lip lesions interfere with eating, foot lesions make the animals so lame that they are losing flesh, or secondary bacterial infections become severe.

Treatment consists of removing the scabs and all necrotic tissue from the ulcers and applying any one of the following preparations: silver nitrate (styptic pencil), strong tincture of iodine, 30% copper sulfate solution, 4% formaldehyde, 5% cresol (sheep dip), or sulfa-urea powder. Foot and lower leg lesions can be treated with copper sulfate or formaldehyde solutions in footbath troughs.

URTICARIA
(Nettle rash, Hives)

A skin disorder characterized by multiple plaque-like eruptions, which are formed by localized edema in the dermis, and often develop and disappear suddenly.

The disease occurs in all domestic animals, but most often in horses (*see also* SWEET ITCH, p 804). Allergic urticaria may be exogenous or endogenous. Exogenous hives may be produced by toxic irritating products of the stinging nettle, the stings or bites of insects, or medications, and may occur more often in warm weather. Chemicals such as carbolic acid, turpentine, carbon disulfide, or crude oil also may be causative. Nonimmunologic factors such as pressure, sunlight, heat, exercise, psychologic stress, and genetic abnormalities may precipitate or intensify urticaria.

Sensitive animals, particularly shorthaired dogs and purebred horses, also may exhibit **dermographism**, a phenomenon wherein rubbing or whipping produces urticaria-like skin lesions. It is of no clinical significance.

Endogenous or "symptomatic" urticaria may develop after inhalation or absorption of ingested allergens, and has been seen mostly in horses and dogs (*see* ATOPIC DERMATITIS, p 427). In horses, it has been noted in the course of GI conditions, particularly severe constipation or inflammation of the intestinal mucosa. A unique form of urticaria has been described, chiefly in the Channel Island breeds of cattle (Jersey, Guernsey), which become sensitized to the casein in their own milk (*see also* p 426). It occurs in cases of milk retention or unusual engorgement of the udder with milk. Urticaria has been observed in bitches during estrus. In young horses, dogs, and pigs, urticaria has been associated with intestinal parasites. **Angioneurotic edema** is a life-threatening variant of urticaria in which there is diffuse subcut. edema, often localized to the head, limbs, or perineum.

Clinical Findings: The wheals or plaques appear within a few minutes or hours of exposure to the causative agent. In severe cases, the cutaneous eruptions are preceded by fever, anorexia, or dullness. Horses often become excited and restless. The skin lesions are elevated, rounded, flat-topped, 0.5-8 in. (1-20 cm) in diameter, and may be slightly depressed in the center. They can develop on any part of the body, but occur mainly on the back, flanks, neck, eyelids, and legs. In advanced cases, they may be found on the mucous membranes of the mouth, nose, conjunctiva, rectum, and vagina. As a rule, the lesions disappear as rapidly as they arise, usually within a few hours.

In sheep, lesions usually are observed only on the udder and hairless parts of the abdomen. In pigs, eruptions have been observed around the eyes, between the hindlegs, and on the snout, abdomen, and back.

In general, the prognosis is favorable. Fatalities are rare and are probably due to anaphylaxis or associated angioedema involving the respiratory passages.

Chronic urticaria is a diagnostic challenge. All allergens in an environment should be considered potential causes, and elimination of exposure instituted, if possible.

Treatment: Acute urticaria usually disappears spontaneously. The rapid-acting adrenocorticosteroids, eg, hydrocortisone sodium succinate, or prednisolone sodium succinate or hemisuccinate are reported to be useful. Dexamethasone (0.1 mg/kg) has been useful in dogs, cats, and horses. Antihistamines are of questionable value, and may induce urticaria if given IV. Epinephrine may be given in life-threatening situations. The lesions promptly disappear, but return rapidly if the allergen is not eliminated. Usually, local treatment of the lesions is not necessary. In especially severe cases, cold packs of water, vinegar, or alcohol (70%) may be applied.

URINARY SYSTEM

URN

URINARY SYSTEM, INTRODUCTION

The urinary system performs metabolic, humoral, and excretory functions. Most abnormalities of the urinary system can be diagnosed by physical examination, urinalysis, and interpretation of a serum chemistry profile. Diagnosis of some conditions may require additional and specific tests and knowledge of renal pathophysiology.

Signalment, history, and physical examination of the animal frequently provide most of the clues necessary to diagnose a urinary tract disorder. The history should include frequency of urination, volume of urine produced, and appearance and odor of the urine. Pollakiuria must be differentiated from polyuria; the presence of polydipsia suggests polyuria.

The physical examination should include palpation of the bladder, examination of the external genitalia, and a rectal examination for evaluation of the distal urethra in both sexes and the prostate in male dogs. A full neurologic examination is required for animals with urinary incontinence.

Urinalysis: This is the most important diagnostic test in evaluation of urinary tract disease. While voided samples are most commonly used for routine urinalysis, urine collected by cystocentesis or catheterization provides more accurate results for quantitative cultures. The latter methods minimize urethral and genital contamination of the urine sample.

A urinalysis should include evaluation of color, turbidity, specific gravity, and pH. The presence of protein, occult blood, glucose, ketones, bilirubin, and urobilinogen may be assessed by a dipstick method. A dipstick cannot differentiate between hemoglobinuria, myoglobinuria, or hematuria; however, examination of the urine sediment can confirm hematuria. The presence of protein in the urine should be evaluated in light of the urine specific gravity; very concentrated urine may have an increased protein concentration without pathologic significance.

Urine sediment examination allows detection of RBC, WBC, epithelial cells, renal casts, crystals, parasitic ova, and bacteria. Exfoliated neoplastic cells may be observed in the urine sediment of animals with a renal or lower urinary tract neoplasm. An active sediment with pyuria, hematuria, and/or crystalluria is highly suggestive of a bacterial urinary tract infection.

Quantitative urine cultures are useful for confirming bacterial urinary tract infections and determining appropriate antibiotic therapy. Voided urine samples with bacterial concentrations >100,000 colony forming units (CFU)/mL of urine are indicative of bacterial infection; >10,000 CFU/mL in a catheterized urine sample, or >1000 CFU/mL in a sample obtained by cystocentesis are evidence of bacterial infection.

Complete collection of urine for a specified time period provides information on fractional excretion of electrolytes, glomerular filtration rate (GFR), and protein excretion. Protein excretion may also be evaluated by obtaining a urine protein to creatinine ratio in a random urine sample. The method correlates well with results obtained using 24-hr urine collections as long as the urine sediment is inactive. The urine protein to creatinine ratio is normally <2 in dogs. A ratio >2 is indicative of a protein-losing nephropathy, and values >10 are frequently associated with renal amyloidosis.

Other Diagnostics: Evaluation of serum chemistries including BUN, creatinine, calcium and phosphorus, and serum electrolytes is required to confirm renal dysfunction. Abdominal radiographs, contrast studies of the upper and lower urinary tract, ultrasonic examination of the kidneys and bladder, cystoscopic examination of the bladder, or renal biopsy may be required to identify a particular urinary tract disorder. Renal biopsies may be obtained via a laparotomy, laparoscopy, or percutaneous methods. While the kidney has a limited range of responses to disease, renal histopathology provides diagnostic and prognostic information.

PRINCIPLES OF THERAPY

See also p 1407.

Diseases of the urinary system may result from a variety of pathological processes that may occur anywhere in the system. Appropriate therapy depends on the location, severity, and etiology of the problem. Therapy should be instituted only after an accurate history, a complete physical examination, and a minimal laboratory data base (complete blood count, serum chemistry analysis, urinalysis, and urine culture) are assessed. The most desirable therapy is removal of the specific cause. Often, this is not possible, and nonspecific or supportive therapy must be instituted.

Acute urinary obstruction is commonly an emergency. Relief is usually accomplished by mechanical manipulation or surgical removal of the cause. Medical therapy is commonly required to alleviate the azotemia by replacing fluid deficits and correcting acidosis and hyperkalemia. Clinical improvement is seen in 24-48 hr since urinary obstruction does not result in permanent parenchymal injury to the kidneys. Treatment of chronic obstruction is more complicated since it requires a thorough search for the site and cause of obstruction; surgery is commonly required to eliminate the cause.

Treatment of acute renal failure requires several days to 2 wk of medical management before it can be determined whether kidney regeneration will be adequate to sustain the animal. Treatment commonly includes parenteral fluids to control fluid balance, and correction of acidosis, hyperkalemia, hyperphosphatemia, and possibly hypertension. In anuria, use of vasodilators such as dopamine or osmotic diuretics may be helpful. If these conservative measures are inadequate, peritoneal dialysis or hemodialysis may be instituted to maintain homeostasis for 1-2 wk while the kidneys are regenerating.

Therapy for chronic renal failure is complex and continually changes as the disease progresses. Special long-term nutritional support may be required to control hyperphosphatemia, restrict protein, maintain calcium balance, maintain vitamin intake, and supply adequate caloric intake in an animal with anorexia and intermittent vomiting. Other considerations may include controlling hypertension, treating acidosis, and using anabolic steroids or recombinant erythropoietin to promote hematopoiesis.

The nephrotic syndrome (qv, p 880) is a therapeutic dilemma, particularly if the animal also has renal failure. If renal failure is absent, treatment can focus on removal of the immunological process or immunosuppression to reduce urinary protein loss. Effective treatment has been rare in animals with glomerulonephritis. Many animals with glomerulonephritis remain in protein balance, which reduces the need for treatment. Plasma transfusions may be given to animals with severe hypoalbuminemia to prevent complications of hypoproteinemia, but the value of protein supplements has not been documented. In animals with a protein-losing nephropathy in renal failure, the need for protein restriction represents a paradox that makes treatment difficult and conflicting. When the cause of the protein loss is amyloidosis, progression is rapid, and treatment is usually unsuccessful.

Simple urinary tract infections are treated initially with a broad-spectrum antibiotic. If the infection persists, antibiotic selection should be based on the results of a culture and sensitivity test. Duration of treatment may vary from 3 wk to several months depending on resistance of the organism and the site of infection. Most urinary tract infections can be effectively resolved within 3 wk. Chronic, recurring infections usually are those associated with pyelonephritis, prostatitis, urolithiasis, or bladder atony.

Medical therapy for urolithiasis is a matter of dissolving calculi, or preventing their recurrence, or both. This is accomplished by creating an undersaturated urine with respect to the type of urolith by use of either diet or specific medication. A mineral-deficient diet has been effective in control of struvite calculi. Other types of uroliths, the so-called metabolic calculi, including cystine, urate, and calcium oxalate, require specific medical treatment.

Renal tubular defects may be treated specifically, depending on the loss or retention of a given solute, eg, the uric acid defect resulting in urate stones responds to treatment with allopurinol. Some forms of tubular defects, eg, renal glycosuria, may not require treatment. Renal tubular acidosis may require bicarbonate therapy depending on the form of acidosis.

CONGENITAL AND INHERITED ANOMALIES OF THE URINARY SYSTEM

Anomalies of the urinary system are uncommon. Defects of the kidneys include cysts, horseshoe kidney, ring kidney, hypoplasia, and aplasia. In dogs and cats, these anomalies may result in progressive azotemia, or may be asymptomatic. Diagnosis is usually made by contrast radiography, ultrasonography, or exploratory laparotomy.

Renal Dysplasia and Hypoplasia: These defects are most common in dogs (Norwegian Elkhound, Lhasa Apso, Shih Tzu, Samoyed, Cocker Spaniel, Doberman Pinscher, and Standard Poodle). The dysplasia may be unilateral or bilateral, and the kidneys are usually small, firm, and pale; some kidneys have a uniformly diminished renal cortex. On histological examination, such kidneys demonstrate primitive and bizarre tubules and glomerular structures, and excess fibrous tissue.

Affected animals usually have polydipsia and polyuria, which precede signs of uremia. Dwarfing occurs if the onset of renal failure occurs within the first few months of life. Changes in the urinalysis, hemogram, and blood chemistry are the same as in other chronic, progressive renal diseases. Uremia is usually present at 6 mo to 2 yr of age. The diagnosis can be suspected based on breed and age of onset, and may be confirmed by renal biopsy. Treatment is as for any other chronic renal failure.

Ectopic Ureter: This defect has been most commonly reported in dogs (usually females) and usually is first noticed at 3-6 mo of age. Continual dripping of urine is the classic sign, although normal voiding may occur in dogs with a unilateral ectopic ureter. A low-grade vaginitis or vulvitis may be present due to urine scalding. The ureter(s) involved may open into the urethra, prostate, or vagina. Diagnosis may be confirmed by an IV pyelogram that traces the course of the ureter. The most successful treatment is transplantation of the affected ureters into the bladder. Animals with ectopic ureters that terminate in the urethra often remain incontinent at a reduced level following surgery, although use of an adrenergic agent such as phenylpropanolamine may minimize the incontinence.

Unilateral Renal Agenesis: This is relatively common in cats and quite rare in dogs. One kidney and its associated ureter are usually absent. Usually, this is an incidental finding in cats, and renal function is normal.

Polycystic Kidneys or Solitary Cysts: Also known as congenital cystic kidneys, multiple cyst formation largely replaces the renal parenchyma. It is relatively uncommon in both dogs and cats. Such kidneys are usually found to be grossly enlarged on palpation. Polycystic kidneys may cause no clinical signs or may lead to progressive renal failure. Diagnosis usually is based on physical and radiographic findings, ultrasonic examination, or exploratory laparotomy. Pyelonephritis is common in such kidneys and may precipitate renal insufficiency.

Miscellaneous Anomalies: Double or multiple renal arteries are seen in ~5% of dogs. Other congenital defects, including renal fusion, persistent urachus, double bladder, and congenital hydronephrosis and hydroureter, are relatively infrequent in both dogs and cats. Nephroblastoma, an embryonal tumor, is rare in domestic animals except pigs; it may cause no problems, but may be very large and cause abdominal distention. While uncommon, the penile urethra may open on the ventral surface of the penis (hypospadias) or on its dorsal surface (epispadias).

INFECTIOUS DISEASES OF THE URINARY SYSTEM, SM AN

Bacterial infections of the urinary tract are common in dogs and uncommon in cats. Cystitis is more common in female than male dogs. *Escherichia coli, Staphylococcus aureus, Proteus* and *Klebsiella* spp, and intestinal streptococci are the most commonly isolated pathogens. In cystitis and pyelonephritis, infections are usually ascending. Predisposing factors include urinary stasis, micturition disorders, acquired or congenital defects of the bladder wall, urolithiasis, catheterization, and immunosuppression. Differentiation of upper tract versus lower tract infection is important prognostically as well as therapeutically. While fungal infections of the urinary tract are rare, candidiasis may occur in animals that are immunosuppressed or have received long-term antibiotic therapy. Systemic mycotic infections, eg, blastomycosis, may involve the urinary tract.

CYSTITIS

Signs are pollakiuria, hematuria, and dysuria; some animals may break house-training. Hematuria may be most prominent in the last part of the voided urine. The bladder wall may be palpably thickened or tender. Infections may be asymptomatic and detected incidentally during routine urinalysis.

Diagnosis: The history and physical findings may be suggestive but are not sufficient to establish a diagnosis. Urinalysis and culture of a urine sample obtained by sterile technique must be performed. Cystocentesis is preferred to catheterization for obtaining a sterile sample. The urinalysis in a typical urinary tract infection reveals elevated Hgb and protein, and increased numbers of RBC, WBC, and bacteria; the pH may be alkaline, especially if the infection is caused by urease-positive bacteria such as *Staphylococcus* or *Proteus* spp. Fungal infections are usually diagnosed by observation of fungal elements in the urine sediment; confirmation is by fungal culture.

Predisposing causes must be considered in chronic or recurrent bacterial cystitis. Persistence of clinical signs despite appropriate antimicrobial therapy suggests additional disease in the lower urinary tract, eg, urolithiasis or neoplasia. Double contrast cystourethrography or ultrasonography is used to diagnose calculi, neoplasia, and anatomic defects. Pyelonephritis (*see* below) should be ruled out. Chronic prostatitis (qv, p 697) in dogs can be diagnosed by cytology and culture of prostatic fluid obtained by ejaculation or prostatic massage. A complete blood count and serum chemistry profile should be done to rule out predisposing systemic diseases, eg, diabetes mellitus or hyperadrenocorticism.

Treatment: First episodes of cystitis should be treated for 2-3 wk with an antibiotic, preferably based on culture and sensitivity; without a culture, broad-spectrum antibiotics that achieve high concentration in the urine should be used. Ampicillin or a trimethoprim-sulfonamide combination may be administered since most urinary pathogens are sensitive to these agents. The drug should be administered following urination, and urination discouraged at other times to lengthen the time medicated urine remains in the bladder. To maximize the rate of absorption, the animal should not be fed for >30 min after the drug is administered. A urinalysis should be performed 3-5 days after cessation of therapy; the urine should be cultured at that time if an active urine sediment is observed. No further treatment is indicated if the sediment is inactive; if the urine culture is positive, a second course of antibiotics is given for a minimum of 3 wk.

If the subsequent urine culture remains positive, the animal should be evaluated radiographically and ultrasonically for predisposing causes. If none are found, antibiotic therapy is reinstituted for 4-6 wk. Urine is cultured again after antibiotics are discontinued. If the culture remains positive, antibiotic suppression therapy may be indicated: a broad-spectrum antibiotic given in the evenings, at one-quarter to one-third the normal daily dose for 4-6 mo, after which urine cultures are repeated. Life-long therapy may be required. Supportive therapy that aids in the mechanical washout of bacteria from the bladder may be useful. The animal should be allowed frequent opportunities to urinate and, for cats, litter boxes should be kept clean and available.

PYELONEPHRITIS

Acute pyelonephritis can cause systemic signs such as fever, anorexia, depression, vomiting, and pain during palpation of the kidneys. Chronic pyelonephritis may be subclinical, cause intermittent fever, anorexia, and depression, or result in uremia if sufficient renal tissue is destroyed. Decreased urine-concentrating ability may cause polydipsia and polyuria. Coexistent cystitis may cause signs of lower urinary tract disease.

Diagnosis: The history and physical findings may be suggestive of acute pyelonephritis, but usually are not helpful in chronic infections. Elevated serum urea nitrogen and creatinine concentrations as well as other laboratory abnormalities associated with renal failure may be present. The urinalysis in most animals is consistent with bacterial infection (see CYSTITIS, above) and yields a positive bacterial culture. Bacterial or WBC casts in the urine are strongly suggestive of pyelonephritis. The urinalysis is normal and urine cultures negative in those few animals in which the infection is localized to the renal parenchyma.

Confirming pyelonephritis can be difficult. Radiographs and ultrasonography may demonstrate enlarged kidneys in acute pyelonephritis, small and irregular ones in chronic pyelonephritis. Evaluation of an IV urogram may reveal evidence of pyelonephritis (dilated, blunted calices) or ureteritis (dilated, tortuous ureters). Renal biopsy and culture are occasionally necessary to definitively diagnose pyelonephritis and identify the pathogen.

Treatment: Antibiotic therapy for a minimum of 4-6 wk is necessary, based on results of urine or renal biopsy culture and sensitivity. Urine culture should be repeated 7-10 days after cessation of antibiotics, and subsequently at 30-day intervals until 3 consecutive negative cultures are obtained. Animals with chronic or recurrent infections should be evaluated for predisposing causes, which should be corrected if possible. Chronic infections can sometimes be controlled with antibiotic suppression therapy (see CYSTITIS, above).

Animals with renal failure secondary to pyelonephritis should be given appropriate fluid and medical therapy (see RENAL FAILURE, p 877).

INTERSTITIAL NEPHRITIS

Acute interstitial nephritis in dogs may be due to leptospiral infections (qv, p 355). Other specific causes of acute or chronic interstitial nephritis are rarely identified. Pollakiuria, hematuria, weight loss, and pain may be caused by kidney worm infection (see below).

CAPILLARIA PLICA INFECTION

This thread-like worm (females to 60 mm long), found occasionally in the pelvis of the kidney, ureter, or bladder of dogs, cats, and other animals, has been reported from North America, Europe, and the USSR. It usually produces no clinical signs. The earthworm is the intermediate host. These worms produce eggs somewhat similar to those of whipworms (but colorless), which are passed in the urine. While neither fenbendazole (50 mg/kg/day for 3 days) nor ivermectin (200 µg/kg) is approved for this use, both have been used effectively for treatment of cystitis in dogs in the rare cases when C plica caused disease. (Note: some sensitive dogs react severely to this dose of ivermectin, qv, p 1493.)

Levamisole seems to be effective for treatment of infections with C felis cati, a similar parasite of the bladder in cats.

GIANT KIDNEY WORM INFECTION IN THE MINK AND DOG

Dioctophyma renale occurs most commonly in mink and occasionally in dogs and many other species, including man. The females are the largest nematodes known, at 75-100 cm long and ≥1 cm in diameter; males are smaller, up to 35 cm long. The adults are red and live in the renal tissues, almost invariably in the right kidney. The renal parenchyma is gradually destroyed as the female worm grows.

Pitted, thick-shelled eggs with bipolar plugs are passed in the urine; if ingested by oligochaete annelids, they hatch, and infective larvae develop. Infection is by ingestion of the annelid or a paratenic host (eg, bullhead, pike) that has fed on infected annelid worms. Larvae migrate from the stomach or duodenum to the peritoneal cavity and, occasionally, the liver before maturing in the kidney. Eggs are passed in the urine 4-6 mo after infection. Reported cases in dogs are relatively few; the incidence in mink is 2-48%.

Clinical Findings and Diagnosis: Signs do not develop until the parasites approach or reach maturity. The sequence involves a marked weight loss, hematuria, frequent urination, restlessness, and evidence of severe abdominal or lumbar pain. Anemia may occur secondary to blood loss. Diagnosis is based on clinical signs and presence of the eggs in the urine. The adult worm may sometimes be detected radiographically or ultrasonically.

Prophylaxis and Treatment: Preventing ingestion of raw fish or other aquatic organisms is recommended, especially in areas where the parasite is known to occur in wild animals. Nephrectomy, in the early stages of infection, leads to rapid recovery.

INFECTIOUS DISEASES OF THE URINARY SYSTEM, LG AN

BOVINE CYSTITIS AND PYELONEPHRITIS
(Contagious bovine pyelonephritis)

A sporadic inflammatory disease of the urinary tract of cattle and sometimes sheep. The causative agent is almost always *Corynebacterium renale*; however, *Escherichia coli, C pyogenes*, streptococci, staphylococci, and unidentified diphtheroid bacilli also have produced urinary tract infections, either as the sole agent involved or in a mixed infection with *C renale*.

Epidemiology: Aberrant *C renale* infections have been reported in horses and dogs. The disease is of economic importance in cattle and occasionally in sheep. Cows are affected more commonly than bulls. *Corynebacterium renale* has been cultured from the vulva, vagina, and penile sheath of apparently normal cattle. It is now recognized as the cause of ulcerative posthitis and vulvitis of sheep (qv, p 699), and a similar disease is seen in pigs (*see* below). Experimentally, the bacteria that have been isolated produce pyelonephritis in mice. The incidence of carrier cows is significantly higher in herds with clinical cases than in herds with no clinical signs of pyelonephritis before a sporadic case appears. Transmission is possibly favored by grooming with contaminated brushes, vulvar contact with urine-soiled bedding, tail switching, and use of improperly sterilized obstetric instruments, particularly urinary catheters. Venereal transmission seems to be a likely means of spread in animals bred by natural service.

Susceptibility to the disease appears to be increased by the stress of heavy feeding, high production, advanced pregnancy, or cold weather.

Clinical Findings: Gradual loss of condition occurs over weeks or months. Animals in the advanced stages are emaciated and dehydrated, and have a poor appetite. Generally, pulse and respiratory rates are normal; temperature may fluctuate. Most cases are progressive, but temporary remissions occur in some.

Restlessness, kicking the abdomen, switching the tail, pollakiuria, and straining are common signs. Frequent passing of bloody urine that contains blood clots is considered to be almost pathognomonic. In advanced cases, it is possible to detect the enlarged painful kidney, ureter, and thick-walled bladder by careful rectal palpation. In early cases showing severe signs, palpation findings may be normal. Palpation of the ureters by the vaginal route in mature cows reveals a cord-like ureter that often contains crepitating blood clots. The ureters are most easily located several inches proximal to their entrance into the neck of the bladder. The stance may resemble that associated with traumatic pericarditis, gastritis, or indigestion.

Lesions: The urethra is inflamed, edematous, and streaked with submucosal ecchymoses. The bladder contains considerable cellular debris, clotted and free blood, and a characteristic "sandy" deposit. The bladder wall is greatly thickened and edematous; its mucosa is hemorrhagic and may be ulcerated, and large vesicle-like swellings usually are present over most of the epithelial surface. The ureters are usually greatly enlarged, from several times their normal diameter up to 2.5 cm; the walls are thickened, edematous, and hemorrhagic; the lumina often are filled with blood clots, pus, and necrotic kidney tissue.

Although the infection may be unilateral, both kidneys are generally involved and may be 2-3 times their normal size. The external cortical lobulations frequently are ill-defined, and the surface may be almost smooth. The capsule may be adherent. The calices are filled with a gray slimy exudate, shreds of necrotic tissue, clotted blood, and urine. Calculi and sand-like precipitate are present, as is a strong odor of ammonia. Numerous abscesses and hemorrhages occur throughout the medulla and cortex. Atrophy of the parenchyma and considerable fibrosis occur in advanced cases. In general, the infection is characterized by an active, extensive, and diffuse necrotizing inflammatory process.

Diagnosis: The signs are reasonably distinctive. Generally, only 1 or 2 animals in a herd are affected at any one time. Herd history may indicate that sporadic infections have occurred in the past. Pyelonephritis should be differentiated from other diseases such as leptospirosis and bacillary or postparturient hemoglobinuria, in which hematuria or hemoglobinuria are constant findings. A stained smear of the sediment of a centrifuged urine sample from an animal with pyelonephritis due to *C renale* contains clumps and parallel arrangements of gram-positive, pleomorphic bacterial rods. Urine from suspected cases may be cultured for *C renale.*

Treatment: If therapy is initiated before enlargement of ureters and kidneys can be palpated, animals infected with *C renale* usually respond dramatically to penicillin therapy, while those infected with *E coli* do not. In all cases, the effectiveness of therapy should be checked by bacteriological examination of the urine sediment. Relapse is common, especially in advanced cases; to avoid it, the course of treatment must be at least 7 days, and 8-15 days is recommended. Treatment should be repeated if the organism is present in urine sediment 1 mo after cessation of therapy. Other antibiotics may be of value, but critical studies of their efficacy have not been reported. In general, the sulfonamides have not proved as valuable as the penicillins.

PORCINE CYSTITIS

While less well characterized than bovine pyelonephritis (*see* above), this condition is occasionally a serious problem, particularly if stress is significant in large piggeries. The cause is *Eubacterium (Corynebacterium) suis*. Although boars may be infected, and in small units a single boar may appear to be the source of infection for all affected sows, it is primarily a disease of mature sows. Sows may die without signs having been observed. Depression, anorexia, and passage of blood-stained urine are characteristic. Indications of pain during urination may be seen. Gross lesions include cystitis and, sometimes, ureteritis and pyelonephritis. Penicillin may be effective if given early enough.

SWINE KIDNEY WORM INFECTION

Etiology: Adult *Stephanurus dentatus* (20-45 mm long and ~2 mm in diameter) are found in the kidneys, walls of the ureters, and perirenal fat. The kidney worm is widely distributed, particularly in tropical and subtropical areas, and is primarily a parasite of pigs raised outdoors. The eggs hatch shortly after being passed in the urine; the larvae reach the infective stage in ~3-5 days and are susceptible to cold, desiccation, and sunlight. The earthworm serves as a paratenic host, and the usual means of infection is via ingestion of the infective larvae of earthworms. Transdermal infections have been reported. They migrate to the liver and, after extensive migration through the liver tissue for ≥ 3 mo, the larvae pierce the capsule and enter the abdominal cavity. The larvae settle in or near the kidney, and occasionally in other tissues or organs. Patent infections in pigs <5 mo old were acquired prenatally.

Clinical Findings and Diagnosis: Heavy experimental infections of kidney worms have an adverse effect on growth. Pleuritis and peritonitis are common. The principal economic loss results from condemnation of organs and tissues affected by migrating worms. The most severe lesions are usually in the liver, which shows cirrhosis, scar formation, extensive thrombosis of the portal vessels, and a variable amount of necrosis. Kidney and lung damage are also common.

When worms are in the kidney or ureter or in cysts that open into the ureter, eggs may be recovered in the urine. Prepatent infections are difficult to diagnose, and a definitive diagnosis depends on demonstration of the worms or lesions at necropsy.

Control: Good control practices are indicated in areas where the worm is known to occur. Because of the long prepatent period, control may be achieved with a "gilts only" breeding program, which prevents patent infection from developing: older boars are replaced with young boars from clean herds, and only gilts are bred and then sold after weaning. Eradication within 2 yr has been reported. Indoor housing or rigorous outdoor sanitation, including provision of a concrete pad under the feeding troughs, also reduces the problem significantly.

Ivermectin (300 μg/kg) and fenbendazole (3 mg/kg/day for 3 days) are effective against *Stephanurus* sp. Experimentally, levamisole (8 mg/kg) stopped egg production in 4 days, and the urine remained free of eggs for the following 6 wk.

NONINFECTIOUS DISEASES OF THE URINARY SYSTEM, SM AN

RENAL FAILURE

Inability of the kidneys to perform their normal functions may be classified as prerenal, renal, or postrenal in origin. Prerenal azotemia is the result of reduced blood flow to the kidney due to such causes as dehydration, congestive heart failure, or shock. Prerenal azotemia may completely resolve with appropriate treatment or may progress to renal disease and failure. Renal azotemia (primary renal parenchymal disease) may occur secondary to acute or chronic renal failure. Postrenal causes of azotemia include tears or ruptures in the urinary tract (usually traumatic in origin) as well as obstruction to urine outflow by calculi, neoplasia, or blood clots.

CHRONIC RENAL FAILURE

A condition resulting from prolonged, significant, and usually progressive loss of functional renal tissue. No sex predilection has been reported. Chronic renal failure usually occurs in older animals, although congenital renal disease may cause renal failure in animals <1 yr old. This condition has been described as chronic interstitial nephritis, but since the term essentially describes the morphological appearance of kidneys with chronic, progressive, and irreversible renal disease, it does not contribute to the understanding of the underlying cause. Identifiable causes of chronic renal failure include pyelonephritis, amyloidosis, chronic obstructive uropathy, congenital lesions, glomerulonephritis, and neoplasia.

Clinical Findings: Polydipsia, polyuria, and occasional vomiting are the early signs. As renal failure progresses over weeks or months to years, anorexia, weight loss, dehydration, oral ulceration, vomiting, and diarrhea are seen. In the terminal stages, severe dehydration, vomiting, convulsions, and coma lead to death. Mucous membranes will be pale if anemia is present. Loose teeth, deformable maxilla and mandible, or pathologic fractures may be seen with renal secondary osteodystrophy. Careful palpation may reveal small, irregular kidneys in animals with end-stage renal disease, or large kidneys in animals with tumors or hydronephrosis.

Diagnosis: The BUN, serum creatinine, and inorganic phosphorus levels are elevated. A moderate to severe nonregenerative anemia, metabolic acidosis, and hypertension develop as renal function decreases. Osteoporosis may be seen radiographically. Urine specific gravity in normal dogs usually is 1.008-1.029; in dogs with renal dysfunction, the specific gravity may be fixed at 1.008-1.012. However, dogs with primary glomerular disease may become azotemic while retaining some urine-concentrating ability. Cats with chronic renal failure usually produce urine with a specific gravity of 1.008-1.034, probably because of their normal ability to produce very concentrated urine.

The polydipsia and polyuria of chronic renal failure must be differentiated from those associated with diabetes (insipidus or mellitus), pyometra, pyelonephritis without renal failure, and hyperadrenocorticism. Adrenal insufficiency may be confused with primary renal failure, since prerenal azotemia may be caused by vomiting, diarrhea, and polydipsia.

Contrast radiography, abdominal ultrasonography, specific renal function tests, urine culture, and renal biopsy may be performed to determine the cause and severity of renal disease. In most cases, however, the advanced stages of renal failure preclude identification of the underlying cause. The condition then is described as end-stage renal disease. Chronic renal failure must be distinguished from acute renal failure, which is potentially reversible. Frequently, this may be accomplished with a careful history, physical examination, and the laboratory findings listed above, although a renal biopsy may be required.

Treatment: Severe loss of renal tissue is a permanently disabling condition. However, animals can survive for long periods with only a small fraction of normal renal tissue. Recommended treatment varies with the severity of signs. Animals with minimal clinical abnormalities (such as occasional vomiting) can be managed medically at home. Fresh drinking water should always be available. Dietary restriction of protein may relieve some of the signs and, in addition, may help slow the inevitable progression of renal failure. High-quality protein, eg, egg or liver, should be fed at a level of 2 g/kg body wt/day for dogs and 3.5 g/kg body wt/day for cats. Commercial diets formulated for cats and dogs with chronic renal failure are available. A protein- and mineral-restricted diet also helps reduce the serum phosphorus concentration, which may be beneficial in slowing progression of the disease. If dietary restriction of protein is unsuccessful in maintaining a normal serum phosphorus level, phosphate-binding gels containing aluminum hydroxide should be administered PO. Administration of an H_2-receptor antagonist such as cimetidine (5 mg/kg, PO, 3-4 times daily) decreases gastric acidity and vomiting, and may reduce parathyroid hormone levels, which decreases serum phosphorus concentration. Sodium bicarbonate, given PO, may be indicated if the animal is acidotic. Multiple B-vitamin preparations should be given (PO) to compensate for urinary losses of water-soluble vitamins. Recombinant erythropoietin or anabolic steroids such as oxymethalone or nandrolone are administered to stimulate RBC production in animals that are anemic; blood transfusions may be required to maintain an adequate PCV. The hypertension seen with chronic renal failure may be at least partially alleviated by feeding a low-salt diet. Change from a normal-salt to a low-salt diet must be gradual to prevent volume depletion. IV fluid therapy (qv, p 1355) is required in animals with severe signs of uremia. Euthanasia may be indicated if fluid therapy does not improve renal function and alleviate signs of uremia.

ACUTE RENAL FAILURE

Acute renal failure occurs when a major insult to the kidneys results in inability to regulate water and solute balance; this may occur with reduced, normal, or increased urine flow. Causes include: toxins, such as heavy metals, ethylene glycol, aminoglycoside antibiotics, methoxyflurane, and phenacetin; vasculitides, including acute glomerulonephritis and lupus erythematosus; prolonged ischemia; infarction due to embolic showers from bacterial endocarditis or disseminated intravascular coagulation; infection, including acute pyelonephritis or leptospirosis; hemoglobinuria or myoglobinuria; and hypercalcemia, which in dogs is usually a paraneoplastic syndrome associated with lymphosarcoma (see HUMORAL HYPERCALCEMIA OF MALIGNANCY, p 285).

Clinical Findings: Signs of acute renal failure include anorexia, depression, dehydration, oral ulceration, vomiting, diarrhea, and hypothermia. Physical findings usually are not remarkable, although pain may be elicited on palpation of the kidneys.

Diagnosis: Affected animals have elevated BUN and serum creatinine and phosphorus concentrations; metabolic acidosis; and hyperkalemia, if oliguria or anuria is present. The history and all clinical and laboratory findings should be evaluated carefully to differentiate acute from chronic renal failure. Animals with prerenal azotemia have concentrated urine, whereas dogs with acute renal failure have urine with a specific gravity of 1.008-1.029, and cats 1.008-1.034. A renal biopsy may be necessary to determine the severity, extent, cause, and potential reversibility of the disease.

Treatment: If the cause of the acute renal failure is known, specific therapy should be instituted, eg, 4-methyl-pyrazole or ethanol for ethylene glycol toxicity (qv, p 1648). Fluid therapy (qv, p 1355) is indicated for all animals with acute renal failure. A polyionic fluid such as lactated Ringer's solution is satisfactory unless hyperkalemia is present, in which case normal saline is recommended. Sodium bicarbonate may be added to the fluid to correct acidosis. Urine production and/or central venous pressure must be monitored closely to prevent overhydration in cases of oliguria or anuria. Therapy to promote urine flow should be instituted if the animal is well hydrated and urine production is <20 mL/kg/day. This may include furosemide (2 mg/kg, IV, which can be doubled and then tripled at 1-hr intervals if urine production does not increase), osmotic diuresis (20% dextrose or mannitol, 0.5, g/kg IV slowly, alternated with infusion of lactated Ringer's solution 30-60 mL/kg, IV), and/or renal vasodilators (dopamine diluted in 5% dextrose, IV infusion to provide 1-5 µg/kg/min). Peritoneal dialysis or hemodialysis is necessary if none of the above measures restores urine production. Fluid therapy is continued until renal function improves and the animal's clinical condition stabilizes.

OBSTRUCTIVE UROPATHY

Even though the kidneys would otherwise be able to function normally, obstruction to urine flow at any point below the level of the kidneys leads to accumulation of metabolic wastes and acute renal failure. Obstruction of the urethra by uroliths in dogs, and by crystalline and mucoprotein plugs in cats is the most common cause, although tumors or blood clots in the urethra or ureters also may be responsible.

Hydronephrosis is characterized by dilatation of the renal pelvis as the result of partial or complete obstruction to outflow of urine from one or both kidneys. When the obstruction is acute, complete, and bilateral, less extensive changes in the kidneys occur because the period of survival is short. In unilateral or partial obstruction, the animal survives long enough to have severe pressure atrophy of the renal parenchyma and cystic enlargement of the affected kidney. Hydroureter is a common accompaniment and is seen when the obstruction occurs lower in the tract. Increased hydrostatic pressure results in atrophy of functional renal parenchyma. The papillae of the medulla disappear first; later, even the cortex may atrophy. The affected kidney eventually becomes a grossly enlarged, functionless sac, filled with urine or serous fluid.

Clinical Findings: Animals with urethral obstruction have strangury, and frequently, hematuria; they may have marked abdominal pain, especially if the obstruction is bilateral. Signs of renal failure develop rapidly and include vomiting, dehydration, hypothermia, and severe depression. The bladder is distended and painful on palpation, and a catheter cannot be passed into it. Bradycardia or cardiac arrhythmias due to acidosis and hyperkalemia may be present. Since compensatory hypertrophy of the nonaffected kidney results in a nonazotemic state, unilateral ureteral obstruction commonly goes undiagnosed unless the enlarged kidney is palpated.

Diagnosis: The history, clinical signs, and physical examination usually provide a straightforward diagnosis of urethral obstruction. An IV pyelogram or abdominal ultrasonography is necessary in ureteral obstruction. Serum potassium levels should be determined immediately in animals with cardiac arrhythmias. An ECG can provide presumptive evidence of hyperkalemia if laboratory results are delayed (bradycardia; tall, peaked T waves; increased P-R interval; widened QRS complex; atrial standstill).

Treatment: The urethral obstruction should be relieved (see UROLITHIASIS, p 885). Fluids are administered IV to improve renal function and correct electrolyte abnormalities. Normal saline is the fluid of choice; sodium bicarbonate is added to correct acidosis and hyperkalemia. In animals with severe hyperkalemia and cardiac arrhythmias, dextrose or regular insulin and dextrose infusions can be given to drive potassium intracellularly. Large quantities of fluids may be required as the animal undergoes a postobstructive diuresis for 1-5 days. Serum electrolytes, body weight, urine output, PCV, and plasma total solids should be monitored daily, and appropriate adjustments made in the type and quantity of fluid administered.

Surgery is necessary for ureteral obstruction. When possible, the obstruction should be removed to reestablish urine flow; however, unilateral nephrectomy is often required.

DISEASE OF THE GLOMERULUS

Animals with primary glomerular disease may have somewhat different clinical and laboratory abnormalities than those with interstitial disease. Damage to the glomerular basement membrane results in albuminuria, which may lead to hypoalbuminemia. Animals may exhibit signs related to hypoalbuminemia rather than uremia. Although uncommon in both cats and dogs, glomerulopathies are less common in cats. No age, sex, or breed predilection has been reported.

Glomerulonephritis is an immune-mediated disease characterized by deposition or *in situ* formation of immune complexes in the glomerular capillary wall, which then incite inflammatory changes (see also p 430.) In cats, it is frequently associated with infection by feline leukemia virus; in some dogs, it has been associated with adenovirus, pyometra, neoplasia, systemic lupus erythematosus (SLE), and heartworm disease. Membranoproliferative glomerulonephritis has been reported in a group of young, related Doberman Pinschers, suggesting a familial disease, and a family of Samoyeds with an X-linked dominant inheritance of glomerular disease has been reported.

Amyloid is the name given to any of several chemically inert fibrillar glycoproteins that can be deposited in tissue and interfere with normal organ function. (*See also* AMYLOIDOSIS, p 319.) All of these proteins are deposited in a β-pleated sheet conformation, which results in the unique appearance and chemical properties of amyloid. In dogs, amyloid usually is deposited in glomeruli; in cats, it is more frequently found in the medullary interstitium.

Clinical Findings: Many animals with renal amyloidosis develop the nephrotic syndrome (massive proteinuria, reduced albumin concentration, and hypercholesterolemia). While a feature of human nephrotic syndrome, edema may or may not be present in other animals. Azotemia is not a consistent finding in the early stages, but most animals with nephrotic syndrome progress to chronic renal failure over a variable time period. Proteinuria (primarily albumin) may lead to weight loss and decreased activity. Hypoproteinemia can result in ascites, dyspnea (due to pleural effusion or pulmonary edema), or occasionally, peripheral edema. Severe or chronic glomerular disease eventually causes renal failure and uremia. Physical findings are usually nonspecific except for ascites or peripheral edema. Protein-losing nephropathies lead to a loss of antithrombin III, which leads to a hypercoagulable state. Severe dyspnea secondary to pulmonary thromboembolism may be seen in dogs with glomerulonephritis or amyloidosis.

Diagnosis: The BUN, and serum creatinine and phosphorus concentrations are elevated variably, depending on the severity of the renal dysfunction at the time of diagnosis. Urine specific gravity may be high or low. Proteinuria is present in all forms of glomerular disease, but it must be quantitated to determine if the loss is significant. Normal 24-hr urine protein loss in dogs and cats is 10-20 mg/kg. Alternatively, the protein:creatinine ratio can be determined in a random urine sample; a value >2 indicates significant proteinuria, and values >10 are frequently associated with amyloidosis.

Abdominal and thoracic radiographs should be obtained to rule out neoplasia and heartworm disease. A renal biopsy is necessary to determine the type of glomerular disease. The degree of proteinuria does not always correlate with the severity of the histological lesions. Tests for SLE (antinuclear antibody titer and LE prep) should be done in dogs with glomerulonephritis. Hypertension occurs in many cases, and a blood pressure determination should be performed in all animals with evidence of glomerular disease.

Treatment: No specific therapy has been shown to be beneficial in dogs with either glomerulonephritis or amyloidosis. Corticosteroids enhance amyloid deposition and should be avoided in these animals. Supportive measures include a small amount of a high-quality-protein diet that is low in sodium to control hypertension, and diuretics to control edema. Changes in dietary sodium levels should be made gradually. Plasma transfusions may be needed in animals with refractory edema or ascites. Animals in renal failure (qv, p 877) should receive appropriate therapy.

RENAL TUBULAR DEFECTS

FANCONI SYNDROME

A constellation of renal tubular defects that leads to excessive loss of many solutes in the urine and results in metabolic disturbances and, in some cases, renal failure. It has been reported as an inherited disease in Basenjis (in adults of both sexes). Renal function studies indicate excessive urinary losses of glucose, sodium, potassium, phosphorus, uric acid, bicarbonate, and amino acids. Blood glucose concentrations are normal. Serum electrolytes are normal early in the disease, but hypophosphatemia, hypokalemia, and metabolic acidosis are seen in the later stages.

Clinical signs include polydipsia, polyuria, and weight loss. Signs of uremia may be present if the animal is in renal failure. Diagnosis is based on documentation of increased urinary fractional excretion of glucose, sodium, potassium, phosphorus, and bicarbonate. Differential diagnoses include simple renal glucosuria and renal disease from other causes. The microscopic renal changes are not remarkable. Some dogs have normal kidneys and others have nonspecific changes. A treatment regimen to reverse the tubular defect has not been described.

Oral supplementation of sodium chloride, potassium, phosphate, and bicarbonate is indicated if the corresponding serum concentration is low. Dogs with renal failure (qv, p 877) should receive appropriate symptomatic therapy. The disease is slowly progressive despite therapy, and eventually causes death from renal failure.

RENAL GLUCOSURIA

Usually a congenital defect in proximal tubular handling of glucose that results in glucosuria despite normal blood glucose concentration. Affected animals may be asymptomatic, have polydipsia/polyuria, or have recurrent urinary tract infections due to bacterial utilization of glucose. Diagnosis is made by demonstrating persistent glucosuria with a normal blood glucose concentration and identifying no other renal abnormality. Although no treatment is available, the condition is not progressive.

RENAL TUBULAR ACIDOSIS

A rare renal tubular defect in dogs that results in hyperchloremic metabolic acidosis. Two types have been described: Type I is characterized by a defect in the distal tubular ability to secrete hydrogen ions; Type II is the result of a reduction in the threshold of bicarbonate reabsorption in the proximal tubule. Type I is more severe and may be associated with demineralization of the skeleton (due to buffering of excess hydrogen ions) and nephrolithiasis (due to hypercalciuria from bone resorption). Diagnosis is based on the presence of hyperchloremic metabolic acidosis without other cause. Type I can be presumptively diagnosed when the urinary pH is inappropriately high for the degree of systemic acidosis. Failure to achieve an acid urine after oral ammonium chloride loading is diagnostic; however, this test is contraindicated in an animal that is already severely acidotic. Type II is diagnosed by demonstrating increased urinary fractional excretion of bicarbonate when plasma bicarbonate levels are normal or decreased. Therapy consists of oral sodium bicarbonate administration sufficient to maintain normal blood pH.

NEOPLASTIC DISEASE

TUMORS OF THE KIDNEY

Tumors of the kidney are uncommon; they have been reported to represent 0.6-1.7% of all canine tumors. Benign tumors are rare, are usually incidental necropsy findings, and are of no clinical significance. Adenomas, lipomas, fibromas, and papillomas have been reported.

Primary malignant renal tumors (except nephroblastomas) are most common in middle-aged to older animals; no breed predilection has been found. The most common primary malignant renal tumor is the adenocarcinoma, which originates from the renal tubular epithelium. Usually, it is unilateral, located at one pole of the kidney, well demarcated, and yellow, white, or gray. Size varies from microscopic to several times that of the normal kidney. Renal adenocarcinomas metastasize early to various organs; the opposite kidney, lungs, liver, and adrenals are involved most commonly.

Nephroblastomas (embryonal nephroma, Wilms' tumor) arise from vestigial embryonic tissue. They occur in young animals, and in dogs are most commonly diagnosed at <1 yr of age. There is no breed predilection, but males are affected twice as commonly as females. Usually, they are unilateral but occasionally bilateral, and can grow to immense proportions: it is not uncommon to have virtually the entire abdomen occupied by tumor. Metastasis occurs to regional lymph nodes, liver, and lungs.

Transitional cell carcinomas, which arise from transitional epithelium of the renal pelvis, ureter, bladder, or urethra, are discussed under TUMORS OF THE LOWER URINARY TRACT, below. Other primary malignant renal tumors include hemangiosarcomas, fibrosarcomas, leiomyosarcomas, and squamous cell carcinomas; all are rare.

The kidneys are a common site of metastatic or multicentric tumors. Metastatic lesions may be unilateral or bilateral. Lymphosarcoma is the most common multicentric tumor involving the kidneys. Up to 50% of dogs and cats with lymphosarcoma have renal lesions, and in some cases only the kidneys are affected. Renal involvement is usually diffuse, interstitial, and bilateral, and results in large, irregular kidneys. Lymphosarcoma in cats frequently is associated with infection by feline leukemia virus.

Clinical Findings: Signs usually are nonspecific and may include weight loss, anorexia, depression, and fever. Bilateral tumors may destroy sufficient renal tissue to cause renal failure and signs of uremia. Astute owners may notice "lumps" in their animal's abdomen or increasing abdominal enlargement. Persistent hematuria, usually microscopic, may occur. Rarely, renal tumors may produce excessive erythropoietin, which results in polycythemia (qv, p 83).

Diagnosis: History and clinical signs may indicate a mass in the area of the kidneys or renomegaly. The location and size of the mass can be confirmed by ultrasonography or radiography, although an excretory urogram or renal arteriogram may be required. Radiographs of the thorax may reveal metastatic disease. Neoplastic cells occasionally can be found in the urine sediment. Histological examination of tissue obtained by needle biopsy or surgical wedge biopsy is necessary to determine the type of tumor. Percutaneous needle aspiration biopsy and cytological examination may be sufficient for the diagnosis of lymphosarcoma in cats and dogs.

Treatment: Treatment of all renal tumors except lymphosarcoma requires surgical removal; unilateral nephrectomy is usually required. Lymphosarcoma is best managed by combination chemotherapy (qv, p 33). Chemotherapy has not been shown to be effective against renal tumors other than lymphosarcoma.

TUMORS OF THE LOWER URINARY TRACT

Tumors of the ureters, bladder, and urethra are uncommon in dogs and rare in cats. The low incidence in cats is thought to be due to a difference in tryptophan metabolism that results in low urinary concentrations of carcinogenic tryptophan metabolites. Older animals are most commonly affected; the mean age of affected dogs and cats is 9 yr.

Benign tumors of the lower urinary tract are uncommon. Papillomas and leiomyomas are diagnosed most commonly, but fibromas, neurofibromas, hemangiomas, rhabdomyomas, and myxomas also occur.

Primary malignant tumors are the most common neoplasm of the lower urinary tract, of which transitional cell carcinomas are diagnosed most frequently. Squamous cell carcinomas, adenocarcinomas, fibrosarcomas, leiomyosarcomas, rhabdomyosarcomas, hemangiosarcomas, and osteosarcomas also can occur. Transitional cell carcinomas may be solitary or multiple papillary-like projections from the mucosa, or may occur as a diffuse infiltration of the ureter, bladder, or urethra. They are highly invasive and metastasize frequently, most commonly to the regional lymph nodes and lungs. Ureteral and bladder tumors can cause chronic obstruction to urine flow with secondary hydronephrosis. Urethral tumors are more likely to cause acute obstructive uropathy. Secondary bacterial urinary tract infections are common with tumors of the bladder and urethra.

Clinical Findings: Hematuria is the most common sign. Animals with ureteral obstruction and unilateral hydronephrosis may show signs of abdominal pain and have a palpable, enlarged kidney. Signs of uremia may be apparent in animals with bilateral ureteral obstruction and hydronephrosis or in those with urethral obstruction. Bladder or urethral tumors may also cause dysuria, strangury, and pollakiuria. The bladder wall may be thickened, and a cord-like urethra may be palpable rectally.

Diagnosis: History and clinical signs are highly suggestive of lower urinary tract disease in animals with tumors of the bladder or urethra. Urinalysis frequently reveals hematuria and evidence of infection. Chronic, uncomplicated urinary tract infections must be differentiated from those associated with tumors. Neoplastic cells may be found in the sediment, particularly with transitional cell carcinomas. A cystourethrogram or ultrasonography is necessary to determine the location and extent of the tumor. Biopsy of the tumor is required for definitive diagnosis.

Treatment: Excision of the tumor is the most beneficial therapy. Transitional cell carcinomas are frequently located at the trigone of the bladder or in the urethra, and may necessitate radical reconstructive surgery of the lower urinary tract. Prognosis is poor for these animals, even with surgery, because recurrence and metastasis occur rapidly. Recent studies suggest that chemotherapy with cisplatinum may prolong the life of affected animals.

DISORDERS OF MICTURITION

Disorders can result from dysfunction of any of the components that control urination. Urinary incontinence is the failure of voluntary control of the urethral sphincter, with constant or intermittent unconscious passage of urine; it can be a failure of urine storage or a disorder of urine voiding, and may be neurologic or non-neurologic in origin. The most common non-neurologic incontinence is attributed to deficiency of sex hormones in neutered animals, particularly females, and may occur as a sequela of ovariohysterectomy.

Incontinent animals may leave a pool of urine where they have been lying or may dribble urine while walking. The coat around the vulva or prepuce may be wet, and perivulvar or peripreputial dermatitis can occur as the result of urine scalding.

Urge incontinence is seen with detrusor irritability, usually associated with cystitis. Destruction of urethral smooth muscle by infection or neoplasia can cause incontinence. Animals with unilateral congenital ectopic ureters may void normally and "dribble" urine intermittently, while animals with bilateral ectopic ureters are less likely to void normally.

Paradoxical urinary incontinence occurs when there is a partial obstruction of the urinary outflow tract. Inability to urinate results in frequent attempts to urinate, strangury, and passage of only small amounts of urine. Occasionally, incontinence may be seen with partial obstruction of the urethra. Animals with complete obstruction rapidly become uremic. Inability to urinate can be due to mechanical obstruction of the urethra by calculi, tumors, or strictures.

Neurologic forms of urinary incontinence are best categorized as upper (UMN) or lower motor neuron (LMN) injuries to the spinal cord. Lesions to the sacral spinal cord, trauma to the pelvic nerve, and detrusor atony lead to LMN signs, which are characterized by a distended, easily expressed bladder. Damage to the thoracolumbar spinal cord, or cerebral, cerebellar, or brain-stem disease lead to UMN signs, which are characterized by a distended bladder that is difficult to express in an animal exhibiting paresis or paralysis. The final form of neurologic urinary incontinence is functional obstruction (reflex dyssynergia), which occurs when there is incoordination of the normal micturition reflex; this is believed to result from overdischarge of sympathetic nerve impulses to the urethral sphincter.

Excitement may cause urinary incontinence in some animals. Idiopathic urinary incontinence in cats has been associated with feline leukemia virus. Iatrogenic urinary incontinence may be created by administration of corticosteroids or diuretics.

Diagnosis: Clinical signs are usually suggestive of a micturition disorder. A thorough physical and neurologic examination is indicated in any animal with urinary incontinence. The history should include age of onset, sexual status of the animal, age at neutering, current medication, and history of previous urinary tract infections. The act of voiding should be observed, and the bladder should be palpated after voiding to estimate residual volume.

The bladder is small to moderately distended in most types of incontinence, and urine can be expressed manually. Animals with LMN incontinence or an atonic bladder have a large distended bladder from which urine can be expressed with minimal pressure. Animals with mechanical or functional obstruction, or UMN lesions to the spinal cord also have a large distended bladder, but urine cannot be expressed. Caution must be exercised when attempting to express urine from these animals to avoid rupture of the bladder. A catheter can easily be passed into the bladder in animals with functional obstruction, but will not pass in animals with mechanical obstruction. Plain and contrast radiography are necessary to determine the type and location of mechanical obstruction.

Treatment: Animals with hormonal incontinence are treated with the appropriate sex hormone—diethylstilbestrol in females and testosterone in males. The dose should be adjusted to the minimum required to maintain continence. Alternatively, an α-adrenergic agonist drug (eg, phenylpropanolamine, 2-4 mg/kg/day in divided doses) can be given. This also may be beneficial in animals with urethral sphincter incompetence. Urge incontinence is treated with anticholinergic drugs such as propantheline (dogs—<20 kg, 7.5 mg daily; >20 kg, 15 mg daily; cats—7.5 mg, q72hr). Cholinergic drugs such as bethanechol are used in animals with detrusor atony. Functional obstruction is treated with sympatholytic drugs (eg, phenoxybenzamine, 2.5-10 mg, 1-3 times daily); cholinergic drugs may also be necessary.

Mechanical obstructions should be relieved by catheterization and retropulsion of the obstructing material into the bladder or by surgery. Animals with detrusor atony from overdistention but without neurological lesions benefit from decompression of the bladder by placement of an indwelling urinary catheter for 3-7 days. Those with neurogenic atony usually do not respond to medical management and require manual expression of the bladder or catheterization several times daily.

UROLITHIASIS

A condition associated with calculi or excessive amounts of crystals in the urinary tract. Subsequent irritation of the mucosal lining results in frequent voiding of often bloody urine, obstruction of the urinary tract, or both. The disease has many names, including urinary calculi, bladder stones, kidney stones, lower urinary tract disease, and in cats, feline urological syndrome (FUS). Urolithiasis is common in cats and dogs; the reported incidence is as high as 2.8% of all dogs, and 10% of hospitalized cats. Large uroliths are common in dogs, whereas in cats, uroliths generally are sand-sized particles or microscopic crystals. Incidence is approximately equal in both sexes of both species, but clinical signs differ due to anatomical differences.

The calculi in all species of animals are composed of some 20 crystalline substances that represent different mineral forms of phosphate, oxalate, urate, cystine, carbonate, and silica. The constituent elements and radicals can be identified by chemical analysis, and the precise crystalline compounds by optical and X-ray crystallography. However, analysis is unnecessary in many cases since the most likely type of calculus can be determined from the species, age, sex, breed, diet, or other clinically available data. In recurring cases, a quantitative, not qualitative, analysis of the calculus should be conducted.

Mechanisms involved in the actual formation of stones are not well understood. Three main theories exist: the matrix hypothesis, which emphasizes the inorganic protein matrix as initiating urolith formation; the crystallization-inhibitor hypothesis, which emphasizes the importance of organic and inorganic inhibitors of crystallization; and the precipitation-crystallization hypothesis, which emphasizes the importance of salt supersaturation. Regardless of which of these, or other, mechanisms may be responsible, calculi cannot be produced without: 1) a sufficiently high concentration of calculi-forming constituents in the urine, 2) adequate time in the urinary tract, and 3) for struvite (magnesium-ammonium-phosphate), cystine, or urate calculi, a favorable pH for crystallization. Anything that enhances or increases any of these factors predisposes to urolith formation. These factors are affected by urinary tract infection, diet, intestinal absorption, urine volume, frequency of urination, and genetics. The importance of each factor in causing or predisposing to urolithiasis, or conversely, in preventing it, differs in different species and for different types of uroliths. The factors involved in urolithiasis in some species for certain types of calculi are well documented: cystine and urate stones of dogs are metabolic in origin; the struvite calculi of dogs frequently are associated with urinary tract infections with urease-producing bacteria.

Prevention is based on chemical composition of the calculi. Once the offending chemical is known, its urinary concentration can be reduced by decreasing dietary intake, increasing urine volume, eliminating infection, changing urine pH, or altering production or excretion with drugs.

Clinical Findings: Signs are caused by the presence and effects of crystals or calculi in the urinary tract. The calculi may cause no noticeable signs; may cause cystitis or urethritis by irritating the lining of the urinary tract; or may obstruct the urethra or, rarely, the ureters. Calculi in the renal pelvis are less common and generally cause no signs unless there is an upper urinary tract infection or sufficient damage to produce renal failure. Occasionally, they may be associated with pyelonephritis, and result in hematuria and fever. Ureteral obstruction may result in hydronephrosis and loss of function of the ipsilateral kidney. Since clinical signs of renal dysfunction may not become apparent until two-thirds of total functional renal parenchyma is lost, signs are not seen unless both ureters are obstructed.

Dribbling urine or urinating in unusual locations by a housebroken animal indicates the possibility of bladder or urethral calculi. The urine may be bloody and have a strong, ammonia-like odor. These signs may begin abruptly and abate within a few days without treatment, only to recur. Generally, they are the only signs observed in females and may be the only signs in many males. However, in males, urethral obstruction is common and may occur suddenly or develop over days or weeks. Initially, there may be frequent attempts to urinate with only drops, a fine stream, or nothing passed. Affected cats may squat, strain, and lick the penis excessively.

Substantial obstruction causes uremia, anorexia, dehydration, lethargy, depression, and occasionally vomiting and diarrhea. If obstruction is complete, coma and death follow within 72 hr. Treatment should begin shortly after obstruction occurs; if delayed until the animal is comatose, chances of survival are greatly reduced. The distended bladder may rupture, although this is more common in ruminants than in dogs or cats. For a short time following rupture, the animal may appear improved because the pain associated with bladder distention has been relieved; however, peritonitis and absorption of waste products occur rapidly and cause depression, abdominal distention, and death. The uremic dog or cat seldom survives surgical repair of a ruptured bladder.

Diagnosis: Calculi >3 mm in diameter are usually visible on radiographs, and some are palpable. Clinical and laboratory findings may be negative, or the only signs may be those of cystitis and urethritis. In urethral obstruction, the bladder is distended or ruptured; if ruptured, it cannot be palpated, and urine can be readily obtained from the abdominal cavity by paracentesis. If the bladder is not ruptured, it is hard, distended, painful, and cannot be expressed.

Abdominal palpation is helpful in detecting cystitis, or cystic or urethral calculi. The bladder wall may be thickened and give a "grating" sensation when palpated. Although palpation may reveal a sufficiently large urolith or multiple calculi by their crepitation, it cannot be depended on to reveal all cases of cystic calculi. Urethral calculi may be detected and located by passing a catheter.

Diagnosis may not be difficult, but since multiple calculi frequently are present throughout the urinary tract, a complete radiographic examination of the tract is indicated. Urinalysis, and culture and sensitivity testing of bacteria in the urine are helpful in determining the type of uroliths present.

CANINE UROLITHIASIS

Breeds predisposed are the Miniature Schnauzer, Dachshund, Dalmatian, Pug, Bulldog, Welsh Corgi, Basset Hound, Beagle, and terriers. Most affected dogs are 2-10 yr old. Urethral uroliths are most common; renal calculi account for 2-8% of cases, and ureteral calculi are rare. Recurrence after treatment is estimated to be 12-75% but varies considerably with the breed, type of urolith, and management. Uroliths of dogs are composed of a predominant chemical that usually identifies the stone as 1 of 4 types: 1) struvite (magnesium-ammonium-phosphate), with or without calcium phosphate (sometimes called double or triple phosphate, depending on the number of cations present); 2) urate, composed of ammonium urate; 3) cystine, consisting of the amino acid cystine; or 4) oxalate, consisting of calcium, magnesium, or ammonium oxalate. The type of urolith can be determined in most cases as described in FIGURE 1. Other less common types consist of silicon dioxide, calcium phosphate, or carbonate and xanthine. Silicate uroliths are most common in German Shepherd Dogs and other large breeds. They generally contain spicules that give them the appearance of children's jacks, and are sometimes referred to as "jack stones".

Figure 1.   Determining Canine Urolith Types

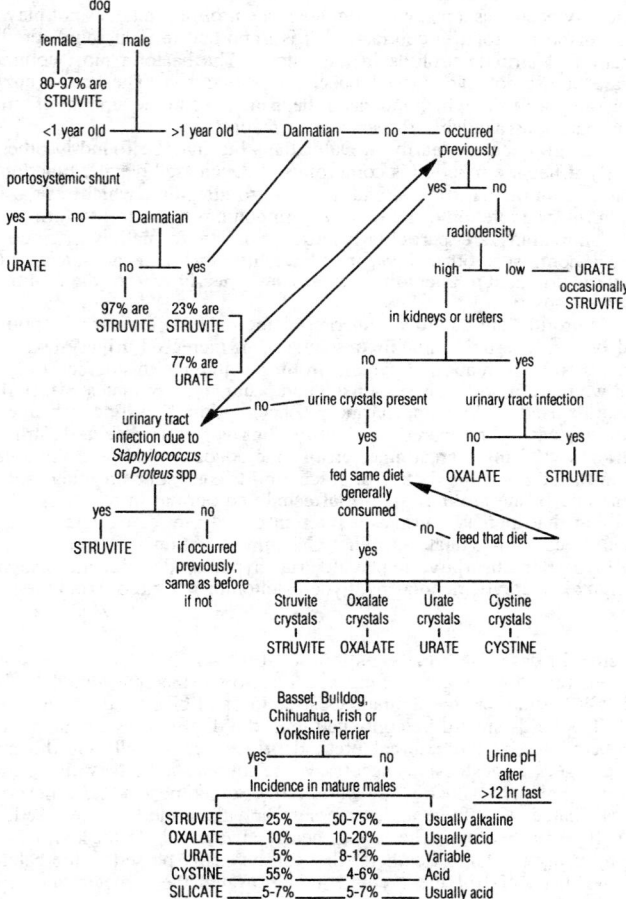

If unsure, obtain a quantitative analysis of urolith or sediment
by centrifuging 25-100 mL of urine in a conical-tipped tube.

The incidence of concomitant urinary tract infection (UTI) varies with the type of urolith: struvite (50-97%), urate (3-80%), and cystine (0-50%); it may be present in dogs with carbonate or silicate uroliths, but is rare in those with oxalate uroliths. UTI generally occurs as a result of nonphosphate uroliths and does not play a causative or predisposing role; in contrast, UTI is important in inducing or predisposing to formation of struvite uroliths in most dogs. The bacteria most commonly involved are urease-positive staphylococci or *Proteus* spp. The urease enzyme enhances urea hydrolysis, which increases the urine pH and the amount of ammonium and phosphate ions available for struvite formation.

Urate calculi occur primarily in Dalmatians but may be found in other breeds, particularly if hepatic function is compromised. Decreased hepatic function impairs conversion of ammonia to urea, and uric acid to allantoin, which results in an increase in urinary excretion of both. Thus, ammonium-urate urolith formation is enhanced. Dalmatians are particularly susceptible to formation of urate uroliths because, in contrast to other dogs, they have little of the hepatic enzyme (uricase) that converts uric acid to allantoin. Nevertheless, nearly 25% of the uroliths in Dalmatians are struvite.

Cystine uroliths are due to an inherited defect in renal tubular resorption of cystine and lysine. The only known consequence of increased urinary levels of these amino acids is the formation of cystine uroliths. Although this defect occurs in both men and women, in dogs it is sex-linked and occurs only in males; affected animals should not be used for breeding. Urinary concentration of cystine or lysine, relative to creatinine, can be measured to identify dogs with this defect. A urine cystine concentration >75 mg/g creatinine, or a lysine concentration >25 mg/g creatinine in the non-fasted dog is predictive of susceptibility to cystine urolithiasis. Excretion of cystine and lysine are the same in affected and normal fasted dogs.

Anything that increases urinary excretion of calcium or oxalate predisposes to formation of calcium oxalate uroliths. Calcium excretion is increased by chronic primary or pseudo-absorptive hypercalciuria, hyperparathyroidism, excessive vitamin D intake, osteolytic neoplasms, hypercalcitoninism, and proximal renal tubular damage.

Treatment: In cases of urinary outflow obstruction, if the dog is visibly dehydrated, lethargic, or comatose, fluid and electrolyte therapy should be instituted immediately to stabilize the animal. Obstruction and bladder distention should be relieved. The fluids should be continued until the dog is drinking and eating well.

An obstruction at the external urethral orifice occasionally can be moved by gentle massage. (If anesthesia is necessary, the animal should be well hydrated first. Generally, inhalant anesthetics are preferred.) Sometimes, when a portion of the urethra is dilated with fluid under pressure and then suddenly released, urethral calculi will be flushed out. The urolith nearly always can be flushed back into the bladder by using the largest catheter that can be easily passed to the calculus, occluding the distal end of the urethral lumen around the catheter, and infusing a sterile mixture of equal parts of isotonic saline solution and an aqueous lubricant. It is sometimes helpful to relieve bladder distention by cystocentesis before hydropropulsion of urethral calculi. The dog should be watched closely for at least 5-7 days for possible re-obstruction; when it is sent home, the owner should monitor urination and look for signs of dysuria for several weeks.

Urolith Removal: For all dogs with nonphosphate or nonurate uroliths, and for pregnant and lactating dogs, surgical removal of the uroliths and flushing of the bladder and urethra with sterile isotonic saline are required. For non-pregnant or non-lactating dogs, struvite and ammonium urate uroliths can be removed surgically or dissolved by feeding a calculolytic diet (available commercially). Dissolution assures that all uroliths are removed; alleviates the risk, time, and aftercare involved with surgery; and is preferred by most owners. Canine uroliths take 2-20 wk (av 8 wk) to dissolve; however, clinical signs generally are alleviated within 1 wk. Immature dogs should be fed the calculolytic diet only until the calculi are no longer visible radiographically; mature dogs should receive the diet an additional 4 wk. If the radiographic size or density of the urolith has not decreased within 2 mo and absolutely nothing but the calculolytic diet and water have been ingested, the uroliths probably are not struvite or ammonium urate and, therefore, should be removed surgically and analyzed.

In adult males, the probable type of urolith (FIGURE 1, p 887) may be determined and treatment selected to remove them and prevent recurrence. Stone analysis is necessary only in recurring cases since 97% of uroliths in males <1 yr old (except Dalmatians) and in all females are struvite, whereas only 23-60% of uroliths in adult males are struvite.

Prevention: Other than those caused by cystine uroliths, only 20-30% of cases of urolithiasis recur, and dietary and medical management for prevention may not be warranted. Following dietary dissolution or surgical removal of recurring uroliths, a mineral- and protein-restricted diet is indicated; during pregnancy or lactation a less-restricted diet will suffice (both diets are commercially available). If there is recurrence when only a restrictive diet and water have been ingested, the following procedures should be instituted: 1) For struvite uroliths, feed a calculolytic diet exclusively thereafter. 2) For urate or cystine uroliths, give 1 g ($\frac{1}{4}$ tsp)/5 kg body wt of sodium bicarbonate PO q6-8hr, and add 2 g ($\frac{1}{2}$ tsp)/10 kg body wt/day of salt to the food. If urate uroliths recur on the restricted diet with added salt and sodium bicarbonate, allopurinol is given at 10 mg/kg, t.i.d. for 1 mo and daily thereafter; if cystine uroliths recur, D-penicillamine is given at 10-30 mg/kg, daily, divided into at least 2 doses and given with food to prevent vomiting.

FELINE UROLITHIASIS AND FELINE UROLOGICAL SYNDROME (FUS)

A common disease that occurs with equal frequency in both sexes. The clinical manifestations may differ: urethral obstruction is common in males, whereas cystitis and urethritis are more usual in females. Most cases occur in cats housed indoors, with the first episode at 1-6 yr of age.

In cats, >90% of uroliths are exclusively, or primarily, struvite (magnesium-ammonium-phosphate), occasionally with smaller amounts of calcium phosphate (apatite), calcium oxalate, or ammonium urate, and 0-5% organic matrix. These calculi may resemble sand. Discrete cystic calculi and nephroliths are less common. From 0.5-3% of the uroliths are urate and oxalate, and 3-5% are gelatinous plugs. The latter differ from uroliths in that they contain a greater amount of organic matrix, which gives them a toothpaste-like compressible consistency, and are found in the urethra, most commonly near the urethral orifice. The mineral in 99% of these plugs is 80-100% struvite; the remaining 1% contain primarily calcium phosphate or calcium oxalate. Calcium carbonate uroliths are rare, and silicate and cystine uroliths have not been reported.

Etiology: Infection, although present in ~5% of the cases, generally is a result of the disease and not a cause. Decreased physical activity, which often decreases water intake and frequency of urination, predisposes to urolithiasis. Factors that decrease physical activity include castration, confinement, adverse weather conditions, illness, and obesity.

Studies indicate that feline urolithiasis can be produced by feeding diets high in magnesium, presumably because they induce struvite calculus formation. Although the role of excessive dietary magnesium in the "naturally occurring" disease remains debatable, and other factors may well be involved, it may be prudent to restrict magnesium intake in cats.

Although it has been reported that urolithiasis is more likely to occur when dry food, rather than canned, is fed, this is not due to differences in water content and is not true for all dry foods. Compared to the average commercial canned cat food the average dry food is lower in fat, digestibility, and calories, and higher in fiber, which increases fecal volume and thus fecal water excretion, thereby decreasing urinary output. The lower the caloric density of a food, the more the cat consumes; this further increases magnesium intake and reduces urine volume, and thus concentrates urinary magnesium. Some dry cat foods are higher in digestibility and caloric content and lower in fiber and magnesium than most canned foods, and therefore may be less likely to induce urolithiasis. Milligrams of magnesium per 100 kcal ME is the best way to evaluate different cat foods.

Treatment: Fluid and electrolyte therapy must be instituted and obstruction relieved as described for the dog (*see* above). Clinical signs in most cases, whether due to urethral obstruction or to cystitis resulting in pollakiuria and hematuria, are due to calculi and crystals in the urinary tract. To alleviate these signs, the calculi must be removed; a calculolytic diet is the best way to do this and is the treatment method preferred by most owners. Such a diet contains ≤15 mg of magnesium/100 kcal, and in the absence of urinary tract infection, maintains urine pH at ≤6, which leads to dissolution of all uroliths. Although in most cases even large calculi are no longer visible radiographically after 1 mo on this diet, it is recommended that the diet be continued for 2-3 mo. Giving urinary acidifiers is contraindicated, and additional salt is not helpful since the diet contains added salt to increase water intake and urine volume. Consumption of vitamin-mineral supplements or any other food slows or prevents calculi dissolution. Urinary tract infection usually does not occur, but if present, should be treated as appropriate (qv, p 871).

Prevention: Urolithiasis affects 1-10% of all cats, and recurs in 50-70% of all previously affected cats fed regular commercial cat foods. However, both occurrence and recurrence can be prevented in most cats by feeding only diets that provide <20 mg magnesium/100 kcal ME and do not increase the urine pH to >6.4. These may be purchased commercially or can be prepared from household foods. (*See* TABLE 1, below).

Table 1.   Homemade Diet for Management and Prevention of Feline Urological Syndrome

1 lb (450 g)	ground beef (not ground chuck) braised lightly and fat retained
¼ lb (110 g)	liver, uncooked or braised lightly
1 cup (230 g)	cooked rice
1 tsp (5 mL)	cooking oil
1 tsp (5 g)	limestone (calcium carbonate), ground eggshells, or 8 "Tums" antacid tablets
2-3 oz (60-90 mL)	water can be added during cooking if the cat prefers moister food.

Combine all ingredients.
Yield: 1.75 lb (800 g).
Feed ¼-½ lb (110-230 g)/cat daily.

Adapted from *Veterinary Medicine/Small Animal Clinician,* **79**:334, 1984.

Perineal urethrostomy, increasing salt intake to increase urine volume, or feeding a urinary acidifier will not prevent recurrence in many cases if dietary management is not instituted, and is unnecessary when a low-magnesium, non-alkalinizing diet is consumed. Continued feeding of a calculolytic diet is needed in the rare case that recurs with preventive diets.

NONINFECTIOUS DISEASES OF THE URINARY SYSTEM, LG AN

UROLITHIASIS, LG AN

See pp 885 and 886, an introduction to urolithiasis in lg an as well as sm an.

UROLITHIASIS IN RUMINANTS

Formation of calculi within the urinary tract of cattle, sheep, and goats is primarily a metabolic disease. The condition is common in ruminants, uncommon in horses, and rare in pigs. Occlusion of the urethra by calculi causes retention of urine, abdominal pain, and distention and rupture of the urethra or bladder, with death from uremia or secondary septicemia. It is an important disease of feeder animals, and a significant number of cases also occur in mature breeding animals. Clinical urolithiasis is seen most frequently during winter in steers and wethers on full feed, or on range where severe weather conditions exist with limited intake of water, especially water that has a high mineral content.

Urolithiasis has no specific geographic distribution, and the different types of calculi reflect the mineral distribution of the feed. Calculi occur in either sex, but urolithiasis occurs primarily in males because of anatomical and hormonal differences. Urolithiasis can occur under a variety of environmental conditions and in animals of all ages.

Etiology and Pathogenesis: Incidence in the USA is highest in the calf, lamb, or kid that has been castrated at an early age and is fed a high-grain diet with nearly a 1:1 calcium to phosphorus ratio, or a diet high in magnesium. Urolithiasis in ruminants is largely nutritional in origin, the struvite calculi being associated with diets high in cereal grains, and the silica calculi with grazing on silica-rich soil.

Under arid range conditions where grass or cereal hay are the primary diet, silicate calculi commonly form. Diets high in calcium, eg, subterranean clover, produce calcite calculi. Plants such as *Halogeton* or tops from the common sugar beet that are high in oxalates may be a factor in calcite or weddelite calculi formation. Examination of the nuclei of the above mentioned calculi suggests that precipitates of the particular mineral involved initiate calculus formation. The most common calculi in feeder animals on high-concentrate rations with poorly balanced mineral composition (high in phosphorus and low in calcium) is the struvite type, which contains calcium, magnesium, and ammonium phosphates. In these cases, mucoprotein, cell casts, or epithelial cells may be involved with calculus formation. The formation of crystals from compounds normally in urine occurs as a consequence of physiochemical factors such as changes in urine concentration and pH. Many components of urine are held in colloidal suspension; disruption of this balance results in precipitation of its components. The mucoproteins and mucopolysaccharides contribute to the formation of calcium carbonate, silica, magnesium ammonium phosphate, and magnesium phosphate uroliths, and may be the key factor precipitating urolith formation.

The mineral composition of water, in concert with the mineral imbalances in the diet, probably contributes more to initiating calculus formation than does the lack of water itself; limiting water intake has not proved to be calculogenic.

Castration of the young male removes the hormonal influence necessary for full development of the penis and urethra. Calculi vary in size and shape from small, smooth, granular material to large, multinucleated stones. When voided, these calculi cause no problem to the female, but may irritate the delicate mucosal lining of the urethra of the juvenile male. The sigmoid flexure of cattle, and the sigmoid flexure and urethral process of sheep and goats are the most common sites for calculi to lodge. Irritation at the site of lodging causes inflammation and restriction, and occludes the urethra. Inclement weather may further constrict an already juvenile urethra.

Clinical Findings: The first clinical sign of either partial or complete occlusion is dysuria manifest by abdominal discomfort. The animal becomes restless, strains, kicks at the belly, and makes frequent attempts to urinate. In sheep and goats, the attempts to urinate are accompanied by rapid twitching of the tail. In steers, the tail is elevated and pulsation of the urethra just ventral to the rectum is frequently observed. In steers, rectal prolapse may be a sequela of straining.

Before complete occlusion, urine may dribble from the urethra, dry on the preputial hairs, and leave mineral deposits. If the condition is uncorrected, the animal will isolate itself, refuse to eat or drink, become uremic, and die. The course of the disease may be 5-7 days.

Lesions: In urethral rupture, the surrounding tissues will be hemorrhagic and necrotic and the subcut. tissues infiltrated with urine. Opening of the urethra may reveal ≥1 calculi; it may be necessary to dissect out the urethra to find the occlusion. In cases of rupture of the bladder, the abdominal cavity will be filled with urine.

Diagnosis: Early clinical signs allow a diagnosis, although acute colic due to other abdominal pain or urinary tract infections must be ruled out by a thorough physical examination. Indigestion, consumption of large quantities of cold water, GI tract stasis or obstruction, primary enteritis, abomasal ulcers, coccidiosis, and other abdominal disorders may cause abdominal pain. Hypersensitivity in the region of the sigmoid flexure may be evident, and deep palpation may locate the swelling resulting from the obstruction. Examination of the urethral process in sheep or goats may identify the occluding calculus. If the early clinical signs are missed, the animal may show only depression and anorexia with subcut. swelling along the penis or a urine-filled abdomen. Abdominal distention due to urine must be differentiated from rumen tympany, diffuse peritonitis, tumors of the peritoneal cavity, and GI tract obstructions. Ballottement allows detection of the fluid, and from behind, the abdomen appears pear-shaped. Confirmation is obtained by examination of the abdominal fluid collected by paracentesis. Subcut. swellings along the prepuce and ventral abdomen due to a ruptured urethra must be differentiated from traumatic injury, subcut. abscesses, and umbilical or ventral hernias. In breeding animals, lacerations of the prepuce, with resultant prolapse and infection of the sheath, and hematoma of the penis must also be differentiated. In these cases, elevated serum creatinine levels or an increase in BUN will help in the differential diagnosis.

Treatment and Control: Surgery for urolithiasis in steers is economically feasible; however, the value of a wether may limit the procedure to simply snipping off the urethral process. The surgical procedure for calculi lodged in the area of the sigmoid flexure is the same for cattle, sheep, or goats. Proper restraint, tranquilization, and a regional anesthetic are necessary. The technique may vary but requires exteriorization of the penis at the proximal portion of the sigmoid flexure. In early cases, the calculi may be palpated and removed by simple incision into the urethra. If the urethra is patent, it can be sutured and returned to normal position with a simple skin closure. In more complicated cases, amputation of the penis proximal to the sigmoid flexure or at the perineal area may be necessary.

In urethral rupture, the subcut. urine must be drained; this is done by lancing the skin overlying the area of accumulated urine. Topical antiseptics and fly repellents may be applied to these ventral lacerations. Parenteral antibiotics are recommended to prevent infection in all surgical cases. Electrolytes or dextrose solutions are given to correct dehydration and promote urine flow if necessary. Treatment for a ruptured bladder requires establishing the ability to urinate, providing for healing of the bladder, and correcting uremia. Use of a trocar to drain the urine from the peritoneal cavity helps relieve the uremia. A urethrostomy should be performed to provide free passage of urine. Attempts to repair the ruptured bladder have been largely unsuccessful. Spontaneous healing of the bladder frequently occurs following urethrostomy and removal of the abdominal fluid, although these animals are best salvaged within 3-4 mo to avoid further complications. Some cases of bladder rupture treated by paracentesis and urethrostomy fail to pass urine within 48 hr following surgery; urine reaccumulates in the peritoneal cavity due to lack of bladder healing. Such animals may be treated by performing a cystotomy, suturing a plastic drain into the bladder, and then exteriorizing the other end of the tube through the posterior ventral abdominal wall. Antibiotic and fluid therapy should follow this procedure to avoid infection and shock. These animals should be salvaged within a few months. Occasionally, neglected animals are examined that have a ruptured bladder and severe uremia. Treatment may be attempted, but the prognosis is poor.

Chemotherapy has met with limited success and must be done before obstruction is complete. In early cases, smooth muscle relaxants plus anti-inflammatory agents may be helpful. Struvite crystals associated with high-grain rations are soluble at a pH of <6.8. Withholding feed for 24 hr in conjunction with oral dosing of ammonium chloride (7-10 g/head/day for a 30-kg lamb or kid, or 56-80 g for a 240-kg steer) can acidify the urine. Acidification of the urine should be maintained for ≥1 wk following surgery due to the probable presence of multiple calculi in the bladder.

An understanding of the composition and etiology of the urolith involved is necessary to establish an appropriate preventive program. The most common calculi in steers, wethers, lambs, and kids in the USA are associated with high-grain rations high in dietary phosphorus. A ration with a 2:1 calcium to phosphorus ratio greatly reduces the incidence of urolithiasis in feeder animals. The addition of 1-4% salt in the ration has proved beneficial. Rations with 9% salt can be fed before feed consumption or rate of gain is affected; alternatively, 2% ammonium chloride can be added. A well-balanced diet that includes adequate amounts of vitamin A along with an ample supply of water is suggested.

UROLITHIASIS IN HORSES

An infrequent metabolic condition characterized by calculus formation, primarily involving the bladder, that produces signs of dysuria and colic. Although it occurs wherever horses are raised, variations in the geographic distribution of minerals and their imbalances (reflected in forages, feed concentrates, and water) may influence the incidence of urolithiasis and the type of calculus formed. In horses, ~99% of cases are due to cystic calculi, most commonly diagnosed in adult males, usually geldings. Anatomical differences between the sexes probably account for the variation in incidence. The urethra of the male is longer and curved, and is constricted at the ischial arch. Obstructions may occur anywhere but are most frequent at the turn of the pelvic inlet.

Etiology: The specific etiology is unknown. Two chemically similar types (calcium carbonate) occur: a rough, spiculated calculus of moderate hardness, and a less frequently seen, much harder, smooth calculus.

Normal equine urine contains significant amounts of mucoproteins and crystals that may serve as a cement substance for the calcium carbonate crystals. Equine urine characteristically is alkaline, and with the high mineral content, this may favor mineral crystallization and precipitation. The nidus for calculus formation may be desquamated epithelial cells or clots of mucus. Dietary influences such as concentrate rations high in phosphorus and low in calcium, which predispose to calculus formation in ruminants, have not been established in horses.

Clinical Findings: The signs depend on location of the calculus. Most calculi are located in the bladder and cause dysuria, hematuria, strangury, and pollakiuria. Hematuria occurs most frequently following exercise or at the end of urination. Other physical signs include a stretching stance while urinating, which may be held for some time following urination and be accompanied by straining and audible groans. The female may dribble urine, which will scald the perineum; geldings and stallions may protrude the penis with intermittent dribbling of urine. Urethral occlusion usually is accompanied by restlessness, varying degrees of colic, and frequent attempts to urinate. The bladder is found distended on rectal examination. In most fatal cases, a single, large urolith, occasionally with smaller ones, is found in the bladder; less frequently, the urolith may be found lodged at the neck of the bladder or ischial arch. Rarely are stones found in the renal pelvis.

Diagnosis: History and clinical signs allow a tentative diagnosis. Confirmation can be made by a combination of rectal palpation, cystoscopy, and catheterization. Locating a firm ovoid mass in and near the neck of the bladder by rectal palpation may be the only procedure necessary. If the bladder is distended, catheterization facilitates palpation; it also may eliminate urethral strictures and smegma impaction of the urethral sinus, or locate the urolith. Cystoscopy will greatly aid in diagnostic and prognostic evaluation.

Treatment: In most cases, cystic calculi must be removed surgically, and good postoperative care is necessary. Antibiotics, diuretics, and urinary acidifiers may aid recovery.

UROPERITONEUM IN FOALS
(Ruptured bladder)

Uroperitoneum occurs in neonatal foals as a result of leakage of urine through tears in the dorsal or ventral wall of the bladder or through the urachus. Rupture may result from parturient trauma to a distended bladder, but usually there is no history of difficult or abnormal birth; some defects may be congenital. The condition is much more prevalent in males.

Clinical signs are usually manifest on the second or third day of life and increase in severity over several days. Foals are depressed and progressively lose their suckling drive. The foal may frequently posture to urinate but pass only small amounts of urine. However, uroperitoneum may be present in foals that appear to urinate normally. Tachycardia and tachypnea may be seen. As the problem progresses, there is increasing abdominal distention. A fluid wave can sometimes be detected by ballottement. Some foals show periodic flank watching. Abdominal paracentesis yields a large amount of clear, pale yellow fluid with low specific gravity and cell count.

The major blood chemistry changes are hyperkalemia, hyponatremia, and hypochloremia. BUN and serum creatinine may be normal or elevated. A positive diagnosis can be made by comparing creatinine levels: in uroperitoneum, the peritoneal fluid creatinine is at least twice the value of the serum creatinine. Another simple diagnostic test is to inject 10 mL of methylene blue solution into the bladder via a urinary catheter and to observe the dye in peritoneal fluid collected by abdominal paracentesis 15 min later. Differential diagnoses include retained meconium, septicemia, and neonatal maladjustment syndrome (qv, p 610).

Treatment is corrective surgery. Because of the hyperkalemia and hyponatremia, life-threatening cardiac arrhthymias are common when foals with uroperitoneum are anesthetized. Fluid and electrolyte imbalances should be corrected before anesthesia. High serum potassium can be lowered by IV administration of normal saline, sodium bicarbonate, and 5% dextrose. Severe cases of hyperkalemia may also require insulin or peritoneal dialysis.

PART II
BEHAVIOR

BEH

BEHAVIOR

MAINTENANCE

Much organized, "standard" behavior is recognized in domestic and laboratory animals as a major part of their genetic programming relating to maintenance. Inherent reactive, ingestive, and kinetic actions represent major behavioral activity; these include reaction, ingestion, body care, motion, exploration, territorialism, rest, and association. They may be expressed regularly, or according to the demands of circumstances, or they can overlap so as to be expressed simultaneously, or substituted, according to the requirements of well-being. This interaction of several ethological modes as a major method of integration between the animal and the environment can be described as an ethosystem.

Maintenance behavior, much of which is genetically determined, is motivated work, a biological factor of paramount importance as a means of tactical existence. Behavioral homeostasis, as much as physique, determines the animal's biological fitness in the environment to which it must adapt. Thus, species-typical behavior contributes to biological fitness so that such fitness and productivity are in considerable association.

Much animal production is maintenance-based. For example, productivity depends on efficient ingestive behavior and self care: selecting for growth may be based largely on selecting for ingestive behavior. Production behavior, however, is not isolated; behavior is a continuum of components. Innate social and spatial behaviors represent other major behavioral activities, which can be viewed as additional ethological needs in the interest of the animal's functional integrity and its harmony with the circumstances of domestication.

GENERAL

The various forms of maintenance behavior serve a number of purposes. Reactions are used by animals as safety precautions, forms of expression, and displays of their presence, status, and hypothetical intention. They are important forms of communication between animals, the basis of a balanced state of understanding. Much consummative behavior, of course, relates to maintenance. Movement is an important component of the balanced stimulation an animal requires. Substantial freedom of movement, use of environment, and association with others are clearly required to produce the range of behavioral activities included in maintenance behaviors.

Maintenance behaviors must be restricted to some degree in protective systems of husbandry; eg, ingestive behavior is inhibited in ungulates, which are genetically coded to graze and forage, whereas confinement prohibits such behavior. Restrictive husbandry also reduces affiliative activity and, as a result, confined animals cannot always harmoniously express organized social behavior. Since food and shelter are provided, animals do not require the use of all maintenance behaviors that are not, or cannot be, shown in these circumstances; however, these still must be recognized in animal production since the question arises whether such normal behaviors can "dam up" when their outlet is blocked, and then be expressed at inappropriate times.

Ethological homeostasis typically involves multisystems tied to behavior, results from varied motivation, and provides successful maintenance (*see* TABLE 1). Self-determining activities are often complex and involve intentional behavior, eg, seeking associates, selecting food, choosing sites for rest and excretion, and developing social arrangements. These activities contribute to the animal's composite function, the purpose of which is integration of the animal with its environment. The manifestations reflect behavioral needs with variability from animal to animal and from time to time.

Animals pursue homeostasis not only to feed, drink, and socialize, but also to render a "boring" environment less monotonous, gain access to social companions when housed in solitary confinement, and avoid pain and environmental extremes.

Table 1. Features of Behavioral Homeostasis Relating to Maintenance

Behavioral Category	Primary Features	Secondary Features	Role in Maintenance
Body care	Grooming, comfort-seeking.	Evacuation, modes of excretory behavior.	Three homeostatic functions of surface hygiene, excretion, and comfort-state are basic to health.
Motion	Changes of position and posture, exercise movements.	Playing and stretching.	Certain processes of movement require regular expression to maintain fitness.
Exploration	Investigative efforts and attentiveness.	Empirical activities in general.	Stimulation, with quantity and variability, needed for sensory satisfaction and learning.
Territorialism	Using individual space for basic functions.	Proprietary behavior in care of home and feeding.	Spatial needs are both quantitative and qualitative for various self-maintenance requirements, eg, nutrition, shelter, defense, reproduction.
Rest	Drowsing, resting, and sleeping in recumbency in diurnal phases.	Idling in various postures.	Physical self-conservation, physiological restoration.
Association	Bonds; positive social acts, eg, affiliation.	Socialization, group affinity.	Social group membership and stability of interaction.

While too much stimulation can act as a stressor, animals also expend effort to avoid too little. It is likely that in some types of husbandry, under-stimulation is as stressful as over-stimulation.

REACTION

Reactive behavior is a primary class of activities utilized by animals to maintain themselves in harmony with their environment and to adjust themselves to sudden environmental changes that are harmful, or potentially so. Included are reflex behavior, communication, avoidance and submissive reactivity, and agonistic behavior. All relate to many routine circumstances as part of the normal management of farm animals.

Forms of behavior that are a result of animals associating with one another are varied, and show the substrate of social activities in livestock life. Because confinement reduces the opportunity for social activities, confined animals may not be able to express their normal highly organized social behavior; thus, such opportunity is an important component of animal welfare.

Sensation of movement is an important requirement of animals in maintaining a functional relationship with their environment. The muscular effort that accompanies voluntary motion is now appreciated as a sensory requirement of animal function. The kinetic sensory system responds to mechanical stress due to gravity acting on the body according to changes in movement and position. This is a component of the supply of stimulation to the animal to create a mixture of the senses.

The overall phenomenon of reactivity is stimulus-dependent behavior, and therefore functions as an important key via the operation of the senses. The sense organs detect specific and general stimuli, and transfer them to inner receptors in the nervous system; when suitably sensitized, directed, and motivated, reactive behavior emerges as motor output. The resulting movement encompasses various forms, from reflex activity at the spinal cord level, to a whole series of conative acts with sensory information processed at the cortical level. Conscious actions are involved in many environmental reactions, such as choosing feed and shelter.

Much reactivity is influenced by the autonomic nervous system. The chief behavioral effects of sympathetic stimulation relate to states of fear or rage, and prepare the animal for "fight or flight". Specific physiological changes resulting from sympathetic stimulation include increased heart rate and blood pressure, expansion of the bronchial tubes, and suppression of GI activity, all of which ensure good oxygenation of musculature for instant action. The autonomic nervous system also acts as a behavioral integrator; its full role is in modulating and molding the intensities of behavioral responses, in general, and emotional behavior in particular.

VARIETIES OF REACTIVE BEHAVIOR

Some reactions are self-determining, others are conspecific; most are bodily responses, some are vocal; some are positive, some are negative. Among various forms, several major classes of reactivity can be recognized, including: 1) reflex action, 2) communication and vocalization, 3) response to specific environmental (including seasonal) factors, 4) avoidance reaction, 5) reproductive reaction, and 6) agonistic reaction. Some reactions involve combinations of these categories.

REFLEX BEHAVIOR

Many forms of reactive behavior occur as simple reflexes, eg, extension or withdrawal of a limb in response to local pain. Reaction to the pain, together with the sensation (in some form), can establish the basis of suffering. Limb reflexes have protective or postural functions. Reflex evacuation (involving sudden defecation or urination) is common, eg, in cattle and sheep following invasion of their individual space. Reflex escape struggles are readily seen in animals placed suddenly in close restraint. Reactive vocalization occurs immediately following the separation of bonded pairs, and in other forms of group disruptions. Orientation reflexes may be negative, as when cattle turn their hindquarters toward driving rain.

The homeostatic role of reactivity collectively comprises a wide range of behaviors that occur as reactive responses.

COMMUNICATION AND VOCALIZATION

Vocal sounds, individually and collectively, can be of considerable use in the adjustments of animals to their circumstances. Communication, which uses body language and phonation to varying degrees, is a major feature of reactivity. Vocalization, particularly in social reactivity, is a feature of communication; eg, vocal signals occur as exchanges between dam and neonate, between breeding male and female, and by bonded individuals when separated. As reactivity increases, vocalizations tend to increase in volume, quantity, and complexity. Deep vocal sounds often accompany the threat displays of mature males. Many vocalizations are incorporated into responses concerned with alarm and threat.

As the main feature of their group associations, dogs, sheep, cattle, and horses maintain visual contact. Pigs use more auditory communications with conspecifics, while cats use both visual and auditory contacts.

AVOIDANCE AND SUBMISSIVE REACTIVITY

During the bunching of groups in natural or high-density situations, individuals may be forced to violate the individual space of others. Reactivity at such close quarters depends on the hierarchical positions of the animals. Hierarchical order, when stable, requires in each animal: 1) recognition of individuals, 2) an initial encounter when the social position is first established, and 3) a durable memory that enables each animal to react to the other according to its established social status.

The notable avoidance reaction is flight, which may be socially controlled or uncontrolled. When herd flight is controlled, the animals flee in their normal traveling order, in which a high-rank individual female is usually the leader. When panic occurs, there is uncontrolled flight without order. The promptness of flight in horses evolved as a vital survival tactic.

Avoidance reactions between individuals can be passive or active in response to threatful approach. Avoidance of an aggressive exchange in the form of social submission has characteristic postures in each species. They may vary from the most common one of slight head depression, with deviation away from the stimulus, to the gross display of hypotonic submission in which the animal assumes recumbency and refuses to rise. This latter behavior is a confusing condition when a concurrent illness contributes to recumbency. Recognition of submissive reactions is essential in handling any sick or "downer" livestock, to ensure that their welfare is given appropriate consideration. General inertia, or submission, is a common feature characterized by an abnormally low level of reactivity to stimuli that usually cause some change of position or posture.

AGONISTIC REACTIVITY

Aggressive behavior is often seen when groups of animals are first formed. Milk production, weight gain, and other physiologic responses can be affected for several days during the resultant aggressive social interactions. Although sheep seldom show overt social dominance, rams compete at the start of each breeding season, and sheep may show aggressive butting if intensive husbandry conditions increase competition over food, space, or bedded areas. Butting in cattle and sheep, biting of the neck or kicking in horses, staring and snarling in dogs, striking by cats, and pushing and biting in pigs are common agonistic activities. Retaliation, avoidance, flight, and submission are dependent reactivities.

Fighting: Species-typical reactivity is notable in the form of fighting. Many "problem" dogs, cats, or horses are considered unpredictable, particularly when aggressive, eg, fear-biters. Their response to an alarm or threat may be flight (or attempted flight) or attack, depending largely on temperament, conditioning, and the specific situation. All livestock react to threats at set distances, which vary with the potential reaction, the individual, and "critical" distances, when the invisibly ringed areas are breached threatfully. Each of these distances is the point at which the given distance between the animal and the advancing subject has been so reduced that the approached animal must react. In flight distance, the animal will flee from the intruder if possible. If, however, the approaching animal reaches the critical distance, the animal will more likely attack. The individual distance immediately surrounds the animal and is reserved for special acquaintances. These distances vary according to the animal's inherent temperament, experience, domesticated training, competition, housing, feeding, etc.

Fighting is most severe when adults are mixed together for the first time. If a strange sow is introduced to an established group, the collective aggressive behavior of the group directed at the stranger is likely to result in severe physical injury. Fighting sessions between cows do not normally last longer than a few minutes, but may take longer if the animals are equally matched. In this case, the animal being attacked from the side turns itself parallel to the other, and pushes its head (and horns) into the region of the other's lower flank. This flank approach often arrests fighting for several minutes before action is resumed. When one animal submits, it turns; if neither submits, fighting may continue until both tire.

Mock Fighting: As a feature of social reactivity, "mock fighting" is seen as a variant of play (qv, p 902). The form is somewhat ritualized, and it occurs in all species of farm animals when they are grouped. The initial activity is one of solicitation, in which the approaching animal usually bounces toward the associate animal with jerky head movements. The following phase is usually a contest in which one pushes or applies weight to the other; it is common for the animals to circle. Such circling motions are a feature of mock fight behavior in foals, calves, and piglets. Mock fights usually terminate without consequence and do not lead to a rout or chasing. Limited fighting may occur as new animals struggle for self-determination in the social and denomination hierarchy of the herd.

INGESTION

Ingestive behavior includes eating, drinking, preferences for food, daily patterns of feeding, and the mechanics of prehension, mastication, consumption, and sometimes, storage of food. Most species have their own characteristics of ingestion. Nursing animals nuzzle onto the teat and suck. Adult ruminants ingest large quantities of vegetation with minimal mastication, but this material is subject to mastication again some hours later during rumination. Carnivorous animals typically have well-developed canine teeth that facilitate the tearing of flesh; consumption is rapid with minimal mastication. Horses and pigs use molars for chewing before swallowing. Rodents typically gnaw and break down food with their incisor teeth. Instant consumption is seen in a wide range of species, including many birds (pecking) and reptiles; the individual item taken into the mouth must be suitable in both appearance and size for consumption.

Feeding behavior is compounded by various associated features: 1) metabolic needs (eg, lactating dams have an increased need), 2) quantitative demands of appetite (ruminants need bulk), 3) diurnal rhythm of eating (cats often eat during night), 4) selectivity of preferred foods (cats and other species can learn food preferences while young), 5) fluid intake (increased in low humidity or high temperatures), 6) digestive requirements (coprophagy by the young may establish intestinal microflora), 7) competition with affiliates (competition can increase consumption, while dominants can cause subordinates to eat less), 8) eating mechanics (dogs gulp, pigs "root", rodents nibble), 9) foraging techniques (ungulates graze large areas, carnivores hunt, poultry scratch), and 10) daily schedules of general activity (herbivores have diurnal peaks, rodents and cats are nocturnal, horses are generally continuous).

Feeding behavior is strongly influenced by learned patterns and preferences, palatability of feed, the environment in which feeding takes place, and the social associations of feeding. Inheritance of feeding behavior also must be considered. Species-specific patterns are inherited, although specific components can have genetic and environmental contributions—how each affects the satiety and hunger centers of the brain is unclear.

Thirst is an occasional feature of the ingestive drive, and the brain centers that control and mediate it are located in the hypothalamic portion of the limbic system. Overall thirst and maintaining a critical level of fluid in the body in all circumstances are regulated by a complex system influenced by hormones, salt intake, moisture content of feed, and environmental factors.

BODY CARE

Behavior of body care is under its own neural control, although motivation is needed to ensure that the needs of the animal are met. The predominance of any given behavior is always temporary and can be preempted by behaviors of greater importance (eg, self-preservation).

Component Features of Body Care: Care of the body is an ongoing system of behavior involved in maintenance. Four main categories can be recognized: 1) skin hygiene, 2) thermoregulation, 3) comfort seeking, and 4) elimination. Scratching, shaking, and licking are frequently recognizable as grooming, the most prominent type of body-care behavior. The primary purpose of such behavior is for proper hygiene of the skin and coat (or feathers). Self-grooming activities are often brief and frequently varied in form, but collectively they represent a significant portion of maintenance. Mutual grooming between closely associating animals is also noteworthy.

"Grooming" can involve natural tools such as teeth or feet, or environmental aids such as tree limbs or dirt. Dry, dusty material that has been worked into the coat can be easily dislodged by vigorous shaking; this also removes natural skin debris. Birds practice preening and dust-bathing behavior for the same reasons.

In thermoregulation, under natural conditions, animals seek shelter, dry resting areas, shade, and ways to cool or warm themselves. Animals use the ground in various deliberate activities aimed at body effect. Before selecting a site on which to lie, they may scrape the surface of the intended area. After this, they often turn their bodies round the intended bed before lying down. They may rub onto the ground surface and roll onto their backs twisting and turning in various ways (eg, horses and dogs). Dogs may rub their bodies in malodorous substances, which greatly enhances individual body odor.

Under warm conditions, some animals will create wet wallows if none are available. Such wallows allow body surfaces to be cooled via both radiation and evaporation, or they may allow the mud to form a protective coat for the skin. Comfort-seeking behaviors are associated with physical care and include behaviors associated with other situations too, such as scratching to relieve an itch and finding a comfortable spot to lie on.

When given sufficient space, animals, except possibly ruminants, normally eliminate in ways that ensure that resting places are not fouled. When evacuating, animals adopt species-specific postures that help keep the tail and hindlimbs clean. In addition, many species use urine (eg, spraying by cats) as an olfactory marker to indicate a territory, leave an identifying message, or help in reproductive "advertising".

Body Care in Illness: In illness, self-maintenance becomes diminished or arrested, and homeostasis is lost; body care behavior is markedly reduced, and animals with persistent illnesses have an unclean appearance. This neglect conserves energy to use with the increased metabolism of fever. Soiling around the eyes, nose, or mouth is a clear indication of poor self-maintenance and ill-health. Body-care behavior returns as convalescence progresses and homeostasis is regained.

MOTION

Movement is vital for free-living animals to find food and shelter. The way in which animals voluntarily engage in nonspecific activities indicates that the behavior of motion has its own motivation. Severe deprivation of kinetic opportunity results in abnormal behavior—even the lack of proper exercise can cause problems. Examples include various forms of abnormal "mouthing" activity. Although affected animals may remain in fair physical condition, their behavioral change(s) indicates unsatisfactory management from a welfare point of view.

Play: Some behavior in animals is in the form of pure movement without obvious purpose. Animals require movement to exercise, which helps maintain healthy musculoskeletal and cardiovascular systems. The need for exercise is greatest in young animals, and they engage in much pure kinetic behavior in the form of play. Young animals play better if they have others of their own kind as company, for much play requires social contact. Although this is not true social behavior, the species-specific activities exploit the availability of affiliate animals as sources of stimulation, which helps motor coordination, nervous system development, and behavior pattern sequencing. (*See also* MOCK FIGHTING, p 900.)

General Kinetic Activities: In general, kinesis takes many species-specific forms such as jumping, running, scurrying, burrowing, climbing, swimming, brachiating, stretching, and scratching at a substrate. The latter is a notable normal behavior of cats. Animals stretch in many ways, including extending the head and neck, arching the neck, straightening the back, and extending the limbs (both fore and hind, often one pair after the other). The forelimbs may be extended singly or together, as when the animal lowers its trunk to the ground while the forelegs are outstretched. The hindlimbs may be stretched as the animal pushes the trunk forward so that eventually the toes of the hindfeet are dragged along the ground for a short distance. Individual hindlegs may be outstretched one after the other, most commonly soon after the animal has risen after resting.

In poultry, much kinetic activity is in the form of pecking and walking. Birds also perform routine stretching activities, eg, vigorous extension of one wing after the other is common. Often, when one wing is outstretched and in a backward direction, the leg on the same side is also extended backwards. Flapping of the wings represents another form of exercise, although many forms of caging prevent this.

EXPLORATORY BEHAVIOR

Animals normally show a strong motivation to explore and investigate their environment. This activity subsides once the environment has become familiar, but it reappears when there is any change or novelty in the environment. This reserve of exploratory behavior allows the animal to adjust its actions considerably when the environment demands adaptation.

The sensory information that results from exploratory and investigative activities alerts the nervous system to produce appropriate forms of behavior in a changing environment. In free-ranging animals, behavior adjusts continuously, and can be considered a basic feature in homeostatic self-maintenance. In confinement, however, exploratory acts decrease and any motivation to explore has limited opportunity for outlet.

In close, chronic confinement—typical of intensive farm animal production and laboratory animal management—exploratory behavior can become redirected and produce alternative behavior. Similarly, chronic confinement can adversely affect the behavior of pets, and may result in repetitious or destructive activities.

Exploratory behavior often takes the form of trial and error activity; this is most evident among neonates. Soon after birth, the animal engages in exploratory and investigative activities involving its immediate environment and its dam. This enables young animals to learn the identities of their dams and other social contacts, such as littermates.

Perceptive Need: The exploratory system in behavior is evident in many activities. The organization of this system can be listed in the following sequence of development: 1) need in the animal to perceive environmental factors that will stimulate its senses; 2) activation of the exploratory behavior, which becomes directed into interactions between the animal and its environment; 3) receipt of sensory feedback from the environment to satisfy the original need; 4) reduction in motivation as a result of sensory satisfaction; 5) return of the cycle to a basal level of readiness, presumably with the prior events in short- or long-term memory.

TERRITORIAL BEHAVIOR

Available space influences animal activities. There are 2 general types of space: 1) actual space is sought as territory to provide adequate boundaries within which the animal can practice the required actions for living; 2) "individual" space is sought for purposes of self-protection, self-determination, and self-care. Some forms of behavior relate jointly to gross territory and to individual (personal) space. Much social behavior is concerned with negotiating space, determining the tenure of space, and practicing spatial privileges. Aggressiveness is a common feature of territorial methods.

Territory: An area that is actively defended, a territory may be established for a specific purpose, eg, reproduction, or it may be used for general daily activities. Not all species use territories, and some may only use them for specific purposes or at certain times of the year.

Individual Space: The most basic and minimal spatial requirement is sufficient room for an animal to lie down, stand up, turn round, groom itself, and stretch. This can be referred to as primary space, and only close associates are allowed within. This basic space must provide an imaginary bubble of space around the animal, and will be defended.

Additional space that relates to comprehensive activity of the individual can be referred to as secondary space. This is needed to permit activities such as avoidance of a neighbor; radical alteration in position, direction, or location; and moving.

Incorporated in the secondary spatial requirement is social space, the minimal distance that an adult routinely keeps between itself and other members of the same species. It is commonly seen as "distance to nearest neighbor" or "social distance". (Many young animals do not create social space for themselves.) Another feature of the same phenomenon is the maximum number of neighbors that an animal will allow within a given radius. When social space is inadequate, crowding results; crowding, in ethological terms, can be defined simply as inadequate social space appropriate to the animal. A further characteristic of individual space is the "flight distance", which is modified when animals become accustomed to manipulation and management.

All forms of individual space can be considered as portable—they tend to go with the animal. Dominance is largely concerned with assertion of one animal over others in acquiring space priority, and thus relates to individual space. Such space priority gives the highest-ranking animal first claim to preferred areas for such activities as feeding and resting. As a result, individual spaces normally become integrated and call for frequent behavioral adjustment to attain spatial harmony.

REST AND SLEEP

Sleep occupies much of the animal's time. Higher animals show types of sleep that correspond to those of man, although the species' characteristics of sleep can be quite distinctive. Rest and sleep allow restoration of the physiological status. During sleep, metabolic recoveries occur in a short time. During rest, the body practices maximal conservation of energy. In the practice of such conservation, rest is used more tactically than sleep.

Different species have different needs for amounts of sleep. Typically, animals of prey sleep less and divide it into numerous short bouts. If these animals live in groups, resting in shifts is a survival tactic that permits lookouts to warn resting or sleeping members.

Forms of Sleep: True sleep occurs in 2 forms, "brain sleep" and "body sleep". In brain sleep, there is an output of slow electrical waves; for this reason, it is usually referred to as "slow wave sleep"—this is a particularly quiet form of sleep.

In body sleep, some electrical currents from the brain are of the same patterns that occur when the animal is awake. Because of this paradox, this form is also referred to as "paradoxical sleep". Because frequently the eyes move rapidly behind closed eyelids, this form of sleep is also known as "rapid eye movement" (REM) sleep. It is the time during which people dream, and dogs vocalize or paddle their feet.

Rest: All species of domestic animals spend much time resting, during which the animal may be drowsy, or simply lying inert but wakeful. Resting postures vary from standing (eg, in the horse) to lateral or sternal recumbency, or a combination in which the front is in sternal recumbency and the rear is in a lateral position. Lateral recumbency is required for REM sleep, unless the animal can prop itself against something.

ASSOCIATION

Animals that live in close groups under natural circumstances are referred to as social animals. Social interactions are important in self-determination and social stability. For this reason, animals held in social isolation usually develop abnormal behavior (eg, pathological mouthing behavior). Their social activities are more restricted than those of others of their kind, and their ability to cope with change is often affected.

Manifestations of associative behavior are extremely varied, numerous, and phenomenal, and provide vital information on group behavior; it is not enough for us to learn the natural behavior of our utilized animals—we must also learn their capabilities, adaptabilities, and limitations. Management of animals as groups rather than individuals has been highlighted recently. Group-use is the major husbandry method in farm animal production and laboratory animal care.

Association serves many purposes; a major product of social behavior, it is motivated by a force that maintains species cohesion. Through association, the dynamic strategies of a species are implemented. Social affiliations transmit learning, and the "group effect" ("social facilitation") influences communal activities. The intimate association of individuals permits organization into homogeneous units, breeding groups, flocks, and colonies. Because individuals are disciplined by the force of association in large groups, the common pursuit of tactics required for living harmony, survival, and proliferation are ensured.

Organized Association: Many forms of behavior are regulated social interactions. The interactions between a balanced, bonded pair are notable. Among closely confined animals, modified social behaviors are seen, dependent on the system of husbandry and the number of animals in a group. *See also* AFFILIATION AND SOCIAL BEHAVIOR, below.

WELFARE ASPECTS OF MAINTENANCE

The behavioral characteristics of self-maintenance are becoming recognized as indicative—and probably definitive—of the range of animal needs in welfare (*see also* p 928). Separation and crowding can be stressful, and cause syndromes of abnormal behavior. Problems have been associated with methods of livestock husbandry, eg, those involved in the intensive production of calves, steers, sheep, pigs, and poultry. Problems are also common in the husbandry of laboratory animals, notably of primates.

Impoverished environments and confinement husbandry have been shown to affect learning abilities in the young and contribute to the development of stereotyped patterns. Deficient stimulation adversely affects the animal's ultimate ability to adjust to its immediate environment and to changes within it. Abnormal behaviors indicate distress and an attempt by the animal to cope with the situation. Ultimately, animal health and well-being cannot be effectively preserved under those conditions. Rational animal husbandry must recognize the ethological needs of intensively utilized animals, meet their behavioral needs, and cushion the impact of confinement stress. The latter factors are interwoven into the complex causes of animal health problems.

Welfare needs, as they are being ethologically conceived, must be met with more than just the provision of food, water, and shelter. The highest priority needs are those that include the fundamental items of reaction and ingestion. The behaviors of body care, motion, exploration, territorialism, rest, and association are the next priority. Each behavioral category represents compound needs that must be considered in welfare.

A return to a free and "natural" environment is not suggested as feasible husbandry since protective management is essential in modern animal production for livestock and for laboratory species. "Freedom" would actually be cruel for many animals. Dairy cattle and rabbits, for example, would encounter a harsh climate, predators, poor diets, and other stressors. Nevertheless, the appreciation of space requirements (*see* TERRITORIAL BEHAVIOR, p 903) as a need is paramount.

AFFILIATION AND SOCIAL BEHAVIOR

Most farm animals and domestic pets are highly social species. The system of husbandry and the size of the group affect the frequency and nature of social behavior. Social interactions, including dominant or subordinate responses, are affected by the relative rank of the animals within the social dominance hierarchy of the group. Similar responses tend to be shown in all encounters between the same animals. Stability of social relationships requires that all group members are able to recognize one another, that group membership is stable (no illness or temporary removals), and that individuals remember their status and act accordingly. Under free-range farming systems, voluntary subgroupings often occur if herds are large enough.

Bunching animal groups in natural or high-density situations may force members to violate the individual space of others. The frequency of social interactions at such close quarters increases, and the outcome depends on the position of the animals in the dominance order. Aggressive encounters between animals in a group are most frequent while the group is developing its own social hierarchy. When the group achieves social stability and has adequate space, aggressive encounters are minimal. An animal newly introduced into a herd will increase the rate of aggressive encounters within the group until its place is established within the heirarchy. This aggression can affect production of the whole group.

Close bonds are a feature of associative behavior between pairs or small groups, and are not confined to the relationship between dam and offspring. Within herds, discrete pairing through mutual selection is common and operates to the advantage of both individuals, particularly in grooming or in agonistic situations involving other dominant animals. From looser associations of individuals arise the organization of family units, breeding groups, herds, flocks, and colonies. Such affiliation ensures the common pursuit of tactics required for reproductive success as well as individual and group survival.

The importance of social behavior to the understanding of many activities in domestic animals needs further elucidation, and some social features of individual species are considered in more detail below (*see* p 906).

Allelomimetic behavior, sometimes called contagious or friendly behavior, refers to common activities shown by most members of groups, flocks, and herds, when they act together. The early bonds formed between parent and young may be generalized to include other species members. Generally, groups are most apt to stay together if the members coexist peacefully. Social dominance hierarchies, leader-follower relationships, associations for mutual grooming, and other social responses are characteristic of farm species and should be considered relative to animal management and welfare.

Leader-follower Relationships: Pigs are reluctant to move across strange ground and must be driven; however, groups of cattle, sheep, and horses, which develop leader-follower orders in free-range conditions, move more readily. In natural flocks of sheep, the oldest ewe generally leads, whereas in herds of dairy cows, the mid-dominant animals lead. Man can train certain ("Judas") animals to lead groups, thus exploiting the natural movement patterns of the species. Sheep, cattle, and horses can be trained to lead, and cattle tied in pairs after weaning teach each other to lead. In dairy cows, the order of movement to the milking area is rather fixed over a season, although the rear animals are more consistent than the "leaders". The milking order is not necessarily the same as the leader-follower order shown when moving between grazing areas. Under free-range conditions, especially in the "follower" species like sheep and horses, older stock can transfer information about seasonal pathways, good pasture areas, and watering points to their offspring if the dam-offspring bond is not disrupted before natural weaning. In this way, home-range areas can be maintained over generations. Large flocks of sheep in pastures of ~250 acres (100 hectare) may establish up to 3 separate home-range areas, and subgroups of the whole flock work with minimal overlap in these regions.

In smaller pastures, dairy bulls 4-5 yr old define individual territories under set-stocking conditions. The sudden attacks of dairy bulls on known handlers may arise from this age-related change to more aggressive territorial behavior.

SOCIAL RELATIONS BETWEEN MAN AND ANIMALS

The basic behavioral traits of each species are altered little through domestication, although the normal social behavior may be transferred to the human caretaker. For example, most dogs fit into families because they react to people as they react to other members of the pack.

During socialization, a young animal learns to accept the presence of its own and other species. This learning process is restricted to a species-specific time period. For example, in altricial species (immature at birth) such as the dog, the optimal time for socialization is 4-6 wk of age (range 3-12 wk). With precocial species (well-developed at birth) such as the sheep, the optimal time is from birth to 4-6 days. If the attachments to man become too exclusive during this time, such hand-raised animals may relate sexually to human beings instead of their own species.

A domestic animal depends on a human caretaker for some or all of its care and well-being, and people become woven into the social reactions of such animals. A leader-follower relationship may occur as the animal follows the person about. In species that develop social dominance hierarchies, the caretaker should be dominant, particularly when the adult animals are potentially dangerous. Increased dominance can be asserted with maturity and growth. The dominant role of man is best established at the appropriate time for the species, usually early in life when little or no punishment may be needed. The social dominance interactions are specific for individuals; that one person can dominate an animal is no guarantee that another will be able to do so (*see also* p 907).

Close interaction of the owner may result in undesirable social behavior. Early and complete isolation of an animal from its own kind can lead to difficulties in later mating, increased aggressiveness or shyness toward strangers, and poor mothering of young. Overcrowding and poor general management also may lead to anomalous social behavior and result in vice, injury, or unthriftiness. A good stockman or veterinarian can predict many of these conditions by assessing the social behavior of the animals and take preventive action or remedial steps before stock condition deteriorates.

SPECIES SOCIAL BEHAVIOR

SOCIAL BEHAVIOR OF DOGS

The social differences between the behavior of dogs and wolves are few. Wolves regularly travel over runways or hunting trails, and urinate, defecate, and scratch the ground as "scent posts" or "marking places". Similarly, free-running dogs move over regular routes using "scent posts". Males travel more extensively than females and are more apt to use the posts. Marking is stimulated by the scent of urine or feces of strange animals while operating within a territory. The "scent post" behavior keeps males informed of what animals have passed by and of the sexual receptivity of the females. During estrus, the urine and vaginal secretions of the bitch have a particular odor that excites males. The female becomes attractive to the male a few days before proestrous bleeding begins, but is not receptive until estrus.

Both wolf parents cooperate to feed the young (by vomiting food) when the pups begin to eat solid food at ~3 wk of age. Weaning takes place at 7-10 wk, and young wolves have been seen hunting with the pack at ~4 mo. The same general timing is seen in domestic dogs. Vestiges of wild parental behavior are seen in bitches that tend to vomit food for their pups.

Like the wolf, the dog is basically a pack animal, and other dogs or people can satisfy this need for companionship. Short periods of isolation of a dog can act as a punishment, and may be useful during some types of training. Pack animals operate within domination-subordination relationships that permit them to live in stable social groups. This helps inhibit fighting in competitive situations, such as those relating to food, living space, and desire for human attention. Size, strength, and sex largely determine social dominance, and these relationships are established among maturing puppies. Strange dogs of the same breed are more often attacked and rejected from a closed social group than are dogs of a different breed, although there are wide breed differences in the tolerance of strangers. There is little evidence that either wolves or dogs develop any strong system of leadership.

Protective and Affiliative Behavior: Adult dogs of certain breeds normally guard the territory around their homes and attempt to keep out strangers by threat or attack. Away from their home territory they are seldom aggressive, and if moved to a new home, take up to 10 days to establish their new territory. Dogs are also likely to attack if members of their pack (or family) are threatened. This is an instinctive reaction and should not be encouraged excessively, for the owners will lose control of the dog when anyone except immediate family is present. A well-trained, well-controlled dog presents few problems.

Abnormal Social Behavior: Although the dog's owner might dominate his pet, a passerby might not—and may be bitten if he attempts to do so. A dog allowed to fight other dogs or people soon develops habits that make it a danger and a nuisance. If severely threatened, a dog may bite from fear; this has become a habit in the typical "fear biter". When a young dog is allowed to persist with seemingly harmless behaviors such as mounting the owner's legs, masturbating against objects, urine marking, and exhibiting separation anxiety (including destructive chewing and digging), such behavior may develop into a more serious problem. If there is a certain degree of internal reward, as in the digging, the problem is difficult to stop. If the problems occur only when the owners are away, delayed punishment is counterproductive.

Man-dog Relationship: Man and dog interact on at least 3 planes: 1) Dependence—beginning in early puppyhood, the dog becomes a perpetual dependent. 2) Social dominance—man must be dominant or risk being threatened or bitten in competitive situations. Dominance is not acquired through severe punishment; controlled but firm restraint is more effective. Most dogs will submit when lifted from the ground by the scruff of the neck, or held in lateral recumbency (owners should take measures to protect themselves if the dog is particularly aggressive). 3) Leader-follower relationship—training is required to produce this in most dogs.

PUPPY BEHAVIOR

House-training: Until puppies begin to eat solid food at ~3 wk, the bitch keeps them clean by licking them and swallowing their excreta. Thereafter, a puppy avoids soiling its bed; it will move away to defecate and urinate but will not begin to use specific areas until ~8 wk. Puppies should be supervised closely from 7 wk to prevent their using improper areas. The puppy can be tied on a short leash, kept in a small crate, or confined to a room between trips to the yard, and may soon be left loose in a room after being outside. They should be given access to toilet areas after awakening, eating, or becoming active. If expected to eliminate outdoors as an adult, it is best to train the puppy to do so; most dogs do not make a transition between paper and grass easily.

Social Development: Dogs of different breeds and strains vary considerably in their behavior. Temperament and "trainability", often cited as important factors when choosing a puppy, are not easy to assess at an early age. Since the most impressionable age to develop a strong relationship between dogs and people is between 3 and 12 wk, the new puppy should be selected at ~6 wk and taken home as soon as possible (*see also* MAN-DOG RELATIONSHIP, above.)

Puppies raised in kennels away from much human association may never be able to adapt to a man-dog relationship if obtained after 12 wk; patience and careful training may help acquaint the dog to a few people, but may be unsuccessful. Such dogs frequently develop a "kennel dog" syndrome; they lack confidence, and may be aggressive, or fear-biters, or be overly submissive. These behaviors may disappear if the dog is returned to its original kennel. Dogs kept in kennels may form their strongest relationships with other dogs, accept the kennel as "home", and thus not make good pets.

Dogs reared exclusively with man may be difficult to mate because they think of man as their own species and do not recognize other dogs. Because dogs are pack animals by nature, their early social experience (before 12 wk of age) should include the kinds of people and breeds of dogs with which they will be in contact in later life.

Fundamentals of Training: All dogs should be taught obedience to commands such as no, sit, stay, come, and heel starting at 8 wk of age. A trained dog willingly does what its owner asks. As little as 10 min a day in training can produce a well-trained dog by 16 wk of age. These lessons should be brief and without interruption, and should start with simple tasks that the puppy can perform. The fundamentals of training are moderate repetition, consistency, praise for good performance given immediately after the desired response, and firmness toward misbehavior within a relationship based on mutual trust and affection. A more formal obedience class at ~6 mo reinforces the concepts and helps refine the early lessons.

SOCIAL BEHAVIOR OF CATS

Cats are asocial animals, and tend to be solitary in their lifestyle. They occasionally form an apparent friendship but will still spend a large amount of time alone. Many feline behaviors center on this solitary life-style, including social, ingestive, and reproductive behaviors. Dominance does not exist in the traditional form. In a group, one cat "owns" the territory, 1 or 2 are extremely low ranking, and the rest share a central social position. This territorial order will vary among the same individuals if in another area. Cats that share a position tend to fight frequently. For successful mating, the male must be present at the appropriate time. Vocalizations are used as an attractant, and induced ovulation guarantees egg and sperm meet at the appropriate time.

Social Development of Kittens: Kittens are social because they depend on the queen for warmth and food, and on their littermates for warmth and, later, play. Social play develops gradually around the third week. These interactions help the kitten develop coordination; learn adult skills for hunting, elimination, and survival; and finish behavioral and physiological maturation.

As the kittens reach 6-8 mo of age, they are capable of surviving on their own. The play bouts become briefer and end in aggressive bouts that become more intense and longer. These tend to drive the litter apart and into the solitary life-style.

Owners often notice a change in their cat's personality at this time, being disappointed that it has become less friendly and perhaps more aggressive.

SOCIAL BEHAVIOR OF LARGE ANIMALS

Herd or Group Structure: Livestock associate together in groups, even under free-range farming systems. Sheep, cattle, and horses maintain visual contact. Pigs spend much time in actual contact with each other, and utilize vocalization. If disturbed, sheep and horses first bunch and, if threatened, then run from the source of disturbance. Pigs and cattle move in a looser group and may stand their ground for danger. During the bunching of animal groups in natural or high-density situations, individuals may be forced to violate the personal space of others. Social interactions at such close quarters depend on the position of the animals in the dominance order. Since aggressive behavior is seen most when groups of pigs, cattle, or horses are first formed, frequent changing of group members should be avoided. Milk production and other physiological responses can be affected for several days while aggressive social interactions are occurring. Although sheep seldom show overt social dominance, subtle but intense interactions do occur, particularly with rams during the breeding season. Agonistic behaviors can take many forms, including butting in cattle and sheep; biting of the rump, neck, or withers in horses; and pushing, biting, and side-ripping with the tusks in boars.

Development of Social Dominance: Piglets show some competitive fighting for preferred nipples of the sow within days of birth; once the teat order is established, the ranking carries over into later dominance positions. Other species do not develop a stable social order until some time after weaning. Social-dominance effects can be important in cases of high stock densities or poor farm layout. Inadequate trough space, narrow races, inadequate space in indoor housing, or lack of feeders can mean that dominant animals command more resources. The subordinates suffer, and health and general production can be affected. In the extremes of dominance, just the presence of the highest-ranking individual can physiologically decrease salivation and hunger. Some subordinate goats have had higher internal parasite loads and a higher death rate during droughts when scarce food was commandeered by dominant stock. There may be an upper limit to the number of group members that can be recognized or remembered by one individual; this could be 50-70 in cattle and 20-30 in pigs.

The horse responds to small changes in stance or skin pressures, and good horsemen use these cues during dominance-subordination interactions. Sometimes tranquilizers have been used to aid social tolerance when strange pigs were penned together, or when wild horses were to be tamed.

SOCIAL BEHAVIOR OF CHICKENS

The chick shows early responses while still in the shell, eg, low-pitched distress calls if cooled, or rapid twittering if warmed. Chicks hatched at slightly subnormal temperatures make distress calls as their moist down dries and they lose contact with the shell. Contact with a broody hen or other warm object prevents these calls. Newly hatched chicks are attracted to the hen by warmth, contact, clucking, and body movements; this attraction is greatest on the day of hatching. They learn to eat, roost, drink, and avoid enemies in the company of the mother hen.

In chicks, the most sensitive period for imprinting to the hen is from 9-20 hr after hatching, and fear is shown by the third day. The attachment to the hen depends primarily on the sound of her voice and her appearance. As the down starts to disappear from their heads, the chicks are rejected by the hen. She pecks at them, and the clutch starts to disperse and become more independent.

Hens and cocks have separate peck orders, with the male order being less stable. The dominance order is most clearly seen in competition for food or mates, and subordinate hens may obtain so little food that production is affected. In a flock kept in a state of social disorganization by removal and replacement, birds eat less, may lose weight or grow poorly, and tend to lay fewer eggs. Additional feed and water troughs distributed about the pen enable subordinate hens to feed undisturbed, and an adequate number of nesting boxes provides these birds better opportunities to lay. Flocks of >80 birds tend to separate into 2 distinct groups, and at least 2 separate peck orders appear to be established.

Flock Behavior: The clutch is the basis of flock organization. A chick reared in isolation tends to stay apart from the flock and does less well than group birds. Flock formation by adults depends on mutual tolerance. Strangers are attacked and only gradually integrated into the flock. Newcomers often are relegated to positions near the bottom of the social order.

SOCIAL BEHAVIOR OF DOMESTIC TURKEYS

Domestic and wild turkeys have similar flocking patterns and social organization, but management practices determine the size and composition of domestic groups. The social dominance order is less stable than that of chickens, particularly for penned males. Certain varieties of turkeys tend to be dominant over others, eg, Black over Bronze over Gray, and in mixed sex groups, males over females.

As with chickens, the most common pair encounter is a simple threat, with one bird submitting to the other. Otherwise, turkeys warily circle each other with wing feathers spread and tails fanned, and each emits a high-pitched trill. Then one or both will leap into the air and attempt to claw the other. The one that can push, pull, or press down the head of the other normally wins the encounter. Bouts usually last a few minutes. Much blood may be shed since highly vascular skin areas may be torn, but actual physical damage is slight and birds do not fight to death. However, an injured, lower-ranking bird should be separated from the group until its wounds heal, since others tend to peck and aggravate the wound.

The poults move freely shortly after hatching and should become socially imprinted to their dam during the first 1-2 days. Normal poults form tightly knit groups that may initially cluster for warmth, but are cohesive even in warm environments. Birds tend to feed or wander as a group, and if they are with the hen, she is the focus of activity. Vocal and visual signals are used by both parent and young to stay in contact until the poults are ≥8 wk old. Fighting is rare before 3 mo of age, but increases to a peak at 5 mo, when social orders are formed.

SOCIAL BEHAVIOR OF DUCKS

Most domestic ducks have originated from 2 species—the mallard (*Anas platyrhynchos*) and the muscovy (*Cairina moschata*). In the muscovy, both sexes have bare skin on the face.

Social Behavior of Muscovies: Muscovies are promiscuous. The adult males, which are twice as heavy as females, are solitary and aggressive toward other males. Their displays are primitive and their calls simple. The female, when alarmed, utters a weak quack; the male uses a hissing noise with tail-shaking, crest-raising, and swinging of the head as both a threat to other males and a sexual display toward females. Since females generally avoid displaying males, they may be chased to exhaustion before the male can mate. Following fertilization, the female retires to her nest site and lays an egg a day. The nest is not continuously occupied until incubation begins with the last or second last egg. Eggs are hatched after 35 days. The male sexually attacks any female he meets, and he plays no part in the selection of the nest, incubation, or care of the young.

Social Behavior of Mallards: Wild mallards are monogamous and stay together from midwinter until the beginning of incubation, a period of 5 mo. In domestic situations, this may not be possible if sex numbers are not balanced.

Sexually stimulated males display singly or in groups toward particular females, which in turn incite the males with a rather formalized display alternating between threatening and submissive gestures with a peculiar call. The threat is toward a strange male and submission is shown to the preferred male, who then swims ahead of the female and turns his nape toward her. Fighting, chasing, and plumage displays are common among males but are not crucial to pairing.

Paired birds leave the flock, but in some domestic situations, females may not be able to avoid attack by unpaired males, and may be drowned or chased to exhaustion. The female is protected by her mate until egg-laying is complete. Incubation takes 28 days, and the young leave the nest after the first day. The female undergoes her annual molt in the 6-8 wk before the brood can fly.

The young normally imprint on their mother during the first few days after hatching. Species recognition occurs more gradually to ensure mating with their own species when mature.

REPRODUCTIVE BEHAVIOR

THE FEMALE

The normal mating state of the female has both behavioral and physiological elements. The term estrus is often reserved to describe the behavioral and not the physiological components. The ovaries can undergo changes associated with estrus without the female showing signs of estrous behavior.

Normal behavioral routines are altered during overt estrus, and typically there is less eating and resting behavior, while locomotor, agonistic, investigative, and vocal behavior increase. These responses are secondary to the essential characteristic of estrus, the female's willingness to stand to be mated.

Mounting behavior between females is typical of estrus of cows in larger groups and is sometimes seen in bitches, but seldom observed in mares, queens, or ewes. The mare in heat often assumes a particular stance, which involves frequent straddling, while urine is spilled in small amounts and the clitoris is exposed by repeated rhythmic eversions. The company of other horses is sought, and particular interest is shown in the male. In the presence of a stallion, the mare in heat will orient her hindquarters toward him and remain still. Sows will begin to follow boars or almost anything that moves.

Estrous periods and cycles vary considerably in mares, possibly because they have been selected to ovulate in early February—an unnatural time of the year. The estrous period generally lasts 4-10 days, and the cycles repeat every 28 days. A period of anestrus typically occurs during the shorter daylight season, although some mares may show behavioral and/or physiological estrus then.

Estrus in most bitches recurs at ~6-mo intervals, irrespective of the time of year. The Rhodesian Ridgeback and Basenji tend to retain the single seasonal breeding per year like their wolf ancestor. Some of the toy breeds cycle 3 times a year. Proestrous bleeding and vulvar swelling are unique characteristics of the bitch. *See also* FALSE PREGNANCY, p 678.

Estrus in the cat has a 3 wk periodicity, with peaks in early spring or summer. Receptivity lasts 4-6 days if mating occurs, or 6-10 days if not. The heat cry vocalization is used to attract toms, and once they are nearby, rolling, rubbing, and lordosis behaviors indicate the queen's hormonal state.

Repeated matings in natural settings tend to shorten the duration of estrus in cattle by as much as 8 hr. Some females "teased" with vasectomized males showed a shorter duration of estrus. These examples substantiate the modern view that estrus is not under endogenous control alone and that its manifestation is subject, in part, to environmental factors, including biostimulation.

The 2 common natural conditions responsible for anestrus are seasonality and pregnancy, eg, in mares and donkeys. As many as 2% of pregnant cows show estrus during pregnancy, almost as many as show silent heats while cycling.

THE MALE

Libido in the male animal develops at puberty and persists, in some degree, throughout life. It depends on the production of testosterone, and its manifestation is determined by inherited characteristics. Libido may be altered as a consequence of physical aging or be inhibited due to adverse experiences. Under natural conditions, a male of low libido leaves few offspring, but in domestic situations, low libido can be perpetuated. Circumstantial and experimental evidence indicates some genetic basis for libido. Nutrition has only a slight influence; however, a high plane of nutrition can inhibit testosterone secretion in some young males, while gross underfeeding can impair libido.

Since there is no significant correlation between sexual behavior and semen quality, an adequate evaluation of the breeding ability of a sire must assess both factors.

Libido manifests itself during male courtship. The "lip-curl", or flehmen, is shown by most ungulates. The male extends the head and neck, contracts the nostrils, and raises and curls the upper lip. This usually occurs after smelling urine or nosing the female perineum, and involves odor testing.

COITAL BEHAVIOR

"Tending" is often shown by the male consorting with the female immediately before and during estrus. Freely associating mating partners may set up a temporary alliance ("tending bond"), which facilitates repeated mating and ensures optimal conditions for fertilization. Nudging in some form occurs in the precoital behavior of most ungulates. By pushing on the hindquarters of the female, the male is able to feel if she moves away, as in proestrus, or stands. This is a common behavior of bulls. Stallions test estrus in the mare by smelling and by biting and nipping areas of the body, working from the hindquarters toward the neck of the mare.

One of the functions of courtship is to orient the male in such a way as to achieve intromission. Appropriate mounting is partly acquired by learning. Males normally mount females of their own species, but stallions will mount female donkeys, and jackasses will mount mares (resulting in mules). Occasionally, sheep and goats will intermate. More rarely, bulls mount mares, stallions mount heifers, and dogs mount various species. Inappropriate imprinting is often cited as the basis for such behavior. Courtship also allows the male to achieve a complete erection, so a long courtship phase is more important in species with a vascular penis, as opposed to those with a fibroelastic one.

The mating phase of male sexual behavior consists of many behavioral components. These include mounting, clasping, pelvic thrusts, intromission, and ejaculation. "False mounts" by the male occur if intromission is not achieved, and more than one attempt may be needed before mating is successful; eg, in stallions, some 2-3 false mounts are normal before effective mating is successful. In bulls, goats, and rams, intromission consists of one or few pelvic thrusts, followed by dismounting. In stallions, there is a longer period of pelvic thrusting before ejaculation. Pigs have a relatively long mating phase, with ejaculation lasting up to 20 min. Mating in cats is terminated quickly; as the tom withdraws his penis, the penile spines stimulate the vaginal epithelium, which often causes the queen to turn and attack the tom. In dogs, a "tie" occurs during intromission as the vulvovaginal musculature tightens behind the bulb of the penis. This tie is maintained for 10-30 min, even if the male dismounts and swings a hindlimb over the back of the female, so as to stand rear to rear.

The postmating phase includes the dismount, genital grooming in some species, and a refractory period when there is no interest in an estrous female. A quicker return to mating readiness is shown by males given opportunity to mate a new female.

Females normally are mated several times during each estrous period. The frequency is influenced by several factors, including the number of estrous females, competing males, prior services, and the degree of receptivity in estrous females. When competition between ewes exists for a limited number of rams, older ewes are usually more successful than "maiden" ones in obtaining repeated matings.

FEATURES OF REPRODUCTIVE BEHAVIOR IN DOMESTIC BIRDS

Sexual Behavior: As the cockerel approaches maturity, testosterone production results in secondary sex characteristics, including the growth of comb and wattles and

Table 2. Coitus, Lg An

Male Reaction Time	Precoital Behavior of Male	Manner of Intromission	Duration of Intromission and Site of Insemination	Repeat Matings
Horses Av 5 min	Noses genital region. Genital olfactory reflex. Bites croup region. Penis erects.	1-4 mounts. Several pelvic oscillations. Terminal inactive phase.	1 min, intracervical	Breeding usually arranged to permit 2-4 services per estrus.
Cattle Mode 2 min Mean 12 min Mean of beef breeds 20 min	Noses vulva. Genital olfactory reflex. Alignment. Licks hindquarters.	Single pelvic thrust coordinated with clasp reflex.	5-10 sec, intravaginal	Free-ranging bulls serve cows 3-10 times in estrous period.
Pigs 1-10 min	Approaches sow giving series of grunts. Noses vulva vigorously. Champs jaw and froths at mouth.	Short protrusions of spiral penis repeated until intromission occurs. Pelvic oscillations followed by somnolent phase.	9 min, intrauterine	Many boars serve a sow 3-7 times in estrous period.
Sheep 30 sec to 5 min	Noses vulva. Genital olfactory reflex. Paws with forefeet. Bleating, stamping with forefoot, rapid locking. Genital olfactory reflex.	Very quick, single pelvic thrust with forelimb clasping.	5 sec, intravaginal	Rams sometimes serve estrous female several times. Some mature rams serve each ewe only once.

crowing. Male courtship activities include "ground pecking", a wing flutter, and waltzing, which leads to copulation. Crowing, which is rare in capons, advertises the location of the male and his territory to prospective mates and warns off other males. Male interference with copulation is common when several males are crowded into small pens with few females.

In the maturing pullet, hormones from the ovarian cortex stimulate the growth of oviducts, inhibit male plumage, and are responsible for the sex crouch when the cock places one foot on the back before mating. Modified wattles and combs also develop.

Parental Behavior: Except in "nonbroody" breeds, incubation commences after a number of eggs have been laid. During sittings, the eggs are turned to prevent adhesions within the shell. A warm, defeathered, highly vascular brood-patch develops on each side of the breast. The broody hen clucks and ruffles her feathers if disturbed. Under feral conditions, an elaborate approach behavior confuses predators and allows hens to return to the nest undetected. During incubation (20-22 days), prolactin reduces ovarian activity and sexual behavior so that egg laying ceases. After hatching, the hen uses brief, repetitive, low-pitched vocalizations to lead the chicks and to indicate food sources. She warns them about ground or overhead predators with cackles or a loud scream.

Turkeys are seasonal breeders; activity peaks in the spring, but with the use of artificial light, they can be kept sexually active throughout the year. Males initiate an elaborate courtship (up to 10 min) with postures and movements, but are ignored by all except receptive hens. This receptivity lasts ~2 days. Such females crouch in response to the male's strutting, sitting down quietly with the head drawn in close to the body. The male approaches slowly, mounts, treads, and makes cloacal contact with the everted oviduct of the female. Ejaculation follows swiftly, the male dismounts, and the female executes a postcopulatory feather ruffling and brief run. Males have a short refractory period and have been seen to mate with as many as 10 females in 30 min. No pair bonds are formed, but range males often gather harems, which they defend against other males. Only higher-ranking males successfully complete a mating. Lower-ranking females are mated more often than high-ranking females, but they lay fewer and smaller eggs. After a single mating, fertile eggs can be laid for 5-6 wk. When eggs are removed routinely, broody behavior is postponed.

BEHAVIORAL STRESS

The control exerted by man on domestic animals continues to increase, and new phases of intensive farming continue to be implemented. There is a growing public demand for veterinarians to assess the management conditions and welfare of the larger number of animals being kept in intensive conditions within artificial environments. Stressors are factors in environments that induce states of distress in livestock. Stress also may be indicated by changes in the behavior of the animal and the strategies it adopts to overcome stressor influences: 1) Animals require some stimulation to overcome stress or "boredom" in a barren environment. 2) The animal can show an effective adaptive response to normal stressors. 3) Beyond a critical level of stress, the animal may be unable to adapt as expected and exhibit abnormal or anomalous responses. Most previous research focused on feeding requirements, health, and hygiene; the behavioral requirements and social needs of the animals were poorly understood. Overcrowding and/or confinement led to various stressor effects, and the resulting behavior patterns have often been designated as "vices". A number of attempts have been made to evaluate the various stressors in an environment and to calculate a stressor index. One difficulty is that a stress to one individual or breed may not be that to another.

Some of the anomalous or abnormal patterns shown by animals in distress as they fall within each behavior system are discussed below.

Table 3. Anomalies of Reactive Behavior

Condition	Animals Involved	Etiology	Clinical Sequelae
Weaving	Horses	Restraint	Condition loss Sore back
Head shaking	Poultry Horses Exotic species	"Frustration"	Not known
Head nodding	Horses	"Frustration" Teeth problems	Not known
Snout (Nose) rubbing	Pigs Dogs Cats	Crowding	Uncertain
Stereotyped pacing	Horses Poultry Dogs Exotic species	Confinement "Frustration"	Condition loss
Pawing	Horses Bulls	Uncertain	Not known
Self-mutilation	Horses Dogs	Confinement "Frustration"	Injuries
Head rubbing	Pigs Cattle	Isolation	Not known
Tail rubbing	Horses	Various	Not known
Displacement activities	All species	"Frustration"	Not known
Chronic standing	Horses Calves	Disability and restriction	Fatigue
Somnolent dog-sitting	Sows Horses Cattle	Various	Usually none Urinary infections Sudden death from kidney failure
Flank sucking	Dogs	"Frustration"	Probably none
Destructive behavior	Dogs Cats Horses	"Frustration"	None

Anomalous Behavior: In the past, comparatively little knowledge was available of the responses of animals kept under intensive systems of management. Many forms of abnormal behavior are related to noxious stimuli or stressors in the environment. Inferior environments appear to be closely linked with anomalous behaviors such as cannibalism, reduction in appetite, stereotyped movements, poor parental care, over-aggressiveness, unresponsiveness, tail-biting, cribbing, destructive chewing, digging, over-grooming, and several others. Behaviors that were formerly regarded as vices are forms of anomalous behavior that arise as an animal attempts to cope with restriction, overcrowding, or a lack of diversionary stimuli in the environment.

Some recent attempts have been made to classify the variety of anomalous behavioral responses seen in domestic animals. Although none is entirely satisfactory, one of these systems is used to make some sense of a difficult field of study. Anomalous behaviors can be characterized by their form, the frequency, and the behavior system under which they occur.

Table 4. Anomalies of Mouth-based Ingestive Behavior

Condition	Animals Involved	Etiology	Clinical Sequelae
Crib-biting	Horses	Confinement	Loss of condition Occasional colic
Licking	Horses Dogs Cats	Confinement Nervousness	Unknown
Tail biting	Pigs Horses Dogs	Complex; involves crowding, poor nutrition, "frustration"	Loss of condition Abscessed hindquarters
Tongue dragging	Horses	Uncertain	Unknown
Bar biting	Pigs	Confinement	Reduced production and subfertility
Prolonged sucking	Calves Piglets Pups Kittens	Early weaning	Hairball (trichobezoars) Trauma to others
Excess grooming	Calves Dogs Cats	Confinement "Frustration"	Hairball Lick granuloma
Wool (Hair) pulling	Sheep Primates	Confinement "Frustration"	Loss of hair or fleece
Tongue rolling	Cattle	Confinement	Unknown
Vacuous chewing	Pigs	Confinement	Marked weight loss and lowered fertility
Feather picking	Poultry	High-density stocking	Loss of feather cover Trauma

Reactive Anomalies: Many of the described anomalous forms of behavior occur while the animal is excited. These anomalies (*see* TABLE 3) include weaving in horses, snout rubbing in pigs, and displacement preening in poultry. They are mostly stereotyped activities of body movement, and often arise as a result of displacement acts.

Anomalous Oral/Ingestive Behavior: Anomalous behavior syndromes involving oral or ingestive responses are another subclass (*see* TABLES 4 and 5). Nutritional deficiencies are only one contributory factor in animals that express mouthing or ingestion anomalies. Pups artificially fed from nipples with large holes continued to suck littermates' ears after the available milk had been ingested. Likewise, bucket-reared calves often develop habits of sucking other calves. Countering such disorders must involve changes to the causal husbandry practices.

Table 5. Anomalies of Ingestive Behavior

Condition	Animals Involved	Manifestations
Wind sucking (Aerophagia)	Horses	Air is repeatedly gulped alone or in association with a biting action.
Wood chewing (Lignophagia)	Horses, Cattle, Sheep	Debarking of tree trunks and chewing at restrictive outdoor and indoor enclosures.
Eating feces (Coprophagia)	Horses, Pigs, Dogs	Normal in rabbits and in young of most species. Also occurs in adult animals, eg, dogs, enclosed horses, and pigs. May follow anal massage activity in pigs.
Hair eating (Trichophagia)	Sheep, Cattle, Horses, Cats, Rabbits	Eating the coat, ie, hair or wool, of self or other. May occur as sequela of excess grooming or body sucking.
Anomalous milk sucking (Galactophagia)	Cattle (Dairy), Lambs, Cats	Cross-sucking by adult animals.
Soil eating (Geophagia)	Horses, Cattle, Cats, Dogs	Ingestion of earth, sand, in substantial amount.
Overeating (Hyperphagia)	Horses, Cattle, Dogs, Cats	Overeating and bolting food as a habit form, or in episodic form.
Excess drinking (Polydipsia)	Horses, Sheep, Pigs, Poultry	Excess consumption of water through frequent drinking, seen in confined animals with *ad lib* water supply. May be a disease process but more frequently is a behavioral disorder.
Pica	Cattle, Sheep, Dogs, Cats	Chewing at foreign objects such as old bones, cloth, etc. Suggests deficiency disease, eg, aphosphorosis.
Litter eating	Horses, Poultry, Kittens	Eating soiled or clean bedding, particularly wood particles or chaff.
Feather eating	Poultry (Hens)	Pecking and swallowing feathers from other birds. Misdirected feeding responses in poultry kept in compact groups on concentrated feeds.
Egg eating	Poultry (Hens) (on litter)	Breaking eggshells by pecking and eating contents.
Body pecking or biting	Poultry, Pigs	Biting or peck-stabbing various body parts such as head, tail, ears, back, vents, toes, and prolapsed viscera.

Reproductive Anomalies: *See* TABLE 6. A number of maladaptive responses relate to sexual, maternal, or neonatal activities. Anomalous responses relating to estrus and libido represent serious problems to the animal industries.

Behavioral Needs: There is much debate as to the importance of ethological needs of farm animals. Do pigs require a wallow when penned indoors, or chickens a

Table 6. Anomalies of Reproductive Behavior

Condition	Animals Involved	Manifestations
Silent heat	Mares, Cows, Bitches	Absence or low levels of behavioral estrus in a female having other physiological features of fertile estrus.
Somnolent impotence	Bulls	Correct male alignment behind estrous female but adoption of inactive somnolent condition; head is often laid on female back.
Coital misalignment	Bulls, Goats	Adoption of a position by the male, in which there is deviation in alignment from the female and no mounting attempt (head mounting).
Intromission impotence	Bulls, Rams	Active mounting, clasping but with little thrusting, and persistent intromission failure.
Monosexual syndrome	Bulls, Rams, Boars, Feedlot steers	Sexual mounting of other males to exclusion of females, eg, in rams raised in dense unisexual groups. Bullersteer syndrome: tolerance by steers of frequent mounting by other steers within confined groups.
Rejection of neonate	All stock	Persistent aggressive reaction toward the newborn or active desertion by dam.
Maternal failure	All stock	Persistent negative maternal reaction toward the newborn, which is not allowed to suck. Failure of milk "letdown".
Stealing other young	Mares, Cows, Ewes	Prepartum efforts by a dam to adopt offspring belonging to others. Often a function of stocking density and synchronized parturition, or high stocking rates.
Low sucking drive	All stock	Failure of newborn to show positive teat-seeking behavior.
Puerperal aggression	Parturient stock	Sudden development (postpartum) of violent aggressive behavior, antisocially directed, occurring temporarily.
Maternal cannibalism	Sows, Ewes, Bitches, Queens	Newly farrowed gilts with their first litters may eat their piglets when agitated. Ewes housed indoors occasionally eat tails and feet of their newborn lambs. Bitches may continue to chew the umbilical stump, rupture the abdominal wall and consume the viscera, occasionally feet, of pups.
Pseudocyesis	Bitches	Bitches with persistent corpora lutea adopt parturient behavior, including nesting and "adoption" of inanimate objects.

Table 7. Anomalies of Agonistic Behavior

Condition	Animals Involved	Manifestations
Strong overt aggression	All farm stock	Rushing, pushing, or charging aggressively at intruding or approaching animals of same or different species (including man).
Excess alarm	All farm stock	Strong overt reactions: stampeding, bolting, hysterical flightiness in poultry.
Threatening	All farm stock	Strong overt threat display, particularly on human approach.
Butting	Ruminants, notably cattle, male goats, rams	Striking with head, goring with horns, poll of the head against competing/intruding/accessible object or person.
Biting	Horses, dogs, cats, pigs	Habitual, antisocial snapping or nipping.
Kicking/Striking		Striking aggressively with a foot or limb
	1. Horses	1. Forward strike with a forefoot.
	2. Horses	2. Lifting hindquarters and lashing out backwards with both hindfeet.
	3. All farm stock	3. Kicking down and back with one hindfoot.
	4. All farm stock	4. Kicking forward with one hindfoot.
	5. Mules, donkeys, cattle	5. Kicking sideward with one hindfoot.
Startle-alarm	All stock, most common in horses	Shying, jibbing, balking, startle reactions. Avoid certain situations, environmental features, or events. Intensive alarm reactions; can include throwing up head, rearing, leaping, turning away sharply.
Freezing (Hypotonia)	All stock, most common in cattle and other ruminants; hens, dogs	Lying, "freezing", and persistent tonic immobility in forms of reactive recumbency. Refusal to rise in response to strong urging. A form of functional inertia or akinesis.

place to dust-bathe when kept in small cages? When conditions allow, pigs will wallow to adjust body temperature or during what seems like recreational play. If a well-housed pig has a comfortable thermal environment, does it have a need to wallow; is there an adverse effect on the pig if a wallow is not provided; will it be frustrated, distressed or even pained? It is often argued that pigs with previous experience of a wallow may have a need for one; would the need be the same if a pig had never experienced a wallow? These subjects are difficult to research, yet may be matters of intense debate.

The veterinarian can respond only out of experience. Some indoor environments may be particularly restrictive and allow few opportunities to groom, stretch, display, or make social contact with other nearby pen members. With limited possibilities for activity, some species tend to adopt oral anomalies. Pigs have a deep-seated urge to root or to mouth materials. The more species-characteristic the behavior response that is thwarted, the more likely it is that an ethological need is not being met. Debate is bound to continue over the importance of behavioral needs of animals and their relationship to animal welfare. It may be found that many of the detailed behavioral needs are not essential, but if fulfilled or alternatives used, the animal may flourish. The studies showing that Tender Gentle Care (TGC) during early handling, talking to indoor animals, etc, have a beneficial effect on growth and production and diminish disease and stress, may reflect the consequences of attention to an animal's ethological needs.

CONTROL OF BEHAVIORAL SYNDROMES

It has been argued that a stress-induced behavioral anomaly (such as repetitive, stereotyped movement) is a sign of adaptation; in other words, behavioral homeostasis has mitigated or eliminated the stress. Others argue that this interpretation, in terms of animal welfare, is illogical. The perseverance of anomalous behavior can be adaptive if the causal factors are still present; however, the behaviors often persist after the stress has been removed. Studies indicate that narcotic antagonists can stop such behavior for a short while, which suggests that these behaviors may release endorphins. Further deterioration, both behavioral and physiological, may follow and affect usability, health, productivity, growth, and disease resistance. The control of behavioral anomalies is ethically and physiologically desirable. Methods of control of behavioral anomalies are indicated, when feasible, below.

SYNDROMES

Weaving: Recognized as a behavioral disorder of caged or confined animals, this is common in horses that have been chronically kept in stalls. The animal stands in one position, but weaves from side to side or may rock back and forth. Once acquired, weaving is extremely difficult to control, and it is believed that the anomaly can be induced in other horses in a stable through association. To some extent, it can be controlled by tying the horse with cross ties so as to limit the lateral movement of its head. Hobbles on the forelimbs also tend to limit the motion in a stall. Without exercise, however, the problem is rarely controlled. Ideally, affected animals should be turned out to pasture, but when this is not possible through lack of space, enforced exercise can be provided by riding, lunging, or use of a mechanical exerciser.

Pawing: Control of pawing is difficult, particularly since the cause is unknown. Since it occurs most frequently in confined and isolated horses, it may be alleviated by turning the affected animal out to pasture with other horses. Hobbles or kick chains have been used on problem horses with limited success.

Stereotyped Pacing: In horses, this is recognized as "stall walking". It is a common behavior in circus and zoo animals that are confined to small spaces. It also occurs in dogs that have been kenneled a long time, and in poultry. In poultry, it appears to be induced by thwarting birds that are both hungry and in a state of high expectation. Affected birds typically show repetitive pacing movements occupying the full range of one side of the pen or cage. Once the condition has become an established behavior of the horse or bird, it cannot be controlled without environmental freedom.

Head Shaking: This is more common in caged birds than in floor-reared hens. It is also seen when the stocking rate of birds is increased. It is reduced when birds are transferred to the fresh environment of a pen of greater space. Horses and zoo animals may also exhibit head shaking.

Head Nodding: Various forms of this behavioral anomaly in horses, which is similar to head shaking, occur as stereotyped behavior. Once established, control is difficult. A heavy fringe on the brow band of a head stall can distract a horse in this practice. The teeth and the fit of the bit should be checked if the behavior is beginning.

Head Rubbing: This is sometimes observed in pigs or cattle subject to chronic confinement within narrow single stalls. Control of this behavior (as with similar somatic, stereotyped actions) seems to require relief of the chronic restraint.

Tail Rubbing: This behavior in horses is nonspecific. To eliminate the possibility of parasitism (qv, p 202), the horse should be examined and given a parasiticide if necessary.

Nose (Snout) Rubbing: This has been observed in certain types of pigs and occasionally in dogs and cats. The anomalous behavior of anal massage by snout rubbing and ingestion of feces, seen in pigs, is a compound anomaly. The condition typically occurs among growing pigs kept in crowded conditions, and has been more noticeable since tail docking has become fairly universal in the control of tail biting.

Easing crowded conditions may control snout rubbing and associated coprophagia (qv, p 925) and is more effective in prevention. Since the anomaly may be induced in adjoining pens by visual association, solid pen walls are useful. Snout rubbing also may be reduced by supplying pens with objects that the pigs can chew and root.

Self-mutilation: Vigorous body friction or flank biting is a serious behavioral anomaly in horses, typically those in confinement and isolation. Dogs show self-mutilation by destructive chewing on their tails or by lick granulomas. Major and minor tranquilizers and, experimentally, narcotic antagonists have been used to stop the behavior. Increasing exercise and minimizing stress is important. Flank sucking in Dobermans and some other dogs is shown during stress; the dog holds its mouth on its loin or flank, leaving a wet spot but rarely causing a problem. While affected animals are not usually found to have any pathological skin condition, parasitism, neuromas, or GI clinical condition, these possibilities should be investigated.

Displacement Activities: Displacement activities are normal behaviors expressed at inappropriate times. A wide range can be recognized in farm animals. These are often in forms in individual units of feeding or grooming behavior, and are shown as "energy shifts" in conflict situations. While all these should not be considered as anomalous behaviors, a high incidence of displacement activity implies such in individual cases.

Chronic Standing: Formerly it was not uncommon for horsemen to provide such animals with a strong chain or timber across the rear posts of a horse stall for the animal to lean its hindquarters against so as to permit rest and sleep.

Dog-sitting: This is seen in breeding sows restrained for most of their pregnancy in narrow single stalls. A form of it is sometimes observed in veal calves after long-term confinement to narrow crates. Also, occasionally, dog-sitting postures are seen in heavy livestock, such as bulls and some horses. Anomalous dog-sitting can be controlled by a change in husbandry; however, since styles of husbandry usually represent prevailing fashions in animal production industries, such a change may be difficult to make.

Reactive Anomalies: Manifestations of anomalous temperament are mostly hyper-reactions of attitude. The reactive etho-anomalies are a particular problem among companion animals, especially dogs. Anomalous reactivity can be determined by observation using clinical judgment. Individual forms of anomalous reactive behavior are given below with reference to control.

Mobile Aggression: Aggressive behavior in a tendency to rush toward an approaching individual is notable in dogs. It is seen also in all farm species from time to time, more commonly in males and in dams of recently born animals. Aggressive rushing is common in dogs with outdoor territory, in mares with young foals, in geese at free range, and in freshly calved cows of certain breeds, eg, Galloway and Brahman. It is also common among stallions and dogs as intermale aggression. Control is in the form of restraint or avoidance.

Mobile Alarm: An abnormal tendency to sudden flight is seen in some animals. Flight is the extensive form of alarm reaction, which is quite normal and adaptive among animals that would be prey in the wild, or even under free-range conditions in domestic animals. Its occurrence within husbandry systems without appropriate stimulation is maladaptive. The tendency to this in poultry is termed "flightiness". Flightiness is a more prominent abnormality in some strains of birds than others (*see* below). It is also seen in other species when they have been penned and energy has accumulated. Horses with this tendency often react to little stimuli and can lose their riders. Control requires eliminating likely stimuli and increasing exercise to eliminate extra energy.

Hysteria: The extensive alarm reaction in poultry is often termed hysteria. Flightiness in the domestic chicken appears in different types of nervous and hysterical behavior in different environments and age groups. Hysteria in the cage-layer is characterized by sudden flying about, squawking, and trying to hide. Control relates to stocking density. Incidence of hysteria in penned poultry is closely related to flock density: flocks of 40 have had 90% incidence, while control flocks of 20 had an incidence of 22%. Toenail removal in birds has been found to reduce hysteria, but this must be considered unethical. For some strains of poultry, caging is favored; undoubtedly this controls hysteria to some extent, although it can spread throughout a flock kept in battery cages.

Threatening: The habit of giving a threat display is a common characteristic of anomalous temperament in some animals, more often in entire males. It takes the form of threat display typical of the species when the animal is in close human association. This is typically of the static type and not the mobile display of aggression considered above. In dogs, threat displays have several common principal features, including muscular tension, pilomotor activity, raising of the head, vocalization, staring, and orientation toward the intruder either directly or obliquely. This may escalate to attack, and is a feature of dominance aggression in dogs. Horses often flatten their ears and bare their teeth when people walk up to their stalls, even with feed. Some rush at a person who attempts to enter the stall. Restraint in the interest of safety should be considered. Punishment for the behavior or rewards for desired behavior can decrease the problem.

Butting: Some ruminants have the habit of striking aggressively with the head, regardless of whether they have horns. The condition can be aggravated by people playing with the animal's head; caution must be used when working around these animals.

Biting: A behavioral vice exhibited occasionally by dogs and horses, biting is usually in the form of snapping and nipping with the incisor teeth directed at another animal or person coming too close. Cats have also been known to bite. The typical biter does so with the warning signals of ears laid flat, lips retracted, and teeth bared, although others may use the behavior only as a playful act. Biting attempts are usually sudden. Muzzling is an effective control. Punishment with each occurrence can also be helpful.

Kicking and Striking: Animals that show anomalous kicking behavior are considered to be hyper-reactive in temperament. Rearing and striking with the forefeet are dangerous habits of some horses, more commonly of stallions and light horses than others, and striking out with one forelimb may be done without rearing. Other horses kick with one or both hindlimbs and may aim at specific targets or just go through the motions. Control of habitual kicking is difficult. Negative conditioning may be attempted by methods that inflict pain on the animal when it kicks, but success depends on having each kick punished in a method that is negative enough for the animal to stop. Hobbles or kick chains have been used. Implicated animals should be managed cautiously.

Shying (Startle/Aversion): Shying is most notable in horses but can occur in other livestock. Control, when deemed necessary, can be partially effected by provision of a companion animal in a pen, for example. Shying is usually the result of an object moving too rapidly for the horse to focus on it; the instinctive reaction that follows is flight. Horses that tend to shy are often fitted with "blinkers" on the bridle, a common aid used during driving, since shying at that time can be dangerous.

Tonic Immobility: Recognition of anomalous tonic immobility (submissive inertia), or tonic dyskinesia, is essential in the rational handling of fallen, or "downer", livestock of all species. The classic of this behavior is shown by the opossum, in which the catalepsy is an instinctive mechanism to not stimulate the prey-chasing responses of predators. Some believe that, in some cases, the downer cow (qv, p 555) may be an example of "tonic immobility" or catalepsy. In such cases, the condition is not so much an inability to rise as a strong unwillingness to try to rise. This unwillingness not only simulates a pathological bodily state but soon establishes one. It is possible that the control of "tonic immobility" in animals lies in the context of differential diagnosis.

Pathological Oral Activity: A major and complex generic syndrome that comprises a variety of manifestations of excessive and abnormally orientated mouthing behavior (*see also* p 901). Most forms of this syndrome are associated with the combined circumstances of chronic restraint, hypostimulation, and perhaps excess energy.

Crib-biting: A "crib-biter" (cribber) grasps the edge of the manger (crib) or some other convenient fixture with the incisor teeth. The upper incisors are often used alone. The animal presses down and raises the floor of the mouth; the soft palate is forced open. Swallowing and gulping of air may also occur. Horses often develop the problem after being wood-chewers (qv, p 925): ("Wind-sucking" [qv, p 925] is a more severe form of this condition, and air is swallowed. It does not require a resting place for the teeth.)

The best approach is to ensure adequate exercise and to pasture the horse. While this is often successful, owners may want a simpler solution, which makes control difficult. The most common measure is to fasten a strap round the throat, sufficiently tight to make arching of the neck uncomfortable. Some types of these have a metal "gullet-piece" that has a recess into which the trachea fits, and which allows the device to be worn without danger of affecting respiration. Such straps usually must be removed during feeding. Other preventive devices are available but are generally painful to the animal. Cribbers may cease the habit if housed in a barewalled loose-box and fed from a trough that is removed as soon as the feed is finished; however, other stereotyped behaviors may be substituted. Surgery to section some of the throat muscles essential to the behavior is sometimes performed as a last resort (*see* AEROPHAGIA, p 925). Narcotic antagonists have shown promise to help these animals.

Tongue Dragging: With this condition, the affected horse repetitiously allows its tongue to hang out of the mouth, often folded longitudinally on itself, for considerable periods. The horse may or may not suck on the tongue. Control methods range from pain to the tongue as while showing in halter classes, to restraining the tongue with a net or spoon bit. Amputation of the tip of the tongue has been used but must be considered unethical.

Crib-whetting (Licking): Some horses subject to chronic confinement draw the body of the tongue slowly but repeatedly across the edge of some part of the stall. In some cases, the provision of a salt block for licking seems to alleviate the habit, which may indicate a need for salt or that excess salt taste inhibits the problem. Occasional dogs, cats (usually feline leukemia positive), and horses lick objects for unexplained reasons. Nervousness can cause horses to lick their handlers, often while being shown.

Tongue Rolling: The bovine equivalent of tongue dragging in horses, this consists of irregular tongue movements inside or outside the mouth. The tongue is typically extruded and rolled back into the open mouth or toward the nostrils in an exaggeration of the normal. There may also be gulping of air. Attempts at control have been only partially successful. Wind-sucking straps or the insertion of a metal ring through the frenulum of the tongue have been tried. In some cases, success has been reported through the provision of salt mixtures. Freedom of movement and forced exercise are also suggested. Tongue rolling may be learned by watching problem animals, and some individuals may inherit the tendency.

Tail Biting: Tail biting in pigs has attracted a great deal of attention. Various conditions are thought to predispose to it, including breed type (eg, Landrace), dense grouping of rapidly growing pigs ~100 lb (45 kg) in body wt, insufficient trough space, insufficient drinking facility, and adverse environmental features (high levels of noise, noxious gas, humidity, temperature). Combinations of these and other factors lead to unrest within the group, which evidently creates irritability, over-excitability, and increased activity. Apart from such apparently inciting factors, intensive grouping in restrictive pens is an impoverished environment with little opportunity for diversive activities.

Amputation of the distal half of the tail has become standard control practice in the contemporary swine industry. The remaining section of the tail is sufficiently sensitive that pigs react effectively when a tail-biting attempt is made on them.

Animals that bite tails should be grouped together, since this usually curtails mutual tail biting. Other potential stresses should also be addressed. Atmospheric factors within the building should receive attention. Pens of growing pigs should be under-populated when the group is first formed, or moved to larger pens often enough to ensure that the pen is of adequate size when the group members have grown to twice or more their original size. General improvement in husbandry is also frequently beneficial in controlling this condition.

Tail biting also occurs in horses, primarily weanlings and yearlings; adequate protein in the diet generally controls the problem. In dogs, tail biting is usually self-directed and part of the tail-chasing behavior; it is considered self-mutilation (qv, p 921).

Bar Biting: This anomalous behavior occurs in breeding sows kept in single crates. It can be partially controlled by environmental enrichment such as by providing straw or sawdust as litter in which the animal can chew or root, or by feeding supplemental roughage, eg, grass, cobs, or pellets.

Vacuous Chewing: Seen in sows, typically in those kept singly in stalls with no litter, the affected animal chews vigorously without oral content. Control is essentially similar to that described for bar biting (see above).

Prolonged Sucking (Cross-sucking): Sucking on another animal or on an object is typically seen in animals that are weaned early or are not able to nurse, as with orphans. (See also GALACTOPHAGIA, p 926.) Best control results are obtained by providing feeding conditions that resemble those of normal ingestive patterns in young animals. Feeding calves through automatic nursers with nipples with sucking periods lasting ~30 min appears to eliminate the problem. Prevention of early weaning in dogs, cats, and pigs also decreases the frequency of the problem. Tying up calves for 1 hr following bucket feeding evidently allows time for the sucking "drive" to diminish. The supply of supplemental roughage, such as a supply of straw, seems to suppress the disorder.

Over-grooming (Self-licking): Excess grooming is probably a stress-related behavior. It occurs commonly in veal calves isolated in single stalls, race stallions confined to stalls, and cats and dogs with major changes in their environment. The excess grooming may create superficial lesions such as lick granulomas (see SELF-MUTILATION, p 921). In cats, the affected areas look as if they have been clipped.

Wool Pulling: An abnormal behavior that occurs in sheep within restrictive enclosure and indoor management systems. Crowding within pens is a contributing factor, but a deficiency of roughage in the diet may contribute too. Control is possible through reduction in pen densities. Pens of ~20 square yards (m) can contain 10 mature sheep, but wool pulling is likely at this stocking level. Reduction to 50% of this density is effective in control; at this level, the anomaly can be eliminated, especially if quality roughage is supplied regularly. Hay is ideal but straw can also be useful; any associated nutritional need appears to relate to inadequacy of structured feed rather than to any specific nutrient factor. Control can also be effected by releasing animals outdoors into extensive husbandry conditions for extended periods. (See also TRICHOPHAGIA, p 926.) Laboratory primates can pull hair out when housed in relatively barren environments. Behavioral enrichment has been useful in eliminating the problems if started early.

Feather Picking: Under conditions of intensive management, this can occur in all ages and many species including chickens, turkeys, ducks, quail, partridges, and pheasants (see also p 928). Control is most commonly effected by debeaking, which involves removal of the anterior part (0.25 in. [6 mm]) of the upper beak.

Although this does not eliminate aggressive picking entirely, or prevent the development of the peck order, debeaked birds are less able to pull feathers. Another control method is to limit the vision of birds by darkening the pens and changing the light to a red hue through the use of infrared lamps or painting window panes red. The vision of each individual bird can be restricted by fixing aluminum rings to the upper beak or applying "poly-peepers" ("blinders"), although the use of such devices is banned in some countries. Where poly-peepers are in general use, feather picking is minimal.

Anomalous Ingestive Behavior: Anomalous ingestive behavior is expressed by various manifestations. In the past, it was felt that these animals had nutritional deficiencies, and they were fed additives (eg, blood, meat meal, bone meal, and horn shavings) in attempts to relieve the disorder. Contemporary knowledge regarding causes is still incomplete. In some cases, this may be due to nutritional deficiencies, but in others it is clear that feeding practice is not a contributing cause. Restrictive confinement serves as a stressor.

Aerophagia: This behavioral abnormality of horses can be distinguished in 2 different forms, viz crib-biting (qv, p 923) and pure **wind sucking**. In both forms, air is ingested abnormally, by swallowing. In pure wind sucking, the horse nods its head and neck several times before making the intake effort. It then jerks its head upwards, opens its mouth, takes in air, raises the floor of the mouth, and contracts the musculature of the pharynx so that air is forcefully swallowed as the neck is flexed. The characteristic wind-sucking sound can occur as some of the air is expelled or as it is swallowed. The action is practiced repeatedly.

As a consequence of persistent aerophagia, the throat musculature undergoes hypertrophy from excess use. Stomach bloating may also occur and this, in turn, can lead to GI catarrh and episodes of colic. Intake of feed may decrease considerably, and these horses become "poor doers".

Control of crib-biting, wind sucking, crib-whetting and tongue dragging is attempted by various methods. Affected horses often improve with an abundance of work and exercise. In the initial stages, wind sucking can be discouraged by removal of all objects about mouth height that can be gnawed, nibbled, or licked. Feeders, mangers, and trough edges can be sheeted over with metal. Taste aversion can also be used, as can the provision of lots of hay.

A common method for preventing aerophagia is use of the wind-sucker strap, which is fastened tightly around the throat, and has a heart-shaped piece of thick leather that sits between the angles of the jaws with the pointed end protruding toward the pharyngeal area. With this device in place, difficulty and apparent discomfort are caused to the horse when its neck is flexed in the attempt to suck wind. Some horses continue in spite of this device and eventually acquire pressure sores where the strap presses.

Various surgical methods have been attempted to stop aerophagia; however, they are generally less than satisfactory. Prevention works best.

Lignophagia (Wood Chewing): Chewing and eating of wood is not uncommon in horses in restrictive quarters or paddocks; of the oral ethopathies in the horse, wood chewing is most common. It is not restricted to stall horses, and can be observed in horses in outdoor enclosures; horses in pastures may debark tree trunks. Adequate nutrition must be provided. Horses should have access to salt and roughage. In studies, severe wood chewing was stopped when hay was provided at 1 lb/100 lb body wt. The inclusion of sawdust in a high-concentrate diet, muzzles, and taste aversion can be considered when access to pasture is not possible. Exercise helps the bored horse.

Coprophagia: A normal form of ingestion in some species, notably rabbits, and in the young of most species, this abnormality is particularly unacceptable to the owner, particularly of dogs. Among dogs, the condition is usually first observed in pups 4-9 mo old. There is great individual variation in the intensity of this behavior when it becomes established. In most cases, however, the habit tends to decrease in intensity after 1 yr of age. Although many outgrow the behavior, others continue to exhibit it periodically and in a few, it persists beyond puppyhood.

Certain clinical conditions are considered to be contributory in dogs. Among these are chronic pancreatic deficiency, malabsorption, heavy parasite loads, and starvation. In disease states that result in undigested food being passed in the feces, it is believed that the material becomes acceptable to the animal for simple ingestive needs. Hydrocephalus may also be a contributing factor. In most cases, however, the condition is recognized as a behavioral abnormality, and the cause of this form is now considered to be anxiety or boredom.

Treatment requires retraining the animal. Emphasis must be placed on preventing the animal from gaining access to feces. Muzzling the dog is a useful beginning in the course of retraining. Other forms of prevention are obvious and include maintaining the dog on a leash and returning it to its home immediately following defecation outdoors. The retraining requires a considerable commitment by the owner. In addition, the animal should receive a good-quality diet, high in protein and low in carbohydrates. In many instances, the addition of vegetable oil to the diet is helpful. Feeding should be b.i.d. on a regular schedule. Such dietary changes maintained for 2 mo arrest this behavior in many cases. However, no definitive treatment for this condition has yet been determined. Animals that fail to respond present a particular ethical problem since the bond between the animal and the owner is often destroyed as a result.

Trichophagia (Hair Eating): This anomaly relates to the ingestion of hair or wool, usually removed from the bodies of associating animals (*see also* p 924). The mildest form is self-grooming during times of normal shedding. Young animals sometimes remove parts of their dam's coats while empirically licking and sucking on parts of her body other than the mammary gland. This anomaly occurs when animals are grouped densely. Among sheep, causal factors may relate to a system of enclosure imposed on the ewe and lamb. Since many of these lambs show preference for soiled wool, there may be an implication of depraved appetite. Phosphorous deficiency is suspected, but unproved.

Hairballs, which are occasional problems in the stomachs of cats, rabbits, and calves, can act as an irritant to cause vomiting or to block passage of food within the GI tract. Hair eating in the horse is an anomaly closely related to wood chewing. Tail chewing can often be stopped by adding protein to the ration. Since nutritional factors are suspect in any animal, careful evaluation of the diet is important. Spatial arrangements are another rational method of control.

Anomalous Milk Sucking (Galactophagia): A behavioral anomaly in which animals suck other than their own natural or foster mothers (*see also* p 924). Cattle that suck herd mates characteristically choose the same lactating animal, which leads to a paired arrangement. Such pairs sometimes mutually suck each other, either simultaneously or alternately.

The anomaly may relate to hereditary predisposition in some cases; however, it is husbandry-related in many others, and it can increase in frequency as a result of imitation. In contrast with the young calf, galactophagia in the adult is more common in open husbandry systems.

The herd should be closely supervised when an adult cross-sucking case has been suspected. By this means, the involved animals can be determined, and endemic spread by mimicry can be arrested. As a preventive measure, increased roughage can be provided in the diet, preferably during times when idling chiefly occurs. Since inheritance is suspect, it may be unwise to breed animals that show the disorder as adults.

In the past, control was attempted by applying pointed-prongs devices to the face and nose region of the sucking animal to ensure an aversive reaction in any animal approached. Unfortunately, some of these devices can hinder the affected animal's natural feeding. Also, if the affected animal is persistent, it can inflict wounds on others. An electrical device secured to the forehead and giving an electrical shock to the wearer when the circuit is closed by face pressure is reported to give results. Since the shock is received by the sucking animal, this method is more appropriate than those in which the aversive stimulation was directed at the receiving animal. In some cases, the affected animal must be culled.

Soil Eating (Geophagia): Horses, cattle, and sometimes dogs and cats may eat soil or other foreign matter. The behavior is related to pica (*see* below). Such animals are susceptible to GI dysfunctions. The condition may be the result of mineral-deficient diets. Phosphorus and iron deficiencies are known to be responsible in some cases, but nutritional deficiencies are not seen in other affected animals. Kittens typically show the behavior within a few days of starting litter box usage.

Control should account for the possibility of mineral deficiency. In addition, affected animals can be examined for anemia and worm burdens, and appropriate treatment provided when indicated. As with other related oral syndromes, affected horses should be provided with enforced exercise.

Hyperphagia (Overeating): Some animals are extremely greedy and rapid eaters, and some may choke in the course of bolting their food. Many were nutritionally deprived when young. Others have been on diets. Since the food is not fully masticated, GI disorders occur in some horses. When these animals gain access to large quantities of food, they consume excess amounts; this can lead to serious and possibly fatal GI illness (*see also* GRAIN OVERLOAD, p 175).

The control of hyperphagia involves tactical feeding. Small amounts of feed can be provided. Spreading the grain in a thin layer in the trough, and placing large smooth stones in the bottom of the trough are methods used to make grain difficult for horses to consume rapidly. Supplying the grain at several different times in the day may be helpful. Feeding hay before grain is most helpful. It is of prime importance to prevent access to large amounts of high-energy grains.

Polydipsia Nervosa: Excess drinking is encountered in various species when in close confinement; water consumption usually is 2-4 times normal. Polydipsia nervosa is seen in some horses that are isolated and confined in stalls with water supplied *ad lib*. Some horses consume ~140 L daily, or ~3-4 times the normal quantity. This may be spread over a period of time or concentrated within 2-3 hr. Polydipsia can also be secondary to excess salt intake, common in stalled horses. Polyuria may be the first indication of the anomaly.

Polydipsia does not appear to become fixed securely in the animal's behavior, and it lends itself to control by appropriate management, which includes the provision of rationed water. Since "boredom" is a contributing factor, the habit can be controlled and broken by an increase in regular exercise. Polydipsia in other stock in confinement apparently can be controlled by an appropriate husbandry change.

Pica: A depraved appetite shown by animals that seek foreign matter for ingestion. The condition is most notable in animals that tend to eat and chew wool, cloth, old bones, and wood. Wool sucking or eating by cats may have a genetic component since it occurs almost exclusively in Siamese and Siamese-crosses.

Nutritional deficiencies, eg, of phosphorus, should be corrected if they exist. Cats that eat or suck wool should be evaluated for low thyroid hormone levels. Usually, though, the problem is controlled by preventing access to favored objects, limiting access to 1 or 2 items, or using taste aversion to break the pattern.

Litter Eating: Confined animals are liable to eat their bedding, even after it has become soiled. Almost every stabled horse eats soiled bedding on occasion, but with some it is habitual. Kittens also eat litter or dirt for a few days before elimination changes from the anogenital reflex to self-initiated. The habit develops in horses and poultry, even when adequate food is available. Generally, litter eating is practiced on wood particles and chaff, so it may represent, to some degree, an appetite for cellulose.

Litter eating in chickens and turkeys is most common when they are reared on chaff or wood litter, with the incidence being highest in flocks that do not have sufficient feed-trough space. Since the incidence is higher in some breeds and strains of birds than others, there may be a genetic predisposition. The condition can be alleviated in many birds by supplying an abundance of grit.

To control litter eating in poultry, there must be abundant feed-trough space so that birds in low positions within the peck order can find secure space at the trough. In horses, control requires appraisal of the feed to ensure adequate quantity, quality, and variety. Feeding and exercise should be maintained on a precise schedule. Horses with worm burdens should receive appropriate treatment.

Feather Eating: Closely related to feather picking (qv, p 924) and to cannibalism (*see* BODY PECKING, below) in chickens. Feather picking marks initiation of cannibalistic behavior in many instances. In feather eating, birds pick out the feathers of others from preferred sites such as the tail and pinions. Although most common in adults, feather picking occurs in all ages from day-old chicks to aged birds. Since the problem is assumed to be misdirected feeding, control is aimed at rectifying feeding and nutrition. Feeding concentrated feedstuffs exclusively may interfere with the activities involved in feed searching, and result in insufficient feed bulk; thus, deprived behaviors leading to feather eating are induced. Therapy can include mixing grain in the feed to increase searching; volume can be improved by adding corn (maize) cobs and green fodder to the diet.

Egg Eating: A habit found in small flocks of chickens kept in pens, this appears to occur equally among flocks on deep litter and on wire mesh floors. The behavior begins with a bird pecking at an egg until it is broken. The contents are then partially eaten. When a bird acquires this habit, it is likely to increase the practice and other birds may also develop the problem. When significant amounts of eggshell are eaten, this may indicate that the diet of affected birds are deficient in grit. Control involves elimination of affected birds, but they may be difficult to identify in a large flock. Concentrated food dye may be injected into an egg to be left lying on the ground; a bird that eats this egg will be marked by coloration about the head. Grit should be provided in long troughs so that all birds can have occasional access to it. To some extent, problems of this nature popularized the introduction of battery caging some decades ago. Caging might still be considered as a method of controlling this condition in small flocks without access to outside runs. Birds with access to free range can be turned out regularly at mid-day, by which time laying should be over.

Body Pecking: In different forms, this occurs as a behavioral vice in poultry under intensive management. In contrast to picking (qv, p 924), the beak is used in body pecking for the combined actions of stabbing and plucking. Ingestion of pecked-out parts also occurs. This is a form of cannibalism that appears in domestic chickens, other gallinaceous birds (eg, turkeys, pheasants, quail), and ducks. Body pecking is often directed at wounds arising when feathers are picked out. Pecking of the toes or back are most common in younger birds. Vent pecking occurs in all ages but is most serious in laying birds, while head pecking is noted in older caged birds.

Appropriate prevention and control of body pecking requires spatial escape opportunity for birds subordinate in peck orders. Debeaking is the most common method of control even though it only addresses the problem, not the cause.

Urine Drinking: This problem has been reported in some dairy herds in Britain and France. Evidently it is practiced during the winter by cows enclosed in cubicle systems and communal yards where concrete flooring allows pools of urine to form. A cow may drink from these pools, or sometimes directly from a urinating cow. The problem becomes evident when the water troughs are too close together or insufficient in number so that dominant cows prevent some subordinates from approaching water troughs or salt licks. When availability of water and salt is evenly distributed in cattle yards, the problem disappears. Also, the behavior ceases when cattle have access to pasture.

ANIMAL WELFARE

INTRODUCTION

The well-being of animals is a prime responsibility of veterinarians. They are called on to oversee and treat animal diseases, develop programs of preventive medicine, and administer a variety of regulations related to hygiene and epidemic control. They should also help owners/operators uphold ethical standards in the industry or the home.

There are a number of definitions of animal welfare, but from a practical stand, the following question can be asked: "Do the methods of handling, housing, and general management adopted impose the least amount of distress (negative side of stress) on animals of this species at this age, weight, stage of development, etc?'' Distress can be gauged by a range of physiological indices and the behavior of the animal(s). Management decisions must be based on this information.

A number of other, deeper issues also are involved in welfare questions: 1) that man has the right to domesticate and use other animals for food, raw materials, research, traction, sport, and companionship; 2) that human intervention must arrange the optimal husbandry by balancing the ideal situation with day-to-day practices in the animal industries; 3) that comprehensive care and control of suffering in animals under various management conditions is an essential responsibility; 4) that total animal health requires a concern for meeting the physical, social, and key ethological needs of the animals; 5) that animal welfare issues and their costs devolve on all of society and not fall solely on owners (an adequate economic return is required to operate any farm unit). There is also pressure from society for cheap food, which implies increasing intensification of the animal industries; however, there is growing pressure from urban dwellers for better welfare for farmed animals, often having expectations that are unrealistic or unnatural for the species involved. Personification can be a problem. If livestock owners become upset and cynical, great hardship may fall on thousands of animals in large-scale production systems or on the consumer in the long term.

In 2 other spheres, veterinarians can assist with issues of well-being of animals. They should encourage animal breeders and husbandrymen to select animals that have the traits and temperament suitable for large-scale intensive farming. Selective breeding is slow—but important if the human population of the world is to be adequately fed. The second is to encourage owners/operators to precondition their animals for future changes. Holding unfamiliar animals in adjacent pens before mixing into a group could reduce subsequent social upheaval. Familiarizing cows with the milking parlor before calving is another example of how careful early handling and conditioning may pay dividends in production and welfare.

The development of welfare regulations, what forms they should take, and how they should be policed are also major concerns of veterinarians. The most positive approach to this area is the encouragement of pride in the way animals are treated. Legislation may have a place in reducing extreme cases of gross cruelty, but the on-going welfare of rural and urban animals is best served by more flexible codes that can be integrated with preventive care programs. Legislation does little to effect a change of heart or re-order the basic motivation of animal owners.

There are times in history when man reexamines his relationship with other animals: the growth of interest in animal welfare indicates that this is one of those times. Veterinarians play an important role in this concern of society since they hold an intermediary role in the owner-animal relationship.

FEATURES

Animal welfare is characterized by definitive features derived from its rational links with ethics, husbandry, and animal health. These are: 1) ethical use of the animal, 2) standards of husbandry and production that meet an attainable level, 3) provision of veterinary care, 4) control of suffering for the well-being of the animal, and 5) ecological management. With the above 5 factors, animal welfare can be incorporated into a unified concept.

As a global, compound discipline, animal welfare has immediate relevance to veterinary medicine, animal research, animal husbandry, and applied animal ethology. As a result, animal welfare is multidisciplinary. It has rational principles using these collateral sciences and is substantially scientific, by virtue of its relationships. In practice it is involved in all spheres of animal industry and carries ethical and regulatory dictates.

As with other applied scientific disciplines, welfare must address practical objectives. The chief objective is avoidance and relief of suffering. Suffering is in the clinical realm and is thus the background of many clinical matters, which is why many welfare considerations are in the domain of veterinary knowledge.

In conditions accompanied by pain, distress, or fear, certain behavioral manifestations are unequivocal evidence of suffering (*see also* p 931). Intense vocalizations, struggling, trembling, passively depressed behavior, and agitated behavior are outward expressions of mental states and reflect states of suffering. It is essential to recognize a relationship between animal behavior and animal welfare. The principal features of animal welfare that provide its definitive framework are as follows.

Ethical Use of the Animal: Even within regions, nations, and cultures, opinions concerning modes of animal use that may be considered ethical (or permissible) are frequently polarized into extremes of a utilitarian or a humanitarian nature. In general, the main body of veterinary opinion is not drawn into polarized extremes. The cultural attitudes relating to acceptable usage of animals may have been derived from history or from the religions prevailing in a given community. By whatever means, community agreement develops about what can be done with and to the animals used for food, clothing, recreation, and work. However, ethical matters are not based on subjective, emotive, or religious bases entirely without regard to objective principles.

Standards of Husbandry and Production: Standards in animal husbandry are taught to students of agricultural science and veterinary medicine. Even normally acceptable standards could often be improved. Husbandry that leads to high levels of morbidity and mortality in livestock is readily recognized as poor. Low standards may be the result of ignorance, gross errors, or deliberate neglect. One aim of animal welfare is to rectify and eliminate poor husbandry levels whether for livestock, pets, laboratory animals, or captive wild animals.

To ensure a balance between the ideal and the basic, some system of surveillance is necessary. This may take the form of a regulatory force of inspectors, or a voluntary society recognized by the community as being a legitimate and concerned organization operating to prevent breaches in welfare. In many countries, both forces operate separately but simultaneously.

Veterinary Care: Development of "herd health" systems for food animals is a specialized branch of veterinary care that is basically preventive medicine. It is in this feature that animal welfare is in its most systematic and scientific form. Systematic welfare practices assure, to both economic and humane interests, that the conduct of the animal-keeping operation is sound, realistically optimal, and wholly consistent with regulatory requirements.

Humane veterinary practice for animals under intensive management, either commercially or experimentally, requires that services be developed to prevent predictable problems in health and welfare. Such services include good hygiene, an appropriate balanced diet and clean drinking water, good sleeping facilities, adequate ventilation, appropriate ambient temperature, and containment within good housing with adequate space. Health should be monitored to provide early detection of any pathological condition. Routine medications and vaccinations are also used to prevent occurrences of predictable disorders. Preventive practice incorporates conventional veterinary attention as is necessary.

Animal health and welfare are obviously related. One of the basic practical objectives in animal welfare is to prevent disease, the specialized domain of veterinary medicine termed Animal Health. An Animal Health program is operated in most countries by a national service that provides the chief monitoring method in animal welfare at the national level. As such services become expanded, consolidated, and sophisticated, the level of welfare contained within them continues to increase and improve proportionately.

Animal Health personnel are veterinarians, so they can advise on management practices, vaccinations, and prophylaxis, with the recognition that stress is a component in the etiology of many diseases in the modern spectrum. Stress alleviation is an additional prophylactic action that calls for increasing consideration.

Control of Suffering: Animal welfare has an implicit role to provide aid for animals in states of crisis, adversity, and suffering. This is the humane component of animal welfare, which ensures managemental or medical aid in any distress. This type of intervention is most frequently done by livestock owners and users themselves, with or without the support of agencies such as a veterinary service. This intervention action is customarily comprehensive; it covers a wide range from relieving difficult birth to provision of humane slaughter. Its aim is to minimize suffering.

Most farm animals have their lives terminated by slaughter. While methods for this vary, the humane objective is dispatch of the animal by a method that renders it insensitive and unconscious as quickly as possible. Preslaughter management and transportation of livestock is also a concern. The modern designs for slaughter plants, which encourage less stressful handling of animals by manipulating their behavior, is a notable frontier of animal welfare.

Although behavioral signs of nonovert suffering are less likely to receive attention, they are identifiable. The more that modern husbandry exerts control over animal maintenance and breeding, the more there is to learn about "behavioral suffering". This also must be of veterinary concern. The 2 main characteristics in the behavior of suffering are depressed or increased activity. But suffering occurs in various forms including illness and stressful circumstances. Many of these are of unexpected occurrence. The forms of welfare at such times may range from first aid, through therapy, to rescue. The animal in pain may need anesthesia, tranquilization, or analgesia. Medical treatment is necessary in addressing the suffering associated with illness.

Ecological Management: Behavioral knowledge can be used to provide the animal with a facility that allows the output of behavior needed for self-maintenance. Systems of ethological homeostasis are recognized that are forms of behavioral work that animals produce to maintain themselves in effective harmony with their environment; these are essentially the behaviors of maintenance (qv, p 896). Because animal production industries have the additional objective of convenience, animal self-care is sometimes compromised.

The broad ecological purpose is integration of the animal with the environment through homeostasis. The basic behavioral processes of utilized animals can be modified only over generations by selective breeding. As this problem becomes more acute for intensively confined animals, the principles of animal welfare create an awareness that these animals possess evolved, ecological, behavioral characteristics that aid in self-maintenance.

OBJECTIVES

Animal welfare has 2 major objectives: to prevent or reduce suffering, and to promote well-being.

Suffering: Avoidance and relief of suffering is obviously the chief objective in animal welfare practice. Undergoing an imposition or enduring a condition that is painful, distressing, or injurious is the general meaning of suffering. Endurance implies an element of continuity. In veterinary medicine, welfare serves as an umbrella term covering all the likely affective features that may coexist with any noxious condition.

A high degree of clinical and ethological judgment is needed for qualitative evaluation of animal suffering. However, a simple system of classification can be used such as acute, subacute, or chronic forms. Chronicity may add to the severity of suffering, but acute suffering that causes changes in behavior can also be severe, if allied to intense pain. Subacute suffering typically takes a transient form, although frequent recurrence may cause this form to acquire real significance, depending on the degree of associated change in behavior.

Pathophysiological conditions commonly provide *prima facie* evidence of animal suffering. Numerous clinical conditions, including disease processes and traumatic incidents, first become apparent through a set of behavioral indicators of suffering. Indeed, behavioral change is the characteristic most likely to indicate level of suffering. Such changes occur when homeostatic activities are arrested completely and replaced by actions of distress, or displaced by persistent aberrant behavior.

When suffering occurs, systematic maintenance behaviors, such as feeding, grooming, or affiliation, are often displaced by agitation, depression, isolation, anorexia, etc. Significant changes in behavior occur and include unusual forms of conduct, unsoundness of bodily movements, reduced activities, and loss of appetite. Such signs are used for diagnostic purposes when the ill or injured animals are being evaluated. They help to determine the nature and extent of the dysfunction of the animal, and the appropriate treatment. Evidence of clinical suffering is so variable and vast that its evaluation requires veterinary expertise. Among features of clinical suffering are abnormal vital signs, physical and behavioral changes, pathological lesions, and altered mood.

Adjunctive suffering is usually addressed indirectly when the clinical dysfunction itself is handled by case management. However, in some instances, eg, trauma, the relief of actual and acute suffering may be an immediate objective before the physical or bodily dysfunction receives specific attention. Outward expressions of mental states in clinical conditions accompanied by pain, distress, or fear (see also p 930) are unequivocal evidence of suffering. If pathophysiological correlates are absent, evidence of suffering may relate to stress.

Since pain is the essence of severe suffering, any conception of suffering must include an appreciation of the variety of features that relate to pain. Pain is a highly variable and subjective experience, but its existence in animals is abundantly evident in typical reactions, eg, inactivity, tucked-up posture, restlessness, flailing or rigid limbs, writhing, self-inflicted bites, and abnormal vocalization. All of these criteria must be considered in conjunction with the nature of any pathological process present. The behavior resulting from pain is easily observed, recognized, and interpreted by anyone with appropriate experience and knowledge with the given species, both in normal states and in illness.

Bio-ethics: While the most imperative objectives in welfare practice relate to the relief of suffering, the promotion of well-being (or the welfare status of, or within, the animal) is an ethical objective. The 2 terms, welfare and well-being, are not synonymous. Well-being is a condition within the animal; it is a state of good health and harmony between the animal and its environment. Welfare certainly incorporates much of the same, but is chiefly an external system of services (which have the state of well-being as one objective). In other words, welfare is exogenous while well-being is endogenous.

Ethics require that the general well-being of animals, used materialistically, should be ensured by adequate standards of welfare. The latter should be provided during the life span of these animals, however short that life span is permitted to be. This is in full accord with the vocational objectives inherent in veterinary medicine. Additionally, ethical practices in the world of animal breeding must bear welfare problems in mind. Physically and behaviorally unsuited breeds, types, or crosses should not have their breeding promoted in the event of a likely stressful outcome, eg, dystocia, stress syndromes, etc. Even common environments on the farm, in the urban situation, or in the laboratory can be stressful to certain breed types.

Animal bio-ethics is a constitution of integrated ethical principles guiding animal welfare practices and serving to control suffering. The 4 broad principles of bio-ethics have been given as: 1) responsible animal management, with appropriate overall husbandry; 2) provision for physical comfort, basic behavioral function, and animal health; 3) prevention or relief of unnecessary pain or suffering; and 4) use of sentient animal life for fully justified reasons. The role of the veterinarian in these matters is obvious and traditional, and a strong veterinary involvement should continue.

PART III

CLINICAL VALUES AND PROCEDURES

CVP

COLLECTION AND SUBMISSION OF SPECIMENS FOR LABORATORY EXAMINATION

Histological Examination: Microscopical examination of adequately prepared sections of tissues from diseased animals is diagnostically valuable. Cellular changes present in diseased tissues are often characteristic for a specific disease or group of diseases. Use of this relatively rapid and inexpensive diagnostic technique often can result in substantial savings in time, money, and animal life. Every clinician should investigate the existence, location, and capabilities of facilities that provide histopathological diagnosis, and make use of their services.

Tissues for histopathological examination should be collected as soon as possible after death to minimize autolysis. They should **not** be frozen before fixation. Specimens of the various organs should be cut <1 cm thick (preferably 7 mm) and placed immediately into ≥10 times their volume of phosphate-buffered 10% formalin for fixation. Thin slices or cubes ensure adequate penetration of the fixative. The tissues should remain in this fixative for ≥24 hr; after this initial fixation, the specimens may be placed in a smaller volume of fresh formalin for shipment. Specimens should be shipped in unbreakable containers and packed in such a way as to prevent spillage during shipment. Fixed tissues should be protected from freezing.

For the brain, when the whole organ may be required, the brain should be placed in concentrated formalin (40% formaldehyde—in which it will float), and water added slowly and mixed until the brain sinks to just below the surface but not to the bottom. To allow faster fixation, a longitudinal incision should be made in the cerebrum to expose the lateral ventricles. The brain should remain in this solution for ≥24 hr, after which it may be removed and placed in a solid container in 10% formalin and mailed (suitably packed), or held until processing is desired. Often, the brain is halved longitudinally and one-half sent unfixed (fresh), properly refrigerated, for microbiological tests.

Tissues collected for histological examination should be representative of the lesion and, if possible, should include some of the apparently normal surrounding tissue. Specimens of all organs should be sent. If the animal exhibited CNS signs, the brain and portions of the spinal cord should be included. Since autolysis occurs rapidly in the GI mucosa, the tissue must be properly fixed. Short sections of gut should be opened lengthwise to allow adequate fixation. Autolyzed tissues generally are useless for histopathological examination.

Biopsy specimens should be fixed in the same manner as necropsy tissues. Small tumors (<1 cm) should be cut in half, and larger tumors into small pieces or several representative samples.

A detailed case history should accompany the specimens to assist laboratory personnel in arriving at a diagnosis. Species, breed, morbidity and mortality, sex, age, and owner should be identified, and clinical signs, gross appearance, size, and location of the lesion(s) should be described. The report should describe previous treatment, if any, and if so, the time of recurrence.

Unfixed specimens should also be submitted for further diagnostic tests (virology, bacteriology, mycology, toxicology, etc). Specimens for microbiological examination should be collected aseptically, as soon as possible after death. Tissues may be frozen before shipment, but freezing is undesirable if specimens can be chilled and delivered directly to the laboratory in a short period. Adequate refrigerant should be provided so specimens will remain chilled until they reach the laboratory.

Toxicological Examination: A successful examination requires appropriate specimens and a thorough history, including signs, treatment, postmortem lesions, and circumstances involved. If a known toxin is suspected, a specific analysis should always be requested—laboratories cannot just "check for poisoning". If mortality is high, potential economic loss should be indicated. A complete description of clinical and epidemiological findings may help differentiate poisoning from infectious diseases that can simulate poisoning.

Tissues or fluids for chemical analysis should be as fresh as possible and kept in a refrigerator or preserved chemically; packing with ice is preferred. A polystyrene refrigerator box, metal can, or stout cardboard box may be used for shipment. Packing must withstand breakage if the ice melts. With dry ice, specimens can be preserved for 72 hr. Packages containing dry ice must be so labeled on the outside and suitably vented to prevent pressure buildup. Adequate refrigeration is of special importance when submitting clean body fluids (readily obtained from an eye) and material for nitrate or nitrite analysis; these salts are rapidly metabolized by microorganisms, and only low or insignificant levels may be found on analysis. Refrigeration impedes microbial growth and helps ensure that the salts are preserved.

For chemical preservation, 95% ethanol, ~1 mL/g of sample, is satisfactory. Denatured alcohol should not be used because the denaturant introduces contamination. Formalin is usually undesirable because it interferes with many tests. The container for packing and transporting specimens should be free of chemicals and prepared beforehand. Plastic containers, both bags and jars, are ideal. Jars with metal screw caps should be avoided, especially when metal poison is suspected. Specimens should be packed individually. Containers must be labeled with all information necessary to identify the specimen, and if mailed, must conform to postal regulations.

If legal action is a possibility, all containers for shipment should be sealed in a way that tampering can be detected, or hand-carried to the laboratory and a receipt obtained. In all legal cases, an accurately documented chain of custody must be maintained. If there is any possibility of legal action, each case should be handled as if it were to be tried in court.

If feed or water is suspected as the source of poisoning, samples of these and any descriptive feed tag should accompany the tissue specimens. If at all possible, a representative composite sample of the feed should be submitted from the lot or shipment involved in the poisoning. In some instances, if an adequate amount of

Table 1. Guidelines for Submitting Specimens for Toxicological Examination

Suspected Poison or Analysis	Specimen Required	Amount Needed	Comments
Ammonia	Whole blood or serum	5 mL	Frozen.
	Urine	5 mL	Frozen.
	Rumen contents	100 g	Frozen (or may add 1-2 drops saturated $HgCl_3$).
Arsenic	Liver	100 g	
	Kidney	100 g	
	Whole blood	15 mL	
	Urine	50 mL	
	Ingesta	100 g	
	Feed	5 lb (2.5 kg)	
Arsenical feed additives	Liver	100 g	
	Kidney	100 g	
	Sciatic nerve		Fixed in formalin.
Carbon monoxide	Whole blood	15 mL	
Chlorates	Stomach contents	100 g	Frozen, in airtight container.
Chlorinated hydrocarbons	Cerebrum	½	Use only glass containers.
	Ingesta	100 g	Avoid contamination. Wrap
	Body fat	100 g	specimens with aluminum
	Liver	100 g	foil.
	Kidney	100 g	
Cholinesterase	Whole blood	10 mL	Heparinized, refrigerated.
	Cerebrum	½	Refrigerated or frozen.
Copper (and Ni, Fe, Co, Cr, and Tl)	Kidney	100 g	
	Liver	100 g	
	Serum	2 mL	
	Feed	5 lb (2.5 kg)	
	Whole blood	10 mL	
	Feces	100 g	
Cyanide	Forage	5 lb (2.5 kg)	Rush to laboratory or ship
	Whole blood	10 mL	promptly, frozen in airtight
	Liver	100 g	container.
Dicumarol	Forage	5 lb (2.5 kg)	
	Liver	100 g	
Ethylene glycol	Serum	10 mL	
	Urine	15 mL	
	Kidneys	Sections	Fixed in formalin.
Fluorides	Bone	20 g	Best to send affected
	Water	100 g	bone(s).
	Forage	100 g	
	Urine	50 mL	
Herbicides (many)	Treated weeds	5 lb (2.5 kg)	
	Urine	50 mL	
	Ingesta	1 lb (500 g)	
	Liver or kidney	100 g	
Lead (also Hg, Mo, Ni, and Tl)	Kidney	100 g	
	Whole blood	10 mL	Heparinized. Do not use
	Liver	100 g	EDTA.
	Urine	15 mL	
Mercury and Molybdenum	Kidney, liver, blood		*See* lead.
	Feed	5 lb (2.5 kg)	
Mycotoxins	Grain, forages	5 lb (2.5 kg)	Consult with laboratory
	Liver, kidney	100 g	personnel on specific tests.

(continued)

Suspected Poison or Analysis	Specimen Required	Amount Needed	Comments
Monensin	Feed	5 lb (2.5 kg)	
	Rumen contents	500 g	
	Heart	Sections	Fixed in formalin.
	Skeletal muscle	Sections	Fixed in formalin.
Nitrate	Forage	5 lb (2.5 kg)	
	Water	100 mL	Boil 2-3 min before shipping.
	Body fluids (eg, aqueous humor)		Consult with laboratory personnel.
Organophosphates (and carbamates)	Feed	5 lb (2.5 kg)	Send also urine, blood, and
	Ingesta	100 g	stomach contents from
	Urine	50 mL	clinically normal animals.
Oxalates	Fresh forage	Plants	Do not macerate; freeze.
	Kidney	Sections	Fixed in formalin.
Phenols	Gastric or rumen cotents	1 lb (500 g)	In airtight container.
Polychlorinated (and polybrominated) biphenyls	Liver	100 g	
	Feed	5 lb (2.5 kg)	
Rumen pH	Ingesta	1 qt (1 L)	Frozen.
Selenium	Whole blood	5 mL	Heparinized.
	Feed	5 lb (2.5 kg)	
	Liver	100 g	
	Hair clippings	10 g	
Sodium (NaCl)	Brain	100 g	Other ½ fixed in formalin.
	Serum	5 mL	
	CSF	1 mL	
	Feed	5 lb (2.5 kg)	
Sodium fluoroacetate (1080)	Stomach contents	All	Frozen.
	Liver	100 g	
Strychnine	Liver	100 g	
	Kidney	Whole	
	Stomach contents	100 g	
Sulfates	Water	1 qt (1 L)	*See* TDS.
	Brain	½	Fixed in formalin.
TDS (total dissolved solids)	Water	1 qt (1 L)	
Triaryl-PO4	Ingesta	100 g	
	Feed	5 lb (2.5 kg)	
Urea	Feed	5 lb (2.5 kg)	*See* ammonia.
Vitamin A (also D and E)	Liver	100 g	
	Serum	10 mL	
Warfarin (also other anticoagulants)	Whole blood	10 mL	
	Liver	100 mL	
	Feed	100 mL	
Zinc	Liver	100 g	
	Kidney	100 g	
Zinc phosphide	Liver	100 g	
	Gastric contents	100 g	

involved feed is available, some of it may be fed to experimental animals in an effort to reproduce the signs and lesions observed in the field cases.

If there is doubt about proper handling, preservation of the specimens, or other essential procedures, a telephone call to the laboratory for instructions is prudent.

Chemical Examination: Most clinical chemistry tests require serum, but an occasional test may require plasma. Anticoagulants present in plasma samples may interfere with tests; therefore, serum should always be sent unless plasma is specifically requested. For serum samples, the blood should be allowed to clot and the sample held at room temperature to allow clot retraction. The serum should then be removed and transferred to a clean tube containing no preservatives. Serum generally does not need to be refrigerated if it will reach the laboratory in a short period. Most commercial laboratories will provide specimen containers and mailers, but government and university laboratories generally do not.

Hematological Examination: Routine studies require a whole-blood sample containing an anticoagulant-preservative and several blood smears. Blood smears should be prepared immediately after collection. Blood samples should not be refrigerated. Coagulation studies and other specialized tests require special handling and containers; the laboratory should be contacted for instructions.

Serological Examination: These tests generally require serum, but plasma is often satisfactory. Samples should be collected as described for chemical tests and should always be free of hemolysis. In some instances, paired samples may be required for an adequate diagnosis. The acute sample should be collected early in the course of the disease and frozen. The convalescent sample should be collected 10-14 days later, and both samples should be forwarded to the laboratory at the same time.

Cytological Examination: Specimens consist of air-dried or alcohol-fixed smears. They may be obtained by aspiration, scraping, or touch preparations. Smears may be prepared from fluids in 2 ways, depending on cellularity. Highly cellular fluids may be smeared directly, but fluids of low cellularity should be centrifuged to concentrate the cells. (*See also* p 943.)

Fluid Analytical Examination: Analysis of fluids usually involves determination of protein content, total cell counts, and cytological examination. Other tests may be performed depending on source (eg, joint fluids) or appearance (eg, chylous fluid). Fluids of low cellularity should be divided into 2 portions; one should be centrifuged to concentrate the cells for smears, the other forwarded to the laboratory unaltered for other tests. Blood or cytological smears should never be mailed to the laboratory in the same package with formalin-fixed tissues because the formalin vapors will produce artifacts in the specimens.

DIAGNOSTIC PROCEDURES FOR THE OFFICE LABORATORY

Numerous laboratory tests can be done in the veterinarian's clinical laboratory, including many that previously had to be sent to an outside laboratory. Because the people performing these tests often have minimal technical training, it is essential that quality control procedures be rigorous. However, the time and care that must be devoted to quality control preclude in-house testing in many practices. Also, errors may occur not only in the actual testing procedures, but in specimen collection and handling and transcription of results.

Commercial laboratories offer a broad panel of inexpensive, accurate biochemical analyses. *See* above for handling of samples; the diagnostic laboratory should be asked for specific instructions before submission of specimens.

CLINICAL CHEMISTRY

Blood-chemical determinations (*see* TABLE 10, p 969) can provide support for or confirm clinical diagnoses. A screening battery of tests may also suggest solutions to differential diagnostic problems. Tests should always be selected based on clinical rationale. Currently, an economic rule of thumb is to use commercial laboratories when >3 tests per animal are required. Private laboratories can provide chemistry profiles of 12-20 tests on automated equipment with much less effort and at considerably less expense. Because availability of private laboratories and their reporting intervals often present problems (eg, nights and holidays), diagnostic screening in blood chemistry by the office laboratory is desirable, if not necessary. Those who purchase a semiautomated or automated chemistry analyzer to conduct chemistry profiles of 12-20 tests should hire an experienced technician to operate it. Dry chemical analytical methods can supply good results for routine chemical analyses, and determination of enzymes and electrolytes. Accurate electrolyte values are most efficiently determined with ion-specific electrode systems. The use of known control sera as a qualitative control procedure insures the accuracy of any analytical blood chemistry system.

For blood chemistry analyses, a centrifuge is essential for separation of blood cells from serum or plasma. Serum or plasma samples are required for chemical and serological assay in contrast to the whole blood needed for hematological analysis. Small quantities of clean serum or plasma that are completely free of hemolysis are a prerequisite of accurate chemical analysis, and multiple determinations can be performed on the same sample.

Lipemia and states of hyper- and hypoglycemia produce misleading assay results. Adept collection of a fasting blood sample and prompt removal of serum from a formed clot avoids such problems. The clot of a 30-min-old blood sample should be rimmed with an applicator stick and centrifuged at no more than 2200 revolutions/min for 10 min. The supernatant serum is aspirated and placed in another clean collection tube for assay or refrigeration. Clear, refrigerated serum samples can be used for chemical analysis up to 5 days after collection if they are warmed to room temperature before use.

BLOOD GLUCOSE

One mL of whole blood collected after a 12-hr fast can be screened for blood glucose levels elevated to >100 mg/dL by 2 simple, semiquantitative, visual, colorimetric tests. The "Dextrotest" is performed with 2 reagent tablets and involves boiling a filtrate. Blood glucose levels of 100, 150, and 200 mg/dL can be estimated by comparing color changes to a color scale supplied with the kit. A more rapid screen can be performed with a glucose oxidase strip and whole blood. A positive visual color change occurs with high glucose levels and is suggestive of diabetes mellitus ($\geq$200 mg/dL) in dogs and cats. Ketoacidosis, which may accompany diabetes mellitus, is detectable with a reagent tablet ("Acetest") that can be used with serum, milk, or urine. Two-fold dilutions of ketoacidotic serum produce a lavender to purple color change of the tablet within 30 sec.

Detection of hypoglycemia requires specific methods for accurately measuring glucose levels. Such methods are used in the various bench-top and automated analyzer systems. Again, the test sample of choice is clear serum that has been obtained after a 12-hr fast and separated from the blood cells within 30 min.

KIDNEY FUNCTION TESTS

Methods of analysis of **BUN** include an enzymatic technique and a colorimetric method. A strip test in the form of a piece of chromatography paper banded with reagents is a rapid (30 min), simple, accurate method for estimating BUN. The test requires 0.2 mL clear serum, one long-tipped pipette, one 10 × 75 mm test tube, and one "Urograph" strip. Normal BUN values are 10-30 mg/dL, and persistently elevated levels are indicative of renal disease more often than of other causes, eg, congestive heart failure. Levels >75 mg/dL can be estimated by diluting the serum sample with a quality control serum standard and repeating the test.

Creatinine is freely filtered by the glomerulus; blood levels are used to estimate the glomerular filtration rate. Muscle tissue contains phosphocreatine, which is converted to creatinine by a nonenzymatic process; this spontaneous degradation occurs at a rather constant rate.

Causes of increases of both BUN and creatinine can be divided into 3 major categories: prerenal, renal, and postrenal. Other diagnostic tests may be helpful in differentiating the causes of the increased BUN and creatinine. (*See* URN, p 869).

Renal proteinuria is most often caused by a glomerular lesion. The degree of proteinuria is used to evaluate the severity of the glomerular lesion, as a basis for formulating dietary therapy, and to assess response to therapy or progression of the disease. Previously, a 24-hr urine collection was done. There is a good correlation between the 24-hr urine protein excretion and the protein:creatinine ratio in a randomly voided urine sample.

LIVER FUNCTION TESTS

The liver performs many functions; thus, several tests are required for evaluation. Clinical signs of icterus, or GI malfunction unresponsive to therapy often suggest which tests will provide the most information. In general, the listed tests measure hepatic catabolism and excretion of biliary pigments, hepatic excretion capability, and serum enzyme concentrations that reflect the release of enzymes from injured hepatocytes.

Serum Bile Pigments: The van den Bergh test can be used to distinguish between hemolytic and obstructive jaundice. The qualitative version is characterized by a color change to reddish purple within 30 sec for a positive direct action (obstructive jaundice), or to pink (intensification) within 15 min after the addition of alcohol for a positive indirect action (hemolytic jaundice). The test can be quantitated with a photoelectric colorimeter to measure concentration differences between total bilirubin and the direct-reacting bilirubin diglucuronide. The difference in concentrations represents the concentration of the indirect-reacting free bilirubin of hemolytic jaundice, especially in the dog and cat. The horse is an exception: it excretes indirect-reacting, unconjugated, free bilirubin in obstructive as well as hemolytic jaundice and other nonhepatic disease conditions (eg, pneumonia and constipation).

Urobilinogen: Excreted bilirubin glucuronide is reduced to urobilinogen by intestinal bacteria. The urobilinogen can be reabsorbed via the portal circulation and recirculated into the intestine via hepatic excretion, or excreted by the kidneys. Fecal urobilinogen is oxidized to the orange-brown urobilin of normal feces. By use of a strip test, urobilinogen is detectable in urine within 1 hr of collection. A 60-sec color change is compared to a color chart. Lack of a positive color change in association with nonpigmented, clay-colored feces indicates bile duct obstruction. Diluted (1:64) urine samples from nonherbivores may produce reddish brown color changes of the strip when large amounts of urobilinogen are produced by hemolytic jaundice or hepatocellular disease. Urobilinogenuria in dogs lacks diagnostic significance—negative tests are not uncommon in normal dogs. Dogs also can excrete high levels of urobilinogen in the urine during bile duct obstruction because normal anaerobic hepatic bacteria, which can produce urobilinogen *in situ*, are present in the canine liver.

Fecal Pigmentation: Urobilin (stercobilin) is a pigmented product of urobilinogen decomposition that contributes an orange color to the feces. Nonpigmented, clay-colored feces of anorectic animals suggest bile duct obstruction. Similar light-colored feces are also associated with pancreatic insufficiency as well as ingestion of bones and some antibiotics. Increased dark orange fecal pigmentation is seen in hemolytic jaundice. Fecal color also may be influenced by many dietary substances.

Sulfobromophthalein Sodium (bromsulfophthalein, BSP) Excretion Test: Excretion of BSP by the liver is delayed in hepatic disease, and the dye can be used to detect nonicteric liver disease. The test requires a continuous block of time and a spectrophotometer. Excretion of 1 g of the dye after IV injection is measured by plasma clearance in large animals. Plasma concentrations of BSP are measured at 2 sequential 4-min time intervals within 12 min of injection. The time required for a 50% reduction of the plasma concentration of BSP is determined by plotting the measured plasma values on semilog paper. The ½ BSP clearance time is 2-3.7 min for healthy mature horses, and 2.5-4.1 min for normal cattle. BSP excretion in small animals is determined by a serum retention value measured 30 min after IV injection. Healthy dogs retain ≤5% of BSP 30 min after injection.

Serum Enzyme Concentration: Hepatocellular damage results in the release of cellular enzymes. Elevated serum levels of certain enzymes indicate damaged liver tissue in some species. ALT (SGPT) is a characteristic liver enzyme of dogs, cats, and primates. The serum concentration of ALT in a clear, nonlipemic sample is stable for up to 1 wk when refrigerated. In large animals, the liver-specific enzymes are generally difficult to assay. Sorbitol dehydrogenase is the enzyme of choice for detecting hepatic lesions in horses, but it must be measured immediately because of its thermolability. Glutamic dehydrogenase is the enzyme of choice for detection of bovine liver disease. Arginase is liver-specific for horses and is found in high concentrations in the liver of cows, sheep, and dogs. Serum arginase levels can be determined within 1 hr by direct colorimetry. Elevations of ornithine carbamyl transferase in the serum is indicative of liver disease in all species, but assays are tedious and time consuming. A simple tablet test is available in kit form for serum alkaline phosphatase (SAP) determinations in dogs and cats. However, there are multiple sources of SAP, including osteoblasts, chondroblasts, the hepatobiliary system, GI mucosa, renal tubules, and the spleen; elevated SAP levels must be interpreted in conjunction with other clinical signs and therapeutic history. The same precaution is advisable in the interpretation of elevated serum levels of other enzymes, especially those that can be drug-induced, including ALT (SGPT).

PANCREATIC FUNCTION TESTS

Acute Pancreatitis: The pancreas is the major source of lipase, and serum levels of the enzyme are elevated in necrotic pancreatitis. Amylase levels are also elevated in acute pancreatitis and can be measured visually by an amyloclastic hydrolysis of starch. Normal serum amylase concentrations are at least doubled in acute pancreatitis. Normal serum amylase values of dogs and cats are 5-10 times higher than that of man.

Chronic Pancreatitis or Atrophy: The loss of functional pancreatic parenchyma may be due to fibrosis or atrophy; the resulting pancreatic enzyme deficiencies are manifest as digestive insufficiencies detectable by fecal examination. Gross inspection of fresh feces reveals a glistening, soft, pale, yellow- to clay-colored, bulky mass that has a rancid odor of steatorrhea (fecal fat). Fat and undigested muscle fibers may be observed by microscopical examination of stained fecal samples, and indicate insufficient pancreatic lipase and trypsin, respectively.

Pancreatic proteolytic enzyme activity can be tested for by a simple radiographic film strip test, and the results can be verified with a gelatin tube test. Feces are added to 9 mL of 5% sodium bicarbonate solution to achieve a total volume of 10 mL. The end of a strip of unprocessed radiographic film is placed in the fecal suspension and incubated at 37.5°C for 1 hr, or for 2½ hr at room temperature; the film strip is then washed gently with tap water and examined to determine if the gelatin emulsion has been digested. Fecal trypsin of a normal dog clears an area on the submerged portion of the film strip (positive test). In contrast, the gelatin emulsion with watermarks persists in pancreatic insufficiency characterized by lack of fecal trypsin. A more sensitive gelatin tube test should be conducted when the film test is positive, because intestinal proteases may clear the film emulsion in 25% of the tests (false positive results). Two mL of 7.5% gelatin is added to each of 2 tubes and liquified by warming to 37°C. Two mL of the 5% sodium bicarbonate fecal suspension is added to one gelatin tube, and 2 mL of 5% sodium bicarbonate solution only is added to the other gelatin tube as a control. The contents of each tube are mixed, incubated at 37°C for 1 hr (or room temperature for 2½ hr), and then refrigerated for 20 min. Gel formation in the tube that contains the fecal suspension indicates a lack of trypsin, which is associated with chronic pancreatic disease.

Pancreatic islet cell function is compromised in 50% of dogs with chronic pancreatic disease. Hyperglycemia and glycosuria are the resulting manifestations of diabetes mellitus (qv, p 267).

CLINICAL MICROBIOLOGY

Collection of samples for identification of bacterial pathogens and/or determination of antibiotic sensitivity must be done before initiation of therapy. The minimum time interval in which identification and sensitivity can be accomplished is the same as that required for bacterial growth, which invalidates the advantage of in-office effort in urban areas where diagnostic laboratories are in close proximity. The details that an independent diagnostic laboratory can provide in confirmation of a clinical infection can be invaluable. In contrast, the minimum capabilities of the office laboratory should include preparation of stained and unstained smears, inoculation of culture (thioglycollate broth) or transport media, preliminary testing for antibiotic sensitivity, and collection of serum samples.

CULTURES

Culture for identification of bacterial pathogens and determination of antibiotic sensitivity requires a stock of dated media, reagents, equipment, and experienced personnel; 4 cultures/day are regarded as the minimum volume to justify the expense and time required. Commercial media kits are available for presumptive identification of up to 18 aerobic pathogens and determination of their antibiotic sensitivity. An alternative is careful aseptic collection of a swab sample or the specimen *per se* for submission to a diagnostic laboratory.

Cultures also may be initiated in appropriate media such as thioglycollate broth, which supports both aerobic and anaerobic bacterial growth. Cultures of samples from the GI tract can be started on selective medium such as MacConkey's agar. Brain-heart-infusion agar and blood agar are 2 examples of all-purpose media. Amies transport medium can be used for shipment of unrefrigerated swab samples directly to a diagnostic laboratory. The various media are commercially available in screw-capped vials and must be refrigerated until used. Initiated (streaked) cultures can be submitted directly to a diagnostic laboratory or incubated for 24 hr at 37°C. If growth occurs, it can be stained and subcultured on blood agar or Mueller-Hinton medium for antibiotic sensitivity testing.

Specific media for culture of dermatophytes are commercially available. The cutaneous lesion should be cleaned with 70% alcohol before hairs and skin scrapings are collected. Selective media contain combinations of inhibitors, supplements, and an indicator to facilitate growth and recognition of various pathogenic fungi, most of which grow at room temperature (25°C) under aerobic conditions. *Trichophyton verrucosum* (bovine ringworm) grows better at 37°C, and some pathogens require 3-4 wk to manifest growth. All growth should be subjected to microscopical examination after staining in a drop of lactophenol cotton blue. Observation of characteristic mycotic structures such as macroconidia and microconidia aid definitive identification.

ANTIBIOTIC SENSITIVITY TESTING

In infectious disease therapy, an antibiotic is chosen with regard to sensitivity of the pathogen and cost. After collection of samples for culture, treatment should be initiated immediately, and be based on clinical experience without actual knowledge of pathogen sensitivity. Subsequent lack of therapeutic response raises the need for such information to a critical level.

Paper disks impregnated with various antibiotics are used to determine *in vitro* sensitivity of bacteria. The disks are placed on the surface of culture plates (blood agar, Mueller-Hinton) that have been streaked with the suspected pathogen. Inhibition of bacterial growth around a disk after 8-24 hr of incubation at 37°C indicates sensitivity to the particular antibiotic impregnated in the disk. The Kirby-Bauer procedure quantitates antibiotic potency into minimal inhibitory concentration (MIC) and minimal bactericidal concentration (MBC).

CYTOLOGY

Cytology can be a useful tool in making a definitive diagnosis. Inflammation, neoplasia, and specific pathogens can be differentiated with routine cytology procedures. Ideally, cytology samples should be one cell layer thick to allow for adequate staining and visualization.

A 22-gauge needle attached to a 6-mL syringe can be used to sample various tissues with minimal discomfort to the animal. To aspirate the tissue, the needle is directed into the mass and suction applied with the syringe. The needle is redirected once or twice, with care to keep the tip of the needle within the tissue. The syringe plunger is gently released before the needle is withdrawn. Often, tissue is not visible within the hub, but diagnostic material is within the needle. The needle should be held over a glass slide as the syringe is removed and filled with air. The syringe is reattached and the specimen in the needle is gently expelled onto the slide. A second slide is used to spread the specimen to make a smear. If the slides are to be stained with Romanoswky-type stains, they are air dried; if by the trichrome method, they are placed immediately in methanol.

Biopsy specimens can also be used for cytology. A freshly cut surface of the biopsy sample should be blotted on a clean paper towel. This surface is then gently touched to a clean glass slide. Several impression smears can be made on the same slide. Cytological specimens must be protected from formalin or its fumes. Formaldehyde alters the staining characteristics of Romanowsky-type stains and hampers diagnostic ability.

Fluid samples should be collected in EDTA tubes to prevent clot formation, which may trap cells, and evaluated by counting the cells and measuring the protein. Smears should be made as soon as possible after collection. A technique similar to that used to make blood smears is used. In samples with few cells, it may be best to concentrate the sample before making a smear.

Cytology is useful to differentiate inflammatory lesions from neoplastic lesions. The etiologic agent of inflammatory lesions, as well as the cellular components of inflammation, may be identified in a cytology sample. Acute inflammatory lesions are usually characterized by a large population of neutrophils with fewer macrophages and lymphocytes. Chronic inflammation tends to have macrophages, giant cells, plasma cells, and a few neutrophils. Special stains may be necessary to help identify infectious organisms such as fungi or bacteria.

Cytologically, neoplasia can be categorized into 3 basic groups: epithelial-glandular tumors, supporting tissue tumors, and a miscellaneous group sometimes referred to as round cell tumors. Cells from the epithelial-glandular group tend to exfoliate in clusters or groups. Cells from malignant tumors tend to vary in size, shape, and nuclear:cytoplasmic ratio. Nuclei may be large with prominent nucleoli. Bizarre mitotic figures and occasionally glandular formations may be seen.

Malignant cells from supporting tissue tumors share many of these cytoplasmic characteristics. Cells from these tumors are much less likely to exfoliate and are usually single cells when they do. The cells are usually ovoid or spindle shaped, with mild to marked variation in size. The cells often appear "wispy" with ill-defined membranes.

Cytology is most useful when evaluating the miscellaneous neoplasms. These include lymphomas, mast cell tumors, histiocytomas, transmissible venereal tumors, and melanomas. Lymphomas are recognized by a fairly uniform population of large, immature lymphocytes. Many have prominent nucleoli and are classified as lymphoblasts. Lymphoma can be diagnosed from aspirates not only from lymph nodes, but also from the liver, kidney, or other organs.

Mast cell tumors are easily recognized by the large population of cells with light blue nuclei and numerous metachromatic-staining granules in the cytoplasm. The granules are so numerous that they may obscure the nucleus. Some quick stains do not adequately stain the granules, allowing easy visualization of the nuclei.

Histiocytomas may exfoliate well or poorly. The round to oval cells vary slightly in size. The cytoplasm is pale blue and moderately abundant. Lymphocytes may be scattered about, and increase in number as the tumor begins to spontaneously regress.

Transmissible venereal tumors can occur at sites other than the urogenital area. The cells readily exfoliate and are fairly large and may vary slightly in size. Mitotic figures are common.

Melanomas have large oval cells with abundant cytoplasm that may contain dark granules (melanin). Occasionally, melanomas contain few or no recognizable granules and may be confused with other tumors.

Vaginal cytology can be used to identify the various stages of the canine estrous cycle. A sample of exfoliated cells is obtained from the vaginal vault cranial to the urethral orifice with a cotton-tipped swab, glass rod, or pipette. The cells are gently rolled onto a glass slide, fixed by a 95% methanol dip, and air dried. The slide film is then stained with a permanent stain for future reference. Various epithelial cell types, RBC, and neutrophils in varying concentrations and ratios characterize the different stages of the estrous cycle. The predominant cells of late proestrus are RBC and noncornified epithelial cells. Estrus is associated with numerous cornified superficial epithelial cells and an increased number of bacteria. In diestrus, the neutrophils and noncornified parabasal and intermediate epithelial cells predominate. The most numerous cell types of anestrus are the noncornified parabasal and intermediate epithelial cells.

FLUID ANALYSIS

Body fluids can be analyzed to aid in diagnosis. Fluid that is normally found in body cavities is characteristically low in protein and contains few cells. It is thought to be an ultrafiltrate of plasma, and the mesothelial lining cell may regulate the fluid flow. When evaluating fluid samples, several parameters should be examined. Since normal body fluids have a low protein content (<3 g/dL), an increase suggests an inflammatory process. Fluids with low protein content are transudates; those with increased protein are exudates. When there is a mild increase in protein and cell number, it is a modified transudate. Distinctions between a modified transudate and an exudate are not always obvious.

Transudates may result from venous stasis, hypoalbuminemia, or lymphatic obstruction. The protein content is <3 g/dL and can be estimated by using a refractometer (specific gravity ≤ 1.015). There are usually few cells (<500 nucleated cells/μL). Smears should be made from the sediment of a centrifuged sample. Cells typically are mesothelial and occasionally inflammatory. The sloughed mesothelial cells may proliferate in the fluid. Since these reactive mesothelial cells do not divide completely, they usually occur in clusters in multiples of 2. Cytoplasm is abundant with nuclei centrally located. The inflammatory cells seen in transudates have the morphology of peripheral WBC.

Modified transudates have a mild increase in protein (3-5 g/dL) and specific gravity (1.018-1.030). The nucleated cell count increases somewhat, but is still $<5000/\mu$L, and most are reactive mesothelial cells. Some of the cell clusters may have mitotic figures and must be differentiated from mesothelial cells. Inflammatory cells, primarily neutrophils, also can be found in the modified transudate.

Exudates are fluid accumulations that have high protein content (>4 g/dL) and cell counts $>5000/\mu$L. The cells vary with the cause of effusion. Chylous effusions result from the leakage of lymph into the body cavities. They have a high lipid content and classically appear milky. Most of the cells are small mature lymphocytes.

Inflammatory effusions can be classified according to the length of time they have been in the body cavity. Neutrophils predominate in acute reactions; if they are degenerate, a bacterial cause is suspect. Chronic inflammatory effusions have higher numbers of macrophages. Even if organisms are not seen, culture should be attempted.

Neoplastic effusions may have characteristic neoplastic cells, eg, lymphosarcomas may cause an effusion with numerous atypical blastic lymphocytes, and tumors of epithelial origin may be singular or in clusters. It is often difficult to differentiate these neoplastic cells from reactive mesothelial cells.

STAINING TECHNIQUES

Exudates, transudates, needle-aspirates, tissue imprints, blood, feces, and urine sediment all can be evaluated microscopically via stained and unstained films. Stains can be used as an aid in identification of bacteria, inflammation, and neoplasia.

Gram's Stain: This stain separates bacteria into 2 taxonomic groups: gram-positive (eg, cocci) stain dark-blue or black, and gram-negative (eg, coliforms and pseudomonads) appear pink. A moderately thin film of the sample is air dried and gently heat-fixed over a flame. The fixed film is covered with Gram's gentian or crystal violet for 1 min, flushed with water, and covered with Gram's iodine for 1 min. It is then decolorized for 5-10 sec with acetone-alcohol, flushed with water, drained, and counterstained with safranin or basic fuchsin for 1 min. After rinsing in water, the film is dried before examination under oil-immersion magnification. In addition to differentiating bacteria into 2 color categories, all fungi stain blue-black, and nuclei of WBC stain pink.

Clear Unstained Films: The following are demonstrable in clear, unstained preparations: mange mites, fungi of dermatomycoses, molds, and yellow granular structures (sulfur granules or ray fungus, which characterize the pus produced by actinomycetes, actinobacilli, and staphylococci). Hair and skin scales are collected from the periphery of a new skin lesion onto a scalpel blade by scraping into the corium layer of the cutis. If for mites, the scraping should be deep enough to cause capillary hemorrhage. Purulent or necrotic tissue debris contains pathogenic molds and "sulfur granules". The collected specimen is placed on a slide, a few drops of 10-40% sodium hydroxide are added, and a coverglass applied. Clearing of the specimen occurs in 30 min and can be facilitated by 5 min of gentle heat. Low-power magnification is used to screen for an area containing hairs and epithelial cells in a single thin layer. High-power magnification and reduced illumination reveal mycotic hyphae and/or spores within or along hair shafts and epidermal cells in dermatomycoses. Gram's stain and cultures can be used for specific identification of granular structures and molds that may be observed as causes of subcut. lesions.

Wright's Stain: This is available in liquid form and is used with phosphate buffer. The slide is covered with stain on a level staining rack for 1-3 min; an equal amount of phosphate buffer is carefully added so as to avoid flow-off and is mixed by gentle blowing until a green metallic scum appears. Optimal staining time is 3-5 min. Stain and scum are floated off with distilled water, and the slide is air dried. A permanent record can be made by applying a coverglass with mounting medium.

Giemsa Stain: Stock solutions are available that are stable and produce consistent results. The slide film is fixed in absolute methanol for 3-5 min and dried. The stain is prepared daily by mixing one volume of stock stain with 15 volumes of distilled water. The fixed, dry, slide film is placed immediately in the diluted stain for 30-60 min, washed in neutral distilled water, air dried, and examined. Permanent records of blood parasites can be made by mounting a coverglass over the stained film.

Fast Convenient Stains: Numerous available commercial stains are quick and easy to use. The manufacturers' directions for use of the various stains should be followed. New Methylene Blue (NMB) is a versatile vital drop stain that reveals reticulocytes, Heinz bodies, nuclei, hemoparasites, and platelets, among other structures. Unlike other stains, NMB does not stain RBC, and cannot be used for a permanent record unless a counterstain has been used.

HEMATOLOGY

Clotting Tests: Hemostasis involves many complex interrelationships among many systems (*see* HEMOSTATIC DISORDERS, p 52). Blood clots when it is removed from normal endothelial-lined vessels. Clotting, or coagulation, is usually divided into 2 major systems, the intrinsic and extrinsic pathways, which terminate in a common pathway; this results in formation of a fibrin plug. Tests have been developed to evaluate both the intrinsic and extrinsic system as well as specific factors within the systems. Some of those tests are best done by commercial laboratories. The blood for these tests requires special handling, and the laboratory should be contacted for specific instructions. However, several coagulation tests can be done in-house.

Bleeding Time: A clear hairless area is chosen for this test (nose, inside of the lip, inner ear). A deep puncture wound is made with a lancet or #11 piercing scalpel blade. The time is noted when blood appears (pressure is not applied). At 30-sec intervals, filter paper, which should not touch the skin, is used to remove the blood. The time at which bleeding stops is noted; for most domestic animals, it is 1-5 min. The bleeding time is prolonged with platelet defects, increased capillary fragility, and von Willebrand's disease.

Activated Coagulation Time (ACT): Whole blood (2 mL) is placed in an ACT tube. This tube contains diatomaceous earth, which serves as an activating agent to shorten clotting time and increase the sensitivity of the whole blood clotting time. Timing begins as soon as the blood is placed in the tube. After mixing, the tube is incubated at 37°C for 1 min. The tube is evaluated at 5-sec intervals for evidence of clotting. This normally occurs within 60-90 sec. Severe thrombocytopenia ($<$10,000 platelets/μL) and defects in the intrinsic system prolong the clotting time.

Fibrinogen: Fibrinogen is essential for blood coagulation. Measurement is accomplished easily by heat precipitation of fibrinogen from a whole blood sample containing an anticoagulant. Two PCV tubes are filled and centrifuged gently for 10 min to clear the plasma. The total solids (mg protein/dL) in the plasma of one tube is determined by use of a refractometer. The other centrifuged PCV tube is immersed in a 57°C water bath for 3 min to precipitate the fibrinogen. It is then recentrifuged, and the total solids of the remaining plasma are determined with the refractometer. The value is subtracted from that of the unheated plasma, and the difference is fibrinogen concentration in mg/dL. The normal range for dogs, cats, and horses is 200-400 mg/dL. For cattle, the range is 450-750 mg/dL, and higher values are a more sensitive indicator of inflammation and neoplasia than the total WBC count. Hypofibrinogenemia may be congenital, or reflect advanced hepatic disease, malnutrition, canine granulocytic leukemia, moribund state, disseminated intravascular coagulation, etc.

The circulating blood cell types vary in number with normal physiological states as well as with pathological conditions. The considerable variation can be influenced by sex, age, nutrition, physical exertion, ambient temperature, and diurnal and sexual cycles. Values listed in TABLE 8, p 967, should be considered as guides rather than rigid criteria.

Blood cell numbers also change in disease states: WBC values rise in acute bacterial infections, neoplastic leukemias, tissue necrosis, trauma, and chemical or metabolic intoxication; however, extreme stages of the same conditions are associated with decreased values. Among the common examples of diagnostic alterations of blood cell numbers is the increase of neutrophils (polymorphonuclear leukocytes) produced by pyogenic bacteria. Elevated numbers of monocytes and lymphocytes are associated with an immune response in a chronic or healing inflammatory process. In contrast, acute viral infections are characterized by leukopenia. Eosinophil counts rise in allergic responses and frequently in association with helminth infections. The anemias of severe parasitism or malnutrition are reflected by smaller numbers of circulating RBC with less Hgb. Numerous immature blood cells with abnormal morphology are often the first indicators of a leukemic neoplastic alteration of the blood-forming tissues.

Collection of the Blood Sample: Blood is collected by venipuncture with a sterile, dry needle and syringe, or an evacuated collection vial containing an anticoagulant (potassium EDTA). Disposable needles, plastic syringes, and collection vials facilitate economical collection of blood by precluding chemical contamination and iatrogenic infections. The size of the animal and the quantity of blood required determine the site of venipuncture. Generally, the largest accessible vein is used. The cephalic, jugular, femoral, and coccygeal veins are sites most often used for companion animals and herbivores. The anterior vena cava is the site of choice for pigs, and the wing (alar) vein is used for birds. Blood samples can be obtained from puppies and kittens by clipping a toenail toward the unguinal bed. The best smears for differential WBC counts are made immediately at the time of collection before exposure to an anticoagulant. Anticoagulant tubes should be inverted gently immediately after blood collection and before use of the blood to ensure uniform mixing. EDTA is the anticoagulant of choice for most hematological procedures if they are performed within 6 hr of collection (the sooner the better). However, EDTA causes shrinkage of RBC and interferes with determinations of nonprotein nitrogen, alkaline phosphatase, creatinine, and carbon dioxide combining power. Hemolysis should be avoided during and after blood collection to avoid interference with several chemical analyses.

Packed Cell Volume (PCV, Hematocrit): The PCV is an accurate, practical evaluation of RBC status, considering the recognized inaccuracy of manual RBC counts and the technical effort required for accurate Hgb determinations. The PCV is most readily obtained by use of a microhematocrit centrifuge. A capillary tube is filled with blood containing an anticoagulant, sealed, and centrifuged. Heparin-coated capillary tubes are available for taking samples directly from the animal (toenail, ear). The centrifuged sample is placed on a hematocrit tube reader, and the percent PCV value is obtained from the underlying scale. Other parameters can be crudely estimated from the PCV. The total RBC count is one-sixth of the PCV, and the Hgb value is one-third of the PCV. The color of the plasma layer in a centrifuged tube may indicate icterus in nonherbivores, anemia, or lipemia. Lipemia is frequently associated with diabetes mellitus, hypothyroidism, acute pancreatitis, and liver disease.

Total WBC Count: The "Unopette" system is a practical, economical, manual system that can be used for determining total numbers of circulating WBC, RBC, platelets, and eosinophils. The system utilizes prefilled, disposable dilution-reservoirs and pipettes, a hemocytometer counting chamber, and a microscope. A 20% margin of error does not diminish diagnostic value of the determinations made with the system.

The laboratory workload should be evaluated before deciding to purchase and maintain the more precise and efficient automated analyzers. Three complete blood counts per day are regarded as minimum economic justification for purchase of an automated instrument. Accuracy of most automated instruments requires recalibration for each species. The use of quality control standards in each test also ensures accuracy.

Differential WBC Count: (*See* TABLE 9 for leukocyte values, p 968.) The best blood smears are made on new glass slides that are electronically clean, dry, and warm, and have beveled edges. A small drop of freshly drawn blood (within 15 min after addition of EDTA) is placed near the end of a slide placed on a flat surface. Another slide held at a 30° angle is slid back on the surface of the stationary slide until it touches the blood drop, which spreads by capillary action along the interface formed by the 2 slides. The angled slide is then pushed forward in a smooth, even motion to form a blood smear on the stationary slide. The smear is air dried rapidly by waving it in room-temperature air or by use of a fan, to prevent cellular distortions or crenation. The dried blood smear should be stained, or fixed in absolute methanol, or stored in a dry dust-free container at room temperature in that order of preference.

The smear is stained with a Wright's or Giemsa-type stain and dried following aqueous flushing of excess stain. The stained smear is screened under low-power magnification for acceptable distribution and staining of WBC. Areas selected for counting should have RBC with central pallor. Cells should be distributed in a single layer. One hundred WBC or multiples thereof (preferred) are classified under high-dry or oil-immersion magnification. The outer margin of the blood smear should be examined uniformly to compensate for uneven distributions of the various cell types. Use of a cell tabulator facilitates the differential count. The total number of each cell type is expressed as a percentage value. Absolute values of each cell type are obtained by multiplying the counted percent value by the total WBC count. The values are used to differentiate actual increases from apparent increases that are relative to reduced numbers of other WBC types. Absolute values ensure accuracy in the interpretation of the differential count.

Hematogenous pathogens (qv, p 949) may be seen while performing differential WBC counts. Platelet numbers can be estimated by counting the number of platelets observed under oil-immersion magnification (*see* below). Four or more platelets are normally present in such fields unless they are in clumps along the edges of the film.

Reticulocyte Count: Clinical signs of anemia may be accompanied by an increased number of RBC that are immature, non-nucleated, and contain basophilic cytoplasmic material. The basophilic material appears as a reticulum or as punctate foci when stained with a vital stain. Equal quantities of blood and 1% New Methylene Blue in saline are placed in a stoppered tube for 15 min at room temperature. A film of the mixture is then prepared on a microscope slide and counterstained as for the differential WBC count. The number of RBC with blue-staining threads or granules per 500-1000 RBC is determined under oil-immersion magnification. The value is expressed in percent, which normally varies from 0% in ungulates to 1% in dogs and cats. Higher values are associated with a regenerative response of bone marrow to anemia in dogs, cats, and cattle. Horses are an exception and do not develop a peripheral reticulocytic response to anemia.

Platelet Count: Platelets (thrombocytes) are fragile, and counts should be performed within 2 hr of blood collection. Platelet counts have large margins of additional inherent error. A "Unopette" system designed for counting WBC and platelets is available. The charged hemocytometer should be covered with a Petri dish for 10 min to allow the platelets to settle before counting the entire RBC area of the chamber under high-dry magnification. An indirect count is simpler and more practical. The number of platelets observed per 100 WBC is recorded during the differential count. This value is divided by 100 and multiplied by the number of WBC/μL (*see* TOTAL WBC COUNT, above). The value obtained is the number of platelets/μL. Platelet counts of <50,000 are associated with spontaneous hemorrhages. A cruder determination of platelet numbers can be made by counting the number of platelets in each microscope field under oil-immersion: the normal average number for 10 fields is 5. Elevated counts are associated with stress, including surgery. Depressed values are associated with hematopoietic diseases and are the most common cause of bleeding disorders in companion animals.

Evaluation of RBC: Both the number and morphology of RBC are subject to change as the result of disease. An increase in the number of RBC is called polycythemia (qv, p 83).

There are many causes of anemia (qv, p 15), but it is rarely a primary disease. Anemias can be classified based on the RBC indices: the mean cell volume (MCV), mean corpuscular hemoglobin (MCH), and mean corpuscular hemoglobin concentration (MCHC). The MCV is determined by dividing the PCV by the RBC count and multiplying by 10; the units used are femtoliters (fL). The MCHC is determined by dividing the Hgb by the PCV and multiplying by 100; the concentration of Hgb per unit volume of RBC is expressed as g/dL. The MCH varies linearly with the MCV. It is calculated by dividing the PCV by the RBC count and multiplying by 10; the result is the mean weight of the Hgb in the RBC and is expressed in picograms. By evaluating the MCV, it can be determined if the RBC are large (macrocytic), small (microcytic), or normal (normocytic). The MCHC indicates if the Hgb content is decreased (hypochromic) or normal (normochromic). It is impossible to have a true elevation of Hgb.

The RBC morphology can be evaluated from the stained smear. Abnormal morphology is most easily recognized in dogs because of the size and biconcave shape of normal cells. The following are descriptive terms used to describe RBC. **Anisocytosis** is variation in size. Macrocytes are larger than normal; they are usually young polychromatophilic cells. Microcytes are smaller than normal cells. **Poikilocytosis** is a general term used to describe alteration in cell shape; it must be evaluated carefully to determine if it is an artifact of slide preparation or due to pathology of the RBC. **Crenated** RBC have a crinkled appearance with short, equally spaced projections from the surface. They are commonly seen in blood smears from pigs, but are usually an artifact of preparation in other species. **Spherocytes** are small, dark cells without central pallor; this is a result of loss of RBC membrane, which causes the RBC to "round up" and lose the biconcave shape. They are seen most frequently in autoimmune hemolytic anemia. **Acanthocytes** (spur cells) have irregular spicular protrusions of the RBC membrane. They may be seen with severe liver disease, vascular neoplasia, and disseminated intravascular coagulation. **Schizocytes** are fragments of RBC. Microangiopathic disorders shear RBC into irregularly shaped pieces. **Leptocytes** are RBC that have an increased membrane or decreased volume. The cell membrane folds or becomes distorted. They sometimes form target cells with a dark peripheral rim and apparent central mass.

Inclusions and infective agents can also be seen in or on RBC. **Howell-Jolly bodies** are small dark-staining inclusions found inside RBC. These are nuclear remnants, and are increased in dogs and cats with regenerative anemia and dogs given glucocorticoids. **Basophilic stippling** may be seen in regenerative anemias in cattle and sheep, and in lead poisoning in dogs. The RBC have multiple, tiny, dark inclusions in normochromic RBC that have been stained with Romanowsky stains. **Siderotic inclusions** are iron-containing granules; they appear similar to basophilic stippling with Romanowsky stains, but can be differentiated with iron stains. **Distemper inclusions** are pieces of viral nucleocapsids that are seen in RBC and WBC; they stain blue or pink.

Evaluation of WBC: Nucleated cells (WBC) of the blood include neutrophils, lymphocytes, monocytes, eosinophils, and basophils. They are differentiated by examining a stained smear. Changes in WBC numbers and morphology are called the leukocyte response. Typical leukocyte responses may aid diagnosis.

Neutrophils: The neutrophil has a segmented nucleus when it is mature and released from the bone marrow. The cytoplasm stains pale pink, with fine granules. With increased need, immature neutrophils, called band neutrophils, are released from the bone marrow. The nuclei of these cells are horseshoe-shaped. With increasing need, more immature cells are released. The younger the neutrophil, the rounder the nuclei.

Lymphocytes: These have round nuclei that may have a slight cleft. Cytoplasm stains blue and is relatively scant. Small pink-purple granules may be present in the cytoplasm of a few of the lymphocytes. Immature cells tend to be larger and have darker cytoplasm.

Monocytes: These have variably shaped nuclei, which may be kidney-bean shaped or lobulated. The cytoplasm is blue-gray. Small vacuoles and/or small pink granules may be present in the cytoplasm.

Eosinophils: These also have segmented nuclei, similar to neutrophils. Different species have characteristically shaped eosinophilic granules: in dogs, these may vary in size within a cell; in cats, they are small and rod-shaped; in horses, they are large and round; in cattle, sheep, and pigs, they are small, round, and uniform.

Basophils: The nuclei of basophils are also segmented. Granules stain purple to blue-black. Dogs have few, horses and cattle have more. Feline basophils have few lavender-stained granules; difficult to see, these may give the nucleus a moth-eaten appearance.

EXAMINATION OF PERIPHERAL BLOOD FOR MICROSCOPIC PATHOGENS

See also BLOOD-BORNE ORGANISMS, POULTRY, p 1544 *et seq.*

Canine heartworm disease (qv, p 73) continues to be a problem of growing magnitude, and feline heartworm is being diagnosed more frequently. The presence of microfilariae in a fresh peripheral blood film of dogs is diagnostic of infection with either the pathogenic *Dirofilaria immitis* or benign *Dipetalonema reconditum*. The microfilariae should be identified before treatment is begun. If the peripheral blood film is negative and heartworm is a consideration in the differential diagnosis, a blood sample should be centrifuged, or filtered using a commercially available kit to increase the probability of finding microfilariae. In the absence of circulating microfilariae, occult heartworm infections can be diagnosed by use of a kit that detects microfilarial antibody by immunofluorescent assay, or adult heartworm antigen by ELISA.

Examination of RBC for Pathogens: Blood films of varying thickness are made on clean slides by varying the size of the blood drop and altering the angle of the spreader slide (qv, p 947). The dried films are fixed in absolute alcohol for 2 min and stained (qv, p 944) with Wright's, Giemsa, or New Methylene Blue stain. The stained films are examined microscopically under oil-immersion for RBC parasites, several of which are included in the following list. The parasitic pathogens usually appear less refractive than artifacts.

Examination of Phagocytes for Pathogens: The buffy coat of a centrifuged blood sample is a source of large numbers of leukocytic phagocytes, including polymorphonuclear leukocytes and monocytes. Smears of buffy coats stained by procedures similar to those for RBC are of diagnostic value for microscopical diagnosis of histoplasmosis, toxoplasmosis, ehrlichiosis, leucocytozoonosis, erysipelas septicemia, etc.

Table 2. Examination of Peripheral Blood for Microscopic Pathogens

Primary Species Affected	Examples of Detectable Hematogenous Pathogens
Dog	*Dirofilaria immitis* *Dipetalonema reconditum* *Ehrlichia canis* *Babesia (Piroplasma) canis* *Haemobartonella* sp *Histoplasma capsulatum*
Cat	*Haemobartonella felis* *Dirofilaria* sp *Cytauxzoon felis* *Histoplasma capsulatum*
Horse	*Ehrlichia* sp *Babesia (Piroplasma) equi* *B caballi*
Cow	*Anaplasma marginale* *Trypanosoma theileri (americanum)*—nonpathogen *Bacillus anthracis*
Pig	*Eperythrozoon suis* *Erysipelothrix rhusiopathiae*
Sheep	*Eperythrozoon ovis*
Duck	*Leucocytozoon simondi (anseris)*
Pigeon	*Haemoproteus* sp

PARASITOLOGY

EXAMINATION FOR ECTOPARASITES

Animals with dermatoses should be evaluated for ectoparasites. The skin is examined for parasites or evidence thereof, eg, fleas may not be seen on a cat or dog, but small black flecks of excrement may be present. If these flecks are placed on a wet paper towel, they produce a bright red stain.

Sometimes the skin must be scraped (eg, with a scalpel blade) to find parasites. A drop of mineral oil is placed on a slide and the blade is run through the oil; the oil holds the scraped debris to the blade. Since some of the parasites (eg, *Sarcoptes, Demodex*) live in burrows and hair follicles, it may be necessary to scrape until a small amount of blood is obtained.

The scraped material is spread in the drop of oil on a slide, and a coverslip placed on top. The entire coverslipped area should be scanned under low-power magnification. Occasionally, it may be necessary to add 2-3 drops of a 10% solution of potassium hydroxide. This clears the debris and allows better visualization.

ESTIMATING INTERNAL PARASITE LOAD

The most common antemortem method of estimating parasite load is the examination of feces for parasite eggs. If possible, fresh fecal samples should be collected from the rectum. A plastic glove is suitable for this, and once sufficient feces have been collected, the glove may be inverted to act as a receptacle. If livestock cannot be gathered, then fecal samples may be obtained from the pasture or floor, again using a plastic glove; only fresh excreta should be collected in this way. A representative number of samples should be collected, and a minimum of 10 is recommended.

Results are more difficult to interpret from older samples in which embryos have developed, or oocysts or eggs have deteriorated, eg, lungworm larvae are most readily identified in fresh feces because larvae of other species may be found in older feces. *Strongyloides* sp are passed as larvae or as eggs that hatch shortly thereafter in dog feces. To prevent such changes, fecal specimens to be submitted to a diagnostic laboratory should be fixed in 5% formaldehyde solution, or maintained chilled but not frozen.

Adult nematodes and tapeworm segments may be detected by gross examination of the feces. Fecal examination usually involves techniques in which the eggs or larvae are concentrated so that small numbers can be detected. A simple direct technique is to dilute a small amount of feces with water and spread the mixture thinly on a microscope slide. A coverslip is then placed on the smear, and the preparation is examined under low power. Adding a few drops of iodine or methylene blue to the smear can facilitate detection of eggs. However, since the fecal material may contain plant cells, grains, or other extraneous matter that can be mistaken for parasite eggs, it is better to use a method that concentrates the eggs and one in which the final preparation is clearer.

These methods are based on the flotation of eggs in solutions with a specific gravity of 1.1-1.2, such as saturated salt (NaCl), magnesium sulfate, or sugar. A saturated NaCl solution is prepared by dissolving as much granulated table salt as possible in water at room temperature. It does not require a preservative and is neither sticky nor attractive to flies. A saturated sucrose solution containing 50 mL of 5% phenol/L is capable of floating the eggs of *Dicrocoelium* and is slower to destroy larvae and delicate oocysts. A number of kits for fecal analysis are available.

About 2 g of feces is placed in a container and ~15 mL of the salt or sugar solution is added. The mixture is stirred until the feces are in suspension, then strained through a clean gauze square into a test tube, using enough solution to fill it to within 0.25 in. (6 mm) of the top. The process of flotation may be accelerated by placing the tube in a centrifuge that is run at low speed (1000-2000 rpm) for ~6 min. When centrifugation is completed, a large drop is lifted from the surface film by means of a beaded glass rod and transferred to a microscope slide, covering a circular area ~1 cm in diameter.

This technique provides a guide to the number of eggs in the sample, but special slides containing chambers with etched areas of known volume are available for estimating the number of eggs per gram of feces (EPG). The strained solution of concentrate (usually saturated salt) is introduced into each chamber with a Pasteur pipette, and the number of eggs counted under low power. A counting slide commonly used is the McMaster slide, which has 2 chambers, each with a volume of 0.15 mL under the etched area. If, eg, 3 g of feces is mixed with 42 mL of concentrate solution, then each egg counted is multiplied by 50 to give the number of EPG of feces. This is calculated by:

$$\frac{42 + 3}{3} \times \frac{1}{0.15 \times 2} = 50$$

The correlation between the EPG and the actual worm burden is often quite good in young animals, although low or negative results can be misleading in adults. Generally, an EPG count of >500 reflects a moderate infection, and >1000 indicates that treatment is required.

SEROLOGY

Brucella canis: A drop of suspect serum is needed for use in a commercial 2-min slide-agglutination test. Positive agglutination indicates presumptive infection with *B canis*, but culturing the pathogen from blood for a positive diagnosis should be attempted, since false positive reactions do occur. (*See also* pp 669 and 1155.) Dogs that test positive should be retested at 1-mo intervals if blood cultures are negative. Negative agglutination tests are generally regarded as valid.

Foal Immunity: Transfer of colostral IgG to the neonatal foal is measured with commercial kits that utilize development of zinc sulfate turbidity or radial immunodiffusion. More rapid latex agglutination test kits have been developed that measure IgG levels in mL quantities of serum or whole blood that has been obtained ≥15 hr after nursing has started. Test results, which can be obtained in 10-15 min, are determined by visual chart comparisons and are expressed in approximate mg of IgG/dL. The same methodology is used to measure IgG concentrations in the mare's colostrum. Foals with low IgG values are predisposed to development of septic infections to 4 wk of age.

ENZYME IMMUNOASSAYS

The use of monoclonal antibodies in combination with enzyme-linked immunosorbent assays (ELISA), known also as enzyme immunoassays (EIA), is being exploited in rapid development of new diagnostic test kits. The advantages of the biotechnical methods are simplicity, speed, sensitivity, and convenience. The latter advantage includes in-office and on-farm capability. Currently, 17 avian pathogens are detectable by ELISA methodology. Classifications of the detectable avian pathogens include 10 viruses, 3 mycoplasmas, *Chlamydia psittaci*, 2 other bacteria, and *Eimeria* spp. In addition to infectious pathogens, mycotoxins and drug residues are also detectable by ELISA.

Feline Leukemia Virus (FeLV): In addition to lymphosarcoma, this virus causes several clinical syndromes in cats, all associated with immunosuppression. ELISA test kits have been developed for detection of serum antibodies to the p27 group-specific protein antigen of FeLV. Less than 1 mL of serum or whole blood is required, and results are determined visually in a short time with minimal effort. Positive reactions (which may occur in 3% of all cats) are indicative of infection, which may be transient, latent, or persistent. Cats that test positive should be isolated and re-tested at 1-mo intervals to determine infection status. It has been suggested that 10-30% of FeLV-infected cats are negative to both ELISA and FA diagnostic tests.

Milk Progesterone Levels: These can be used to determine the reproductive status of cattle: milk is assayed in 1 hr to differentiate between follicular (estrus) and luteal (pregnancy) ovarian phases. Progesterone concentrations decrease to <5 ng/mL during estrus and increase to >10 ng/mL during pregnancy. ELISA kits have been developed for this test, and values are determined by visual color comparisons to controls. Results to date indicate that the greatest value of the test will be detection of estrus.

DIAGNOSTIC IMAGING

COMPUTED TOMOGRAPHY
(CT, Computerized axial tomography, CAT scan)

The animal is placed on a platform that moves by controlled increments through the circular aperture of a gantry that supports the X-ray tube and detectors. Accurate positioning of the animal and absence of motion during the scan are essential. At each incremental position, the X-ray tube rotates quickly around the animal as it emits X-rays. Detectors on the opposite side of the gantry register attenuation of the X-ray beam by the animal for each rotation position. The raw attenuation data is recorded on a computer and, through a variety of reconstruction algorithms, is converted into a cross-sectional image of the slice.

Sensitivity is considerably better than for conventional radiography, which allows differentiation of various soft-tissue densities. Incremental movements provide multiple slices of the body section of interest. Most modern machines also allow reconstruction of various sagittal views, provided sufficient numbers and density of transverse slices have been obtained. Hard-copy images are recorded on a multiformat imager, and raw data and/or processed images are stored on magnetic tape for later recall or analysis.

CT scanning is particularly valuable for areas that are difficult to reach using conventional radiography and ultrasonography, eg, the brain, nasal cavity and paranasal sinuses, mediastinum, and retroperitoneal and intrapelvic spaces. Cross-sectional scanning of the limb bones, head, and cervical spine in horses also has been valuable. Contrast techniques also can be employed to accentuate (enhance) tissues affected by certain types of pathological processes, eg, some brain tumors.

Due to the high cost of equipment and maintenance, CT in veterinary medicine is limited to larger institutions. Several veterinary schools now have CT scanners and a number of others have access to CT facilities in neighboring medical schools.

MAGNETIC RESONANCE IMAGING
(MRI, Nuclear magnetic resonance)

Although comparatively new as a clinical diagnostic tool, magnetic resonance analysis has been used as a chemical technique in laboratory and industrial settings for >30 yr.

The part of the body to be imaged is subjected to an intense magnetic field and simultaneous pulses of energy in the form of radio waves. The chemical composition of tissues determine the rate at which they absorb and release the radiofrequency energy. Emerging radiofrequency waves are detected on receiving coils, and the signal strengths converted by complex computer algorithms into an image of a particular section of the body. Appearance of the image (brightness or darkness) depends on the proton density and chemical composition of the tissue. By using radiofrequency with different pulse sequences, minor chemical differences between similar tissues can be shown as differences in image intensity.

Advantages of MRI are the extreme sensitivity (gray and white matter can be differentiated), the fact that ionizing radiation is not used, and the ability to make "cuts" in any plane of the area examined—a feature not shared by other cross-sectional scanning techniques. The magnetic field strengths used in medical MRI have no known adverse effects. A major disadvantage is the high cost of such equipment; as a result, MRI for animals is usually performed in medical institutions.

RADIOLOGY

RADIOGRAPHY

Equipment: The basic equipment for satisfactory radiography is a diagnostic-type X-ray machine with adequate protective housing. For small animals, such a machine should have a capacity of 100 kilovolt peak (kVp) and 100 milliamperes (mA). A machine of greater capacity, in a well-planned fixed installation, is necessary for use on large animals. However, a light, mobile unit with a highly movable, well-shielded head, with a capacity of 85-90 kVp and 30 mA is satisfactory for radiography of the extremities of large animals.

A filter in the useful beam of ≥2 mm of aluminum, and an interval timer capable of $^1/_{60}$ of a second with the larger unit and $^1/_{10}$ of a second with the mobile unit are essential.

All units must be equipped with a beam-limiting device. A collimator with adjustable lead shutters and an illuminated field effectively limits the primary beam, reduces the hazard from primary radiation and secondary scatter, and improves radiographic technique.

Whenever the part to be radiographed is >10 cm in thickness, the use of a grid improves detail. A grid with a 6:1 ratio and 60 lines/in. (2.5 cm) is satisfactory for most diagnostic needs in large- and small-animal radiography. Additional equipment should include at least two 10 × 12 in. (25 × 30 cm) and two 14 × 17 in. (35 × 43 cm) cassettes with high-speed screens, film hangers, a film-marking device, calipers to measure the part thickness, a tape for measuring focus-film distance, 2 film illuminators, and darkroom supplies. Film badges and protective aprons and gloves of ≥0.5 mm lead equivalent should be provided for all persons involved in radiographing animals.

Darkroom: The darkroom must be lightproof, and should be designed to provide separate wet and dry working surfaces. The room should be equipped with a 3-compartment tank (developer, water rinse, and fixer) capable of handling 14 × 17 in. films. Temperature of the solutions must be maintained at 60-74°F (15.5-23°C), preferably at 68°F (20°C), by running water or refrigeration. Since the rate of development varies with developer temperature, the temperature of solutions should be checked before use, and a time-temperature chart should be referred to at temperatures other than 68°F (20°C). Manufacturer's instructions should be followed, but as a rule, the developing time for screen film is 5 min, and fixing requires 10 min. Films should be washed for 30 min in running water before drying in a dust-free atmosphere.

During processing, films should be removed from the solutions quickly and the excess solution not permitted to drain back into the tank. Fluid loss should be replaced by replenisher from stock solutions, which maintains the strength as well as the fluid level of the developer and fixer. Replenishing cannot be continued indefinitely, and the solutions should be discarded when the volume of replenisher used equals 3 times the original quantity of developer. In any event, the solutions should be discarded after 3 mo because of oxidation. Developing solutions must not be replenished while films are being processed. Solutions should be covered when not in use to prevent oxidation and contamination with dirt.

Automatic processors are available in the size and price range of most large practices. These small processors can be installed in existing darkrooms. In new construction, the cost of a processor may be offset by reduction in the space normally allocated to the darkroom. Processors reduce processing time, provide radiographs ready for interpretation, and by virtue of their consistent processing technique, eliminate common darkroom errors.

Essential Factors in Radiography: The following factors contribute to the production of a satisfactory radiograph: 1) correct kVp for satisfactory penetration, 2) sufficient mA per sec to ensure proper density, 3) time of exposure short enough to stop motion, 4) proper target-to-film distance to obtain maximum photographic detail, 5) close approximation of the part radiographed to the film, 6) uniform sensitivity of screens and films, 7) standard darkroom technique, and 8) standard positions for exposure.

The **kVp** is the peak measurement of the pulsating voltage output of the generator, and indicates the energy level in the X-ray beam; when the value is high, the penetrating power of the beam is greater, the contrast on the film is diminished, and the quality of the beam is said to be "hard". When the kVp is lower, the beam is said to be "softer" and, because absorption is greater, contrast is improved while penetration is diminished. Good radiographic technique requires the selection of a beam with sufficient energy to penetrate the thickness of the tissue examined, while providing suitable contrast for visual separation of the various tissues involved.

The **mA** is a measurement of current flowing across the X-ray tube. The amount of current directly determines the total film exposure or density. Good technique requires careful selection of time and amperage to achieve satisfactory density under the conditions of the examination. The mA required to produce a given radiographic density is directly proportional to the square of the focal-film distance when other factors are constant.

The use of a higher kVp with a reduction in mA results in less radiation exposure to the animal without significantly detracting from film quality.

To reduce the loss of detail by motion of the animal, short exposure times are desirable. Motion may be further reduced or eliminated by sedation or anesthesia. To minimize image distortion caused by divergence of the X-rays, the part to be radiographed should be in close contact with the cassette. As previously recommended, high-speed screens increase the photographic effect with little loss of detail.

To consistently obtain satisfactory radiographs, a technique chart should be developed using thickness of the part measured in centimeters, relating each change in thickness to a corresponding change in kVp or mA. For parts >10 cm, a grid should be employed.

Positioning: Correct positioning of the animal is essential, and 2 views at right angles to each other should always be taken. Whenever possible, positioning should be accomplished using foam rubber blocks, leg ties, sandbags etc, always with care to minimize human exposure. Rotation of the part is to be avoided, particularly in radiographs of the thorax, skull, and pelvis.

Whenever a joint is radiographed, the beam should be projected directly across the articular surface so that the intra-articular space and articular facets can be assessed. The beam should be perpendicular to the film to minimize distortion.

Standing lateral projections using a horizontal beam are useful in demonstrating free fluid in the thoracic cavity or the multiple fluid levels and gas caps seen in stasis of the bowel.

Radiographic Interpretation: Immediately following processing, the radiograph should be examined for technical quality and a preliminary diagnosis may be made. Definitive diagnosis should await a thorough study of the dried radiograph.

In assessing the image for pathological changes, a systematic analysis is made of each anatomical part. Gross pathological changes usually fall into one or more of the following categories:

Alteration in the position of an organ or part: These may be the result of a congenital anomaly, inadequate support, passive displacement by enlargement of adjacent viscera, or rotation of viscera as in gastric torsion.

Alteration in size: Increase in size of an organ may indicate hypertrophy, hyperplasia, neoplasia, congenital anomaly, etc. Reductions in size occur with atrophy, hypoplasia, scarring, malformation, etc.

Alteration in contour: Contour changes may affect a localized portion or the entire organ silhouette. They may result from malformation, trauma, scarring, loss of tone, neoplasia, necrosis, etc.

Alteration in density: Increases in density of normally radiolucent soft tissues are frequently due to calcification. Mineralization commonly indicates poorly nourished or necrotic tissue, precipitation around a nidus or due to altered tissue pH, and metaplasia or neoplasia. Other dense mineral deposits include renal and cystic calculi and fecal concretions. Decreases in soft-tissue density are usually due to the abnormal presence of air or gas in tissues as in gangrene, subcut. emphysema, or ileus of the small intestine.

In assessing bone with diminished radiographic density, 2 major causes should be considered: disturbance in mineralization and disturbance of osteoid formation. The former includes rickets and related nutritional deficiency states, whereas the latter is defined as osteoporosis and may be due to endocrine disturbances, disuse atrophy, protein deficiency, etc.

Increases in bone density may result from increased mineral deposition within the substance of the bone proper (sclerosis) or from periosteal proliferation. The pattern of periosteal new bone may be classified as layer-like, lace-like, spiculated, or amorphous, and may be indicative of the cause.

Productive and destructive changes may occur in the same bone, as in osteomyelitis and neoplasia.

Alteration in architecture: Recognition of architectural changes requires familiarity with normal anatomy and its variations. When in doubt about a particular radiographic finding, comparison with the opposite normal limb or a radiograph of a normal animal is often helpful.

Alterations in alignment or function: Alignment of bones and joints is usually demonstrated on plain radiographs; stress radiographs may sometimes be necessary to determine the extent of abnormality. Dynamic phenomena may be studied by means of fluoroscopy.

Artifacts arising as a result of film processing, positioning, foreign material, etc, should always be considered during interpretation.

Contrast Media: Selective delineation of an organ or body cavity may be accomplished by use of contrast media. Basically, there are 2 types of contrast media: 1) negative media such as air, carbon dioxide, and oxygen, which outline the structure by increasing blackness on the film, and 2) positive media such as insoluble salts of heavy metals or inorganic iodides, which are opaque and appear white on the film.

Negative media are commonly used when radiographing the bladder, peritoneum, or colon. Barium sulfate, a positive medium, is ideal for visualization of all parts of the GI tract. The bladder can be defined by introduction of opaque iodides, and when used in conjunction with air, the double contrast effect is excellent for defining intraluminal lesions. Numerous commercially prepared, soluble organic iodides are available for urography, angiocardiography, etc. For detailed instructions on radiographic contrast techniques, the reader is referred to texts on radiology.

FLUOROSCOPY

Fluoroscopy is an excellent means of studying the dynamic function of an organ or part, but it must be used judiciously. Unfortunately, the diagnostic units in most veterinary hospitals are not designed for safe operation as fluoroscopes, and in such cases the technique should be avoided. For details of equipment standards, the National Council on Radiation Protection, Publication No. 36, should be consulted.

The eyes of the fluoroscopist should be dark-adapted for 20 min before examining the animal, and protective aprons and gloves must be worn. Only persons actively participating in the procedure should be in the room. If possible, the animal should be anesthetized or sedated to expedite the procedure.

The inherent disadvantages and hazards of fluoroscopy have been largely overcome by electronic image intensification, in which the fluorescent screen image is detected by a light-sensitive photocathode and the light pattern converted to low-energy photoelectrons. By accelerating and focusing the photoelectrons onto an output phosphor screen, the image produced is considerably brighter, although reduced in size. The image may be viewed directly by the operator or indirectly on a television monitor through a system of lenses and mirrors. This technique has the added advantage of allowing permanent recording on videotape, cine film, or spot films. However, image intensifiers are expensive, and the radiation risk to personnel operating the equipment is increased.

RADIATION THERAPY

There are few diagnostic or portable X-ray units used in veterinary practice capable of safely delivering the radiation dose required for therapy. Because of the large amounts of radiation required, and the safety risk to the tube and operator, it is questionable whether the general practitioner should attempt radiation therapy of neoplastic or even inflammatory lesions. Since veterinary radiation therapy centers are becoming established, animals requiring this form of therapy should be referred to such specialists.

RADIATION PROTECTION

According to the 1977 recommendations of the National Council on Radiation Protection and Measurements, the maximum permissible dose equivalent of X-ray or gamma radiation from external sources for radiation workers is 0.1 rem (1 mSv) per week. All persons using equipment that produces such radiation should wear film badges routinely, and the amount of exposure should be checked regularly. Hands and other parts of the body must be kept out of the primary beam, and leaded gloves and aprons must be worn for protection against stray radiation.

Users of ionizing radiation are referred to the National Council on Radiation Protection, Publication No. 36, "Radiation Protection in Veterinary Medicine", and reports numbered 17, 22, 33, 34, and 35.

ULTRASONOGRAPHY
(Echography, Sonography)

A technique that utilizes painless and harmless sound waves (frequencies of 2.5-10 megahertz [Mhz]) to provide information about the structure and function of various internal organs and organ systems. Combined with information gained from physical examination, laboratory data, and other imaging techniques such as radiography, ultrasonography has improved diagnostic capabilities in all species of animals. Sonograms should be performed by highly trained individuals with extensive knowledge of the many sonographic artifacts and physical properties of the sound beam used to create the ultrasonographic images.

Image formation relies on the pulse echo principle. A short pulse of ultrasound is emitted into the animal, and small portions of this beam are reflected back when structures of different density are encountered. The interface between soft tissue and air causes a large echo and provides no information beyond this interface. The same situation occurs at a soft-tissue/mineral interface. However, at mineral interfaces, a portion of the sound beam is absorbed, which causes an acoustic shadow that can be useful in determining the presence of calculi. No evidence of significant adverse biological effects has been demonstrated, probably because of the small amount of sound entering the animal and the short duration of the pulse phase when compared to the echo phase.

Images displayed during a sonogram are most often in brightness (B) mode. The brightness of the display is determined by the amplitude of the echo, which in turn is determined by the difference in density of the 2 adjacent tissues. "Real-time scanning" refers to the fact that the image is updated so frequently that motion of the tissues being scanned is detectable on the screen. This makes sonography particularly helpful in examining the heart (echocardiography).

The 2 image formats used are sector scan and linear array. Linear array is most commonly used during transrectal pregnancy examinations in mares. Sector scanners are the instruments of choice in all other applications due to their small area of contact with the surface of the animal.

Sonograms are usually interpreted at the time of the examination; however, they can also be stored on video tape, multi-image camera, or polaroid film.

ABDOMINAL SCANNING

Since stress can cause aerophagia, which interferes with diagnostic image production, sonography should be performed before other routine procedures. Barium might interfere with sound transmission, and thus, administration of barium should not precede abdominal ultrasonography. Organic iodide contrast agents do not have the same effect on ultrasound transmission and can be used concurrently.

The animal's position during ultrasonic evaluation is less important than keeping the animal comfortable to avoid ingestion of air. The examination usually begins with the animal in dorsal recumbency. Tranquilization is rarely needed as the procedure is painless. The standing position can be used if bowel gas interferes with the procedure.

Ideally, the abdominal hair should be clipped before examination. Acoustic coupling gel is then placed on the skin to facilitate sound beam penetration and to avoid air pockets between the transducer and skin.

Imaging the Cranial Abdomen: When imaging the cranial abdomen, the diaphragm is very echogenic (appears bright white on a black background) because of the interface between lungs (air) and diaphragm (soft-tissue density). The liver parenchyma displays a uniformly echogenic pattern interrupted by the gallbladder and vascular structures. Liver parenchymal echogenicity is slightly greater than renal cortex but somewhat less than that of the spleen. Portal vessels can be traced into liver parenchyma; they can be distinguished from hepatic veins by the characteristic echogenic pattern of the former, attributed to fat and the high fibrous content of their walls. Except for hepatic veins near their origin at the caudal vena cava, hepatic veins in general do not have echogenic walls.

The gallbladder appears as an anechoic (black on most real-time units) area with regular, smooth margins. The size of the gallbladder varies in normal animals according to diet and feeding schedule. Fluid-filled structures such as the gallbladder have bright echoes on their far wall and increased echogenicity (acoustic or distant enhancement), a characteristic of all true cystic structures. Bile ducts normally cannot be seen in the healthy animal.

Hepatomegaly is best diagnosed by palpation and radiography. To date, there are no accurate methods for quantitating liver size in animals. Diffuse liver disease does not have clearly defined borders; as a result, echogenicity is either increased (cirrhosis or fatty infiltration) or decreased (edema or lymphocytic infiltration). In diffuse liver disease, biopsy is necessary for a definitive diagnosis.

Imaging the Midabdomen: The spleen, left kidney, and small intestines can be seen in the midabdominal region. The pancreas is not visible under normal circumstances because of surrounding bowel gas. The adrenal glands and the mesenteric lymph nodes are visible only when enlarged.

The spleen is located close to the skin surface, which makes near-field adjustments mandatory to acquire good diagnostic images. The margins of the spleen should be smooth, and the parenchyma should be slightly more echogenic than the liver. The splenic vein and its branches are easily observed at the hilum.

Normal kidneys are the least echogenic of the major abdominal organs, and many types of renal pathology can be diagnosed with ultrasonography. Kidney size, shape, and echogenicity should be evaluated. Renoliths and nephrocalcinosis are easily diagnosed; acoustic shadows usually can be seen, even if the stones are very small. As with the liver and spleen, sonographically guided biopsy should be performed to arrive at a definitive diagnosis.

Normally not visible in the midabdomen, the uterus occasionally appears as an enlarged tubular-shaped mass with a hypoechoic center. Various amounts of cellular debris within the uterus may be noticed following gentle manipulation of the abdomen.

Imaging the Caudal Abdomen: The bladder can be clearly visualized caudally, and its size, shape, and contents are easily examined. The interior of the bladder should be anechoic with no evidence of debris floating in the urine following gentle agitation. Cystic calculi appear as echo-dense structures with acoustic shadowing. Tumors are seen as tissue densities attached to the bladder wall.

The normal prostate gland is difficult to image because it lies within the pelvic canal. When diseased, it often shifts cranially into the caudal abdomen, making it easier to image. Benign hypertrophy causes symmetric enlargement of the gland, with uniform echoes observed throughout. Cysts, abscesses, and tumors can be seen sonographically.

ECHOCARDIOGRAPHY

Two-dimensional, M-mode, and Doppler echocardiography have had a major role in the improved diagnostic capabilities in veterinary cardiology. The structure and function of the heart can be thoroughly examined painlessly and noninvasively.

The thickness of chamber walls, the degree of contractility, chamber size, valvular structure and range of motion, and the pericardial sac are all visible in real-time. Both congenital and acquired diseases are more accurately diagnosed with use of echocardiography. Doppler echocardiography, enhanced by color mapping, is mainly a research tool with little clinical advantage over 2-dimensional echocardiography in its present state. (*See also* p 40.)

EQUINE TENDONS

Sonographic evaluation of equine tendons has greatly increased ability to evaluate the extent and nature of soft-tissue injury. The ability to distinguish the various causes of soft-tissue swelling as well as determine the progress of therapy in an easily repeated and noninvasive manner has improved diagnostic and prognostic capabilities.

OCULAR EXAMINATION

Examination of both chambers of the eye as well as the retrobulbar area are possible using both direct contact with the eyelid and with stand-off devices. Higher frequency transducers (5-7.5 Mhz) are recommended for these techniques.

DISPOSAL OF DEAD ANIMALS AND DISINFECTION OF PREMISES

When animals die or are slaughtered on farms, disposal of carcasses or parts that are unfit for use as food, and cleaning of the premises should be done in a manner that prevents any infectious or toxic health hazard to domestic or wild animals or man. Information on the safe and lawful disposal of dead animals may be obtained from local environmental protection agencies. When circumstances under which death has occurred suggest a possible disease or toxic hazard, the nearest available animal health official should be notified immediately.

General Precautions: Persons handling carcasses and disinfectants should wear protective clothing and be properly equipped to complete the tasks of disposition and disinfection. The handling and disposition should preclude contamination of soils, air, or water. Hides and other parts of animals that have died from infectious diseases should be destroyed and not retained for use.

Rendering: Rendering is a safe, rapid, convenient, and economical method of disposition when the service is available and the situation permits. Renderers ordinarily are required to use trucks, equipment, and practices that prevent health hazards.

Burial: Burial is the preferred method of disposal. In selecting a site, it is well to consider the soil depth and presence of underground cables, water, gas pipes, septic tanks, water wells, etc. The trench should be ≥7 ft wide and 9 ft deep (2.3×3 m). At this depth, 14 sq ft (1.3 m²) of floor space is required for each mature bovine carcass, or each 5 mature pigs or sheep. Soil conditions may require a deeper trench. For each additional 3 ft (1 m) in depth, the number of animals per 14 sq ft of floor space may be doubled. Contaminated bedding, soil, manure, feed, milk, or other materials should be placed in the trench with the carcasses and covered with ≥6 ft (2 m) of soil. The covering soil should not be packed. Decomposition and gas formation causes cracking, bubbling, and leaking of fluids from a packed trench. The soil should be mounded and neatly graded.

Burning: Burning should be used only when conditions such as a high water table, excessive rock, or public health considerations prevent burial, and local laws and ordinances permit. In selecting a site, one should consider the proximity to buildings, stored materials, overhead cables, underground pipes, and prevailing winds that may carry smoke and odors. Burning requires that the carcass be placed on a combustible platform that may include oil, wood, coal, straw, tires, etc. The fire burns better if the platform is at right angles to the wind; it should be tended to ensure that all material is destroyed and to prevent dissemination of contaminated material by animals or birds.

To prepare the fire: stake out the area of the firebed allowing 3 ft (1 m) of length for each cattle carcass; lay 3 rows of straw or hay bales lengthwise along the line of the firebed, with rows 12 in. (30 cm) apart, and 12 in. (30 cm) between bales in a row; place loose straw between bales; place large timbers lengthwise on each row; place more timbers across rows with 6-12 in. (15-30 cm) between timbers; place old tires and kindling on timbers; spread loose straw over wood and tires; spread coal at a rate of 500 lb/yard (225 kg/m) over wood and tires to make a level bed; place carcasses on the firebed on their backs; place loose straw on and between carcasses; pour or spray on liquid fuel (**not gasoline**); start fire along the full length of the firebed.

Under favorable conditions, burning should be complete in 48 hr. Additional fuel may be needed. When the fire has died out, the ashes should be buried and the area cleaned, graded or plowed, and prepared for seeding.

Cleaning and Disinfection: Cleaning and disinfection should be appropriate for the suspected agent. For infectious agents, cleaning requires that all manure and litter be removed and buried as previously described; dirt floors be scraped down to clean soil; any material—such as wood—that cannot be thoroughly cleaned, be removed and buried or burned; buildings be thoroughly cleaned—ceilings, floors, walls, and all other surfaces; and all equipment used in material removal—such as manure loaders, shovels, brushes, and scrapers—be cleaned thoroughly. A cleansing agent must be used in the water; trisodium phosphate and sodium carbonate are excellent for the purpose. They are readily available, inexpensive, safe to use, and do not interfere with disinfectants. Sodium hydroxide (lye) causes the precipitation of colloids, which protects organisms from disinfectants and is not recommended. All cleaned facilities and equipment should be rinsed with clean water, and a liberal amount of an appropriate disinfectant applied. Disinfectants recommended for general use on surfaces free of organic matter are sodium hypochlorite (1200 ppm available chlorine) and calcium hypochlorite (1200 ppm available chlorine).

Disinfectants vary according to their chemical composition, and their effectiveness is limited by the temperature and other conditions under which they are applied. Label instructions for application should be followed. The label should bear the approval statement of the US Environmental Protection Agency, or of a similar agency in other countries.

EXAMINATION OF ANIMALS PRIOR TO SALE
(Prepurchase examination, Soundness examination)

Whenever ownership of animals changes and they are moved to other premises, animal health comes under serious consideration. The purchaser wants assurance that the health of the animals is such that they can fulfill the purpose for which they are intended, and that they do not introduce disease into the new herd. Animal health regulatory officials want assurance that new diseases are not introduced into their area of jurisdiction, or transferred from one herd to another. When purchases are made in foreign countries, federal animal health regulatory officials want assurance that diseases of any kind, especially exotic ones, if present in the exporting country, are not likely to be introduced into the importing country.

The USA also has health regulations that must be met before animals can be exported. These regulations have been developed to protect foreign purchasers by assuring them that the animals are healthy and can be added to their herds with confidence.

Animal health requirements vary with the country, species, age, sex, intended use of the animal, and specific demands of the purchaser. Therefore, it is not possible to list specific regulations that apply to all situations; this description is limited to some general requirements for animal movement in the USA. Local animal disease regulatory officials should be contacted for regulations that apply to the specific situation.

When breeding cattle are sold, they must be certified to be free of brucellosis and tuberculosis. The certificate, which must be signed by the seller and a veterinarian, certifies that the veterinarian has inspected the animals and that they are not showing signs of infectious and/or communicable disease. Pregnancy status of breeding-age females is usually determined, and semen is usually evaluated when breeding-age bulls are sold. When breeding pigs are sold, they must be tested for (and found free of) brucellosis and pseudorabies. Horses usually can be sold and moved to new intrastate premises in the USA without any tests or veterinary inspection; however, interstate movement usually requires testing for infectious diseases. A detailed examination often is required for valuable breeding or racing animals.

The prospective purchaser may insist on selecting another veterinarian to perform an additional inspection.

In the examination of any animal prior to sale, several points should be emphasized: 1) The veterinarian is working for the person paying the fee and reports only to that person. The person responsible for compensating the veterinarian should be informed of the cost before the inspection. 2) The purpose for which the animal is to be used should be clearly established before the examination. 3) The examining veterinarian must be knowledgeable in the care and treatment of animals that are used for the established purpose.

The examination is divided into 3 parts: history, clinical examination, and special examinations or diagnostic procedures.

Although all abnormalities in race horses are noted and recorded, the musculoskeletal and respiratory systems are given special attention. Since legal action against veterinarians has become much more common recently, many veterinarians are refusing to provide a written report for equine examinations. However, a written record of their findings should be made as it may be needed at some future date. The prospective purchaser is given an oral report of all identified abnormalities. The veterinarian may render an opinion if the horse will be suitable for the intended purpose but will rarely, if ever, recommend purchase. The responsibility of the veterinarian is to supply information; the prospective purchaser must make the decision whether to purchase.

History: A complete history should be obtained by questioning the seller, examining his/her records, and observing the rest of the herd and the management conditions. The animal's breed, sex, age, color, markings, tattoos, ear tags, or brands should be noted; its registration papers checked; and its identity definitely established. For a breeding animal, the records of its sire and dam also should be considered, eg, their breeding ability, the possibility of heritable defects in the strain to which each belongs, and the cause of their deaths (if dead). Also, breeding records of the animal itself should be reviewed to determine its fertility. Breeding records of the herd of origin of the animal should be examined for evidence of diseases likely to affect reproduction. If the animal is an adult female, the service dates and stage of pregnancy, if applicable, should be noted.

Records should be examined to determine whether the animal has had any previous diseases, injuries (and their severity), or surgical procedures. Any previous vaccinations, their type, and date of administration should be noted. The health of the herd of origin and possible contacts with other animals before the sale should be determined, if possible, since animals so exposed could be in the incubation period of disease. It should also be established, if possible, if the animal had received any drugs or medication that could alter its normal state. If this cannot be established in the history, it may be necessary to include assays for suspected medication within the special test section of the examination.

Clinical Examination: No area of the body or any function should be overlooked: the clinical examination should establish the current state of the animal's health and condition of each body system.

Special Examinations or Diagnostic Tests: Certain special diagnostic tests are routinely performed at the time of sale; others may be desired by the buyer, or may be indicated by the findings of the clinical examination. If the animal is to be shipped into another state or country after purchase, the required tests or inoculations either must be performed before the sale, or the sale may be subject to the satisfactory passing of these tests by the animal. Therefore, the regulations of the state or country to which the animal is to be sent must be thoroughly understood.

Purchasers of valuable racing animals often demand numerous diagnostic procedures (in addition to the physical examination), including endoscopy, ultrasonography, rectal examination, nerve blocks, hematology, microbiology, high speed cinematography, biopsies, radiography, electrocardiography, and drug testing.

MEAT INSPECTION

Inspection of meat by qualified individuals to eliminate from the food supply unwholesome meat and adulterated or mislabeled meat or meat products helps to protect consumers from the infectious, toxic, and physical hazards that may originate in food animals, the environment, or human beings. Inspection activities are divided into antemortem, postmortem, and processing inspection.

ANTEMORTEM INSPECTION

Antemortem inspection is conducted at the abattoir on the day of slaughter to detect and condemn animals that are unfit for slaughter and to note signs or lesions of disease that may not be apparent after slaughter, such as rabies, listeriosis, and heavy metal poisoning. Animals with signs or lesions that do not warrant immediate condemnation can be identified as "suspects" so that their carcasses and viscera can be inspected separately. Certain animals may be retained for minor diseases, or confined for a period of time sufficient for the depletion of harmful residues.

The animals are confined for inspection in a lighted enclosure so that they can be clearly observed at rest and in motion. Gates, chutes, and equipment must be available to segregate abnormal animals for closer examination, and for proper identification.

POSTMORTEM INSPECTION

Animals should be inspected immediately after slaughter and evisceration for possible changes and lesions that indicate unsuitability of the meat for food. Postmortem examination requires observation of all parts of the carcass, dressing procedures, and environmental conditions to prevent contamination of edible parts. The inspector must make sure that condemned carcasses and parts are disposed of safely.

A routine postmortem examination should include the following procedures:

Cattle—Head: 1) Incise and examine the left and right mandibular, parotid, atlantal, and suprapharyngeal lymph nodes. 2) Examine 2 incised layers of both masseter muscles. 3) Examine and palpate tongue. **Viscera:** 1) Examine mesenteric lymph nodes and abdominal viscera. 2) Examine and palpate ruminoreticular junction. 3) Examine esophagus and spleen. 4) Incise and examine anterior, middle, and posterior mediastinal, and right and left bronchial lymph nodes. 5) Examine and palpate costal and ventral surfaces of the lungs. 6) Incise heart from base to apex through interventricular septum, and examine and cut inner and outer surfaces. 7) Incise and examine hepatic (portal) lymph nodes. 8) Oȶen bile duct in both directions and observe contents. 9) Examine and palpate ventral and dorsal surfaces and renal impression of the liver. **Carcass:** 1) Examine exposed internal and external surfaces. 2) Palpate superficial inguinal or supramammary, and internal iliac lymph nodes. 3) Examine and palpate kidneys and diaphragm.

Calves and Veal—Head: Incise and examine suprapharyngeal lymph nodes. **Viscera:** 1) Examine and palpate lungs, bronchial and mediastinal lymph nodes, and heart. 2) Examine spleen. 3) Examine and palpate dorsal and ventral surfaces of the liver, and palpate portal lymph nodes. 4) Examine abdominal viscera. **Carcass:** 1) Examine exposed inner and outer surfaces. 2) Palpate internal iliac lymph nodes and kidneys.

Sheep and Goats—Viscera: 1) Examine abdominal viscera, esophagus, mesenteric lymph nodes, omental fat, and spleen. 2) Examine bile duct and contents and express gallbladder. 3) Examine and palpate liver, and costal and ventral surfaces of lungs. 4) Palpate bronchial and mediastinal lymph nodes. 5) Examine and palpate heart. **Carcass and Head:** 1) Examine outer surfaces and body cavities. 2) Examine and palpate kidneys. 3) Palpate prefemoral, superficial inguinal or supramammary, and popliteal lymph nodes. 4) Palpate back and sides of carcass. 5) Palpate prescapular lymph nodes. 6) Examine neck, shoulders, and head. 7) Incise lymph nodes when required to rule out caseous lymphadenitis.

Pigs—Head: 1) Examine head and cervical muscles. 2) Incise left and right mandibular lymph nodes. **Viscera:** 1) Examine and palpate spleen and mesenteric lymph nodes. 2) Palpate portal lymph nodes. 3) Examine dorsal and ventral surfaces of the liver. 4) Palpate right and left bronchial and mediastinal lymph nodes. 5) Examine and palpate dorsal and ventral surfaces of the lungs. 6) Examine and palpate heart. **Carcass:** 1) Examine internal and external surfaces and cut where abnormalities are suspected. 2) Examine and palpate kidneys.

Horses—Head: 1) Examine surfaces. 2) Palpate, incise, and examine mandibular, pharyngeal, and parotid lymph nodes; guttural pouches; and tongue. **Viscera:** 1) Examine and palpate lungs and bronchial and mediastinal lymph nodes (incise when abnormal). 2) Examine and palpate spleen, liver, and portal lymph nodes. 3) Open hepatic duct. 4) Examine remaining viscera. **Carcass:** 1) Inspect as for cattle. 2) In addition, examine and incise when necessary the internal abdominal walls for encysted parasites; spinous process of thoracic vertebrae, supraspinous bursa, and first 2 cervical vertebrae for fistulous conditions; and axillary and subscapular spaces of white and gray horses for melanosis.

Poultry: 1) Examine external surfaces for dressing defects, bruises, and disease lesions. 2) Palpate tibia for bone diseases. 3) Examine internal surfaces, lungs, and kidneys in place. 4) Examine viscera and palpate liver, heart, and spleen.

CONDEMNATIONS (GENERAL)

Carcasses with the following abnormalities should be disapproved for use as food: 1) contaminated by infectious, toxic, or hazardous physical agents; 2) generalized conditions or disease processes, including malignant tumors, that have so altered the normal characteristics of the meat as to cause it to be inedible, or sufficiently abnormal to be reasonably considered unfit for food. 4) Localized conditions that do not affect the wholesomeness of the entire carcass should be removed by trimming so that the remainder of the carcass can be used for food.

Special Considerations—Tuberculosis: The entire carcass should be condemned when there is evidence of tuberculosis: 1) an active lesion; 2) the animal is cachectic; 3) a lesion occurs in muscle, intermuscular tissue, bone, joint, abdominal organs other than the GI tract, or in a lymph node associated with these parts;

4) extensive lesions occur in the thoracic or abdominal cavity; 5) lesions are multiple, acute, and actively progressive; or 6) the nature or extent of lesions does not indicate localization. An organ or part should be condemned when it or its corresponding lymph nodes contain lesions. When lesions in pigs are localized and occur at only one primary site of infection, such as the cervical lymph nodes, the unaffected parts are acceptable for food after condemnation of the affected organ or part. Even though federal and state regulations permit the commercial cooking of certain carcasses minimally affected with tuberculosis, this procedure is not recommended for other than commercial use.

ABATTOIR SANITATION

The buildings, equipment, personnel, and operating procedures should assure the continued wholesomeness and freedom from adulteration of carcasses and meat. Floors, walls, and ceilings should be constructed of materials and in a manner that allow sanitary operations and thorough cleaning. An ample supply of hot and cold water and cleaning materials should be conveniently available for slaughtering, cleaning, and personal hygiene. Water at 180°F (82°C) should be available for sanitizing tools and equipment after cleaning. Equipment, knives, and other utensils that have contacted diseased carcasses should be cleaned and sterilized before being used again. Drainage, with proper trapping and sewage disposal, should be adequate to maintain the abattoir in a sanitary condition. Ventilation should ensure that edible product areas are free of obnoxious odors. Flies, rodents, and other vermin should be excluded. Lighting should be maintained at an intensity adequate for cleaning and inspection. Equipment should be of such material and so constructed as to be readily and thoroughly cleaned and should be properly maintained. Separate, clean containers for edible and inedible materials should be provided at convenient locations. Tables or racks should be provided for heads. Personnel should wear clean garments.

DETECTION OF UNWHOLESOME MEAT

Meat for human consumption should be prepared from animals that were healthy and have been exsanguinated. Animals having infectious, toxic, or physical agents in their tissues that may be hazardous to human health or that are otherwise unhealthy should not be used for food. Fitness for food can be determined by a comprehensive evaluation that may include organoleptic, histological, microbiological, chemical, and toxicological examinations.

Meat should be examined under light of adequate intensity. Foreign objects on the surface or visible within the tissue can be collected for further examination. Items such as feathers, hair, fibers, parasites, or insect larvae may provide valuable data on the species, origin, and handling of the meat.

Texture, color, and odor should be noted. Meat should be firm, and cut surfaces should be glossy. Gray or green discolorations may indicate bacterial action. Dark-red meat may result from the postmortem collection of blood in animals that were not exsanguinated. A stable, bright-red color in old meat is sometimes produced by the addition of sulfite. Rodent urine and substances produced by certain spoilage bacteria fluoresce under ultraviolet light. Areas of bruising, hemorrhage, or inflammation should be readily recognized. Odors from chemicals, urine, fish, or other sources may be present. Some of these can be accentuated by boiling or frying the meat.

Histological examination often can detect abnormalities caused by infectious or toxic agents, or foreign matter. Microbiological examination of meats for spoilage organisms or those capable of causing infectious or toxic illness in the consumer, and serological examination to determine species require laboratory methods. Chemical and toxicological examinations should be made when the presence of adulterative or toxic substances is suspected.

SOME PHYSIOLOGICAL VALUES

Table 3. Basal Body Temperature of Various Species, Related to Weight

Body
Temperature
(°F)

110

Sparrow Lark
Crow
Cardinal Titmouse
Starling Pigeon
Thrush
Waxwing

(In general, the very large and very small
mammals have low body temperatures.)

108

Grouse
Blackbird Falcon
Heron
Pheasant
Ibis Hawk
Curassow
Guinea Hen
Woodpecker Duck
Chicken
Gannet Goose

106

Parrot Cormorant
Gull Crane
Murre Turkey
Pelican
Flamingo
Owl Swan

104

Peahen
Penguin
Hedgehog
Petrel
Macaque
Rabbit Raccoon
Dog Goat Reindeer
Emu
Sheep

102

Guinea Pig Pig
Cat Panther
Fruit Bat Cassowary
Ocelot
Seal Cow
Jackal Donkey
Rat Horse

100

98

Ground Squirrel Man Tiger
Camel
Prairie Dog
Mouse

Bat

Elephant

96 Shrew

0.01   0.1   1.0   10   100   1000   10,000
Body Weight (lb)

Adapted from *Science* **111**: 465, 1950.

Table 4. Rectal Temperatures

Species	°F ± 1°F	°C ± 0.5°C
Beef cow	101	38.3
Dairy cow	101.5	38.6
Cat	101.5	38.6
Dog	102	38.9
Goat	102.3	39.1
Mare	100	37.8
Stallion	99.7	37.6
Pig	102.5	39.2
Rabbit	103.1	39.5
Sheep	102.3	39.1

Adapted from Andersson, B.E., Temperature Regulation and Environmental Physiology, in *Duke's Physiology of Domestic Animals*, 10th ed., Swenson, M.J., Ed., 1984, by permission of Cornell University Press.

Table 5. Heart Rates (beats/min)

Species	Av	Range	Species	Av	Range
Ass	50	(40-56)	Hamster	450	(300-600)
Bat	750	(100-970)	Horse	44	(23-70)
Camel	30	(25-32)	Lion	40	
Cat	120	(110-140)	Monkey	192	(165-240)
Chick		(350-450)	Mouse	534	(324-858)
Chicken (adult)		(250-300)	Pig		(55-86)
Cow		(60-70)	Rabbit	205	(123-304)
Dog		(100-130)	Rat	328	(261-600)
Elephant	35	(22-53)	Sheep	75	(60-120)
Giraffe	66		Skunk	166	(144-192)
Goat	90	(70-135)	Squirrel	249	(96-378)
Guinea pig	280	(260-400)			

Table 6. Resting Respiratory Rates (breaths/min)

Species	Rate	Species	Rate
Cat	26	Horse	12
Chicken	13	Monkey	40
Cow	30	Pigeon	26
Dog	22	Rabbit	39
Guinea pig	90	Rat	97
Hamster	74	Sheep	19

Table 7. Urine Volume

Species	mL/kg body wt/day
Cat	10-20
Cow	17-45
Dog	20-100
Goat	10-40
Horse	3-18
Pig	5-30
Sheep	10-40

The data in the above tables (TABLES 5-7) were adapted in part from *Duke's Physiology of Domestic Animals*, 9th ed., Swenson, M.J., Ed., 1977, by permission of Cornell University Press, and from other sources.

Table 8. Hematological Reference Ranges (Approximate)

Determination	USA Conventional Units	SI Units	Canine	Feline	Bovine	Equine	Porcine	Ovine	Caprine
Hematocrit (PCV)	%	×10⁻²L/L	37-55 (25-34)[a]	30-45 (24-34)[a]	24-46	32-48[b]	36-43 (26-35)[a]	27-45	22-38
Hemoglobin (Hgb)	g/dL	×10 g/L	12-18	8-15	8-15	10-18	9-13	9-15	8-12
Red Blood Cell (RBC)	×10⁶/μL	×10¹²/L	5.5-8.5	5-10	5-10	6-12	5-7	9-15	8-18
Reticulocyte	%	%	0-1.5	0-1	0	0	0-12	0	0
Mean Corpuscular Volume	fL	fL	60-77	39-55	40-60	34-58	52-62	28-40	16-25
Mean Corpuscular Hgb	pg	pg	19.5-24.5	13-17	11-17	13-19	17-24	8-12	5.2-8
Mean Corpuscular Hgb Concentration	g/dL	×10 g/L	32-36	30-36	30-36	31-37	29-34	31-34	30-36
Platelet Count	×10⁵/μL	×10¹¹/L	2-9	3-7	1-8	1-6	2-5	2.5-7.5	3-6
White Blood Cell (WBC)	×10³/μL	×10⁹/L	6-17	5.5-19.5	4-12	6-12	11-22	4-12	4-13
Segmented Neutrophil	×10³/μL	×10⁹/L	3-11.4	2.5-12.5	0.6-4	3-6	2-15	0.7-6.0	1.2-7.2
	%	%	(60-70)	(35-75)	(15-45)	(30-75)	(20-70)	(10-50)	(30-48)
Band Neutrophil	×10³/μL	×10⁹/L	0-0.3	0-0.3	0-0.12	0-0.1	0-0.8	0	rare
	%	%	(0-3)	(0-3)	(0-2)	(0-1)	(0-4)		
Lymphocyte	×10³/μL	×10⁹/L	1-4.8	1.5-7	2.5-7.5	1.5-5	3.8-16.5	2-9	2-9
	%	%	(12-30)	(20-55)	(45-75)	(25-60)	(35-75)	(40-75)	(50-70)
Monocyte	×10³/μL	×10⁹/L	0.15-1.35	0-0.85	0.025-0.85	0-0.6	0-1	0-0.75	0-0.55
	%	%	(3-10)	(1-4)	(2-7)	(1-8)	(0-10)	(0-6)	(0-4)
Eosinophil	×10³/μL	×10⁹/L	0.1-0.75	0-0.75	0-2.4	0-0.8	0-1.5	0-1	0.05-0.65
	%	%	(2-10)	(2-12)	(2-20)	(1-10)	(0-15)	(0-10)	(1-8)
Basophil	×10³/μL	×10⁹/L	rare	rare	0-0.2	0-0.3	0-0.5	0-0.3	0-0.12
	%	%			(0-2)	(0-3)	(0-3)	(0-3)	(0-1)
Myeloid/Erythroid Ratio			0.75-2.4:1	0.6-3.9:1	0.3-1.8:1	0.9-3.8:1	1.2-2.2:1	0.8-1.7:1	0.7-1.0:1
Plasma Proteins[c,d]	g/dL	×10 g/L	6-7.5	6-7.5	6-8	6-8.5	6-8	6-7.5	6-7.5
Plasma Fibrinogen[e]	g/dL	×10 g/L	0.15-0.3	0.15-0.3	0.1-0.6	0.1-0.4	0.2-0.4	0.1-0.5	0.1-0.4

Adapted from Duncan, J.R. and Prasse, K.W., *Veterinary Laboratory Medicine*, 2nd ed., Iowa State University Press, 1986.

[a]5- to 6-wk old pups, kittens; 3- to 45-day old pigs.
[b]Lower in foals and cold-blooded horses.
[c]Refractometry.
[d]Lower in young animals.
[e]Heat precipitation.

Table 9. Leukocyte Values*
(Approximate ranges × 10³/µL or × 10⁹/L)

	Leukocytes	Neutrophils	Immature Neutrophils	Lymphocytes	Eosinophils	Monocytes
Horse	5-15	3-7	0-0.1	1.5-5.5	0-0.5	0-0.8
Cow	5-13	0.6-4	0-0.12	2.5-7.5	0-2.4	0.25-0.84
Sheep	5-13	0.7-6	rare	2-9	0-1	0-0.75
Goat	5-13	1.2-7.2	rare	2-9	0.05-0.65	0-0.55
Pig	7-20	3.2-10	0-0.8	4.5-13	0.5-2	0.25-2
Dog	8-18	3-12	0-0.3	1-4.8	1-1.3	0.15-14
Cat	8-25	2.5-13	0-0.3	1.5-7	0-1.5	0-0.85
Rabbit	6-13	2-6	rare	0.2-0.5	0-0.5	0.1-1
Rat	5-25	0.001-5	rare	7-13	0-1	0-1
Mouse	4-12	0.5-4	rare	3-9	0-0.05	0-1
Chicken	9-56	3-17	—	10-30	0-0.5	0-5

*For RBC counts, PCV (%), and Hgb levels, *see* ANEMIA, p 15.

Table 10. Serum Biochemical Constituents (Reference Ranges)

	Dog	Cat	Horse	Cow	Sheep	Pig	Goat	Units
In conventional (USA) units:								
ALT(SGPT)	8.2 - 57.3	8.3 - 52.5	2.7 - 20.5	6.9 - 35.3	14.8 - 43.8	21.7 - 46.5	15.3 - 52.3	u/L
Amylase	269.5 - 1462.4	371.3 - 1192.6	46.7 - 188.1	41.3 - 98.3	140.0 - 270.0	43.5 - 88.0		u/L
Alk phos	10.6 - 100.7	12.0 - 65.1	70.1 - 226.8	17.5 - 152.7	26.9 - 156.1	41.0 - 176.1	61.3 - 283.3	u/L
AST(SGOT)	8.9 - 48.5	9.2 - 39.5	115.7 - 287.0	45.3 - 110.2	49.0 - 123.3	15.3 - 55.3	66.0 - 230.0	u/L
CPK(CK)	13.7 - 119.7	17.0 - 150.2	34.0 - 165.6	14.4 - 107.0	7.7 - 101.0	65.7 - 489.4	16.3 - 47.7	u/L
GGT	1.0 - 9.7	1.8 - 12.0	2.7 - 22.4	4.9 - 25.7	19.6 - 44.1	31.0 - 52.0	20.0 - 50.0	u/L
LDH	24.1 - 219.2	35.1 - 224.9	102.3 - 340.6	308.6 - 938.1	83.1 - 475.6	159.6 - 424.7	78.5 - 265.3	u/L
SDH	3.1 - 7.6	2.4 - 6.1	1.2 - 8.5	6.1 - 18.4	3.5 - 20.6	0.5 - 4.9	9.3 - 20.7	u/L
Bicarbonate	18.1 - 24.5	16.4 - 22.0	21.7 - 29.4	20.7 - 28.9	20.3 - 26.7	18.0 - 27.0		mEq/L
Calcium	8.7 - 11.8	7.9 - 10.9	10.4 - 13.4	8.4 - 11.0	9.3 - 11.7	9.3 - 11.5	9.0 - 11.6	mg/dL
Chloride	102.1 - 117.4	107.5 - 129.6	97.2 - 110.1	95.7 - 108.6	100.8 - 113.0	97.1 - 106.4	100.3 - 111.5	mEq/L
Phosphorus	2.9 - 6.2	4.0 - 7.3	2.3 - 5.4	4.3 - 7.8	4.0 - 7.3	5.5 - 9.3	3.7 - 9.7	mg/dL
Magnesium	1.7 - 2.7	1.9 - 2.8	1.8 - 2.7	1.7 - 3.0	2.0 - 2.7	2.3 - 3.5	2.1 - 2.9	mg/dL
Potassium	3.8 - 5.6	3.8 - 5.3	2.8 - 4.7	4.0 - 5.8	4.3 - 6.3	4.4 - 6.5	3.8 - 5.7	mEq/L
Sodium	140.3 - 153.9	145.8 - 158.7	133.3 - 147.3	134.5 - 148.1	141.6 - 159.6	139.2 - 152.5	136.5 - 151.5	mEq/L
Bilirubin	0.1 - 0.6	0.1 - 0.5	0.3 - 3.0	0.0 - 0.8	0.0 - 0.5	0.0 - 0.5	0.1 - 0.2	mg/dL
Cholesterol	115.6 - 253.7	71.3 - 161.2	70.9 - 141.9	62.1 - 192.5	44.1 - 90.1	81.4 - 134.1	64.6 - 136.4	mg/dL
Creatinine	0.5 - 1.6	0.5 - 1.9	0.9 - 2.0	0.6 - 1.8	0.9 - 2.0	0.8 - 2.3	0.7 - 1.5	mg/dL
Glucose	61.9 - 108.3	60.8 - 124.2	62.2 - 114.0	42.1 - 74.5	44.0 - 81.2	66.4 - 116.1	48.2 - 76.0	mg/dL
Urea nitrogen	8.8 - 25.9	15.4 - 31.2	10.4 - 24.7	7.8 - 24.6	10.3 - 26.0	8.2 - 24.6	12.6 - 25.8	mg/dL
Albumin	2.6 - 4.0	2.4 - 3.7	2.5 - 3.8	2.8 - 3.9	2.7 - 3.7	2.3 - 4.0	2.3 - 3.6	g/dL
Alb/Glob	0.7 - 1.9	0.6 - 1.2	0.5 - 1.5	0.6 - 1.3	0.4 - 0.8	0.4 - 0.7	0.6 - 1.1	ratio
Globulin	2.1 - 3.7	2.4 - 4.7	2.4 - 4.6	2.9 - 4.9	3.2 - 5.0	3.9 - 6.0	2.7 - 4.4	g/dL
Protein	5.5 - 7.5	5.7 - 8.0	5.7 - 7.9	6.2 - 8.2	5.9 - 7.8	5.8 - 8.3	6.1 - 7.4	g/dL

(continued)

Table 10. Serum Biochemical Constituents (Reference Ranges) (continued)

	Dog	Cat	Horse	Cow	Sheep	Pig	Goat	Units
In SI units:								
Bicarbonate	18.1 - 24.5	16.4 - 22.0	21.7 - 29.4	20.7 - 28.9	20.3 - 26.7	18.0 - 27.0		mmol/L
Calcium	2.2 - 3.0	2.0 - 2.7	2.6 - 3.3	2.1 - 2.8	2.3 - 2.9	2.3 - 2.9	2.3 - 2.9	mmol/L
Chloride	102.1 - 117.4	107.5 - 129.6	97.2 - 110.1	95.7 - 108.6	100.8 - 113.0	97.1 - 106.4	100.3 - 111.5	mmol/L
Phosphorus	1.0 - 2.0	1.3 - 2.4	0.7 - 1.7	1.4 - 2.5	1.3 - 2.4	1.8 - 3.0	1.2 - 3.1	mmol/L
Magnesium	0.7 - 1.1	0.8 - 1.2	0.7 - 1.1	0.7 - 1.2	0.8 - 1.1	0.9 - 1.4	0.9 - 1.2	mmol/L
Potassium	3.8 - 5.6	3.8 - 5.3	2.8 - 4.7	4.0 - 5.8	4.3 - 6.3	4.4 - 6.5	3.8 - 5.7	mmol/L
Sodium	140.3 - 153.9	145.8 - 158.7	133.3 - 147.3	134.5 - 148.1	141.6 - 159.6	139.2 - 152.5	136.5 - 151.5	mmol/L
Bilirubin	0.9 - 10.6	1.2 - 7.9	5.4 - 51.4	0.7 - 14.0	0.7 - 8.6	0.3 - 8.2	1.7 - 4.3	μmol/L
Cholesterol	3.0 - 6.6	1.8 - 4.2	1.8 - 3.7	1.6 - 5.0	1.1 - 2.3	2.1 - 3.5	1.7 - 3.5	mmol/L
Creatinine	44.3 - 138.4	48.6 - 165.0	76.8 - 174.5	55.8 - 162.4	75.8 - 174.3	69.6 - 207.7	59.7 - 134.8	μmol/L
Glucose	3.4 - 6.0	3.4 - 6.9	3.5 - 6.3	2.3 - 4.1	2.4 - 4.5	3.7 - 6.4	2.7 - 4.2	mmol/L
Urea nitrogen	3.1 - 9.2	5.5 - 11.1	3.7 - 8.8	2.8 - 8.8	3.7 - 9.3	2.9 - 8.8	4.5 - 9.2	mmol/L
Albumin	25.8 - 39.7	24.5 - 37.5	25.3 - 37.6	27.5 - 39.4	26.7 - 36.8	22.6 - 40.4	23.5 - 35.7	g/L
Alb/Glob	0.7 - 1.9	0.6 - 1.2	0.5 - 1.5	0.6 - 1.3	0.4 - 0.8	0.4 - 0.7	0.6 - 1.1	ratio
Globulin	20.6 - 37.0	24.4 - 47.0	23.5 - 45.8	28.9 - 48.6	32.3 - 50.0	39.5 - 60.0	27.0 - 44.3	g/L
Protein	55.1 - 75.2	57.5 - 79.6	57.1 - 79.1	61.6 - 82.2	58.9 - 78.1	58.3 - 83.2	61.0 - 74.5	g/L

Adapted from Boyd, J.W., The interpretation of serum biochemistry test results in domestic animals, in *Veterinary Clinical Pathology*, Veterinary Practice Publishing Co., Vol. XIII, No. II, 1984.

READY REFERENCE GUIDES

Table 11. Atomic Weights (Approximate) of Some Common Elements

Ion	Atomic Weight	Valence
Hydrogen (H)	1	1
Carbon (C)	12	4
Nitrogen (N)	14	3
Oxygen (O)	16	2
Sodium (Na)	23	1
Magnesium (Mg)	24	2
Phosphate (P)*	31	3,5
Chlorine (Cl)	35.5	1
Potassium (K)	39	1
Calcium (Ca)	40	2

*as phosphorus, inorganic

Table 12. Celsius-Fahrenheit Equivalents

Conversion:			
To convert degrees F to degrees C, subtract 32, then multiply by $5/9$ (0.5555)		To convert degrees C to degrees F, multiply by $9/5$ (1.8), then add 32	
°Celsius	°Fahrenheit	°Celsius	°Fahrenheit
Freezing (water at sea level):		Clinical Range	
0	32	36.0	96.8
		36.5	97.7
Boiling (water at sea level):		37.0	98.6
100.0	212.0	37.5	99.5
		38.0	100.4
−40	−40	38.5	101.3
		39.0	102.2
Pasteurization (holding), 30 min at:		39.5	103.1
61.6	143.0	40.0	104.0
		40.5	104.9
Pasteurization (flash), 15 sec at:		41.0	105.8
71.1	160.0	41.5	106.7
		42.0	107.6

Table 13. Clinical Chemistry SI Conversion Factors

Component	Conventional (USA) Units (with examples)	Conversion factor	SI Unit (with examples)
Alkaline phosphatase	30-150 u/L	1.00	30-150 u/L
ALT (SGPT)	0-40 u/L	1.00	0-40 u/L
Albumin	2.8-4.0 g/100 mL	10.0	28-40 g/L
Ammonia (NH_4)	10-80 μg/100 mL	0.5871	5-50 μmol/L
Amylase	200-800 u/L	1.00	200-800 u/L
AST (SGOT)	0-40 u/L	1.00	0-40 u/L
Bilirubin	0.1-0.2 mg/100 mL	17.10	2-4 μmol/L
Calcium	8.8-10.3 mg/100 mL	0.2495	2.20-2.58 mmol/L
Carbon dioxide	22-28 mEq/L	1.00	22-28 mmol/L
Chloride	95-100 mEq/L	1.00	95-100 mmol/L
Cholesterol	100-265 mg/100 mL	0.02586	2.58-5.85 mmol/L
Copper	70-140 μg/100 mL	0.1574	11.0-22.0 umol/L
Cortisol	2-10 μg/100 mL	27.59	55-280 nmol/L
Creatine kinase	0-130 u/L	1.00	0-130 u/L
Creatinine	0.6-1.2 mg/100 mL	88.40	50-110 μmol/L
Fibrinogen	200-400 mg/100 mL	0.01	2-4 g/L
Glucose	70-100 mg/100 mL	0.05551	3.8-6.1 mmol/L
Iron	80-180 μg/100 mL	0.1791	14-32 μmol/L
Lactate	5-20 mg/100 mL	0.1110	0.5-2 mmol/L
Lipase			
Sigma Tietz (37°C)	<1 ST u/100 mL	280	<280 u/L
Cherry Crandall (30°C)	0-160 u/L	1.00	0-160 u/L
Lipids, total	400-850 mg/100 mL	0.01	4-8.5 g/L
Magnesium	1.8-3 mg/100 mL	0.4114	0.80-1.2 mmol/L
Mercury	<1 μg/100 mL	49.85	<50 nmol/L
Osmolality	280-300 mOsm/kg	1.00	280-300 mmol/kg
Phosphate (as inorganic phosphorus)	2.5-5 mg/100 mL	0.3229	0.80-1.6 mmol/L
Potassium	3.5-5 mEq/L	1.0	3.5-5 mmol/L
Protein, total	5-8 g/100 mL	10.0	50-80 g/L
Sodium	135-147 mEq/L	1.00	135-147 mmol/L
Testosterone	4-8 mg/mL	3.467	14-28 nmol/L
Thyroxine (T_4)	1-4 μg/100 mL	12.87	13-51 nmol/L
Urea nitrogen	10-20 mg/100 mL	0.3570	3.57-7.14 mmol/L (Urea)
Urobilinogen	0-4 mg/24 hr	1.693	0-6.8 μmol/L
D-xylose	30-40 mg/100 mL	0.0666	2-2.71 mmol/L
Zinc	75-120 μg/100 mL	0.1530	11.5-18.5 μmol/L

Adapted from *The SI Manual in Health Care*, Metric Commission, Canada, 1981.

Table 14. Comparative Linear Measures

1 meter (m)	=	39.37 inches (in.)
1 centimeter (cm)	=	0.39 in.
1 millimeter (mm)	=	0.039 in.
1 yard (yd)	=	91.44 centimeters (cm)
1 foot (ft)	=	30.48 cm
1 inch (in.)	=	2.54 cm

Table 15. Household Measures (Approximate)

1 drop[1]	1/20 mL
1 teaspoon	5 mL
1 tablespoon	15 mL
1 cup	250 mL

[1]official dropper size for H_2O at 15°C, or ~1/45 mL for alcoholic liquids.

Table 16. Metric and Apothecaries' Equivalents[1]

1 milligram (mg)	=	$^{1}/_{65}$ grain ($^{1}/_{60}$)
1 gram (g)	=	15.43 grains (15)
1 kilogram (kg)	=	2.20 pounds (avoirdupois)
1 milliliter (mL)	=	16.23 minims (15)
1 grain (gr)	=	0.065 gram (60 mg)
1 ounce (oz)[2]	=	31.1 grams (30 g)
1 minim	=	0.062 mL (0.06)
1 fluid ounce (oz)	=	29.57 mL (30)
1 pint (pt)[3]	=	473.2 mL (500)
1 quart (qt)[3]	=	946.4 mL (1000)
1 gallon (gal.)[3]	=	3785.6 mL (4000)

[1]approximate values
[2]avoirdupois, 1 ounce = 28.4 grams
[3]In the Imperial system: 1 pint = 200 fluid ounces
1 quart = 40 fluid ounces
1 gallon = 160 fluid ounces

Table 17. Metric System Prefixes and Symbols

Factor	Prefix	Symbol	Factor	Prefix	Symbol
10^{18}	exa	E	10^{-1}	deci	d
10^{15}	peta	P	10^{-2}	centi	c
10^{12}	tera	T	10^{-3}	milli	m
10^{9}	giga	G	10^{-6}	micro	μ
10^{6}	mega	M	10^{-9}	nano	n
10^{3}	kilo	k	10^{-12}	pico	p
10^{2}	hecto	h	10^{-15}	femto	f
10^{1}	deca	da	10^{-18}	atto	a

Table 18. Metric System Weights and Measures*

1 kilogram (kg)	=	1000 grams (10^{3})
1 milligram (mg)	=	0.001 gram (10^{-3})
1 microgram (μg)	=	0.000001 gram (10^{-6})
1 liter (L)	=	1000 mL (10^{3})
1 milliliter (mL)	=	0.001 L (10^{-3})
1 microliter (μL)	=	0.000001 L (10^{-6})

*commonly employed terms

Table 19. Milligram-Milliequivalent Conversions

The milliequivalent (mEq) is the unit of measure often used for electrolytes. It indicates the chemical activity, or combining power, of an element relative to the activity of 1 mg of hydrogen. Thus, 1 mEq is represented by 1 mg of hydrogen (1 mole) or 23 mg of Na^+, 39 mg of K^+, 20 mg of Ca^{++}, or 35.5 mg of Cl, etc.

$$mEq/L = \frac{(mg/L) \times valence}{molecular\ weight}$$

$$mg/L = \frac{(mEq/L) \times molecular\ weight}{valence}$$

Table 20. SI Metric System Base Units

Physical Quantity	Base Unit	SI Symbol
Length	meter	m
Mass	kilogram	kg
Time	second	s
Amount of substance	mole	mol
Thermodynamic temperature	kelvin	K
Electrical current	ampere	A
Luminous intensity	candela	cd

Most laboratory values are expressed as amount/liter, eg, mol/L, mg/L, cells/L. In the SI system, if the molecular weight is known, it is preferable to express the amount of a substance as the amount in moles per liter, eg, mol/L, mmol/L, μmol/L, nmol/L.

Example: to convert 10.5 mg/100 mL Ca to mmol/L

$$10.5\ mg/100\ mL = \frac{mg/100\ mL \times 10}{molecular\ weight}$$

$$= \frac{10.5 \times 10}{40} = 2.62\ mmol/L$$

Table 21. Weight Equivalents for Feed Additives

grams	Additive per Ton*		
	percent	ppm	mg/kg**
1	0.00011	1.1	1.1
5	0.00055	5.5	5.5
10	0.0011	11	11
100	0.011	110	110
pounds (avoirdupois)			
1	0.05	500	500
2	0.10	1000	1000

*2000 lb or 907.2 kg; note 1 metric ton (1000 kg) = 2204.6 lb.
**for SI units, convert to moles when molecular weight is known.

Table 22. Conversion Formulas

Gallons into Pounds: Multiply the specific gravity of the liquid by 8.33* (weight in pounds of 1 gallon of water); then multiply this result by the number of gallons, to obtain the weight in pounds.

Pounds into Gallons: Multiply the specific gravity of the liquid by 8.33* (weight in pounds of 1 gallon of water); then divide the number of pounds by the result, to obtain the volume in gallons.

Milliliters into Grams: Multiply the specific gravity of the substance by the number of milliliters, to obtain the weight in grams.

Grams into Milliliters: Divide the number of grams by the specific gravity of the substance, to obtain the volume in milliliters.

Milliliters into Pounds: Multiply the number of milliliters by the specific gravity of the substance; then divide the product by 453.59 (equivalent in grams of 1 avoirdupois pound), to obtain the weight in pounds.

Pounds into Milliliters: Multiply the number of pounds by 453.59 (equivalent in grams of 1 avoirdupois pound); then divide the product by the specific gravity of the substance, to obtain the volume in milliliters.

Milliliters into Ounces: Multiply the number of milliliters by the specific gravity of the substance; then divide the product by 28.35 (equivalent in grams of 1 avoirdupois ounce), to obtain the volume in ounces.

Ounces into Milliliters: Multiply the number of ounces by 28.35 (equivalent in grams of 1 avoirdupois ounce); then divide the product by the specific gravity of the substance, to obtain the volume in milliliters.

Grains, Drams, and Ounces into Grams (or mL): 1) Divide the number of grains by 15; or 2) multiply the number of drams by 4; or 3) multiply the number of ounces by 28.35. The result in each case equals the approximate number of grams (or mL).

Kilograms into Pounds: Multiply the number of kilograms by 2.2046, or multiply the number of kilograms by 2 and add 10% to the product.

Pounds into Kilograms: Divide the number of pounds by 2.2046, or multiply by 0.4536.

*10 for imperial gallons

PART IV

FUR, LABORATORY, AND ZOO ANIMALS

AQUACULTURE SYSTEMS

Although aquaculture is an ancient science, it has not kept pace with the technological development of intensive methods of plant and animal production. Successful management of aquaculture systems depends on the same general principles as agriculture. For efficient mass animal production, these include breeding of genetically and nutritionally standardized animals in a well-managed environment. The latter includes maintenance of optimal stocking densities for each stage of production, and programs to prevent and control diseases specific for each aquaculture species.

While there are many similarities, there are some important differences between aquaculture and agriculture. Aquaculture relies on the aquatic, rather than the terrestrial environment. A basic understanding of water qualities, in relationship to aquatic animal health, is required. Agriculture has developed standardized management methods for a few select species of genetically and nutritionally defined domestic farm animals for mass production. In sharp contrast, the needed management standards for aquaculture are only currently being developed. Aquaculture relies heavily on wild animal breeding stocks.

Optimal genetic, nutritional, and environmental standards for each of the many animal candidates for aquaculture are being defined. Many such species have complicated life cycles, and require greater understanding of their reproductive physiology and management strategies for economically feasible mass production.

Outbreaks of serious diseases are not uncommon in aquaculture: the most common causes are related to alterations of the physical and chemical aquatic environment. The environment must be constantly monitored for hazardous conditions, eg, oxygen depletion, hyperthermia and hypothermia, and accumulation of metabolic wastes (eg, ammonia and nitrites). The environment also may be contaminated by industrial or agricultural chemicals. Feral aquatic organisms may act as intermediate or transport hosts, or carriers of disease. Pathogens are difficult to manage in the aquatic environment due to constant recycling of susceptible animal stocks.

Knowledge of specific diseases is required for prevention, control, and eradication. A great variety of vertebrate and invertebrate aquatic animals are produced in

FLZ

aquacultural or maricultural systems. Some of the more important commercial finfish species cultured for food are salmon, trout, catfish, tilapia, eel, and carp. Tropical, ornamental, and bait fish are also important aquacultural industries. Among the more important invertebrate species are molluscs (oysters, clams, scallops, abalone) and crustacea (shrimp, lobsters, and crayfish ["crawfish"]).

Although there is great variation in life cycles and management of each species cultured, all can be divided into the following stages of production: breeding and hatchery, and growout operations.

Breeding and Hatchery Operations: There are 2 types of hatcheries. One relies on artificial control of the reproductive cycle, in which breeding and spawning are regulated for larval production. The other depends on the harvest of ova and sperm from wild adults (eg, shrimp and lobsters) or the capture of larvae from the wild (eg, eels).

In the first type, breeding and spawning can be artificially induced by regulation of water temperature and light, nutrition, and chemical substances. Crude pituitary extracts and human chorionic gonadotropin are injected into some finfish breeders to induce spawning in aquaria. Management of unfertilized or fertilized ova and sperm in the hatchery is critical, and the techniques vary with the species cultured. For artificial fertilization of ova with sperm, the ratio, dilution, temperature, and timing of fertilization are important steps. Proper methods of sanitation, and preparation of a cultural medium that is physically and chemically compatible with the embryonating eggs are required. Once fertilized, the embryonating eggs are washed, diluted, and resuspended. Hatching and embryo development are monitored at regular intervals. Each aquaculture species has its own hatchery management needs. Most aquaculture species have great fecundity. An oyster may produce as many as 110 million ova during one spawn. Finfish produce many less, but are still prolific by mammalian standards. Female catfish produce ~4000 ova/lb (0.45 kg) body wt.

During the development of embryos and larvae in the hatchery, many aquaculture species undergo metamorphic changes that require special methods and management. Larval bivalve molluscs (oysters, clams, and scallops) lose their mobility and become attached to substrates (shells, rocks, etc) following a process of metamorphosis ("settlement stage"). Settlement tanks should be provided for this purpose.

Specific diseases may develop during these stages of development and include congenital, metabolic, nutritional, and infectious diseases. Many of the congenital diseases are genetic or due to infections in cultured or wild breeding stocks. Infections transmitted in the aquatic culture media to embryos and larvae spread rapidly. Overcrowding in the culture vessels or aquaria exacerbate disease processes. Mortalities tend to be higher in hatchery-reared larvae due to such rapid dispersion of pathogens in the aquatic environment, the lack of larval immunity, and the specific retention of larval pathogens that are continuously recycled in great numbers within the hatchery system.

Freshwater or seawater pumped into the hatcheries may contain larval pathogens that proliferate rapidly at certain times of the year. These include many bacteria, eg, *Aeromonas, Pseudomonas,* and *Vibrio* spp. Larval foods also may be contaminated with such pathogens.

Hatchery water and food supplies require routine monitoring for bacterial pathogens and toxic substances. A hatchery health program should include routine pathological and microbiological examinations of larval cultures, water supplies, and larval foods utilized during production.

In addition to infectious diseases, rapid growth of undesirable, contaminating competitive organisms may occur in larval cultures, and result in starvation of the desirable cultured animals. Some accidentally introduced undesirable organisms may be toxic, predacious, or parasitic, or may interfere with the vital processes (fouling) of the cultured animal.

Finfish hatcheries can be examined and certified as being free of specific known pathogens. Such certification is needed to define SPF breeding stocks suitable for interstate transport or export. Since the knowledge of the diseases of many species utilized in aquaculture is extremely limited, more research and regulatory measures are needed for production of pathogen-free breeding stock.

Growout Operations: Once the hatchery phase of production is complete, finfish fingerlings, metamorphosed crustacea, or juvenile bivalve molluscs require growout facilities that provide more space and food for growth to market size or adult breeders. The type of growout facility is determined by the needs of the particular species and the availability of land, water, and foods for economic production.

In the case of finfish (salmon, trout, catfish, tilapia, carp, and others), growout operations may be in raceways, tanks, ponds, and net or wire pens or cages in open bodies of water. Saltwater species may be reared in pens or cages placed in estuaries or seawater ("sea ranching").

Ponds utilized for aquaculture may be either natural or constructed. For some herbivorous cultured finfish or invertebrates, ponds are artificially fertilized to promote the growth of vegetation, which is utilized as food by the cultured organism (eg, catfish, crayfish, shrimp). In addition to pond vegetation, supplemental commercial or farm-formulated rations may be fed. Commercial finfish formulated rations are available and can be used in raceways or tanks. Salmonid fish are reared in freshwater raceways, ponds, or are sea-ranched in net or wire pens, and receive formulated feeds.

Oyster juveniles ("spat" or "seed oysters") are placed in estuaries, saltwater rivers, and ponds for growout. If the seed oysters are attached to shells or shell fragments, they may be placed in trays of submerged rafts, or in netted bags, or broadcast individually in the growout area. Clams may be planted in raceways or submerged trays, and motile juvenile scallops may be suspended in lantern-like nets in seawater. Since oysters, clams, mussels, and scallops are filter feeders, their foods consist of natural planktonic blooms of algae and diatoms available in seawater.

Bivalve molluscs may ingest toxic planktonic algal blooms (that are harmful for man and molluscs—eg, paralytic shellfish poisoning) in addition to beneficial algal foods that are present.

CARE OF ZOO ANIMALS

The health and well-being of captive wild animals depends on their enclosure design, management, and medical care. The natural-looking enclosures with soil and vegetation, which are more appealing to the public, make sanitation and parasite control programs difficult, and complicate handling. Exhibits with different species can create problems of disease transmission, aggression, and design of feeding stations to assure proper food consumption.

Preventive medicine is the backbone of any medical program in a zoo due to inherent problems in diagnostic procedures and treatment of wild animals. Preventive medical procedures are recorded and become the start of the animal's medical record. Complete records are essential to all medical programs, and zoo animals are no exception.

Animals entering the collection must undergo quarantine. The quarantine facility should be isolated and designed to allow handling of the animals and proper cleaning and sanitizing of the enclosures. It should be serviced by separate keepers who are skilled at recognizing signs of stress and disease, and will carefully monitor food intake and fecal characteristics. Quarantined animals often require specialized care, including force-feeding during initial acclimation to new surroundings and diets.

During the quarantine period, the animal should receive the appropriate vaccinations and diagnostic tests (eg, tuberculosis). Before release from quarantine, the animal should be free or greatly relieved of parasite loads and receive a physical examination, which can include radiographs and blood sampling for hematology and clinical chemistry. Some sera should also be frozen for future reference and possible epidemiological studies.

Wild animals are vulnerable to a wide variety of endo- and ectoparasites, similar to those of domestic animals. Impact of parasites on individuals is variable, but probably is greatest at the time of shipment and arrival at the zoo. During this period of extreme stress, many normally commensal parasites, especially protozoa, appear to be capable of causing disease. Acute diarrhea may result from massive infections of *Trichomonas, Giardia,* or *Balantidium* spp. Amebiasis is fairly common in primates and reptiles, and can be fatal.

The skin and pelage and fecal specimens should be examined during quarantine. Ecto- and endoparasites should be treated appropriately. Parasites with indirect life cycles pose a problem less frequently if the exhibit area is clean and free of intermediate hosts. If ectoparasites are found on newly received animals, the shipping crate and its contents should be sprayed before the crate leaves the quarantine area. Quarantine facilities may require barriers against ingress of potential vectors and vermin.

Preventive medicine programs continue with booster vaccinations, periodic fecal examinations and treatments for parasites, and screening procedures. Intestinal parasites are a major ongoing problem in many species kept in naturalistic exhibits on dirt substrate, especially in warmer climates. Continuous vigilance is necessary to control the level of infection, especially in young and stressed individuals. As in domestic species, anthelmintic resistance may develop and necessitate a change in medication. Animals should receive medical screening to ensure that they are healthy before being shipped to other zoos. Necropsies of all dead animals help evaluate medical, management, and nutritional programs, and help identify underlying problems that may require immediate action to safeguard the rest of the collection. Variations in anatomy should be recorded since such observations can aid diagnostic procedures and therapy in future problems with the species.

Pest control is often neglected; a successful control program requires a concerted effort to minimize harborage and food for pests in addition to mechanical and chemical methods of control. Access of the agent to animals and the chance of secondary poisoning is minimized by choice of agent and its storage. Common zoo pests are important vectors of disease: cockroaches are intermediate hosts for GI parasites of primates; rodents can harbor and spread listerosis and leptospirosis; and foxes and raccoons can devastate waterfowl collections, and be important in rabies outbreaks. Raccoons are also capable of transmitting *Baylisascaris procyonis* to other species in which it causes fatal neuropathy. Pigeons and starlings are potential reservoirs for avian diseases, and consume or contaminate animal food and deposit droppings everywhere.

Mammalian tuberculosis (TB) remains a potential problem, and routine screening of primates, hoofstock, and keeper staff is indicated. Interpretation of intradermal tuberculin tests creates uncertainty in some nondomestic species. When a test is suspicious or positive, additional diagnostic tests may be indicated, such as gastric and bronchial lavage for cytology and culture.

Avian TB is a chronic problem in many bird collections. Control measures are difficult since antemortem tests are unreliable. Aggressive sanitation and culling of exposed birds help control the disease but will not eliminate it. Marsupials and young primates also develop avian TB when exposed to infected birds or contaminated environments such as in a mixed exhibit. The disease in marsupials usually is manifest by bone lesions and is resistant to most therapy. The disease in primates is often benign, but causes equivocal tuberculin test reactions.

Vaccination of exotic carnivores is essential because of their susceptibility to various diseases such as feline panleukopenia, feline rhinotracheitis, feline calicivirus, canine distemper, and parvovirus. Previously, only killed virus vaccines were recommended, but recent studies have shown that some modified live vaccines are safe for use in some species; further studies are required. Rabies vaccination is controversial and depends on the circumstances of each collection; if indicated, only killed products should be used. Vaccines are available for other diseases shared by domestic and wild species. The decision to vaccinate wild species for less common diseases for which a vaccine may be of questionable value is decided on an individual basis. (*See also* VACCINATION OF EXOTIC MAMMALS, p 1083.)

Management Practices: The mainstay of a medical program is a qualified and dedicated keeper staff that observes the animals daily for abnormalities such as anorexia, inactivity, abnormal feces, and changes in behavior that may reflect early medical problems. Overzealous reporting of observations is preferable to indifference. Since many exotic species instinctively mask overt signs of illness until the problem is well advanced, it is necessary to make keepers aware of what may seem to be trivial changes. Past associations with the veterinarian may arouse the animal's responses to the veterinarian's presence, which will mask subtle changes noticeable to keepers.

The animal's environment should approximate its natural environment and enhance the visual experience of the visitor. Many healthy mammals or birds can tolerate a fairly wide temperature range if given access to shade and water in hot weather, and a dry draft-free shelter with a warm spot and ample food to meet increased energy requirements in winter. The key to making this work is to ensure that each animal has access to the protected environment and that one dominant individual does not exclude others from shelter, food, or water. Such exclusion can result in frostbite or even death due to exposure. Feed receptacles should be designed to avoid fecal contamination.

For introduction to new enclosures, caution and forethought are necessary to prevent self-induced trauma in frightened animals, which may crash into barriers or glass fronts. Visual barriers such as canvasses suspended from the fences or cage walls, or obscuring the glass windows with soap offer some protection against such accidents.

With larger numbers of birds or mammals, and especially in mixed exhibits, several watering and feeding stations should be established at appropriate elevations to reduce injuries and death resulting from territorial invasions. The timing of feedings is important; in many species it is best to feed small amounts throughout the day for a more active animal and a better display.

Handling of Animals: The treatment of disease in captive wild animals does not differ substantially from that of domestic species once the diagnosis is made, except in the method of restraint and drug administration. Most wild animals resent being handled and usually fight manual restraint. Struggling with an animal to administer treatment may do more harm than can be offset by the treatment.

Physical restraint is indicated in some species for minor manipulation or close observation. The squeeze cage or chute is frequently used in larger and dangerous species. While the dimensions and construction of these cages vary, all operate by movement of one wall to restrain the animal against the other. The squeeze cage has openings to allow safe access to the animal. Useful procedures on an unanesthetized animal so confined include limited physical examination, giving injections, administering anesthetics, obtaining blood samples, trimming malformed claws, and applying topical medication. Ideally, squeeze cages are designed as part of the animal's regular quarters. Whenever possible, animals should be enticed rather than forced into the cage. The cage can be located in a normal shifting area where the animals enter it daily. It is helpful if exhibits contain nest boxes or catch pens equipped with doors that can be operated remotely to catch the animal. From these catch pens, the animal can be transferred to a squeeze cage, anesthetic chamber, or shipping crate. Weighing facilities are essential.

Small animals and birds may be caught and restrained in long-handled hoop nets. These nets must be deep enough that the animal can be dropped into a blind end, and the upper part twisted to prevent escape.

Personnel participating in capture or restraint procedures should understand their role and be aware of the behavioral characteristics and armamentarium of the animal. Such coordination is essential to help ensure safety. Heavy gloves are used to protect the handler from teeth and claws when animals are manually held after capture. Care must be used to avoid excessive pressure on the animal, since the gloves hinder dexterity and the perception of the pressure being exerted. Gloves are also difficult to clean, and can be a fomite for transmitting infections.

Drug Administration: Few drugs are approved for use in other than domestic species or man. This presents a dilemma, but it is commonly recognized that to provide adequate medical care to zoo animals, these drugs must be used even though basic knowledge of therapeutic benefit, dosage, treatment schedule, contraindications, and toxicity is lacking. Therefore, it is necessary to extrapolate. In general, zoo animals can be placed in 5 recognized metabolic groups: passerine birds, non-passerine birds, placental mammals, marsupial mammals, and reptiles. The veterinarian should endeavor to extrapolate dosage within such groups when data are available.

Antibiotic therapy in exotic species has been empirical. Doses have been extrapolated from other mammals, but little consideration has been made of the different metabolic rates of the animals, eg, snakes versus birds. It is important to recognize that dosages are generally higher in small animals and lower in large animals of a metabolic group. An animal that is 15 times the size (body wt) of a smaller animal may require only half the dose rate of the smaller animal when both belong to the same energy or metabolic group.

The pharmacokinetics of drugs in the various species is important. When prescribing, these factors must be kept in mind if therapy is to be beneficial, especially in drugs with potential organ toxicity.

Drug administration can be challenging. Oral medication has the advantage of minimal disturbance to the animal, but the problem is to ensure adequate intake; this may be accomplished by mixing it with favorite foods or treats. IM injection with a hand syringe can be difficult unless a squeeze cage or other means of physical restraint is used. Remote IM injections may be made by firing a projectile syringe from a gun. These injections are painful and add the trauma of the dart impact, especially when delivering large volumes (eg, 10 mL) over long distances (60 m). Practice with projectile darts is mandatory before their clinical use because marksmanship as well as familiarity with the weapon is essential; such weapons in the hands of a novice can be fatal. Other less traumatic methods of IM injection, over a shorter distance, include a syringe pole or blow gun.

Safe immobilization and anesthesia in wild animals are of special concern. Many procedures, routinely accomplished on domestic animals with minimal restraint, require chemical immobilization for the welfare of both the zoo animal and handler.

Ketamine alone or in combination with tranquilizers or xylazine is a common anesthetic agent for small to medium-sized mammals and birds. A tranquilizer in combination speeds induction, minimizes excitement, increases muscle relaxation, and provides a smoother anesthetic procedure than does ketamine alone.

Tiletamine-zolazepam, a dissociative anesthetic, is relatively safe in most species, has a rapid induction, and can be concentrated to 500 mg/mL, which allows a small delivery volume.

Etorphine, alone or in combination with other agents (acepromazine, xylazine) is used extensively for immobilization of ungulates, elephants, and rhinoceroses. One advantage of etorphine is that a rapid-acting antagonist, diprenorphine, can be given IV. The potency of etorphine creates potential dangers to people administering the drug; procedures to follow after accidental human injection should be established. Carfentanyl is related to etorphine and also has a rapid induction, but due to its long half-life, renarcotization occurs following reversal with diprenorphine, which can make it undesirable for field use.

Xylazine alone produces adequate immobilization in some species of ungulates, mainly bovids. Its sedative effects can be antagonized by yohimbine. It should not be used as the sole anesthetic agent in dangerous carnivores because they may appear sedated, but can respond aggressively when stimulated.

The factors that affect response to immobilizing drugs include age, sex, stage of reproductive cycle, general nutritional status, and mental state of the animal before drug administration. Variations are marked between species as well as individuals, and between different collections of the same species. An excited animal usually requires more drug and, once immobilized, has a greater tendency for hyperthermia and acidosis. When anesthesia must be prolonged, inhalation anesthetics such as halothane, methoxyflurane, or isoflurane can be used. The nature of an enclosure in which animals are to be chemically immobilized can be critical. Prey species that are darted may dash themselves against fences and other barriers.

Reproduction: The nature of the animal and its social behavior must be understood to promote successful breeding programs. Species should be maintained alone, in pairs, or in groups, depending on their established social system; eg, in mixed species groups in Artiodactyla, it is possible to establish estrous cycles by species and thus have only one male in the enclosure at a time. The other males can be rotated to coincide with the estrous periods of the females of their species. Such measures reduce injuries from interaction of breeding males. At parturition, the males of some species should be removed for several weeks to prevent attack on the postpartum females or their offspring. In colder climates, males should be introduced at a time that will allow births to occur during warm weather.

An emerging problem in zoos is animals that reproduce and overload the carrying capacity of the exhibit, the zoo, and other zoos. Such successful species are competitive for limited resources and can compromise other programs. Control of the population size may require euthanasia or, preferably, birth control measures such as surgical intervention or hormonal suppression of reproduction, or separating males and females.

Other Procedures: Bone fractures are repaired under general anesthesia. Since maintaining a splint on a wild animal is often difficult, rigid internal fixation is preferable whenever possible. For best results, any fracture fixation should be rigid, strong, and require minimal postoperative care. When a cast is applied, freedom of movement and a minimum of discomfort must be assured since the cast must be left on for 3-4 wk. Newer lightweight, strong, waterproof casting material is especially applicable in zoological medicine as are other orthopedic appliances and techniques.

Prevention of flight in birds is readily accomplished by amputating one wing just distal to the radiocarpal joint or performing a tenectomy and fusing the radiocarpal joint. Other pinioning methods used can be found in the literature. Pinioning of young birds is easier and more successful than the same procedure in adults. (*See also* p 999 *et seq.*)

Dentistry in zoo animals presents unique problems. The roots of canine teeth in primates and carnivores are more extensive than the exposed crown, and it is not possible to remove such a tooth intact by simple traction and rotation; dislodging with a dental elevator is essential. A small electric drill or bone chisel may be used to remove a section of maxilla around the labial margin of the root. The incisor teeth of rodents, such as beavers, porcupines, and capybaras, grow continually throughout life; unless these animals are supplied with coarse feed or logs to gnaw on, their incisors grow excessively long and interfere with their ability to feed. Periodontal disease in exotic species is treated by routine cleaning and providing adequate chewing substances to supplement the soft prepared diets fed many animals.

Care of Orphaned Native Birds and Mammals: It is critical to determine if the animal is truly orphaned. In many cases if the bird is returned to its nest or the mammal is left alone and monitored, the parent returns to care for it. Handling of baby birds to return them to their nest does not preclude the parents from accepting them. If an animal or bird is taken for hand-rearing, warmth, hydration, and energy are critical.

Since most orphans initially cannot maintain or regulate their body temperature, supplemental heat must be provided with the aid of heating pads, hot water bottles, or incandescent light bulbs. The orphan must be insulated from the heat to prevent thermal burns. Electric coil heating devices can develop hot spots when worn or damaged. The initial temperature range should be 80-90°F (26-32°C). A hypothermic orphan should not be fed until the body temperature is near normal. During this rewarming phase, hydration and energy requirements can be met with oral saline and 10-20% dextrose solutions.

Various diets are used to feed altricial birds; they generally contain ⅓ cooked egg yolk, ⅓ meat (dog food) and ⅓ baby cereal (pabulum), which is mixed with a milk replacer or whole milk in a 1:1 ratio to make a slurry that is fed through a medicine dropper. A few drops of pediatric multivitamins are added to all formulas for orphans. Young birds should be stimulated by rustling the nest or tapping them on the upper beak to stimulate gaping. The food is then delivered to the back of the mouth; the bird will stop gaping when it is full. For the first few feedings it is best to keep the bird hungry and not overfed, which can create digestive problems. The bird should be fed q15min for 1-2 hr; then hourly for 12 hr during the day.

The diet for pigeons and doves is different and consists of dry dog food soaked in evaporated milk and water (1:1) to form a slurry.

Hand-rearing of orphan skunks, foxes, and raccoons is inadvisable because of the potential rabies hazard and local regulations. For raising squirrels and opossum, a milk replacer should be fed q3hr for 18 hr a day. Rabbits are very difficult to raise; they can be offered this formula 2-3 times a day.

DISEASES OF FISH

Fish are poikilotherms, and their growth and metabolic rates and inflammatory and immunological responses are greatly influenced by water temperature. In freshwater, the internal tissues of fish are hyperosmotic; in saltwater, they are hypoosmotic. Skin surface injuries make osmoregulation more difficult and may be of serious consequence, since loss of fluid balance and circulatory collapse may occur.

Fish lack organized lymph nodes and Kuppfer's cells. Phagocytic tissue is located in the hematopoietic tissue of the spleen and kidney and often in the atrium of the 2-chambered heart. The structure of the fish kidney varies with the species; generally, it is divided into 2 regions, an anterior "head" kidney and a "caudal" kidney, located retroperitoneally, ventral to the vertebral column. Hematopoietic, renal, and endocrine tissues are found in the kidney. Divalent ions are excreted principally from the kidney, and monovalent ions and nitrogenous excretions from the gills. Accordingly, lesions of the gills and kidney may seriously interfere with respiration, excretion, and fluid balance.

The swim bladder in bony fish, which originates as an appendage of the foregut, regulates body buoyancy and may also be employed for sound production. Gas is either secreted or absorbed into the swim bladder to maintain the needed buoyancy or specific gravity and balance in specific water conditions. A sensory lateral line system along the sides of the body and head receives stimuli from the aquatic environment and mediates adaptive responses through the CNS.

A humoral antibody system occurs in all fish but varies considerably between classes. Although antibody production often is temperature dependent, specific serum antibodies can be demonstrated. B lymphocytes, found in the spleen and liver, are responsible for production of immunoglobulins found in the serum and tissue fluids of fish. However, fish lack the potent immunoglobulins similar to IgG of higher animals. Fish do increase production of IgM, similar to those of higher animals, when responding immunologically to many infectious agents. Unlike higher homeotherms, poikilothermic fish depend on increases in environmental temperature for efficient antibody production during infections (or vaccination), when most pathogens are replicating at a more rapid rate. The optimal temperature for antibody production varies with the species of fish (coldwater or warmwater). Extreme environmental temperature elevations (above that of the natural habitat) inhibit antibody production. T lymphocytes of fish, like those of higher animals, are responsible for cell-mediated immunity. Immunity is not as age dependent in fish as it is in higher animals; young fish are usually immunologically competent, and can be vaccinated successfully. Antibodies are found in the mucus of the fish skin and GI tract.

While anamnestic immunological responses have been demonstrated in fish, the duration of acquired immunity appears limited. Individual parenteral administration of antigens apparently gives longer lasting immunity when compared to mass bath methods. Although vaccination of fish against specific diseases has been economically important in preventing losses, needs for better methods are realized.

Fish culture has evolved from production of ornamental pond fish, food-fish production, and restocking sport fisheries. Currently in the USA, channel catfish, trout, salmon, bait, and ornamental fish farming are profitable finfish industries; shellfish aquaculture is developing rapidly. While much interest has been shown, technical difficulties have delayed development of lobster and shrimp culture. In some countries, carp and tilapia food-fish farming continues to be important. In developing countries needing protein foods, underutilized aquatic resources are being developed rapidly for food-fish farming and culture of ornamental fish for export. Technical development of all of the above forms of aquaculture is needed to make them efficient and economically competitive with commercial fisheries and agricultural animal production. As with other forms of domestic animal production, diseases in intensive aquacultural systems (qv, p 978) are responsible for serious economic losses.

While the general range of infectious, parasitic, nutritional, genetic, toxic, and neoplastic diseases is found in cultured aquatic animals, the relationship of these diseases to the aquatic environment and aquacultural practices requires greater understanding. In addition to signs of disease, emphasis also must be given to the physical and chemical qualities of the aquatic environment that may be related to cause, duration, and resolution of disease: temperature, pH, salinity, oxygen availability, gas pressures, and suspended solids are water qualities that affect fish health and are easily measured. These water qualities often are interrelated: eg, an increase in water temperature decreases its oxygen-carrying capacity; as pH rises, ionized ammonium is converted to free ammonia, which is highly toxic. The most common aquatic animal intoxications are related to the hydrolysis and oxidation of nitrogenous wastes, food, and decomposition products within the aquaria, which results in high levels of ammonia, nitrite, and nitrate.

Species requirements vary, but water quality can be regulated by controlling pH, temperature, population densities, salt and organic content, rate of water flow or dilution, and chemical and biological filtration. Salmonids require cool water and high oxygen levels (8-12 ppm); in contrast, cultured pond fish require warm water and can tolerate lower oxygen levels (4-6 ppm). High water temperatures and hypoxia are common causes of mortality in cultured fish during summer.

Supersaturation of aquarium and pond water with gases can lead to "**gas bubble disease**", in which free gas accumulates in the eye, gill, blood vessels, and skin. The condition can be recognized easily by observing bubbles in the affected tissues. It can occur when fish are moved from cold to warm water, gas is introduced under pressure into aquaria by defective pumps, or when there are air leaks in water lines.

While the same principles are employed in necropsy of fish as in other animals, greater emphasis is placed on an accurate history, antemortem signs, fresh necropsy material, and direct microscopical examination of fresh tissue smears and squash preparations. Fish decompose quickly and many saprophytic microorganisms reproduce rapidly in the decaying tissues, which complicates isolation of pathogens unless samples are collected immediately after death. Fresh smears are valuable for observing living motile pathogens in tissues; they are easily seen and often provide a rapid diagnosis. Many laboratories are equipped to help with diagnosis of fish diseases, but permission should be sought before material is submitted.

Drugs are administered in aquacultural systems by a number of methods. Mass treatments are currently the most popular, and delivery of drugs in the water is most commonly practiced due to reduced cost, uniform delivery within the system, and ease of control.

Water treatments are indicated in external parasite infestations of the skin and gills, in which the drug acts directly on the parasite. Water treatments can be applied in aquaria, tanks, raceways, and ponds as continuous, intermittent, or single treatments. Within aquaria, such treatments may be given as a dip or bath, or as a continuous flush with the drug at a constant level.

Although a wide range of "unapproved" drugs and antibiotics have been employed in both vertebrate and invertebrate aquatic animals, both the Environmental Protection Agency (EPA) and the Food and Drug Administration (FDA) of the USA have instituted or are considering regulatory measures for these industries. Therapeutic, disinfectant, sterilizing, osmoregulatory, and anesthetic agents have been used extensively to reduce costs and enhance production. Concern regarding the safety of drugs or chemicals has been greatest in fish produced directly for human consumption, such as salmonids and catfish. Use in sport fish or other hatcheries that produce juveniles to supplement natural stocks of sport fishes, molluscs, and crustacea are also of concern, since ultimately they may be consumed by man. Before using any drug, especially in food fish, current local regulations should be checked since they vary from country to country, as well as from time to time.

Table 1. Drugs for Use in Aquaculture
(See precaution note above.)

Drug	Species	Dose	Indications	Use Limitations	Withdrawal Time
Oxytetracycline	Salmonids	2.5-3.75 g/100 lb (45 kg) fish in feed	Furunculosis, bacterial septicemias	10 days 48°F (9°C)+	21 days
	Catfish	as above	Bacterial septicemias	10 days 62°F (17°C)+	21 days
	Lobsters	1 g/lb (0.45 kg) feed	Gaffkemia	5 days	30 days
Sulfamerazine	Trout Brown Brook Rainbow	10 g/100 lb (45 kg) fish daily in feed	Furunculosis	Not more than 14 days	21 days
Sulfadimethoxine + ormetoprim (5:1 ratio) "Romet-30"	Salmonids	50 mg/kg of fish daily in feed	Furunculosis	5 days	42 days
	Catfish	as above	*Edwardsiella ictaluri* infection	5 days	3 days
Formaldehyde solution (Formalin)	Salmonids	Up to 200 ppm up to 1 hr	Control of protozoa and monogenetic trematodes	Above 50°F (10°C): up to 170 ppm in tanks and raceways; 15-25 ppm in ponds; may be repeated in 5-10 days	none
	Catfish	as above	as above	Below 50°F (10°C): up to 250 ppm; in ponds 15-25 ppm	none
	Eggs Salmonid Esocid	Up to 2000 ppm up to 15 min	Control of fungi	—	none
"Tricaine"	Salmonids, catfish, other fishes, amphibia, and poikilotherms	15-330 mg/L	Anesthesia, sedation	Hatcheries and laboratories only	21 days

For internal infections or vaccinations, drugs or vaccines may be injected, most often IP. Since such parenteral injections are stressful, labor intensive, and costly, other methods are employed. Systemic infections are most commonly treated by delivering drugs mixed in the feed. Vaccines are most commonly administered in the water, in hyperosmotic solutions or under pressure.

The effects of drugs on the filtration systems of aquaria should always be considered before their use. Their antibacterial properties may inhibit or destroy the beneficial bacteria required for biological filtration (oxidation of nitrogenous substances) and thus render such systems useless, which results in the accumulation of ammonia and nitrite and intoxication of the fish following therapy. If possible, filters should be removed from the aquarium, or the fish moved to another aquarium for treatment. Following treatment, the aquarium should be flushed or the fish placed in an aquarium with operational filters.

BACTERIAL DISEASES

Epidemics of bacterial diseases are common in dense populations of cultured food or aquarium fish. Predisposition to such outbreaks frequently is associated with poor water quality, organic loading of the aquatic environment, handling and transport of fish, marked temperature changes, hypoxia, and related stressful conditions. High concentrations of water-borne bacteria are normally found in ponds and aquaria. Many of these aquatic bacteria are opportunistic facultative pathogens, being activated by an adverse environment, a debilitated host, or a primary pathogen. In sharp contrast, obligatory bacterial pathogens of finfish require the finfish for replication, and are unable to survive alone for long in the aquatic environment.

Most bacterial pathogens of fish are aerobic gram-negative rods. Diagnosis is by isolating the organism in pure culture from infected tissues, and identifying the bacterial agent.

One of the most common bacterial diseases associated with stressful conditions in freshwater, pond culture, or aquaria is *Aeromonas hydrophila (liquefaciens, punctata)* infection. *Pseudomonas* spp (*P fluorescens* and *P putida*) also are facultative, freshwater finfish pathogens similiar to *A hydrophila*. All species of freshwater fish seem susceptible. Nutritional deficiencies, traumatic injuries, parasitism, and sharp seasonal temperature changes appear to be predisposing. The acute form is characterized by signs of a septicemic infection with external reddening, and hemorrhages are found in the peritoneum, body wall, and viscera. Control of the disease is directed toward removing predisposing factors. Oxytetracycline administered in the food (to provide 60-75 mg/kg of fish body wt, daily for 10 days) is helpful (withdrawal time 21 days).

Aeromonas salmonicida is a gram-negative, nonmotile, pigment-producing rod originally described as the cause of a septicemic disease of salmonids (**furunculosis**) and goldfish (**ulcer disease**). It is also a serious pathogen of many other freshwater and marine fishes, and may produce high mortality. In the acute form, hemorrhages are found in the fins, tail, muscles, gills, and internal organs. In more chronic forms, focal areas of swelling, hemorrhage, and tissue necrosis develop in the muscles. These lesions progress to crateriform abscesses that discharge from the skin surface (furuncles). Liquefaction necrosis occurs in the spleen and kidney. Diagnosis is made by isolating a pure culture of the organism from infected tissue and identifying it. Avoidance is the most effective prevention, since *A salmonicida* is an obligatory fish pathogen. Fish and fish eggs should be obtained from disease-free sources. Infected stocks should be depopulated and wild-fish reservoirs eliminated. Eyed fish eggs may be treated for 10-15 min in a solution containing 100 ppm iodine at a pH of 7 and a temperature of 10-15°C, although the drug is not approved for use on food-fish eggs. Eggs should be rinsed immediately after treatment. Sulfamerazine at 200 mg/kg of fish weight for 14 days is approved for treating salmonids (withdrawal time 21 days).

Vibriosis is a serious common systemic disease of many cultured, aquarium, and wild marine and estuarine fishes; it is less common in freshwater fish. *Vibrio anguillarium* and other *Vibrio* spp are responsible for the disease, which produces systemic manifestations, including skin, fin, and tail hemorrhages and ulcerations; and hemorrhagic and degenerative changes of internal organs. Diagnosis requires identification of pure isolates from infected tissues. Preventive measures are directed toward avoiding crowding and minimizing stress. **Coldwater vibriosis** (Hitra disease), a serious problem in sea farming of salmonids, is characterized by high mortality, resistance to drug therapy, and stress mediation. The etiologic agent is *V salmonicida*, a newly described strain. Since *Vibrio* spp are ubiquitous in marine environments, avoidance is difficult. Preventive vaccination with formalin-killed *Vibrio* is now used commercially. Sulfamerazine at 17 g/100 kg of fish for 10 days has effectively controlled the disease (withdrawal time 21 days).

Yersiniosis (enteric redmouth disease) is a serious acute or chronic bacterial disease of intensively cultured salmonids. The etiologic agent is *Yersinia ruckeri.* Signs are darkening and hemorrhage of the mouth (red mouth), skin, anus, and fins. Chronic signs are associated with inappetence, exophthalmia, and swelling and degenerative changes of internal organs. Diagnosis is by isolation and identification of pure cultures of the organism obtained from the internal organs of infected fish.

Depopulation of infected fish and avoidance of introduction of infected fish can be recommended, but preventive vaccination is the normal procedure in affected areas. The disease has been treated successfully with a combination of sulfamerazine at 20 g/100 kg of fish/day for 5 days, followed by oxytetracycline at 5 g/100 kg of fish/day for 3 days (withdrawal time 21 days).

Edwardsiella ictaluri and *E tarda* produce high mortality and serious economic losses in cultured catfish and eels. This enterobacterial septicemic disease is characterized by its seasonal incidence (summer), putrefactive and emphysematous subcut. tissue alterations, and liquifaction necrosis ("abscesses") of muscle. Prevention is related to depopulating infected fish, avoiding introduction of infected fish, and eliminating sources of fecal contamination from reptilian or human sources. The disease can be controlled by feeding oxytetracycline in the diet at 55 mg/kg of fish/day for 10 days (withdrawal time 21 days).

The order Cytophogales (Myxobacterales, slime bacteria) includes an important group of opportunistic fish pathogens that are common soil and water inhabitants. The gram-negative, rod or filamentous bacterium has a distinctive gliding motility and carotenoid pigmentation, and forms palisading masses on infected fish tissues. Skin or gill lesions have slimy or cotton-like surface exudates, which usually cover surface necrosis, ulcerations, and marginal hemorrhages. *Flexibacter columnaris,* the member of this group responsible for **columnaris disease** (cottonmouth disease, saddleback), occurs most commonly in warm water and warmwater species of fish. The disease can be prevented by lowering water temperature, reducing organic loading, and avoiding traumatic injuries. *Cytophaga psychrophila,* responsible for **coldwater** (peduncle) disease and **fin and tail rot,** most commonly infects coldwater fish, but can be found in warmwater fish subjected to low temperatures. The lesions are especially common on the dorsal, posterior surface of the fish under the dorsal fin, but may be found on any part of the body. Advanced cases show necrosis and ulceration of the peduncle. Both *Flexibacter* and *Cytophaga* infections can be controlled by oxytetracycline in the feed at 60 mg/kg of fish/day for 10 days (withdrawal time 21 days).

Bacterial gill disease is a disease complex most frequently reported in young cultured salmonids and aquarium fish. It may be initiated by crowding and poor water quality, including organic loading, high ammonia levels, and silt. Opportunistic bacteria such as *Flexibacter, Aeromonas,* and *Pseudomonas* spp may follow as secondary invaders of traumatized gill tissue. Signs of the disease are related to respiratory embarrassment due to impaired gill function. Gills appear swollen and mottled with patchy areas of bacterial growth, which can be confirmed by microscopical examination of direct gill smears. Hyperplasia, adhesions, and deformity of the gill lamellae can be observed. Young fish affected with the disease are subject to high mortality and sustained morbidity. Prevention is directed toward improving water quality and avoiding overstocking. Antibacterial drugs are helpful for secondary infections.

Bacterial kidney disease (corynebacterial kidney disease) is economically important in cultured salmonids. It also has been reported in other species of fish including wild, cultured, and aquarium fish. A gram-positive, small rod, *Renibacterium salmoninarum,* is the etiological agent. Infected fish remain carriers, and the obligatory pathogen can be transmitted congenitally. Characteristic signs are grayish, localized, or conglomerate granulomata in the viscera, especially the kidney or body wall; exophthalmia; blindness; and emaciation. Diagnosis requires isolation and identification of the bacteria. Because of the chronic carrier state, chemotherapy is not recommended. Avoidance by obtaining disease-free stock and preventing contamination by infected wild stocks are the best preventive measures. Infected premises should be depopulated.

Fish tuberculosis (mycobacteriosis) is a chronic or acute, systemic, granulomatous disease principally of aquarium fish, less commonly of cultured fish. The causative bacteria can be any number of species of *Mycobacterium*, including *M piscium*, *M platypoecilus*, and *M fortuitum*. They are gram-positive, acid-fast, nonmotile bacteria that are difficult to grow. Signs are variable and often resemble those of other diseases; they include emaciation, ascites, skin ulceration and hemorrhages, exophthalmos, paleness, and skeletal deformities. On necropsy, gross lesions of viscera consist of grayish white, necrotic foci (tubercles) that sometimes have coalesced to form tumor-like masses. Diagnosis can be made by isolating and identifying the bacteria. Because the disease can produce skin lesions and an allergic dermatitis in man, and because treatment does not eliminate the disease, infected fish should be destroyed. An aquarium should be disinfected before other fish are added. Infected fish or contaminated fish products should not be added to the aquarium.

A wide range of other less commonly recognized bacterial diseases has been described in fish. These include pasteurellosis, streptococcosis, *Haemophilus piscium* infection (ulcer disease), flavobacteriosis, *Eubacterium* infection (fish meningitis), and others. Diagnosis of these diseases requires isolation and identification of the specific bacterial agent.

MYCOTIC DISEASES

Aquatic fungal diseases often are considered secondary tissue invaders that follow environmental insults such as traumatic injuries, poor water quality, and other infectious agents. Once fungi have successfully invaded fish tissues, they continue to grow, produce progressively enlarging lesions, and may cause death. Since many fungi grow on decaying organic matter, they are especially common in the aquatic environment. Fish egg masses, which usually contain tissue debris and other dead ova or embryos, are especially vulnerable. Iodophors of varying iodine concentrations are used to prevent mycotic infections of non-food-fish eggs, which can be disinfected by a 100 ppm iodine bath for 10-15 min. This solution is toxic for hatched fish, and only eggs should be treated. Formaldehyde, up to 2000 ppm for 15 min, can be used to treat eggs of food fish (salmonid and esocid) for the control of fungi.

Saprolegnia **infections** are among the most common fungal infections of fish and fish eggs. Gross signs are grayish white, cotton-like growths on the skin, gills, eyes, or fins that may invade deeper tissues of the body. Microscopically, saprolegniasis can be recognized by making direct smears from the infected tissues and observing the nonseptate hyphal elements and mycelia. The sexual stages of the fungus can be observed only in cultures of the organism and are required for specific identification. Prevention of the disease is directed toward removing the predisposing causes—dead infected fish and decaying organic material.

Zinc-free malachite green employed as a bath at concentrations of 0.1-5 ppm of aquarium water for ≤1 hr has been successful. It is not approved for use in food fish, and normal fish should not be exposed to the drug. Sick fish should be treated separately in a protected environment without the competitive pressures of normal fish.

Ichthyophonus is a common fungal infection in wild fish and aged cultured and aquarium fish. The disease usually is chronic and progressive. It usually is detected on necropsy when the characteristic spherical cyst stages are observed microscopically in the smears of granulomatous lesions of the heart, liver, spleen, kidney, skin, and muscle. Prevention is directed toward removing infected fish and avoiding feeding fish products that contain the organism.

Branchiomycosis is a fungal disease of gill tissue characterized by respiratory distress and gill necrosis. The causative agents are *Branchiomyces sanguines* and *B demigrams*, which are opportunistic pathogens found in decaying organic materials in the aquatic environment. A diagnosis can be made from direct smears or stained histological sections of affected gill tissue. The disease is of greatest importance in cultured European food fish, in which mortality is severe. Zinc-free malachite green has been employed for treatment as indicated above, but it is not approved for food fish in the USA.

Many other less common mycotic infections have been reported in fish (*Achyla, Aphanomyces, Dermocystidium, Ichthyosporidium, Basidiobolus, Phoma, Candida, Cladosporium, Fusarium, Penicillium, Ichthyochytrium* spp, and others). Many of these organisms have questionable status as fungi and require laboratory culture of their complete life cycle for accurate diagnosis.

PARASITIC DISEASES

All of the major groups of animal parasites are found in fish, and apparently healthy wild fish often carry heavy parasite burdens. Parasites with direct life cycles are important pathogens of cultured and aquarium fish; parasites with indirect life cycles frequently utilize fish as intermediate hosts. Knowledge of specific fish hosts greatly facilitates identification of parasites with marked host and tissue specificity, while others are recognized because of their common occurrence and lack of host specificity. Knowledge of the key morphological features of major parasite groups aids greatly in diagnosis and treatment of parasitism. Examination of direct fresh smears that contain living parasites often is diagnostic.

PROTOZOAN PARASITES OF THE SKIN AND GILLS

CILIATES

One of the most common fatal infections of the skin and gills of fish is **"ich"** or **"white spot"** caused by *Ichthyophthirius multifiliis*. This round, ciliated protozoan is easily recognized by its large size (50 μm to 1 mm), horseshoe-shaped macronucleus, and constantly rotating motion. The young stages penetrate the mucous coat to the epidermis and gills, and feed on epithelial and blood cells extracted from the superficial capillaries. After reaching maturity, the organism leaves the host and sinks to the bottom of the aquarium or pond where it divides within a cyst-like structure, producing 500-1000 tomites (a small, potentially infective stage). Sudden mortality may be the first evidence of disease. In more chronic infections, resistance to infection is manifest by skin inflammation and development of localized granulomas, which increase in size and enclose the parasite. The encysted organisms can be seen as white spots on the surface of the fish. If the gills are involved, respiratory distress may occur. The disease can be prevented by avoiding infective material (carrier fish; contaminated water, plants, or ornaments). If the fish are tolerant of higher temperatures, the best treatment is to raise the water temperature to 86°F (30°C). Increased aeration helps protect fish during increases in water temperature. Although no drug can safely penetrate and kill the encysted parasite in the skin, some commonly employed drugs kill the organism in the water. Only formalin has been approved by the FDA for treatment of ichthyophthiriasis in food fish. Treatment must conform to the recommended procedures and withholding period before marketing. Some commonly employed nonapproved drugs that kill the organism in water are: quinine hypochloride, 10 ppm; sodium chloride, 30,000 ppm; and nifurpirinol, 0.05-0.2 ppm. A vaccine for "ich" is currently being studied. The infective stages are short-lived, so that aquaria without fish for ≥3 days are safe. The marine form of "ich" is caused by a similar ciliate, *Cryptocaryon irritans*.

Chilodonella and *Brooklynella* spp are related freshwater and marine finfish pathogens, respectively. **Chilodonelliasis** is especially common in cyprinid fish (goldfish, barbs, and related species) and cyprinodont fish (killifish, guppies, swordtails, platys, and many other common aquarium species). Although the disease is found in virtually all species of freshwater aquarium fish, epidemics are observed most frequently in crowded aquaria and fishfarm ponds. The acute form primarily affects the gills and is characterized by sudden death without any prodromal signs. In more chronic forms, there may be respiratory signs, paleness, weakness, and uncoordinated swimming motions. Chronic forms also are characterized by generalized or patchy skin changes with increased mucus production. It can be diagnosed rapidly by demonstrating the causative agent in direct fresh smears of unfixed skin or gill. *Chilodonella* sp (50-70 μm) can be identified by its characteristic ciliate motility, flattened heart shape, and its distinctive organelles (protrusible, striped, basket-shaped cytostome, and rows of cilia).

Infected fish should be isolated since they remain carriers. The organism can be eliminated from the aquarium by emptying the tank and allowing it to dry completely. Reducing the density of fish stocks and increasing water flow may aid in prevention and control.

Formalin (*see* TABLE 1, p 987) is the only approved drug for treatment of chilodonelliasis in food fish and hatcheries. A commonly used, but unapproved, drug for aquarium fish is acriflavine at 10 ppm in the water for 10 hr (some commercial establishments object to its use because it stains the water, aquarium, and objects in the tank). Salt (NaCl) can be used at 2000 ppm in freshwater aquaria for an indefinite period of time.

Trichodinids are peritrichous ciliates that include various finfish pathogens (*Trichodina, Trichodinella, Tripartiella, Vauchomia* spp, and others). These organisms are 40-100 μm long. Their bodies may be cylindrical, hemispherical, or discoid. Members of this group are characterized by an attaching disk with a horny corona of denticles on the adoral sucker surface. The most common trichodinid pathogen for marine or freshwater finfish is *Trichodina* sp. Microscopically, it is bell-shaped and can be observed swimming freely in direct smears of the skin and gills. When attached to tissues, *Trichodina* becomes flattened as the adoral sucker compresses the organism to the surface. If on the gills in great numbers, it may produce respiratory embarrassment and death by limiting respiratory surfaces, especially with low oxygen tension in the aquatic environment. Increasing the rate of water flow and oxygen tension tends to overcome the anoxia. Formalin, at 200 ppm in the water for 1 hr, has been approved by the FDA for treatment of trichodinid infestations in food fish (salmonids, catfish, and bluegills). Since many aquarium fish are more sensitive to the drug, baths of 1 part of formalin to 4000 parts of water for 1 hr are recommended.

Tetrahymena corlissi is an important pear-shaped, 10-20 μm long protozoan pathogen of aquarium and pond fish. It has longitudinal rows of cilia and inconspicuous cytostomes. Although the organism can be found in direct smears from the skin surface of affected fish, it is capable of invading and reproducing in the deep muscular tissues and viscera. Disease outbreaks are associated with overstocking and excess nitrogenous wastes. Progressively developing areas of depigmentation and hemorrhages in the body wall associated with increased mortality are signs of the disease. No treatment has been reported. Prevention and control should be related to reducing stocking densities and organic content of the water.

FLAGELLATES

The parasitic dinoflagellates *Oodinium* and *Amylodinium* spp are responsible for "**velvet, rust, gold-dust,** or **coral disease**" in marine and freshwater aquarium fish, less commonly in pond fish. The pathogenic stages of the organism are pigmented, photosynthetic, nonflagellated, nonmotile algae that attach to and invade the skin and gills during their parasitic existence. When mature, these parasites give rise to cysts that contain numerous flagellated, small, free-swimming stages that are capable of initiating new infections. If the parasitic stages are abundant in skin and gill tissues, they can be detected grossly by altered skin pigmentation; hence, their common names. Gill infection is far more serious than skin infection. Progress of the disease can be delayed by reducing lighting, and by lowering temperature and organic loading of the aquarium. Treatments with drugs are limited to aquarium fish (not approved for food fish), and include copper sulfate at 0.5-1 ppm in aquarium water. Copper is extremely toxic and solubility rates may vary in specific environments. Treated fish should be observed carefully, and treatment discontinued if signs of toxicity appear. In contrast, methylene blue treatment, 5 ppm in aquarium water, is relatively safe, even for young fish.

Ichthyobodo (Costia) spp are some of the smallest (~15 × 5 μm) flagellated protozoan parasites of the skin and gills. They are flattened, pear-shaped organisms with 2 flagellae of unequal lengths. The organisms move in a jerky, spiral pattern, and can be identified easily in direct smear preparations of the diseased skin or gill. The affected skin often has a steel-gray discoloration. Acute signs of **costiasis** are those of hypoxia, with fish flashing to the surface frequently. In chronic cases, fish appear weak and thin, and are off feed. The disease affects aquarium, pond, and marine fish. It can be controlled by increasing rate of flow and oxygenation of water. One of the most common treatments for aquarium fish is dips of 500-2000 ppm of glacial acetic acid for 30-60 sec.

INTERNAL PROTOZOAN PARASITES

Hexamita, Octomitus, and *Spironucleus* spp are common, small (~9 × 4 μm), bilaterally symmetrical, flagellated (4 pairs), protozoan parasites. These organisms are similar, but differ slightly in the position and shape of their nuclei (2 within one organism). They can be found in great numbers in the intestinal tract, skin lesions, or degenerating soft tissues of finfish, but their pathogenicity is variable. Some are normal inhabitants of the body cavities of finfish; others are associated more frequently with debilitating diseases in young fish and chronic ulcerative skin lesions ("hole in the head") of older aquarium fish. Infected fish remain carriers, and the water in which they are kept remains contaminated. Metronidazole at 10,000 ppm in the feed for 5 days, or 2-amino-5-nitrothiazole at 2000 ppm for 3 days, are recommended for treatment of aquarium fish, but are not approved for food fish.

Cryptobia and *Trypanosoma* spp are slender, elongated, actively motile, biflagellated protozoa, 6-20 μm long, and are easily detected in fresh blood and tissue smears of both marine and freshwater finfish. *Trypanosoma* have a well-developed undulating membrane, *Cryptobia* do not. Blood forms are considered pathogenic; those found in the intestinal tract are not. Signs of disease usually are inapparent, although inappetence, emaciation, and circulatory disturbances are reported. The disease can be prevented by removing leech infestations in finfish.

SPOROZOANS

Coccidiosis, while common in freshwater or marine finfish, is rarely diagnosed in live fish. Many species of finfish are affected. The life cycles of many fish coccidia are unknown, and some involve >1 host to complete their development. In addition to intestinal infection, the internal organs also are commonly affected; sporulated *Eimeria*-like oocysts and sexual and asexual stages commonly are found in direct smears and histological sections of the internal organs. Sulfamethazine, at 22-24 g/100 kg of fish wt/day in the feed for 50 days at 50°F (10°C), is used to treat food fish (21-day withdrawal time) in some countries. For aquarium fish, 10 ppm in the aquarium water once a week for 2-3 wk is prophylactic.

The **myxosporidia** are common fish parasites. The myxosporidian spore consists of 2 valves, a suture line, and 1-4 polar capsules that contain coiled, extensible filaments and an infective central body called the sporoplasm. Evidence suggests that these organisms have indirect life cycles and employ other aquatic organisms such as annelids as intermediate hosts. Hence, myxosporidial infections are more common in, and more pathogenic for, wild fish or fish reared intensively in outdoor fish ponds. The organisms tend to be host- and tissue-specific. Accordingly, expression of the disease is related to the specific pathogen and host. *Myxosoma cerebralis*, an important pathogen of young salmonids, produces skeletal deformity by infecting the cartilaginous structures. Nervous signs and abnormal pigmentation accompany the skeletal alterations. Recovered fish remain carriers and adults do not show signs. The disease can be prevented by purchasing uninfected breeding stock and maintaining them in an environment free of the intermediate hosts. *Ceratomyxa* infects the musculature and visceral organs of salmonids.

Many species of myxosporidians produce nodular or cystic lesions in the skin, gills, muscle, or visceral organs of fish, depending on their host species and tissue preference. *Henneguya* is found commonly in white, cystic skin lesions of cultured channel catfish and aquarium fish; it is easily identified by the "forked-tail" appendage of the spore observed microscopically. If ponds are dried and limed heavily, infection can be eliminated, apparently by reduction of the intermediate hosts. Aquarium infection can be self-limiting in the absence of intermediate hosts.

Renal dropsy of goldfish is a specific myxosporidian (*Sphaerospora auratus*) infection of pond-reared goldfish, characterized by renal degeneration and ascites. It usually is diagnosed by identification of spores in histological sections of the kidney. Newly purchased pond-reared goldfish placed in aquaria may show signs of the disease with mortality. No practical treatment is available. The **carp-dropsy complex** is a disease of carp and goldfish characterized by dropsy and exophthalmia. It is associated with *Sphaerospora angulata* infection and may be complicated by viral infections, such as spring viremia of carp or carp swim-bladder disease, or bacterial septicemias. Mortalities may be acute or occur over a 6-mo period. The response to drug treatment is generally poor.

Microsporidians are tiny, intracellular, spore-forming organisms with single polar filaments that are common host- and tissue-specific parasites of finfish. They also are capable of infecting helminth parasites of fish. The spores are extremely resistant. Golden shiners (baitfish) frequently are affected with *Pleistophora*, which are transmitted congenitally. Aquarium infection with *Pleistophora* and *Nosema* spp also is common in certain species of aquarium fish, eg, "**neon-tetra disease**". Affected fish appear pale. The spores are easily detected microscopically in direct smears of affected organs as masses of opaque, dense, tiny, oval or round bodies that rupture from affected host cells. No successful treatment is known. Infected fish should be removed, and disease-free stock should be placed in uninfected environments.

Proliferative kidney disease (PKD) affects salmonid fish; renal lesions are attributed to an unclassified myxosporean agent. PKD is characterized by proliferation of the renal hematopoietic and fibrous tissues. No treatment has been described. Avoidance is the best preventive measure, although losses may be minimized by reduced disturbance and enhanced husbandry. Infected stocks in nonendemic areas should be depopulated, premises should be sanitized, and disease-free stock obtained for replacement.

HELMINTHIASIS

Helminths are common in both wild and cultured fish. Fish frequently serve as intermediate or transport hosts for larval parasites of many animals, including man. Helminths with direct life cycles are most important for dense populations, and heavy parasite burdens are common in aquarium or cultured fish.

Monogenetic trematodes, which have direct life cycles, are common, highly pathogenic, obligatory parasites of the skin and gills. They are ~0.1-0.8 mm long and are best seen microscopically. The worms can be identified by their characteristic hold-fast organ, the haptor, which is armed with large and small hooks. Aquarium and cultured fish are subject to a rapid buildup of parasites by continuous infection and worm transfer to other fish in the tank or pond. Although many species are host-specific, the more common types observed in aquariums are less selective. The 2 most common genera are *Gyrodactylus* and *Dactylogyrus*: the former give birth to living young, which can be seen within the body of the adult worm, and frequently are skin parasites; the latter lay eggs and are principally parasites of the gills. Infected fish show hyperactivity and erratic swimming, often flashing above the water surface or rubbing the sides of their bodies against an object in the aquarium to dislodge the worms. Fish become pale as colors fade. They breathe rapidly and distend their gill covers, exposing swollen pale gills. Localized skin lesions appear with scattered hemorrhages and ulcerations. Mortality may be high. To prevent the disease, introduction of infected fish should be avoided. Treatment must be started early to be successful. Formaldehyde, up to 200 ppm in water for 1 hr, is the only drug approved for use in food fish. This can also be used in aquarium fish; however, doses should be reduced to 25 ppm due to the greater sensitivity of some species. Organophosphates (eg, trichlorfon at 0.25 ppm) in the water for 1 wk have been employed for aquarium fish, but are not approved by the FDA. Marine infections (*Benedinia* and *Microcotyle*) can be controlled by dipping infected fish into freshwater for 1-5 min, depending on the tolerance of the aquarium fish.

Digenetic trematodes have complicated life cycles, with several larval stages that infect one or more hosts. With rare exceptions, the first intermediate host is a mollusc, without which the life cycle generally cannot be completed. A diagnosis usually can be established by gross or microscopical examinations that reveal the cercarial, metacercarial, or adult worm in any of the tissues or body cavities of the fish. Fish tend to encyst the parasites by forming pigmented tissue encapsulations around the trematode. Depending on the color of the cysts in the skin, the condition is called **black, white,** or **yellow spot disease.** Heavily parasitized fish often are weak, thin, inactive, and feed poorly. Treatment is not recommended.

Tapeworms in both the larval and adult forms are common in fish. Larval forms encyst in visceral organs and muscle, while adults usually are found in the intestinal tract. Aquatic crustacea are the most common intermediate host for fish; accordingly, wild and cultured pond fish may be heavily infected. *Diphyllobothrium latum*, the broad fish tapeworm infection of man, is acquired by eating larval tapeworms in the flesh of food fish. Aquarium fish may be purchased with heavy cestode infections, but have limited exposure once in the aquarium, unless fed infected intermediate hosts. There is no safe, effective treatment for larval tapeworm infections. Fish can be treated for adult tapeworms by feeding di-n-butyl tin oxide at 250 g/kg of fish for 3 days; however, it is not approved for use in food fish.

Acanthocephala (thorny-headed worms) are common in wild fish, both as larval tissue stages, or as adult intestinal parasites. They are more common in salmonid and marine fish. Arthropods are the first intermediate host. Adult acanthocephala are easily recognized by their protrusible proboscis, armed with many recurrent hooks.

Nematodes are common in wild fish that are exposed to the intermediate hosts. Fish may be definitive hosts for adult nematodes or they may act as transport or intermediate hosts for larval nematode forms (anisakids, eustrongylids, and others) that infect higher vertebrate predators, including man. Encysted or free nematodes can be found in almost any tissue or body cavity of fish. Some are grossly visible on the body, face, tail, or fin surfaces in the subcut. tissues as coiled or extended worms that contrast with the surrounding tissues by their shape, color, and movement. Aquarium and cultured pond fish may be heavily infected if crustacean intermediate hosts are present. *Cyclops* and *Daphnia* spp are common intermediate hosts for *Philometra* sp, a nematode that is pathogenic for guppies and other aquarium fish. These blood-red worms can be seen in the swollen abdominal cavity and protruding from the anus of affected fish (**red worm disease**). *Capillaria* spp are commonly found in aquaria fish, and heavy infections may be harmful.

In addition to being parasitic blood suckers, **leeches** can transmit blood parasites of fish (eg, *Trypanosoma, Cryptobia,* and haemogregarines); they can produce a debilitating anemia due to chronic blood loss and disease. Leech infestations are most common in wild fish, but aquarium and pond infestations can occur by introduction of infested fish, plants, etc. Trichlorfon (0.5-1 ppm in aquarium water) is effective but is not approved for use in food fish. Avoidance of leeches and depopulation of infested aquarium fish are methods of prevention.

COPEPODS

Some copepods, during specific stages of their complicated life cycle, are obligatory parasites of finfish. They lose their copepod form, including their appendages, and become rod- or sac-like structures specifically adapted for piercing, holding, feeding, and reproducing. Grossly, they appear as barb-like attachments to the skin or gills, where they feed on blood and tissue fluids. They are capable of causing hemorrhage, anemia, and tissue destruction, as well as providing a portal of entry for other pathogens. Many different species of these parasites can be found on freshwater and marine fish. The anchor worms, *Lernea* spp, are commonly found in a wide variety of aquarium- and pond-reared fish, including goldfish and other cyprinids. *Ergasilus* spp are common gill parasites. Lice (*Branchiura*) are related to the parasitic copepods and have flattened bodies that are adapted for rapid movement over the skin surface. By means of hooks and suckers, they periodically attach for feeding by inserting the piercing mouth part (stylet) into the skin. *Argulus* spp are lice commonly found on aquarium, pond-reared, and wild fish.

Trichlorfon at 0.25 ppm of aquarium water is the drug of choice for treating infested fish but is not approved for use in food fish. Infested fish should not be introduced.

VIRAL DISEASES

Fish virology is a relatively new science. Viral diseases of economically important cultured fish have received the greatest attention. While viruses of higher homeothermic animals are cultured at uniform temperatures, fish viruses have a wider, but specific, temperature tolerance in fish cell cultures at lower temperatures. Because of the relatively defined temperature range, variation in temperature may enable control, although often it merely induces latency. Because many viral diseases of fish are geographically limited, regulatory agencies and fish farms in disease-free areas recognize them as exotic diseases and require certification of introduced stocks. Many produce high mortality in young fish and little or no losses in adults, which may become carriers. For these reasons, avoidance of carriers, and certification of SPF replacement stocks frequently are required. Specific testing procedures are available. Vaccines are not yet commercially available and drugs are not effective. Drugs and antibiotics are employed to control secondary bacterial infections that frequently follow viral diseases.

Channel catfish virus disease is an acute, virulent herpesvirus infection of fry and fingerlings that often causes mortality of >80% at water temperatures ≥77°F (25°C). There is evidence of vertical transmission. Signs are ascites, exophthalmia, and hemorrhages in fins. Originally known only from the southern USA, the virus has been transported as far west as California and as far south as Central America. It is isolated readily in cell cultures from members of the freshwater catfish family. It induces syncytia and intranuclear inclusions. Serum neutralization is used for identification.

Herpesvirus disease of salmonids is a viscerotropic infection of young rainbow trout and kokanee salmon in the USA. It requires temperatures ≤50°F (10°C) to develop, and death occurs ~1 mo after infection. The virus produces anemia, exophthalmia, and ascites; mortality is ≥50%. It is isolated readily in salmonid cell cultures and produces syncytia and intranuclear inclusions. Identification is presumptive and based on cell culture changes.

Herpesvirus disease of turbot is a condition of wild and cultured turbot that causes massive hypertrophy and fusion of epithelial cells of the skin and gills of young fish. Mortality is associated with heavy gill infections and poor water quality. High levels of oxygenation are essential for such fish with respiratory distress. Diagnosis is by examination of skin scrapings or histological sections for the characteristic fusion of giant cells.

Infectious hemopoietic necrosis is an acute rhabdovirus infection of salmonids that is vertically transmitted and, at a temperature of ≤54°F (12°C), produces high mortality in fry and fingerlings. Affected fish darken, have pale gills and exophthalmia, and shed thick fecal pseudocasts. Renal hemopoietic and excretory tissues are necrotic, as are pancreatic acinar cells and granular cells of the intestinal stratum compactum. The virus is readily grown in various fish cells, if incubated at ≤59°F (15°C). Identification is by the serum neutralization test.

Infectious pancreatic necrosis (IPN) is an acute systemic contagious disease of salmonid fry and fingerlings caused by a birnavirus. Reported worldwide, it is vertically and horizontally transmitted, is widespread, and produces the greatest mortalities in young trout (fry and fingerlings). The disease is either subclinical or inapparent in older salmonids, which may act as carriers. It is one of the most common fish viruses in the aquatic environment and exists as multiple strains that vary in virulence and serological responses. IPN-like viruses have been isolated from other animals, including molluscs and crustaceans. Symptomatic fry and fingerlings exhibit whirling about their long axis and may have a whitish exudate (but no food) in their stomachs and intestines. Pancreatic acinar cells and intestinal mucosal cells show severe cytolytic necrosis. Most fish cell lines are susceptible, and the virus is identified by serum neutralization, FA, complement fixation, and ELISA tests.

Pike fry rhabdovirus disease is an acute hemorrhagic infection of young northern pike, thus far known only in Europe. Affected fry have pale gills, exophthalmia, and hydrocephalus. Kidney tubules show degeneration and necrosis. The causal agent is readily isolated in a variety of cell cultures. Identification is by the serum neutralization test.

Spring viremia of carp is an acute, virulent, usually hemorrhagic disease of cultured carp caused by a rhabdovirus. It can cause death in adults as well as in the young. Affected fish lose motor control, have ascites, and show petechiation of the skin, gills, and visceral mass. This disease is known to occur only in Europe and the USSR. The virus is readily isolated on common fish cell lines and identified by serum neutralization and FA tests. It forms part of the carp-dropsy complex (qv, p 994). Prophylaxis against possible secondary aeromonad infections, which often are responsible for high mortality, may be achieved by IP injection of oxytetracycline at 1.5 mg/100 g of fish body wt, just before the spring temperature rise and outbreaks of the disease are anticipated. Also, the drug can be administered in the feed at 60 mg/kg of fish wt per day for 10 days (withdrawal time 21 days).

Viral hemorrhagic septicemia (Egtved disease) is an acute, virulent disease of rainbow trout of all ages, caused by a rhabdovirus; it is found in Europe. Typical outbreaks occur at water temperatures ≤50°F (10°C). Affected fish become dark and show exophthalmia and severe anemia due to the petechial or more extensive hemorrhages that can develop, particularly within the abdomen and musculature. There is necrosis of the liver and renal, hemopoietic, and excretory tissues. Cell culture isolations are made at ≤59°F (15°C), and identification is by a serum neutralization test.

Lymphocystis disease is a unique, typically chronic, viral infection of many wild or captive marine and freshwater species. It results in development of benign growths that are characteristically external and composed of enormously hypertrophied dermal fibroblasts. Feulgen-positive cytoplasmic inclusions and a hypertrophied nucleus are pathognomonic. The causal agent is an icosahedral DNA virus ~300 nm in diameter, of the same group (Iridoviridae) as African swine fever virus.

Viral erythrocytic necrosis (VEN, PEN) is a recently recognized blood dyscrasia of salmon, herring, cod, and other marine species. RBC show a cytoplasmic inclusion, karyorrhexia, and icosahedral virions—presumably DNA. The impact on the host is deleterious. The agent has not been isolated but is suspected to be a member of the Iridoviridae.

Fishpox is a term applied to diseases of fish characterized by pox-like skin lesions. These diseases are not caused by poxviruses, but are associated with a herpesvirus infection. Carp are affected most commonly, and their skin lesions typically appear as benign, non-necrotizing, epidermal, hyperplastic, circumscribed skin elevations. Many other species of fish evidence similar lesions that appear to be associated with herpesvirus-like infections. Walleyes manifest similar lesions associated with a herpesvirus infection; however, other viral infections have been described in walleyes. The latter include **walleye dermal sarcoma virus** and **epidermal hyperplasia retrovirus** infections.

A number of viruses have been isolated from eels. These include several strains of rhabdoviruses of questionable pathogenicity, isolated from both diseased and apparently normal eels. An orthomyxovirus-like agent has been isolated from eels with stomatopapillomas (**cauliflower disease**). A birnavirus (Eel Virus European), serologically related to IPN, has been isolated from cultured European, Taiwanese, and Japanese eels. The virus produces an acute virulent disease characterized by lesions of the kidney and other visceral organs. Japanese eel iridovirus has been isolated from diseased cultured immature (leptocephali and elvers) Japanese eels.

NUTRITIONAL DISEASES

Although different species of fish vary as to their food requirements, there is a remarkable similarity to higher vertebrates in terms of protein, energy, and vitamin requirements. Wild fish exhibit fewer signs of dietary deficiencies than do cultured food fish or aquarium fish. Wild fish have a greater variety of foods, while cultured or aquarium fish consume formulated diets of restricted ingredients that may be subject to spoilage, commonly including fat rancidity. Many of the observed nutritional diseases of fish are complex and do not result from single deficiencies. They may be expressed in composite generalized signs of anemia, skeletal deformities, nervousness, poor growth, and retrograde changes in internal organs. Therapy should be directed toward general dietary improvements. Some of the specific changes associated with pure vitamin deficiencies in finfish are as follows: Vitamin A deficiency produces poor growth and retinal atrophy. Acute thiamine deficiency results in convulsions and death; chronic deficiencies result in loss of equilibrium, edema, and poor growth. Riboflavin deficiencies are characterized by vascularization of the cornea, hyperpigmentation, and clouding and hemorrhage of the eyes. Pantothenic acid deficiency is associated with gill disease. Niacin, biotin, and pyridoxine deficiencies are responsible for nervous signs, such as spasms and convulsions. Choline, inositol, and folic acid deficiencies are associated with poor growth. Ascorbic acid deficiencies produce skeletal deformities, including lordosis and scoliosis. Vitamin E deficiencies are related to myopathies, including muscular deformities. Similiar muscular lesions are related to dietary fat rancidity and selenium deficiencies.

The National Academy of Sciences (USA) has published the nutritional requirements for trout, salmon, catfish, warmwater fishes, and aquarium fish.

MISCELLANEOUS NONINFECTIOUS DISEASES

Much emphasis has been given to monitoring wild fish populations for detection of toxic pollutants. According to many sources, the industrial and domestic production of sulfur dioxide fumes from the combustion of fossil fuels has been responsible for acid rain and the resultant high mortalities in fish in natural bodies of water. The formation of toxic aluminum compounds in acid waters also has been incriminated as a cause of fish morbidity and mortality. The discharge of many toxic substances into natural waters has resulted in fish kills; some pollutants are being investigated as carcinogens because of a high incidence of tumors in fish in defined bodies of water, both marine and freshwater. Higher incidences of tumors have been found in bottom-dwelling species and are thought to be related to carcinogens in the sediment. **Ulcerative dermatitis** and **fin and tail rot** have been described in marine fishes such as flounder, salmon, sea trout, and others. Although aquatic pollutants have been incriminated, the etiology of these conditions remains obscure.

Cultured, pond-reared food fish also are subject to environmental pollutants due to such factors as industrial pollutants, fertilizers, pesticides, road salt, and other run-offs from surface drainage into fish ponds. Aquarium fish also have environmental problems due to accidental or intentional introduction of toxic substances, including drugs for medication, disinfectants, soaps, and aerosol sprays.

As indicated, feed intoxications of fish are commonly due to spoilage and rancidity. A dramatic food intoxication is **aflatoxicosis,** which results from ingestion of fish feeds contaminated with aflatoxin produced by *Aspergillus flavus.* Other toxin-producing molds can produce similar intoxication. Rainbow trout and other salmonids are particularly susceptible to aflatoxicosis, which results in the induction of rapidly growing hepatomas and high mortality.

Pansteatitis and **swim-bladder thickening** due to toxic cottonseed in fish meals incorporated in a diet low in vitamin E have been reported to be associated with high mortality in cultured fish. Contaminated binders, used in making pelleted fish feeds, and salt contamination have been reported. The latter may result from errors in feed formulation or from contamination with seawater during storage. Heavy metals, plastics, oil, phenolic compounds, and other organic substances have been reported to be toxic for fishes. Fish are commonly employed for bioassays of such toxic substances, and have become standard laboratory animals for this purpose.

Neoplastic diseases similiar to those found in other animals are found in fish. Their incidence frequently is higher in some geographic areas and in certain species of fish. Some tumors are genetically mediated, such as the malignant melanoma of the gypsy-swordtail cross, and possibly the pseudobranch tumor of cod, thyroid tumors, malignant lymphosarcoma of northern pike, and fibromas or sarcomas of goldfish. Sharks, skates, and rays have a reported low incidence of tumors.

Coloration anomalies and **yolk-sac anomalies** or deformities are common in cultured fish and may be of genetic or environmental origin. For example, blue-sac disease, a condition of larval rainbow trout, is believed to be associated with unsuitable hatchery water, and pseudoalbinism in cultured flatfish, with excess light levels shortly after hatching.

Sunburn can occur in surface swimming fish or can be induced even in bottom dwellers by feeding photodynamic drugs such as phenothiazine, although ultraviolet light penetrates water poorly.

Nephrocalcinosis and **visceral granuloma** are found particularly in salmonid culture, induced supposedly by a high level of carbon dioxide in the water; this produces a metabolic acidosis, and urinary and tissue precipitation of calcium, around which extensive granulomata develop.

MANAGEMENT AND DISEASES OF CAGED BIRDS

In part because birds appear to compensate well for organic dysfunction, and in part because bird owners tend to be less knowledgeable about their pets than are dog or cat owners, frequently disease is advanced in caged birds when they are first noticed to be ill. Fortunately, preventive medicine is becoming more important in avian practice, with "new bird" examinations or routine procedures aiding in the education of the owner. Also, pet retailers are taking advantage of comprehensive veterinary programs in increasing numbers.

Transport, mixing or crowding, inadequate heat or excessive air conditioning, and poor nutrition are common stresses associated with clinical problems in the recently acquired bird. Infectious disease is the most frequent expression of such stress, particularly since groups of birds are often housed and fed under contaminated conditions. Neoplastic and nutritional diseases and trauma are more common in established pets. The increased use of diagnostic aids, including clinical pathology and radiology, and advances in microsurgery and anesthesiology are rapidly raising the level of expertise in avian medicine. Knowledge of basic husbandry and careful nursing techniques contribute greatly to success in this expanding field.

History: The bird should be brought in its own cage for critical examination of the environment, food, and droppings. Cold weather is a frequent excuse for reluctance in bringing a pet bird to a clinic. Exposure to cold air can be avoided easily by wrapping the cage in a large blanket. Some owners also have reservations about the handling or examining of a sick bird, but inadequate treatment at home may be more harmful than stress encountered in the clinic.

When evaluating a bird, history should include how long it has been with the present owner, as much information as possible about its source(s), and history of other birds in the owner's collection. Careful questioning and examination of seed debris are necessary before drawing conclusions about nutrition. Feed offered to a bird by way of seed types, vitamin supplements, mineral sources, etc, is not necessarily the same as what is actually eaten. Most illnesses are described by owners as "sudden" because feathers effectively mask even severe emaciation or abdominal distention. Also, some birds continue to eat (or simulate eating behavior) even when close to death.

Physical Examination: Sick birds do not tolerate long handling times well; any drugs or diagnostic procedures should be anticipated, and all items ready for immediate use. A strong light source, gram scale, and magnification device are basic equipment. Safety for the handler usually requires use of one or more towels for restraint of larger birds (cockatiels and larger). Extra assistance also shortens handling times.

External surface, respiratory rate, movements, and behavior must be noted before handling, as these are altered once the bird is caught. Perches should be carefully removed from the cage before capture. Darkening the room facilitates the capture of small birds and reduces stress associated with a chase. Once caught, most birds are best held in a towel, with the base of the lower mandible or beak used to control movements of the head. Wings and feet must be restrained, but the chest left free for respiration. Smaller birds such as parakeets may be held without a towel, but the head must be controlled to avoid painful bites. Physical condition should be assessed first. Feet should be held carefully when examining chest or abdomen (or when giving IM injections), as they are often strong and capable of a great range of movement. If the bird is ataxic in the cage, and thin and weak in hand, it can tolerate little additional stress; a short examination and tentative diagnosis are obviously preferable to death during a thorough examination.

Eyes, nostrils, external ear openings, beak, and oral cavity (mouth can be opened using gauze strips, or "teased" open by tapping on upper mandible) should be examined. The crop must be palpated to detect thickening or foreign bodies (bird should be held upright during this procedure). Evidence of vomitus can be seen as dried mucus on the feathers above the nostrils, on the forehead, and sometimes at the sides of the mouth. A nasal discharge also stains feathers above the nostrils. The sternum should be traced from upper to lower end to check for deviations. Body condition can be assessed by palpating the pectoral muscles. Normal birds should have musculature that is somewhat convex in relation to the keel. Accurate weighing of the bird is recommended and is essential for monitoring an illness. The abdomen of most birds in dorsal recumbency is distinctly concave, and the pubic bones are easily felt just in front of the vent. The vent is examined, then the feet, legs, and wings. Fractures of the proximal long bones (humerus, femur) may be found more easily if joints are palpated while moving the limb. Feathers may mask swelling or discoloration, but crepitus and fracture movement are often detected during careful manipulation. Alcohol, if applied in moderation, is helpful in visualizing abnormalities normally hidden by feathers. Plucking may tear delicate skin if not performed cautiously. The back and the uropygial gland also should be examined.

Routine Procedures: Until recently, vaccines for pet birds have not been commonly available. Vaccines for parrotpox (qv, p 1009) and Pacheko's disease (qv, p 1008) have now been introduced to the market.

Wing clipping is a frequent request from owners. It can be a taming aid and prevent loss of birds allowed outside the cage. Owners should be warned about unexpected flight after the wing clip, particularly outside in a breeze. Clipping all of the primaries on both wings is frequently done, as any "outside" primaries left tend to become unsightly through wear and breakage. It may be best to clip only the 8 primaries, from the outside inward. Unilateral wing clips may result in unpredictable falls or flights. Pin feathers (growing feathers) must not be cut, or hemorrhage results. Pin feathers are frequently bitten or broken by the bird, and immediate removal by pulling out the remaining quill and applying pressure until the bleeding stops is the best treatment.

Nail trimming is often requested and generally easy to do. Silver nitrate or similar hemostatic agents should be available for application, with pressure, to a bleeding nail bed. Hobby drills with sanding bits are good for use on macaws and cockatoos. They are also excellent for corrective beak trimming, but should be sterilized between trims. Because normal birds rarely require beak trims, requests for such may well be an indication of pathology.

Many birds are leg banded, either for individual identification or to indicate a proper quarantine history. Bands present certain hazards to the bird, but removal also entails some risk. Open (gap present), rolled, steel rings are extremely strong and generally require a full-size bolt cutter. Caution is indicated lest a projectile piece of metal injure operator or spectator, and obviously, care is needed to avoid injuring the bird. Aluminum bands should be stabilized with hemostats and then cut with side-cutters or pin-cutters.

Hematology and blood chemistry are especially important in birds, since physical examination tends to be less revealing than in other animals. A cleaned nail is the common blood collection site of the small bird (capillary tubes should be held horizontally to collect), although the (right) jugular vein is occasionally used. Hemostatics should always be used after collection attempts on nails even if blood flow appears to have stopped. TABLE 2 lists some guidelines for volumes that may be taken. In larger birds, usually blood is collected from the median ulnar vein (alcohol applied topically can reveal it as it crosses the inside of the elbow). Wing veins require careful hemostasis using local pressure. The medial tarsal vein of larger parrots is also sometimes used. Flushing a syringe with an anticoagulant before collection may be helpful.

Table 2. Recommended Maximum Amount of Blood that Can be Drawn from Common Avian Species

Finch (~10 g)	0.1 mL
Budgerigar (~30 g)	0.25 mL
Cockatiel (~85 g)	0.75 mL
Amazon (~400 g)	3 mL
Macaw (~950 g)	5 mL

Treatment Methods: IM injections are readily given into the pectoral muscles, although the use of alcohol for visualizing the site is highly recommended. Placing the needle at an acute angle and applying pressure following withdrawal minimizes hemorrhage. Subcut. injections are also simplified when the skin can be seen clearly. An insulin syringe (50 u or 0.5 mL) with a 27-gauge needle is invaluable in accurate dosing. IV injections are becoming more common in pet birds as the practice of bolus fluid administration becomes popular. Some common IV fluid volumes are listed in TABLE 3. Indwelling catheters (20-gauge needle with stylet) seated in the lateral, distal surface of the ulna are also becoming popular in avian medicine; intraosseous fluids are rapidly absorbed and easy to start. Crop-tubing (gavage) may be used to maintain hydration in selected birds. In small birds, a metal (ball-tipped) crop needle is gently lowered into the crop, or a very small blunt-ended stomach tube can be used. Extending the neck is the key to rapid entry into the crop, particularly in large birds. A speculum of some type should be used in large birds, or they may bite and swallow part of the stomach tube. The tube must not be forced as tissues are thin and fragile, especially in smaller birds. Crop tubes are easily palpable in the neck, and as the entry to the trachea is anterior, placement of the tube can be checked by looking in the mouth with a penlight.

Table 3. Initial Amounts of IV Fluids for Bolus Administration in Common Avian Species

Finch	0.5 mL
Budgerigar	1 mL
Cockatiel	2 mL
Amazon	8 mL
Macaw	12 mL

Oral medications may be given in some commercial feeds (impregnated millet, pellets, premixes for soft mash) or directly dosed into the mouth. Water medications are only indicated in special circumstances, as dosing, stability, and palatability factors make this route undesirable in most cases. Food and water treatments are effective only if ingested; therefore, close monitoring is essential.

Sedation is sometimes desirable for diagnostic or treatment procedures. Even severely ill birds can usually be safely anesthetized with ketamine IM (2-3 mg for a budgie, 6 mg for a cockatiel, 15 mg for a 450-g parrot), but the extremely rough recoveries tend to negate the safety advantages. Isoflurane anesthesia can safely sedate stressed or debilitated birds, and provides an extremely rapid recovery (premedications generally are not recommended).

Any severely ill bird benefits greatly from an increase in temperature and humidity. A warm environment can be created by wrapping clear plastic film (cling-wrap) around a cage except for the door, and placing the cage on an electric heating pad (all but one perch should be removed to facilitate future capture attempts). A household thermometer in the cage allows monitoring of the temperature. A quiet location is best, although anorectic birds may benefit if they can see other birds feeding.

BACTERIAL DISEASES

The gram-negative Enterobacteriaceae are common pathogens, although many are regarded as opportunists. *Escherichia coli, Serratia marcescens,* and *Salmonella, Klebsiella, Enterobacter, Proteus,* and *Citrobacter* spp are frequently isolated. Salmonellosis has been associated with African gray parrots (recently stressed). Other important gram-negative organisms include *Pasteurella, Pseudomonas, Aeromonas,* and *Acinetobacter* spp, *Mycobacterium avium,* and *M tuberculosis. Pasteurella* has been reported as a possible septicemic agent in birds attacked by pet cats or rats. Avian tuberculosis is a common problem in the gray-cheeked parakeet and other *Brotogeris* spp. Staphylococci and streptococci (especially hemolytic strains), and *Bacillus* spp also may be responsible for disease in psittacines. Staphylococci are often isolated from bumblefoot-like lesions of pet budgerigars or cockatiels. TABLE 4 lists some antibacterials frequently recommended for caged birds. Excess portions of reconstituted drugs are often stored frozen in syringes, although permissible storage times are unknown.

The GI flora of healthy psittacines is predominantly gram-positive (streptococci and *Staphylococcus epidermidis* with a variable number of *Bacillus* and *Lactobacillus* spp), but gram-negative bacteria predominate as pathogens. Stressed or diseased birds frequently shed potential pathogens such as *E coli,* although the exact clinical significance varies from case to case.

CHLAMYDIOSIS
(Psittacosis, Ornithosis)

A reportable, widespread, zoonotic disease, caused by *Chlamydia psittaci.* It is not limited to newly imported psittacines, but also is seen in breeding collections (especially cockatiels and budgerigars) and in birds sold from retail outlets. Birds can carry the organism for years before developing disease under stress. When possible, birds should be obtained from breeding establishments known to be free of infection.

Clinical Findings: Most have weight loss, depression, transient anorexia, chartreuse or lime-green urates, and loose feces; many are emaciated when examined. Respiratory signs are sometimes present and usually related to an airsacculitis. Psittacosis is frequently complicated by accompanying bacterial infections. WBC counts in affected birds are very high; 25-95 $\times$ 10^3/μL values are not uncommon. Normal WBC counts are <13 $\times$ 10^3/μL.

Diagnosis: Diagnosis is by isolation of the causative organism in chick embryos or by cell culture. Frankly ill birds usually shed the organism continually, and normal "contact" birds may do so intermittently. Diagnosis is aided by the direct complement fixation test: titers <1:8 are considered negative; 1:16, suspicious or equivocal; and those >1:16, positive. Titers usually remain elevated for an extended period after treatment. Testing by latex agglutination may prove helpful but is not yet widely available. ELISA-based tests for antigen in feces may be helpful, provided that the method used has been properly designed and evaluated. Specially stained impression smears of air sac, spleen, liver, and pericardium may reveal intracellular elementary bodies of chlamydia, and are aids in presumptive diagnosis, as are history, clinical signs, hematology, and radiography.

Table 4. Antibacterials Recommended for Use in Caged Birds*

Agent	Dosage	Route, Frequency, Duration
Amikacin sulfate	15 mg/kg	IM, b.i.d. × 7 days
Carbenicillin	150 mg/kg	IM, b.i.d. × 7-10 days
Cefotaxine sodium	100 mg/kg	IM, b.i.d. × 7 days
Chloramphenicol succinate	80 mg/kg	IM, b.i.d. × 7 days
Chloramphenicol palmitate	50 mg/kg	PO, t.i.d. × 7 days
Chlortetracycline premix, 100 g/lb	100 g/20 lb (9 kg) oral mash	sole food source
Chlortetracycline seeds	0.5% mg/g of seed (0.05%)	sole food source for 45 days
Chlortetracycline pellets	4-10 mg/g (0.4-1%)	sole food source for 45 days
Doxycycline suspension	50 mg/kg 25 mg/kg	PO, daily for macaws, cockatoos; PO, b.i.d. for others; all × 45 days
Doxycycline 20 mg/mL, injectable**	100 mg/kg	IM (divided) once weekly × 6 treatments
Enrofloxacin, oral or injectable	12 mg/kg	PO or IM, b.i.d., × 5 days
Gentamicin	10 mg/kg	IM, daily or b.i.d., × 5 days
Nitrofurazone (9.3% soluble powder)	1 mL/L	drinking water × 7-10 days
Oxytetracycline (6.2% soluble powder)	2 mL/L	drinking water × 7 days or more; change b.i.d. (unstable); no calcium source
Piperacillin	100 mg/kg	IM, b.i.d. × 7 days
Spectinomycin 50 mg/mL	5 mL/L	drinking water × 7-10 days
Trimethoprim/sulfamethoxazole, oral suspension	75 mg/kg	PO, b.i.d. × 7 days
Trimethoprim/sulfamethoxazole, injectable suspension	50 mg/kg	IM, b.i.d. × 7-10 days
Tylocine, soluble powder (tylosin tartrate)	1 mL/L	drinking water × 7-10 days
Tylocine, injectable	35 mg/kg	IM, b.i.d. × 5 days

* Most of these are unapproved (off-label) uses and caution is indicated.
**Not presently available in USA.

Lesions: Hepatomegaly, splenomegaly, air-sac changes (opacification, thickening, caseation), and fibrous pericarditis may occur. The liver may have necrotic areas with mixed inflammatory cell infiltrates and bile stasis. Inflammation tends to be suppurative if there is secondary bacterial infection. The air sacs are thickened by fibrinous exudate with mixed inflammatory cells; the lungs may be congested and edematous.

Transmission is primarily by inhalation of nasal exudates, expired aerosols, or fecal dust. Removal of food and water containers during cleaning operations, and attention to minimizing scatter of cage-bottom debris help minimize transmission.

Treatment and Control: Although chlortetracycline (CTC) in the feed of all imported psittacines during the 30-day quarantine is required by law in the USA, this may not eliminate all cases within a flock. Therapy includes CTC premix in food for 45 days (large psittacines), CTC-containing pelleted feeds, or hulled millet impregnated with CTC. Individual treatments with doxycycline (50 mg/kg body wt, PO, once daily) are extremely effective and avoid ''starve-outs'', but require 45 days of therapy. Tetracyclines such as oxytetracycline may be used (in a flock situation) in the drinking water until more effective forms of therapy can be instituted. Antibiotic in the water alone is not an effective cure if used as the sole method of treatment. Approved therapies in the USA include the CTC premix and CTC-impregnated millet.

MYCOTIC DISEASES

CANDIDIASIS

The causative yeast is *Candida albicans*. Young birds are most susceptible, although adults of some species (especially lovebirds) are also frequently affected. Prolonged antibiotic therapy, vitamin A deficiency, and spoiled feed are predisposing factors. Some consider the yeast to be part of the normal flora, but disease results when overgrowth occurs. (*See also* THRUSH, p 1562.)

The infection usually involves the crop mucosa; with secondary bacterial infection, it is a common cause of crop stasis and death in newborn psittacines. Affected birds are unthrifty, underweight, and may vomit; adults have increased appetites with concurrent weight loss. The crop is thickened and empties slowly in newborn birds; regurgitation may occur. There are raised, white lesions on the oral mucosa. If the yeast invades the intestinal mucosa, a malabsorption syndrome may develop. The eyes and lungs also may be affected. Diagnosis is based on culture and identification of the yeast.

Nystatin, ketoconazole, topical iodine, and supplemental vitamin A are effective treatments. *See also* TABLE 5.

ASPERGILLOSIS

A systemic fungal disease caused by *Aspergillus fumigatus*. It is common in raptors, penguins, and waterfowl but not among psittacines. When it does occur in the latter, it usually is associated with poor husbandry, stress, concurrent or previous illness, or immunodeficiency. Dusty or damp environments or exposure to moldy food or nesting material may increase the incidence. Transmission is by inhalation of spores. (*See also* p 1613.)

In psittacines, dyspnea of acute onset may occur, or a chronic debilitating disease complicated by one or more pathogenic bacteria may develop. In the acute form, findings may be limited to small caseous plugs within the distal trachea or small plaques on one or more of the air sacs, which may also appear thickened. In chronic cases, there is usually a visible fungal growth on the air sacs, often overgrowing onto the serosal surfaces of adjacent organs; other organs also may be involved.

Table 5. Antifungals for Use in Caged Birds: Dosage, Route, and Frequency

Agent	Dose	Route and Frequency
Amphotericin B	0.001 mg	Given intratracheally daily until asymptomatic, or can be nebulized, or a portion given IP
5-Flucytosine	0.25 mg	b.i.d. via gavage
Ketoconazole*	200-mg tablet	Pulverize and add to 1 qt (1 L) of water and give for 7-14 days
Nystatin oral suspension (100,000 u/mL)	1 mL/350 g body wt	PO, b.i.d. for 7 days
Nystatin premix (20 g/lb)	2 tsp/5 lb mash	Feed for 10-14 days

* For nystatin-resistant candidiasis, mix 0.2 mL of 1N HCl, 0.8 mL of water, and 50 mg of ketoconazole; dose PO, b.i.d. × 14 days: King parrots, 0.05 mL; Amazon parrots, 0.07 mL; umbrella cockatoos, 0.1 mL.

Transtracheal wash with culture and cytology, and laparoscopy afford a diagnosis. Radiography may aid in a presumptive diagnosis. Serology is unreliable. Aspergillosis should be considered when a respiratory disease has been refractory to therapy that was based on culture and antibiotic sensitivity testing.

Treatment may be rewarding in acute cases, but often is unsuccessful in chronic cases. Surgical debridement of air sacs has been described. Amphotericin-B (IV or IP) in combination with oral flucytosine or ketoconazole is helpful; nebulization also may be employed. Levamisole has been used as an immunostimulant. TABLE 5 lists some antifungals popular for use in caged birds. An autogenous vaccine has been used with some success.

PARASITIC DISEASES

See also POULTRY section, p 1541 *et seq.*

PARASITES OF THE INTEGUMENTARY SYSTEM

MALLOPHAGA

Various species of biting (chewing) lice parasitize many birds; aviary cockatiels and canaries are infested most commonly. Clinical signs are mild or absent; heavy infestations signal concurrent disease problems. Pyrethrin sprays or carbaryl powders, 1-2 applications 7-10 days apart, are usually effective treatments.

SCALY FACE (LEG) MANGE MITE

Cnemidocoptes (Knemidocoptes) pilae is common on budgerigars, rare on all other psittacines. Passerines also are parasitized, but have different clinical signs. Stress plays a role in the expression of both psittacine and passerine mange.

In budgerigars, white, porous, proliferative encrustations involving the corners of the mouth, cere, eyelids, and beak are typical. The beak may grow outward in an unusual fashion. In passerine birds (particularly the European goldfinch), long smooth crusts form on the plantar surfaces of the digits ("tassel foot"). The mites can be recovered from facial scrapings of budgies; interference with the base of any large crusts on passerines can result in hemorrhage and is not recommended.

Ivermectin at 200 μg/kg (0.2 μg/g [1-2 injections, 1-2 wk apart]) is usually curative. Mineral oil, used sparingly, hastens relief.

GRAY-CHEEKED PARAKEET MANGE MITE

Myialges (Metamicrolichus) nudus or *Megninia* sp are most frequently found on the gray-cheeked parrot. Either is presumed to be very contagious. Lesions tend to be limited to the head and neck; treatment with ivermectin (200 μg/kg) has been effective.

FEATHER MITES

Although the overall rate of infestation in caged birds is low, *Dermanyssus gallinae* (red mites) may be encountered in canaries and their young. Feather mites are a common complaint of psittacine owners as they frequently perceive a relationship between mites and feather picking. This is rarely the case; psychological or systemic disease factors are more often related to feather loss. Signs are restlessness (especially at night), anemia, and death. Diagnosis is by visual inspection and microscopical confirmation. Covering the cage at night with a white sheet and looking for mites the following morning on the underside of the cover aids in mite collection.

For individual birds, pyrethrin sprays or ivermectin have been effective treatments. For flocks, Vapona (dichlorvos) strips are sometimes used. The cage should be cleaned thoroughly (with close attention to cracks and crevices where mites hide during the day).

PARASITES OF THE RESPIRATORY SYSTEM

AIR SAC MITES

Sternostoma tracheacolum parasitizes the entire respiratory tract, most frequently of canaries and Lady Gouldian finches, rarely of psittacines. All stages of the mite are found within the respiratory tissues. The life cycle is poorly understood.

In mild infections, birds usually are asymptomatic; in heavy infections, audible dyspnea (high-pitched noises and clicking), tail bobbing, and open-mouth breathing are noted. Signs are exacerbated by handling, exercise, and other stresses. Mortality can be high.

Transillumination of the trachea in a darkened room occasionally reveals the presence of the mite. There may be absolute basophilia and/or eosinophilia. Response to treatment can also help in reaching a diagnosis, which is confirmed at necropsy.

For treatment, parenteral ivermectin (200 µg/kg) may be given twice, 1-2 wk apart. Subcut. or oral treatments are preferable to the IM route, particularly in finches.

GAPEWORM

Syngamus trachea (*see also* p 1614) sometimes parasitizes gallinaceous birds and passerines; it is extremely rare in caged birds.

PARASITES OF THE GASTROINTESTINAL SYSTEM

See also POULTRY section, p 1541 *et seq.*

GIARDIASIS

An intestinal protozoal disease, caused by *Giardia psittaci*, seen most often in aviary cockatiels and budgerigars. Unlike the disease in mammals, giardiasis may be fatal, particularly in nestling budgerigars; adult birds may be latent carriers. Transmission is presumably direct (ingestion of infective cysts).

Cockatiels exhibit intense feather pulling and vocalization, and the plumage appears oily. The droppings are light in color, increased in volume, and loose or pasty. Budgerigars have voracious appetites, but become anorectic and emaciated, and die. The changes in their droppings are similar to those seen in cockatiels.

Microscopical examination of a saline mount of fresh feces may reveal motile trophozoites. Since the presence of cysts is variable, serial tests are advised. A drop of Lugol's iodine solution added to the preparation aids in detection of the cysts.

Ipronidazole (0.5 g/gal. of drinking water [~125 mg/L], changed daily) as the sole source of drinking water for 7-14 days is an effective treatment. Dimetridazole has been used in drinking water to treat groups of birds (0.02-0.04% for 5 days); individuals can be intubated (0.05 mg/g, q12hr for 3 doses).

TRICHOMONIASIS

Trichomonas gallinae (*see also* p 1562) causes **frounce** (diptheritic membranes covering the oropharynx and sides of the mouth) in birds of prey and **canker** in columbiformes. It is occasionally seen in canaries, finches, and budgerigars.

White-yellow caseous lesions, well adherent to the mucosae of the oropharynx, crop, and esophagus, cause anorexia and dysphagia; weight loss and death result. Transmission is by direct (parents feeding young) or indirect contact (ingestion of contaminated food and water); raptors may become infected by ingesting infected pigeons or doves.

Microscopical examination of a saline mount of material from lesions reveals the flagellated organism.

Metronidazole (40-60 mg/kg, PO once daily for 5 days) is recommended for treatment.

OTHER PROTOZOAL DISEASES

Other protozoan parasites such as coccidia are much more common in gallinaceous or columbiform birds, although coccidial oocysts have been reported in budgerigars and some finches. Poultry water treatments are probably suitable for use in these species. Atoxoplasmosis is a highly pathogenic protozoal disease that causes hepatomegaly and splenomegaly in canaries, with coccidia-like oocysts being shed in the feces. (*see also* PARASITES OF THE HEMATOPOIETIC SYSTEM, below). Sarcocystosis has recently been diagnosed as a cause of mortality in parrots housed outdoors in the southern USA (exposure or contamination of food with opossum feces).

ROUNDWORMS

Psittacines (especially Australian parakeets and Amazon parrots) are the species most often parasitized by *Ascaridia* spp. Transmission is direct via ingestion of embryonated ova.

Clinical findings include loss of condition, weakness, emaciation, and death; intestinal obstruction is common in heavy infections. Diagnosis of intestinal nematode infection is by fecal flotation or necropsy. Levamisole (13.65% injectable) at 2 mL/L of drinking water for 3-5 days, repeated in 2 wk, has been recommended. Australian parakeets may be treated individually with ivermectin (200 μg/kg, subcut.) or mebendazole (gavage, 50 mg/kg, PO). These treatments are probably also effective for such parasites as *Capillaria* (crop worm) and *Spiroptera* (gizzard worm), although these are rarer.

CESTODES

Cestodiasis is most common in cockatoos, African gray parrots, and finches; tapeworms of the *Raillietina* and *Hymenolepis* spp are incriminated. Life cycles are indirect. Intermediate hosts are most likely insects of various types, earthworms, and slugs. Clinical signs are rarely present, but proglottids are sometimes recognized in the droppings of affected birds.

Niclosamide has been given at 250 mg/kg by gavage for psittacines, 500 mg/kg for finches, and repeated in 10-14 days. Praziquantel is effective at 0.85 mg/100 g body wt. Preventing access to intermediate hosts provides control.

PARASITES OF THE HEMATOPOIETIC SYSTEM

See also BLOOD-BORNE ORGANISMS, POULTRY, p 1544.

PROTOZOA

Imported cockatoos, birds of prey, and some types of passerines are most frequently parasitized by blood protozoa such as *Haemoproteus, Leucocytozoon, Plasmodium*, and *Atoxoplasma* spp.

Haemoproteus is commonly seen on blood smears from clinically normal cockatoos, and appears as an intraerythrocytic gametocyte that partially encircles the nucleus of the host cell. *Leucocytozoon* is a large intranuclear parasite that may inhabit RBC, and not WBC as the name suggests. It has a characteristic "winged" appearance on the blood smear. Treatment for these conditions is probably best directed at any concurrent disease, stress, or nutritional problems.

Plasmodium is a much more serious infection (malaria), best known for causing mortality in canaries, although psittacine deaths have been reported. Affected birds have hepatomegaly, splenomegaly, and depression; the intraerythrocytic gametocytes and schizonts can be seen next to the host nucleus. Treatment is difficult, but quinacrine hydrochloride at 250 mg/kg, PO (gavage), once daily for 5 days (repeated in 10 days) has been used.

The life cycles of these parasites are indirect, usually employing a mosquito or biting fly.

Less common blood parasites include *Atoxoplasma* (which is sometimes recognized as an intracytoplasmic inclusion in circulating lymphocytes), trypanosomes, and various microfilariae.

FILARIDS

Imported psittacines may harbor adult filarial worms (*Pelecitus* sp, *Paraprocta* sp, and others) in a number of locations (feet, air sacs, body cavity, connective tissue locations) and do not always show signs of illness. However, for swollen feet, hocks, or toes on South American species, filarid worms should be considered. Microfilariae may be seen in tissue or peripheral blood.

Treatment by surgical removal and/or ivermectin injection at 200 µg/kg (probably repeated in 2-3 wk) has been recommended.

VIRAL DISEASES

VISCEROTROPIC VELOGENIC NEWCASTLE DISEASE (VVND)

VVND (qv, p 1591), caused by a paramyxovirus, is a significant threat to the poultry industry. Various less pathogenic strains of the virus exist; a paramyxovirus group 3 infection has been reported in cockatoos and is suspected in other species. "Twirling" and "shaker" syndromes both have been linked with possible paramyxovirus group 3 in Australian grass parakeets, cockatoos, and finches. Cockatiels and cockatoos are highly susceptible to paramyxoviruses in general; Amazon parrots and conures are less so. Macaws, lories, African gray parrots, finches, and canaries are relatively resistant. Transmission is by respiratory aerosols, fecal contamination of food/water, direct contact with infected bird(s), and fomites.

Birds may be asymptomatic or die acutely. Signs include depression, anorexia, weight loss, sneezing, nasal discharge, dyspnea, conjunctivitis, bright yellow-green diarrhea, ataxia, head bobbing, and opisthotonos. In prolonged cases, uni- or bilateral wing and leg paralysis, chorea, torticollis, and dilated pupils also may be seen.

Lesions include hepatomegaly, splenomegaly, petechial or ecchymotic hemorrhages on serosal surfaces of all viscera and air sacs, airsacculitis, and excess straw-colored peritoneal fluid. Diagnosis is by virus isolation.

Only symptomatic treatment is possible and thus is not advisable: if suspected, VVND must be reported to authorities. Vaccination is prohibited in birds entering the USA because it does not eliminate the carrier state and hampers the detection of virus during quarantine.

PACHECO'S PARROT DISEASE

A highly contagious, acute disease of psittacines caused by a herpesvirus. It is associated with stress, which can cause healthy carriers to shed virus and initiate infection in susceptible birds. It is spread by direct contact, and aerosol or fecal contamination of food or water.

Amazon parrots, macaws, cockatoos, and a few conures, eg, peach-fronted, are highly susceptible. Morbidity in Asiatic and Australian parakeets is usually only sporadic. Most conures are relatively resistant. Nanday, Patagonian, and white-eyed conures may be natural hosts in the wild, and certain individuals among them may be asymptomatic shedders of the virus when stressed. Most of the other species probably can act as carriers.

Signs include acute death (carcasses well fleshed), bright yellow urates with scant feces, anorexia terminally, and visible icterus (some macaws). At necropsy, affected birds have an enlarged liver that may be mottled or have other color changes. Petechiae are sometimes found on the coronary band of the heart, the ventriculus, and the mesenteric fat. Edema of the mesenteric fat and ascites also occurs occasionally. Eosinophilic intranuclear inclusion bodies are found in the liver and spleen. Primary differentials are acute salmonellosis and psittacine reovirus. Reovirus infection is similar to herpesvirus hepatitis, but is better known for affecting African gray parrots, Timneh gray parrots, and cockatoos. No inclusion bodies are seen, and serology is used for diagnosis. No treatment is available for either disease, although IM injections of acyclovir have been used in a few herpes cases. The most prudent course of action is to immediately divide the flock into several smaller groups and house in separate rooms or buildings. Strict hygiene and preventing contamination of food and water are helpful. A new vaccine is available (conditional license in the USA) and has been recommended for the more susceptible parrot species in open breeding collections or flocks.

POX DISEASE

The most important poxviruses of pet birds are canarypox, parrotpox, agapornis pox (lovebirds), and pigeonpox.

Clinical Findings: Signs depend on host susceptibility and virulence of the virus. There are 3 clinical forms: 1) Cutaneous—discrete papules, pustules, or crusty scabs (depending on stage of infection) develop on unfeathered parts of the body. Mortality is low, and the infection usually is self-limiting. 2) Diphtheritic—extensive fibrinonecrotic lesions develop on mucous membranes of the oropharynx, upper respiratory tract, and esophagus (occasionally conjunctivae). Mortality is high. 3) Acute—onset of general signs, including depression, cyanosis, anorexia, and rapid death, is sudden. Transmission is by direct contact with infected birds or fomites, and insects may act as mechanical vectors.

Canarypox may occur in the acute form with respiratory signs and death in 1-3 days, or as a chronic infection with proliferative dermal lesions around the eyes, mouth, nostrils, or feet. The virus causes eosinophilic, intracytoplasmic inclusion bodies (Bollinger's bodies).

Parrotpox is common among Amazon parrots (especially blue-fronted), *Pionus* spp, lovebirds, Australian parakeets, and rosellas. Lovebirds are apparently susceptible to both parrotpox and agapornis pox. Poxvirus may cause high mortality in lovebirds.

Most signs involve the periocular tissues. Early in the course, unilateral blepharitis and conjunctivitis usually are present and lead to palpebral edema, which causes the affected eye to close; ulcers and scabs at the medial or lateral canthus follow. The serous ocular discharge becomes mucoid, and ocular lesions may develop (keratitis, ulcerative keratitis, anterior uveitis, possibly endophthalmitis). Scarring of eyelids and small opacifications of the cornea are common sequelae, although permanent damage is relatively minor compared to the original lesions. Dermal lesions include scaly papules at the commissures of the mouth, margins of the cere, and around or within the external nares. Superficial, raised plaques in the choanal area, at the base of the tongue, in the posterior pharynx, and within the esophagus also are seen. Anorexia, sneezing, dyspnea, and occlusion of nostrils may result. Death sometimes occurs and can be related to septicemia, pneumonia, or starvation. Secondary fungal infections are not uncommon.

Diagnosis: Diagnosis is by virus isolation and typical histological findings (epidermal hyperplasia with ballooning degeneration, intraepithelial vesicles, and eosinophilic intracytoplasmic inclusion bodies).

Treatment and Control: Parenteral vitamin A, ophthalmic ointments, heat, humidity, parenteral antibiotics, daily cleansing of the affected eye, and attention to diet is recommended. A vaccine for parrotpox has been released under conditional license in the USA, and may become a routine vaccination for such species as lovebirds or blue-fronted Amazons. Whenever such birds are boarded, or a new bird is brought into the household, they are at risk. Canarypox vaccine has been used for many years in Europe. Commercial pigeon- and fowlpox vaccines are not effective in psittacines, and conventional fowlpox vaccines do not protect chickens against parrotpox.

AVIAN INFLUENZA VIRUSES

Avian influenzas are caused by orthomyxoviruses. Hemagglutinating viruses are found often in passerine birds (especially African finches), but less frequently in psittacines. (*See also* p 1618.)

BUDGERIGAR FLEDGLING DISEASE

A viral syndrome (papovavirus-psittacine polyomavirus) best known for its role in psittacine nestling mortality, originally of budgerigars and now described with increasing frequency in newborn parrots. Although surviving budgerigar young often show feathering abnormalities, this syndrome may be distinct from classical "French moult". French moult is usually described as a delayed or abnormal eruption of wing and tail primaries in second-clutch budgerigar young, and has a possible association with another viral syndrome, psittacine beak and feather disease (*see* below).

Signs in affected nestlings include delayed feathering, diarrhea, dehydration, swollen abdomen/ascites, erythematous skin, subcut. hemorrhages, and death. High mortality is seen in birds 1-3 wk old. Growth of some feathers may be delayed in budgies that survive >2 wk; feathering may vary in survivors of other species but is usually normal. Asymptomatic adults may be carriers, and the infection possibly is egg-transmitted.

The kidneys and liver are enlarged and may be pale, congested, mottled, or have pinpoint white foci. Petechial or ecchymotic hemorrhages may be present, particularly on organs and in the subcut. tissues of the neck and trunk. The heart is enlarged, with hydropericardium, and the surface may possess multiple pinpoint white foci. Intranuclear inclusion bodies are seen in the liver, kidneys, heart, spleen, bone marrow, uropygial gland, skin, feather follicles, and elsewhere.

PSITTACINE BEAK AND FEATHER DISEASE (PBFD)

A debilitating disease that can be reproduced in cockatoos and budgerigars given homogenates of feather follicles from affected birds. Basophilic intracytoplasmic inclusions are found in follicular epithelium, and recently a small virus particle has been found.

Although principally a disease of cockatoos, many other psittacines with typical lesions have been reported. Classical "French moult" (*see also* p 1014) also has been linked with the virus. The natural infection appears to occur primarily in birds <5 yr old.

Typical findings include feather loss, abnormal pin feathers (constricted, clubbed, or stunted), abnormal mature feathers (blood in shaft), and varying degrees of beak abnormality. Beaks have been described as shiny, overgrown, broken, or with palatine necrosis. Birds may have feather lesions, beak lesions, or both; all lesions are progressive without treatment. Immunosuppression is part of the syndrome. Diagnosis is based on gross appearance of the bird and biopsies of affected feather follicles showing basophilic intracytoplasmic inclusions.

The contagious nature of PBFD and its probable terminal outcome warrant euthanasia in most cases. Strict hygiene, screening protocols, and lengthy quarantines are recommended highly in cockatoo breeding colonies. The removal of all eggs for cleaning and incubation may also be helpful.

NEOPLASTIC DISEASES

Many forms of cancer are common in pet birds; the most notable is renal adenocarcinoma in budgies, a leading cause of death in males. Lameness in a young male budgie with concurrent weight loss and a palpable abdominal mass are typical findings. Females occasionally develop renal tumors, but more often, a mass in a female bird is an ovarian tumor. Testicular tumors are also common in male budgies, and may produce changes in cere color.

Lameness caused by sciatic nerve pressure is not as common in gonadal tumors but does occur. Constipation and/or fecal pasting are seen in advanced cases. Radiographs are helpful in diagnosis (ventrally displaced ventriculus). These tumors rarely metastasize; microsurgery occasionally has been used in early cases. Radioactive implants (iodine 125) also have received some attention in experimental therapy. Most pet birds are treated with long-acting prednisolone (methylprednisolone, 1 mg/budgie, IM). Gonadal tumors are frequently cystic, and draining of fluid also provides some relief. Euthanasia is warranted in advanced cases.

Fibrosarcomas are often seen in pet birds, with an affinity for wings, legs, and face. Wing fibrosarcomas are best treated with amputation, as local invasion tends to preclude removal of the mass. Leg amputations tend not to have the same success.

Lymphosarcoma and avian leukosis-like syndromes are commonly reported in caged birds. Splenomegaly in canary flocks (with mononuclear infiltrates in liver and spleen) must be carefully distinguished from atoxoplasmosis.

NUTRITIONAL DISEASES

Calcium/Phosphorus/Vitamin D_3 Imbalance: Seed diets are well known for their problems with calcium (Ca) and phosphorus (P) metabolism. Sunflower seeds, which tend to be selected preferentially by most psittacines, are low in Ca and high in fat. Vitamin D_3 sources are also not always available in sufficient quantities to pet birds not receiving a supplement or varied diet. Removing sunflower seed and offering safflower seed, or even hulled sunflower seed, often promotes experimentation and expansion of diet.

Some well-known expressions of mineral inadequacies in pet birds include egg binding, acute hypocalcemia (especially African grays), and pathologic fractures/osteoporosis. Rickets and "splay-leg" are frequently seen in nestlings (especially doves, cockatiels, budgerigars) when their parents cannot provide them with correct nutrients. "Splay-leg" has also been linked to genetic and substrate factors.

Egg binding is occasionally related to problems other than insufficient Ca intake, but response to Ca therapy in many cases is dramatic. History usually indicates an acute collapse or weakness; females frequently go down on the floor of the cage, or they may support themselves against cage bars with the beak. Gentle palpation usually reveals an egg in the abdominal cavity. If radiographs must be used for diagnosis, Ca injections should be given first, as hypocalcemic birds rarely have well-calcified eggs. Immediate Ca therapy is recommended in any case, along with increases in temperature and humidity. Heat may be transferred rapidly in an emergency by placing the bird on a plastic bag filled with warm water.

After the bird has stabilized ($\sim$1 hr), gentle manipulation can be used to attempt to "milk" out the egg. Percutaneous aspiration followed by lateral pressure to collapse the egg is another treatment. Laceration of the oviduct rarely occurs. Supportive antibiotic therapy is recommended for most egg-bound birds. If the bird appears to be in shock, steroids can be given. Calcium is given IM, and subcut. if diluted (0.5-1 mL/kg of a 5 mg/mL calcium gluconate + 5 mg/mL calcium lactate solution), and maintained with an oral supplement. Oxytocin is also given in many cases (0.01-0.1 mL, IM).

Acute hypocalcemia in African grays and cockatiels is characterized by weakness, tremors, and seizures. The exact etiology is unknown, as some birds appear to be relatively well nourished. However, parenteral Ca effects an immediate improvement, and blood Ca levels are consistently low. Differential diagnosis includes lead poisoning.

Vitamin A Deficiency: This is frequently unrecognized in its subclinical forms in pet birds, although poorly nourished birds may have overt lesions. Also, use of the vitamin in treatment of various diseases is increasing.

White plaques (hyperkeratosis) in and around the mouth, eyes, and sinuses are typical. Chronic epithelial conditions such as bumblefoot, sinusitis, and conjunctivitis that have been refractory to other treatments may warrant vitamin A therapy.

Parenteral vitamin A can be given IM (100,000 u/kg). Diets of all caged birds should be evaluated for vitamin A.

Iodine Deficiency: Goiter, or thyroid hyperplasia, is a serious problem of pet budgerigars in certain areas. The normal thyroid glands of budgies are ~3 mm long, but enlarge to ≥1 cm. Classical signs include a respiratory stertor, wheeze, or click due to the pressure of the thyroid on the syrinx. Regurgitation is seen in some severe cases, and the (right) jugular vein may be engorged; these signs are related to mechanical obstruction of the thoracic inlet. Affected birds tolerate stress poorly; diagnosis is sometimes expedited by a test injection of sodium iodide (0.01-0.02 mL/budgie, IM). Response to therapy (by diminished respiratory stertor) is usually seen in <24 hr.

Hypothyroidism and thyroid neoplasia are possible sequelae in chronic cases. Cockatiels are occasionally affected with thyroid hyperplasia, but thoracic inlet obstruction has not been reported.

Iodized calcium blocks (pink) or specially iodized seed mixes (hulled carrier) are the easiest methods of preventing this syndrome. Lugol's iodine can be used in the drinking water, but long-term owner compliance is poor.

Stunting: A syndrome of young, hand-raised psittacines caused by inadequate feeding formulas and/or insufficient caloric intake. Signs include a head large in proportion to the body; thin feet, toes, and wingtips; pale skin; misdirected or delayed feathering; and inadequate weight gains. Treatment includes careful scrutiny of the formula, feeding frequency, and amounts fed.

Iron Storage Disease: Hemochromatosis is a common problem in pet mynahs and toucans as well as in certain zoo birds such as the bird-of-paradise. Hemochromatosis is believed to be related, in part, to excessive intake of dietary iron. However, not all birds become affected when kept on similar diets. Some believe a maintenance diet containing iron at <40 ppm (mg/kg) may prevent the disease. Low-iron diets and blood-letting have been helpful in treatment of mild cases. Recommending low-iron diets for pet mynahs is prudent. Mixing 2 parts cooked rice to one part canned cat food usually forms a low-iron base; low-iron fruits (eg, apples, bananas) and an iron-free vitamin/mineral supplement should also be provided separately.

TOXICITIES

Contrary to popular belief, houseplant toxicities and mysterious "fume" deaths are rarely encountered in clinical practice. However, polytetrafluoroethylene (nonstick bakeware coating) may give off a lethal gas if pans are allowed to overheat. Much more common is lead poisoning; paint remains a significant source, usually "old" paint. Tiffany lamps, stained glass leading, lead curtain weights, and other lead metal objects are frequently sampled by pet birds.

Clinical signs of lead poisoning include vomiting, liquid pink or brown droppings (common with hemoglobinuria), weakness, ataxia, and seizures. Radiographs often show the abnormally dense material contained within the ventriculus. Surgical removal is recommended in birds large enough to make this practical. Calcium EDTA (30-50 mg/kg, IM, t.i.d. until asymptomatic) is indicated in all cases, and response to therapy is usually rapid. Feline laxatives can be administered to help dislodge lead particles residing in the gizzard. Prognosis is guarded in chronic cases.

TRAUMATIC INJURY

Traumatic injuries in caged birds are generally rewarding to treat. Fractured legs are often found in pet budgies, and generally involve the tibiotarsal bone. Sedation with isoflurane and application of a tape "sandwich" cast is effective. Perches should be padded for birds required to bear weight on one leg (all nails should be trimmed). Tape solvent is helpful in removing such splints and casts, but should be used only in well-ventilated areas.

Injuries inflicted by cats are relatively uncommon but always warrant antibiotic therapy (*see* BACTERIAL DISEASES, p 1002). Gangrenous necrosis of the toes is a traumatic injury seen in finches and canaries. Dust-like fibers or threads become wrapped around the digits of nesting adults and nestlings. Careful hemostasis and magnification are required for safe removal. Burn injuries are frequent in free-flying pets (usually the feet are affected), and are becoming a major problem in hand-raised newborn parrots. Food heated in a microwave and not mixed before feeding may produce "spot" burns of the crop. Conservative surgical therapy usually is successful.

DISEASES OF UNCERTAIN ETIOLOGY

Macaw wasting disease or **proventricular dilatation syndrome** is characterized by chronic weight loss, regurgitation, and an enlarged proventriculus. Macaws, cockatoos, and other psittacines have been reported with typical findings, including multifocal lymphocytic leiomyositis and the absence of normal myenteric plexi on histological section of the proventriculus. Successful treatment has not been described.

Cockatiel conjunctivitis is prevalent in recently shipped or purchased cockatiels. A characteristic erythematous anterior swelling of the conjunctiva is noted. Localized chlamydial infections and mycoplasma infections have both been suspected. Remission is most rapid with tetracycline ophthalmic ointment in conjunction with nutritional support.

Cloacal papillomas are thought to be transmissible, yet a viral agent has never been recovered. It does tend to occur as a flock problem, particularly in breeding colonies of macaws. Prolapsed tissue is erythematous and originates from the inside rim of the cloaca. Spread to the mouth and upper GI tract is not uncommon. Surgical removal (electrocautery) is indicated but cannot be regarded as a permanent cure. Relapses may occur (infrequently) from year to year, and autogenous vaccines may or may not be helpful.

Lipomas in budgerigars have been linked to neoplasia, hypothyroidism, genetic factors, and simple obesity. Weight control is recommended in management of affected birds.

Diabetes mellitus is seen in pet birds and causes fairly typical signs of polyuria, polydipsia, and high blood and urine glucose levels. Treatment with insulin is effective but may not be practical.

Gout is the source of some confusion because of the 2 different expressions of uric acid crystallization that are produced. Articular gout is a disease of uncertain etiology, and is a distinct entity from visceral gout. Visceral gout is an antemortem event related to dehydration with or without terminal renal failure. The relationship of articular gout to high protein levels or renal failure has never been clearly documented. However, birds with gout should have uric acid levels run, and they should be placed on a low-protein diet. Articular gout is best diagnosed with an aspirate, which shows the characteristic spindle-shaped crystals. Distal joints of wings and legs are affected first in most birds. The tophi can be seen through the skin and resemble subcut. abscesses/granulomas. Surgical intervention is controversial and not generally recommended. Allopurinol (30 mg/kg, b.i.d., PO) in combination with a pain reliever (acetylsalicylic acid) has been the traditional treatment, although it is known only to stop production of additional lesions or deposits. However, a new drug regimen (colchicine/probenicid) shows much more promise in reversing lesions. Although findings are still preliminary, the colchicine regimen is the first to demonstrate actual remission. A combination tablet (0.5 g probenicid and 0.5 mg colchicine) is diluted in dextrose or glucose powder (15 mL), and 0.5 mL of the resulting mix may be given (in syrup) b.i.d. to a 100-g bird. Other dose protocols have also been reported; ataxia and other nervous signs may occur in overdose.

Feather cysts are ingrown feathers that result in a granulomatous mass, and as such, are easy to treat. Unfortunately, certain breeds of canaries (Norwich, border) are often burdened with hundreds of abnormal feathers in pectoral and dorsal tracts.

Surgical removal of the entire feather tract or regular removal of encysted feathers may be helpful. A viral etiology is not suspected. **"Feather dusters"** are almost certainly the result of a lethal gene, as affected budgerigars do not survive for longer than a few months. Feather dusters are so-called because of their large mop-like appearance (not found in other species). **French moult** is suspected to be a viral disease and may encompass more than one pathological process (*see* p 1010).

Feather picking is a multifactorial syndrome that was formerly attributed only to boredom. Important factors (depending on species) may include boredom, sexual or social stress/frustration, stress associated with fear or nervousness, and residual habit after resolution of other psychological factors. Infectious disease or other pathology is also involved in some types of self-mutilation. Giardiasis (qv, p 1006) in cockatiels is suspected to influence feather-picking in this species. Cockatiels and parrots such as cockatoos may respond to medroxyprogesterone therapy (30 mg/kg, IM), but repeated doses are not recommended. Elizabethan collars (X-ray film is best) are sometimes useful in breaking the feather-picking habit, but should be reserved for the most severe cases. Their repeated use is not recommended; rather, the owner should be counselled to accept the bird's appearance and protect it from cold stress.

Provision of safe, chewable toys, branches, and twigs on a continuing basis helps divert the bird's chewing habit away from feathers. A cagemate may also distract the bird, and installing a nesting box or hiding area is recommended.

MANAGEMENT, HUSBANDRY, AND DISEASES OF FOXES

MANAGEMENT

The importance of cleanliness in raising foxes (*Vulpes* spp) cannot be overemphasized. Pens with raised, woven-wire bottoms should be used for ranch foxes. These pens disrupt the life cycle of many parasites because the feces drop through the wire. Usually, foxes are kept in individual pens with an attached kennel.

The ration for ranch-raised foxes is roughly the same as that fed mink, which consists of a commercial cooked cereal with chicken, beef by-products, and fish (qv, p 1240). Fox pellets are available commercially and have given satisfactory performance. The vixen usually shows signs of estrus in late January and February. The period varies between silver and blue foxes. Most farmers use a polygamous mating system, taking the female to the pen of the male. Most females are in standing heat for 2-3 days and are bred 2 or 3 times during this period. Many ranchers utilize vaginal cytology or electronic "rut gauges" to determine the proper time for best mating. Considerable research is being done on artificial insemination, which is becoming widely used on larger ranches. The gestation period is ~52 days. Foxes have one litter per year. Blue foxes should average 6-7 pups per litter, silver foxes 3-5 pups. Foxes are usually pelted in November and December.

DISEASES OF FOXES

Distemper: Foxes are susceptible to canine distemper virus (qv, p 408). The virus is easily transmitted between dogs, mink, ferrets, raccoons, and other susceptible species. Because of the high population density in confinement, and the high transmissibility of the virus, mortality on unvaccinated farms may be 50% in the breeding stock and 75% in the pups. The diagnosis is based (as in dogs) on clinical signs; histological lesions, including the presence of inclusion bodies; and FA procedures. The most effective control procedure during an outbreak is to immediately destroy all foxes showing signs of the disease, and to vaccinate all others. All dead animals should be incinerated, and all equipment thoroughly disinfected.

Since there are no licensed distemper vaccines for foxes, mink vaccine is used. Some of the current dog distemper vaccines may lead to post-vaccinal encephalitis in foxes. Vaccination of weaned pups at 12-13 wk of age is suggested. Annual vaccination of breeder foxes is recommended.

Fox Encephalitis: This disease, caused by the same virus that causes infectious canine hepatitis (qv, p 418), may cause serious losses when unvaccinated foxes are raised in high concentration. Mortality may be 2-40% on affected ranches.

In contrast to distemper, fox encephalitis has a rapid course. Signs include loss of appetite, bloody diarrhea, depression, and often, nervous signs such as convulsions and paralysis; death occurs in a few hours to a few days. The virus invades the endothelial lining of small blood vessels, and cells in the liver and kidneys. Signs and death are due to hemorrhage of small vessels throughout the body, including the brain. Diagnosis is confirmed by demonstrating typical intranuclear inclusion bodies in liver, kidney, and endothelial cells; virus isolation; or FA technique.

An inactivated vaccine is available. Pups from unvaccinated vixens are vaccinated at weaning, and others when 10-12 wk old. Breeders should be given booster vaccinations in December or January.

Salmon Poisoning: This disease (qv, p 414), caused by *Neorickettsia helminthoeca*, is the result of eating salmon, trout, or steelhead that harbor the vector fluke, *Nanophyetus salmincola*. Signs are similar to those of dogs and include fever, inappetence, vomiting, lethargy, and diarrhea. In untreated foxes, death usually ensues.

Botulism: Improper handling and storage of food is the usual source of botulism in foxes as well as in mink (qv, p 1051). Storage of meat by-products in metal drums, in which anaerobic conditions prevail, is an excellent medium for production of botulism toxin. In almost all instances, type C toxin has been incriminated. The signs are similar to those seen in mink. Affected animals show flaccid paralysis and abdominal breathing, usually followed by death. Because vaccines approved for foxes are not available, those approved for mink are used.

Canine Parvovirus: While canids in zoological parks have succumbed to canine parvoviral infection, there have been no reported outbreaks of canine parvovirus (qv, p 249) on commercial fox farms; however, the prospect of an outbreak should be kept in mind. Some fox farmers routinely vaccinate with inactivated mink viral enteritis or canine parvovirus vaccines.

Parasites: Both internal and external parasites are controlled by means essentially the same as those recommended for dogs.

Fleas (*Ctenocephalides canis*) infest foxes, and cause skin irritation and sometimes severe anemia. They are particularly harmful in pups. Ear mites (*Otodectes cynotis*) are common in ranch-raised foxes. Infected foxes shake their heads and dig at the base of the ears with their front paws. Secondary bacterial or mycotic otitis may result. Some foxes hold their heads to one side. (For treatment *see* FLEAS, p 795, and OTITIS EXTERNA, p 309.)

Sarcoptic mange (*Sarcoptes scabiei*) may cause serious economic loss in ranch-raised foxes. Clinical signs are similar to those seen in dogs. Ivermectin at 200 μg/kg, subcut., has been used successfully to treat outbreaks, but reports of idiosyncratic reactions in dogs at this dosage suggest caution in use of this product in foxes.

Hookworms (*Uncinaria stenocephala*) occur in commercially raised foxes, and can be responsible for deaths in pups. Fox pups are infected by larvae in the vixen's milk. Pups begin to die at 12 days of age with profound anemia. Fecal samples from these pups often are negative for eggs, and death may occur before the infection becomes patent. Pups with milder infection may grow poorly, appear emaciated, and have a marginal anemia. Treatment involves worming pups at 10 and 21 days with pyrantel pamoate. The vixen also should be wormed when the pups are 21 days old.

Foxes are commonly infected with ascarids (*Toxocara canis*), which may cause vomiting, diarrhea, abdominal distention, lethargy, and occasionally, intestinal obstruction. Ascarid larvae migration may cause parasitic pneumonia. Fox pups may be infected *in utero* or after whelping by ingesting eggs. Treatment involves worming pups at 10 and 21 days of age with pyrantel pamoate or piperazine.

Two lungworms, *Capillaria aerophila* and *Crenosoma vulpis*, infect foxes. Lungworm infection and the consequent chronic bronchitis or pneumonia may cause death in ranch-raised foxes.

Foxes may be infected with coccidia, the most common being *Isospora bigemina*. The signs are mild to bloody diarrhea, loss of appetite, and death. Foxes may be treated as dogs are (qv, 717).

Dermatomycosis: Although the condition appears to be rare in the USA, *Trichophyton mentagrophytes* has been incriminated in an outbreak. It is reported to be common in foxes in the USSR.

Nutritional Diseases: Rickets may occur in young foxes shortly after weaning. Affected pups appear bow-legged due to curvature of the long bones and joint enlargement. Distortion of the facial bones and enlargement at the costochondral junction sometimes occur. Rickets is treated by correcting the calcium-phosphorus ratio in the diet and supplementing with vitamin D.

Chastek paralysis (qv, p 1055) is a vitamin B_1 deficiency induced by feeding certain types of raw fish that contain the enzyme thiaminase. Early in the course of the disease, a few foxes may have an abnormal gait as though their legs were stiff; within 12-36 hr, they have extensive spastic paralysis and are unable to rise. Convulsions often occur shortly before death. Raw fish should be removed from the diet and daily injections of 100 u of thiamine given. Cooking of all fish before mixing prevents the deficiency.

Biotin deficiency also has occurred in foxes. Preventive measures are described for the disease in mink (qv, p 1242).

Cardiac myopathy is observed only when fox pups are fed certain commercial pellets. Some factor(s) is deficient in the pup's early growth phase, which results in an enlarged right ventricle. The condition can be prevented if the ration is supplemented with liver or muscle meat.

MANAGEMENT, HUSBANDRY, AND DISEASES OF LABORATORY ANIMALS

This discussion is of the more important diseases of those animals used in the largest numbers for research purposes: mice, rats, guinea pigs, hamsters, as well as ferrets, various nonhuman primates, and amphibians. Diseases of other domestic species that are also widely used in research, such as dogs, cats, rabbits, and chickens, are dealt with elsewhere in the MANUAL.

THE GUIDE FOR THE CARE AND USE OF LABORATORY ANIMALS, DHHS, PHS (NIH, Publication 85-23), is a primary reference for information on basic principles and standards. In addition, regulations promulgated under authority of PL 89-544 (1966), as amended by PL 91-579 (1971), PL 94-279 (1976), and PL 99-198 (1985), should be consulted for detailed federal (USA) legal requirements.

MANAGEMENT AND HUSBANDRY

Laboratory rodents that are disease- and pathogen-free and that do not possess antibodies indicative of past infection are readily available from commercial vendors. Procuring such animals from high-quality sources, transporting them in filtered shipping containers, and maintaining them in facilities with both physical and procedural barriers to the introduction of infectious agents are effective measures in colony disease prevention.

However, although there are colonies of some species of primates that are free of most agents that cause infectious disease in these species, most primates used are wild-caught. For this reason, a strict quarantine and isolation program should be implemented in addition to the program followed in the importers' facilities.

For proper management, the animal care and research staff must be responsible, well trained, highly motivated, sensitive to the animals' health and well-being, and diligent in performing their duties and responsibilities. Standard operating procedures must be determined, and training and supervision provided to assure a consistently applied and uniformly high level of animal care. Research staff must also be properly trained in the humane care and use of laboratory animals. Research facilities must have carefully controlled environmental conditions that, along with conscientiously applied programs of animal care and use, provide the best possible conditions for conducting research.

Housing: Cages, pens, or runs should provide adequate 3-dimensional space to allow for normal postural adjustments and species-specific behavior. When possible, compatible groups of animals should be housed together. Primary enclosures should be constructed of durable materials, be easily cleaned and sanitized, and designed for comfort and safety.

Temperature, humidity, ventilation rates, and lighting conditions (quality, quantity, and photoperiod) should be carefully controlled at all times. In general, temperature should be maintained at 66-79°F (19-26°C) for most rodents and 64-84°F (18-29°C) for primates. Within these ranges, the systems should be capable of maintaining temperatures ± 2° of the set point. Relative humidity should be maintained at 40-70% for most rodents, 40-60% for rabbits, and 30-70% for primates, preferably within 5% of the set point. Ventilation rates should be 10-15 air changes/ hr. Air should not be recirculated unless it has been treated to remove particulate and gaseous contaminants. Lighting intensity should be evenly distributed, and adequate to permit inspection of the animals and maintenance of sanitation and personnel safety, and most importantly, animal well-being. Diurnal or day:night cycles, as determined by a given species' requirements, should be controlled by automatic timers to maintain circadian and neuroendocrine regulation. The microenvironment within certain types of caging may be very different from that of the macroenvironment of the room. Carefully conducted research is needed to define the optimal environmental conditions for each species or group of species at the cage level.

Feeding: Feed should be of adequate quantity, palatable, free of contaminants, and nutritionally adequate, according to specific species requirements. Feeds specifically manufactured for research animal use are more likely to be uniformly constituted, free of contaminants, and mill dated. Food should be manufactured, transported, stored, and used in ways that minimize its deterioration, contamination, or infestation. Most small animals are fed *ad lib*; rabbits, laboratory carnivores, and primates may be restricted to measured quantities of feed each day. In addition to commercially prepared and usually pelleted diets, semisynthetic or completely synthetic diets can be prepared for use in certain kinds of research. Autoclavable or irradiated diets are available for rodents, and may be used when sterilization of feed is desired.

Bedding: Bedding materials should be nonirritating, absorbent, free of chemical contamination and pathogens, and nonpalatable. Adequate quantities should be used to keep animals dry and clean between changes of bedding or caging. Hardwood bedding products and others not made with softwoods are recommended since softwood products contain volatile oils that may alter hepatic enzyme systems and affect certain kinds of research.

Water: Potable, uncontaminated water should be provided in adequate quantities to meet particular species requirements. Quality assurance programs that measure pH, hardness, chemical content, and microbial load are recommended. Highly purified, deionized, acidified, chlorinated, or sterile water may be required under certain experimental or husbandry conditions. Water is usually provided *ad lib* in manually filled or automatic watering devices.

Sanitation: A uniformly high level of sanitation is mandatory. Housing rooms and ancillary support space should be cleaned and sanitized as often as necessary to keep them free of dirt, debris, and potentially harmful contamination. Primary enclosures also should be cleaned and sanitized as often as necessary to keep animals clean and dry. For rodents in solid-bottom cages, usually 1-3 changes/wk will suffice; for rodents in suspended cages over excreta pans, biweekly changes should be adequate. For larger animals, excreta and soiled bedding should be removed daily, and primary enclosures cleaned and sanitized at least biweekly. Water bottles and other watering or feeding devices should be cleaned and sanitized at least weekly. Automatic watering devices on cages, racks, or in rooms should be drained, rinsed, and sanitized at regular, frequent intervals. Heating cages and other equipment to 180°F (82.2°C) and/or using appropriate chemical disinfection, eg, hypochlorite solutions, kills nonspore-forming pathogenic bacteria and viruses. All caging and other equipment should be rinsed thoroughly following treatment with detergents and/or disinfectants.

Vermin Control: Professionally directed programs to prevent, identify, and eradicate or control insects, or escaped or feral rodents must be instituted. The use of pesticides should generally be confined to areas not used for animals or storage of feed or bedding. Relatively inert substances, such as silica aerogel or boric acid powder, are recommended and are useful in control of crawling insects, eg, cockroaches.

COLONY MONITORING

While most commercially reared rodents, some rabbits, and relatively fewer dogs, cats, and primates can be obtained as SPF animals, resident animal colonies must be monitored for naturally occurring disease as a measure of the effectiveness of the prevention and control program. Investigators should be informed regularly as to the health status of their research animals. In addition to monitoring for infectious disease, a quality assurance program should monitor for genetic integrity, especially for inbred mouse strains that are bred and maintained in the research facility, as well as environmental factors (feed, water, and bedding quality, efficacy of sanitation programs, air handling and quality, lighting, noise, etc) that can affect colony health.

Colony health monitoring consists of a defined program of regular physical and laboratory evaluations of animals within a unit, as well as a morbidity and mortality reporting system that enables timely identification of potential problems. Thorough investigations of illnesses and deaths in a colony are essential components of such a program.

While certain general principles apply, a health monitoring program must be specifically developed for each species maintained in a facility, eg, generally all primates are quarantined and isolated on arrival. Physical examinations, tuberculin testing, baseline hematological and other clinical pathological tests should be performed. In addition, serological evaluation for herpesvirus B, simian AIDS, and other specific agents may be performed, depending on the species of primate. Primates should be released from quarantine only when both the health status and suitability for use are determined. Furthermore, primates should have quarterly, semiannual, and annual health surveillance screens, each consisting of defined elements.

For colony-bred rats and mice, programs for disease monitoring can consist of any or all of the following: 1) vendor surveillance, 2) quarantine and isolation evaluation, 3) ongoing clinical and postmortem evaluation during the course of studies, 4) sentinel animal program, and 5) evaluation at termination of the study. In addition, all transplantable tumors, cells, or other biological products to be introduced should be screened for murine and zoonotic pathogens. Of particular concern to colony health is the occasional and justifiable need to obtain animals from less well-defined sources, such as an investigator's colony or other nonapproved source. The presence of infectious agents either in transplantable tumors or noncommercial animal sources can pose a substantial threat to resident colonies and personnel.

DISEASES OF RATS AND MICE

Therapeutic intervention may be practical for individual pets, but may not be in rodent colonies and under certain research conditions. As outlined above, a disease-prevention program is essential in mouse and rat colonies.

BACTERIAL DISEASES

Corynebacterium kutscheri **Infection (Pseudotuberculosis):** Infection by this opportunistic pathogen most commonly is inapparent but may cause nasal and ocular discharge, dyspnea, arthritis, or skin abscesses. Lesions are variable, but usually include focal abscesses in the liver, kidneys, lungs, and lymph nodes, and occasionally, purulent arthritis. Abscesses usually appear as discrete, gray to yellow nodules up to 15 mm in diameter. Diagnosis depends on finding characteristic lesions and isolation of the organism or serology (agglutination or complement fixation, or ELISA). Treatment with penicillin (4500 u/100 g body wt, IM) for 7-10 days may prevent clinically apparent disease, but will not eliminate the carrier state.

Murine Respiratory Mycoplasmosis: A relatively common chronic disease syndrome characterized by inflammation of the respiratory tract and middle ear. Signs include chattering and dyspnea in mice, and nasal discharge, sneezing, snuffling, rales, dyspnea, head tilt, incoordination, and circling in rats. Lesions include suppurative bronchitis and bronchopneumonia, mucopurulent rhinitis, and otitis media and interna. The primary etiological agent is *Mycoplasma pulmonis*; however, *Pasteurella pneumotropica, Corynebacterium kutscheri, Bordetella bronchiseptica,* cilia-associated respiratory bacilli (CAR bacillus), streptococci, or viruses may act in concert with the primary agent. Diagnosis depends on lesions and isolation of the etiological agent or demonstration of antibodies against the agent. ELISA tests to detect rat serum IgG to *M pulmonis* are available. The condition can be prevented by keeping an infection-free colony behind a microbiological barrier. Outbreaks can be controlled to a limited extent by providing oxytetracycline in the drinking water at 2-5 mg/mL in sweetened (5% sucrose) water for 10-14 days. The solution should be made fresh every other day.

Pasteurella **Infection:** *Pasteurella pneumotropica,* an opportunistic pathogen, exists in a latent, carrier state in some rodent colonies. When other diseases such as Sendai virus infection of mice or *Mycoplasma pulmonis* infection of rats are present, severe pneumonia or otitis media may result. In addition, when rodents are stressed, abscesses may occur in skin, uterus, lymph nodes, or urinary system. Oxytetracycline (500 mg/L) or chloramphenicol (1 g/L) in the drinking water for 10-14 days may be effective in treating clinically apparent disease but will not eliminate the carrier state.

Pseudomonas **Infection:** Pseudomonads are part of the normal intestinal flora but may cause early deaths in stressed, irradiated, or otherwise immunosuppressed mice. *Pseudomonas aeruginosa* may also cause otitis media and interna in nonirradiated mice. Prevention and control are best accomplished by acidification (pH 2.5) or chlorination (10-12 ppm) of the drinking water.

Salmonellosis (Paratyphoid): *Salmonella* spp, usually *S typhimurium* or *S enteritidis,* may cause enteritis and septicemia with focal necrosis of the liver or spleen in rats and mice. Although rarely a problem in commercially bred rodents, salmonellosis can be introduced into a colony by feral or wild rodents, or contaminated feed or bedding products. Clinical signs include anorexia, rough coat, weight loss, conjunctivitis, and sporadic deaths. Subclinical carriers make elimination of the infection difficult. Because of the public health hazard, infected rodents should be eliminated. (*See also* p 148.)

Transmissible Murine Colonic Hyperplasia: This syndrome, caused by *Citrobacter freundii* variant 4280, primarily affects 2- to 4-wk-old mice. Clinical signs are nonspecific and include hunched posture, rough coat, rectal prolapse, dehydration, perineal staining, and loose unformed feces. At necropsy, a thickened descending colon due to mucosal hyperplasia is characteristic. Oxytetracycline (500 mg/L drinking water) reduces the clinical signs but will not eliminate the carrier state. Neomycin sulfate (2 g/L drinking water) reportedly will eliminate the bacteria from the host.

Tyzzer's Disease: This endemic disease is widespread in laboratory mice in Europe and Japan, and outbreaks have been reported in a wide variety of laboratory animals in the USA. (*See also* pp 152 and 1062.) The causative organism is a slender gram-negative rod, *Bacillus piliformis*. Although the disease is usually subclinical, stress, or cortisone injections or other immunosuppressant drugs may precipitate epidemics. Signs include diarrhea, humped back, poor coat, and sudden deaths, especially in young animals. Lesions usually include focal necrosis of the liver and inflammation of the terminal ileum. Diagnosis depends on histological demonstration of the bacilli in bundles within the hepatocytes surrounding the focal areas of necrosis; an ELISA-based test is effective in detecting antibodies in rats and mice. The organisms stain well with Giemsa, periodic acid-Schiff, and silver stains. Outbreaks may be controlled by isolation of affected animals and implementation of strict hygienic procedures; however, elimination of *B piliformis* from a facility is difficult because of the resistant spores. A 0.5% hypochlorite solution is effective in killing spores; quaternary ammonium compounds generally are ineffective.

Miscellaneous Bacterial Infections: *Staphylococcus aureus* causes skin and facial abscesses in nude athymic mice. *Klebsiella pneumoniae* may rarely cause bronchopneumonia, pleuritis, and abscesses in various organs of mice. *Streptococcus pneumoniae* is a cause of acute bronchopneumonia, pleuritis, pericarditis, meningitis, and splenic infarcts in rats. *Streptobacillus moniliformis* is a gram-negative, highly pleomorphic bacillus frequently found in the nasopharynx of asymptomatic rats; it may rarely cause arthritis, pericarditis, and focal necrosis of the liver and spleen of mice housed in the same room. It also causes rat-bite fever or Haverhill fever in man. *Bordetella bronchiseptica* is a common inhabitant of the respiratory tract of rats and mice. Although its role as a primary pathogen in rats and mice is uncertain, it has been identified as a primary cause of pneumonia. *Pasteurella multocida* may occasionally cause pneumonia or abscesses in rats and mice. Diagnosis of these infections depends on isolation of the organism. Therapy is based on culture and antibacterial sensitivity tests.

MYCOTIC DISEASES

For ringworm, *see* RINGWORM IN GUINEA PIGS, p 1028. Histoplasmosis, coccidioidomycosis, sporotrichosis, cryptococcosis, and phycomycosis usually do not pose significant problems in laboratory colonies; however, they may occasionally disrupt research because of an overwhelming effect on animals in which resistance has been diminished by radiation or immunosuppressive drugs.

PARASITIC DISEASES

Blood Parasites: Several blood parasites have been reported in rats and mice. These include *Plasmodium berghei*, *P vinckei*, *Trypanosoma lewisi*, *T cruzi*, *Hepatozoon muris*, *Babesia muris*, *Haemobartonella muris* (primarily rats), and *Eperythrozoon coccoides* (primarily mice). These organisms usually do not cause clinically apparent disease unless the animals are splenectomized or severely stressed. Blood-sucking ectoparasites may transmit these parasites.

Cestodes: The dwarf tapeworm (*Hymenolepis nana*) occurs in the small intestine of rats and mice, and is transmissible to man. The life cycle may be direct or indirect. *Hymenolepis diminuta* occurs in the anterior ileum of rats and mice. A flea, beetle, or cockroach may act as an intermediate host. The treatment of choice for tapeworms is niclosamide (100 mg/kg, PO). Rats and mice may also harbor the intermediate forms of *Taenia taeniaeformis (Cysticercus fasciolaris)* in the liver, and *T (Coenurus) serialis* in the connective tissue. Their presence indicates probable fecal contamination of the food supply by the definitive host(s).

Ectoparasites: In mice, the mites *Myobia musculi* and *Radfordia affinis* may cause hair loss and scabby lesions over the head, neck, and shoulders. The effect in different strains of mice varies greatly. Breeding males seem to be affected most severely. *Myocoptes musculinus* and *Trichoecius (Myocoptes) romboutsi* also may cause hair loss and dermatitis. *Psorergates simplex* causes chronically inflamed epidermal cysts that are visible only on the inner surfaces of the pelt or skin at necropsy. Mites that affect rats include *Laelaps echidninus* and *Radfordia ensifera*, which cause dermatitis, and *Notoedres muris*, the ear mange mite. Lice and superficial mites are most easily and consistently diagnosed by identification of parasites on the skin and hair with a magnifying glass or dissecting microscope. Migration may be hastened by first placing the carcass or skin in the refrigerator, then examining it after return to room temperature. The burrowing mite, *P simplex*, can be diagnosed by examining the pelt for the subcut., pinpoint, white focal lesions.

Infestation of laboratory rats or mice with fleas, such as *Xenopsylla cheopis, Nosopsyllus fasciatus*, or *Leptopsylla segnis*, is uncommon. Infestation with lice, *Polyplax spinulosa* (rats) or *P serrata* (mice), is more common than flea infestation, and can cause hair loss and pruritus.

Ectoparasites can be eliminated only by cesarean derivation procedures. Clinical control may be achieved by placing 2 sq in. (13 cm^2) of resin strip containing dichlorvos on cage tops for 24-48 hr every 2 wk for 2-3 treatments. Restriction of air flow in the room or cage during treatment increases effectiveness. Ivermectin at 200 μg/kg body wt, PO or parenterally, has been recommended.

Nematodes: *Heterakis spumosa* is found in the cecum and colon of rats and mice. No lesions have been reported. Diagnosis is based on identification of ova in the feces. *Nippostrongylus muris* occurs in the small intestine of rats and mice. Clinical signs include unthriftiness, diarrhea, and dyspnea. Lesions include pneumonia and pulmonary hemorrhage due to larval migration through the lungs. Characteristic eggs are passed in the feces. *Gongylonema neoplasticum* occurs in the epithelium of the stomach, esophagus, and tongue. There is little tissue reaction; infection does not produce neoplasms. The intermediate host is the cockroach. Embryonated eggs are passed in the feces. Adult *Trichinella spiralis* (qv, p 386) are found in the duodenum of rats and many other animals. The pinworms *Aspicularis tetraptera* and *Syphacia* spp occur in the cecum and colon of rats and mice. Impaction by worms, colonic intussusception, or rectal prolapse may result. *Aspicularis* eggs are passed in the feces; *Syphacia* eggs are deposited on the perianal region by the female worm. Diagnosis can be made by fecal flotation (*Aspicularis*) or by the cellophane-tape method (*Syphacia*). Control is difficult because of reinfection due to the presence of eggs on fomites and in air currents; however, ivermectin, piperazine, or pyrantel pamoate may be helpful. *Capillaria hepatica* occurs in the liver parenchyma of mice and rats. Eggs cause yellow streaks and patches in liver due to the local chronic inflammatory response. Eggs are liberated only when the liver is eaten by some other animal. The eggs are then passed in the feces to develop on the ground to become infective. The nematode *Trichosomoides crassicauda* lives in the bladder, renal pelvis, and ureters of rats. Operculated eggs are passed in the urine. Larvae migrating through the lungs may cause focal granulomas. A thorough cleaning of the facility followed by disinfection with formaldehyde gas may be necessary to kill ova.

Acanthocephala: The thorny-headed worm (*Moniliformis moniliformis*) inhabits the small intestine of rats, mice, and other rodents. The thorn-like hooks on the head may cause enteritis, ulceration, and occasionally, intestinal perforation with subsequent peritonitis.

Protozoa: At least 4 species of coccidia (*Eimeria* spp) can infect the intestinal tract of laboratory rats, and 8 species can infect mice. One species (*Cryptosporidium muris*) occurs in the stomach. Diagnosis is based on identification of oocysts after fecal flotation, or by finding organisms in the epithelial cells of the intestinal tract. Renal coccidiosis due to *Klossiella muris* occurs in mice. Oocysts are passed in the urine. Coccidial infections of the intestine, stomach, or kidney rarely cause lesions or clinical signs. The principal intermediate host of the coccidian parasite *Toxoplasma gondii* (qv, p 365) is the mouse; other intermediate hosts are rats and other mammals, including man.

Spironucleus (Hexamita) muris, an opportunistic flagellated protozoan, may cause diarrhea, weight loss, and sporadic deaths, primarily in weanling mice. Lesions include duodenitis with crypts dilated by numerous hexamitae. Diagnosis is based on microscopic lesions and demonstration of organisms in saline mounts and fixed smears from the duodenum. Transmission occurs by ingestion of the encysted, environmentally stable stage of the parasite. *Hepatozoon muris* occurs in the hepatic cells of rats and mice. *Pneumocystis carinii* may be found in the lungs of mice and rats; respiratory signs may result from stress or immunosuppression.

VIRAL DISEASES

Ectromelia (Mousepox): A highly contagious disease of laboratory mice, caused by ectromelia virus. It may remain latent, or cause low-grade endemic disease or violent epidemics. Inbred mouse strains vary widely in susceptibility. In the acute systemic form, deaths with no lesions can occur. In more chronic cases there may be facial swelling; conjunctivitis with a secondary rash; and ulcerating or scaly lesions of the head, tail, or extremities. Occasionally, extremities become necrotic and slough. Other lesions include focal necrosis of the liver, spleen, pancreas, and lymph nodes, and intestinal hemorrhage. Eosinophilic cytoplasmic inclusion bodies may be found in hepatocytes, pancreatic acinar cells, or in swollen epidermal cells in areas of cutaneous inflammation. Diagnosis is based on characteristic lesions, serology, and confirmation of poxvirus morphology with electron microscopy.

Outbreaks sporadically occur in research colonies, especially those used in immunogenetic research. While animals from commercial breeders are free of the virus, mice that come from abroad or other research colonies in the USA should be screened carefully for ectromelia. Newly received mice should be isolated and observed for 2-3 wk before they are introduced into the colony.

Infected colonies generally should be destroyed, the facility and equipment thoroughly disinfected, and all biological materials derived from infected mice screened for virus, eg, by the mouse antibody production (MAP) test. However, in small colonies of irreplaceable mice, control can be achieved by vaccinating all susceptible animals with the IHD-T strain of vaccinia virus in concert with the above measures.

Mouse Hepatitis Virus (MHV) Infection: A widespread, highly contagious coronaviral infection of mice that is often difficult to control. Infection is usually endemic and subclinical, or epidemic; different inbred strains vary markedly in susceptibility. Many different strains of virus exist; each possesses a characteristic tissue tropism and ability to express itself differently in different inbred strains of mice. Depending on strain of virus and strain of mouse, clinical signs may include diarrhea, neurological signs, weight loss, jaundice, and death. Clinical disease may be precipitated by any immunosuppressant drug or procedure, or concomitant infection with K virus or *Eperythrozoon coccoides*. Susceptible suckling mice are generally more severely affected, but older mice may lose weight, have decreased breeding efficiency, and die. MHV infection alters a wide variety of immunological parameters and, as such, presents a threat to research studies. Infection with enteropathogenic strains of MHV in suckling mice produces a syndrome previously known as lethal intestinal virus of infant mice. Histological lesions include focal hepatic necrosis and syncytial cell formation in the intestinal epithelium. Diagnosis is based on serology (complement fixation or ELISA) and characteristic lesions. There is no effective treatment; however, cessation of breeding and of introduction of new susceptible mice into a colony for 8-15 wk has been reported to arrest the infection. Recovered mice are thought to regain normal immunocompetence, reportedly no longer shed virus, and may be considered suitable for some research studies.

Rotavirus Infection: Known previously as **epizootic diarrhea of infant mice**, rotavirus infection affects young mice 1-3 wk old. Affected mice have soft yellow feces that stain the perineum, dry around the anus, and may cause obstipation and death. Diagnosis is based on the clinical signs and history, and confirmed by electron microscopy or immunofluorescent identification of rotavirus in diarrheic feces. The only effective treatment is removal of obstructing feces from the anus and perineum. Infection can be prevented by procurement of uninfected mice and use of both physical and procedural barriers to prevent transmission of the agent.

Sendai Virus Infection: An infection that usually remains subclinical in rats and hamsters but is the most significant cause of respiratory disease in mice, in which it can cause violent epidemics with high mortality. As with mouse hepatitis virus, this produces profound changes in the immune system, and therefore, may have serious consequences for many kinds of research. The signs are due to pneumonia and include weight loss, dyspnea, chattering, and increased mortality. Usually suckling, weanling, and young mice are affected. Diagnosis is based on characteristic histology of pneumonic lesions and serology (hemagglutination inhibition, ELISA) of exposed or recovered animals. The characteristic histological lesions are interstitial pneumonitis, proliferation of bronchial epithelium with atypical cells, then squamous metaplasia, and finally, alveolar bronchiolization with focal collections of macrophages. The disease is highly contagious and difficult to control. Since weanlings serve as a reservoir population in a closed colony, an outbreak may be controlled by exclusion of young animals from the colony for 1-2 mo. Vaccination provides short-term protection of susceptible stocks.

Sialodacryoadenitis (SDA): A common coronaviral infection that causes severe, self-limiting inflammation and necrosis of the salivary and nasolacrimal glands of rats, especially the young. Highly contagious, it causes high morbidity but low mortality in susceptible colonies. Signs are exophthalmos, squinting, excessive blinking, chromodachryorrhea (red tears), and swollen face and neck. Lesions in the lacrimal duct may result in corneal drying with severe secondary ocular lesions. The disease is self-limiting, and most lesions resolve within 2 wk. Transmission is by respiratory aerosol and direct contact with respiratory secretions. During the acute phase of SDA, a high incidence of anesthetic deaths may occur.

Other Viral Infections: A number of viruses can be isolated from seemingly clinically normal rats and mice. Often, these viruses do not pose significant clinical disease problems in laboratory colonies; however, they may seriously disrupt research by directly affecting results or causing disease in animals that have had their resistance diminished by experimental procedures. (*See* TABLE 6, OTHER VIRAL INFECTIONS, below.)

Table 6. Other Viral Infections of Rats and Mice

Disease	Agent	Lesions	Diagnosis	Comments
Mouse adenovirus infection	Adenovirus	Focal necrosis of heart. Intranuclear inclusions in heart, kidneys, adrenals.	CF*.	Very rare. Contaminates mouse tumors or tissue cultures.
Cytomegalovirus infection	Herpesvirus	Intranuclear inclusions in salivary duct epithelium.	Lesions.	Rats and mice have species-specific infections.
K-virus infection	Papovavirus	Interstitial pneumonia with proliferation of endothelial cells.	HI**, CF; intranuclear inclusions in endothelial cells.	Dyspnea and death in suckling mice. Contaminates mouse tumors or tissue cultures.
Kilham rat virus (Rat virus)	Parvovirus	Cerebellar necrosis in suckling rats. Fetal resorption. Congenital malformations.	HI, ELISA.	Affects mitotically active cells. A teratogen. Contaminates transplantable tumors and cell lines.
Lactic dehydrogenase (LDH) virus infection	Unclassified RNA virus	Experimental polio-encephalomyelitis in immunosuppressed mice.	Elevation of plasma LDH in mice.	Causes elevated plasma enzyme levels. Contaminates transplanted tumors.
Lymphocytic choriomeningitis (LCM)	Arenavirus	Lymphocytic choriomeningitis. Necrosis of liver and lymphoid tissue.	Guinea pig or LCM-free mouse inoculation. CF, FA***.	Clonic convulsions, transplacental infection. Transmissible to man.
Mouse mammary carcinoma	Bittner agent; RNA virus	Mammary adenocarcinomas, adenocanthomas, carcinosarcomas.	Lesions.	Virus in milk of infected dam.
Minute virus of mice	Parvovirus	Cerebellar hypoplasia.	HI, FA.	Contaminates transplanted tumors. Also affects hamsters and rats.

Disease	Agent	Lesions	Diagnosis	Comments
Theiler's mouse encephalomyelitis (GD-VII)	Picornaviruses	Necrosis of brain stem, spinal cord.	HI. Rats also may have antibody.	Flaccid posterior paralysis, virus carried in intestine.
Mouse thymic virus infection	Herpesvirus	Thymic necrosis.	Inoculation of new-born mice.	Affects newborn only.
Pneumonia virus of mice infection (PVM)	Paramyxovirus	Interstitial pneumonia, pulmonary edema.	HI, ELISA. Inoculation of PVM-free mice.	May also affect rats and hamsters.
Polyoma virus infection	Papovavirus	Experimental tumors at various sites.	HI, CF.	Natural infection seldom produces tumors.
Rat coronavirus infection	Coronavirus	Experimental pneumonia.	CF, ELISA.	Occurs naturally in rats. Cross reacts with sialodacryoadenitis virus.
Reovirus infection	Reovirus type 3	Necrosis of liver, myocardium, pancreas. Neuronal degeneration. Encephalitis.	HI, ELISA. Rats also may have antibody.	Jaundice, yellow feces, oily coat and skin, neurological signs in mice.
Toolan HI infection	Parvovirus	Cerebellar lesions.	HI, ELISA.	Occurs naturally in rats.

*Complement fixation **Hemagglutination inhibition ***Fluorescent antibody

NONINFECTIOUS DISEASES

Age-associated Diseases: Rats and mice are used widely in gerontological research. Maximal longevity of many rat stocks and strains is 36-40 mo, with a 50% survival time of ~30 mo. For mice, the comparable range is 21-40 mo, with 50% survival time of 14-30 mo, depending on the strain. Genetic and environmental factors clearly influence longevity and the prevalence of age-associated diseases. When rats or mice are to be used in aging research, they should be reared and maintained under barrier conditions to prevent exposure to infectious diseases. The principal age-associated, non-neoplastic lesions of rats and mice have a degenerative, inflammatory, or autoimmune basis, and include chronic glomerulonephropathy, polyarteritis nodosa, myocardial degeneration, and radiculoneuropathy. Among the most common neoplasms are pituitary or pulmonary adenomas, pheochromocytomas of the adrenal gland, hepatocellular pancreatic islet cell tumors, testicular interstitial cell tumors, and leukemias. Prevalence or severity of lesions in both rats and mice increases after 1 yr of age. The differentiation of naturally occurring lesions of aging is a major challenge in experimental gerontology. The use of diagnostic screening procedures in selecting old rats and mice for research may be helpful in culling animals bearing lesions that could add to the variability of research results, or in selecting for specific lesions of research interest.

Fighting: Trauma due to fighting is often a significant cause of morbidity and mortality in male mice. Fighting usually occurs at night and results in bite and scratch wounds over the head, perineum, and lumbosacral skin. Frequently, these lesions become infected. A high incidence of secondary amyloidosis has been reported in animals that have chronic lesions stemming from fighting. Fighting can be prevented by separating males or, preferably, by grouping males at weaning rather than a later time.

Hair Chewing (Barbering): Partial alopecia due to chewing of their hair by cagemates is most common in pigmented mice. The earliest indication of hair chewing is loss of whiskers from some of the mice. Alopecia of the muzzle, head, and middorsum of the trunk typically follows. There is no dermatitis, but the skin may become increasingly pigmented. Usually, the chewing mice in a cage can be identified as those that have normal whiskers and coats. When the hair chewers are removed from the cage, regrowth of hairs on the remaining mice is usually complete in 2-3 mo. In black mice, the regrown hair may be gray.

Nutritional Diseases: Standardized balanced rations for rats and mice are commercially available. Most manufacturers provide separate diets for maintenance, breeding, and other specific purposes. Diets should be stored properly, protected from contamination, and fed within 180 days of the milling date. If colonies are fed fresh diets manufactured by a reputable company, the possibility of clinically apparent nutritional deficiency is remote. However, long-term *ad lib* feeding of presently available stock diets to rats and mice can lead to obesity, increased prevalence or severity of certain age-associated lesions, and reduced longevity. Feeding of natural vegetable supplements is neither necessary nor desirable since they may be contaminated with *Salmonella* spp, *Yersinia* spp, or *Bacillus piliformis*. Control of these problems is complex, but long-term restriction of caloric intake, reduced protein intake, or both, may be helpful.

Ringtail: A condition of young rats and mice characterized by annular constriction and later, edema, necrosis, and sloughing of the tail. The condition in rats can be produced experimentally by lowering the ambient relative humidity. The disease can be controlled by providing a relative humidity of ≥50%, and housing in solid-bottom plastic cages with deep bedding.

DISEASES OF GUINEA PIGS

Antibiotic-induced Toxicity: Guinea pigs and hamsters are highly susceptible to the toxic effects of many commonly used antibiotics. Toxicity results from overgrowth of *Clostridium difficile* and subsequent elaboration of toxins. This causes enterocolitis, with diarrhea and death in 3-7 days. Antibiotics with a primarily gram-positive spectrum (eg, penicillin, lincomycin, erythromycin, tylosin) should not be used in guinea pigs and hamsters. Broad-spectrum antibiotics should not be used PO because of their direct effect on the intestinal flora, but may be used parenterally with caution. If ingested, topical antibiotic ointments also may induce the syndrome.

Conjunctivitis: Conjunctivitis frequently is caused by *Chlamydia psittaci* in guinea pigs, although *Salmonella* spp, *Streptococcus* spp, *Staphylococcus aureus*, and *Pasteurella multocida* also can be involved. Clinical signs include conjunctival hyperemia and chemosis and a purulent ocular exudate. Diagnosis is based on demonstration of the agent in conjunctival smears or isolation and identification of the causative organism. Treatment with appropriate ophthalmic antibiotics should be effective.

Lymphadenitis: Inflammation and enlargement of the cervical lymph nodes is common in guinea pigs. The causative organism is usually β-hemolytic *Streptococcus zooepidemicus*, although other bacteria also may cause the condition. The organisms may gain entry to the lymphatics from abrasions of the oral mucosa or from the upper respiratory tract. Clinical findings are large, often unilateral swellings or abscesses in the ventral region of the neck. Otitis media and panophthalmitis also may be associated with cervical lymphadenitis. Microscopically, there is suppuration of the cervical lymph nodes. Diagnosis is based on clinical signs and isolation and identification of the causative organism. The use of abrasive materials in feed or litter should be avoided. In addition, upper respiratory tract infections should be prevented and controlled. Affected animals should be culled since organisms from the draining abscesses may infect others in the colony. Antibiotic therapy generally is unrewarding because of the adverse effects of many antibiotics (*see* above). Cephaloridine (25 mg/kg body wt, IM, daily) is reported to be effective in controlling and eliminating the disease.

Metastatic Calcification: Although usually clinically inapparent, this occurs most often in male guinea pigs >1 yr old. Signs include stiff joints and high mortality. At necropsy, calcium deposits are seen in the lungs, liver, heart, aorta, stomach, colon, kidneys, joints, and skeletal muscles. There are conflicting reports concerning the etiology; however, most agree that when animals are fed diets low in magnesium and potassium, the calcific lesions increase with the phosphorus content of the ration. The condition may be minimized or prevented by feeding diets that contain adequate magnesium (0.35%), a calcium:phosphorus ratio of 1.3-1.5:1, and not more than 6 IU of vitamin D/g.

Muscular Dystrophy: Guinea pigs are exquisitely sensitive to vitamin E deficiency. Signs are stiffness, lameness, and refusal to move. Microscopic lesions include coagulative necrosis, and inflammation and proliferation of nuclei in skeletal muscle fibers. Diets should provide vitamin E at 3-5 mg/100 g body wt/day.

Parasitic Diseases: Several protozoa (*Toxoplasma gondii, Eimeria caviae, Encephalitozoon (Nosema) cuniculi*), nematodes (*Paraspidodera uncinata*), and lice (*Gyropus ovalis, Gliricola porcelli*) may infect guinea pigs. (*See* PARASITIC DISEASES OF RATS AND MICE, p 1020 *et seq*, for control and treatment of nematodes and ectoparasites.)

Pneumonia: Caused in guinea pigs by several bacteria (*Bordetella bronchiseptica, Streptococcus zooepidemicus, S pneumoniae, Klebsiella pneumoniae*, or *Pasteurella pneumotropica*), clinical signs are of respiratory distress. Diagnosis is based on signs, pneumonic lesions, and isolation and identification of the causative organism. Prevention and control depend on maintenance of good husbandry and culling of affected animals. Treatment with antibiotics should be approached cautiously since most commonly used antibiotics are toxic for guinea pigs (*see* above). Treatment with tetracycline PO or parenterally, or chloramphenicol parenterally may be helpful.

Pregnancy Toxemia or Ketosis: A metabolic disorder similar to that observed in sheep before parturition (qv, p 456). Predisposing factors are obesity and any stress that might induce temporary anorexia during the late stages of pregnancy. Relative uterine ischemia in obese sows and/or those with a larger than normal litter size may also contribute to the development of this condition. Clinical findings are anorexia, adipsia, muscle spasms, coma within 48 hr of onset, and death within 4-5 days, unless the course is interrupted by parturition. Laboratory findings are aciduria, proteinuria, and hyperlipemia. Microscopically, there is fatty degeneration of parenchymatous organs. Control may be achieved by preventing obesity, avoiding stress during late pregnancy, and providing a high-quality ration during pregnancy. Early treatment with propylene glycol PO, calcium gluconate IP, or parenteral corticosteroids may be helpful, although the prognosis remains poor.

Ringworm: In guinea pigs, this dermatomycotic infection is usually caused by *Trichophyton mentagrophytes*, less frequently by *Microsporum gypseum*. It causes patchy alopecia, usually starting at the head, characterized by crusty, flaking lesions on the skin. Facial lesions are usually prominent, but the disease may spread over the posterior portions of the back. Diagnosis is based on lesions, and isolation and identification of the causative agent in/on infected hairs. The disease usually is self-limiting if good husbandry and sanitation are maintained. Long-term feeding of griseofulvin (2.5 mg/100 g body wt) is effective. Isolated skin lesions may be treated effectively with tolnaftate cream applied daily for 2-4 wk. The disease is contagious to man and other animals.

Salmonellosis: In guinea pigs, this is similar to the disease in other animals (*see* p 148).

Scurvy (Vitamin C Deficiency): Guinea pigs require a continuous dietary supply of ascorbic acid (vitamin C) because they lack the enzymes necessary for conversion of L-gulonolactone to L-ascorbic acid and cannot store the vitamin to any appreciable extent. Signs of vitamin C deficiency are unsteady gait, painful locomotion, hemorrhage from gums, swelling of costochondral junctions and joints, and emaciation. Lesions include hemorrhages in the subcutis, in the skeletal muscle around joints, and on all serosal surfaces. Microscopically, there is disarray of cartilage columns and fibrosis of the marrow in areas of active osteogenesis. The condition may be prevented by providing 15-25 mg/day of ascorbic acid. When commercial guinea pig diets are properly stored after milling, the vitamin C is stable for 3 mo. Diets manufactured for laboratory use have milling dates imprinted on the bag, but diets destined for the pet trade may not. Supplementation should be considered if the milling date is unknown; marginal diets should be supplemented with vitamin C in the drinking water. Vegetables high in vitamin C, such as parsley, cabbage, green pepper, and kale may be used but can serve as a source of infection for Tyzzer's disease, salmonellosis, etc. Lettuce (frequently used by pet owners) is a poor source of vitamin C.

Slobbers (Ptyalism): Several conditions characterized by wet, matted hair around the mouth, chin, and ventral neck. Drooling occurs whenever mastication or deglutition is impaired, which is usually due to dental abnormalities; however, subacute scurvy (vitamin C deficiency) also may cause ptyalism due to mandibular deformity, as may folate deficiency or excess dietary fluoride. The incisors of guinea pigs, like those of other rodents, grow continuously. Thus, malocclusion may result in tooth overgrowth and difficult mastication. When ptyalism is noted, the mouth should be evaluated carefully. Incisor teeth can be clipped or cheek teeth filed to improve occlusion, but if malocclusion continues, dental prophylaxis at monthly intervals may be necessary. If scurvy has resulted in mandibular deformity, the prognosis is poor.

DISEASES OF HAMSTERS

Golden or Syrian hamsters (*Mesocricetus auratus*) are susceptible to infection by a number of common bacteria, including streptococci, salmonellae, leptospires, staphylococci, and pasteurellae. Clinical signs and lesions are similar to those seen in other animals. Antibacterial therapy should be given cautiously since hamsters are highly susceptible to antibiotic-associated enterocolitis. For antibiotic toxicity, *see* the discussion under DISEASES OF GUINEA PIGS, p 1026.

Hamsters may occasionally be infected by the tapeworm *Hymenolepis nana*, and the pinworm *Syphacia obvelata*. (*See* PARASITIC DISEASES OF RATS AND MICE, p 1020 *et seq* for lesions and therapy.)

Two species of demodectic mites, *Demodex criceti* and *D aurati*, are commonly found on hamsters, usually those >18 mo old. Dermatitis and alopecia over the back and rump may result. Diagnosis is by identification of the mites in a skin scraping. The condition responds to treatment with acaricides that are used on dogs (qv, p 1500). Ronnel, 4% solution in propylene glycol, applied daily for several weeks has been effective. Dermatitis of the ears, face, feet, and tail may be caused by *Notoedres* sp mites. Ivermectin at 200 μg/kg body wt has been recommended.

Hamsters are very sensitive to vitamin E deficiency, which leads to skeletal muscular dystrophy. Balanced diets formulated specifically for hamsters are commercially available; however, hamsters also thrive on commercial rat and mouse diets.

Amyloidosis is common in hamsters >1 yr old, and the prevalence increases with age. It is usually subclinical until renal function is impaired by amyloid deposits. When azotemia results, signs include anorexia, ruffled fur, hunched posture, and depression. There is no effective treatment.

Naturally occurring lymphocytic choriomeningitis (LCM) has been reported in both laboratory and commercial breeding colonies. Wild mice usually serve as the reservoir in nature, but transplantable tumors or other cell lines contaminated with the virus are the source in laboratory outbreaks. Generally the disease is subclinical in hamsters, but large quantities of virus are shed in the urine and may serve as a source of human infections.

Hamsters are susceptible to other viruses that produce mild clinical disease or subclinical infection (*see* TABLE 6, OTHER VIRAL INFECTIONS OF RATS AND MICE, p 1024).

Proliferative ileitis is a specific, apparently infectious disease of uncertain etiology, although *Campylobacter jejuni* has been implicated. It is also called wet tail, regional enteritis, or transmissible ileal hyperplasia. The disease is endemic in some laboratory and commercial colonies, and may reach epidemic proportions. Acute clinical signs are diarrhea (wet tail), dehydration, anorexia, depression, and death within 48 hr. Weanling animals (3-8 wk old) are most often affected. Lesions include ileitis or typhlitis or both, and colitis with marked hyperplasia of the ileal epithelium. This epithelial hyperplasia results in marked thickening and rigidity of the ileal wall with partial stenosis of the lumen that may lead to ileal obstruction, intussusception, or impaction. The condition may respond to therapy with tetracycline (400 mg/L in drinking water for 10-15 days) and oral kaolin-pectin suspension. It has been reported that 0.5 g erythromycin phosphate/gal. (3.8 L) of drinking water reduced mortality in a large breeding colony. While this may predispose to antibiotic-associated enterocolitis, it may be attempted in selected cases. Vigorous therapy for dehydration and acidosis is also usually necessary. Affected animals should be isolated under cage filter covers and both facility and procedural barriers maintained in contaminated rooms.

DISEASES OF FERRETS

Ferrets should be routinely vaccinated against canine distemper with modified live virus or chicken-embryo tissue culture origin only. Modified live canine distemper virus vaccines of ferret culture origin should not be used because of vaccine-induced disease. Inactivated distemper virus vaccine produces questionable immunity. Vaccination should begin at 8-10 wk of age (4-6 wk if the dam has no titer) and repeated at 10-12 wk, then q2-3yr. An inactivated rabies virus vaccine of murine origin may be administered subcut. to ferrets ≥3 mo old, and repeated annually. Commercially raised ferrets are usually vaccinated when 6-8 wk old with *Clostridium botulinum* type C toxoid, but pet ferrets need not be vaccinated if they are fed fresh food such as canned or dry cat or dog food. Ferrets are not susceptible to feline panleukopenia, feline rhinotracheitis, feline calicivirus, canine parvovirus, infectious canine hepatitis, or mink enteritis virus under natural conditions; vaccination against these diseases is not required.

Bacterial Diseases: *Staphylococcus aureus* causes mastitis, dermatitis, abscesses, and vulvar infections during estrus. *Streptococcus zooepidemicus* causes abscesses, pneumonia, metritis, and vulvar infections. *Escherichia coli* causes mastitis, metritis, vulvar infections, pneumonia, and septicemia. *Campylobacter* spp and *Campylobacter*-like organisms have been associated with proliferative colitis and gastric ulcer disease. Treatment is the same as for dogs and cats. Ferrets are also susceptible to botulism and to avian, bovine, and human strains of tuberculosis. Intradermal tuberculin injections are undiagnostic in ferrets.

Canine Distemper: Ferrets are susceptible to infection with canine distemper virus (CDV). Transmission is by aerosol and direct contact with CDV-infected secretions. Exposed animals appear normal until 7-10 days after exposure, when anorexia and a rash at the chin and inguinal area are evident; 1-2 days later, mucopurulent ocular and nasal discharges are characteristic. The ferret usually deteriorates until death occurs 12-14 days after exposure. Antibacterial and supportive therapy may be helpful, but the prognosis is grave. Ferrets that initially survive may die of a neurotropic form of the disease weeks to months later.

Influenza: Ferrets are susceptible to infection with human influenza virus. Persons shedding the virus should wear gloves and face masks when handling ferrets. Infected ferrets may exhibit anorexia, depression, and fever. Sneezing and purulent nasal discharge may accompany the fever for 1-2 wk. Typically, recovery is rapid after the fever subsides. Immunity is conferred against the homologous strains for 4-6 wk. Vaccination with attenuated live virus affords little protection against nonhomologous strains. The virus may be transmitted from ferrets to man.

Mycotic Infections: Ringworm (*Microsporum canis*) has been reported in ferrets. Lesions are similar to those in cats. Griseofulvin (25 mg/kg) PO for several weeks is effective.

Parasites: Ferrets may have sarcoptic mange mites, fleas, ear mites, heartworms, and GI helminths. Treatment of these conditions is the same as for cats.

Miscellaneous Diseases: Aplastic anemia caused by estrogen-induced bone marrow depression is commonly associated with prolonged estrus in unbred female ferrets. Females are induced ovulators and remain in estrus up to 6 mo if not bred. The syndrome may be avoided by spaying females when 6-8 mo old. Prognosis is guarded in clinically affected jills. Once the animal is stabilized by blood replacement and/or estrus terminated by IM administration of 20 μg of gonadotropin-releasing hormone or 50-100 IU human chorionic gonadotropin, ovariohysterectomy is recommended.

Lymphoid system tumors, most commonly lymphosarcoma, are the tumors most often reported in ferrets. Ferret parvovirus (Aleutian disease virus) and a ferret retrovirus are suspected etiologic agents. Reproductive tract tumors (eg, leiomyoma of the ovary) and skin and subcut. tumors (eg, squamous cell carcinoma) are the next most commonly reported tumors of ferrets.

Seasonal weight loss in the spring, up to 30-40% of body wt, normally occurs in both sexes when subcut. fat stores from the fall are absorbed. Testicles descend into the scrotum only from December through July when spermatogenesis occurs.

Neonate eyes open at 34 days of age, and weaning occurs at 6-8 wk, although solid food may be consumed by 2 wk. Ferrets are fed a combination of commercial dog and cat food. They are extremely susceptible to heat prostration; optimal environmental temperature is 40-65°F (4-18°C) with 40-65% humidity. Coat colors include albino, sable, or fitch (black guard hair), siamese (brown guard hair), silver mitt (sable with white chest and feet), and siamese silver mitt. Anesthetics used in cats may be used in ferrets.

Table 7. Some Physiological Data of Laboratory Animals

Species	Approx. Gestation Period* (days)	Approx. Litter Size	Age at Sexual Maturity (Body wt)	Total RBC ($\times 10^{12}$/L)	Total WBC ($\times 10^9$/L)	Average Body Temp. (°C)	Approx. Water Consumption** (per day)
Mice	19-21	6-10	6 wk (20-30 g)	7-11	4-12	37	4-7 mL
Rats	21-23	6-14	3 mo (0.2-0.3 kg)	7-10	5-15	38	30 mL
Guinea pigs	68	1-4	3-4 mo (0.4-0.5 kg)	5-7	7-14	39	150 mL
Hamsters, golden	16	4-10	2 mo (85-110 g)	6-7	7-10	38	30 mL
Gerbils	25	2-9	3 mo (60-100 g)	7-8	8-11	39	4 mL
Rabbits	30	4-12	5-6 mo (3-4 kg)	5-7	6-12	40	300-700 mL
Squirrel monkeys	170	1	3-5 yr (0.6-1.1 kg)	8.3	8.2	39	70-110 mL
Rhesus monkeys	165	1-2	3-5 yr (5-11 kg)	4-6	10-20	38	0.2-1 L
Chimpanzees	225	1	8-12 yr (40-50 kg)	4-6	6-14	37	0.6-1.5 L
Baboons	154-183	1	3-6 yr (11-30 kg)	4-5	5-9	39	0.3-0.5 L

*See also REPRODUCTIVE PHENOMENA, p 640.

**Varies with number of animals per cage, moisture in feed, temperature, etc.

DISEASES OF NONHUMAN PRIMATES

The primate species most widely used in research are *Macaca mulatta* (rhesus monkey), *M fascicularis* (cynomolgus monkey), *M nemestrina* (pig-tailed monkey), *Cercopithecus aethiops* (African green monkey, vervet), *Papio* spp (baboons), *Saimiri sciureus* (squirrel monkey), *Aotus trivirgatus* (owl monkey), *Cebus* spp (capuchins), *Ateles* spp (spider monkeys), *Saguinus* spp (marmosets), and *Callithrix* spp (tamarins, marmosets).

Increased restrictions on exportation or availability of primates from countries of origin have led to decreased inportation and increased domestic production, with an attendant increase in the cost of primates. Importation of primates into the USA is prohibited except for scientific, educational, and exhibition purposes.

Primates are susceptible to, or may carry, numerous infectious diseases, many of which are anthroponoses and zoonoses. They should be quarantined before use for 1-3 mo, to permit adequate evaluation of their health status, and adaptation to the laboratory environment.

BACTERIAL DISEASES

Intestinal Diseases: The bacteria most commonly associated with intestinal disease in primates are *Shigella*, *Salmonella*, and *Yersinia* spp, *Campylobacter jejuni*, and occasionally, enterotoxigenic *Escherichia coli*, *Pseudomonas aeruginosa*, and *Aerobacter aerogenes (hydrophila)*. Primates may be intermittent, asymptomatic carriers of any of these organisms.

Diarrhea is a major problem in primates. Clinical signs include watery or mucoid blood-tinged feces, and rapid dehydration, emaciation, and prostration. Rectal prolapse is an occasional sequela. Helminths or protozoa may be a complicating factor. Mortality can be extremely high in acute outbreaks unless treatment is instituted promptly to restore and maintain normal fluid and electrolyte balance. The most common lesions at necropsy are hemorrhagic enteritis, enterocolitis, colonic ulcers, or simply colitis.

Clinical signs and death are generally due to dehydration, hypokalemia, and metabolic acidosis. Affected primates should be treated individually. Hydration should be maintained with parenteral lactated Ringer's solution. Potassium, B vitamins, electrolytes, and antibacterial agents can be administered PO or by nasogastric tube in most primates. Widespread intensive use of broad-spectrum antibiotics may lead to development of resistant strains of organisms. The combination of trimethoprim (4.4 mg/kg body wt) and sulfamethoxazole (17.6 mg/kg of body wt), administered as a total daily oral dose for 10 days is useful in treating active shigellosis and may aid in eliminating the organism from carriers. Erythromycin (5 mg/kg, b.i.d., IM) for 7-14 days is recommended for treating *Campylobacter*-associated diarrhea.

Pneumonia: Upper respiratory disease and pneumonia of bacterial origin can cause widespread illness and mortality, particularly in newly imported primates. Causative agents include *Streptococcus pneumoniae*, *Klebsiella pneumoniae*, *Bordetella bronchiseptica*, *Haemophilus influenzae*, and various species of streptococci, staphylococci, and pasteurellae. Pneumonia may accompany or follow primary disease elsewhere, eg, pneumonia and dysentery often occur together. Clinical signs may include coughing, sneezing, dyspnea, mucoid or mucopurulent nasal discharge, lethargy, anorexia, and unthriftiness. The principal lesions seen at necropsy are those of broncho- or lobar pneumonia.

Antibiotic therapy generally is helpful in treating primate pneumonias. Cultures from pharyngeal swabs or transtracheal lavage are useful in isolating the causative agent and determining the specific antibiotic sensitivity. Treatment of animals at risk with a long-acting penicillin or a broad-spectrum antibiotic is appropriate. Intensive nursing and other supportive therapy, such as fluid and oxygen administration, may also aid recovery in selected cases.

Tuberculosis: All primates are susceptible to tuberculosis, although species differences exist; eg, Old World primate species such as rhesus monkeys are very sensitive to infection, while New World species such as squirrel monkeys appear to be less susceptible. Clinical signs are not a reliable indication of the extent of tuberculosis in monkeys. An animal that appears healthy may have extensive miliary disease involving thoracic and abdominal organs; signs of debilitation may appear only shortly before death. A testing program is mandatory. Tuberculin tests should be performed on all primates on arrival at the facility and at 2-wk intervals thereafter until at least 3 consecutive negative tests have been recorded for the entire group.

The time from initial infection to skin-test conversion is 3-4 wk in rhesus monkeys. Late in the disease, anergy can result in a negative skin test. After their release from quarantine, all primates should be skin-tested at least semiannually, and quarterly testing is recommended. The test consists of injecting mammalian tuberculin or Old Tuberculin (15 mg or 1500 tuberculin units in 0.1 mL of water) intradermally into the upper eyelid or the shaved abdominal skin. The animal is examined at 24, 48, and 72 hr. A positive hypersensitivity reaction is marked by edema, induration, or erythema. Radiographic examination of the chest may aid diagnosis in well-established cases, but is unreliable, since lesions rarely calcify or cavitate as they do in man. The tuberculin skin test is the primary diagnostic method for routine surveillance. Other diagnostic tests, such as culture and staining of a gastric lavage sample, ELISA, and comparative testing with avian and atypical tuberculins, may aid in diagnosis. Due to the public health risk, euthanasia is recommended for all positive reactors. Tuberculosis should then be confirmed by necropsy. Personnel working in primate facilities should have semiannual skin tests.

Isoniazid is an effective tuberculostat when administered daily at 5-10 mg/kg body wt on a sugar cube or incorporated in the feed of valuable, endangered primates such as great apes. However, it may suppress the skin-test reaction. There is no evidence that the continuous use of isoniazid leads to development of isoniazid-resistant mycobacteria.

MYCOTIC DISEASES

See also FUNGAL INFECTIONS, p 340.

Microsporum and *Trichophyton* spp affect primates. Topical treatment of ringworm with undecylenic acid ointment or 1% tolnaftate cream b.i.d. for 2-3 wk, or administration of griseofulvin (25 mg/kg, PO, for 3-4 wk) is recommended. *Candida* sp is a common saprophyte of the skin, GI tract, or reproductive tract, and acts as a facultative pathogen in debilitating conditions. Ulcers or white, raised plaques may be seen on the tongue or mouth; the fungus may also attack fingernails. Oral lesions must be differentiated from those of trauma, monkeypox, or herpesvirus infections. A topical cream containing nystatin is effective in superficial infections. Oral nystatin (200,000 u, q.i.d., continued for 48 hr after clinical recovery) is effective for GI tract candidiasis. *Dermatophilus congolensis* has been reported in owl monkeys. Papillomatous lesions are seen on the face and extremities. The infection is transmissible to man. Aspergillosis may occur in various primate species, and the organism usually is a facultative pathogen.

PARASITIC DISEASES

Newly imported primates harbor numerous parasites. Some are commensal; others can be made self-limiting by strict sanitation and good husbandry. However, some can cause serious diseases or debilitation and should be removed by specific treatment.

Arthropods: Pulmonary acariasis (*Pneumonyssus* sp) is common in wild-caught Asian and African primates, particularly rhesus monkeys and baboons. Infection is rare in laboratory-raised primates. The life cycle of *Pneumonyssus* sp is not well understood. Infestations usually do not produce serious disease, although they may cause sneezing and coughing. Lesions include dilation and focal chronic inflammation of terminal bronchioles. The gross lesions may occasionally be confused with tuberculous granulomas. Ivermectin (200 μg/kg body wt, subcut.) has been used for treatment in closed breeding colonies.

Mange mites (*Psorergates* spp, *Sarcoptes scabiei*) or sucking lice (*Pedicinus obtusus [longiceps]*) are seen occasionally and may produce dermatoses. Topical treatment of affected animals with pyrethrin, repeated after 3 days, if necessary, is recommended. Use of more toxic parasiticides should be avoided because of the possibility of ingestion during grooming.

Helminths: *Oesophagostomum* may cause characteristic granulomatous nodules in the large bowel associated with development of the worms and with an immune reaction of the host. The nodules may rupture and cause peritonitis. *Strongyloides* and *Trichostrongylus* are invasive; adults may cause enteritis and diarrhea; larvae may cause pulmonary lesions during migration. These helminths, as well as *Trichuris*, can be treated effectively with thiabendazole (100 mg/kg body wt), administered PO at intervals of 2-4 wk. *Prosthenorchis* are filarid worms, common in Central and South American primates, that burrow into the mucosa of the ileocecal junction and sometimes perforate the bowel, or cause obstruction when present in large numbers. Cockroaches are intermediate hosts, and their elimination, along with strict sanitation, is essential if infection is to be controlled. *Dipetalonema* and *Tetrapetalonema* occur in the peritoneal cavity of New World species; large numbers may be present without apparent harm to the host. *Filaroides* are found in the lungs.

Protozoa: Primates may serve as hosts of various intestinal amebae. *Entamoeba histolytica* is the principal pathogenic form in nonhuman primates as it is in man. In a heavy infection it may cause severe enteritis and diarrhea, and cysts may be demonstrated in the feces in large numbers. *Giardia* inhabit the upper small intestine and may cause diarrhea. Treatment with metronidazole (50 mg/kg, PO, daily for 5-10 days) is recommended.

Blood parasites, such as *Plasmodium*, *Leishmania*, and *Trypanosoma* spp also occur. Generally, there is an equilibrium between the parasite and the natural host, but serious reactions may result from cross-infections. Transmission of simian malarias to man has occurred in areas where the appropriate mosquito vectors are present. The disease usually does not pose a clinical problem in primate colonies. Some primate species, such as owl monkeys, are excellent models for malarial research.

Naturally occurring toxoplasmosis (*T gondii*) has been reported more frequently in Central and South American primates than in African or Asian primates. Clinical signs of infection tend to be nonspecific (lethargy, anorexia, diarrhea). Hepatic focal necrosis and fibrinous pneumonia with edema are common histological findings. *Toxoplasma* can be demonstrated in blood smears in acute cases.

VIRAL DISEASES

Many herpesviruses affect primates; some exist as latent or subclinical infections in reservoir hosts, but cause severe disease or death when transmitted naturally to other hosts. All macaques are considered to be potential shedders of herpesvirus simiae (herpesvirus B). The infection is generally subclinical or mild (conjunctivitis or oral vesicles) in *Macaca* spp, but may cause a fatal encephalitis and encephalomyelitis in man. Transmission may occur through a bite, by contamination of a superficial wound with infected saliva, conjunctival secretion, or by aerosol. Fatalities in handlers of primates due to herpesvirus B encephalitis emphasize the importance of preventing direct or indirect contact with secretions and body fluids from macaques.

Herpesvirus T (H tamarinus, H platyrrhinae) causes mild herpetic lingual ulcers and stomatitis in squirrel monkeys (*Saimiri sciureus*), but fatal epidemics have followed natural transmission to owl monkeys (*Aotus trivirgatus*) and marmosets (*Saguinus* spp). **"Herpesvirus hominis"** (Herpes simplex virus 1) causes a mild infection in man and certain other primates, but owl monkeys, gibbons, and tree shrews (*Tupaia glis*) are highly susceptible and may die; signs may include mucous membrane or skin ulcerations, conjunctivitis, meningitis, or encephalitis.

Man may transmit to chimpanzees the virus of infectious hepatitis (**hepatitis A virus**). Elevated AST (SGOT) and ALT (SGPT) values are of diagnostic significance. High levels of antibody to hepatitis A virus have been demonstrated in laboratory-maintained owl monkeys, suggesting that this species also is susceptible to natural infection.

Table 8. Nonhuman Primate Therapeutics

Antibiotics	
Amoxicillin	11 mg/kg, IM or subcut., daily
	11 mg/kg, PO, b.i.d.
Gentamicin	5 mg/kg, IM or subcut., daily
Trimethoprim-sulfadiazine 24%	1 mL/9 kg, subcut., daily
Trimethoprim-sulfamethoxazole syrup	TMP 4 mg/kg, PO, b.i.d.
	SMZ 20 mg/kg, PO, b.i.d.

Parasiticides	
Ivermectin	200 μg/kg, IM or subcut.
Fenbendazole	50 mg/kg, PO daily for 3 days, repeat in 2 wk
Mebendazole	22 mg/kg, PO daily for 3 days, repeat in 2 wk
Metronidazole	50 mg/kg, PO daily for 5 days
Thiabendazole	100 mg/kg, PO once, repeat in 3 wk

Anesthetics/Analgesics	
Ketamine hydrochloride	10 mg/kg, IM, restraint only; with diazepam 0.5 mg/kg, IM, for additional muscle relaxation
Maintenance of surgical plane anesthesia: a) Inhalant gas (isoflurane, methoxyflurane, halothane) or b) Sodium pentobarbital	25 mg/kg, IV, given slowly to effect
Banamine (analgesic)	1 mg/kg, IV, b.i.d.
Meperidine	1-4 mg/kg, IM, q4-6hr
Pentazocine	1-5 mg/kg, IM, q3-4hr

Because vaccines are not available to protect primate colony personnel or the primates against herpes and hepatitis viral infections, exposure should be prevented. This is best accomplished by carefully training personnel in the handling of primates; use of protective clothing, face masks or shields, and gloves; separating primates in species-specific rooms; and strict attention to hygienic standards.

Several other viruses commonly produce clinical disease in newly imported primates. **Rubeola infection** (measles) can assume epidemic proportions. The virus causes a nonpruritic, exanthematous rash on the chest and lower portions of the body; it may also cause interstitial giant-cell pneumonia, rhinitis, and conjunctivitis. There is no specific treatment. Vaccination of infant rhesus monkeys, other macaques, and marmosets with human measles vaccine is recommended. **Monkeypox** may occur in primate colonies. It is characterized by a maculopapular rash and variolous pustules. Affected monkeys usually survive; after recovery, they are immune to challenge with vaccinia virus.

Simian acquired immunodeficiency syndrome (SAIDS) is caused by at least 4 distinct viral isolates, none of which has been shown to infect man. Two type D retroviruses and 3 different lentiviruses may produce an immunodeficiency-related complex of diseases such as atypical mycobacteriosis, intestinal cryptosporidiosis, pneumocystis pneumonia, and candidiasis in colonies of macaques, African green monkeys, and sooty mangabeys. There is great host-interspecies variation in clinical signs and susceptibility from virus to virus. Transmission between primates is via direct or indirect contact with infected blood and other body fluids. Prognosis is grave in clinically affected animals.

NUTRITIONAL DISEASES

See also NUTRITION: EXOTIC AND ZOO ANIMALS, p 1210.

All laboratory primates are susceptible to vitamin C deficiency. Vitamin-C-deficient animals usually succumb to infectious diseases before clinical signs of the deficiency appear. Commercial monkey diets contain vitamin C that is stable for 3 mo after the diet is milled and packaged, if properly stored. Supplemental sources are citrus fruits. Orally administered pediatric vitamin preparations that contain ascorbic acid are readily accepted. Daily intake of vitamin C at ~4 mg/kg body wt prevents scurvy. Primates require vitamin D to prevent rickets and osteomalacia. Asian and African primates can utilize provitamin D_2 (in plant materials); Central and South American primates cannot—they require provitamin D_3. Animal proteins and fish-liver oils provide an adequate source of D_3, or as little as 1.25 IU/g of diet can be added to the ration. Without adequate D_3, New World primates may develop osteodystrophia fibrosa (qv, p 483).

MISCELLANEOUS DISEASES

Acute Gastric Dilatation: This occurs sporadically in primate colonies, and may be associated with feed or water restriction, and accidental overfeeding or overwatering. Etiological factors may include intragastric fermentation associated with *Clostridium perfringens* and abnormal gastric function. Clinical findings are similar to those seen in small animals (*see* p 234). The condition often is fatal unless emergency treatment is given. The stomach must be evacuated and fluids replaced, in like volume, with lactated Ringer's solution given parenterally. Shock and dehydration usually occur, and require prompt treatment. Periodic evacuation of the stomach may be necessary for several days until GI function is normal. Metabolic alkalosis may result from continued loss of hydrochloric acid. Adequate sodium, chloride, and potassium must be provided via parenteral fluid therapy.

Trauma: Trauma from cagemate aggression or self-mutilation (biting or hair pulling) may occur occasionally, as may thinning of the hair due to self-induced alopecia. Measures to enhance the psychological well-being of primates, eg, group housing, exercise pens, and cage toys, are currently being evaluated.

DISEASES OF AMPHIBIANS

The most widely used amphibians are leopard frogs (*Rana pipiens*), bullfrogs (*R catesbiana*), African clawed frogs (*Xenopus laevis*), marine toads (*Bufo marinus*), salamanders (*Ambystoma* spp), and Mexican axolotls (*Seridon mexicanum*). Most laboratory specimens are collected in the wild, but several breeding colonies exist. Malnutrition, parasitism, and certain bacterial and viral diseases are common. Good husbandry and adequate feeding are key elements in managing amphibians intended for laboratory use. However, individual or mass treatment of diseased amphibians can be used selectively in management of certain diseases.

Bacterial Diseases: Saprophytic, gram-negative organisms such as *Aeromonas hydrophila*, and *Pseudomonas, Proteus*, and *Citrobacter* spp can cause the so-called "red-leg" syndrome (bacterial septicemia). Malnourished, newly received amphibians maintained in poor-quality water are particularly susceptible. Clinical signs may include lethargy; emaciation; ulcerations of the skin, nose, and toes; and characteristic cutaneous pinpoint hemorrhages of the legs and abdomen. Hemorrhages may also occur in skeletal muscles, tongue, and nictitating membrane. In acute cases, these signs may be absent. Histological evidence of systemic infection may include inflammatory or necrotic foci in the liver, spleen, and other coelomic organs. Tank treatment with nifurpirinol may be helpful. Individual treatment with oxytetracycline (150 mg/kg body wt, b.i.d.) or chloramphenicol (50 mg/kg body wt, b.i.d.) may be effective. The antibiotics should be administered in a small volume of distilled water (0.2 mL to a 30-g frog) by stomach tube for ≥5 consecutive days. Prognosis is guarded. Prevention is best accomplished by maintaining optimal husbandry and caging conditions, avoiding overcrowding, and using circulating filtered water or flowing water.

Amphibian mycobacteriosis occurs principally in debilitated animals and usually is not a colony problem. "Cold water" mycobacteria are widely present in aquatic environments, and the usual portal of entry is thought to be the skin. Accidental infection from unsterile parenteral injections may occur. Affected animals may exhibit typical tuberculous granulomas in the liver, kidneys, spleen, lungs, and other coelomic organs. Specific treatment is not feasible.

Chlamydia psittaci infection has occurred in *Xenopus laevis*. Affected frogs die peracutely or exhibit lethargy, disequilibrium, cutaneous depigmentation, petechiae, and edema. Histologically, intracytoplasmic basophilic inclusion bodies can be identified in sinusoidal lining cells of the liver and spleen. Antibiotic treatment as described for other bacterial diseases of amphibians may be effective.

Parasitic and Mycotic Diseases: Helminth parasites, protozoa, and ectoparasites are common in wild-caught amphibians, but heavy parasite loads are detrimental. Gavaging amphibians with thiabendazole and prevention of reinfestation by disinfection or replacement of substrate is said to be effective. Inflammatory reactions to parasitism are often imperceptible. Laboratory-reared animals have a strikingly lower incidence of helminths than those collected in the field. The parasite loads of wild-caught amphibians can be reduced markedly by maintaining good husbandry and nutrition in the laboratory.

Fonsecaea sp and *Cladosporium* sp are among the genera of brown-pigmented septate fungi that cause chromomycosis. The fungi are ubiquitous opportunistic pathogens. Gross and microscopic lesions are similar to mycobacteriosis, but are differentiated by the presence of pigmented fungal forms. Adequate sanitation of holding tanks, good nutrition, and maintenance of environmental homeostasis aid in preventing infection.

Viral Diseases: Renal adenocarcinomas (Lucké tumors) are relatively common in *Rana pipiens* wild-caught in the northeastern and northcentral USA. Few tumor-bearing frogs are seen in the summer since viral replication is temperature dependent. Virus particles and inclusion bodies are seen when frogs are in hibernation, at 41-50°F (5-10°C). Metastasis of the tumor to liver, lungs, and other organs is common; both the primary and metastatic tumors can become very large. There is no treatment. The neoplasm is a model of herpesvirus-induced cancer.

Nutritional Diseases: Long-term laboratory maintenance of most amphibians requires live food. Rickets is one example of a nutritional deficiency that may occur in frogs (*Rana* spp). Amphibians should be fed live food such as crickets, sow bugs, meal worms, or flies as a part of a balanced diet that includes dog- or monkey chow. Coating the insects with powdered multiple-vitamin preparations that includes vitamin D and calcium is one way to supplement a natural diet.

MANAGEMENT, HUSBANDRY, AND DISEASES OF MARINE MAMMALS

Marine mammals are a diverse group of species placed together primarily because they depend on marine environments for survival. In the USA and its territories, the Marine Mammal Protection Act of 1972 protects cetaceans, pinnipeds, sirenians, sea otters, and polar bears as marine mammals. The cetaceans include 2 major groups with different physiology and anatomy—toothed whales (Odontocetes) and baleen whales (Mysticetes). The pinnipeds include 3 major groups—true seals (Phocidae), eared seals (Otariidae), and walruses (Odobenidae). Sirenians (Sirenidae) are a single family, which includes manatees and dugongs. The sea otter is a marine member of the Mustelidae, and the polar bear is the only member of the Ursidae considered marine.

Few pharmaceuticals or vaccines have been approved for use in marine mammals. Many recommendations can be made based on personal experience or published reports; however, sufficient documentation for official approval is unlikely, and caution is indicated.

HUSBANDRY

The general rule in maintaining marine mammals in captivity is to duplicate their natural environment as closely as possible. Most cetaceans live in marine habitats, although some species migrate into freshwater, and a few are adapted to river habitats. Baikal seals have adapted completely to freshwater. Marine cetaceans should be kept in water with a salinity of 25-35 g/L. Preferably this "salt" water should consist of balanced sea salts although captive animals have survived for long periods, in apparent health, in simple sodium chloride solutions. The pH of mid-ocean waters is 8-8.3; water for captive marine cetaceans should be maintained as close to this as possible. Freshwater cetaceans also require water similar to that of their natural habitat. In the USA, the Marine Mammal Protection Act specifies that coliform bacterial counts of water for captive marine mammals must be ≤1000 MPN (most probable number per 100 mL).

The temperature tolerance range of each species of cetacean can be fairly wide, but the optimal temperature range is narrower. Temperature requirements should be evaluated carefully for any cetacean in captivity. Animals kept in the extremes of their temperature tolerance range are more susceptible to environmental and infectious disease. Inappropriate combinations of display animals can result in compromises in which one or all species are held at temperatures that jeopardize their well-being but not their immediate survival.

Good air quality, especially in indoor facilities (10-20 air changes/hr) is as important as good water quality. Photoperiods, light spectral and intensity requirements, sound tolerances, and flight distance requirements are not well established for any cetacean. They undoubtedly vary between species with widely diverse habitats, and among individuals. Extremes in any of these factors should be considered detrimental in the absence of specific data for the species in question.

Most pinnipeds live in marine habitats. Their environmental requirements are similar to those of cetaceans except that pinnipeds can "haul out" on land. Although captive pinnipeds can be kept in freshwater if given additional salt in their diet, saltwater pools that meet the specifications listed above for cetaceans are preferred. Most pinnipeds obtain their metabolic water requirements in food and do not require access to freshwater if provided fish with a high-fat content. However, it is common practice to allow pinnipeds access to fresh water.

Most pinnipeds are much more tolerant of cold temperatures than excessive heat. The considerations of cetaceans are equally valid for pinnipeds. Pools for captive pinnipeds should provide shelter from wind and some shade. Haul out requirements are different for each species, and some pinnipeds, eg, the northern fur seal, require very specific timing of access to land only at the pupping season.

Sirenians have similar water requirements to those of cetaceans, although the most common sirenian in the USA, the manatee, migrates between marine and freshwater environments seasonally. It does better in captivity if salinity is changed seasonally to match migrations in the wild. It is a warmwater species.

The natural habitat of the sea otter is the Pacific northwest from northern California to Alaska. In captivity, it thrives best in a cold marine water system. Since the fur of the sea otter is its major protection against hypothermia, the water must be kept completely free of oils and organic material that could mat or damage the coat.

The polar bear naturally lives on arctic and subarctic ice. It has successfully adapted to captivity even in subtropical climates, but is more susceptible to disease in warm climates. Polar bears traditionally have been provided with freshwater in captivity. Proper attention to filtration and water quality is beneficial.

RESTRAINT

Marine mammals must be restrained for detailed examinations. Trained cetaceans and pinnipeds can be taught behaviors that facilitate examination and collection of diagnostic samples. For these animals, the presence of familiar attendants is important.

For complex procedures or untrained animals, the safest approach to restraining a cetacean is to remove it from the water. Captive enclosures should allow water drainage so cetaceans can be stranded without the use of nets. As the animal begins to lose buoyancy in the draining water, it should be positioned over thick foam pads to minimize struggling and injury. Nets are an alternative for corralling or catching small cetaceans kept in sea pens or encountered in the wild; however, experienced personnel are required to minimize the risk of drowning or injury to the animal or staff. Netted cetaceans are placed on foam or specially designed stretchers that can be suspended above water level to support and restrain the animal.

Restraint of cetaceans on the foam depends on the procedure to be performed and the animal. Small cetaceans (dolphins) can often be restrained by the weight of 3 or 4 attendants—one person controls the peduncle of the tail fluke and the others apply weight to the animal's body. The pectoral fins should be placed alongside the animal in a physiologic position to avoid permanent damage. In larger cetaceans (whales), the powerful tail fluke may need to be secured with a loop over the tail stock.

Capturing pinnipeds is generally easier on dry ground; small ones can be captured in the water with end-release hoop nets, but larger animals should not be netted in water. They must be coaxed or driven from the water or have the water drained from their pool. On land, hoop nets can be used on larger animals, but cargo nets, baffle boards, and "come-along" poles also can be helpful. Once captured, small seals can be restrained for some procedures by an experienced handler sitting on the seal's back, holding the head. Larger pinnipeds or more complex procedures require an appropriately designed squeeze cage.

Sirenians are generally relatively docile; problems in restraint center on their bulk and weight, and caution is recommended as they tend to roll. They can be handled in much the same way as cetaceans. Sea otters can be restrained like most other large mustelids. Hoop nets can be used for removing them from pools. Once out of the water, restraint bags, squeeze boxes, or other restraint devices for small wild carnivores can be used. Polar bears are large and dangerous; manual restraint is not advised.

ANESTHESIA

Tranquilizers, sedatives, and anesthetics should be used only by experienced personnel. Physiological adaptations to diving and marine environments make general anesthesia of cetaceans and pinnipeds difficult. Anesthetic drugs commonly used in other animals often have narrow margins of safety or cause unexpected reactions in marine mammals. Specialized anesthestic machines and respirators are required for cetaceans. Sirenians rarely require general anesthesia or tranquilization for treatment. Sea otters can be sedated with diazepam (0.2 mg/kg body wt) or tiletamine-zolazepam (1 mg/kg). Surgical anesthesia can be obtained with higher doses of tiletamine-zolazepam (2 mg/kg) or with halothane and nitrous oxide. Polar bears are routinely immobilized with etorphine, tiletamine-zolazepam, and other IM agents. The required dose is highly dependent on the individual animal and environment.

BACTERIAL DISEASES

Actinomycetes: Nocardiosis (*Nocardia* spp) is commonly reported in debilitated marine mammals. It has been diagnosed in the pilot whale, harbor porpoise, killer whale, false killer whale, spinner dolphin, and leopard seal. Infections due to *Actinomyces* spp also have been diagnosed in bottlenosed dolphin. Successful treatment has not been reported, but the treatment of choice would be sulfonamide therapy, except in killer whales, in which sulfonamides are contraindicated.

Clostridial Myositis: Severe myositis due to infections with *Clostridium* spp has been diagnosed in captive killer whales, pilot whales, bottlenosed dolphins, California sea lions, and manatees. All marine mammals are probably susceptible. The disease is characterized by acute swelling, muscle necrosis, and accumulations of gas in affected tissues, accompanied by a severe leukocytosis. Untreated, it can be fatal. Diagnosis is based on detection of gram-positive bacilli in aspirates of the lesions, and confirmed by anaerobic culture and identification of the organism. Treatment includes systemic and local antibiotics, surgical drainage of abscessed areas, and flushing with hydrogen peroxide. Commercially available inactivated clostridial bacterins are used routinely in some facilities, although efficacy in marine mammals has not been studied.

Pneumonia: The chief cause of death in captive marine mammals is believed to be pneumonia. It is not common in polar bears. Most cases of marine mammal pneumonia have significant bacterial involvement, and most organisms cultured from terrestrial species have been identified in marine mammals. The disease can be considered the result of mismanagement. Marine mammals require good air quality, including high rates of air exchange at the water surface in indoor facilities. Tempered air or acclimation to cold temperatures is also important to prevent lung disease, even in polar species. Animals acclimated to cold temperatures are usually quite hardy; however, sudden transition from warm environments to cold air, even with warmer water, can precipitate fulminating pneumonias, particularly in nutritionally or otherwise compromised animals. Clinical signs include lethargy, anorexia, severe halitosis, dyspnea, pyrexia, and marked leukocytosis. The disease can progress rapidly. Diagnosis is usually based on clinical signs and confirmed by response to therapy. Treatment consists of correction of environmental factors and intensive antibiotic and supportive therapy. The initial antibiotic is usually broad-spectrum, commonly cephalexin (40 mg/kg, t.i.d. or q.i.d.); adjustments are based on cultures and sensitivities from blowhole or tracheal samples.

Erysipelas (Diamond Skin Disease): Erysipelas can be a serious infectious disease of captive cetaceans and pinnipeds. The organism, *Erysipelothrix rhusiopathiae (insidiosa)*, which causes erysipelas in pigs and other domestic species, is a common contaminant of fish. A septicemic form of the disease in marine mammals can be peracute or acute; affected animals die suddenly with no prodromal signs, or with only sudden depression, inappetence, and/or fever. A cutaneous form that causes typical rhomboidal skin lesions is usually a more chronic form of the disease. Animals with this form usually recover with timely antibiotic treatment.

Necropsy of peracute cases generally fails to reveal grossly discernable lesions other than widespread petechiation. Diagnosis is based on culture of the organism from the blood, spleen, or body cavities. Arthritis has been found in animals that have died with the chronic form of the disease.

Treatment of the peracute and acute forms has rarely been attempted because the absence of prodromal signs obscures the diagnosis. Animals with the dermatologic form usually recover with administration of penicillins, tetracyclines, or chloramphenicol, and supportive treatment.

Control seems primarily related to the provision of high-quality fish, properly stored and handled. Vaccination is controversial and not implemented in many aquaria because of problems with the bacterin. Vaccine breaks are common. Vials of killed erysipelas bacterin should be cultured for surviving organisms before use in marine mammals. Modified live bacterins should be avoided for the initial vaccination. Fatal anaphylaxis can occur on revaccination. For this reason, some vaccination programs have been reduced to one-time administration even though antibody titers fall below the presumed effective level.

If cetaceans are to be revaccinated, sensitivity tests should be performed by injecting a small amount of bacterin submucosally on the lower surface of the tongue. Hypersensitive animals develop swelling and redness at the injection site within 30 min. No more than 3-5 mL of the vaccine should be used at any one site since it is extremely irritating, even in nonsensitive mammals. A long needle ($\geq$2 in. [5 cm]) should be used to assure that the vaccine is deposited in the muscle and not between muscle and blubber, or a sterile abscess may result. Bacterin should be administered in the dorsal musculature anterior and lateral to the dorsal fin. Administration posterior to the dorsal fin can immobilize the animal for several days from the severe tissue reaction. To maintain high antibody titers, a booster after 6 mo and annual revaccination is required.

Leptospirosis: This has been diagnosed in otarid pinnipeds and bears. In seals, the disease is characterized by depression, reluctance to move, polydipsia, and pyrexia. It may also cause abortions and neonatal deaths in California sea lions and Northern fur seals. Lesions include a severe, diffuse, interstitial nephritis, with renal tubules packed with spirochetes. The gallbladder may contain inspissated black bile, but hepatitis may not be apparent grossly. Hyperplasia of Kupffer's cells, erythrophago-cytosis, and hemosiderosis are seen histologically. Gastroenteritis can be a feature. Antibodies to various serovars (*canicola, icterohaemorrhagiae, autumnalis,* and *pomona*) have been identified in affected animals by FA techniques; however, only *Leptospira pomona* has been isolated from marine mammals. Treatment in pinnipeds is similar to that in dogs (qv, p 355). Control in captive situations requires serological examination of new animals during quarantine. Captive animals can be vaccinated in endemic areas. Leptospira can infect man, and appropriate precautions should be taken.

Tuberculosis: Marine mammals are susceptible to various mycobacteria. Unconfirmed tuberculosis has been reported in a stranded wild bottlenosed dolphin in the Mediterranean; otherwise, mycobacteriosis has been a disease of captivity. Pinnipeds, cetaceans, and sirenians have developed disease due to *Mycobacterium bovis, M smegmatis, M fortuitum, M chelonei,* and *M marinum.* Cutaneous and systemic forms are seen. There are strong indications that immunosuppression may be involved in the development of infections by the atypical mycobacteria. Intradermal testing with high concentrations of bovine or avian purified protein derivative (PPD) tuberculin can be used to screen exposed animals; however, anergy occurs. In pinnipeds, injections in the webbing of the rear flippers should be read at 48 and 72 hr. ELISA screening has identified antibodies in seals, but requires further evaluation before it can be considered a screening test. Diagnosis is made by culture and identification of the organism from lesion biopsies, tracheal washes, or feces. Tuberculosis in marine mammals probably is of public health significance.

Miscellaneous Bacterial Diseases: Marine mammals are probably susceptible to the entire range of pathogenic bacteria. Bacteria other than those discussed above cause significant disease in marine mammals. *Pasteurella multocida* has caused several outbreaks of hemorrhagic enteritis with depression and abdominal distress leading to acute death in dolphins and pinnipeds. It has also been reported to cause pneumonia in pinnipeds. In dolphins, *P haemolytica* has been incriminated in hemorrhagic tracheitis that responded to chloramphenicol therapy.

Plesiomonas shigelloides has been responsible for gastroenteritis in harbor seals. *Pseudomonas pseudomallei* has caused serious fatal outbreaks of disease in various marine mammals in captivity in the far east. *Salmonella* spp have caused fatal gastroenteritis in manatee and beluga whales. Staphylococcal septicemia has caused the death of a dolphin with osteomyelitis of the spine (pyogenic spondylitis). Another case of intradiskal osteomyelitis, due to *Staphylococcus aureus,* was treated successfully with a prolonged course of cefazolin sodium and cephalexin. *Staphylococcus aureus* also has been incriminated in a fatal pneumonia in a killer whale. *Vibrio* spp infect slow-healing wounds of cetaceans managed in open sea pens.

MYCOTIC DISEASES

Captive marine mammals seem particularly prone to fungal infections. There is no definitive evidence of horizontal transmission of most of these; they appear to be secondary to stress, environmental compromise, or other infectious disease. Some systemic mycoses have distinct geographic distributions. Diagnosis is based on clinical signs and confirmed by identification of the organism in biopsy or, preferably, culture. Wet mounts in lactophenol or cotton blue may render an immediate diagnosis with some of the morphologically distinct fungi. Tissue smears cleared in warm 10% potassium hydroxide can be examined to identify characteristic fruiting bodies or hyphae.

Topical medication of pinnipeds for dermatophytosis is feasible. Smaller cetaceans can be kept out of water in a sling for 2-24 hr, provided areas of the body not being treated are kept moist. Otherwise, systemic therapy is employed.

Aspergillosis: Fatal pulmonary aspergillosis has been diagnosed in bottlenosed dolphins and a California sea lion. Cutaneous aspergillosis has been seen in gray seals with concomitant mycobacteriosis. The respiratory form has been a postmortem diagnosis. Cutaneous lesions respond to topical povidone iodines with ketoconazole therapy (10 mg/kg, PO, daily).

Candidiasis: A common mycotic disease in captive cetaceans, candidiasis occurs secondary to stress, unbalanced water disinfection with chlorines, or indiscriminate antibiotic therapy. The lesions usually are found around body openings. At necropsy, esophageal ulcers are often observed, particularly in the area of the gastroesophageal junction. Diagnosis is based on identification of the yeast in cultures or biopsy. Candidiasis generally responds well to ketoconazole (6 mg/kg, PO, daily) along with correction of any environmental deficits. Early detection and treatment is usually successful. Another opportunistic yeast, *Cryptococcus neoformans*, has been diagnosed in fatal advanced pulmonary disease in a bottlenosed dolphin.

Dermatophytosis: Mycotic dermatitis due to *Trichophyton* spp or *Microsporum canis* generally responds to topical povidone iodines and/or oral griseofulvin.

Streptothricosis (Dolphin Pseudopox, Cutaneous Dermatophilosis): Streptothricosis (*Dermatophilus congolensis*), a subcut. mycosis, has been reported in pinnipeds. It must be distinguished from sealpox. Simultaneous infections of streptothricosis and pox have been recorded in sea lions. Cutaneous streptothricosis usually manifests as sharply delineated nodules distributed over the entire body, and usually progresses to death. Diagnosis is based on demonstration of the organism in biopsies or culture. Treatment with systemic antifungal drugs has been unsuccessful. *Sporothrix schenckii*, the cause of another subcut. mycosis, has been reported in a Pacific white-sided dolphin.

Systemic Mycoses: The systemic mycoses of marine mammals pose a zoonotic risk. Precautions should be taken to prevent infection when handling dead and diseased animals. Keloidal blastomycosis (Lobo's disease) has been reported only in man and dolphins. Blastomycosis has caused fatal disease in California sea lions, a Stellar sea lion, and northern fur seals. Lobomycosis due to infection with *Loboa loboi* is seen in Atlantic bottlenosed dolphin. Fatal systemic histoplasmosis has been reported in a captive harp seal. Coccidioidomycosis has been found in the California sea lion and sea otter. Blastomycosis has been successfully treated with intensive management including 70 days of itraconazole (3.5 mg/kg, PO, daily) combined with antibiotic and supportive therapy when indicated.

Zygomycetoses: *Mucor* spp and *Entomophthora* spp have caused fatal disease in the bottlenosed dolphin and harp seal. *Fusarium* dermatitis occurs in California sea lions and gray seals. These should be considered diseases of debilitated animals; the underlying cause of the low host resistance to these opportunistic infections must be corrected if therapy is to be successful. Amphotericin B is the therapy of choice for zygomycete infections, but newer imidazoles warrant consideration.

PARASITIC DISEASES

Marine mammals are susceptible to all of the major groups of parasites, including various nematodes, trematodes, cestodes, mites, lice, and acanthocephalans. Clinical experience with many of these is limited, while others are commonly seen in recently captured specimens.

Acariasis: Nasal and lung mites are found in phocid and otarid seals. Lung mites cause rattling coughs. Nasal mites cause nasal discharge but apparently little discomfort. Diagnosis is made by identifying the mite in nasal secretions or sputum. The life cycles of these mites are unknown. Infections have been cleared rapidly with 2 injections of ivermectin (200 µg/kg) 2 wk apart. Treatment of infected animals eliminates the problem in captive enclosures without environmental treatment. Mites have been associated with large, roughened lesions of the laryngeal area of cetaceans, but their overall significance or treatment is unknown.

Demodectic mange has been diagnosed in California sea lions. Nonpruritic, alopecic lesions with hyperkeratosis, scaling, and excoriation occur on the flippers and other body surfaces that contact the substrate. Diagnosis is made by deep skin scrapings and identification of the mite. Secondary bacterial infection that results in pyoderma occurs in chronic cases. Treatment is the same as in dogs. Predisposing factors in pinnipeds are unknown. The disease is not readily transmitted among contact animals.

Heavy infestations of sucking lice are common in wild pinnipeds and can cause severe anemia. The lice can be seen grossly and are readily transmitted. They are highly sensitive to chlorinated hydrocarbon insecticides. Rotenone powder is also effective. The affected animal must be removed from the water, allowed to dry before being dusted, and kept out of the water ≥12 hr. Treatments must be repeated in 10-12 days. Animals in captivity can be freed of parasites, provided that no new sources of infestation are introduced.

Lungworm: Lungworms are common in all pinnipeds. Sea lions have *Parafilaroides decorus*, while true seals are usually parasitized by *Otostrongylus circumlitus*. The latter parasite is also found in the hearts of some phocids; however, it does not produce a microfilaremia. There are at least 4 species of lungworms in various cetacean hosts.

Lungworm infection can be diagnosed by examination of feces or bronchial mucus. Anorexia, coughing, and sometimes, blood-flecked mucus are the first signs of pulmonary parasitism. Treatment of *P decorus* infection consists of mucolytic agents administered intratracheally, antibiotics to treat any concomitant bacterial pneumonia, and levamisole phosphate (15 mg/kg) daily for 5 days. Treatment of *O circumlitus* has been intratracheal administration of levamisole phosphate (5 mg/kg) daily for 5 days. Cetacean lungworms probably are also susceptible to levamisole and ivermectin.

Lungworm infections often remain asymptomatic for long periods; when an animal becomes debilitated for other reasons, clinical signs may appear. In captivity, lungworm infections are usually self-limiting if larvae are not introduced in fresh fish intermediate hosts. Feeding frozen fish prevents reinfection.

Heartworm: Heartworms of the genus *Dipetalonema* are a common necropsy finding in pinnipeds but have not been reported in cetaceans or sirenians. Phocid seals are affected by *D spirocauda*, and otarids are infected subcut. by *D odendhali*. Both groups of pinnipeds can be infected with the canine heartworm *Dirofilaria immitis* in endemic areas; however, phocid seals are abnormal hosts. Dirofilariasis is diagnosed by identifying microfilariae in the blood. Transmission is by the same mosquitoes that bite dogs. A high-dose levamisole phosphate regimen (40 mg/kg, daily for 1 wk) has successfully cleared infection in captive pinnipeds, with the advantage of oral administration. Prevention in endemic areas has been successful with daily administration of diethylcarbamazine at 3.3 mg/kg body wt in food during the mosquito season. This drug is also effective as a larvicide.

Other Nematodes: Members of the Anasakidae are very pathogenic nematodes found in the stomach of marine mammals. They cause granuloma formation at their attachment sites and can lead to blood loss, ulceration, and ultimately, perforation and peritonitis. Raw fish is most often incriminated as the source of infection. Infections with *Contracaecum* spp are common in wild cetaceans and pinnipeds. Polar bears in captivity are prone to heavy ascarid infection. Gastric nematodes can be successfully treated with oral dichlorvos (30 mg/kg), fenbendazole (11 mg/kg), or mebendazole (9 mg/kg) given twice, 10 days apart. Ivermectin may be considered.

Hookworms (*Uncinaria* spp) are found in pinnipeds. Severe infections are known only in the fur seals. Newborn pups are infected via colostrum. Disophenol (12.5 mg/kg) or ivermectin (100 μg/kg) injected subcut. are effective against these parasites.

Many species of a large spirurid nematode (*Crassicauda* spp) infect the cranial sinuses, major vessels, kidneys, and mammary gland ducts of cetaceans. Successful treatments are not documented, but are potentially possible with systemic parasiticides.

Cestodiasis: The cestode *Diphyllobothrium pacificum* is commonly found in sea lions, and heavy infection is thought to cause intestinal obstruction. Niclosamide (160 mg/kg) or praziquantel (10 mg/kg) are effective treatments. Other cestodes commonly seen include *Diphyllobothrium lanceolatum* in phocid seals, *Diplogonoporus tetrapterus* in all pinnipeds, and *Tetrabothrium forsteri* and *Strobilocephalus triangularis* in cetaceans. Cetaceans are also commonly infected with subcut. tapeworm cysts throughout the blubber. These usually are the larval forms of tapeworms of sharks.

Trematodiasis: A common problem in pinnipeds and cetaceans. *Nasitrema* spp are found in the nasal passages and sinuses of cetaceans. Ova of these trematodes have been associated with necrotic foci in the brains of animals showing behavioral aberrations, and have been incriminated as a cause of localized pneumonia in cetaceans. Infections are often accompanied by halitosis, brown mucus around the blowhole, and occasionally coughing. Diagnosis is based on demonstration of typical operculated trematode ova in blowhole swabs or feces. Treatment with oral praziquantel (10 mg/kg, twice 1 wk apart) is usually effective. Reinfection can be controlled by not feeding fresh or live fish.

Zalophotrema hepaticum is an important hepatic trematode of the California sea lion; it causes biliary hypertrophy and fibrosis of the liver. Signs are usually seen in adults and include icterus, lethargy, and anorexia. Bilirubinemia and elevated serum hepatic enzymes are common. Diagnosis is based on identification of trematode ova in the feces. Treatment with bithional at 20 mg/kg body wt has been successful.

Various other trematodes infect the stomach, intestines, liver, pancreas, and other abdominal organs of marine mammals. Pancreatic fibrosis due to trematodiasis is a common necropsy finding.

Coccidiosis: Coccidia (*Eimeria phocae*) have been found in harbor seals with a fatal, bloody diarrhea. These coccidia are probably susceptible to anticoccidial drugs used against other species, eg, amprolium. There have been no reports of coccidiosis in other marine mammals.

VIRAL DISEASES

Adenovirus: Adenovirus has been isolated from a sei whale and bowhead whales and observed in livers from 6 young stranded California sea lions (*Zalophus californianus*) with hepatitis. No disease was noted in the cetaceans. Pinnipeds developed weakness, emaciation, photophobia, polydipsia, abdominal splinting, blood-tinged diarrhea, and eventually posterior paresis, and exhibited a relative lymphopenia and monocytosis. All pinnipeds developed pneumonia and died 1-28 days after initial observation.

The most prominent histological lesion in all cases was hepatic necrosis. Massive coagulation necrosis without apparent zonal distribution occurred in some animals. Basophilic intranuclear inclusions in hepatocytes or granular amphophilic intranuclear inclusions in Kupffer's cells were seen. No evidence of adenovirus was detected in the lungs. Adenovirus from California sea lions is not known to cause disease in man.

Caliciviruses (San Miguel Sea Lion Virus): Caliciviruses have been isolated from otarid seals, walrus, Atlantic bottlenosed dolphin (*Tursiops truncatus*), and opaleye fish (*Girella nigricans*). The marine caliciviruses appear to be serotypes of vesicular exanthema of swine virus (VESV, qv, p 388). Several species of mysticete cetaceans have antibodies to different serotypes of VESV. By 4 mo of age, most California sea lions have neutralizing antibodies to one or more of the serotypes. Opaleye fish are probably responsible for the endemic status of caliciviruses in marine mammals that inhabit the coastal waters of California. To date, infections have not been diagnosed in marine mammals in the Atlantic ocean.

The most consistent lesion in marine mammals is skin vesicles. In pinnipeds, the vesicles are most prevalent on the dorsal surfaces of the fore flippers. In dolphins, vesicular lesions have been observed in association with "tattoo" lesions and old scars. Vesicles are 1 mm to 3 cm in diameter. They usually erode and leave shallow fast-healing ulcers, but occasionally vesicles regress and leave plaque-like lesions. Skin lesions usually resolve without any supportive treatment. Infection may cause premature parturition in pinnipeds. Affected pups have interstitial pneumonitis and encephalitis, and fail to thrive.

Inoculation of marine caliciviruses into pigs causes vesicular lesions identical to those seen in vesicular exanthema. There is no evidence that marine caliciviruses cause clinical disease in man, but heavy exposure can result in neutralizing antibodies, and recent isolation of calicivirus from a clinically ill primate indicates that these viruses should be handled carefully.

Herpesvirus: Herpesviruses have been isolated from neonatal harbor seals (*Phoca vitulina*), a California sea lion (*Zalophus californianus*), and a gray seal (*Halichoerus grypus*). Herpesvirus-like particles have been demonstrated in skin lesions from beluga whales (*Delphinapterus leucas*). Herpesvirus-like lesions occur in a wide variety of other pinnipeds and cetaceans.

Harbor seals develop nasal discharge, inflammation of the oral mucosa, vomiting, diarrhea, and fever followed by coughing, pneumonia, anorexia, and lethargy that can result in death in 1-6 days. Morbidity can approach 100% in stressed seals in crowded conditions; mortality is ~50%. The incubation period appears to be 10-14 days.

In the California sea lion and gray seal, recurring circumscribed areas of alopecia ~0.5 cm in diameter were the primary sign of infection. Systemic disease, including pneumonia, can occur. Herpetic lesions in beluga whales are generally circular, up to 2 cm in diameter, and may appear slightly depressed with a target appearance or be raised and proliferative. The centers of some lesions are necrotic or may contain verrucous growths. Systemic infections have not been documented in the whales.

Necropsy findings include interstitial pneumonia, hepatomegaly with massive coagulation necrosis, and small erosions of the oral mucosa and skin. Intranuclear inclusions may be seen in biopsies of early skin lesions. In seals, interstitial pneumonia caused by herpesvirus must be distinguished from bronchial pneumonia caused by influenza virus. Other infectious organisms, eg, bacteria and parasites, may complicate herpesvirus pneumonia. Herpesvirus hepatitis must be differentiated from adenovirus hepatitis, which has intranuclear inclusion bodies.

In systemic infection, therapy is supportive. In a documented epidemic, oral acyclovir did not eliminate the infection but appeared to significantly shorten clinical signs in primary infections. Vaccination with 1 mL of trivalent poliovirus vaccine to control recrudescence of suspected herpesvirus lesions has been used with some success; although it reduced the severity of recrudescence in seals, there is a potential public health risk since live poliovirus may be shed following vaccination. Stress and immunosuppression are associated with recrudescence of latent infections. There is no evidence that the herpesviruses of pinnipeds or cetaceans are zoonotic.

Influenza Virus: Two different influenza A viruses have been isolated from stranded harbor seals (*Phoca vitulina*) and 2 other subtypes from a stranded pilot whale (*Globicephala melaena*). Infection is probably common. Clinical signs in seals are dramatic; even well-nourished animals become weak, incoordinated, and dyspneic, with occasional white or bloody nasal discharge. Swollen necks due to fascial trapping of air escaping through the thoracic inlet is common. The single pilot whale had difficulty maneuvering, was extremely emaciated, and was sloughing skin. The incubation period during epidemics is ≤3 days. Many factors probably contributed to the explosive nature of the epidemics in the harbor seals. High population densities and unseasonably warm temperatures contribute to high mortality.

In the seals, pneumonia was characterized by necrotizing bronchitis and bronchiolitis, and hemorrhagic alveolitis. In the pilot whale, the lungs were hemorrhagic and a hilar node was greatly enlarged. For differential diagnosis, *see* HERPES-VIRUS, above.

The virulence of epidemics has precluded attempts at serious supportive care. Persons whose eyes were contaminated while doing necropsies, or by being sneezed on by affected seals have developed keratoconjunctivitis within 2-3 days, and identical virus has been recovered. All affected people have recovered completely within 7 days without developing any antibody titers, which suggests that the reaction was local, as occurs with Newcastle disease virus.

Paramyxovirus: Phocid seals are susceptible to canine distemper virus. Generally, young seals are affected and show depression, anorexia, crusting conjunctivitis, nasal discharge, and dyspnea. Pneumonia develops and mortality can be high in previously unexposed populations. Recent outbreaks in wild harbor seals have been extensive in the North Sea. Experimentally, captive seals have been vaccinated with canine distemper vaccine and rendered immune to challenge with the virus (suspension of organ material) obtained from dead wild seals.

Poxvirus: Poxvirus has been identified morphologically in skin lesions of both captive and free-ranging pinnipeds and cetaceans. Lesions in California sea lions (*Zalophus californianus*), harbor seals (*Phoca vitulina*), and gray seals (*Halichoerus grypus*) probably are due to parapoxviruses. Lesions in South American sea lions (*Otaria byronia*) and Northern fur seals (*Callorhinusus*) probably are not. An unclassified poxvirus is also associated with skin lesions in Atlantic bottlenosed dolphins (*Tursiops truncatus*), and in a stranded Atlantic white-sided dolphin (*Lagenorynchus acutus*).

Outbreaks typically occur in postweanling pinnipeds recently introduced into captivity. The incubation period is 3-5 wk. A break in the epithelial surface may be required to start an infection. Lesions can recur. Small, cutaneous, raised nodules (0.5-1 cm in diameter) occur on the head, neck, and flippers of affected pinnipeds. These may increase to 1.5-3 cm in diameter during the first week, and may ulcerate or develop satellite lesions during the second week. After the fourth week, lesions begin to regress, although nodules are reported to persist as long as 15-18 wk. Areas of alopecia and scar tissue may remain after resolution.

Cutaneous poxvirus infections in cetaceans can occur on any part of the body, but are most common on the head, pectoral flippers, dorsal fin, and tail fluke. They range from ring or pinhole lesions to black, punctiform, stippled patterns ("tattoo" lesions). Ring or pinhole lesions appear as solitary, 0.5-3 cm, round or elliptical blemishes, which sometimes coalesce. They are usually light gray and may have a dark gray border, although the reverse color pattern is also seen. Lesions may persist for months or years without any apparent ill effects to the animal.

Major differentials include cutaneous streptothricosis and calicivirus. Poxvirus has not been isolated from pinnipeds or cetaceans. Diagnosis is based on the presence of eosinophilic, intracytoplasmic inclusion bodies in lesion biopsies, and is confirmed by identification of typical poxvirus particles by electron microscopy.

Poxviruses of marine mammals do not appear to cause systemic infections. Although animals with cutaneous poxvirus lesions have died, other factors were responsible. Therapy to control secondary bacterial infections is indicated only when skin lesions suppurate. The parapoxviruses of pinnipeds can cause isolated lesions on the hands of persons not wearing gloves when in contact with infected animals.

Miscellaneous Viruses: A ringed seal in Norway was wounded and appeared confused; its overall condition deteriorated over 5 days, and it became aggressive. Rabies was confirmed by immunofluorescent examination of the brain. At the time, there was an epidemic of rabies in foxes in the area.

The only retrovirus identified to date in a marine mammal was a spumavirus isolated from recurring skin lesions in a California sea lion that subsequently died of *Pasteurella* pneumonia complicated with herpesvirus.

An enterovirus of unknown pathogenicity was isolated from a rectal swab of a California gray whale. Antibodies, unassociated with disease, against human influenza virus (after challenge) and poliomyelitis virus were found in *Tursiops truncatus*.

Severe enteritis and vomiting in a captive beluga whale was suggestive of parvovirus enteritis. Death was rapid; however, no virus was isolated.

ENVIRONMENTAL DISEASES

Corneal Edema: Corneal opacity occurs frequently in captive pinnipeds kept in either fresh- or saltwater; it is also seen in captive cetaceans, but is rare in wild animals. It can be due to various environmental problems. Transient cases can be caused by simply moving an animal to fresh- from saltwater, or vice versa. Lack of shade and excessive bright light have been implicated. Unsanitary water conditions with high bacterial loads and over-use of oxidative disinfectants in the water also have been associated with the disease. Nutritional deficiencies have been suggested as causes, but response to supplementation of vitamin C or A has not been dramatic. The condition is usually self-limiting if the underlying insult to the cornea is removed.

Corneal Ulcers: These occur frequently in captive pinnipeds and cetaceans. They can be the sequelae of unresolved or untreated cases of corneal edema, or initiated by direct trauma. Diagnosis is by observation of epithelial defects on corneas stained with fluorescein. Small lesions can be treated topically in trained animals. In untrained animals, subconjunctival injections of antibiotics and steroid are required. Extensive lesions benefit from protection by suturing the eyelids. Deep ulcers or lacerations in danger of eroding Descemet's membrane should be stabilized with a thin methylacrylate patch. As in corneal edema, successful resolution and prevention of recurrence depend on removal of the underlying cause.

Foreign Bodies: Many captive marine mammals develop the vice of swallowing objects dropped into their pools. In cetaceans, the opening to the second compartment of the stomach is small, and foreign objects remain in the first compartment. In pinnipeds, the small pylorus prevents passage of most foreign bodies. Frequently, no clinical signs are evident. On occasion, anorexia, regurgitation, or lethargy may be observed. Gastric foreign bodies, however, should be considered a hazard to the animal, and all efforts should be made to prevent their ingestion or to remove them once ingested. Sharp objects may cause gastric perforation. Other objects, including coins, can initiate ulceration, which can culminate in perforation. Diagnosis is often made by observing the animal swallow an object. Smaller animals can be radiographed, and small cetaceans can be palpated via the esophagus to establish the presence of foreign bodies. Animals occasionally regurgitate foreign bodies; however, assisted removal is usually indicated. Removal of the objects is usually best performed by gastroscopy, which is also used as a method of confirmation. Training animals to retrieve for reward as a displacement to swallowing foreign objects is thought to be beneficial.

Gastrointestinal Ulceration: GI ulcers are a significant problem in captive marine mammals. Ulcers of the first compartment of the cetacean stomach are a common necropsy finding and pose less severe clinical problems than ulcers of the pyloric region or proximal duodenum. Gastric ulcers in pinnipeds frequently progress to perforation, which results in peritonitis and subsequent death. Gastric ulcers also occur in sirenians. Although ulcers in cetaceans perforate less frequently than in pinnipeds, they should be treated as a serious clinical problem. Various etiologies have been suggested, including parasitic damage and increased histamine content of spoiled fish, but the disease must be considered primarily an environmental or stress-related condition. Dramatic environmental changes, including changes of personnel or companion animals, can precipitate serious GI ulceration in cetaceans or pinnipeds.

Clinical signs include lethargy, partial anorexia, abdominal splinting, pallor, and occasionally regurgitation. Cases with bleeding ulcers show anemia and possibly a leukocytosis. Diagnosis generally is based on identification of mammalian RBC in gastric washes; confirmation is by endoscopic visualization of the lesions. Palliative treatment of nonperforating ulcers consists of administration of cimetidine (6 mg/kg, t.i.d.) and alumina-gel-based antacids with or without simethicone, along with frequent small meals. The underlying cause must be identified and corrected if treatment is to be successful long term. Management of perforating ulcers with resulting peritonitis must include intensive broad-spectrum antibiotic and fluid therapy. As in man, once marine mammals develop stress-induced GI ulcers, they become more prone to develop ulcers than ones that have not.

Trauma: Many traumatic lesions (cuts, wounds from gunshots or propeller blades) are found on marine mammals. Propeller injuries are a major problem in manatees, which commonly enter heavily navigated recreational waters in Florida. Traumatic wounds should be cleaned, debrided, and generally allowed to heal as open wounds unless body cavities are breached. Antibiotics should be administered during convalescence to prevent gross infection. Maintenance of good water quality and a high plane of nutrition is beneficial to uncomplicated healing. Large wounds frequently heal uneventfully.

NEOPLASIA

Tumors in marine mammals are infrequent and of little consequence except for malignant lymphoma in harbor seals, in which horizontal transmission can occur in a closed population. A wide variety of tumors has been reported in marine mammals.

NUTRITION AND NUTRITIONAL DISEASES

In captivity, animals that eat solely or primarily fish are generally provided dead fish that have been frozen. The logistics and difficulty in providing this fish can lead to some special nutritional concerns. All fish are not of equal nutritional value; diets consisting of a single species of fish are unlikely to provide balanced nutrition for any animal. Similarly, one diet will not serve all piscivores equally. Only fish suitable for human consumption should be fed. (*See also* p 1220.)

Frozen fish pose the added risks of improper storage and thawing; these procedures must be monitored carefully. Feed fish should be held at $<30°F$ ($-1°C$) to reduce deterioration of their nutritional value through oxidation of amino acids and unsaturated lipids. Dehydration of frozen fish can also be a problem for animals that obtain their water from their food. Fatty fish should not be stored >6 mo. Few fish, with the possible exception of capelin, should be stored >1 yr. To retain optimal vitamin content and reduce moisture loss, frozen fish should be thawed in air under refrigeration. Thawing in water leaches away water-soluble vitamins. Thawing at room temperature encourages bacterial growth and spoilage.

The energy requirements of marine mammals vary with age, environmental temperatures, and condition. Young growing dolphins and smaller pinnipeds generally require 9-15% of their body wt in high-quality fish per day. Older animals may need only 4-9% of their body wt for maintenance. Larger species (whales, elephant seals) generally require less food (2-5% of body wt) as adults.

Sirenians thrive on a diet of hydroponic grass and various lettuces and vegetables, supplemented with high-protein monkey chow, carrots, bananas, and multivitamin-mineral supplements used particularly to balance calcium/phosphorus ratios.

It is thought that sirenians ingest considerable animal protein incidentally during grazing in the wild. Intake requirements have been estimated at 7-9% of body wt daily. Sirenians are generally fed several times a day to accommodate their grazing feeding pattern.

Sea otters are usually fed diets consisting of various invertebrates (echinoderms, molluscs, occasional crustaceans) and fish. Adult animals require ~25-30% of their body wt in food each day.

Polar bears in the wild have high-lipid diets, particularly in winter when they subsist heavily on seals. They are considered to have an exceptional dietary requirement for vitamin A, and some dermatological conditions respond to daily supplementation of 20,000-1,000,000 IU in the diet. Polar bears are commonly fed large amounts of fish in captivity, and for these, the precautions for fish-eating animals should be followed.

Neonatal Nutrition: Young marine mammals are frequently encountered in strandings. Often they are not weaned and must be fed a diet resembling their dam's milk. In captivity, neonates may be abandoned by their parents and require artificial rearing. Marine mammals have high-lipid-content milks. Most species are carbohydrate intolerant, and neonates fed formulas with carbohydrates develop severe, life-threatening, bacterial gastroenteritis. Most neonatal marine mammals also require immense caloric density in replacement milks.

Phocid and otarid seals can be reared on the same formula, made by grinding 340 g of headless, tailless herring to a paste in 100 mL of water. This is put through a ricer to produce a fish mash, which is supplemented with a mixture of 150 mL lactated Ringer's, 1¼ tsp (8.3 g) sodium chloride, 400 mg thiamine, 400 IU vitamin E, ¼ tsp (1.3 g) calcium gluconate powder, 250 mg vitamin C, 1 tsp (5 mL) safflower oil, 1 tsp (2.5 g) lecithin with 0% carbohydrates, and 1 powdered human multivitamin tablet. The mix is then blended with 200 mL of heavy whipping cream that has been treated with lactase enzymes at least several hours before. This formula can be stored refrigerated for up to 24 hr.

Pinniped pups should be fed q4hr in their first week of life; gradually, the amount of formula fed should be increased and the feedings dropped to 5 per day. Harbor seal pups should be tube fed until 2-3 wk old before weaning to small pieces of fish. Elephant seal pups require tube feeding until they are 4 wk old, when weaning can begin. California sea lion pups can be force fed fish as early as 4 wk of age and be free feeding by 6 wk.

Neonatal walruses have been reared on whipping-cream-based formulas extended with ground molluscs (clams) rather than fish, and seem to tolerate carbohydrates reasonably well. These animals have a much longer nursing period than other pinnipeds.

Neonatal cetaceans have longer nursing periods than pinnipeds. Success at bottle-rearing has been minimal. The fat content of cetacean milks varies considerably: bottlenosed dolphin milk is ~17% fat (half that of most pinniped milks); beluga whale milk, 27%; harbor porpoise milk, 46%; and mysticete blue whale milk, 42% fat. Formulas similar to the pinniped formula, adjusted for fat content with oils should be successful in neonatal cetaceans if the logistics of delivery are solved.

Neonatal sirenians begin to nibble sea grasses shortly after birth but may continue to nurse up to 18 mo. They can be reared on artificial milks with early weaning. Neonatal sea otters also have been reared successfully from birth on artificial formulas. Neonatal polar bears are extremely altricial and are a challenge because of an apparently immature immune system. Polar bear milk is high in fat (31%) and contains minimal lactose. Polar bears have been successfully reared on whipping-cream- and oil-based formulas.

Thiamine Deficiency: This can be seen in any piscivorous animal. Thiamine in the food is destroyed by the activity of thiaminase enzymes or antithiamine substances in the fish being fed. These active enzymes also destroy supplemental thiamine that is placed in fish if it sits for long periods before feeding. Clinical signs of thiamine deficiency are primarily of CNS disturbances. Affected animals may show anorexia, regurgitation, or ataxia. The condition can progress to seizures, coma, and death.

Clinical cases of thiamine deficiency respond rapidly to IM injection of thiamine hydrochloride (up to 1 mg/kg body wt), followed by oral supplementation. Control usually involves supplemental thiamine at 25 mg/kg food, preferably administered 2 hr before a main feeding.

Vitamin E Deficiency (Steatitis, White Fat Disease): The antioxidant properties of vitamin E are believed to play an important role in maintaining the integrity of cellular membranes. Oxidative processes during the storage of fish destroy vitamin E and other antioxidants. Steatitis has been induced experimentally in phocid seals, and relationships between vitamin E deficiency and hyponatremia are suspected. Captive piscivores commonly are supplemented PO with vitamin E at a rate up to 100 mg/kg of feed, which generally maintains high serum levels of the vitamin. This does not appear necessary if fish is properly stored and thawed.

Hyponatremia: (Salt Deficiency, Addison's Disease): Hyponatremia in pinnipeds is closely related to adrenal exhaustion and development of Addison's disease, which links the syndrome to environmental stressors rather than a simple primary salt deficiency. It is most common in pinnipeds maintained in freshwater exhibits, but can be seen in animals kept in saltwater. It is more common in phocid seals, but occurs in otarids and other marine mammals. Signs include periodic weakness, anorexia, lethargy, incoordination, tremor, and convulsions. Serum sodium levels can fall to <140 mEq/L. Severe cases may collapse in Addisonian crisis, which can be fatal.

Emergency therapy consists of sodium chloride infusion and replacement corticosteroids. Long-term management of advanced cases requires mineralocorticoid supplementation in conjunction with oral sodium chloride supplements and periodic monitoring of serum sodium levels. Control consists of provision of saltwater pools or supplementation of sodium chloride (3 g/kg food) in the diet of captive pinnipeds maintained in freshwater pools. Animals on salt supplementation should have continuous access to freshwater.

Histamine Toxicity (Scombroid Poisoning, Mackerel Poisoning): Scombroid fish (mackerel, tuna) and other dark-fleshed fish have a short shelf life, even when frozen at low temperatures. They have a high histidine content, which is converted to histamine by bacteria as the fish deteriorates. Ingestion of one of these fish can cause histamine toxicity in marine mammals. It is most common in pinnipeds but is seen in other marine mammals. Clinical signs include anorexia, lethargy, a red inflamed mouth or throat, conjunctivitis and increased lacrimation, and occasionally vomiting, diarrhea, pruritus, urticaria, and postures indicative of abdominal pain. Antihistamines may provide symptomatic relief, but the condition is generally self-limiting and the animal begins feeding within 2-3 days. Control consists of avoiding scombroid fish in the diet or careful attention to their quality, storage, and handling when used.

MANAGEMENT, HUSBANDRY, AND DISEASES OF MINK

MANAGEMENT

Mink (*Mustela vison*) ranches should be located on well-drained soil, well away from urban areas. Good husbandry and proper, regular manure disposal help control flies and odors. A guard fence around the farm aids in preventing the escape of mink, and keeping out feral or wild animals. Many wild species such as skunk (*Mephitis mephitis*) or raccoon (*Procyon lotor*) may act as vectors for diseases such as distemper.

Mink are housed individually in wire mesh pens raised above the ground. A nest box with a hole for entry is attached outside or placed within the pen. Wood used for the nest box should not be painted or treated with wood preservatives. Soft, awn-free marsh hay, chopped straw, untreated wood shavings, or fine wood-wool make suitable nest material. Nest boxes should be cleaned and nest material replaced as required, especially before whelping, and during cold weather.

Sheds are used throughout the year. They should admit sufficient natural light to supply normal daylight hours, and there should be plenty of air circulation in the warmer months.

Mink feed may be supplied as a wet gruel placed on top of the wire or as a commercially prepared, dry, pelleted ration placed in feed hoppers. During the weaning and postweaning periods, food is supplied on feeding trays placed on the floor of the pen for small kits that cannot reach the top of the pen. Fresh water should always be available. Watering cups fastened to the outside of the pen with a lip protruding inside are commonly used. Automatic watering systems with individual nipples or flotation cups are used in sheds, temperature permitting.

Cold storage facilities are necessary to freeze and store the meat portion of the ration. A day's supply of fish and meat by-products is thawed, commercial cereal added, and the combined ration mixed with water to a consistency that will remain on the wire of the pen without dropping through. Ready-mixed feeds may be delivered daily, ready to feed, or may be in frozen blocks that are thawed as required. Dry pelleted diets are used on some ranches for part or all of the year. (*See also* NUTRITION: MINK, p 1240.)

Pelting usually is done in November or December. The most humane way to kill mink is with carbon monoxide.

Ranchers usually keep one male for each 5 female breeders. Mink are seasonal breeders, with sexual activity controlled by increasing periods of daylight. Artificial lights in the sheds must be used with caution since they may adversely affect photoperiod and interfere with the normal reproductive cycle. In the Northern Hemisphere, the breeding season begins in late February-early March and lasts ~4 wk. Mating should occur within 1 hr after the female is placed in the male's pen. If fighting ensues, they should be separated. Ovulation is induced by coitus. Females mated before mid-March are usually mated again after 7-8 days, often with an additional mating the following day; thus, individual females may be mated 2-3 times. Ova from 2 matings have been known to contribute to the same litter. Implantation of the fertilized ova is delayed, so the apparent gestation period is 40-75 days.

Mink have one litter a year of 1-12 kits (av 4). Most are born during the last week in April and the first 2 wk in May. Kits are blind, hairless, and weigh ~10 g when born, but grow rapidly throughout the summer to reach a weight of ~800 g (females) or 1600 g (males) by October. Kits are weaned at ~6-8 wk of age, and may be separated shortly thereafter and housed in single pens. Adult mink are extremely agile, strong, and vicious. Handling requires the use of special leather gloves or wire catching cages.

BACTERIAL DISEASES

Botulism: Botulism (qv, p 328) occasionally causes heavy losses in unvaccinated mink that consume feed that contains type C toxin. Usually, many mink are found dead within 24 hr of exposure to the toxin, while others show varying degrees of paralysis and dyspnea. Postmortem findings are nonspecific and are related to death from respiratory paralysis. Diagnosis is confirmed through inoculation of serum or filtered tissue from affected mink into mice. The immunotype of the botulism toxin is type C in almost all outbreaks.

Toxic feed should be removed, and stored feed or ingredients examined for the toxin. Recovered mink are not immune to further challenge. Annual vaccination of kits and breeders with botulism (type C) toxoid is recommended to prevent outbreaks.

Hemorrhagic Pneumonia: *Pseudomonas aeruginosa* may result in serious losses. Mink of all ages are affected, particularly during the stress of fall molt. Mink are usually found dead with no prodromal signs. A bloody nasal exudate may be observed at the time of death. Gross lesions include a severe hemorrhagic pneumonia with swelling and consolidation of one or more lung lobes. Treatment involves immediate vaccination of the entire herd or a "buffer zone" of animals around the focus of infection with a *Pseudomonas* bacterin, and immediate administration of sodium sulfathiazole (1 oz/150 lb [410 mg/kg] of wet mixed feed) and an equivalent quantity of sodium bicarbonate for 1 wk as a herd treatment. Care must be taken with dosage since sulfonamides are potentially toxic for mink. The mink should have ample water. *Pseudomonas* bacterins are available for ranch vaccination.

Tuberculosis: Mink, particularly Aleutian types, are susceptible to infection with avian, bovine, and human tubercle bacilli. Infection is usually food-borne, and the disease has become endemic on some ranches. Signs include weight loss and, in some cases, abdominal distention. Affected mink are severely emaciated and have enlarged spleen and lymph nodes. There may be miliary involvement of the lungs, liver, and other organs. The diagnosis is confirmed by identifying acid-fast intracellular organisms in smears from affected tissues. There is no treatment, and control consists of culling visibly affected mink and feeding meat products from inspected processing plants. Tuberculin tests are generally ineffective in detecting infected mink.

Urinary Infections and Urolithiasis: Urinary tract infections, commonly called "plum bladders", cause serious losses in females in late spring (during pregnancy and lactation) and in males in late summer and autumn (during the rapid-growth and furring period). Several predisposing factors have been suggested: contamination of food, cages, or nest boxes by pathogenic bacteria; decreased water intake; or increased ash intake.

Mink may die without showing signs, or they may have difficulty in urinating, dribble urine, and occasionally have hematuria. Gross postmortem findings include acute hemorrhagic cystitis or pyelonephritis, or both, usually associated with calculi (magnesium ammonium phosphate) in the bladder or kidneys. Various organisms, including staphylococci, coliforms, and *Proteus* sp have been isolated.

In severe outbreaks, culture and antibiotic sensitivity tests should be done, and medication added to the feed. Good sanitation to reduce environmental contamination, increasing the water supply, and pelting out of families in which the condition is seen help to prevent the condition. When a continual problem exists (with magnesium ammonium phosphate calculi), feed-grade (75%) phosphoric acid may be added to the feed (0.8 lb/100 lb [8 g/kg] of wet mixed feed) from March to early June and from mid-July to October, to reduce the pH of the urine; phosphoric acid should not be used in young mink. Salt (NaCl, 0.5%) may be added to the diet to increase water consumption.

Mastitis: One of the most economically important diseases on commercial mink farms, a variety of bacteria but mainly staphlococci, streptococci, and *Escherichia coli* are involved. Staphylococcal mastitis typically results in abscessation of affected glands, or subclinical disease noticed only by mild diarrhea in the kits. *Escherichia coli* causes a peracute, necrotizing mastitis similar to that seen in dairy cattle. Predisposing factors include poor nest box and cage sanitation, rough or sharp edges to the entrance of nestboxes, and high bacterial contamination of feed. Treatment and prevention involve improving management, and treating individual animals or the herd with the appropriate antibiotic based on sensitivity testing.

Miscellaneous Bacterial Diseases: Various diseases or signs of disease, including septicemia, pneumonia, purulent pleuritis, abortions, abscesses, cellulitis, and enteritis occur sporadically on mink ranches; occasionally, they may become herd problems. Many bacteria, including *Proteus, Klebsiella*, and *Campylobacter* spp, coliforms, streptococci, staphylococci, and salmonellae, have been isolated.

Treatment should be selected based on antibacterial sensitivity tests. Drugs may be administered parenterally or in the feed and water. Dosage can be estimated on the basis of body wt—female mink weigh ~1¾-2 lb (0.8-1 kg), and males ~4-4½ lb (1.8-2.1 kg). Dosages recommended for cats should be used and adjusted for weight. However, some sulfonamides, eg, sulfaquinoxaline and sulfamethazine, and streptomycin should not be used in mink.

The source of infection should be determined and eliminated. Enteritis often is caused by contaminated or spoiled feed, and abscesses by injury from wire or splintered wood in the pens, awns in hay or straw used for bedding, or spicules of bone in the feed. Outbreaks of tularemia, anthrax, brucellosis, and clostridial infections have been caused by feed contaminated with tissue of animals that have died or are carriers of these infections. Careful selection of feed ingredients, and disinfection of equipment and pens are important in the prevention and control of many infections of mink. "Dead stock" should not be used as mink feed.

VIRAL DISEASES

Aleutian Disease (AD, Plasmacytosis): A slow virus infection of mink, characterized by poor reproduction, gradual weight loss, oral and GI bleeding, renal failure and uremia, and high mortality. All color phases of mink may be infected with AD, but light color phases genetically derived from the Aleutian color phase are most susceptible. The cause is a parvovirus not related to mink viral enteritis (*see* below). Transmission occurs *in utero* and by direct or indirect contact with infected mink.

Following infection, mink frequently respond with marked increases in immunoglobulin levels. Immunoglobulins are unable to neutralize the AD virus; immune complexes form and deposit in various tissues, resulting in immune-complex glomerulonephritis and arteritis. Gross pathological changes include splenomegaly; kidney changes, varying from swelling and petechiation to atrophy and pitting; and enlargement of mesenteric lymph nodes. Histological lesions include plasma cell infiltration in the kidneys, liver, spleen, lymph nodes, and bone marrow; bile duct proliferation; membranous glomerulonephritis; and fibrinoid arteritis. Kits from AD-negative dams may die from acute interstitial pneumonia.

The disease is controlled through a test-and-slaughter program. Positive mink are identified by blood testing for specific antibody by counterimmunoelectrophoresis. All positive mink should be culled. Mink that are to be kept for breeding stock are tested in late fall (before selection of breeding stock, and pelting) and in January or February (before breeding). New introductions to the herd should be tested.

There is no vaccination or effective treatment; positive females and their litters should be separated from the rest of the herd and pelted in season. The virus is present in the saliva, urine, feces, and blood of infected animals. Pens should be steam cleaned, and dipped in or sprayed with 2% sodium hydroxide. Equipment should be disinfected after handling, vaccinating, or testing mink on infected farms. Wild birds and flies may serve as vectors, and their control is essential.

Distemper: Mink of all ages are susceptible to canine distemper virus. The incubation period is 9-14 days. The virus may be recovered from infected mink 5 days before clinical signs appear. Mink that appear to have recovered may continue to shed the virus for several weeks. Transmission may be direct (through contact or aerosol) or indirect (the virus may persist ≥1 day in the environment).

Clinical signs include nasal and ocular discharge; hyperemia, thickening, and crustiness of the skin on the muzzle, feet, and ventral abdominal wall; neurological signs (convulsions and "screaming fits"); or a combination of these. Histological or FA examination may reveal intracytoplasmic or intranuclear inclusions or distemper antigen in epithelial cells of the bladder, kidneys, bile ducts, intestine, lungs, trachea, and occasionally brain. Nonsuppurative encephalitis may be present in mink with neurological signs.

In outbreaks, affected animals should be culled and the balance of the herd vaccinated as soon as possible. Kits should be vaccinated prophylactically when 9-10 wk old with a modified live vaccine (parenteral or aerosol route). Ordinarily, adults are vaccinated at the same time, although some believe that vaccination of adults in alternate years will suffice.

Mink Viral Enteritis: A highly contagious disease caused by a parvovirus related to, but not identical with, that of feline panleukopenia. All ages are susceptible, but the disease is most serious in kits. Transmission usually occurs by the fecal/oral route; the incubation period is 4-8 days.

Clinical signs include sudden anorexia; depression; watery, mucoid, blood-tinged diarrhea; dehydration; and death. Characteristic gross lesions include a flaccid, dilated, hyperemic small intestine, with liquid fetid contents. Some mink may die suddenly with no gross lesions. Intestinal lesions are characterized by erosion of surface mucosa, blunting and attenuation of villi, and cryptal dilation. Ballooned epithelial cells may contain inclusion bodies similar to those of feline panleukopenia. Splenic and lymph node lesions include lymphoid depletion and necrosis.

Early in an outbreak, all mink showing signs should be culled or isolated, and all clinically normal mink should be vaccinated immediately with a formalinized tissue-culture vaccine. Affected mink can be treated PO with a mixture of kaolin, pectin, and neomycin. Mink viral enteritis can be prevented by vaccination. All mink should be vaccinated when 7-8 wk old with a combination mink viral enteritis/botulism vaccine. Annual vaccination is recommended. If females have experienced an outbreak or have been vaccinated against mink viral enteritis in January or February, their kits born in May and June should not be vaccinated until they are 12 wk old.

Aujeszky's Disease (Pseudorabies): This occurs occasionally in mink fed pork products contaminated with pseudorabies virus. Mortality may be high, and clinical signs are referable to the CNS (tonic and clonic convulsions; excitement, alternating with depression; and, in some cases, self-mutilation). The diagnosis is confirmed by virus isolation or serology. Since contaminated pork is the usual source of infection, all pork products should be cooked before they are fed to mink.

Transmissible Mink Encephalopathy (Mink Scrapie): Scrapie in mink is rare but has potential to cause high mortality in adults. The incubation period in experimental infections is ≥8 mo. Clinical signs are similar to those in sheep (qv, p 622) and include hyperirritability, ataxia, compulsive biting, somnolence, coma, and death. Histologic lesions in brains of affected mink are similar to those of scrapie in sheep. Although mink have been infected experimentally by intracerebral inoculation of brain material from scrapie-infected sheep, and by feeding tissues from infected sheep, the means of natural transmission is unknown. Control measures are not known, except to exclude sheep (and probably cattle) by-products from the ration in endemic areas.

Epizootic Catarrhal Gastroenteritis: Millions of mink have been affected by an agent (most likely a virus) that causes an acute catarrhal gastroenteritis. The disease usually occurs in adult dark mink. Outbreaks occur most frequently during stress, ie, during early fall molting, spring mating, and whelping seasons. The clinical signs (mucus in the feces and partial anorexia) rarely last longer than 5-6 days. Death may occur if the affected mink is immunosuppressed by the Aleutian disease virus. There are no commercially available vaccines. Treatment is symptomatic and of questionable value. It is important to differentiate this condition from mink viral enteritis.

NUTRITIONAL DISEASES

Steatitis (yellow fat disease, qv, p 551) occurs in young, rapidly growing mink as a result of excessive rancid unsaturated fatty acids or a deficiency of vitamin E in the diet. Affected mink may be found dead, or they may exhibit slight locomotor disturbances followed by death. Necropsy findings include yellow, edematous internal or subcut. fat that contains an acid-fast pigment. Control consists of removal of the source of the rancid fats and proper storage of feed. Stabilized vitamin E may be administered in the feed (15 mg/mink) for 2 wk, and affected kits should be injected parenterally with 10-20 mg vitamin E for several days. The condition can be prevented by feeding a nutritionally sound diet.

Chastek paralysis (thiamine deficiency) results from feeding certain raw fish that contain the enzyme thiaminase. These include whitefish, freshwater smelt, carp, goldfish, creek chub, fathead minnow, buckeye shiner, sucker, channel catfish, bullhead and minnow, white bass, sauger pike, burbot, and saltwater herring. Affected mink gradually lose their appetite and weight, and die after terminal convulsions and paralysis. Fish that contain high levels of thiaminase should be thoroughly cooked at 181°F (83°C) for ≥5 min, or fed raw as a portion of the diet only on alternate days. Mink injected subcut. with 50 mg of thiamine hydrochloride recover rapidly. Adequate thiamine (brewer's yeast) should be included in the ration.

Because of the rapid growth of mink kits, **rickets** occurs when rations are deficient in vitamin D, calcium, or phosphorus. Affected kits usually crawl unsteadily in a frog-like posture, have rubbery bones, and are smaller than normal. The diet should be supplemented as required, and severely affected kits may be treated individually.

Nursing disease is a metabolic disease that affects lactating mink ~40 days after whelping. It is characterized by rapid dehydration, serum electrolyte imbalances, renal shutdown, and death. Treatment can be successful if affected females are identified, as soon as they begin refusing feed, and rehydrated with intraperitoneal or subcut. sterile fluids. The disease is multifactorial; although there appears to be a genetic predisposition in certain light color mutations, it is more severe in females with large litters and during hot weather. Often affected females have concurrent subclinical mastitis. Adequate water, environmental cooling systems, fostering kits from large litters to make litter size more manageable for the female, and early weaning help prevent this condition.

Cotton underfur usually indicates anemia, and may be caused by certain fish (Pacific hake, coalfish, whiting) that interfere with iron metabolism in the mink, which interferes with melanin pigment formation. This condition can be prevented by thoroughly cooking the offending fish at 181°F (83°C) for ≥5 min, or by feeding it on alternate days.

Gray underfur and loss of guard hair occurs when high levels of uncooked eggs, particularly turkey eggs, are fed. Avidin, a factor present in eggs, inactivates biotin, a vitamin required for pigmentation and hair growth. Affected mink may be injected with 1 mg biotin twice weekly for 4 wk, and biotin may be added to the ration. Biotin deficiency can be prevented by cooking eggs at 196°F (91°C) for 5 min. (*See also* p 1242.)

POISONING

Lead poisoning may occur in mink that have ingested lead-containing paints from wire or other equipment. Affected mink gradually lose weight and die within 1-2 mo with clinical signs consistent with either gastroenteritis or CNS disturbance. Individual mink may be treated with calcium EDTA as a chelating agent. All sources of lead should be removed.

Insecticides other than pyrethrum, piperonyl butoxide, and rotenone may be highly toxic to mink. Even these insecticides should not be used on mink under 8 wk old, or where such mink can contact them (eg, nest boxes). Other insecticides should be avoided whenever possible.

Wood preservatives (chlorinated phenols, cresols) cause mortality of kits in the first 3 wk of life and, occasionally, of older mink. They should not be used where mink can chew on treated wood (pens, nest boxes, or nest litter). Shavings used as nest-box litter should not contain wood preservatives.

Diethylstilbestrol-containing products cause reproductive failure and a high incidence of urinary tract infections in mink, and should not be included in the ration. Similarly, **thyroid** and **parathyroid** glands included in meat trimmings fed to mink may result in reproductive failure if present at high levels.

Chlorinated hydrocarbons and **polychlorinated biphenyls** (PCB) contained in the ration have caused reproductive failure in mink. Mink appear to be exquisitely sensitive to **polybrominated biphenyls** (PBB); 1 ppm in the ration has caused litter size and offspring viability to decrease.

DMNA: In the past, addition of sodium nitrate as a preservative to herring meal resulted in formation of dimethylnitrosamine (DMNA), which is hepatotoxic in mink. It causes hepatic degeneration, ascites, and extensive internal hemorrhage.

Sulfaquinoxaline upsets normal blood-clotting mechanisms of mink and causes extensive internal hemorrhage, which results in serious losses. **Streptomycin** is toxic to mink.

MISCELLANEOUS DISEASES

Fur-clipping and **tail-biting** are common vices of mink, and may be related to abnormal behavior patterns of captivity. Fur-clipping decreases the value of the pelt, and tail-biting frequently results in fatal hemorrhage. There is no effective treatment—all mink demonstrating these vices should be pelted.

Urinary incontinence (wet-belly disease) is a nonfatal condition that usually affects obese males in the late summer and autumn. It is characterized by dribbling of urine and staining of the pelt around the urinary orifice. Since affected areas of the pelt must be discarded, the condition is of economic importance. The cause is unknown, but at least 3 factors, including the genetic strain, high dietary fat level, and obesity, appear to have the greatest influence on incidence. Affected animals should have an ample water supply.

Starvation and **chilling** cause death in mink fed inadequate fat, or provided with too little feed during the winter and early spring. Affected mink are thin, and may run until they collapse and die, or they may be found dead in their cages. Such deaths usually occur after a sudden decrease in environmental temperature, especially in the early spring when mink are being brought into breeding condition. Necropsy reveals emaciation and an absence of body fat, in some cases accompanied by hepatic lipidosis and gastric ulceration. This management disease must be differentiated from infectious diseases.

Gray diarrhea in mink clinically resembles chronic pancreatic necrosis in dogs, and is characterized by a ravenous appetite and the passage of large amounts of gray, fetid feces. Affected mink appear to die of starvation. No pancreatic abnormalities, viruses, bacteria, or parasites have been demonstrated to be causes. Treatment is of questionable value.

Gastric ulcers and **hepatic and renal lipidosis** are common in mink, and usually are associated with high levels of dietary fat or with other diseases or stresses that result in several days of inappetence. This condition usually occurs during late gestation, the period of weaning kits, or the fall period of furring up.

Hereditary diseases such as hydrocephalus, hairlessness, "screw neck", "bobbed tails", Ehlers-Danlos syndrome, hemivertebrae, and tyrosinemia occur occasionally and must be controlled by pelting the sire, dam, and littermates of the affected mink.

Coccidiosis occasionally causes losses in young mink. Affected animals have diarrhea, dehydration, and weight loss. Coccidiostats may be used to control outbreaks. Coccidiosis can be prevented through good sanitation and regular manure removal.

Myiasis: Females of *Wohlfahrtia* spp lay maggots directly on the skin of the kits. The larvae penetrate the skin and produce inflammation and lesions that resemble abscesses. Affected kits become restless, lose condition, and may die. Malathion dust (5%) placed beneath the litter in the nest boxes beginning a few days before the occurrence of the flies may help prevent infestation. It should not be used before whelping or until the kits are 1 wk old. Treatment may be repeated once after a 2-wk interval. The above treatment can also be used for flea control. (*See also* CUTEREBRA INFESTATIONS, SM AN, p 785, and INSECTICIDE AND ACARICIDE TOXICITIES, p 1658.)

Flea infestations are common in mink and may cause itching, fur chewing, and subsequent economic losses.

MANAGEMENT, HUSBANDRY, AND DISEASES OF RABBITS

MANAGEMENT AND HUSBANDRY

Consistent application of the principles of sanitation, reproduction, nutrition, and disease control makes the difference between success and failure in raising rabbits. Use of proper equipment in the rabbitry also is of prime importance. The following is an outline of these principles primarily as they apply to rabbits kept as pets, and used for commercial production of pelts, fur, and meat.

Housing: The housing requirements for rabbits depend on climate. Minimal housing (an "A-frame" roof without sides) can be used in moderate climates, while a climate-controlled rabbitry may be necessary in areas with excess heat or cold. Rabbitries should be located on nearly level ground and utilize well-drained soil or tile-drained pits for manure. Shade should be provided over as much of the rabbitry as possible. Good ventilation at all times is imperative. Narrow buildings of modular construction offer the advantages of easy ventilation and expansion as needed.

Cages and Ancillary Equipment: All-wire cages are preferred. The standard size is 30 × 36 in. (75 × 90 cm) with a height of 16-18 in. (40-45 cm). A "Quonset" style (rounded top) with the door in front makes all corners of the cage accessible when reaching inside. Cages should be constructed of 1 × 2 in. (2.5 × 5 cm) mesh welded wire for the top and sides, with 0.5 × 1 in. (1.25 × 2.5 cm) mesh welded wire for the floors. Cage dividers can be made of the same material as the top and sides or a type of wire called "baby saver", in which the mesh size of 1 × 2 in. (2.5 × 5 cm) is progressively reduced to 0.5 × 2 in. (1.25 × 5 cm). This prevents neonates born on the wire from crawling between cages. During its manufacture, wire may be galvanized before or after welding; the latter type is more expensive but has considerably greater longevity. Wood should be avoided in cage construction since it can be chewed and cannot be sanitized adequately.

The cage should be equipped with a feed hopper and a watering system. Feed hoppers are best constructed of sheet metal with holes or a screen in the bottom for removal of "fines" (small broken feed particles). Automatic watering systems are used in large rabbitries and consist of a series of connecting pipes with individual watering valves for each cage. Rabbits often chew on the watering valve and eventually destroy it unless it is made of stainless steel or has a stainless centerpiece. Water bottles with sipper tubes are preferred, but crocks and cans are also used in small rabbitries. Contamination of open crocks and cans needs to be monitored carefully; its effects can be lessened by washing and disinfecting the containers daily.

Nest boxes should be constructed so that they can be easily placed in the cage and later removed for cleaning and disinfecting between litters. Disinfecting the nest box twice, once after cleaning and again just before placing it in the cage, helps reduce the incidence of disease. The box should be large enough to prevent crowding, but small enough to keep the kits warm. The standard size of nest box for medium-sized rabbits is 16 × 10 × 8 in. high (40 × 25 × 20 cm). Wooden nest boxes seem to work best, but welded-wire nest boxes with disposable cardboard liners are becoming popular. Nesting material consisting of straw, wood shavings, or shredded sugarcane serves well in either warm or cold weather.

Breeding Stock: Selection of breeding stock is vital to successful reproduction. The genetic potential of the individual buck and doe contributes to the overall output of the rabbitry. Good-quality stock is best obtained from successful breeders. The type of breeding stock to select depends on the purpose of the grower: meat, wool, or show. Common meat breeds are the New Zealand White and the Californian. The common wool breeds are the English, French, and German Angora. For rabbit shows, ~40 breeds are recognized by the American Rabbit Breeders Association.

Reproduction: Rabbit breeds of medium size are sexually mature at 4-4½ mo; giant breeds at 6-9 mo; and small breeds, such as the Polish Dwarf and Dutch, at 3½-4 mo of age. The rabbit is an induced ovulator, but contrary to popular belief, rabbits have a cycle of mating receptivity; they are receptive to mating ~14 of every 16 days. The degree of mating receptivity is indicated by the color of the vaginal orifice and amount of moisture on the labia. The vaginal color cycle runs from a pale whitish pink to a reddish purple. A doe is most receptive when the vagina is purple and moist. Does that are not receptive have a whitish pink vaginal color with little or no moisture. Many breeders test mate the doe 16 days after breeding, as a means of detecting and successfully breeding does that had undergone a false pregnancy following the initial breeding.

A ratio of 1 buck to 10 does is common practice, but many commercial growers find that 1 buck to 20-25 does is more economical. Bucks can be used daily without decreasing fertility; more frequent use requires periods of rest. The doe is always taken to the buck's cage for breeding. The breeding program should continue year round. Does that have experienced long periods of rest between litters tend to become obese and difficult to breed. Does that are constantly in gestation and lactation may become underweight, and their receptivity to the buck and fertility decrease dramatically.

The gestation period is ~31-33 days. Does with a small number of fetuses (usually 4) seem to have a longer gestation period than does that produce larger litters. If a doe has not kindled by day 33 of gestation, 1-2 IU of oxytocin should be given to induce parturition; otherwise a dead litter is almost always delivered sometime after day 34. Occasionally, pregnant does abort or resorb the fetuses due to nutritional deficiencies or disease.

Abdominal palpation 10-12 days following breeding is a valuable technique to detect fetuses in the uterus, and does not damage the young. Does not pregnant are returned to the buck for rebreeding.

Nest boxes are added to the cages 28 or 29 days after breeding. If boxes are added too soon, the does foul the nests with urine and feces. A day or 2 before parturition (kindling), the doe pulls fur from her body and builds a nest in the nest box. The young are born naked, blind, and deaf. They begin to show hair on the second or third day following birth, and by 10 days their eyes and ears are open. Rebreeding can occur anytime following parturition. Some commercial operators use accelerated breeding schedules and rebreed 7-21 days after kindling, while most people raising for show or home use rebreed 35-42 days after parturition.

Most medium-size female rabbits have 8-10 nipples; however, it is not uncommon for them to kindle 15-18 young. Such a doe is generally unable to nurse all the young effectively, so some young are "fostered". Young are removed from the nest box during the first 3 days and given to a doe with a small litter (eg, 8) of about the same age. If the fostered young are mixed with the doe's own kits and covered with hair of the doe, they are generally accepted.

Nutrition: Feeding is an important management practice in the rabbitry. It is easy to over- or underfeed does and fryers. The amount to feed depends on the age of the young rabbits, or the stage of pregnancy or lactation of the does. A general rule in feeding growing, adolescent rabbits (fryers) is to feed all that can be consumed in 20 hr with the feed hopper empty ~4 hr each day. Does are usually fed *ad lib* once they kindle. The general practice is to bring the doe from restricted to full feed slowly during the first week of lactation. Does that are bred to kindle 5 times during the year generally have their feed restricted between litters; those bred intensively should be on full feed continously once they begin the first lactation. Feeding rabbits has been greatly aided by scientifically compounded commercial pelleted diets, most of which are nutritionally complete. (*See* NUTRITION: RABBITS, p 1277.)

When they are unobserved, usually in the early morning or at night, rabbits ingest part of their feces by contorting themselves so that the mouth touches the anus. They ingest only the soft matter that has been processed in the cecum. Coprophagy or pseudorumination is normal in rabbits and not a sign of nutritional deficiency. It serves an important nutritional function by supplying the animal with intestinally synthesized B vitamins and protein. Stability of the normal intestinal microflora may depend on normal coprophagy. Wire-mesh cage flooring does not prevent coprophagy.

Sanitation: Sanitation is important in any livestock enterprise, but especially in rabbit production. Because poor sanitation leads to disease and deaths, cleaning and sanitizing must be constant. Nest boxes must be disinfected between uses. Cages, feeders, and watering equipment should be sanitized periodically. An effective and inexpensive sanitizing solution is sodium hypochlorite (household chlorine bleach) added to water (1 oz/1 qt [30 mL/1 L]).

An active rabbitry constantly experiences a loose hair problem. Does pull hair from their bodies to make nests, and some of this hair becomes airborne. It sticks to cages, ceiling, lights, and almost any other surface and must be removed periodically. The most effective ways to remove it from cages are by washing, or use of a propane torch or flame. Washing, brushing, sweeping, and vacuuming also are effective in other parts of the rabbitry.

Manure removal is essential. Excess manure causes unacceptable levels of ammonia in the air, which predisposes to respiratory disease. Either an efficient pit system must be constructed for composting the manure, or it must be removed periodically (daily is best).

Other Management Techniques: Rabbits may be carried by grasping the loose skin over the shoulders with one hand and placing the other under the rump to support the weight. If they are not held properly and securely, fractures or luxations of lumbar vertebrae may follow struggling; also, the claws on the rear limbs may severely scratch handlers' unprotected arms. Some breeders tattoo or place ear bands on their animals for identification purposes. For show purposes, the right ear is reserved for registration marks applied by American Rabbit Breeders Association registrars.

Sex can be determined at birth; however, it usually is done at weaning. By depressing the external genitalia, the mucous membrane can be exposed. In males, the mucous membrane protrudes and forms a circle; in females, it extends and forms a slit. Castration has no advantage for meat-type rabbits; the growth for males and females is about the same until after market age. Angora rabbits kept for >6 mo are sometimes castrated. The technique is similar to that of castrating cats, although it should be noted that the testes in the scrotum are lateral to anterior to the penis, as in marsupials, and not as in most other placental mammals.

Although most techniques suitable for dogs and cats may be applied to rabbits for physical examination and restraint, general anesthesia of rabbits with barbiturates is often accompanied by significant mortality. Inhalation agents, eg, halothane, are safer. Use of such preanesthetic agents as chlorpromazine hydrochloride (25 mg/kg), diazepam and propiopromazine (5 mg/kg), or fentanyl and droperidol (a combination product [0.22 mL/kg]) allays apprehension, may reduce the dosage of general anesthetic by 50%, and often prolongs anesthesia. Ketamine (35-60 mg/kg) and xylazine (5-10 mg/kg), given together, result in adequate general anesthesia.

BACTERIAL AND MYCOTIC DISEASES

PASTEURELLOSIS

A highly contagious disease, common in domestic rabbits, transmitted either by direct or indirect contact. The etiologic agent is *Pasteurella multocida*. Apparently, rabbits develop little immunity following infection; many are asymptomatic carriers and perpetuate the disease in the rabbitry. An indirect FA test for use on nasal swabs is effective in identifying carriers, which may constitute 30-90% of apparently healthy rabbits in conventional colonies.

A pediatric nasopharyngeal swab technique that utilizes small, saline-moistened swabs has proved superior to the standard, larger nasal swab. The swab is directed medially through the external nares past the turbinates and onto the dorsal surface of the soft palate. The swab can then be retracted and used in the FA test or plated onto a culture medium. A newly developed ELISA test for detecting antibodies against *P multocida* may also prove beneficial in detecting carriers. Infections may be manifest as any of the following: rhinitis (snuffles), pneumonia, otitis media, conjunctivitis, abscesses, genital infections, or septicemia.

Diagnosis is based on clinical signs and by isolation of *P multocida*. Treatment is difficult and does not eradicate the organism. Antibiotics seem to provide only temporary remission, and the next stress (eg, kindling) may cause relapse. Since an effective vaccine has not been developed, the best method of control is strict culling. Barrier colonies of *Pasteurella*-free laboratory rabbits are in widespread use.

Rhinitis (snuffles or nasal catarrh) is a *Pasteurella*-induced, acute, subacute, or chronic inflammation of the mucous membranes of the air passages and lungs. The initial sign is a thin, serous exudate from the nose and eyes that later becomes purulent. The fur on the inside of the front legs just above the paws is matted and caked with dried exudate as a result of pawing at the nose. Infected animals usually sneeze and cough. Snuffles, in general, occurs when the resistance of the rabbit is low. Those animals that seem to recover remain carriers. Pneumonia (*see* below) can ensue.

Abscesses caused by *Pasteurella* may be found in any part of the body or head. All ages are susceptible. When bucks are penned together, their fight wounds frequently develop into abscesses. In most instances, it is advisable to eliminate rather than to treat the affected rabbit. The condition may terminate in septicemia and death within 48 hr. Necropsy may reveal bronchial congestion, tracheitis, splenomegaly, and subcut. hemorrhages.

A troublesome **genital infection** is often caused by *Pasteurella*, but several other organisms also may be involved. Manifest by an acute or subacute inflammation of the reproductive tract, it most frequently is found in adults, more often in does than bucks. If both horns of the uterus are affected, the does often become sterile; if only one horn is involved, a normal litter may develop in the other. The only sign of pyometra in does may be a thick, yellowish gray vaginal discharge. Bucks may discharge pus from the urethra, but usually orchitis is noted. Chronic infection of the prostate and seminal vesicles is most likely and since venereal transmission may ensue, it is best to cull the animal. The contaminated hutch and its equipment should be thoroughly disinfected. For a valuable breeder, antibiotics may be used to combat the infection; however, the prognosis is poor.

Pneumonia, not uncommon in domestic rabbits, may occur in adults or may infect the young while they are in the nest box. Frequently, it is a secondary and complicating factor in the enteritis complex. The cause is bacterial, with *P multocida* accounting for the greatest number of cases. Other bacteria involved may be *Klebsiella pneumoniae*, *Bordetella bronchiseptica*, and pneumococci. Upper respiratory disease (**snuffles**) is often a precursor of pneumonia. Inadequate ventilation, sanitation, and nesting material are predisposing factors. The number of cases of pneumonia is directly proportional to the level of ammonia in a rabbitry. The rabbits usually succumb within 1 wk after signs appear. Affected rabbits are off feed, and have fever (104°F [40°C]), dyspnea, and lassitude. Necropsy reveals bronchopneumonia, pleuritis, pyometra, or pericardial petechiae. Diagnosis depends on signs and lesions. Treatment consists of oxytetracycline, chlortetracycline, or penicillin. Combinations of penicillin and streptomycin are also useful and may be effective for such mixed infections. However, treatment often fails because the pneumonia is advanced before it is detected.

Mature bucks and young rabbits seem particularly susceptible to **conjunctivitis** (weepy eye) caused by *P multocida*; however, the incidence is low. Transmission is by direct contact or fomites. Affected rabbits rub their eyes with their front feet, and the exudate may vary in consistency and color. Any of the common ophthalmic ointments containing sulfonamides, antibiotics, or antibiotics and a steroid are satisfactory for treatment, but recurrence is common. In deep-seated infections, injections of penicillin should be given. Flushing the lacrimal duct with an antibiotic solution is often beneficial in chronically affected show rabbits. Conjunctivitis also accompanies rabbitpox (qv, p 1067) and myxomatosis (qv, p 1065).

LISTERIOSIS

A sporadic septicemic disease characterized by sudden deaths or abortions, or both. Poor husbandry and stress may be important in initiating the disease. Clinical signs are variable and nonspecific, but include anorexia, depression, and weight loss. In contrast to the disease in cattle and sheep, listeriosis seldom affects the CNS in rabbits but spreads via the blood to the liver, spleen, and gravid uterus. At necropsy, the liver consistently contains multiple, pinpoint, gray-white foci. Since antemortem diagnosis is rarely made, treatment is seldom attempted. The causal agent is *Listeria monocytogenes*, which can infect many animals, including man.

STAPHYLOCOCCOSIS

Staphylococcus aureus infection is common in animals, including man. In domestic and wild rabbits, it is manifest as a fatal septicemia of young rabbits (usually in the nest box) or a suppurative inflammation of older rabbits involving almost any organ or tissue, often skin or mammary glands. The organism is transmitted by direct contact or aerosol but is a skin commensal of universal distribution. Rabbits may be colonized but show little or no clinical disease unless resistance is decreased. Abscesses develop in chronic infections. In acute septicemia there is usually fever, depression, and anorexia terminating in death. Diagnosis depends on isolation of the bacteria. Since *S aureus* is resistant to many antibiotics, sensitivity testing should precede antibiotic treatment whenever possible. Thorough disinfection of the nest box both before and after use helps prevent the septicemic form in neonatal rabbits.

MASTITIS
(Blue breasts)

A common disease in commercial rabbitries and occasionally seen in smaller units. It affects lactating does and may spread throughout the rabbitry if sanitation is poor. Mastitis may expand to a septicemia and rapidly kill the doe. Generally, it is caused by staphylococci, but streptococci and other bacteria have been isolated. The mammary glands become hot, reddened, and swollen; later, they may become cyanotic, hence the common name. The doe will not eat, but may crave water. Fever $\geq 105°F$ (40.5°C) is often noted. The condition can be treated with penicillin by parenteral injection. If treatment is started early (the first day the doe goes off feed), the rabbit may be saved and damage limited to 1-2 mammary glands. If >2 glands are lost, it may not be economical to keep the doe. Since penicillin often causes diarrhea in rabbits because of a resulting microbial imbalance in the GI tract, does should be treated only after the pelleted ration has been replaced with hay or some other high-fiber diet. Kits should not be fostered to another doe, since they spread the infection to the foster mother. Hand-rearing of infected young may be attempted, but is difficult. The incidence can be reduced if nest boxes are sanitized both before and after use.

TREPONEMATOSIS
(Vent disease, Syphilis, Spirochetosis)

A specific venereal disease of domestic rabbits characterized by appearance of denuded or scab-covered areas about the external genitalia and caused by the spirochete *Treponema cuniculi*. It occurs in both sexes, and is transmitted by coitus and from the doe to offspring. It is not transmissible to other domestic animals or man. Small vesicles or ulcers are formed, which ultimately become covered with a heavy scab. These lesions usually are confined to the genital region, but the lips and eyelids may be involved. Infected animals should not be mated. Diagnosis depends on detecting the lesions on the genitalia and observing the spirochete by darkfield microscopy. Hutch burn (*see* below) is a diagnostic problem.

Benzathine penicillin G-procaine penicillin G (42,000 IU/kg body wt, subcut.) at weekly intervals for 3 wk is necessary to eradicate treponematosis from a herd. All rabbits must be treated even if no lesions are present. Lesions usually heal within 10-14 days, and recovered animals can be bred without danger of transmitting the infection. A potential side effect of penicillin treatment is diarrhea and the possibility of an enteritis outbreak due to proliferation of gram-negative bacteria in the gut. Rabbits treated with penicillin should be switched to hay and treated with antidiarrheals immediately if needed.

INTESTINAL DISEASE

Intestinal disease is the major cause of death in young rabbits. Previously, most diarrheal diseases were lumped together (as the enteritis complex) or were simply called mucoid enteritis. More recently, specific diseases have begun to be delineated.

Enterotoxemia is an explosive diarrheal disease, primarily of rabbits 4-8 wk old. It occasionally affects adults and junior stock. Signs are lethargy, rough coat, a perineal area covered with greenish brown fecal material, and death within 48 hr. Often, a rabbit looks normal in the evening and is dead the next morning. Necropsy reveals the typical lesions of enterotoxemia, ie, a fluid-distended intestine with petechiae on the serosal surface. One recognized cause is *Clostridium spiroforme*, which produces an iota toxin. Little is known about transmission of the organism; it is assumed to be a commensal that is normally present. The type of diet seems to be a factor in development of the disease. Less enterotoxemia is seen when high-fiber diets are fed. Because of the rapidity of death, treatment is seldom attempted. Lincomycin and related antibiotics induce *Clostridium*-related (eg, *C difficile*) enterotoxemia due to their selective effect on the normal gram-positive bacteria, and are contraindicated in rabbits. These diarrheas remarkably mimic those that occur naturally and that are described above as enterotoxemia. Feeding hay or straw is often helpful. Reducing the amount of feed helps in prevention. Changing to a new brand of feed may also help. Diagnosis depends on history, signs, and lesions.

Mucoid enteropathy is a diarrheal disease of rabbits of any age. While the etiology is still largely unknown, it is basically the result of constipation. Impaction of the cecum or terminal part of the small intestine, or both, is a common necropsy finding. This, along with a gelatinous mucus found in the colon, is almost pathognomonic. The clinical signs are gelatinous or mucus-covered feces, anorexia, lethargy, subnormal temperature, dehydration, rough coat, and often, a bloated abdomen due to excess water in the stomach. The perineal area is often covered with mucus and feces. The impaction can be palpated through the abdominal wall in young rabbits. The disease is chronic in nature; rabbits may live for ≥1 wk. Diagnosis is made on clinical signs and necropsy findings. Treatment is not very successful. Rehydration with electrolytes is sometimes beneficial. Changing the dietary formula usually prevents the condition.

Tyzzer's disease (qv, pp 152 and 1020), caused by *Bacillus piliformis*, has been recognized as a cause of severe diarrhea and death in rabbits 6-12 wk old. It is characterized by profuse diarrhea, anorexia, dehydration, lethargy, and death within 1-3 days. The lesions consist of necrotic enteritis along with focal necrosis in the liver and heart. Infection occurs by ingestion and is associated with poor sanitation and stress. Diagnosis is made histologically; special stains (eg, Giemsa or silver) show the characteristic intracellular bacterium. Culturing is impractical because the bacterium does not grow on artificial media. No cases have been reported in man, but it does affect other species of animals.

SALMONELLOSIS

Although not common in rabbits, the number of reports is increasing. It may be characterized by septicemia and rapid death but more often is asymptomatic. The most common causal agent is *Salmonella typhimurium* or *S enteritidis*. Young rabbits and pregnant does are most susceptible, which suggests that stress has an important role in the disease. Transmission is by direct contact and ingestion of food or water contaminated with feces. Nonspecific clinical signs consist of anorexia, depression, fever, and sometimes, diarrhea. Often, only a dead rabbit is found. In peracute cases, lesions of septicemia are present (vascular congestion is seen in most organs with petechiae on the surface of abdominal and thoracic organs). In acute cases, pinpoint areas of necrosis are seen in the liver, and the spleen is enlarged. Diagnosis depends on isolation and identification of the specific agent. Treatment is rarely attempted since treated rabbits might become carriers. Suspect animals are best eliminated. Prevention depends primarily on sanitation. Since salmonellosis is seen in many animal species, including man, good hygiene should be exercised in an outbreak in rabbits.

RINGWORM
(Dermatophytosis)

An uncommon disease of domestic rabbits, generally associated with poor husbandry. The lesions usually appear first on the head and may spread to any area of the skin. Affected areas are circular, raised, reddened, and capped with white, bran-like, flaky material. The most common cause is *Trichophyton mentagrophytes* var *granulare*, which also affects man, guinea pigs, mice, and rats. Because rabbits with active infections are infectious for man and other animals, they should be isolated and treated, or killed. A degree of control can be obtained by application of powdered sulfur to all nest boxes before kindling, or by use of topical agents such as those containing salicylic and benzoic esters of propylene glycol, aqueous solutions of sodium caprylate, and tinctures containing tannic, benzoic, and salicylic acids. Griseofulvin at an individual dose of 12 mg/lb (25 mg/kg) body wt daily for 2 wk or in the feed at 375 mg/lb (825 mg/kg) of feed is effective, but is not approved for use in rabbits; it should not be used in those intended for human consumption.

MISCELLANEOUS

Tuberculosis and tularemia are uncommon infections of rabbits, now largely of historical interest. Systemic mycotic infections are rare, although individual cases have been reported.

PARASITIC DISEASES

COCCIDIOSIS

A common and worldwide protozoal disease of rabbits. Animals that recover frequently become carriers. There are 2 anatomic forms: hepatic, caused by *Eimeria stiedae*, and intestinal, the cause of which may be *E magna, E irresidua, E media, E perforans,* or other *Eimeria* spp. Transmission of both the hepatic and intestinal forms is by ingestion of the sporulated oocysts, usually in contaminated feed or water.

Hepatic Coccidiosis: Severity of disease depends on the number of oocysts ingested. There may be an infection with no apparent signs, or infrequently, death may follow a short course. Young rabbits are most susceptible. Affected animals may exhibit anorexia and a rough coat. Growing rabbits may fail to make normal gains, but the condition is most often subclinical. The animals usually succumb within 1 mo after a severe experimental exposure. At necropsy, the lesions usually are recognized easily. Small, yellowish white nodules are found throughout the hepatic parenchyma. They may be sharply demarcated in the early stages, while in the later stages, they coalesce. The early lesions have a milky content; older lesions may have a more cheese-like consistency. Microscopically, the nodules are composed of hypertrophied bile ducts. A large number of oocysts is seen. This form of coccidiosis is diagnosed from the gross and microscopic changes along with demonstration of the oocysts in the bile ducts. An impression smear of a lesion in the liver examined under light microscopy often reveals oocysts. The oocysts may also be demonstrated easily by fecal flotation.

Sulfaquinoxaline administered continuously in the drinking water (0.04% for 30 days) prevents clinical signs of hepatic coccidiosis in rabbits heavily exposed to *E stiedae.* Sulfaquinoxaline may also be given in the feed at 0.025% for 20 days, or for 2 days out of every 8, until marketing. Feed-grade sulfaquinoxaline has become difficult to obtain. Withdrawal time is 10 days for rabbits used for food. Rabbits that are treated successfully are immune to subsequent infections. The above treatments will be of no avail unless a sanitation program is instituted simultaneously. Feed hoppers and water crocks should not become contaminated with feces. Hutches should be kept dry, and the accumulated feces removed frequently. Wire cage bottoms should be brushed daily with a wire brush to help break the life cycle. Some chemicals, such as 10% ammonia solution, are lethal to oocysts and may be used to disinfect cages or ancillary equipment exposed to fecal material.

Intestinal Coccidiosis: This form of the disease can occur in rabbits receiving the best of care, as well as in rabbits raised under unsanitary conditions. Typically, infections are mild and no clinical signs are observed. In early infections, there are few lesions; later, the intestine may be thickened and pale. All of the responsible coccidia develop in the intestine. While a good sanitation program can eliminate hepatic coccidiosis, the same program does not seem to eliminate the intestinal form. Intestinal coccidiosis is generally diagnosed by fecal flotation and microscopical identification of the oocysts (species). Treatment is the same as for hepatic coccidiosis.

LARVAL TAPEWORM INFECTION

Although adult tapeworm infections are rare in domestic rabbits, the discovery of larval tapeworm cysts on the serosal peritoneum is not uncommon. Rabbits are intermediate hosts for 2 species of dog tapeworm, *Taenia pisiformis* and *T serialis*. Although *T serialis* is rare in domestic rabbits, it is somewhat more common in wild ones. The larval stage of *T pisiformis* is a cysticercus. Most are found attached to the mesenteries. Before forming these fluid-filled cysts, the young larvae migrate through the liver, where they leave white, tortuous subcapsular tracts. Generally, no clinical signs are associated with this condition. Diagnosis occurs at necropsy. Treatment is not attempted, but control is accomplished by restricting access of dogs to the area in which food and nesting material are stored. Dogs should not be fed infected dead rabbits since this perpetuates the cycle.

MITE INFESTATION

The ear mite *Psoroptes cuniculi* is a common parasite of rabbits throughout the world. Head shaking and ear flapping, along with scratching at the ears are common signs. Torticollis and spasms of the eye muscles may be observed. Affected rabbits lose flesh, fail to produce, and succumb to secondary infections, which frequently damage the inner ear and may reach the CNS. The mites irritate the lining of the ear, and cause serum and thick crusts to accumulate. Under good restraint or even general anesthesia, the brown crumbly exudate should be removed with cotton soaked in dilute hydrogen peroxide, and treated with any of the miticides approved for use in dogs and cats, or even with light mineral oil alone. Those products containing a cerumenolytic agent are particularly useful in removing the heavy, crusty material. The medication should be applied around the external ear and down the side of the head and neck as well. Application must be repeated in 6-10 days. Additional treatments may be necessary. The hutches used by the affected rabbits must be carefully cleaned and disinfected. Incidence is much lower in wire than in solid cages. The mite is readily transmitted by direct contact.

Infrequently, rabbits are infested with either *Sarcoptes scabiei* or *Notoedres cati*. The rabbits scratch themselves almost continually. There is loss of hair on the chin, nose, head, base of the ears, and around the eyes. The condition is extremely contagious and can be transmitted to man. It is difficult to eliminate the parasites on domestic rabbits. Owners should be advised to destroy the animals unless they are valuable breeders. They may be dipped in a lime-sulfur preparation, or rotenone may be rubbed into the lesions.

Fur mite infestations are common; 2 species are found worldwide: *Cheyletiella parasitovorax* and *Listrophorus gibbus*. These live on the surface of the skin (unlike the sarcoptic mites, which burrow in the skin). They do not cause the intense pruritus seen in sarcoptic mange. Fur mite infestations usually are asymptomatic unless the animal becomes debilitated. Occasionally, small scabs and sores are seen on the neck of adult rabbits. Diagnosis is accomplished by skin scraping and light microscopy. These mites do not seem to affect man. Transmission is by direct contact, and treatment is seldom done except for pets or show animals. A solution of 0.5% malathion used twice as a dip with a 1-wk interval is effective in control. Ivermectin shows promise in controlling both ear and fur mite infestations; however, it is not approved for use in rabbits.

NOSEMATOSIS

Encephalitozoon (Nosema) cuniculi is a widespread protozoal infection of rabbits and occasionally of mice, guinea pigs, rats, and dogs. Usually, no clinical signs are seen. It is mildly contagious in a rabbitry and is believed to be spread in the nest box from shedder does to the sucklings. At necropsy, the most significant lesion is pitting of the kidneys. Microscopical lesions consist of focal granulomas and pseudocysts in the brain and kidneys. Sometimes a severe, focal, interstitial nephritis is seen. Diagnosis is made by identifying the lesions (pseudocysts) and observing the organisms when stained with special stains. Several serological and skin tests are helpful in screening rabbits for antibodies to the organism. Treatment has not been attempted. Prevention entails good sanitation and, perhaps, serological screening of breeding stock with elimination of positive reactors. One case of nosematosis has been reported in man.

PINWORMS

Passalurus ambiguus, the rabbit pinworm, usually is not clinically significant but often is upsetting to owners. It is common in many rabbitries and is distributed worldwide. It is not transmissible to man. Transmission is by ingestion of contaminated food or water. The adult worm lives in the cecum or anterior colon. Diagnosis is made by observing the adults at necropsy or finding the eggs during examination of the feces. Single treatments are not very effective, since the life cycle is direct and reinfection common. Treatment of pet rabbits with piperazine citrate in water (3 g/L) for alternating 2-wk periods is effective. Experimentally, ivermectin shows promise in the treatment of pinworms.

VIRAL DISEASES

Viruses are not important causes of clinical disease of rabbits in the USA. Those listed include the infectious fibromas, papillomatosis, rabbit pox, myxomatosis, and a herpesvirus infection (Virus III). Recently, there has been speculation about the possible role of viruses in enteritis outbreaks in rabbitries. Rotavirus infection has been suggested, but the reports are preliminary and inconclusive.

The infectious fibromas of *Sylvilagus* cottontail rabbits are composed of connective tissue and consist largely of fibroblasts and their products. They are located under, rather than in the skin, in which respect they differ from the papillomas. Two main syndromes of infectious fibrotic tumors occur naturally: the loose, areolar lesions of infectious myxomatosis and the Shope fibroma. Both are viral and restricted to rabbits.

INFECTIOUS MYXOMATOSIS

Myxomatosis is a fatal disease of all breeds of domestic rabbits, and *Oryctolagus cuniculus* (the European wild rabbit). Cottontail (*Sylvilagus*) and jackrabbits are quite resistant. All other mammals are refractory. Myxomatosis virus, a member of the poxvirus group, is transmitted by mosquitoes, biting flies, and direct contact. Several strains are pathogenic.

In the USA, myxomatosis is restricted largely to the coastal area of California and Oregon, where epidemics occur infrequently. These areas represent the geographic distribution of the California brush rabbit (*Sylvilagus bachmani*), the reservoir of the infection. Losses may reach 25-90% in rabbitries. All ages are susceptible, although young up to 1 mo old appear more resistant than adults.

The first characteristic sign is conjunctivitis that rapidly becomes more marked and is accompanied by a milky ocular discharge. The animal is listless and anorectic, and the temperature frequently reaches 108°F (42°C). In acute outbreaks, some animals may die within 48 hr after signs appear. Those that survive become progressively depressed and develop a rough coat; the eyelids, nose, lips, and ears become edematous, which gives a swollen appearance to the head. In females, the vulva becomes inflamed and edematous; in males, the scrotum swells. A characteristic sign at this stage is drooping of the edematous ears. A purulent nasal discharge invariably appears, breathing becomes labored, and the animal goes into a coma just before death, which usually occurs within 1-2 wk after clinical signs appear. Occasionally, a rabbit survives for several weeks; in these cases, fibrotic nodules appear on the nose, ears, and forefeet. Rabbits inoculated experimentally with laboratory strains of the virus invariably develop small nodules at the point of injection after several days; these are followed by development of similar nodules on other parts of the body, particularly the ears.

Few characteristic lesions are found at necropsy. The spleen is occasionally enlarged and is almost always devoid of lymphocytes when examined histologically. The seasonal incidence of the disease, clinical appearance of infected rabbits (especially the swollen genitalia), and high mortality are all of diagnostic significance. Large, eosinophilic, cytoplasmic inclusion bodies in the conjunctival epithelial cells are also helpful.

An attenuated vaccine prepared from a myxomatosis virus has protected both field- and laboratory-infected animals. This vaccine is not available in the USA, and since there is no effective treatment, euthanasia and burying or burning of affected rabbits is indicated.

THE SHOPE FIBROMA

The Shope fibroma occurs under natural conditions in the cottontail only, although the domestic rabbit can be infected by inoculation of virus-containing material. The disease may occur in domestic rabbits in areas where it is endemic in wild rabbits and where husbandry practices allow contact with arthropod vectors.

The cause of this tumor, which occurs on the legs, feet, and ears, is a fibroma virus, a member of the poxvirus group. The earliest lesion observed in an infected rabbit is a slight thickening of the subcut. tissues, followed by development of a clearly demarcated soft swelling. These tumors may persist for several months before regressing, leaving the rabbit essentially normal. No control measures for this disease have been developed, since it is of little significance in domestic rabbits.

PAPILLOMATOSIS

Two types of infectious papillomas are recognized in domestic rabbits in the USA. The most important clinically, and of highest incidence, is caused by the oral papilloma virus (papovavirus). The lesions consist of small, grayish white, pedunculated nodules or warts on the under surface of the tongue or the floor of the mouth (oral papilloma virus). The second type, produced by the Shope papilloma virus, and characterized by horny warts on the neck, shoulders, ears, or abdomen, is primarily a natural disease of cottontail rabbits. Shope papilloma virus is transmitted by arthropod vectors. The oral papilloma virus is distinct from the Shope papilloma virus (which is also distinct from the Shope fibroma virus). Skin tumors caused by the Shope papilloma virus never occur in the mouth. Neither type of papillomatosis is treated.

RABBITPOX

An acute, generalized disease of laboratory (*Oryctolagus*) rabbits (apparently it has not been recognized in wild rabbits [*Sylvilagus*]), characterized by pyrexia, nasal and conjunctival discharge, and skin rash. The mortality varies but is always high. A few outbreaks have been reported in the USA since 1930. The causative virus is closely related to vaccinia virus, and some outbreaks may have been caused by a virulent strain of vaccinia. The virus may be isolated or diagnosed serologically by methods appropriate to vaccinia. (*See* POX DISEASES, p 823). Spread through a rabbitry is rapid, but rabbits inoculated with smallpox vaccine (vaccinia virus) are immune. Rabbitpox virus does not infect man.

The most characteristic lesions seen at necropsy are a skin rash, subcut. edema, and edema of the mouth and other body openings. Small gray areas of necrosis are often seen throughout the parenchyma of the liver, spleen, lungs, testicles, ovaries, and uterus. A "pockless" type of rabbitpox has been described and, because of the edematous condition, may be confused with myxomatosis.

VIRAL HEMORRHAGIC DISEASE
(VHD, Necrotic hepatitis)

An acute, highly contagious infection, primarily of domestic lagomorphs. First described in 1984 in China, Korea, and Germany, it has since been reported in other European countries and Mexico.

Etiology and Transmission: The causative agent is believed to be a parvovirus antigenically related to porcine parvovirus and mouse and rat parvoviruses, although some suggest that it may belong to the Caliciviridae or Picornaviridae families.

Aerosol transmission seems to be important, although all secretions and excretions may also be sources of infection. Mechanical transmission by fomites, rodents and other vermin, rabbit by-products, and man can be important. Insects do not seem to be important vectors.

The disease most often occurs in domestic rabbits. Lactating and gestating females are most susceptible, followed by other adults; young rabbits (<2 mo old) are the most resistant. Existence of carriers in surviving domestic animals and in the wild has yet to be determined, but is suspected to occur.

Clinical Findings: The incubation period is short (24-72 hr). Typically, the rabbits are found dead, with no prior indication of illness in the colony. In more protracted cases, dyspnea, congestion of the eyelids, orthopnea, abdominal respiration, tachycardia, and increased uneasiness can be seen. Before death, there is violent cage activity, with rapid turns and flips, which resemble convulsions or mania. High shrills followed quickly by collapse and death are sometimes the only signs reported. In some instances, a blood-tinged nasal discharge can be seen. Blood-stained floors under the cages where animals have died have also been reported. Morbidity is estimated at 30-80%, with mortality up to 80-90%.

Lesions: Due to the rapid course, animals found dead are usually in good condition. Gross lesions are subtle and generally limited to congestion of the respiratory tract and liver. The respiratory tract appears to be most affected, with intense congestion of the trachea and lungs. The trachea may be filled with froth, sometimes blood-tinged. Hemorrhages in the thymus are common. Mild to marked congestion and enlargement of the liver, spleen, and kidneys can be seen. The liver may have yellow-brown surface areas. Congestion of the meninges has been reported. Distention of the distal bowel with gas has been seen, even when necropsy was performed immediately after death. The proximal areas of bowel are usually completely filled with ingesta.

Histologically, there is submassive to massive, focal, coagulative hepatic necrosis. In the lungs, hemorrhages into clusters of alveoli can be seen. Lesions in the spleen vary from simple congestion to necrosis and hemorrhage. Multiple focal areas of necrosis of the myocardium also can be seen. In field cases, severe necrosis of the crypts of the small intestine has been documented; this same finding was more subtle in inoculated laboratory rabbits.

Diagnosis: The peracute course of the disease is the most salient feature. This, with respiratory distress, high mortality, and rapid spread, suggest a presumptive diagnosis. Tissue suspensions of liver, spleen, and lung hemagglutinate human RBC, type O. Serum from convalescent rabbits inhibit this agglutination. FA tests and immunostaining techniques also have been used to identify the viral antigen; liver, spleen, and lung are the specimens of choice since they contain high concentrations of virus. These should be shipped to the laboratory using ice, or dry ice if the shipment is expected to take >48 hr.

VHD should be differentiated from the acute forms of other rabbit diseases such as pasteurellosis, atypical myxomatosis, enterotoxemia, and poisonings.

Prevention: Absolute quarantine measures must be applied to rabbits entering from countries where VHD is present.

The documented increased resistance of young rabbits may be due to passive immunity acquired from ingesting colostral antibodies against the apathogenic lapine parvovirus. A vaccine that confers protection for 6 mo has been developed in various countries, and recently marketed in Spain. The vaccine should be used only where the disease is already widespread and eradication efforts are difficult to employ. Vaccines have been used to complement control efforts, but this may be a disadvantage if the vaccine masks the infection or helps induce a carrier state in the vaccinates.

NONINFECTIOUS DISEASES

Broken Back: Fracture or dislocation of lumbar vertebrae with compression or severing of the spinal cord is common in both pet and commercial rabbits. Common signs include posterior paresis or paralysis, and urinary and fecal incontinence due to loss of sphincter control. Initial signs of paralysis often resolve within 3-5 days as swelling around the cord resolves. Paralysis after 3-5 days, or incontinence, indicates a grave prognosis and warrants euthanasia.

Cannibalism: Young does may kill and consume their young for any of a number of reasons, including nervousness, neglect (failure to nurse), and severe cold. Cannibalism of the dead young occurs as a natural, nest-cleaning instinct. Dogs or predators entering a rabbitry often cause nervous does to kill and eat the young. If all management practices are proper and the doe kills 2 litters in a row, she should be culled.

Dental Malocclusion: The incisors, premolars, and molars of rabbits grow throughout life. The normal length is maintained by the wearing action of opposing teeth. Mandibular prognathism (malocclusion, brachygnathism) probably is the most common inherited disease in rabbits, and leads to overgrowth of incisors with resultant difficulty in eating and drinking. Temporary correction can be effected by cutting the overgrown teeth from time to time with bone or wire cutters. Occasionally, the cheek teeth overgrow and cause severe tongue or buccal lesions. Because it is generally considered to be inherited, rabbits with this condition should not be bred. However, young rabbits can damage their incisor teeth by pulling on the cage wire, which results in misalignment and possibly malocclusion as the teeth grow. This condition cannot be differentiated from genetic malocclusion, and these rabbits also should be culled.

Hair Chewing and Hairballs: The rabbit is a constant groomer, and often the stomach contents contain hair, which is normally passed through the GI tract and excreted with the fecal pellets. The hair or wool (Angora) becomes a problem only if excess amounts are consumed or if it accumulates in the stomach and blocks the pylorus. If this happens, the rabbit becomes anorectic, loses weight, and dies within

3-4 wk. Daily currying to remove loose hair effectively prevents this condition. Mineral oil and laxatives are not effective in removing the hair mass. Surgical removal might be attempted with valuable animals.

Pineapple juice contains the digestive enzyme bromelain, and has been used to treat early cases of trichobezoar or hairballs; an adult is given 10 mL of fresh or frozen juice through a stomach tube or intubation needle once daily for 3 days. Both the fluid and the enzyme help to break up the matrix of the hairball. Hay or straw should be fed during the treatment. This roughage helps to carry the hair fibers through the GI tract and out with the feces.

Hair chewing causes another problem in fryer rabbits. The pelt is damaged due to loss of hair and becomes worthless. This type of hair chewing is generally a result of low fiber in the diet and can be corrected by increasing the fiber or feeding hay along with the pellets. Adding magnesium oxide to the diet at 0.25% also may be helpful. In some cases, hair chewing is a result of boredom. Placing distractions in the cage, eg, soda pop cans or metal rings, often halts this vice.

Heat Exhaustion: Rabbits are sensitive to heat. Hot, humid weather, along with poorly ventilated hutches or transport in poorly ventilated vehicles, may lead to death of many rabbits, particularly pregnant does. Affected rabbits lie on their sides and breathe rapidly. They should be immersed in cool water. Hutches should be constructed so that they can be sprinkled in hot, humid weather. Free access to cool water should be provided. When the environment can be controlled, optimal criteria are: temperature 50-70°F (15.5-21°C), relative humidity 40-60%, with 10-20 air changes per hour. Wire cages are preferable to solid hutches.

Hutch Burn (Urine Burn): A disease often confused with treponematosis that can be truly differentiated only by the absence of spirochetes on darkfield microscopy and the lack of antibodies to *Treponema cuniculi*. It affects the anus and external genitalia, and is caused by wet and dirty hutch floors. Also, rabbits that lack adequate sphincter control of the bladder constantly dribble urine, and may be affected. The membranes of the anus and genital region become inflamed and chapped. The area soon becomes secondarily infected with any of a number of pathogenic bacteria. Brownish crusts cover the area and a hemorrhagic, purulent exudate may be present. Keeping hutch floors clean and dry, and applying nitrofurazone or an antibiotic ointment to the lesions hastens recovery.

Hydrocephalus: This condition, occasionally seen in neonatal rabbits, is characterized by an enlarged head. The top of the skull appears dome-shaped, and the fontanelle is wider than normal. Most affected rabbits are born dead, but occasionally they live for several weeks. However, they generally exhibit neurological signs. At necropsy, the brain is enlarged; on cut section, the ventricles are greatly enlarged and filled with CSF. The cause can be either genetic, or result from dietary deficiency or excess of vitamin A. If it is the result of a dietary deficiency or hypervitaminosis, poor reproduction (low fertility, small litter size, abortion, etc) also is observed in the breeding herd.

A correct assessment of vitamin A becomes critical in treatment. Both serum and liver should be analyzed for vitamin A. A deficiency causes the serum level of vitamin A to decrease below normal (2.6-4.2 IU/mL). In a toxicity, the serum level can be normal, but the liver vitamin A is very high (>4000 IU/g). Treatment of the deficiency involves increasing the carotene content of the diet or adding vitamin A supplement. Treatment of hypervitaminosis A requires reducing the vitamin A in the diet. Control of genetic hydrocephalus requires culling both parents, since it seems to be a genetic recessive.

Ketosis (Pregnancy Toxemia): A rare disorder that may result in death of does at or 1-2 days before kindling. Predisposing factors include obesity and lack of exercise. The disease is more common in first-litter does. The signs are dullness of eyes, sluggishness, anorexia, respiratory distress, prostration, and death. The most significant lesions are fatty liver and kidneys. The probable cause is starvation. For some reason, not well understood, there is anorexia. The body mobilizes fat and transports it to the liver to be broken down for energy, thus the fatty liver. Diagnosis depends on clinical signs and necropsy lesions. Injection of fluids that contain glucose may be helpful in correcting the disease. Breeding junior does early, before they become too fat, is also helpful.

Milkweed Poisoning: This type of poisoning is caused by feeding hay that contains woolly pod milkweed, *Asclepias eriocarpa*, reported only from the Pacific southwestern USA. Sometimes, it is called "head down disease", inasmuch as the affected rabbits develop paralysis of the neck muscles and loss of coordination. If the animal has not consumed too much of the weed and the paralysis has not progressed too far, treatment may be attempted. The head of the rabbit is held so that it can drink water and consume food. Leafy greens and carrots should be fed. Hay and bedding must be free of this weed for prevention. The poisonous principle is a resinoid; consumption of ~0.25% of an animal's weight of green plant is lethal.

Moist Dermatitis (Wet Dewlap): Female rabbits have a heavy fold of skin on the ventral aspect of the neck. As the rabbit drinks, this skin may become wet and soggy ("slobbers"), which leads to inflammation. Factors that may contribute to this condition include dental malocclusion, open water crocks, and damp bedding. The hair may slip and the area become infected or fly blown. The area often turns green if infected with *Pseudomonas* sp. Automatic watering systems with drinking valves generally prevent wet dewlaps. If open water receptacles are used, they should have small openings or be elevated. Once the area is infected, the hair should be clipped and antiseptic dusting powder applied. In severe cases, parenteral antibiotics may be necessary.

Ulcerative Pododermatitis (Sore Hocks): This disease does not involve the hock but the metatarsal and, less commonly, the metacarpal-phalangeal region. The cause is pressure on the skin from bearing the body weight on wire-floored cages, or trauma to the skin from stamping, with secondary infection of the necrotic skin. Several factors, including accumulation of urine-soaked feces, nervousness, posterior paralysis following spinal cord injury, and the type of wire, may influence its development. Genetics are also involved. Heavy-breed rabbits such as the Flemish Giant and Checkered Giant are more susceptible. Pododermatitis is a major problem in the Rex rabbit because of a poorly developed foot pad. Affected rabbits sit in a peculiar position with their weight on their front feet, or if all 4 feet are affected, they "tip-toe" when walking. There is no effective method of treatment, and affected animals should be culled. Since these traits are hereditary, selection of breeding stock for big feet and thick foot pads can reduce the incidence of pododermatitis.

MANAGEMENT, HUSBANDRY, AND DISEASES OF REPTILES

Reptiles can be recognized readily by their horny or scaly integument. The class Reptilia comprises 4 orders. The tuatara is the sole species in the order Rhynchocephalia; Crocodilia includes the alligators, caimans, crocodiles, and gavials; the tortoises and turtles are members of Chelonia; and the order Squamata contains the lizards and snakes. Knowledge of the many physiological and anatomical characteristics of reptiles is essential for successful management of these animals in captivity. Most reptiles are ectothermal poikilotherms, while most mammals and birds are endothermal homeotherms. Structurally, reptiles other than the crocodilians have an incomplete ventricular septum, yet functionally, the heart acts more like a 4-chambered heart. A renal portal system exists in addition to the hepatic portal system. Internal fertilization occurs, and the embryo develops within an amnionic egg, either externally (oviparity) or internally (viviparity). There are many other morphological and biological differences between the reptiles and other vertebrates.

HUSBANDRY

Reptiles maintained in captivity should be kept in an environment similar to that of their native habitat. Specific requirements in the captive environment correspond to many natural variations (temperature, rainfall, photoperiod, food availability, etc) seen in the wild. These requirements necessitate a thorough understanding of the natural history and biology of the herpetofauna to ensure a high quality of life in captivity.

Temperature: Most reptiles are ectotherms; the heat generated from metabolic activity is limited, and they lack control mechanisms for retaining the heat produced. However, many reptiles overcome this by seeking out cool or warm areas to control the daily fluctuations in body temperature. In their natural habitat, they are quite adept at maintaining a relatively narrow range of body temperature, compared to the ambient. Therefore, the cage or enclosure used to house reptiles should provide a thermal gradient (within the preferred temperature optimum for each species), which provides for both physiological and psychological well-being. Tropical species generally prefer temperatures of 80-100°F (27-38°C); temperate species, 68-95°F (20-35°C); semiaquatic turtles prefer a slightly lower range. Lethal temperatures for some species may be within 10°F (5°C) of the upper limits of the preferred range. Reptiles become inactive at lower temperatures (torpor). This is a normal seasonal event for temperate species and may be required for optimal captive reproduction. Temperature extremes and rapid fluctuations of temperature in the animal unit should be avoided.

Photoperiod: Photoperiod requirements for reptiles are based on circadian and circannual activity requirements. For temperate species, variations in photoperiod are utilized as environmental cues to synchronize reproductive cyclicity with optimal environmental conditions. For tropical species, photoperiod variations are less of a primary consideration in synchronizing reproductive cyclicity, while other factors (seasonal humidity/rainfall, droughts, changes in food availability, population density, etc) assume greater importance as seasonal environmental cues. Fluctuations in photoperiod of ~10 hr of daylight for winter months to ~14 hr of daylight for summer months are common for tropical areas. Temperate areas experience changes in photoperiod ranging from ~8 hr of daylight during the winter to ~16 hr during the summer. Seasonal alterations in light intensity have proved beneficial for reproduction in captivity. Full-spectrum light is recommended; this requires use of fluorescent tubes with spectral qualities similar to natural sunlight, including ultraviolet. Improved feeding behavior and reproduction have been observed with full-spectrum light. Incandescent bulbs can be used for light and heat in reptile cages, but direct contact should be avoided to prevent thermal burns. Heat lamps may be used to provide hot spots within an enclosure but should be protected, and should be placed ≥18 in. (45 cm) from the substrate.

Water/Humidity: Semiaquatic species require enough water to allow complete immersion. Feeding, reproduction, and social interaction occur in the water in many species. Water quality should be controlled through filtration and aeration to prevent accumulation of toxic organic wastes and overgrowth of pathogenic organisms. For estuarine species, water salinity should be considered. Water pH for some species of aquatic turtles may need to be adjusted to that of the natural habitat.

Requirements for water intake are linked to availability in the natural habitat. Aquatic and semiaquatic species tend to be ureotelic (urea excretors), which results in significant water loss. Species from drier environments tend to be uricotelic (uric acid excretors), which acts to conserve water. Loss of water through the skin occurs in many species when deprived of soaking areas, with a loss as high as 20% of body wt occurring in crocodilians. Likewise, transcutaneous absorption of water has been documented. Many species drink readily from pools or bowls, but a number of small lizards (anoles and true chameleons) drink by lapping water droplets that accumulate through condensation. Misting the environment provides options for water intake.

The humidity should closely mimic that of the natural environment. Excessively low humidity (<35%) may result in abnormally dry skin and dysecdesis, especially in species that are not adapted to an arid environment. Excessively high humidity (>70%) may result in bacterial and/or fungal blooms, and predispose to cutaneous infections.

Enclosure Design: Many reptiles appear nervous and insecure in captivity. This can be minimized by providing appropriate cage furniture and hiding spaces. Arboreal species should be provided with tree branches or other appropriate climbing material in a vertical orientation. Terrestrial species usually require more horizontal space. Many terrestrial/fossorial species require hiding places; these can be in the form of boxes, tree trunks, rocks, or other objects. For some species, a solid black border painted on the glass wall 8 in. (20 cm) from the cage bottom provides added security. Community housing of highly social, diurnal species often requires placing several stations for basking, eating, and drinking that are all out of the view of dominant conspecifics and any human observers. Overcrowding must be avoided to reduce stress and competition for food, water, basking sites, mates, etc. Aggressive species may have to be separated during feeding to prevent injury to cagemates. Fighting can be reduced significantly by housing compatible specimens together.

Substrates: Cage substrates should be disposable, inexpensive, nontoxic, nonabrasive, provide minimal areas for microbial growth, and facilitate cage cleaning. Newsprint, sand, peat moss, potting soil, wood shavings, and artificial (nylon) turf have all been used successfully for most snakes. Snakes should not be fed while on shavings since the shavings accumulate around the mouth (predisposing to stomatitis) and may be swallowed (predisposing to intestinal impaction). The pungent volatile substances in cedar shavings can cause mucosal irritation as well as neurological problems. Sand, potting soil, and leaf litter are adequate substrates for many species of lizards and tortoises. Crocodilians and aquatic turtles can be maintained on a combination of sand, gravel, and cement substrates if basking areas are provided. Rice hulls and ground corn cobs are readily available, but these are relatively expensive and often contain mites that proliferate rapidly if the litter is moistened. These mites can be eliminated if the litter is heated to ~250°F (121°C) for 1 hr before use.

Sanitation: Sanitation is essential for long-term maintenance of reptiles. Cages should be kept free of excreta, and uneaten food should be removed daily. Tools used for removing wastes should be disinfected with a quaternary ammonium compound before use in each cage to reduce the possibility of disease transmission. Aquatic and terrestrial environments should be disassembled and disinfected q6mo. Turtles appear to tolerate chlorine in treated water reasonably well, but the effects of chloramine are undetermined.

RESTRAINT

Most lizards can be restrained manually for examination by grasping them near the shoulder girdle and gently surrounding the body. Covering the eyes with cloth facilitates the procedure. Many lizards shed the tail when grasped distal to the pelvic girdle (autotomy). Some of the small species are too delicate to be handled, and should be coaxed into small screen boxes for visual examination or induction of chemical restraint; larger ones should be grasped behind the head and at the pelvic girdle.

Small nonvenomous snakes can be restrained by grasping the neck just behind the head and supporting the body with the other hand. Many snakes can be moved by use of a snake hook positioned near the center of the body; these snakes balance on the hook, and physical contact is not necessary. Aggressive snakes may be gently pinned just behind the head for initial handling. Large constrictors require more than one person for adequate restraint. The head is draped with a moist cloth to obscure the snake's vision. The area just behind the head is grasped and other individuals then restrain the coils of the body.

Venomous reptiles should be handled with extreme caution, only by experienced personnel, and never by one person alone. Clear plexiglass tubes with one end blocked can be safely used for examining and treating venomous species. This is accomplished by placing the tube of suitable diameter (large enough for the snake to enter, but too small for it to turn its head around) held by a pair of pilstrom tongs in front of the snake. When half the snake has entered the tube, the open end of the tube and the snake are grasped together and held as a unit. This type of restraint permits examination, administration of medication, and even minor treatment procedures.

Chelonians are restrained by grasping the shell. Several species (snapping turtles and soft-shelled turtles) are aggressive biters, and caution should be exercised.

Restraining large crocodilians requires chemical immobilization, although smaller ones can be restrained with a snare. The snare is placed around the head, the handle brought back over the pelvis, and the snare handle and pelvis grasped together. This prevents the animal from turning. The eyes are covered with a cloth and the mouth forced closed and taped shut. Specimens >5 ft (1.5 m) long require 2 people to provide adequate restraint. Even small crocodilians can inflict serious wounds with the tail as well as the mouth.

ANESTHESIA

Although protocols for anesthesia in reptiles have been inconsistent in the past, research and clinical experiences are providing more sound approaches. Before elective surgery, the animal should be acclimated to a temperature within the preferred range, with induction and recovery occurring at the same temperature. Enzyme systems function best when at the optimal temperature, and consistency is best achieved with temperature control.

A number of anesthetic techniques are inappropriate for use in reptiles. Hypothermia reduces movement but does not induce analgesia, and therefore is unacceptable. Barbiturates have been used in reptiles but are not recommended: the duration of action is prolonged, and depth of anesthesia is difficult to assess and manage.

Ketamine hydrochloride can be used for induction of anesthesia or for minor procedures of short duration. Tranquilizing effects are seen at lower doses. Smaller specimens may require proportionally slightly higher doses. The amount needed for anesthesia varies considerably by species. Dosages of 40-100 mg/kg are appropriate for induction, while 5-30 mg/kg reduce aggression and slow striking reflexes. Recovery occurs in 2-72 hr, depending on dose and temperature.

Tiletamine-zolazepam can be used to induce anesthesia. As with ketamine, the degree of analgesia is often inadequate for major procedures. Doses are 3-30 mg/kg, IM.

SEX DETERMINATION

Sex can be determined in snakes by using a cloacal probe of appropriate size. The end of the probe must be smooth and rounded to avoid injury to the delicate cloacal tissues. The lubricated probe is inserted into the cloaca and directed caudally just lateral to the midline. In females, the probe will enter 2-4 subcaudal scales; in males, it will enter 8-12 subcaudal scales. Some species of lizards show sexual dimorphism; for species that do not, the male's hemipenis can be extruded from the vent by placing pressure with the thumb caudal to the vent and rolling the thumb cranially. Some species of lizards can be probed in a similar fashion to that used with snakes. Helodermatids and some Scincids are difficult to sex reliably; some may require use of ultrasonography or laparoscopy. The penis of the male crocodilian can be identified by deep digital palpation of the cloaca.

The male turtle has a longer tail than the female; in semiaquatic species, the male is smaller and has longer claws. Males also may possess a spur on the hindlegs. Tortoises show distinct differences in the shape of the plastron. The plastron of the male is concave, while that of the female is flat. Some male tortoises also possess an enlarged gular scale pair.

NUTRITION

The nutritional requirements of reptiles are poorly defined. Research in the area is limited, and most recommendations are empirical. The level of macronutrients, protein, carbohydrates, and fat in the diet are qualitatively similar to the requirements of mammals. The reduced metabolic rate of ectotherms allows them to feed less frequently. Feeding behavior, digestion, and assimilation are related to environmental temperature and activation of the associated enzyme systems. Humidity, light source, population density, and type of food also affect feeding behavior. In turtles and some herbivorous lizards, the color of the food contributes to food acceptance; red and yellow are preferred colors. Some reptiles habituate to certain foods and are unwilling to accept alternatives. Providing a variety of foods at each feeding may alleviate this problem.

Quality is important when feeding whole animal foods. Goldfish, mealworms, crickets, wax moth larvae (*Galleria* sp), mice, or rats intended for use as reptile food should be fed a complete and balanced diet to provide adequate nutrients. Herbivores and omnivores also require balanced rations. Many vegetable diets are deficient in calories, protein, and calcium. Insects and grubs are deficient in available calcium, and supplementation is required. A common technique to supplement insect prey with vitamins and calcium is to place the insects in a plastic bag with a small amount of a powdered vitamin/mineral supplement. Shaking the bag coats the insects with the powder, and they should be fed immediately to the reptile. The limitations of this technique are: 1) many reptiles shake the insects in the process of ingestion, causing much of the powder to fall off the insect; and 2) if not eaten immediately, the powder falls off the insect prey in the course of normal locomotion. The addition of calcium to the diet of crickets and wax moth larvae intended as prey items for insectivorous animals increases their calcium:phosphorus ratio to a more acceptable level.

Protein content of the diet should be ~18-20% for carnivores and 11-12% for herbivores. Amino acid requirements are identical to those of mammals, with the addition of histidine in reptiles. Inadequate protein levels cause weight loss, muscle wasting, increased susceptibility to secondary infections, failure to reproduce, and slower healing following injury. Any nonresponsive infectious process can be the result of a primary nutritional deficiency. Most protein deficiencies are seen in herbivorous species on "salad-type" diets or in anorectic individuals. Herbivore diets may be supplemented with alfalfa sprouts, bean sprouts, soy beans or meal, invertebrates, or soft-moist or canned cat food; the overuse of high-protein diets prepared for carnivores has been incriminated in disease production in tortoises. Anorectic specimens may require force-feeding, environmental alteration, or sufficient variety in the diet to identify a preferred food item.

Carbohydrates do not appear to be essential to carnivorous species but, in many cases, caloric requirements can be met by addition of carbohydrates to the diet or through gluconeogenesis of dietary protein. Crocodilians appear unable to assimilate certain polysaccharides. Blood glucose values are variable for each order and may remain elevated for as long as 1 wk after a meal. Blood glucose is elevated during breeding seasons, especially in males.

Clinical hypoglycemia has been reported in captive crocodilians. Signs include mydriasis, tremors, opisthotonos, loss of the righting reflex, and death. Overcrowding and stress with the prolonged release of adrenergic compounds is thought to be causative. Hypoglycemia without clinical signs is normally observed in alligators during the winter.

In large land tortoises and other herbivorous species, the addition of roughage in the form of hay has eliminated chronic malodorous diarrheas. Fiber is required for the normal functioning of the digestive tract.

Specific fatty acid requirements have not been determined for reptiles, but 0.2% linoleic acid in the diet is recommended. Deficiencies have not been reported. Reduced stores in the visceral fat bodies have been associated with small clutch size during the breeding season. Atherosclerosis has been reported; restriction of cholesterol may be an important long-term dietary consideration in captive reptiles.

Water is essential for normal hydration. The ability of the arid species to conserve water is not indicative of a reduced intake requirement. In several species, reduced water availability has resulted in lowered growth rates without apparent changes in the physiologic status of the animals.

Mineral deficiencies are seen frequently in captive reptiles. A vitamin/mineral supplement should be added to the diet of every captive reptile; many of those commercially available for use in birds and small domestic mammals are suitable.

A calcium:phosphorus (Ca:P) ratio of 1.2:1 is generally recommended. However, in some situations (females laying large numbers of calcareous eggs, or rapidly growing juveniles) a ratio approaching 2:1 is more appropriate. As food sources, skeletal muscle has a Ca:P ratio of ~1:25; beef heart and liver, ~1:44. The chitinous exoskeleton of insects is devoid of calcium. Vitamin D is required for proper metabolism and calcium balance. Vitamin D_3 and/or access to ultraviolet light have been recommended as sources for this vitamin/hormone. Commonly used sources of ultraviolet light are the Vitalite, Grolux, and Black Light fluorescent tubes. These tubes are often used together for reptiles. Inadequate levels of vitamin D or an inappropriate Ca:P ratio can result in nutritional secondary hyperparathyroidism, fibrous osteodystrophy, osteomalacia, cystic calculi, cloacal calculi, and rickets. Pathological fractures, bone deformities, and soft or deformed shells in turtles may be observed. Terminal signs may include tetanic seizures. Treatment consists of correcting the Ca:P ratio and injecting vitamin D_3 at weekly intervals. Advanced metabolic bone disease rarely responds to treatment. Excessive supplementation of vitamin D has resulted in soft-tissue calcification in reptiles. While specific requirements for vitamins in reptiles have not been adequately studied, supplemental dietary vitamin D at 100 IU/kg body wt/wk has been recommended. Good sources of calcium for reptiles include crushed or powderized cuttlebone, Neo-Calglucon, crushed chicken eggshell, crushed oyster shell, and crushed or pulverized calcium lactate tablets.

Lethargy and an abnormal swelling at the thoracic inlet (goiter) may indicate an iodine deficiency. Feeding of goitrogenic compounds, including certain green forages, may precipitate the problem. The imbalance is corrected by supplementation with a balanced vitamin-mineral mixture (1 g/kg body wt) or iodized salt (0.5% of the diet).

Iron and copper deficiencies associated with anemia have been reported in turtles.

Hypovitaminosis A is seen frequently in captive turtles, in which it has been associated with palpebral edema, chronic respiratory disease, and renal disease. Squamous metaplasia of epithelial structures is characteristic. Palpebral edema is characterized by occluded Harderian glands, swollen eyelids, and subsequent inability to locate food. Chronic respiratory disease and skin problems, including hyperkeratosis, frequent dysecdesis, and ulceration, may occur. Treatment consists of weekly vitamin A injections of 2500 IU/kg body wt.

Diets containing fish with high thiaminase levels can cause a vitamin B_1 deficiency, and exogenous supplementation is required. Weight loss with adequate food intake is characteristic. Goldfish are low in thiaminase activity, while smelt are extremely high. Posterior paresis progressing to flaccid paralysis has been seen in iguanas, and is associated with a B-complex deficiency. Deficiencies of the water-soluble vitamins often involve more than one vitamin, and require treatment with a multivitamin preparation.

Biotin deficiency, associated with the feeding of unfertilized, uncooked chicken eggs, has been reported in the Helodermata, some varanids, tegus, and larger skinks. Anorexia and weakness are the primary signs. Avidin, an antibiotin substance, is found in ovalbumin. Feeding fertilized eggs reduces the amount of avidin in the egg, and biotin supplementation reduces the frequency of the condition.

Endogenous production of vitamin C by the reptile kidney has been documented. Ascorbic acid deficiency has been incriminated in cases of infectious stomatitis, and oral or injectable supplementation of vitamin C (daily or as needed administration of from 25 mg to several g of vitamin C, depending on the size of the individual) has been suggested as an adjunct to treatment, especially in the presence of renal disease.

Vitamin-K-responsive coagulopathies characterized by prolonged gingival bleeding after loss of deciduous teeth have been reported in crocodilians. Treatment with vitamin K at 0.5 mg/kg body wt has been suggested.

Steatitis has been reported in crocodilians fed mackerel and tuna, and in snakes fed obese rats. Ceroid deposition was observed postmortem. Vitamin E supplementation at 100 IU/day has been recommended as a preventive, but more important is to avoid feeding fish that has been frozen and thawed improperly, stored too long, or left uneaten for ≥ 1 day.

Anorectic animals may require force-feeding to correct severe deficiencies. Initial feedings should include electrolyte solutions with amino acids and simple carbohydrates, followed by blended mixtures of electrolytes, raw egg, and dog or cat food. Solid whole-animal food should be provided only after the digestive system and tissues are showing signs of recovery.

Two procedures are frequently used to force-feed captive reptiles. In one, soft tubing is lubricated and introduced down the esophagus for approximately one-third the body length; a food slurry or solution is then injected using a drenching syringe or caulking gun. Regurgitation can be avoided by feeding small amounts. Care should be exercised not to damage oral structures when removing the tube. The second technique involves placing small whole animals, lubricated with egg white, a small distance down the esophagus. The bolus is then massaged manually into the stomach. In addition to oral force-feeding, parenteral administration of fluids such as dextrose (2.5-5%) and lactated Ringer's solution either subcut. or intracoelomically has been recommended. Environmental factors (ie, temperature, light, humidity, etc) should be optimized for all anorectic specimens.

BACTERIAL DISEASES

Bacterial diseases are seen in all reptilian orders. Opportunistic infections caused by gram-negative bacteria are common. In all bacterial or fungal infections, the nutritional and environmental status of the animal should be considered and deficiencies corrected. Culture and sensitivity are essential in determining appropriate therapy. Cultures should be incubated at 73°F and 98°F (23°C and 37°C).

Treatment with antibiotics is best accomplished by parenteral injection; the degree of absorption of drugs through the intestinal wall from clinically abnormal animals is variable, and regurgitation is frequent. Supportive multiple vitamin therapy is indicated in most infectious diseases. Fluids, such as half-strength normal saline and 5% dextrose, may be given via intracoelomic injection. Sanitation and environmental control improve the chances of success. Environmental temperatures should be maintained near that preferred by the species to enhance immune function. Higher metabolic rates may necessitate force-feeding of anorectic specimens.

Antibiotics frequently used include: ampicillin trihydrate, IM or subcut., at 5 mg/kg, daily; potassium penicillin at 50,000 u/kg, IM or subcut.; benzathine penicillin with procaine penicillin at 10,000 u/kg, IM, q24-72hr; carbenicillin at 400 mg/kg/day at 86°F (30°C) constant body temperature; ticarcillin at 20 mg/kg, IM, daily; and ceftazidime at 20 mg/kg, IM, q72hr at a constant body temperature of 30°C. Tetracycline at 25-50 mg/kg/day, IM or subcut.; chlortetracycline at 200 mg/kg/day, PO; and oxytetracycline at 6-10 mg/kg, IM, IV, or PO have been recommended for infections of *Arizona* and *Salmonella* spp in lizards and chelonians. Sulfaméthazine at 1 oz of a 33% solution per gal. of drinking water (8 mL/L), and sulfadimethoxine at 30 mg/kg, PO, on the first day and at 15 mg/kg/day for 3 days has also been suggested. Trimethoprim-sulfadiazine at 15 mg/kg, daily, has been used. For gram-positive, penicillin-resistant organisms, cephalothin sodium, 30 mg/kg, IM, daily, and cephaloridine, 7 mg/kg, daily, can be used. Chloramphenicol succinate is recommended for many infections at 40 mg/kg, IM, daily, at 75°F (24°C) constant body temperature. Tylosin (25 mg/kg, IM, daily) and lincomycin (6 mg/kg, IM, daily) may be beneficial.

The aminoglycosides are used frequently for the multitude of gram-negative organisms found in reptiles. Neomycin can be used PO for intestinal infections, or to flush abscesses or wounds, but is not recommended systemically. Systemic aminoglycosides may require concurrent administration of fluids to prevent toxic damage to the kidneys and liver. Streptomycin sulfate and kanamycin sulfate have been recommended at 10 mg/kg, IM, daily. Gentamicin sulfate has been recommended at 2.5 mg/kg, subcut., q72hr for snakes and terrestrial tortoises at 24°C constant body temperature. The recommended dose for gentamicin in aquatic turtles is 10 mg/kg, q48hr at 79°F (26°C) constant body temperature, for a maximum of 2 wk. In alligators, gentamicin at 1.75 mg/kg, q96hr at 71.5°F (22°C) was reported to be effective. Amikacin has been recommended at an initial dose of 5 mg/kg, IM, followed by 2.5 mg/kg, q72hr.

A number of infectious conditions are similar in appearance regardless of species and are considered together. **Septicemia** is a common cause of death. The systemic disease may be preceded by trauma, local abscessation, parasitism, or environmental stress. *Aeromonas* and *Pseudomonas* are frequently isolated; the former may be transmitted by the snake mite, *Ophionyssus natricis*. Death may be peracute or chronic. Signs frequently seen are respiratory distress, lethargy, convulsions, and incoordination. Petechiae may be found on the ventral abdomen, and chelonians show erythema of the plastron. Sanitation and husbandry can be significant factors in reducing outbreaks. Affected reptiles should be isolated and antibiotic therapy initiated.

Clostridium novyi has been isolated from a turtle that died of septicemia. *Clostridium botulinum* causes "floppy flipper" disease in sea turtles, which is characterized by incoordination, loss of equilibrium, and drowning.

Septicemic cutaneous ulcerative disease (SCUD) in turtles is often caused by *Citrobacter freundii*. *Serratia* sp may act synergistically by facilitating entry of *C freundii* into the turtle. The scutes are pitted and may slough with an underlying purulent discharge. Anorexia, lethargy, and petechial hemorrhages on the shell and skin are seen; liver necrosis is common. Systemic antibiotics are recommended. Good sanitation is paramount in prevention.

Another shell disease of turtles is caused by *Beneckea chitinovora*, a common infectious agent of crustaceans. Erythema and pitting of the shell with ulceration is seen. Septicemia is uncommon. Treatment with topical iodine is recommended.

Ulcerative dermatitis (scale rot) is seen in snakes and lizards. High humidity may be predisposing. Secondary infection with *Aeromonas* spp, *Pseudomonas* sp, and a number of other bacteria may result in septicemia and death if left untreated. Erythema, necrosis, and ulceration of the dermis, and an exudative discharge are common. Treatment with systemic antibiotics and improved hygiene and husbandry are essential.

Abscesses caused by traumatic injury, bite wounds, or poor environmental quality are seen in all orders. Subcut. abscesses are seen as nodules or swellings. Differential diagnoses include parasitic nodules, tumors, and hematomas. Isolates of the anaerobic organism *Peptostreptococcus,* and of the aerobes *Pseudomonas, Aeromonas, Serratia, Salmonella, Micrococcus, Erysipelothrix, Citrobacter freundii, Morganella morganii, Proteus, Staphylococcus, Streptococcus, Escherichia coli, Klebsiella, Arizona,* and *Dermatophilus* have been recovered from reptilian abscesses, often in combinations. Localized abscesses should be excised and followed with aggressive local wound treatment. Appropriate systemic antibiotics may also be indicated (*see* above).

Visceral abscessation may occur as a result of hematogenous infection. Abscesses of the female reproductive system are common and may result in peritonitis. Surgical intervention is indicated; systemic antibiotics alone are rarely successful.

Subspectacle abscessation is seen in snakes, and conjunctivitis in the other orders. Severity ranges from mild inflammation to panophthalmitis and may occur as a result of infectious stomatitis. Topical antibiotic ointments are applied in turtles, lizards, and crocodilians. In snakes, drainage is achieved by surgically removing a small wedge from the spectacle and flushing with an antibiotic solution (neomycin or streptomycin). All cases should be treated with supplemental vitamin A.

Infectious stomatitis is seen in snakes, lizards, and turtles; it is characterized early by petechiae in the oral cavity. Caseous material develops along the dental arcade as the condition worsens. In severe cases, infection extends into the bony structures of the mouth. *Aeromonas* and *Pseudomonas* spp, normal oral inhabitants, are most frequently isolated, along with a variety of gram-negative and gram-positive cocci. Respiratory or GI infection may occur in poorly managed cases. Debridement, irrigation with antiseptics and/or antibiotics, systemic antibiotics, and supportive therapy are indicated. In severe cases with ulceration or granuloma formation, surgery may be indicated. Vitamin supplementation, especially with vitamins A and C, is recommended.

Respiratory infections are common; the incidence can be influenced by respiratory and/or systemic parasitism, unfavorable environmental temperatures, unsanitary conditions, concurrent disease, and malnutrition. Open-mouth breathing, nasal discharge, and dyspnea are frequent signs. *Aeromonas* and *Pseudomonas* spp are frequently isolated, but many respiratory infections are mixed. Septicemia may occur in severe or prolonged cases. Treatment consists of improving the environment, systemic antibiotics, and vitamin A supplementation at 5000 IU weekly. Nebulization therapy with antibiotics diluted in saline, in combination with dimethyl sulfoxide and/or acetylcysteine, has been used in combination with parenteral antibiotics to treat bacterial pneumonia.

Middle and inner **ear infections** occur in turtles, most frequently in box turtles. Marked swelling is seen at the tympanic membrane, and caseous material is present. *Proteus* sp, *Pseudomonas* sp, *Citrobacter* sp, *Morganella morganii, Enterobacter* sp, and other bacteria have been isolated. Drainage and systemic antibiotics are appropriate. This condition may be secondary to hypovitaminosis A; parenteral and dietary supplementation of vitamin A may be beneficial.

Infectious cloacitis is characterized by edema and hemorrhagic discharge. The cause may be traumatic. Cloacal calculi may form in vitamin/mineral imbalances and should be manually removed and followed by dietary correction. *Escherichia coli* and *Pseudomonas* and *Staphylococcus* spp have been isolated. Pericloacal abscesses often involve migration of the infection cranially by subcut. or coelomic tissue pathways. Ascending urinary or genital tract infections are common sequelae. Aggressive therapy, including surgical debridement, local wound treatment, and appropriate systemic antibiotics, is indicated.

Mycobacterial infections are often associated with chronic wasting and are seen as granulomatous lesions at necropsy. Chelonians generally exhibit pulmonary involvement, while lizards, snakes, and crocodilians show visceral granulomas. There is no known treatment for reptilian tuberculosis. The species isolated are *Mycobacterium ulcerans, M chelonei,* and *M thamnophis.* All are cultured at reduced temperatures and may require long periods for growth.

Salmonella, Arizona, and *Edwardsiella* spp are isolated from clinically normal turtles. The zoonotic nature of these organisms must be considered when handling or treating turtles. Attempts to eliminate these microorganisms from infected animals and their eggs have been unsuccessful.

ECTOPARASITIC DISEASES

Except in wild and on newly acquired specimens, a limited number of ectoparasites are seen. The mite *Ophionyssus natricis* is distributed worldwide, and most reptilian species are affected. Reduced vitality and, in heavy infestations, death due to anemia may occur. Skin of affected animals appears coarse, and dysecdesis is frequent. The mite is <1.5 mm long and is often found near the eyecaps. It may be associated with the mechanical transmission of *Aeromonas hydrophila*, and result in septicemia or pneumonia. Treatment consists of placing dichlorvos pest strips near the cage for 4 days. Direct contact of the strips with the animal should be avoided. Cages may be treated by spraying with a 0.1-0.2% solution of trichlorfon. Large reptiles also may be sprayed with this solution. Silica-gel preparations have been recommended as a topical dessicant. Care must be exercised when smaller specimens are treated with silica preparations.

The larvae of trombiculid mites (chiggers) are seen occasionally, but are not considered to be pathogenic.

Ixodid ticks are frequently found on reptiles, and heavy infestations may result in anemia. Argasid ticks may cause paralysis, with muscle degeneration at the site of the bite. The transmission of green-lizard papilloma-associated virus, several hemogregarines, and the filarid worm *Macdonaldius oscheri* has been associated with ticks. Ticks can be removed manually.

Leeches have been found on a variety of turtles and crocodilians—on the legs, head, and neck, and in the oral cavity.

Turtles are frequently seen with cutaneous myiasis, around the cloaca and commissures of the mouth.

Ectoparasites are best prevented by thorough screening and quarantine of all new animals entering a collection.

ENDOPARASITIC DISEASES

In captivity, reptiles are at greater risk for pathological lesions due to internal parasites. The stress of captivity coupled with a closed environment favors a heavy parasite load. Every effort must be taken to rid specimens of parasite burdens, and the environment of intermediate hosts.

Pathogenic trematodes infect the vascular system of turtles, and the oral cavity, respiratory system, renal tubules, and ureters of snakes. Chemotherapeutic agents have not been effective in eliminating these parasites.

Tapeworms are found in all orders, but rarely in crocodilians. Reptiles may act as the definitive, paratenic, or intermediate hosts for a large number of species. Although most species are nonpathogenic, weight loss and death have been reported. The complex life cycle of cestodes and restricted geographic range of intermediate hosts limit the number of cases in captive animals. When present, proglottids may be found around the cloaca, or typical cestode ova may be isolated from feces. Treatment is with praziquantel, 7.5 mg/kg; bunamidine hydrochloride, 25-150 mg/kg, PO, q2wk; or niclosamide, 150-300 mg/kg, once monthly. Plerocercoids of the genus *Spirometra* may be found as soft swellings in the subcutis. These larval stages may be removed surgically.

Nematodes are found in all orders of reptiles; several genera are important. *Strongyloides* spp frequently inhabit the intestinal tract of reptiles; larvae are seen in the respiratory tract and nasal exudate. In snakes, the larvae have been observed within granulomas distributed throughout the body wall, suggesting that the larvae may be capable of penetrating the skin. Overwhelming parasitism is common when poor hygiene results in highly contaminated environments. *Rhabdias* and related species have been found in the lungs in a variety of snakes; embryonated ova may be found in the oral cavity and in lung aspirates. Embryonated ova and free larval forms may be seen in the feces. Larvae resembling *Rhabdias* also have been observed in the gingiva of snakes with stomatitis. Infections often are subclinical, but may be associated with secondary bacterial pneumonia. In severe cases, death may result.

Stomach worms of the genus *Physaloptera* are seen in lizards. Gastric ulceration may occur in severe infections. Ova are elliptical and may be embryonated. Numerous snakes are infected by *Kalicephalus* sp. This hookworm prefers the upper GI tract and causes erosive lesions at sites of attachment. Ova are similar to those of *Physaloptera* spp. Large granulomas caused by the above species have also caused GI obstruction in snakes.

Ascarids frequently infect reptiles. Ova are similar to those of ascarids from mammalian hosts. Severe lesions and death may be seen in infected snakes. Clinically infected snakes frequently regurgitate partially digested food and/or adult nematodes, and are anorectic. The major lesions are large granulomatous masses in the GI tract, which may abscess. The intestinal wall may perforate.

Many other nematode species may be found in reptiles. Capillarid, trichurid, and oxyurid ova may be found on fecal examination. The nonpathogenic larval and oval forms of parasites of prey items (eg, *Syphacia obvelata*, the mouse pinworm) may be found when infected prey is consumed. In captive specimens, treatment should be attempted when evidence of parasitism is present.

Some of the larval forms of nematodes are suspected or confirmed to penetrate the skin, bypassing the oral reinfection route. The subtle nature of reinfection by this route often goes unnoticed by the hobbyist until the reptile is overwhelmed by parasites. Close attention to the immediate removal of excreta and good sanitation help to reduce parasite burdens in captivity.

These parasites can be treated PO with mebendazole, 20-25 mg/kg; thiabendazole, 50-100 mg/kg; or fenbendazole, 50-100 mg/kg; with the dose repeated in 2 wk. Levamisole, 10-50 mg/kg, via intracoelomic, IM, or subcut. injection, and 200 mg/kg, PO, has been reported to be effective for *Rhabdias* sp. Ivermectin has been used safely in snakes and lizards at 0.2-0.4 mg/kg. In turtles, ivermectin toxicity was evident as paresis at doses as low as 0.025 mg/kg, and it is therefore not recommended for use in turtles.

Dermal lesions caused by a spirurid worm, *Dracunculus* sp, may be seen. Numerous species of spirurids infest the mesentery, peritoneal cavity, and blood vessels. The requirement for a mechanical vector reduces the incidence of these worms in captive-bred specimens or long-term captives. Treatment consists of increasing the environmental temperature to 95-98°F (35-37°C) for 24-48 hr. However, some "cool-adapted" reptiles may not tolerate this treatment.

Acanthocephalans and pentastomes are found in reptiles and are variably pathogenic. Pentastomids are occasionally associated with pneumonic signs. No effective treatment for these parasites has been reported.

MYCOTIC DISEASES

Excessively high humidity, low environmental temperature, concurrent disease, malnutrition, and stress from poor husbandry may be factors in the development of mycotic diseases in reptiles, which develop over a long period. Little is known about the pathogenesis of systemic mycoses, but maintaining good sanitation and husbandry reduces the frequency of infection. *Aspergillus, Metarhizium, Mucor, Paecilomyces,* and *Penicillium* spp are a few of the organisms that have been isolated from reptiles suffering from systemic mycoses. Reports of successful treatment of systemic mycoses in reptiles are few. Suggested treatments for deep fungal infections include amphotericin B, 5 mg/kg body wt, nebulized in 150 mL of saline for 1 hr, b.i.d.; and thiabendazole, 50 mg/kg, and ketoconazole, 50 mg/kg in combination, administered PO daily. For superficial or localized mycotic infections, surgical removal of the granuloma with local wound treatment is advised. *Basidiobolus* sp, pathogenic for mammals, is found in feces of normal reptiles.

Dermatophytosis has been described in all orders. *Geotrichum, Fusarium,* and *Trichosporon* are the genera most frequently isolated. In most cases, cutaneous injury precedes a secondary fungal infection. Chelonians with fungal infections of the shell can be treated by local debridement and application of Lugol's solution or povidone-iodine topically. Griseofulvin, at 20-40 mg/kg, PO, q72 hr for 5 treatments, has been recommended for mycotic skin infections. Topical 1% tolnaftate cream has also been effective. Exposure to ultraviolet light also may be beneficial.

Ulceration of GI tissues has been associated with infections by *Mucor* and *Fusarium* spp. Chronic visceral granulomatous disease of liver, kidneys, and spleen has been caused by *Metarhizium* and *Paecilomyces* spp. Few signs other than weight loss are observed before death. Animals may continue to feed until a few days of death.

The most frequent sites of mycotic infection are the skin and respiratory tract. *Metarhizium, Mucor,* and *Paecilomyces* spp are frequent isolates. *Aspergillus* sp has been isolated from pulmonary lesions in the chuckwalla (*Sauromalus obesus*). Most infections involve granuloma or plaque formation with resultant signs of respiratory distress before death.

Candidiasis in large snakes has been treated with nystatin, 100,000 u, PO, for 10 days.

PROTOZOAL DISEASES

Numerous protozoans exist in reptiles; many are harmless commensals. The most serious protozoal pathogen of reptiles is *Entamoeba invadens*. Clinical signs are anorexia, weight loss, vomiting, mucoidal or hemorrhagic diarrhea, and death. Entamebiasis may be epidemic in large snake collections. Herbivores appear less susceptible than carnivores; infection may be severe in snakes, turtles, and tortoises. Transmission is by direct contact with the cyst form. Hepatic abscesses containing numerous *E invadens* trophozoites are common in chronic cases. At necropsy, gross lesions may extend from the stomach to the cloaca. The intestine shows areas of ulceration that tend to coalesce, caseous necrosis, edema, and hemorrhage. Multifocal abscesses in a swollen, friable liver are seen with the hepatic form. Identification of trophozoites or cysts in a wet preparation of fresh feces or tissue impressions, or in histological sections is diagnostic. Turtles and snakes should not be housed together.

Entamoeba invadens is best treated with metronidazole, 160 mg/kg, PO for 3 days, with a total daily maximum dose of 400 mg. The indigo snake, *Drymarchon* sp, and king snake, *Lampropeltis* sp, appear sensitive to metronidazole; doses of 40 mg/kg and 100 mg/kg, respectively, have been safe. Dimetridazole may be given PO for 10 days at 40 mg/kg. Emetine hydrochloride may be given IM or subcut. at 2.5-5 mg/kg as a single dose daily for 10 days. Tetracycline and paromomycin have been used, but are considered ineffective against the hepatic form.

Flagellates, especially *Hexamita* sp, have been reported to cause urinary tract disease in chelonians, and intestinal disease in snakes. The "giardia" seen in some cases of enteritis in snakes may actually be *Hexamita*, or one of the relatively nonpathogenic flagellates that inhabit the intestinal tract of snakes. Expertise is required to distinguish between the different species, and special preservatives and stains are required to identify most of these organisms. Dimetridazole at 40 mg/kg, PO, for 5 days, and metronidazole at 125-275 mg/kg, PO, repeated in 2 wk, have been used to treat flagellates.

Several coccidial organisms have been reported: *Klossiella* from the kidney, *Isospora* from the gallbladder and intestine, and *Eimeria* from the gallbladder. The severity of disease varies with the organism and affected species. Treatment with sulfamethoxydiazine has been suggested; a 20% solution is administered IM or subcut. at an initial dose of 80 mg/kg, then 40 mg/kg for the next 4 days. Sulfamethoxine has been used at a dose of 90 mg/kg the first day, then 45 mg/kg for the next 5 days, by stomach tube.

Plasmodial (malarial) organisms, as well as other intracellular "hemic" protozoans, have been reported in reptiles. Cryptosporidiosis is frequently reported in association with postprandial regurgitation. The organism affects the GI mucosa, resulting in marked thickening of the rugae and loss of segmented motility. A mass in the gastric region is palpable, and contrast radiographs reveal rugal thickening. Mucosal thickening occurs as a result of invasion by numerous cryptosporidial organisms. There is no effective treatment.

VIRAL DISEASES

Few viruses have been clearly defined as etiological agents of disease in reptiles, but they have been associated with various disease conditions. In snakes, an outbreak of fatal respiratory disease in captive *Bothrops* sp was found to be associated with a paramyxovirus, designated Fer-de-lance virus. A retrovirus was isolated from a sarcoma in a Russell's viper and designated viper virus. A related virus was isolated in a corn snake from a rhabdomyosarcoma, and designated cornsnake retrovirus.

Progressive anemia in Australian geckos has been linked to an iridovirus. Benign papillomas from the green lizard, *Lacerta viridis,* contained viral particles similar to herpesvirus, reovirus, and papovavirus. In Bolivian side-neck turtles, papovaviruses have been linked to papillomatous growths. A nonpathogenic herpesvirus was isolated from the common iguana, and 2 nonpathogenic rhabdoviruses from the lizard *Ameiva* sp.

A herpesvirus was associated with an outbreak of "gray patch disease" in green sea turtles hatched in captivity. Papular skin lesions with epidermal necrosis was observed. Affected animals had 5-20% mortality. Fatal hepatitis in 2 Pacific pond turtles was associated with a herpesvirus.

Parvoviruses, picornaviruses, adenoviruses, and herpesviruses have been found within the intestinal tract of snakes, but their exact role is unknown.

A poxvirus-like virus has been isolated from circumscribed cutaneous lesions in a caiman.

ENVIRONMENTAL DISEASES AND TRAUMATIC INJURIES

Abnormal beak growth, which inhibits adequate feeding, occurs occasionally in turtles and tortoises. Treatment consists of trimming the mouthparts into a more normal conformation. The condition usually recurs due to primary malocclusion.

Aggression at mating and feeding is common in crocodilians and some semi-aquatic turtles. Injuries to cagemates can be severe and are best avoided by separation at feeding and reducing the number of animals allowed in a breeding group.

Blister disease, a common cutaneous infection, can be caused by high humidity and prolonged exposure to moist or contaminated bedding. Moist, contaminated bedding allows bacterial and fungal growth which, when coupled with exposure to fecal degradation products, can predispose to small cutaneous erosions. Cutaneous infection results in rapidly enlarging erosions and ulceration. Left untreated, septicemia and death can result. Initial treatment requires a clean, dry environment. Secondary infections are treated with appropriate antibiotics.

Bone fractures due to trauma are seen in all species. Long-bone injuries may be repaired with splints or internal fixation devices. Injury to the spinal column must be assessed on an individual basis; when clear displacement is not evident, radiographic evaluation should be done. Spinal injuries caudal to the vent may be tolerated, but injuries cranial to the vent frequently result in constipation and retention of urates.

Burns (associated with the use of incandescent lights or other heat sources) are treated by cleansing the site, applying antibiotic ointments, and placing the reptile in a clean, dry environment. In severe burn cases, intracoelomic or subcut. administration of fluids may be needed to prevent dehydration.

Crush injuries to turtles may result in fractures to either the plastron, the carapace, or both. These wounds should be cleansed topically, realigned under light anesthesia, and the defect repaired using an epoxy resin. Healing is slow and may require >1 yr.

Dysecdesis refers to an incomplete or inadequate shed. Low humidity and other stresses, including decreased thyroid function, ectoparasitism, nutritional deficiencies, infectious diseases, and lack of suitable abrasive surfaces have been incriminated as contributing factors in dysecdysis. Often, eye caps and/or annular bands on the tail or digits are retained. Treatment is best accomplished by soaking the animal in warm (77-82°F [25-28°C]) water for several hours and then applying gentle friction with a gauze sponge. After softening the retained spectacle with water, glycerol, or a similar softening agent, the eye caps may be removed with a pair of fine forceps; the retained portion is grasped by the edge and gently teased away from underlying tissues.

Ecdysis (shedding) is the hormonally mediated process by which reptiles shed the outer keratinized skin in response to growth or wear. In snakes and some lizards, the process results in shedding the entire layer of skin as a single piece. Crocodilians and many lizards shed small sections of skin intermittently. Turtles follow this pattern on scaled regions and shed skin coverings from individual scutes one at a time. Large, moderately abrasive rocks or other articles for reptiles to rub on during ecdysis facilitates a normal shed. Before shedding, snakes become anorectic, and their color becomes mildly translucent, which is especially evident over the eye caps (opaque). Increased irritability and aggressiveness is frequently seen at this time. The shed is initiated around the mouth, and the old skin is everted as it is shed.

Maladaption syndrome, the inability of a reptile to adapt to its environment in captivity, is characterized by lethargy, anorexia, cachexia, and death. Manipulation of environmental variables and/or diet may reverse the condition, but most often it is fatal. Misting the enclosure before offering food may induce feeding. Likewise, increasing the environmental temperature may stimulate appetite, as may full-spectrum light. Vitamin B_{12} injections are reported to increase appetite and feeding behavior. Individuals refusing food over long periods at preferred temperatures sometimes start to self-feed after a forced 3-wk long dormancy fast. The temperature should be lowered to 60-65°F (15-18°C), then slowly raised to the preferred level. This technique should not be used in reptiles that are cachectic.

Rodent bites, inflicted by uneaten prey, frequently cause traumatic injuries; secondary infection and abscessation are common sequelae. When possible, frozen/thawed, or freshly sacrificed rodents should be offered to prevent injury to the reptile (dead prey should be discarded after 24 hr if left uneaten). Fresh bite wounds may be treated by cleansing and saturating with povidone-iodine (diluted 1:4). Parenteral antibiotics based on sensitivity should be utilized. Untreated wounds frequently abscess (qv, p 1077) and are seen as a swelling that may be soft or hard. The abscess, including the fibrous capsule, should be removed surgically, and the defect sutured. Open or draining abscesses should be curetted, flushed with a povidone-iodine or Lugol's solution, and parenteral antibiotics administered. Antibiotic ointments with proteolytic enzymes may be helpful.

METABOLIC DISEASES

Gout is seen in all orders; visceral and articular forms have been reported. Radiographs often reveal tophi in affected organs and joints. The accumulation of urates occurs in organs and may be associated with dehydration, severe catabolic states (starvation), disturbances of protein metabolism, high-protein diets, and renal disease. Environmental and psychological stressors may play a role in the development of this disease. Allopurinol (15 mg/kg) with colchicine may be beneficial if the diagnosis is made early. Renal tubules obstructed with urates are frequently seen at necropsy. A history of anorexia with concurrent dehydration is common.

Endocrine diseases are not often documented in reptiles, although diabetes mellitus has been reported in chelonians: polyphagia may or may not be apparent, and glucosuria and hyperglycemia are the primary clinicopathological findings. The etiology is as yet undetermined; pancreatectomy in lizards may result in hypoglycemia, implying that other hormones, such as glucagon or somatotropin, may play a role in the pathogenesis of diabetes mellitus in reptiles.

Hypothyroidism and/or thyroid hyperplasia have been reported mainly in tortoises from the Galapagos Islands. It has been speculated that high amounts of dietary iodine in the natural diet may play a significant role in this disease. Feeding goitrogenic foods to tortoises has been incriminated in development of this condition. The primary clinical sign in this complex is subcut. edema.

NEOPLASTIC DISEASES

Neoplasia should always be included in the differential diagnosis of disease in reptiles. In addition to spontaneously developing neoplastic diseases, tumors have been associated with parasitism and oncogenic viruses. Techniques such as radiography, ultrasonography, cytology, histopathology (biopsy), and viral isolation provide improved diagnostic capabilities. Once neoplasia is diagnosed, treatment protocols similar to those used in other animals could be adapted.

VACCINATION OF EXOTIC MAMMALS

A number of diseases of domestic animals also infect certain wild animals; therefore, immunization of captive exotic mammals is desirable when they are at risk of exposure. However, since claims of efficacy and safety for commercial vaccines can be made only for the species in which adequate research has been performed, recommendations for use in exotic mammals are based on limited published data and anecdotal experiences. In general, inactivated viral or bacterial vaccines are preferable to their modified live counterparts; modified live virus (MLV) vaccines may be insufficiently attenuated to be nonpathogenic in exotic species, even though they are avirulent in domestic counterparts. In certain instances,

MLV vaccines are recommended in exotic species, based on considerable experience in zoos with satisfactory safety results and limited serological data; however, studies evaluating protection against virulent virus challenge generally are not done.

In general, animals with active clinical illness should not be immunized.

Canine Distemper: All members of the families Canidae, Procyonidae, Mustelidae, and some members of Viverridae are considered susceptible. The susceptibility of Hyaenidae and Ursidae is questionable, even controversial. Clinical distemper in exotic carnivores usually resembles that in dogs, but often appears primarily as a neurological disease that results in the affected animal losing its fear of man, thus the disease can be confused with rabies.

Caution is advised in vaccinating wild-caught animals because they may be incubating the disease. There is marked variation between species and individuals in their reaction to MLV vaccines, and different MLV vaccines vary considerably in their degree of attenuation. While a killed virus vaccine would be preferred, one is not currently available. Several MLV vaccines of chick-embryo or tissue-culture origin have been used safely by zoo veterinarians for several years. Avian (chick embryo)-origin MLV vaccines appear to be the best attenuated and therefore safest, based on limited studies in foxes. It is prudent to consult a zoo veterinarian for recommendations of specific products, although there are differences in experiences with specific vaccines. MLV vaccines marketed for use in mink generally are more highly attenuated, and are recommended for use in all Mustelidae. Ferret-origin MLV vaccines are poorly attenuated and therefore contraindicated for use in any nondomestic carnivores. Single doses of MLV vaccines are administered subcut. or IM to young animals after weaning, with monthly booster doses up to 4 mo of age, and annual revaccination thereafter.

Canine Parvovirus and Feline Panleukopenia: Canine parvovirus, raccoon parvovirus, and feline panleukopenia virus are closely related antigenically and pathogenetically. Wild Canidae, Felidae, most Mustelidae, Procyonidae, and Viverridae are considered susceptible to one or more of the above parvoviruses. Caution should be exercised when vaccinating, since some MLV products safe for one species may be insufficiently attenuated for others. Inactivated vaccines of tissue or tissue-culture origin are preferred. Recommendations for dosage and frequency of vaccination have been arrived at somewhat empirically: for small species, one standard small animal dose (1 or 2 mL) is given subcut. or IM; for larger species, 2 mL/10 lb (4.5 kg) body wt to a maximum of 10 mL. A booster dose should be given at 10-14 days, and vaccination repeated at 6- to 12-mo intervals. Combination vaccines containing MLV canine distemper, canine adenovirus 2, canine parainfluenza, and feline panleukopenia or canine parvovirus have been used in wild Canidae without adverse effects, but experience of zoo veterinarians has been variable. Similarly, there are combination MLV feline vaccines that contain feline panleukopenia, feline rhinotracheitis, and feline caliciviruses. Most zoo veterinarians report good results with such vaccines in exotic felids, but a few report conflicting results. Combination killed feline panleukopenia, feline rhinotracheitis, and feline calicivirus vaccines are preferred.

Equine Encephalomyelitis—Eastern, Western, Venezuelan: Wild Equidae are susceptible to the 3 equine encephalomyelitides. Vaccination should follow guidelines recommended for domestic horses in endemic areas. Inactivated trivalent (EEE, WEE, VEE) or bivalent (EEE, WEE) vaccines, or combinations of these with tetanus toxoid, are administered according to manufacturers' instructions, usually intradermally or IM, depending on the product used. Initial immunization consists of 2 doses, 1-2 wk apart. Annual boosters consist of 2 similarly spaced injections with intradermal products, and usually a single injection with combination IM products.

Equine Herpesvirus 1 Infection: This can cause abortion in exotic Equidae. Only killed virus vaccines are recommended since it is not known if MLV vaccines are adequately attenuated. A single vaccination should be given to foals at 3-4 mo of age, and at 4-mo intervals up to 1 yr. Mares should be immunized q4mo to maintain adequate protection against abortion, because even following recovery from natural infection, protective immunity lasts only ~4 mo.

Erysipelas: *Erysipelothrix rhusiopathiae* is pathogenic for wild Suidae, Tayassuidae (peccaries), and cetaceans, especially dolphins. Erysipelas bacterin is administered as a 2 mL subcut. dose at 2-3 mo of age with a repeat dose in 3-5 wk, and a single annual booster (*see also* p 335).

Feline Caliciviruses: Exotic felids are susceptible to feline caliciviruses. As with feline rhinotracheitis virus, vaccines against this disease are contained in combination feline vaccines. Vaccination recommendations are the same as for feline rhinotracheitis (*see* below).

Feline Herpesvirus Rhinotracheitis: Feline viral rhinotracheitis has emerged as a serious disease threat in exotic Felidae. Vaccines currently available are killed or MLV, usually in combination with other agents (*see* CANINE PARVOVIRUS AND FELINE PANKEUKOPENIA, above). These are given IM or subcut. in a single dose at weaning. Doses are then given at monthly intervals to 4 mo, and annually thereafter.

Infectious Canine Hepatitis (Canine Adenovirus 1 [CAV-1]): All Canidae are susceptible. In foxes, the disease is called **fox encephalitis** due to a predominant neurotropism and neurological signs. Recently, evidence has emerged that Ursidae may be susceptible to CAV-1 infection. No killed virus vaccines are commercially available. MLV vaccines that contain combinations of canine distemper and CAV-1 or CAV-2 are used. The CAV-2 MLV is considered less likely to cause adverse postvaccinal reactions than the CAV-1 MLV, and therefore is preferred for immunization against diseases caused by CAV-1 or CAV-2. These viruses are closely related antigenically and provide cross-protection. Single doses of such combination vaccines are administered subcut. or IM at weaning and thereafter as for canine distemper.

Leptospirosis: Leptospirosis is occasionally seen in exotic Canidae, Procyonidae, Ursidae, Mustelidae, Suidae, Tayassuidae, and in Cervidae and other ruminants of the families Bovidae, Camelidae, Giraffidae, etc. Bacterins that contain immunogens against *interrogans, canicola,* and *icterohaemorrhagiae* serovars are used in the carnivores listed above. Ruminants, pigs, and peccaries are immunized with bacterins that contain *pomona, hardjo, icterohaemorrhagiae, canicola,* and *grippotyphosa* serovars. Carnivores are vaccinated with a 1 or 2 mL dose, IM or subcut, at 6-8 wk of age and repeated in 14 days. Boosters are given q6mo. Hoofed animals are immunized with 5 mL of pentavalent bacterin IM. Annual or, preferably, semiannual boosters are recommended.

Vaccination does not necessarily prevent shedding of the causal organism(s).

Measles, Mumps, Rubella: Pongidae are immunized against measles, mumps, and rubella at 2-3 mo of age with 0.5 mL of MLV human vaccine injected subcut. This vaccination is also recommended for monkeys. Annual booster doses are given.

Parainfluenza 3: Wild sheep and goats are susceptible to pneumonia similar to shipping fever pneumonia of domestic sheep. Parainfluenza 3 (PI-3) is recognized as an important primary component, along with stress and *Pasteurella haemolytica*. Modified live virus PI-3 vaccines, particularly those intended for intranasal administration, have been useful in reducing lamb pneumonia. Vaccine is administered at 3-4 mo of age, 1 mL in each nostril, and repeated 3-4 wk before anticipated shipment, and annually.

Poliomyelitis: Primates, particularly the Pongidae (great apes) are susceptible to poliomyelitis. Oral trivalent MLV poliomyelitis vaccine is preferred over parenteral inactivated vaccine because of ease of administration. A single human dose (0.5

mL) is given PO on a sugar cube after 6 mo of age, and annually thereafter. Vaccinated animals should not have contact with unvaccinated people or nonhuman primates for 1 mo after inoculation.

Rabies: All wild mammals are susceptible. In areas where the incidence of rabies in free-living wildlife is high, mammals in zoos or kept as pets may be at high risk of exposure. In such cases, vaccination is recommended. However, this recommendation is contrary to the stated position of the National Association of State Public Health Veterinarians (NASPHV) regarding wildlife vaccination: "Vaccination of wildlife is not recommended because no rabies vaccine is licensed for use in wild animals. Neither wild nor exotic animals susceptible to rabies should be kept as pets. Offspring of wild animals bred with domestic dogs or cats are considered wild animals." (Compendium of Animal Rabies Control, JAVMA 196:1, 1990). When vaccination is considered necessary, only killed virus vaccine should be used. Several inactivated vaccines prepared of nervous tissue (eg, murine, ovine, or caprine) or tissue-culture have been found satisfactory in terms of safety and immunogenicity, the latter based on limited tests that demonstrated adequate antibody responses in some exotic carnivores. These vaccines should be administered by deep IM injection. Young animals are vaccinated at 3-4 mo of age, and vaccinations must be repeated annually. MLV rabies vaccines licensed for domestic animals should **never** be used in exotic animals since they are often insufficiently attenuated and may produce clinical rabies and death. Evaluation of vaccines intended to control rabies in wildlife continues in several countries.

Wild-caught animals, especially foxes, raccoons, and skunks, even when very young, may have been exposed to rabies and may be in the incubative phase. Since the incubation period can be quite prolonged (up to 1 yr), a short observation period for such animals is inadequate. The NASPHV recommends that wild-caught animals that will have public contact in zoos should be quarantined for ≥180 days.

Because of the potential danger of rabies, keeping wild animals as pets, especially wild-caught carnivores, should be discouraged and is, indeed, illegal in many jurisdictions. There are, of course, many other reasons for discouraging the use of wild animals as pets.

Tetanus: Exotic Equidae, Proboscidea (elephants), Pongidae, Cervidae (deer), and wild sheep and goats should be immunized against tetanus. Exotic Equidae and elephants are immunized on the same schedule as domestic horses: primary immunization at 3-4 mo of age consists of 2 IM injections of tetanus toxoid, 1 mo apart. A single booster dose is given annually.

Pongidae are immunized against tetanus using the diphtheria, tetanus toxoid, and phase 1 pertussis (DPT) vaccines intended for use in human children. Primary immunization should begin at 2-3 mo of age and consist of 0.5 mL vaccine injected IM on 3 occasions at 4- to 6-wk intervals with a reinforcing dose 1 yr after the third injection. Thereafter, booster immunizations of 0.5 mL of diphtheria-tetanus toxoid are given q10yr.

Wild sheep and goats and cervids are usually immunized with multivalent clostridial bacterin-toxoids containing immunogens for *Clostridium tetani, C perfringens* (types B, C, D), *C septicum, C chauvoei, C novyi, C sordellii,* and *C haemolyticum* beginning at 10-12 wk of age. The initial dose is 5 mL followed in 6 wk by a 2-mL dose, administered subcut. A 2-mL booster dose should be given annually.

Miscellaneous: A number of infectious diseases, eg, bovine viral diarrhea (BVD), bluetongue, malignant catarrhal fever (MCF), and epizootic hemorrhagic disease (EHD) of deer, may appear as serious local problems but are not widespread in zoos.

Inactivated BVD vaccines are recommended in situations in which BVD has been a problem. Annual vaccination with one standard bovine dose IM should begin at 3 mo of age.

Satisfactory vaccines for bluetongue, EHD, and MCF are not currently available but are needed for exotic ruminants in many regions of the USA.

For ease of reference, vaccination recommendations (excepting rabies [*see* above]) for exotic mammals are summarized in TABLE 9, by taxonomic categories.

Table 9. Vaccinations Recommended for Exotic Mammals

Animal Group	Disease/Product	Vaccine Type (K*/MLV**)	Vaccination Frequency
Primates (especially Pongidae) monkey, ape	Poliomyelitis	MLV	A[1]
	Measles	MLV	A
	Mumps	MLV	A
	Rubella	MLV	A
	DPT or Tetanus	K	A
Canidae fox, wolf, coyote, wild dog	Canine distemper	MLV[2]	A
	Canine adenovirus-2	MLV	A
	Canine parvovirus	K	A
	Canine parainfluenza	MLV	A
	Leptospira bacterin-CI[3]	K	A
Felidae exotic cats	Feline panleukopenia	K/MLV	A
	Feline rhinotracheitis	K/MLV	A
	Feline caliciviruses	K/MLV	A
Mustelidae/Viverridae/ Procyonidae raccoon, skunk, ferret, coati, genet, otter, weasel, mink, kinkajou	Canine distemper	K/MLV[2]	A
	Feline panleukopenia	K/MLV	A
	Canine adenovirus-2	K/MLV	A
	Leptospira bacterin-CI	K	A
Ursidae bear	Canine adenovirus-2	K	A
	Leptospira bacterin-CI	K	A
Hyaenidae hyena, aardwolf	Canine distemper[4]	K/MLV	A
	Feline panleukopenia[4]	K/MLV	A
Artiodactyla/Ruminantia deer, sheep, cattle, goat, antelope	BVD (in endemic areas)	K	A
	8-way *Clostridium* bacterin	K	A
	5-way *Leptospira* bacterin	K	A or q6mo
	Parainfluenza-3	MLV	A
Perissodactyla Equidae—ass, zebra	Tetanus	K	A
	EEE	K	A
	WEE	K	A
	Equine rhinopneumonitis	K	q4mo
Suidae/Tayassuidae pigs, peccaries	5-way *Leptospira* bacterin	K	A
	Erysipelas bacterin	K	A

*Killed.
**Modified live virus.
[1] Annual.
[2] Not ferret origin; avian origin preferred.
[3] *canicola/icterohaemorrhagiae.*
[4] Controversial—some believe hyaenids are not susceptible.

PART V
MANAGEMENT, HUSBANDRY, AND NUTRITION

MHN

MANAGEMENT, HUSBANDRY, AND NUTRITION, INTRODUCTION

Although it is commonly accepted that viruses, bacteria, and other microorganisms are the basic causes of disease in domestic animals, errors in management, husbandry, and nutrition are significant predisposing factors. Many disease outbreaks could be minimized or totally prevented with proper management, husbandry, and nutrition.

Even though most who are in animal husbandry are aware of the importance of these factors, they constantly seek a cure-all for disease problems. For a time, many believed that antibiotics were the answer. Antibiotics were added to rations beginning shortly after birth, and sometimes continued throughout the animal's life. Initially, they were quite effective. However, even though larger amounts have been added to rations, higher dosages have been administered parenterally, and newer and more effective antibiotics have been developed (both to cover a broader spectrum and to cope with developing bacterial resistance), they have not provided the complete solution. Diseases in farm animals still cause annual losses of billions of dollars, a large portion of which is attributable to deaths, treatment costs, and reduced feed efficiency and growth rate.

Not only do antibiotics have limits to their efficacy, there is also widespread concern about drug residues in food of animal origin and development of super-resistant bacteria capable of affecting man as well as livestock. Laws have been proposed that would eliminate low-level feeding of antibiotics and prohibit the therapeutic use of some antibiotics in animals. Use of some antibiotics has already been prohibited and further prohibition is virtually certain. In the future, livestock producers will be forced to rely even more heavily on good management.

Management has long been emphasized as a means of lowering labor costs and of increasing feed efficiency and rate of gain, but these are not its only roles. Intensive production methods have made good management more important than ever. When many animals, whatever species, are confined in a small area, both direct and indirect contact is increased. This bears a direct relationship to disease incidence; each animal introduced into a group potentially can introduce disease to every other animal in the group. As the size of the group increases, the individual attention that each animal receives tends to decrease—and disease is more likely to become well established before it is recognized and treated. As a result, treatment is less likely to be effective. Managing a large group of animals is much more demanding than managing a small one.

Additionally, as production methods in farm animals are intensified, the period from birth to marketing or reproduction is shortened; efficiency of conversion of feed to meat, milk, or wool is increased; and stresses are introduced that increase the potential for disease.

Although the specific enterprise must be considered when making management recommendations, some general recommendations apply to all situations: 1) Provide adequate space. 2) Provide adequate ventilation (qv, p 1106). 3) Prevent undue exposure to extreme temperature changes. 4) Practice good sanitary procedures at all times. Remove feces as often as practicable. 5) Follow an "all-in/all-out" concept when feasible. 6) Thoroughly clean and disinfect the premises during the interval between removal of one group and introduction of the next group. 7) Provide adequate potable water at all times. 8) Provide adequate total nutrients, including vitamins and minerals. 9) Prevent fecal contamination of feed and water. 10) Make certain that newborn animals nurse shortly after birth and receive adequate colostrum. 11) Do not feed damaged or spoiled feed. If such feed must be fed, mix it with good-quality feed. 12) Separate age groups as much as is practical. 13) Do not mix species. 14) Wait to breed females until they are of proper size. 15) Provide assistance at parturition if needed. 16) Immunize young animals against diseases that are endemic in the area. 17) Control internal and external parasites. 18) Keep animals under close surveillance to identify early signs of disease. 19) Begin treatment of diseased animals as soon as possible. 20) Provide adequate nursing care for diseased animals. 21) Isolate diseased animals.

Management also becomes extremely important in preventing disease when new animals are added, or when animals removed from the group are permitted to contact animals from other premises and then are returned to the original premises. Isolation of such animals for ≥ 2 wk after arrival or return provides an essential period to observe for signs of disease. If disease appears, isolation is continued until the disease has run its course. Although newly arrived animals can introduce numerous diseases, respiratory disease and neonatal diarrhea are among those most costly and feared. The following classes represent the greatest risk of introducing disease into an established group: neonates, weanlings, naturally bred females that fail to conceive and are rebred, males that have served females with unknown reproductive disease status, females that have aborted, and animals with a history of undiagnosed diarrhea. The best safeguards against introduction of disease, in addition to isolation, are careful inspection of the remaining animals at the site of origin, a reputable seller, and (if obtainable) an official certificate of inspection signed by a licensed veterinarian and the seller and approved by state and/or federal animal health officials (*see also* p 960).

Management is always important in disease prevention but is especially so at birth when both dam and fetus are at increased risk (*see* THE NEONATE, below).

Faulty nutrition causes many disease problems; lack of nutrients is one of the major reasons why many animals do not realize their potential and are prone to disease. Despite the known influence of nutrition, numerous animals are fed rations deficient in both quantity and quality. Overfeeding also can be a problem when animals are being fed for extremely high production or condition. Adequate amounts of roughage must be included in a ruminant's ration to prevent severe GI disturbances and secondary disease such as laminitis. Many foot problems are the end result of indigestion and acidosis caused by overfeeding of concentrates and limited roughage.

Rations should contain all of the essential vitamins and minerals and a balance of protein, carbohydrates, and fats. Age, gestation, lactation, and physical activity of an animal must be considered when formulating a ration and determining the amount to be fed. Care should be taken that toxic plants or chemicals are not included. Toxic materials not only affect the health of the animal ingesting the material but may produce anomalies in the fetus.

THE NEONATE

Proper care of the neonate is essential if an enterprise is to grow and prosper. Whenever practical, the dam should be isolated at parturition in quarters that are spacious, well lighted, clean, and disinfected. An attendant should be on hand, particularly in the case of primiparous animals, but should be aware that birth is a physiological process that usually occurs without outside intervention. Many reproductive tracts have been permanently injured, and neonates injured or killed by an over-anxious attendant. A reasonable period of labor must be permitted to prepare and dilate the cervix, vagina, and vulva for passage of the fetus. For more involved cases, the attendant should secure professional help. Cesarean sections save many fetuses that would not survive delivery through the birth canal, particularly in fat or immature dams.

After delivery, the neonate's respiratory tract should be cleared immediately. A portion of the placenta may be covering the nostrils, or enough fluid may have been inhaled to block air passages. Artificial respiration and, in large animals, elevation of the neonate's rear parts often assist in initiating respirations; small animals can be held head down and, while carefully supported, be swung through a small arc to promote drainage of the respiratory tract. Brisk rubbing with a towel stimulates respiration. Prompt insertion of a tube into the trachea and applications of suction save some animals that would otherwise die.

If birth was normal and the umbilical cord was not ruptured in the process, the cord should be left intact for ~5 min; contraction of the uterus forces placental blood into the neonate, thus increasing its chances of survival. After the cord is broken, tincture of iodine should be applied to the stump; in areas where screwworms are a problem, repellent should be applied. Some dams, especially primiparous ones, may be apprehensive and injure their offspring by butting, striking, kicking, or biting.

The neonate should be examined for abnormalities soon after birth. Early recognition and euthanasia of a hopelessly deformed neonate will save an owner the expense of prolonged care and treatment. Although many birth defects are heritable, it is often extremely difficult to differentiate between those that are and those that are not. Surgical correction of some abnormalities is possible but usually not desirable when the breed's future is considered. (*See also* the tables of contents of the sections in PART I for discussions of specific congenital and inherited diseases.)

Animals should receive colostrum as soon after birth as possible, preferably within the first hour. They should be observed closely to make certain that they nurse; assistance may be required. If the neonate is too weak to nurse, colostrum should be fed via stomach tube. When the dam does not provide colostrum, it should be secured from another animal or from a previously frozen supply.

Ingestion of colostrum that contains adequate amounts of IgG, IgM, and IgA is essential if a neonate is to survive in a hostile environment. These immunoglobulins protect the neonate against systemic and GI diseases when absorbed through the gut wall and when occupying the gut lumen. The amount of colostrum ingested, the concentration of immunoglobulins in the colostrum, and the absorptive capability of the gut wall determine its effectiveness in disease prevention and control.

Vaccines against endemic neonatal intestinal diseases should be administered to the gravid dam or to the young at birth. If commercial products are ineffective, consideration should be given to producing autogenous bacterins that may be more effective. Additional immunization procedures should be applied as the disease problems of the premises and the area dictate. If newborn animals become sick, diagnosis and treatment must be prompt, since they have little reserve and die quickly. Although proper nursing care often determines whether a sick animal will live or die, it is often neglected.

GI diseases are the most frequently identified disease problems in neonates. Diarrhea can be a problem during any time of the year but appears to take a greater toll during cold winter months when low temperatures can be an added stress.

Although most newborn livestock can withstand very cold temperatures once they are dried (piglets are an exception—*see* NEONATAL HYPOGLYCEMIA, below), their extremities may freeze if they are born into a cold environment. In climates where winter temperatures drop to low levels, protection should be provided. If economic conditions make this unfeasible, animals should be bred to give birth later in the winter or early spring when temperatures are higher.

Every effort should be made to maintain body heat during inclement weather. For large animals, it usually is not practical or advisable to heat a large barn to maintain the temperature during extremely cold environmental temperatures. In such cases, it is advisable to partition small areas that can be more economically heated for severely stressed animals. If used, artificial heat should be regulated to meet the needs of the species of animals being managed. Piglets require a much warmer environment than calves or foals. A heat lamp placed out of the animal's reach probably is the most effective method of maintaining body heat in sick animals or in neonates.

(*See also* DISEASE-MANAGEMENT INTERACTION and MANAGEMENT OF REPRODUCTION for each of the common species.)

NEONATAL HYPOGLYCEMIA

Although also known to occur in calves and lambs, this is best documented in piglets <1 wk old. A final pathway to death in many diseases, it accounts for 15-35% of total piglet mortality. The discussion below centers on piglets.

Etiology: With only partial gluconeogenic ability, limited energy reserves, and essentially no brown fat, newborn piglets rely on glycogen reserves and, most importantly, frequent nursing. Predisposition to piglet hypoglycemia occurs with any disease of the sow that decreases or inhibits milk production or letdown. Large litter size with an inadequate number of teats precludes proper nursing; improper placement of the farrowing crate's lower rail, which impairs access to the udder, can lead to inadequate milk intake and hypoglycemia.

Critical temperature for newborn piglets is ~95°F (35°C). Piglets have an effective metabolic response to cold and fully functional peripheral vasoconstriction, but their lack of insulating subcut. fat (until 1-2 wk old) allows marked heat loss. In drafty or wet environments, on cold floors, or in low ambient temperatures, maintenance of body temperature demands rapid glucose utilization, which depletes glycogen reserves; if milk intake is impaired, hypoglycemia and death result.

Clinical Findings: One or more piglets in a litter may be involved. Initially, behavior changes from vigorous sucking or play alternating with sleep, to solitary lassitude. Affected pigs wander aimlessly with faltering gait, cry weakly, and are gaunt with pale, cold, clammy skin; they are hypothermic, have poor muscle tone, and are unresponsive to external stimuli. As incoordination increases, piglets may stand with legs splayed, and sternal or lateral recumbency follows. Terminally, they exhibit convulsions with jaw champing, salivation, opisthotonos, nystagmus, forelimb and hindlimb contraction, coma, and death. Many affected piglets are crushed by the sow.

Blood glucose levels fall from a normal of 90-130 mg/dL to as low as 5-15 mg/dL; affected piglets usually manifest clinical signs when levels are <50 mg/dL.

Diagnosis: Any condition that impairs food intake by neonatal pigs is a potential diagnostic problem. Generally, however, hypoglycemia can be diagnosed by examination of the sow and environment for predisposing factors, and by the piglet's response to glucose therapy.

Treatment and Prophylaxis: Treatment is 15 mL of 5% glucose given IP. Treated pigs should be placed under a heat lamp or in an equivalently warm environment. Response follows within 5-10 min with shivering and more activity. Severely hypoglycemic and hypothermic piglets may not respond. Sustained energy intake must be provided to avoid relapse.

If oxytocin fails to promote milk letdown in the sow, 20 mL of 5% dextrose, cow's colostrum, or evaporated milk diluted one-half with water can be administered intragastrically to each piglet through a small plastic cannula (with care to avoid damage to the pharyngeal diverticulae), or IP glucose can be repeated q4-6hr. Active piglets learn quickly to drink from a dish. Foster-suckling of piglets is possible in batch farrowing units; most sows accept piglets introduced quietly during the milk letdown period. Distribution of uneven-sized litters may reduce mortality from starvation and hypoglycemia. Any primary disease of the sow should be treated effectively and any faults within the environment corrected. Piglets should be held in a draft-free creep area heated to 95°F (35°C) during the first week of life. Cold-stressed and marginally hypoglycemic piglets are more susceptible to intestinal and other neonatal diseases.

APPETITE AND CONTROL OF FOOD INTAKE

Physiological control of appetite and food intake are mediated through the CNS, which plays a primary role in feeding behavior and regulation of energy balance.

Specific sites in the hypothalamus have critical effects. Destruction of the ventromedial hypothalamus results in overeating and eventual obesity. Lesions in the lateral hypothalamus generally result in complete anorexia for up to 2 wk. Stimuli at either of these levels may override stimuli from other levels. Thus, while destruction of the ventromedial hypothalamus results in overeating, stimulation of this same area causes cessation of feeding.

In addition to control by CNS centers, appetite and feeding behavior can be altered by many internal and external influences. Certain internal factors may result in feedback mechanisms that control appetite and intake.

Signals from the mouth and upper GI tract can alter feeding response. Taste of food can affect length of the feeding period, with bitter food generally reducing total intake time. Most species prefer sweet tastes. Gastric distention has a strong influence on feeding behavior. Generally, gastric loading and distention, even with non-nutritive substances, result in significantly less consumption. However, increased osmolarity in the duodenum also influences satiety, and animals respond to hypertonic solutions introduced into the duodenum by rapid reduction in food intake. Plasma glucose level is an important controlling factor; it is monitored and mediated by receptors in the ventromedial and lateral hypothalamus as well as the liver and possibly the duodenum. Certain monoamines such as noradrenaline, dopamine, and serotonin may influence feeding behavior and satiety. While the interrelationships and absolute effects of these monoamines are not fully understood, stress, nutrition, or disease can influence their output and probably influence feeding behavior and appetite. Sex hormones are influential in determining the amount of food eaten by animals, as are pancreatic and pituitary hormones. The role of opiate peptides is still unclear. No single feedback mechanism alone is responsible for complete induction of satiety or control of appetite; in normal animals, several are interrelated to maintain a homeostatic balance between hunger and food intake.

Factors related to food or feed itself may alter feeding response and appetite. **Palatability** is a general term that considers taste, aroma, nutritional value, and physical form of food. In some cases, specific hungers for nutrients such as proteins, amino acids, or salt may influence apparent palatability. However, nutritional quality alone is not sufficient to ensure that these feeds will be consumed. In fact, a pleasant tasting but deficient food may be consumed in preference to a nutritionally balanced one; this may continue until death occurs from nutritional deficiency. Conversely, dietary factors expected to reduce food intake include: 1) increased digestible energy and caloric density, 2) markedly reduced feed concentration of protein or essential amino acids, 3) increased dietary salt (NaCl), and 4) mineral imbalances, especially deficiencies of calcium and magnesium in ruminants. Thus, it is doubtful that animals can adequately balance their own diet by free-choice selection. Palatability may be affected by temperature of food and decreases as temperature of the food falls. Physical form may also alter palatability. Pelleted feeds are sometimes preferred to meals, while ruminants may consume more hay in long-stemmed than in pelleted form. Intake of some feeds is increased when particle size is reduced. Digestibility of food is not strongly associated with taste preference.

External influences, including management practices, photoperiod, weather variations, ambient temperature, monotony, and frequency of feeding may alter food intake. Photoperiod and diurnal rhythms may alter feeding behavior. Pigs consume more feed in daylight than dark. This is generally true for cattle, except during hot weather when eating increases during darkness. In poultry, a longer photoperiod increases food intake and thus growth; in cattle, longer photoperiods stimulate growth, which is followed by increased intake. Reduced ambient temperature almost invariably causes large increases in food consumption, while elevated ambient temperature causes a reduction. Adverse weather conditions such as storms may cause severe short-term restriction in food intake. Restricted water consumption strongly influences feeding behavior, with food intake reduced in direct proportion to limited water intake. Monotony induced by continued offering of very similar feeds has been suggested to affect palatability and intake. For monogastrics, high-quality proteins and commercial flavor enhancers appear to positively influence total food intake and acceptance, although few flavors have been tested systematically. In most species, socialization and group feeding may increase food intake, while for certain animals (eg, cats) competition in group feeding may have a negative effect on food intake. Estrus may cause depressed food intake, while pregnancy increases nutrient needs and voluntary food consumption. Food intake is generally low on the day of parturition.

Anorexia may be caused by pain, fever, stress, learned aversion to available food, metabolic disorders, and other unknown causes. Food refusal or reduced food intake is a special problem that may confront owners of food-producing livestock, performance animals, or pets. In the absence of illness or obvious environmental influences, food refusal may be affected by palatability or by taste aversion. Palatability is a direct sensory response. Taste aversion, which is delayed at least by several hours or more, and depends on offering an offensive food ≥ 2 times, is both a sensory and a learning response. It is sensory since taste is involved in recognizing an offending agent in the food, and it is a learning process since the animal associates a particular taste or ingestion of food with an unpleasant event such as nausea, vomiting, pain, or other environmental stress. Thus, any circumstances that associate food consumption with unpleasant experiences may induce taste aversion. In pigs, the mycotoxin deoxynivalenol, and in dogs, the inorganic arsenic compounds may cause taste aversion. As a learned response it has some residual effects, and several feedings may be required before an animal learns to fully accept a food formerly associated with an unpleasant event. Careful observation and test feeding of foods that are refused may be necessary to properly judge whether palatability or aversion are factors in food refusal.

In ruminants, factors that alter ruminal production of volatile fatty acids can affect feed intake. For example, the ionophore drugs monensin and lasalocid alter propionic acid balance and slightly reduce voluntary feed consumption.

Stimulation by frequent presentation of small amounts of palatable feeds and reduction of pain, fever, or stress often override the negative feedback generated by the disease process. Chemical stimulation by benzodiazepine derivatives (at extremely low doses) or anabolic steroids may be of benefit in cats.

Obesity (qv, p 450) usually results from disruption of the normal feeding pattern by presentation of various palatable foods (eg, table scraps), inactivity, learned preferences for high-caloric foods, or metabolic dysfunction. The only way to treat obesity caused by feeding pattern and diet is to reduce caloric intake and/or increase exercise. Low-calorie "reducing" diets for dogs are commercially available.

Engorgement occurs when animals gain sudden access to a highly palatable feed and eat until pathological distention or fermentation, or both, begin to occur. The only way to prevent feed engorgement in domestic animals is to prevent access to large amounts of palatable feed. If a large amount of palatable feed is to be made available (pasture or feedlot), feeding the animal 1 hr before access may reduce subsequent intake and the chance of engorgement. Gradual introduction of the free-choice situation is also effective, eg, with the cow or horse allowed free access to a lush pasture for only 30 min on the first day and for gradually increasing periods on subsequent days.

The performance animal often has tremendous food expenditures and must consume great amounts of food to maintain a certain body weight. The diet may be "bulk-limiting" in this situation, and horses, dogs, or lactating dairy cows may be physically incapable of consuming amounts adequate for their needs. High-caloric "stress" diets for dogs are commercially available. The addition of fat to racehorse diets may positively influence performance.

BREEDING SOUNDNESS EXAMINATION OF THE MALE

Many examination techniques are applicable for particular animals and economic circumstances. These include the history, physical examination (including the reproductive organs), evaluation of serving behavior, semen examination in the field and in the laboratory, tests for infectious and inherited diseases, and cytogenetic and endocrine examinations. Results permit an evaluation of breeding soundness; however, fertility is a continuous variable.

When normal structure and function with respect to reproductive efficiency are found, the conclusion is warranted that the animal is sound for breeding, and fertility should be normal. If an abnormality is diagnosed, its severity and relationship to fertility are assessed. A prognosis is given, often based on serial examinations.

Male fertility is estimated by services per pregnancy, non-return rates, diagnosable pregnancy rates, and progeny born. However, since females can influence these figures, they are imperfect estimates. A bull that gets 95% of 50 cows pregnant over 9 wk, most of them in the first 3 wk, can be called highly fertile; figures below this reflect degrees of reduced fertility.

Interpretation of examination results requires consideration of the many factors that may influence reproductive function. Genetic factors are important; eg, in bulls, testicular size and therefore sperm production, as well as serving capacity, are highly heritable. Results of the examinations can be influenced by environmental factors such as high temperature (all species), photoperiod (rams, goats, and horses), and scrotal frostbite (bulls). Recent mating activity, sexual rest, nutritional plane, stress, and concurrent disease are other factors that need to be considered. The results may also be influenced by the techniques used, particularly semen characteristics, which may be influenced by method of collection. If the quality of the first sample is poor, additional samples are needed to determine if the first sample truly reflects the animal's reproductive capacity; it is important to collect a representative sample of semen.

For all species, the fertilizing capacity of semen appears to depend primarily on the morphology, number, motility, and viability of the spermatozoa, and secondarily on the volume and physical and biochemical properties of the seminal plasma. For any species, average standards for normal semen under stated conditions such as age of donor, frequency of service, time in relation to breeding season, and methods of collection and examination can be defined. Obvious deviations from these standards can be recognized and may be associated with reduced fertility. However, as the range between normal and abnormal semen characteristics narrows, the difficulty of accurately assessing fertility increases and, for any individual animal, the semen findings must be interpreted with caution and in light of the results of other examinations. Similarly, the interpretation of serving behavior is based on the prevailing conditions at the time of the examination.

The examiner's report should include the reason for the examination, techniques used (materials and methods), results, diagnosis, relationship of the diagnosis to fertility, prognosis or the possible basis for a prognosis, and advice on management of the case.

The scope of evaluation varies considerably. Packages of examination techniques are constructed for particular purposes and particular clients; however, they should be cost effective. Members of a bull team in a beef herd may be subjected to a general clinical examination that concentrates on structural soundness, palpation of the scrotal contents and measurement of the scrotal circumference, examination of the internal genitalia, inspection of the penis and prepuce, and a serving capacity test. An individual bull examined for sale is likely to be subjected to a full range of serological tests and a detailed semen examination.

Since more is known about breeding soundness examination of bulls than for males of other species, examination of the bull will be described specifically. Equivalent standards for other species have not been established as definitively. (For related discussions, see the chapters on MANAGEMENT OF REPRODUCTION of the various species, below, and the REPRODUCTIVE SYSTEM, p 638 et seq.)

The following recommendations and procedures are useful for evaluating the bull to be used for natural service.

THE PHYSICAL EXAMINATION

At least part of the physical examination should be performed before the semen sample is collected. In this way, bulls with undesirable physical characteristics or abnormalities can be identified and eliminated before useless attempts at collection are made. Proper handling and examination of the bull avoids excitement and facilitates collection. If an artificial vagina is used, semen collection is usually attempted before restraint and physical examination.

The bull should be observed free of restraint in the pasture or corral, noting general body condition (including nutritional status), condition of the coat, masculinity, and conformation. Particular attention is given to locomotion; the stride should be free with no signs of lameness. Abnormal conformation of the rear limbs is especially detrimental.

Following observation, the bull is confined to a suitable chute for the physical examination and collection of semen. The bull is identified and the information recorded. The head and mouth and feet and legs are examined. Any condition of the hooves or any defect that may produce lameness should be noted. The penis is palpated through the external sheath and protruded manually. Protrusion is easier if the glans is grasped with cotton gauze. A gloved hand inserted into the rectum makes protrusion of the penis much easier. Preputial samples may be taken for culture of *Campylobacter* or *Tritrichomonas* spp. The scrotum and its contents are palpated, and position and consistency noted. A normal testicle is firm and resilient; deviations vary from extremely fibrotic to flaccid. Conditions such as testicular degeneration or hypoplasia or orchitis affect the consistency and size of the testicles and result in abnormal semen characteristics.

Scrotal circumference is probably the best single indicator of a bull's ability to produce spermatozoa. The measurement is made by encircling the neck of the scrotum with the hand and using the fingers to push the testicles ventrally to eliminate wrinkles in the scrotal skin. The operator's thumb is placed on one lateral surface and the forefinger on the other (placement on the cranial or caudal surface of the scrotum forces the testicles laterally, resulting in errors in measurement). The Colorado metal tape is passed over the scrotum and tightened snugly at the point of greatest circumference, which is recorded in centimeters. When properly performed, this measurement is highly repeatable. Yearling bulls should have a circumference ≥30 cm; however, those of *Bos indicus* breeding tend to mature at an older age and their scrotal circumference (as yearlings) may be smaller.

Table 1. Scrotal Circumference Evaluation of Bulls
(*Bos taurus* and Crossbred Bulls)

Age (mo)	Scrotal Circumference* (cm) and Classification		
	Very Good	Good	Poor
12-14	>34	30-34	<30
15-20	>36	31-36	<31
21-30	>38	32-38	<32
>31	>39	34-39	<34

* Average scrotal circumference may vary considerably according to breed; for one example, *see* below.

Scrotal Circumference Measurements
(Holstein Bulls)

Age (mo)	Scrotal Circumference Means (cm)
7-12	28.4
13-18	34.9
19-24	37.1
25-30	38.7
31-36	39.3
37-42	40.6
43-48	41.2
49-54	41.2
55-60	42.0
61-72	42.8
73-84	42.2
85-96	42.0
97-168	42.9

The positive relationship between scrotal circumference and testicular size and sperm production has been demonstrated in dairy and beef bulls. In addition, bulls with small testicles tend to produce a higher percentage of abnormal spermatozoa. Degeneration of the testicles, eg, if it is mild and affects spermatocytes and spermatids only, may result in reduced fertility for 10-14 days (epididymal passage time) after the degenerating influence. Recovery may then occur as the spermatogenic epithelium regenerates over the next 5-6 wk. If spermatogonia are damaged, regeneration takes ≥2 mo before normal fertility is restored.

If an artificial vagina (AV) is used, **examination per rectum** of the internal genitalia and associated tissues in the bull should be done after semen is collected. If massage is used, the examination is done during semen collection. Abnormalities of the accessory sex organs are not uncommon and are often associated with poor semen quality.

COLLECTION OF SEMEN

In bulls, semen may be collected by use of an AV, an electroejaculator or, less preferably, massage of the accessory sex glands. The AV is used universally in artificial insemination centers. Bulls are induced to mount a teaser animal, and the erect penis is directed into the AV by the collector. With experience, bulls soon become accustomed to this procedure; inexperienced bulls may respond more slowly, but reluctance to mount can often be overcome by having them watch other cows or bulls mount. Teasing of bulls in these ways also increases the number of spermatozoa per ejaculate.

In preparing the AV for use, nonspermicidal lubricant is used, and the temperature, which is a critical factor in stimulating ejaculation, is maintained between 105 and 107°F (40.5 and 42°C). Temperatures up to 118°F (48°C) may assist collections in untrained bulls. On each collection day, up to 3 services may be permitted, yielding ~10-20 mL (total) of semen. For maintenance of normal semen quality, collections from dairy bulls can be made ~6 times/wk, usually 2 ejaculates of semen daily 3 days/wk. Data from beef bulls are lacking. "Normal fertility" is probably maintained well after sperm concentration begins to fall.

Electrical stimulation of ejaculation is a valuable means for collecting semen from bulls that are unable to mount. It is commonly used for collecting samples for diagnostic purposes from larger numbers of yearling beef bulls. The rectal probe has a series of banded electrodes and is connected to a variable current and voltage source. The bull to be ejaculated should be restrained in a chute because the stimulation results in vigorous contraction of various muscle groups, particularly those of the back. The rectum is emptied, and the entire probe is inserted with the electrodes placed ventrally. A hand-operated rheostat permits intermittent pulses of current to be given as the voltage is gradually increased. The response varies considerably, but it is common to use 2- to 4-sec pulses repeated at 5- to 7-sec intervals. After a variable number of such stimulations, erection and protrusion of the penis occur, followed by a flow of seminal fluid, the latter part of which is rich in spermatozoa. The semen may be collected by any convenient method; some operators use a modified AV and others an insulated bottle. In some bulls, ejaculation occurs only after a final series of momentary pulses at 1- to 2-sec intervals. Older bulls usually require a higher voltage for semen emission. A few bulls ejaculate within the prepuce. Semen collected by electrical stimulation appears to be as fertile as that collected with an AV.

An alternative method is used in South America: the electrodes of the electroejaculator terminate in finger rings rather than in a solid rectal probe. A ring is placed on each of the first and third fingers of the gloved hand, the hand is inserted in the rectum, and the techniques of electroejaculation and massage are combined.

Erection seldom occurs during collection by massage of the accessory sex glands. If semen is to be used for artificial insemination, the sheath should be cleaned by douching with 500 mL of sterile saline solution containing 1 million u of penicillin and 1 g of streptomycin. After completely emptying the rectum, the vesicular glands are massaged with a backward motion until a few mL of fluid drop from the sheath. The ampullae are then massaged, and an assistant collects the semen with a glass funnel and vial. This method is not always successful, and the quality of the semen is usually lower than that collected by the other 2 procedures. Frequently, samples for diagnostic purposes may be obtained, but it depends on the individual bull and skill of the operator.

The volume of ejaculate is 4-8 mL, and the concentration 1-1.5 billion sperm/mL.

EVALUATION OF THE SEMEN SAMPLE

Evaluation of the quality of the semen sample should begin as soon as possible after collection. A suitable laboratory should be prepared before obtaining the sample; it may be improvised, but should be clean and provide environmental control to ensure that ambient temperature does not adversely affect the semen. All surfaces with which the semen has contact must be warm (102°F [39°C]) and free of water or chemicals that may be toxic to spermatozoa. Required laboratory equipment includes: 1) microscope capable of 100X, 400X, and 1000X magnification, 2) slide and microscope stage heater, 3) module heater or water bath to maintain the sample at 98°F (37°C) during evaluation, 4) sperm stain such as Hancock's or Blom's eosin-nigrosin stain, 5) fresh isotonic diluting solution such as physiologic saline or phosphate-buffered 2.9% sodium citrate, 6) cell counter, and 7) microscope slides and coverslips.

Numerous criteria have been employed to evaluate bovine semen; those below are useful for clinical evaluation of bulls for breeding soundness.

Wave motion (mass activity, swirl), a characteristic of semen observed by placing a drop on a warm glass slide and observing it under low power, is a function of the activity of the spermatozoa and their concentration. The intensity of wave motion may be divided into 4 categories: very good—intense swirling, rapid dark and light waves; good—slower swirling, waves not as intense; fair—slow movement with fewer waves; poor—very little or no swirl activity.

Very good wave motion is seen in samples of high concentration with a high proportion of spermatozoa moving actively forward. Spermatozoa characteristically move against a current. Eddies set up in the drop create synchronous movement of groups of cells and lead to dark and light bands and further eddies. Motility is the proportion of spermatozoa moving actively forward; it is estimated as a percentage under the 400X power of the microscope after placing a cover slip on a small drop of semen. Wave motion may be lowered because of a reduction in concentration or motility, or both. Dilution with warm, fresh isotonic saline solution may be necessary to observe individual movement. Abnormal spermatozoal movement, eg, circular or backwards, may be noted. Motility may be classified as: very good—80%, good—60-80%, fair—40-60%, poor—20-40%, or very poor—<20%.

The concentration or **density** of a semen sample may be estimated visually: 1) Very good—thick, creamy or white, opaque and viscid; samples may have a yellow tinge (flavins), which is normal for some bulls; concentration is 1-2 billion/mL. 2) Good—creamy white and opaque, but less viscid; 500 million to 1 billion/mL. 3) Fair—milky; more dilute, approaches translucency; pours freely; 250-400 million/mL. 4) Poor—watery, gray, pours freely; <250 million/mL.

In addition to the above criteria, several factors can influence semen quantity and quality. Concentration may be lowered as a result of reduced spermatogenic function, recent intensive use, or collection technique. Motility may be lowered through poor spermatogenic function, abnormal function of the duct system, the presence of foreign material (eg, WBC), recent sexual rest, poor collection technique, and environmental factors such as water in the sample or cold shock.

The presence of cells other than spermatozoa in the sample should be investigated while estimating motility. RBC, WBC, and excess numbers of round epithelial cells and developing forms of spermatozoa indicate genital tract abnormality. On initial examination of a sample, the origin of round cellular elements in the ejaculate cannot be determined accurately. WBC tend to be similar in size and are about the same diameter as the length of a sperm head. Examination of the stained semen helps, but still may not be conclusive. In most cases, a thorough physical examination will reveal the source of foreign cells in the ejaculate.

WBC are found in the semen when the vesicular glands are inflamed. Motility of the spermatozoa may range from good to poor, depending on the etiology of the inflammation. Inflammation in the epididymides or ampullae of the vas deferens has a much more serious effect on motility than does inflammation of the vesicular glands. To assess its effect on fertility, it is important to locate the affected site and determine the etiology. Until this is done and the inflammation resolved, caution must be exercised, although some bulls with WBC in the semen do have good fertility.

Of all the criteria, a careful analysis of spermatozoan **morphology** has the best correlation to fertility, and the highest repeatability. Increased spermatozoal abnormalities are associated with decreased pregnancy rates. Morphology reflects the functional condition of the testes, and to some degree, the excurrent duct system.

Abnormalities of the head, midpiece, and tail assist in identifying the site of dysfunction in the reproductive system and its severity. Normal bull semen contains some abnormal sperm cells and approximate limits are given below, together with an indication of the sites of formation of the defects.

Table 2. Bovine Sperm Abnormalities

Abnormality	Upper Limit of Normal Range (%)	Site of Formation
Abnormally shaped heads including acrosome defects, double formations, and extreme undeveloped forms	20	testicle
Structural abnormalities of midpiece	2	testicle
Tightly double bent and folded tails	4	testicle
Abaxial attachment of midpiece	2	testicle
Proximal protoplasmic droplets	4	testicle or epididymal head
Distal protoplasmic droplets	4	epididymis, testicle
Tailless heads	15	testicle, duct system
Singly bent	8	testicle, duct system, or after ejaculation
Coiled tails	3	testicle, duct system, or after ejaculation

A stained smear is prepared by mixing a small amount of semen (the amount depending on concentration of the sample) with a suitable stain (eg, Hancock's or Blom's eosin-nigrosin). A drop of stain is placed on a clean, warm, glass slide, and the corner of a second slide is dipped into a drop of semen. The stain and semen are mixed for 7-10 sec by gently rocking the second slide. The second slide is then used to spread the smear by slowly pulling it across the first slide at an angle of 30°. With practice, a slide can be prepared that is not excessively stained and in which the spermatozoa are spaced to allow accurate differentiation among normal cells and those with primary and secondary abnormalities. The stained slide is allowed to dry and examined under oil immersion (1000X). A minimum of 100 cells are evaluated from 4 or 5 randomly selected areas of the slide. If many abnormal cells are encountered, ≥200 cells should be evaluated.

EVALUATION OF SERVING BEHAVIOR

This evaluation can be done during natural service or during collection of semen with an AV. Libido, protrusion of the penis, seeking movements, intromission, ejaculatory thrust, and body position are assessed. Such an examination establishes a bull's serving ability, ie, that he is willing and able to serve normally. Reduced libido needs to be interpreted in light of the test conditions, eg, a stallion that had good serving behavior on one property may develop behavioral problems and reduced fertility in response to poor management on another property. Abnormalities of serving behavior include deviations of the penis, patent corpus cavernosum defects, inability to protrude due to adhesions, retained frenulum, and poor seeking and thrusting referable to abnormalities of the vertebrae, limbs, joints, or feet.

Under standardized conditions, a quantitative estimate of serving capacity may be made in a 40-min yard test with restrained estrous heifers. When properly done, the number of services in this test is highly correlated with the number of services obtained in a paddock mating situation.

TESTS FOR INFECTIOUS AND INHERITED DISEASES

An abnormal neonate may be the result of genetics, environmental factor(s), or both. It has been estimated that 0.2-3.5% of all calves born have defects, and >80 inherited diseases are known. Congenital defects of genetic origin reduce the value of the related animals; if an inherited disease is suspect, it is prudent to communicate with the breed association. Serological tests are available to aid in the detection of infectious diseases such as brucellosis, leptospirosis, and infectious pustular vulvovaginitis. Preputial scrapings or washes can be cultured for *Campylobacter* and *Tritrichomonas* spp. A semen sample obtained by massage, and collected aseptically through the relaxed penis is the method of choice for finding the cause of upper genital infections in bulls.

Chromosomal examination is useful in boars for revealing translocations associated with low litter size. This examination may also assist in reaching a diagnosis in infertile stallions when conventional examinations fail to reveal a cause.

Endocrine examinations are used to detect the presence of a retained testicle when stallion-like behavior occurs in horses that appear to be geldings. Estrogen assays or the testosterone response to human chorionic gonadotropin injection are most useful.

CYTOGENETIC AND ENDOCRINE EXAMINATIONS

Chromosome spreads prepared from short-term WBC cultures are used to evaluate karyotype in cattle. The technique is used mainly to screen bulls for the 1/29 translocation that is associated with increased embryonic death in some populations.

Endocrine examinations are rarely used in bulls. In experimental work, leutinizing hormone, follicle-stimulating hormone, and testosterone levels, and responses to gonadotropin-releasing hormone are being studied to evaluate the usefulness of this information.

CLASSIFICATION

Any system of classification must be based on: 1) properly recorded observations and measurements; 2) interpretation of these data in terms of normality or abnormality with emphasis on the reproductive system; 3) a decision about the site and severity of any dysfunction and the extent to which it will interfere with fertility now or in the future; 4) a consideration of the genetic implications of any abnormalities; and 5) formulation of a prognosis, or the basis on which a prognosis might be given (eg, additional examinations).

When practicality precludes performing part of the examination, conclusions must be suitably modified.

If no abnormalities are found that could interfere with reproductive efficiency, the bull is classified as a satisfactory potential breeder; if abnormalities are found, the bull is classified as an unsatisfactory potential breeder. When the classification is in doubt, further tests or examination may be necessary.

The principles of examination apply to all species. Some details with respect to each species are worth noting: The ram is similar to the bull except for the semen characteristics; rams produce less volume, but it is of higher concentration. Serving capacity tests in rams are available, but they have not been adapted for field use to the same extent as in bulls. In boars, testicle size is measured by the length and width of each testicle or total scrotal width. The semen is of relatively high volume and low concentration, and contains a copious gel fraction. It is collected by using the gloved hand to hold the penis firmly in a manner simulating the sow's cervix. Serving behavior is assessed during collection or natural service. In stallions, the greatest scrotal width with the 2 testicles held side by side produces a good estimate of testicular size. The semen is collected in a large AV, and serving behavior can be assessed at the same time. The semen is of high volume and low density and contains a gel fraction. The greatest scrotal width is also applicable to dogs as a record of testicular size. The presence of a bitch in heat facilitates semen collection. The semen is of low concentration relative to that of bulls and rams.

Culture of semen for microorganisms is used in most species when upper genital tract infection is present. The sample should be collected with as little contamination from the prepuce as possible.

EMBRYO TRANSFER IN FARM ANIMALS

In farm mammals, pre-attachment embryos can be removed from their dam (the donor) and transferred to other females (recipients) for development to term. Commercialization of embryo transfer has led to rapid technical advances and simplification of procedures so that transfers are now widely practiced on farms and to a lesser extent in large-scale embryo transfer units.

Proliferation of selected individuals remains the principal direct contribution of embryo transfer to animal production. Others are: identifying potential artificial insemination (AI) bulls through contract matings, disease control (eg, to introduce new bloodlines into SPF pig herds), importation and exportation of livestock, rapid screening of AI sires for genetically recessive characteristics such as syndactyly, and treatment or circumvention of some types of infertility. Other useful applications include genetic improvement programs such as multiple ovulation and embryo transfer (MOET) and juvenile MOET programs for genetic gain, and the use of MOET programs to genetically test new AI sires.

Embryo transfer also is a useful research tool to: 1) investigate the degrees to which the dam and fetus control characteristics such as gestation length, birth weight, fleece qualities, and immunoglobin absorption from colostrum; 2) elucidate the interrelationships between the embryo, uterus, and ovary, which are essential to establish and maintain pregnancy; and 3) manipulate embryos to produce specialized experimental animals such as twins, chimeras, and fetuses of known sex. Further, embryo transfer is an indispensable component of the new "biotechnology", which includes efforts to improve the results of *in vitro* fertilization and nuclear transfer in farm species, and to emulate the dramatic results obtained in laboratory mammals by injecting genetic material into uncleaved, newly fertilized oocytes.

Meticulous attention to detail, practice, and dexterity are required to achieve consistently good results with embryo transfer in cattle. Donors are induced to superovulate with gonadotropin treatments during the luteal phase (about day 9-14) of the cycle. Gonadotropin treatments may include a single IM injection of ~2500 IU of pregnant mare serum gonadotropin (PMSG, also called equine chorionic gonadotropin [eCG]), which may or may not be followed by an IV injection of an antibody to PMSG at the time of first insemination, or b.i.d. injections of a pituitary extract that contains high levels of follicle-stimulating hormone (FSH). Normally, a luteolytic dose of prostaglandin (PG) $F_{2\alpha}$ is administered 48-72 hr after initiation of gonadotropin treatment, and estrus should occur 36-48 hr later. Cows are normally inseminated twice with high-quality semen, 12 and 24 hr after onset of estrus. Cows that are cycling abnormally can be superovulated on an artificial luteal phase by utilizing a progestogen implant or progesterone-releasing intravaginal device. The implant or device is usually removed 12 hr after the $PGF_{2\alpha}$ injection. Sixty to 90% of cows have been reported to respond to superovulatory treatments; however, 20-30% of cows produce no transferable embryos. An average of 5-6 transferable embryos can be expected from each donor cow, but variability in response to superovulatory treatments is high. Induction of superovulation is particularly difficult in old or high-yielding, lactating dairy cows and may even lead to loss of milk. Some practitioners use repeated single embryo collections during successive untreated cycles while others superovulate and collect embryos from donor cows just before breeding to maintain close to a 365-day calving interval. A cow can be successfully superovulated every 50-60 days.

In commercial practice, embryos are collected transcervically, usually 6-8 days after estrus and insemination. Many practitioners favor the use of a Foley- or Rusch-type catheter, which is introduced through the cervix and into one uterine horn with the aid of a removable stylet in the catheter lumen. Others prefer to use a 3-way catheter, which is introduced through a cervical cannula. In all cases, the cuff of the catheter is inflated to seal off the uterine horn and hold the catheter in place. Phosphate-buffered saline (PBS) medium, enriched with antibiotics and heat-inactivated serum or bovine serum albumin (BSA), is used to wash embryos from the uterine horn by way of a gravity-feed, continuous flow technique, or alternatively a syringe technique. The medium is introduced into the uterine horn until it is mildly distended (which is confirmed by rectal palpation of the horn during the collection procedure), and then the medium is collected from the horn. Each horn is flushed several times using the same catheter. The ova/embryos are easily located as they settle out in the bottom of the collection vessel, or after being separated from the collection medium by commercially available or home-prepared plankton filters. Ova/embryos are located using a dissecting microscope at ~10X magnification.

Once embryos are located, they are transferred to a smaller volume of fresh medium with up to 20% serum or 0.4% BSA, and examined morphologically at 50-100X magnification to evaluate their quality. Those selected as being viable and of transferable quality are held in the medium at room temperature until they are transferred to recipients or prepared for bisection ("splitting"), freezing, or more specialized treatment, such as sex determination. Alternatively, embryos can be held in PBS culture in the refrigerator with no loss of viability.

Splitting embryos into identical halves by microsurgery is now practiced by many commercial embryo transfer teams. The number of embryos to be transferred can be doubled with only a minor depression in pregnancy rates. This technique has other applications, eg, the production of identical twins, use in sexing, genetic testing, etc. However, techniques of freezing manipulated embryos still need to be improved.

Cryopreservation of embryos in liquid nitrogen is now in common usage for all species except pigs. Techniques for freezing and thawing bovine embryos in ampules or straws have been simplified to the point that careful use of published procedures for good-quality embryos produces pregnancy rates that approach those obtained by transferring fresh embryos; therefore, commercial use of cryopreservation for the bovine species is routine. The most widely used cryoprotectant is glycerol at a concentration of ~1.5 M in PBS. Normally, embryos (in straws) are placed in the freezing chamber of a biological freezer at or near 19.4°F (-7°C). After seeding (the induction of ice crystals), cooling is resumed at 0.3-0.5°C/min and straws are plunged in liquid nitrogen between -30°C and -35°C. Straws are normally thawed in a water bath between 20°C and 35°C, or in air at room temperature. Glycerol is removed before transfer by a 6-step dilution procedure taking up to 60 min, or by a 10-min exposure to a nonpermeating cryoprotectant, eg, sucrose, at a concentration of 0.25-1 M in PBS. Others have reduced the 6-step dilution procedure to 3 steps utilizing 0.3 M sucrose. Newer, experimental, fast-freezing procedures utilize combinations of permeating and nonpermeating cryoprotectants. Vitrification is one such approach in which high concentrations of various cryoprotectants are used. Freezing results in the formation of a "glass" rather than ice crystals; thus, freezing injury is expected to be reduced. Procedures for fast-freezing of bovine embryos may soon be as simple as those for freezing semen.

Progress in embryo sexing has not been rapid. Chromosomal analysis of trophoblastic cells removed from hatched 12- to 15-day bovine embryos, or of half-embryos obtained by splitting at day 7, produces reliable results but is unsuitable for widespread application because of its complexity and because ~1/3 of embryos produce inadequate chromosome spreads. Immunological detection of the H-Y (male) antigen on the surface of entire embryos seems a more promising approach, but again, ~20-25% of embryos cannot be accurately sexed because of the subjectivity of the procedure. A more recent approach is the use of a Y-chromosome-specific DNA probe, which also requires the recovery of embryonic cells by micromanipulation; although the procedure is reported to be 95% accurate, ~1/3 of embryos cannot be sexed because of insufficient DNA from embryonic cells. However, recent advances in the technique of DNA amplification may substantially improve this situation.

Generally, embryos are transferred nonsurgically to recipient cows with a Cassou AI-type gun threaded through the cervix or, less commonly, surgically via a flank incision to introduce the embryo in a minimal volume of medium through a puncture in the uterine horn. In cows, single embryos are transferred to the horn adjacent to the ovary bearing the corpus luteum.

To successfully establish pregnancy, the recipients and donors must have closely synchronized estrous cycles (preferably ± 24 hr). If fresh embryos are being transferred, a large herd of cattle may be required to provide the appropriately synchronous recipients. Alternatively, the estrous cycles of the recipients can be artificially synchronized with that of the donor by injecting recipients with $PGF_{2\alpha}$ ~18 hr before the donor. Also, frozen embryos can be used to make more efficient use of recipients.

Following direct transfer of single fresh embryos to the uterine horn adjacent to the corpus luteum, ~60% of recipients become pregnant; frozen embryos result in 40-50% pregnancy rates. When 2 embryos are transferred to each recipient, the pregnancy rate is 60-90%, with 40-60% embryo survival. Twin transfers are rarely used commercially because of the risks of causing calving difficulties and of producing freemartins when the twins are not of the same sex. Splitting of embryos would overcome the latter problem.

Techniques and results in sheep and goats are basically similar to those in cattle, except that surgical or laparoscopic methods are almost always used for collection and transfer. Recently, a nonsurgical (transcervical) method of collecting embryos has been reported. This seems to work well in goats, but it is much less reliable in sheep. Sheep have been, and continue to be, useful models in which to develop procedures and applications for other ruminants.

Embryo transfer in pigs is done surgically, although a nonsurgical technique has been reported recently. When transfers are done within 5 days of ovulation, embryo survival rates are reported to be similar to those occurring naturally. Although pigs can be readily superovulated, unstimulated donors normally are collected repeatedly. Methods of synchronization are more complicated than in cattle. Although swine embryos have been refractory to attempts to preserve them by freezing, some success in cooling has been reported.

The mare has been especially difficult to superovulate, but the easily dilated, simple cervix lends itself well to nonsurgical collection and transfer methods. Normally, a single, and occasionally twin, equine embryo(s) is collected nonsurgically 6-8 days after ovulation. Synchronization of ovulation is possible using oral progestogens, combinations of progesterone and estrogen, or prostaglandins with human chorionic gonadotropin. However, the need for synchrony between donor and recipient in mares apparently is less rigid than in cows. Initial results in progesterone-treated, ovariectomized recipients suggest that a universal recipient produced in this way is much more practical and economical. Practical application of embryo transfer in horses is limited by the registration requirements of most breed societies.

Because embryo transfer procedures are costly, they are not used to the same extent as AI. However, rapid and continuing progress in techniques justifies its use in meeting many current and future production and research requirements in farm species. In addition, the new technologies, such as in vitro fertilization, cloning, and the production of transgenic animals, offer tremendous potential in the production of uniquely different animals, which may be designed to meet the needs of a changing agriculture.

HORMONAL CONTROL OF ESTRUS

Hormones, natural or synthetic, can be used either to induce or delay the onset of estrus. Administration of progesterone or synthetic progestins for long periods maintains serum progesterone concentrations, which mimics the action of the corpus luteum (CL) during the luteal phase; when the progesterone therapy is withdrawn, estrus follows in a few days. Administration of a luteolytic substance during the luteal phase destroys the CL (luteolysis) and ends the luteal phase, and an ovulatory estrus follows within a few days.

In mares that are cyclic or showing prolonged estrus, estrus can be suppressed with daily IM injections of progesterone in oil for 7-10 days. Following the last injection, an ovulatory estrus occurs within 7 days. Synthetic progestins, eg, altrenogest (0.44 mg/kg, PO, daily for 15 days), have a similar effect. Prostaglandin (PG) or prostaglandin-analog injection into mares with a functional CL results in luteolysis, and an ovulatory estrus occurs in 2-4 days. Prostaglandin treatment does not influence the estrous cycle of mares when administered during the first 4 days after ovulation or during seasonal anestrus. Injection of estrogen or synthetic estrogen into mares during anestrus induces behavioral but anovulatory estrus lasting 24-96 hr. Administration of human chorionic gonadotropin (HCG) or gonadotropin-releasing hormone (Gn-RH) during estrus in mares may induce ovulation of a preovulatory follicle within 48 hr. When administered during early estrus, it hastens ovulation, and thereby shortens the duration of estrus.

In cows, both progesterone and prostaglandin have been used to synchronize estrus. Progesterone in oil, oral progestins, and progestin-impregnated implants or intravaginal devices have been used. The period of administration is usually 10-14 days, and estrus occurs a few days after cessation of progesterone treatment. Conception rate at the estrus following treatment may be low; however, the second estrus also is synchronized and conception rate is normal. A regimen that combines an IM injection of 5 mg estradiol valerate, 3 mg norgestomet, and an ear implant of 6 mg norgestomet that is left in for 9 days has been used to synchronize estrus in cows; normal conception rates follow mating at the synchronized estrus. Administration of $PGF_{2\alpha}$ (25 mg, IM) or prostaglandin analogs (cloprostenol [500 μg, IM] or fenprostalene [1 mg, subcut.]) to cows with a functional CL results in estrus within 2-7 days. The treatment is effective only in cows 6-16 days after ovulation. Two PG injections given 11 days apart will synchronize estrus in most cows.

In goats and sheep, progestogen-impregnated vaginal pessaries have been the most widely used agents for control of ovulation. Progestogen treatment (usually fluorogestrone acetate) has been administered for 10-14 days in sheep, and 21 days in goats, followed by an injection of pregnant mare serum gonadotropin (PMSG) at the time of removal of the pessaries. A successful program of artificial insemination using frozen semen from genetically superior bucks has recently been practiced in France. All insemination is performed after estrus synchronization, beginning in June, using vaginal pessaries that are left in place for 11 days. On day 9, an injection of PMSG (400-600 IU) and cloprostenol (100-200 μg) is administered. Insemination is performed on days 12 and 13. During the breeding season, 2.5 mg $PGF_{2\alpha}$ or 175 μg cloprostenol is effective for inducing luteolysis in goats 5-16 days after ovulation.

In bitches, mibolerone (an androgen) and progestins are used to suppress estrus for indefinite periods of time; progesterone treatment may induce cystic endometrial hyperplasia and pyometra. Progestins may also cause obesity, diabetes mellitus, and neoplasia of the uterus and mammary glands. Mibolerone may cause skin, vaginal, and clitoral changes. Estrus may be suppressed for long periods in queens by using megestrol acetate, a progestin. Maximum treatment time of queens with megestrol is 18 mo. Mibolerone should not be used in queens. Estrus has been induced in bitches and queens with PMSG and follicle-stimulating hormone. Dose and treatment regimen depend on the product used. Ovulation should be induced by administration of a luteinizing hormone product, usually given at mating.

Administration of a combination of PMSG and HCG induces estrus in gilts with delayed puberty. Exogenous PG induces luteolysis of the porcine CL only after day 12 of the estrous cycle, and therefore is not a practical agent for estrous cycle control.

Some of the above treatments currently lack regulatory approval; label instructions should be checked.

VENTILATION
(Airborne noxious agents)

Inhalation of a variety of agents may cause toxic or allergic reactions. Historically, the reaction usually was due to accidental exposure or was allergic, and involved individuals or small groups. However, confinement housing associated with intensive agricultural practices of animals has decreased the space allotted per animal, and thereby increased the concentration of microbes, noxious gases, and irritating dust particles in the environment. Each of these undesirable elements may contribute to disease in animals and in their caretakers. In improperly ventilated buildings, over half the personnel may sustain some form of lung disease, typically with a night fever, lung congestion, an irritating hacking cough, and hoarseness with frequent "clearing" of the throat. This syndrome may last a few days or longer, depending on the individual's immune mechanism and the size of inoculum in repeated exposures. In properly ventilated buildings, disease processes associated with noxious gases have not been evident.

Although the value of treatment has long been recognized, the influence of environmental management with respect to animal and caretaker health has been given less attention. Medical treatment often is attempted as a substitute for environmental management, but with minimal success.

Carefully planned ventilation, mechanical or natural, based on sound engineering and medical principles, is an important key to a profitable livestock operation.

Livestock buildings can be divided into 2 broad categories: insulated and mechanically ventilated, with the minimum temperature maintained at $\geq40°F$ (4°C); and those with little or no insulation, with the inside temperature approximating the outside temperature, and with air movement caused by natural forces.

MECHANICAL VENTILATION

To be of maximal benefit, a mechanical ventilation system must be correctly planned, and properly installed, managed, and maintained. A poorly ventilated barn that has a foul-smelling and damp atmosphere is conducive to a high incidence of disease.

Functions of the ventilation system are to: 1) remove the expired moisture (~3 gal./1000 lb [15 L/500 kg] body wt/day at 50°F [10°C]), 2) dilute pathogens that are shed by the animals, 3) maintain a reasonably uniform temperature in winter (40-45°F [4-7°C]), and 4) prevent the temperature in summer from rising more than ~5°F (3°C) above the outside temperature. To maintain an acceptable inside temperature in winter and to prevent condensation from occurring on even well-insulated walls and ceilings, the barn must be filled to capacity. In mechanically ventilated calf barns or farrowing barns, supplemental heat usually must be provided.

When the outside temperature reaches about −10°F (−23°C), some condensation or frost can be expected on the surfaces where the cold outside air and the warm inside air meet. These conditions must be tolerated; a system that would eliminate them would be impractical.

Successful ventilation requires proper insulation. In northern USA, R-values of ~15 for the walls and 25 over flat ceilings are recommended. (R-value is a measure of resistance to the passage of heat; the higher the R-value, the better the insulation.) Because windows have a low insulation value compared to walls, their area should be limited. Likewise, height of the exposed foundation should be kept as low as possible to prevent heat loss.

The fresh-air inlet system and the exhaust system are equally important.

Exhaust System Design: Calculation of a ventilation system's capacity for moisture removal and temperature control in winter has commonly been based on weight of the animals housed. Their exact weight is seldom known and does not remain constant. A simpler method of determining exhaust capacity is based on a minimal continuous number of air changes needed per hour to remove moisture and to maintain reasonable air purity in cold weather. A practical maximum exhaust capacity is also necessary to control temperature in summer. The minimal continuous air exchange rate is 4 air changes per hour. This air is removed at a point ~15 in. (38 cm) above the floor, through a duct constructed around the continuous fan (or fans) that provide this capacity. Minimal fan capacity (in ft^3/min) required is determined by dividing the volume of the animal housing compartment by 15. In barns with connected manure storage, that volume must be included when calculating ventilation capacity; the total continuous exhaust capacity must be removed from the connected manure storage. Mechanically ventilated barns constructed with underfloor manure storage (slat-floored units) should be designed to allow one-half of the total ventilation capacity to be removed from the pit before any wall fans begin to operate. In summer, an exhaust capacity of 40 air changes per hour (10 times the winter capacity) is necessary to prevent the temperature in the building from rising more than ~5°F (3°C) above the outside temperature.

The total exhaust capacity is then made up of the continuously operating fan or fans, plus a number of thermostatically controlled fans that turn on and off to regulate the barn temperature. About one-half of the total capacity should be considered the winter, spring, and fall part of the system; the remaining half is for summer or mild weather use only.

An exhaust rate of >40 air changes per hour makes little difference in summer barn temperature, and is not economical.

When the inside temperature is >70°F (21°C), human and animal comfort may be increased by providing strategically placed, manually controlled air-circulating fans in the housing compartment. When winter temperatures fall to about −10°F (−23°C), the continuous air exchange rate may have to be reduced slightly for short periods to prevent the inside barn temperature from falling below 40°F (4°C). This can be done by turning off one fan when there is more than one in continuous operation; it also can be accomplished by throttling the airflow through the duct to a single continuous fan.

Fans used for animal shelter ventilation should be designed specifically for that purpose. All fans should be certified as being capable of delivering the required airflow, at ⅛ in. (0.3 cm) static pressure. This is approximately equivalent to the pressure created by a 15 mile (24 km) per hour wind blowing against the operating fan. Wind substantially affects the output of ventilating fans, as does the resistance to airflow created by an insufficient air intake.

Fans that exhaust air from connected manure storage pits must have performance characteristics that at least equal those of the wall fans; otherwise, the wall fans may overcome the manure storage fans and draw air through the manure pit into the barn, which would increase odor and health hazards to animals and caretakers.

As a general rule, properly selected single-speed fans should be used. Variable-speed fans are not recommended because of their general inability to develop the recommended static pressure of ⅛ in. at low speed. Thus, if a wind of ~15 miles per hour is blowing against a variable-speed fan operating at low capacity, air may actually blow back through the fan and effectively cause the exhaust to become an air intake.

Fresh Air Necessary: Poor fresh-air intake design is one of the most common causes of unsatisfactory ventilation performance. A fresh-air intake system that can distribute incoming air uniformly without causing undue drafts in winter is essential. It must have sufficient capacity to prevent the negative static pressure in the building from rising >⅛ in. (0.3 cm) of water. High static pressure indicates resistance to airflow. It can be measured with a portable inclined column manometer. However, a readily available guide is the barn door: if the door slams shut, or if the sound of the fans changes when the door is open, fresh-air intake is inadequate.

The slot inlet system is an efficient and economical means of bringing fresh air into any mechanically ventilated livestock housing unit. It is sometimes disregarded because of its low cost and simplicity of construction, but experience indicates that no other system outperforms it.

During the summer, the inside barn temperature should be prevented from rising appreciably above the outside temperature. Thus, it is an obvious advantage to draw in the coolest air available. The north side of the barn is least affected by the sun; next coolest is the east side. Continuous doors or slide-regulated openings (6 in. [15 cm]) should be built into the underside of boxed-in eaves.

These are opened in summer to allow outside air from the shaded area beneath the eaves to enter the slot inlet. In winter, these eave openings must be closed. Then, all air entering the barn through the slot inlet is supplied by large attic louvers built high in the gable at each end of the barn.

NATURAL VENTILATION

Natural ventilation is accomplished by the forces of nature—wind and gravity (stack effect). No mechanical equipment is used, except in rare instances for air circulation in very wide buildings, or on hot, still summer days.

Since the force of gravity is a primary mover of air through the building (warm air rises and cold air falls), buildings with a gable roof should have a continuous, unobstructed opening at the peak 2 in. (5 cm) wide for each 10 ft (3 m) of building width, and the full length of the building. Such buildings should be oriented on an east-west axis when possible. They may have the south side open with continuous, or nearly continuous, adjustable ventilation openings in the north wall, or they may have both long walls closed, with adjustable openings the full length of both sides and at the ends, unless large doors are provided. Permanently fixed openings in one or both walls are also desirable to permit minimal air entry at all times. This may be accomplished by leaving the space between the top of the plate and the underside of the roof open, or by providing a narrow full-length opening in both long walls.

When buildings are located in unprotected areas subject to high winds, closure of even these openings on the windward side may be necessary under extremely adverse conditions.

The temperature inside the building should closely follow the outside temperature. Attempting to maintain a higher temperature in winter, usually to prevent manure from freezing, causes severe moisture and subsequent respiratory and other health problems. Fog, condensation, or frost forms when the building is not ventilated properly.

Hot, muggy, summer weather can cause great environmental stress with subsequent reduction in productivity. Adequate sidewall openings and roof insulation can be important in reducing animal stress. During these times, air movement across the animals may be of value. Vertically mounted circulating fans can be spaced 20-30 ft (6-9 m) apart to move air in a circular pattern around the livestock housing compartment. When the roof structure permits, fans can be placed horizontally at approximately the same intervals to blow air down on the animals.

DISEASE-MANAGEMENT INTERACTION: CATTLE

When attempting to identify the etiology of disease, initial efforts are often directed toward identifying a specific virus, bacterium, or other microorganism. Isolation and identification of infectious agents are frequently productive and necessary, but if management errors are not considered, control of the outbreak and prevention of future outbreaks may be difficult or even impossible.

Management is especially important when animals are being added to or removed from the herd, or permitted to contact those from other herds and then returned. Such animals should be isolated for ≥ 2 wk, or if disease appears, until the disease has run its course. Although numerous diseases can be spread by new animals, some of the most serious are brucellosis, tuberculosis, paratuberculosis, respiratory disease, and neonatal diarrhea. Also important are careful inspection of the individual animal and the herd of origin, a reputable seller, and a signed and dated certificate of inspection. (*See also* p 960.)

Animals most likely to introduce disease into a herd are neonatal or newly weaned calves, naturally bred cows that return to heat and are naturally bred in the new herd, bulls that have served naturally in herds of unknown reproductive disease status, cows that have aborted, and animals with a history of undiagnosed diarrhea.

BEEF CATTLE

Despite advances in veterinary medicine, disease continues to take a tremendous toll in beef herds. Management efforts have been directed toward improving rate of gain and feed efficiency, but the role of management must be emphasized if intensive beef operations are to return a profit and survive. Disease-management interactions are important in all beef operations but especially so in intensive ones. Application of effective management procedures would eliminate a major portion of disease losses. Some significant procedures are discussed below.

When large numbers of animals are confined in a small area, both direct and indirect animal contact is increased. Adding animals to a herd increases disease probability geometrically since each added animal has the potential of introducing disease to every other animal in the herd. Also, when herd size is increased, the individual attention that each animal receives is usually lessened, and disease is more likely to become well-established before it is recognized and treated. As a result, treatment is less likely to be effective, and mortality is increased unless management is improved.

Breeding and feeding practices that accelerate the growth of animals (and shorten the period from birth to market or to reproduction) tend to increase the potential for disease. Although many medicaments (especially antibacterials) have been developed and are currently used to treat disease in cattle herds, therapy has not been the complete answer: losses due to deaths, growth inefficiencies in recovered animals, and cost of treatments continue to be great. Management is important in preventing any departure from a state of health, but is especially so at birth. (*See also* MANAGEMENT OF REPRODUCTION: CATTLE, p 1127.) Cows giving birth and calves being born into an unfavorable environment are prone to develop disease. Cows are most likely to develop infections of the uterus and udder, and calves of the GI tract (*see* DIARRHEA IN NEONATAL RUMINANTS, p 181). The value of vaccination in preventing salmonellosis in calves is questionable, but vaccination against colibacillosis, coronavirus infection, and rotavirus infection is widely accepted and practiced in herds in which those diseases have been identified. Rotavirus and coronavirus vaccines are usually administered to calves at birth but also can be administered to pregnant cows. Calves should receive the vaccine at birth or within the first 12 hr. Cows should receive the first dose several months after conception, and the second 1 mo before parturition. Vaccinating either cows or calves is effective, but vaccinating both has created some problems suggestive of isoerythrolysis. In field trials, vaccination reduced morbidity from 48% to 28% and mortality from 19% to 3%. Since colibacillosis affects calves <1 wk old, this vaccine is administered to the dam before parturition. Two doses, 3 wk apart, are recommended; the first given ≥6 wk before parturition. (*See also* TABLES 6 and 7, p 1134.)

Newborn calves should receive an adequate amount of fresh colostrum within a few hours after birth and for the first 3 days. They should receive an amount equivalent to 5% of their body weight in the first 6-8 hr after birth, and again over the next 18-20 hr. On each of days 2 and 3, they should receive an amount equivalent to 8% of their body weight, which will help control pathogens in the gut even if absorption of antibodies has ceased. If necessary, colostrum (50-80 mL/kg body wt) can be given by gravity tube to newborn calves. Once ingested and absorbed, the half-life of IgG is considered to be ~16 days; IgM, 4 days; and IgA, 3 days.

Since the amount of immunoglobulin in colostrum is highly variable and it is difficult to determine the amount ingested, it is frequently helpful in problem herds to determine the amount of gamma globulins that have been passively transferred to the calf. Three tests—zinc sulfate turbidity, total protein, and radial immunodiffusion—are available. The guidelines in TABLE 3 are used for interpreting those tests.

Table 3. Guidelines for the Interpretation of Tests for Passive Transfer of Colostral Immunoglobulins

Test	Failure of Passive Transfer	Preferred Value
Radial immunodiffusion IgG$_1$	<5 mg/dL	≥15 mg/dL
Zinc sulfate turbidity	<10 ZST units	≥30 ZST units
Refractometer		
serum	<5 g/dL	≥6 g/dL
plasma	<5.5 g/dL	≥6.5 g/dL

Adapted from Gay C. and Besser T., *Animal Nutrition & Health*, April, 1985, Watt Publishing Co., Mt. Morris, Illinois.
For more information on colostrum, *see* p 1112.

Control of lice is important throughout the year, but especially during the winter when many animals are confined in a small area and grow long coats. Lice cause irritation and blood loss, and there is also some evidence that they may be carriers of viral diseases. Numerous effective pediculicides are available; timing and proper application are more important than selection of the product, although some injectable products are less effective against biting lice than against sucking lice.

Internal parasites depress rate of gain and feed efficiency in young animals, but evidence also indicates that in at least some herds, administering anthelmintics to nursing cows significantly increases weaning weight of their calves. Both coccidiosis and cryptosporidiosis are recognized with increasing frequency as a problem in animals up to 1 yr old and occasionally even in older animals. Although liver flukes were once thought to be restricted to the far west and southeastern USA, they have been found in many areas of the country. In the past, lungworms have not been considered a serious problem in many parts of the USA, but are being diagnosed more often. Although heavy lungworm infection is a problem in itself, the increased susceptibility to pneumonia may be even more important. Periodic fecal examinations for both intestinal parasites and lungworms are important; flotations usually detect intestinal parasites, but sedimentation is required to detect lungworms and liver flukes. Some of the newer anthelmintics are very effective for both GI parasites and lungworms. Treatment for cattle grubs (*Hypoderma* spp) is effective and safe if administered before the time the larvae are in the esophagus or spinal cord (the date after which treatment should not be administered varies between different areas).

A basic management concept that minimizes internal parasite problems and other diseases such as paratuberculosis is prevention of fecal contamination of feedstuffs. Confined cattle should not be fed on the ground, and feed bunks should be constructed to minimize contamination.

Diseases of the respiratory system are responsible for major losses in beef cattle. All breeds and ages are susceptible, but by far the greatest loss occurs when cattle are moved from the breeding herd to the feedlot. Stresses, viruses, and bacteria are the basic causes of shipping fever that occurs shortly after cattle arrive in the feedlot. Calves lead a relatively stress-free life on the ranch until they are sold as feeders, at which time their lives suddenly change drastically: they are taken from their dam (a major stress in itself) and castrated, dehorned, placed in a dusty pen, and expected to find water in an unfamiliar tank. Their ration is changed from milk and green grass to dry hay and grain; they run the pen fences seeking their dams, stir up dust that is inhaled, tire themselves to the point of exhaustion, and bawl until their throats are irritated. They may be moved long distances in drafty crowded vehicles, and environmental temperature may vary as much as 100°F (38°C) between points of origin and destination.

Management, not medication, is the answer to many respiratory problems. Numerous preconditioning programs have been devised to prepare calves for the transition from the breeding herd to the feedlot, with variable results.

Lameness (qv, p 494) is a serious problem in intensive beef operations. Many lamenesses are a result of failing to select breeding stock for sound feet and legs. Contributing factors are close confinement, improper foot care, and feeding high-concentrate rations for rapid weight gains at an early age, which place excessive stress on developing feet and legs. When an animal inherits a predisposition toward interdigital skin hyperplasia or corkscrew claw, the likelihood of the abnormality being manifest is increased if the animal is overfed and confined and its feet permitted to grow long. High-concentrate rations with limited roughage often produce laminitis and horizontal and vertical fissures. Tarsitis frequently develops in "post-legged" cattle, and necrobacillosis results from improperly maintained floor surfaces and filth.

Hoof trimming should be a basic management procedure in intensive beef breeding enterprises. Overgrowth of the hoof occurs either when the animals are confined on surfaces that do not wear the hoof sole, or under extremely dry conditions when the hooves become very hard and fail to wear. In either case, the hoof wall and heel bulb elongate, which puts abnormal strain on the suspensory system of the limb.

Aberrations of the hoof horn other than overgrowth and deformity are encountered in intensively managed dairy cows. These take many forms: heel erosions, double or split soles, ulcers, and abnormalities of the abaxial white line. If hoof trimming is instituted as a routine annual procedure, it is claimed that the functional life of a dairy herd is increased by ≥ 1 yr.

For restraint, beef cattle and bulls may require sedation. Tipping tables are used routinely. Hoof trimming of dairy cattle is most easily done with the animal standing. Stocks should be used for large herds. Other devices are available, such as the "hoof nack", that provide mechanical advantage in elevating the limb. Hoof-trimming devices should not be used in the milking parlor lest subsequent interference with milk letdown result. A hindlimb may also be elevated with a rope, one end of which should be applied with a slip knot around the Achilles tendon, the other run over a beam above the hip of the animal.

Inadequate and/or poorly maintained equipment makes hoof trimming extremely laborious and may account for the widespread inadequacy of hoof care. Two each of left- and right-handed, narrow-bladed hoof knives are basic equipment. A triangular file should be used to sharpen the concave edge of the blade, and a chain saw file to sharpen the hook. Small-handled, small, flat-bladed, stainless steel hoof cutters are also required. An electric, rotary angle grinder with a steel blade is useful for paring the extremely hard horn encountered in beef cattle.

There are 2 objectives in hoof trimming: to restore normal hoof balance and to correct defects of the hoof. The first step is to correct lateral balance. If one heel is longer than the other, excess horn should be removed to equalize the height. Lateral claws are usually higher than the medial claw; when this abnormality is present, the hocks turn inward. The longitudinal balance is dealt with next. Using the pincers, cutting commences at the abaxial sole heel junction (abaxial groove). Very little wall should be removed at this point; more is removed as the paring proceeds toward the toe. The sole is pared next, and must be reduced to a point at which it will not bear weight: the most important principle of hoof trimming is to ensure that weight is borne by the abaxial wall. Digital pressure should be applied frequently to the sole to determine its thickness.

DAIRY CATTLE

Much of the discussion under beef cattle (*see* above) also applies to dairy cattle.

Management influences the occurrence, severity, and prognosis of many diseases. The newborn calf should be born into a disease-free environment and receive colostrum as soon as possible after birth, preferably within the first 30 min.

Most dairy cows produce colostrum far in excess of the calf's requirement. First-calf heifers can yield 32 kg of colostrum in the first 4 days after parturition, mature cows 40-50 kg. Calves consume, at the maximum, only about one-third of the colostrum available from dairy cows. There may be sufficient surplus colostrum to feed calves 2-3.5 kg daily from 3-16 days of age, or longer. If bull calves are sold early, there may be sufficient colostrum to feed heifer calves for 4 wk.

Colostrum obtained from the first milking is of the highest quality, and colostrum from mature cows contains a higher level of antibodies and is considered to be of higher quality than that from first-calf heifers. The concentration of immunoglobulin gradually decreases over the first 3 days.

Colostrum can be frozen for several months with almost no deterioration; it must be thawed using tepid (not hot) water. It also can be stored at ambient temperatures for extended periods, in which case, the following recommendations apply: 1) It should be handled in a sanitary manner to prevent contamination. 2) Fermented and chemically treated colostrum should be stored in plastic-lined containers with lids. Corrosion of metal containers occurs following acid additions or acid production during fermentation. Plastic liners allow easy cleanup of empty containers. 3) Extremely bloody colostrum should not be fermented. 4) Daily stirring of stored colostrum counteracts separation of solids. A more uniform diet for calves can be obtained by stirring colostrum immediately before feeding. 5) Unfermented colostrum may be added to fermented colostrum without appreciably altering composition. 6) Colostrum not preserved with chemicals should be stored at cool temperatures. Use of chemical additives is recommended for warm temperatures. Formaldehyde may be added at 0.05% (wt/volume). Propionic acid may be added at 1% (wt/wt). 7) Chemical additives should be incorporated into fresh colostrum before placing in storage containers. Waiting until all colostrum has been added to a storage container may allow initiation of undesirable fermentation. 8) Colostrum should be fed within a few weeks of collection, since nutrient content continues to decline throughout storage. However, fermented colostrum has been fed successfully after 84-100 days of storage. The ideal temperature range for the storage of fermented colostrum is 50-70°F (10-21°C). Colostrum that has been stored at such temperatures has resulted in greater weight gains in calves than has feeding milk replacer.

Table 4. Some Physical Characteristics and Composition of Colostrum and Whole Milk

	Colostrum (No. of postpartum milkings)					Milk
	1	2	3	4	5	
Specific gravity	1.056	1.040	1.035	1.033	1.033	1.032
Total solids (%)	23.9	17.9	14.1	13.9	13.6	12.9
Fat (%)	6.7	5.4	4.9	4.4	4.3	4.0
Solids-not-fat (%)	16.7	12.2	9.8	9.4	9.5	8.8
Total protein (%)	14.0	8.4	5.1	4.2	4.1	3.1
Vitamin A (µg/100 mL)	295	190	113	76	74	34

Adapted from Foley, J.A. and Otterby, D.E., *Journal of Dairy Science*, **61**, 1978.

The generally recommended guideline for feeding liquid diets to dairy calves, particularly replacement heifer calves, is that calves receive 8-10% of body wt as whole milk equivalent daily. Colostrum, with a higher solids content than whole milk, can be fed at reduced rates (~6% of body wt) to supply approximately the same amount of dry matter.

Colostrum can be diluted to approximate the solids content of whole milk. It has been diluted with whole milk, reconstituted skim milk, and milk replacer, but the most popular diluent is water. Dilution with water allows a given amount of colostrum to replace more than an equal weight of whole milk in calf-feeding programs. To approximate the solids content of whole milk (12%), colostrum with 18% solids can be diluted 2 to 1 (colostrum to water), and colostrum with 16% solids can be diluted 3 to 1. When the colostrum is diluted to approximate a whole-milk diet, it should be fed at 8-10% of body wt. Most calves that initially refuse fermented colostrum adjust within a few days. Under conditions of warm ambient temperatures, refusals may be a problem.

In dairy herds in which rotavirus or coronavirus infections are a problem in calves 5-14 days old, feeding stored or fermented colostrum daily from the third day of life until ~14 days of age assists in the control of those diseases. The colostrum may be fed fermented and diluted with water as recommended above, or fed fresh or fermented mixed (1:1) with cow's whole milk or milk replacer for calves 3-14 days old.

Neonatal Veal Calves: Almost all veal calves are dairy calves, and they are fed, housed, and managed similarly; however, disease problems are often more severe in veal calves because they originate from many different farms and may be severely stressed before arriving at the feeding facility. A bull calf intended for veal may receive little attention at the farm of origin because of limited value and change of ownership shortly after birth. He may not even receive colostrum, which severely limits his chances of survival. In addition, he is exposed to calves from many different farms, confined in a holding area for a variable time until a truckload is accumulated or a purchaser is found, and then transported long distances to the veal feeder's facility. During this time he may be poorly nourished or overfed, and exposed to wide variations in temperature. Although the situation improves dramatically at the veal feeder's facility, morbidity and mortality are often high due to previous stresses that lead to diarrhea and pneumonia. Proper sanitation, careful attention to mixing feed, supplying feed of good quality and in satisfactory amounts, parasite control, and adequate ventilation and environmental temperature control are essential management factors in controlling veal calf diseases. (*See also* BOVINE RESPIRATORY DISEASE COMPLEX, p 721; DIARRHEA OF NEONATAL RUMINANTS, p 181; and VENTILATION, p 1106.)

Individual calf hutches have become popular for raising dairy calves, and the most frequently observed calf diseases (gastroenteritis and pneumonia) have practically disappeared when hutches were properly used. Calves should be placed in the hutches within the first day of life and kept there for ~2 mo. The calves should have a dry place to rest, be protected from wind chill, have access to water, receive good-quality hay, and be started on grain at an early age so they can readily make the transition from milk or milk replacer to dry feed at 6-8 wk of age. (*See also* MANAGEMENT OF REPRODUCTION: CATTLE, p 1127.)

When dairy calves are removed from calf hutches and grouped in pens with calves of similar ages, they should receive adequate nutrients and be vaccinated against endemic diseases. Dairy heifer calves in the USA should be vaccinated (even in areas where the risk of disease is limited) against brucellosis, since many states will not permit unvaccinated females to be moved into their state or from one herd to another within the state. To prevent injury by larger animals and exposure to many diseases at an earlier, more susceptible age, young heifers should not be permitted to associate with the adult herd until after parturition when they are added to the milking herd. Proper sanitation, grouping of animals of similar age, and preventing fecal contamination of feed prevents most GI and respiratory parasite problems.

Mastitis (qv, p 686) is the most costly disease in dairy cattle, and management beginning at birth is important in prevention. Calves should not be permitted to nurse each other's udders, especially if milk from cows with mastitis is being fed. It is also harmful to permit nursing of the developing heifer's udder at any time before parturition. Supernumerary teats should be removed early, since pathogens occasionally gain entrance through them. Overfeeding of the preparturient heifer not only leads to excessive deposition of fat in the udder and limited development of milk secretory tissue, but predisposes to breakdown of udder support and mammary edema. Prefreshening milking has little effect on udder edema but is frequently practiced in an effort to prevent breakdown of udder support tissues. Sanitation is important in the calving environment and throughout the cow's lactation, since practically all mastitis organisms gain entrance through the teat end.

Cattle fed for high milk production are prone to develop **GI problems.** The basic cause is overfeeding of grain to an animal with a GI tract that evolved primarily for digestion of forages. Abruptly increasing grain or feeding high amounts for long periods results in clumping of rumen villi and decreased tone of the abomasal wall. Gastroenteritis, bloat, abomasal ulcers, and abomasal displacement may result. Gradually increasing grain, adding a buffer such as sodium bicarbonate, feeding long dry hay (0.5 lb/100 lb [500 g/100 kg] body wt/day), supplying long cut (≥0.5 in. [1.25 cm]) silage, and feeding little or no grain during the dry period prevents many GI disturbances.

Paratuberculosis (qv, p 399) is becoming increasingly apparent in US dairy cattle, and many herds are infected. Since infection almost always occurs during the first few weeks of life, separating the heifer calf from the cow herd immediately after birth and not returning it until after lactation has begun (~2 yr) often results in a paratuberculosis-free herd. This is especially true if long-term fecal culture and removal of positive animals is also practiced.

Proper pasture management and a sound antiparasite program are useful aids in controlling **GI parasitism**. (*See also* GASTROINTESTINAL PARASITES, CATTLE, p 205.)

Lameness (qv, p 494) has become a significant problem due to confinement and excessive grain feeding. Feet grow approximately twice as fast as usual in free-stall barns, in which they are constantly moist from urine and feces. (*See also* HOOF TRIMMING, p 1111.) In addition, feeding excessive grain frequently results in laminitis, and feet grow abnormally and require frequent trimming. Foot baths of copper sulfate or formalin aid in preventing and controlling many foot infections.

DISEASE-MANAGEMENT INTERACTION: GOATS

HUSBANDRY

Management of goats depends on the type (eg, dairy, pygmy, meat, mohair, or cashmere) and the reasons for which they are kept (eg, companionship or commercial enterprise). However, all are ruminants, and the basic principles of livestock husbandry are applicable. Dairy goats and pygmies usually are raised intensively, with most of the feed being brought to the animals. Meat goats and Angoras mainly are raised extensively with most of the diet coming from browse, and occasionally from high-quality pasture at times of highest nutritional need, such as the first 18 mo of life and the last 6 wk of gestation. A pregnant Angora doe will continue to grow mohair without adequate energy and protein, even if stressed until she aborts.

Mature bucks develop a powerful characteristic odor that is most intense in the breeding season, and personnel are reluctant to handle them. This often leads to neglect of feet and failure to recognize heavy parasite loads. The sebaceous glands on top of the head can be removed surgically at any age, or can be cauterized at the time of disbudding; however, this does not render the buck totally odorless. Does are attracted by this smell, and may refuse to be bred by a descented buck if there is an odoriferous one nearby; therefore, the glands should not be removed inadvertently at the time of disbudding if male kids are to be kept for breeding. The habit of urinating on the face, beard, and forelegs also contributes to buck odor and often leads to ulcerating sores in cold weather. During the breeding season, most bucks lose weight; however, this is not necessarily due to breeding too many does; many lose weight when housed close to does in heat, even when breeding is not allowed. The only way to manage this is to get the bucks into prime physical condition before the breeding season. The dominant male in a group of bucks is in much better condition than some of the others.

The genetically homozygous polled doe usually is anatomically an intersex, and therefore, infertile. Aberrations vary from a slightly enlarged clitoris visible only after puberty, to a buck-like conformation, with a scrotum, penis (often shortened), and ovo-testes. Some phenotypically male pseudohermaphrodites show male libido with breeding activity. Since these animals are infertile, early recognition and culling is advisable. Some homozygous polled males may be capable of siring kids, but are likely to develop sperm granulomas as they mature. Most owners reduce the incidence of homozygous polled animals by never mating 2 polled animals. While most hermaphrodites are polled, similar anatomical aberrations occasionally can occur in horned goats. These would most probably be chimeras (freemartins), the result of anastomoses occurring *in utero* between males and females. Such chimeras in goats are rare (considering the high frequency of twins in goats) when compared with cattle.

Of all farm animals, goats have the strongest social hierarchy; thus, adequate feeder space should be provided so that the dominant animals cannot guard the feeders and prevent others from eating. The amount of floor space available per doe affects the amount of aggressive behavior. A goat can become so subordinated by its pen mates that it does not eat and loses condition. This psychological component must be considered in cases of wasting goats. For maximum longevity, and to avoid fighting injuries, adult males should be fed and housed individually. However, they should be housed either close to other goats, or have a companion such as a dry doe in the pen.

Goats are adventurous and are natural climbers, and efforts should be made to control them; the ultimate control would be high-tensile, electric fences. Goats stand and push on other fences and can be very destructive. Hazards that might contribute to broken legs and strangulations should be removed. Tethering goats is potentially dangerous since they are vulnerable to dog attacks, and if chained too close to another goat, invariably one will strangle. Goats chew on painted surfaces, and lead poisoning is a potential hazard in old barns. An efficient layout of pens, easy access to well-designed feeders, and effective control minimize management-related problems.

It is extremely difficult to keep goats' feet, urine, and feces out of many types of grain feeders, hay racks, and waterers. Goats refuse to eat soiled feed or water, hay that has fallen on the floor, and grain contaminated with urine and feces of farm pets or vermin. Hay feeder design is critical to reduce feed wastage. Most dairy and pygmy goats are bedded on wasted hay. Wet bedding contributes to development of coccidiosis in kids and staphylococcal impetigo on the udder, commonly but erroneously known as "goat pox". Under similar conditions, joint-ill and navel infections of the newborn are likely. In certain areas, kids are susceptible to white muscle disease, which can be controlled by injection of vitamin E/selenium to the pregnant doe and/or newborn, and selenium supplements in the diet.

Housing of goats affects disease patterns. Angoras in the south and west of the USA are given access to shelter only during severe storms or for a few weeks after the twice yearly shearing, without which they die of cold weather stress. Goats in the northern states are housed in the winter, perhaps more for the owners' comfort than for optimal health of the goats. Intensive management of adult dairy goats may promote horizontal transmission of the virus of caprine arthritis-encephalitis (CAE, qv, p 393). Combinations of manure packs, overhead hay-mows, or uninsulated ceilings lead to dampness and ammonia buildup, especially if the barn is closed tightly. Warm, wet barns are conducive to development of neonatal navel infections, mastitis, enteritis, pneumonia, and coccidiosis. The disease known as "abscesses", caused by *Corynebacterium pseudotuberculosis (ovis)*, spreads rapidly in closely confined animals (*see also* p 64). The slow-growing, nonpainful lymph node abscesses eventually rupture and contaminate all the feeders, walls, and other animals. The infection is spread by contact with the pus, and the organism can penetrate intact skin. Isolating affected animals, preferably culling them, and preventing environmental contamination is important. In Australia, a vaccine is available.

For foot care, *see* LAMENESS IN GOATS, p 503.

PERINATAL MANAGEMENT

A common problem is extra teats, double teats, and fish-tail teats with double orifices. In cattle, extra teats can be snipped off with impunity, but in dairy goats there is often a functional milk gland behind the spare teat.

Newborn goats must be fed colostrum, and if CAE is a problem, pasteurization is essential for control. Later, they can be fed (in decreasing order of desirability) goat's milk, goat-milk replacer, lamb-milk replacer, or cow's milk. Any fresh milk fed should be pasteurized or from stock known to be free of CAE virus, mycoplasma, and paratuberculosis. Newborn goats should be fed at 10-12% of their body wt per day. On average, they are fed 1 pt (500 mL) of milk b.i.d., but often they are overfed.

Kids should have access to hay and a grain-based creep feed as early as 1 wk of age. They can be weaned when they are readily eating a large handful of grain per day; this should occur no later than 8 wk of age in dairy breeds, and at 6 wk in others. Weaning is delayed in many goat operations because there is no commercial outlet for doe's milk other than to feed it to kids.

Disbudding of dairy goats should be done as soon as the kid has good muscle tone. For bucks of the Swiss breeds, it is important to disbud at 1-2 days of age to have the best chance of inhibiting horn growth or subsequent development of abnormal regrowth (scurs). Nubian doe kids have the least vigorous horn growth, and disbudding can be delayed for 2-3 wk. Hot iron disbudding is the method of choice, using either a restraint box and nerve block, or general anesthesia such as xylazine (1-2 mg/kid). Excessive applications of heat lead to brain damage or subsequent death of the kids. Disbudding kids with caustic paste is not recommended.

Angora goats are not disbudded in range operations, since the horns are thought to be helpful against predators, and owners handle the goats by their horns. Where goats are housed in winter, disbudding is advantageous; it reduces trauma and prevents accidents in which animals are trapped by their horns in feeders and fence lines. Pygmies can be disbudded according to the owner's preference; it is not a cause for disqualification or discrimination in the show ring. Dairy goats generally are disbudded, and horned animals usually are barred from the show ring. Tetanus can occur after disbudding (or other means of infection) and, as a precaution, antitoxin (150 u/kid) can be given.

Castration of dairy goats and pygmy bucks is done in the first few weeks; Angoras are castrated later, after they have attained good horn growth. Males to be kept as pets should have castration delayed to allow maximal urethral development, which reduces the likelihood of urolithiasis. To improve their desirability as pets, these goats also should have the scent glands removed along with the horns.

NUTRITION

Dairy goats can and should be fed similarly to dairy cattle (*see* p. 1171). A good-quality hay, preferably alfalfa, should be the basis of the ration, and a 14-16% protein concentrate should be fed as a supplement during lactation. Silage is not a common dietary constituent because most goats are kept in small groups, which does not justify the equipment. A common problem is overfeeding grain to does in late lactation. Goats store fat preferentially in the abdominal cavity, and by the time fat is grossly obvious, the internal deposits are substantial; this can lead to problems at parturition and to pregnancy toxemia.

Loose trace mineral salt (TMS) should be fed rather than block salt; its composition varies with the area of the country, eg, iodine and selenium supplements are necessary in midwestern USA. Goats are highly susceptible to copper deficiency and, unlike sheep, fairly resistant to copper toxicity. Therefore, cattle TMS, rather than sheep salt with no copper, should be offered.

Pet wethers fed on substantial amounts of grain are prone to develop urinary calculi. Reducing grain consumption, adding ammonium chloride to the diet, keeping the calcium:phosphorus ratio ~2:1, and keeping the magnesium level low will help. A urethrostomy helps such animals, but recurrences and urethral scarring necessitate euthanasia for many. To encourage water consumption, clean loose TMS should be fed, and fresh water offered b.i.d.. To increase water consumption, especially for high-yielding does, their water should be fresh and warm in winter, and fresh and cool in summer.

COMMON DISEASES

Rotating all the kids through 1 or 2 pens is dangerous; adult goats shed coccidia and infect the newborn. As infection pressure builds up in the pens, morbidity in kids born later is increased. Goat kids harbor several species of coccidia, but not all have clinical coccidiosis. Signs are diarrhea or pasty feces, loss of condition, general frailness, and failure to grow. Peracute cases die with no signs. To help prevent coccidiosis in artificially reared dairy goats, the kids should be put in small, age-matched groups in outside portable pens that are moved to clean ground periodically. Eradication is not feasible, but control through management is. Coccidiostats added to the water or feed are adjuncts to a management control program and not substitutes. Chronic coccidiosis is one of the main causes of poor growth in kids, and is responsible for the uneconomical practice of delaying breeding for a year until the goat has reached adequate size (70 lb [32 kg]). In Angora goats kept extensively, the problem occurs at weaning, when the kids are kept in smaller lots and fed supplement on the ground.

Clostridium perfringens type D can be fatal, and it is not always associated with the classical "change in quality and quantity of feed". In problem herds, vaccination q4-6mo may be necessary. Vaccination prevents the acute death syndrome, but occasionally even vaccinated animals may develop acute enteritis. Affected goats develop severe diarrhea and profound depression; milk yield drops abruptly and they may die in 24 hr. Treatment involves fluid therapy, correction of acidosis, and antibiotics.

Contagious ecthyma (soremouth) vaccination is not indicated unless the disease exists in the herd. The main problems with infected kids are difficulty in nursing, spreading lesions to the does' udders or the assistants' hands, and not being allowed to attend goat shows. Live virus vaccine is used by scarifying the skin (eg, inside the thighs or under the tail) and painting on the vaccine. Both natural lesions and those resulting from vaccination may last as long as 4 wk, but after the scabs have dropped off, the animals can go to shows.

Culling is vital to the overall productivity of the herd. "Wasting disease" occurs quite frequently; it is not a single disease, but a syndrome. Generally, if a goat is well fed, kept in a stress-free environment, and has good teeth and a low parasite load, it should thrive and produce. If it does not, and begins "wasting", it should be culled immediately. The major causes of wasting disease, in addition to poor nutrition, parasitism, and dental problems, are paratuberculosis, internal visceral abscesses due to *Corynebacterium pseudotuberculosis (ovis)* or *C pyogenes*, locomotor problems (particularly arthritis due to retrovirus infection [CAE virus]), and any chronic hidden infections (eg, metritis, peritonitis, or pneumonia). Tumors occur rarely. None of these diseases is treatable, and many are contagious; this is the basis for the strict culling policy. Paratuberculosis in goats differs from that in cattle in that there is no profuse diarrhea, and gross postmortem lesions are rare. Consequently, many cases may go undiagnosed at necropsy. The ileocecal node is the most rewarding tissue for bacteriological culture and histopathology. Agar gel immunodiffusion is a useful serological test, but it can be used only on a herd basis for test and cull. Availability is limited, and it will not function as a pre-purchase screening test. The control program for paratuberculosis in goats is similar to that in cattle.

(*See also* MASTITIS IN GOATS, p 691.)

DISEASE-MANAGEMENT INTERACTION: HORSES

Knowledge of equine management has increased tremendously in recent years, and many losses due to disease and injury are now preventable. The 2 major management rules for an equine facility, regardless of size or number of horses, are not to overcrowd and to maintain cleanliness. Unfortunately, many facilities do not meet these criteria, which frequently are compromised in favor of economics.

In most instances, the veterinarian is asked to attend to a sick or injured animal, or to administer prophylactic agents; rarely is advice requested regarding management. However, because management plays a major role in the prevention of disease and injury, the veterinarian must understand and be aware of medical and physical management practices.

In horses, the single most important factor contributing to disease and injury is overcrowding. Prevention of disease and injury can best be achieved through nutritional management, adequate housing, vaccination programs, parasite control, cleanliness, and general equine husbandry.

Proper nutrition is important in maintaining health. Nutritional demands vary with age, size, use, and pregnancy (*see* NUTRITION: HORSES, p 1225); they are usually met with good-quality forages and roughages combined with grain concentrate or protein supplement. Free-choice salt is recommended. Vitamin supplementation is generally not necessary except when roughage is of low quality. Constant availability of clean water is essential. When horses are fed in groups, adequate amounts of feed should be spaced so that every horse can eat comfortably.

Housing requirements are also quite variable. When stalls are used, they should be of adequate size and proper construction to minimize chances of injury to the horse. Stalls that are 12 ft × 12 ft (3.7 m × 3.7 m) are adequate for most horses, although larger ones are preferred for pregnant mares (especially at foaling) and breeding stallions. Walls should be free of protruding bolts, nails, etc, and should be constructed to withstand kicking. Doors should be wide enough (≥4 ft [1.2 m]) to allow easy entry and exit without risk of injury, especially to the shoulders or tuber coxae. Individual hay and grain feeding equipment and watering facilities should be provided. Flooring should have good footing and, ideally, allow for drainage of urine and water.

Proper ventilation is important: respiratory problems are aggravated by ammonia and dusty conditions in the stable. Overhead storage of hay and straw can contribute to dust in the environment and should be avoided if possible. Feed should be stored in an area not accessible to horses to prevent accidental grain overload, and in bins or containers to prevent rodent contamination. Manure- and urine-soaked bedding should be removed daily to prevent conditions such as thrush, and buildup of ammonia. If manure is spread on pastures, it should first be allowed to compost to reduce contamination with parasite ova. Stabled horses not in a regular training program should be allowed adequate exercise to help prevent development of vices (*see* BEHAVIOR, p 895 *et seq*) and to maintain general health.

Bands of horses not being used daily may be housed satisfactorily in open sheds. If halters are left on horses while on pasture, they should be leather; if a halter becomes caught on an object while on the horse, leather is more apt to break readily than is nylon, which may prevent self-inflicted trauma. Paddock and pasture fencing should provide a secure enclosure free of objects that can cause lacerations. Well-constructed wooden fences, steel pipes, or tightly woven wire fences kept in good repair are generally adequate. Wood and woven wire should be secured to posts from the inside. Fences should be ~5 ft (1.5 m) high and, ideally, have 12 ft (3.7 m) spacing between adjacent paddocks or pastures. Narrow corners should be avoided to prevent injury to other horses by the dominant individual. Overcrowding should be avoided to minimize injuries due to kicking and fighting.

An important but often overlooked method of disease prevention is avoiding exposure. Horses are commonly mingled at shows, sales, trail rides, race meets etc. Animals so exposed should be isolated for ≥2 wk to minimize risk of spreading disease to other animals in the stable or on the farm. Separate feeding and watering equipment and tack also should be provided. Likewise, people caring for isolated horses should minimize contact with other horses on the farm. Good insect control and proper manure disposal also can help prevent spread of disease.

Many believe that routine administration of mild enemas to newborn foals is advisable to prevent retention of meconium (*see also* COLIC IN FOALS, p 172).

VACCINATION

Vaccines are available for many of the serious infectious diseases, including tetanus, encephalomyelitis, influenza, rhinopneumonitis, strangles, and viral arteritis. Vaccines for equine encephalomyelitis (eastern, western, and Venezuelan) are effective and long-lasting; high antibody titers are produced and persist >1 yr.

Equine encephalomyelitis vaccines are commonly combined with tetanus toxoid. Two initial vaccinations are recommended (1 mo apart), followed by annual revaccination. It is important that the vaccine be administered before the mosquito season begins.

Influenza and equine herpesvirus 1 (rhinopneumonitis) vaccines produce low titers of short duration (~2-3 mo). Therefore, frequent vaccination is recommended for high-risk groups of young horses if protection is to be maintained. Vaccination of high-risk animals for influenza, using a bivalent vaccine (influenza virus A_1 and A_2) should be repeated q3mo. Vaccinations should not be administered immediately before performance events due to injection site reactions. For low-risk horses, annual vaccination before the season of use may be adequate. Foals should be vaccinated at ~3 mo of age followed by a booster 2-3 mo later.

There are 2 types of vaccines for equine herpesvirus 1. Although not licensed in all countries, a modified live vaccine, used to prevent respiratory and neurologic forms of the disease, may be administered initially in 2 doses (1 mo apart) followed by boosters at 6-mo intervals. The interval may be reduced to 3 mo in high-risk horses. The killed vaccine, used primarily in broodmares to prevent abortion, is given at 5, 7, and 9 mo of pregnancy.

Young horses (6 mo to 3 yr) should be vaccinated against common respiratory diseases such as influenza and rhinopneumonitis ~2 wk before expected gathering dates at sales, shows, training stables, etc.

Vaccination for strangles is recommended if exposure is likely (public stables, breeding farms, etc). Horses require 3 vaccinations (2-wk intervals) during the initial series. Revaccination should be annual or any time exposure is likely. In facilities where exposure to the organism is likely, pregnant mares should be vaccinated ≥1 mo before foaling. Vaccination for viral arteritis is used primarily in breeding animals, and its use is restricted in some states. The initial vaccination should be followed by an annual booster. All breeding horses, including mares after foaling, should be vaccinated ≥3 wk before breeding.

Appropriate vaccination is helpful, but no vaccine is effective in every case. Good management must constantly be practiced to prevent stress, which can precipitate disease even in vaccinated animals. Vaccination of mares ~1 mo before expected foaling date can enhance protection of newborn foals against bacterial and viral infection via passively derived colostral antibodies. Age of foals at vaccination is also an important consideration. Vaccinating too early may not be effective due to interference from maternal antibodies. The duration of maternal antibodies in newborn foals varies for each specific disease entity; therefore, recommendations should be followed strictly.

PARASITE CONTROL

Internal parasitism is one of the most serious of all equine disease problems. Parasitism is commonly associated with poor coat and general unthriftiness, and is also associated with a high incidence of colic. The most severe problems are caused by large strongyles and roundworms in younger horses. Less severe problems are caused by small strongyles, pinworms, stomach worms, bots, and tapeworms. *See also* p 201.

Stable and pasture management can be helpful in parasite control. Stalls should be cleaned regularly, and manure should be composted before being spread on pastures where horses graze. Pastures should not be overstocked and should be rotated regularly. Young horses should be separated from older horses after weaning. New animals should have fecal examinations and receive appropriate anthelmintics before addition to pastures. Fecal contamination of feed and water should be avoided.

Under many conditions, foals up to 1 yr old should be treated with an effective anthelmintic at 2-mo intervals. Rotation between different groups of anthelmintics is helpful in preventing development of resistance. Periodic examination of feces can help evaluate anthelmintic efficacy and adequacy of management procedures.

TRANSPORTATION

Horses are frequently injured during transportation. Many of these injuries are due to improper preparation of the animal before loading. Trailers and vans should be free of protruding objects, and should be of adequate height. When appropriate, protective devices such as helmets, leg wraps, boots, blankets, and tail wraps can further protect the animal from injury.

Available hay in the trailer helps prevent boredom during transit. Suitable flooring (rubber mats, straw, shavings, or a combination of these) should be available on long transits. Appropriate rest stops should be planned: when trips are ≥24 hr, an overnight rest stop and fresh water should be given; on shorter trips, a walking rest stop with water should be adequate. Tranquilizers should be used carefully since they may result in incoordination, intestinal stasis, and penile paralysis in stallions. Administration of mineral oil may help prevent intestinal stasis during long trips.

DENTAL CARE

The teeth should be checked periodically and floated when necessary. Young horses should be examined for proper tooth eruption, caps on the upper molars, and other abnormalities. These problems should be corrected as soon as possible. (*See* DENTISTRY, LG AN, p 115).

FOOT CARE

Proper foot care is essential to maintain normal health of the foot and to prevent lameness. The hooves should be trimmed regularly, usually at 3- to 6-wk intervals depending on the use of the horse and the ground surface the horse is running on. When horses are shod, the same interval for shoeing or resetting is usually appropriate.

The feet should be cleaned frequently. For stabled horses, clean dry bedding should be maintained to help prevent thrush. Excessive dryness of the hoof should be avoided.

DISEASE-MANAGEMENT INTERACTION: PIGS

Proper management can increase reproductive performance and feed utilization, and reduce mortality. Disease in farm animals is often the end result of inadequate management. Independent of management, pigs are susceptible to many devastating infections; however, sensible control of their contact with people, and adherence to the closed herd principle will minimize the risk of infection. Management of the pig-people-environment interaction has the greatest effect on disease expression and on productivity. In many cases, clinical disease is merely the indicator of failure in one or more of these interactions. Treatment of disease through chemotherapy is a first step in disease control, but elimination of the underlying environmental or management problem is the most important one.

When large numbers of pigs are housed together, pig-to-pig and pig-to-environment interactions are enhanced and manager-to-pig interaction is diminished. These are the basis of disease problems on intensive swine farms, and an understanding of their consequences is necessary to reduce health-related losses in modern pig enterprises. The losses in extensive production units due to management and environmental factors may be even greater than those on intensive farms, but are not discussed here.

On poorly managed farms, ~30% of pigs do not survive to market weight: ~6% are stillborn; ~20% die before weaning, 2% in the nursery, and 2% during the grower-finisher stages of production. The stillbirth rate increases with size of the litter (and thus with parity of the sow) and with any other factor that prolongs parturition. Since both parity distribution and farrowing speed are influenced by management, their role in stillbirth problems must be investigated thoroughly. There are, of course, some infections that increase the stillbirth rate, eg, leptospirosis, encephalomyocarditis virus, and parvovirus infections.

Once the piglet is born, its survival past the first 4 days depends on 3 major factors: 1) adequate intake of energy, 2) suitable environmental temperature, and 3) immunity to intestinal colibacillosis, the major infectious cause of diarrhea in neonatal piglets.

Since piglets are born with limited glycogen reserves, they need to replace and add to their energy reserves within hours of birth. If energy (colostrum) is not acquired, mortality due to hypoglycemia will follow. Hypoglycemia (qv, p 1093) probably is the most common cause of piglet death. Several management procedures may reduce these starvation losses.

Piglets that are below average weight at birth have a much higher mortality than do heavier pigs. These losses are affected mainly by variation in birthweight and environmental temperature, both of which can be altered by management practices. Older sows have larger litters and greater variation in birthweight within each litter. There are also small pigs in many younger sows' litters. The intense competition among newborn piglets results in smaller pigs being relegated to poorly producing or nonproducing mammary glands; this leads to decreased energy intake, accentuation of hypothermia and hypoglycemia, and for many, death. Equalizing piglet weights within litters by cross-fostering in the first few hours of life eliminates or markedly reduces losses, and can have a dramatic effect on overall mortality rates. Small pigs, having greater surface area per kg of body wt than larger pigs, suffer greater heat loss, are more sensitive to low environmental temperatures, and die from hypoglycemia more rapidly than do larger pigs. Piglets should be born and maintained for 1 wk in environmental temperatures of 86-93°F (30-34°C).

In addition to its vital role in supplying energy, colostrum supplies piglets with antibodies to protect them against common infections. The most common fatal infection is intestinal colibacillosis; this can be reduced by vaccinating the sow, which provides antibodies to the piglet via the colostrum and milk.

Any disease of the sow that results in reduced milk production increases susceptibility to *Escherichia coli* diarrhea, as does low environmental temperature, which slows gut motility. (*See also* MASTITIS, p 692, and MMA, p 657.) Slower passing of milk and its antibodies through the intestines enables *E coli* to adhere more readily to the intestinal wall; they then produce enterotoxins that cause excess secretion of the intestinal cells and diarrhea. Other bacterial infections, notably of *Streptococcus suis*, may present problems in the neonatal period. Great care in dipping umbilical cords in iodine soon after birth, and tails after docking, is important in minimizing these conditions.

Significant numbers of piglets die from crushing in the first few days after birth. The sow is likely to lie on piglets if she is clumsy, if the warmest spot in the farrowing pen is next to her, or if the piglets are hypoglycemic and sleepy. Suitably designed farrowing crates and correctly placed heat lamps can minimize losses from crushing, though they are unlikely to completely eliminate them.

Careful attention to these management factors usually reduces neonatal mortality to 5-10%. Even in extensive systems, at least some of the neonatal pig mortality is management-induced, and to this extent, avoidable.

After weaning, fewer pigs die: 1-2% mortality is considered acceptable on a commercial basis, but 0.5% is attainable. The major infectious disease is diarrhea, but starvation and inadequate growth are also problems. Weaning is a particularly stressful period due to a change in diet and also in surroundings and often in social order. Generally, the earlier the weaning, the more important management becomes. At weaning, piglets should have enough trough space to allow them all to eat at the same time. They should have ready and continuous access to fluids, but should be fed little and often with highly palatable feed. Ideally, they should be kept in their litter groups. Each of these procedures is aimed at minimizing the changes from their preweaning environment. Environmental temperature is critical, and pigs maintained in suboptimal temperatures frequently succumb to diarrheal disease. Depending on the age of pigs to be weaned, environmental temperatures should be maintained at 77-80°F (25-27°C). Size at weaning is as important as age; small pigs are more likely to starve or have diarrhea because their digestive enzymes are not fully developed. Postweaning diarrhea may be associated with immune sensitization to dietary antigens during the neonatal period, but work is needed to substantiate this before creep-feeding practices are modified. Oral fluid therapy is a good adjunct to antibiotics in the prevention and treatment of postweaning diarrhea.

In warm environments, skin diseases such as greasy pig disease and sarcoptic mange seem to be more prevalent and should be dealt with promptly. *Streptococcus suis* infection occurs in intensively maintained, recently weaned pigs, especially in overcrowded situations. Mulberry heart disease is becoming more common where environmental conditions are good and the pigs are growing rapidly; this requires increased selenium and/or vitamin E for the sows and, in some circumstances, injection of selenium at weaning.

The greatest economic losses due to inadequate management occur in the grower-finisher stage of production. Respiratory diseases such as atrophic rhinitis and enzootic pneumonia, and intestinal diseases such as porcine intestinal adenomatosis and swine dysentery significantly reduce growth rate and efficiency of feed utilization.

With good ventilation and spacing, pigs in many herds with endemic respiratory infections, eg, enzootic pneumonia, grow at rates almost identical to those free of the infection. Most herds could improve growth efficiency in environments that permit the pigs to contain the respiratory infection themselves, rather than having to rely on antibiotic prophylaxis.

Swine dysentery is a costly disease that justifies the strictest quarantine procedures to ensure that the causative organism, *Treponema hyodysenteriae*, does not gain entrance to herds free of the disease. Most farms have inadequate quarantine facilities and containment procedures. Reliance is usually placed on the development and recognition of clinical signs in purchased animals. Use of sentinels and serological testing of purchased and sentinel animals at intervals of 3-4 wk before permitting them to join the main herd are minimal precautions necessary to prevent the introduction of certain infections. Prevention of introduction of swine dysentery, transmissible gastroenteritis, campylobacteriosis, mange, streptococcosis, etc, relies on the purchase of healthy stock from a reputable breeding unit.

Management practices greatly influence reproduction. Simply maintaining an optimal average sow age benefits reproductive efficiency, especially litter size. After 6-8 litters, the number of live-born pigs is only ~1 more than for a gilt. Since the cost of feeding a sow exceeds that of feeding a gilt by about the value of 1 pig, it is economically sound to maintain the sows in the herd with parities of 3-6. This necessitates a culling rate of ~30% annually: if the culling rate is greater than this, average litter size may be reduced because of the larger number of gilts; if culling is <30%, litter size may be reduced through an increase in stillbirths.

Insufficient energy intake during lactation results in reduced conception rates and reduced subsequent litter size, especially between the first and second parities. Infertility at this time is a common cause of culling. The second most important cause of sow culling is lameness, and this is often management-induced; rough or slippery concrete floors in combination with excessive moisture can soften the hooves, as will a shortage of biotin in the early growing period.

In addition to direct traumatic hoof injury, other lamenesses are associated with fighting injuries that occur when sows are mixed after weaning. This is especially common when small first-litter sows are mixed with larger ones.

DISEASE-MANAGEMENT INTERACTION: SHEEP

The major products from sheep are meat and wool; hides and milk are important in some areas of the world. Sheep are raised in many different environments, with great variation in efficiency. The type of system in any area depends on many factors, including breed of sheep, type of breeding program, terrain, weather, availability of nutrients, predators, land and building costs, shelter, availability of skilled labor, and interrelationships with other livestock or cropping systems.

In North America, the 4 major production systems are: 1) total confinement, in which sheep are housed in facilities with light and temperature control, and with minimal access to outdoor pens or pasture; 2) semiconfinement, in which open-front buildings are used for lambing, and sheep have access to pastures for 6-8 mo of the year; 3) range lambing with shelter; and 4) range lambing with minimal observation. The size of farm flocks varies greatly, and many units consist of <100 breeding ewes. Each system requires different management skills and controls, and the productivity potential varies greatly among the systems. Furthermore, disease incidence can vary dramatically, depending on the production system.

The roles of management, nutrition, and disease in sheep flocks are closely interrelated; a multifaceted epidemiological approach to identifying specific factors that limit either health or production is likely to be more rewarding than a one disease/one agent/one drug (or vaccine) approach. Thus, periodic reviews of flock health status are likely to be cost effective. When possible, problems should be investigated from a flock standpoint, and resolution attempted only after a complete history has been taken, representative animals have been examined, and laboratory or necropsy findings reviewed.

The efficiency of an operation is aided by accurate recording of health and production data, provided that individual animals are appropriately identified, weighed, or condition scored at intervals, and results of lambing, cause of losses, and other health-related events recorded. For larger flocks, a computerized system has marked advantages, particularly for detecting suboptimal performance and identifying animals for culling. Adequate physical facilities for yarding, segregating, weighing, lambing, examining, dipping or spraying, and medicating individual animals are required.

PREGNANCY AND LAMBING

Preparturient losses (abortions) may be caused by infections, including campylobacteriosis, salmonellosis, toxoplasmosis, chlamydiosis, listeriosis, and leptospirosis. When there is a history of campylobacteriosis or chlamydiosis, ewes should be vaccinated before breeding. Sheep seropositive for toxoplasmosis are unlikely to abort, so if depopulation or removal of cats is not practical, ewes should be exposed before their first mating. Recently purchased ewes should be lambed separately, and aborting ewes should be isolated. Listeriosis has been associated with feeding corn silage. Vaccination of pregnant ewes may be indicated when there is a risk of parturient infections (eg, *Clostridium septicum* or *C chauvoei*), or when it is desirable to passively protect the newborn lamb (eg, from enterotoxemia or tetanus).

Lambing management is critical to minimize losses. Selection for ewes that lamb unassisted and within a short period is recommended. Depending on season and shelter, lambing can occur indoors or out. Good environmental hygiene is essential to minimize the risk of perinatal infections. When possible, newborn lambs should have their navels clipped and dipped in aqueous iodine to reduce the risk of infection. Ewes should be checked carefully for mastitis and patency of teat ducts. Starvation is a major factor in many lamb deaths. If maternal colostrum is unavailable, a supplemental frozen supply (caprine or bovine colostrum may be substituted) should be available, and the lamb should receive $3^{1}/_{2}$-$6^{1}/_{2}$ oz (100-200 mL) by stomach tube during the first 24 hr.

A bonding period of at least 24-36 hr in small pens or cubicles, as well as branding of ewes and lambs, is recommended to avoid subsequent mismothering problems. Various techniques promote fostering of orphan lambs (<3 wk old) by ewes that have lost a lamb. These include applying vaginal discharges from the foster ewe to the lamb or covering the lamb with the hide of the dead lamb. Poorly bonded or weak lambs can be fatally injured by aggressive ewes; this can be minimized by keeping ewes and lambs in small groups before moving to larger mixing pens.

Excess lambs can be reared on milk replacer diets containing 25% crude fat, 25% protein, 25% lactose, 6-7% ash, and 0.5% fiber. Calf milk replacers are not recommended.

Lambs usually are castrated and docked within the first 10 days of life. A variety of methods are available: sectioning by knife, electrocautery, and pressure by "burdizzo" type instruments or "elastrator" rubber rings. The latter methods reduce the risk of hemorrhage in larger lambs, but "elastrator" rings carry an increased risk of tetanus. Whichever method is used, clean techniques and equipment are essential.

Lambs usually are vaccinated at 10-14 days against enterotoxemia (*Clostridium perfringens* types C and/or D); vaccination should be repeated at least once (2-4 wk later), and preferably again when the lambs are put on concentrate rations. If contagious ecthyma is endemic in the flock, this vaccine should be given soon after birth.

PERINATAL LOSSES

Selection for "easy care" sheep that require minimal attention during or after lambing appears to offer the best solution to this problem, since rearing ability is both repeatable and heritable. Dead lambs should be necropsied to establish the major causes of deaths. Probably the most important cause of perinatal mortality is the starvation-mismothered-exposure complex, a major component of which is birth injury to the CNS. Prolonged parturition, often as a result of feto-pelvic disproportion, appears to be a major cause of birth injury.

Prenatal nutrition affects perinatal survival through its effect on lamb birthweight. During the last trimester, overfeeding causes increased birthweight, particularly of single lambs, and subsequent dystocia; underfeeding results in low birthweight, particularly of multiple lambs, and increases the risk of hypothermia. The survival rate is highest when lamb birthweight is 7-11 lb (3-5 kg).

Shearing provides a suitable opportunity to treat all ewes for both ecto- and endoparasites, if necessary.

Pneumonia and enteritis can cause high morbidity and mortality, particularly in flocks raised in confinement. Inadequate ventilation, overcrowding, colostrum deprivation, and unhygienic conditions in the lambing area all significantly increase the risk of these diseases. Prompt antibiotic or anticoccidial treatments help reduce losses.

NUTRITION

(*See also* p 1278.) Feed costs (ewe and lambs) constitute 60-70% of production expenses in intensive systems, and the ewes' annual feed costs represent about two-thirds of these. Feeding should be adjusted for the given stage of production so as to reach predetermined target liveweights. For example, depending on the type of breeding ewe in the flock, reasonable objectives are 60-70 lb (27-31.5 kg) for a 70-day weaning weight, 100-130 lb (50-60 kg) at mating for ewe lambs, and 140-160 lb (64-73 kg) at mating for ewes ~18 mo old (or 2 tooth).

Computerized programs to formulate least-cost rations are becoming more widely used in confinement operations. In grazing operations, the use of appropriate forages and grazing techniques, such as use of electric fences, can significantly increase production per unit area. Any poisonous plants in the area should be noted and appropriate precautions taken, particularly when grazing pressures and seasonal influences may increase potential risks.

In late pregnancy, ketosis (pregnancy toxemia) is an important cause of losses in both lambs and ewes, particularly in ewes that are overly fat or thin in early pregnancy, or are carrying multiple fetuses. Ewes should be introduced to concentrates or high-quality forages in the last 6 wk of pregnancy and be fed at least daily to avoid ruminal acidosis. Adequate trough space should be provided, and it may be expedient to separate ewes in poorer condition and "shy" feeders from the rest of the flock. However, ewes fat at lambing are more likely to experience dystocias or vaginal prolapses.

Ideally, lambs should have access to good legume-based pasture or be creep fed from an early age. Creep feeding can be encouraged by using a palatable, high-protein ration in a well-lighted area with several openings for lambs. Medication with lasalocid (20-30 g/ton of feed [15-70 mg/head/day]) to reduce the risk of coccidiosis is recommended.

After weaning, lambs are destined for slaughter at varying liveweights (up to 120 lb [54 kg]), or to be breeder replacements. Range producers often sell lambs as feeders for subsequent finishing in feedlots. Recently moved animals require careful adaptation to their new surroundings; season, geographic origin and distance traveled, weather, and available shelter must be considered. If lambs cannot be finished and sold before hot weather, they are best shorn. Animals should be adjusted gradually to concentrate feed to avoid ruminal acidosis (*see* GRAIN OVERLOAD, p 175). Ionophores in the ration may assist in this regard. A free-choice, untreated, accessible water supply is desirable for maximal growth. Reluctant feeders or ill animals should be segregated and treated appropriately.

After weaning, ewes need to regain weight lost during lactation and to maintain wool growth. Older or thinner ewes and rams should be fed separately. Feed additives are used to promote growth in finishing lambs; these include antibiotics, ionophores, and anabolic agents. Recommended withdrawal times should be observed before animals are slaughtered. In finishing rams or wethers, and occasionally in older animals, urolithiasis can be a significant problem, especially if high-concentrate rations with inappropriate calcium:phosphorus ratios are fed. The latter should be adjusted to 2:1 with powdered limestone, a urinary acidifier such as ammonium chloride added to the ration (0.2-0.5%), and ample water provided.

Sheep usually are supplied with free-choice, trace mineralized salt; selenium and iodine are commonly incorporated. Copper also may be needed, but all ages of sheep are highly susceptible to copper toxicity and, as with selenium, the need should be defined before the addition is made.

Wool chewing in lambs or adult sheep under confinement conditions can be minimized by providing more roughage, such as long-stemmed hay.

INFECTIOUS DISEASE CONTROL PROCEDURES

Vaccination programs should consider the probabilities of the diseases occurring either on the farm or in the general area, the economics of vaccination, and the class of animal to be protected (adult, fetus, or newborn). The following vaccines, bacterins, or toxoids are usually available, either singly or in various combinations: *Clostridium tetani* toxoid, especially to protect young lambs following docking and castration; *C perfringens* (types C and D) toxoids to protect newborn lambs passively or older lambs actively; *Bacteroides nodosus* vaccine to prevent contagious foot rot in all age groups; *Campylobacter fetus* bacterins to prevent abortion in late pregnancy; *Chlamydia psittaci* vaccine to prevent ovine enzootic abortion in late pregnancy; *Brucella ovis* vaccine to prevent epididymitis; contagious ecthyma vaccine (live) to prevent disease in lambs and adults; rabies vaccine (inactivated); bluetongue vaccine (modified live) for use in endemic areas; and *Corynebacterium ovis* bacterins.

Vaccines intended for use in other species occasionally are used in sheep, eg, *Leptospira* spp bacterins and parainfluenza 3 (live) vaccine. *Listeria monocytogenes* bacterins are available for experimental use.

FOOT CARE

Infectious foot rot (qv, p 541) is one of the more difficult diseases of sheep to control or eradicate. A regular system of foot care, including careful trimming and inspection of any lameness, is necessary for early detection. Noninfected flocks should be protected by isolation and careful inspection of any introduced animals. Foot abscesses, usually of one digit, are relatively common in some flocks, and need to be differentiated from foot rot.

PARASITISM

Management practices in relation to both endo- and ectoparasite control are an integral component of any sheep production system. The prevalence and epidemiology of parasitic species vary greatly depending on the climate, geographical region, and production system. (*See also* pp 98 and 209.)

CULLING AND PURCHASING PRACTICES

Assuming that adequate records are available and adult animals are identifiable, culling of surplus animals, usually after weaning, is an important management practice. The ability of a ewe to give birth unassisted to 2 or more lambs, and raise them successfully to weaning should ensure her retention in the flock. While younger ewes may produce more lambs than older ones, the latter are usually better mothers and, especially under confinement or semiconfinement systems, can reproduce successfully until 8-10 yr old. Systematic culling of inferior and aging ewes and retention of superior young ewes keeps the flock permanently young.

Indications for culling include udder abnormalities (eg, mastitis, nonpatent teats, injuries), mouth or tooth problems (eg, missing incisors, excessive or abnormal wear of incisors, over- or undershot jaws, periodontal disease), and reproductive problems (eg, repeated dystocias, vaginal or uterine prolapses). Aborting ewes, especially younger ones, may well be retained on the assumption that they will develop some degree of immunity to whatever agent may have been involved, although the cause should be sought if abortions are more than sporadic. Rams with evidence of infectious epididymitis are best culled, as are animals with chronic foot problems.

Replacement ewes or rams are best purchased directly from the farm of origin. If large numbers are being purchased, a random sample should be examined carefully, and particular attention paid to any abnormalities of teeth, feet, or udders. A 1-mo quarantine for new arrivals is recommended, during which time the animals can be treated for parasitism, shorn if necessary, and observed for signs of infectious disease.

PREDATOR CONTROL

The sheep industry has to cope with predation by both feral and nonferal species. While no single control method is universally effective, various techniques have been developed and evaluated: the 2 most promising are electric fences and livestock guard dogs. The former, if properly designed and operated, have excellent potential for predator exclusion; the use of dogs appears to be more successful in flocks of <1000 sheep, and less so when sheep are widely scattered.

DISEASE-MANAGEMENT INTERACTION: SMALL ANIMALS

Proper management to prevent and control disease is as important in dogs and cats as in any other species; it is no less important to the owner of 1 or 2 pets than it is to the owner of a kennel or cattery. However, the household pet frequently shares its owner's residence, and usually is not subject to the wide range of environmental factors that may affect a kenneled population.

The owner of a household pet should be instructed in the basic responsibilities of pet ownership: 1) routine care and grooming, 2) preventive medicine, 3) parasite control, 4) nutrition, 5) common sense prevention of household accidents and hazards, and 6) environmental and housing needs.

Routine care is an aid to good health; personal attention during grooming of the animal provides the owner an opportunity to assess general condition, detect skin lesions, etc. Attention should be given to the coat, ears, nails, and teeth. If the nails are not trimmed periodically they may cause the feet to splay, or cause discomfort; excessively long nails may grow into the foot pads and cause lameness.

Preventive medicine: Most pets run the risk of exposure to various infectious diseases. Dogs should be vaccinated against distemper, hepatitis, leptospirosis, parvovirus, coronavirus, rabies, and tracheobronchitis; and cats against panleukopenia, rhinotracheitis virus, calicivirus, leukemia, and rabies. The exact diseases and immunization schedule vary with the risk, immune status of the dam, etc.

Parasite control is especially important in the young; intestinal infections acquired *in utero* or at nursing can become overwhelming by 3-4 wk of age. Activation of hypobiotic larvae in the dam makes neonatal infection virtually certain. Ectoparasites may cause severe disease, or serve as vectors of others. Periodic fecal exams and a strong preventive program based on sanitation are recommended. In endemic areas, a heartworm preventive program is essential.

Nutrition often is poorly understood by owners; although many feed a commercially prepared diet, others feed only scraps, others over-supplement the diet, and still others (with misguided good intentions) restrict the diet to a single category, eg, fish or organ meats. Prolonged malnutrition causes various clinical manifestations, depending on the nutrients involved. Signs usually are first noted in the skin and coat, or the skeletal system.

Specially formulated diets for particular circumstances (growth, stress, lactation, etc) are available. Feline urological syndrome may be amenable to dietary control. Some dogs are predisposed to gastric dilatation, and owners should be advised of the spatial relationship between eating, exercise, and dilatation. Sudden changes in diet often cause a transient diarrhea.

Water quality is often ignored since many areas are on carefully controlled municipal water supply systems. However, a water analysis should not be overlooked when trying to determine the cause of illness in a kennel or cattery. Excessive levels of nitrates have been incriminated in some kennels. Heavy metal and pesticide screens may be indicated as well.

Household hazards: Owners should be reminded of the obvious potential dangers when pets have access to electrical cords, household supplies, poisonous plants, etc. Less obvious hazards may include slippery floors or stairs, which may exacerbate arthritic conditions or locomotor difficulties.

Housing needs are more applicable in a kennel or cattery; improper design or construction can cause myriad problems. Good ventilation is essential: feline respiratory disease and canine infectious tracheobronchitis are common in confined populations, but the incidence is dramatically lower when ventilation is adequate.

Porous surfaces are difficult to clean and may harbor infectious agents, including parasite ova, as well as urine or cleaning agents that may irritate the skin. Run surfaces should provide good drainage and, ideally, provide secure footing but not abrade the foot pads. Large breeds of dogs are prone to develop hygromas over bony prominences when they are not provided soft bedding. Similarly, cages must be nonporous and easily cleaned; flooring should be such that nails and foot pads will not be torn or become stuck. Dogs confined on wire flooring frequently develop interdigital cysts. Some painted surfaces, cages, and glazed ceramic bowls may contain lead and eventually result in lead poisoning.

MANAGEMENT OF REPRODUCTION: CATTLE *

Reproductive performance can be improved by properly identifying animals; keeping records that enable determination of important herd indices, such as percent calf crop, pregnancy rate, length of calving season, culling rates, calf mortality, breeding efficiency of bulls, and performance production information; meeting the nutritional requirements of various classes of livestock in the herd, emphasizing the nutritional needs and cost efficiencies; establishing a breeding program for heifer replacements and cows; practicing bull selection and reproductive management; adopting an immunization program for the cow/calf herd, bulls, and calves; evaluating all abortions; giving careful attention at calving; providing adequate facilities; and ensuring that the calf is well cared for at birth, and receives adequate colostrum.

The national (USA) calf crop average is ~70%. A realistic and major goal of every cow/calf operator and dairyman should be to raise or market 95 calves per 100 cows, every year. A workable record-keeping system is imperative if progress is to be attained in reproductive performance. Records that allow calculation of herd indices such as pregnancy rate, length of calving season, culling rate, and calf mortality are invaluable in assessing performance and determining what changes are

---

*Adapted from a joint effort by the National Cattlemen's Association and the American Association of Bovine Practitioners.

needed. Individual animal identification is equally important when culling and selecting.

NUTRITION

Nutrition is the most important management factor in maintaining the desired short calving season every year in beef breeding herds. The limiting nutrient related to reproduction in beef cattle is usually **energy**, but this is not as significant in dairy cattle since most are fed rations that supply adequate energy during lactation. The level of energy before calving primarily influences when a cow returns to estrus, while level of energy after calving primarily influences conception rate. Feed requirements vary during the reproductive cycle (*see* NUTRIENT REQUIREMENTS OF BEEF CATTLE, TABLE 14, p 1179).

Period 1 (interval from calving to breeding—82 days) is the period of greatest nutritional demand. The cow is at maximal milk flow, recovering from the stress of parturition, and by the end of the period she is expected to be ready to breed.

Period 2 (interval from rebreeding to weaning the calf—123 days [beef cows]). Periods 2 and 3 overlap in dairy cows and are not as easily separated as in beef cattle. The beef cow should gain weight while still milking. Although some dairy cows maintain body weight, most high producers lose weight during this period.

Period 3 (weaning to 50 days before calving—110 days). The beef cow has only to maintain her condition and develop a fetus. Her needs are the least of any stage of the cycle. The dairy cow should gain body weight during the last few months of lactation.

Period 4 (a critical stage preceding calving—50 days). During the last 50 days of pregnancy, 75% of fetal growth occurs. Cow condition at calving is critical to rebreeding; the onset of estrus after calving is delayed in cows that lose weight or are thin and not gaining during late pregnancy.

The dairy cow (*see* NUTRITIONAL REQUIREMENTS OF DAIRY CATTLE, p 1182) is usually fed for maximal milk production throughout her 10-mo lactation. It is assumed that she will lose weight during heavy lactation and regain the loss during the remainder of lactation. The dairy cow should not be overfed during the dry period because of the fatty liver syndrome (qv, p 444).

The amount of cow feed required per pound of calf weaned is fairly constant, although larger cows require more feed than smaller cows. Cows that give more milk require more feed with a higher level of protein. Increased milk is produced at the expense of reproduction when feed is not adequate to meet all needs.

The **protein** requirement of young growing stock and heavy milkers is often a limiting factor, while mature dry cows are often overfed protein. Heifers must be fed adequately from weaning to breeding if they are to calve at 2 yr of age.

To do a proper job of providing the essential nutrient requirements during various stages of the reproductive cycle, major roughages and homegrown grains should undergo analysis to monitor true nutrient content and actual dollar value. Variation in amounts of trace minerals is common between and within different geographic areas, which further supports the need to use specific feed analysis information.

Two systems used to determine energy levels of the ration are the Total Digestible Nutrient System and the California Net Energy System. Both are commonly used, and application should be tailored to fit the individual operation. (For nutrient requirements of cows of various weights and by period, *see* TABLE 16, p 1184.)

Even within nutritional need categories, cattle benefit from feeding and handling in subgroups: lightweight heifers at weaning need to gain more than heavier heifers to reach puberty by breeding season; first-calf heifers require special attention from both an energy and competition standpoint if they are expected to be rebred. These heifers are still growing, as well as lactating, and they may not have the rumen capacity to meet postcalving energy needs on roughage alone. Supplemental feeding of both high-energy and high-protein feeds to first-calf heifers may be required to realize optimal reproductive potential. Many operators wean calves from first-calf beef heifers 30-40 days earlier than from cows in the main herd to allow the heifer more time to grow and recover from demands associated with lactation.

Thin, old, and small cows may not compete favorably with heavier cows within the same herd and often benefit from being fed as a separate subgroup.

Lactating dairy cattle are usually fed according to milk production. They may be fed concentrate on an individual basis or divided into groups according to milk production and fed an appropriate complete blended ration.

BREEDING PROGRAM—HEIFER REPLACEMENTS AND COWS

If a cow is to calve consistently, she must be early with her first calf. Puberty is a function of breed, age, and weight. Heifers that are bred at 14 mo and calve at 23 mo have 2 advantages: 1) they get closer attention by calving before the main herd starts to calve, and 2) they have the extra time needed to rebreed. For heifers to breed at 14 mo, they should have attained at least 65-75% of their projected mature weight; therefore, adequate nutrition of the growing heifer is of major importance. The breeding season for virgin beef heifers should start 3 wk before that of the main cow herd. Since dairy cattle calve throughout the year, the above considerations do not apply to them.

To compensate for the greater attrition rate usually experienced with virgin heifers, a greater number should be bred than is needed. The cost of energy, protein and mineral supplementation, interest rates, and expected value of surplus heifers must be considered when these decisions are made.

IRREGULARITIES OF ESTRUS AND ANESTRUS

Obviously, breeding will not occur if the cow is anestrous, or if estrus is undetected. Anestrus or irregular estrous cycles in the cow may result from a number of factors, including poor management or nutrition, disease, injury, or disturbances in endocrine functions. One of the most important of the management factors in artifically bred herds is failure to observe estrus. The average duration of estrus is 18 hr, but in many cows it is appreciably shorter. A systematic program for observing cows in estrus is important if they are to be bred at the right time. A husbandryman must be familiar with signs of estrus. Cows given an androgen, steers, or bulls altered so they cannot inseminate cows make excellent estrus detectors and are used in many artificially bred herds. Aids in heat detection, such as chalk marks on the tailhead, a device attached to the tailhead of the cow that reveals when other cows have been riding, or a vaginal probe that measures the electrical conductivity of the vaginal mucus, are valuable adjuncts to the heat-detection program. Accidental access of bulls to cows and failure to keep proper breeding records often result in pregnancy without a service history.

Silent heat refers to normal follicular development and ovulation without the behavioral signs of estrus; its frequency decreases as lactation progresses, so that incidence is low by 4 mo postpartum. Those with true silent heats may be detected only through rectal palpation of the ovaries or the use of progesterone assay in milk or plasma.

The 21-day cyclic changes in the ovary, particularly in the 3-4 days before ovulation, at the time of ovulation, or 3-4 days after ovulation, generally can be recognized and the time of the cycle estimated. The corpus luteum (CL) regresses 1-2 days before the onset of estrus; it becomes smaller in size and changes from a diestrous, liver-like to a more fibrous consistency. Estrus is determined by the presence of a palpable follicle, an absent or regressed CL, and firm uterine tone. The vaginal mucosa is edematous, the cervix is relaxed and hyperemic, and a variable amount of clear serous mucus is frequently observed at the vulva, which is puffy and swollen. The immediate postovulatory period is characterized by blood in the mucous discharge and an ovary with a corpus hemorrhagicum, which on palpation is recognized as a soft area (5-15 mm in diameter) in the ovary. The CL is detectable by day 4 or 5 as a small and somewhat softer structure than the mature CL, which reaches maximum size by day 7.

During almost half the cycle, the examiner can predict the next estrus with reasonable accuracy. Thus, the cow can be watched closely for the next anticipated estrus. In cows that are approaching ovulation, the appropriate time can be estimated and the cow bred, regardless of whether she shows behavioral signs or not. Should the esti-, mate be in error and the cow exhibit signs a few days later, she can be rebred. Because these cows lack only behavioral signs of estrus, endocrine treatments are not indicated.

Regimens have been developed for the administration of prostaglandins and their analogs to synchronize estrus and reduce the dependence on observation. Prostaglandins are effective only if a cow has a functional CL. For estrus synchronization, the prostaglandin or its analog is administered to all animals. In those in days 5-18 of the cycle, the CL will regress and estrus will occur in 2-7 days. The others may either have been in estrus recently or will be in a few days. Eleven days later all animals will be between days 5 and 18 of their cycle, and prostaglandin is administered a second time. Most animals will be in estrus in 2-3 days and ovulate in 4-5 days. Breeding is done either on signs of estrus, or heifers are bred once at 60 hr and lactating cows are bred once at 72 hr after injection of the prostaglandin.

A cystic CL is not a cause of anestrus; only ~25% of cows with cystic ovarian follicles are anestrous.

Under certain circumstances, nonfunctioning ovaries are encountered. They can be recognized as smooth, small, bean-shaped structures on a single examination, or reveal no activity or change after several examinations over a period of 3 wk. The most common cause is low total energy intake during late winter.

The stress of chronic or severe disease, injury, or ovarian tumors may interrupt ovarian activity and result in anestrus. Congenital defects, such as freemartinism and ovarian hypoplasia, result in estrual failure. The treatment for inactive ovaries is correction of the basic cause; they usually do not respond to gonadotropic or steroid hormone treatment.

BULL REPRODUCTIVE MANAGEMENT

A desirable goal for beef producers is a 95% calf crop dropped within 45-65 days, with the optimal weaning weight obtained at the most efficient cost. Bull selection, management, and evaluation of performance are integral aspects of beef improvement. The bull can affect calving percentage as well as quality of calves. The use of performance-tested bulls (beef and dairy) is recommended for both natural breeding and artificial insemination.

Table 5. Recommended Disease Control Program for Bulls

Diseases to be Checked Before Using Bull	Diseases to Vaccinate Against	Breeding Soundness Examination
Brucellosis, Tuberculosis, Paratuberculosis (from a herd free of that disease)	IBR, BVD, Clostridial group, *Haemophilus*, Campylobacteriosis-Leptospirosis Administer at 6 mo and 1 yr of age. Repeat yearly, 1 mo before breeding season.	Examine at most economically advantageous period for producer (usually 1 mo before start of breeding season); *see* details below.

Bulls previously used in other herds, particularly herds in which disease status is not known, may spread diseases, particularly campylobacteriosis and trichomoniasis. Such animals should be checked for these diseases, as well as those mentioned above.

All bulls should be on the premises 2 mo before the breeding season to allow them to adapt to the environment. Isolation of all new additions to the herd (bulls or cows) is recommended for proper adaptation and preparation. A breeding soundness examination consisting of a thorough physical examination, measurement of testicles, and microscopical examination of semen should be conducted ~1 mo before the breeding season (*see also* p 1095).

During the breeding season, the bull should be watched closely for mating behavior. The standard recommendation is 25 cows for a 1- to 2-yr-old bull. There are some variations in this ratio, depending on the breeding soundness and libido of individual bulls, differences in terrain, and length of breeding season.

The weight loss that occurs in bulls during the breeding season should be restored during the off-period, but overconditioning avoided.

BREEDING

Artificial insemination (AI, *see* below) has been available for some time; it is widely used in dairy cattle and increasingly in beef cattle. When the nutritional program and heat detection are properly managed, satisfactory results are obtained. Failure to detect estrus is the major reason for unsuccessful AI. When cows are properly inseminated with good-quality semen at the proper time, 50-60% conceive on first service, the same percentage on second service.

Embryo transfer (qv, p 1102) is frequently used to increase the number of progeny from the most valuable beef and dairy cows. Cloning of embryos and sexing of spermatozoa and embryos are all being developed and may soon be adapted to field usage.

Before breeding, the following points should be considered: 1) Heifers should be bred according to size and age at puberty; at first breeding they should be 65-75% of their projected mature body weight. 2) The breeding program may be either AI or natural service. AI offers a range of bulls known to sire calves that have low birth weights. Selection of natural service bulls should be based on likely size of the calf at birth; the bull's own birth weight (not his adult weight) is a useful guide. 3) Heat synchronization of heifers and cows is now possible, but such programs depend on adequate management and cooperation. Also, sufficient skilled labor to breed and assist during calving is essential.

ARTIFICIAL INSEMINATION (AI)

In cattle, AI is utilized primarily for genetic improvement of livestock, although there are several other conditions that warrant its use. The worldwide adoption of AI for genetic improvement in dairy cattle was made possible by development of a progeny test system and subsequent utilization of milk production records as an objective measure of performance on which to select superior bulls, technique for freezing semen, and liquid nitrogen storage refrigerators.

The development of objective systems to measure economic traits in beef cattle, such as growth rate, carcass conformation and composition, and efficiency of feed conversion, and thus the more accurate selection of sires, led to an increase in usage of AI in beef cattle. With control of the estrous cycle becoming practical, the use of AI in beef cattle has gradually increased.

Processing of frozen semen is a highly specialized technique. Attention to detail at each step is important to maintain semen quality. There is variation between bulls in the freezability of semen. However, semen that is of high quality generally freezes well. Best results are obtained when semen is processed in a properly equipped laboratory by experienced staff at an AI center.

Collection and Handling of the Semen Sample: (*See* p 1098.) The artificial vagina is the method of choice. Electroejaculation and massage of the seminal vesicles and ampullae can be used in special circumstances. So long as the sample is of high quality, freezability and fertility should be normal. These techniques should not be used if the bull is unable to serve for reasons that could be genetic.

Most cattle AI today is performed with frozen semen. Frozen semen may be maintained for years, and extenders permit more insemination doses to be processed from one collection of semen, maintain its fertility longer, protect the spermatozoa from sudden temperature or pH change, and prolong their viability. Semen is usually extended with citrate-buffered egg yolk or heat-treated skim milk plus glycerol, sugars, enzymes, and antibiotics. Final extension is designed to package 0.5 mL of semen containing 20-30 million spermatozoa at time of freezing.

Extenders are often divided into fraction A and fraction B. The initial extension of semen is done with fraction A at the same temperature, eg, 86°F (30°C). The extended semen is then cooled to 41°F (5°C) over 40-50 min, or more slowly. Holding the extended semen at this temperature for 3-4 hr enables the antibiotics in fraction A to complete their action before being inhibited by the cryoprotectant glycerol. Fraction B contains glycerol (eg, 14%) and is added at 5°C in equal quantity to the extended semen. Each AI center has its own standard extenders and processing procedures. Glycerol (11-13%) may be used with milk-based diluents. Four to 18 hr of storage at 5°C before freezing is recommended.

For freezing, bull semen is usually packaged in appropriately identified plastic straws (0.25 or 0.5 mL). Optimal freezing rates are now known for many cells, and spermatozoa can withstand a wide range of rates. In practice, extended semen is frozen in liquid nitrogen vapor before being plunged into liquid nitrogen at −320°F (−196°C). Storage in liquid nitrogen tanks is safe for ≥20 yr, and semen is transported in such tanks. The level of liquid nitrogen in tanks must be monitored to avoid semen losses, which occur when the tanks become defective.

Because spermatozoa do not survive for long after thawing, the semen should be used immediately. Thawing is best done as quickly as possible without damaging the semen by overheating. In practice, straws may be thawed in warm water (95°-98°F [35-36.5°C]) for ≥30 sec but not >15 min. Recommendations by the laboratory that processed the semen should be followed.

Insemination Procedure: The rectovaginal method is now used almost exclusively. After thoroughly cleaning the external genitalia with disposable toweling, one hand (with disposable glove) is introduced into the rectum and grasps the cervix. The insemination pipette is introduced through the vulva and vagina to the external cervical os. By manipulating the cervix, along with light cranial pressure on the pipette, it is advanced through the annular rings of the cervix to the junction of the internal cervical os and the body of the uterus. The semen should be expelled slowly (5 sec) to avoid sperm loss. Deposit of semen into one uterine horn is to be avoided since lower pregnancy rates occur. If insemination records and consistency of the cervical mucus suggest possible pregnancy, the pipette should be advanced less than one-half of the way through the cervix, and the semen expelled. The optimal time to inseminate is between the last half of standing estrus and 6 hr thereafter.

If fertility problems arise when AI is being used, the semen is one of the factors to be investigated, although many factors other than semen are involved in attaining high fertility. Post-thaw motility is an important criterion, but a more critical factor is the availability of an adequate number of motile spermatozoa at the time of insemination. Morphological examination helps assess the role of semen in infertility cases only when fresh semen is available. Within-herd comparisons of diagnosable pregnancies resulting from the suspect semen and from semen from other bulls may be useful. Evaluating inseminator proficiency is useful. This includes an evaluation of thawing temperature, time of thawing in relation to actual insemination, temperature changes from thawing to insemination, site and speed of semen deposition, and sanitary procedures. Estrus detection continues to be the most important factor that influences AI efficiency. This factor should be investigated first, and inseminator proficiency second. If semen is purchased from a reputable supplier, it is unusual for the cause of the infertility to be poor-quality semen.

PREGNANCY DETERMINATION

Pregnancy determination is recommended to maximize efficiency in the well-managed herd. In beef herds, the breeding season (natural service or AI) is terminated in 60-70 days. This gives the average cow 2 or 3 services to conceive. Cows that are not pregnant or were bred late should be identified; if kept in the herd, they will upset the program by calving late in the season. Maintenance costs are significant although they vary widely between farms and from year to year.

Pregnancy determination of beef cows should be done shortly after the breeding season is over; if the breeding season starts June 1 and ends early in August, then it can be done during late September while the cows still have plenty of flesh from summer pasture. It is then possible to profitably market nonpregnant animals before expensive winter feeding starts.

Dairy cows should be examined within 1 mo after calving and again 2-3 mo after breeding.

Other herd health examinations should be considered while the cows are being checked for pregnancy. These include an accurate evaluation of the reproductive tract, teats and udder, feet and legs, teeth, and early cancer-eye lesions. Vaccinations, grub and louse control, and processing of beef calves also can be done at this time.

EMBRYONIC DEATH, ABORTION, AND ABNORMAL FETAL DEVELOPMENT

Pregnancy may be terminated prematurely by early death of the embryo or by abortion. Abnormal development of the fetus may also result in abortion or in calves that die soon after birth.

Etiology: Infection results when viruses, bacteria, molds, rickettsiae, chlamydiae, or other infectious agents attack the placenta or the fetus, or both. Some of these microorganisms reach the uterus hematogenously; others (such as venereal infections) are contracted during mating.

Infectious abortion may be sporadic or a herd problem. Herd problems usually are associated with significant losses and may be caused by infectious bovine rhinotracheitis, bovine viral diarrhea, brucellosis, leptospirosis (various serotypes), campylobacteriosis, trichomoniasis, anaplasmosis, ureaplasmas and mycoplasmas (their role as infectious agents capable of causing abortion and other infertility problems is still under investigation), and possibly others, not yet identified.

Mycotic abortion usually is caused by *Aspergillus* or *Mucor* spp, which reach the uterus hematogenously and cause abortion in late gestation. In many of these fetuses, the skin is not affected; in others, ringworm-like lesions are seen. The placenta frequently is severely affected with necrosis of the cotyledons and thickening of the intercotyledonary areas. Diagnosis is based on identification of the fungus through culture of the fetal or placental tissues, histological examination of these tissues, or direct examination of cotyledons after clearing with potassium hydroxide solution. These abortions are almost always sporadic, and the only means of control is to reduce exposure to the fungi.

Sporadic losses may result from *Listeria* sp (a bacterium occasionally present in silage when pH is >7), miscellaneous bacteria such as *Haemophilus* sp, *Corynebacterium pyogenes, Staphylococcus aureus, Chlamydia* sp, and others, or viruses (eg, bluetongue).

Noninfectious causes of abortion are numerous; the most common are: 1) recessive or lethal genes (or both), hydrocephalus, osteopetrosis ("marble bone" disease), arthrogryposis ("crooked calf" syndrome), and several others, some not fully identified; 2) poisons, eg, excessive nitrates from feed or water, certain pine needles, poisonous plants (eg, lupine, locoweed), mycotoxins (moldy feeds); 3) hormonal imbalances in the pregnant dam; 4) injuries affecting the pregnant cow; and 5) nutritional deficiencies, particularly vitamin A, vitamin E or selenium (or both), iodine, and manganese.

Many cases of bovine abortion cannot be diagnosed. In addition to the specific causes mentioned above, numerous other agents such as *Bacillus cereus, Pasteurella multocida, Pseudomonas aeruginosa, Corynebacterium pyogenes, Streptococcus bovis,* and *Staphylococcus aureus* have been isolated from sporadically aborted fetuses.

Diagnosis: Accurate diagnosis of causes of reproductive loss should be used to provide a cumulative herd history, thus enabling implementation of preventive measures. Laboratory assistance is needed in most cases. Carefully selected, properly preserved, quality specimens should be submitted to a diagnostic laboratory for analysis. Even with these, the exact cause of an abortion may not be detected, especially if it is noninfectious. Many infectious causes can be ruled out, however, which assists in formulating a preventive strategy. Laboratory diagnosis of abortion requires examination of the fetus and placenta, and serology. For the latter, paired blood samples should be collected from the aborting dam, the first sample taken at the time of abortion and the second, 10-14 days later. An absolute diagnosis may be impossible since, in many cases, the causative toxins ingested by the cow a few weeks or months earlier may no longer be available when abortion occurs.

Defective newborn calves can be recognized only by a thorough examination, and sometimes not until time has passed.

Prevention and Control: Several factors are critical to prevent and control abortion and production of defective calves. A balanced nutritional program helps control losses associated with mineral or vitamin deficiencies and poor-quality feeds, including moldy grain and forages. Genetic selection and a functional record-keeping system help to detect and eliminate bloodlines that prove to be carriers of recessive or lethal genes. Adequate facilities for housing, handling, and environmental control lower the incidence of accidents and provide an environment conducive to health. The cattleman and veterinarian need to establish a positive working relationship to assess the herd's reproductive performance, tailor a vaccination program to the herd's specific needs, and assist in the diagnosis and control of potential herd problems on an ongoing basis.

Regular Immunizations: Infectious diseases in a herd can disrupt and reduce reproductive efficiency by causing embryonic or fetal death, abortion, or illness and death of neonates. A complete vaccination program will not eliminate reproductive problems, but will prevent losses associated with specific infections. The following tables summarize the vaccines and bacterins available:

Table 6. Immunization Program to Protect Against Prepartum Diseases of the Breeding Herd That May Affect Production

	Disease	When to Immunize
Heifers	Brucellosis	Calfhood
	IBR BVD	Before weaning and before breeding
	Campylobacteriosis Leptospirosis	Before breeding
Cows	IBR BVD	May booster early before breeding
	Campylobacteriosis Leptospirosis	Each year, before breeding
Bulls	IBR BVD	Calfhood and booster before first breeding
	Campylobacteriosis Leptospirosis	Each year, before breeding

Table 7. Immunization Program to Protect Against Diseases of the Neonatal Calf

	Disease	When to Immunize
Heifers and Cows	Rota- and coronaviruses E coli bacterins Clostridial bacterins	As on label As on label As on label
Calves	Rota- and coronaviruses (if indicated)	As on label

CALVING MANAGEMENT

The expected occurrence of dystocia is ~10-15% in first-calf heifers and 3-5% in mature cattle. It may not be eliminated from a herd, but the incidence can be greatly reduced by management decisions made before the breeding season and during gestation.

NUTRITION

Heifers and cows should be gaining weight before calving, but overconditioning will cause excess fat deposition in the udder and result in lower milk production. Excessive fat deposition in the pelvis also may result in dystocia. Good body condition will aid in calving and also milk production. If a cow is placed on a ration to maintain or increase body weight after calving, breeding will be more uniform and the breeding season shorter.

CALVING FACILITIES

Calving facilities may be needed in certain areas. They should be in good repair and functional before the calving season starts. Weather conditions, geographical differences, and local experience usually dictate how much attention and individual care calves will need immediately after birth. Calving sheds, small pastures, or other calving arrangements must be clean, dry, and protected from the weather. A clean area to handle dystocia problems is also needed. Calving in a clean area, separated from the rest of the herd helps to reduce calfhood diseases, scours in particular. In large herds, it is desirable to have several small calving pastures to allow weekly rotation to avoid buildup of disease-causing organisms. When calving stalls are used during inclement weather, they should be cleaned and disinfected between calvings.

CALVING

Close observation of labor is necessary to determine when a delivery should be assisted. Labor is divided into 3 stages: 1) It begins with uterine contractions and dilation of the cervix. Stage 1 may last 1-24 hr, with 1-4 hr being normal. 2) The calf starts to enter the birth canal and the "water sac" usually breaks. Birth should be expected within 1-4 hr for heifers. A mature cow should calve in <3 hr if the presentation of the calf is normal; if no progress is seen within 1 hr, assistance may be required. 3) Stage 3 starts with birth of the calf and involves the initiation of uterine shrinking and loss of the placenta, which normally occurs within 12 hr after parturition.

Feeding preparturient cows at 11:00 am-12:00 noon and again at 9:30-10:00 pm causes 75% of cows to calve between 7:00 am and 7:00 pm, a period when a problem is more likely to be identified and assistance more likely to be available.

Parturition is often difficult for both fetus and dam. Many factors influence the degree of difficulty: breed, age, nutrition, and pelvic area of the dam; breed and genotype of the sire; gestation length; and sex, size, position, and presentation of the fetus. Some, though not all, of these factors are directly influenced by management. The herd manager has control over the age and size of the dam. There are breed differences to consider, but most heifers should be ≥14 mo old and weigh ≥650 lb (300 kg) before breeding.

A small, live calf is always preferable to a large dead calf. The breed of both sire and dam, as well as the sire's genotype, are subject to control; also, it is practical to determine pelvic size before breeding and cull heifers with a very small pelvis. When the above procedures are ignored or are unsuccessful in preventing dystocia, survival of both dam and calf depends on proper assistance, which requires identification of the problem, proper facilities, and adequate help. When dystocia occurs, a delay in assisting may mean the loss of the calf, or injury and even death of the cow. However, caution should be exercised since it is important to allow sufficient time for the dam to dilate before applying traction. Before assisting the delivery, the position of the fetus must be determined accurately, and any abnormal presentation corrected. If the calf is simply too large to pass through the birth canal without danger to the cow or calf, a cesarean section or other surgical assistance may be necessary. Dystocias tend to repeat in individual cows, and many cattlemen routinely cull cows that have had a dystocia.

MANAGEMENT AFTER CALVING

Muddy lots, crowding, filth, chilling, and inclement weather make the calf more vulnerable to disease organisms and may result in sickness and possibly death for both dam and calf. *See also* pp 1109 and 1111.

MANAGEMENT OF REPRODUCTION: GOATS

PUBERTY AND ESTRUS

In theory, goats cycle at 21-day intervals. Most dairy goats and Angoras are seasonal breeders and come in heat in the fall. Pygmies and some individuals of other breeds (particularly Nubians) can cycle at other times of the year. Heat detection is based on behavioral signs, bleating, flagging of the tail, reddened vulva, vaginal discharge (which causes the tail hairs to stick together), and occasional "riding" by other does, although this last sign is far less common than in cattle. Shorter cycles can occur at the onset of the breeding season, and sometimes can be provoked by prostaglandin induction of estrus. Longer cycles occur later in the season. Goats can show overt signs of estrus while pregnant; natural service will not interfere with pregnancy, but these does should not be artificially inseminated. Most dairy goat females can be bred at 70 lb (30 kg) or 7 mo, if they are born early in the year. Late-born kids may not cycle in the first season. Angora kids frequently are not bred until they are 1½-2½ yr old. Puberty in well-grown bucks can occur as early as 4 mo.

BREEDING SOUNDNESS EXAMINATION

The external genitalia of does should be examined for abnormalities that suggest intersex, a condition common in homozygous polled females. These include an enlarged clitoris and a hypotrophic vulva. Occasionally, a doe has a shortened vagina and no cervix, and segmental aplasia of various parts of the tract can occur.

Physical examination of the buck before the breeding season should include evaluation of the penis and prepuce. The goat is set on his rump and the shoulders pushed down to curve the spine convexly; this makes it easier to protrude the penis. Shearing wounds, especially in Angoras, prior balanoposthitis, and old fly-strike wounds and scarring around the prepuce may make it impossible to do so. Based on data from other species, it would seem wise to eliminate those animals with testicles smaller and softer than their seasonal age-matched counterparts. Prior amputation of the urethral process to prevent obstruction by a calculus has no apparent deleterious effect on breeding ability. Occasionally, bucks develop functional udders but this does not preclude their siring kids.

Caseous lymphadenitis (qv, p 64) and spermatic granulomata and calcification of the testicles (which also may be due to *Corynebacterium pseudotuberculosis [ovis]* infection) all reduce or eliminate the buck's fertility.

Anemia due to heavy parasite infections, chronic debilitating diseases (commonly pneumonia), and foot problems lead to loss of libido. Bucks suffering from caprine arthritis and encephalitis virus infection (CAE, qv, p 393) may have painful, enlarged stifles; they may mount does, but the pain makes them reluctant to ejaculate.

ARTIFICIAL INSEMINATION (AI)

AI is practiced in the dairy goat industry, but most is done by the owners rather than by dairy cow inseminators. Deep intracervical or intrauterine insemination is considered to give better conception rates than insemination just into the first cervical ring or onto the cervical os. There are multiple rings in the goat cervix, and the pipette generally must be maneuvered past each one. Frozen semen in 0.5 mL straws generally is purchased directly from buck owners or custom collectors. There is no legislation or industry-wide standard in North America that governs the collection, processing, and sale of frozen semen. Natural service is the easiest, and most systems have the bucks running with the does. Most hobby operations have a low doe:buck ratio (5:1) because of multiple breeds and different bloodlines. Bucks have a strong libido and can breed far more does than this, although as they get older, and especially during the off-season, they are less efficient.

Semen can be collected in an artificial vagina. Most bucks will mount a doe in estrus and ejaculate; with training they will ejaculate year round, and will even mount wethers. Old bucks are often reluctant to breed does that have had estrus induced outside the normal breeding season; therefore, collections are more successful when young bucks are used.

INDUCTION OF ESTRUS

Estrus can be induced in several ways, depending on the time of year and the relationship to the doe's natural breeding season. Out-of-season breeding is of interest to dairy goat owners to reduce seasonal fluctuation in the herd's milk production.

The sudden introduction of an odoriferous buck often advances the onset of cycling by a few weeks, and the does also may show some synchronization. The buck should be housed well away from the does (out of their sight and smell) for ≥3 wk before introduction. Even if the whole group does not cycle, this method can get a few to conceive in the theoretically out-of-season period.

If the corpus luteum is functional, 2.5 mg prostaglandin (PG) $F_{2\alpha}$ will induce estrus (but it is not effective during anestrus); it also may provoke short cycles, which tend to occur normally at the beginning of the season.

Providing 20 hr of light/day in January and February (northern USA), with a sudden return to available daylight on March 1, will bring goats into heat several weeks later. In this system, it is more difficult for the owner to pick out the does that are in heat; consequently, running a young, vigorous buck with the does gives the highest conception rate.

If a portion of the herd is artificially synchronized, some of the remaining does also may come into heat.

Progestogen treatment, combined with follicle-stimulating hormone (FSH) or pregnant mare serum gonadotropin (PMSG), will cause out-of-season estrual activity. Good conception rates can be achieved with this system, and fixed-time insemination is feasible, but these products are not approved for use in this species. Progestogen treatment can be in the form of injections with an oily base every 3 days, impregnated vaginal sponges, or CIDR's—a form of impregnated plastic for vaginal use. A more readily available and popular, but also nonapproved, product now being widely used in conjunction with PMSG is a norgestomet ear implant (designed for cattle).

PREGNANCY TESTING

With the rectal Doppler ultrasound machine, pregnancies can be diagnosed early with no false positives. The external Doppler can be used from mid to late gestation. The sonic pregnancy machine also can be used; it may give false positives in midgestation, and it is not effective in late gestation.

Ultrasound scanners as used for sheep and racehorses are very accurate with a skilled operator. These are best used between 50 and 90 days of pregnancy, and multiple pregnancies are diagnosed with 95% accuracy. Such scanning units are expensive. Routine radiography can be used with 100% accuracy after day 70 and detect kid numbers after day 75.

The progesterone test can be done on milk or serum, but samples must be collected precisely one cycle after the animal was bred. The progesterone test is good at detecting non-pregnancy, but is not a positive pregnancy test because it cannot differentiate between midcycle, true pregnancy, or false pregnancy. The estrone sulfate test, performed on milk or urine, can determine pregnancy. Between 40 and 50 days after conception, the level of estrone sulfate rises substantially and stays elevated throughout pregnancy. Abortion, fetal death, or resorption causes a drop in the estrone sulfate level; therefore, the test also is a useful measure of fetal viability.

Precocious milking is common in heavy-milking strains of goats, and can occur in a virgin doe, or during her first pregnancy. Therefore, udder development is no guarantee of pregnancy.

False pregnancy is a problem in dairy goats. It can be shorter or longer than a true pregnancy. Usually, the udder enlarges, but true filling does not occur, and the doe may show behavioral signs of impending parturition; she may even call or search for the nonexistent kid. Many of these does conceive the next year, but many are dried off and are economic losses for 1 yr.

OBSTETRICS

Parturition or kidding occurs 145-155 days (av 150) after breeding. Generally, first-kidding goats have 1-2 kids, and in subsequent kiddings, ≥2. Quadruplets are not uncommon, especially in large, well-fed, heavy milkers. Quintuplets and sextuplets are rare. The flock average for range Angora goats in the USA and South Africa is ~100% but is higher in Australasia; the weaning average varies with the harshness of the environment, including the existence of predators. Induction of parturition is a useful technique to increase survival in dairy goat kids, and to obtain colostrum-free kids in CAE- and mycoplasma-control programs. Cloprostenol (125 mg) or $PGF_{2\alpha}$ (10 mg) given on day 143 usually results in delivery of kids on day 144, ~30-35 hr after injection.

Retained placentas are uncommon in goats and usually are associated with the birth of a mummy or rotten fetus, or a difficult delivery.

Pregnancy toxemia syndrome is similar to that in sheep. Hypocalcemia or milk fever occurs, but not nearly so frequently, nor as severely as in cattle. Often, there is only a tendency to fall off the milk stand. Lactational ketosis occurs.

In extremely cold weather, newborn kids should be dried (especially the ears) to prevent frostbite. Heat lamps are not necessary if the kids are dry, well fed, and out of a draft. Kids born in intensive systems should have their navels dipped in tincture of iodine to prevent infection. Angora, pygmy, and meat kids are raised on the dams. Dairy goat kids often are removed at birth and fed from a bottle or nipple-pail.

MANAGEMENT OF REPRODUCTION: HORSES

All breeding animals should be regularly dewormed and maintained on a routine vaccination program to minimize infectious diseases (*see* DISEASE-MANAGEMENT INTERACTION: HORSES, p 1117).

BREEDING SOUNDNESS EXAMINATION OF THE FEMALE

Evaluation of a mare should begin with a good history of her reproductive record. It should include number of foals produced and date of last foaling. Information about dystocias as well as retained fetal membranes is important because the uterus or cervix may have been damaged. Information concerning the mare's cyclic activity, the method of breeding, and any previous treatments should be obtained.

A general physical examination should be done before the reproductive evaluation. The reproductive examination should include the procedures discussed below.

Estrus Detection: "Teasing" is the most common method for detecting estrus in mares. Using an aggressive male is important, and accurate interpretation of a mare's reaction to a teaser is essential for a successful breeding program. Teasing information can be helpful in diagnosis of erratic cyclic activity, such as prolonged estrous periods, which are common early in the breeding season, or such conditions as prolonged luteal activity. Failure to return to estrus after breeding also can be used as an indicator of pregnancy. Adequate exposure to the teaser should be allowed to evaluate the mare's response. Mares in estrus raise their tail, squat, uri-nate, evert the clitoris, etc, whereas mares in diestrus usually squeal, kick, and bite. Mares in seasonal anestrus may remain passive to the teaser. Some mares with foals by their side may not exhibit estrus to the teaser due to their protective nature. In some cases, application of a twitch may be helpful in evaluating a mare's response to the teaser. The findings of teasing are confirmed by examination.

Visual Examination of Perineum: The perineal area should be examined for conformation of the vulva, evidence of vaginal discharge, injuries, previous sur-gery, or other apparent problems.

Rectal Examination: The ovaries, uterus, and cervix should be evaluated by rec-tal palpation to determine correlation with teasing information. During the physiological breeding season, mares in estrus should have one or more palpable follicles, which are usually 3-4 cm or more in diameter and, in many cases, soften detectably before ovula-tion. Follicles as large as 8-10 cm in diameter are not uncommon; however, 2 adjacent follicles may appear as one large follicle on rectal palpation. Ultrasonography may be the only way to distinguish between one large follicle and 2 adjacent follicles. Recent ovulations may be detected as a depression on the ovarian surface, and some mares show signs of discomfort when these areas are palpated.

A corpus hemorrhagicum or corpus luteum may be difficult to differentiate from a follicle; however, palpation of the cervix or teasing may help. During estrus, the cervix becomes detectably softer and is easily flattened against the floor of the pel-vis. After ovulation, however, the cervix becomes more tubular under the influence of progesterone. The uterus should also be palpated to determine size, tubularity, tone, and possible accumulation of fluid or purulent material. Enlargements of the uterus may be caused by myometrial atrophy, endometrial cysts, uterine tumors, or lymphatic lacunae. Other conditions that may be detected by rectal palpation in-clude ovarian tumors and hematomas, fimbrial or paraovarian cysts, and pyometra. Ultrasonography may confirm many of the above findings.

Examination by Vaginal Speculum: After properly cleaning the perineal area, a speculum is passed into the vagina, which is examined for purulent discharge, urine or fluid pooling on the vaginal floor, scars, or adhesions that may indicate a previous dystocia. Examination of the cervix can also aid in determining the stage of the cycle. During estrus, the cervix is relaxed, edematous, and hyperemic; in diestrus, it is pale and tightly closed. The cervix should also be examined for adhesions and torn muscu-laris; digital examination can determine its patency and confirm suspected damages. Inability to insert a speculum into the vagina may be caused by a persistent hymen. In such cases, the hymen can be incised and reflected against the vaginal wall.

Endometrial Culture: Although a "clean" culture does not always correlate with breeding soundness, a culture can be a helpful diagnostic tool. It also can be misleading if not interpreted properly. Positive cultural findings without clinical signs of disease and a positive cytology are of questionable value. Assessment of the amount and classification of the organism(s) isolated is essential.

The endometrial culture can be obtained through a speculum or by manual introduc-tion of a guarded culture instrument into the uterus. The use of a guarded instrument is important to prevent contamination before introduction into the uterus. Organisms con-sidered pathogenic include *Streptococcus zooepidemicus, Pseudomonas* spp, *Klebsiella* spp, hemolytic *Escherichia coli*, and *Taylorella (Haemophilus) equigenitalis*.

Endometrial Biopsy: This enhances the diagnosis of many pathological condi-tions of the uterus, which includes an estimation of fertility in mares. In most in-stances, it does not indicate whether a mare is capable of conceiving, but should indicate whether she is capable of carrying to term. Acute endometritis is character-ized by infiltration of neutrophils, whereas chronic endometritis is characterized by predominance of lymphocytes and/or plasma cells with underlying periglandular fi-brosis. Severity of endometrial fibrosis is a major criterion for prognosis of repro-ductive potential. Severe periglandular fibrosis can be associated with embryonic loss. Endometrial biopsies also can be used to evaluate the success of a treatment.

Cytology: Cytological examination of an endometrial swab also can aid in diag-nosis of endometritis. In acute endometritis, neutrophils are observed. The presence of WBC supports the diagnosis when pathogenic bacteria are recovered from an endometrial culture.

BREEDING SOUNDNESS EXAMINATION OF THE MALE

The breeding soundness examination should begin with a good history, including information concerning libido, mating ability, fertility (if the stallion has bred in the past), prior illness or injury, and any medication received. A general physical examination should be done, noting lameness (particularly of the hindlimbs) and heritable conditions that may affect breeding ability or desirability as a sire.

The genital organs should be evaluated thoroughly. The penis and prepuce should be free of lesions. The testes and epididymides should be evaluated for size, shape, and consistency. The testes should be freely movable within the scrotum. The internal genitalia are evaluated by rectal examination after adequate restraint.

The stallion should attain an erection soon after exposure to a mare in estrus. Libido can vary depending on the time of year.

Semen Collection: A mare in estrus is used for collection of semen from most stallions. The mare should be adequately restrained by breeding hobbles or twitch, the tail wrapped, and the perineal area washed.

Once the stallion attains an erection, the penis should be thoroughly washed with water or a mild, nonresidual soap. If soap is used, the penis should be rinsed thoroughly and dried. The urethra is then cultured for pathogenic bacteria, and is recultured following ejaculation.

The preferred method of semen collection is the artificial vagina. This gives the most representative semen sample. The most common types of artificial vaginas available are the Missouri, Colorado, and Japanese models.

The artificial vagina should have an internal temperature of 113-118°F (45-48°C) at the time of collection. It should be lubricated with sterile, nonspermicidal lubricant just before collection. The stallion is allowed to mount the mare, and the penis is directed into the artificial vagina. The stallion will begin thrusting, and ejaculation can be detected by "flagging" of the tail and by placing the hand on the ventral side of the penis to feel urethral pulsations that accompany ejaculation. After ejaculation, the stallion dismounts, and the second urethral culture is obtained.

The collection bottle is removed from the artificial vagina and placed in an incubator water bath (37°C) to maintain viability of the semen. If a filter is not used in the collection bottle at the time of collection, the gel is aspirated from the sample with a sterile syringe before the semen is evaluated. All equipment used to evaluate the semen should be maintained at 37°C to prevent temperature shock. The total volume of gel-free semen should be recorded.

Motility is estimated promptly after collection by placing a drop of semen on a warm slide and examining it microscopically. Concentrated samples may be diluted with semen extender or saline to evaluate motility. Concentration can be determined with a hemocytometer or a spectrophotometer; the total number of sperm ejaculated can then be calculated. Morphology can be evaluated by microscopical evaluation of stained smears or preferably by phase-contrast microscopy of semen fixed in buffered formalinized saline. If the pH of the semen is measured, it should be done immediately after collection; the normal pH is 7-7.5.

The urethra and semen almost always contain a resident bacterial flora. However, if consistent heavy growth of potential pathogens such as *Pseudomonas* spp, *Klebsiella pneumoniae*, or *Streptococcus zooepidemicus* occurs, and there is a history of repeated infection in mares bred, it may be necessary to breed by artificial insemination, using antibiotic-treated semen extender. If natural service is required, antibiotic-treated extender may be infused into the uterus before servicing. If *Taylorella (Haemophilus) equigenitalis*, the cause of contagious equine metritis (qv, p 693) is present, the stallion should not be used for breeding. Stallions with lesions of coital exanthema should not be used for breeding until such lesions heal.

IRREGULARITIES OF ESTRUS

During the transitional period of the breeding season, mares tend to have irregular estrous cycles, especially prolonged estrous periods. Since these irregularities diminish as the physiological breeding season arrives, no treatment is required in most cases. However, irregular cycles can be controlled with the oral progestin allyltrenbolone. After administration of this compound for 15 days, most mares exhibit normal estrous periods. A combination of progesterone and estradiol 17 β-cypionate in oil injections, given daily for 10 days, and followed by one dose of prostaglandin produces similar results.

Normal cycles may be initiated earlier in the year by the use of artificial light. By providing 16 hr of light each day, for 60 days beginning in December, many mares establish normal cycles by February. For the average stall (12 ft × 12 ft [3.7 m × 3.7 m]), 200 watts of incandescent light is effective.

Prostaglandins or their analogs can be used in mares with functional corpora lutea. Luteolysis results in estrus 2-4 days after treatment, with ovulation usually occurring 7-9 days after treatment. Prostaglandins are not effective when used within 4 days after ovulation.

Administration of human chorionic gonadotropin during early estrus induces ovulation, usually within 24-48 hr.

BREEDING METHODS

The most commonly used method of breeding is natural service. The proper time to breed is determined by teasing and rectal palpation, which detect estrus and the presence of a well-developed follicle, respectively. Mares should be bred (naturally or artificially) beginning on day 2 or 3 of estrus and every other day until ovulation occurs. The mare should be adequately restrained by using a twitch and/or breeding hobbles. A tail wrap should be applied, and the perineal area of the mare adequately cleaned. The stallion's penis also should be washed before breeding to remove smegma and minimize contamination of the mare's reproductive tract. During breeding, the stallion should be controlled adequately to prevent injury to the mare. A muzzle may be necessary for some stallions to prevent savaging of the mare during breeding. After breeding, the penis should be rinsed to remove contamination that may have occurred during breeding.

ARTIFICIAL INSEMINATION

Semen is collected, motility and concentration are determined (*see* above), and the insemination dose is calculated. Semen may be used raw or added to an appropriate extender.

The mare is prepared for insemination by application of a tail wrap and thorough washing of the perineal area. If soap is used, it should be rinsed thoroughly to remove any residue.

Mares should be inseminated with ≥500 million progressively motile, morphologically normal spermatozoa. Insemination is accomplished by depositing the semen into the body of the uterus using a sterile, plastic insemination pipette. Disposable equipment is recommended to prevent contamination. Sperm cells can be expected to remain viable in the mare's reproductive tract for ≥48 hr.

EMBRYO TRANSFER

Embryo transfer (qv, p 1102) has limited application in horses due to registration restrictions of most breed associations. Advances in the technique have been made in recent years; nonsurgical collection and transfer methods are resulting in acceptable success rates. Synchronization between donor and recipient is critical to success and can be accomplished by using progesterone and/or prostaglandins to synchronize estrus, and human chorionic gonadotropin to synchronize ovulation.

PREGNANCY DETERMINATION

Pregnancy can be determined by rectal palpation as early as 18 days. In early pregnancy, diagnosis is based on increased tone of the uterus and cervix; after 30-35 days, the uterus enlarges due to development of the chorionic vesicle. The fetus can be palpated by ballottement of the uterus from day 110 to term. Ultrasonography permits a tentative diagnosis of pregnancy as early as 12 days. Pregnancies are usually confirmed when fetal heart beat is detected at 24-25 days. Ultrasonography is beneficial in the early detection of twin pregnancies as well as determining fetal viability.

Biological pregnancy tests in mares are based primarily on detection of pregnant mare serum gonadotropin, which is produced by the endometrial cups. The tests are generally reliable from about day 40-100 of pregnancy. However, false positives may result if abortion or embryonic death occur after the cups begin to function. Estrone conjugate values of urine or serum are also an aid to diagnosis of pregnancy from about day 40 to term.

ABORTION

See also INDUCED ABORTION AND PARTURITION, p 650.

The most common cause of abortion in mares is infection by equine herpesvirus 1 (qv, p 734). These abortions occur predominantly in the last trimester and usually are not associated with a respiratory infection. Equine viral arteritis (qv, p 376) causes abortion less frequently than does equine herpesvirus, but it is a problem in some areas of the USA. Vaccines are available for both of these diseases.

Sporadic abortions can be caused by bacterial and mycotic infections of the placenta. These are predominantly ascending infections acquired through the cervix. Bacteria involved include *Streptococcus zooepidemicus, Escherichia coli, Klebsiella pneumoniae, Pseudomonas aeruginosa, Staphylococcus aureus, Rhodococcus equi,* and *Actinobacillus equuli.* Mycotic organisms include *Mucor* and *Aspergillus* spp. These abortions can be prevented by good breeding hygiene, treatment of genital disease before breeding, and corrective surgery (Caslick's operation) to prevent pneumovagina.

Many twin pregnancies result in abortion. This may be due to insufficient placental attachment and subsequent fetal malnutrition. Abortions due to twinning may be prevented by manual crushing of the smaller of the 2 embryos during the early stages (22-25 days) of gestation following confirmation of twins by ultrasonography. Torsion of the umbilical cord is also considered as an occasional cause of abortion in mares.

POSTPARTUM COMPLICATIONS

Hematomas or bruising of the vagina are common during foaling; usually, these are not serious and resolve over several days. Postpartum metritis can occur; it is usually accompanied by uterine discharge and may be associated with fever and laminitis. Treatment includes intrauterine and/or parenteral antibiotics, nonsteroidal anti-inflammatory drugs, and oxytocin. Uterine prolapse may occur postpartum or after abortion, and requires immediate care, which includes thorough cleaning and replacement. Uterine infusion with antibiotics may be helpful, and oxytocin may aid in uterine involution.

Retained fetal membranes are common in mares. In most cases, they can be successfully treated with oxytocin (40-50 IU, IM, or added to saline and given as a slow IV drip). Distention of the intact placenta with a dilute povidone-iodine solution via a nasogastric tube in the uterus also has been successful. If manual removal is attempted, force should not be excessive; care must be taken to avoid injury to the endometrium and retention of tightly adhered placental fragments.

MASTITIS

Mastitis (qv, p 691) is uncommon in mares, but occasionally one or both glands may be involved. It is usually caused by group C streptococci or staphylococci. The udder is swollen and painful, and fever and depression may be present. Treatment may include parenteral antibiotics or intramammary infusions following attempted removal of milk from the affected glands. When intramammary infusions are used, they should be inserted into both teat orifices.

AGALACTIA

Agalactia is seen sporadically, usually in maiden mares; it can be a serious problem in mares grazing on endophyte-infected fescue pastures. Mares should not be grazed on fescue during the last trimester of pregnancy. If agalactia occurs, 10-20 IU of oxytocin, IM, may be given to stimulate initial release of milk. If not successful, *see* CARE OF THE ORPHAN FOAL, p 1239.

MANAGEMENT OF REPRODUCTION: PIGS

Management of the swine breeding herd involves a thorough understanding of reproductive physiology, genetics, nutrition, immunology, disease control, environment, and other factors. (*See also* ABORTION IN PIGS, p 650.) The closed-herd concept, with emphasis on immunization of the dam, minimizes the risk of disease loss if sound nutrition and genetic selection are integrated. The breeding program must be evaluated at specified intervals to ensure that progress in efficiency is being made. The parameters of litters/sow/year, weaning-to-conception interval, stillborn and early postpartum losses, and preweaning losses can be evaluated if good records are maintained on individual sows and litters, as well as the herd as a whole (TABLE 8). The postweaning performance can be measured by feed efficiency, total days to market, and postweaning death loss.

Table 8. Breeding Herd Record Parameters Used to Detect Reproductive Problems

Parameter Target	Level	Interference Level
Sow inventory	Weekly farrowing × 26	—
Gilt inventory	Gilt breedings per wk × 1.2 to 1.5 × wk in gilt pool*	—
Boar inventory	Female inventory ÷ 20	—
Number bred per week	Expected farrowings ÷ farrowing rate	—
Sows	80-85% of total breedings	—
Gilts	15-20% of total breedings	—
Percentage of sows in estrus by 10 days postweaning	90%	85%
Regular returns	4%	10%
Delayed returns	1%	2.5%
Negative pregnancy diagnosis	4%	Should be less than the per cent of regular returns
Abortion	1%	2.5%
Not-in-pig	1%	2.5%
Farrowing rate	90%	85%
Live births/litter	10.5	10
Stillbirths	5%	8%
Mummies	0.5%	1%
<8 pigs/litter	10%	15%
Weaned/litter	9.5	9
Preweaning mortality	8%	12%
Litters/sow/year	2.2	2
Pigs/sow/year	20	18

* Factor of 1.2 to 1.5 depends on the percentage of selected gilts that are eventually serviced.

From Thacker, B.J.: Detection and diagnosis of swine reproductive failure, In: *Current Therapy in Theriogenology 2*, Morrow D.A. (ed.), W.B. Saunders Co., Philadelphia, 1986.

BREEDING SOUNDNESS EXAMINATION OF THE FEMALE

Selection: Gilt selection should be based on growth rate, disease status, sexual development, reproductive history (including dam's performance as to litter size, milking ability, and pigs weaned), conformation, and underline (including teat number and placement). Of potential replacements, ~40% are culled because of problems such as delayed puberty, defective teats, locomotor problems, vulval abnormalities (indicative of intersexuality or genital hypoplasia), or failure to conceive. Those selected can be fed grower-finisher ration until they reach 200-220 lb (90-100 kg) or are 5-6 mo old. At that time they should be separated from growing pigs and limit-fed a 16% protein ration balanced with minerals and vitamins.

Gilts selected for breeding should not have excessively straight legs or muscling, the external genitalia should be well developed by 5 mo of age, their udders and milk pads should be well developed (6 pairs of evenly spaced nipples), and they should reach puberty by 6-8 mo, when they should weigh 200-250 lb (90-110 kg).

Disease Precautions: Parvovirus, pseudorabies, enteroviruses, brucellosis, leptospirosis, and other diseases can affect reproductive performance. Gilts and sows should be vaccinated against leptospirosis (5 strain), parvovirus (gilts), and erysipelas. Brought-in gilts should be isolated for 21 days, during which serological tests for exposure to brucellosis and pseudorabies can be done. This should be followed by ≥21 days of exposure to the breeding herd and boars by through-the-fence contact and manure exchange before sexual contact. This allows natural exposure to endemic herd pathogens, which provides some protection against parvovirus and enteroviruses that cause stillbirths, mummified fetuses, embryonic deaths, and infertility (SMEDI), as well as other infectious agents that can cause reproductive failure.

Puberty: First estrus occurs between 6 and 8 mo of age depending on genotype, liveweight, nutritional status, and exposure to the boar. Male contact is the final trigger. Pheromones produced by the boar provide potent sensory stimulation to the gilts. Gilts should be exposed to the boar by 140-190 days of age; daily exposure for 30 min is adequate. Boar exposure is effective in inducing estrus when combined with a change of environment.

If first estrus has not occurred by 8 mo, the gilt should be culled or treated with a gonadotropin. In the latter case, the progeny should not be kept for breeding. Gilts are not served until their second or third estrus to ensure maximum ovulation rate and litter size. Timing of estrus can be controlled by adding a progestogen to the feed (eg, allyltrenbolone at 15-20 mg/day for 14-18 days). Estrus will occur in 60-80% of the gilts 2-8 days following the last feeding. This allows gilt estrus to be synchronized with a batch of weaned sows, or formation of a group of gilts that will farrow together.

BREEDING SOUNDNESS EXAMINATION OF THE MALE

The importance of male fertility in swine breeding is often ignored in herd health programs. Boars should be examined before breeding and whenever they show lack of libido or inability to copulate, or if an increased number of served females return to estrus 3 wk later. A breeding soundness evaluation should include history, general physical examination, genital examination, and semen evaluation.

Selection: Boars are usually selected for the breeding herd at ~6-8 mo, at which time they are sexually immature. A 40-50% cull rate due to locomotor dysfunction, poor libido, low conception, and poor semen quality is seen in young boars selected for breeding. The genetic background of the boar should be consistent with the intended use. Heritable defects such as scrotal hernias and poor underlines can be avoided by careful analysis of the records. Production records that accurately document average daily gain, feed efficiency, and backfat thickness should be considered when evaluating the boar's potential. Testicular development and spermatogenesis occur by ~127 days, and sperm numbers increase greatly between 5 and 8 mo of age. The increase is not affected by sexual rest or frequent ejaculation, but is a function of age and testicular growth. Since age and testicular weight are important factors in sexual development, boars should be ≥8 mo old before they are used for breeding.

History: A complete history should be taken of each animal and include the age and origin of the boar, immunizations, previous disease problems, exposure to other animals and premises, as well as the time spent in isolation and exposure to the present premises and its breeding animals. It should also include a description of the boar's previous libido, mating behavior, conception rates, litter size, and performance of relatives and other boars in the herd. For young boars, observations of previous sexual behavior are also useful. Exposing the boar to several cycling market gilts during the isolation period can be used as an indicator of his breeding potential, which is based on libido and breeding performance, the 21-day return or nonreturn of the gilts to estrus, and inspection of the gilts at slaughter to determine pregnancy status.

Physical and Genital Examinations: A general physical examination should be part of every fertility evaluation. Attention should be given to body condition and conformation, including the back and legs and locomotor function. Osteomalacia, osteoarthrosis, and arthritis, which may result in lameness and reluctance to mount or bear weight on the rear legs, are serious problems.

The testicles, epididymides, and scrotum should be examined for size, symmetry, consistency, and pathological changes; the penis and prepuce for abnormalities during semen collection. Testicular size is directly correlated with the age and weight of boars between 142-282 days of age and 185-375 lb (84-171 kg) body wt.

The testicles are affected by diseases such as brucellosis, and are vulnerable to trauma by handlers, other animals, and improperly maintained facilities; they should contain no nodules or soft masses. The initial reaction of testicles to trauma or infection is swelling, while the long-term result is reduction in size, increased firmness, and loss of resiliency. Asymmetry, as a result of unilateral reduction in resiliency and size or swelling, is potentially deleterious to fertility, and semen evaluation may reveal azoospermia or reduced sperm numbers and morphological changes indicative of testicular damage. Azoospermia may also indicate congenital testicular hypoplasia.

Semen Collection: Collection allows evaluation of libido and ability to mate and ejaculate; in addition, it provides a sample ejaculate. Precopulatory behavior involves visual and olfactory stimulation. The boar grunts rhythmically ("courting song"), salivates, and typically engages in head-to-head contact with the sow, followed by nuzzling her flanks and attempts to mount. These activities should be observed because aberrant sexual behavior may result in infertility. Head mounting is a common problem with inexperienced boars.

Libido can be affected by psychological as well as physical events. Fighting and domination by older boars and sows can inhibit libido in young boars. Breed and strain differences are also seen: the tendency to be timid, nervous, and nonaggressive can be influenced by selection in a breed over several generations, and result in boars with poor libido. Pain from genital lesions or orthopedic problems can have a strong negative effect. Libido may be impaired by an unfamiliar environment, the presence of a feared person, or distractions such as available feed.

Once mounting is achieved, erection and protrusion of the penis occur as the boar searches for the vulva. Close observation of these events is necessary to notice injuries and lesions of the penis and improper erection. Congenital and genetic problems include incomplete erection, masturbation in the diverticulum, and persistent frenulum.

There are 3 methods of semen collection: the gloved-hand method, use of an artificial vagina, and electroejaculation. To obtain a satisfactory ejaculate, the gloved-hand method is preferable and easy to learn. The boar is allowed to mount an estrous female and attempt to copulate. Boars used for artificial insemination (AI) are usually trained to mount a dummy sow. The boar should then be approached quietly from the rear without being touched or frightened, and on the same side as the hand being used for collection (ie, right side for the right-handed person). The back of the gloved hand is placed against the ventral abdomen of the boar just cranial to the preputial orifice, and the penis is allowed to thrust into the gloved hand. Digital pressure is applied to the distal 2-3 cm of the penis only, being careful not to close the entire hand too tightly over the penis, which causes most boars to dismount. The boar fully extends the penis and becomes very quiet when adequate pressure is applied. This is followed immediately by ejaculation. Once the tip of the penis is firmly in the hand and ejaculation has begun, it continues for 3-7 min. If the boar dismounts when the attempt is made to grasp the penis, he should be allowed to make several false mounts until he is aggressively attempting intromission again.

A nervous boar may not allow the penis to be locked into the hand, even after several attempts. Collection can be made from many such boars by allowing them to achieve intromission and lock the penis into the cervix to begin the ejaculation, then quickly retrieving the penis and locking it into the hand. The boar will continue to ejaculate, and the major portion of the ejaculate can be collected.

A prewarmed vacuum bottle (37°C) is a convenient and economical collection vessel. The presperm fraction, consisting of 5-15 mL of clear fluid, is usually ejaculated first, followed by varying amounts of thick, tenacious gel. The gel fraction is filtered out by a double layer of coarse gauze (placed over the mouth of the vacuum bottle) because it coagulates into a semisolid mass that can interfere with evaluation of semen quality. Ejaculation of the milky-to-cream-colored, sperm-rich fraction follows the gel fraction, either all at once or interrupted by several jets of presperm fluid as well as beads of gel. Care should be taken to collect all of the ejaculate possible and to let the boar complete the ejaculation, voluntarily withdraw the penis from the hand, and dismount.

Semen Evaluation: To evaluate semen quality, the adverse influences of rapid temperature change, sunlight, osmotic shock, pH change, water, and disinfectants must be avoided. Vacuum bottle, gloves, slides, stain, and glassware should all be clean, dry, and warm (37°C). Motility of the spermatozoa should be observed microscopically as soon as possible after collection and assessed in terms of the "wave motion", a phenomenon due to the concentration and motility of sperm cells. A scale from 0 to 4 is commonly used. Estimation of individual sperm cell motility requires dilution of the ejaculate with isotonic saline or buffered 2.9% sodium citrate.

Stained slides of diluted and undiluted semen should be prepared immediately after collection. A 5% nigrosin-eosin stain has been used to determine the percentage of live sperm cells, but there is wide variation between slides; progressive motility is a more accurate indication of viability. New Methylene Blue or nigrosin-eosin can be used for morphological evaluation. Phase-contrast microscopy after fixation by buffered formalinized saline provides a more accurate and repeatable assessment of sperm morphology.

Estimates of concentration can be made by observing color, which ranges from watery to creamy (creamy, 1×10^9/mL; milky, 300-500 $\times 10^6$/mL; watery, 50-200 $\times 10^6$/mL). The use of the WBC "Unopette" to achieve a 1:100 dilution, and a hemocytometer make counting sperm relatively easy and accurate. A spectrophotometer also can be used for counting cells (1:50 dilution).

The volume is important in calculating total cells in the ejaculate, and although it has not been shown to affect fertility in natural mating, it is important in AI. The normal volume for young boars (8-12 mo) is 100-300 mL; for those >12 mo, 100-500 mL. The total number of cells ranges from 10×10^9 to as high as 40×10^9 (in mature boars). The minimum number of sperm cells (of which >70% must be motile) necessary for maximum fertility in AI is 2-3 $\times 10^9$ per insemination dose.

Ejaculates of <10 × 10⁹ total cells are thin and watery, and indicative of azoospermia, oligospermia, or failure to collect the entire ejaculate. The semen should be free of blood, pus, and foreign material, and should have no more than 10% abnormal sperm heads, 5% proximal cytoplasmic droplets, 5% acrosome abnormalities, 5% abnormal midpieces, and 25% single-bent sperm cells.

Interpretation of Findings: Boars that fail to meet acceptable semen values are not necessarily subfertile or infertile, since frequency of use, age, environment, disease, genotype, and method of sperm cell fixation can affect these values. Boars <9 mo old can change dramatically over a short period of time and should not be culled on the evaluation of a single ejaculate. Breed differences in onset of puberty, libido, mating ability, and conception rate have been demonstrated.

Environment can affect fertility over a short period of time. Cold temperatures do not significantly influence semen quality or fertility, but high ambient temperatures of 92°-100°F (33.4°-37.7°C) for 4-7 days have adversely affected fertility rate without affecting semen volume, sperm concentration, or sperm output. Prolonged exposure to temperatures >88°F (31°C) adversely affects sperm motility, percentage of normal sperm, and total sperm cell output, as well as embryonic survival and pregnancy rate.

Boars ill after exposure to pseudorabies virus have increased numbers of immature sperm cells and spermatozoa with proximal droplets. Semen quality was not affected in boars with subclinical pseudorabies infection. Any disease that raises body temperature has the potential to cause temporary infertility.

Infertility can occur shortly after heat stress, disease, or interference with spermatogenesis, but frequently there is a delay of 20-45 days because of the length of the spermatogenic cycle and epididymal transport time, which are ~35 days and 10 days, respectively.

Guidelines for Boar Evaluation: Libido, mating ability, semen quality, and breeding results (conception rate and litter size) must be considered. Boars with <10 × 10⁹ total cells per ejaculate, and >30% morphologically abnormal sperm cells (those with acrosomal damage, defects of the head and midpiece, and proximal cytoplasmic droplets) are recommended for reexamination or test-mating with a limited number of sows. Boars with azoospermia on 2 complete ejaculates or inability to achieve complete erection should be culled. Those that have penile lesions or blood in the semen should be sexually rested for 1-2 wk and reevaluated. For boars with persistent frenulum or that habitually masturbate in the diverticulum, surgical correction is recommended, and the progeny should not be kept for breeding because these conditions may be heritable. All results of the fertility examination must be considered in relation to age, disease history, environmental stress, prior breeding usage, mating system, and the techniques of semen collection and handling.

BREEDING MANAGEMENT

Estrus: The estrous cycle is 18-24 (av 21) days in sows and gilts. Sows are usually anestrus during pregnancy, but many show a nonovulatory estrus 3-4 days after parturition. This is due to residual effects of fetoplacental estrogens in the absence of progesterone. Ovulatory estrus usually is not seen during lactation except under conditions of group rearing, high feed levels, and boar contact. Partial weaning or gonadotropin treatment can induce estrus during lactation, but the results are inconsistent and not economical. Normal uterine physiology is reestablished by 20-25 days postpartum. Most sows exhibit estrus 3-7 days after weaning.

Gonadotropins have been used to reduce the number of anestrus sows following weaning: pregnant mare serum gonadotropin and human chorionic gonadotropin are effective when used in combination to induce estrus in weaned sows.

Estrus lasts 1-5 (av 2) days and is characterized by a swollen red vulva, and seeking out the boar. Vulval changes are more marked in gilts than sows and commonly develop 2-3 days before estrus. In response to the sight, sound, and attention (nuzzling and grunting) of the boar, the sow or gilt assumes a rigid, immobile, receptive stance. Vulval changes are often unreliable, so the ultimate criterion of estrus is either standing to the boar or a positive response to the "riding test" (an attendant applies pressure with the hands in the loin area, then gently sits on the pig's back to elicit the standing reaction). This test must be conducted in the presence of a boar (eg, in an adjacent pen) or after exposing the sow to a synthetic boar-odor aerosol.

Table 9. Factors Affecting Ovarian Activity in Pigs

Proved or Suspected Factors	Stage of Breeding Affected		
	Puberty	After weaning	After service
Insufficient male stimulation	+[1]	+	-[2]
Housing/social environment	+	+	-
High ambient temperature	+	+	+
Season of year (summer/fall)	+	+	+
Photoperiod	+	?[3]	-
Genotype	+	+	-
Nutrition	+	+	+
Short lactation	-	+	-
Large litter reared	-	+	-

[1]Effect has been demonstrated
[2]No evidence for effect
[3]Effect uncertain
Adapted from Meredith M.J., *Pig News and Information* **5**, 1984.

Anestrus is a common problem; failure to detect estrus must be distinguished from true cases of ovarian inactivity. First-litter sows are particularly vulnerable to postweaning anestrus as a consequence of excessive weight loss during the first lactation. At this time, the young sow has to support her own growth as well as maintenance and lactation while her feed intake capacity is not yet fully developed. The problem can be avoided by breeding only gilts in good condition, not overfeeding in the first gestation, and encouraging energy intake during the first lactation by *ad-lib* feeding, high-energy diets, wet feeding, and avoiding high temperatures in the farrowing quarters.

Ovulation occurs 36-42 hr after onset of estrus, and 15-25 ova are released. Ovulation rate increases over the first 3 parities so that the fourth to sixth litters tend to be the largest. The ovulation rate decreases when gilts are undernourished, and it can be increased by ~2 ova by "flushing", ie, increasing energy intake for 10 days before estrus.

Breeding: The 3 methods of breeding are pen mating (boar run with females), hand mating (supervised), and artificial insemination (AI). The optimal time for insemination is 24-36 hr after onset of estrus. In natural service, the female is mated twice during estrus, with the first service on the first day that standing estrus is detected, and the second 24 hr later. Many commercial producers breed the sow or gilt once daily as long as she will accept the boar. The use of 2 different boars can increase by one the number of pigs per litter but may mask infertility in one of the boars. When AI is used, the female should be tested for estrus twice daily. The first semen dose is given 8-16 hr after first detection of standing estrus and the second 12-24 hr later. Some experienced users of AI obtain satisfactory results with a single dose. The recommended dose is ≥ 2 billion live sperm cells (2×10^9) in a minimum volume of 50 mL.

Overuse of the boar should be avoided. In pen mating, 8-10 sows per mature boar (>1 yr of age) or 4-6 gilts per young boar (<1 yr) per 21-day breeding period is recommended. If sows are weaned in groups, a sow-to-boar ratio of 4:1 for mature boars and 2:1 for young boars is recommended. In hand mating, a mature boar should be used for no more than 2 breedings per day, nor more than 5 days per week. With AI, up to 30 sows can be inseminated with one ejaculate.

Pregnancy: Sperm cells reach the oviducts within 30 min of mating, and fertilization can occur within 2 hr. Fertilization rates approach 100% in sows, but embryo mortality as high as 30-40% accounts for the usual litter size of 10-12 pigs. Intrauterine mixing and distribution of embryos occur by day 9-11. Attachment begins by day 13 and is complete by day 18. A minimum of 5 embryos must be present at the time of attachment for the pregnancy to continue; if 1-4 embryos are present, the sow is likely to return to estrus with a delayed cycle length of 25-30 days. The embryonic period ends at day 35, and calcification of the skeleton begins. Thus, fetal deaths after day 35 result in expulsion or retention of recognizable piglets. Retained dead fetuses become mummified and may be expelled with normal fetuses at farrowing. The average gestation length is 114 ± 2 days and is somewhat shortened in sows with large litters.

The embryo is at greatest risk during the first 30 days, and efforts should be directed toward removing stresses (eg, overfeeding, heat, handling or moving, and immunization) during this period. Avoiding exposure to outside animals reduces disease risk. If the gilts have been flushed for breeding, the feed intake should be reduced to the limit feeding level of 4-5 lb (~2 kg) immediately after breeding to avoid embryo loss due to high energy intake. Farrowing of <5 piglets is indicative of embryo death after the time of attachment.

Infertility may occur if the sow's ration is contaminated with estrogenic toxins as a result of mold infection. Molds of the *Fusarium* group are commonly found in corn (*see* ESTROGENISM AND VULVOVAGINITIS, p 1685).

Table 10. Pregnancy Tests for Pigs

Test	Days After Service			Special Merits or Problems
	Earliest	Latest	Optimum	
External physical signs	42	Term	>55 (gilts) >84 (sows)	Inexpensive confirmation of late pregnancy.
Non-return to estrus	Daily testing 18-24	-	Daily testing 18-30	Anestrus and delayed returns result in problems.
Rectal palpation	18	Term	28-term	Gilts too small. Can check genital organs of empty sows.
Blood progesterone	17	Term	17-20	False positives can be a problem.
Estrone sulfate	18	77-term	25-29	Also useful to diagnose death of embryos.
A-mode ultrasound	23	85	30-70	Quick, easy test. False positives a problem.
Doppler ultrasound Uterine artery pulse	21	Term	30-40	Prolonged use distressing to ears.
Fetal pulse	28	Term	42-term	Can confirm fetal viability and predict farrowing date.
Real-time ultrasound	19	Term	24-term	Can detect mummified fetuses. Fetal age/health information. Expensive.

Adapted from Meredith M.J., *In Practice,* **10**, 1988.

To increase colostral antibodies, the gilt or sow can be immunized during the last 6 wk of gestation. The immunization program can include transmissible gastroenteritis, *Escherichia coli*, atrophic rhinitis, erysipelas, and other vaccines appropriate to the disease situation on the individual farm.

Parturition: Parturition is initiated by elevated cortisol levels, which also stimulate release of prostaglandin (PG) $F_{2\alpha}$ from the uterus. $PGF_{2\alpha}$ causes luteolysis of the corpora lutea and release of relaxin, which causes relaxation of the birth canal and cervix. Oxytocin is released from the pituitary gland, which causes uterine contractions and onset of labor. Piglets should be delivered at frequent intervals (15-20 min). The stillbirth rate usually is 5-10%; intrauterine deaths are due to infection, incorrect position in the uterine horn during delivery, or anoxia. Anoxia occurs when the umbilical cord ruptures or becomes constricted because of the extreme length of the uterine horn, or delay in the birth canal. Stillbirths and weak piglets also may be due to low temperatures in the farrowing house or low Hgb levels (<9 g/dL) in the sow. Any increase in the interval between pigs born (eg, due to exhaustion and atony of the uterus as a result of a fetus lodged in the birth canal) increases the risk to the piglets still in the uterus. Assistance can be provided in the form of oxytocin injections and manual removal of piglets. Walking the sow for a few moments also can be helpful. The number of pigs born alive can be increased by ~1 per sow if an attendant is present to assist delivery and immediately remove piglets to a warm, dry, creep area.

Farrowing can be induced by IM injection of 10 mg $PGF_{2\alpha}$ or equivalent dose of synthetic analogs. Nearly all treated sows farrow 12-36 hr later, and most within 22-32 hr. This can be used so that most farrowings occur in working hours and to avoid weekend or holiday farrowing; however, it requires good management practices and certain precautions. Good records are essential, and average days of gestation for the sow herd and individual breeding dates for each animal must be known. The drug must be used within 72 hr of the expected farrowing date to prevent an increase in stillbirths. The slightly premature piglets require good environmental conditions, particularly in winter.

Farrowings can be concentrated into an even shorter period by injecting 20 IU of oxytocin 15-24 hr after the prostaglandin injection. This shortens the interval to parturition, but can be accompanied by an increase in dystocia.

Poor lactation is a significant cause of impaired productivity in pigs (*see* AGALACTIA SYNDROME, p 656).

Weaning: The sooner piglets are weaned, the earlier the sows can be rebred and the greater will be the number of pigs reared per sow per year. However, earlier weaning requires better diets and housing and generally higher levels of management. The most common times for weaning are 3-6 wk after farrowing. Depriving the sow of water or feed is unnecessary and may impair estrus and ovulation rate. Sows should be weaned and served in groups so that they will farrow in batches, and litters can be weaned in batches. Batch farrowing facilitates cross-fostering and "all-in/all-out" cleaning and disinfection of farrowing rooms.

MANAGEMENT OF REPRODUCTION: SHEEP

Both genetic and nongenetic factors can markedly affect the reproductive performance of sheep flocks. Breed differences have been recorded in anestrous periods, conception rates, semen quality, embryo mortality, birth and weaning weights, percentage of multiple births, ovarian response to hormones, and adaptation to environmental stress. Rapid improvements can be achieved by crossbreeding, provided that the crosses are appropriate for the local conditions, eg, in the USA, the introduction of Finnsheep (crosses) has resulted in significant increases in the number of live lambs produced per ewe. This is particularly advantageous under intensive or semi-intensive conditions in which multiple births are of maximum advantage.

Nongenetic factors that influence reproductive efficiency include nutrition, disease, management techniques, and environmental factors such as weather. Obviously, several of these factors may operate and interact in a flock to cause losses at specific stages of the reproductive cycle. Reproductive efficiency in sheep usually is measured by weaning percentage (number of lambs surviving to weaning, divided by the number of ewes mated). Acceptable figures depend on the type of operation and range from 80-85%, under range conditions with minimal shelter, to 170-200% under intensive confinement systems.

REPRODUCTIVE PHYSIOLOGY

The ewe is seasonally polyestrus, cycling every 16-17 days during the breeding season. The major environmental factor controlling this annual reproductive cycle is the photoperiod. Geographical location and environmental temperatures also modify the length of anestrus, as does the breed of sheep. Fine-wooled breeds (eg, Rambouillet, Merino) and the Dorset have a shorter anestrous period than other breeds such as the Suffolk, Hampshire, and Columbia. Regardless of this breed-related variation in the length of the breeding season, all breeds are most fertile in the fall.

The length of estrus (~30 hr) is also influenced by the breed and age of the ewe, and the season; the estrous periods occurring in the fall are longer and more intense, and maiden ewes have a shorter and less intense estrus than mature ewes. The optimal time to mate (naturally or artificially) ewes is in the first half of the estrous period. Heat detection requires the presence of a ram, since ewes show no overt signs of estrus. In general, a ewe's reproductive performance is maximal at 4-5 yrs.

The age at puberty of ewe lambs varies greatly and is influenced by breed, nutrition, and season of birth. Well-grown ewe lambs, particularly in the meat breeds, can be mated at 7-8 mo of age and 90-100 lb (41-45 kg) body wt. This practice is desirable because ewes that cycle as lambs tend to have higher twinning rates as adults; therefore, selecting such ewes for replacements increases the prolificacy of the flock. Also, ewes that breed as lambs are able to produce more lamb crops than those bred as 2-yr-olds.

The ovulation rate, which is a major determinant of fertility, is influenced by age, breed, nutrition, and season. Ewe lambs have a lower ovulation rate than mature ewes, and breeds such as the Finnsheep consistently have multiple ovulations. Ovulation rates tend to be higher for all breeds in the fall. The effect of nutrition on ovulation rate is complex and appears to be influenced primarily by the actual weight of the ewe at mating and, to a lesser extent, by the weight changes that are occurring at mating. Heavier ewes generally have more ovulations than lighter ewes. Nutritional supplementation aimed at increasing weight before mating ("flushing") may result in high ovulation rates, but it is difficult to separate this effect from the static effect of having ewes heavier at mating. Phytoestrogens, such as are present in some strains of subterranean clover, cause infertility by reducing the ovulation rate, lowering the incidence of estrus, and impairing sperm transport.

ESTRUS SYNCHRONIZATION

Estrus can be synchronized to a degree by using either teaser rams, progestogen-containing pessaries or implants, or prostaglandins.

Teaser Rams: When rams are suddenly introduced into the ewe flock just before the normal breeding season, most ewes ovulate within a few days and have a normal fertile estrus at their next cycle, or following a second short silent heat. Mating teaser rams (vasectomized or epididymectomized) with ewes for 2 wk before the introduction of entire rams results in a compact lambing period.

Progestogens: Progesterone, medroxyprogesterone acetate, and flurogestone acetate have been used in intravaginal pessaries. Silastic implants of progestogens are used subcut. The pessaries or implants are removed 12-15 days after insertion, and estrus should occur within 72 hr.

Prostaglandins: Prostaglandin F_2 and its synthetic analogs induce estrus in ewes by terminating the functional activity of the corpus luteum. IM administration between days 5 and 14 of the estrous cycle induces estrus within 3-4 days.

Estrus synchronization with either progestogens or prostaglandins may decrease fertility by impairing sperm transport.

OUT-OF-SEASON BREEDING

Accelerated lambing programs such as 3 lamb crops in 2 yr, and 2 lamb crops per year have been proposed as a possible method of increasing reproductive efficiency. The most common method to induce estrus involves long-term progestogen therapy (as for estrus synchronization, *see* above), followed by pregnant mare serum gonadotropin (PMSG) or administration of follicle-stimulating hormone (FSH) at progestogen withdrawal. Other possibilities include artificial control of the photoperiod and use of melatonin.

The response to treatment varies greatly, depending on factors such as breed of sheep, time of year when therapy is instituted, nutritional status of the ewes, and whether the ewes are lactating.

PRENATAL LOSSES

Embryo mortality is the death of embryos up to the end of implantation—about day 40 in sheep. It is the main source of loss during pregnancy; deaths during the fetal period usually are few. Because most of the deaths occur sufficiently early in the pregnancy to allow at least one more service before the rams are removed, embryo mortality does not usually cause a dramatic fall in lambing percentages; however, it delays lambing, increases its time distribution, reduces twinning rates, or leaves a few ewes barren. Embryo death before day 12 does not disturb the normal cycle length, whereas embryo death after this time increases cycle length.

The basal level of embryonic mortality (ie, that occurring in the absence of recognized stress) has been estimated to be 20-30%. The cause(s) of this loss is unknown, although environmental factors such as severe undernutrition, selenium deficiency, and high temperatures may increase embryonic loss above this basal level. Ureaplasmosis also may contribute to embryonic mortality.

Fetal death results most commonly from infectious processes, and the organisms responsible almost invariably have their effect in middle and late pregnancy. (*See also* DISEASE-MANAGEMENT INTERACTION: SHEEP, p 1122.)

PREGNANCY DIAGNOSIS

Accurate pregnancy diagnosis may increase the efficiency of sheep operations by allowing the separation of pregnant ewes for supplementary feed and the culling of open ewes. Plasma progesterone levels, laparoscopy, and ultrasonography are all accurate, but each requires special handling facilities, highly trained technicians, or considerable time per ewe. Rectal-abdominal palpation can be accurate after 65 days of gestation but has been associated with damage to the rectal wall and peritonitis. Use of an external ultrasound device has consequently become popular since it is quick and safe. False negative findings are the most common error; it is most accurate if used to test ewes 50-110 days after they have been exposed to rams.

The ultrasound transducer is placed anterior and lateral to the mammary gland in the woolless area of the right flank, and the beam is directed forward and upward toward the last rib of the left side. The ewe should be considered pregnant only if the pregnancy signal can be sustained for 3 sec. Pregnancy also can be determined accurately by using a portable 50 megahertz real-time ultrasound unit. Transabdominal scanning of ewes between 51 and 75 days of gestation accurately differentiated single and twin lambs.

RAM MANAGEMENT

To achieve maximum fertility, rams should be carefully screened for fitness by physical examination to detect any abnormalities (eg, lameness) that may limit mating. The circumference of the scrotum should be measured, and its contents and the penis carefully examined. Any palpable lesions, particularly of the epididymides, should be considered potentially contagious (eg, *Brucella ovis* and *Actinobacillus seminis*), and appropriate tests performed to establish a flock diagnosis. Semen collected by electroejaculation, and examined for motility and morphology, also can be advantageously incorporated into the screening of potential sires, particularly in single-sire mating systems. All screening procedures should be done 2-3 wk before mating to allow purchase of replacement rams if some rams are found to be potentially unsatisfactory breeders.

Mating activity can be monitored by using a breeding harness on the rams and changing the crayon color every 16-17 days. When fewer than expected ewes are marked, poor ram libido, a low ram/ewe ratio, or anestrus is suggested. When ewes are marked with different colors, conception failure or early embryonic death is suspected.

Under flock conditions with multi-sire matings, mature rams usually make up 1.5-3% of the flock; single sires are used for stud flocks. Flock dispersion should be avoided at mating. Since younger ewes have a shorter, less intense estrous period, they are better mated separately with mature rams.

ARTIFICIAL INSEMINATION

Collection of Semen: Of the 2 methods available for collection of ram semen, the artificial vagina is used more commonly. It is prepared for collection by the introduction of warm water (107-113°F [42-45°C]) and air between the outer casing and inner sleeve, lubrication with petrolatum or paraffin in the end where intromission of the penis will occur, and attachment of a collecting glass at the opposite end. The rams should have been trained previously to mount a ewe, preferably one in estrus and restrained.

The second method is by electroejaculation, for which the ram may be restrained on its side. The moistened bipolar electrode is inserted into the rectum. The withdrawn penis may be held with a piece of gauze to facilitate insertion of the glans into a 10- to 15-cm graduated collecting tube. Ejaculation occurs after a few short electrical stimulations; "stripping" of the urethra may be helpful when expulsion of semen seems incomplete. In general, electroejaculation is less reliable than the artificial vagina; the specimens vary in quality and can be contaminated with urine.

The volume of semen collected with the artificial vagina is 0.5-1.5 mL, and the concentration of spermatozoa is 2.5-6 $\times$ 10^9/mL. Semen obtained by electroejaculation generally is of larger volume but lower concentration.

Examination, Dilution, and Storage of Semen: Immediately after collection, the volume of semen, and motility and concentration of spermatozoa are assessed. The collected semen may be extended 5-fold, depending on the initial concentration. The most common extenders are whole, skimmed, or reconstituted cow's milk that has been heated for 8-10 min in a water bath, and egg yolk/glucose/citrate (15% egg yolk; 0.8% glucose, anhydrous; 2.8% sodium citrate dihydrate; in glass-distilled water). The number of motile spermatozoa and volume of an insemination dose for the ewe depends on the site of insemination. For vaginal insemination, 0.3-0.5 mL with $\geq$300 million motile spermatozoa is used; for cervical insemination, 0.05-0.2 mL is used with 100, 150, and 180 million for fresh, liquid-stored, and frozen-stored semen, respectively. Intrauterine insemination by laparoscopy requires 0.05-0.1 mL per uterine horn and a total of 20 million motile spermatozoa.

The semen may be stored for up to 24 hr by cooling the extended semen to 35-41°F (2-5°C) over 90-120 min and by holding at this temperature. Although a portion of the chilled spermatozoa may remain motile for up to 10 days, fertility decreases rapidly after 24 hr and generally is quite low by 48 hr.

Freezing and storage of ram semen at liquid nitrogen temperature (-320°F [-196°C]) is not as successful in maintaining fertility as it is for bull semen, but considerable progress has been made by freezing in pellet form or in synthetic straws. Extenders used are TRIS or lactose-based media that are slightly hypertonic. Use of thawed semen may result in a lambing rate of >50%.

Insemination Technique: Estrus may be controlled in the ewe by suitable progestogen treatment, preferably with associated injection of 400-600 IU pregnant mare serum gonadotropin (PMSG) at cessation of treatment. If PMSG is used, estrus occurs 36-60 hr later, and ewes may be inseminated at a fixed time, usually at 48 hr. If PMSG is not used, insemination is recommended at the next estrus, 17-20 days after cessation. Ewes in estrus are identified by vasectomized rams carrying some suitable "marker" device on their briskets. Ewes should be inseminated while the vaginal mucus is copious, thin, and clear to cloudy in appearance.

For cervical insemination, the ewe is restrained to limit movement and to present the hindquarters at a convenient height for easy access to the vagina. After cleaning the vulvar region, the cervix is located with the aid of a speculum and suitable illumination, and the insemination made as deeply as possible into the cervical canal. For this purpose, a graduated syringe (1-2 mL) attached to a long, thin inseminating tube is preferred; alternatively, a semiautomatic inseminating device can be used. The relatively long, tortuous, and firm-walled cervical canal of the ewe usually precludes penetration by the tube for >1 cm. In old multiparous ewes, as a consequence of distortion of the cervical tissues, the difficulty increases and the semen can be deposited only about the posterior folds of the cervix. In maiden ewes, in which insertion of the speculum and dilation of the vagina is difficult and can cause injury, the semen should be deposited into the anterior vagina. All these difficulties can be minimized with experience.

For intrauterine laparoscopic insemination, the ewe must be deprived of food and water for ≥12 hr. Special cradles are used to restrain the ewes, first in dorsal recumbency for clipping and surgical preparation of the abdomen. The cradle is then raised at the posterior end of the ewe so she is tilted upside down at ≥45° with the abdomen presented to the operator. Local anesthetic is injected subcut. at 3 sites: 4 cm on each side of the ventral midline ~6 cm anterior to the udder, and another site just posterior to one of the previous sites. The first 2 anesthetized sites allow for entrance of the trocars and cannulae, while the third allows cannulation for insufflation to distend the abdomen with carbon dioxide. The trocars and cannulae are inserted, and semen is deposited through a fine-tipped glass pipette into each uterine horn.

MANAGEMENT OF REPRODUCTION: SMALL ANIMALS

BREEDING SOUNDNESS EXAMINATION OF THE FEMALE

Examination begins with the history, which should include previous cycles, pregnancies, breeding management, dystocia, abortion, etc. A thorough physical examination, with particular attention given to the genitalia and mammary glands, should be performed. Congenital defects of the breed should be identified, which may require other techniques, eg, radiography and ophthalmoscopy. Digital examination and vaginoscopy of the bitch is advised to detect strictures or other defects of the vulva or vagina that may hinder copulation or delivery. Culture of the pericervical area, using a guarded culture instrument of appropriate length, is advisable if there is a history of infertility. This requires sedation in cats. Routine vaginal cultures are of little value since the vagina normally harbors a wide variety of bacteria, including β streptococci. Bitches should be tested for brucellosis before each estrus when breeding is planned. Queens should be tested annually for feline leukemia virus and feline immunodeficiency virus.

Before an anticipated breeding, females should be vaccinated against the common infectious diseases. If a modified live virus is employed, this should be given ≥1 mo before estrus so that maximal replication of the vaccine virus will not coincide with early embryogenesis. Deworming should be performed far enough in advance so that the parasite burden is well controlled without having to administer medication during pregnancy. Use of heartworm disease preventives during pregnancy appears to be safe.

BREEDING SOUNDNESS EXAMINATION OF THE MALE

Breeding soundness examination of the male begins with the history of breeding management, number of litters sired, and general health. A thorough physical examination is performed, with particular attention given to heritable defects and to the genitalia. The penis should be fully protruded from the prepuce and examined. This may require sedation in toms. If hair accumulates around the base of the cat penis, it can prevent copulation and should be removed. Prostate size and symmetry should be assessed by simultaneous abdominal and rectal palpation. This is not necessary in toms since prostate disease is rare. Mild balanoposthitis is common in dogs, and requires no treatment, but severe cases should be treated appropriately and the condition resolved before mating. (*See also* DISORDERS OF THE MALE, p 682.)

Collection of semen for evaluation is difficult in toms unless the cat has been trained to ejaculate into an artificial vagina, or electroejaculation equipment is available. Collecting a vaginal wash immediately after copulation can determine if a cat is producing sperm. (Sperm disappear from the vagina within 1-2 hr of copulation.) Warm saline is flushed into the vagina of the queen and aspirated, the sample is centrifuged, and the sediment examined (New Methylene Blue or routine hematological stains are adequate). Fine needle aspiration of the testes can also be used to demonstrate spermatogenesis, but both methods provide crude information.

Semen is readily collected from most dogs by manual stimulation; presence of a teaser bitch may be helpful. All equipment should be warm and free of contaminants, including chemical disinfectants. The canine ejaculate consists of 3 fractions: the first is sperm-free, the second is sperm-rich, the third and largest fraction is prostatic fluid. The concentration of spermatozoa depends on the amount of prostatic fluid collected. Nevertheless, enough prostatic fluid should be collected to assure that the entire sperm-rich fraction has been ejaculated and collected.

Semen is then evaluated for number of spermatozoa, and their motility and morphology. Because the sperm-rich fraction is diluted by a variable amount of prostatic fluid, the number of spermatozoa is reported as sperm per ejaculate, rather than sperm per mL. Normal dogs reportedly have $300\text{-}500 \times 10^6$ sperm per ejaculate. Sperm production is related to testicular size, so larger dogs should produce more sperm than small dogs. The sperm count (number of sperm per dL or per mL) is usually determined with a hemocytometer or by spectrophotometry. This number is then converted to sperm per ejaculate by multiplication with the volume of semen collected. Motility is evaluated as soon as the sample is collected; $\geq 80\%$ of sperm should show rapid, steady, forward progression. Several commercially available stains are suitable for morphology examination; eosin-nigrosin is used most commonly. Morphologic defects are categorized into primary and secondary abnormalities. The percentages of defects are calculated on 200 sperm. Normal canine semen should have $<25\%$ abnormal spermatozoa.

INFERTILITY

The causes of reproductive failure (*see also* p 647) can be classified as genetic, infectious, hormonal-metabolic, management-related, or anatomic. The latter may be congenital or acquired.

A common infectious cause of infertility is low-grade bacterial endometritis. There are no external signs and hemograms are normal. A presumptive diagnosis of endometritis is based on the history of normal cycles and proper breeding management, and normal physical examination and recovery of large numbers of one type of bacteria from a pericervical culture. The normal flora of the vagina is usually a mixed population and produces a light growth. Endometrial biopsy is necessary to confirm the diagnosis. If mating is planned, the culture should be taken in early proestrus so that antibiotic therapy can be started before estrus. Parenteral therapy with semisynthetic penicillins, cephalosporins, and macrolides is usually safe for the conceptus. Chloramphenicol, tetracyclines, sulfonamides, aminoglycosides, and nitrofurans should be avoided. Douches are of questionable value in the treatment of uterine disease, and the material may be spermicidal.

Bacterial vaginitis may cause infertility, presumably by spermicidal action of the bacteria and their metabolic products. This should be treated vigorously with parenteral antibiotics and douching, but the latter should be stopped several days before mating. Vaginitis in bitches may also be caused by a herpesvirus for which there is no treatment. The diagnosis of herpes vaginitis is based on biopsy of the lesions, which are small vesicles that progress to pustules or shallow ulcers.

Brucella canis (qv, p 669) is a highly contagious disease that causes abortion and infertility in bitches, and infertility in males. A rapid slide agglutination test (RSAT) kit to detect serum antibodies is commercially available. If the RSAT is negative and there is no history of exposure or abortion, the bitch is presumed to be *Brucella*-free; if positive, the serum is treated with 2-mercaptoethanol (2ME) to eliminate nonspecific antibodies and the RSAT repeated. If the 2ME-RSAT is positive, the bitch is presumed to be infected and further tests are indicated (agar-gel diffusion and blood and vaginal cultures).

In cats, infectious causes of infertility include toxoplasmosis, leukemia virus, infectious peritonitis, and viral rhinotracheitis. These may cause abortion, neonatal death, fetal resorption, and apparent infertility.

Hypothyroidism (qv, p 280) is a common hormonal cause of infertility in some breeds of dogs. Affected animals may or may not show any of the signs commonly associated with hypothyroidism. It may cause infertility, abnormal heat cycles, poor libido, and/or abnormal semen in males. It is uncommon in cats.

Prolonged anestrus may be congenital or acquired; some large breeds may not have their first estrus until ≥2 yr old; some individuals and some breeds typically are in estrus once each year. Congenital forms of anestrus may be due to lack of function of the hypothalamic-pituitary axis or ovarian dysgenesis. The diagnosis of congenital anestrus is based on exclusion of all other possible causes (including chromosomal defects, endocrine disorders, and previous oophorectomy) and age of the animal. Induction of fertile estrus in the bitch is difficult: one reported method is to give porcine pituitary follicle-stimulating hormone (FSH, 0.75 mg/kg, IM, daily for 10 days); and then to induce ovulation by an IM injection of luteinizing hormone (LH [human chorionic gonadotropin, HCG], 500-1000 IU) at day 10-12, or gonadotropin-releasing hormone (Gn-RH, 50-200 µg). Since cyclicity in queens is determined by photoperiod, proper lighting should be available for several months before congenital anestrus is diagnosed and exogenous hormones are administered. One reported method for estrus induction in cats is FSH at 2 mg/cat, IM, daily until signs of estrus appear, but not >5 days.

Acquired anestrus may result from previous oophorectomy, exogenous hormonal treatment (including glucocorticoids), or ovarian disease (cysts or neoplasia). Diagnosis is usually based on history, physical examination, biochemical evaluation, and laparotomy.

Prolonged estrus may be caused by estrogen-producing ovarian cysts, functional ovarian tumors, or exogenous estrogens. Exogenous hormones should be discontinued. If HCG or Gn-RH fails to induce ovulation and resolve the persistent estrus, laparotomy is indicated. Tumors should be removed surgically.

Anatomic defects may be congenital or acquired. The heritability of congenital defects, except cryptorchidism, is poorly understood. Stricture of the vagina or vestibule is common in the bitch, and usually prevents copulation, but if pregnancy ensues from mating with an "outside tie" or from artificial insemination (AI), dystocia results. Diagnosis is based on palpation and vaginoscopy. Treatment is surgical.

For a discussion of vaginal hyperplasia, *see* p 681.

Fibrosis of the oviducts or uterine horns, probably a result of inflammation following infection or trauma, leads to infertility. Diagnosis is via laparotomy with dye studies. There is no reliable treatment, although microsurgery may be attempted.

Other causes of inability to copulate include vaginal foreign bodies, hematomas, intersex states, and neoplasia. Diagnosis is based on physical examination and vaginoscopy. Exploratory surgery and biopsy are needed to confirm the diagnosis of intersex.

Cryptorchidism is a common genital defect in males. Unilateral cryptorchidism does not result in infertility. In dogs it appears to be hereditary, and affected animals should not be bred. Since retained testes have a higher incidence of neoplasia, castration is recommended. If either or both testes are not present in the scrotum at puberty, the diagnosis of cryptorchidism is warranted; testicles normally descend into the scrotum as early as 2 wk of age. Attempts at medical therapy with gonadotropins and/or testosterone have been unsuccessful. Orchiopexy is considered unethical. Failure of one testis to develop (true monorchidism) may occur in dogs, but the prevalance and heritability are unknown.

Persistent penile frenulum prevents protrusion of the penis from the prepuce and thus copulation. Treatment is surgical. Deviation of the penis is uncommon. These animals require assistance in breeding or may be bred via AI. Hypospadias prevents normal sperm transport from the testes to the glans penis and is easily detected by physical examination. Small defects may close spontaneously, but some type of reconstructive surgery entailing urethrostomy and penile amputation is usually necessary.

Stenosis of the preputial opening may be congenital or result from chronic inflammation (trauma or bacterial dermatitis). It results in phimosis (qv, p 683). Any underlying cause should be treated and then, if necessary, the opening enlarged surgically.

Testicular neoplasia usually causes infertility. Castration of the affected testis may allow the contralateral testis to regain its ability to produce sperm, but the prognosis is guarded.

High environmental temperature can induce either temporary or permanent hypospermia. Kennel or cattery management should allow for breeding males to remain cool during the summer.

HORMONAL CONTROL OF ESTRUS

The estrous cycles of dogs and cats are not as easily manipulated as in other species. Although onset of a particular cycle may be delayed, return to normal cycling is highly variable. Estrus induction (*see* above) is expensive, unreliable, and rarely justified; it can succeed only in normal, anestrus animals.

Ovariohysterectomy is the best method to prevent estrus in the bitch and queen. Long-term suppression of estrus in the bitch may be accomplished with mibolerone, a synthetic androgen. The dose is 3 μg/kg/day except for German Shepherd Dogs and their crosses, which require 6 μg/kg/day. Therapy must begin ≥1 mo before proestrus. Common side effects are clitoral hypertrophy, vaginitis (especially in prepubertal bitches), increased activity of skin sebaceous glands, mild epiphora, and alterations in hepatic function studies. Return to estrus following cessation of therapy is variable, but is ~70-90 days. Conception rates are reportedly normal by the second cycle after treatment. If given to pregnant bitches, the urogenital system of female puppies will have severe developmental anomalies. Mibolerone should not be given to cats.

Temporary control of estrus can be accomplished with megestrol acetate, a synthetic progestogen. In bitches, megestrol stops (prevents) estrus if given at 2.2 mg/kg/day for 8-10 days beginning during the first 3 days of proestrus. Efficacy is ~93%. Return to estrus is variable, but often is ~2 mo earlier than expected, presumably a result of preventing the normal luteal phase. To postpone an anticipated estrus, the drug is given at 0.55 mg/kg/day for 32-40 days beginning ≥7 days before onset of proestrus. Efficacy is ~97%. Return to estrus is variable, but if timed properly, approximates the next regularly anticipated cycle. Side effects include increased appetite, weight gain, and personality changes (usually more docile). Cystic endometrial hyperplasia may also develop. Rarely, lactation occurs.

Megestrol is not approved for use in cats in the USA, but European data indicate it is efficacious for estrus suppression. In addition to the side effects described above for bitches, cats may develop diabetes mellitus during treatment.

Ovulation can be induced in estrual queens physically or, more reliably, hormonally to produce a luteal phase (diestrus or metestrus) of ~45 days. Physical methods include mating with a vasectomized tom (very effective) or insertion of a sterile swab or glass rod into the vagina. The latter should be performed repeatedly for best results. Hormonal ovulation can be achieved by HCG at 500 IU/cat or GnRH at 25 μg/cat. Both are given IM, daily for 2 days.

The use of progestogens, especially repositol injectables, should be discouraged in both dogs and cats because of development of cystic endometrial hyperplasia and subsequent pyometra, mammary neoplasia, and diabetes mellitus.

The use of injectable testosterone, as is practiced commonly in racing Greyhounds, frequently leads to future difficulties with fertility.

NATURAL MATING

The bitch should be taken to the stud. Mating should occur in a place familiar to him without excess distraction. She should arrive before her optimal breeding dates to become familiar with the area. The breeding area should be one that is not used for training purposes since the male may develop negative behavior about such areas and perform poorly. Good footing should be provided. Some breeds require physical support to facilitate mating; any such device should be constructed to be as comfortable as possible. With the bitch already in the breeding area, the stud should be introduced and their interactions observed. Since mate selectivity may occur in dogs, desired matings may not be accomplished naturally. Aggression on the part of either dog warrants intervention.

Breeding the bitch every other day from the first to the last day of estrus ensures that sperm are present both before and after ovulation, and ensures adequate time for the ova to shed their polar bodies and for sperm capacitation. If only 2 matings are allowed, the first should be on the first day of estrus, the second ≥3 days later. Vaginal cytology (qv, p 943) can be employed to determine onset of estrus by maximal cornification/maturation of the epithelial cells. For bitches with "average" or "typical" cycles, the first day of estrus occurs 10 days after onset of proestrus. Vaginoscopy to determine crenation or angulation of the vaginal mucosal folds may also help determine the stage of the estrous cycle. The mucosa is sharply angulated in mid to late estrus; it is rounded with pronounced wrinkling in early estrus and early diestrus. After copulation, the male should be examined to ensure that the penis has retracted fully into the prepuce. Both animals should be returned to quiet areas.

The queen also should be taken to the tom. A quiet breeding area with good footing and a minimum of interference should be supplied. The "courtship" should not be interrupted unless there is concern for the safety of either cat. Males have been known to mate to the point of physical exhaustion, but the queen will normally go through a period of rolling and grooming following a breeding and not let the tom remount for a period of time. Since ovulation is induced by vaginal-cervical stimulation, multiple breedings over 3 days is advised. Periods of separation between matings prevent exhaustion and diminish the chances of fighting.

The stress of shipping may adversely affect estrus and early pregnancy, especially in animals not accustomed to being transported. Potentially pregnant animals should not be shipped until pregnancy can be determined.

ARTIFICIAL INSEMINATION (AI)

Various breed registry organizations and studbooks have regulations concerning AI. Likewise, the interstate or international shipment of semen may be regulated. AI may be performed with fresh, chilled, or frozen semen. All instruments should be sterile and free of any chemical contamination. Collection of semen has been described above. After collection and evaluation, the semen should be deposited in the anterior vagina of the bitch using a rigid insemination pipette of appropriate length; semen may be diluted and refrigerated for later use (within 24 hr), or diluted and frozen for long-term storage. Phosphate-buffered egg yolk diluent or TRIS-buffered diluent is used most often. Canine semen is frozen as pellets or in straws, and stored in liquid nitrogen. Chilled semen should be warmed, and frozen semen thawed as directed by the shipper, and immediately inseminated. Current recommendations are that each inseminate contain $\geq 125 \times 10^6$ normal, motile sperm.

In the belief that this will improve sperm transport, some recommend that following insemination, a sterile glove be donned and lubricated with sterile jelly; the index finger is then inserted into the vagina and the dorsal wall gently stroked in an attempt to induce muscular contractions of the tubular genitalia.

EMBRYO TRANSFER

Embryo transfer has been accomplished in dogs, but collection of embryos and implantation into the recipient require invasive surgical techniques that do not seem readily applicable to practice.

PREVENTION OF PREGNANCY

Unplanned and unwanted mating of cats and dogs is common. Postcoital douches are of no value in preventing unwanted pregnancy. Although estrogens, when administered appropriately, can prevent pregnancy, their use involves great risk for serious side effects including pyometra and potentially fatal bone marrow suppression. They must be administered soon after copulation, before potentially fertilized ova reach the uterus. Estrogens should never be administered during diestrus because the risk of pyometra is much greater; vaginal cytology should be performed before administration to determine whether the animal is still in estrus. Generally, nonsteroidal estrogens (eg, diethylstilbestrol 0.4-0.5 mg/kg, PO once daily for 5 days) are less toxic than other compounds, but they are also less effective in preventing pregnancy. Estradiol cypionate (ECP) is the most commonly used estrogen for pregnancy prevention. The dose of ECP for bitches is 0.02 mg/kg, IM, not to exceed 1 mg total dose. The dose of ECP for queens is 0.25 mg/cat, IM. Only one dose is given. Behavioral estrus will be prolonged. The risks and signs of pyometra should be explained to the owner, and the animal reexamined ~1 mo later. Bone marrow suppression may be reflected by bleeding due to thrombocytopenia, lethargy or weakness due to anemia, or septicemia due to neutropenia.

Ovariohysterectomy prevents pregnancy. There should be no increased risk to animals <4 wk pregnant, but the risks increase with advancing pregnancy. Some recommend that clotting studies be performed before surgery, since both estrogen and progesterone can aggravate certain bleeding disorders (eg, von Willebrand's disease) or cause abnormal platelet function.

PREGNANCY DIAGNOSIS

Fertilization in both the bitch and queen occurs in the oviducts. Implantation of zygotes in the uterus occurs at ~18 days in the bitch and 14 days in the queen. This is accompanied by the formation of small swellings along the uterine horns (deciduomata) by ~21 days. These are palpable, assuming the animal is cooperative, at this time. Fetal growth is rapid during early pregnancy, and these swellings double in diameter every 7 days. After day 35-38, they become indistinct, and palpation becomes difficult until late pregnancy when fetal heads and rumps are palpable as firm, nodular structures in the ventral posterior abdomen.

Although calcification of the fetal skeleton begins as early as day 28, it is not detectable by routine radiography until about day 42-45 and is quite prominent by day 47-48. Radiography at this time is not teratogenic.

Ultrasonography is also useful in pregnancy determination, especially after 35 days. Before 21 days, "false negative" results occur. Doppler-type instruments allow one to "hear" the fetal heart, which beats 2-3 times faster than that of the dam. Placental sounds may also be heard. Ultrasonography is especially helpful in differentiating pregnancy and pyometra.

Currently there are no biological tests that accurately determine pregnancy in either the bitch or queen. External observation of the teats is unreliable, especially in multiparous animals. Generally, weight gain and abdominal distention are not obvious until the last third of gestation, and could occur in the absence of pregnancy because of progesterone or false pregnancy.

INDUCTION OF PARTURITION, ABORTION

Precise induction of parturition in the bitch and queen is not presently possible. Further, a routinely safe and efficacious abortifacient has yet to be developed. After day 40 of pregnancy, prostaglandin (PG) $F_{2\alpha}$ at ~10 μg/kg, t.i.d. for 2 days, has induced abortion in ~60% of bitches treated. Cats pregnant ≥40 days can be aborted with $PGF_{2\alpha}$ at 0.5-1 mg/kg, daily for 2 days, provided they have been "stressed" or are pretreated with adrenocorticotropic hormone. Higher doses have many undesirable side effects.

Dexamethasone has produced intrauterine fetal death and resorption when given to bitches at 0.5 mg/kg, IM, b.i.d. for 10 days. The same treatment after day 45 produced abortion. The effect of dexamethasone on cats has not been reported.

POSTPARTUM CARE

The first need is to determine (by palpation and, if necessary, radiography) if all pups have been delivered. The routine postpartum administration of oxytoxin and/or antibiotics is unnecessary in healthy dams with nursing neonates. The dam's body temperature and the character of the lochia and milk should be monitored. Normally, the lochia is dark green to black and is heavy for the first few days after parturition. It is not necessary that the dam consume the placentas. Disinfection of the navel with tincture of iodine or merthiolate helps prevent bacterial infection. The neonate should be weighed accurately as soon as it is dry, and daily for the first week. Any weight loss during the first 24 hr should be regarded as a sign of a potential problem and should be given immediate attention.

PERIPARTURIENT PROBLEMS

Retention of a placenta or its remnants usually leads to metritis. Signs are continued straining as if in labor, the presence of a fusiform mass associated with the uterus, abnormal vulvar discharge, fever, and lethargy as the infection develops. Oxytocin may cause passage of the placenta. If not, it should be delivered via hysterotomy.

The principal metabolic disease associated with pregnancy is eclampsia, or puerperal tetany (qv, p 457). It is rare in cats and most common in dogs weighing <20 kg.

Some dystocias respond to parenteral calcium preparations along with oxytocin. Presumably these are due to moderately low serum calcium.

Anatomical abnormalities associated with pregnancy and parturition include uterine prolapse, uterine torsion, and vaginal strictures. Except for vaginal strictures, these are rare. They usually produce a maternal dystocia (qv, p 677).

Bacterial infection of the uterus may occur postpartum (metritis, qv, p 677) or during the luteal phase (pyometra, qv, p 679).

Postpartum uterine hemorrhage is rare. Treatment with ergonovine (15 mg/kg, IV) may be tried; if it fails to stop the hemorrhage, surgery must be performed.

Uterine subinvolution is most common in young, primiparous bitches. In affected animals, the lochia appears normal, but may persist for 8-10 wk or longer. Treatment is unnecessary because the condition resolves spontaneously. Future fertility is unaffected.

Agalactia (other than that caused by severe illness) is uncommon in dogs and cats. When it does occur, it often responds to oxytocin administered by injection or intranasally. Body weight of the newborn should be monitored carefully to determine if milk flow is adequate; newborn pups and kittens should show daily weight gains.

Mastitis is more common in bitches than in queens. Diagnosis and treatment are similar to these in other species.

Bitches and queens should deliver in a familiar area where they will not be disturbed. Unfamiliar surroundings or strangers may impede delivery, interfere with milk letdown, or adversely affect the maternal instinct. This is especially true in young or primiparous animals. The dam's apprehension or nervousness may subside in a few hours, but in the meantime the neonates must receive colostrum and be kept warm.

A nervous dam may ignore the neonates or give them excess attention. The latter may result in nearly continuous licking and biting at the umbilical stump, which may cause hemorrhage, or the abdominal wall may be damaged, which may lead to evisceration. Excess grooming of the neonate may prevent it from nursing. If the dam's maternal instinct is blocked, she may assume sternal recumbency and not allow nursing, or she may leave the neonates unattended.

It is not unusual for the dam to pick up the pups and to rearrange them in the box, especially following delivery of each pup; however, she should then assume the normal nursing position.

NUTRITION: CATS

The cat is a true carnivore; however, it can meet its nutritional needs from a wide variety of diets. Requirements for many nutrients are increased during growth, pregnancy, lactation, and fever. TABLES 11 and 12 list some of the nutrient requirements and allowances for cats. Close association with man has led to significant modification of eating patterns in cats (eg, easy access to food can lead to excessive food intake). Its ability to conserve water has led to the myth that the cat does not

Table 11. Estimated Daily Food Allowances for Cats

	Body wt (kg) (approx.)	Dry Type (90% dry matter)		Semimoist (70% dry matter)		Canned (25% dry matter)	
		(g/kg body wt)	(g/cat)	(g/kg body wt)	(g/cat)	(g/kg body wt)	(g/cat)
Kitten							
10 wk	0.9-1.1	78	70-86	83	75-91	227	204-250
20 wk	1.9-2.5	41	78-103	43	82-108	118	224-295
30 wk	2.5-3.8	31	78-118	33	83-125	91	228-346
40 wk	2.9-3.8	25	73-95	27	78-103	73	212-277
Adult cat[1]							
Inactive	2.2-4.5	22	48-90	23	51-99	64	141-288
Active	2.2-4.5	25	55-113	27	59-122	73	160-329
Gestation	2.5-4.0	31	78-124	33	83-132	91	228-364
Lactation[2]	2.2-4.0	78	172-312	83	182-332	227	499-908

[1] Fifty weeks old or older.

[2] Queens nursing 4-5 kittens in wk 6 of lactation.

Adapted, with permission, from *Nutrient Requirements of Cats*, 1986, National Academy of Sciences. Published by National Academy Press, Washington, DC.

Table 12. Minimum Requirements for Growing Kittens (u/kg of diet, dry basis)

Nutrient	Unit	Amount[1]	Nutrient	Unit	Amount[1]
Fat			Sodium	mg	500
Linoleic acid	g	5	Chloride	g	1.9
Arachidonic acid	mg	200	Iron	mg	80
Protein (N × 6.25)	g	240	Copper	mg	5
Arginine	g	10	Iodine	µg	350
Histidine	g	3	Zinc	mg	50
Isoleucine	g	5	Manganese	mg	5
Leucine	g	12	Selenium	µg	100
Lysine	g	8	Vitamins		
Methionine plus cystine	g	7.5	Vitamin A (retinol)	mg	1 (3333 IU)
(total sulfur amino acids)			Vitamin D (cholecalciferol)	µg	12.5 (500 IU)
Methionine	g	4	Vitamin E (α-tocopherol)	mg	30 (30 IU)
Phenylalanine plus tyrosine	g	8.5	Vitamin K (phylloquinone)	µg	100
Phenylalanine	g	4	Thiamine	mg	5
Taurine	mg	400	Riboflavin	mg	4
Threonine	g	7	Vitamin B_6 (pyridoxine)	mg	4
Tryptophan	g	1.5	Niacin	mg	40
Valine	g	6	Pantothenic acid	mg	5
Minerals			Folacin (folic acid)	µg	800
Calcium	g	8	Biotin	µg	70
Phosphorus	g	6	Vitamin B_{12} (cyanocobalamin)	µg	20
Magnesium	mg	400	Choline	g	2.4
Potassium	g	4			

[1] Based on a diet with an ME of 5 kcal/g dry matter.

Adapted, with permission, from *Nutrient Requirements of Cats*, 1986, National Academy Press, Washington, DC.

require much water. Because it can produce a hypertonic urine, withholding water or limiting water intake can lead to a much more concentrated urine than normal, which can exacerbate feline urinary disorders (*see* UROLITHIASIS, p 889).

Nutrient requirements in early life are tied to growth. The growth rate is exceptionally rapid for the first 3-4 mo but begins to plateau at ~150-160 days of age. The average mature (450-day) weight of domestic toms is ~7 ± 2 lb (3.2 ± 0.9 kg), and of queens, 6 ± 1 lb (2.75 ± 0.5 kg). Maximum growth is completed within 200-220 days for both sexes.

Healthy cats eat a variety of foods. While odor, consistency, taste, and learned dietary habits determine which foods a cat prefers, how much it will eat is determined by such things as noises, lights, food containers, the presence or absence of man or other animals (including other cats), physiological state, and disease. Cats dissatisfied with their diet may starve themselves to death.

Dietary modifications are required by changes in the life cycle, environment, and body weight, and by disease. Growth, pregnancy, and lactation greatly increase nutrient intake (*see also* p 1167). Growing kittens and pregnant and lactating queens should be fed *ad lib* or several times a day to meet their daily needs. Variations in temperature may require a cat to eat more during the winter, especially if it remains outdoors year-round or at night. The diet must supply a balanced nutrient intake, and a properly reduced or augmented energy intake is necessary to correct obesity or an underweight condition. Numerous diseases may require dietary changes. Diseases unrelated to nutritional imbalances, such as parasitic, renal, pancreatic, hepatic, GI, and most metabolic disorders, may produce a more subtle but equally important dietary need.

NUTRITIONAL REQUIREMENTS

Energy: Cats require sufficient energy to allow for optimal utilization of proteins and to provide for growth, maintenance, activity, pregnancy, and lactation. This amounts to a range between 75 kcal/kg body wt for average inactive adults, to 250 kcal/kg in growing kittens, and to as much as 300 kcal/kg in lactating queens. The most useful measure of energy is metabolizable energy (ME), or that part of the energy component of the diet that is retained within the body. The precise ME values for many feedstuffs are not known for cats, although it is believed that the factors used for dogs may apply. They are: carbohydrate, 3.5 kcal/g; fat, 8.5 kcal/g; and protein, 3.5 kcal/g. The values of 4, 9, and 4 used for man are too high for cats. The precise impact of environmental temperature is not well known since most of the research has been done under thermoneutral (68-72°F [20-22°C]) conditions; however, food intake increases as the temperature falls below 68°F (20°C).

Protein: The cat has a higher protein requirement than most species. Healthy adults need ~5 g of protein of high biological value per kg body wt/day. Optimal diets should contain at least 28-29% ME as protein for growing kittens, and ≥21% for adult cats. Growing kittens are more sensitive to the quality of dietary protein and amino acid balance than adults. Protein suitable for cats must supply ≥500 mg of taurine/kg diet dry matter. Unless essential amino acids are added, some animal protein is necessary in the diet to prevent taurine depletion and development of feline central retinal degeneration or dilated cardiomyopathy.

Fats: As much as 60% of the calories in a cat's diet may come from fat, and diets that contain 8-40% fat on a dry-matter basis have been fed successfully; however, the higher fat levels in a palatable diet tend to produce obesity if consumption is unlimited. The recommended fat intake of cats is nearly twice that of dogs. If there is insufficient antioxidant protection from vitamin E in the diet, too much polyunsaturated fat may lead to steatitis (qv, p 551). Adding a small amount of fat usually improves acceptability of diets. Cats cannot convert linoleic acid to linolenic acid or arachidonic acid, which must be obtained from animal sources; recommendations include both linoleic acid and arachidonate at 5 g and 0.2 g/kg diet, respectively.

Carbohydrates: These apparently are not essential in the diet when ample protein and fats supply glucogenic amino acids and glycerol, but carbohydrates afford a less expensive source of energy than does fat or protein. If starches are not cooked, they will be digested poorly and may result in flatulence and diarrhea. Except for the occasional case of lactose or sucrose intolerance, most cooked carbohydrates are well tolerated.

Vitamins: The vitamins recommended for cats are listed in TABLE 12. Most commercial cat foods are fortified with vitamins to levels that meet requirements. Cats require vitamin A in their diet and cannot use carotene as a precursor. The thiamine requirement of cats is 5 times that of dogs.

Minerals: Limited evidence exists for the recommendations of dietary mineral requirements made in TABLE 12; many are based on the mineral content of successfully fed diets. There is evidence that magnesium levels >0.3% (dry-matter basis) may be detrimental if the diet is too alkaline. Likewise, amounts of calcium and phosphorus much greater than recommended may have a negative impact on metabolism.

CAT FOODS

Commercial cat foods are available in 3 different forms: canned, dry, and semimoist. As with all food products, comparisons should be made on a dry-matter or caloric basis. Dog foods are not satisfactory for cats since most dog foods are lower in protein, often do not contain taurine, and are not designed to produce a urinary pH of ≤6.5 (which helps prevent the crystallization of struvite or magnesium-ammonium-phospate in the urinary tract [which may create blockage]). Also, some cat foods are not satisfactory, especially those derived from a single food item.

All commercial cat foods are legally required to have information on the label including name of product, guaranteed analysis, ingredient guarantee, net weight, and name and address of manufacturer or distributor. Ingredients are listed in descending order of quantity. In the USA, all pet foods sold must be registered with the state feed control officials and must contain approved ingredients generally regarded as safe (GRAS), unless they are for specialized purposes such as the amelioration or prevention of disease. These foods designed to "cure" ailments are considered by the Food and Drug Administration to be drugs and must be approved by them.

Good commercial cat diets are formulated to provide adequate quantities of each required nutrient without an intolerable excess of any nutrient. Supplementation of commercial cat foods should be done carefully and only with appropriate justification.

Dry-type cat foods contain 90-94% dry matter, semimoist foods usually contain ~70% dry matter, and most canned foods contain ~22% dry matter. This helps explain why owners may be alarmed when cats changed from canned to semimoist or dry foods consume more water than previously, or why those eating canned foods consume so little water. Normally, cats consume about twice as much water by weight as they consume dry matter. Thus, when eating canned food containing 78% water, their moisture intake is usually considerably more than is required. This is an expensive method of providing water, but helpful in diluting cat urine and avoiding feline urological syndrome.

NUTRITIONAL DISEASES

Nutritional diseases are rarely seen in cats fed good-quality commercial rations or homemade diets following nutritionally balanced recipes. Some instances of malnutrition have been noted in cats fed "natural" or "organic" diets concocted by their owners. This is true particularly of raw freshwater fish, which can induce thiamine deficiency, or an excess of raw egg whites, which causes a deficiency of available biotin. Neglect, including failure to control parasites, is a frequent etiological factor in malnutrition. Many nutritional diseases may be the result of some pathological condition; the primary etiology may be elusive in cases of apparent nutritional disease.

PROTEIN AND ENERGY

Without sufficient energy from dietary fat or carbohydrate, some dietary protein that ordinarily would be utilized for growth or maintenance of body functions is converted to energy. Feedstuffs that contain insufficient amounts of fat or digestible carbohydrate or are deficient in water-soluble vitamins can be considered energy-deficient. Too little high-quality protein in the diet, relative to the energy density, can cause an apparent protein deficiency.

The signs produced by protein deficiency or an improper protein:calorie ratio may include any or all of the following: weight loss, dull unkempt coat, anorexia, reproductive problems, persistent unresponsive parasitism or low-grade microbial infection, unexplained "breaks" in vaccination protection, rapid precipitous weight loss after injury or during disease, and failure to respond properly to treatment of injury or disease.

The amino acids required for cats are listed in TABLE 12, p 1162.

FATS

Cats require linoleic and arachidonic acids in their diet. Essential fatty acid deficiencies induce one or several signs, such as a dry, scaly, lusterless coat, inactivity, or reproductive disorders (such as anestrus, testicular underdevelopment, or lack of libido), and are reflected in the fatty acid composition of tissues and membranes.

FAT-SOLUBLE VITAMINS

Vitamin A: Unlike most other mammals, cats cannot convert β-carotene to vitamin A; they require a preformed source in their diets such as that supplied by liver, fish liver oils, or synthetic vitamin A. Cats exhibit a vitamin A deficiency in much the same way as other species except that classical xerophthalmia, follicular hyperkeratosis, and retinal degeneration occur rarely and usually are associated with concomitant protein deficiency. Nonetheless, cats fed experimental diets deficient in vitamin A have been reported to exhibit conjunctivitis, xerosis with keratitis and corneal vascularization, retinal degeneration, photophobia, and slowed pupillary response to light; certain of these alterations also result from the retinal degeneration that occurs in taurine deprivation.

Hypovitaminosis A may exhaust vitamin A reserves of the kidneys and liver, and affects reproduction, causing stillbirths, congenital anomalies (hydrocephaly, blindness, hairlessness, deafness, ataxia, cerebellar dysplasia, intestinal hernia), resorption of fetuses, and the same changes in epithelial cells noted in other animals. Squamous metaplasia of the respiratory tract, conjunctiva, endometrium, and salivary glands has been noted. Changes such as subpleural cysts lined by keratinizing squamous epithelium and extensive infectious sequelae are frequent in the lungs and are occasionally noted in the conjunctiva and salivary glands. Focal dysplasia of pancreatic acinar tissue and marked hypoplasia of seminiferous tubules, depletion of adrenal lipid, and focal atrophy of the skin have been noted.

Borderline deficiency is more common, especially in chronic ill health. Dietary levels of 6000 IU (1.2 mg) retinol/kg diet should meet the needs of gestation and lactation and exceed the needs of the growing kitten.

Excessive consumption of liver can lead to hypervitaminosis A and may produce skeletal lesions including deforming cervical spondylosis, osseocartilagenous hyperplasia, osteoporosis, epiphyseal plate damage, and gingivitis with tooth loss.

Vitamin D: Classical signs of rickets are rare in cats and usually are confined to kittens born in winter or from queens fed vitamin-D-deficient rations, those kept permanently in dark quarters, or those fed improperly formulated homemade diets. Rickets has been reported in kittens fed vitamin-D-deficient diets, even though they contained normal amounts of calcium and phosphorus.

Overdosing should be avoided. As with other species, hypervitaminosis D causes hypercalcemia and may result in premature ossification, soft-tissue calcification, and even death. Rodenticides that function via vitamin D intoxication can be lethal to cats directly, or indirectly if they consume the poisoned rodent.

Vitamin E: Steatitis results from a diet high in polyunsaturated fatty acids, particularly from marine fish oils when these are not protected with added antioxidants. Kittens or adult cats develop anorexia and muscular degeneration; depot fat becomes discolored by brown or orange ceroid pigments. Lesions occur in cardiac and skeletal muscles and are similar to those described for other species (qv, p 551).

Vitamin K: Vitamin K requirements have not been established in cats; however, kittens have developed petechial hemorrhages that resolved with the addition of vitamin-K-active supplements.

WATER-SOLUBLE VITAMINS

Thiamine: Deficiency generally does not occur in cats if fed properly prepared commercial diets. Thiaminase, which tends to be high in uncooked freshwater fish, can produce a deficiency by rapid destruction of dietary thiamine. Although canned commercial cat foods may contain fish, the heat associated with canning is sufficient to destroy thiaminase. Destruction of thiamine has also resulted from treatment of food with sulfur dioxide or overheating during drying or canning, but deficiencies are not encountered with modern cat foods. Thiamine-deficient cats develop anorexia, an unkempt coat, a hunched position, and with time, convulsions that become more severe, leading later to prostration and death. At necropsy, small petechiae may be found in the cerebrum and midbrain. Diagnosis can be confirmed in the early stages by giving thiamine PO or IM; recovery occurs in minutes to hours. If the diet is not supplemented following this treatment, relapse can be expected.

Thiamine deficiency may cause a number of other neurological disorders: impairment of labyrinthine righting reactions as shown by head ventroflexion and loss of the ability to maintain equilibrium when moving or jumping, impairment of the pupillary light reflex, and dysfunction of the cerebellum (suggested by asynergia, ataxia, and dysmetria). Cardiac disorders such as sinus bradycardia are also noticed.

Riboflavin: Deficiency causes fatty liver, testicular hypoplasia, cataracts, and periauricular alopecia with epidermal atrophy. Riboflavin is light-sensitive; direct sunlight for 1 hr will destroy the riboflavin content of milk.

Niacin: Deficiency has been reported to result in nonspecific signs such as weight loss, anorexia, and apathy. The oral cavity may be ulcerated, with a reddish margin near the midline. Unkempt fur and diarrhea may be noted. These animals are subject to respiratory disorders that may be fatal. However, niacin is ubiquitous in foodstuffs, and deficiency is seldom, if ever, encountered.

Pantothenic Acid: Deficiency is marked chiefly by emaciation and moderate to severe fatty infiltration of the liver. Giant, blunted villi are noted in the intestine, and some of the villi show infarct necrosis. Hematological disorders and graying of the hair have not been reported in cats.

Vitamin B$_6$ (pyridoxine): Deficiency in cats is marked by weight loss and various other lesions, including a mild, microcytic, hypochromic anemia that does not respond to iron or copper therapy. There may be convulsions. The kidneys may show areas of irreversible tubular atrophy and fibrosis, as well as intratubular deposition of calcium oxalate. The urine of cats deficient in vitamin B$_6$ contains large quantities of oxalate.

Biotin: Severe, experimental biotin deficiency may be marked by bloody diarrhea, anorexia, and emaciation. Scaly dermatitis about the nose and mouth, generalized alopecia, and hypersalivation are noted. Kittens have depressed growth after ~150 days on a biotin-deficient diet.

Choline: A choline deficiency depends on the dietary methionine level since methionine can substitute for choline as a methyl donor and actually facilitate its biosynthesis. Fatty infiltration of the liver, depressed growth, and hypoalbuminemia have been reported in experimental deficiency.

MINERALS

Calcium and Phosphorus: The requirements for dietary calcium (Ca) and phosphorus (P) are increased during growth, pregnancy, and lactation. The ratio of Ca to P is important. Insufficient supplies of Ca or excess P decrease Ca absorption and may result in nutritional secondary hyperparathyroidism (*see also* p 284). Irritability, hyperesthesia, and loss of muscle tone with temporary or permanent paralysis have been reported. Skeletal demineralization, particularly of the pelvis and vertebral bodies, may be associated with Ca deficiency; by the time it can be confirmed radiographically, the condition is severe. Often, there is a history of feeding a diet composed almost entirely of meat, liver, fish, or poultry. The condition can be corrected by feeding a diet designed for growth that provides a near equal Ca:P ratio and adequate vitamin D.

Iodine: Deficiency may occur when high-meat diets are fed, but rarely when diets containing saltwater fish or commercial rations are used. The deficient kitten shows signs of hyperthyroidism (qv, p 284) in the early stages, with increased excitability, followed later by hypothyroidism and lethargy. Abnormal calcium metabolism, alopecia, and fetal resorption have been reported. The condition can be confirmed by thyroid size (>12 mg/100 g body wt) and histopathology at necropsy. (In older cats that develop hyperthyroidism with elevated blood thyroxine and triiodothyronine, the etiology is unknown.)

Iron and Copper: The iron and copper found in most meats are utilized efficiently. Nutritional deficiencies are rare except in animals fed a diet composed almost entirely of milk or vegetables. Occasionally, deficiencies result from GI disorders. Deficiency of iron and/or copper is marked by a microcytic, hypochromic anemia and, often, a reddish tinge to hair that otherwise would be white.

Zinc: The metabolism of zinc appears to be connected with that of copper and iron. Deficiency of zinc produces emesis, keratitis, achromotrichia, retarded growth, and emaciation.

Manganese: Deficiency of manganese in other species results in bone dyscrasias. Excess dietary manganese may reduce fertility. Manganese toxicity has been reported to produce albinism in some Siamese cats.

WATER

Dehydration is a serious problem in disorders of the GI, respiratory, and urinary systems. During anorexia, 1% glucose/saline or similar solutions, 20-30 mL/lb (44-66 mL/kg) body wt/day (30-40 mL/lb [66-88 mL/kg] in kittens), given PO or parenterally, help maintain normal fluid balance and urine flow. (*See also* FLUID THERAPY, p 1355.)

FEEDING THE SICK CAT

The nutritional requirements of sick cats are qualitatively the same as for healthy ones; however, they differ either in the amounts required or by the need to restrict or eliminate certain nutrients. Nutrition is an important part of disease management, even though few disorders can be cured with diet.

Gestation and Lactation: Although not pathological conditions, these are times of nutritional stress. During the latter third of gestation, the amount of food and level of nutrient intake normally increases by 25%. The queen requires 2-3 times the normal food intake during lactation, depending on litter size.

To meet the demands of gestation and lactation, the diet should be highly digestible and contain at least 10% fat and 30% protein on a dry-matter basis. These requirements can be met by feeding high-quality cat foods. Lactating queens should be fed *ad lib*. Supplementing an already balanced diet is not encouraged. Some queens may decrease food intake early in gestation and again immediately before parturition. These lapses in appetite are normal and should be of concern only if prolonged.

Allergies: Allergy should always be considered in the differential diagnosis of diseases of the skin or GI tract, and it is not uncommon for cats to be allergic to one or more dietary ingredients. The technique for determining if allergies are at issue is to feed a diet composed of ingredients not commonly found in commercial cat foods, such as mutton and rice (a hypoallergenic diet), which is balanced by adding vitamins and minerals to maintenance levels. In some cases, chicken has been as effective as mutton in hypoallergenic diets. The customary diet is replaced with the hypoallergenic diet for 1-4 wks, and the cat observed to determine if the condition improves. If it does, other components of the diet may be restored, one at a time, until the allergen is identified, or the hypoallergenic diet may be fed indefinitely providing that vitamins and minerals have been balanced.

Anemia: Iron and/or copper deficiency is the major cause of hypochromic, microcytic anemia. A folic acid deficiency also produces anemia. Chronic steatitis from vitamin E deficiency may be accompanied by hemolytic anemia. Good commercial diets have more than required amounts of iron and copper, so a secondary cause such as hemorrhage or heavy parasite infection should be investigated. Feeding large amounts of table scraps or bizarre diets also may result in anemia.

The objective of treatment is to support the blood-forming system in the body with an improved nutrient supply to assure that it is not a limiting factor. Ample amino acids must be available for the synthesis of Hgb, iron for heme synthesis, and copper for the proper mobilization of iron. Folic acid and vitamin B_{12} are necessary to support normal cell division. Supplemental dietary liver is a major source of all of these nutrients and an excellent source of protein. (*See also* p 15 *et seq.*)

Anorexia: Anorexia, which accompanies many disorders or may be a reaction to changes in environment or diet, requires stimulation of the normal appetite and food intake; one alternative is either tube- or forced feeding—which may be stressful. Before treatment of anorexia, it is essential to establish the cause. If tube- or forced feeding is required, the diet should be highly digestible and provide sufficient water, nutrients, and energy to meet normal requirements (*see* TABLES 11 and 12, pp 1161 and 1162), plus any additional requirements imposed by fever or other special conditions. A tube-feeding preparation can be made by homogenizing (in a home blender) a high-quality canned cat food with sufficient water to make it flow easily. Additional energy should be added as corn oil at the rate of 1 tbsp per 6.5 oz (185 g) of canned cat food. Sometimes, anorectic cats can be persuaded to eat by adding highly flavored substances to the diet (eg, meat drippings, fish juices, or certain vitamin preparations).

Since cats can become habituated easily to a particular food, they may resist any dietary change. New food should be introduced slowly by mixing increasing amounts of the new with the old over a period of several days or weeks until the diet is entirely new. Sometimes cats must be exposed to this "starter" program several times. If the animal is to be switched from a canned to a dry diet, it may be useful to moisten the product by adding sufficient warm water, and also to release the odor and flavor components by heating briefly. Some cats prefer their food dry, and others prefer the same food moistened.

Cachexia: Cachexia has a number of causes and appears to be a response to stress or extreme physical demands. In many cases, cachexia is observed in animals with "normal food intake". It is clear from the deterioration of the animals' condition that their nutritional requirements are not being met, either because those requirements have been increased beyond the normal capacity of the animal to consume, or because the diet does not contain nutrients in sufficient balance or density. The chief means of treating this disorder is to change the diet or increase the caloric density and palatability of the food while meeting the animal's requirements for protein and other nutrients. It should be established also that the animal is not suffering from some pathological condition other than stress. In that event, dietary considerations should be altered accordingly.

The usual management of cachexia is to feed smaller amounts of nutritionally dense food more frequently (3-6 meals/day). The form of food (dry or canned) that the cat prefers should be fed. The caloric content of the diet can be increased by adding 1 tbsp (15 mL) of corn oil per cup (275 mL) of dry cat food or 1 tsp (5 mL) per 15 oz can of canned cat food (½ tsp/6 oz of "gourmet" canned cat food).

Vitamin-fortified, high-calorie preparations for administration PO are available and generally well accepted. Most cats readily consume a small amount placed on their paws.

Congestive Heart Failure (CHF): One objective in managing CHF (qv, p 11) is to reduce water retention; restricting sodium intake and lowering sodium levels encourage diuresis. Sodium restriction requires a special diet: all processed meats, cheeses, bread, heart, kidney, liver, salted fats, whole eggs, and snack foods should be avoided. Foods that are reasonably low in sodium include beef, rabbit, chicken, horsemeat, lamb, freshwater fish, oatmeal, corn, and rice. Two levels of dietary sodium restriction are used: severe restriction is 240 mg sodium/100 g dry-matter diet; mild restriction is 400 mg sodium/100 g. Typical commercial cat foods have a sodium content of 0.45-0.90% (450-900 mg sodium/100 g dry matter). Clearly, commercial cat diets do not fall into even the mild sodium restriction category, and commercially prepared low-sodium diets or recipes must be used that employ low-sodium foods from the list above. Because failed contractility may contribute to CHF, a taurine supplement should be provided to rule out a possible depletion of this amino acid in cardiac muscle.

Obesity (*see* below) can be a contributing factor in CHF. Such animals should be placed on a weight management program together with sodium restriction. In some instances, edema may give the appearance of obesity and conceal emaciation; body weight should be evaluated when the edema is resolved. If the animal is underweight, the food intake should be increased or the caloric content of the diet increased by adding 1 tbsp (15 mL) of corn oil and the protein content increased by adding 1-2 oz (30-60 g) of either beef, horse, lamb, or rabbit to the diet. If renal failure (qv, pp 877 and 878) is also present, protein and phosphorus intake must be restricted.

Constipation: This results from impaired peristalsis and increased water absorption from the large gut. The objective in management is to provide a balanced diet that is reasonably high in fiber to increase intestinal volume, stimulate peristalsis, and hold water within the colon. Animals should be fed at least b.i.d. The use of mineral oil in this condition is not encouraged because it impairs the absorption of fat-soluble vitamins. Administration PO of 1 tsp (5 mL) of petroleum jelly once weekly or more often is helpful in preventing constipation, particularly in cats prone to hairball production. (*See also* p 228.)

Diabetes Mellitus: Most cases of diabetes (qv, p 267) in cats are Type II (mature onset) and are thought to reflect insulin insensitivity that should respond to weight reduction. Thus, the objective in dietary management of diabetes in cats is the same as in man: to reduce food consumption and to balance energy intake (especially carbohydrate) with insulin dosage, while slowing the rate of carbohydrate absorption. A feline reducing diet is usually elevated in protein and lower in fat and carbohydrates, which helps in diabetes mellitus management. To ensure a reasonably constant intake of carbohydrates, or nutrients that contribute available carbohydrate, it is recommended that only one food be fed. Since both fat (triglycerides) and carbohydrate (glucose) depend on insulin for their removal from circulation, their blood concentration affects the amount of insulin required. Meals should be timed to coincide with peak insulin release; this may require more than 1 or 2 meals/day. Many diabetic cats are overweight and benefit from a weight management program (*see* obesity, below).

Diarrhea: This results from either altered fluid secretion into, or reabsorption from, the colon, or from increased water retention in the feces. The etiology should be established and any intestinal infection treated. Most normal animals should receive a highly digestible diet that contains <1.5% crude fiber and >15% fat on a

dry-weight basis. If dehydrated, the animal should be rehydrated with oral or parenteral fluids, and lost electrolytes replaced. In general, low-residue, high-fat, low-
fiber diets (dry or canned) are recommended for animals with diarrhea. For certain
noninfectious diarrheas, a higher level of fiber (eg, a 10% load of wheat bran mixed
into a canned diet) can be fed to bulk the feces and help control the diarrhea, especially if the condition is caused by the inability of the colon to reabsorb water. The
fiber acts to retain the water in this case. Prolonged modification (>1 mo) of the
diet is not advised, since this may adversely alter nutrient availability and absorption.

Feline Urological Syndrome (FUS): This is marked by the accumulation of magnesium-ammonium-phosphate crystals in the urinary tract, together with mucus-like
material. Etiology is by no means certain, but providing the animal with a diet that
maintains a urine pH of <6.4 helps limit the development of FUS.

Since FUS prevention depends largely on dietary control of urine dilution and
whole body acid-base balance, management is an important aid. Watering dishes
and litter boxes should be cleaned daily, excluding any phenolic disinfectants or
phenolic-based soaps, to encourage maximum water intake and urination. If more
than one cat uses the litter box, pheromones or other odors may tend to repel one
cat; thus with multiple cats confined together, multiple litterboxes may be helpful in
controlling FUS. (*See also* UROLITHIASIS, p 885.)

Fever: Fever increases energy requirements due to increased metabolic activity; in
general, a 1°F (0.5°C) rise causes an increase in caloric need of ~7 kcal/kg body
wt/day. A highly palatable diet should be fed in quantities that can be consumed
easily, and the caloric content should be increased by feeding a high-fat diet or
administering ~1 tsp (5 mL) of corn oil/day/°F of fever. This provides ~45 kcal
and is sufficient for the average cat. The diet should be very palatable because the
animal may have a diminished desire to eat; it may be necessary to offer smaller
meals more frequently. Personal attention also may help stimulate intake. If the
fever is prolonged, or if there is proteinuria, it may be helpful to feed a quality
"growth" diet or add a hard-cooked egg/day to a good maintenance diet to increase
protein and energy intake.

Hepatic Disease: Liver disorders (qv, p 138) are managed by reducing the need for
liver function. In general, the diet should provide a protein source of high biological
value, and be limited to an amount consistent with the animal's maintenance needs.
It should provide sufficient energy in the form of fat and carbohydrate and moderately restrict sodium intake. This minimizes transamination and deamination, and
reduces toxic nitrogenous waste products. Foods that contain purines and uric acid,
such as shellfish, fish meal, spleen, thymus, liver, brain, etc, should be restricted in
a further effort to decrease the load of uric acid precursors, which require hepatic
metabolism.

Frequent feeding of small meals (up to 6/day) lowers the amount of nutrients
or metabolites requiring transformation by the liver at one time to more manageable levels. In general, protein sources equivalent to egg or milk protein are used
and provided at levels of 2-3 g/kg body wt. If ascites or edema is present, the
animal should be placed on a restricted diet that contains ~240 mg sodium/100 g
diet (dry matter). If blood ammonia levels are increased (hepatic encephalopathy), the protein intake should be restricted to 1-1.5 g protein/kg body wt. In
practice, protein intake is reduced, and the serum ammonia levels are monitored
until they return to normal. The level of arginine in the diet is important in converting ammonia to urea. Good commercial diets contain adequate arginine.

Animals suffering from liver disorders are frequently anorectic (*see* ANOREXIA,
above).

Obesity: It is estimated that 40-50% of cats seen by veterinarians are overweight, and many are obese. Dietary management requires the reduction of caloric intake to slightly less than the caloric expenditure of an animal until its
"ideal" or normal weight is achieved. In treating obesity, the normal or ideal

weight for the animal should be estimated, as should the animal's maintenance energy requirement, and enough high-quality food provided to meet 60-70% of this requirement. The burden of resisting the constantly begging cat under these circumstances can be lessened by feeding small amounts (1 tbsp) several times a day and carefully monitoring future food allotments once the desired body weight is attained. (*See also* p 450.)

Pancreatic Insufficiency: The pancreas (*see also* p 122) produces most of the intestinal enzymes required for food digestion. Treatment of pancreatic insufficiency requires that the diet be highly digestible. Foods should contain easily digestible carbohydrates such as glucose, corn starch, rice flour, or other cooked and available carbohydrates. High-quality protein such as cheese, egg, or muscle meat is recommended, and the food should contain low dietary fiber. In addition, a pancreatic enzyme extract may be added to the diet. The food may have to be offered in 5 or 6 smaller meals daily.

Pansteatitis: Animals suffering from steatitis (*see also* p 551) should receive diets restricted in unsaturated fatty acids. The diet of choice is dry, commercial food to which supplemental vitamin E (100 mg/kg) has been added. Foods that contain large amounts of unsaturated fatty acids or fatty fish such as tuna or mackerel should be avoided (this precludes many commercial canned foods).

Renal Failure: The objective of dietary management in renal failure (qv, p 877) is to lessen the "workload" on the kidney and to diminish the production of metabolic end-products that cannot be readily excreted. This can be done by several means. The first consideration is to ensure normal water equilibrium. Regardless of whether the animal is polyuric, oliguric, or anuric, water should always be readily available. Elevated BUN is lowered by reducing those components in the diet that, in the process of deamination, produce nitrogen (urea). This is done by supplying energy primarily from highly digestible fats and carbohydrates. The amount of protein in the diet should be the minimum that meets the requirements imposed by turnover of enzymes and tissue repair. In addition, phosphorus intake should be restricted. The diet dry matter should contain ~28% protein of high biological value and not more than 0.4-0.6% phosphorus and 0.2-0.4% sodium. These amounts are less than those ordinarily found in many commercial diets, which suggests that special diets are indicated. If renal failure becomes more advanced, ie, the BUN levels can no longer be maintained at normal, 1-2 tsp of vegetable oil or fat drippings should be added to the diet. This helps the cat to meet its energy needs with less total food consumed, and therefore less protein.

Stress: Cats are subjected to a variety of stresses, such as extremes of heat and cold, hospitalization, other changes in environment, or to changes in diet, any of which may cause food intake to decrease abruptly. A highly palatable, high-fat, balanced diet should be provided 2-3 times/day or *ad lib* to maintain normal body weight. The food can be warmed to release odors and encourage consumption.

NUTRITION: CATTLE

NUTRITIONAL REQUIREMENTS OF BEEF CATTLE

Beef cattle production, whether on range, improved pasture, or in the feedlot, is most economical when roughages are used effectively. Young growing grass or other pasture crops usually supply ample nutrients, and mature and growing cattle can consume sufficient good-quality mixed pasture for normal growth and maintenance. However, mature and weathered pasture, crop residues, or other forage crops harvested in such a fashion that excessive losses occur due to shattering, leaching, or spoilage may be so reduced in nutritive value (particularly protein, phosphorus, and pro-vitamin A) that they are suitable only as a maintenance ration for adult cattle. Such feeds should be supplemented if they are to be used for other than maintenance.

Furthermore, the major- and trace-mineral content of pasture and forage crops may be influenced by corresponding levels in the soil or by excess minerals that reduce the availability of other minerals. Mature forage may also be lower in mineral content, especially phosphorus. Normally, supplemental minerals are supplied in a free-choice mineral mix.

Certain nutrients are required by beef cattle in the daily ration; others can be stored in the body, and a deficiency is improbable over short periods. When body stores of a nutrient are high (eg, vitamin A), dietary supplementation is not necessary until these stores become reduced.

The following are dietary requirements for maintenance and successful growth, finishing, and reproduction in beef cattle:

WATER

An abundant supply of good water is needed at least once daily. Range cows consume a minimum of 2.5 gal. (9.5 L) of water/head/day in winter and up to 12 gal. (45 L)/head/day in summer. When salt is fed with a protein concentrate to control protein intake, more water is needed to aid in excreting the excess salt. Breeding cows, yearlings, and 2-yr-old steers need ~10 gal. (38 L) of water daily, and finishing calves drink 6-8 gal. (23-30 L). With fresh succulent feeds or silage, less water is required.

ENERGY

Except for young calves, beef cattle can meet their maintenance energy requirements from roughage, if it is of reasonable quality. A shortage of energy occurs on overstocked pastures, with inadequate feed allowance or poor-quality forages, or during a drought. For production, additional energy from concentrates may be necessary, especially when fair- or poor-quality forages are consumed.

Especially in cold weather, roughages of varying quality may have similar maintenance energy values. Heat released during digestion and assimilation contributes to the maintenance of body temperature for wintering stock cattle when little productive energy is required. For finishing, reproduction, and lactation, however, additional productive energy is needed, thus, the necessity for good-quality feeds, including concentrates.

The energy requirement for wintering, mature, pregnant beef cattle is 130-180 kcal digestible energy per 100 lb (45 kg) of body wt. For growing calves, lactating cows, or finishing cattle, the requirement is much greater.

PROTEIN

Although digestible protein in the daily ration is essential, protein quality is considered relatively unimportant and, except in young animals, beef cattle can thrive on protein from a single feed source. The protein from some feeds has good "by-pass" qualities, ie, it "by-passes" the rumen and is digested in the lower digestive tract, which may result in better protein utilization. Except for energy deficiency due to low feed intake, protein deficiency is the most common deficiency that limits growth, milk production, and reproduction. Protein deficiencies of long duration eventually depress appetite with consequent weight loss and unthriftiness, even when ample energy is available.

Feeds vary greatly in protein digestibility; eg, the protein of common grains and most protein supplements is ~75-85% digestible, that of alfalfa hay ~70%, and that of grass hays is usually 35-50%. The protein of low-quality feeds such as weathered grass hay or range grass and cottonseed hulls is digested poorly. Thus, total protein intake may be "adequate" but digestible protein intake insufficient.

Lack of protein in the ration also adversely affects the microbial population in the rumen, which in turn, reduces the utilization of low-protein feeds. Much of the potential nutritive value of roughages (especially energy), therefore, may be lost if protein levels are inadequate. Since there is little storage of available protein in the body, it must be present in the daily ration for best results.

The requirement for digestible protein varies with body weight and stage of development (growth, finishing, and reproduction). Growing beef calves require about as much digestible protein as mature, nonpregnant beef cows. Steers on a full-feed of grain, making maximal gains, have a much higher requirement than cattle of the same age and weight that are making only moderate gains. The digestible protein requirement for maintenance of beef cattle is ~0.6 lb/1000 lb (0.6 g/kg) body wt daily; for rapid growth and finishing, it is nearly double this amount. Cows nursing calves need about twice as much digestible protein as dry cows.

Urea is used commonly in commercial protein supplements to supply one-third or more of the total nitrogen. It is utilized well at this level, provided the ration has ample phosphorus, trace minerals, sulfur, and soluble carbohydrates. The amount of crude protein (N × 6.25) supplied by nonprotein nitrogen must be stated on the feed tag. Toxicity is not a serious problem when urea is fed at the recommended levels and mixed thoroughly with the feed. However, rapid ingestion of urea at levels >20 g/100 lb (45 kg) body wt may lead to toxicity. Several urea-molasses liquid supplements, which may contain nearly 10% urea, currently are self-fed to beef cattle. Caution should be exercised when cattle are started on these supplements. Such supplements should be fed in a licker-type self-feeder to avoid overeating, or mixed in the complete ration for bunk feeding. (*See also* p 1693.)

MINERALS

Qualitatively, the mineral requirements of beef cattle are essentially the same as those of dairy cattle; quantitatively, however, they generally are much lower than for high-producing dairy cows. The minerals most likely to be deficient in beef cattle rations are sodium (as salt), calcium, phosphorus, and magnesium. (*See* NUTRITIONAL DISEASES OF CATTLE AND SHEEP, p 1194.) In some areas, including the interior of the USA, iodine may be deficient in rations for pregnant cows. Natural feeds usually contain adequate amounts of the other required mineral elements, viz, potassium, magnesium, sulfur, iodine, iron, copper, cobalt, manganese, selenium, and zinc. Under certain conditions, feedstuffs may not provide adequate amounts of some essential minerals, and it becomes necessary to supplement the diet. Such deficiencies usually are area problems rather than widespread. The actual method of supplementation is determined largely by the type of husbandry. Under intensive systems of stocking, calcium, phosphorus, potassium, and magnesium can be applied as fertilizer to the pasture; in addition to supplying the necessary minerals to the animal, this practice may well increase the total yield of forage. Copper and cobalt also may be added to the fertilizer mixture. Perhaps the most economical and widely used method of supplementation in the USA is to add a calcium and phosphorus source to trace mineral salt, preferably in the loose form.

The **salt** (NaCl) requirements of beef cattle are not well established. Beef calves wintered on dry roughage and a small amount of protein supplement make slower and more expensive gains than others receiving salt. In contrast, calves full-fed grain gain as rapidly and efficiently with no salt as others fed salt. Similar comparisons have not been made in the USA with grazing cattle, but when salt is provided free choice, cattle on pasture consume more salt than those in drylot. Range cattle usually consume 2-2.5 lb (1 kg) of salt/head/mo when forage is succulent, and 1-1.5 lb/mo with mature and drier forage. When salt is added to protein feeds to limit the protein intake, beef cows may eat >1 lb salt/day over long periods without adverse effects, if they have plenty of water.

In Australia and New Zealand, cattle grazing on good pasture rarely are fed salt, and there is some question whether the amounts provided in the USA (where it is usually fed free choice) are really necessary.

Calcium is relatively high in most roughages, but low in cereal hays and silages, corn silage, sorghum hays and silages, cereal residues, corn and sorghum residues, and concentrates. Legume hay is a richer source than grass hay, but even nonlegume roughages often supply sufficient for maintenance. When the roughage is produced on soil exceptionally low in calcium, or when cattle are full-fed grain with corn or sorghum silage or a limited amount of nonlegume hay, a calcium deficiency may develop. Finishing rations are more apt to be deficient in calcium than are growing rations. Since the beef cow produces less milk than the dairy cow and usually is consuming more roughage, a deficiency of calcium is unlikely. However, it is good husbandry to supply a free-choice mineral mix at all times. This may consist of two-thirds dicalcium phosphate and one-third iodized or trace mineralized salt. In addition, iodized or trace mineralized salt should be supplied free choice. A commercial mineral supplement also can be provided free choice or included in the total ration. The total ration should provide a calcium:phosphorus ratio of ~2:1, although it appears that wider ratios are tolerated if the minimum requirements for each element are met and adequate vitamin D is available. Range cattle should be provided a mineral supplement that has as much or more phosphorus than calcium.

Phosphorus (P) may be deficient in ordinary beef cattle rations since it is often low in roughages. Soils in many beef-producing areas are low in available P. Further, when weathered native range grass is the only roughage, or when such feeds as cottonseed hulls, stover, or cobs are fed, the P level may drop precariously low. As forages mature, their P content declines, and when it is <0.16%, maximal performance is not attained. For best utilization of feeds, the P level in the ration should be ~0.2%. Most protein feeds are relatively good sources of P; therefore, when such feeds are given in amounts necessary to supplement protein-deficient roughages, P intake is adequate. However, a mineral mix offered free choice is recommended. Steamed bone meal, mono- and dicalcium phosphate, defluorinated rock phosphate, mono- and disodium phosphate, sodium tripolyphosphate, and ammonium polyphosphate are good sources of P. Since most grains are fair to good sources, feedlot cattle usually receive sufficient P from grain, although the phytic acid chelation of P in grain may render up to one-half of it unavailable. An intake of P of 2-3 g/100 lb (44-66 mg/kg) body wt is considered ample for finishing cattle.

Cobalt deficiency in beef cattle is usually a consequence of soil deficiency. Such deficiencies are known in many parts of the world.

With some of the other minerals, eg, iodine, copper, selenium, and possibly zinc, the explanation is not so clear. There may be a simple deficiency in the soil, and therefore in the plant. Further, the level in the feed may be reasonably high, but the animal is unable to utilize the particular element because of unusual amounts of other minerals or substances in the diet. Therefore, induced deficiencies develop, but fortunately can be overcome by suitable supplements. Selenium deficiency may be a more widespread problem in the USA than previously recognized. These conditions are described under NUTRITIONAL DISEASES OF CATTLE AND SHEEP, p 1194.

VITAMINS

While cattle probably have a metabolic requirement for all the known vitamins, a dietary source of vitamins C and K and the B complex is not necessary. In all but the very young, vitamin K and B vitamins are synthesized in sufficient amounts by the ruminal microflora, and vitamin C is synthesized in the tissues of all cattle. However, if rumen function is impaired, as by starvation, nutrient deficiencies, or excessive levels of antimicrobials or medicaments, synthesis of these vitamins may be impaired.

Vitamin A: Since most beef cattle are raised in range and semiarid regions and are finished on large amounts of grain and limited quantities of roughage, a shortage of vitamin A is always a potential danger. Many stocker cattle and pregnant cows are wintered on low-quality roughages low or devoid in β-carotene, the precursor of vitamin A. Except for newly harvested yellow corn, grains and other concentrates are almost devoid of vitamin A precursors. However, cattle on green pastures have the ability to store large quantities of vitamin A and carotene in their liver; thus, depending on the amount of green feed obtained during the previous grazing season, weaner calves may have sufficient liver stores to last 80-140 days on low-carotene rations before showing evidence of deficiency, yearling cattle ~100-150 days, and mature cattle ~180-240 days. Newborn calves, which have small stores of vitamin A, depend on colostrum and milk to meet their needs. If the dam is fed a ration low in carotene during gestation and nursing, severe deficiency signs may become apparent in the young suckling calf within 2-4 wk of birth, while the dam appears normal.

It is sound practice to supply 2-5 lb (1-2 kg) of early-cut, good-quality legume or grass hay, or 0.5-1 lb (0.25-0.5 kg) of dehydrated alfalfa pellets in the daily ration of stocker cattle and pregnant cows as insurance against vitamin A deficiency. Most commercial protein and mineral supplements are fortified with dry, stabilized vitamin A. When certain trace minerals are added, vitamin A must be protected against destruction. Access to green pasture, even for short periods, is the ideal method of preventing a deficiency. The daily requirement for beef cattle appears to be ~5 mg of carotene or 2000 IU of vitamin A/100 lb (45 kg) body wt. Lactating cows may require twice this amount to maintain high vitamin A levels in the milk.

Vitamin A deficiency under feedlot conditions has caused considerable loss to cattle feeders, especially if high-concentrate and corn silage rations low in carotene have been fed. Destruction of carotene during hay storage or in the GI tract, or the failure to convert carotene to vitamin A, all may increase the need for vitamin A supplementation. Growing and finishing steers and heifers fed low-carotene rations for several months require 1000 IU of vitamin A/lb (2200 IU/kg) of air-dry ration. Commercial vitamin A supplements are not expensive and should be used when such rations are fed and any danger of a deficiency exists. An alternative method is by IM injection; in nonpasture situations, injection of 5 million IU of vitamin A once yearly will suffice.

Vitamin D deficiency is comparatively rare in beef cattle since they are usually outside in direct sunlight and fed sun-cured roughage. In northern latitudes during long winters, or in show calves that are kept in the barn or turned out only at night, a deficiency is possible. Direct exposure to sunlight, feeding sun-cured roughage, or supplementary vitamin D (300 IU/100 lb [45 kg] body wt) will protect against a deficiency.

The interrelationships of **vitamin E** and selenium in reproduction and in the etiology of various myopathies are discussed under MYOPATHIES, p 547.

FEEDING AND NUTRITIONAL MANAGEMENT

Feeds for beef cattle vary widely in quality, palatability, and essential nutrient content. The composition of some common feeds for beef cattle is shown in TABLE 20, p 1192. To be most effective, any supplement must be patterned to fit the kind and quality of roughage available. Chemical analyses of roughages are very useful to determine their nutrient deficiencies and adequacies. Under certain systems of management, beef cattle are wintered as economically as possible on low-quality roughages, and thus may not receive the recommended nutrients for optimal performance. This may not be undesirable if no severe deficiency develops and the cattle can make up for poor winter gains on abundant summer pasture. However, when maximal performance is desired (cows nursing calves, rapid growth of calves, steers on full feed), an attempt should be made to meet or exceed the nutrient requirements as shown in the following tables.

Feeding and nutritional management for 3 systems of beef production are discussed separately. (See also DISEASE-MANAGEMENT INTERACTION: BEEF CATTLE, p 1109.)

THE BREEDING HERD

In most areas, producers follow a spring calving program (February to May in the USA), depending on available feed, growth of early spring pasture, and prevailing climate. Fall calving is on the increase, particularly in the south, and wintering the lactating cow presents a much greater nutritional problem than does wintering the pregnant cow. Spring-born beef calves commonly are weaned at 6-8 mo, and their dams bred again while on summer pasture. Heifers may be bred to calve first as 2-yr-olds (24-27 mo) if good winter feeding is practiced to assure maximal development and prevent high death losses at parturition. Heifers (British breeds) should weigh at least 600-650 lb (275-300 kg) at breeding time (exotic crossbreds should be heavier) and should be fed well thereafter to allow for continued growth, good milk production, and early re-breeding. It is good practice to breed the heifers to calve 2-4 wk ahead of the cow herd; then they can receive more attention at calving and have a longer interval from calving to breeding, which improves conception rate as 3-yr-olds.

Older cows have greater body reserves and lower nutrient requirements than heifers; therefore, they can be wintered on poorer quality rations. Usually, they are fed all the hay, fodder, silage, or dry grass they will consume. Their ration should provide a minimum of 5.9% total or crude protein in the dry matter; if it does not, then 1-2 lb (0.5-1 kg) of a 20-30% protein supplement or its equivalent should be fed daily. A mineral mix and salt should be provided.

Mature beef cows may lose ≥150 lb (67 kg) of body wt from fall until after calving in the spring. This weight loss does not impair reproductive performance if spring and summer pastures are adequate. Under most profitable systems of management, a cow will maintain her weight from fall to fall. Lactation requires more nutrients than gestation. However, feeding beef cows more than is necessary for satisfactory production, such as frequently occurs in purebred herds, is undesirable. Large accumulations of body fat may lead to low conception rates, difficult calving, a lower calf crop, and a shorter life span.

Often, a system of "creep feeding" is practiced whereby suckling calves are allowed access to a grain mixture in a self-feeder in an enclosure. A creep-feed mixture might contain 6 parts corn, 3 parts oats, and 1 part protein supplement. The mixture should be ground as coarsely as possible. A commercial 12-14% protein creep feed could be fed also.

Growing bull calves and yearlings should receive ~2 lb (1 kg) of protein supplement, 3-5 lb (1.5-2 kg) of grain, and good-quality roughage. Mature bulls commonly are wintered in the same manner as the cow herd, with a greater feed allowance during the late winter. Highly fitted show bulls may have to be "let down" by gradual reduction in the ration and much exercise before they are suitable for pasture mating. Breeding stock should have adequate nutrients in their ration and be gaining weight before and during breeding. Several nutrient deficiencies, especially carotene, phosphorus, energy, and protein, reduce fertility. These nutrients should be present in adequate amounts in the ration at least 6-8 wk before breeding.

STOCKER CATTLE

It is common practice to feed calves or yearlings to make moderate gains in winter, with faster and cheaper gains on summer pasture. Such cattle may be sold as feeders in the spring or finished out in drylot the following fall. The cost of winter gain on harvested feeds invariably is higher than summer gain on grass; hence, it is advisable to winter cattle so as to make the greatest possible gain on grass. To maintain good health, weanling calves should gain ≥1 lb (0.5 kg)/day. Two pounds (1 kg) of grain plus 1-2 lb (0.5-1 kg) of protein supplement are recommended in addition to nonlegume roughage. If legume roughage is fed, no protein supplement is needed. Older cattle, particularly if they enter the winter in fleshy condition, may do well to maintain their fall weight. A free-choice mineral mix and trace mineralized salt should be supplied. Limited amounts of grain fed to yearling cattle on pasture during the late summer may increase their market value.

Table 13. Nutrient Requirements of Growing and Finishing Beef Cattle*
(Nutrient Concentration in Diet Dry Matter)

Weight, lb (kg)	Daily gain kg	Daily gain lb	Dry matter intake, kg	Total protein, g	Total protein, %	NE_m, Mcal/kg	NE_g, Mcal/kg	TDN, %	ME, Mcal/kg	Ca, %	P, %
			Steer Calves and Yearlings, Medium to Large Frame								
300 (136)	0.45	1.0	3.9	440	11.3	1.19	0.62	56.0	2.03	0.46	0.23
	0.68	1.5	4.1	529	12.9	1.30	0.73	59.5	2.16	0.58	0.27
	0.91	2.0	4.3	628	14.6	1.41	0.84	63.5	2.29	0.70	0.30
	1.13	2.5	4.4	717	16.3	1.54	0.97	67.5	2.45	0.85	0.34
	1.36	3.0	4.3	774	18.0	1.70	1.08	72.0	2.60	0.99	0.39
500 (227)	0.45	1.0	5.8	551	9.5	1.19	0.62	56.0	2.03	0.33	0.19
	0.68	1.5	6.1	634	10.4	1.30	0.73	59.5	2.16	0.39	0.21
	0.91	2.0	6.3	718	11.4	1.41	0.84	63.5	2.29	0.46	0.24
	1.13	2.5	6.4	794	12.4	1.54	0.97	67.5	2.45	0.55	0.25
	1.36	3.0	6.4	858	13.4	1.70	1.08	72.0	2.60	0.63	0.28
700 (318)	0.45	1.0	7.4	636	8.6	1.19	0.62	56.0	2.03	0.27	0.19
	0.68	1.5	7.8	718	9.2	1.30	0.73	59.5	2.16	0.31	0.19
	0.91	2.0	8.1	794	9.8	1.41	0.84	63.5	2.29	0.36	0.21
	1.13	2.5	8.2	861	10.5	1.54	0.97	67.5	2.45	0.40	0.22
	1.36	3.0	8.2	910	11.1	1.70	1.08	72.0	2.60	0.45	0.23
900 (408)	0.45	1.0	9.0	720	8.0	1.19	0.62	56.0	2.03	0.23	0.18
	0.68	1.5	9.4	799	8.5	1.30	0.73	59.5	2.16	0.27	0.18
	0.91	2.0	9.7	863	8.9	1.41	0.84	65.5	2.29	0.29	0.20
	1.13	2.5	9.9	921	9.3	1.54	0.97	67.5	2.45	0.31	0.20
	1.36	3.0	9.8	960	9.8	1.70	1.08	72.0	2.60	0.36	0.21
1100 (500)	0.45	1.0	10.5	809	7.7	1.19	0.62	56.0	2.03	0.21	0.18
	0.68	1.5	10.9	872	8.0	1.30	0.73	59.5	2.16	0.23	0.18
	0.91	2.0	11.3	938	8.3	1.41	0.84	63.5	2.29	0.25	0.18
	1.13	2.5	11.5	978	8.5	1.54	0.97	67.5	2.45	0.26	0.18
	1.36	3.0	11.5	1024	8.9	1.70	1.08	72.0	2.60	0.29	0.19

(continued)

Table 13. Nutrient Requirements of Growing and Finishing Beef Cattle* (continued) (Nutrient Concentration in Diet Dry Matter)

Weight, lb (kg)	Daily gain kg	Daily gain lb	Dry matter intake, kg	Total protein, g	Total protein, %	NE_m, Mcal/kg	NE_g, Mcal/kg	TDN, %	ME, Mcal/kg	Ca, %	P, %
Heifer Calves and Yearlings, Medium to Large Frame											
300 (136)	0.45	1.0	3.8	429	11.3	1.28	0.71	59.0	2.16	0.45	0.24
	0.68	1.5	4.0	520	13.0	1.43	0.86	64.0	2.31	0.58	0.25
	0.91	2.0	4.0	584	14.6	1.63	1.01	69.5	2.51	0.69	0.30
500 (227)	0.45	1.0	5.6	526	9.4	1.28	0.71	59.0	2.16	0.30	0.20
	0.68	1.5	5.9	608	10.3	1.43	0.86	64.0	2.31	0.38	0.20
	0.91	2.0	5.9	661	11.2	1.63	1.01	69.5	2.51	0.44	0.24
700 (318)	0.45	1.0	7.2	597	8.5	1.28	0.71	59.0	2.16	0.25	0.18
	0.68	1.5	7.5	675	9.0	1.43	0.86	64.0	2.31	0.29	0.19
	0.91	2.0	7.6	730	9.6	1.63	1.01	69.5	2.51	0.33	0.20
900 (408)	0.45	1.0	8.7	687	7.9	1.28	0.71	59.0	2.16	0.22	0.18
	0.68	1.5	9.1	746	8.2	1.43	0.86	64.0	2.31	0.23	0.18
	0.91	2.0	9.2	791	8.6	1.63	1.01	69.5	2.51	0.26	0.18

*The concentration of vitamin A in all diets for finishing steers and heifers is 2200 IU/kg dry diet.

Total or crude protein; NE_m, net energy for maintenance; NE_g, net energy for gain; ME, metabolizable energy.

Adapted, with permission, from *Nutrient Requirements of Beef Cattle*, 1984, National Academy of Sciences. Published by National Academy Press, Washington, DC.

Table 14. Nutrient Requirements of Beef Cattle Breeding Herd*
(Nutrient Concentration in Diet Dry Matter)

Weight, lb (kg)	Daily gain kg	lb	Dry matter intake, kg	Total protein, g	Total protein, %	NE_m, Mcal/kg	NE_g, Mcal/kg	TDN, %	ME, Mcal/kg	Ca, %	P, %
Pregnant Yearling Heifers, Last Third of Pregnancy											
700 (318)	0.64	1.4	7.2	648	9.0	1.32	0.75	60	2.18	0.33	0.21
	0.86	1.9	7.2	706	9.8	1.54	0.95	67	2.43	0.33	0.21
800 (363)	0.64	1.4	7.9	695	8.8	1.30	0.73	60	2.16	0.33	0.21
	0.86	1.9	7.9	735	9.3	1.52	0.93	66	2.38	0.35	0.21
900 (408)	0.64	1.4	8.6	731	8.5	1.28	0.71	59	2.14	0.30	0.21
	0.86	1.9	8.7	783	9.0	1.50	0.90	65	2.36	0.32	0.21
Dry Pregnant Mature Cows, Middle Third of Pregnancy											
800 (363)	—	—	6.9	490	7.1	0.93	NA	49	1.76	0.17	0.17
1000 (454)	—	—	8.2	574	7.0	0.93	NA	49	1.76	0.18	0.18
1200 (544)	—	—	9.4	649	6.9	0.93	NA	49	1.76	0.19	0.19
1400 (635)	—	—	10.6	731	6.9	0.93	NA	49	1.76	0.20	0.20
Dry Pregnant Mature Cows, Last Third of Pregnancy											
800 (363)	0.91	2.0	7.6	623	8.2	1.12	NA	55	1.96	0.26	0.20
1000 (454)	0.91	2.0	8.9	703	7.9	1.10	NA	54	1.94	0.26	0.20
1200 (544)	0.91	2.0	10.1	788	7.8	1.08	NA	53	1.92	0.26	0.21
1400 (635)	0.91	2.0	11.3	859	7.6	1.06	NA	53	1.90	0.26	0.21

(continued)

Table 14. Nutrient Requirements of Beef Cattle Breeding Herd* (continued)
(Nutrient Concentration in Diet Dry Matter)

Weight, lb (kg)	Daily gain kg	Daily gain lb	Dry matter intake, kg	Total protein, g	Total protein, %	NE_m, Mcal/kg	NE_g, Mcal/kg	TDN, %	ME, Mcal/kg	Ca, %	P, %
Cows Nursing Calves, Average Milking Ability, First 3–4 Mo Postpartum											
800 (363)	—	—	7.8	796	10.2	1.26	NA	58	2.12	0.30	0.22
1000 (454)	—	—	9.2	883	9.6	1.21	NA	57	2.05	0.28	0.22
1200 (544)	—	—	10.4	967	9.3	1.17	NA	56	2.01	0.27	0.22
1400 (635)	—	—	11.6	1044	9.0	1.12	NA	55	1.98	0.27	0.22
Cows Nursing Calves, Superior Milking Ability, First 3–4 Mo Postpartum											
800 (363)	—	—	7.1	1008	14.2	1.87	NA	77	2.80	0.48	0.31
1000 (454)	—	—	9.3	1144	12.3	1.54	NA	67	2.43	0.39	0.27
1200 (544)	—	—	10.8	1242	11.5	1.43	NA	64	2.31	0.36	0.26
1400 (635)	—	—	12.1	1331	11.0	1.37	NA	62	2.23	0.35	0.26
Bulls, Maintenance and Slow Rate of Growth (Regain Body Condition)											
1300 (590)	0.45	1.0	11.5	874	7.6	1.17	0.62	56	2.03	0.22	0.19
1500 (680)	0.45	1.0	12.8	947	7.4	1.17	0.62	56	2.03	0.21	0.19
1700 (771)	0.23	0.5	13.4	938	7.0	1.04	0.49	52	1.87	0.20	0.19
1900 (862)	0.23	0.5	14.6	1007	6.9	1.04	0.49	52	1.87	0.20	0.20
2100 (953)	—	—	14.7	1000	6.8	0.90	NA	48	1.74	0.22	0.22

*The concentration of vitamin A in all diets for pregnant heifers and cows is ~2800 IU/kg dry diet; for lactating cows and breeding bulls, ~3900 IU/kg. Total or crude protein; NE_m, net energy for maintenance; NE_g, net energy for gain; ME, metabolizable energy.

Adapted, with permission, from *Nutrient Requirements of Beef Cattle*, 1984, National Academy of Sciences. Published by National Academy Press, Washington, DC.

FINISHING CATTLE

This phase of beef production consists of full feeding of grain with limited amounts of roughage until market weight is reached. Older cattle may finish on pasture alone, or with a few pounds of grain/day or 60-90 days in the feedlot on high-grain rations to improve market grade. Weanling calves commonly are shipped direct to the feedlot for a 120-150 day warm-up program followed by finishing rations for 100-150 days; yearlings require ~150 days, and older steers 100-125 days. Grain consumption of cattle on full feed is ~2-2.5 lb/100 lb (1 kg/45 kg) body wt. Roughage consumption usually is limited to about one-fourth to one-third of the total grain intake after cattle are on full feed. Cattle consume ~3% of their body weight daily when self-fed mixed rations. For calves, ~1.5-2 lb (<1 kg) of 30-35% protein supplement is required daily for best gains and market grades when nonlegume roughage is fed.

The grain allowance for finishing cattle should be increased gradually. Feeding too much grain early in the period may lead to lactic acidosis, founder, severe scouring, and cattle that go off feed. About 3 wk is required to get calves on a full feed of grain; a shorter period is required for older cattle. Self-fed, mixed rations should contain ≥50% roughage as cattle are started on feed.

Corn or sorghum silages are very palatable, and cattle of lower grade may be finished principally on silage supplemented with protein. Alfalfa or grass silage is relatively high in protein, carotene, and minerals, but is lacking in available energy, especially when no grain or molasses is added as a preservative. Alfalfa hay is an excellent roughage, but may cause bloat in calves if fed as the only roughage. Grains for finishing cattle have about the same relative value as is indicated by their TDN content. Plant sources of protein are equal in value and can be replaced in part by feeding commercial supplements that contain urea. These supplements are also fortified with minerals, vitamins, and feed additives. A small amount of molasses (1 lb [0.5 kg]/head/day) may improve rations that contain low-quality roughages, such as corn cobs, weathered hays, or cottonseed hulls.

A number of non-nutrient hormone or hormone-like compounds are used to increase gains in finishing cattle, either as feed supplements (melengesterol acetate) or as injectable implants. (*See also* p 1532.) The use of these, eg, estradiol, zeranol, progesterone-estradiol benzoate, testosterone propionate with estradiol benzoate, or trenbolone acetate, commonly results in appreciable improvement in rates of gain and feed efficiency, but strict compliance with manufacturers' directions is indicated. Antibiotics also improve gains and feed efficiency.

Cattle fed monensin and lasalocid consume 10% less feed but gain comparably and more efficiently due to increased production of propionic acid in the rumen. They may also help to control bloat.

The use of tranquilizers to reduce stress and weight loss during weaning or shipment has not proved consistently beneficial. Various means of processing rations, such as pelleting, roasting, flaking, and high-moisture ensiling, have been beneficial in some situations.

CONDITIONING FEEDER CATTLE AFTER SHIPMENT

A daily oral dose of 350 mg each of chlortetracycline (CTC) and sulfamethazine (SMZ) for feeder cattle (especially calves) for 2-3 wk immediately following shipment has significantly lowered the incidence of shipping fever syndrome and also resulted in more rapid regain of shrinkage suffered during shipping and/or weaning. Size of the animal as related to levels of CTC and SMZ is not critical. Some animals may not respond to this treatment and should be isolated for individual attention. The nutritional program recommended for such cattle is a full feed of medium-quality roughage plus 1-2 lb (<1 kg)/head/day of a 32% protein supplement that derives at least two-thirds of its protein from natural sources. Thus, the prescribed daily dose of CTC and SMZ for one animal may be incorporated into each 1-2 lb (0.5-1 kg) of the protein supplement.

NUTRITIONAL REQUIREMENTS OF DAIRY CATTLE

The specific dietary needs of dairy cattle are greatly modified by rumen activity. For their first 3-5 wk, calves are essentially monogastric animals, have dietary requirements similar to those of pigs and dogs, and must obtain these nutrients from milk or a milk replacer. They require high-quality, easily digested feeds to supply available energy, essential amino acids, essential minerals, and nearly all of the vitamins. Soon after 1 mo of age, as roughage and grain consumption increases, microorganisms in the rumen become increasingly active in synthesizing the essential amino acids and B vitamins and in digesting cellulose. Mature dairy cattle, therefore, can survive largely independently of a dietary supply of essential amino acids or high-quality protein and the B vitamins. However, for high-producing dairy cows early in lactation, degradability of dietary protein in the rumen should be considered. Supplemental niacin may be beneficial under some conditions. In common with other ruminants, mature cattle utilize coarse feeds, high in cellulose and hemicellulose, which are less useful for nonherbivores. Veal calves, which are fed solely a milk or milk-replacer diet and no dry feed, exist as nonruminants in terms of their nutritional requirements.

For daily nutrient requirements of dairy cattle, see TABLE 15 for growing cattle and TABLE 16 for lactating and pregnant cows. Specific requirements are shown for large breeds for total feed, energy, total protein, calcium, phosphorus, and vitamins A and D. TABLE 17 summarizes the concentration of all the known nutrients in the diets recommended for different classes of dairy cattle. When maximum tolerances are known, these are also included.

WATER

Since dairy cattle suffer more quickly from an inadequate water intake than from a deficiency of any other nutrient, clean fresh drinking water should be available at all times. Milk production and feed intake will be depressed if free access to water is not allowed. Cows will consume 3-5 kg of water for each kilogram of dry matter consumed plus additional water for milk production. Thus, cows yielding 80 lb (36 kg) of milk may drink >300 lb (136 kg) per day. On succulent feeds, water consumption is less. In winter, cows will drink more water if it is warmed slightly; in warm weather, intake may be trebled. Calves during the latter part of the milk-feeding period, heifers, and bulls should be offered water ad lib.

ENERGY

The principal use of feed by the body is as a source of energy. All organic nutrients, eg, protein, carbohydrates, and fats, supply energy; thus, the energy values of the organic components of a feedstuff are combined and expressed as total digestible nutrients (TDN), digestible energy (DE), metabolizable energy (ME), or net energy (net energy—maintenance, NE_m; net energy—gain, NE_g; net energy—lactation, NE_l). TDN and DE account for energy losses in the feces; ME from the feces, urine, and combustible gases from the gut; and NE equals ME minus the heat increment or energy losses from the metabolism of feed nutrients for specific purposes. The latter connotation reflects a truer value of the feedstuffs for productive purposes and more accurately compares concentrates with roughages. Consequently, it is the most commonly used method for calculating the energy value of feeds. In many laboratories, NE values are calculated from acid detergent fiber. Thus, if added fat sources are used in a ration, these must be accounted for separately.

Insufficient intake of energy is a more frequent cause of retarded growth, delayed puberty, or depressed milk production than probably any other nutritional deficiency. The energy requirements (TABLES 15-17) serve primarily as guides. Lower intakes than suggested reduce growth rates and decrease milk production. Larger intakes increase growth rates and may increase production or fat deposition, or both, in lactating cows.

Table 15. Daily Nutrient Requirements of Growing Dairy Cattle and Mature Bulls

Live Weight (kg)	Gain (g)	Dry Matter Intake (kg)	Energy					Protein			Minerals		Vitamins	
			NE$_m$ (Mcal)	NE$_g$ (Mcal)	ME (Mcal)	DE (Mcal)	TDN (kg)	UIP (g)	DIP (g)	CP (g)	Ca (g)	P (g)	A (1000 IU)	D (1000 IU)
Growing Large-Breed Calves Fed Only Milk or Milk Replacer														
40	200	0.48	1.37	0.41	2.54	2.73	0.62	—	—	105	7	4	1.70	0.26
45	300	0.54	1.49	0.56	2.86	3.07	0.70	—	—	120	8	5	1.94	0.30
Growing Large-Breed Calves Fed Milk Plus Starter Mix														
50	500	1.30	1.62	0.72	5.90	6.42	1.46	—	—	290	9	6	2.10	0.33
75	800	1.98	2.19	1.30	8.98	9.78	2.22	—	—	435	16	8	3.20	0.50
Growing Veal Calves Fed Only Milk or Milk Replacer														
50	400	0.57	1.62	0.57	2.39	2.63	0.59	—	—	125	9	5	2.10	0.33
75	900	1.36	2.19	1.47	4.82	5.39	1.21	—	—	300	16	9	3.20	0.50
100	1250	2.00	2.72	2.26	6.22	7.06	1.58	—	—	440	20	11	4.20	0.66
150	1100	2.72	3.69	2.29	8.46	9.60	2.15	—	—	598	24	15	6.40	0.99
Large-Breed Growing Females														
100	700	2.82	2.72	1.44	7.54	8.72	1.98	346	75	452	18	9	4.24	0.66
150	700	3.75	3.69	1.71	9.76	11.33	2.57	307	173	600	19	12	6.36	0.99
200	700	4.68	4.57	1.95	11.87	13.84	3.14	274	267	686	21	14	8.48	1.32
300	700	6.66	6.20	2.39	16.00	18.81	4.27	223	452	799	24	18	12.72	1.98
400	700	8.92	7.69	2.80	20.23	24.00	5.44	190	641	1070	26	20	16.96	2.64
500	600	10.93	9.09	2.69	23.32	27.96	6.34	175	785	1311	28	20	21.20	3.30
600	600	14.11	10.43	3.00	28.23	34.24	7.77	193	1007	1694	28	20	25.44	3.96
Large-Breed Growing Males														
100	800	2.80	2.72	1.42	7.48	8.66	1.96	401	65	448	18	10	4.24	0.66
300	1000	6.73	6.20	2.80	16.70	19.53	4.43	323	464	884	26	20	12.72	1.98
500	900	10.48	9.09	3.25	23.76	28.19	6.39	233	786	1257	29	22	21.20	3.30
700	800	15.16	11.70	3.46	31.14	37.59	8.52	219	1124	1820	29	22	29.68	4.62
Maintenance of Mature Breeding Bulls														
500	—	7.89	9.09	—	15.79	19.15	4.34	161	472	789	20	12	21.20	3.30
900	—	12.27	14.13	—	24.53	29.76	6.75	135	854	1227	36	22	38.16	5.94
1300	—	16.16	18.62	—	32.32	39.21	8.89	108	1196	1616	53	32	55.12	8.58

NE$_m$, net energy for maintenance; NE$_g$, net energy for gain; ME, metabolizable energy; DE, digestible energy; TDN, total digestible nutrients; UIP, undegraded intake protein; DIP, degraded intake protein; CP, crude protein.

Adapted, with permission, from *Nutrient Requirements of Dairy Cattle*, 1989, National Academy of Sciences. Published by National Academy Press, Washington, DC.

Table 16. Daily Nutrient Requirements of Lactating and Pregnant Cows

Live Weight (kg)	Energy				Total Crude Protein (g)	Minerals		Vitamins	
	NE$_l$ (Mcal)	ME (Mcal)	DE (Mcal)	TDN (kg)		Ca (g)	P (g)	A (1000 IU)	D (1000 IU)
Maintenance of Mature Lactating Cows[a]									
400	7.16	12.01	13.80	3.13	318	16	11	30	12
500	8.46	14.20	16.32	3.70	364	20	14	38	15
600	9.70	16.28	18.71	4.24	406	24	17	46	18
700	10.89	18.28	21.00	4.76	449	28	20	53	21
800	12.03	20.20	23.21	5.26	486	32	23	61	24
Maintenance Plus Last 2 Mo of Gestation of Mature Dry Cows[b]									
400	9.30	15.26	18.23	4.15	875	26	16	30	12
500	11.00	18.04	21.55	4.90	978	33	20	38	15
600	12.61	20.68	24.71	5.62	1074	39	24	46	18
700	14.15	23.21	27.73	6.31	1165	46	28	53	21
800	15.64	25.66	30.65	6.98	1254	53	32	61	24
Milk Production—Nutrients Per Kg of Milk of Different Fat Percentages									
(% Fat)									
3.0	0.64	1.07	1.23	0.280	78	2.73	1.68	—	—
3.5	0.69	1.15	1.33	0.301	84	2.97	1.83	—	—
4.0	0.74	1.24	1.42	0.322	90	3.21	1.98	—	—
4.5	0.78	1.32	1.51	0.343	96	3.45	2.13	—	—
5.0	0.83	1.40	1.61	0.364	101	3.69	2.28	—	—
5.5	0.88	1.48	1.70	0.385	107	3.93	2.43	—	—

NE$_l$, net energy for lactation; ME, metabolizable energy; DE, digestible energy; TDN, total digestible nutrients.

[a]To allow for growth of young lactating cows, increase the maintenance allowances for all nutrients except vitamins A and D by 20% during the first lactation and 10% during the second lactation.

[b]Values for calcium assume that the cow is in calcium balance at the beginning of the last 2 mo of gestation. If the cow is not in balance, then the calcium requirement can be increased from 25 to 33%.

Adapted, with permission, from *Nutrient Requirements of Dairy Cattle*, 1989, National Academy of Sciences. Published by National Academy Press, Washington, DC.

Table 17. Recommended Nutrient Content of Diets for Dairy Cattle

Cow Wt (kg)	Fat (%)	Wt Gain (kg/day)
400	5.0	0.220
500	4.5	0.275
600	4.0	0.330
700	3.5	0.385
800	3.5	0.440

	Lactating Cow Diets (Milk Yield, kg/day)					Early Lactation (wk 0-3)	Dry Pregnant Cows	Calf Milk Replacer	Calf Starter Mix	Growing Heifers and Bulls[a]			Mature Bulls	Maximum Tolerable Levels[b]
										3-6 mo	6-12 mo	>12mo		
Milk Yield (kg/day)	7,8,10,12,13	13,17,20,24,27	20,25,30,36,40	26,33,40,48,53	33,41,50,60,67									
Energy														
NE_l, Mcal/kg	1.42	1.52	1.62	1.72	1.72	1.67	1.25	2.40	1.90	1.70	1.58	1.40	1.15	—
NE_m, Mcal/kg	—	—	—	—	—	—	—	1.55	1.20	1.08	0.98	0.82	—	—
NE_g, Mcal/kg	—	—	—	—	—	—	—	—	—	—	—	—	—	—
ME, Mcal/kg	2.35	2.53	2.71	2.89	2.89	2.80	2.04	3.78	3.11	2.60	2.47	2.27	2.00	—
DE, Mcal/kg	2.77	2.95	3.13	3.31	3.31	3.22	2.47	4.19	3.53	3.02	2.89	2.69	2.43	—
TDN, % of DM	63	67	71	75	75	73	56	95	80	69	66	61	55	—
Protein equivalent														
Crude protein, %	12	15	16	17	18	19	12	22	18	16	12	12	10	—
UIP, %	4.4	5.2	5.7	5.9	6.2	7.0	—	—	—	8.2	4.4	2.1	—	—
DIP, %	7.8	8.7	9.6	10.3	10.4	9.7	—	—	—	4.6	6.4	7.2	—	—
Fiber content (min.)[c]														
Crude fiber, %	17	17	17	15	15	17	22	—	—	13	15	15	15	—
Acid detergent fiber, %	21	21	21	19	19	21	27	—	—	16	19	19	19	—
Neutral detergent fiber, %	28	28	28	25	25	28	35	—	—	23	25	25	25	—
Ether extract (min.), %	3	3	3	3	3	3	3	10	3	3	3	3	3	—
Minerals														
Calcium, %	0.43	0.51	0.58	0.64	0.66	0.77	0.39[d]	0.70	0.60	0.52	0.41	0.29	0.30	2.00
Phosphorus, %	0.28	0.33	0.37	0.41	0.41	0.48	0.24	0.60	0.40	0.31	0.30	0.23	0.19	1.00
Magnesium, %[e]	0.20	0.20	0.20	0.25	0.25	0.25	0.16	0.07	0.10	0.16	0.16	0.16	0.16	0.50
Potassium, %[f]	0.90	0.90	0.90	1.00	1.00	1.00	0.65	0.65	0.65	0.65	0.65	0.65	0.65	3.00
Sodium, %	0.18	0.18	0.18	0.18	0.18	0.18	0.10	0.10	0.10	0.10	0.10	0.10	0.10	—
Chloride, %	0.25	0.25	0.25	0.25	0.25	0.25	0.20	0.20	0.20	0.20	0.20	0.20	0.20	—
Sulfur, %	0.20	0.20	0.20	0.20	0.20	0.25	0.16	0.29	0.20	0.16	0.16	0.16	0.16	0.40
Iron, ppm	50	50	50	50	50	50	50	100	50	50	50	50	50	1000
Cobalt, ppm	0.10	0.10	0.10	0.10	0.10	0.10	0.10	0.10	0.10	0.10	0.10	0.10	0.10	10.00
Copper, ppm	10	10	10	10	10	10	10	10	10	10	10	10	10	100
Manganese, ppm	40	40	40	40	40	40	40	40	40	40	40	40	40	1000
Zinc, ppm	40	40	40	40	40	40	40	40	40	40	40	40	40	500

(continued)

Table 17. Recommended Nutrient Content of Diets for Dairy Cattle (continued)

Cow Wt (kg)	Fat (%)	Wt Gain (kg/day)	Lactating Cow Diets — Milk Yield (kg/day)					Early Lactation (wk 0-3)	Dry Pregnant Cows	Calf Milk Replacer	Calf Starter Mix	Growing Heifers and Bulls[a] 3-6 mo	6-12 mo	>12 mo	Mature Bulls	Maximum Tolerable Levels[b]
400	5.0	0.220	7	13	20	26	33									
500	4.5	0.275	8	17	25	33	41									
600	4.0	0.330	10	20	30	40	50									
700	3.5	0.385	12	24	36	48	60									
800	3.5	0.440	13	27	40	53	67									
Iodine, ppm[h]			0.60	0.60	0.60	0.60	0.60	0.60	0.25	0.25	0.25	0.25	0.25	0.25	0.25	50.00[i]
Selenium, ppm			0.30	0.30	0.30	0.30	0.30	0.30	0.30	0.30	0.30	0.30	0.30	0.30	0.30	2.00
Vitamins[j]																
A, IU/kg			3200	3200	3200	3200	3200	4000	4000	3800	2200	2200	2200	2200	3200	66,000
D, IU/kg			1000	1000	1000	1000	1000	1000	1200	600	300	300	300	300	300	10,000
E, IU/kg			15	15	15	15	15	15	15	40	25	25	25	25	15	2000

NOTE: The values presented in this table are intended as guidelines for the use of professionals in diet formulation. Because of the many factors affecting such values, they are not intended and should not be used as a legal or regulatory base.

a The approximate weight for growing heifers and bulls at 3-6 mo is 150 kg; at 6-12 mo, it is 250 kg; and at >12 mo, it is 400 kg. The approximate average daily gain is 700 g/day.

b The maximum safe levels for many of the mineral elements are not well defined and may be substantially affected by specific feeding conditions.

c It is recommended that 75% of the NDF in lactating cow diets be provided as forage. If this recommendation is not followed, a depression in milk fat may occur.

d The value for calcium assumes that the cow is in calcium balance at the beginning of the dry period. If the cow is not in balance, then the dietary calcium requirement should be increased by 25-33%.

e Under conditions conducive to grass tetany, magnesium should be increased to 0.25 or 0.30%.

f Under conditions of heat stress, potassium should be increased to 1.2%.

g The cow's copper requirement is influenced by molybdenum and sulfur in the diet.

h If the diet contains as much as 25% strongly goitrogenic feed on a dry basis, the iodine provided should be increased ≥2 times.

i Although cattle can tolerate this level of iodine, lower levels may be desirable to reduce the iodine content of milk.

j The following minimum quantities of B-complex vitamins are suggested per unit of milk replacer: niacin, 2.6 ppm; pantothenic acid, 13 ppm; riboflavin, 6.5 ppm; pyridoxine, 6.5 ppm; folic acid, 0.5 ppm; biotin, 0.1 ppm; vitamin B_{12}, 0.07 ppm; thiamine, 6.5 ppm; and choline, 0.26%. It appears that adequate amounts of these vitamins are furnished when calves have functional rumens (usually at 6 wk of age) by a combination of rumen synthesis and natural feedstuffs.

Adapted, with permission, from Nutrient Requirements of Dairy Cattle, 1989, National Academy of Sciences. Published by National Academy Press, Washington, DC.

Under rigid experimental conditions, calves have been shown to require essential fatty acids; however, under usual feeding conditions, even when low-fat milk replacers are used, the deficiency does not occur. A specific dietary fat requirement for ruminating cattle does not appear to exist or at least is met by normal feedstuffs. Fats in the form of whole cottonseed, soybeans, etc, are frequently added to rations of high-producing cows to improve energy balance and should be limited to a maximum of 0.5 kg/cow/day.

FIBER

While fiber is the most undigestible portion of the ration of a dairy cow, it is necessary as part of the overall feeding program. The actual amount to be included depends on several factors including body condition, level of production, type of fiber fed, and physical characteristics of the fiber. Animals that are producing large amounts of milk are fed rations with less fiber, while those producing less milk, or during the growing or dry periods are fed diets with more fiber. The amount and type of fiber that is fed can have a great effect on rumen function, which affects the amount of rumination, saliva production, rumen pH, and milk fat level.

The amount of fiber is expressed in terms of acid detergent fiber (ADF) or neutral detergent fiber (NDF). ADF consists of cellulose, lignin, acid-detergent-insoluble nitrogen, and acid-insoluble ash; NDF consists of the same plus hemicellulose. Generally, the ADF content of a ration is thought to be a good indicator of the overall digestibility of the diet, while the NDF content is considered to correlate well with total dry-matter intake. However, because both chemical and physical properties of feeds affect the fiber determination, it is difficult to completely predict the fiber quality and energy value of feeds.

Published recommendations for the levels of ADF and NDF vary widely. In general, it appears that levels of ADF in lactating cow rations should be ~21% on a dry-matter basis, while the level of NDF should be ~28%. Further, it is recommended that ~75% of the NDF should be present in the forage fraction of the total ration.

It is thought that, in general, cows will consume ~1.2% of their body wt/day as NDF. Thus, given a level of 28% NDF in a given ration, a 1300-lb (600-kg) cow might be expected to consume ~55 lb (25 kg) of feed dry matter per day. If her production level suggests a higher or lower level of dry-matter intake is appropriate, reformulation of the feed, including the concentration of NDF, may be in order. TABLE 17 lists recommended percentages of ADF and NDF for various classes of dairy cattle.

PROTEIN

The total crude protein values in TABLES 15-17 represent the approximate minimum requirements. Additional protein may result in a marginal increase in milk production. However, gross excess of protein (>19%) in the ration of dry pregnant cows or lactating cows may prolong days open and services per conception following parturition. Feeding excess protein to dry cows has also been implicated in the alert downer syndrome of parturient dairy cows (qv, p 555).

Dairy cattle, like other animals, require essential amino acids that must be absorbed from the small intestine. These amino acids are derived from microbial protein produced in the ruminoreticulum and digested in the small intestine, as well as from dietary protein that escapes degradation in the rumen but is digested to amino acids postruminally. Under normal feeding conditions, in which total crude protein requirements are met, growing heifers, dry cows, and cows in mid to late lactation can meet amino acid needs from microbial protein produced in the rumen. The amount of microbial protein synthesis depends on factors such as the level of nonstructural carbohydrate in the diet, physical density and form of the diet, level and frequency of feeding, availability in the rumen of sulfur and branched-chain fatty acids, and especially on the amount of rumen-degradable intake protein (DIP). High-yielding cows, however, have amino acid requirements in excess of what can be supplied by rumen microbes even at high rates of synthesis. Consequently, the diet of such cows should include proteins of relatively low degradability in the rumen that will escape breakdown until they reach the small intestine. This escape protein is known as undegraded intake protein (UIP). Estimates of UIP and DIP requirements are listed in TABLES 15 and 17. Since feedstuffs vary considerably in proportions of degradable and undegradable proteins, TABLE 18 lists some selected values for use in balancing diets.

Urea may be used in the ration to meet part of the DIP requirement of older heifers, dry cows, and low-producing cows as long as adequate energy in the form of non-structural carbohydrate is present in the rumen. Some urea may occasionally be justified in diets of high-yielding cows when their diet is otherwise high in UIP. Urea should be introduced to the diet gradually over a 3-wk period and mixed thoroughly with palatable feeds, preferably in ways that will avoid excessive intakes over short periods of time. (*See also* p 1693.) Common recommendations are to add urea at rates up to 7.5 kg/ton of corn silage, or up to 1% of the concentrates for a maximum intake of 0.23 kg of urea daily. If urea is added to a ration already more than adequate in degradable protein, it is not only wasted but can adversely affect feed intake, health, and production. Conversely if rations are relatively high in UIP and starches, urea or other nonprotein nitrogen such as ammonia may be used to meet the needs of rumen microorganisms for nitrogen.

Table 18. Estimates of Ruminal Undegradability of Protein in Common Feedstuffs

Feed	Value	Feed	Value
Alfalfa hay	0.28	Distillers dried grains	0.54
Alfalfa silage	0.23	Fishmeal	0.60
Barley	0.27	Grass silage	0.29
Brewers dried grains	0.49	Linseed meal	0.35
Bromegrass	0.44	Rapeseed (canola) meal	0.28
Corn	0.52	Meat and bone meal	0.49
Corn gluten feed, dry	0.22	Soybean meal	0.35
Corn gluten meal	0.55	Soybeans, raw	0.26
Corn silage	0.31	Wheat	0.22
		Wheat bran	0.29

Adapted, with permission, from *Nutrient Requirements of Dairy Cattle*, 1989, National Academy of Sciences. Published by National Academy Press, Washington, DC.

MINERALS

Dairy cattle need a dietary source of calcium, phosphorus, magnesium, sulfur, potassium, sodium, chlorine, iron, iodine, manganese, copper, cobalt, zinc, and selenium. A few of the minerals needing special attention in practical feeding are discussed below.

Table 19. Some Good Sources of Calcium and Phosphorus (As Fed)

Feed	Calcium %	Phosphorus %
Alfalfa hay (early vegetative)	1.91	0.27
Clover hay (early bloom)	2.03	0.34
Dried skim milk	1.17	0.97
Dried whey	0.91	0.75
Wheat bran	0.11	1.17
Cottonseed meal	0.16	1.21
Distiller's solubles	0.35	1.37
Bone meal	29.0	13.2
Defluorinated rock phosphate	31.7	13.7
Dicalcium phosphate	22.7	18.0
Limestone	38.0	0.02

Ordinary feeds do not supply **salt** (sodium chloride) in amounts sufficient to meet the needs of dairy cattle, with the possible exception of good pasture. The preferred method of feeding salt is to include it in concentrate mixtures or complete feeds at 0.46% of total ration dry matter for lactating cows and at 0.25% of total ration dry matter for dry cows and other nonlactating cattle. Allowing animals free access to salt is a practical way of meeting the requirement of animals not receiving concentrates. Loose or block salt should be protected from the weather.

Calcium and phosphorus must be added to almost all dairy cattle diets. The calcium and phosphorus contents of certain feeds and supplements are shown in TABLE 19. Alfalfa and clover hays are rich in calcium but somewhat low in phosphorus, as are most legumes. Nonlegume forages are poor in calcium.

Concentrate feeds used for dairy cattle are relatively deficient in calcium. Wheat bran, distillers' solubles, and cottonseed meal are the common feeds rich in phosphorus, but they are low in calcium. Bone meal, defluorinated phosphates, and dicalcium phosphate are the most common supplements of calcium and phosphorus. Limestone (feed grade) is the least expensive single source of calcium. Both the ratio of calcium to phosphorus and the presence of vitamin D affect calcium and phosphorus utilization. The NRC recommends (TABLE 17) a calcium:phosphorus ratio of ~1.5:1 for growth, maintenance, and milk production. Mature bulls receiving 3-5 times their calcium requirement have developed a high incidence of osteoporosis, which markedly reduces their ability to walk and to mount. Milk fever has been reduced by decreasing calcium intake to ~30 g/day 2 wk before calving and increasing it to 150-200 g/day after calving. To guarantee satisfactory intakes, mineral supplements should be incorporated in the concentrate or total mixed ration at levels calculated to meet requirements. Although free-choice feeding of minerals to yearlings and dry cows not receiving concentrates is a common practice, cattle will not balance their diets in this way.

Iodine is required for the synthesis of iodothyroglobulin and thyroxine, by which the thyroid gland exercises a degree of control over the basal metabolic rate and growth, reproduction, and lactation. In the newborn calf, simple goiter (qv, p 283) is evident when maternal iodine intake is deficient. The iodine requirement is increased by goitrogenic substances in feeds, such as raw soybeans, linseed, certain clovers, and cruciferous crops in general. Pasture plants vary greatly in their ability to take up iodine from the soil. The only feeds naturally rich in iodine are the saltwater fish meals and dried kelp, so that deficiency is more readily prevented by providing stabilized iodized salt containing 0.01% iodine as part of a trace mineral mixture in the concentrate.

Since the thyroid can store iodine, the daily requirement does not have to be met each day. However, excessive quantities fed over short periods give rise to signs of iodism. Iodine deficiency (qv, p 1196) occurs on deficient soils such as around the Great Lakes and westward to the Pacific coast.

Cobalt is required for normal ruminal metabolism. When the intake of cobalt is inadequate, the bacterial population in the rumen is altered and the synthesis of vitamin B_{12} is greatly lowered. In some areas, particularly the southeastern seacoast (USA), the soil, and hence the forages, are deficient in cobalt. Usually, legumes are richer than grasses. Corn (maize) appears to have a low content, while linseed meal is a rich source. When the forage contains <0.07 ppm of cobalt (dry basis), signs of deficiency (qv, p 1197) may occur. Effective supplementation of the ration of dairy cattle can be achieved by adding 2 g of cobalt sulfate to each ton of concentrate mixture.

Copper is required as a constituent or activator of certain enzyme systems concerned with Hgb synthesis, melanin production, hair growth, and the functional integrity of bone and nervous tissues. Except in general terms, it is not possible to set a uniform copper requirement for all areas because it is markedly influenced by the level of other dietary constituents, particularly molybdenum, inorganic sulfate, and phosphorus. The levels of these minerals being normal, the daily requirement of copper for dairy cattle may be satisfied by forage that contains not less than 10 ppm (dry basis).

There are many areas in the USA where, either because of a low copper content of the herbage or the presence of complicating factors such as high molybdenum, the copper content of the ration must be supplemented to maintain normal health, growth, production, and reproduction in dairy cattle (*see* p 1197).

VITAMINS

Calves up to 4-5 wk old should receive all of the known vitamins in their feed except niacin and ascorbic acid. Niacin is synthesized from dietary tryptophan, and synthesis of ascorbic acid in the liver is adequate. Milk, cereal grains, and other feeds consumed by young calves contain sufficient B vitamins to meet their needs before rumen synthesis begins. Milk replacers should probably contain all the added B vitamins (*see* TABLE 17).

As bacterial function develops in the rumen, the B vitamins are synthesized in large amounts and need not be supplied in the diet thereafter. However, evidence suggests that under some conditions, high-yielding cows in early lactation may be less prone to ketosis when fed supplemental **niacin**. Supplementation of 6-12 g of niacin/day from 2 wk before calving and continued 8-12 wk after calving may be beneficial in dairy herds with an above average incidence of ketosis and overconditioned cows. Some response in both milk yield and fat test may be seen in rations containing all-natural protein supplemented with niacin.

Vitamins A, D, and E: A deficiency of any of these vitamins is relatively rare for cattle receiving natural mixtures of high-quality feeds. White muscle disease (qv, p 548) due to a deficiency of vitamin E or selenium is not uncommon in dairy and beef calves and lambs in areas where the soil is low in selenium.

When cows are fed poor-quality, bleached roughage for long periods, they may show reproductive failure from vitamin A deficiency, or they may produce milk low in vitamin A. Under such conditions, supplementation with synthetic vitamin A is desirable. Fresh pasture in summer is an excellent source of carotene, the precursor of vitamin A. Because even high-quality, properly cured hay or silage loses its vitamin A value with storage over time, most commercial concentrates now contain several thousand IU of vitamin A per kg as assurance against deficiency.

All natural feeds except sun-cured hay have a low vitamin D content. Animals that are exposed to sunlight for as little as 1 hr/day synthesize ample vitamin D in the skin and do not require high levels in their feed. Vitamin D deficiency may be observed in young calves that are confined with inadequate light, and do not consume sun-cured roughage. Whole milk and skim milk are always low in vitamin D. Concentrate mixtures are also naturally low in the vitamin. As little as 300 IU of vitamin D/kg feed is an adequate amount for calves. Feeding sun-cured hay *ad lib* to young calves prevents vitamin D deficiency. Since vitamin D is relatively inexpensive and cattle may be exposed to little sunlight, it is commonly included in calf and cow rations.

Vitamin E has been added to dairy concentrates at the level of 500 mg/cow/day to minimize oxidized flavor in milk.

Although the use of vitamins A, D, and E in dairy concentrates is widespread, appearance of a frank deficiency in the field when they are not supplemented is unlikely. Injections of vitamins A, D, and E at the time of drying off were of no value to cows fed normal diets. Milk replacers should be fortified with vitamins A, D, and E.

β-carotene has been suggested to be of value in minimizing reproductive problems, especially when blood levels are low in cows and heifers. However, research data are limited and conflicting.

Vitamin K is ordinarily synthesized in the rumen in ample quantities, although *see* SWEET CLOVER POISONING, p 1733.

FEEDING AND NUTRITIONAL MANAGEMENT

Dairy cattle require some concentrates until the age of 8-12 mo, although forage can supply an increasing percentage of the ration after ~4 mo. In addition, concentrates are needed for lactating cows and as a supplement to poor-quality, unpalatable, sparse forage. However, concentrates do not completely compensate for lack of quality in forages fed to high-yielding cows.

Table 20. Estimated Nutrient Content of Some Feeds for Dairy and Beef Cattle (Dry-matter Basis)

Feedstuff	DE	ME	NE_m	NE_g	NE_l	TDN	Crude Protein	Crude Fiber	NDF	ADF	Ca	P	Vitamin A	Dry Matter
		Mcal/kg				%	%	%	%	%	%	%	1000 IU/kg	%
Dried roughage														
Alfalfa hay														
good (early bloom)	2.65	2.22	1.31	0.74	1.35	60	18	23	42	31	1.41	0.22	56	90
poor (full bloom)	2.43	2.00	1.14	0.58	1.23	55	15	29	50	37	1.25	0.22	26	90
Bermuda grass hay	2.21	1.78	0.97	0.42	1.11	50	12	33	76	38	0.32	0.20	—	93
Other legume hay	2.43	2.00	1.14	0.58	1.23	55	16	29	46	36	1.53	0.25	8	89
Grass hay														
early cut	2.87	2.45	1.47	0.88	1.47	65	15	31	61	34	0.27	0.34	15	89
late cut	2.38	1.96	1.11	0.55	1.20	54	8	37	72	45	0.26	0.30	8	91
Corn stover	2.21	1.78	0.97	0.42	1.11	50	6	34	67	39	0.57	0.10	2	85
Cottonseed hulls	1.98	1.55	0.78	0.25	0.98	45	4.1	47.8	90	73	0.15	0.09	—	91
Silages														
Corn, well eared	3.09	2.67	1.63	1.03	1.60	70	8.1	23.7	51	28	0.23	0.22	18	33
Sorghum	2.65	2.22	1.31	0.74	1.35	60	7	28	—	38	0.35	0.21	6	30
Grass	2.87	2.45	1.47	0.88	1.47	65	15	31	61	34	0.27	0.34	15	33
Alfalfa	2.78	2.36	1.41	0.83	1.42	63	20	20	38	28	1.80	0.35	—	38
Concentrates														
Barley	3.70	3.29	2.06	1.40	1.94	84	13.5	5.7	19	7	0.05	0.38	1	88
Beet pulp, dried	3.44	3.02	1.88	1.24	1.79	78	9.7	19.8	54	33	0.69	0.10	—	91
Brewers grains, dried	2.91	2.49	1.51	0.91	1.50	66	25.4	14.9	46	24	0.33	0.55	0	92
Citrus pulp, dried	3.40	2.98	1.86	1.22	1.77	77	6.7	12.7	23	22	1.84	0.12	—	91
Corn, ears, ground	3.66	3.25	2.03	1.37	1.91	83	9	9.4	28	11	0.07	0.27	2	87
Corn, grain	3.75	3.34	2.10	1.43	1.96	85	10	3	9	3	0.02	0.32	1	88

(continued)

Table 20. Estimated Nutrient Content of Some Feeds for Dairy and Beef Cattle (continued) (Dry-matter Basis)

Feedstuff	DE	ME	NE$_m$	NE$_g$	NE$_l$	TDN	Crude Protein	Crude Fiber	NDF	ADF	Ca	P	Vitamin A	Dry Matter
	Mcal/kg					%	%	%	%	%	%	%	1000 IU/kg	%
Corn, shelled, high moisture	3.88	3.47	2.18	1.50	2.04	88	10	3	9	3	0.02	0.32	1	78
Corn gluten feed	3.66	3.25	2.03	1.37	1.91	83	25.6	9.7	45	12	0.36	0.82	3	90
Cottonseed meal	3.35	2.93	1.82	1.19	1.74	76	45.6	14.1	26	19	0.22	1.21	—	91
Cottonseed, whole	4.23	3.82	2.41	1.69	2.23	96	25	17.2	37	26	0.12	0.54	—	90
Corn distillers grains	3.88	3.47	2.18	1.50	2.04	88	25	9.9	44	18	0.15	0.71	1	92
Linseed meal	3.44	3.02	1.88	1.24	1.79	78	38	10	25	19	0.43	0.89	—	90
Milk, whole	5.69	5.29	3.34	2.16	3.04	129	26.7	—	—	—	0.95	0.76	—	12
Molasses, cane	3.17	2.76	1.69	1.08	1.64	72	5.8	—	—	—	1.00	0.11	—	75
Oats	3.40	2.98	1.86	1.22	1.77	77	13.3	12.1	32	16	0.07	0.38	—	89
Sorghum, milo	3.53	3.12	1.94	1.30	1.84	80	9.7	2	18	9	0.04	0.34	—	87
Soybean meal	3.84	3.42	2.16	1.48	2.01	87	55.1	3.7	8	6	0.29	0.70	—	90
Wheat	3.88	3.47	2.18	1.50	2.04	88	16	2.9	—	8	0.04	0.42	1	89
Wheat bran	3.09	2.67	1.63	1.03	1.60	70	17.1	11.3	51	15	0.13	1.38	—	89

DE, digestible energy; ME, metabolizable energy; NE$_m$, net energy maintenance; NE$_g$, net energy gain; NE$_l$, net energy lactation; TDN, total digestible nutrients; NDF, neutral detergent fiber; ADF, acid detergent fiber.

Adapted, with permission, from *Nutrient Requirements of Dairy Cattle*, 1989, National Academy of Sciences. Published by National Academy Press, Washington, DC.

In determining the amount and kind of concentrate mixture needed, it is essential to know what types and amounts of roughage are available; a concentrate can then be selected that will supply the amounts of additional nutrients needed at lowest cost. As an aid in formulating a concentrate mixture, the nutrient requirements stated as amounts per kg of feed are shown in TABLE 17. (Note: These data are for total feed, including forage and concentrates.)

The amounts of nutrients furnished by some common cattle feeds are listed in TABLE 20. Hays and silages of the same species vary greatly in composition, depending on the stage of maturity at the time of cutting and curing, and preservation methods. However, although the precise value of a hay or silage cannot be known without chemical analysis (or even a feeding experiment), its approximate value can be estimated from TABLE 20, and a concentrate mixture of appropriate composition can be made or purchased to balance the roughage available. Forage-testing services available either through Cooperative Extension or local feed companies can give more precise information as to composition, and should be used whenever possible.

High-protein feeds, such as soybean meal, cottonseed meal, linseed meal, and canola meal, usually are higher in price than the cereal grains. Therefore, it is generally good economy to use concentrate mixtures as low in protein as will supply an adequate amount of total protein. Simple mixtures are as effective as complex ones provided some thought is given to ruminal degradability of protein. Feed companies provide significant economies by using by-product feeds in complex mixtures.

Palatability and nutrient content rather than the number of ingredients in a mixture largely determine the value of feeds for dairy cattle.

Calves should receive colostrum for at least the first 3 days, and then milk at the rate of 10% of body wt/day during the first few weeks after birth. A milk replacer or fermented colostrum (2:1 with water) are also excellent liquid feeds.

Milk from cows with mastitis or other illness is satisfactory as well. Calves usually can be weaned at 4-6 wk of age or when they are regularly consuming 1-2 lb (0.5-1 kg) of starter daily. During the first week, starter containing ≥18% protein and hay should be placed before calves. The calf should be allowed all the starter it will eat up to a maximum of 5 lb (2.3 kg)/day. Calves do not like finely ground and dusty feeds. They readily consume coarsely cracked or rolled grains or feeds in which the "fines" are pelleted. While often economical, hay is not required during the first 2 mo. With a coarse starter, calves begin to ruminate within 2 wk. If hay is fed, early-cut, green, leafy, soft-stemmed material is the best kind for calves. They can be offered all the hay they will eat. After 4-6 mo of age, the calf starter can be replaced with a less expensive grower ration or regular dairy cow ration containing 16% total protein. Hay crop or corn silage can be fed to young calves, although they will consume it more effectively after 4 mo of age.

Well-grown heifers and young stock normally do not need concentrates after 8-12 mo of age if fed high-quality forage. More rapid gain or improved condition, if desired or needed, results from the addition of 2-3 lb (1-1.5 kg) of concentrates. It is advisable to feed 5-6 lb (2-3 kg) daily if the forage is of poor quality or scanty.

Pregnant cows and heifers should receive as much attention just before calving as after. If too fat, they are predisposed to ketosis. If they are in good condition, and fed at a high level after calving, ketosis tends to be reduced. During most of the dry period, cows in good condition fed good-quality grass hay or pasture require no concentrates. All-corn silage (plus protein and calcium) often results in too-fat cows at parturition and an increased incidence of left-displaced abomasums. Two weeks before parturition, cows and heifers should be offered grain (alone, in a complete feed, or as a part of corn [maize] silage [50% corn grain]) up to 6-10 lb (3-4 kg)/day by calving time to allow the rumen to adjust. On calving, cows should be encouraged to increase feed intake as rapidly as possible to minimize negative energy balance and to produce to their potential. Abrupt changes in types and amounts of feed offered should be avoided. Off-feed problems are less likely with complete feeds (total mixed rations). A forage:concentrate ratio of 1:1 can be offered with complete feeds immediately on calving. If grain is fed separately, an increase at the rate of 1-1.5 lb (0.5-0.7 kg)/

day to a maximum of 30-36 lb (14-16 kg) is fast enough to generate production but not so fast as to produce GI upsets or inappetence. For poor eaters, greater intakes are possible if cows are fed concentrates more often, ie, 3 times a day, and roughage several times in between.

After the peak of lactation, the amount of concentrate should be adjusted gradually and be based on the amount and fat content of the milk produced and the quality of the forage consumed. Size of the cow and her feed intake capacity as well as age must be considered in deciding on concentrate allowance. Computer programs that consider all these factors are widely used to provide optimal levels of nutrition. Cows fed complete feeds should be grouped by age and production and offered rations ranging from a maximum of 60% concentrate, 40% roughage (dry basis) for fresh cows, to 20% concentrate, 80% roughage for the low-producing group. When corn silage is a major feed ingredient, a 50% concentrate, 50% roughage diet is adequate for high-producers. For maximum fat test, the total ration should contain at least 17% crude fiber or 21% acid detergent fiber (ADF) or 28% neutral detergent fiber (NDF). However, the optimal levels of ADF or NDF depend on level of milk production and type of forage being fed. Caution should be exercised in following recommendations for NDF (TABLE 17), since only limited information is available on the interaction of NDF with other factors affecting the fat test. Protein levels of concentrates that meet the requirements for different forage qualities are: nonlegume, including all-corn silage, 23%; mixed legume-nonlegume, 16%; all-legume, 12-14%. Feed consultants, company representatives, and Cooperative Extension personnel can assist in determining least-cost concentrate feeds to use in a local area. All dairymen are encouraged to join some type of testing association as a means of evaluating their herd and its feeding and management program.

NUTRITIONAL DISEASES OF CATTLE AND SHEEP

Nutritional deficiencies involving energy, protein, certain minerals, and vitamins A, D, E, and K have been reported for ruminants under natural conditions. Experimentally, it has been possible to produce and study deficiencies of thiamine, riboflavin, biotin, choline, and pantothenic acid in preruminant dairy calves.

A simple uncomplicated deficiency, as observed in carefully controlled experiments, is rarely if ever seen in the field. More likely, a deficiency of several nutrients contributes to the signs observed. Many signs of nutrient deficiencies are nonspecific and often are the result of a low plane of nutrition. Further, interactions of one nutrient with another and with other dietary constituents in the development of deficiencies usually are not defined clearly. This is illustrated well by the interrelationship of copper, molybdenum, and sulfate; of vitamin E and selenium; of zinc and calcium; and of iodine and the various goitrogens.

ENERGY

Given a balanced high-energy diet, ruminants will consume feed until they satisfy some physiological need for energy. In the strictest sense, most ruminants are energy deficient (for maximal performance) since they are not fed *ad lib*, eg, dry cows, growing heifers, mature cattle, or sheep on pasture or stovers. Others, eg, veal calves, cows in high production, or finishing steers, are fed *ad lib*. The most common energy deficiency is due to inappropriate allotment of feed, which reduces production efficiency. Generally, this is unintentional or thought to be "economical", or there may be no choice because of drought; poor pastures; or low-quality, highly lignified, unpalatable forage.

A caloric deficiency often is subclinical and results in lowered production, retarded growth, delayed puberty, and lowered reproductive performance. In severe cases, often it is complicated with other deficiencies, particularly of vitamin A, protein, and phosphorus. Young ruminants may be stunted temporarily or permanently, and mature animals become thin and unthrifty. Milk production decreases rapidly relative to the deficiency, and nonfat milk solids decrease. Pregnant animals may produce weak young and have inadequate milk to support the newborn. Continually underfed surviving calves and lambs often do not do well and are unthrifty at weaning time.

Livestock are more likely to consume toxic plants if they are grazing on poor pastures, and those in poor physical condition are more susceptible to the ravages of weather and parasites.

Overfeeding of potential breeding stock in early life produces unnecessarily fat animals that often have trouble conceiving and lactating. It is better to allot enough energy to allow dairy and beef cows to reach the breeding stage at 12-15 mo. (*See* also BREEDING PROGRAM—HEIFER REPLACEMENTS AND COWS, p 1129.) Even when cattle are underfed until 2½ yr of age, they are able to recover most of the loss in size and produce normally when fed well, although their first production cycle may be delayed. Under current livestock conditions in the USA, dramatic underfeeding by design is not justified; growing animals should progress at a steady rate but not be allowed to become too fat.

The energy requirement for maintenance is 25-100% greater when grazing than when stall fed.

PROTEIN

A deficiency of protein often is associated with an energy shortage and may be the first limiting factor in practical feeding when cattle and sheep are on poor pasture. Nonlegume forages, if fertilized poorly with nitrogen often are too low in protein for optimal performance, whereas legume forages usually contain ample protein. Adequate amounts of protein (or nitrogen) are required, not only by the animal itself, but also by the rumen microflora, the composition and function of which may be altered markedly on a low-protein diet. If feeds are low in protein, feed intake is depressed and growth is severely retarded. Other signs may be similar to those encountered with insufficient energy. Weight gains and condition of finishing cattle and sheep are reduced, and milk production is lowered; if severe or prolonged, animals become thin and emaciated, and serum protein and BUN are low. Weight losses may occur even though ample energy is available. In addition, with sheep, growth of the wool fiber is restricted and "breaks" occur in the fleece.

Pregnant cows or ewes on a low-protein diet may lose considerable body weight and become weak. Estrus becomes irregular and conception may be delayed. Such females may have difficult parturition and retained placenta, milk poorly, and produce offspring that have poor chances of survival or, at best, are small and thin at weaning. Such unthrifty stock are susceptible to adverse weather, disease, and parasites.

MINERALS

Sodium Chloride (Salt): This is an essential component of the acid-base mechanism in the body and is needed for maintenance of proper osmotic pressure. Animals adjust to low-salt diets by reducing urinary sodium excretion. Continued deprivation results in an intense craving for salt in which animals chew and lick various objects such as wood, metal, and dirt, a condition known as pica. Feed consumption declines, and body weight and milk production drop. Feed efficiency is poor. As death approaches, milking cows shiver and show incoordination, weakness, and cardiac arrhythmia.

A trace mineralized salt block or loose salt should be available throughout life. Following a deficiency, salt should be offered gradually. Salt intoxication, however, is unlikely if adequate water is available.

Calcium: The bones and teeth contain ~99% of the body calcium (Ca) and serve as a reservoir of this element. The remaining 1% is found mainly in the extracellular fluid and is essential for proper nerve function, cardiac and other muscular activity, and blood clotting. A dynamic equilibrium exists between these 2 pools.

Calcium deficiency in the young prevents normal bone growth and may lead to spontaneous fractures. General growth and development is retarded. Pure rickets is seen only in phosphorus deficiency. If bone reserves are substantial in the adult, a lengthy depletion period is required before bone mineral loss is sufficient to result in fragile bones. Under these conditions, milk yield is depressed, but not its Ca content. Blood Ca will be low only after an extended period of deficient intake. For positive diagnosis, Ca content of the feed should be checked.

Under practical feeding conditions, Ca deficiency is a possibility except when milk or legume forage is used extensively. Almost all concentrates and nonlegume forages, including corn silage, are Ca deficient. Heavily lactating animals have the greatest need due to significant Ca secretion in the milk. During early lactation, a high-producing cow is always in negative Ca balance (relying on bone resorption for adequate Ca to support milk production) but restores her reserves in late lactation if fed adequately. Animals fed heavily on concentrates with little forage need supplemental Ca. Milk fever (qv, p 451) is characterized by a reduced blood Ca but is not due to a Ca deficiency *per se*.

Ground limestone, steamed bone meal, and dicalcium phosphate are excellent sources of Ca. Addition of lime to soil may increase the potential to grow legumes and hence provide more feed Ca.

Phosphorus: About 75% of the body phosphorus (P) is present in the bones and teeth. The remaining 25% is present in the soft tissues in the form of phosphoprotein, nucleoprotein, phospholipids, and hexose phosphate, which are essential in organ structure, nutrient transport, and energy utilization.

Phosphorus deficiency in the young results in slow growth, poor appetite, and unthriftiness, and has produced rickets (qv, p 487) in lambs. Energy utilization is reduced. In adults, milk production declines, bones become fragile, and feed intake is poor. The animals may become lame and stiff. Anestrus and low conception rates may occur. The P content of the milk does not decline. While pica has long been recognized as occurring with a P deficiency, this sign is not specific. Many wellnourished animals engage in this vice.

In contrast to calcium (Ca), blood P declines rather quickly on a P-deficient diet.

Forages produced on deficient, unfertilized soils may be marginal in P content, and deficiencies occur when these roughages form the entire ration. Over much of North America, pasture and especially range forage have a low P content. Most of the winter range areas of the west are deficient in P, particularly those ranges that are predominantly dry leached grass. Phosphorous fertilizers markedly increase crop yields in these areas and also may raise the percentage of P in the forage. Fortunately, grains, protein supplements, and by-product feeds usually are adequate in P and may supplement low-phosphorus roughages effectively.

Phosphorus deficiency can be corrected or prevented most easily by feeding supplements; eg, bone meal, dicalcium phosphate, and defluorinated rock phosphate contain ~14, 18, and 14% P, respectively. Colloidal clay phosphates (so-called "soft" phosphates) contain P in a relatively unavailable form and also may have a considerable fluoride content. Wheat bran, cottonseed meal, linseed meal, and soybean meal are rich in P, and their use in concentrate mixtures insures adequate P intakes. The Ca:P ratio may vary widely in natural feeds, but wide ratios are tolerated by growing calves; the desirable ratio is ~1.4:1. A ratio of <1:1 is highly undesirable. Vitamin D is essential for absorption and utilization of both Ca and P. In cows prone to milk fever, low Ca intake is recommended before parturition (*see* NUTRITIONAL REQUIREMENTS OF DAIRY CATTLE, p 1182).

It is critical that sheep do not receive excess P or magnesium, since these are associated with urinary calculi.

Iodine: About 80% of the body iodine is stored in the thyroid gland. A simple iodine deficiency results in enlargement of the thyroid gland (goiter, qv, p 283) but with a reduction of thyroxine secretion leading to cretinism in the young or myxedema in the adult. Iodine deficiency occurs in areas where soil (hence, plants and water) iodine is low, eg, around the Great Lakes and in the northwest, ie, away from the seacoast. Some plants, eg, cabbage, soybeans, and yellow turnips, may promote goiter development because they contain substances (goitrogens) that inhibit thyroxine production. The goitrogenic effect of raw soybeans is only partially destroyed in processing.

Iodized salt is an effective source of iodine and is used widely. The iodine in the salt should be stabilized, since weathering can reduce the content. The same is true for trace mineralized salt. In both types of salt, 0.007% iodine (0.01% potassium iodide) is usually added. Neither iodized nor trace mineralized salt should be added to a concentrate supplement as a means to limit feed intake.

Cobalt: While cobalt is considered a dietary essential, the tissues actually require vitamin B_{12}, which contains cobalt and is synthesized by rumen microorganisms. Vitamin B_{12} will alleviate signs of cobalt deficiency.

Cobalt deficiency develops rapidly since little is stored. Deficient animals have a normocytic normochromic anemia with concomitant anorexia, retarded growth, general emaciation, rough coat, and loss of milk production. While herbage and liver analyses are helpful in diagnosis, the proof is prompt improvement in feed intake after cobalt is fed.

Forages containing <0.07 ppm of cobalt usually are considered deficient for sheep and cattle; regions where this may occur are found in Florida, Michigan, Wisconsin, New Hampshire, New York, western Canada, Scotland, South Africa, Australia, and New Zealand.

Drenches of ~1 mg of cobalt, given twice weekly, have corrected the deficiency syndrome in sheep. In cattle, feeding 5-15 mg of cobalt daily cures cobalt deficiency, and as little as 1 mg prevents it. Inclusion of 15-30 g of cobalt chloride or sulfate per 100 lb (45 kg) of salt usually is adequate to prevent deficiency in both cattle and sheep. The use of such trace mineralized salt is the most common method of supplying cobalt to ruminants in the USA. In New Zealand and other intensively farmed areas, cobalt is applied to the soil annually at the rate of 5 oz of cobalt sulfate per acre (371 g/hectare), either as a spray or as part of the phosphate fertilizer. A cobalt "bullet" (90% cobalt oxide baked hard in 10% clay) given PO dissolves slowly over many months in the rumen, and has been successful. This "bullet" is used extensively under range conditions where other methods of oral administration are not practical. In ~5% of sheep, the bullet is regurgitated and lost, and in a further small percentage, it is covered with a deposit that prevents dissolution of the cobalt. Injections of cobalt are not effective since B_{12} synthesis occurs in the rumen. Extremely large doses of cobalt (300 times the requirement) may be toxic.

Copper and Molybdenum: Copper is involved at the functional level in the formation of the porphyrin nucleus of Hgb and in maintaining the function of bone osteoblasts providing collagen (lysyl oxidase). It is essential also in melanin production and in keratin (wool) formation. General signs of deficiency include anemia, brittle or fragile bones, loss of hair or wool pigmentation, and poor wool growth in sheep characterized by loss of crimp (steely wool).

Poor growth, anemia, bone fragility, diarrhea, and myocardial fibrosis occur in cattle. Ends of leg bones become enlarged, and the hair loses its color. Milk production and body condition are poor, fertility is low, and calves may show congenital rickets. Anemia and depressed growth are less common in sheep. Demyelination of certain tracts in the fetal and neonatal CNS results in incoordination, immobilization, blindness, and death. The disease is known as swayback (qv, p 596) or enzootic ataxia. Bone fragility also may occur.

In many cases, copper deficiency can be a simple deficiency of the element (primary); in other areas where excessive molybdenum and sulfates are in the feed, these elements act to reduce copper solubility in the GI tract and induce a secondary copper deficiency.

A normal level of sulfate in the diet counteracts the effects of molybdenum toxicity by increasing its rate of excretion. However, higher sulfate levels appear to enhance molybdenum intoxication with a detrimental effect on copper utilization. Frank cases of molybdenum toxicity (qv, p 1677) occur on pastures that contain an excess of the element; they are characterized by profuse scouring and can be alleviated by supplying 0.25 g of copper sulfate per 100 lb (45 kg) body wt daily.

The requirement for copper is ~5 ppm of the dry diet for sheep and 10 ppm for cattle. Adequate intake can be met by providing feed with this level or 0.5% copper sulfate in a trace mineralized salt. In cattle, toxic levels are ~10 times the minimum requirement, but sheep are much more susceptible—2 times the requirement causes toxicity in some cases. Since copper is extensively used in poultry diets, sheep rations that are supplemented with poultry litter may contain toxic amounts of copper.

Iron: Normal Hgb formation requires iron as a component of the heme molecule. Most feedstuffs contain adequate iron, and deficiency in adult cattle is rarely a problem. Young calves or lambs on a low-iron (milk) diet and prevented from consuming dry feed develop a microcytic, normochromic anemia. Providing 30 ppm iron prevents anemia in milk- and milk-replacer-fed calves. On normal feeding regimes in which dry feeds are offered from birth, no special iron supplements are needed.

Magnesium: The normal calcium:magnesium ratio is ~55:1. About 60% of the tissue magnesium is found in the bones, where it is relatively difficult to mobilize. A variable amount (15-50%) is bound to serum proteins. It plays a vital role as an activator of many enzyme systems involved in energy exchange. It also is involved in maintaining normal nerve irritability and function. Signs of magnesium deficiency are always accompanied by low blood magnesium (≤ 1 mg/dL). However, blood concentrations this low are not always accompanied by clinical signs.

Magnesium deficiency has been produced in calves by feeding rations deficient in magnesium, or by giving whole milk as the only food for 8-10 mo. (*See* HYPOMAGNESEMIC TETANY OF CALVES, p 446.)

During a cool spring, adult lactating cows on early spring pasture that has been fertilized with nitrogen or potassium, or both, may develop signs of "grass tetany" (qv, p 445). While this is clearly due to low blood magnesium, and animals respond to magnesium drench or infusion, it is not a simple dietary magnesium deficiency. The etiology is complex and not well understood. Fertilizing pastures to provide sward containing 0.25% magnesium on a dry-matter basis prevents the condition.

Sulfur: All ruminants require sulfur to synthesize the sulfur-containing amino acids, cystine and methionine. Sulfur deficiency results in poor growth and a marked impairment of wool growth in sheep. In cattle, it results in reduced feed intake, lower digestibility, slower gains, and depressed milk production. If the diet is adequate in natural proteins, sulfur intake will be satisfactory. If high levels of nonprotein nitrogen (NPN) such as urea are used, sources of inorganic or organic sulfur should be added. Elemental sulfur is satisfactory but less well utilized. An NPN:sulfur ratio of 12:1 is recommended for cattle. Sulfur is a cofactor of many enzymes and an integral part of others. It should be ~0.2% of the diet on a dry-matter basis.

Manganese: In cattle, manganese deficiency results in delayed estrus, reduced fertility, abortions, and skeletal abnormalities in calves. Calves have deformed legs with "over-knuckling" and enlarged joints and grow poorly. Newborn calves often exhibit ataxia. Deficient dairy heifers are slower to exhibit estrus and to conceive.

Most feeds are adequate in manganese, but since corn grain (maize) is relatively low (5 ppm), beef cattle on high-concentrate diets may need supplementation. A level of 40 ppm in the diet is adequate.

Zinc: Many enzymes that are distributed widely throughout the body contain zinc, eg, carbonic anhydrase, many dehydrogenases, and alkaline phosphatase. Zinc probably is related intimately to the processes of cell division. Signs of zinc deficiency have been produced experimentally with highly specialized diets. In lambs, such a diet produced slipping of wool, swelling and lesions around the hooves and periorbital regions, excessive salivation, anorexia, wool-eating, general listlessness, and reduced growth rate. Beef calves develop parakeratosis, and the mouth becomes inflamed; they are stiff in the joints and unthrifty. Dairy calves show alopecia, general dermatitis of the neck and head, listlessness, reduced testicular growth, and swollen feet. Wounds fail to heal properly. Calves adjust quickly to varying dietary levels of zinc but can become deficient in 3 wk. The toxic level is at least 10-30 times the minimum daily requirement (40 ppm, dry-matter basis).

Selenium: Selenium is an integral part of glutathione peroxidase, which acts to eliminate the effect of free radical damage from fatty acid peroxidation. Its function is inextricably involved with that of vitamin E. The predominant deficiency disease in ruminants is nutritional muscular dystrophy or white muscle disease (qv, p 548). Prevention and cure has been effected under field conditions by supplementation with either vitamin E or selenium. The incidence of retained placentas in cattle has been reduced with selenium treatment.

Selenium deficiency is related to geography; it is found in many parts of the world where the soil contains inadequate amounts, eg, New York, Ohio, and the Pacific northwest. Striking responses to selenium therapy in lambs suffering unthriftiness have been reported from New Zealand. Selenium may be injected, or incorporated into the feed at 0.3 ppm or in the salt-mineral mixture at 90 ppm on a dry-matter basis.

A dietary level of 0.3 ppm is adequate for ruminants. Levels of 3-5 ppm are toxic and result in anorexia, loss of hair from the tail, and sloughing of hoofs, and may be fatal. Some plants are selenium accumulators when grown on soils high in selenium such as are found in parts of South Dakota, Wyoming, and Utah. (*See also* p 1727.)

VITAMINS

Vitamin A: This vitamin serves to maintain the integrity of all epithelial tissues, including germinal epithelium, as well as its well-known role in vision. It is also required for normal bone metabolism. Thus, in addition to reducing the efficiency of the epithelium *per se*, a deficiency permits much of this tissue to be exposed to secondary invasion by indigenous pathogens. Most signs of deficiency can be traced to this function. Since vitamin A is related to epithelium and not metabolism, the requirements are generally related to body weight.

Tissue vitamin A may be derived from either provitamin A (carotene), a yellow pigment in plants that is converted in the intestinal wall to vitamin A, or from preformed vitamin A *per se*.

Carotene is destroyed when roughage is dried and bleached; hence, a deficiency may occur in cattle and sheep under drought conditions or when they are fed old, weathered roughage for long periods. Carotene is abundant in growing pasture, silage, and well-cured hay that has been stored <6 mo; grains (except for yellow corn) and cereal by-products contain little or none.

Usually, the first signs of deficiency are excessive lacrimation, thin or watery diarrhea, nasal discharge, coughing, and pulmonary involvement. Night blindness may develop in the early stages; in fact, this sign has been used experimentally to establish minimum carotene requirements. Vitamin A levels in the blood decline to <8-10 μg/dL of plasma in calves, and <12-15 μg in yearlings and older cattle. Considerable individual variation, however, often is observed in plasma vitamin A levels: in vitamin-A-deficient cattle, blood levels of carotene are consistently low and are indicative of insufficient carotene intake. Sheep have only traces of carotene in the blood even when carotene intake is high.

Calves and lambs have low vitamin A blood levels at birth and depend on colostrum (a rich source of vitamin A) to protect them against a deficiency until sufficient vitamin A or carotene from other sources can be obtained. Calves and lambs from dams with vitamin A deficiency may be born dead or so weak that they die within a few days; females may abort during the latter stage of pregnancy. Injury to the optic nerve as a result of stenosis of the optic foramen may occur in growing animals. CSF pressure is elevated and frequently results in staggering gait, muscular incoordination, and convulsions ("fainting" of feedlot cattle). Anasarca often is observed in finishing cattle, and opacity and cloudiness of the cornea and xerophthalmia with subsequent infection and blindness may result.

Young bulls and rams may become sterile due to aspermatogenesis. Vitamin-A-deficient mature bulls show muscular incoordination and are unable to mount. This occurs before spermatogenesis is altered.

While normal plasma carotene levels differ little among the major beef breeds, they differ considerably among dairy breeds because of variation in the ability to metabolize carotene to vitamin A. Colored breeds have high carotene levels. The liver can store large quantities of vitamin A, and most animals off good pasture have a 200-day reserve in their liver.

Except for irreparable changes in the eye or bone tissues, signs of vitamin A deficiency can be corrected rapidly by high intake of vitamin A. Treatment should be by injection of preformed vitamin A at ~2000 IU/100 lb (45 kg) live wt; up to 100 times this level is not detrimental as a single curative dose. Changing to diets adequate in carotene or vitamin A is imperative. The rate of conversion by ruminants is considered to be 400 IU of vitamin A from 1 mg β-carotene, but this fluctuates widely and unpredictably. It is lower than in monogastrics. Therefore, many commercial feeds are now fortified with dry stabilized vitamin A, and supplements are used to fortify home-grown rations. Such a source of vitamin A may be more economical and dependable than carotene from natural feeds. The vitamin A requirement is 47 IU/kg body wt. Single injections of 1 million IU of vitamin A apparently protect from a deficiency for 2-4 mo.

Vitamin D: Calcium, phosphorus, and vitamin D are related closely in metabolism. Vitamin D, which is produced in the skin as vitamin D_3 or eaten in the diet as vitamin D_2, is essential for adequate absorption of calcium and phosphorus. In the liver, it is converted to 25-hydroxycholecalciferol; thereafter it is transported to the kidney where it is hydroxylated to 1,25-dihydroxycholecalciferol (1,25[OH]$_2$D). This then stimulates the synthesis of a calcium-binding protein in the intestinal mucosa, which is involved in enhanced calcium absorption. The effect of 1,25(OH)$_2$D on phosphorus absorption is by a different mechanism. Vitamin D also is necessary for proper mineralization of the cartilaginous matrix that develops at the epiphyses. Poor mineralization results in cartilaginous overgrowth and disorganization, leading to swollen leg joints and beaded ribs (rickets). In the absence of the active forms of vitamin D, plasma calcium and phosphorus decrease, and serum phosphatase increases. An absolute or relative deficiency of calcium, phosphorus, or vitamin D results in rickets (qv, p 487). Vitamin D deficiency in adult cattle has not been well defined.

In practice, vitamin D deficiency is possible but not probable, even for the young. Milk is not especially rich in vitamin D, but the calf or lamb can obtain adequate amounts by skin irradiation if exposed daily to sunlight for 1-2 hr. Sun-cured forage is the best natural source of vitamin D_2. Even silages have sufficient dead leaves (thus sun-cured) to provide ample vitamin D_2 to calves that are housed indoors. Probably, however, it is prudent to provide a vitamin D supplement to young calves in their milk replacer and starter until they are turned out or are consuming adequate forage, ie, at 6-8 wk. Older ruminants consuming normal forages should need no added vitamin D. It is important to realize that vitamin D_3 is much more potent in dairy cattle than is D_2.

Vitamin E: Most natural feeds contain vitamin E, but oxidation destroys it rapidly so that old hay or ground grain may be poor sources. A deficiency of vitamin E or selenium is recognized as a common cause of muscular dystrophy (qv, p 547) in calves and lambs. Vitamin E does not seem to be associated with reproductive failures in ruminants; thus, it is of practical importance only for young animals. Milk replacers should be fortified.

Vitamin K: This vitamin is synthesized by rumen bacteria and is distributed widely in green, leafy forages. A deficiency is seen only in sweet clover disease (qv, p 1733).

B Vitamins: Deficiencies have not been observed in ruminants 1-2 mo old or older, except when they have been restricted to special diets. Rumen bacteria can synthesize all the B vitamins if other necessary factors are present (eg, cobalt in B_{12} synthesis). Niacin (nicotinic acid), synthesized from tryptophan within the tissues of even young calves, together with that synthesized in the rumen, fully meets the needs of ruminants. Most of the other B vitamins are essential in the diet of calves before rumen function becomes established. However, milk and other natural feeds contain adequate amounts to meet the needs of young calves and lambs. Milk replacers should be fortified.

Two conditions have been identified in cattle that may be related to a relative **thiamine** deficiency. Apparently some corn silages contain thiaminase, which causes a condition known as "circling disease". Also, wet corn gluten feed may contain residual sulfate or sulfite ions, which destroy thiamine. Such ions are a "carryover" from the first stages of the processing of corn with weak sulfurous acid to help soften the corn seed coat. Polioencephalomalacia (qv, p 614) is a thiamine deficiency disease that occurs in older calves related to development of a thiaminase in the rumen. The cause of the development of this thiaminase is unknown.

The ruminant depends on bacterial synthesis for B vitamins and might actually undergo a shortage of these if it goes off feed for long periods. Further, low-protein diets or mineral-deficient feeds may depress the number of bacteria and their synthesis mechanisms. Administering certain B vitamins or yeast preparations to ruminants that have been off feed for a considerable period has been tried with apparent success in the field.

Vitamin C (Ascorbic Acid): Since it is synthesized in the tissues of even young ruminants, deficiencies do not occur and it is not required in the diet.

NUTRITION: DOGS

Feeding is one of the most important management practices of the dog owner. Nutritional management is increasingly recognized as an integral part of both preventive health care and treatment protocols for medical and surgical patients. Advances in biotechnology, ie, enteral and parenteral nutrition, better biochemical assessments of nutritional status, and "fine tuning" of macro- and micronutrient needs are also focusing more attention on nutrition.

The interaction between illness, health, and nutritional status is multifactoral and complex. Therefore, the initial nutritional evaluation of an animal requires integration of the history, physical examination, anthropometric measures, and laboratory data. In many dogs, dietary therapy is an integral component of disease management, complementing or even replacing drugs or surgery in some cases.

Pet owners are inundated with books, articles, testimonials, and advertisements proclaiming advantages of certain nutritional practices while denouncing the life-threatening properties of others. The 2 most common questions asked by owners are 1) what kind of food? and 2) how much to feed?

Daily feeding recommendations are usually based on energy calculations (*see* TABLES 21 and 22) or feeding tables established by the food manufacturer. This amount should be considered an estimate or starting point and should be modified based on continual evaluation of the animal's body weight and condition, and any other existing physiological or pathological conditions.

Table 21. Equations to Estimate Canine Resting Energy Requirement (RER) in kcal of ME

Allometric: RER = 70 (body wt in kg)$^{0.75}$
Linear (>2 kg body wt): RER = 30 (body wt in kg) + 70

Table 22. Equations to Estimate Canine Maintenance Energy Requirement (MER) in kcal of ME

MER = 2 × RER	=	132 (body wt in kg)$^{0.75}$
	=	144 + 62.2 (body wt in kg)
Growth	=	1.5-2 × MER
Lactation	=	2-4 × MER
Sedentary	=	0.8 × MER
Last 3 wk gestation	=	1.1-1.3 × MER
Moderate work	=	1.1-1.5 × MER
Heavy work/stress	=	1.5-4 × MER
Surgery/trauma	=	1.25-1.75 × RER

At best, these equations are estimates of energy needs and should be viewed as starting points. The individual animal's body weight and condition must be reevaluated continually, and the energy intake adjusted as necessary.

The diet should not be changed abruptly; new food should be introduced gradually over at least 7-10 days. When changing diets, it is better to offer slightly less than the calculated new food dose. Overindulgence and abrupt changes frequently initiate GI disorders or diet refusal.

Small, firm, dark feces suggest superior nutrient digestion and absorption. Large volumes of pale feces indicate less than optimal utilization. Dry-matter digestibilities for dog food vary from 60% to 90% due to ingredient quality, crude-fiber content, processing, and level of intake. Maintenance of body weight, condition, coat, and general attitude and activity are also reliable means of evaluation.

DIET SELECTION/RECOMMENDATION

Although palatability is the characteristic most owners use to judge a food, it does not relate well to nutritional value. The initial step in diet selection is to determine the approximate needs of the dog by a history and physical examination. The level of performance desired must be considered, ie, working, showing, or sedentary. After establishing requirements, a product choice must be made; this should be based on the nutrient profiles and feed management characteristics of the different commercial products available. Commercial foods cannot be compared accurately on the as-fed basis listed on pet-food labels; instead, they should be compared on a dry-matter (see TABLE 23) or energy basis. Because the energy density of dog foods varies from 2.5 to >5 kcal/g dry matter, general feeding recommendations should not be given; each food must be evaluated individually.

Table 23. Conversion of Nutrient Expression on an As-fed Basis to a Dry-matter Basis

Nutrient	% As Fed
Protein	8.0
Fat	6.0
NFE (soluble carbohydrate)	13.0
Fiber	0.5
Ash	1.5
Moisture	71.0
	100%

Note: 100 − moisture = % dry matter
100 − 71 = 29%
% protein dry matter = protein % as fed/% dry matter
27.5% = 8.0%/29%
% fat dry matter = fat % as fed/% dry matter
20.6% = 6.0%/29%

TYPES OF COMMERCIAL DOG FOOD

Commercial dog foods are sold as 5 general types—dry, canned, soft-moist, treats, and frozen. Several types have recently appeared on the market, which are mixtures of dry and soft-moist foods. The classification depends on the processing method and water content more than on the ingredient content or nutrient profile.

Dry Dog Food: More dry foods are sold than any other; they generally contain ~90% dry matter and 10% moisture. About 95% of dry dog foods are extruded; ie, they are made by combining ingredients (grains, meat and meat by-products, fats, minerals, and vitamins) and cooking, and forcing the mixture through a die. During cooking and extrusion, a temperature of ~150°C converts the starches into a form more easily digested, destroys toxins and inhibitory substances, and flash sterilizes the product. It is then enrobed with fat and/or digest (material derived from controlled degradation of animal tissues, eg, chicken digest) during drying to increase palatability. Advantages of dry food include a lower cost than canned or soft-moist food, and refrigeration of unused portions is not required. Dry food may also provide beneficial massage of the teeth and gums to help decrease periodontal disease.

Canned Dog Food: Canned dog foods contain 68-78% water and 22-32% dry matter. Ingredients determine whether the food is ration type, animal tissue, chunk style, or stew. Chunk style and stew are ration types, with stew containing more water than chunk style. Ration type contains a mixture of cereals, meat, and meat by-products, which are blended together in different physical forms for packaging. The animal tissue foods do not contain cereals but commonly contain meat as well as organ tissues (lungs, udders, and other animal by-products) and adipose tissue. All these types of food need to be properly supplemented with minerals and vitamins to be a balanced diet. Advantages of canned food include a long shelf life in a durable container and high palatability. Disadvantages include no beneficial effect on the teeth and gums, and increased cost.

Soft-Moist Dog Food: Soft-moist dog foods contain 25-40% water and 60-75% dry matter. They do not require refrigeration and are preserved using humectants—substances that bind water so that it is unavailable for bacteria and mold growth. They include simple sugars (usually sucrose), sorbitol, propylene glycol, and salts. Some recent reports of an increased risk of Heinz body anemia in cats that consume soft-moist foods preserved with propylene glycol have raised some questions concerning the use of this ingredient in pet foods. Many soft-moist foods are acidified using phosphoric, malic, or hydrochloric acid to further retard spoilage. Advantages include convenience, high energy digestibility, and palatability. Disadvantages include higher cost and no beneficial effect on the teeth and gums.

HOME-COOKED DIETS

Dogs can be successfully maintained on properly formulated home-cooked diets. Advantages include the use of fresh, high-quality ingredients. Disadvantages include time commitment of the owner, higher cost, and necessary nutritional skill of the person balancing the diet. Many home-cooked diets have been high in protein and caloric density, while being inappropriate with regard to calcium/phosphorus ratio and inadequate with regard to calcium, copper, iodine, fat-soluble vitamins, and several of the B vitamins.

PET-FOOD LABELS

Labels are not in themselves of great assistance in selection of a food based on a pet's nutrient requirements, although they provide a guaranteed analysis, an ingredient list, and a statement of nutritional adequacy.

Guaranteed Analysis: This lists the minimum level of crude protein and crude fat and the maximum amounts of water and crude fiber on an as-fed (not dry-matter) basis. It does not guarantee that the product contains the amount listed, but rather that its protein and fat levels are not less than, and the water and crude fiber contents are not more than, a certain level. It is not the same as a chemical proximate analysis report, which lists actual levels of nutrient in a food. Two foods may have identical guaranteed analyses but very different proximate analyses. A guaranteed analysis for protein may list a minimum level of 25%, while the product could contain anywhere from 25 to 50% protein. If possible, the label guaranteed analysis should not be used for diet evaluation; instead, the manufacturer should be contacted for the average chemical profile.

Ingredient List: Ingredients are listed in descending order of weight, on an as-fed basis in the food. A food ingredient may be listed first, eg, chicken, but because that ingredient is 75% moisture, it may be only a small percentage of the actual food dry-matter. In addition, an ingredient such as corn may be listed by individual components, ie, flaked corn, ground corn, screened corn, kibbled corn, etc, so that corn is moved further down on the ingredient list. No reference to quality or grade of an ingredient is allowed to be listed. Therefore, it is difficult to evaluate a product on the basis of ingredient list alone.

Statement of Nutritional Adequacy: This indicates that when fed as the sole diet without any other food or supplement, the product meets or exceeds the published National Research Council (NRC) requirements or is nutritionally adequate for one or more of the following: gestation, lactation, growth, maintenance, or all life stages. Products exempted from this requirement include those intended for intermittent or supplemental feeding (supplements, snacks, treats), or those intended for use under the direction of a veterinarian. The statement "complete and balanced for all dogs" indicates the product has a growth-type diet profile. The claims must be substantiated by successfully completing feeding trials conducted according to protocols approved by the American Association of Feed Control Officials (AAFCO), or by containing at least a minimum amount of each nutrient recommended by the NRC publication *Nutrient Requirements of Dogs*, 1985, which cautions "against the use of these requirements (levels) without demonstration of nutrient availability". Some of the requirements are based on studies in which the nutrients were supplied by purified ingredients, and are not representative of ingredients in commercial dog foods.

The AAFCO is considering the controversial Policy Statement 21 which "is intended to assure the consumer that the finished product has been tested by feeding trials which have demonstrated the nutrients are present not only in sufficient quantities to support the desired physiologic demands but in forms that are bioavailable to the dog". If this policy is adopted, submitting a chemical profile that meets or exceeds the minimum nutrients recommended by the NRC would no longer be sufficient because it does not address the bioavailability issue.

ENERGY AND THE NUTRIENT GROUPS

Energy: The energy requirement of an individual dog is the level that will support metabolism during the various physiologic states: growth, maintenance, gestation, lactation, old age, or disease. Resting energy requirement (RER) is the largest component of energy expended by an animal under fasting, thermoneutral, nonambulatory conditions. It is closely correlated with lean body mass. RER is commonly estimated by any one of several empirically derived estimation equations (*see* TABLE 21). Maintenance energy requirement is a function of RER depending on the individuals "life-style" (*see* TABLE 22). It is highly variable between individuals and requires continual adjustment based on body condition.

Of the 6 nutrient groups, only protein, fat, and carbohydrate provide energy; vitamins, minerals, and water do not. To offer the appropriate amount of food to an animal each day, the caloric density of the food must be estimated accurately. When a feedstuff is oxidized completely, the heat given off is considered to be the gross energy (GE). This measure is a starting point for determining the value of the food.

In dogs, the unit of measure most commonly used to discuss food energy is metabolizable energy (ME). The ME content of a food is estimated by subtracting the energy of the feces and urine from the GE. The ME values for many dog-food ingredients have not been experimentally determined and are often borrowed from other monogastric species (often pigs) or calculated using Atwater physiologic fuel values modified for use with typical dog-food ingredients. In addition to supplying the proper total number of ME calories/day, the optimal range of ME derived from fat, carbohydrate, and protein varies depending on physiologic or pathologic state.

Carbohydrate: The carbohydrates added to pet foods are mainly in the form of polysaccharides (starch and cellulose), disaccharides (sucrose and lactose), and monosaccharides (glucose and fructose). Properly cooked nonfibrous carbohydrates are utilized well by dogs. Except for the lactating bitch, there appears to be no dietary requirement for carbohydrate. Gluconeogenesis from alanine and lactate can supply any need for glucose.

Crude Fiber: There are several chemical methods to determine the fiber level of a food: all extract the components of fiber to different degrees, which results in different estimates of fiber level for the same feedstuff. Dog-food labels list a maximum content of crude fiber on an as-fed basis. Crude fiber consists mainly of cellulose and lignin, and is a portion of food that is resistant to hydrolysis by mammalian digestive secretions. It is not, however, an inert traveler through the GI tract. Increased levels of crude fiber in dog rations increase fecal output, normalize transit time, depress digestibility of diet dry matter, alter colonic microflora and fermentation patterns, alter glucose and insulin kinetics in diabetic animals, and affect hepatic and peripheral metabolism of lipoproteins.

Fats: Dietary fat consists mainly of triglyceride with varying amounts of sterols and phospholipids, and is a concentrated source of energy, yielding ~2.25 times the amount of ME (as an equal dry-weight portion) of soluble carbohydrate or protein. In general, as the fat content of a diet increases, so does the caloric density and palatability. Fats serve as a carrier for the fat-soluble vitamins A, D, E, and K, and as a source of essential fatty acids (EFA), which maintain functional integrity of cell membranes and are precursors of prostaglandins and leukotrienes. Dogs have a dietary requirement for linoleic acid, an unsaturated EFA, which is found in appreciable amounts in corn and soy oil. High-quality fats are the most digestible component of the diet, and dogs can tolerate quite high levels. However, in addition to the problem of supplying an excessive amount of energy with high-fat diets, caution must be used to avoid suboptimal intakes of protein, minerals, and vitamins.

Triglycerides are divided into short, medium, and long chain based on the number of carbon atoms in the fatty acid chain. Fatty acids are either saturated, indicating there are no double bonds, or unsaturated, indicating there are one or more double bonds. Coconut and palm kernel oil are particularly rich sources of medium-chain triglycerides. Their principal difference from long-chain triglycerides is that they are more water soluble, and relatively independent of pancreatic lipase, bile salts, and enterocyte transformation during the digestion and absorption process.

Fat content of commercial foods varies widely based on the diet purpose (*see* TABLE 24); work, stress, growth, and lactation require higher levels than maintenance. Fat supplements containing unsaturated fatty acids are often recommended for animals with dry flaky coats, which may be fed diets marginal in those fatty acids.

Table 24. Diet Profile Ranges for Selected Physiological Conditions in Dogs (% dry matter)

Physiological Condition	Crude Protein	Crude Fat	Crude Fiber	Ca*	P	Na
Growth Last third gestation Lactation	28-35	20-30	0-5	1.0-1.8	0.8-1.6	0.3-0.7
Maintenance (adult)	20-28	10-20	0-5	0.5-0.9	0.4-0.9	0.25-0.5
Sedentary Obesity prevention	20-25	8-12	5-15	0.5-1.0	0.4-0.9	0.25-0.5
Old age	15-25	10-20	0-5	0.5-0.85	0.4-0.75	0.25-0.4
Work/stress Convalescence	25-30	25-30	0-5	0.7-1.4	0.7-1.4	0.3-0.7

*Calcium:phosphorus ratios should be between 1:1 and 2:1.

Protein: The primary function of dietary protein is as a source of amino acids. Essential amino acids must be dietary constituents because they cannot be synthesized within the dog's body. Nonessential amino acids are made within the body from carbon and nitrogen precursors. Amino acids supply nitrogen for the synthesis of all other nitrogenous compounds and supply a variable amount of energy when catabolized. Dietary protein is enzymatically digested and passes into the bloodstream as free amino acids. The dietary requirement for protein is satisfied when the dog's metabolic need for amino acids and nitrogen is satisfied. The quality of the protein (biologic value/bioavailability) varies directly with the number and amount of essential amino acids it contains. The higher the biologic value of a protein, the smaller the amount of protein needed in the diet to supply the essential amino acid requirements. Amino acid requirements as a percent of diet generally decline from birth to maturity.

Protein requirements of animals vary with age, activity level, temperament, growth rate, reproductive and health status, stress level, etc (*see* TABLE 24).

Most commercial dog foods have a combination of cereal and meat proteins. Protein digestibility in dog foods varies from ~75% to 90%. Digestibility is less for poor-quality protein ingredients and poor-quality diets. If excessive heat is used in processing, proteins can become chemically unavailable for digestion and absorption.

Minerals: In animal nutrition, minerals can be classified into 3 major categories: those the body stores in large quantities (Na, K, Ca, P, Mg), the trace minerals of known importance (Fe, Zn, Cu, I, F, Se, Cr), and other trace minerals important in laboratory animals but that have an unclear role in companion animal nutrition (Co, Mo, Cd, As, Si, V, Ni, Pb, Sn).

A balanced amount of the necessary dietary minerals in relation to the energy density of the diet is important. As intake of a mineral exceeds the requirement, an excessive amount may be absorbed, which may be detrimental, or a large amount of the unabsorbed mineral may prevent the absorption of adequate amounts of another mineral. Indiscriminate mineral supplementation should be avoided since it may cause serious mineral imbalances. The most commonly used (often inappropriately) mineral supplement is a calcium/phosphorus mix with vitamin D in growing dogs. This is generally not necessary in dogs receiving a diet balanced for growth.

Mineral deficiency is uncommon in well-balanced diets. Exceptions include diets rich in meat, which are therefore rich in phosphorus and poor in calcium; diets high in phytates or calcium (>2.5% dry-matter basis), which inhibit absorption of trace minerals; and poor-quality foods with low digestibility and bioavailability.

Manipulation of dietary intake of Ca, P, Na, Mg, and Cu for therapeutic effect is common.

Vitamins: Vitamins are divided into 2 groups: fat soluble (A, D, E, and K) and water soluble (C, and the B vitamins). Because water-soluble vitamins are usually readily excreted if excess amounts are consumed, they are thought to be less likely to cause toxicity or side effects when ingested in megadose amounts. Fat-soluble vitamins, except vitamin K, are stored to an appreciable extent in the body, and when ingested in large amounts over a period of time, toxic reactions may be observed, especially with vitamins A and D.

FEEDING THE HEALTHY DOG

Growth, Late (last third) Gestation, and Lactation: An enhanced level of protein, fat, and minerals is required to meet the increased demands of growth, fetal development, and milk production. A diet with increased nutrient density, digestibility, and bioavailability is desired to provide nutrients necessary in a small volume of food. Supplementation of calcium, phosphorus, and vitamin D over levels present in good-quality diets designed for these functions is usually not necessary, and may be containdicated if the calcium level is raised to >2.5% on a dry-matter basis. The calcium to phosphorus ratio should be in the range of 1:1 to 2:1. Overfeeding during growth may contribute to obesity as well as increased growth rate, which is incompatible with proper skeletal development. Offering energy levels 2-4 times maintenance is often required for the lactating bitch to avoid excessive loss of body condition.

Maintenance: After an animal has reached ~90% of its expected adult weight, a diet less nutrient dense than the growth-type diet is desirable. A diet that is highly digestible, low in residue, and of high nutrient availability is indicated. Moderate levels of protein, fat, calcium, phosphorus, and sodium should be fed. Providing excessive calories compared to energy expenditure is the most common error in feeding adult dogs, and results in obesity.

Old Age: A continued moderation of intake of energy, protein, phosphorus, and sodium in older adult dogs (5-8 yr old or older), while maintaining the characteristics of high digestibility, bioavailability, and low residue is recommended. These animals should be monitored in a preventive health program since the incidence of chronic degenerative organ disease increases as dogs age. Chronic diseases are a unique challenge for nutritional management.

Work/Stress: The nutritional needs of working or stressed animals may exceed the ability of the maintenance-type diet to meet them. Most work/stress diets have increased levels of high-quality fats, with the other nutrients balanced to the increased energy density. At extreme levels of stress, many recommend not only increasing the percent ME from fat, but also increasing the percent ME from protein, while minimizing the contribution of carbohydrate.

FEEDING RECOMMENDATIONS FOR SELECTED PATHOLOGICAL STATES

In therapeutic dietary management, general diets are altered to provide optimal health in normal dogs or to help manage a disease process (*see* TABLE 25). If the diet is altered as a part of the disease management, the dog's nutritional status should be monitored frequently and the diet modified as the clinical condition of the animal changes. Diets are usually best accepted in multiple, small meals.

Chronic Renal Disease: In oliguric chronic renal disease, various metabolic abnormalities occur that modify nutritional status: impaired clearance of nitrogenous products of protein metabolism; impaired regulation of sodium, potassium, and phosphorus; impaired vitamin D metabolism; and often anorexia. The diet should be high in energy density, with a moderate to restricted level of high-quality protein (13-16% ME, 15-20% dry matter), phosphorus, magnesium, and sodium with a balanced calcium level. Levels of water-soluble vitamins should be increased.

Chronic Liver Disease: Because anorexia is common, a diet high in fat and low in residue should be selected initially, although fat restriction may be necessary to maintain normal feces. Dietary fats are not a source of short-chain fatty acids, which may exacerbate hepatic encephalopathy. Calories from protein should be moderated, and those from carbohydrate should be from highly available sources (not cereal by-products). Ingredients high in uric-acid precursors (eg, organ meats) should be avoided, and copper should be restricted in dogs at risk of developing copper-induced hepatopathy. Often, ascites and edema can be controlled by moderating sodium intake, and water-soluble vitamins should be increased above maintenance levels. Lipotrophic agents such as choline should be avoided. The effectiveness of manipulation of branched chain and aromatic amino acids in chronic disease has not been demonstrated.

Chronic Heart Disease: Optimal body weight can be achieved by feeding a moderate- to high-fiber diet to animals that require weight reduction, and a high-fat, low-residue, calorie-dense diet to animals with cardiac cachexia. A moderate quantity of high-quality protein should be offered. B vitamins and potassium should be supplemented at levels above maintenance to maintain body pools of these nutrients. The diet should be moderately restricted in sodium.

Diabetes Mellitus: In addition to traditional insulin replacement therapy, dietary management is useful to optimize the care of diabetic animals. The diet should enhance glycemic control, and should be high in complex carbohydrates, low in soluble carbohydrates, high in crude fiber, low to moderate in dietary fat, and have moderate to high biologic-value protein. To control hyper- and hypoglycemias, the feeding schedule should be constant, with meals coordinated to match insulin action.

Weight Loss/Weight Control: Obesity (qv, p 450) is the most common type of malnutrition in dogs. The usual cause is excessive caloric intake in relation to energy expenditure. The nutritional goals are to produce a caloric deficit (60-70% of maintenance energy requirement at optimal body weight) while delivering adequate quantities of protein, vitamins, and minerals. These goals can be accomplished by feeding a diet that contains 15-25% crude fiber and <10% fat. A high-fiber ration induces satiety at a lower total caloric intake. After reaching a desired body weight, animals are most effectively managed with a moderate level of dietary crude fiber (7-15%) and moderate dietary fat (10-15%). Repetitive cycles of weight gain and weight reduction increase the risk of obesity and should be discouraged.

Intestinal Lymphangiectasia: This is the most common cause of protein-losing enteropathy in dogs; it results from an obstruction of lymph flow, followed by distention and rupture of lacteals. Clinical signs include varying degrees of diarrhea and weight loss, edema, ascites, and vomiting. For successful management, the diet should be low in fat (<10%), high in crude fiber (>15%), and high in protein (25-30%). If animals cannot maintain desirable body weight, caloric supplementation with medium-chain triglyceride oil has been used successfully.

Neoplasia: Unlike in people, high-fiber diets have not been reported to have preventive effects against certain cancers in dogs and cats. Confusion has developed between proposed cancer prevention hypotheses for high-fiber diets and their inappropriate use in debilitated animals. Debilitated animals generally require diets with minimal crude fiber (<2%), a low percentage of energy from carbohydrate, and a high level of dietary fat and protein.

Constipation: Constipation usually involves the large bowel. Increased levels of crude fiber (10-25%) increase fecal bulk and water content (decreasing fecal density), and hasten transit time, while eliciting a strong defecation reflex and easing evacuation.

Colitis: Many dogs with idiopathic colitis respond to rations high in crude fiber (>10%) and moderate to low in fat (10-15%). Increasing the fiber levels slows transit time in animals with abnormally fast transit times and may decrease intracolonic pressure. These animals should be offered small, frequent meals (3-6/ day). If the animal does not respond within 3-6 wk, a highly digestible, moderate to high fat (20-30%), low-residue, hypoallergenic diet should be tried. The latter recommendations may also be of benefit for animals with histologically identified lymphocytic-plasmacytic enteritis.

Food Hypersensitivity: Food allergy, which is ranked as the third most common cause of allergic skin disease in dogs, may occur concurrently with other types of allergies. Throughout life, most dogs are offered a mixture of different meats, cereals, and vegetables, each of which contains many antigenic components that are potential sensitizing agents. Pruritic allergic hypersensitivity to ingested allergens can occur suddenly for the first time at any age, but is rarely seen in dogs <4 mo old. Generally, food hypersensitivity is not associated with a history of a recent dietary change; in fact, most of the dogs have been eating the same diet for >2 yr. Concurrent GI signs occur in a small percentage of animals.

When an allergic response to an ingested allergen is suspected, a detailed history of past dietary intake should be obtained, followed by the feeding of a "hypoallergenic diet" exclusively for 3 wk, along with distilled water. A diagnosis is made by observing a decline in pruritus and recurrence of clinical signs when the original diet (or ingredients composing that diet) is reintroduced. Unless concurrent allergies (if present) are properly managed, results may be less than optimal.

Suitable hypoallergenic diets should contain a limited number of dietary components (additives, protein sources, etc) that previously have not been a part of the animal's diet, or are not common ingredients in commercial pet foods. Simply changing brands or flavors is not acceptable; all treats, supplements, and unnecessary medications should be avoided since they often contain meat protein sources for palatability. Commonly used protein sources include lamb or mutton, rabbit, fish, cottage cheese, or egg; sources of carbohydrate include rice, pasta, or potatoes. Properly balanced (with vitamins, essential fatty acids, and minerals) and prepared home-cooked diets can be individualized for each animal from the ingredients above. The final concentration of protein in the diet should be moderate (20-25%). Commercially prepared hypoallergenic diets that are balanced are convenient, and also can be used. Labels on hypoallergenic foods should be checked carefully, since some contain beef, milk, chicken, wheat, etc, which would render that diet inappropriate for this use.

Malabsorption/Maldigestion: Diseases of the small intestine and pancreas often lead to the vague clinical syndrome of weight loss, vomiting, diarrhea (often with steatorrhea), and changes in appetite. The recommended diet is low in fiber (0-5%), low residue, highly digestible, has moderate levels of fat (10-15%) and protein (20-25%), and carbohydrate from noncereal by-product sources. Levels of water-soluble vitamins should be elevated. In pancreatic exocrine insufficiency, supplementation with a powdered enzyme supplement on the food immediately before feeding should be considered. (*See also* p 122.)

Debilitation/Cachexia/Sepsis: Many severely ill animals exhibit suboptimal body condition, which indicates depleted body reserves. These animals (irrespective of their primary problem) have cumulative negative net energy balance, altered energy needs, and handle metabolic fuels differently than fed or fasted normal animals. Hormones stimulated by stress enhance lipid catabolism, which suggests that lipids are efficiently utilized in compromised states. In contrast, studies in some starvation-stressed people and animals have documented abnormal carbohydrate metabolism often referred to as a "diabetic-like syndrome".

A diet rich in high-quality protein and fat and minimal carbohydrate is indicated. The caloric intake and energy-yielding nutrient contributions (percent ME from protein, fat, and carbohydrate) should be based on individual response. Caloric intake can be supplied by several routes (in order of preference): voluntary oral, forced enteral, mixed enteral and parenteral, and total parenteral.

Gastric Dilatation (Bloat): To date, there is no evidence to suggest that certain nutritional practices (eg, feeding diets that contain soy protein) lead to development of gastric dilatation in susceptible dogs. (*See also* p 234.) Anecdotally, certain practices have been reported to reduce the incidence and recurrence; eg, avoid offering food and water immediately before and after exercise, and feed frequent small meals of a low-residue (0-5% crude fiber) diet that is high in energy density and dry-matter digestibility.

Struvite Urolith Dissolution: A medical protocol using antimicrobials and a calculolytic diet is an effective alternative to surgical intervention for removal of struvite uroliths. (*See also* p 885.) The diet profile includes a reduced amount of high-quality protein (7-8%), calcium, phosphorus, and magnesium; the salt level is enhanced. The urine pH of dogs fed this diet is acidic (<6). This type of diet should be used with caution in growth, lactation, gestation, azotemic primary renal failure, congestive heart failure, liver disease, and prolonged adult maintenance.

Hyperlipidemia: This can be primary or secondary to hypothyroidism, pancreatitis, hepatic disease, diabetes mellitus, nephrotic syndrome, or hyperadrenalism. The condition is present when blood lipids are elevated with or without gross lipemia and probably results from abnormalities in the synthesis or degradation of plasma lipoproteins. In primary hyperlipidemia, the abnormalities might be genetic, as has been suggested in Miniature Schnauzers. Some animals with hyperlipidemia are asymptomatic. Clinically affected animals may have recurrent seizures, depression, abdominal tenderness, vomiting, acute blindness, corneal opacity, and xanthogranulomas. The goal of dietary management is to decrease the digestion and absorption of fat by feeding a diet restricted in fat (<10%).

Table 25. Diet Profile Ranges for Selected Pathological Conditions in Dogs (% dry matter)

Pathological Condition	Crude Protein	Crude Fat	Crude Fiber	Ca*	P	Na
Chronic oliguric renal failure	15-20	20-30	0-5	0.5-0.85	0.2-0.4	0.2-0.4
Chronic liver insufficiency	15-25	15-30	0-5	0.5-1.4	0.2-1.2	0.2-0.4
Obesity/weight loss	22-28	8-12	15-25	0.5-1.4	0.3-1.2	0.25-0.5
Struvite urolith dissolution	7-8	25-27	0-5	0.2-0.3	0.1-0.2	1.2-1.3
Chronic congestive heart failure	15-25	15-30	0-5	0.5-0.85	0.2-0.6	0.05-0.3
Hyperlipidemia	15-28	8-12	0-25	0.5-1.4	0.3-1.2	0.25-0.5
Constipation	15-28	10-20	10-25	0.5-1.4	0.3-1.2	0.25-0.5
Colitis, idiopathic	15-28	8-12	10-25	0.5-1.4	0.3-1.2	0.25-0.5
Lymphocytic-plasmacytic infiltrative intestinal disease	20-28	20-30	0-3	0.7-0.9	0.4-0.85	0.25-0.5

*Calcium:phosphorus ratios should be between 1:1 and 2:1.

NUTRITION: EXOTIC AND ZOO ANIMALS

The nutrition of exotic and zoo animals has advanced significantly in the last 25 yr. Greater knowledge of nutrient requirements and the availability of commercially prepared diets have substantially reduced the incidence of improperly nourished animals in zoos. Information on exotic pets is now available to help prevent, detect, and treat such previously common nutritional problems as nutritional secondary hyperparathyroidism and deficiencies of vitamin A, thiamine, and selenium/vitamin E. Although much is still unknown, information is now available for adequate nutritional management of most exotic species in captivity.

All species require specific nutrients and energy in a metabolizable form rather than specific foods. The nutrients and energy must be properly balanced and correctly "packaged" to suit each species' particular tastes and digestive system. Diets for exotic and zoo animals have been developed by considering food habits in the wild, oral and GI morphology, nutrient requirements established for domestic and laboratory animals and man, nutritional research on exotic species, and practical experience. The ultimate criteria for evaluating the suitability of a diet for a species are growth, reproductive success, and longevity.

Wild animals require the same basic nutrients as their domestic counterparts. For many exotic species that have closely related domestic counterparts (eg, ungulates, mustelids, canids, felids, rodents, primates, lagomorphs, gallinaceous birds, anseriform birds, freshwater fish), nutrient requirements established by the National Research Council (NRC) for domestic and laboratory animals can be a guide to minimum nutrient concentrations in the diet. Although less directly applicable to other species, NRC requirements can still serve as a useful general reference for evaluating the nutritional adequacy of diets for any bird or mammal. The nutritional adequacy of diets for reptiles and amphibians is much more difficult to evaluate, since there are no good domestic animal models. In addition, because they are poikilothermic, their metabolic rates fluctuate with changes in ambient temperature.

Although NRC guidelines can help establish nutrient concentrations in the diet, they provide little or no information on the types of foods and diets that are suitable for exotic animals, nor how the food should be presented to account for the physical or behavioral attributes of the species. Following are brief discussions of the feeding of different types of animals, and examples of diets used for some species.

All food should be of good quality. Spoiled or moldy foods, or foods stored for long periods (generally >1 yr for most bagged feeds and 6-12 mo for most frozen foods) should not be fed. Clean, fresh water should always be available to nonmarine species. Usually, it is desirable to have trace mineral salt blocks, bricks, or "spools" available free choice to most mammals and psittacine birds. Cafeteria-style feeding is strongly discouraged; given a wide selection of foods, captive animals are unlikely to select a balanced diet. Belief in "nutritional wisdom" has resulted in many malnourished animals. In most cases, a nutritionally complete commercial product or in-house mixture that cannot be sorted should make up the bulk of the diet with components such as meat, fruit, and seeds making up only a small percentage. Muscle and organ meats, fruit, most grains and seeds, and many insects are low in calcium, and overconsumption can result in calcium deficiency. Oversupplementation of some nutrients (eg, vitamins A or D, selenium, copper) can be just as harmful as deficiency. Obesity is a problem more often than inadequate intake. Care should be taken not to overfeed ungulates, carnivores, primates, and other species that can quickly become overweight when excess amounts of a high-quality diet are offered, particularly when activity is limited. Rapid growth rates in some birds increase the incidence of leg and wing problems. Animal weights should be taken and recorded whenever possible. Nothing can substitute for the watchful eye of a conscientious keeper or pet owner in monitoring the health of their animals.

BIRDS

Nutrient deficiencies in birds often do not become obvious unless breeding is attempted, or during molt. Feather problems frequently are related to inadequate nutrition. Deficiencies of vitamin A, protein in general and sulfur amino acids in particular, calcium, zinc, folic acid, and pantothenic acid, as well as other nutrients, can cause abnormal and ragged feathering. Some birds (eg, flamingos, ibises, trogons, tanagers, woodpeckers) depend on dietary carotenoid pigments for natural feather coloration. Suitable pigment sources include carrots, carrot extract, alfalfa meal, shrimp meal, brine shrimp, and synthetic pigments such as canthaxanthin. Although most captive birds are fed the same diet year-round, many birds in the wild have evolved with diets that vary greatly with seasons. Little is known about the influence of seasonal dietary changes in the reproduction of exotic birds. Fruits and vegetables should always be washed thoroughly to remove residual pesticides. Uneaten soft foods should be discarded daily to prevent bacterial contamination. Birds do not use vitamin D_2 efficiently; vitamin D_3 should be used when vitamin D is added to avian diets. Seed-eating species should always have grit available for proper gizzard function.

AQUATIC BIRDS

Penguins in the wild feed primarily on fish, crustaceans, and squid. In captivity, smelt, herring, mackerel, and whiting are commonly fed. One of the most important aspects of feeding penguins and other fish-eating birds is fish quality (*see* MARINE MAMMALS, p 1220). All penguins should receive a mixed diet consisting of ≥2 fish species to ensure proper nutrition. Supplements commonly given to penguins include salt, polyunsaturated fatty acids, and vitamins. Dietary salt (NaCl) is provided to birds in freshwater exhibits to help maintain proper functioning of the salt glands; 0.5-1 g salt/bird/day should be adequate for most species. Providing a supplemental source of essential fatty acids has been recommended during reproduction and molting when monotypic diets of smelt are fed: 2-3 mL of corn oil/bird/day has been satisfactory. Thiamine and vitamin E supplementation (25 mg thiamine and 100 IU vitamin E/kg of fish, as fed) is recommended whenever fish that have been frozen are fed. Vitamin D_3 supplementation (250-500 IU/kg of fish, as fed) may be beneficial for birds not exposed to direct sunlight. Providing calcium carbonate or dicalcium phosphate to females during reproductive periods is a common practice to ensure proper eggshell formation. Penguins should be fed individually by hand to ensure that each bird receives the proper amounts of supplements, and to better monitor intake. Generally, intake is 0.5-2 kg fish/day depending on the species of penguin, fat content of the fish, and molt status.

Recommendations for feeding other fish-eating birds (eg, pelican, cormorant, heron, gull, tern, loon, grebe, petrel) are similar to those for penguins. Some species will accept commercial bird-of-prey diets, trout pellets, and/or mice in the diet, as well as fish.

Flamingos can be fed commercial flamingo diets or a mixture of trout pellets (#4 size), duck-grower or game-bird pellets, dry dog food, and a carotenoid pigment source (eg, canthaxanthin, carrot oil extract). Lack of a suitable pigment source in the diet results in faded feather coloration. Dry ingredients should be mixed with water, forming a slurry to permit natural filter feeding.

Most waterfowl can be fed commercial duck or game-bird pellets along with chopped lettuce or hydroponic grass. Dry dog food (<10% fat, dry-matter basis) or trout pellets are readily consumed by many species, particularly diving ducks, and can be included in the diet. Scratch grains can be fed in moderation (<25% of the diet dry matter) but are no substitute for a nutritionally complete pelleted product.

GALLINACEOUS BIRDS

Most gallinaceous birds (eg, pheasant, quail, turkey, grouse, partridge) do well on commercial game-bird diets. Starter, grower, maintenance, and layer diets are available. Grit should always be available free choice. Chopped lettuce, hydroponic grass, or other green vegetation also can be provided. Some herbivorous grouse species are difficult to maintain in captivity and may require specific natural foods such as willow, heather, or blueberry leaves and buds. Artificial diets that have been used successfully for grouse often contain higher levels of fiber (eg, 10% crude fiber, dry basis) than rations for poultry and game birds. Growing chicks of some grouse species appear to require a dietary source of vitamin C. Diets of most young gallinaceous birds may be supplemented with crickets and mealworms to provide variety and to serve as a feeding stimulus.

HUMMINGBIRDS

Captive hummingbirds readily adapt to artificial nectar mixtures (for examples of formulas, *see* TABLE 26, p 1214). Nectar should always be available to satisfy their extremely high energy requirements. Satisfactory commercial nectar dry mixes that are fortified with protein, vitamins, and minerals also are available. Commercial nectar mixes that are simply sugar and food coloring are not adequate. A nutritionally complete nectar should be offered early each morning. At the end of each day, the morning nectar should be discarded to prevent bacterial contamination and fermentation; in hot weather, it may need to be changed during the day. In the afternoon, morning nectar can be replaced with a sugar-water mixture that is less likely to sour overnight. Nectar can be dispensed in commercially available tube-type hummingbird feeders. Common backyard hummingbird feeders are not recommended for captive hummingbirds because they tend to clog with morning nectar and are difficult to clean. Feeding tubes should be colored (usually red) and must be an appropriate size and shape to accommodate the hummingbird's bill. Feeders should be cleaned thoroughly each day. Coloration of hummingbirds is not influenced by dietary pigments; therefore, pigmented nectars are not necessary. Fruit flies also should be included in the diet. Screen-covered containers (with screens of suitable size to permit fruit flies to exit, but exclude insect pests) with fruit-fly cultures can be placed in the birds' enclosures and replaced as the flies are depleted.

PASSERINES

Passerines can be grouped into 5 categories depending on their primary natural food habits: insect feeder, fruit eater, nectar feeder, seed eater, and omnivore. Insectivorous birds (eg, warbler, flycatcher, shrike) can be fed artificial insectivore mixtures supplemented with crickets, mealworms, maggots, house flies, and/or fruit flies. Many insectivore mixes have been devised; for one that has been used successfully, *see* TABLE 26, p 1214. Insects can be placed on top of the insectivore mixture to stimulate feeding. Frugivorous birds (eg, waxwing, bellbird) can be fed fruit mixtures fortified with protein, minerals, and vitamins. Examples of frugivore mixes that have supported reproduction in various bird species are shown in TABLE 26. Nectar feeders (eg, sunbird, honeycreeper) can be maintained in captivity using artificial nectars. (*See* HUMMINGBIRDS, above, and TABLE 26.) Most nectar-feeding species will also eat insects, insectivore mix, and/or frugivore mix. Seed eaters (eg, finches, sparrows, cardinals) can be offered seed mixtures (primary seeds include canary seed and yellow, white, and red millet; secondary seeds include oat groats, flax, and niger or thistle). Chopped green vegetables, insects, insectivore and frugivore mixes, peanut butter, and cooked egg yolk also are readily accepted by most species, and should be included in addition to seeds to provide a balanced diet. Cuttlebone and grit should be available free choice to seed-eating birds. Omnivorous species (eg, corvid, tanager, starling, mynah, oriole, manakin, bird of paradise) can be fed frugivore and insectivore mixes in equal portions. Insects, chopped green vegetables, peanut butter, cooked egg yolk, or bird-of-prey diet also can be offered to most species. Commercial soft-pelleted diets are available for mynahs. Some omnivorous passerines (eg, blackbird, meadowlark, horned lark) will also eat seed and grain mixtures.

PIGEONS AND DOVES

Seed-eating pigeons and doves can be fed commercial pigeon pellets and pigeon grains (wheat, milo, corn, Canada peas [field peas], and millet). Fruit-eating pigeons and doves can be fed a large-frugivore mixture (TABLE 26, p 1214).

PSITTACINES

Large seed-eating species (eg, macaw, parrot, cockatoo) commonly are maintained on diets of seeds (sunflower, hemp, millet, canary, safflower, oats), peanuts, monkey biscuits, dry dog food, fruits (apple, banana, grape, orange), vegetables (green vegetables, carrot, ear corn, sweet potato), and various supplements (cooked egg yolk, vitamins, minerals, wheat germ). The percentage of each ingredient fed varies widely; eg, some breeders have reported good success on diets consisting almost entirely of monkey biscuits, while others have recommended that no more than 10% of the diet consist of monkey biscuits. For an example of a mixed diet that has been used successfully for large psittacines, *see* TABLE 26, p 1215. Intake of each ingredient should be monitored closely whenever mixed diets are fed. Many birds show a pronounced preference for certain items such as sunflower seeds and peanuts, and will select an improper diet if given the opportunity. When certain items are selected in unduly high amounts, they should be decreased in the diet to force consumption of other foods. Vitamin and mineral premixes can be added to the drinking water, and dusted over fruits and vegetables that have been cut into pieces that are easy for the birds to handle. Several commercial diets are available for large psittacines. Some are simply mixes of seeds and other ingredients that still permit sorting by the birds. Others are fortified, pelleted, or extruded products that ensure the birds consume a specific concentration of nutrients. Although the pelleted or extruded diets are often more complete and easier to feed than mixed diets, it can be difficult to switch birds accustomed to mixed diets to these products. Smaller seed-eating psittacines (eg, cockatiel, budgerigar, lovebird) can be fed commercial seed mixtures (canary seed; red, yellow, and white millet; oat groats) along with chopped greens, bread, and fruit. There are also commercial diets (complete feeds) available in small sizes to accomodate these types of birds; these are more likely to provide well-balanced diets. Vitamin and mineral supplements can be added in the same manner as with the larger species. Unlike most psittacines, lories and lorikeets are primarily frugivorous. Various fortified fruit mixtures have been used successfully for these species.

Cuttlebone or a mineral block should be available free choice to all psittacines. Daily food intake is usually ~10-15% of body wt for most species, with higher relative intakes occurring in smaller birds.

Table 26. Avian Diets

Morning Nectar

Protein powder (soy-based)	25 g
Protein supplement (casein-based)	10 g
Multivitamin drops*	2.4 mL
Calcium, phosphorus, vitamin D_3 supplement	6.5 g
Canthaxanthin	0.5 g
Sugar	400 g
Water	1920 mL

Remove remaining nectar at the end of each day and discard. Canthaxanthin is optional and is not required for birds that do not depend on carotenoids for feather pigmentation (eg, hummingbirds).

Evening Nectar

Sugar	400 g
Multivitamin drops*	2.4 mL
Water	1440 mL

Insectivore

Ground dog food	23%
Steamed bone meal	5%
Ground trout pellets	4%
Protein supplement (casein-based)	2%
Ground mynah bird pellets	8%
"Super Caradee"	6%
Frozen bird-of-prey diet	52%

Thaw bird-of-prey diet and thoroughly mix all ingredients. Final product should have a crumbly texture. Refrigerate or freeze for storage.

Small Frugivore

	g/kg of diet
Apple	470
Grape	110
Banana without skin	100
Currant	70
Tomato	50
Papaya	50
Blueberry	50
Frugivore basemix (*see* below)	100

Place apples and grapes in a food processor and mix until in small pieces but not soupy. Drain in a colander. Place tomato, papaya, and banana in food processor and blend. Pieces should be small, but the mixture should not be soupy. Combine all ingredients and mix thoroughly. Mixture can be refrigerated for up to 3 days. Calculated analysis (dry-matter basis): 24% dry matter, 26% crude protein, 4% fat, 3.6% crude fiber, 7.7% ash, 1.49% Ca, 0.76% P.

Large Frugivore

	g/kg of diet
Apple	480
Banana without skin	200
Grape	100
Raisin (seedless)	50
Blueberry	50
Frugivore basemix (*see* below)	120

Chop apple and banana into pieces ~15 mm wide. Combine all ingredients and mix thoroughly until blended to a thin applesauce-like consistency. Calculated analysis (dry-matter basis): 31% dry matter, 24% crude protein, 3.7% fat, 2.6% crude fiber, 7.2% ash, 1.4% Ca, 0.71% P.

Table 26. Avian Diets (continued)

Frugivore Basemix — g/kg of basemix

Corn gluten meal (60% CP**)	359
Calcium caseinate	280
Soybean protein concentrate (70% CP)	100
Dicalcium phosphate	75
Corn oil	50
Brewer's yeast, dehydrated	45
Calcium carbonate	38
Iodized salt (NaCl)	13
L-lysine monohydrochloride	5.5
DL-methionine	4.5
Frugivore vitamin premix***	16
Frugivore mineral premix****	14

Large Psittacine

Seeds and nuts	20%
Fruit	25%
Greens	15%
Yellow vegetables	25%
Monkey biscuit or dry dog food	15%
Cuttlebone or mineral block	free choice

Kiwi (per adult)

Rolled oats	20 g
Water	160 mL
Vegetable oil	2.5 mL
Wheat germ	2 g
Vitamin-mineral premix*****	2 g

Trim fat off beef heart and slice into thin, worm-like strips. Cook oats in water, and combine all ingredients to make a gruel. Feed from a shallow dish. Earthworms also can be offered.

*Multivitamin drops (per mL): 1500 IU vitamin A, 400 IU vitamin D, 5 IU vitamin E, 0.5 mg vitamin B_1, 0.6 mg vitamin B_2, 8 mg niacin, 0.4 mg vitamin B_6, 1.5 μg vitamin B_{12}, 35 mg vitamin C.

**CP = crude protein

***Frugivore vitamin premix (g/kg of premix): 33.3 g retinyl acetate mix (30,000 IU/g), 0.4 g cholecalciferol mix (500,000 IU/g), 18.1 g dl-α-tocopheryl acetate mix (276 IU/g), 576 g choline chloride mix (60% choline chloride), 1.38 g thiamine HCl (87.5% B_1), 1.3 g riboflavin (96% B_2), 10.1 g niacin (99.5% niacin), 1.55 g pyridoxine HCl (80.65% B_6), 5.43 g d-Ca pantothenate (92% pantothenate), 2.5 g biotin mix (2% biotin), 1.25 g folic acid mix (20% folic acid), 1.89 g vitamin B_{12} mix (600 mg/lb), 0.76 g menadione sodium bisulfite complex (33% menadione), and 346 g soybean protein concentrate.

****Frugivore mineral premix (g/kg of premix): 7 g $CuSO_4$ • $5H_2O$ (25.2% Cu), 42 g $ZnSO_4$ • H_2O (35.5% Zn), 60 g $MnSO_4$ • $5H_2O$ (28% Mn), 17 g $FeSO_4$ • H_2O (30% Fe), 150 g sodium selenite mix (0.02% Se), and 724 g calcium caseinate.

*****Vitamin-mineral premix for kiwis (per kg): 320 g calcium, 2.7 g iron, 2.7 g zinc, 2.7 g manganese, 0.27 g copper, 27 mg iodine, 27 mg cobalt, 16 mg selenium, 800,000 IU vitamin A, 60,000 IU vitamin D, 6000 IU vitamin E, 0.43 g vitamin B_1, 0.32 g vitamin B_2, 0.27 g vitamin B_6, 40 g choline, 10.6 g inositol, 5.3 g ascorbic acid, 2.13 g nicotinic acid, 1.6 g pantothenic acid, 0.43 g vitamin K, 0.11 g folic acid, 21 mg biotin, 2.7 mg vitamin B_{12}, 1.06 g butylated hydroxy toluene.

RAPTORS

Vultures, hawks, falcons, and owls can be fed whole-animal diets. Commonly fed items include chicks up to 5 wk old, coturnix quail, mice, rats, and pigeons. Feeding a variety of prey items is preferred, although some species more readily accept certain kinds of prey, depending on natural food habits. Fish can be included in the diet of piscivorous species (eg, osprey, sea eagle, bald eagle), and fortified insects can be given to kestrels and falconettes. If fish or day-old chicks are fed, thiamine supplementation (30 mg/kg feed, as-fed basis) on alternate days is recommended. To ensure a nutritionally complete diet, prey items should not be eviscerated before feeding. Commercial bird-of-prey diets also can be used successfully by many species and often provide a simpler, more economical alternative to live-prey diets. A commercial diet suitable for a variety of species is 55-60% moisture and contains (dry-matter basis) 45-50% crude protein, 18-20% ether extract, 2.2-2.5% crude fiber, and 1-1.5% calcium and 0.7-1% phosphorus. Due to the soft consistency of these diets, usually it is desirable to provide whole-prey items twice a week to help prevent impaction and beak overgrowth as well as to provide added insurance of a complete diet. Small raptors can eat as much as 25% of their body wt/day; large species may eat as little as 4%. Captive raptors should be weighed regularly to monitor weight gain and loss, and food intake should be adjusted accordingly.

RATITES

All large ratite birds (emu, cassowary, ostrich, rhea) can be fed commercial pelleted ratite diets. Diets suitable for growth and maintenance contain 20-24% crude protein, 12-19% crude fiber, 1.2-2% calcium, 0.6-1.1% phosphorus, 10,000-15,000 IU/kg vitamin A, and 1500-2500 IU/kg vitamin D_3 (dry-matter basis). Breeding diets are similar except for a higher level of calcium (eg, 2.8% Ca in the pellet, or oyster shell free choice). Mixtures of pelleted poultry or duck feed, dry dog food, rabbit pellets, and oyster shell also have been used. Green, leafy vegetables and, for cassowarys, chopped apple can be added to the diet. Young ratites are particularly susceptible to leg abnormalities that appear to be nutritionally related. Reducing the growth rate by feeding diets lower in ME and higher in fiber appears to reduce the incidence of spraddled leg syndrome in young birds. A diet using beef heart cut into worm-like strips as a base item has been used successfully for kiwis (*see* TABLE 26, p 1215).

MISCELLANEOUS BIRDS

Most large, fruit-eating softbills, eg, hornbill, toucan, toucanet, and touraco, will eat a large-frugivore mixture (*see* TABLE 26, p 1215) along with insects, greens, and dry dog food or bird-of-prey diet. Gelatin-based diets also have been used successfully for hornbills and toucans. Placing diet ingredients in gelatin obviates sorting but requires careful formulation to compensate for the low tryptophan content of the gelatin. Frogmouths and kookaburras will eat mice and commercial bird-of-prey diets.

MAMMALS

Handrearing Mammals: Successful nutrition of handreared mammals requires: 1) selecting a formula that will support adequate growth and not cause GI upset; 2) offering it at proper intervals, in proper amounts, and in the proper way to ensure acceptance, and prevent overfeeding or underfeeding, or aspiration into the lungs; and 3) keeping all feeding utensils clean and disinfected. If success is judged in terms of survival and not in comparison with maternal-raised growth and health, most precocial species maintained in captive collections have been handreared successfully. Handrearing more altricial species (eg, marsupials, rodents, rabbits) generally has met with more limited success unless the young have been dam-raised to a more advanced stage.

Whenever possible, data on milk composition and handrearing case histories should be consulted before attempting to bottle-raise a species for the first time. Unfortunately, milk composition data are not available for most species, and some of the published data are of dubious value. Lactose content of milk varies widely between different species. Those animals (eg, pinnipeds, rabbits) that normally consume milk low in lactose generally produce little lactase and often develop severe GI problems and diarrhea when fed a high-lactose milk, eg, bovine. Similarly, adding sucrose to milk formulas is often contraindicated because many neonates produce little sucrase. Many species have been raised using diluted evaporated milk or commercial calf, lamb, foal, or doe milk replacers (eg, most ungulates), commercial dog milk replacer (eg, canids, procyonids, bears, bats, edentates, mustelids, rabbits, rodents), commercial cat milk replacer (eg, felids), human infant formulas in general (eg, most primates), and soy-based human milk replacers in particular (eg, rabbits, some marsupials). In some cases, these basic formulas can be modified to better suit the needs of a particular species by the addition of ingredients such as egg yolk, butterfat, and casein. Supplementation with vitamin and mineral products may be warranted.

Some species (eg, ungulates, marsupials, mink) must receive colostrum within 48 hr of birth to acquire immunoglobulins necessary for survival. Including some colostrum in the diet of ungulates for up to 2-3 wk after birth may provide additional local gut protection. Domestic cow colostrum has proved satisfactory for many exotic ruminants and can be frozen for storage. Many neonates (eg, artiodactyls, rodents, carnivores) must be stimulated to defecate and urinate by gently rubbing anal and genital areas.

Table 27. Diets of Selected Mammals

Freshwater Otter Diet	%
Ground horsemeat	38
Ground beef heart	20
Ground dry cat food	13
Beet pulp	2.9
"Mirra Coat"	1.9
Calcium carbonate	0.8
Poultry fat	4.9
Water	16.9
Lactose	0.04
Yogurt	0.72
Mineral-vitamin mix (eg, "Theralin")	0.84

Combine all ingredients in a large mixer. Divide into daily portions and freeze. Add lactose for lactobacilli in yogurt to help maintain freshness. Lactose and yogurt are optional.

Liquid Diet for Bats	
Dry mix:	%
Mixed baby cereal	20.7
Wheat germ	4
Nonfat dried milk powder	9
Calcium caseinate	15.8
Sugar	45.5
Protein supplement (casein-based)	3
Mineral-vitamin mix (eg, "Pervinal Powder")	2

Mix 100 g of the dry mix with 540 mL of canned peach nectar, 260 mL water, and 6 mL corn oil. Feed along with peeled bananas.

Aardvark	%
Water	61
Horsemeat, ground	12
Beef heart, ground	6
Dry mix	21
Dry mix:	
Nonfat dried milk	28.15
Ground dry dog food (21% CP*)	28.3
Mixed baby cereal	5.7
Soybean protein concentrate (7 % CP)	11.4
Alfalfa meal, dehydrated (17% CP)	8.1
Sodium caseinate	5.7
Soybean oil	5.9
Whole egg powder	2.6
Calcium carbonate	1.15
Mineral-vitamin mix (eg, "Theralin")	3

Mix all ingredients into a gruel.

(continued)

Table 27. Diets of Selected Mammals (continued)

Giant Panda (per adult)	
Powdered cottage cheese	0.25 lb (100 g)
Mineral premix**	10 tsp (50 g)
Vitamin premix***	4 tsp (20 g)
Soybean oil	1 tbsp (15 mL)
Honey	2 tbsp (30 mL)
Water	1 qt (1 L)
Canned feline diet (eg, "Zu/Preem")	7 oz (210 g)

Mix all ingredients into a gruel. Feed along with 430 g of carrots, 340 g of apples, and 11 kg of bamboo.

Large Herbivore Pellet	%
Wheat middlings	30
Alfalfa hay, sun-cured, ground (16% CP)	22
Corn grain, ground	19.1
Soybean meal without hulls (48% CP)	11.4
Alfalfa meal, dehydrated (17% CP)	10
Sugarcane molasses	5
Soybean oil	1
Phosphorus supplement (eg, "Biofos")	0.8
Sodium chloride	0.5
Mineral premix**	0.1
Vitamin premix***	0.1

* CP = crude protein

** Mineral premix (mg/kg of premix): 75,000 Zn, 50,000 Fe, 30,000 Mn, 10,000 Cu, 800 I, 200 Se, and 100 Co.

*** Vitamin premix (per kg of premix): 5,000,000 IU vitamin A, 400,000 IU vitamin D_3, 200,000 mg vitamin E, 500,000 mg choline, 40,000 mg niacin, 20,000 mg pantothenic acid, 4000 mg riboflavin, 20 mg vitamin B_{12}.

Calculated composition (dry-matter basis): 89% dry matter, 19% crude protein, 4.3% fat, 16% acid detergent fiber, 12% crude fiber, 0.75% Ca, 0.7% P.

Frequency of feeding and the amount fed depends on natural nursing behavior, formula composition, and the desired rate of gain as well as practical man-hour restrictions. As a general guide, most newborns should be fed q2-4hr, and daily ME intake (kcal) should be ~210 × body wt $(kg)^{0.75}$. Appetite, condition of feces, and general health should be monitored closely. Body weights should be recorded at frequent intervals. Smaller, more altricial species often must be fed by stomach tube.

BATS

Captive insectivorous bats frequently are fed diets consisting primarily of mealworms; crickets, fruit flies, blowfly larvae, and other insects also are commonly offered. Because insects typically are low in calcium, they should be maintained on a calcium-enriched diet so that the bat will consume the insect's high-calcium gut contents. A suitable mealworm diet can be formulated using 40% wheat middlings, 40% ground dry dog or cat food, and 20% ground calcium carbonate. Alternatively, calcium and vitamin supplements can be dusted on the insects just before feeding, and vitamin drops can be added to drinking water. Often, captive insectivorous bats must be fed by hand when flying insects are not available. Some bats can be trained to accept insects from a food dish by being placed directly on the live food. Various artificial diets have been used with insectivorous bats with mixed success.

Many frugivorous and insectivorous bats can be maintained successfully in captivity using artificial liquid or solid diets. See TABLE 27, above, for one example of a widely used liquid diet. Liquid diet can be placed in shallow plastic trays positioned near wire or branches for the bats to land on and hang from while feeding. Leftover liquid diet should be replaced daily. Solid diets usually include bananas as the major ingredient. Additional ingredients frequently offered include papaya, apple, pear, melon, grape, and cooked carrot and sweet potato. Fruit can be rolled in a supplement mixture that contains powdered milk, protein powder, corn oil, and a vitamin-mineral mix. Canned cat or dog food, chopped eggs, and mealworms also have been fed with the fruit.

CARNIVORES

Most zoos in the USA now use nutritionally complete commercial diets for feeding exotic felids, canids, mustelids, and viverrids rather than attempting to prepare diets in-house. The incidence of nutritional problems in captive exotic carnivores has greatly declined, and problems previously commonplace when meat diets were fed (eg, calcium, vitamin A, and iodine deficiencies) have virtually been eliminated. Most commercial diets are based on horsemeat and its by-products, but diets based on beef and poultry are also available. Typical lesser ingredients include fish meal, soybean meal, beet pulp, and ground corn, as well as mineral and vitamin supplements.

Exotic feline diets are usually higher in fat, protein, and vitamin A than canine diets. A diet suitable for most cat species contains 45-50% protein, 30-35% fat, 3-4% crude fiber, 1.2-1.5% calcium, 1-1.2% phosphorus, and 20,000-40,000 IU of vitamin A/kg diet (dry-matter basis). From available evidence, it appears that exotic cats share with domestic cats the inability to convert carotene to vitamin A, tryptophan to niacin, and linoleic acid to arachidonic acid. Like domestic cats, they also probably cannot synthesize adequate taurine (a taurine deficiency has been reported in leopards) and would be susceptible to ammonia toxicity if fed an arginine-deficient diet. Therefore, these nutrients should be considered dietary essentials for all cats. Frozen and canned cat foods usually are more palatable to exotic cats than dry ones. Many zoos prefer frozen diets over canned products because generally they are less expensive, and large quantities are easier to feed. The soft, hamburger-like consistency of commercial diets can result in excess calculus deposits and, ultimately, periodontal disease if hard or unprocessed items are not provided in the diet. It is recommended that all cats fed a soft diet receive bones with some meat intact 2 times/wk. Horse or beef shank bones are suitable for large cat species; oxtails, rib bones, or whole rodents can be used for smaller cats. Mice, rats, and chicks are frequently included in the diets of smaller cats. Rodents, poultry, fish, and organ and chunk muscle meats can be offered as occasional treat items to administer medication or to stimulate appetite, but generally are not required as dietary staples for large cats fed commercial diets.

Canids can be fed frozen, canned, or dry canine diets. Although most canids are less particular than cats, frozen and canned foods are generally preferred over dry ones. Bones should also be included in the diet when soft foods are fed. Small amounts of fruits and vegetables can be included in the diets of foxes and coyotes.

Most mustelids and viverrids do well on frozen feline diet or canned cat foods. Many species readily accept small amounts of fruits, vegetables, and cooked egg. Mice, fish, and chicks can be offered as occasional treat items and to stimulate appetite and activity. Rib bones can be given 1-2 times/wk to promote dental health. Ferrets can be fed dry cat food or commercial dry ferret diets. A diet used successfully for freshwater otter species is shown in TABLE 27, p 1217.

Procyonids can be fed diets similar to those offered to small canids. Feeding a good-quality dry dog food along with apple, banana, and carrot is satisfactory for raccoons, and helps minimize obesity problems that commonly result when frozen or canned diets are fed. The red or lesser panda has been maintained successfully on a gruel diet consisting of mixed baby cereal, evaporated milk, egg yolk, honey, applesauce, beet pulp, water, and mineral-vitamin supplements. Apple, banana, and bamboo also are offered.

Bears can be fed frozen canine diet, dry dog food, fish, and commercial omnivore biscuits. Polar and Kodiak bears do well on a diet of 25% frozen canine diet, 25% fish (eg, smelt), 15% dry dog food, 15% omnivore biscuits, 10% bread, and 10% apples. Commercial diets formulated especially for polar bears are available. Other bear species can be fed less fish and more omnivore biscuits, bread, and produce. Bananas and green vegetables can be included in the diet of sun, sloth, spectacled, and black bears. Food intake of captive bears varies widely with season. Maximum intakes generally occur during summer and early fall, minimum intakes during winter. The herbivorous food habits of the giant panda require a more specialized diet (*see* TABLE 27, p 1218).

INSECTIVORES, EDENTATES, AND AARDVARKS

Most shrews, hedgehogs, tenrecs, and moles can be fed frozen cat food supplemented with mealworms, earthworms, crickets, and mouse pups. Ground meat fortified with minerals and vitamins, canned dog food, cooked egg, and small amounts of fruits and vegetables also are readily accepted by many species. Armadillos will eat frozen feline diet, moistened dry cat food, canned dog food, or ground meat fortified with minerals and vitamins. Milk, chopped egg, cooked sweet potato, diced banana, and other fruits also are consumed. Vitamin K supplementation of armadillos has been recommended to help prevent hemorrhaging: 5 mg of menadione sodium bisulfite/kg dry diet should be adequate. Two-toed sloths will eat a variety of diced vegetables and fruits (eg, lettuce, kale, spinach, celery, green beans, carrot, cooked sweet potato, banana, apple) in combination with frozen feline diet, moistened dry dog food, canned primate diet, and/or monkey biscuits. Food pans should be placed such that the animal can hang from a perch while feeding. In captivity, aardvarks, lesser anteaters, and giant anteaters readily accept semiliquid diets in place of termites, ants, and other natural foods. Artificial diets typically consist of milk, water, ground meat, and/or a meat-based product such as frozen feline diet, mink chow or dry dog food, hard-boiled egg, protein powder, baby cereal, and a mineral-vitamin supplement. All ingredients are mixed in a blender to the consistency of a thick gruel. Adult giant anteaters may develop loose feces when fed a semiliquid diet. In this case, milk and water can be withdrawn gradually from the formula. As a precaution, vitamin K often is added to all edentate diets. An example of an aardvark diet is listed in TABLE 27, p 1217.

MARINE MAMMALS

Fish are the primary food of captive marine mammals except for the herbivorous sirenians. The purchasing and subsequent proper storing and handling of good-quality fish (*see also* p 1048) are the most important aspects of feeding cetaceans and pinnipeds. On receipt, fish should always be inspected for quality; the following are useful for evaluation: 1) the boxes should be checked to see if catch dates are indicated; 2) overall appearance of the fish should be good; 3) gills should be red (light pink gills indicate considerable time may have elapsed before the fish were frozen after being caught); 4) eyes should not be sunken, indicating dehydration; 5) flesh of thawed fish should be firm, skin should be intact and not discolored, and there should not be a bad odor; 6) there should not be excess water and blood pooled in the bottom of frozen cases, which indicates the fish have thawed and been refrozen; and 7) ideally, the lenses of frozen fish should be cloudy, which indicates the fish have been properly stored at or below $-30°C$ before purchase (higher temperatures often result in clear lenses). To minimize peroxidative damage and nutrient destruction, fish should be stored at or below $-30°C$. Most fish species should not be stored >6 mo if at all possible (a maximum of 3-4 mo is recommended for fatty fish such as mackerel; lean fish such as smelt may remain in good condition for up to 9 mo). Ideally, fish should be thawed overnight under refrigeration. If this is not possible, thawing at room temperature is preferable to thawing in water, which can cause significant nutrient leaching. Individually quick frozen fish are preferred by many zoos because proper quantities can be thawed without leftover waste.

As a general rule, marine mammals should be given marine fish. Composition of marine fishes can vary greatly between species and even within species depending on age, season, and catch location. Fish that have been used successfully include Atlantic and Pacific herring; Atlantic, Pacific, and Spanish mackerel; bluerunner; capelin; and anadromous smelt. Squid are readily consumed by many pinnipeds, and clams can be included in walrus diets. No commercial substitute for fish has been developed that will be accepted by cetaceans, but such products have been used with some success for pinnipeds. The regular diet of any marine mammal should consist of ≥2 fish species to help ensure a balanced diet.

The possibility of thiamine destruction by thiaminases occurring in several fish species and associated bacteria make addition of this vitamin a recommended part of any marine mammal feeding program: 25 mg/kg fish, as fed, twice weekly is considered adequate, although daily supplements of similar quantity are often given. Supplemental vitamin E helps compensate for oxidative destruction of natural vitamin E in fish during storage, and helps protect against the deleterious effects of peroxides formed in stored fish. Oily fish such as mackerel, which are high in unsaturated fatty acids, are particularly susceptible to vitamin E destruction and peroxidative damage. Vitamin E at 100 IU/kg fish, as fed, per day is generally recommended.

Salt (NaCl) supplementation of pinnipeds maintained in freshwater is recommended to prevent hyponatremia; 3 g salt/kg fish is adequate. Although supplemental vitamin C is frequently given to captive cetaceans, there is no conclusive evidence it is beneficial. Recent evidence indicates liver vitamin A levels in captive dolphins are often much lower than in their wild counterparts. Although specific recommendations cannot be made, vitamin A supplementation of some captive cetacean diets may be desirable.

Food intake in marine mammals can vary considerably, depending on fat content of fish, water temperature, and activity. Performing Atlantic bottle-nosed dolphins generally eat 7-10 kg fish/day. Adult seals and sea lions consume ~5-8% of their body wt in fish/day. Captive sirenians can be maintained on a diet of lettuce, cabbage, alfalfa, and aquatic plants (eg, water hyacinth).

MARSUPIALS

Most didelphid marsupials can be fed dry or canned dog or cat food, or frozen dog food. Smaller species can be fed canned primate diet. Hard-boiled egg, green vegetables, carrot, sweet potato, apple, and banana also can be offered. Dasyurids (eg, marsupial "mice", native-cats, and Tasmanian devil) and bandicoots can be fed canned or frozen feline diet. In addition, crickets, mealworms, and mouse pups can be given to smaller species; larger species can be given mice and shank or rib bones. Wombats and the larger macropod marsupials can be fed a combination of large herbivore pellets and rabbit pellets. Rat kangaroos will eat a combination of mouse pellets and rabbit pellets. In addition, green vegetables, carrot, sweet potato, apple, and banana can be offered to all herbivorous and omnivorous marsupials. Because of potential problems with lumpy jaw, feeding hay to macropods is generally discouraged unless high-quality, leafy hay that is free of weeds, awns, and coarse stems is available. Currently, captive koalas can be fed successfully only on leaves of certain species of eucalyptus.

PRIMATES

Most primates can be fed a diet based on commercial monkey biscuits and/or canned primate or marmoset diet. Moderate amounts of assorted green vegetables, carrot, sweet potato, apple, banana, and orange also can be offered. It is recommended that monkey biscuits and the canned products make up ≥50% of the dry-matter intake of most species, and that fruits and treat items comprise ≤25%. High-protein monkey biscuits (25% crude protein) should be fed to New World primates to ensure that their higher protein requirements are met. Regular or high-protein monkey biscuits can be fed to Old World species depending on other components in the diet. Monkey biscuits can be made more palatable for some species by soaking them in water or fruit juice. To prevent leaching of nutrients, the biscuits should be placed in a thin film of liquid such that the liquid is drawn up into the biscuit. Other items commonly included in primate diets include hard-boiled egg, yogurt, skim milk (milk should be introduced gradually to prevent diarrhea), and bread. Grapes, raisins, peanuts, crickets, mealworms, and mouse pups are treat items well liked by most species. Sunflower seeds, instant rice, cracked corn, and shredded coconut can be scattered around exhibit or holding areas to promote foraging activity. Hay should be provided for nesting materials, diversion, and to act as a foraging substrate. Many zoos offer meat to their great apes. Although meat is often relished by the animals, there is no evidence it is necessary if the diet is properly balanced. For most primates, meals should be offered in the morning and afternoon.

New World primates utilize vitamin D_2 poorly. It is particularly important that these species receive an adequate source of stabilized vitamin D_3 (cholecalciferol) in their diet if they are not exposed daily to direct sunlight. Marmosets require up to 4 times the amount of vitamin D_3 required by other New World primates. Because of potential vitamin D toxicity, commercial marmoset diets should be fed only to marmosets.

All primates require a source of vitamin C. Because (except for a recently available, more stable form) vitamin C added to commercial monkey biscuits can begin undergoing significant destruction within 6 mo of milling, a supplementary source should be included in the diet (eg, green vegetables, oranges, multiple vitamins, fruit juice, or fruit juice powders with added vitamin C).

Members of the subfamily Colobinae are perhaps the greatest challenge in the proper feeding of captive primates. Pregastric fermentation, similar to that in ruminants, occurs in the complex stomach of these species. In the wild, leaves make up a major part of the diet of most colobines (the more frugivorous red colobus is an exception). Therefore, natural diets are usually moderately high in fiber, and animals spend much time foraging. Offering a rich, rapidly consumable diet of monkey biscuits and fruit in captivity presents a situation quite different from that typically occurring in the wild and may be partly to blame for the frequent GI problems reported in these species. Also, some evidence suggests that a high percentage of colobus monkeys may be sensitive to gluten. A commercial, gluten-free, high-fiber monkey biscuit (25% neutral detergent fiber) has recently been developed for feeding captive colobines. A diet consisting of 50% high-fiber biscuit, 40% green vegetables and fresh browse, and 10% fruit is recommended for most colobines. Alfalfa pellets or good-quality alfalfa hay can be provided free choice. If a suitable high-fiber biscuit is not available, fresh browse and/or high-fiber green vegetables such as kale, mustard greens, broccoli, celery, spinach, green beans, lettuce, and escarole should make up ≥50% of the diet, with regular monkey biscuits and canned primate diet comprising ~25% of the diet dry matter. If a gluten-sensitive enteropathy is suspected, any product that contains wheat, barley, rye, or oats should be removed from the diet. Diet changes always should be made gradually in colobines to allow adaptation of their stomach microflora.

RODENTS AND LAGOMORPHS

Most rodent and lagomorph species do well on diets based on commercial laboratory rodent pellets and/or rabbit pellets. Rabbits, hares, pikas, marmots, and prairie dogs can be maintained on rabbit pellets, alfalfa or grass hay, and assorted vegetables. Most other sciurids can be fed rat pellets and a mixture of sunflower seeds, millet, corn, and rolled oats. Ground squirrels can also be offered green leafy vegetables, carrot, and apple. Most murids, cricetids, gophers, dormice, and jerboas do well on rat pellets or, for smaller species, mouse pellets, a seed and grain mix, green leafy vegetables, carrot, and apple. Hay should be made available to voles and lemmings. Muskrats, agoutis, and capybaras will eat a combination of rat and rabbit pellets along with alfalfa hay, carrot, and apple. Porcupines can be fed rat pellets, rabbit pellets, and dry dog food in equal portions along with some apple, carrot, and bread; evergreen and willow branches should be made available whenever possible. Beavers will eat a combination of rabbit pellets, large herbivore pellets, and dry dog food, regularly augmented with willow, poplar, aspen, or alder branches. Guinea pigs can be offered commercial guinea-pig pellets along with greens and carrot. Although guinea pigs and cavies are the only rodents known to require a dietary source of vitamin C, lagomorphs and rodents may benefit from it.

SUBUNGULATES AND UNGULATES

Hay comprises the bulk of the diet for most ungulates in captivity and should be available for most of the day rather than fed at intervals as meals. As a general rule, a leafy legume hay, eg, alfalfa, should be used for those species that ꞏre primarily browsers (eg, Giraffidae, Cervidae, sitatunga, bongo, duiker, black rhinoceros, tapir, etc), whereas a good-quality grass hay is satisfactory for most grazers or bulk feeders (eg, zebra, elephant, bison, buffalo, wildebeest, camel). Legume hays are higher in nitrogen and calcium and, if of good quality, are more digestible than grass hays. Hay should be leafy and green, free of mold, dirt, excess weeds, and other foreign matter, and should not be over-mature. Hay analysis can be very useful for evaluating quality and designing proper feeding programs.

In addition to hay, a pelleted diet that contains protein, minerals, and vitamins in concentrations adequate to meet the needs of domestic species and those wild species for which data are available (eg, white-tailed deer) should be offered. Most products manufactured for cattle are not appropriate for zoo ungulates. In the frequent situation in which animals are fed as a group rather than as individuals, it is preferable to use a pelleted diet that is not excessively high in digestible energy (~3 kcal DE/g dry matter is suggested) and that contains sufficient fiber to support proper rumen and/or colon function. This precaution reduces the possibility of untoward effects (eg, rumen acidosis, colic, obesity) caused by the overconsumption of concentrates. Some zoos prefer to use 2 pelleted diets: one high in fiber for grazers or bulk feeders, and one lower in fiber for browsers. Other zoos prefer to use one pelleted diet for all grazing and browsing species. In the latter case, the type of hay fed along with the pellet, and the percentage of pelleted diet offered, are used to adjust for differences between grazing and browsing species. A pelleted diet that has been used successfully for various grazing and browsing ungulates and subungulates is shown in diets of selected mammals, TABLE 27, p 1217. A 3/16 in. pellet size is satisfactory for most artiodactyls, whereas a 1/2 in. (~13 mm) pellet or cube size helps minimize waste when fed to larger perissodactyls and subungulates. Alternatively, commercial equine pellets often can be used satisfactorily for most nonruminant species (eg, elephant, rhinoceros, hippopotamus, zebra), although vitamin E supplementation may be needed. Commercial omnivore biscuits are readily consumed by tapirs and can be used in combination with commercial hog pellets for peccaries.

As a general rule, most large ungulates (>250 kg) consume 1.5-2% of their weight in dry matter daily. Smaller species (<250 kg) generally consume 2-4%. Offering a pelleted diet at 25-50% of the dry-matter intake is adequate for most species if good-quality hay is fed. As hay quality declines, or for more delicate species, the percentage of pellets should be increased. Hay should be fed from a rack rather than off the ground for most species (elephants are an exception). Hay racks should be located at eye levels for tall browsers such as giraffes and gerenuks. Pellets can be offered from a covered trough or rubber feed pans. Regularly feeding the pelleted diet in an animal's holding area can facilitate close observation and easy capture. At least 2 widely separated feeding stations may be necessary to reduce conflict and ensure that subordinate animals get their share.

Water should be freely available 24 hr/day. Also, in addition to hay and pelleted diet, assorted fruits, vegetables, and hydroponic grass often are fed to exotic ungulates. For most species, these items usually are not necessary except as an occasional treat. The exception might be those species that regularly feed on fruits and succulents in the wild. It may be advisable to include some fruits and vegetables (~0.5 kg/100 kg body wt) in the diet of species such as okapi, duikers, dik diks, bongo, and tapirs. Day-old bread, if readily available, can be included in moderate amounts in the diets of most species. Fresh or frozen browse is consumed avidly by most captive ungulates and subungulates, and can be offered to relieve boredom.

REPTILES

Maintaining reptiles in a proper environment is essential for overall management, including proper nutrition. Ambient temperature and humidity must be carefully controlled for proper feeding and digestion. Photoperiod, substrate, and cage props also can affect their feeding behavior. Ideally, enclosures should be designed to provide environmental gradients so reptiles can select their own microenvironment. For those species offered vertebrate prey, the food animal should be killed or stunned just before feeding. This protects the reptiles from bites and reduces the chance of injury caused by striking walls of the enclosure. Familiarity with a species' food habits in the wild is essential if proper foods are to be offered. Whenever possible, it is usually desirable to provide a diverse diet to reptiles to ensure a proper balance of nutrients and minimize dependence on a single food or prey species. Single-prey dependence frequently occurs in snakes and can be unavoidable. Commercial diets for reptiles are available; generally these have not been widely accepted by owners or, in many cases, by the reptiles themselves. They do, however, offer a potentially simpler and more economical alternative to feeding live prey. Acceptability is better when the commercial diets are offered to young reptiles.

CROCODILIANS

Captive alligators and crocodiles can be fed a combination of rodents, poultry, fish, and meat-based diets. A varied diet is recommended. Diets consisting primarily of fish should be supplemented with 30 mg of thiamine and 50-100 IU vitamin E/kg of fish, as fed.

LIZARDS

As a group, lizards display diverse food habits. Many are primarily insectivorous (eg, night lizards, alligator lizards, whiptails, most small and juvenile iguanids), but carnivores (eg, monitor lizards, gila monster, Mexican beaded lizard), herbivores (eg, marine iguana), and omnivores (eg, most large adult iguanids) are all represented. Insectivorous species are commonly fed mealworms and crickets in captivity. If unsupplemented, a diet based on these foods can result in a calcium (Ca) deficiency because of the low Ca content and inverse Ca to phosphorus ratio. The Ca level can be increased by maintaining the insects on a high-Ca diet (eg, 8% Ca as calcium carbonate) and/or dusting them with a Ca mixture (calcium carbonate or calcium gluconate) before feeding. In addition, it is desirable to feed the insects a nutritious medium that will be in their gut when they are consumed by a lizard. A satisfactory diet for crickets can be made using 29% wheat middlings, 10% corn meal, 40% ground dry cat or dog food, and 21% calcium carbonate. (See BATS, p 1218, for mealworm diet.) Some insectivorous lizards will also eat mouse pups, cooked egg yolk, earthworms, and small amounts of vegetable mixes. Depending on their size, carnivorous lizards can be fed mouse pups, mice, rats, chicks, chickens, and eggs. Omnivorous lizards can be fed a combination of insects and/or vertebrate prey (some iguanas will also eat chopped smelt) and a chopped vegetable mixture. (See TURTLES AND TORTOISES, below, for vegetable mix.) Most lizards should be fed daily or every other day. Different food items are often fed on different days. Large carnivorous species can be fed 1-2 times/wk.

SNAKES

Snakes feed almost exclusively on vertebrate and/or invertebrate prey. A few species are specialized for feeding on eggs. Most boids, pythons, vipers, colubrids, crotalids, and elapids can be fed mouse pups, mice, chicks, hamsters, rats, guinea pigs, chickens, ducks, and rabbits. Some species (eg, king cobra, hognose snake, garter snake) feed primarily on other ectotherms in the wild. Some of these species can be switched, at least in part, to endothermic prey (which is often more readily available and less expensive) by rubbing the scent of preferred foods on the new food item, stuffing preferred foods with the new food, or sewing the new food to preferred foods. Anoles, yellow rat snakes, frogs, and smelt, depending on natural food habits, can be fed when endotherms are not accepted. Prey size usually is proportional to snake size and, in general, should not be much larger in diameter than the snake's head. Snakes that are routinely handled can be fed in a separate feeding tank to minimize biting. To reduce the chance of regurgitation, snakes should not be handled for 3 days after feeding. Most species should be fed q1-2wk. Some large, less active snakes may typically go ≥4 wk between feedings. Force-feeding should be used only as a last resort. Animals can be force-fed whole prey that has been lubricated with egg white by gently inserting the food a few inches down the throat using forceps. Tube feeding is also possible using ground prey.

TURTLES AND TORTOISES

Most freshwater and terrestrial turtles and terrapins do well when fed a vegetable mixture consisting of chopped lettuce or escarole, spinach, hydroponic grass, banana, apple, cooked sweet potato, trout pellets, a vitamin-trace mineral mix, a calcium supplement, vegetable oil, and cod liver oil. This mixture can be fed along with smelt, insects, earthworms, mouse pups, and/or supplemental ground meat. Alligator-snapping turtles will eat a variety of prey, including fish, mice, and chicks. Fish that have been frozen should be supplemented with 30 mg of thiamine and 50-100 IU vitamin E/kg, as fed. Tortoises are primarily herbivorous and do well on vegetable mix and chopped alfalfa hay or pellets. Chopped smelt, flower blossoms, dandelions, and small amounts of dry dog food also can be offered to many species. Oyster shell and pea gravel should be included in the diets of tortoises. Herbivorous tortoises and lizards may not receive enough micronutrients if fed inadequately supplemented vegetable mixes. Herbivore pellets may be adequate as the base diet for some, but such pellets may not contain enough vitamin D. Another alternative is to combine moistened, dry dog food as 20-25% of the dry matter with vegetables and chopped alfalfa.

NUTRITION: HORSES

The feeding recommendations given below are based on both practical experience and scientific research. Horses are kept for a much longer time than most farm animals, and feeding programs must support the development of sound feet and legs to sustain a long and athletic life.

NUTRITIONAL REQUIREMENTS

Although horses obviously utilize hay and other roughage more efficiently than do other nonruminants such as poultry or pigs, the anatomy of the equine GI tract limits this ability as compared with the ruminant. The site of fermentation in horses is the cecum and large intestine, where large numbers of microorganisms digest hemicellulose and cellulose, utilize protein and nonprotein nitrogen, and synthesize certain vitamins. Some of the products of fermentation, such as volatile fatty acids and some of the vitamins, are absorbed and used. Microbial protein synthesized from nitrogen entering the cecum and colon undergoes only limited proteolysis, and the supply of essential amino acids from an unbalanced dietary nitrogen source is not satisfactorily balanced by microbial amino acids for optimal growth. Horses, therefore, depend more on the quality of the diet than do ruminants.

WATER

Water requirements depend largely on environment, amount of work being performed, nature of the feed, and physiological status of the horse. Daily consumption by an adult horse typically is 5-12 gal. (19-45 L). Clean, fresh water should be provided *ad lib* for all horses. As physical activity increases, water consumption increases. If a horse is hot following exercise, it should be allowed to cool before given unlimited access to water.

Table 28. Daily Nutrient Requirements of Growing Horses and Ponies

Age	Body Weight	Fraction of Adult Weight	Daily Gain	Daily Feed[1]	Digestible Energy	Crude Protein	Ca	P	Vitamin A[2]
Mo	kg		kg	kg	Mcal	g	g	g	IU (thousands)
Growing ponies 200 kg adult weight									
3	60	0.30	0.40	2.10	6.44	404	22	12	2.7
6	95	0.48	0.30	2.60	7.55	488	22	11	4.3
12	140	0.70	0.20	3.50	8.71	392	12	7	6.3
18	170	0.85	0.10	3.80	8.34	375	10	6	7.7
24	185	0.92	0.05	3.90	7.93	337	9	5	8.3
Growing horses 400 kg adult weight									
3	125	0.31	0.85	4.38	12.05	562	29	16	5.6
6	180	0.45	0.65	4.95	13.95	698	28	16	8.3
12	265	0.66	0.40	6.63	15.56	700	23	13	11.9
18	330	0.82	0.25	7.42	15.90	716	21	12	14.9
24	365	0.91	0.15	7.76	15.30	608	18	10	16.4
Growing horses 500 kg adult weight									
3	155	0.31	0.90	5.43	13.35	668	35	19	7.0
6	215	0.43	0.80	5.91	16.65	883	34	21	10.4
12	325	0.65	0.55	8.13	19.70	887	31	19	14.6
18	400	0.80	0.35	9.00	19.85	893	27	17	18.0
24	450	0.90	0.20	9.56	18.83	759	23	15	20.3
Growing horses 600 kg adult weight									
3	170	0.28	1.00	5.95	14.61	711	37	21	7.7
6	245	0.41	0.85	6.74	18.10	905	37	21	11.9
12	375	0.63	0.70	9.38	23.53	989	34	19	17.3
18	475	0.79	0.45	10.69	23.94	995	30	17	21.4
24	540	0.90	0.30	11.48	23.49	915	28	1	24.3

[1]90% dry matter.

[2]One mg of β-carotene equals 400 IU of vitamin A for the horse.

Adapted, with permission, from *Nutrient Requirements of Horses*, 1989, National Academy of Sciences. Published by National Academy Press, Washington, DC.

Table 29. Daily Nutrient Requirements of Mature Horses and Ponies

Body Weight	Daily Feed[1]	Daily Nutrients Per Animal					Daily Milk Production
		Digestible Energy	Crude Protein	Ca	P	Vitamin A[2]	
kg	kg	Mcal	g	g	g	IU (thousands)	kg
Mature Horses and Ponies, Maintenance							
200	3.50	7.4	296	8	6	6	—
400	7.00	13.4	536	16	11	12	—
500	8.75	16.4	656	20	14	15	—
600	10.50	19.4	776	24	17	18	—
Mature Horses and Ponies, Last 90 Days Gestation							
200	3.50	8.58	378	16	12	12	—
400	7.00	15.54	684	30	22	24	—
500	8.75	19.02	837	36	27	30	—
600	10.50	22.50	990	43	32	36	—
Mature Horses and Ponies, Lactating Mare, First 3 Months							
200	5.0	13.74	688	27	18	12	8
400	10.0	22.90	1141	45	29	24	12
500	12.5	28.28	1427	56	36	30	15
600	15.0	33.66	1711	67	43	36	18
Mature Horses and Ponies, Lactating Mare, 3 Months to Weaning							
200	4.5	12.15	528	18	11	12	6
400	9.0	19.74	839	29	18	24	8
500	11.25	24.32	1048	36	22	30	10
600	13.50	28.90	1258	43	27	36	12

[1]90% dry matter.

[2]One mg of β-carotene equals 400 IU of vitamin A for the horse.

Adapted, with permission, from *Nutrient Requirements of Horses*, 1989, National Academy of Sciences. Published by National Academy Press, Washington, DC.

ENERGY

Energy requirements may be classified into those needed for maintenance, growth, pregnancy, lactation, and work. Studies with light horses have resulted in equations to estimate energy requirements at any state of performance or production. Such estimates are provided in TABLES 28 and 29. The need for energy differs considerably among individuals; some horses are "easy keepers", while others require prodigious amounts of feed. Thus, these formulas provide only a sound basis for estimating energy needs, not the energy needs of any individual horse.

Maintenance: To maintain body weight and support normal activity, the daily digestible energy (DE) requirement (in Mcal) of the nonworking horse weighing 200-600 kg is $1.4 + (0.03 \times$ body wt [in kg]); for horses weighing >600 kg, daily DE requirements are $1.82 + (0.0383 \times$ body wt$) - (0.000015 \times$ body wt$^2)$.

Growth: The DE requirements for growth (to be added to that for maintenance) are estimated from the following equation in which X equals age in months and ADG equals average daily gain in kg.

DE growth (Mcal/day) = $(4.81 + 1.17X - 0.023X^2) \times$ ADG

Pregnancy: Maintenance energy intakes are adequate until the last 90 days of gestation, when most of the fetal tissue growth occurs. During gestation months 9, 10, and 11, DE requirements are estimated by multiplying maintenance requirements by 1.11, 1.13, and 1.20, respectively. Voluntary intake of roughage decreases as the fetus gets larger, and it may be necessary to increase the energy density of the diet by using some concentrate.

Lactation: The NRC has estimated that 792 kcal of DE/kg of milk produced per day should be added to maintenance needs to support lactation. This level of energy intake has produced increased body weight gain in lactating ponies, indicating that it may exceed the minimum requirement for lactation. Some data on average milk production of mares are listed below. Condition of the mare determines desirability of increasing grain.

Table 30. Average Milk Production of Mares

Months after foaling	Average Daily Milk Production (kg)		
	Draft Horse	Light Horse	Shetland Pony
0-1	15.4	13.9	10.3
1-2	16.8	14.7	11.8
2-3	18.2	16.9	12.5
3-4	17.0	15.1	9.5
4-5	14.7	10.9	9.1

Work: Many factors such as type of work, condition and training of the horse, fatigue, environmental temperature, and skill of the rider or driver can influence the energy requirements of work. An accurate evaluation of the intensity of effort is important in predicting the energy requirement of exercising horses. Studies indicate that as the duration of exercise increases and level of activity is maintained, the DE requirement per unit of time decreases. For these reasons, DE requirements for various activities of light horses shown below are given on a daily basis and should be adjusted to meet individual needs.

Table 31. Energy Requirements of Work, Horses (200-600 kg body wt)

Activity	DE (Mcal/day)
Idle (maintenance)	$1.4 + (0.3 \times$ body wt [in kg])
Halter competition, pleasure trail riding	1.25 (maintenance DE)
Performance show (Park English and Western Pleasure youth activity), equestrian instruction	1.50 (maintenance DE)
Ranch work, show cutting and roping, barrel racing, endurance trail ride, 3-day event (hunt course, stadium jumping, dressage)	1.75 (maintenance DE)
Polo, race training, and competitive racing	2.00 (maintenance DE)

PROTEIN AND AMINO ACIDS

Although some amino acid synthesis occurs in the cecum and large intestine, it is not sufficient to meet the amino acid needs of growing, working, or lactating horses; therefore, the protein quality of the feed is important. Weanlings require 2.1 g, and yearlings 1.9 g, of lysine/Mcal DE/day. While other dietary amino acid requirements have not been established, the feed recommendations presented in TABLES 28, 29, 32, and 33 contain an adequate distribution of those amino acids considered essential for nonruminants.

Nitrogen needs expressed as crude protein (CP) are presented in TABLES 28 and 29. Growing horses have a considerably greater need for protein than mature horses. Also, the protein requirements of growing horses of the heavier breeds are higher at the same body weight than those of the lighter breeds. Fetal growth during the last fourth of pregnancy increases protein requirements somewhat, while lactation increases requirements still further. Work apparently does not increase the protein requirement, provided that the ratio of crude protein to digestible energy in the diet remains constant and the increased energy requirements are met. However, :f the energy requirement is not met, body fat and then muscle is metabolized, which results in a net nitrogen loss.

MINERALS

Because the skeleton is of such fundamental importance to performance of the horse, mineral requirements deserve careful attention. Excessive intakes of certain minerals may be as harmful as deficiencies; therefore, mineral supplements should be based on composition of the basic feeds in the diet. For example, if the horse is consuming mostly roughage with little grain, phosphorus is more likely to be in short supply than is calcium. However, if little roughage and much grain is being consumed, a shortage of calcium is more likely. The total mineral contribution and availability from all parts of the diet (roughage, grain, commercial products, and supplements) must be considered in evaluating the mineral intake. Aside from actual feeding trials, no suitable test for availability of minerals now exists. Some caution is necessary in interpreting mineral requirements.

Calcium and Phosphorus: See TABLES 28 and 29. The need during growth is much greater than for maintenance of the mature animal. Work does not increase requirements as a portion of diet. The last fourth of pregnancy and lactation increase the need appreciably. Aged horses may require 30-50% more calcium (Ca) and phosphorus (P) than is required for maintenance of younger horses. However, an excess of dietary Ca interferes with utilization of magnesium, manganese, iron, and probably zinc. The Ca:P ratio should be maintained at not <1:1. A desirable ratio is ~1.5:1 although if adequate P is fed, foals tolerate a ratio of 3:1 and mature horses a ratio of 6:1. Phosphorus levels should be evaluated carefully because of phytate forms of P, which are estimated to be only 45-50% available.

Sodium and Chlorine: Salt requirements are markedly influenced by perspiration losses. Fifty to 60 g of salt may be lost daily in the sweat, and 35 g in the urine of horses at moderate work. Supplemental salt may be provided at 1% of the grain ration plus extra salt ad lib to replace the losses during hard work and hot weather. If more convenient, the entire salt needs may be met ad lib; salt poisoning is unlikely unless a salt-deprived animal is suddenly exposed to an unlimited supply of salt, or water is not available.

Magnesium: The daily magnesium (Mg) requirement for maintenance has been estimated at 6.8 mg/lb (15 mg/kg) body wt. For the growing foal, Mg at 0.57 g/lb (1.25 g/kg) body wt gain must be added to the maintenance requirement. Working horses require 10 to 25% more Mg for light to moderate exercise, respectively. Outbreaks of tetany that respond to magnesium therapy have been reported from humid grassland areas. Addition of 5% magnesium oxide to the salt mixture has been protective.

Potassium: Foals require up to 1% potassium in a purified diet, while mature horses require ~0.4% potassium in a natural diet (27 mg/lb [60 mg/kg] body wt). Since most roughages contain ≥1.5% potassium, a diet containing ≥35% roughage provides sufficient potassium. Protein supplements also are high in this element. Horses receiving diuretics need more potassium.

Sulfur: It is doubtful that sulfur, beyond that in methionine, is a dietary essential. If the protein requirement is met, the sulfur intake of horses usually is ≥0.15%— a level that is apparently adequate.

Iodine: Most iodized salts provide the dietary iodine requirement (estimated to be 0.6 ppm). The iodine should be in a stable but available form. Pentacalcium orthoperiodate, calcium iodate, cuprous iodide, ethylenediamine dihydroiodide (EDDI), and stabilized potassium iodide are generally satisfactory. Iodine is poorly available from diiodosalicylic acid. Iodine toxicity has been noted in pregnant mares consuming as little as 40 mg of iodine/day. Goiter due to excess iodine was noted in both mares and their foals, and several cases were associated with large amounts of dried seaweed (kelp) in the diet.

Cobalt: The dietary requirement for cobalt is apparently <0.05 ppm. It is undoubtedly incorporated into vitamin B_{12} by the microorganisms in the cecum and colon. Absorption of the synthesized vitamin is probably sufficient to obviate any need for preformed vitamin B_{12}.

Table 32. Required Nutrient Concentrations in Diets for Horses and Ponies[1]

	Digestible Energy Mcal/kg	Crude Protein %	Ca %	P %	Vitamin A[2] IU/kg	Example Diet Proportions			
						Hay Containing 2.0 Mcal DE/kg[3]		Hay Containing 1.8 Mcal DE/kg[4]	
						Concentrate[5]	Roughage	Concentrate[5]	Roughage
Mature horses and ponies, maintenance	1.80	7.2	0.21	0.15	1650	0	100	0	100
Mares, last 90 days of gestation	2.15	9.5	0.41	0.31	3280	20B	80	25A	75
Lactating mares, first 3 mo	2.35	12.0	0.47	0.30	2480	40A	60	50A	50
Lactating mares, 3 mo to weaning	2.20	10.0	0.33	0.20	2720	30B	70	40A	60
Stallions, breeding season	2.15	8.6	0.26	0.19	2370	25A	75	30A	70
Creep feed	2.80	16.0	0.65	0.35	1800	70A	30		
Foal (3 mo old)	2.70	14.0	0.65	0.35	1500	70A	30	80A	20
Weanling (6 mo old)	2.60	13.1	0.55	0.30	1680	60A	40	70A	30
Yearling (12 mo old)	2.50	11.3	0.40	0.22	1950	40B	60	50A	50
Long yearling (18 mo old)	2.35	10.4	0.32	0.18	2050	30B	70	40B	60
Two year old (light training)	2.40	10.1	0.31	0.17	2380	40B	60	50B	50
Mature working horses (light work)[6]	2.20	8.8	0.27	0.19	2420	25B	75	35B	65
(moderate work)[7]	2.40	9.4	0.28	0.22	2140	40B	60	50B	50
(intense work)[8]	2.55	10.3	0.31	0.23	1760	50B	50	60B	40

[1] 90% dry matter.

[2] One mg of β-carotene equals 400 IU of vitamin A for the horse.

[3] Good quality legume-grass hay.

[4] Grass hay.

[5] Concentrate containing 3.2 Mcal DE/kg. A or B refers to suitable concentrates (see TABLE 33).

[6] Western pleasure, bridle path hack, equitation.

[7] Ranch work, roping, cutting, barrel racing, jumping.

[8] Race training, polo.

Adapted, with permission, from *Nutrient Requirements of Horses*, 1989, National Academy of Sciences. Published by National Academy Press, Washington, DC.

Table 33. Concentrates Satisfactory for Use with Hays as Indicated in Table 32

Ingredient[1]	Formula	
	A	B
Corn[2] or sorghum grain, rolled or cracked	45	55
Oats[2], rolled or crimped	24	24
Soybean meal (44% CP)	20	10
Cane molasses[3]	8	8
Limestone (34% Ca)	0.5	0.5
Calcium phosphate, monobasic (16% Ca, 22% P)	1.5	1.5
Trace mineral salt[4]	1	1
	100	100
Analysis		
Digestible energy, Mcal/kg	3.2	3.2
Crude protein, %	16	12
Digestible protein, %	12	8.5
Calcium, %	0.60	0.58
Phosphorus, %	0.67	0.62

[1] Except for the cane molasses, all figures are on 90% dry-matter basis.

[2] Barley may be used to replace the corn or sorghum and the oats, by using weights of barley equal to the combined weights of the grains replaced.

[3] Cane molasses is not an essential part of a concentrate mixture, but it may help to minimize separation of "fines" and reduces dustiness.

[4] Providing NaCl, Fe, Cu, Mn, Co, I, Zn plus Se (from sodium selenite) to provide 0.2 mg selenium/kg concentrate.

Copper: The dietary copper requirement for horses probably is not >10 ppm. The presence of 1-3 ppm of molybdenum in forages has interfered with proper copper utilization in ruminants, but has not been shown to cause problems in horses. A proposed inverse cause and effect relationship between copper concentration in weanling diets and incidence of metabolic bone disease is unproved.

Iron: The dietary maintenance requirement for iron is estimated to be 40 ppm. For rapidly growing foals and pregnant and lactating mares, the requirement is estimated to be 50 ppm. Work in other species suggests that ferric oxide and ferrous carbonate are not effective iron supplements, and ferrous sulfate is the compound of choice. Only horses receiving milk are apt to have iron deficiency since iron is so widespread in soils. Concentrations in forages and grains are relatively high.

Manganese: Requirements for horses have not been established; amounts found in the usual forages (40-140 ppm) are considered sufficient.

Zinc: The zinc requirement is estimated to be 50 ppm of the ration. This mineral is relatively innocuous and intakes several times the requirement are considered safe, although very large intakes have induced copper deficiency.

Fluorine: Rock phosphates, when used as mineral supplements for horses, should contain ≤0.1% fluorine. Fluorine intake should not exceed 50 ppm in the diet or 0.45 mg/lb (1 mg/kg) body wt. Excessive ingestion can result in fluorosis (qv, p 1651).

Molybdenum: Although an essential cofactor for xanthine oxidase activity, no quantitative requirement for horses has been demonstrated. Excessive levels may interfere with copper utilization.

Selenium: The requirement for selenium is inversely related to the vitamin E content of the diet. The dietary requirement probably is not >0.2 ppm, but there are regions of the world (including the lower Great Lakes states, the Pacific Northwest, the Atlantic Coast, Florida, and part of New Zealand) where soils are deficient. In other areas (including parts of North and South Dakota), feeds may contain 5-40 ppm of selenium and produce toxicity (qv, p 1727). Selenium and vitamin E may be instrumental in preventing cellular damage from increased oxygen metabolism as a result of strenuous exercise. Exercise increases glutathione peroxidase (selenium-containing enzyme) activity within the RBC and may indicate an increased need for supplementation in heavily exercised horses.

Supplemental Minerals: Perhaps the most satisfactory method of providing supplemental calcium, phosphorus, and salt is to furnish mineral salt on one side of a 2-compartment box and a mixture of one-third trace mineral salt and two-thirds dicalcium phosphate on the other. If relatively more phosphorus than calcium is desired, dicalcium phosphate may be substituted for monobasic calcium phosphate. The mineral box should always be protected from rain.

VITAMINS

Carotene and Vitamin A: The vitamin A requirement of horses can be met by carotene, a precursor of vitamin A in plants, or by the vitamin itself. Fresh green forages and good-quality hays are excellent sources of carotene. However, because of breakdown due to oxygen and light, the carotene content decreases with storage, and hays that are stored ≥1 yr may not furnish sufficient vitamin A activity. Horses convert dietary β-carotene to vitamin A so that 1 mg is equivalent to ~400 IU. Horses that have been consuming fresh green forage usually have sufficient stores of vitamin A in the liver to maintain adequate plasma levels for 3-6 mo. The NRC has suggested that diets for all horses should provide 30-60 IU vitamin A/kg body wt (13.6-27.2 IU/lb). These requirements expressed per kg of feed may be found in TABLE 32. Prolonged feeding of excess vitamin A may cause bone fragility, hyperostosis, and epithelial exfoliation.

Vitamin D: Grazing horses or horses that exercise regularly in sunlight or consume sun-cured hay normally satisfy their requirements for vitamin D. For horses deprived of sunlight, suggested dietary vitamin D concentrations are 365-455 IU/lb (800-1000 IU/kg) for early growth, and 227 IU/lb (500 IU/kg) for later growth and other life stages. Vitamin D toxicity is characterized by general weakness; loss of body weight; calcification of the blood vessels, heart, and other soft tissues; and bone abnormalities. Dietary excesses as small as 10 times the requirement may be toxic and are aggravated by excessive calcium intake.

Vitamin E: No minimum requirement has been established. Selenium and vitamin E work together to prevent nutritional muscular dystrophy (white muscle disease, qv, p 550). Evidence of vitamin E deficiency is most likely to appear in the foal nursing a mare on dry winter pasture or given only low-quality hay unsupplemented with grain. Horses forced to exert severe physical effort are also likely to develop deficiency signs if they are fed low-vitamin-E diets grown in low-selenium areas. If selenium intakes are 0.15 ppm of the diet, it is likely that 40-60 IU of vitamin E per kg of diet is adequate for most stages of the life cycle and moderate activity. Levels up to 100 IU/kg diet may help prevent myopathy associated with exercise.

Vitamin K: This vitamin is synthesized by the microorganisms of the cecum and colon, probably in sufficient quantities to meet the normal requirements of the horse. However, consumption of moldy sweet clover hay may induce a deficiency (qv, p 1733).

Ascorbic Acid: Mature horses synthesize adequate amounts of ascorbic acid for maintenance. Despite suggestions that stressed horses may need supplemental ascorbic acid, no controlled studies demonstrating such have been conducted.

Thiamine: Although thiamine is synthesized in the cecum and colon by bacterial action and ~25% of this may be absorbed, thiamine deficiency has been observed in horses fed poor-quality hay and grain. While not necessarily a minimum value, 25 µg of thiamine/lb (55 µg/kg) body wt per day (~1.4 mg/lb [3 mg/kg] diet) has maintained peak food consumption, normal gains, and normal thiamine levels in skeletal muscle. As much as 2.3 mg/lb (5 mg/kg) diet may be necessary for horses that are exercising strenuously. Occasionally, horses are poisoned by consuming certain plants that contain thiaminases or antithiamines (*see* BRACKEN FERN POISONING, p 1641).

Riboflavin: Under certain conditions, riboflavin may be required in the diet. Early reports implicated riboflavin deficiency in equine uveitis (qv, p 302) but this has not been substantiated. The dietary riboflavin requirement likely is not >0.9 mg/lb (2 mg/kg).

Vitamin B$_{12}$: Intestinal synthesis of this vitamin is probably adequate to meet ordinary needs, provided sufficient cobalt is in the diet; deficiencies of cobalt in horses have not been reported. Absorption of vitamin B$_{12}$ from the cecum has been established, and the feeding of a B$_{12}$-free diet had no effect on the normal hematology of adults. Vitamin B$_{12}$ injected parenterally into race horses has been rapidly and nearly completely excreted.

Niacin: This vitamin probably is synthesized in adequate quantities by the bacterial flora of the cecum and colon, and is synthesized in the tissues from tryptophan.

Folacin, Biotin, Pantothenic Acid, and Vitamin B$_6$: All these vitamins are probably synthesized in adequate quantities in the intestine.

FEEDS AND FEEDING PRACTICES

The horse is an athlete; for top performance, it must be properly nourished and appropriately trained. Proper nourishment implies more than simply providing essential nutrients; these should be provided in an appropriate form at the proper time. Horses do best when fed regularly and, because their capacity for roughage at any one time is relatively limited, they may need to be fed frequently. For a hard-working horse in harness or under saddle, this may mean 3 or more feedings a day. Under these circumstances, "feeding a little at a time and often" is a good principle. A horse should not be worked on a loaded stomach, and if 3 meals a day are offered, the daily roughage ration should be split between the morning and evening meals and should be offered at least 1-2 hr before work starts. The noon feeding should be light and 1-3 lb (0.5-1.5 kg) of grain should suffice. An alternative to this would be to feed one-fourth of the hay ration in the morning, a second fourth at noon, and the remaining half at night.

Hot horses should be offered only small amounts of water until they are cool. Water should be clean and fresh.

Because horses are particularly sensitive to toxins found in spoiled feeds, all grains and roughages should be of good quality and free of mold. Grains should be stored at a moisture content of <13%; in humid areas, processed feeds should contain a mold inhibitor to preclude spoilage. Likewise, dusty feeds should not be fed because they tend to initiate or aggravate respiratory problems.

FEEDS

Pasture: The use of good pasture makes an ideal feeding program because it provides both nutrients and the opportunity to exercise. The pasture should be kept free of weeds. Old, excessively mature growth should be clipped. A legume-grass mixture is ideal because it offers the advantages of good nutrient supply, a long grazing season, and a long-lived stand. Alfalfa and smooth bromegrass make a good combination for many parts of the world, although many choices exist. Most grasses are improved by the presence of legumes.

In sandy areas, horses should be provided with supplemental roughage when pasture is short due to overgrazing. If roughage is not provided, sand accumulates in the GI tract and results in sand colic. Feeding wheat bran at 5-10% of the grain ration resolves the problem.

Hay: The same species that make good pasture usually make good hay. Exceptions are low-growing plants, such as bluegrass and ladino clover. Hay should be harvested at the vegetative state (before bloom). Legume-grass mixtures are generally high-yielding and contain considerably more protein, minerals, and vitamins than do grasses alone. However, they may be more difficult to cure in a humid climate, and moldy hay should be avoided.

Concentrates include the grains and by-product feeds high in energy or protein. Processing them before feeding is often desirable to improve nutrient availability and to increase bulkiness (volume per unit of weight). The bulkier concentrates are less apt to produce intestinal impaction and colic. Also, the speed of digestion in the upper GI tract is important. If a large volume of undigested grain reaches the lower gut, excessive fermentation can occur and the consequences (eg, laminitis) can be serious. Horses should be acclimated to concentrate over a period of 3 wk. Ruptured stomachs or "grain founder" may occur in horses that have overloaded on concentrates. Most difficulties can be avoided if grain is fed according to weight rather than volume; this accounts for density of grains.

Oats, perhaps the grain of choice, may be fed whole, but rolling or crimping increases the bulk 20-30% and improves digestibility. Newly harvested oats may be dangerous due to development of molds if moisture content is >13%.

Barley is a good grain for horses; it is higher in energy than oats but lower than corn. It may be fed as the only grain to horses that have a high energy need. It should be rolled or crimped.

Corn (maize) is a high-energy feed, useful for horses that are working hard or being fattened. It is low in bulk and more prone to produce colic than oats or barley if carelessly used. A good method of feeding is on the cob. This promotes salivation and the horse cannot bolt the grain. To maximize digestibility, shelled corn may be cracked or rolled, but the moisture level should be low enough to avoid spoilage during storage. Grains that are cracked or rolled may become "stale" and should be processed as close to feeding as possible.

Sorghum grain and **wheat** should be fed with care to avoid colic. These grains should be cracked or rolled. **Wheat bran** is a bulky, mildly laxative feed that is well liked by horses. However, it is excessively high in phosphorus, and the proper calcium:phosphorus ratio should be maintained when wheat bran is added to the diet, especially of young horses. Wheat bran is an expensive substitute for hay.

Soybean meal is a palatable protein supplement with good amino acid balance for use with grains. It may be fed when pastures or hay are low in protein and are of poor quality or when protein requirements are greatest, such as during early growth or lactation. **Linseed meal** or **cottonseed meal** should not be used as a protein supplement for young foals because of amino acid imbalances. Linseed meal imparts sheen to the coat, but is not as effective as unsaturated oils. Cottonseed meal also may be used as a protein supplement, but it is also low in lysine. In addition, it contains gossypol, which may be toxic in excess (qv, p 1652), although horses seem less susceptible than pigs.

Cane molasses is frequently used to stimulate the appetite of poor eaters. It also minimizes separation of "fines" and reduces dustiness of concentrate mixtures. The sugar increases the desire for water. The readily fermentable carbohydrate and the moisture that cane molasses contains may increase mold growth in hot weather.

Fats may be added to the diet to increase the energy density. Horses seem to prefer corn oil. However, feed-grade animal fats may provide an inexpensive source for horses with high-energy demands. Diets containing 5-10% added fat have been associated with improved performance in some types of exercise. Fat should be fresh and not rancid.

Limestone of a high grade (38% calcium [Ca]) may be used as a supplemental source of Ca when this element alone is needed, which may occur when poor-quality grass pasture or grass hay is the only roughage provided. Grains, being low in Ca, do not help. When both supplemental Ca and phosphorus (P) are needed, dicalcium phosphate, steamed bone meal, or defluorinated rock phosphate is recommended. Dicalcium phosphate is particularly good because the cost per unit of P is low, the elements are quite available, and there is no danger of anthrax, as there might be in improperly processed bone meal. Monocalcium-dicalcium phosphate mixtures supply relatively more P than Ca, and are recommended when the need for supplemental P is greater than that for Ca. A supplement of both Ca and P may be needed when poor-quality grass pasture or grass hay is provided without grain. Grain, which contains appreciable P, tends to correct any deficiency of this element.

Salt (NaCl) should be provided in a block or in loose granular form *ad lib.* It may be desirable to use a trace mineralized salt that contains added iodine, iron, copper, cobalt, manganese, zinc, and selenium. The need for these additional minerals varies with the locality, but trace mineral salts are readily available and not costly. They may provide some nutritional insurance in areas where trace element deficiencies are a problem.

Succulent feeds: These feeds are high in water, somewhat laxative, and tend to stimulate the appetite. They should be introduced gradually when offered for the first time. Carrots are the safest and most satisfactory. A daily allowance of 1-3 lb (0.5-1.5 kg) is a desirable feeding rate. An artificial succulent feed can be made by soaking dried beet pulp in water sweetened with cane molasses. Well-preserved silage of good quality and free of mold affords a highly nutritious succulent forage during the winter. Horses fed good-quality hay and water *ad lib* have no need for succulent forages. Since horses are much more susceptible to mold, botulism, and GI disturbances than are cattle and sheep, only choice fresh silage should be fed. Mechanical silo unloaders may blend good and spoiled silage together, and the spoilage may go undetected until GI disturbances develop. Various types of silages may be used successfully, but corn silage and grass-legume silage are the most common. Silage should not replace more than one-third to one-half of the roughage ration, considering that 6 lb (2.7 kg) of wet silage is approximately equivalent to 2 lb (1 kg) of hay. Thus, the silage allowance usually does not exceed 10-15 lb (4.5-7 kg) daily for a mature animal, although in some instances much larger amounts have been fed satisfactorily.

RATE OF FEEDING

Individual differences in the need for energy and nutrients make it difficult to generalize about the amount of feed to provide. The following guidelines usually satisfy the requirements; however, there is no substitute for observation and good judgment.

Horses at light work: Allow ~0.5 lb (0.25 kg) of concentrate and 1.25-1.5 lb (0.6-0.75 kg) of hay per 100 lb (45 kg) body wt.

Horses at moderate work: Allow ~1 lb (0.5 kg) of concentrate and 1-1.25 lb (0.45-0.6 kg) of hay per 100 lb (45 kg) body wt.

Horses at intense work: Allow ~1.25-1.5 lb (0.6-0.75 kg) of concentrate and 1 lb (0.45 kg) of hay per 100 lb (45 kg) body wt.

The total allowance of concentrates and hay falls within the range of 1.25-2.75 lb (0.6-1.25 kg) daily per 100 lb (45 kg) body wt. No grain should be left from one feeding to the next, and all edible forage should be cleaned up at the end of each day.

The need for grain while on pasture depends on pasture quality, but is more important for young horses and lactating mares than for mature horses. It is desirable to creep-feed nursing foals, and they frequently eat good-quality hay even when on pasture. They may be given free access to a concentrate mixture if accustomed to this regime gradually.

SUGGESTED RATIONS

Example proportions of roughage and concentrate are listed in TABLE 32 (p 1230), with concentrate formulas in TABLE 33 (p 1231). While these generally meet the needs of the horses for which they were designed, many other choices exist. It is logical to use feeds that are locally available and, in certain areas of the world, several of the feeds suggested are not grown or are too expensive. Alternatives should be chosen on the basis of nutrient composition, palatability, and general suitability for horses.

Complete pelleted feeds, incorporating both concentrate and roughage, have been developed for horses. They have the advantage of uniform quality, complete control over nutrient intake, suitability for horses with bad teeth, less dustiness (which reduces respiratory problems), and reduced bulk for storage and transport. Pellets should be ≥½ in. (13 mm) in diameter. Because these feeds can be eaten so quickly, confined horses may exhibit increased boredom, and stable vices (eg, wood-chewing) may be aggravated. This can be minimized by feeding some long hay. Damage to stable and fences can be reduced by treating wood with creosote or by covering or replacing wood with metal in vulnerable areas.

NUTRITIONAL DISEASES

Descriptions of uncomplicated nutrient deficiencies in horses are rare. The natural feeds typically consumed are most likely to be deficient in protein, calcium, phosphorus, sodium, chlorine, iodine, and selenium, depending on age, productive level of the horse, and geographic area. Dried, weathered forages may be very low in carotene, and if fed for long periods, vitamin A deficiency may develop. Thiamine deficiency has been produced experimentally.

Signs of deficiency are frequently nonspecific, and diagnosis may be complicated by a simultaneous shortage of several nutrients. The consequences of increased susceptibility to parasitism and bacterial infections may superimpose still other clinical signs. The signs of deficiency noted in horses are discussed below; when these are not seen, the most likely signs, as suggested by research with other species, are described.

ENERGY

Many nonspecific changes found in horses with nutritional deficiencies are related to caloric deficiency, and result from inadequate intake of a well-balanced diet or from poor utilization of the diet that follows development of a specific deficiency. In partial or complete starvation, most internal organs exhibit some atrophy. The brain is least affected, but the size of the gonads may be strikingly decreased, and estrus may be delayed. Hypoplasia of lymph nodes, spleen, and thymus leads to a marked reduction in their size. The adrenal glands are usually enlarged. The young skeleton is extremely sensitive, and growth slows or may completely stop. In adults, the skeleton may become osteoporotic. A decrease in adipose tissue is an early and conspicuous sign, not only in the subcutis, but in the mesentery; around the kidneys, uterus, and testes; and in the retroperitoneum. Low fat content of the marrow in the long bones is a good indicator of prolonged inanition. The ability to perform work is impaired, and endogenous nitrogen losses increase as muscle proteins are metabolized for energy.

PROTEIN

A deficiency of dietary protein may represent either an inadequate intake of high-quality protein or the lack of a specific essential amino acid. Synthesis by microorganisms in the gut plus proteolysis of microbial protein is not adequate to meet the essential amino acid needs of horses. The effects of deficiency are generally nonspecific, and many of the signs do not differ from the effects of partial or total caloric restriction. In addition, there may be depressed appetite, and decreased formation of Hgb, RBC, and plasma proteins. Edema is sometimes associated with hypoproteinemia. Milk production is decreased in lactating mares. The following liver enzymes have shown decreased activity: pyruvic oxidase, succinoxidase, succinic acid dehydrogenase, D-amino acid oxidase, DPN-cytochrome C reductase, and uricase. Corneal vascularization and lens degeneration have been noted. Antibody formation is impaired.

MINERALS

Calcium: Young, growing horses or lactating mares fed poor-quality grass hay or pasture are most likely to develop calcium deficiencies. Serum calcium levels may be depressed while serum inorganic phosphorus levels may be elevated; however, single samples of blood are generally not diagnostic. Serum alkaline phosphatase activity is usually elevated. Clotting time may be prolonged slightly. Young, growing bone is frequently rachitic and brittle. Fractures may be common and heal poorly. Adult bone may be osteomalacic.

Phosphorus: A deficiency is most likely in horses being fed poor-quality grass hay or pasture without grain. Serum inorganic phosphorus levels may be depressed and serum alkaline phosphatase activity increased. Occasionally, serum calcium levels may be elevated. An insidious shifting lameness may be seen. Bone changes resemble those described for calcium deficiency. Adult horses may consume large quantities of soil before other signs are visible.

Sodium and Chlorine: Horses are most likely to develop signs of sodium chloride (salt) deficiency when worked hard in hot weather. Perspiration and urinary losses are appreciable. Horses deprived of salt tire easily, stop sweating, and exhibit muscle spasms. Anorexia and pica may be evident. However, pica is not a specific sign of salt deficiency. Milk production of lactating mares seriously declines. Hemoconcentration and acidosis may be expected.

Potassium: Deficiency results in decreased rate of growth, anorexia, and hypokalemia.

Magnesium: Foals fed a purified diet containing 3.6 mg/lb (8 mg/kg) exhibited hypomagnesemia, nervousness, muscular tremors, and ataxia followed by collapse, with hyperpnea, sweating, convulsive paddling, and death.

Iron: Deficiency may be secondary to parasitism and results in microcytic, hypochromic anemia.

Zinc: Deficiency in foals is accompanied by reduced growth rate, anorexia, cutaneous lesions on the lower extremities, alopecia, lowered blood levels of zinc, and reduced plasma alkaline phosphatase activity.

Copper: An apparent relationship between low serum copper levels and bleeding in aged parturient mares suggested reduced copper absorption with age or reduced ability to mobilize copper stores. Deficiency may cause aortic aneurysm, contracted tendons, and improper cartilage formation in growing foals.

Iodine: Deficiency is an endemic problem in many areas (*see* GOITER, p 283).

Cobalt: Deficiency is apparently rare in horses; they have been known to thrive on pastures so low in cobalt that sheep and cattle wasted and died.

Selenium: Deficiency results in reduced serum selenium, elevated AST (SGOT) activity, white muscle disease, alopecia, yellow-brown fat, and numerous small hemorrhages. (*See also* NUTRITIONAL MYOPATHIES, p 547.)

VITAMINS

Vitamin A: A deficiency may develop if dried, poor-quality roughage is fed for a prolonged period. If body stores are high, signs may not appear for several months. The deficiency is characterized by nyctalopia, lacrimation, keratinization of the cornea, susceptibility to pneumonia, abscesses of the sublingual gland, incoordination, impaired reproduction, capricious appetite, and progressive weakness. Hooves are frequently deformed, the horny layer unevenly laid down and unusually brittle. Metaplasia of the intestinal mucosa and achlorhydria have been reported. Genitourinary mucosal metaplasia may be expected. Bone remodeling is defective. The foramina do not enlarge properly during growth, and skeletal deformities are evident. The latter may be seen in foals of deficient mares.

Vitamin D: If sun-cured hay is consumed or the horse is exposed to sunlight, it is doubtful that a deficiency of vitamin D will develop. Prolonged confinement of a young horse offered only limited amounts of sun-cured hay may result in reduced bone calcification, stiff and swollen joints, stiffness of gait, irritability, and reduced serum calcium and phosphorus.

Thiamine: Signs of experimental deficiency include anorexia, weight loss, incoordination, lowered blood thiamine, and elevated blood pyruvate. At necropsy, the heart is dilated. Similar signs have been observed in bracken fern poisoning (qv, p 1641). Under normal circumstances, the natural diet plus synthesis by microorganisms in the gut probably meet the thiamine need.

Riboflavin: Although natural feeds plus synthesis within the gut normally provide adequate riboflavin, limited evidence indicates an occasional deficiency when the diet is of poor quality. The first sign of acute deficiency is catarrhal conjunctivitis in one or both eyes, accompanied by photophobia and lacrimation. The retina, lens, and ocular fluids may deteriorate gradually and result in impaired vision or blindness. Equine uveitis (qv, p 302) has been linked to riboflavin deficiency, but may be a sequela of leptospirosis or onchocerciasis.

Vitamin B$_{12}$: While the normal feedstuffs of horses generally contain very little vitamin B$_{12}$, the horse can synthesize this vitamin in the gut, from which it is absorbed.

FEEDING THE SICK HORSE

Nutrition is an important part of the management and treatment of sick horses. Stresses, eg, surgery, severe orthopedic problems, or infection, can significantly increase an animal's caloric needs. This increase is due to an increase in catabolism. In addition, anorexia or dysphagia can lead to inadequate intake of the proper nutrients. If proper nutrition is not provided, the consequences include impairment of the immune system, delayed wound and fracture healing, hypoproteinemia, muscle wasting, and weakness. Generally, supportive nutritional therapy should be considered if the adult horse has been hypophagic for ≥ 3 days. Neonatal foals require some energy source within 24 hr of decreased intake.

The order of nutrient priorities is water, electrolytes, energy, and protein. Some water-soluble vitamins are poorly stored in the body and should be supplemented. The basal energy requirement (BER) can be calculated by the following formula: BER = 70 (body wt [in kg])$^{0.75}$ = kcal/day. For example, BER is ~6800 kcal daily for a 450-kg horse and 1300 kcal for a 50-kg foal. Illness significantly increases these needs.

There are several methods of providing nutritional support to a sick horse. The simplest method is to encourage the animal to eat on its own. Unusual feed preferences may be seen. Offering a variety of feeds and letting the horse choose can best determine what is most palatable to the animal. Many horses will eat fresh, green grass even though they refuse other feeds. Alfalfa hay is more palatable than grass hays. Whole oats and sweet-feed mixtures of rolled grains and molasses are the most appetizing of grains. Bran mashes are low in palatability, but the addition of molasses and salt may increase their acceptance.

When horses are experiencing pain or fever, analgesics can improve food intake; nonsteroidal anti-inflammatory drugs, such as dipyrone, flunixin meglumine, meclofenamic acid, and phenylbutazone, can be used. Prolonged use of phenylbutazone should be avoided because of the side effects of gastric and small intestinal ulceration and renal papillary necrosis.

Tube feeding is a second method of providing nutrition to horses that will not (or cannot) eat voluntarily. A normal stomach tube may be passed several times a day or may be sutured to the nostril and left as an indwelling feeding tube. This is an effective method of providing nutrients to sick neonates. It is also an inexpensive method of replacing fluid and electrolyte losses. Enteral nutritional supplements used in human medicine are particularly useful in providing sufficient caloric intake to adult horses. These products have a known caloric content, which facilitates calculation of the animal's needs. Soaking a complete feed in water can make a slurry for tube feeding. Problems that arise from feeding a slurry include the inability to provide enough nutrient and frequent clogging of the stomach tube with feedstuff. Neonatal foals should be fed mare's milk or a mare's milk supplement.

The third method of providing energy and protein to sick horses is through use of total or partial parenteral nutrition (TPN or PPN). IV fluid administration is a means of maintaining hydration in horses that are either unable to drink or absorb fluids. Common replacement solutions include sodium chloride, lactated Ringers, and 5% dextrose. The nutritional value of these fluids is insignificant. The components of parenteral nutrition are glucose, amino acids, lipid, trace minerals, and multivitamins. The resultant solution is hypertonic and is delivered by constant infusion through a jugular catheter. Delivery is optimized through use of a fluid pump. Blood and urine glucose should be monitored b.i.d. to regulate the rate of infusion. TPN is costly and requires intensive care and monitoring, which limits it usefulness in adults.

NUTRITION FOR SPECIFIC DISEASES

Chronic pulmonary disease: Horses with chronic pulmonary disease, such as heaves (qv, p 733), are frequently sensitive to the dust and molds found in normal hay. They often improve when hay is removed from their diet and they are placed on a complete ration that is pelleted or contains a roughage source such as beet pulp. They do best on pasture. Another source of dust-free roughage is haylage.

Dental disease: Older horses often lose weight due to dental wear. Their teeth lose the grinding surface, which results in poor mastication of food. Feeding a moistened, complete pelleted ration may aid these animals.

Diarrhea: Diarrhea in horses is primarily a colonic disease. Traditionally, affected horses are fed less grain and more hay. This increase in dietary fiber can bind water and may result in better formed feces. If weight loss is a concurrent problem, it may be better to maintain grain intake. Grain is digested mainly in the small intestine, and hay in the large intestine. Unless the small intestine is also affected, feeding more grain helps maintain body mass. (*See also* pp 172 and 184.)

Liver disease: The role of nutrition in horses with liver disease (qv, p 138) is to provide adequate energy, thus easing the liver's role in energy production and decreasing the amount of metabolic waste to which the liver is exposed. Parenteral or enteral glucose administration may be important as an energy source in anorectic horses. In the animal that is eating, cereal grains should provide adequate carbohydrates. High-protein feeds, such as alfalfa hay, should be avoided because of their role in GI ammonia production.

CARE OF THE ORPHAN FOAL

Irrespective of the circumstance in which a foal becomes an orphan, it is important to determine whether it has received colostrum. If it has not received colostrum from its dam, it must receive colostrum from another mare, or frozen-stored colostrum within 24 hr of birth—preferably within the first 3-12 hr, since the foal absorbs best during this period. If colostrum is not available, plasma should be administered IV.

A nurse mare, preferably with a good disposition, is best for the overall care of an orphan foal. The amnion and/or placenta of a mare who has lost a newborn foal can be placed over the orphan foal in hopes of deceiving the foster mare. The 2 should not be left unattended until the mare has accepted the orphan; physical or chemical restraint of the mare may be required initially and repeated on several occasions before she will accept. Patience may be required for a time-consuming effort. Occasionally, a high-milk-producing mare with a good disposition and with a foal already at its side will accept and rear an additional foal successfully. If a mare is not available, a goat mounted on a bale of straw may serve as an alternative. This method, however, also requires constant monitoring and participation by the individual in charge of the foal since the foal must be fed frequently, particularly in the first few days of life.

Artificial mare's milk diets, goat's milk, and commercially available calf milk replacers have been used successfully. Foals should be fed at 1- to 2-hr intervals for the first day or 2 of life, then at 2- to 3-hr intervals for the following 2 wk at the rate of ½-1 pint (250-500 mL) per feeding with a warmed milk container and an artificial nipple. Of the various artificial nipples available, those designed for use by lambs are best suited for foals. The feeding intervals may be lengthened gradually after 2 wk; however, the amount per feeding also should be increased so that the foal consumes 8-10% of its body wt/day. A foal should be encouraged to drink freshly prepared milk out of a bucket, *ad lib*, early in life. If this can be achieved, it is more convenient for both the foal and the individual in attendance. The foal can then be encouraged to eat digestible grain with ≥18% crude protein, and good-quality hay. Fresh water should be available to the foal at all times from the day it is born.

A heat lamp in an enclosed stall should be available, particularly for the first few weeks of life so that the foal may rest in a warm environment (68°F [20°C]). Another alternative during cold weather is a comfortably fitted down vest.

A companion animal such as a goat or pony of excellent disposition also may be beneficial to the well-being of the foal. As soon as it can maintain itself, the foal should be placed with other weaned foals to complete its socialization.

NUTRITION: MINK

Adequate nutrition is important to the success of fur-production operations: it is an area of economic concern to the mink rancher, as well as an effective basis for maintaining health of the animals. The basic principles of mink nutrition are similar to those for other animals but there are important differences, based on the characteristics of mink. Mink are carnivorous and able to sustain themselves from animal food sources. Such feeds, usually given fresh, need careful storage and sanitation to avoid problems with food-borne pathogens. They may also contain antimetabolites, which interfere with metabolic processes in ways not usually exhibited by heated or dried feeds. Because the GI tract of mink is simple and short, and feed passage is rapid, the diet must be highly digestible to be effective. Beyond these anatomical differences, mink have an extremely rapid growth rate (newborn kits double their birthweight in 3 days, and reach 10 times their birthweight in 3 wk), which increases nutritional stress of the females during lactation and of the kits during early postnatal growth.

Table 34. Nutrient and Energy Requirements of Mink: Percentage or Amount Per Kilogram of Dry Matter

Constituent		Growth		Maintenance (Mature)	Gestation	Lactation
		Weaning to 13 wk	13 wk to Maturity			
Energy						
males	kcal ME[a]	4080	4080	3600	—	—
females	kcal ME	3930	3930	3600	3930	4500
Crude protein	%	38[b]	32.6-38.0	21.8-26.0	38	45.7
Fat-soluble vitamins						
Vitamin A	IU	5930	c	c	c	c
Vitamin E	mg	27	c	c	c	c
Water-soluble vitamins						
Thiamine	mg	1.3	c	c	c	c
Riboflavin	mg	1.6	c	c	c	c
Pantothenic acid	mg	8.0	c	c	c	c
Vitamin B_6	mg	1.6	c	c	c	c
Niacin	mg	20.0	c	c	c	c
Folic acid	mg	0.5[d]	c	c	c	c
Biotin	mg	0.12	c	c	c	c
Vitamin B_{12}	μg	32.6	c	c	c	c
Minerals						
Calcium	%	0.4	0.4	0.3	0.4	0.6
Phosphorus	%	0.4	0.4	0.3	0.4	0.6
Ca:P ratio		1:1 to 2:1	1:1 to 2:1	1:1 to 2:1	1:1 to 2:1	1:1 to 2:1
Salt	%	0.5	0.5	0.5	0.5	0.5

[a] E is gross energy; ME is metabolizable energy.

Nutrient requirements are based on an energy level of 5300 kcal E, or 4080 kcal ME.

Nutrient requirements increase with higher ME levels and decrease with lower ME levels.

[b] Based on average-quality protein with calculated digestibility of 83%.

Higher-quality protein and higher digestibility decrease the requirement; lower-quality protein and lower digestibility increase the requirement.

[c] Quantitative requirement not determined but dietary need demonstrated.

[d] May not be minimum but known to be adequate.

Adapted, with permission, from *Nutrient Requirements of Mink and Foxes*, 1982, National Academy of Sciences. Published by National Academy Press, Washington, DC.

Conventional, modern mink diets are generally composed of 80-90% fresh ingredients that are stored frozen, thawed just before mixing, and fed with the balance in the form of a dry meal mix; this is commonly called "cereal", and serves as a source of carbohydrate energy, a diet binder to improve consistency, and a convenient carrier for supplemental nutrients and medicaments. The fresh ingredients have included horsemeat, beef liver, and whole fish, but in the interests of availability and economy, many other materials are now used, including packing house by-products, cull poultry (both chicks and older birds), poultry by-products (largely viscera, without heads and feet), fish scrap, cottage cheese, and cooked eggs. The dry meal component is usually composed of finely ground cereal grain, supplemented with liver, or meat or fish meals, as appropriate. Because carbohydrates are not well digested by mink, some form of heating the cereal ingredients is often practiced. Steaming, extruding, and popping processes have been used with some success.

The nutrient requirements for mink, as far as they are presently known, are listed in TABLE 34. Protein requirements are higher than for most other animals because of the need to support both rapid body growth and fur production. Quality of protein is important too, since the sulfur amino acids, cystine and methionine, are needed for fur growth. Dietary protein levels should be consistent with the energy supply, much of which usually comes from fat. A common guide is for the protein level to be 10% greater than fat (eg, a minimum of 35% crude protein in a diet containing 25% fat, each measured on a dry-matter basis). The relationship of energy supply to the contents of various essential nutrients is important since the energy concentration tends to regulate diet intake. Low-energy diets increase the volume of feed that must be handled daily, while high-energy diets may result in deficient consumption of certain nutrients. Adequate minerals for skeletal growth usually are available if the fresh ingredients in the diet include such items as bone-in meat by-products, whole poultry, or fish and fish-fillet scrap.

The National Research Council (NRC) recommends an after-weaning protein requirement of 25% on a dry-matter basis; most practical diets provide 35-40% protein in combination with 20-25% fat and 25-35% carbohydrate. A lean, high-protein diet with emphasis on cooked eggs, liver, and muscle meats is used for the breeding/reproduction period from January into early May. Higher energy levels may be used during the lactation/early growth period (May-June) with higher levels of protein added to the high-caloric density diets. For the late growing period (July-August), good growth and minimal feed volume may be achieved with a diet containing 20% fortified cereal in combination with 25% fat and 35-37% protein on a dry-matter basis. For the fur production period (September-December), many ranchers use a "leaner" diet (20-22% fat on a dry-matter basis) and feed more quality proteins of animal origin, eg, cooked eggs and muscle meats.

Diets containing 35-40% of bone-in products should provide adequate calcium and phosphorus. Extra salt supplementation (0.5% NaCl) may be used from May 15 to late June to help prevent a dehydration problem of nursing females known as nursing anemia.

Generally, there is no need for vitamin fortification of mink diets formulated from quality ingredients, especially if these include fresh liver. There are some exceptions. If high levels of unsaturated fat are fed, as in diets with a high proportion of high-fat fish, fish-fillet scrap, or horsemeat, the vitamin E should be increased. When metabolic antagonists are suspected in the diet (eg, thiaminase for vitamin B_1, or avidin for biotin), addition of the affected vitamins is prudent. If the rancher is formulating his own cereal, he may use commercial vitamin supplements with vitamin concentrations in the diet similar to those recommended by the NRC Subcommittee on Fur Animal Production. Vitamin A must be provided as the vitamin and not as β-carotene, which is inefficiently utilized by mink.

Proper preparation and storage are extremely important, both to retain nutritional values and avoid bacterial contamination. Freezing was the method most used with fresh feedstuffs in the past: the material is commonly frozen in blocks 3-4 in. (8-10 cm) thick, and protected in multi-wall paper sacks. Broad-spectrum antibiotics may be added to prevent bacterial contamination, and antioxidants, eg, vitamin E, are used to restrict fat rancidity. Fresh materials are sometimes preserved by acidification, usually with phosphoric acid, and so-called "fish silage" has been fed widely in the Scandinavian countries. Sometimes hydrolysates are prepared from fresh by-product feeds, using inherent or added enzymes followed by acid-stabilization. Such products are quite liquid, which restricts their use to mixtures with dry materials that improve their consistency. Use of dried meals and other feed ingredients has been practiced by some ranchers, usually to lower costs of labor in feeding and of refrigeration in prolonged storage. Dried feed mixes can be rehydrated and fed on the cage wire in the usual way, or pelleted and offered free choice in special feed hoppers. Some mink producers use dry feeds on weekends and fresh feeds during the week; some feed dry feeds only during the less demanding periods of late summer and early fall; others use them year-round. Whenever dry feed mixes are used, a watering system that is functioning properly is important, since mink usually fill much of their water requirements from the fresh mix. Water can be provided by cups, troughs, or automatic pressure nipples.

The quantity of feed offered may be restricted during February, March, and early April to keep animals trim through the breeding season; however, feed for males should not be too restricted because of their large body size and intense breeding activity. The periods of lactation for the females and early growth of the kits (mid April-early July) are nutritionally critical. A poor diet during this time adversely affects the health of the females and survival and growth of the young. Some ranchers feed b.i.d. or even t.i.d. during this critical time to ensure that the high nutritional demands are met. At ~3 wk of age, the nursing kits should begin to receive solid food supplementation. This is usually mixed to a thinner, porridge-like consistency to help meet needs for both food and water, and is offered on boards placed on the cage floor. At other times of the year, once-daily feeding is practiced.

Several other items besides the nutrient content of the diet need attention for a successful, practical mink feeding program. These include bioavailability of the nutrients, palatability, digestibility, and presence of substances in the feed ingredients that may interfere with and impair normal metabolism.

Bioavailability, which includes digestibility, is particularly important for mink because of their simple GI system and rapid food passage. Certain types of feeds, eg, meals made from hair or feathers, although they test very high in protein, are unavailable because of low digestibility. Availability of some amino acids may be low in overheated meat meals subjected to poor feed-processing methods.

Since the demands of rapid growth and dense fur production require a high rate of food consumption, palatability is important. While early ranchers thought that only fresh, animal-source feed ingredients would be accepted, mink will also accept some plant-source materials. Mink can be induced to eat diets that are less attractive by adding highly palatable materials; fresh liver is sometimes used for this purpose, or to tempt the appetites of animals that have gone off feed for some reason. Many ranchers feed 5-10% fresh liver routinely, from March 1 to early June.

The presence of interfering factors in feeds has received a good deal of attention. Some fresh materials fed to mink may contain interfering enzymes that would be inactive in the dried feeds given other classes of livestock. A well-known example is thiaminase, an enzyme found in the flesh of a number of species of fish (including bullheads, carp, herring, and ocean smelt), which destroys dietary thiamine and causes anorexia and Chastek paralysis in mink. Certain other fishes, usually from the cod family, generate formaldehyde or trimethylamineoxide (TMAO), which interferes with iron metabolism and causes severe anemia and development of a whitish underfur ("cotton fur"). Raw eggs, which are otherwise an excellent protein source, contain a substance called avidin that binds with and inactivates dietary biotin. The consequent biotin deficiency causes achromotrichia and alopecia in severe cases. When enzymes cause these nutritional problems, they can be inactivated by heating; however, this adds expense to the diet preparation. Cooking at 91°C for ≥5 min inactivates avidin. Alternatively, diets known to contain these interfering substances can be supplemented with the deficient nutrient(s).

Ingredient contamination with hormonal or other growth stimulants is a concern; high-potency residues of pellet implants may remain in portions of the carcass sold for mink feed. Diethylstilbestrol residues were a case in point, and interfered with normal reproduction in mink before such practices were disallowed. Thyroactive iodine compounds can also be troublesome. The best defense against such problems is strict quality control, which includes free exchange of information between vendors and users of animal waste products.

Spoilage of feed before or during storage can also be troublesome. Slaughterhouse offal exposed to temperatures >60°F (15°C) and anaerobic conditions may contain toxin produced by *Clostridium botulinum*. Mink are extremely sensitive to this toxin. They can be protected by vaccination, but once botulism (qv, p 1051) is seen, it may be too late for such remedial treatment. Rapid cooling of offal products after slaughter, washing, and sanitary storage are preventive.

A diet with rancid fats can lead to "yellow fat" or steatitis (qv, p 1054) and often death in mink that consume it. Highly unsaturated fats, such as fish oils, are most susceptible to oxidative rancidity, which can be prevented by addition of vitamin E (~50 IU/kg mixed feed) or some other effective antioxidant. Very high levels of fat in the diet, whether spoiled or not, have been associated with "wet belly disease" (qv, p 1056) in which soiling of the inguinal region may lower pelt value.

NUTRITION: PIGS

NUTRITIONAL REQUIREMENTS

Advanced technology contributes to the many phases of modern swine production. This is most evident in nutrition as formulation of synthetic diets becomes more precise and economical.

Maintenance requirements should be distinguished from therapeutic doses of many times the normal needs, administered singly or over short periods to correct deficiencies. Factors such as stress, availability of nutrients, or variability in animals may increase the levels of some nutrients for optimal performance. Natural diets may contain more of some nutrients than the table recommends, but the effect is minimal except in extreme cases of imbalance. Ingredient concentration should be modified to prevent serious imbalances.

Table 35. Nutrient Requirements of Swine Allowed Feed *Ad Lib*
(90% Dry Matter)

Intake and Performance Levels	Swine Liveweight (kg)				
	1-5	5-10	10-20	20-50	50-110
Expected wt gain (g/day)	200	250	450	700	820
Expected feed intake (g/day)	250	460	950	1900	3110
Expected efficiency (gain/feed)	0.800	0.543	0.474	0.369	0.264
Expected efficiency (feed/gain)	1.25	1.84	2.11	2.71	3.79
Digestible energy intake (kcal/day)	850	1560	3230	6460	10,570
Metabolizable energy intake (kcal/day)	805	1490	3090	6200	10,185
Energy concentration (kcal ME/kg diet)	3220	3240	3250	3260	3275
Protein (%)	24	20	18	15	13

(continued)

**Table 35. Nutrient Requirements of Swine Allowed Feed *Ad Lib* (continued)
(90% Dry Matter)**

Nutrient	Requirement (% or amount/kg diet)*				
Essential amino acids (%)					
Arginine	0.60	0.50	0.40	0.25	0.10
Histidine	0.36	0.31	0.25	0.22	0.18
Isoleucine	0.76	0.65	0.53	0.46	0.38
Leucine	1.00	0.85	0.70	0.60	0.50
Lysine	1.40	1.15	0.95	0.75	0.60
Methionine + cystine	0.68	0.58	0.48	0.41	0.34
Phenylalanine + tyrosine	1.10	0.94	0.77	0.66	0.55
Threonine	0.80	0.68	0.56	0.48	0.40
Tryptophan	0.20	0.17	0.14	0.12	0.10
Valine	0.80	0.68	0.56	0.48	0.40
Linoleic acid (%)	0.1	0.1	0.1	0.1	0.1
Mineral elements					
Calcium (%)	0.90	0.80	0.70	0.60	0.50
Phosphorus, total (%)	0.70	0.65	0.60	0.50	0.40
Phosphorus, available (%)	0.55	0.40	0.32	0.23	0.15
Sodium (%)	0.10	0.10	0.10	0.10	0.10
Chlorine (%)	0.08	0.08	0.08	0.08	0.08
Magnesium (%)	0.04	0.04	0.04	0.04	0.04
Potassium (%)	0.30	0.28	0.26	0.23	0.17
Copper (mg)	6.0	6.0	5.0	4.0	3.0
Iodine (mg)	0.14	0.14	0.14	0.14	1.14
Iron (mg)	100	100	80	60	40
Manganese (mg)	4.0	4.0	3.0	2.0	2.0
Selenium (mg)	0.30	0.30	0.25	0.15	0.10
Zinc (mg)	100	100	80	60	50
Vitamins					
Vitamin A (IU)	2200	2200	1750	1300	1300
Vitamin D (IU)	220	220	200	150	150
Vitamin E (IU)	16	16	11	11	11
Vitamin K (mg) (menadione)	0.5	0.5	0.5	0.5	0.5
Biotin (mg)	0.08	0.05	0.05	0.05	0.05
Choline (g)	0.6	0.5	0.4	0.3	0.3
Folacin (mg)	0.3	0.3	0.3	0.3	0.3
Niacin, available (mg)	20.0	15.0	12.5	10.0	7.0
Pantothenic acid (mg)	12.0	10.0	9.0	8.0	7.0
Riboflavin (mg)	4.0	3.5	3.0	2.5	2.0
Thiamine (mg)	1.5	1.0	1.0	1.0	1.0
Vitamin B_6 (mg)	2.0	1.5	1.5	1.0	1.0
Vitamin B_{12} (μg)	20.0	17.5	15.0	10.0	5.0

NOTE: Knowledge of nutritional constraints and limitations is important for the proper use of this table.

* These requirements are based on the following types of pigs and diets: 1- to 5-kg pigs, a diet that includes 25-75% milk products; 5- to 10-kg pigs, a corn-soybean meal diet that includes 5-25% milk products; 10- to 110-kg pigs, a corn-soybean meal diet. In the corn-soybean meal diets, the corn contains 8.5% protein, the soybean meal contains 44%.

Adapted, with permission, from *Nutrient Requirements of Swine*, 1988, National Academy of Sciences. Published by National Academy Press, Washington, DC.

The nutrients required by pigs are classified as water, energy (chiefly carbohydrates and fat), protein (amino acids), minerals, and vitamins. In TABLE 35, nutrient requirement values are expressed per kg of total air-dry diet; those in TABLE 36 are expressed as daily needs. Certain antibiotics and chemotherapeutic agents added to swine diets to increase the rate and efficiency of gain are not considered nutrients.

WATER

Pigs should have free and convenient access to water, beginning before weaning. The amount required varies with age, type of feed, environmental temperature, status of lactation, fever, high urinary output (as from high salt or protein intake), or diarrhea. Normally, pigs consume 2-5 kg of water/kg dry feed. Their total intake is 7-20 kg of water/100 kg body wt daily, or even more.

ENERGY

The amount of feed consumed by growing pigs fed *ad lib* is controlled principally by the energy contents of the diet. If diets contain excessive amounts of fiber (>5-7%) without commensurate increases in fat, the rate and, especially, the efficiency of gain are adversely affected. Energy requirements of pigs are expressed in terms of kilocalories (kcal) either as digestible energy (DE), metabolizable energy (ME), or net energy (NE). Most swine nutritionists use ME values.

FEEDING LEVELS

Estimates of daily feed intake for growing-finishing pigs (*see* TABLE 35) are useful as a guide in projecting total feed requirements or prescribing in-feed medication.

The feeding levels set forth by the National Research Council (NRC) provide a daily intake of 4.2 lb (1.9 kg) for pregnant gilts and sows. Sows and gilts need little more energy during pregnancy than is required for maintenance of body weight and good health. The diets on which these recommendations are based would be classified as high-energy diets (corn-soybean meal type) with no oats, alfalfa meal, or other energy diluent. Heavy-milking sows may need to be fed more (up to 6 lb [2.7 kg]/day) during the last 30 days of gestation to prevent excessive weight loss during lactation. Voluntary intake by pregnant pigs is difficult to limit even with a high-fiber or a high-mineral level and, invariably, both excess intake and weight gain occur.

A feeding method for pregnant gilts and sows that is widely accepted is to feed only every third day, but to offer the total 3-day amount of feed (eg, feed 5.7 kg every third day instead of 1.9 kg daily). The feed is spread out to allow opportunity for individuals to eat simultaneously. Sows may also be self-fed a complete diet for a limited time (8 hr) every third day.

During lactation the NRC recommends 9.7 lb (4.4 kg), 11.7 lb (5.3 kg), and 13.4 lb (6.1 kg) of feed daily for sows producing 11, 13.8, and 16.5 lb (5, 6.25, and 7.5 kg) of milk daily, respectively. High-energy diets should be self-fed during lactation. If sows become too thin, top-dressing the feed with additional fat should be considered. If problems still exist, more energy should be provided during the last trimester of pregnancy.

PROTEIN AND AMINO ACIDS

Amino acids, normally supplied by proteins, are required for maintenance, growth, gestation, and lactation. Many amino acids are synthesized in the animal; however, some must be provided in the diet to achieve normal growth. The essential amino acids for growing pigs are arginine, histidine, isoleucine, leucine, lysine, methionine, phenylalanine, threonine, tryptophan, and valine. The suggested feeding levels for crude protein in TABLE 35 are guidelines that will provide the required levels of amino acids when diets are based on corn and soybean meal (or for young pigs on corn, soybean meal, and milk products). The essential amino acid requirements of pigs are given, in part, in the tables. Further research is needed to clarify the amino acid requirements, particularly for boars.

Table 36. Daily Nutrient Intakes and Requirements of Intermediate-weight Breeding Pigs

Intake and Performance Levels	Mean Gestation or Farrowing Weight (kg) of:	
	Bred Gilts, Sows, and Adult Boars	Lactating Gilts and Sows
	162.5	165.0
Daily feed intake (kg)	1.9	5.3
Digestible energy (Mcal/day)	6.3	17.7
Metabolizable energy (Mcal/day)	6.1	17.0
Crude protein (g/day)	228	689
Requirement (amount/day)		
Nutrient		
Essential amino acids (g)		
Arginine	0	21.2
Histidine	2.8	13.2
Isoleucine	5.7	20.7
Leucine	5.7	25.4
Lysine	8.2	31.8
Methionine + cystine	4.4	19.1
Phenylalanine + tyrosine	8.6	37.1
Threonine	5.7	22.8
Tryptophan	1.7	6.4
Valine	6.1	31.8
Linoleic acid (g)	1.9	5.3
Mineral elements		
Calcium (g)	14.2	39.8
Phosphorus, total (g)	11.4	31.8
Phosphorus, available (g)	6.6	18.6
Sodium (g)	2.8	10.6
Chlorine (g)	2.3	8.5
Magnesium (g)	0.8	2.1
Potassium (g)	3.8	10.6
Copper (mg)	9.5	26.5
Iodine (mg)	0.3	0.7
Iron (mg)	152	424
Manganese (mg)	19	53
Selenium (mg)	0.3	0.8
Zinc (mg)	95	265
Vitamins		
Vitamin A (IU)	7600	10,600
Vitamin D (IU)	380	1,060
Vitamin E (IU)	42	117
Vitamin K (menadione) (mg)	1.0	2.6
Biotin (mg)	0.4	1.1
Choline (g)	2.4	5.3
Folacin (mg)	0.6	1.6
Niacin, available (mg)	19.0	53.0
Pantothenic acid (mg)	22.8	63.6
Riboflavin (mg)	7.1	19.9
Thiamine (mg)	1.9	5.3
Vitamin B_6 (mg)	1.9	5.3
Vitamin B_{12} (μg)	28.5	79.5

Adapted, with permission, from *Nutrient Requirements of Swine*, 1988, National Academy of Sciences. Published by National Academy Press, Washington, DC.

The 3 amino acids of greatest practical importance are lysine, tryptophan, and threonine. Corn, the basic grain in most swine diets, is markedly deficient in lysine and tryptophan. The other principal grains for pigs (sorghum, barley, and wheat) are low in lysine and threonine. The limiting amino acid in soybean meal is methionine, but sufficient is provided when soybean meal is combined with cereal grains into a complete diet containing the recommended level of protein. Cows' milk protein is well balanced in essential amino acids, but usually is too expensive to be used in swine diets, except for very young pigs. Diets based on corn and animal protein by-products (tankage, meat, meat meal, and bone meal) are inferior to corn-soybean meal diets, and can be improved significantly by adding tryptophan or supplements that are good sources of tryptophan.

MINERALS

The requirements for calcium, phosphorus, salt, and other essential minerals are listed in TABLES 35 and 36.

Calcium and Phosphorus: Although used primarily in skeletal growth, Ca and P play important metabolic roles in the body, and are essential for gestation and lactation. Pregnant animals should receive a minimum of 16 g Ca and 13 g P daily, and lactating sows should receive 50 g Ca and 40 g P daily. The NRC dietary requirements are 0.6% Ca and 0.5% P for the growing pig, and 0.5% Ca and 0.4% P for finishing pigs. These levels were established with semi-purified diets and, although adequate for maximal growth (rate of gain), they do not allow for maximal bone mineralization. The usual recommendation for such diets is to continue feeding 0.5% P to market weight. Even higher levels of P (0.6%) may be required to maximize bone strength of growing boars. The use of feedstuffs such as tankage, meat, meat meal, bone meal, and fish meal that are rich sources of Ca and P may preclude the need to add a P supplement. Calcium sources normally used in swine diets (limestone and oyster shell) have a high biological availability. Steamed bone meal, defluorinated phosphate, soft phosphate, or dicalcium phosphate may be used to increase both dietary Ca and P. There is some variation in the biological availability of the P in these supplements.

Sodium Chloride: The recommended salt allowance is 0.25% of the total diet. Animal and fish by-products, as well as certain cereal by-products, contribute appreciable amounts of salt.

Iodine: Iodine is used by the thyroid gland to produce thyroxine, which affects cell activity and metabolic rate. The iodine requirement of pregnant sows is ~0.3 mg daily. Growing pigs require 0.14 mg/kg of diet. Stabilized iodized salt that contains 0.007% iodine, fed to meet the salt requirement, will meet the iodine needs of pigs.

Iron and Copper: These are necessary for Hgb formation and, therefore, to prevent nutritional anemia. For the first 3 wk after birth, 15 mg of iron per pig daily will maintain normal Hgb levels. The requirement for copper is listed by the NRC as 3-6 mg/kg total diet. It has been reported that 11 mg/kg body wt daily will prevent signs of copper deficiency. Because the amount of iron in milk is very low, suckling pigs should receive supplemental iron. Piglet anemia (qv, p 18) can be prevented with injectable iron compounds, which is the preferred method; 100-200 mg of iron, in the form of iron dextran, iron dextrin, or gleptoferron, given in the first 3 days of life, will suffice (however, see IRON DEXTRAN TOXICITY, p 1673). Feeding iron and copper salts to, or injecting iron dextran into, pregnant or lactating sows does not prevent anemia in neonatal pigs. Iron can also be supplied PO to the suckling pig by mixing ferric ammonium citrate with water in a piglet waterer or periodically dropping a mixture of iron sulfate and a carrier, such as corn, on the floor of the farrowing stall.

Cobalt: Cobalt is present in the vitamin B_{12} molecule, and does not need to be added to swine diets in the elemental form.

Manganese: Although essential for normal reproduction and growth, the quantitative requirement for manganese is unknown. It seems that 4-10 ppm in the diet is adequate for growth, gestation, and lactation.

Potassium: When practical diets are fed, no deficiency is encountered because natural feedstuffs contain adequate amounts of potassium.

Magnesium: A dietary essential for growing pigs, the requirement for magnesium is 400 ppm in the complete diet. Because of the content of this mineral in ordinary feedstuffs, a deficiency is unlikely under practical conditions. Magnesium oxide supplementation has been used to prevent cannibalism, but controlled studies do not support this practice.

Zinc: Supplemental zinc at 50-100 ppm is recommended to prevent parakeratosis (qv, p 818). When diets contain excessive calcium (ie, $\geq 1\%$), 80-130 ppm zinc is recommended.

Selenium: The selenium content of soils and, ultimately, crops is quite variable. In general, areas west of the Mississippi River contain considerable amounts of selenium, while areas east of the river tend to yield crops deficient in selenium. Under practical conditions, 0.1-0.3 ppm selenium added in the diet should meet the minimum requirements, provided the diet is supplemented with vitamin E.

VITAMINS

Requirements for vitamins are given in TABLES 35 and 36, above.

Vitamin A: The use of stabilized vitamin A is common in manufactured feeds and in vitamin supplements or premixes. Concentrates containing natural vitamin A (fish oils most often) may be used to fortify diets, but both natural vitamin A and carotene, a precursor of vitamin A from plants, are rather easily destroyed by air, light, high temperatures, rancid fats, and certain mineral elements. For these reasons, less reliance is placed on natural feedstuffs as sources of vitamin A activity for pigs. The NRC suggests that for pigs, 1 mg of β-carotene is equal to ~200 IU of vitamin A. Green forage is an excellent source of carotene, as are high-quality legume hays. Dehydrated alfalfa meal is available as a standard feed ingredient and can be purchased with a guaranteed carotene content. Corn is not a reliable source.

Vitamin D: This antirachitic, fat-soluble vitamin is necessary for proper bone growth and ossification. Pigs can use vitamin D_2 (irradiated plant sterol) and vitamin D_3 (irradiated animal sterol) to meet their vitamin D requirement. Vitamin D needs can be met by exposing pigs to direct sunlight for a short period each day. Sources of vitamin D include irradiated yeast, sun-cured hays, activated plant or animal sterols, fish oils, and vitamin A and D concentrates.

Vitamin E (α-tocopherol): Required by pigs of all ages, it is interrelated with selenium and is included at 11-22 IU/kg of diet where selenium and vitamin E deficiencies have been reported. Vitamin E supplementation can only partially obviate a selenium deficiency. Green forage, legume hays and meals, cereal grains, and especially the germ of cereal grains contain appreciable amounts of vitamin E. Vitamin E activity seems to be reduced in feedstuffs stored under high-moisture conditions. Grinding grains and including high levels of copper (125-250 ppm) in mixed diets greatly reduce the stability of naturally occurring α-tocopherol.

Vitamin K: This fat-soluble vitamin is necessary to maintain normal blood clotting time. Hemorrhages have been reported in newborn as well as growing pigs, perhaps indicating deficiencies of vitamin K in pigs fed practical diets. Supplemental vitamin K should be added at 2 mg/kg diet as an insurance measure.

Thiamine: This water-soluble vitamin is not of practical importance in diets commonly fed to pigs because grains and other feed ingredients supply ample amounts to meet the requirement of ~1.1-1.5 mg/kg of total diet.

Riboflavin: The requirement of breeding stock and lightweight pigs is 3-4 mg/kg of diet. For ≥ 20-kg growing pigs, 2-2.5 mg/kg diet is required. Riboflavin is a constituent of several enzyme systems in the body. Swine diets are normally deficient in this vitamin, and the crystalline form is added in premixes. Natural sources include green forage, milk by-products, brewer's yeast, legume meals, and some fermentation and distillery by-products.

Niacin (nicotinic acid): The requirement for available niacin is 15 mg/kg diet for the 10-kg pig, and 10 mg/kg diet for ≥ 20-kg pigs. Niacin is a component of coenzymes concerned with utilization of carbohydrates. Pigs inefficiently convert some tryptophan to niacin. Corn contains niacin at 9-10 mg/lb, but the niacin from corn and other cereal grains seems to be unavailable to pigs. Swine diets are normally deficient in this vitamin, and the crystalline form is added in premixes. Natural sources of niacin include fish and animal by-products, brewer's yeast, peanut meal, and distillers' solubles.

Pantothenic acid: The requirement for panthothenic acid is 12 mg/kg of feed for pigs <10 kg, 9 mg for pigs ≥10 kg, and ~12 mg for breeding animals. Pantothenic acid is necessary for reproduction in sows. Swine diets are normally deficient in this vitamin, and the crystalline form is added in premixes. Natural sources of pantothenic acid include green forage, legume meals, milk products, brewer's yeast, fish solubles, wheat bran, peanut meal, and rice polishings.

Pyridoxine (vitamin B_6): The requirement for pyridoxine is 1.5 mg/kg diet for 5- to 20-kg pigs, and 1 mg/kg diet for heavier pigs. It is important in amino acid metabolism, and is present in plentiful quantities in the feed ingredients usually fed to pigs.

Choline: Essential for the normal functioning of all tissues, pigs can synthesize some choline from methionine in the diet. The requirement for choline is listed as 500 mg/kg of feed for 5- to 10-kg pigs and 400 mg/kg for 10- to 20-kg pigs. Recent evidence indicates that the requirement is not >330 mg/kg of feed for starter pigs. Corn-soybean diets are not deficient in choline for starting, growing, or finishing pigs. Supplemental choline chloride at 440-770 mg/kg of feed increases litter size in gilts and sows. Natural sources of choline include fish solubles, fish meal, soybean meal, liver meal, brewer's yeast, tankage, and meat meal.

Vitamin B_{12}: The requirement for vitamin B_{12} is 20 μg/kg diet for 1- to 10-kg pigs; 15 μg/kg diet is suggested for breeding stock. Vitamin B_{12} potency of natural feed sources is quite variable. Swine diets are often deficient in this vitamin, and the crystalline form is added in premixes.

Biotin: This is an essential nutrient. There is evidence that sorghum-soybean meal and barley-soybean meal diets fed to breeding animals may be deficient in available biotin. Conflicting evidence has been published regarding the biotin status of corn-soybean meal diets. Biotin supplementation of these diets may increase litter size and decrease foot-pad lesions in adult pigs.

Folic acid and ascorbic acid: Folic acid is a dietary essential vitamin for pigs, but ascorbic acid (vitamin C) is synthesized by the pig at a rapid enough rate to meet its needs. Evidence indicates no need to supplement practical swine diets with ascorbic acid. Recent research indicates that supplemental folic acid in pregnancy diets increases the number of pigs born.

FEEDING PRACTICES

Swine Feeding Plan: A fundamental principle of the economics of pork production is to feed the most economical cereal grains and to correct the deficiencies by supplementation. Dependable mineral and vitamin premixes or complete manufactured supplements are available.

The consumption of creep-feed before 3 wk of age is minimal. Litters nursing beyond this age should be self-fed a palatable starter diet until weaning. Supplemental feed is needed for optimal performance because milk production peaks at 3-4 wk of age while the pig's nutrient needs are increasing rapidly.

Preparation and Feeding of Farm Grains: An improvement in weight gain and, particularly, in feed efficiency can be expected from grinding grain; the older the pig, the greater the response. Grain should be reduced to a medium-fine particle size. Excessive particle size reduction may lead to an increased incidence of gastric ulcers. Pelleting of diets may result in a small improvement in gain and especially feed efficiency. In general, the greatest benefit is realized with pelleted diets containing high levels of fiber.

Corn (maize): This is the most widely used grain for feeding pigs in North America. It is high in metabolizable energy (ME) but relatively low in crude protein.

Oats: Because of the relatively low energy content of oats, they should not account for >20% of the cereal grain in the diet. On that basis, finely ground oats can replace corn on a pound-for-pound basis. Rolled oats (dehulled) are often used in starter diets; they have a somewhat higher energy density than corn.

Wheat: Although wheat contains 2-3% more protein than corn, little or no increased substitutive value is gained because the lysine content is only slightly greater than in corn. The ME values of wheat and corn are nearly identical. Wheat should be coarsely ground before feeding.

Barley: Ground or rolled barley has ~90% the feeding value of corn even though it usually contains 2-3% more protein. Pelleted diets that contain high levels of barley result in improved performance over similar diets fed in meal form. Scabby barley should not be fed. Pelleted barley diets that contain adequate amounts of all required nutrients are nearly equal to diets based on ground yellow corn and the necessary supplements.

Sorghum: This grain has become a major energy source for pigs in western and southwestern USA. The protein content varies from 9 to 13%, depending on whether the crop was grown on irrigated or nonirrigated land and whether the soil was fertilized. In general, sorghum can be substituted for corn on an equal-weight basis, but because the ME value is slightly lower than that of corn, a poorer feed conversion should be expected.

Nutritional Management of Sows and Litters: Profit can be increased by preventing pig fatalities; ~20% of all pigs die before weaning. The following help reduce this loss: 1) Produce healthy pigs by feeding gestation diets adequate in all nutrients. The more vigorous a pig is at birth, the better its chances of survival. 2) Make sure the sow is in good condition at farrowing and does not need a laxative feed, which is primarily a reflection of feeding during gestation. Constipation problems are minimal if the sow is limit-fed throughout gestation. After farrowing, the sow should be allowed to return to feed as she chooses. 3) Make sure that each pig has nursed. If necessary, the milk flow (or letdown) may be stimulated in some sows by administering oxytocin. If the sow is slow in coming to milk, weak pigs may benefit from receiving artificial milk, but success depends on good management and sanitation. 4) Prevent nutritional anemia. 5) Provide a palatable pig starter diet from 3 wk of age until weaning. (*See also* DISEASE-MANAGEMENT INTERACTION: PIGS, p 1120, and MANAGEMENT OF REPRODUCTION: PIGS, p 1143.)

Nutritional Management of Growing Pigs: Pigs weaned at an early age (3-4 wk) perform best if fed a complex starter diet for 2 wk. Typically, this starter diet contains milk products and refined carbohydrates. The nutritional needs of growing-finishing pigs are best met by a full-feeding program. Limited feeding reduces the rate of gain, but may improve feed efficiency and the carcass quality of finishing pigs. Proper design and adjustment of self feeders is necessary to prevent feed wastage or restricted growth.

Space recommendations for growing pigs given herein are adapted from a report by the Nutrition Council of the American Feed Industry Association. When maintained on slatted floors, each growing-finishing pig should be provided 4-6 sq ft of floor space from 50-125 lb, and 8 sq ft from 125-200 lb body wt (*see* TABLE 37).

Growth Stimulants: Antibiotics and other chemotherapeutic agents are commonly added to swine diets to promote growth. In general, antibiotics have resulted in a larger and more consistent response than the arsenicals when added to growing-pig diets. The levels of antibiotics fed and drug withdrawal requirements should be in accordance with manufacturers' recommendations and legal restrictions.

The inclusion of effective antibiotics in diets for starter pigs (<23 kg) tends to increase the rate of gain by ~15% on the average, and the feed efficiency by ~7%; for grower-finisher pigs, improvements of ~4% in rate of gain and ~2%

in feed efficiency can be expected. The feed additives commonly used are penicillin (alone or in combination with streptomycin), chlortetracycline, oxytetracycline, bacitracin, tylosin, carbadox, bambermycins, and virginiamycin. For best results, the antibiotic should be included in the diet throughout the growing-finishing period. It may help to reduce the number of runts and unthrifty pigs and cause such pigs to make more rapid and efficient gains. It helps to prevent and control scours and certain forms of enteritis. (This advantage may be lost if resistant strains of enteritis-causing organisms develop.) Several studies indicate that feeding antimicrobial agents at breeding time and at farrowing usually results in improved reproductive performance. The greatest response to feed additives is usually seen in starter diets. The inclusion of such agents in pig starters may be of value in controlling scours and overcoming the added stress imposed by weaning. Feeding antimicrobials to pigs will not substitute for good management.

Table 37. Space Needs of Growing-finishing Pigs

	Weaning to 75 lb (<34 kg)	75-125 lb (34-57 kg)	25 lb to Market Size (>57 kg)
Sleeping space or shelter per pig, square feet	4	5-6	8
Pigs per linear foot of self-feeder space (or per hole)			
On dry lot..................	4	3	3
On pasture	4-5	3-4	3-4
Percent of feeder space for protein supplement			
On dry lot..................	25	20	15
On pasture	20-25	15-20	10-15
For hand-feeding or hand-watering, running feet of trough per pig*	3/4	1	1 1/4

*Access from one side.

New growth promotants commonly referred to as "repartitioning agents" may be available soon; β-agonists, such as cimaterol and ractopamine, and porcine somatotropin are examples. These compounds improve feed conversion and result in a leaner carcass. They affect nutrient requirements, particularly increasing the requirements for protein and amino acids.

NUTRITIONAL DISEASES

Diagnosis of nutritional deficiencies by observation of signs is difficult. Quite often, the clinical signs are the result of a complex of mismanagement and infectious diseases, including parasitism, as well as malnutrition. For most nutritional deficiencies, the signs are not specific, eg, poor appetite, reduced growth, and unthriftiness are common to deficiencies of most nutrients. Deficiency of a single nutrient may bring about inanition; the subsequent starvation may cause multiple deficiencies. Then, too, a nutritional deficiency may exist without the appearance of definite signs. In the field, the deficiency may be only slight or borderline, which makes the diagnosis difficult.

Diagnosis of a deficiency by observing the response to nutritional therapy is not always clear-cut, particularly for long-term deficiencies, the lesions of which may be irreversible. A nutritional deficiency should be diagnosed positively only after observance of several of the clinical signs expected, and a careful review of the dietary, disease, and management history of the animals.

PROTEIN

Protein deficiency, which may result from suboptimal feed intake or an imbalance of one or more of the essential amino acids, causes reduced gains, fatter carcasses, and poorer feed conversion. For optimal utilization of protein, all essential amino acids must be liberated during digestion at rates commensurate with needs. Therefore, protein supplement should not be hand-fed at infrequent intervals, but should be mixed with the grain or be available at all times with grain on a free-choice basis.

No evidence has been presented to support the theory of "protein poisoning". Diets containing as much as 34-51% protein have proved laxative, but not harmful, and no toxic effects were noted.

FAT

A semipurified diet containing 0.06% fat produced such deficiency signs as hair loss, scaly dermatitis, areas of skin necrosis on the neck and shoulders, and an unthrifty appearance in growing pigs; however, a level of 1-1.5% fat seemed ample to furnish the essential fatty acids. With practical diets, a specific fat or fatty acid deficiency is unknown.

MINERALS

The clinical signs of deficiencies of the more important mineral elements are briefly discussed below.

Calcium and Phosphorus: Deficiencies of Ca and P result in rickets (qv, p 487) in growing pigs, and osteomalacia in mature pigs. Signs include deformity and bending of long bones and lameness in young pigs, and fractures and posterior paralysis in older pigs. Deficient sows produce weak pigs, and usually show a posterior paralysis, sometimes as a result of fractures in the lumbar region. Sows with a marginal deficiency often farrow strong and vigorous pigs that grow normally. However, after nursing the pigs for ≥3 wk, such sows may develop posterior paralysis. A deficiency of vitamin D also causes these signs, especially if the dietary Ca or P differs markedly from the recommended feeding level.

Sodium and Chlorine: Pigs fed low-salt diets show slow growth, reduced appetite, and poor hair and skin condition.

Iodine: Bred females fed diets deficient in iodine produce hairless pigs that are weak or stillborn. With a borderline deficiency, the newborn pigs may only be weak at birth, but their thyroids are enlarged and have histological abnormalities. (*See also* GOITER, p 283.)

Iron and Copper: Deficiency of these 2 elements reduces the rate of Hgb formation and produces typical nutritional anemia. Signs of nutritional anemia in suckling pigs include low Hgb and RBC count, pale mucous membranes, enlarged heart, an edematous condition of the skin about the neck and shoulders, listlessness, and rapid breathing (thumps).

Zinc: A relative lack of this element results in parakeratosis (qv, p 818) in growing pigs, particularly when diets contain more than the recommended amount of calcium. The exact mode of action of zinc in the prevention of parakeratosis is not known.

Selenium/Vitamin E: Sudden death of young, rapidly growing pigs may be observed due to a deficiency of these nutrients (*see* HEPATOSIS DIETETICA and MULBERRY HEART DISEASE, p 550).

VITAMINS

Signs resulting from deficiency of the vitamins of greatest practical importance are briefly discussed below.

Vitamin A: Deficiency results in disturbances of the eyes and the epithelial tissues of the respiratory, reproductive, nervous, urinary, and GI systems. Reproduction is impaired in sows, and vitamin-A-deficient sows may farrow blind, eyeless, weak, or malformed pigs. Herniation of the spinal cord in fetal pigs is reported as a unique sign of vitamin A deficiency in pregnant sows. Growing pigs, deficient in vitamin A, show incoordination and develop night blindness and respiratory disorders.

Vitamin D: Deficiency signs include rickets, stiffness, weak and bent bones, and posterior paralysis.

Riboflavin: In riboflavin-deficient pigs, reproduction is impaired; post-pubertal gilts fail to cycle but show no other clinical signs. Deficient sows are anorectic and farrow dead pigs 4-16 days prematurely. The stillborn pigs have very little hair, often are partially resorbed, and may have enlarged forelegs. Growing pigs fed low-riboflavin diets gain weight slowly, and have a poor appetite, a rough coat, an exudate on the skin, and possibly cataracts.

Niacin: Niacin-deficient pigs have inflammatory lesions of the GI tract. The pigs exhibit diarrhea, weight loss, rough skin and coat, and a dermatitis on the ears. Intestinal conditions may be due to niacin deficiency, bacterial infection, or both. Deficient pigs respond readily to niacin therapy, and although it is not a cure for infectious enteritis, adequate dietary niacin probably allows the pig to maintain its resistance to bacterial invasion.

Pantothenic Acid: Growing pigs and pregnant sows develop a typical "goose-stepping" gait, ataxia, and a noninfectious bloody diarrhea when maintained on pantothenic-acid-deficient diets. When the deficiency becomes severe, anorexia develops.

Choline: Choline-deficient pigs exhibit incoordination and an abnormal shoulder conformation. At necropsy, they may have fatty livers and usually show kidney damage. Choline-deficient sows have a slightly smaller litter size ($\sim$0.5 pig), but show no clinical signs of deficiency.

Vitamin B_{12}: Neonatal pigs fed synthetic diets low in vitamin B_{12} show hyper-irritability, voice failure, and pain and incoordination in the hindquarters. Histological examination of the bone marrow reveals an impairment of the hemopoietic system. Fatty livers are also noted at necropsy. Under farm conditions, weanling pigs fed practical diets low in vitamin B_{12} do not show the above signs, but merely gain weight more slowly than pigs receiving adequate B_{12}.

NUTRITION AND MANAGEMENT: POULTRY

NUTRITIONAL REQUIREMENTS

Poultry rank high in their ability to convert feed into food products, and this efficiency has been greatly increased in recent decades. The nutrient requirement figures published in NUTRIENT REQUIREMENTS OF POULTRY (National Academy of Sciences, 1984) are derived from experimentally determined levels found, under ideal laboratory conditions, to be adequate for normal growth, health, productivity, and quality of product. However, under practical conditions, genetics, energy content of the diets, environmental temperatures, type of floor, availability of nutrients from various feedstuffs, destruction or loss of nutrients in the gut, pro-oxidants, intestinal parasites, mycotoxins, diseases, and many other stresses may increase these nutrient requirements. Thus, many practical diets add a margin of safety to the nutrient requirements shown.

ENERGY, PROTEIN, AND AMINO ACIDS

Metabolizable energy (ME) values used by most poultry nutritionists are not corrected for metabolic fecal or endogenous energy losses, and therefore represent "apparent" metabolizable energy (AME) rather than "true" metabolizable energy (TME). The AME values serve well as the assessment of the available energy content of feedstuffs.

Chickens and other fowl can adjust their feed intake over a considerable range of feed energy levels to meet their daily energy needs. Thus, energy "requirements" are given as a range, usually ~2500-3400 kcal/kg of diet. Because energy content of the diet influences feed intake, protein and amino acid levels are usually given in relation to the energy content. Since protein nutrition is really amino acid nutrition, the calorie:protein ratio concept extends also to amino acids. Some of the amino acid figures in the tables were established by direct experimentation, while other values were calculated, assuming the amino acid requirements to be proportional to protein requirements. The amino acids shown in these tables are considered essential for poultry. Poultry can synthesize glycine, but often not in sufficient amounts. Cystine and tyrosine are considered essential, even though they can be synthesized from methionine and phenylalanine, respectively.

In practical feed formulation, methionine can spare choline as a methyl donor, and tryptophan can be used to synthesize niacin. These relationships are important since the 2 vitamins can be supplied in diets more economically than the 2 amino acids.

Table 38. Protein and Important Amino Acid Requirements of Chickens as Percentages of Diet

Nutrients*	Starting and Growing			Laying and Breeding***
	Weeks			
	0-6	6-12	12-20	
Protein	20	17	14**	17**
Arginine	1.05	0.85	0.72	0.88
Lysine	1.05	0.76	0.63	0.76
Methionine	0.42	0.34	0.30	0.35
Cystine	0.33	0.27	0.24	0.28
Threonine	0.72	0.60	0.52	0.60
Tryptophan	0.19	0.15	0.14	0.16

* Assuming all diets contain 2900 kcal ME/kg.

** These figures apply in a moderate climate. For warm environmental temperatures, all values for the developing diets and for layers and breeders should be increased ~10%. Similarly, in cold houses, the above nutrients may be reduced as a percentage of the diet.

*** These requirements apply to Leghorns. Brown-egg strains may consume ~10% more feed/day, and thus their diets can be proportionately lower in these nutrients.

Table 39. Protein and Important Amino Acid Requirements of Broilers as Percentages of Diet

Energy Base kcal ME/kg Diet[a] →	Wk 0-3 3200	Wk 3-6 3200	Wk 6-8 3200
Protein	23	20	18
Arginine	1.44	1.20	1.00
Glycine + Serine	1.50	1.00	0.70
Histidine	0.35	0.30	0.26
Isoleucine	0.80	0.70	0.60
Leucine	1.35	1.18	1.00
Lysine	1.20	1.00	0.85
Methionine + Cystine	0.93	0.72	0.60
Methionine	0.50	0.38	0.32
Phenylalanine + Tyrosine	1.34	1.17	1.00
Phenylalanine	0.72	0.63	0.54
Threonine	0.80	0.74	0.68
Tryptophan	0.23	0.18	0.17
Valine	0.82	0.72	0.62

[a] These are typical dietary energy concentrations.

Adapted, with permission, from *Nutrient Requirements of Poultry*, 1984, National Academy of Sciences. Published by National Academy Press, Washington, DC.

Table 40. Protein and Amino Acid Requirements of Turkeys as Percentages of Diet

	Age (wk)							
Energy Base kcal ME/kg Diet[a] →	M: 0-4 F: 0-4 2800	4-8 4-8 2900	8-12 8-11 3000	12-16 11-14 3100	16-20 14-17 3200	20-24 17-20 3300	Holding 2900	Breeding Hens 2900
Protein	28	26	22	19	16.5	14	12	14
Arginine	1.6	1.5	1.25	1.1	0.95	0.8	0.6	0.6
Glycine + Serine	1.0	0.9	0.8	0.7	0.6	0.5	0.4	0.5
Histidine	0.58	0.54	0.46	0.39	0.35	0.29	0.25	0.3
Isoleucine	1.1	1.0	0.85	0.75	0.65	0.55	0.45	0.5
Leucine	1.9	1.75	1.5	1.3	1.1	0.95	0.5	0.5
Lysine	1.6	1.5	1.3	1.0	0.8	0.65	0.5	0.6
Methionine + Cystine	1.05	0.9	0.75	0.65	0.55	0.45	0.4	0.4
Methionine	0.53	0.45	0.38	0.33	0.28	0.23	0.2	0.2
Phenylalanine + Tyrosine	1.8	1.65	1.4	1.2	1.05	0.9	0.8	1.0
Phenylalanine	1.0	0.9	0.8	0.7	0.6	0.5	0.4	0.55
Threonine	1.0	0.93	0.79	0.68	0.59	0.5	0.4	0.45
Tryptophan	0.26	0.24	0.2	0.18	0.15	0.13	0.1	0.13
Valine	1.2	1.1	0.94	0.8	0.7	0.6	0.5	0.58

[a]These are typical ME concentrations for corn-soya diets. Different ME values may be appropriate if other ingredients predominate.

Adapted, with permission, from *Nutrient Requirements of Poultry*, 1984, National Academy of Sciences. Published by National Academy Press, Washington, DC.

Table 41. Nutrient Requirements of Pheasants[a] and Bobwhite Quail[b] as Percentages or as Milligrams per Kilogram of Diet

		Pheasant			Bobwhite Quail	
Energy Base kcal ME/kg Diet[c] →	Starting 2800	Growing 2700	Breeding 2800	Starting 2800	Growing 2800	Breeding 2800
Protein %	30	16	18	28	20	24
Glycine + Serine %	1.8	1	—	—	—	—
Lysine %	1.5	0.8	—	—	—	—
Methionine + Cystine %	1.1	0.6	0.6	—	—	—
Linoleic acid %	1	1	1	1	1	1
Calcium %	1.0	0.7	2.5	0.65	0.65	2.3
Phosphorus, available %	0.55	0.45	0.40	0.55	0.45	0.50
Sodium %	0.15	0.15	0.15	0.15	0.15	0.15
Chlorine %	0.11	0.11	0.11	0.11	0.11	0.11
Iodine mg	0.3	0.3	0.3	0.3	0.3	0.3
Riboflavin mg	3.5	3.0	—	3.8	—	4.0
Pantothenic acid mg	10	10	—	13	—	15
Niacin mg	60	40	—	30	—	20
Choline mg	1500	1000	—	1500	—	1000

[a] For values not listed, see REQUIREMENTS FOR TURKEYS as a guide (TABLES 40 and 43).

[b] For values not listed, see REQUIREMENTS FOR LEGHORN-TYPE CHICKENS as a guide (TABLES 38 and 42).

[c] These are typical dietary energy concentrations.

Adapted, with permission, from *Nutrient Requirements of Poultry*, 1984, National Academy of Sciences. Published by National Academy Press, Washington, DC.

Body weight and composition are important factors in rearing pullets of any strain for maximum egg production. Most strains of White Leghorn chickens have relatively low body weights and do not tend, under normal feeding, to become obese. Feed should not be restricted with this type of bird lest they fail to reach adequate body weights at onset of lay. There may be times when, for various reasons, pullets are to be delayed in coming into production. Under such circumstances, feed restriction is necessary to restrict body weight gain of the pullets. For brown-egg strains of chickens, some degree of restriction is often practiced (~90% of *ad lib* feeding). Some type of feed restriction program is particularly important for broiler-strain pullets, which tend to become very obese if fed *ad lib*. The broiler breeder also is restricted in feed intake during the laying period.

Pullets now come into production and reach peak production weeks earlier than they did several years ago. This is true both for commercial layers and broiler breeders. Thus, it is of utmost importance that the starting, growing, and developer feeds are fully adequate for development of strong pullets of normal body weight at onset of lay.

VITAMINS

Vitamin requirements are presented in the following tables in terms of mg/kg of diet except for vitamins A, D, and E, which are given in International Units (IU).

One IU of **vitamin A** activity is equivalent to 1.3 μg of pure retinol (or 0.344 μg of retinyl acetate). In chickens, 0.6 μg of β-carotene is considered equivalent to 1 IU of vitamin A. However, young chicks are not efficient in utilizing β-carotene. The vitamin A requirements recommended herein are based on use of stabilized vitamin A preparations, and thus are somewhat lower than previously recommended levels.

Requirements for **vitamin D** are expressed in IU. Birds use vitamin D_3 from fish oils and irradiated animal sterols quite effectively, but cannot use vitamin D_2. Metabolic forms of vitamin D have been isolated and synthesized; these are 25-hydroxy vitamin D_3, which is synthesized in the liver, and 1,25-dihydroxy vitamin D_3, which is synthesized in the kidneys. One IU of vitamin D represents the vitamin D activity of 0.025 μg of pure vitamin D_3.

One IU of **vitamin E** is equivalent to 1 mg of synthetic dl-α-tocopherol acetate. Vitamin E requirements vary with the type and level of fat in the diet, the levels of selenium and trace minerals, and the presence or absence of other antioxidants.

Choline is required as an integral part of the body phospholipids, as a part of acetylcholine, and as a source of methyl groups. The growing chicken can use betaine as a methylating agent, but betaine cannot replace choline in preventing perosis. Betaine is widely distributed in practical feedstuffs and may be important in sparing choline. Adequate dietary vitamin B_{12} helps the pullet develop the ability to biosynthesize choline. The choline requirement values presented are applicable to diets containing the specified levels of vitamin B_{12}.

MINERALS

The calcium requirement of laying hens is difficult to define. Too much dietary calcium interferes with the utilization of several other minerals as well as fat, and tends to reduce palatability. For laying, the recommended level of 3.25% is adequate in most cases for early egg production, but hens >42 wk old, and especially those subjected to high environmental temperature, may require levels up to and perhaps >3.75%.

UNIDENTIFIED NUTRIENTS

The chick has requirements for 40 nutrients, together with an adequate level of ME. Some unidentified growth and hatchability factors may be required for maximum performance under certain stress conditions.

Table 42. Linoleic Acid, Mineral, and Vitamin Requirements of Leghorn-type Chickens as Percentages or as Milligrams or Units per Kilogram of Diet

Energy Base kcal ME/kg Diet[a] →		Growing			Laying		Breeding
		Wk 0-6 2900	Wk 6-14 2900	Wk 14-20 2900	2900	Daily Intake/Hen (mg)[b] 1100	2900
Linoleic acid	%	1	1	1	1	1	1
Calcium	%	0.80	0.70	0.60	3.40	3750	3.40
Phosphorus, available	%	0.40	0.35	0.30	0.32	350	0.32
Potassium	%	0.40	0.30	0.25	0.15	165	0.15
Sodium	%	0.15	0.15	0.15	0.15	165	0.15
Chlorine	%	0.15	0.12	0.12	0.15	165	0.15
Magnesium	mg	600	500	400	500	55	500
Manganese	mg	60	30	30	30	3.30	60
Zinc	mg	40	35	35	50	5.50	65
Iron	mg	80	60	60	50	5.50	60
Copper	mg	8	6	6	6	0.88	8
Iodine	mg	0.35	0.35	0.35	0.30	0.03	0.30
Selenium	mg	0.15	0.10	0.10	0.10	0.01	0.10
Vitamin A	IU	1500	1500	1500	4000	440	4000
Vitamin D	IU	200	200	200	500	55	500
Vitamin E	IU	10	5	5	5	0.55	10
Vitamin K	mg	0.50	0.50	0.50	0.50	0.055	0.50
Riboflavin	mg	3.60	1.80	1.80	2.20	0.242	3.80
Pantothenic acid	mg	10.0	10.0	10.0	2.20	0.242	10.0
Niacin	mg	27.0	11.0	10.0	10.0	1.10	10.0
Vitamin B_{12}	mg	0.009	0.003	0.003	0.004	0.00044	0.004
Choline	mg	1300	900	500	?	?	?
Biotin	mg	0.15	0.10	0.10	0.10	0.011	0.15
Folacin	mg	0.55	0.25	0.25	0.25	0.0275	0.35
Thiamine	mg	1.8	1.3	1.3	0.8	0.088	0.80
Pyridoxine	mg	3.0	3.0	3.0	3.0	0.33	4.50

[a]These are typical dietary energy concentrations.

[b]Assumes an average daily intake of 110 g of feed/hen daily.

Adapted, with permission, from *Nutrient Requirements of Poultry*, 1984, National Academy of Sciences. Published by National Academy Press, Washington, DC.

Table 43. Linoleic Acid, Mineral, and Vitamin Requirements of Turkeys as Percentages or as Milligrams or Units Per Kilogram of Feed

		Age (wk)							
Energy Base kcal ME/kg Diet[a] →		M: 0-4 F: 0-4 2800	4-8 4-8 2900	8-12 8-11 3000	12-16 11-14 3100	16-20 14-17 3200	20-24 17-20 3300	Holding 2900	Breeding Hens 2900
Linoleic acid	%	1.0	1.0	0.8	0.8	0.8	0.8	0.8	1.0
Calcium	%	1.2	1.0	0.85	0.75	0.65	0.55	0.5	2.25
Phosphorus, available	%	0.6	0.5	0.42	0.38	0.32	0.28	0.25	0.35
Potassium	%	0.7	0.6	0.5	0.5	0.4	0.4	0.4	0.6
Sodium	%	0.17	0.15	0.12	0.12	0.12	0.12	0.12	0.15
Chlorine	%	0.15	0.14	0.14	0.12	0.12	0.12	0.12	0.12
Magnesium	mg	600	600	600	600	600	600	600	600
Manganese	mg	60	60	60	60	60	60	60	60
Zinc	mg	75	65	50	40	40	40	40	65
Iron	mg	80	60	60	60	50	50	50	60
Copper	mg	8	8	8	6	6	6	6	8
Iodine	mg	0.4	0.4	0.4	0.4	0.4	0.4	0.4	0.4
Selenium	mg	0.2	0.2	0.2	0.2	0.2	0.2	0.2	0.2
Vitamin A	IU	4000	4000	4000	4000	4000	4000	4000	4000
Vitamin D[b]	IU	900	900	900	900	900	900	900	900
Vitamin E	IU	12	12	10	10	10	10	10	25
Vitamin K	mg	1.0	1.0	0.8	0.8	0.8	0.8	0.8	1.0
Riboflavin	mg	3.6	3.6	3.0	3.0	2.5	2.5	2.5	4.0
Pantothenic acid	mg	11	11	9	9	9	9	9	16
Niacin	mg	70	70	50	50	40	40	40	30
Vitamin B$_{12}$	mg	0.003	0.003	0.003	0.003	0.003	0.003	0.003	0.003
Choline	mg	1900	1600	1300	1100	950	800	800	1000
Biotin	mg	0.2	0.2	0.15	0.125	0.100	0.100	0.100	0.15
Folacin	mg	1.0	1.0	0.8	0.8	0.7	0.7	0.7	1.0
Thiamine	mg	2	2	2	2	2	2	2	2
Pyridoxine	mg	4.5	4.5	3.5	3.5	3.0	3.0	3.0	4.0

[a]These are typical ME concentrations for corn-soya diets. Different ME values may be appropriate if other ingredients predominate.

[b]These concentrations of vitamin D are satisfactory when the dietary concentrations of calcium and available phosphorus conform with those in this table.

Adapted, with permission, from Nutrient Requirements of Poultry, 1984, National Academy of Sciences. Published by National Academy Press, Washington, DC.

Table 44. Nutrient Requirements of Pekin Ducks as Percentages or as Milligrams or Units per Kilogram of Diet[a]

Energy Base kcal ME/kg Diet[b] →		Starting (0-2 wk) 2900	Growing (2-7 wk) 2900	Breeding 2900
Protein	%	22	16	15
Arginine	%	1.1	1.0	—
Lysine	%	1.1	0.9	0.7
Methionine + Cystine	%	0.8	0.6	0.55
Calcium	%	0.65	0.6	2.75
Phosphorus, available	%	0.40	0.35	0.35
Sodium	%	0.15	0.15	0.15
Chlorine	%	0.12	0.12	0.12
Magnesium	mg	500	500	500
Manganese	mg	40	40	25
Zinc	mg	60	60	60
Selenium	mg	0.14	0.14	0.14
Vitamin A	IU	4000	4000	4000
Vitamin D	IU	220	220	500
Vitamin K	mg	0.4	0.4	0.4
Riboflavin	mg	4	4	4
Pantothenic acid	mg	11	11	10
Niacin	mg	55	55	40
Pyridoxine	mg	2.6	2.6	3.0

[a] For nutrients not listed, *see* REQUIREMENTS FOR CHICKENS (TABLE 42) as a guide.
[b] These are typical dietary energy concentrations.
Adapted, with permission, from *Nutrient Requirements of Poultry*, 1984, National Academy of Sciences. Published by National Academy Press, Washington, DC.

Table 45. Nutrient Requirements of Geese as Percentages or as Milligrams or Units per Kilogram of Diet[a]

Energy Base kcal ME/kg Diet[b] →		Starting (0-6 wk) 2900	Growing (after 6 wk) 2900	Breeding 2900
Protein	%	22	15	15
Lysine	%	0.9	0.6	0.6
Methionine + Cystine	%	0.75	—	—
Calcium	%	0.8	0.6	2.25
Phosphorus, available	%	0.4	0.3	0.3
Vitamin A	IU	1500	1500	4000
Vitamin D	IU	200	200	200
Riboflavin	mg	4.0	2.5	4.0
Pantothenic acid	mg	15	—	—
Niacin	mg	55	35	20

[a] For nutrients not listed, *see* REQUIREMENTS FOR CHICKENS (TABLE 42) as a guide.
[b] These are typical dietary energy concentrations.
Adapted, with permission, from *Nutrient Requirements of Poultry*, 1984, National Academy of Sciences. Published by National Academy Press, Washington, DC.

ANTIBIOTICS

Antibiotics at low levels (5-25 mg/kg of feed, depending on the antibiotic) are used in poultry feeds to improve growth rate and feed efficiency. However, in some countries regulations now restrict this usage for certain antibiotics.

FEEDING AND MANAGEMENT PRACTICES

Feed and the length of time required for attaining certain weights in pullets and turkeys are presented in the growth and feed tables. These figures can be used as a guide in estimating the amount of feed required. Considerable variation from these figures may occur due to differences in the nutrient density of feed, strain or breed of bird, amount of feed wasted, and environmental temperature.

Most diets used in feeding poultry are nutritionally "complete" diets that are commercially mixed, ie, prepared by feed manufacturing companies, most of which employ trained nutritionists. The formulation and mixing of poultry feeds requires knowledge and experience in purchasing ingredients, experimental testing of formulas, laboratory control of ingredient quality, and use of computers. Improper mixing can result in vitamin and mineral deficiencies, lack of protection against disease, or drug toxicity.

The physical form of the feed influences the expected results. Most feeds for starting and growing birds are sold as crumbles or pellets. In the pelleting process, the mash is treated with steam and then passed through a suitably sized die under pressure. The pellets are then cooled quickly and dried by means of a forced air draft. The conditions under which pelleting occurs have an important effect on the nutritional quality of the pellets, or the crumbles that are produced by crushing the pellets.

Table 46. Vaccination Program for Broilers*

Age	Vaccine	Route	Type
1 day	Marek's disease	Subcut.	Turkey herpesvirus (HVT)
1 day	Newcastle disease	Coarse spray	B1
or 14-21 days	Newcastle disease	Water or coarse spray	B1 or LaSota
1 day	Infectious bronchitis	Coarse spray	Massachusetts
or 14-21 days	Infectious bronchitis	Water or coarse spray	Massachusetts
14-21 days	Infectious bursal disease	Water	Intermediate

* This is a typical vaccination program. Individual programs are highly variable and reflect local conditions, severity of challenge, and individual preferences.

Notes:

SB-1 (an avirulent strain of the virus that causes Marek's disease) is mixed with turkey herpesvirus (a closely related, avirulent virus) in some areas.

A mild strain of tenosynovitis is mixed with HVT in some areas. This vaccine may interfere with immunity against Marek's disease.

Mild strain of fowlpox vaccine is mixed with HVT in some areas. This vaccine may interfere with immunity against Marek's disease.

Infectious bursal disease vaccine may be combined with HVT.

Connecticut strain often combined with Massachusetts. Bronchitis vaccine is usually combined with Newcastle.

Other bronchitis strains such as Arkansas 99 and Florida 88 are included in some areas.

14-21 day vaccinations are optional. A single drinking water application for Newcastle/bronchitis is common also.

METHODS OF FEEDING

For newly hatched birds of any species, a "complete" feed in crumble form is the program of choice, regardless of other considerations. A "complete" feed program for growing stock, particularly for laying and breeding stock, is also highly recommended. Advantages of the "complete" feed program over the "mash and grain" system include the simplicity of feeding, accuracy of medication, improved balance of dietary nutrients, and superior feed conversion efficiency.

Regardless of the system of feeding, recommendations of the feed manufacturer should be followed with regard to the feeding of extra calcium, grit, or whole grain. Fresh, clean water should be available *ad lib*.

MANAGEMENT OF GROWING CHICKENS

Heated brooders for chicks are surrounded by a chick guard to keep the birds near the heat source. As the birds become older, the brooder temperature is lowered and the chick guard is moved out until the birds finally have the run of the whole pen. Ample space should be provided for feeders and waterers, which should be well distributed in the pen.

Table 47. Vaccination Program for Broiler Breeders*

Age	Vaccine	Route	Type
1 day	Marek's disease	Subcut.	Turkey herpesvirus (HVT)
6-7 days	Tenosynovitis	Subcut.	Live (Mild)
14-21 days	Newcastle/infectious bronchitis	Water	B1/Mass
14-28 days	Infectious bursal disease	Water	Intermediate
4 wk	Newcastle/infectious bronchitis	Water or coarse spray	B1/Mass
6-8 wk	Tenosynovitis	Subcut.	Live (Mild)
8-10 wk	Infectious bursal disease	Water or coarse spray	Live
8-10 wk	Newcastle/infectious bronchitis	Water or coarse spray	B1 or LaSota/Mass
10-12 wk	Encephalomyelitis	Wing web	Live, chick-embryo origin
10-12 wk	Fowlpox	Wing web	Modified live
10-12 wk	Laryngotracheitis	Intraocular	Modified live
10-12 wk	Tenosynovitis	Parenteral	Inactivated
10-12 wk	Fowl cholera	Parenteral	Inactivated
or	Fowl cholera	Wing web	Live (CU or M9)
12-14 wk	Newcastle/infectious bronchitis	Water or aerosol	B1 or LaSota/Mass
14-18 wk	Fowl cholera	Parenteral	Inactivated
or	Fowl cholera	Wing web	Live CU or M9
16-18 wk	Infectious bursal disease	Parenteral	Inactivated
16-18 wk	Tenosynovitis	Parenteral	Inactivated
16-18 wk and every	Newcastle/infectious bronchitis	Water or aerosol	B1 or LaSota/Mass
60-90 days	Newcastle/infectious bronchitis	Water or aerosol	B1 or LaSota/Mass
or 18 wk	Newcastle/infectious bronchitis	Parenteral	Inactivated

*This is a typical vaccination program. Individual programs are highly variable and reflect local conditions, severity of challenge, and individual preferences.

Notes:

SB-1 may be combined with HVT in some areas (*see* TABLE 46).

Vaccination for fowlpox and laryngotracheitis depends on local requirements.

Other strains of infectious bronchitis (Connecticut, Arkansas 99, Florida 88, etc) are included in some areas.

At least 3 in. (7.5 cm) of suitable litter, clean for each brood, and spread to an even depth, should be provided at the start. Litter must be free of mold; it should absorb moisture without caking, be nontoxic, and of large enough particle size to discourage consumption. Chicks are started with 24 hr of light for several days; thereafter, light is reduced. Both length of day and intensity of light are important. Lighting programs vary widely depending on whether housing is windowless or open-sided, and should comply with recommendations of major breeders in similar situations.

Feeding systems are often combined with day-length control during rearing to influence the rate at which birds mature. Under certain conditions, pullets may be debeaked at 4-7 days of age. In controlled environment housing, day lengths are controlled more precisely, and with dim lights, debeaking may be delayed until later in the growing period.

Pullets should be treated for external and internal parasites as required. Vaccination should be used to control problem diseases of the area (*see* the POU section, p 1541 *et seq* and TABLES 46, 47, and 48).

Table 48. Vaccination Program for Commercial Layers*

Age	Vaccine	Route	Type
1 day	Marek's disease	Subcut.	Turkey herpesvirus (HVT)
14-21 days	Newcastle/infectious bronchitis	Water	B1/Mass
14-21 days	Infectious bursal disease	Water	Intermediate
4 wk	Newcastle/infectious bronchitis	Water or coarse spray	B1/Mass
8-10 wk	Newcastle/infectious bronchitis	Water or coarse spray	B1 or LaSota/Mass
10-12 wk	Encephalomyelitis	Wing web	Live, chick-embryo origin
10-12 wk	Fowlpox	Wing web	Modified live
10-12 wk	Laryngotracheitis	Intraocular	Modified live
10-14 wk	*Mycoplasma gallisepticum*	Intraocular or spray	F strain
or 18 wk	*M gallisepticum*	Parenteral	Inactivated
12-14 wk	Newcastle/infectious bronchitis	Water or aerosol	B1 or LaSota/Mass
16-18 wk and every	Newcastle/infectious bronchitis	Water or aerosol	B1 or LaSota/Mass
60-90 days	Newcastle/infectious bronchitis	Water or aerosol	B1 or LaSota/Mass
or 18 wk	Newcastle/infectious bronchitis	Parenteral	Inactivated

*This is a typical vaccination program. Individual programs are highly variable and reflect local conditions, severity of challenge, and individual preferences.

Notes:

SB-1 may be combined with HVT in some areas (*see* TABLE 46).

Vaccination for infectious bursal disease, laryngotracheitis, and fowlpox depends on local requirements.

Other strains of infectious bronchitis (Connecticut, Arkansas 99, Florida 88, etc) are included in some areas.

Mycoplasma gallisepticum and *Haemophilus gallinarum* (coryza) are used only on infected, multi-age premises.

Many pullets are reared in cages. The cage manufacturer usually supplies specific instructions regarding heating, bird density, feeding space, etc. Most commercial rations are fortified with sufficient nutrients to meet the requirements of cage-reared birds.

MANAGEMENT OF LAYING CHICKENS

Most laying pullets are housed in cages and should be moved to these facilities ≥1 wk before egg production commences. Breeders moved from a growing house to an adult house should also be given ≥1 wk to adjust to their new environment before the stress of egg production commences. Beaks should be retrimmed as necessary, and culls removed at the time of housing.

Feeders and waterers should be of the proper type, size, and height for the stock and management system. Feeders that are too shallow, too narrow, or lacking a lip or flange on the upper edge may permit excess feed waste. Uneven distribution of waterers or lack of water space results in reduced intake and thus reduced performance.

Artificial Lights: Day length should be increased gradually as the pullets come into egg production, and should reach a 14- to 16-hr light period daily at peak production for both market-egg and hatching-egg layers. An intensity of at least one foot-candle of light (10 lux) at the feed trough should be provided; this is about equal to one 60-watt light bulb to each 100 sq ft (~9 sq m), hanging 7 ft (2.1 m) above the birds. Production may decrease if day length or light intensity is reduced during the laying period. With cage systems of all types, illumination is more even if smaller wattage bulbs closer together are used rather than large bulbs suspended over the center of each aisle. With 2- or 3-tiered cages, the bulbs are suspended 6-7 in. (15-18 cm) above the level of the top cage.

Table 49. Vaccination Programs for Turkeys[1]

Age (wk)[2]	Market Turkeys	Breeder Hens	Breeder Toms
2-3	Newcastle disease (ND), B1-B1[3] or LaSota, DW[4] or spray	ND, B1-B1 or LaSota, DW or spray	ND, B1-B1 or LaSota, DW or spray
4	Hemorrhagic enteritis, DW	Hemorrhagic enteritis, DW	Hemorrhagic enteritis, DW
6	Fowl cholera[5], DW (live) or subcut. (inactivated)	Fowl cholera, DW (live) or subcut. (inactivated)	Fowl cholera, DW (live) or subcut. (inactivated)
9-10	ND, LaSota, DW or spray	ND, LaSota, DW or spray	ND, LaSota, DW or spray
12	Fowl cholera, DW (live) or subcut. (inactivated)	Fowl cholera, DW (live) or subcut. (inactivated)	Fowl cholera, DW (live) or subcut. (inactivated)
15	ND, LaSota, DW or spray	ND, LaSota, DW or spray	ND, LaSota, DW or spray
18	—	Fowl cholera, DW (live) or subcut. (inactivated)	Fowl cholera, DW (live) or subcut. (inactivated)
21	—	ND, LaSota, DW or spray	ND, LaSota, DW or spray
24	—	Fowl cholera, DW (live) or subcut. (inactivated)	Fowl cholera, DW (live) or subcut. (inactivated)
26	—	Erysipelas, DW (live) or subcut. (inactivated) Pox, WW[4]	Erysipelas, DW (live) or subcut. (inactivated) Pox, WW
28	—	ND, subcut. (inactivated) Fowl cholera, DW (live) or subcut. (inactivated) Encephalomyelitis, DW	ND, subcut. (inactivated) Fowl cholera, DW (live) or subcut. (inactivated) Encephalomyelitis, DW

[1] Recommendations are for production areas where the diseases listed are common. In addition, other vaccinations may be advisable if previous experience indicates prevalence of certain diseases in the area. These may include: turkey bordetellosis eye drop vaccine at 1 day old and in water or spray at 14 days old, or bacterin; paramyxovirus 3 and influenza A (prevalent hemagglutinin) at 26-28 and 40 wk old; erysipelas—live or killed products might be required for market turkeys, and repeated vaccinations might be required for breeders; and salmonellosis bacterins at 24 and 28 wk old.

[2] Recommended age at vaccination is an approximation.

[3] Spray ND vaccines should not be used for birds suffering from respiratory disease; in such cases and at that age, the mild B1-B1 strain vaccine could be used in water. Timing of vaccination depends on maternal antibody levels.

[4] DW = drinking water; WW = wing web stab.

[5] Live fowl cholera vaccines should be used only in healthy flocks.

Record Keeping: Successful intensive poultry keeping requires good records of all flock activities, including hatch date, regular body weights (to ensure that the pullets will have reached optimal body wt when they are brought into egg production), lighting program, house temperatures, disease history, medication and vaccination dates, quantity and type of feed given (important in calculating efficiency of feed utilization), and mortality.

Table 50. Vaccination Program for Duck Breeders

Estimated number of weeks before onset of egg production*	Duck Hepatitis Virus (DHV)		Duck Virus Enteritis (Duck plague)
	Type I** (Classic)	Type III***	Live Chick Embryo Attenuated Strain
12	X	X	X
8	X		
4	X	X	
After onset of egg production			
Every 3 mo	X		
Every 6 mo		X	
Yearly			X

* White Pekin breeder ducks normally start egg production at 28 wk of age. Egg production can be accelerated or delayed. Breeder vaccination should be before onset of egg production to optimize parenteral immunity. The vaccines are administered subcut. in the neck.

** A modified live virus vaccine of chick-embryo origin, provided as a frozen concentrate and sterile diluent, which are mixed together just before use. Used mainly for vaccination of breeder ducks to obtain immune offspring, it also can be used for early vaccination of ducklings susceptible to DHV.

*** A modified live virus vaccine of duck embryo origin, provided as a frozen concentrate and a sterile diluent, which are mixed together just before use. Used mainly for vaccination of breeder ducks to obtain immune offspring.

Table 51. Vaccination Program for Domestic Ducklings

Age	Bacterin		Vaccine
	Pasteurella* anatipestifer	Pasteurella** anatipestifer and Escherichia coli	Pasteurella*** anatipestifer live vaccine
1 day old			X
2 wk	X	X	
3 wk	X	X	

* A suspension of formalin-killed whole cultures of 3 major serotypes of *P anatipestifer*. It is recommended for preventive immunization on farms where the disease is endemic or epidemic; 2 injections are necessary.

** A suspension of formalin-killed whole cultures of 3 serotypes of *P anatipestifer* and one of *E coli*.

Both should be shaken before use, and stored at 35-45°F (2-7°C), without freezing. Ducklings should not be vaccinated within 21 days of slaughter.

*** A live, avirulent vaccine consisting of 3 major serotypes of *P anatipestifer*. Administered by aerosol to 1-day-old ducklings.

Floor Space, Feeding, and Watering Requirements: Egg-production type birds usually spend their entire lives in cages. While some broiler breeders are similarly housed, most are reared on litter floors or in pens where up to two-thirds of the floor is slatted. For egg-strain pullets that are reared in cages, there is little chance of altering the feeding and watering space available, but periodic checks are necessary to ensure that feed and water are being continuously supplied. With the success of

Table 52. Space Requirements for Egg-strain Birds

Cages

Age in wk	Floor area per bird		Straight trough feeder space per bird not less than		Waterers		Trough space per bird	
	sq in.	sq cm	in.	cm	Birds per nipple	Birds per cup	in.	cm
0-6	25	161	1	2.5	15	25	1	2.5
7-18	43	277	2	5	8	12	1	2.5
19 onward	60	387	3	7.5	8	12	2	5

Litter and Slats

Age in wk	Floor area—litter only or combined with slats		Straight trough feeder space per bird		Pans (15 in. [38 cm] diameter) per 100 birds		Waterers	Trough space per bird	
	sq ft/ bird	birds/sq meter	in.	cm	Full fed	Restricted	Birds per fount	in.	cm
0-6	0.5	20	1	2.5	3	—	100	1	2.5
7-13	1	10	2	5	4	5	50	1	2.5
19 onward	1-1.5	7-10	3	7.5	4	—	30	2	5

nipple- and cup-waterers and the various types of automatic feeding systems, it becomes more difficult to give specific recommendations for feeding and watering space. Decisions must be made about optimal floor space and feeding and watering requirements based on advice from equipment manufacturers, careful observation, and past experience as to productivity. The space requirements for egg-strain and meat-strain birds presented in TABLES 52 and 53 are meant simply as a guide. Environmental housing and various types of ventilation may alter these specifications.

Table 53. Space Requirements for Meat-strain Birds

Age	Floor Space	Feeder Space*	Cups or Founts* (per 1000 birds)
From day 1	Heated area 5 sq ft (0.46 sq m) of brooder/100 chicks	10 trays/1000 (feed little and often)	8
From wk 1	1 sq ft/bird (10-11 birds/sq m)	2 in. (5 cm)/bird	20
From wk 8	2 sq ft/bird (5-6 birds/sq m)	4 in. (10 cm)/bird	30
Mated adults	All litter: 3 sq ft/bird (3.6 birds/sq m)	4 in. (10 cm)/bird	30 (60 in hot weather)
	½ to ⅔ slats: 2¼ sq ft/bird (4.3 birds/sq m)		

* For feeder and drinking trough space, count both sides of the trough. Drinking trough space (all ages) is 1 in. (2.5 cm) per bird, except double this for adults in hot weather.

Pen size: The smaller the pen population, the better the average flock performance. The ideal flock size depends on several factors, including labor and cost, and can be determined only by the individual poultryman.

NUTRITIONAL DISEASES

A nutritional deficiency may be simple or multiple, ie, the total feed consumed may contain an inadequate quantity of one or more essential nutrients. A given deficiency may be borderline, marked, or absolute. About the only observable result of a borderline deficiency is poorer feed utilization, or slightly decreased growth, egg production, or hatchability. An absolute deficiency of any essential nutrient can result in cessation of production or growth, and eventually, death. A marked deficiency of one or more essential nutrients leads to overt disease.

Since many deficiency diseases result in the same clinical signs (eg, retarded growth, poor feathering, and weakness), in most instances, a correct diagnosis can be made only by obtaining complete information about the diet and management of the birds, clinical signs in the affected living birds, and necropsies of at least a few birds soon after death. Because they are difficult to diagnose, chronic deficiencies may be more costly than acute ones.

The composition of individual ingredients in a diet is variable, and some nutrients are comparatively unstable while others are unavailable as they occur naturally in feeds. A diet that, by analysis, appears to contain just enough of one or more nutrients may actually be deficient to some degree in those nutrients. Stress (bacterial, parasitic, and viral infections; high or low temperatures; low humidity; drugs) may either interfere with absorption of a nutrient or increase the quantity required. Thus, a toxin, microorganism, etc, may destroy, or render unavailable to the bird, a particular nutrient that is present in the diet at normally adequate levels.

Only deficiencies occurring in practical diets in the field are discussed below.

PROTEIN AND AMINO ACID DEFICIENCIES

The optimal level of balanced protein intake for young growing chicks is ~18-23% of the diet; for young growing poults and gallinaceous upland game birds, ~26-30%; and for young growing ducklings and goslings, ~20-22%. If the protein content of the diet is below these levels, the birds tend to grow more slowly. Even when a diet contains the above specified quantities of protein, satisfactory growth requires sufficient quantities and proper balance of all the essential amino acids. With a lowering of the available protein in the diet, the calorie:protein ratio usually increases, which can reduce egg production or growth, and increase fat deposition in the bird.

Few specific signs are associated with a deficiency of the various amino acids, except for a peculiar cup-shaped appearance of the feathers in arginine-deficient chickens, and loss of pigment in some of the wing feathers in bronze turkeys with lysine deficiency. All deficiencies of essential amino acids result in retarded growth, or reduced egg size or egg production.

MINERAL DEFICIENCIES

CALCIUM AND PHOSPHORUS IMBALANCES

A deficiency of either calcium (Ca) or phosphorus (P) in the diet of young growing birds results in abnormal bone development even though the diet contains adequate vitamin D. This condition, rickets, can also be caused by a dietary deficiency of vitamin D (qv, p 1272) because vitamin D is necessary for absorption of Ca. A deficiency of either Ca or P results in lack of normal skeletal calcification. Rickets is seen mainly in young growing birds; Ca deficiency in adult laying hens usually results in osteoporosis. This wasting of bone structure causes a disorder that is commonly referred to as "cage layer fatigue". When Ca is mobilized from bone to overcome a dietary deficiency, the cortical bones become too thin to support the weight of the hen.

Etiology: The bones of the newly hatched chick or poult have a much lower Ca:P ratio than those of adults. Hence, the newly hatched bird requires an immediate supply of dietary Ca. If the diet is markedly deficient in either Ca or vitamin D, the osteoporotic condition becomes more pronounced. However, osteoporotic conditions are not common in young chicks. Rickets is by far the most common skeletal problem seen in chicks. In addition to the causes mentioned above, a high level of dietary Ca ties up P and renders it unavailable to the bird, and results in rickets.

Clinical and Laboratory Findings: The first signs of a deficiency of Ca or P, or both, in young growing birds are similar to those of vitamin D deficiency. All 3 deficiencies typically cause a stiff gait, retarded growth, and ruffled feathers. The beaks and leg bones are rubbery, and the joints tend to be enlarged. In Ca deficiency, some birds may become paralyzed.

If a hen in heavy egg production does not obtain enough Ca from its feed, "cage-layer fatigue" occurs; a few thin-shelled eggs and also eggs with low hatchability are produced, and then production ceases. If Ca is not supplied following paralysis, death follows within 1-3 days.

In both rickets and osteoporosis, ash content of the bones is decreased. If dietary Ca is low, the blood level of Ca may be approximately normal, but the level of P may be increased due to the breakdown of labile bone.

Prophylaxis and Treatment: Diets must provide adequate quantities of Ca and P to prevent deficiencies. However, feeding diets that contain >2.5% Ca during the growing period produces a high incidence of nephrosis, visceral gout, calcium urate deposits in the ureters, and at times, high mortality.

Eggshell strength can be improved by feeding ~50% of the dietary Ca supplement in the form of oyster-shell flakes or coarse limestone, with the remaining half as ground limestone. Oyster shell or any other form of Ca supplement should never be added without an equivalent reduction in the amount of limestone; feeding too much Ca reduces feed consumption and egg production. Offering the coarse supplement permits the birds to satisfy their requirements when they need it most, or allows the coarse material to be retained in the gizzard and the Ca to be meted out continuously.

A readily assimilable Ca supplement is effective if started very soon after paralysis develops from Ca deficiency.

MANGANESE DEFICIENCY

A deficiency of manganese in the diet of young growing chickens is one of the causes of perosis, and of thin-shelled eggs and poor hatchability (*see also* CALCIUM AND PHOSPHORUS IMBALANCES, above, and VITAMIN D DEFICIENCY, p 1272). It may also cause chondrodystrophy.

Etiology: Most poultry feedstuffs are poor sources of manganese. Perosis caused by manganese deficiency is exacerbated by excess calcium (Ca) and phosphorus (P) in the diet. Birds reared on wire or slatted floors are more susceptible to perosis than those reared on litter. All commercial poultry diets are now supplemented with a source of available manganese, eg, manganese sulfate. Since manganese deficiency is now rare, other possible causes should be considered when perosis is encountered (*see* TWISTED LEG, p 1604, CHOLINE DEFICIENCY, p 1274, and NIACIN DEFICIENCY, p 1275).

Clinical Findings: Perosis is a malformation of the hock joint; usually the joint is swollen and flattened, and sometimes the Achilles tendon slips from its condyles. The tibia and the tarsometatarsus of one or both legs may bend near the joint and rotate laterally. A shortening and thickening of the long bones of the legs and wings may be apparent. Signs in poults, ducklings, and goslings are similar to those in chicks. Perosis has been observed in various wild birds, including pheasants, grouse, quail, and sparrows.

Adult chickens fed a diet deficient in manganese have no observable changes in their leg joints, but the shells of their eggs tend to become thinner and less resistant to breakage. If the deficiency is sufficiently marked, both egg production and hatchability are reduced. The reduced hatchability results from an increase in embryonic mortality that occurs after day 10 of incubation and peaks at about day 20-21. The embryos that die after day 10 usually are chondrodystrophic; they have short thickened legs, short wings, "parrot beaks", a globular contour of the head, protruding abdomen and, in the most severe cases, retarded development of the down. The few chicks that hatch usually have very short leg bones (micromelia), and the bones may be deformed as in chicks in which perosis develops after hatching. Manganese deficiency is not likely to occur in adult birds raised by conventional methods on commercial starting, growing, and developing rations; these rations are fortified with manganese salts, and the birds can store enough manganese to provide for the small needs of this element for egg production over a long period of time.

Prophylaxis and Treatment: Prevention of perosis requires a diet adequate in all necessary nutrients, especially manganese, choline, niacin, biotin, and folic acid. Deformities cannot be corrected by feeding. Effects of manganese deficiency on egg production are fully corrected by an adequate diet that contains 30-40 mg/kg of manganese, provided that the diet does not contain excess Ca and P. Ca intake may be excessive if Ca supplements are provided free choice. When meat meal or meat-and-bone meal is used as the principal source of protein, the feed may contain excess P.

IRON AND COPPER DEFICIENCIES

A microcytic, hypochromic anemia with no change in the number of RBC can be produced by iron or copper deficiency. A deficiency of iron, due to its role in RBC synthesis, has a direct causative effect on anemia. The anemia of copper deficiency is more indirect. A copper deficiency can cause depigmentation of feathers.

Since copper is essential in the synthesis of elastin tissue, a deficiency can result in weak or thin blood vessels and, hence, has been suggested as a cause of dissecting aneurysm in poultry, especially turkeys (qv, p 1548). However, experiments have shown no benefit of added copper for prevention of aortic rupture in turkeys. Most practical diets for poultry contain adequate iron and copper. Nevertheless, most feed manufacturers add small amounts as an insurance measure.

IODINE DEFICIENCY

Few cases of goiter, or enlarged thyroids, have been observed in poultry, probably because commercial poultry diets are almost universally fortified with iodine, either as iodized salt or in the mineral premix. Goiter has been produced experimentally in laying hens by feeding a diet exceedingly low in iodine (~0.025 ppm). Some of the older varieties of rapeseed meal, which were high in goitrogenic factors, invariably resulted in birds with enlarged thyroids if significant quantities were fed. Iodine deficiency in poultry is obviated easily by supplementing the feed with as little as 0.35 mg of iodine/kg.

MAGNESIUM DEFICIENCY

Magnesium deficiency seldom occurs in poultry fed practical diets. It may be produced experimentally by feeding a diet of highly purified feedstuffs. In young chicks, such a diet causes poor growth and feathering, decreased muscle tone, ataxia, progressive incoordination, and convulsions followed by death.

POTASSIUM DEFICIENCY

Most feedstuffs and many of the by-product feedstuffs used in commercial poultry rations contain more potassium than is needed; therefore, deficiencies are not ordinarily seen. An exception occurred in Australia when meat meal, low in potassium, supplied the major portion of the supplemental protein.

SALT DEFICIENCY

The salt (NaCl) requirement of chickens, and presumably other kinds of poultry, is low. Sodium is required in appreciably larger quantity than chlorine, and diets with <0.13% sodium retard growth in young chicks. Egg production and hatchability in laying chickens are depressed when the sodium level is <0.1%. A high level of potassium appears to increase the requirement for sodium and *vice versa*. Most practical poultry diets require the addition of 0.25-0.35% of salt to prevent a deficiency.

Inasmuch as nearly all feedstuffs contain some salt, and a few contain 1-4.5% or more (eg, whey, fish meal, meat meal, condensed fish solubles), an excess of salt is possible. An excess causes the droppings to be loose and watery. Chickens may be raised on diets that contain as much as 3% salt if clean drinking water is available, but growth is retarded and feed efficiency is reduced. The bird can tolerate much less salt in the drinking water since, as the level rises to 0.9%, the bird cannot get rid of excess salt by drinking more water.

ZINC DEFICIENCY

When a diet is deficient in zinc, growth is retarded and feather development is poor. The hock joints may become enlarged, and the long bones shortened and thickened. Slipping of the tendons does not occur. On occasion, the skin on the foot pads becomes dry, thickened, and fissured, and hyperkeratosis develops.

In mature hens, zinc deficiency reduces egg production and hatchability. Embryos show a wide range of skeletal abnormalities including micromelia; curvature of the spine; and shortened, fused thoracic and lumbar vertebrae. It is usual practice to include a zinc supplement in all practical poultry diets.

SELENIUM DEFICIENCY

A deficiency of selenium in growing chickens causes exudative diathesis. The early signs (unthriftiness, ruffled feathers) usually occur at 5-11 wk of age. The edema results in weeping of the skin, which is often seen on the inner surface of the thighs and wings. The birds bruise easily; large scabs often form on old bruises. In laying hens, the tissue damage is unusual, but egg production, hatchability, and feed conversion are adversely affected.

In most countries it is now legal to add selenium to starter and grower diets. In most cases, 0.1 ppm is permitted in chicken diets and 0.2 ppm in turkey diets. The commonly used forms are sodium selenate and sodium selenite. Feeds grown on high-selenium soils may be used in poultry rations and are good sources of selenium. Fish meal and dried brewer's yeast are also good sources. Availability of selenium varies considerably in different feedstuffs. Even with adequate vitamin E, rations must contain selenium at 0.15-0.2 mg/kg of feed. Eight to 10 mg/kg is toxic.

VITAMIN DEFICIENCIES

VITAMIN A DEFICIENCY

Vitamin A is required for normal development and repair of epithelial structures and for normal development of bones. It helps combat disease by maintaining the "first line of defense", the epithelial structures.

Vitamin A and its several precursors (α, β, and γ-carotene and cryptoxanthin) are relatively unstable. Feeds stored for a long time may lose a large portion of their vitamin A activity, especially if they contain sources of unstabilized polyunsaturated fats.

Clinical Findings: When young chicks are fed a diet markedly deficient in vitamin A, their growth rate becomes subnormal after ~3 wk and then declines rapidly. Other early characteristic signs are droopiness, ataxia, and ruffled feathers. If the chicks survive another week, the eyes may become inflamed and there may be a discharge from the nostrils; in some chicks, swelling around the eyes develops and a sticky exudate accumulates beneath the lids. When the diet is not markedly deficient in vitamin A, the first signs may not appear until the chicks are 4-6 wk old, in which case, a larger proportion of the chicks eventually develop eye lesions and marked nervousness.

Signs of vitamin A deficiency in poults are similar to those in chicks, but tend to be more acute. In mature chickens and other poultry, signs develop more slowly than in young birds, but the inflammation of the nose and eyes is much more pronounced. A borderline deficiency results in decreased egg production and hatchability.

Lesions: In mature birds, vitamin A deficiency produces lesions resembling pustules in the mouth, pharynx, and esophagus; in young growing birds, these lesions are less frequent. Often, there are white or grayish white urate deposits in the kidneys and ureters; they occur more frequently in young chickens than in poults. Sometimes, there are urate deposits on the surfaces of the heart, liver, and spleen. Usually, urate or urate-like deposits are found in the thickened folds of the bursa of Fabricius.

In general, there is keratinization of the epithelial cells of the olfactory, respiratory, upper alimentary, and urinary tracts. In severe cases, especially in mature birds, virtually all organs may be affected. Also, degenerative changes in both the central and peripheral nervous systems occur.

In marked vitamin A deficiency in chickens, the uric acid content of the blood may increase 8-9 times. The accumulation of uric acid in the blood and deposits in the ureters, kidneys, and elsewhere probably are due to failure of repair of the epithelial structures, especially those of the kidneys.

The nasal structures may be used in diagnosing borderline deficiencies. In all degrees of vitamin A deficiency, there are true squamous metaplasia of the secretory and glandular epithelium, and secondary inflammatory or obstructive changes. In absolute deficiency, atrophy, squamous metaplasia, and hyperkeratinization occur.

Prophylaxis and Treatment: While the naturally occurring vitamin A precursors tend to be unstable (oxidize) in stored feed, most feed manufacturers include an antioxidant to prevent this. Also, since stabilized, dry, vitamin A supplements are almost universally used today, it is unlikely that a deficiency will be encountered.

However, if a deficiency does develop through inadvertent omission of the vitamin A supplement or because of poor mixing, 3-4 times the normally recommended level should be fed for ~2 wk. The dry, stabilized forms of vitamin A are the feed supplements of choice. Forms that can be administered through the drinking water are available, and usually result in faster recovery than medication of the feed.

VITAMIN D DEFICIENCY

Abnormal development of the bones has been discussed under calcium and phosphorus deficiencies and manganese deficiency (*see* above). Vitamin D is required for the normal absorption and metabolism of calcium and phosphorus. Thus, a deficiency can result in rickets in young growing chickens and osteoporosis and poor eggshell quality in laying hens, even though the diets may be well supplied with calcium and phosphorus.

Etiology: The rickets and osteoporosis encountered in practical production of poultry most frequently are due to a deficiency of vitamin D. Most poultry reared in strict confinement need a higher dietary level of vitamin D than those that have access to sunshine.

Mycotoxins in the feed or litter may cause a vitamin D deficiency, apparently by interfering with absorption of the vitamin (as well as of fat and the other fat-soluble vitamins).

Clinical Findings: The first signs in young chickens and turkeys are a tendency to rest frequently in a squatting position, a disinclination to walk, and a stiff gait. These are distinguished from the clinical signs of vitamin A deficiency in that birds with a vitamin D deficiency are alert rather than droopy and walk with a lame rather than a staggering gait. Other signs, in the usual order of occurrence, are retarded growth, enlarged hock joints, beading at the ends of the ribs, and marked softening of the beak. As in many other nutritional diseases, the feathers soon become ruffled.

In red or buff-colored breeds of chickens, a deficiency of vitamin D causes an abnormal black pigmentation of some feathers, especially those of the wings. If the deficiency is marked, the blackening becomes pronounced, and nearly all feathers may be affected. When adequate vitamin D is supplied, the new feathers and the newer part of the older feathers are normal in color; the discolored portion remains black.

When laying chickens are deficient in vitamin D, the first sign is thinning of their eggshells. If the deficiency is marked, there is a prompt reduction of egg production and hatchability. Embryos frequently die at 18-19 days of age. After a time, the breast bones become noticeably less rigid, and there may be beading at the rib ends.

Lesions: In young chickens and turkeys, there are marked changes in the bones and parathyroid glands, and variable changes in the calcium and phosphorus content of the blood. The bones may be moderately to quite soft. The epiphyses of the long bones usually are enlarged. The parathyroid becomes enlarged, sometimes to ~8 times its normal size, as a result of hypertrophy and hyperplasia.

In adult chickens, a deficiency of vitamin D eventually produces changes in the parathyroid similar to those produced in young chicks. The bones tend to become rarefied (osteoporotic) rather than soft.

Treatment: Enough vitamin D is added to commercial diets to provide 3 times the normally recommended level for a period of ~3 wk. Dry, stabilized forms of vitamin D_3 are recommended.

In severe cases of mycotoxicosis, a water-miscible form of vitamin D is administered in the drinking water to provide ~3 times the amount normally supplied in the diet.

VITAMIN E DEFICIENCY

Chicks deficient in vitamin E may show one or more of 3 classical disorders, viz, encephalomalacia, exudative diathesis, and muscular dystrophy. Various dietary changes unrelated to the vitamin E content of the diet can completely prevent any one of these diseases without affecting the course of the other two. Thus, synthetic antioxidants can prevent encephalomalacia, inorganic selenium can prevent exudative diathesis, and cystine can prevent muscular dystrophy. It appears that no common metabolic defect can account for all 3 disorders. Vitamin E is required for normal reproductive performance in the hen and for normal fertility in the mature male.

Etiology: Although both selenium and antioxidants can spare the requirements of vitamin E for certain functions, practical poultry diets should still contain vitamin E. Encephalomalacia occurs when diets borderline in vitamin E also contain polyunsaturated fats such as fish oils or vegetable oils that oxidize and become rancid. Since vitamin E deficiency is related to peroxidation of fats, it may be prevented with vitamin E or a suitable antioxidant, eg, ethoxyquin. Exudative diathesis is common when birds are fed corn and soybean meal diets that were grown on soils deficient in selenium; both vitamin E and selenium are necessary to prevent it. Nutritional muscular dystrophy, not ordinarily a commercial problem, is found only when the diet is deficient in both vitamin E and sulfur amino acids. Because of the importance of sulfur amino acids for growth and feed efficiency, they are usually present in adequate levels in practical diets.

Clinical Findings: Signs of encephalomalacia are sudden prostration, with legs outstretched and toes flexed, and retraction of the head. In early stages, the gait may not be coordinated. At necropsy, lesions are found in the cerebellum and sometimes in the cerebrum. In some birds, necrotic, reddish or brownish areas are on the surface of the cerebellum.

Exudative diathesis is a severe edema produced by a marked increase in capillary permeability (*see* SELENIUM DEFICIENCY, p 1271). Broilers are often severely downgraded because of the yellow staining inside the thighs caused by leakage of plasma into the subcut. tissues.

Nutritional muscular dystrophy in chicks is characterized by degeneration of the muscle fibers, especially of the breast, but also occasionally of the leg. There is perivascular infiltration, with marked accumulation of eosinophils, lymphocytes, and histiocytes. Large numbers of free nuclei are evident.

In mature chickens, no outward signs of vitamin E deficiency are apparent even after a prolonged period. However, degenerative changes in the testes may occur, which leads to loss of fertility. Egg production appears not to be affected, but hatchability is markedly reduced. During incubation, growth and differentiation are slow, and many embryos die during the first few days of incubation due to circulatory failure.

Prophylaxis and Treatment: Only stabilized fat should be used in feed. When feed is stored for >2 wk, a chemical antioxidant should be used. High ambient temperatures and high humidity accentuate destruction of vitamin E.

Signs of exudative diathesis and muscular dystrophy due to vitamin E deficiency can be reversed provided that treatment is begun early by administering vitamin E by oral dosing or through the feed. Oral administration of a single dose of 300 IU of vitamin E per bird usually causes remission. Old feed should be replaced with fresh that is amply fortified with vitamin E.

VITAMIN K DEFICIENCY

Vitamin K deficiency reduces the prothrombin content of the blood. For some time there has been a tendency to reduce the quantity of alfalfa meal, which is a rich natural source of vitamins K and E, in poultry feeds. There also has been a trend toward use of solvent-extracted soybean meal and other seed meals, and better quality but less putrefied fish meals, which are lower in vitamin K than the original expeller meals and putrid fish meals. Thus, it is now common practice for all commercial diets to contain added synthetic vitamin K.

Clinical Findings: In young chicks deficient in vitamin K, blood coagulation time begins to increase after ~5-10 days of age and becomes greatly prolonged in 7-12 days. After ~1 wk, hemorrhages often occur in any part of the body, either spontaneously or as the result of an injury or bruise. The only external signs are the resulting subcut. hematomas. Necropsy usually reveals accumulations of blood in various parts of the body; sometimes there are petechiae in the liver, and almost invariably there is erosion of the gizzard lining. When hemorrhagic disease is encountered under practical conditions, the signs usually are observed after 3 wk of age.

Prophylaxis and Treatment: The inclusion of menadione at 1 mg/ton of feed is effective and is now a common practice. If signs of vitamin K deficiency are encountered, the level should be doubled. A number of stress factors increase the requirements for vitamin K, eg, coccidiosis and other intestinal parasitic diseases. Dicumarol, sulfaquinoxaline, and warfarin are antimetabolites of vitamin K.

VITAMIN B_{12} DEFICIENCY

The vitamin B_{12} requirement of poultry is exceedingly low; an adequate allowance is only a few μg/kg of feed. Vitamin B_{12} is produced by many bacteria and, in general, is present in feedstuffs of animal origin and in feces. Vitamin B_{12} is now included in most commercial poultry feeds, thus making a deficiency unlikely. It is required for growth and hatchability.

Marked vitamin B_{12} deficiency is difficult, if not impossible, to produce in birds that have free access to their droppings. However, such birds may not receive optimal vitamin B_{12} levels and may fail to grow at a maximal rate. While few truly characteristic signs of vitamin B_{12} deficiency have been reported, it is one of several causes of retarded growth, decreased feed efficiency, and reduced hatchability. It is easily prevented and cured by feeding a diet containing feedstuffs of animal origin or a commercial cobalamin supplement.

CHOLINE DEFICIENCY

Choline has several physiological functions in poultry. In addition to being necessary for the prevention of perosis, it plays a role in growth, methylation, and regulation of the synthesis and transport of lipids. A deficiency of choline in the diet, even when quantities of manganese, biotin, folic acid, and niacin are adequate, results in perosis (*see* MANGANESE DEFICIENCY, p 1269) and retarded growth. There is some evidence that choline is required for maximal egg production, high hatchability, and prevention of fatty livers. However, laying hens have considerable ability to synthesize choline, and practical diets may provide enough for their needs.

Diets that contain appreciable quantities of soybean meal, wheat bran, and wheat middlings are unlikely to be deficient in choline because soybean meal is a good source of choline, and wheat bran and middlings are good sources of betaine, which can perform the methyl-donor function of choline. Other good sources of choline are distillers' grains, fish meal, liver meal, meat meals, distillers' solubles, and yeast. A number of commercial choline supplements are available, and choline is routinely added to a number of poultry feeds, especially in turkey starter diets, in which the requirement is quite high.

NIACIN (NICOTINIC ACID) DEFICIENCY

There is good evidence that poultry—even chick and turkey embryos—can synthesize niacin, but at a rate that is too slow for optimal growth. It has been claimed that a marked deficiency of niacin cannot occur in chickens, unless there is a deficiency of tryptophan, a niacin precursor.

Niacin deficiency has been observed in chicks, ducks, geese, and turkey poults when certain practical-type diets were fed. Diets high in corn (maize) and soybean meal are particularly amenable to improvement by inclusion of supplemental niacin. Ducks, turkeys, and geese have considerably higher requirements for niacin than chicks. Most of the niacin present in practical feedstuffs, such as corn, is unavailable to poultry. Mature birds are better able to synthesize niacin than young ones.

Clinical Findings: In a borderline deficiency in chicks, the only sign is retarded growth. Chicks and poults fed a deficient diet develop a hock disorder similar in appearance to perosis, with swollen hocks and bowed legs. Goslings and ducklings develop abnormalities of the legs, which have been referred to as perosis and bowed legs, respectively. Laying chickens fed a diet deficient in niacin exhibit weight loss and reduced egg production and hatchability. (*See also* MANGANESE DEFICIENCY, p 1269.)

Prophylaxis and Treatment: Niacin deficiency in chickens may be prevented by feeding a diet that contains ~27 mg niacin/kg, but many nutritionists recommend 2-2½ times as much. An allowance of 55-70 mg/kg of feed appears to be satisfactory for ducks, geese, and turkeys. Ample niacin should be provided in poultry diets so that the birds do not have to synthesize it from tryptophan, which may be difficult to supply.

PANTOTHENIC ACID DEFICIENCY

Although most poultry feedstuffs are fairly good sources of pantothenic acid, diets composed largely of cereal grains and containing some meat meal, fish meal, or both, may not contain enough of this vitamin. Kiln-dried corn (maize) tends to have lower amounts, and in general, pantothenic acid in feedstuffs is destroyed by dry heat.

Clinical Findings: When chicks are deficient, growth is retarded and the feathers appear ragged. Within 12-14 days, the eyelid margins become granulated and, frequently, a viscous exudate causes the eyelids to stick together. Crusty scabs appear at the corners of the mouth; the skin on the bottoms of the feet often becomes thickened and cornified. After 4-5 mo of chronic deficiency, feathers are lost from the head and neck. Depigmentation of the feathers has been reported.

Signs in young turkeys are similar to those in young chickens and include general weakness, keratitis, and sticking together of the eyelids. Young ducks do not show the usual signs seen in chickens and turkeys, except retarded growth; however, mortality is high.

When the diet of laying chickens is deficient in pantothenic acid, hatchability is greatly reduced. The few chicks that hatch grow slowly, and their mortality is high.

Lesions: In chicks, lesions of the spinal cord are characterized by myelin degeneration of the medullated fibers. Degenerating fibers may be found in all segments of the spinal cord down to the lumbar region. Involution of the thymus, a fatty liver, and acute nephritis also have been reported.

Prophylaxis and Treatment: While it is easy to formulate feed mixtures that are fully adequate in pantothenic acid, it is often more economical to add calcium pantothenate (~5-5.5 mg/kg of feed). Sometimes, half-grown chickens fed practical diets develop a scaly condition of the skin, the exact cause of which is not known, but treatment with both calcium pantothenate (2 g) and riboflavin (0.5 g) in the drinking water (50 gal. [190 L]) for a few days has been successful in some instances.

RIBOFLAVIN DEFICIENCY

Only a few poultry feedstuffs contain enough riboflavin to meet the requirement of young growing chicks, poults, or ducklings. Hence, if the ingredients of a poultry feed are not carefully selected, or if a special supplement is not included, a deficiency may result. Since riboflavin is generally added to practical rations, its deficiency is now relatively uncommon.

The characteristic sign in the chick is "curled toe" paralysis; however, when the deficiency is absolute or marked, the chicks die before it appears. Three degrees of severity of "curled toe" paralysis have been described: the first is characterized by a tendency of the chicks to rest on their hocks and the toes are only slightly curled; the second, by marked weakness of the legs and a distinct curling of the toes on one or both feet; and the third, by toes that are completely curled inward or under, and a weakened condition of the legs that compels the chicks to walk on their hocks.

Other signs are stunting, diarrhea after 8-10 days, and high mortality after ~3 wk. Feather growth apparently is not impaired; on the contrary, the main wing feathers often appear disproportionately long.

Signs of riboflavin deficiency in poults and ducklings differ from those in chicks. In poults, dermatitis appears in ~8 days; the vent becomes encrusted, inflamed, and excoriated; growth is retarded or completely stopped by about day 17; and deaths begin to occur about day 21. Ducklings usually have diarrhea and growth ceases.

When laying hens are fed a diet deficient in riboflavin, egg production and hatchability are reduced, roughly in proportion to the degree of the deficiency. Embryonic mortality typically peaks on days 4 and 20 of incubation, and often on day 14. Most embryos are dwarfed and have pronounced micromelia; some are edematous. The down fails to emerge properly, which results in a typical abnormality, termed "clubbed" down, which is most common around the neck and vent.

Riboflavin deficiency in young poultry produces specific changes in the main peripheral nerve trunks. In acute cases, the nerve trunks hypertrophy and exhibit readily observable changes. Degenerative changes also appear in the myelin of the nerves. Congestion and premature atrophy of the lobes of the thymus may also be observed.

THIAMINE AND PYRIDOXINE DEFICIENCIES
(Vitamin B_1 and B_6 deficiencies)

Although the amount of thiamine and pyridoxine in most poultry feedstuffs is more than adequate, thiamine deficiency has been reported in poults and chicks due to its destruction in the crop or proventriculus. Raw fish contains a thiaminase capable of breaking down thiamine into 2 nonactive forms. A similar breakdown occurs in the presence of sulfite. If signs suggestive of thiamine deficiency are observed, the diet should be examined for the presence of raw fish, and the drinking water tested for sulfites.

FOLIC ACID (FOLACIN) DEFICIENCY

Until recently it was believed unlikely that folic acid deficiency would occur in chicks or turkeys under field conditions. However, today, many feeds contain no alfalfa. Also, fish meal and meat meal are rather poor sources. While much of the folic acid in feedstuffs is present in conjugated form, young chicks can utilize it well.

Clinical Findings: In young chicks, the chief signs are retarded growth, poor feather formation, feather depigmentation in colored breeds, and mortality. The outward signs are accompanied by a macrocytic, hypochromic anemia. In turkey poults, growth rate is reduced, and a characteristic cervical paralysis develops in which the birds extend their necks and appear to gaze downwards. Since field cases usually have been in young poults, it is possible that the breeder hens were fed deficient diets. In breeding chickens, folic acid deficiency reduces egg production and hatchability. Deficient embryos show bending of the tibiotarsus, mandibular defects, syndactyly, and hemorrhages.

Prophylaxis and Treatment: When fish meal and meat meal are used as major sources of protein, or the feed is pelleted, it may be advisable to supplement breeder diets with synthetic folic acid. Many feed manufacturers also supplement turkey starter diets with folic acid at ~0.5-1 g/ton. When signs occur in young poults, the vitamin may be added to the drinking water at 150-200 mg/gal. (40-50 mg/L). In birds that are down, injection of 150 mg of folic acid per bird usually results in recovery within a few days.

BIOTIN DEFICIENCY

This vitamin is necessary to prevent perosis in chicks and poults, and a fatty liver and kidney syndrome in chickens. Deficiencies have been reported in turkey poults and young chicks. While the exact cause of such a deficiency has not been elucidated, there is some evidence that certain disease conditions in poults can increase the requirement for biotin. A deficiency is more likely to occur on diets high in wheat or barley than if corn is being fed. The availability of biotin from these and several other cereals is quite low. Good sources of biotin include liver, dried brewer's yeast, molasses, and green leafy plants. Cereals, meat meal, and fish meal are poor sources. Some of the biotin in natural feeds occurs in bound form that is poorly available to the bird. An abnormal intestinal flora can increase the bird's requirement.

Clinical Findings: In poults, typical signs include broken flight feathers, bending of the metatarsus, and a dermatitis affecting the bottoms of the feet, the corners of the mouth, and the edges of the eyelids. Egg hatchability is reduced in turkeys and chickens. Signs in embryos include "parrot beak", chondrodystrophy, micromelia, and syndactyly. Dermatitis in mature birds similar to that in chicks and poults has not been reported.

Prophylaxis and Treatment: A number of factors increase biotin requirements, including oxidative rancidity of feed fat, competition by intestinal microorganisms, and lack of carryover into the newly hatched poult. Since the best feed sources of biotin are often expensive or difficult to obtain and not completely available to the bird, it is good practice to add 150-200 mg of synthetic biotin to turkey breeder and starter diets. Certain antibiotics added to the feed spare the need for biotin, presumably by fostering a less competitive intestinal flora. Raising the feed level of materials such as dried brewer's yeast, or adding synthetic biotin to the feed or water are effective means of counteracting existing cases of biotin deficiency.

NUTRITION: RABBITS

The rabbit is a nonruminant herbivore. Its large cecum supports a population of microorganisms that uses nutrients that are not digested in the small intestine. Separation of digesta on the basis of particle size occurs in the hindgut. Peristaltic action rapidly moves large particles, primarily ligno-cellulose, through the colon and excretes them as hard fecal pellets. Antiperistaltic action moves small particles and solubles into the cecum, where they undergo fermentation. At intervals, the cecal contents are expelled as "soft feces" and consumed by the rabbit directly from the anus. This reingested material provides microbial protein, vitamins (including all the B vitamins needed), and small quantities of volatile fatty acids. However, since amino acids obtained in this manner make only a minor contribution to the rabbits' protein needs, particularly for young growing animals, the diet must supply the additional amino acids, although essential amino acid requirements have not yet been defined.

Rabbits digest fiber poorly because of the selective separation and rapid excretion of large particles in the hindgut. They do need a generous amount of fiber in the diet

(~15% crude fiber) to promote intestinal motility and minimize intestinal disease. Fiber may also absorb toxins of pathogenic bacteria and eliminate them via the "hard feces". Diets low in fiber promote an increased incidence of intestinal problems, eg, enterotoxemia. This may be a result of the higher starch content of low-fiber diets. Starch is a substrate for the proliferation of pathogenic bacteria such as *Clostridium spiroforme*, which produce a potent toxin. High-fiber diets (>20% crude fiber) may result in an increased incidence of cecal impaction and mucoid enteritis. Volatile fatty acids produced in the cecum are important metabolites since they aid in the control of pathogenic organisms by helping to maintain a low pH in the cecum.

A dietary supply of vitamins A, D, and E is necessary. Bacteria in the gut synthesize vitamin K and B vitamins in adequate quantities; thus, dietary supplements are unnecessary. Disease and stress may increase the daily vitamin requirements. Oxidation destroys vitamins A and E more readily than the other vitamins. Feed preparation and storage must be done in a manner that will reduce losses from oxidation. Diets containing ≥30% of alfalfa meal generally provide sufficient vitamin A. Levels of vitamin A in the diet must be >5000 IU/kg and <75,000 IU/kg. Levels out of this range may cause abortion, resorbed litters, and fetal hydrocephalus. Rabbits voluntarily adjust their feed intake to meet their energy needs when appropriate feed is available. Pelleted rabbit feeds largely have supplanted homegrown feeds and provide good nutrition at reasonable cost. TABLE 54 provides a summary of suggested requirements. Fresh, clean water should always be available. Rabbits fed hay (alfalfa or clover) and grain (corn, oats, barley) should be provided with a trace mineral salt block.

Table 54. Requirements of Rabbits for Some Nutrients

	Protein		Fat %	Fiber %	Digestible Carbohydrates (NFE, %)	Total Digestible Nutrients %
	Total %	Digestible %				
Maintenance	12	9	1.5-2	14-20	40-45	50-60
Growth and Finishing	16	12	2-4	14-16	45-50	60-70
Pregnancy	15	11	2-3	14-16	45-50	55-65
Lactation (with litter of 7 or 8)	17	13	2.5-3.5	12-14	45-50	65-75

NFE = nitrogen-free extract

NUTRITION: SHEEP

The economical and efficient production of lamb and wool is contingent on maximum production per ewe. Economical maintenance of breeding animals, a high percentage of the lamb crop weaned, continuous and rapid growth of lambs, heavy weaning weights, and a heavy fleece weight are important to efficiency. All of these are influenced by nutrition.

Quantifying the nutritional requirements for maintenance, reproduction, growth, finishing, and wool production is complex because sheep are maintained under a wide variety of environmental conditions.

NUTRITIONAL REQUIREMENTS

An adequate diet must include water, energy (carbohydrates and fats), proteins, minerals, and vitamins (*see* TABLE 55). These amounts generally are sufficient to promote optimal growth and production. Under field conditions of particular stress, additional nutrients may be needed.

Table 55. Daily Nutrient Requirements of Sheep

Body Wt		Wt Change/Day		Dry Matter per Animal			Energy[b]				Nutrients per Animal		Ca (g)	P (g)	Vitamin A Activity (IU)	Vitamin E Activity (IU)
											Crude protein					
(kg)	(lb)	(g)	(lb)	(kg)	(lb)	(% body wt)	TDN (kg)	TDN (lb)	DE (Mcal)	ME (Mcal)	(g)	(lb)				
Ewes[c]																
Maintenance																
50	110	10	0.02	1.0	2.2	2.0	0.55	1.2	2.4	2.0	95	0.21	2.0	1.8	2350	15
60	132	10	0.02	1.1	2.4	1.8	0.61	1.3	2.7	2.2	104	0.23	2.3	2.1	2820	16
70	154	10	0.02	1.2	2.6	1.7	0.66	1.5	2.9	2.4	113	0.25	2.5	2.4	3290	18
80	176	10	0.02	1.3	2.9	1.6	0.72	1.6	3.2	2.6	122	0.27	2.7	2.8	3760	20
90	198	10	0.02	1.4	3.1	1.5	0.78	1.7	3.4	2.8	131	0.29	2.9	3.1	4230	21
Nonlactating — First 15 wk gestation																
50	110	30	0.07	1.2	2.6	2.4	0.67	1.5	3.0	2.4	112	0.25	2.9	2.1	2350	18
60	132	30	0.07	1.3	2.9	2.2	0.72	1.6	3.2	2.6	121	0.27	3.2	2.5	2820	20
70	154	30	0.07	1.4	3.1	2.0	0.77	1.7	3.4	2.8	130	0.29	3.5	2.9	3290	21
80	176	30	0.07	1.5	3.3	1.9	0.82	1.8	3.6	3.0	139	0.31	3.8	3.3	3760	22
90	198	30	0.07	1.6	3.5	1.8	0.87	1.9	3.8	3.2	148	0.33	4.1	3.6	4230	24
Last 4 wk gestation (130-150% lambing rate expected) or last 4-6 wk lactation suckling singles[d]																
50	110	180 (45)	0.40 (0.10)	1.6	3.5	3.2	0.94	2.1	4.1	3.4	175	0.38	5.9	4.8	4250	24
60	132	180 (45)	0.40 (0.10)	1.7	3.7	2.8	1.00	2.2	4.4	3.6	184	0.40	6.0	5.2	5100	26
70	154	180 (45)	0.40 (0.10)	1.8	4.0	2.6	1.06	2.3	4.7	3.8	193	0.42	6.2	5.6	5950	27
80	176	180 (45)	0.40 (0.10)	1.9	4.2	2.4	1.12	2.4	4.9	4.0	202	0.44	6.3	6.1	6800	28
90	198	180 (45)	0.40 (0.10)	2.0	4.4	2.2	1.18	2.5	5.1	4.2	212	0.47	6.4	6.5	7650	30
Last 4 wk gestation (180-225% lambing rate expected)																
50	110	225	0.50	1.7	3.7	3.4	1.10	2.4	4.8	4.0	196	0.43	6.2	3.4	4250	26
60	132	225	0.50	1.8	4.0	3.0	1.17	2.6	5.1	4.2	205	0.45	6.9	4.0	5100	27
70	154	225	0.50	1.9	4.2	2.7	1.24	2.8	5.4	4.4	214	0.47	7.6	4.5	5950	28
80	176	225	0.50	2.0	4.4	2.5	1.30	2.9	5.7	4.7	223	0.49	8.3	5.1	6800	30
90	198	225	0.50	2.1	4.6	2.3	1.37	3.0	6.0	5.0	232	0.51	8.9	5.7	7650	32

(continued)

Table 55. Daily Nutrient Requirements of Sheep (continued)

Body Wt (kg)	Body Wt (lb)	Wt Change/Day (g)	Wt Change/Day (lb)	Dry Matter per Animal[a] (kg)	(lb)	(% body wt)	Energy[b] TDN (kg)	TDN (lb)	DE (Mcal)	ME (Mcal)	Crude protein (g)	(lb)	Ca (g)	P (g)	Vitamin A Activity (IU)	Vitamin E Activity (IU)
First 6-8 wk lactation suckling singles or last 4-6 wk lactation suckling twins[d]																
50	110	-25 (90)	-0.06 (0.20)	2.1	4.6	4.2	1.36	3.0	6.0	4.9	304	0.67	8.9	6.1	4250	32
60	132	-25 (90)	-0.06 (0.20)	2.3	5.1	3.8	1.50	3.3	6.6	5.4	319	0.70	9.1	6.6	5100	34
70	154	-25 (90)	-0.06 (0.20)	2.5	5.5	3.6	1.63	3.6	7.2	5.9	334	0.73	9.3	7.0	5950	38
80	176	-25 (90)	-0.06 (0.20)	2.6	5.7	3.2	1.69	3.7	7.4	6.1	344	0.76	9.5	7.4	6800	39
90	198	-25 (90)	-0.06 (0.20)	2.7	5.9	3.0	1.75	3.8	7.6	6.3	353	0.78	9.6	7.8	7650	40
First 6-8 wk lactation suckling twins																
50	110	-60	-0.13	2.4	5.3	4.8	1.56	3.4	6.9	5.6	389	0.86	10.5	7.3	5000	36
60	132	-60	-0.13	2.6	5.7	4.3	1.69	3.7	7.4	6.1	405	0.89	10.7	7.7	6000	39
70	154	-60	-0.13	2.8	6.2	4.0	1.82	4.0	8.0	6.6	420	0.92	11.0	8.1	7000	42
80	176	-60	-0.13	3.0	6.6	3.8	1.95	4.3	8.6	7.0	435	0.96	11.2	8.6	8000	45
90	198	-60	-0.13	3.2	7.0	3.6	2.08	4.6	9.2	7.5	450	0.99	11.4	9.0	9000	48
Replacement ewe lambs[e]																
30	66	227	0.50	1.2	2.6	4.0	0.78	1.7	3.4	2.8	185	0.41	6.4	2.6	1410	18
40	88	182	0.40	1.4	3.1	3.5	0.91	2.0	4.0	3.3	176	0.39	5.9	2.6	1880	21
50	110	120	0.26	1.5	3.3	3.0	0.88	1.9	3.9	3.2	136	0.30	4.8	2.4	2350	22
60	132	100	0.22	1.5	3.3	2.5	0.88	1.9	3.9	3.2	134	0.30	4.5	2.5	2820	22
70	154	100	0.22	1.5	3.3	2.1	0.88	1.9	3.9	3.2	132	0.29	4.6	2.8	3290	22
Replacement ram lambs[e]																
40	88	330	0.73	1.8	4.0	4.5	1.1	2.5	5.0	4.1	243	0.54	7.8	3.7	1880	24
60	132	320	0.70	2.4	5.3	4.0	1.5	3.4	6.7	5.5	263	0.58	8.4	4.2	2820	26
80	176	290	0.64	2.8	6.2	3.5	1.8	3.9	7.8	6.4	268	0.59	8.5	4.6	3760	28
100	220	250	0.55	3.0	6.6	3.0	1.9	4.2	8.4	6.9	264	0.58	8.2	4.8	4700	30

| Body Wt | | Wt Change/Day | | Dry Matter per Animal[a] | | | Energy[b] | | | | Nutrients per Animal | | | | | |
| | | | | | | | | | | | Crude protein | | Ca | P | Vitamin A Activity | Vitamin E Activity |
(kg)	(lb)	(g)	(lb)	(kg)	(lb)	(% body wt)	TDN (kg)	(lb)	DE (Mcal)	ME (Mcal)	(g)	(lb)	(g)	(g)	(IU)	(IU)
					Lambs finishing—4-7 mo old[f]											
30	66	295	0.65	1.3	2.9	4.3	0.94	2.1	4.1	3.4	191	0.42	6.6	3.2	1410	20
40	88	275	0.60	1.6	3.5	4.0	1.22	2.7	5.4	4.4	185	0.41	6.6	3.3	1880	24
50	110	205	0.45	1.6	3.5	3.2	1.23	2.7	5.4	4.4	160	0.35	5.6	3.0	2350	24
					Early weaned lambs—Moderate growth potential[f]											
10	22	200	0.44	0.5	1.1	5.0	0.40	0.9	1.8	1.4	127	0.38	4.0	1.9	470	10
20	44	250	0.55	1.0	2.2	5.0	0.80	1.8	3.5	2.9	167	0.37	5.4	2.5	940	20
30	66	300	0.66	1.3	2.9	4.3	1.00	2.2	4.4	3.6	191	0.42	6.7	3.2	1410	20
40	88	345	0.76	1.5	3.3	3.8	1.16	2.6	5.1	4.2	202	0.44	7.7	3.9	1880	22
50	110	300	0.66	1.5	3.3	3.0	1.16	2.6	5.1	4.2	181	0.40	7.0	3.8	2350	22

[a] To convert dry matter to an as-fed basis, divide dry matter values by the percentage of dry matter in the particular feed.

[b] One kg TDN (total digestible nutrients) = 4.4 Mcal DE (digestible energy); ME (metabolizable energy) = 82% of DE.

[c] Values are applicable for ewes in moderate condition. Fat ewes should be fed according to the next lower weight category and thin ewes at the next higher weight category. Once desired or moderate weight condition is attained, use that weight category through all production stages.

[d] Values in parentheses are for ewes suckling lambs the last 4-6 wk of lactation.

[e] Lambs intended for breeding; thus, maximum weight gains and finish are of secondary importance.

[f] Maximum weight gains expected.

Adapted, with permission, from *Nutrient Requirements of Sheep*, 1985, National Academy of Sciences. Published by National Academy Press, Washington, DC.

WATER

The usual recommendations are ~1 gal. (3.8 L) of water/day for ewes on dry feed in winter, 1½ gal./day for ewes nursing lambs, and ½ gal./day for finishing lambs. In many range areas, water is the limiting nutrient; even when present, it may be unpotable because of filth or high-mineral content. For best production, range sheep should be watered daily during warm weather. However, the cost of supplying water often makes it economical to water range sheep every other day. When soft snow is available, range sheep do not need additional water except when dry feeds such as alfalfa hay and pellets are fed. If the snow is crusted with ice, the crust should be broken to allow access.

ENERGY

Because so much of the diet can depend on grass and forage that is either sparse or of poor quality, the provision of adequate energy is important. Poor-quality forage, even in abundance, may not provide sufficient available energy for maintenance production. The energy requirement of ewes is greatest during the first 8-10 wk of lactation. Since milk production declines after this period and the lambs have begun foraging, the requirement of the ewe is reduced to a level equivalent to that of ewes 1 mo before lambing. This is of considerable economic importance.

PROTEIN

Good-quality forage and pasture generally will provide adequate protein for mature sheep. However, sheep do not digest poor-quality protein as efficiently as do cattle, and there are instances when a protein supplement should be fed with mature grass, hay, and winter range.

Sheep can convert nonprotein nitrogen, such as urea, ammonium phosphate, and biuret, into protein in the rumen but possibly not as efficiently as beef cattle. This source of nitrogen can provide at least a part of the necessary supplemental nitrogen in high-energy diets with a nitrogen:sulfur ratio of 10:1. In lamb-finishing diets, the inclusion of alfalfa and utilization of approved growth stimulants enhance nitrogen utilization.

MINERALS

Sheep require the major minerals: sodium, chlorine, calcium, phosphorus, magnesium, sulfur, and potassium; and the trace minerals: cobalt, copper, iodine, iron, manganese, molybdenum, zinc, and selenium. Trace mineralized salt provides an economical method of preventing deficiencies of sodium, chlorine, iodine, manganese, cobalt, copper, iron, and zinc. Selenium is approved by the Food and Drug Administration of the USA for inclusion in salt mixtures. Since sheep diets usually contain sufficient potassium, iron, magnesium, sulfur, and manganese, these minerals are not discussed.

Salt: In the USA, except on certain alkaline areas of the western range and along the seacoast where forage and soil are high in salt, sheep are provided with salt (sodium chloride). Sheepmen in the USA and Canada believe that sheep need salt to remain thrifty and make economical gains. However, salt supplements rarely are fed to sheep on good pasture in Australasia. Mature sheep will consume ~0.02 lb (9 g) of salt daily and lambs one-half this amount. Range operators commonly provide 0.5-0.75 lb (225-350 g) of salt/ewe/mo. Recent research indicates that 0.2% of the dry matter of the sheep diet as salt is adequate.

Calcium and Phosphorus: In plants, generally the leafy parts are relatively high in calcium (Ca) and low in phosphorus (P), whereas the reverse is true of the seeds. Legumes, in general, have a higher Ca content than grasses. As grasses mature, P is transferred to the seed (grain). Furthermore, the P content of the plant is influenced markedly by the availability of P in the soil. Therefore, low-quality pasture devoid of legumes and range plants tends to be naturally low in P, particularly as the forage matures and the seeds fall; characteristically, the range soil also is deficient in P. Consequently, sheep subsisting on mature, brown, summer forage and winter range sometimes develop a P deficiency (qv, p 1196). Sheep kept on such forages or fed low-quality hay with no grain should be provided a P supplement.

Since most forages have a relatively high Ca content, particularly if there is an admixture of legumes, natural feeds usually supply adequate amounts of this element. However, when corn silage or other feeds from the cereal grains are fed exclusively, ground limestone should be fed daily at the rate of 0.02-0.03 lb (9-14 g).

Sheep seem to be able to tolerate wide Ca:P ratios as long as their diets contain more Ca than P. However, an excess of P may be conducive to development of urinary calculi or osteodystrophy; a Ca:P ratio of 1.5:1 is appropriate for feedlot lambs. For pregnant ewes, the diet should contain $\geq 0.18\%$ P and, for lactating ewes, $\geq 0.27\%$. A content of 0.2-0.4% Ca is considered adequate.

Iodine: Sometimes, either as a consequence of low availability of iodine from the soil, or goitrogenic substances in the food (which interfere with the utilization of iodine by the thyroid), the iodine requirements of sheep are not met in the natural diet, and iodine supplements must be fed. Regions naturally deficient are known throughout the western USA, in the Great Lakes area, and in many other parts of the world. A deficiency of iodine (qv, p 1196) can be prevented by feeding stabilized iodized salt to pregnant ewes. A deficiency of iodine manifests itself as goiter in the adult and as wool-lessness in the young. The young of iodine-deficient ewes often are born dead.

Cobalt: Sheep require ~0.1 ppm of cobalt in their diet. Normally, legumes have a higher content than grasses. Since cobalt levels of the feedstuffs are seldom known, a good practice is to feed trace mineralized salt that contains cobalt.

Copper: Pregnant ewes require ~5 mg of copper daily; normally this amount is provided when the forage contains ≥ 5 ppm. However, the amount of copper in the diet necessary to prevent a copper deficiency (qv, p 1197) is influenced by the intake of other dietary constituents, notably molybdenum and inorganic sulfate. High intake of molybdenum in the presence of adequate sulfate increases the requirement for copper. Since sheep are more susceptible than cattle to the toxic effects of copper, care must be taken to avoid copper toxicosis. Toxicity may be produced in lambs by continued feeding of diets with 10-20 ppm of copper. This is true particularly where the molybdenum and sulfate contents in soil and feed are low.

Selenium: Selenium is effective in at least partially controlling nutritional muscular dystrophy (*see* p 548). Areas east of the Mississippi River and in the northwestern USA appear to be low in selenium. It can be provided by IM injections or oral feeding. The dietary requirement is ~0.3 ppm. Levels of 7-10 ppm or higher may be toxic.

Zinc: Growing lambs require ~30 ppm of zinc in the diet on a dry-matter basis. The requirement for normal testicular development is somewhat higher. Since many feeds do not contain this much zinc, the possibility of a deficiency is real. Furthermore, a high-calcium intake increases the need for zinc.

VITAMINS

Sheep diets usually contain an ample supply of vitamins A (provitamin A), D, and E. Under certain circumstances, however, supplements may be needed. The B vitamins and vitamin K are synthesized by the rumen microorganisms and, under practical conditions, supplements are unnecessary. However, polioencephalomalacia sometimes occurs; apparently it is due to destruction of thiamine in the rumen, and animals respond to supplements. Vitamin C is synthesized in the tissues of sheep.

On diets rich in carotene, such as high-quality pasture or green hays, sheep can store large quantities of vitamin A in the liver, often sufficient to meet their requirements for 6-12 mo. Daily supplies are unnecessary and deficiencies (qv, p 1199) rarely are a problem.

Vitamin D_2 is derived from sun-cured forage and vitamin D_3 by exposure of the skin to ultraviolet light. When exposure of the skin to sunshine is reduced by prolonged cloudy weather or confinement rearing, and when the vitamin D_2 content of the diet is low, the amount supplied may be inadequate. The requirement for vitamin D is increased when the amounts of either calcium or phosphorus in the diet are low or when the ratio between them is wide. Fast-growing lambs kept in sheds away from intense sunlight or maintained on green feeds (high carotene) during the winter months (low irradiation) may suffer impaired bone formation and show other signs of vitamin D deficiency (qv, p 1200). Normally, sheep on pasture seldom need vitamin D supplements because of exposure to the sun.

The major sources of **vitamin E** in the natural diet of sheep are green feeds and the germ of seeds. A deficiency of this vitamin, therefore, is uncommon in mature sheep. Vitamin E deficiency in young lambs may contribute to nutritional muscular dystrophy (*see*, p 548) if selenium intake is low.

FEEDING PRACTICES

FEEDING FARM SHEEP

See TABLE 55 (p 1279) for nutrient requirements of sheep. Using these data and the results of practical experience, suggestions for feeding sheep are outlined below.

Specialized Sheep Production: Much information has been compiled concerning larger sheep units under a confined system of management. Such innovations as early weaning or artificial rearing of lambs, slotted floors, accelerated lambing, synchronization of breeding, and production testing are being used. It is questionable if the extensive use of pasture for lambs in the midwestern and eastern USA will expand.

Use of Forage: Good hay is a highly productive feed; poor hay, no matter how much is available, is suitable only for maintenance unless improved by some processing method. Hay quality is determined primarily by: 1) its botanic composition, eg, a mixture of palatable grasses and legumes—brome/alfalfa or bluegrass/clover; 2) the stage of maturity when cut, eg, the grass before heading and alfalfa before one-tenth bloom; 3) method and speed of harvesting since they affect loss of leaf, bleaching by sun, and leaching by rain; and 4) spoilage and loss during storage and feeding. In general, the same factors influence the quality of silage. Sheep make excellent use of high-quality roughage stored either as hay or low-moisture, grass-legume silage or occasionally chopped green feed.

FEEDING EWES

The period from weaning to breeding of the ewe is critical if a high rate of twinning is desired. Ewes should not be allowed to become excessively fat but should make a slight daily gain from weaning to breeding. The rate of gain depends on the desired weight gain. If pasture production is inadequate, ewes may be confined and fed high-quality hay and, if necessary to make the desired gain, a small amount of grain. Since there is evidence that breeding while grazing legume pastures, particularly red clover, tends to depress the size of the lamb crop, mixed pasture 2 wk before and during breeding is preferred.

After mating, ewes can be maintained on pasture, thus allowing feed to be conserved, if necessary, for other times of the year. Good pasture for this period will allow the ewes to enter the winter feeding period in good condition. One of the rations outlined in TABLE 56 may be used when pasture is unavailable.

During the last 6-8 wk of pregnancy, growth of the lamb is rapid; from a nutritional viewpoint, this is a critical period, particularly for ewes carrying more than one fetus. Commencing 6-8 wk before lambing, the plane of nutrition should be increased gradually and continued without interruption by the addition of supplements such as those described in TABLE 57. The amount offered depends on the condition of the ewes. If ewes are in fair to good condition, 0.5-0.75 lb (225-350 g) daily usually is sufficient. The roughage of the ration should provide all the protein required by ewes for most efficient feeding of the farm flock. If necessary, the ewes may be classified according to age and condition and divided into groups for differential treatment.

Table 56. Rations For Pregnant Ewes up to 6 Weeks Before Lambing

Feed	Ration No.			
	1	2	3	4
	lb (kg)	lb (kg)	lb (kg)	lb (kg)
Legume hay, such as alfalfa, clover, or lespedeza	3.0-4.5 (1.36-2.04)	1.5-2.0 (0.68-0.91)	—	—
Corn or sorghum silage	—	4-5 (1.81-2.27)	—	—
Legume grass, low-moisture (50%) silage	—	—	6-8 (2.72-3.63)	—
Cottonseed, soybean, linseed, or peanut meal 90%; limestone 10%	—	—	—	0.25 (0.112)
Minerals[a]	ad lib	ad lib	ad lib	ad lib

[a]Mineral mix: 2 parts dicalcium phosphate to 1 part trace mineralized salt.

Table 57. Grain Mixture for Pregnant Ewes

Feed	Mixture No.			
	1	2	3	4
	%	%	%	%
Whole barley, corn, or wheat	60	75	75	50
Whole oats	30	—	25	50
Beet pulp, dried	—	25	—	—
Wheat bran	10	—	—	—

Lactating Ewes: Succulent pasture furnishes adequate energy, protein, vitamins, and minerals for ewes and lambs; no added grain is necessary. When pasture is not available or not used under confinement rearing, ewes should be fed one of the rations outlined for pregnant ewes in TABLE 56, and 1-1.5 lb (450-675 g) of one of the grain mixtures in TABLE 57. Ewes should have access to trace mineralized salt and dicalcium phosphate. Ewes with twin lambs should be separated from those with single lambs and fed more grain. Ewes nursing twin lambs produce 20-40% more milk than those with singles. Under confinement rearing or accelerated lambing, lambs are commonly weaned at 2 mo of age. The ewe's milk production declines rapidly after this period and, since the lambs are consuming feed from a creep, it results in more efficient use of feed.

FEEDING LAMBS

From ~2 wk of age, the lambs should have free access to creep feed, unless they are born on succulent pasture. If pasture is to be used later, they should be creep-fed for 1-2 mo until it is available. If it will not be available until the lambs are 3-4 mo old, they should be finished in dry lot. The grain should be ground coarse or rolled at first, but may be fed whole later. At first, small amounts are fed, and the feed is kept clean and fresh. The amount is raised gradually until the lambs are on full feed.

Feeding lambs from birth to market in dry lot, together with early weaning at 2-3 mo of age, has become more popular throughout the USA. A complete diet of hay, grain, and supplement is ground, mixed, and either fed in this form or made into 3/16- or 3/8-in. (5 or 10 mm) pellets. Such lambs usually reach market weight in 3 1/2-4 mo. Some examples of creep ration used in dry-lot feeding are shown in TABLE 58.

Table 58. Creep Ration for Suckling and Early-weaned Lambs

Feed	Mixture No.			
	1	2	3	4
	%	%	%	%
Alfalfa hay, leafy ground	25	30	40	—
Dehydrated alfalfa leaf meal	53.5	—	20	48
Corn, shelled	—	—	—	35
Corn or wheat	—	55	—	—
Oats or barley	—	—	20	—
Soybean, linseed, or cottonseed meal	19	10	10	10
Molasses	—	3.5	8.5	5.5
Bone meal or dicalcium phosphate	1	1	1	1
Limestone	1	—	—	—
Trace mineralized salt	0.5	0.5	0.5	0.5
Antibiotic	—	—	0.002	0.002

Rearing Lambs on Milk Replacer: In intensified sheep production, lambs such as orphans, extras, or those from poor-milking ewes should be raised on milk replacers. They should first receive colostrum, if not from a ewe, then from a frozen supply from cows. Milk replacers designed specifically for lambs are available. They contain ~30% fat, 25% protein, and a high level of antibiotic. It is advisable to inject such lambs with vitamins A, D, and E; a combination of penicillin and streptomycin; and selenium.

Multiple nipple pails or containers are used, and the milk should be offered cold after the first week. Cold milk replacer can be used by older lambs, which will nurse more often, and the milk will not sour as quickly. The lambs should be given water in addition to the milk when a creep ration is offered at 9-10 days of age. They can be weaned from the milk abruptly at 4-5 wk of age if consumption of creep feed and water intake is at a reasonable level.

FINISHING FEEDER LAMBS

Preconditioning the lambs before they leave the producer's property should be encouraged. This includes starting on feed, vaccinating, worming, and under some conditions, shearing. If this is not done, the lambs should be rested for several days and fed dry, average-quality hay after arrival at the feedlot. Following this rest, the above-mentioned practices should be performed. (*See also* DISEASE-MANAGEMENT INTERACTION: SHEEP, p 1122.)

Feeding Method: There is no best method or diet for finishing lambs. They may be finished on alfalfa or wheat pasture with no grain. They may be started on pasture or crop aftermath and fed grain later. When fed in dry lot, usually they are self-fed. These diets may be completely pelleted, ground and mixed, a mixture of alfalfa pellets and grain, or a high-concentrate type. Self-feeding means more efficient use of labor, and allows the size of the operation to be increased. Self-feeding usually results in maximum feed intake and gain. Hand-feeding can be mechanized with an auger system or self-unloading wagon. It involves feeding at regular intervals so that the lambs clean up the feed before they are fed again. Feed consumption and gain can be controlled. Corn silage should be hand-fed.

Starting on Feed: Feeders who feed lambs year-round or feed heavy lambs usually prefer to place the lambs on full feed as soon as possible. This means full feeding within 10-14 days. Lambs can be started safely on self-fed, ground, or pelleted diets containing 60-70% hay. Within 2 wk the hay may be reduced to 30-40% when the ration is not pelleted. Other roughages such as cottonseed hulls or silage can be used in a similar manner. Lambs can be started and finished on pelleted rations that contain less grain than needed for nonpelleted rations. Digestive disturbances usually are reduced also. Feed cost may be higher depending on processing charges.

Table 59. Recommended Formulas for Finishing Lambs*
(lb/ton or kg/metric ton)

	Starter 10-day period		High Roughage		High Concentrate	Corn Silage
	Loose	Pelleted	Loose	Pelleted		
Grain-corn, barley or milo**	500	200	780	400	1500	540
Alfalfa hay	1280	1700	1000	1400	200	
Molasses	100	100	100			
Oil-seed meal	100		100			100
Urea					45	
Beet pulp			200	200		
Silage						1350
Limestone	10				35	10
Trace mineralized salt	10		20	20	35	
Antibiotic (g)	50	20	20	10	20	10
Vitamin A (IU/ton)						1,000,000

* Feeder lambs should have ~14% crude protein in rations (dry basis).

** Wheat can be substituted for other grains, but allow a period of time for adaptation.

Vaccination against enterotoxemia and feeding tetracyclines at 25-30 mg/lamb/ day are helpful in starting lambs on feed more rapidly and in feeding diets that may consist entirely of concentrates.

Feeds: Corn, sorghum, or alfalfa silage can replace about half the hay with hand-feeding, but finish and yield will be decreased to some extent. Rations that may be used in self-feeding are given in TABLE 60. Corn, barley, milo, wheat, or a mixture of these are used; 0.5% salt and 0.5% bone meal or equivalent should be added to the grain. Pelleting of rations for finishing lambs is beneficial when low-grade roughages or high-roughage rations are used. Caution should be used when feeding large amounts of wheat; lambs not adapted to it are more apt to develop acute indigestion than if fed grains such as corn, sorghum, or barley.

Mineral supplements, including salt, should be offered separately whether or not they are included in the grain mixture. Approved growth stimulants usually increase growth rate 10-15% and feed efficiency 8-10% but may decrease carcass quality.

FEEDING MATURE BREEDING RAMS

Mature breeding rams should be grazed on pasture when available, or fed rations 1, 2, or 3 outlined in TABLE 56. If rams are in a thrifty condition at breeding time and the ewes are on a good flushing pasture, it should not be necessary to grain-feed the rams while with the ewes. When daytime temperatures are >90°F (32°C), rams should be shorn before mating and turned out with the ewes at night only.

FEEDING RANGE SHEEP

The condition of the sheep, the amount and kind of forage on the range, and the climatic conditions determine the kind and amount of supplement to feed. Supplements usually consist of high-protein pellets or cottonseed meal and salt, medium-protein pellets, low-protein pellets or corn, alfalfa hay, and minerals.

When the diets of sheep on the western winter range are supplemented properly, the lamb crop can be increased 10-15% and wool production increased by ~1 lb (400-500 g) per ewe. Each operator needs to determine if the increased production will more than cover the cost of supplementation. One recommended practice is to feed ~0.25 lb (115 g) of high-protein (36%) supplement or 0.33-0.5 lb (150-225 g) of medium-protein (24%) pellets ~3 wk before and during the breeding season, during extremely cold weather, and for ~1 mo before green feed starts in the spring (TABLE 56). In addition, small lambs, small yearling ewes, old ewes with poor teeth, and thin ewes should be separated from the main flock and fed one of the above supplements from about December 1 until shearing time. In many instances, the old ewes, lambs, and yearlings from more than one band can be herded together in a special flock.

When sheep are unable to obtain a full ration of forage because of deep snow, 1-3 lb (450-1350 g) of alfalfa hay and 0.2-0.3 lb (90-150 g) of a low-protein pellet mixture (TABLE 60) or corn should be fed. If alfalfa hay is not available, 0.5-1 lb (225-450 g) per head of a low-protein pellet mixture should be fed daily for emergency feeding periods.

Table 60. Pattern for Range Supplements for Sheep

Main Groups	Subgroups	Feedstuff	Suggested Maximum	Recommended Amount of Protein high	Recommended Amount of Protein medium	Recommended Amount of Protein low
			%	%	%	%
Energy feeds	Grains	Barley	75		33.0	57.5
		Corn	60	5.0	10.0	15.0
		Wheat	60			
		Milo	60			
		Oats	15			
		Screenings No. 1	10			
	Mill feeds	Wheat mixed feed	10			
		Shorts	10			
		Molasses	15	5.0	5.0	10.0
		Beet pulp	10			10.0
Protein supplements	30-40% Protein feeds	Cottonseed meal	75	62.5	32.5	5.0
		Linseed meal	25			
		Soybean meal	75	10.0	10.0	
		Peanut meal	25			
	20-30% Protein feeds	Corn gluten feed	15			
		Corn distiller's dried grains	10			
		Wheat distiller's grains	10			
		Brewer's dried grains	5			
		Safflower meal	25			
		Cull beans	15			
Mineral supplements		Bone meal or defluorinated phosphate		4.0	3.0	2.0
		Dicalcium phosphate		1.0	0.5	0.5
		Disodium phosphate				
		Monocalcium phosphate				
		Monosodium phosphate				
		Salt or trace mineralized salt				
Vitamin supplements		Dehydrated alfalfa meal	20	12.5	6.0	
		Sun-cured alfalfa meal	20			
		Vitamin A and carotene concentrates				
Total				100.0	100.0	100.0
Suggested composition						
Total crude protein, %				36.0	24.0	12.0
Phosphorus, %				1.5	1.0	0.5
Carotene, mg/kg				35.0	17.0	—
Rate of feeding, g/day — ewes				115	150 to 255	90 to 450

Deficiencies of Range Forages: Deficiencies most apt to occur among range forages are protein, energy, and phosphorus. These are most prevalent as the forages approach maturity or are dormant, and they may appear singly or in combination. Range sheep often travel long distances and are exposed to cold weather. This results in a higher energy requirement. Protein supplements such as soybean or cottonseed meal increase digestibility and utilization of forage, and provide needed protein and phosphorus. Most ranges used for winter grazing are considered adequate in carotene because most browse species, even in the dormant stage, furnish as much carotene as sun-cured alfalfa hay. However, when sheep are required to graze dry-grass ranges for >6 mo without intermittent periods of green feed, vitamin A supplements are recommended.

Mineral Mixtures: On the range, portable mineral boxes are convenient for sheep. Suggested mineral mixtures high in phosphorus are given in TABLE 61. One of these mineral mixtures should be fed free choice along with salt in a 2-compartment mineral box. Mixture 1 is used if there are no iodine or trace-mineral deficiencies, Mixture 2 when an iodine deficiency exists, and Mixture 3 if deficiencies of trace minerals are present.

Table 61. Suggested Mineral Mixtures for Sheep

| Ingredient | Mixture No. | | |
	1	2	3
	%	%	%
Salt	50	—	—
Iodized salt	—	50	—
Trace mineralized salt	—	—	50
Bone meal or phosphorus supplement	50	50	50

Under winter range conditions, the amount of phosphorus supplement that should be added to range pellets varies with the type of range forage available, the rate of feeding, and the ingredients used in the pellets. It is suggested that 36, 24, and 12% protein pellets contain 1.5, 1.0, and 0.5% phosphorus, respectively. It is assumed that the 36% protein pellets will be fed at the rate of 0.25 lb (115 g) per head daily, the 24% protein pellets at 0.33-0.5 lb (150-225 g), and the 12% protein pellets at 0.2-0.5 lb (90-225 g), together with alfalfa or clover hay.

PART VI
PHARMACOLOGY

PHM

BASIC CONCEPTS IN PHARMACOTHERAPEUTICS

Once a diagnosis has been established, there are 4 main options: 1) do nothing, 2) medical treatment, 3) surgical intervention, 4) euthanasia. An additional important responsibility is to make provision for the care, comfort, feeding, and alleviation of pain or suffering of the affected animal(s). When medical treatment is deemed necessary, safe and effective pharmacological agents that possess the appropriate actions should be selected. Also to be considered are the dose rates and frequencies of administration of the chosen drugs, the optimal routes for delivery, the particular pharmaceutical forms to be used, any public health or environmental implications, and regulatory constraints. Proper concern also must be given for the handling, storage, stability, incompatibilities, bioavailability, and potential drug or nutrient interactions with pharmaceutical products; failure to do so may result in therapeutic failures.

Following administration of the selected agent(s), a complex series of events occur, which govern in large measure the disposition of the drugs and the ultimate clinical success (or failure) of the regimen selected. An understanding of the fundamental pharmacological principles involved, together with an appreciation of the major attributes of each class of drug, form the basis of rational pharmacotherapeutics.

To avoid repetition, not all classes of drugs are discussed under each subsection; eg, for discussion of clinical pharmacology of drugs used to treat diseases of the respiratory system, it is necessary to refer to several subsections such as the respiratory system itself, antibacterial agents, antiviral agents, anti-inflammatory drugs, antiparasitic drugs, and antifungal drugs. Additionally, more specific information may be found in the section of the MANUAL that refers to diseases of the particular system, or under discussions of specific diseases thereof.

It is important to be aware of relevant legal restrictions, which may vary with time; also, a drug use approved in one country may not be in another. Departures from label instructions may be desirable or even necessary, eg, in "minor" species, but pertinent laws and regulations must be observed. In all instances, it is important to read carefully the label instructions for use of specific drugs. Each extra-label usage must be undertaken with a clear understanding of legal as well as medical ramifications.

DISPOSITION AND FATE OF DRUGS

Once a drug has been dosed orally, injected, or applied topically, it probably is absorbed into the bloodstream from the site of administration. The agent then is distributed into various body fluids and tissues to a greater or lesser degree; the objective is to attain an effective concentration of the drug for a (variable) period of time at a site of action or infection to effect a beneficial response. Subsequently, the drug is inactivated and/or eliminated from the body, generally by metabolic transformations (usually hepatic) and excretion (mainly renal and biliary routes); the effectiveness of these processes, with respect to time (pharmacokinetics), varies with the particular drug and species of animal, but may also be influenced by the disease or lesions present and the effects of concurrently administered agents (drug interactions). The principles that govern the absorption and disposition of drugs, their modes of action, and the factors that may modify these processes should be considered to make optimal use of the extensive therapeutic armamentarium available.

DRUG DOSAGE FORMS

Common **oral dosage forms** include tablets, capsules, boluses, powders, granules, syrups, solutions, suspensions, and pastes. Powders, granules, and pellets are used for medicating feeds, and soluble powders and liquid forms for medicating drinking water. These preparations use various inert fillers, binders, lubricants, disintegrants, vehicles, and diluents. These adjuvants and excipients may influence the chemical stability of the formulation and the clinical effectiveness of the drug. The rates of disintegration and dissolution of solid dosage forms within the GI tract are also determined by these ingredients and may vary among different manufacturers' products. Such discrepancies in pharmaceutical availability can lead to generic or therapeutic inequivalence between supposedly identical preparations. This problem is well recognized, and in large measure has been rectified by regulatory requirements. The bioavailability of the drugs in self-compounded concoctions is, however, always open to question.

In addition to the standard dosage forms for oral (PO) administration, a number of specialized delivery systems are also available. These include enteric-coated tablets and sustained-action or controlled-release preparations. These time-release formulations provide delayed or gradual escape of active ingredient in several ways: special coating of granules, microencapsulation, embedding in a slowly eroding matrix or inert carrier, formation of poorly soluble chemical complexes, and the use of ion-exchange resins. Several types of extended-action boluses are employed in ruminants (in which the loss from the ruminoreticulum through the rumination reflex may be troublesome). The blood levels obtained from such specialized drug dosage forms are not always reliable. Many factors may be responsible for unpredictable absorption, but the pronounced differences between the GI tracts of the various species play an important role.

The most common **parenteral dosage form** is a stable aqueous solution. Less frequently, the active components may be dissolved in an inert vegetable oil, which delays absorption. Other kinds of prolonged-release preparations include subcut.

implants of solid dosage forms, and relatively insoluble salts and esters as suspensions in various vehicles. Examples of long-acting formulations are preparations of penicillin G, oxytetracycline, insulin, adrenocorticotropic hormone, corticosteroids, anabolic steroids, and sex steroids. When these special parenteral controlled-release dosage forms are used, it is important to appreciate the basic differences between these and standard pharmaceutical preparations. Initial concerns revolve around the route of administration, since accidental IV administration can lead to serious and even fatal effects due to microembolism. Second, persistent drug residues in food animals and race horses have ethical and legal ramifications. The stability of solutions intended for parenteral administration usually is quite delicate and depends on pH, temperature, and the presence of stabilizers, solubilizers, and preservatives. Indiscriminate mixing of such products for the sake of convenience (eg, single versus multiple injections) should be avoided unless there is proof that the formulations are physically and chemically compatible. Currently, several novel approaches for the parenteral delivery of drugs are being developed. Included among these are microspheres, microcapsules, liposomes, microsponges, resealed carrier erythrocytes, and projectile biodegradable missiles. Additionally, monoclonal antibodies have been utilized to carry highly selective, bound drugs to specific target tissues or even cells. New implantable controlled-release drug delivery systems include pellets composed of various polymeric forms, and silicone capsules. Several implantable devices also have been introduced that permit constant systemic delivery of a drug within the body. The best known of these include osmotically or propellant-driven pumps and minipumps.

Dosage forms intended for administration via the respiratory tract include inhalant anesthetic gases and vapors, fine mists produced by nebulization, aerosols, and sprays. Drugs in the gaseous state readily reach the alveolar surfaces, whereas only particles <2 μm (produced by nebulization) are inspired into the terminal ducts and alveoli. Particles <5 μm may reach the respiratory bronchioles, and those 5-10 μm in size, the upper respiratory tract and larger airways. Aqueous solutions of antibacterial drugs intended for injection are also frequently delivered intratracheally. Absorption usually, but not always, occurs from the respiratory tract.

Local or topical administration of drugs usually is restricted to readily accessible organs and structures such as the skin, eyes, body orifices, body cavities, and mammary glands. Many dosage forms have been developed to deliver active principles to the site of application to produce local effects. However, in many instances, absorption into the systemic circulation also occurs. A large variety of preparations are available for dermal application. These include ointments, creams, pastes, dusting powders, lotions, sprays, liniments, and poultices. Systemic effects may occur due to licking of the applied medication or to percutaneous drug absorption, which often occurs—especially when the skin is damaged or inflamed (burns, ulcers, wounds, dermatitis). Absorption through the skin can also be enhanced by occlusive dressings, inunction, or the use of dimethylsulfoxide (DMSO) as a carrier. Several drugs are deliberately applied to the skin with the anticipation of systemic effects following transdermal absorption, eg, external parasiticides available as "pour-on" formulations, medicated ear tags, nitroglycerine ointment, and scopolamine in a transdermal patch device.

Drugs are applied locally to mucous membranes (eyes, mouth, throat, urethra, vagina, uterus, rectum, bladder) to achieve anti-infective, anti-inflammatory, decongestant, astringent, or anesthetic effects. Absorption through mucous membranes may be sufficient to produce systemic effects. Drug forms most frequently administered by the mucosal route include solutions, suspensions, and suppositories; less commonly used forms include creams, ointments, tablets, powders, sponges, and tampons.

Intramammary infusion of antibacterial and anti-inflammatory ointments is frequently employed for the treatment of bovine mastitis. Again, absorption into the bloodstream may occur from the udder.

Whatever drug dosage form is used to treat a particular animal, it is imperative to have an appreciation of the makeup of the pharmaceutical formulation, of the factors that may alter the efficacy of the product, and of how to derive optimal therapeutic benefit from the agent without jeopardizing its bioavailability or pharmacological action.

ROUTES OF DRUG ADMINISTRATION

Choice of the route and technique of administration is generally based on several factors. The most important of these include the physicochemical properties of the drug and the formulation to be used, the therapeutic indication, the pathophysiology of the disease, the species of animal involved and any special physiological or other considerations, the ease of handling and controlling the animal, and economic factors (especially for repetitive dosing or mass medication of a herd or flock). The manufacturer's recommendations should always be followed carefully unless it is explicitly known that a proposed deviation will not adversely alter the activity or kinetic fate of the principal ingredients.

Oral Administration: Drugs administered PO are exposed to low pH ranges, digestive enzymes, intestinal microflora, and ingesta that vary greatly among species. Moreover, when a drug is absorbed from the GI tract, it enters the portal circulation and passes through the liver before reaching the systemic circulation. During this time a high degree of metabolic transformation may occur—the "first pass" effect. The advantages of oral dosage are that it is usually convenient and safe, sterility is not a requirement, and the danger of acute drug reaction is not great. The disadvantages include a slower onset of action, and unpredictability and inconsistency of absorption. Additionally, a transit time may be modified by GI disturbances, a larger dose may be required, the procedure may be difficult in fractious animals, poor technique or dysphagia may lead to intratracheal delivery and subsequent bronchopneumonia, and inactivation may occur within the GI tract.

Various techniques, each more or less appropriate for the respective species, include use of a nasogastric or stomach tube, probang, dosing or drench gun, nurser, or dropper. Drugs can be placed directly into the mouth, or in a salt block, feed, or drinking water.

Parenteral Administration: The most frequently used parenteral routes are intravenous (IV), intramuscular (IM), and subcutaneous (subcut.). Common but less frequently employed routes include epidural, intradermal, intratracheal, and intraperitoneal (IP). Occasional routes of injection include intra-arterial, intramedullary, intrathecal, intrathoracic, subarachnoid, intracardiac, subconjunctival, and intratesticular. Intralesional injection is a way of attaining high concentrations of a drug at the target site. In all cases, solutions for injection must be sterile, techniques must be aseptic, the dose must be accurate, and a painful reaction is a possibility.

For the IV route, aqueous solutions are preferable, which lead immediately to predictably high blood levels with a rapid onset of action. Irritating and nonisotonic solutions can be injected IV—if done slowly and carefully. The disadvantages of IV administration include the short duration of action, adverse effects usually are more severe, and there is no redress once the injection has been made.

The IM route can be used for aqueous or oleaginous suspensions, or solutions, as well as other depot preparations. Absorption occurs either hematogenously or via lymphatics and usually is fairly rapid except for long-acting preparations. Moderately irritating preparations can be injected IM, but tissue reaction and necrosis may become evident with time. The duration of drug action is longer than for IV injection, but most often is a little shorter than for subcut. administration; however, this is not always predictable. A disadvantage of the IM route is the possibility of improper deposition in nerves, blood vessels, fat, or between muscle bundles in connective tissue sheaths.

The advantages of the subcut. route are similar to those of the IM route, although irritant preparations and oily vehicles should be avoided due to possible undesirable reactions. The rate of absorption from subcut. injection sites may be unpredictable and depends on several factors. The most important of these is blood flow, and the presence of vasoconstrictors or vasodilators can substantially alter rates of absorption. Usually, the rate of absorption is slightly slower than from IM sites.

The other parenteral routes of administration are generally used for the following purposes: epidural and subarachnoid—spinal analgesia and myelography; intradermal—testing for hypersensitivity and for vaccination; intratracheal—treatment of respiratory tract infections; intra-arterial—with simultaneous venous constriction produces high concentrations of the drug in the dependent area for a short time, which occasionally is necessary in cancer chemotherapy and special radiographic or other imaging techniques; intramedullary—blood transfusion directly into the bone marrow when other routes are awkward, as in neonates; intrathecal (cisterna magna)—for treatment of meningoencephalitis and myelography; intrathoracic (intrapleural or intrapulmonary)—not commonly used today, once used for injectable anesthetics and euthanasia; intracardiac—for emergencies, especially cardiac arrest.

The techniques and actual sites favored for the parenteral administration of drugs are often based on personal preference.

Inhalation (Pulmonary Route): Gases, volatile agents, and fine particles usually are rapidly absorbed from the airways and alveoli into the pulmonary circulation. Delivery into the respiratory passages is done by standard anesthetic machines in the case of inhalation anesthetics, or by vaporization or nebulization for the local delivery of expectorants, bronchodilators, and anti-infective agents.

Topical Administration (Local Application): Drugs can be applied locally to the skin and its adnexa or to a variety of mucous membranes. The routes that may be employed include: sublingual, intranasal, intravaginal, intrauterine, intracystic, rectal, preputial, ocular, and aural. The intramammary route is a special case of local application.

ABSORPTION OF DRUGS

Passage of Drugs Across Cellular Membranes: Regardless of the route of administration, a drug usually must traverse a number of membranes before it reaches its site of action. Membrane barriers may be composed of several layers of cells (eg, skin, vagina, cornea, placenta), a single layer of cells (eg, enterocytes, renal tubular epithelial cells), or may consist only of a boundary less than one cell in thickness (eg, single cell membrane, mitochondrion, nucleus). In general, the composition and architecture of all membranes involves a lipoproteinaceous barrier that has a small but significant number of dynamic aqueous channels that are associated with the globular protein components of the membrane. The outside surfaces of biological membranes are hydrophilic and the inside consists of a lipid bilayer, which prevents the free entry of water and many solutes.

Drugs and other molecules can cross cellular membranes by several processes. Passive transfer or simple diffusion is the most important for xenobiotics, although specialized transport systems are used for a limited number of therapeutic agents.

In simple diffusion, movement of the drug is due to and directly related to its concentration gradient across the membrane. In the case of lipid diffusion, lipid-soluble substances dissolve in the lipid phase of the membrane and diffuse down their concentration gradients into the aqueous phase on the other side of the barrier. Thus, the ability of a compound to traverse a membrane by simple lipid diffusion is a function of its degree of lipid solubility (lipid-to-water partition coefficient). The molecular mass of the drug, the thickness of the membrane(s), and the surface area available also influence the rate of diffusion.

Many agents of pharmacological interest are weak organic electrolytes. At physiological pH, these weak acids or bases may be present partly in the ionized (dissociated) and partly in the nonionized (undissociated) form. The concentration of the respective forms depends on the drug's dissociation constant (pK_a) and the pH of the solution in which it is dissolved. The nonionized fraction may penetrate biological membranes by lipid diffusion and become distributed across the membrane according to 1) the degree of ionization on each side of the membrane, and 2) the extent to which the drug is bound to proteins or other macromolecules in the solutions bathing either side of the membrane. Membranes are more permeable to the undissociated molecule than to the ionized form, simply because the nonionized form is much more lipid soluble. However, although a compound may be nonionized, it also may be so poorly soluble in lipids that it penetrates biological membranes only to a limited extent. A degree of aqueous solubility is also necessary for a drug to be in solution in the body fluids on either side of a cellular membrane. Occasionally, 2 lipid-insoluble polar drugs complex together, which reduces their water solubility and increases their lipid solubility to the point that they can then diffuse across membranes in a dimeric form. This process is known as augmented diffusion.

It is supposed that aqueous pores exist in lipoproteinaceous biological membranes. Lipid-insoluble compounds can easily diffuse through these pores as well as directly through the membrane at rates that depend on their molecular masses and concentration gradients. However, with ions or other polar compounds, the speed of transfer is determined by both the charge and molecular dimensions of the drug. When a hydrostatic or osmotic pressure difference exists across a membrane, water will flow through the aqueous pores; this bulk fluid movement will carry or "drag" solute molecules through the pores in the moving stream, provided the dimensions of these solute molecules are less than those of the aqueous channels. This passive movement of drugs is known as filtration, hydrodynamic flow, or solvent drag, depending on the forces involved.

A number of specialized transfer processes account for the passage of certain organic ions and other large lipid-insoluble substances across biological membranes. Certain membrane proteins act as selective but saturable carrier-transport systems that may or may not require direct metabolic energy to function. Active transport, facilitated diffusion, and exchange diffusion are 3 distinct types of carrier-mediated conveyance used for moving specific substances across cellular membranes. In active transport, the process requires energy and, characteristically, the movement is against an electrochemical gradient. The highly selective carrier-mediated systems are principally utilized for transporting nutrients and natural substrates across biological membranes.

Pinocytosis is an important transport process in mammalian cells, particularly intestinal epithelial cells and renal tubular cells. Drugs that exist in solution as molecular aggregates, have large molecular masses themselves, or are bound to macromolecules may be transferred across membranes by pinocytosis.

Absorption of Drugs from the GI Tract: Absorption can occur throughout the GI tract. However, the physicochemical properties of each drug, the GI physiology of the species involved, alterations of the normal structure and function of the GI tract, and a number of pharmaceutical considerations may all play a role in determining the major site of absorption and, more particularly, the rate of absorption from the GI tract.

The rate of absorption of nonelectrolytes such as simple alcohols, polyhydric alcohols, amides, and ethers is governed primarily by the degree of lipid solubility of the compound. Generally, substances with higher lipid-to-water partition coefficients diffuse across GI epithelium more rapidly. These neutral compounds are absorbed by simple lipid diffusion, which is independent of the pH of GI fluids.

The gastric epithelium is also preferentially permeable to the lipid-soluble nonionized form of a drug, but the relative epithelial surface area is much less than that of the small intestine. Weak acids (pK_a 3-10), such as nonsteroidal anti-inflammatory drugs, barbiturates, sulfonamides, nalidixic acid, and nitrofurantoin, which are mainly undissociated in gastric juice, are readily absorbed from the stomach and upper small intestine. However, weak bases (pK_a 5-10), such as opioid analgesics, quinidine, ephedrine, and other alkaloids that are highly ionized in acidic environments with pH values of 1-4, are poorly absorbed from the monogastric stomach. In fact, the marked difference in pH between gastric juice and plasma leads to an uneven distribution of both weak acids and bases between the 2 fluid compartments. Basic drugs, such as levorphanol, strychnine, and many others, become more concentrated in gastric juice than in plasma because the ionized form present in the gastric lumen cannot be reabsorbed. This is an example of a phenomenon known as "ion-trapping".

The degree of ionization and lipid solubility of weak electrolytes also determines their rates of diffusion through the intestinal mucosa. The epithelial surface area available for absorption is much greater in the small intestine because of its villous structure. In the normal intestine, acidic drugs with pK_a >3 and basic drugs with pK_a <7.8 are usually well absorbed. Outside these limits the absorption of the stronger acids and bases occurs slowly. It seems that the pH in the microenvironment of the absorbing surface of the intestinal mucosa is ~5.3, which is more acidic than the usual content of the small intestinal lumen. Absorption from the colon is less rapid than from the small intestine but occurs by the same mechanisms. Drugs administered by enema or suppository are often well absorbed.

The absorption of natural substrates, such as L-amino acids, glucose, and uracil, from the small intestine occurs by specific active transport processes. Foreign compounds that structurally resemble natural substrates may be transferred by these mechanisms. The best known examples of this phenomenon include the absorption of a few unnatural sugars by the glucose transport mechanisms and 5-fluorouracil by the uracil carrier system.

Factors Affecting the GI Absorption of Drugs: Although the basic principles governing the absorption of drugs from the GI tract are understood, many confounding factors may play a role in modifying the process, and erratic responses may result. Some of the more important factors to be considered are: 1) molecular size and shape of the drug and its concentration, 2) degree of ionization at specific pH values (depends on pK_a of the drug), 3) lipid solubility of the neutral or nonionized form of the drug, 4) chemical or physical interactions with co-administered drug preparations or even food constituents, 5) the pharmaceutical preparation and characteristics of the dosage form (especially the disintegration and dissolution rates of solid dosage forms), 6) morphological and functional differences of the GI tract among the various animal species, 7) gastric motility and secretion as well as the rate of gastric emptying, 8) intestinal motility and secretions as well as the intestinal transit time, 9) fluid volume within the GI tract, 10) osmolality of intestinal content, 11) intestinal blood and lymph flow, 12) disruption of the structural and functional integrity of the gastric and intestinal epithelium, and 13) drug biotransformation within the intestinal lumen by microflora, or within the mucosa by host enzyme systems.

Bioavailability: Sometimes also called "pharmaceutical availability", this term is used to define the rate and extent to which a drug administered in a particular dosage form enters the systemic circulation intact. All of the considerations outlined above, as well as the particular product used, can influence bioavailability. Biotransformation by intestinal epithelial cells, and particularly by liver cells, can substantially reduce the amount of unchanged drug that enters the systemic circulation following administration PO. This is known as the "first pass" effect and is significant for a number of drugs.

Absorption of Drugs from Topical Sites of Application: Drugs may be absorbed through the skin following topical application. The intact skin allows the passage of small lipophilic substances, but efficiently retards the diffusion of water-soluble molecules in most cases. Lipid-insoluble drugs generally penetrate the skin slowly in comparison with their rates of absorption through other body membranes. Absorption of drugs through the skin may be enhanced by inunction or more rarely by iontophoresis if the compound is ionized. Certain solvents may facilitate the penetration of drugs through the skin. The best known of these solvents is dimethyl sulfoxide (DMSO). Damaged, inflamed, or hyperemic skin allows many drugs to penetrate the dermal barrier much more readily.

The same principles that govern the absorption of drugs through the skin also apply to the application of topical preparations on epithelial surfaces.

Many drugs traverse the cornea at rates that are related to their degree of ionization and lipid solubility. Thus, organic bases, such as atropine, ephedrine, and pilocarpine, often penetrate quite readily, whereas the highly polar antibiotics generally penetrate the cornea poorly.

Absorption of Drugs from the Tracheobronchial Surfaces and Alveoli: The volatile and gaseous anesthetics are the most important group of drugs administered by inhalation. These substances enter the circulation by diffusion across the alveolar membranes. Since they all have relatively high lipid-to-water partition coefficients and generally are rather small molecules, they equilibrate practically instantaneously with the blood in the alveolar capillaries.

Particles contained in aerosols can be deposited, depending on the size of the droplets, on the mucosal surface of the bronchi or bronchioles, or even in the alveoli. Most drugs are usually absorbed quite rapidly from these sites according to the same principles as discussed above.

Absorption of Drugs from Parenteral Delivery Sites: After a drug has penetrated the skin, GI epithelium, or other absorbing surface, or has been deposited by injection into a body tissue, it comes into the immediate vicinity of capillaries, which it must enter to exert a systemic effect. Solutes traverse the capillary wall by a combination of 2 processes: diffusion and filtration. Diffusion is the predominant mode of transfer for lipid-soluble molecules as well as for small lipid-insoluble molecules and ions. Hydrodynamic flow predominates for large lipid-insoluble molecules, for which the rates of diffusion across the capillary endothelium are, however, relatively slow. All drugs, whether lipid-soluble or not, cross the capillary wall at rates that are extremely rapid compared with their rates across other body membranes. In fact, the movement of most drug molecules in various tissues is limited by the rate of blood flow rather than by the capillary wall. However, some endothelial cells have much tighter intercellular junctions than others, and diffusion through these capillary beds, eg, the blood-brain barrier, is significantly more restrictive.

Aqueous solutions of drugs are usually absorbed from an IM injection site within 10-30 min, provided blood flow is unimpaired. Faster or slower absorption is possible, depending on the concentration and lipid-solubility of the drug, vascularity of the site (there are differences between various muscle groups), the volume of injection, the osmolality of the solution, and other pharmaceutical factors. Substances with molecular weights >20,000 are principally taken up into the lymphatics.

Absorption of drugs from subcut. tissues is influenced by the same factors that determine the rate of absorption from IM sites. Some drugs are absorbed as rapidly from subcut. tissues as from muscle, although absorption from injection sites in subcut. fat is always significantly delayed.

Increasing blood supply to the injection site by heating, massage, or exercise hastens the rate of dissemination and absorption. Spreading and absorption of a large fluid volume that has been injected subcut. may be facilitated by including hyaluronidase in the solution.

The rate of absorption of an injected drug may be prolonged in a number of ways, including immobilization of the site, local cooling, a tourniquet, incorporation of a vasoconstrictor, an oil base, and implant pellets and other insoluble "depot" preparations. Among these depot preparations are drugs that are converted to less soluble salts (eg, procaine and benzathine penicillin) or less soluble complexes (eg, protamine zinc insulin), or that are administered as insoluble microcrystalline suspensions (eg, methylprednisolone acetate).

DISTRIBUTION OF DRUGS IN THE BODY

After absorption into the bloodstream, drugs become disseminated to all parts of the body. Compounds that permeate freely through cell membranes become distributed, in time, throughout the body water, both extracellular and intracellular. Substances that pass readily through and between capillary endothelial cells, but do not penetrate other cell membranes, are distributed into the extracellular fluid space. Occasionally, the drug molecule may be so large (>65,000 daltons) or so highly bound to plasma proteins that it remains in the intravascular space following IV administration. Drugs may also undergo redistribution in the body after initial high levels are achieved in tissues that have a rich vascular supply, eg, the brain. As the plasma concentration falls, the drug readily diffuses back into the circulation to be quickly redistributed to other tissues with high blood-flow rates, such as the muscles; then, over time, the drug also becomes deposited in lipid-rich tissues with poor blood supplies, such as the fat depots. Most drugs are not distributed equally throughout the body, but tend to accumulate in certain specific tissues or fluids. The general principles that govern the passage and distribution of drugs across biological membranes (see above) are applicable. Basic drugs tend to accumulate in tissues and fluids with pH values lower than the pK_a of the drug; conversely, acidic drugs concentrate in regions of higher pH, provided that the free drug is sufficiently lipid-soluble to be able to penetrate the membranes that separate the compartments. Even small differences in pH across boundary membranes, such as those that exist between CSF (pH 7.3) and plasma (pH 7.4), milk (pH 6.5-6.8) and plasma, renal tubular fluid (pH 5.0-8.0) and plasma, and inflamed tissue (pH 6.0-7.0) and healthy tissue (pH 7.0-7.4), can lead to unequal distribution of drugs with pK_a values close to those of the pH of the fluid. Only freely diffusible and unbound drug molecules are able to pass from one compartment to another. Binding to macromolecules such as protein components of cells or fluids, dissolution in adipose tissue, formation of nondiffusible complexes in tissues such as bone, incorporation into specific storage granules, or binding to selective sites in tissues all impede movement of drugs in the body and account for differences in the cellular and organ distribution of particular drugs. Therapeutic agents may also be transported by carrier-mediated systems across certain cellular membranes, which leads to higher concentrations on one side than the other. Examples of such nonspecific transport mechanisms are found in renal tubular epithelial cells, hepatocytes, and the choroid plexus.

Drugs tend to become associated with several blood constituents. Binding to plasma proteins or to components in RBC facilitates absorption into the bloodstream by lowering the concentration of free drug in plasma. It is only the unbound or free fraction of a drug that can diffuse out of capillaries into tissues. The most important binding of drugs in circulation is to plasma albumin, although the globulins and, especially, α-1 acid glycoprotein (for bases) may also play a significant role. A drug may become bound to plasma proteins to a greater or lesser degree, depending on a number of factors, eg, plasma pH, concentration of plasma proteins, concentration of the drug, the presence of another agent with a greater affinity for the limited number of binding sites, and the presence of acute phase proteins during active inflammatory conditions. Acidic drugs are generally more highly bound than basic drugs. Highly lipid-soluble substances are almost always carried in the plasma in association with plasma proteins; hydrophilic polar compounds are generally freely soluble in plasma water. The degree of plasma-protein binding and the affinity of a drug for the nonspecific protein-binding sites is of great clinical significance in some instances and much less so in others. For example, a potentially toxic compound (such as dicumarol) may be 98% bound, but if for any reason it becomes only 96% bound, then **double** the concentration of the free active drug becomes available in the plasma with potentially harmful consequences. The concentration of a drug administered in overdose may exceed the binding capacity of the plasma protein and lead to an excess of free drug, which can diffuse into various target tissues and produce exaggerated effects. Several drugs are so water insoluble that, except for protein binding, they would either precipitate out or become insoluble microemboli. Of equal importance is the readiness with which drugs dissociate from plasma proteins. Those that are more tightly bound tend to have much longer elimination half-lives since they are released gradually from the plasma protein reservoir. The long-acting sulfonamides are good examples of this phenomenon.

Drugs become associated with or bound to specific or selective tissue components through a number of ways. This is often a characteristic of a drug or class of drugs. Examples include: arsenic and griseofulvin are taken up by keratinous tissues; tetracyclines are deposited in growing bone and teeth; exogenous biogenic amines may be captured and stored in specific vesicles, together with endogenous neurotransmitters or autacoids; iron accumulates in ferritin deposits in the intestine, liver, and spleen; aminoglycoside antibiotics are transported into proximal tubular epithelial cells, where they interact with organelle membranes and become trapped in the cell; adipose tissue can accept considerable quantities of highly lipid-soluble drugs, although slowly because of poor blood supply, before their release for ultimate elimination. Characteristically, many drugs and their metabolites may be found predominately in the principal organs of elimination, the liver and kidneys.

During distribution in, and elimination from the body, a drug may or may not penetrate certain "physiological" (the blood-brain, placental, and mammary) barriers.

A drug may gain access to the CNS by 2 distinct routes, viz, the capillary circulation and the CSF. Drugs penetrate into the cortex more rapidly than into white matter, probably because of the greater delivery rate of drug via the bloodstream to the tissue. Certain specialized areas are also penetrated unusually well, but whether because of a rich blood supply or exceptionally permeable capillaries, or both, is not clear. These include part of the fourth ventricle, the pineal body, and the posterior lobe of the hypophysis. In the brain, the capillaries have tight junctions and are much less permeable to a variety of water-soluble substances. Another structural feature associated with decreased permeability of capillaries in the CNS is the close application of the glial connective tissue cells (astrocytes) to the basement membrane of the capillary endothelium. This glial sheath is ~85% complete. Predictably, the permeability characteristics of the brain capillaries are rather like cell membranes elsewhere in the body and not like the permeability characteristics of the usual capillary structure. Thus, the "blood-brain barrier" is not absolute but represents a quantitative, rather than qualitative, difference in capillary permeability as compared with other tissues. Drugs enter the CSF either via the choroid plexus or by diffusion directly across capillaries into the interstitial fluid. They leave the CSF by bulk flow into the venous sinuses, diffusion back into the capillaries within the CNS, absorption or transport back into the systemic circulation at the choroid plexus, or diffusion into the neuronal cells. The heavy myelinization of white matter significantly impedes the entry of drugs. However, in neonates, myelinization may not be complete, and drugs (as well as bilirubin) can penetrate in large quantities in some species, especially primates. Factors that determine the rate of penetration of a drug into brain and CSF include the concentration of free drug in plasma and lipid solubility of the agent.

The pharmacological factors and consequences of the diverse rates of entry of different drugs into the CNS include the following: 1) water-soluble ionized drugs will not enter the CNS; 2) low ionization, low plasma-protein binding, and a fairly high lipid-water partition coefficient confer ready penetration; 3) direct injections into the CSF often produce unexpected effects; and 4) meningoencephalitis can substantially alter the permeability of the blood-brain barrier.

The placental barrier should be considered when selecting an agent to treat a pregnant animal. The potential teratogenicity of any drug needs to be known before its administration, and if it is to be used during late gestation, its effects on the fetus and on the process of parturition should be considered. Nutrients, such as glucose, amino acids, minerals, and even some vitamins, are actively transported across the placenta. The passage of drugs across the placenta is largely by lipid diffusion, and the factors discussed above play a role. Species differences must also be considered. The distribution of drugs within the fetus follows essentially the same pattern as in the adult, with some differences with respect to the volumes of drug distribution, plasma-protein binding, blood circulation, and greater permeability of interceding membranous barriers.

The mammary gland epithelium, like other biological membranes, acts as a lipid barrier, and many drugs readily diffuse from the plasma into milk. The pH of milk varies somewhat, but in goats and cows it is generally 6.5-6.8 if mastitis is not present. Weak bases tend to accumulate in milk because the fraction of ionized, nondiffusible drug is higher. The opposite is true for acidic drugs. Agents delivered by intramammary infusion can diffuse into plasma to a greater or lesser degree by the same processes noted earlier.

BIOTRANSFORMATION OF DRUGS

Drugs and other foreign chemicals (collectively known as xenobiotics) that may be present in the body generally fall into 2 basic categories: 1) polar water-soluble compounds that usually are not metabolized to any appreciable extent (although they may undergo hydrolysis if they are esters) and are excreted unchanged, principally by the kidneys; 2) nonpolar lipid-soluble compounds that first must be metabolically transformed to more polar and water-soluble forms that only then can be efficiently excreted in urine or bile.

The general principle is that xenobiotics are converted by enzymatic processes to compounds of ever-increasing water-solubility until they can be excreted via one or several of the routes available. Metabolism or biotransformation and the subsequent excretion of drugs is known as "elimination".

There are several possible consequences of the biochemical transformation of drugs: 1) inactivation, during which an active drug is converted to an inactive metabolite(s); 2) activation, during which an inactive drug (or pro-drug) is converted to a pharmacologically active primary metabolite; 3) modification of activity following the conversion of an active drug to a metabolite that also possesses pharmacological activity; 4) conjugation (or detoxification), through which a molecule that is usually much more polar is attached to the parent compound or to its metabolites with a marked increase in overall water-solubility and a complete loss of pharmacological activity; or 5) lethal synthesis (or intoxication), in which a drug is incorporated into a normal cellular metabolic pathway that ultimately leads to failure of the reaction sequence because of the presence of spurious substrate (cellular death will then occur).

Many drugs are metabolized in the body in 2 basic phases. The first phase is asynthetic, and the reactions that occur include oxidations, hydroxylations, deaminations, and N-dealkylations. Hydrolysis of esters and amides also can occur. These reactions result in the introduction or unmasking of functional groups, rendering a nonpolar compound polar—or a polar compound even more polar—and, hence, more readily excreted than the original compound. These functional groups often act as the center for the second phase of biotransformation, in which a synthetic step occurs so that the metabolite is conjugated with endogenous molecular groups (such as methyl, acetyl, sulfate), glucuronic acid, or one of a number of amino acids. These conjugated metabolites are usually excreted in the urine and bile. Most drugs are biotransformed by both Phase I and Phase II reactions. However, there are some drugs, particularly compounds that already possess a functional group, that often only undergo Phase II reactions. The basic scheme for drug biotransformation is as follows:

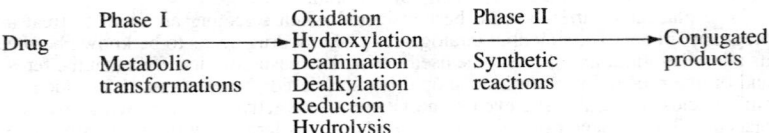

Several enzymatic systems may be involved in these metabolic transformations and conjugations; the most important are the microsomal mixed function oxidase (MFO) enzymes principally located in the smooth endoplasmic reticulum of the hepatocytes, although these enzymes may also be active in the intestinal wall, kidneys, and lungs. Microsomal enzymes are specific for functional groups but not for substrates.

The first functional component of the MFO system consists of multiple forms of 2 hemoproteins (cytochrome P_{450} and P_{448}) that act as oxygen-activating enzymes as well as sites of substrate interaction for oxidative transformations of various compounds. Another hemoprotein, cytochrome b_5, also plays a role in some MFO-mediated reactions, acting as a carrier of electrons from NADH and NADPH for specific fatty acid desaturation. A third component of the MFO system is NADPH-cytochrome c reductase, which is an inducible flavoprotein; its primary physiological role is to transfer electrons from NADPH to cytochrome P_{450} during microsomal hydroxylations. Several phospholipids, especially phosphatidylcholine, are also thought to be essential for the microsomal electron transport system. Certain short-lived, highly reactive, intermediate metabolites, such as epoxides, are potentially toxic in a number of ways. Their rapid conversion to the benign end-product metabolite is often of cardinal significance. Acetaminophen toxicity in cats exemplifies this hazard. Some oxidation and reduction reactions are not mediated by hepatic microsomal enzymes but by enzymes present in the soluble and mitochondrial fractions of the liver, plasma, kidneys, placenta, intestinal mucosa, and gut flora. Drug metabolism by hydrolysis is restricted to esters and amides. Esterases are found in plasma and in the soluble fraction of the cells of many tissues. The amidases are also non-microsomal enzymes and are found mainly in the liver. Phase II or conjugation reactions include glucuronide synthesis; acetylation; glycine and glutamine conjugation; mercapturic acid formation; synthesis of ethereal sulfates; and N-, O-, and S-methylation. These synthetic reactions generally require an "active" intermediate, usually a nucleotide, and a transferring enzyme that may or may not be located in the microsomal fraction of hepatic and other cells.

Several aspects of the biotransformation of drugs have direct clinical significance. These include microsomal enzyme induction and inhibition, nutritional state, age, disease conditions, and species differences.

Many drugs may stimulate hepatic microsomal enzymes, which lead to the synthesis of new protein with an increase in the amount of smooth endoplasmic reticulum and other components of the microsomal system within the hepatocytes. A microsomal enzyme inducer shortens the plasma half-life of a co-administered agent by hastening its biotransformation and excretion. This effect generally reduces the pharmacological action of the second drug. The exception, however, is seen when activation of a pro-drug is required. In these cases, toxicity may result from the rapid conversion of an inactive drug to a primary active metabolite. This possibility exists with malathion and cyclophosphamide. Clinically, concern for the possibility of enzyme induction arises with long-term administration of therapeutic agents. Continued use of phenobarbital and other barbiturates, rifampin, phenytoin, benzodiazepines, phenylbutazone, griseofulvin, and chlorinated hydrocarbon insecticides may induce microsomal enzymes. Microsomal enzyme induction usually develops over several days or weeks, and may persist for a similar period following withdrawal of the inducing agent.

A number of agents are capable of effectively blocking the activity of the microsomal enzymes, most often by substrate competition. The result is an exaggerated or prolonged reaction to the second agent and an increased risk of toxicity. The plasma half-life may be markedly prolonged. Chloramphenicol is a potent microsomal enzyme inhibitor with a rapid onset of action (within hours) and a long residual effect. Other microsomal enzyme inhibitors include cimetidine, quinidine, dicumarol, sulfaphenazole, oxyphenbutazone, and several phenothiazine neuroleptics.

Severe hypoproteinemia, avitaminosis B, or energy deficiency lead to a depletion of hepatic glycogen, and to exaggerated drug responses due to a functional impairment of microsomal enzyme activity.

Because drug biotransformation is negligible in early life, the neonate is much more sensitive to lipid-soluble drugs than is the adult of any species. The postnatal development of drug-metabolizing enzymes in the liver appears to be biphasic, consisting of a rapid and nearly linear increase in activity during the first 3-4 wk, followed by slower development up to the tenth week postpartum; dose rates for the very young must be reduced accordingly. A decrease in hepatic mass and hepatic blood flow, as well as diminishing microsomal enzyme activity, may occur in older animals.

Many disease states impair the normal activity of the hepatic microsomal enzyme system, which in turn prolongs the half-lives of many drugs administered to such animals. Frank hepatotoxicity, acute hepatitis, or other extensive liver lesions invariably depress enzyme activity. Changes in hepatic blood flow, with similar consequences, may be encountered in congestive heart failure, circulatory shock, and cirrhosis. Hypothyroidism tends to reduce microsomal enzyme function, and hyperthyroidism tends to increase activity.

Species variations in the biotransformation patterns of lipid-soluble drugs are common. Differences in the duration of action of these drugs in various species frequently can be attributed to differences in their rates of biotransformation. This must be remembered when either dosages or withdrawal times are extrapolated from one species to another.

EXCRETION OF DRUGS AND THEIR METABOLITES

The concentration of a drug in the plasma or at its receptor sites may be reduced in 3 basic ways: 1) distribution or redistribution into various tissue compartments, 2) metabolic inactivation, and 3) excretion from the body via one of several possible routes. The kidneys are the principal organ of excretion but the liver, GI tract, and lungs also may play important roles. Milk, saliva, and sweat are usually of less importance, although the presence of an active drug in milk may affect suckling young.

Renal excretion of foreign compounds involves glomerular filtration, passive diffusion into and out of the tubular lumen, and carrier-mediated secretion, mainly in the proximal convoluted tubule. Only unbound molecules <66,000 daltons are readily filtered through the glomerular membranes into the tubular lumen. The amount of compound in the filtrate depends on the degree of binding to plasma proteins and the glomerular filtration rate. Since water is reabsorbed throughout the length of the nephron, filtered drugs tend to concentrate in the tubular fluid, which favors their reabsorption into the peritubular capillaries. Because reabsorption depends on the factors that govern the transmembrane passage of molecules, the tubular epithelium is permeable only to lipid-soluble molecules. Highly ionized or polar agents are not reabsorbed, and the degree of ionization depends on the pK_a of the compound, whether it is an acid or a base, and on the pH of the tubular fluid. Tubular reabsorption via nonionic diffusion becomes a factor for acidic drugs when their pK_a values are between 3 and 8 and the urine is acidic. For basic drugs when the urine is alkaline, the pK_a values need to be between 6 and 11 to significantly affect the tubular reabsorption process. Acidification or alkalinization of the urine may alter the rate of excretion of some drugs because of ion-trapping in the tubular fluid.

Tubular secretion of both acidic and basic drugs occurs in the proximal convoluted tubule by saturable carrier-mediated transport processes. The compounds are delivered to the renal tubule cells by the peritubular capillary network and then are transported into the tubular fluid. Characteristically, the molecules are ionized or polar and are either parent compounds or metabolites. The transport systems are energy-dependent and nonspecific, but may be competitively inhibited by drugs with similar chemical properties. Binding to plasma proteins usually does not hinder tubular excretion of drugs because of the dynamic equilibrium that exists between free and bound drug. As free drug is removed and transported across the tubular epithelium, immediate dissociation of the drug-albumin complex usually occurs. Concurrent administration of either acidic or basic drugs that are substrates for carrier-mediated secretion processes prolongs the elimination of the drug that has the lesser affinity for the carrier sites, thus increasing its duration of action.

Drugs and their metabolites may also be excreted either passively or actively by hepatocytes into the bile canaliculi, and ultimately into the duodenum in the bile. Examples of drugs that are actively secreted in bile include stilbestrol, morphine, chloramphenicol, cefamandole, and cefoperazone. If the properties of such compounds are favorable for intestinal absorption, or if a water-soluble conjugate such as glucuronic acid is cleaved by bacterial hydrolysis within the gut so that the drug once again becomes lipid-soluble, it will be reabsorbed and an enterohepatic cycle may become established. During such a cycle, biliary secretion and intestinal reabsorption continue until metabolic degradation or urinary excretion eventually eliminate the agent from the body. Enterohepatic cycles often account for prolonged half-lives of drugs that are primarily excreted in bile.

The main role of the biliary route is to eliminate certain organic ions that cannot be reabsorbed from the intestinal tract because they are ionized at the prevailing pH.

These drugs generally have a molecular weight above ~400 daltons, although somewhat smaller molecules also may be eliminated by the biliary route in some species. There are nonspecific carrier-mediated transport systems for both acids and bases located in the hepatocytes. Drugs with molecular masses less than ~300 daltons generally diffuse passively into bile.

The other routes of excretion are of lesser clinical importance. However, several drugs may diffuse directly into the GI tract and then be eliminated in the feces. The ruminoreticulum also can act as a drug reservoir or "sink". The tracheobronchial tree also may represent a potential avenue of excretion. Many drugs that are administered parenterally are found in bronchial secretions. Alveolar elimination is of major significance when inhalant anesthetics are used. The main factors governing elimination by this route are the same as those determining the uptake of inhalant anesthetics, viz, the concentrations in plasma and alveolar air, and the blood/gas partition coefficient. Excretion of drugs by mammary and salivary glands occurs by nonionic passive diffusion. The process is determined by pH/pK_a relationships, lipid solubility, and concentration gradients. The salivary route of excretion is important in ruminants because they secrete such voluminous amounts of alkaline saliva.

If the excretory functions of those organs concerned with drug elimination are impaired or altered in any way (disease, very young or very old animal), prolonged elimination patterns result. Moreover, several nutritional and pharmacokinetic interactions have the potential to change the rates of drug excretion.

When urinary excretion is an important route of elimination, renal failure results in decreased drug clearance, and thus slower removal of the drug from the body. A usual dosage regimen in such cases tends to lead to accumulation and, ultimately, toxicity. A number of disturbances may occur within failing kidneys, all of which may influence the excretion of drugs: renal ischemia, glomerular involvement, tubular damage, impaired intrarenal perfusion, functional disabilities of the tubular cells, failed homeostatic mechanisms, and obstructive lesions in the tubules or collecting ducts (or even the ureters or urethra). Changes in the pH of the filtrate also alter the excretion rates of drugs with appropriate pK_a values. In addition to the direct effect on renal excretory mechanisms, pathological changes in the kidneys can influence the disposition and elimination of drugs. In most instances, drug toxicity is increased. The binding of many drugs to plasma proteins is decreased in uremic animals. The rates of many metabolic reactions are also often depressed in renal failure, and this may impair effective elimination of agents that require biotransformation. Associated clinical signs and pathophysiological changes, often encountered in renal failure, can also alter pharmacodynamic responses to particular drugs. Derangements of acid-base balance, hyper- and hypokalemia, hyper-and hyponatremia, dehydration, and hyper-and hypotension are examples of systemic conditions that may radically modify a drug's fate or action.

The normal urinary pH of dogs and cats is acidic (5.5-7), while that of herbivorous animals tends to be alkaline (7-8). Dietary constituents may alter urinary pH, which in turn may influence the renal excretion of drugs. Acidification can occur in monogastric animals with a protein intake containing a high concentration of sulfur-containing amino acids, or with high levels of acidifying salts such as calcium and ammonium chloride, or sodium hydrogen phosphate.

Although less often of clinical significance, impairment of the excretory functions of the hepatocytes or obstruction of bile flow due to any cause interferes with the biliary excretion of drugs. Dose rates should then be adjusted accordingly. The normal kinetics of a drug's enterohepatic cycle may change in such cases, or may be modified by disruption or elimination of the intestinal flora.

A number of potential pharmacokinetic interactions that modify the excretion of drugs have been recognized. Agents that increase glomerular filtration rate generally enhance renal elimination, and the converse is true for those drugs that reduce glomerular filtration rate. Diuretics tend to increase the renal elimination of some drugs; furosemide is the most potent in this regard. Urinary acidifying agents facilitate the excretion of some weak bases such as morphine, meperidine, procaine, and several antihistaminic agents, and by this action shorten their elimination times. The excretion of certain acidic drugs is enhanced by urinary alkalinization, or delayed by acidification. Competition for the renal tubular transport systems for organic ions can occur among concurrently administered drugs. Weak acids that may competitively inhibit the system include the penicillins, cephalosporins, certain sulfonamides, phenylbutazone, probenecid, salicylates, indomethacin, furosemide, ethacrynic acid, acetazolamide, thiazide diuretics, and glucuronic acid conjugates. Weak bases, such as procainamide, dopamine, trimethoprim, and tolazoline, may also compete for the nonspecific transport system, but these interactions are less often of clinical importance.

Choleretics or a high fat intake promote bile flow and therefore, biliary excretion, and enhance the hepatic secretion of drugs. Broad-spectrum antibacterial agents are expected to diminish the hydrolytic action of intestinal flora, and thus may prevent effective enterohepatic cycles.

PHARMACOKINETICS

To produce a therapeutic effect, a drug must enter the systemic circulation and be delivered in sufficient amount to the target cells in an organ or tissue so that it can combine with specific receptors to initiate its pharmacological action. Between the time of administration and onset of action, various pharmacokinetic and pharmacodynamic processes occur that continue throughout and even beyond the duration of the drug's clinical effects. The pharmacokinetic characteristics of a particular drug (rates of absorption, distribution, biotransformation, and excretion) determine its concentration in the plasma, which is generally proportional to the concentration at the drug's specific receptors (biophase). Because the intensity of the tissue response is usually determined by the concentration of the drug in the direct environment of the receptors, a drug's concentration in plasma is generally assumed to be correlated with the time course of its action. Dosage regimens are derived from pharmacokinetic studies in normal animals but often require modification in diseased, young, old, obese, thin, or pregnant animals. A large number of pharmacokinetic measures can be determined from time-course studies of drug concentrations in plasma, but only the more clinically useful features and values are emphasized below.

CONCENTRATION OF DRUGS IN BLOOD

Drugs administered PO or parenterally are absorbed into the systemic circulation, distributed throughout the body, and then eliminated. Their concentrations in the blood can be determined and graphed against time. In most instances, the time course of a drug's concentration in the plasma correlates well with the onset, intensity, and duration of the pharmacologic effect. Thus, the measurement of sequential plasma concentration of drugs following their administration is used to establish dosage regimens that are likely to produce the desired therapeutic levels for appropriate periods of time, without the risk of drug failure or toxicity.

Single-dose Concentration Curves (Extravascular Administration): When a drug is administered by an extravascular route, it usually appears in the plasma within a short time, and its concentration rises steadily until a peak level is reached. Once absorbed into the circulation, it is subjected simultaneously to distribution, biotransformation, and excretion. During the initial period, the rate of absorption and distribution exceeds the rate of elimination. The peak plasma concentration is reached when absorption and elimination rates are equal. Thereafter, the elimination rate exceeds the rate of absorption because less drug remains available at the site of administration, and plasma drug levels begin to fall. When the concentration of a drug in plasma is determined at appropriate time intervals following a single dose, a characteristic curve is obtained as is illustrated in FIGURE 1:

**Figure 1. Typical Plasma Concentration Versus Time Curve (linear scale)
Following Extravascular Administration of a Drug**

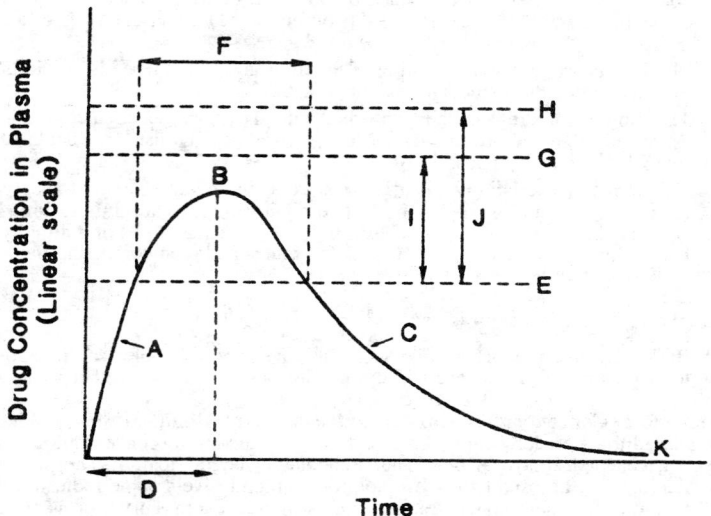

Key: A = absorption and distribution phase
      B = peak plasma concentration (Cp [max])
      C = elimination phase (biotransformation and excretion)
      D = time to attain peak concentration
      E = minimal effective plasma concentration (MEC)
      F = duration of clinical effect
      G = potentially toxic plasma concentration
      H = maximum tolerated plasma concentration (MTC)
      I = therapeutic zone
      J = effective zone or "therapeutic window"
      K = last measurable plasma concentration

The clinically useful information that can be obtained from this curve is as follows:

1) The slope of the ascending limb of the plasma curve reflects the rate of drug absorption and the rate of its distribution to tissues. The steeper the slope, the more rapidly the drug is absorbed and/or the more slowly it is distributed.

2) The peak of the curve indicates the Cp (max) obtained after a single dose, and the time required for this to occur can also be determined.

3) The slope of the descending limb reflects the rate of distribution, biotransformation, and excretion. The steeper the slope, the more rapidly a drug is eliminated.

4) The action of a drug generally becomes evident when the plasma level reaches the MEC and persists as long as the plasma level remains above the MEC. The intensity of the therapeutic effect is also usually proportional to the height of the plasma concentration curve. By increasing plasma concentrations, potentially toxic levels are reached before signs of frank toxicity first become evident at the MTC. The difference between the MTC and the MEC of a drug in plasma is known as the "therapeutic window".

5) The last measurable concentration of the drug in plasma depends on the limits of detection of the particular analytical method used.

6) The amount of drug actually absorbed into the systemic circulation can be estimated from the area under the curve (AUC). This can be calculated by several different methods.

7) The term "bioavailability" is used to express the rate and extent of absorption of a drug, usually from the GI tract following administration PO. Bioavailability (F) is determined by administering equal doses of a drug by the IV (absorption effectively 100%) and PO routes and then comparing the areas under the 2 curves.

The following equation is used: $F = \dfrac{AUC, PO}{AUC, IV}$

Bioavailability is expressed as a percent. The same principles can be applied to calculation of the bioavailability of drugs administered by other routes.

Single-dose Concentration Curves (Intravascular Administration): When a drug is administered by rapid IV injection, the maximum concentration in the blood is reached almost at once and immediately begins to fall. The profile of this decline can be established by monitoring blood levels at periodic intervals and then plotting these concentrations against time. Several curve forms are possible, but the one most typically obtained (2-compartment open model) is illustrated in FIGURE 2.

Figure 2. Typical Plasma Concentration Versus Time Curve (semilogarithmic scale) Following IV Administration of a Drug (2-compartment open model)

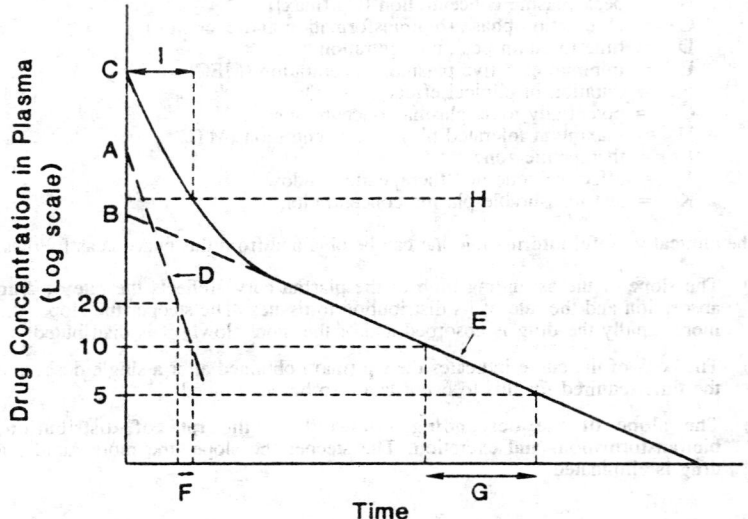

Key: A   = zero time intercept of distribution phase
          B   = zero time intercept of elimination phase
          C   = plasma concentration immediately following IV administration of
               bolus dose ($C^{o}p$)
          D   = distribution or α phase, slope of line = $-\alpha/2.3$
          E   = elimination or β phase, slope of line = $-\beta/2.3$
          F   = distribution half-time ($t_{1/2}\alpha$)
          G   = elimination half-life ($t_{1/2}\beta$)
          H   = minimal effective plasma concentration (MEC)
          I   = duration of clinical effect

Useful information that can be obtained from this curve is as follows:

1) The zero-time plasma drug concentration intercepts for the biphasic disposition curve (A for the distribution line and B for the elimination line).

2) The plasma drug concentration immediately following the IV injection of a single dose ($C^{o}p$).

3) The hybrid rate constants of the biphasic disposition curve. Values of α and β are related to the slopes of the distribution ($-\alpha/2.3$) and elimination ($-\beta/2.3$) phases, respectively. Alpha (α) is the overall distribution rate constant reflecting the diffusion of the drug from the central to the peripheral (tissue) compartment. Beta (β) is the overall elimination rate constant. The unit used for elimination rate constants is reciprocal time.

4) The distribution half-time ($t_{1/2}\alpha$) and the elimination half-time or plasma half-life of the drug ($t_{1/2}\beta$) in minutes or, more commonly, in hours.

From the information obtained above, a number of additional pharmacokinetic parameters can be calculated. Only the more significant of these are outlined and their usefulness noted.

Transfer rate constants: First-order transfer rate constants for drug distribution between the central and peripheral compartments (k_{12}, k_{21}, k_{13}, k_{31}, etc) are values used to determine the first-order elimination rate constant (k_{el}) for the disappearance of drug from the central compartment.

Elimination half-life: The expressions $0.693/k_{el}$ or $0.693/\beta$ represent the half-life of a drug that undergoes first-order (exponential) elimination: in the first case, for a one-compartment open-model; and in the second, for a 2-compartment open model. The plasma half-life ($t_{1/2}$) of a drug has important clinical significance ($t_{1/2} = 0.693/k_{el}$ or $t_{1/2} = 0.693/\beta$).

APPARENT VOLUME OF DISTRIBUTION

When a drug is introduced into an animal's body, it diffuses through various membrane barriers into the tissues and body fluids where it may bind to proteins to a greater or lesser degree. Such processes occur at various rates depending on the physicochemical characteristics of the drug as discussed earlier. Consequently, a drug produces a characteristic plasma-tissue distribution pattern. A high plasma concentration implies significant retention in the blood, whereas a low plasma concentration suggests notable diffusion from the vascular bed and retention of the drug in tissues. The pharmacokinetic measure used to indicate this pattern, as well as the size of the compartment into which a drug would seem to have distributed in relation to its concentration in plasma, is known as the apparent volume of distribution (Vd). The units used for Vd are liters (L). Since the concentrations of a drug in various tissues and body fluids usually differ greatly, the volume of the compartment derived from the concentration of a drug in plasma does **not** reflect a real body volume, except in the rare circumstance in which a drug is uniformly distributed in all body compartments. Thus, the apparent Vd is a proportionality constant that relates the plasma concentration of a drug to the amount of drug in the body, assuming that no elimination has occurred. More commonly, the Vd is corrected for the body weight of the animal and is then known as the apparent specific volume of distribution (V'd), and the units employed are L/kg. The Vd, or V'd, of a drug is an important pharmacokinetic value with significant clinical applications.

Several methods are employed to estimate the Vd. Since the concentration of a drug in the plasma can be measured and the dose is known, the apparent Vd can be calculated from the formula:

$$Vd = \frac{\text{dose (D) of the drug (= amount of drug in body or Ab)}}{\text{concentration of the drug at zero time } (C^{\circ}p)}$$

$$\text{or Vd} = \frac{Ab \text{ (or D)}}{C^{\circ}p}$$

Because drugs in the blood are subject to biotransformation and excretion, the amount of drug in the body and the concentration in the plasma must be determined at zero time, assuming thorough mixing in the body fluids and before any elimination has occurred. A zero-time concentration cannot be determined experimentally and must be obtained by extrapolation of the plasma concentration-time curve back to the ordinate. This is fairly accurate for a one-compartment model but not for 2-compartment models, in which the intercept B is used (*see* FIGURE 2), and Vd (B) is calculated neglecting the α or distributive phase of drug disposition. Values determined by the extrapolation method are usually erroneously high for the apparent Vd.

The apparent Vd can also be computed by the area method in which Vd = $\frac{Ab \text{ or } D}{AUC}$ AUC is the area under the concentration-time curve following IV injection of the drug. The values of Vd obtained by this method are independent of the model employed.

The apparent Vd for a drug is determined by its degree of water or lipid solubility, the extent of plasma- and tissue-protein binding, and the perfusion of tissues. Low Vd are encountered for drugs that tend to maintain high concentrations in the plasma because of low lipid solubility, extensive binding to plasma proteins, and diminished tissue binding. The reverse is true for drugs with high apparent Vd. The value of Vd or V'd is characteristic for a drug and is usually constant over a wide dose range for a given species of animal. However, a number of clinically significant factors can influence the Vd. Included among these are age; functional status of the kidneys, liver, and heart; fluid accumulations; concentration of plasma proteins; acid-base status; inflammatory processes or necrosis; and any other causes for alteration in the degree of plasma-protein binding.

The specific Vd can be used to determine dosage. A desired plasma concentration can be calculated from the formula D = C × V'd × kg body wt, in which D is the dose and C is the required plasma concentration for a given drug.

DRUG CLEARANCE (ELIMINATION)

Once a drug is absorbed and distributed among the tissues and body fluids, it is then eliminated, or cleared, mainly by the liver and kidneys. Consequently, the plasma concentration of a drug decreases steadily, although at different rates for various drugs in different species. Following a single dose, only ~3% of a given dose remains in the body after 5 half-lives, since 96.87% has been cleared by this time. Drug clearance (Cl) is defined as the volume of plasma that would contain the amount of drug excreted per minute or, alternatively, the volume of plasma that would have to lose all of the drug that it contains within a unit of time (usually 1 min) to account for an observed rate of drug elimination. Thus, clearance expresses the rate or efficiency of drug removal from the plasma but **not** the amount of drug eliminated. The concept of drug clearance is of great clinical significance.

Total body clearance (Cl_B) is the sum of individual clearances by various organs but mainly by the liver (Cl_h) through biotransformation and biliary excretion, and by the kidneys (Cl_r) through filtration and/or tubular secretion. Generally, $Cl_B = Cl_h + Cl_r$.

Organ clearance expresses the efficiency with which a specific organ removes a drug from the perfusing blood. The extent of this reduction is expressed as the extraction ratio (E), which can be determined from the following formula: $E = \dfrac{Ca - Cv}{Ca}$, in which Ca is the arterial and Cv is the venous plasma concentration of the drug. If the plasma flow through an organ is Q (in mL/min), then the volume of the plasma from which the drug is completely removed per unit time (or its clearance, Cl) is equal to $E \times Q$. If the extraction ratio for a drug is high (eg, renal excretion of p-aminohippurate or hepatic extraction of propranolol), then clearance becomes primarily a function of organ blood flow.

Renal clearance is defined as the volume of plasma that is totally cleared of a drug in 1 min during passage through the kidneys. Its value depends on the degree of glomerular filtration, tubular secretion, and tubular reabsorption of the drug. At constant plasma concentration, the renal clearance of a drug is determined by the following equation: $Cl_r = \dfrac{Cu \times V}{Cp}$, in which Cu is the mean concentration of unchanged drug in the urine during the collection interval, Cp is the plasma concentration at the midpoint of the collection interval, and V is the urine flow rate. This equation is used to determine renal clearance when a steady state is achieved by IV infusion over a time interval equivalent to ~5 half-lives of the drug.

To measure renal clearance after a single IV injection, the following equation is used: $Cl_r = \dfrac{Cu}{AUC}$, in which Cu is the cumulative amount of unchanged drug in the urine during the collection period, and AUC is the area under the plasma concentration-time curve during the collection period.

The renal clearance of drugs depends on urine pH, extent of plasma-protein binding, and renal plasma flow. These factors may vary from animal to animal as well as among species, because of differences in diet, environmental temperature, physical activity, many diseases, and concomitant use of certain drugs. For drugs that are excreted primarily by glomerular filtration, the animal's creatinine clearance may serve as an indicator of drug clearance because creatinine undergoes complete glomerular filtration while being subjected to minimal tubular reabsorption. Consequently, creatinine clearance rate can be used for adjusting dosage schedules of some drugs in animals with impaired renal function.

Hepatic clearance is defined as the volume of plasma that is totally cleared of drug in 1 min during passage through the liver. Most drugs, except highly hydrophilic compounds, are cleared from the plasma mainly by biotransformation in the liver, although biliary excretion can also contribute to the hepatic clearance of a drug. The main factors that determine hepatic clearance include hepatic blood flow (delivery of drug to the liver), uptake of the unbound drug by the hepatocytes from the blood, metabolic transformation of the drug by microsomal or other enzyme systems, and rate of biliary secretion. One equation that reflects these relationships is $Cl_h = Q \times (\dfrac{f \times E}{Q + f \times E})$, in which Cl_h is the hepatic clearance fraction of drug present in the blood, and E is the liver's extraction ratio for the particular drug (representing the efficiency of enzyme activity and biliary secretion if present).

Typically, 2 groups of drugs are recognized. The first is those that are readily biotransformed with high extraction ratios, eg, lidocaine, propranolol, and nitroglycerine. The hepatic clearance of this group depends mainly on blood flow and is only rarely limited by diminished enzyme activity because of the high intrinsic ability of the liver to metabolize them. The second is those drugs, eg, the benzodiazepines, procainamide, and theophylline, with very low extraction ratios because of the poor intrinsic ability of the liver to metabolize them. In these instances, hepatic clearance depends more on the efficiency of the enzyme systems and the degree of plasma-protein binding rather than the adequacy of hepatic blood flow.

Some drugs undergo substantial removal from the portal circulation by the liver following administration PO. This "first pass" effect can significantly reduce the amount of parent drug that reaches the systemic circulation. A number of factors can modify the magnitude of the first pass effect for a particular drug. Hepatic clearance can be impaired by liver disease, biliary stasis, decreased hepatic blood flow, and drugs that inhibit microsomal enzyme systems. Microsomal enzyme inducers often increase hepatic clearance of a concurrently administered drug. There is no reliable liver function test to assess the impediment of hepatic clearance of drugs (as creatinine clearance does for the kidneys). The dose rates for drugs used in animals suffering from liver disease must be adjusted on clinical judgement alone.

Relationship Between Body Clearance, Volume of Distribution, and Plasma Half-life: Since only the free drug present in plasma can be removed during passage through an organ responsible for biotransformation and/or excretion, the overall rate of drug elimination from the body must be related to the apparent volume of distribution (Vd). Moreover, for first-order processes this overall rate of removal from the central compartment (plasma and readily exchangeable tissues and fluids) is given by the elimination rate constant or k_{el}. Thus,

$$Cl_B = k_{el} \times Vd, \text{ or } k_{el} = \frac{Cl_B}{Vd}$$

The fraction $\frac{Cl_B}{Vd}$ is also known as the fractional elimination constant.

The actual rate of elimination at any given time can be determined by $k_{el} \times$ amount in the body (Ab), or by $Cl_B \times Cp$, in which Cp is the plasma concentration. As noted above, $k_{el} = \frac{0.693}{t_{1/2}}$: therefore, $Cl_B = \frac{0.693\ Vd}{t_{1/2}}$ or $t_{1/2} = \frac{0.693\ Vd}{Cl_B}$

This important relationship clearly shows that a drug's plasma half-life is determined by both clearance and its Vd: the $t_{1/2}$ of a drug is directly proportional to its Vd and has an inverse relationship with the body clearance of the drug. Thus, the plasma $t_{1/2}$ of a drug may be shortened because of increased clearance, or lengthened because of decreased clearance. Many factors may influence both hepatic and renal clearance rates as noted earlier. Also, the plasma $t_{1/2}$ of some drugs is shortened when their Vd is reduced, but when their Vd is large or expanded, elimination generally proceeds slowly.

An understanding of these 3 pharmacokinetic parameters ($t_{1/2}$, Vd, Cl_B) and their relationship to each other is fundamental to pharmacotherapeutics.

Steady State Plasma Concentration (Repeated Administration or Constant IV Infusion): In some cases, the desired therapeutic effect of a drug is produced with a single dose. However, to achieve a satisfactory response, it is frequently necessary to maintain drug concentrations longer in the therapeutic range. Rather than administering large doses, which could be potentially toxic, repeated safe doses at regular intervals or continuous IV delivery are generally necessary.

When a drug is infused IV, the plasma concentration continues to rise until elimination equals the rate of delivery into the body. Thereafter, if the infusion rate is constant, it is continually balanced by elimination, and a plateau concentration of the drug is attained in the plasma. The plateau concentration achieved is a function of the rate of infusion; the time required to reach the plateau concentration is determined solely by the drug's elimination rate constant (k_{el}).

The infusion rate for a drug (R_i) can be calculated from $R_i = Cp \times Vd \times k_{el}$, or $R_i = Cp \times Cl_B$, or $R_i = D \times k_{el}$, in which Cp is the plasma concentration, Vd is the apparent volume of distribution, k_{el} is the elimination rate constant, Cl_B is the clearance, and D is the usual therapeutic dose. The units for amount, volume, and time must be consistent when infusion rates are calculated.

If a drug is infused IV for a period of time equal to its $t_{1/2}$, 50% of the plateau concentration will be attained. Similarly, for 2, 3, and 4 half-lives, 75%, 87.6%, and 93.6% of the plateau concentration will be reached, respectively. For practical purposes, steady state is achieved by 5 half-lives.

When a drug is administered intermittently rather than by constant infusion, the relationship between plasma concentration and the dose given at each dosing interval can be expressed as $D = C_{p(av)} \times Cl_B \times T$, in which D is the dose, $C_{p(av)}$ is the average plasma concentration, Cl_B is body clearance, and T is the dosage interval.

For orally administered drugs that are not completely absorbed, the calculated dose must be corrected by the fraction (F) of the drug that reaches the systemic circulation. Thus, in this case, $D = \dfrac{C_{p(av)} \times Cl_B \times T}{F}$

The time required to reach steady state depends only on the drug's $t_{1/2}$. The shorter the $t_{1/2}$, the more rapidly steady state is reached. The size of the dose and the route of administration have little effect. Consequently, whether a drug is delivered by constant or intermittent IV injection, by other parenteral routes (provided there is not pharmaceutical manipulation to delay absorption), or orally, a steady state concentration is reached after at least 5 half-lives.

When a drug normally requires some time to reach a steady state level, and some haste is necessary, plasma levels may be achieved more rapidly by the administration of a loading dose or doses. This entails the administration of a single large dose or smaller doses at frequent intervals to bring the concentration in plasma quickly to the level desired during the steady state. The loading dose required to achieve the plasma levels present at steady state can be determined from the fraction of drug eliminated during the dosing interval and the maintenance dose. Thus, $D_L = \dfrac{100}{f_{el} \times D_M}$, in which D_L is the loading dose, f_{el} is the fraction of drug eliminated per dosing interval, and D_M is the maintenance dose. Maintenance doses are frequently 50% of the loading dose, and replace the amount of drug lost during the dosing interval.

The steady state volume of distribution (Vd) of a drug can be used to estimate the amount of drug in the body at infusion equilibrium (plateau) and during steady state on repetitive dosing.

An appropriate dosing interval for most drugs should usually be equal to the drug's plasma half-life. Shorter dosing intervals increase the risk of drug-induced toxicity because of increased blood levels. Prolonged dosing intervals diminish the drug's efficacy since plasma concentrations fall below the MEC. Often, however, dosing intervals equal to the half-lives are impractical for drugs with short half-lives, and in most cases, either high doses of a relatively nontoxic drug are given to produce therapeutic concentrations for a sufficient time period, or potentially harmful drugs are administered by careful IV infusion. Another approach is to employ dosage formulations or devices that allow for a more gradual release of the active principle into the systemic circulation.

PHARMACOKINETIC MODELS

Zero and First-order Processes: Following administration, a drug passes through various cells, tissues, and extracellular spaces until eventually it is completely excreted. The physicochemical and biological principles governing the fate of drugs in the body are reviewed above. However, in pharmacokinetics, the transfer of drugs is not described in physicochemical terms but is represented by equations that describe the rates at which drugs are absorbed, distributed, and eliminated.

For most drugs, the absorption, distribution, and elimination processes follow first-order kinetics. In a first-order process, the rate of change of drug concentration is directly proportional to the concentration of the drug at the time. Thus, the process may be described by an exponential function, eg, the rate of drug elimination is described by $\dfrac{dC}{dT} = -kC$. This means that the rate of change of the concentration of the drug in blood is equal to a proportionality constant times the concentration at time t. The constant k really represents the fraction of a drug that diminishes per unit time and has the dimension of reciprocal time. If the above differential equation is integrated, we obtain $C = C_o e^{-kt}$, in which C is the plasma concentration at time t, C_o is the initial concentration, and k is the first-order rate constant.

If a drug is eliminated from the plasma by first-order kinetics, a plot of the log of the concentration in plasma versus time yields a straight line, the slope of which is

$-k/2.3$, and the intercept with the ordinate yields the zero time plasma concentration. The application of this concept is illustrated in the elimination phase of the graph in FIGURE 2, p 1312.

Less frequently, the absorption, biotransformation, or excretion of a drug may follow zero-order kinetics, which is then characterized by a constant rate of change, irrespective of the drug's concentration. A zero-order process is expressed by the equation: $\dfrac{dC}{dT} = k$, in which k is the zero-order rate constant with dimensions of amount per unit time (eg, mg/min). The differential rate equation in this case is solved as follows: $C = C_0 - kt$, in which C is the plasma concentration at any time t after drug administration, and C_0 is the theoretical concentration at zero time. In this case, a linear plot of plasma concentration versus time yields a straight line.

The elimination of some important drugs (eg, phenytoin, aspirin, phenylbutazone, dicumarol, and ethanol) does not follow first-order kinetics within therapeutic ranges. For these drugs, the rate of elimination is not constant, but fluctuates as levels in the body are altered by changes in dose or reduced by elimination. This pattern of elimination is said to be dose-dependent or capacity-limited, and occurs when processes other than simple diffusion play a major role. Drug metabolism, carrier-mediated transport, and plasma- and tissue-protein binding are saturable processes that may exhibit a limited capacity for the amount of drug that can be handled. For drugs with this kinetic characteristic, increases in the dose above saturation levels can be accompanied by disproportionately large increments in plasma and tissue levels that substantially increase the risk of toxicity.

Theoretical Compartments: The disposition and elimination of a drug is a complex process based on many interdependent and kinetically controlled events. When all of these steps follow first-order kinetics, the resultant pharmacokinetic model (semilogarithmic) is accepted as a linear model.

Generally, it is the plasma (or central compartment) time curves that are determined, which may then reflect 1, 2, 3, or even more exponential decay functions. These, in turn, suggest that the body may be regarded as a single compartment or as 2, 3, or more interconnecting compartments. This mathematical concept of compartments is entirely theoretical and often bears no relationship to any real physiological space or compartment.

Pharmacokinetic models that describe various kinetic patterns of drug disposition are available, and a set of experimental data points collected from animals may be fitted to the best model, usually by making use of a suitable computer program.

The simplest pharmacokinetic model for a drug depicts the body as a single compartment with a certain constant volume in which the drug equilibrates at a fast rate. A drug is eliminated from this one compartment at a certain rate that is described by a rate constant, k_{el}, as defined above. A steady concentration of a drug in the plasma can be achieved by infusing the drug at a rate identical to its elimination rate.

Most drugs, however, distribute at different rates into and out of tissues and various body fluids. Most commonly, a drug appears to almost instantaneously distribute into a volume called the central compartment, which in most cases is probably represented by the blood, extracellular fluid, and the well-perfused organs (liver, heart, kidneys, and lungs). Equilibration with the second space is much slower because this peripheral compartment generally represents the more poorly perfused tissues such as fat, bones, and skin. The rate of diffusion of drug from the central to the peripheral compartment is represented by a distribution constant (k_d) and the reverse process by a redistribution rate constant (k_{rd}). The elimination of drugs occurs from the central compartment and is an irreversible process characterized by an elimination rate constant (k_{el}).

More complex models also can be established. For example, the aminoglycoside antibiotics characteristically follow a 3-compartment model, suggesting a third "deep" compartment with extremely slow equilibration with the central compartment.

Comparisons between the duration of action of related drugs can be readily obtained from such pharmacokinetic models. Moreover, they can be predictive, and tissue or plasma concentrations of a drug at any particular time can be estimated fairly accurately to allow dosage regimens to be established for individual animals. However, the important role of pathophysiological processes has now been recognized, and pharmacokinetic models need to be developed for particular populations suffering from specific disease conditions.

CLINICAL APPLICATION OF PHARMACOKINETICS

Therapy may be optimized by measuring and interpreting plasma drug levels. There are a number of drugs and therapeutic situations for which a pharmacokinetic approach is of considerable benefit. These include: 1) drugs with a low therapeutic index, 2) drugs with effects that are not readily monitored clinically, 3) drugs with dose-dependent kinetics, 4) suspected interactions in animals receiving several drugs, 5) unexplained therapeutic failures, 6) unexpected development of toxicity, 7) prophylactic therapy, 8) disease states (eg, renal, liver, cardiovascular, and GI diseases), and 9) treatment of neonatal or very old animals.

These factors may influence the plasma half-lives, volumes of distribution, and plasma clearance of drugs—particularly those with low therapeutic indices. Unfortunately, much of this specific information is not yet readily available for clinical application in veterinary medicine.

MECHANISMS OF DRUG ACTION

GENERAL CONCEPTS

Drugs do not induce different actions in the body; rather, they enhance or modify existing general or specific cellular functions, which usually return to their predosage states when the drug is removed. A thorough understanding of the biochemical and physiological effects induced by drugs is essential for their rational use.

Therapeutic agents are applied topically (externally) or used systemically (internally), and may then exert either a local or a general effect. The tissue responses may be immediate or delayed and can be due to the unchanged drug itself or to one or more of its metabolites. In addition, the desired therapeutic effect may result from a direct action on a target organ, or from a response elicited in another part of the body with indirect beneficial consequences for the affected organ.

A drug's effects may lead to an increase in cellular or tissue responsiveness (stimulation) or may limit or depress cellular functions (inhibition). A biphasic reaction is possible in which initial stimulation is followed by depression. This type of response is quite common when CNS depressants are used. The therapeutic effect sought from some agents is the actual destruction of cells—either of the host (eg, corrosives, blisters, antineoplastic agents) or of invading pathogens (eg, antimicrobial agents, parasiticides). Certain pharmaceutical preparations may contain hormones, enzymes, vitamins, minerals, or electrolytes that are needed to correct deficiency states. Such replacement therapy may also be appropriate for diseases in which there is an intrinsic lack of a neurotransmitter (eg, the use of DOPA as a dopamine precursor to treat Parkinsonism in man).

The drugs employed in veterinary medicine fall into 2 broad general categories: pharmacodynamic and chemotherapeutic. Pharmacodynamic agents exert their actions directly on the host in one way or another to achieve the desired beneficial effects. Chemotherapeutic agents produce toxic effects in pathogenic organisms or neoplastic cells without causing undue harm to the host. However, many chemotherapeutic drugs also possess pharmacodynamic properties, particularly at higher dosages.

BASIC MECHANISMS OF DRUG ACTION

The sites of action vary considerably for the various classes of therapeutic drugs. Many produce effects in the extracellular fluids as well as on cutaneous and mucosal surfaces without any direct involvement with the cellular constituents of the body. Some drugs affect cellular functions through interactions with constituents of cell membranes, thereby altering the membrane's permeability and functions. Drugs may also act intracellularly on specific macromolecular structures to achieve their typical effects. Membrane and intracellular sites of drug action (receptors) are mainly composed of protein subunits arranged in a highly stereospecific fashion.

Noncellular Mechanisms of Drug Action: Drug reactions that occur extracellularly and that involve noncellular constituents include the following.

Physical Effects: Examples include the protective, adsorbant, and lubricant properties of locally active agents that are applied to cutaneous and membrane surfaces.

Chemical Reactions: A number of drugs produce their effects through a chemical union with an endogenous or foreign substance. Examples include the inactivation of heparin (an organic acid) by protamine (an organic base), the chelation of lead by calcium disodium edetate, neutralization of hydrochloric acid in the stomach by antacids such as aluminum hydroxide or sodium bicarbonate, treatment of alkali poisoning with weak acids, the conversion of Hgb to methemoglobin by nitrites for the treatment of cyanide poisoning, the binding of bile salts in the intestinal tract by cholestyramine and colestipol, the precipitation of protein by astringents on the skin surface, and oxidation reactions initiated by certain antiseptics and disinfectants.

Physicochemical Mechanisms: Certain drugs act by altering the physicochemical or biophysical properties of specific fluids or even components of cells (*see* below). Examples of the former include the surface-active agents, or surfactants. Surfactants reduce the tension of the interface between 2 immiscible phases because their molecules contain 2 localized regions, one being hydrophilic in nature and the other hydrophobic. Detergents or emulsifiers, antifoaming agents, and several antiseptics and disinfectants possess surfactant properties.

Modification of the Composition of Body Fluids: Several therapeutic manipulations involve the administration of substances that exert osmotic effects across particular cellular membranes. Examples of osmotically active agents used in this manner include magnesium sulfate as a purgative, mannitol as a diuretic, hypertonic poultices applied on the skin, and the use of dextran 40 and dextran 70 as plasma-volume expanders. In addition, acid-base and electrolyte derangements, which occur in the extracellular fluid in many diseases, can be corrected by the appropriate and judicious use of various electrolyte solutions. Also, acidifying or alkalinizing salts may be administered to alter the pH of the urine for specific therapeutic purposes.

Cellular Mechanisms of Drug Action: Most of the responses elicited by drugs occur at the cellular level and involve either functional constituents or, more commonly, specific biochemical reactions.

Physicochemical and Biophysical Mechanisms: As noted above, certain drugs appear to act by altering the physicochemical or biophysical characteristics of specific components of cells. Examples include the effect of general inhalant anesthetics on the lipid matrix (membrane expansion theory), and perhaps the hydrophobic proteins in neuronal membranes within the CNS. Cisplatin reacts with DNA of tumor cells and forms both intrastrand and interstrand crosslinks, which then inhibit transcription and translation (another example of a biophysical mechanism of drug action).

Modification of Cell Membrane Structure and Function: Various drugs may influence either the structure or specific functional components of cell membranes and thereby initiate their characteristic effects. These mechanisms of action may also involve enzyme systems or receptor-mediated reactions (*see* below). A few examples serve to illustrate how cell membranes can represent a site of action. Local anesthetics bind to components of the sodium channels in excitable membranes and prevent depolarization. Calcium-channel blockers, eg, verapamil, nifedipine, and diltiazem, inhibit the entry of calcium into cells or its mobilization from intracellular stores. Insulin facilitates the transport of glucose into cells. Neurotransmitters characteristically increase or decrease sodium ion permeability of the excitable membranes that are in apposition to their sites of release and thereby either stimulate or inhibit neurotransmission, respectively. Polyene antifungal antibiotics disrupt the sterol component of fungal cell membranes and lead to loss of integrity and fatal cell leakage.

Mechanisms Associated With Neurohumoral Transmission: A number of drugs interfere with the synthesis, release, effects, or re-uptake of neurotransmitters. Once again, enzyme-and/or receptor-mediated effects may be responsible. For example, reserpine blocks the transport system of adrenergic storage granules, while amphetamine displaces norepinephrine from axonal terminals. Botulinum toxin prevents the release of acetylcholine from cholinergic terminals, and bretylium inhibits the release of norepinephrine from adrenergic terminals. Many drugs can also selectively stimulate or block neurotransmitter receptor sites.

Enzyme Inhibition: Certain drugs exert their effects by inhibiting the activity of specific enzyme systems either in the host animal or in invading pathogens. This inhibition may be competitive (with normal substrate) or noncompetitive. Noncompetitive enzyme inhibition may be reversible or irreversible. Allosteric inhibition is also possible when the drug influences enzymatic function by interacting with a part of the enzyme remote from its usual active site. There are many examples of drug action mediated through the inhibition of various enzyme systems. A few examples noted here illustrate the diversity of this type of drug action:

Acetylcholinesterase	— neostigmine (reversible), organophosphate inhibitors (irreversible)
Membrane Na^+/K^+-ATPase	— digitalis glycosides
Phosphodiesterase	— methylxanthines
Carbonic anhydrase	— acetazolamide
Cyclooxygenase	— nonsteroidal anti-inflammatory drugs
Converting enzyme	— captopril
Xanthine oxidase	— allopurinol
Vitamin-K-sensitive enzymes for clotting factor synthesis	— warfarin and other coumarins
Plasminogen-activating enzymes	— aminocaproic acid
11 β-Hydroxylase in corticosteroid biosynthesis	— metyrapone
Thymidine kinase (viral)	— acyclovir
Transpeptidase (bacterial)	— β-Lactam antibiotics
Dihydrofolate synthetase (bacterial)	— sulfonamides
DNA-dependent RNA polymerase (bacterial)	— rifampin
Thymidylate synthetase (fungal)	— flucytosine metabolite
Dihydrofolate reductase (protozoal)	— pyrimethamine

Regulatory Molecule Activation or Inhibition Through Receptor-mediated Effects: In addition to the ability of certain drugs to react with enzymes and to interfere with their function, it is also possible for drugs to interact with another set of specific cellular proteins, commonly known as receptors. In this case, activation or inhibition of a sequence of biochemical events is usually initiated. Receptors may be located either on the cell membrane or in the cytosol (steroid hormone receptors mainly). The normal role of receptors is initially to interact with endogenous regulatory ligands (substances that bind to receptors), such as hormones, neurotransmitters, and autacoids, and thereby to propagate appropriate signals within the target cell. The effects may be direct or may depend on the synthesis and release of other intracellular regulatory molecules, often called second messengers. These second messengers then interact with closely associated cellular proteins (protein kinases) and ultimately activate one or several enzyme systems, which then finally initiate the appropriate response. The arrangement constitutes a receptor-effector system. Receptors with their associated effector and coupling proteins may also act as integrators of extracellular information for the cell.

The basic mechanisms through which ligand-receptor interactions may initiate cellular responses are as follows: 1) The receptor proteins themselves may be part of an ion channel across the plasma membrane. The ion channels open or close in response to a drug-receptor interaction and thereby change the cell's membrane potential and possibly its ionic equilibrium. Examples include the receptors for several neurotransmitters such as acetylcholine, γ-aminobutyric acid, and glycine. 2) Membrane proteins may act as receptors for agents that either stimulate or inhibit adenylate cyclase. This leads to either an increase or a decrease in the intracellular concentration of cyclic AMP (cAMP). The regulation of adenylate cyclase activity depends on distinct guanosine triphosphate (GTP)-binding regulatory proteins. Cyclic AMP acts in the cell to stimulate cAMP-dependent protein kinases, which in turn catalyze the activation of numerous intracellular enzymes, thus producing the specific effects associated with the endogenous ligand or exogenous drug. A number of drug responses are mediated through adenylate cyclase mechanisms. 3) The concentration of calcium ion plays a major role in the regulation of many intracellular events. Calcium entry into cells through the plasma membrane is controlled by a distinct set of receptors. In some cases, the calcium ion itself regulates reactions directly; in other instances, calcium plays a role only when it is bound to an intracellular calcium-dependent regulatory protein known as calmodulin. Calmodulin also controls several cell functions directly and others through distinct protein kinase systems. A number of drug reactions are mediated through calcium-dependent mechanisms. 4) Stimulation of certain membrane receptors leads to the formation of inositol-triphosphate and diacylglycerol from membrane phospholipid. Inositol triphosphate in turn leads to the release of calcium from intracellular stores which, in conjunction with diacylglycerol, activates a distinct protein kinase with resultant increased specific enzyme activity and responses. 5) Several membrane-bound proteins are themselves protein kinases that can be activated by specific agents to produce their effects. Insulin receptors are of this type. 6) Perturbation of the plasma membrane or the release of calcium ions may bring about the activation of membrane-associated phospholipases. This leads to the genesis of prostaglandins, leukotrienes, and related eicosanoids, which then play a major role in local cellular regulation. Several drugs may initiate the prostaglandin cascade in their target tissues—either as a primary effect or because of cellular disruption. 7) Oxidative events in some cells, potentially produced by a variety of pathways, lead to the activation of guanylate cyclase with consequent elevation of the intracellular concentration of cyclic GMP (cGMP). This cyclic nucleotide is an activator of yet another set of protein kinases. Several endogenous and exogenous substances can modulate cellular levels of cGMP. 8) Steroid hormone receptors are responsive to both endogenous ligands and to synthetic congeners. They occur in the cytoplasm of the cells in the target tissues for the specific steroid hormone. The steroid ligands bind with a measurable affinity to the cytoplasmic receptor protein. Following some modification, the steroid-receptor complex is converted to a form that is translocated to the nucleus, where binding of the steroid-protein complex to chromatin occurs. As a result, specific mRNA and proteins (enzymes) are synthesized, which then lead to the characteristic steroid-hormone-induced effects for the particular tissue. All steroid hormones used as drugs exert their primary effects through this mechanism.

Drugs are capable of either stimulating or inhibiting receptor-mediated effects provided their molecular structure is analogous, at least in part, to the physiological ligands that usually interact with specific receptors. This is the basis of modern receptor theory.

DRUG RECEPTORS AND PHARMACODYNAMICS

Most drugs are effective in extremely low concentrations and generally elicit predictable responses that depend on the concentration of the drug and of the receptors at the site of action. These reactions are usually mediated through the interaction of the drug with specific macromolecules (receptors) in the target cell, which activates or inhibits one or more of the various mechanisms discussed above. Only the basic tenets of modern receptor theory, as they apply to clinical pharmacology, are briefly reviewed here to provide a foundation for the understanding of drug actions and reactions.

Nature of Drug Receptor Interactions: The selective action of a drug depends on its combination with a specific set of receptors. The receptor sites are almost invariably composed of proteins. They may be regulatory proteins, enzymes, transport proteins, and rarely structural proteins. Drug-receptor interactions are usually reversible and are governed by the Law of Mass Action schematically represented as follows:

$$\text{receptor} + \text{drug} \rightleftarrows \text{drug-receptor complex} \rightarrow \text{effect}$$

The binding of drugs to receptors may involve all types of molecular interactions—van der Waals forces; hydrophobic interactions; and hydrogen, dipole, ionic, and covalent bonds.

Besides receptor proteins, drugs may also become bound in a similar fashion to other proteins. However, in these cases, no pharmacodynamic response is initiated ("silent receptors"). Examples of such drug acceptors include plasma proteins, intracellular proteins, and membrane protein fractions. These macromolecules represent sites of drug loss or storage.

Drugs that are capable of reacting with specific receptors and then produce a defined response are said to possess affinity as well as intrinsic activity, and are termed "agonists". In contrast, certain drugs are capable of combining with the same receptor complex, thus possessing affinity, but they lack intrinsic activity, and no response occurs. These agents are termed pharmacological "antagonists". Antagonists may act in several different ways. It is also possible for some drugs to interact with the same receptors as a full agonist, but the response may be limited and less than maximal. These agents then possess affinity for the receptor but only intermediate activity, and are termed "partial agonists". Finally, there are some special drugs that at certain concentrations act as agonists on one type of receptor population but as antagonists on other subsets of the receptor. These agents are known as "agonist-antagonists".

Properties of Agonists: Receptor agonists have several typical properties. The **affinity** of a ligand (drug or endogenous substance) for a receptor is a measure of its capacity to bind to the receptor. Affinity may vary greatly among agonists (as well as antagonists).

Intrinsic activity is a measure of the ability of the agonist-receptor complex to initiate the observed biological response. A full agonist has an intrinsic activity value (α) of 1.

Maximal efficacy reflects the upper limit of the dose-response relationship without toxic effects being evident. Agonists differ from each other in this regard.

Potency refers to the range of concentrations over which an agonist produces increasing responses. Highly potent drugs produce their effects at lower concentrations; this may impart an advantage to their clinical use, provided the increase in potency is not accompanied by an increase in toxicity.

Selectivity and specificity: Few agonists are so specific that they interact only with a single subtype of receptor. However, several agonists (and antagonists) do show evidence of selectivity for certain subpopulations of receptors.

Structure-activity relationships: The affinity of an agonist (or antagonist) for a receptor as well as the agonist's intrinsic activity are intimately related to the chemical structure of the drug. The relationship is usually quite stringent, and minor modifications in the drug molecule can result in significant differences in its pharmacological properties. Often, congeners of a parent drug molecule are developed for therapeutic use because of advantages in their therapeutic effects or reduced toxicity.

Drug-receptor theories: Whatever its actual nature, the conformational change that occurs when a receptor is occupied by an agonist is only one of several steps necessary for the expression of a full pharmacological response. The transduction process between occupancy of receptors and the drug response is called "coupling". Receptor-effector coupling is influenced by the ionic environment, several coupling factors, and the receptor itself. A number of theories have been advanced to explain how agonist-receptor interactions lead to effective receptor-effector coupling and the specific pharmacological response observed. The Occupancy Theory, based on the Law of Mass Action, suggests that one drug molecule occupies one receptor site and, if the concentration of the drug in the medium is sufficiently large, it remains effectively constant during the binding process. The Rate Theory suggests that the biological response depends on the rate of agonist-receptor interaction. The Induced-Fit Theory proposes that in the process of agonist-receptor interaction, a conformational change occurs that generates the active receptor site. The Perturbation Theory differentiates between specific conformation changes induced by agonists versus nonspecific perturbations produced by antagonists. The Activation-Aggregation Theory proposes that receptors exist in dynamic equilibrium between different functional states, and that agonists shift the equilibrium toward the activated forms of the receptor.

Properties of Antagonists: Many receptor antagonists are used therapeutically. However, different forms of drug antagonism occur and have direct clinical implications.

Competitive antagonists combine reversibly with the same receptor site as agonists and progressively inhibit the response to agonists. Competitive antagonists may even possess greater affinity for the receptor site than pure agonists. Typically, the blockade can be overcome by increasing the concentration of the agonist in the biophase.

Noncompetitive antagonists may act reversibly or, more commonly, irreversibly. Characteristically, high concentrations of agonist cannot completely overcome the antagonism, and a maximal response cannot be produced. Several types of noncompetitive antagonism are recognized. The binding may occur to the same receptor and produce blockade. If covalent bonds are formed, receptor inhibition becomes permanent and the synthesis of new receptors is required for complete reversal of the antagonist's effects. This form of irreversible noncompetitive antagonism is encountered with some organophosphates and cholinergic receptors. Binding of noncompetitive antagonists to a different part of a receptor macromolecule may lead to deformation of the active receptor site and a diminution in the affinity for the usual agonists. This effect is similar to allosteric inhibition of enzymes. Antagonists may also bind to an extrareceptor area in a membrane but, because of their molecular configuration, may obscure the receptor sites for one or more agonists. The phenothiazine neuroleptics appear to be multipotent receptor blockers of this type.

Physiological or functional antagonists are, in fact, agonists that elicit physiological responses that directly oppose those of the first drug administered by stimulating a different class of receptors. Examples of physiological antagonism include the reversal of histamine's effects (histaminergic receptors) by epinephrine (adrenergic receptors), and the stimulation of intestinal smooth muscle by acetylcholine (cholinergic receptors) following its inhibition by norepinephrine (adrenergic receptors).

Properties of Partial Agonists and Agonist-Antagonists: Partial agonists, eg, nalorphine and pentazocine, produce a lower than maximal response at full receptor occupancy notwithstanding high receptor affinities in many cases. They also act as competitive antagonists in the presence of pure agonists. Agonist-antagonists that are used clinically include the opioid analgesics that possess selective affinity and intrinsic activity for certain of the opioid receptor types but act as competitive antagonists at others, thus reducing some of the undesirable features of full opioid agonists. Butorphanol and nalbuphine are regarded as opioid agonist-antagonists.

Properties of Receptors: It is extremely difficult to isolate and study receptors obtained from living cells. However, much progress in characterizing these macromolecules has been made by use of receptor-specific, radio-labeled ligands. Only a few of the general functional features of receptors are presented below.

Specificity: A receptor's specific molecular shape, form, and ionic configuration determine whether an agonist (or antagonist) with complementary molecular size, shape, and electrical charge will bind with avidity to the site. Receptors are responsible for the selectivity of drug action.

Number of Receptors: The number of functional receptors in a tissue or cell is not necessarily fixed. Receptors may be induced ("up-regulation"), eg, thyroid hormones increase the number of β-adrenergic receptors in cardiac muscle. Certain agonists can promote a decrease in the number ("down-regulation") or coupling efficiency of receptors. The long-term use of select antagonists may actually raise the number of receptors by preventing down-regulation. This leads to the "overshoot" phenomenon with exaggerated responses following withdrawal of the drug. Steroid receptors present in the cytoplasm of target cells are both inducible and mobile.

Spare Receptors: In many cases, only a limited percentage of the receptors available need to be occupied by an agonist to produce a maximal response. The extras are known as spare receptors. The sensitivity of tissues that possess spare receptors can be altered by changes in the receptor's concentration. Agonists with low affinities can still produce maximal responses at low concentrations when spare receptors are present in the target tissue.

Classification of Receptors: A number of major receptor types have been identified. Moreover, several subtypes also have been defined according to ligand affinity as well as by the reactions produced by either agonists or antagonists. These differences between the responses elicited through various receptor subtypes are quantitatively selective but are rarely absolute for either agonists or antagonists. A selection of receptor types and subtypes that are clinically important is listed below.

Receptor	Types	Subtypes
Cholinergic	Muscarinic	M_1 and M_2
	Nicotinic	skeletal muscle and autonomic ganglia
Adrenergic	Alpha	α_1 and α_2
	Beta	β_1 and β_2
Dopaminergic	DA_1	
	DA_2	
Serotonergic	$5\text{-}HT_1$	
	$5\text{-}HT_2$	
Histaminergic	H_1	
	H_2	
GABAergic	$GABA_1$	
	$GABA_2$	
Adenosine	A_1	
	A_2	
Opioid	μ κ	
	μ_1 δ	
Steroid	Progesterone	
	Estrogen	
	Testosterone	
	Glucocorticoid	
	Mineralocorticoid	
Peptide hormones and amino acids	Wide variety	

Dose-Response Relationship: The ultimate concentration reached by a drug at its receptor site in the biophase depends on the dose administered. The response of the target tissue, in turn, is determined directly by the amount of drug at the receptor site. Thus, a direct relationship exists between drug dose and tissue or organ response. Two major forms of dose-response are recognized. First, a graded response may occur in which the target tissue (or even animal) shows a progressively greater response with increasing doses of drug, ultimately reaching a maximum response. A plotted graph of a graded response is a hyperbola on a linear scale and a sigmoid curve on a semilogarithmic scale. Second, a quantal or all-or-none response may be evident. In this case the target tissue, or animal, reacts either maximally or to a specified end-point within the therapeutic dosage range. The plotted graph of a quantal response is usually a sigmoid curve on both linear and semilogarithmic scales.

From studies on dose and toxicity response curves for a particular drug, several important clinical characteristics can be established: 1) Median effective dose (MED or ED_{50}), which is the dose of the drug at which 50% of animals exhibit a specified quantal effect. The ED_{50} of drugs that produce the same effect can be used to compare relative potencies. 2) Median toxic dose (MTD or TD_{50}), which is the dose required to produce a specified toxic effect in 50% of the animals receiving the drug. 3) Median lethal dose (MLD or LD_{50}), which is the dose required to produce death in 50% of the animals that have received the drug. 4) Therapeutic index, which is a measure that relates the dose of a drug needed to produce a desirable effect to the dose required to produce a toxic or even lethal effect. The therapeutic index of a drug is obtained by dividing the TD_{50} (or LD_{50}) by the ED_{50}. Therapeutic ratios are also useful indices of drug safety, but in this case the steepness of the dose response curves are also considered. Therapeutic ratios are often calculated by dividing the LD_{25} by the ED_{75}. 5) Comparative potency, maximal efficacy, selectivity, and variability of response may also be determined from either graded or quantal dose-response curves for drugs that have the same action.

FACTORS MODIFYING THE ACTION AND FATE OF DRUGS

Following the selection of a specific therapeutic agent to treat a disease that has been diagnosed in a particular animal, an appropriate pharmaceutical form of the drug is administered by a predetermined route at the recommended dose rate and frequency. The desired pharmacological response is expected to occur for a known time period without any extraneous reactions. However, unanticipated effects can occur following administration of almost any drug. Drug-induced reactions may be exaggerated (hyperresponsiveness) or of reduced magnitude (hyporesponsiveness) compared with those that would normally result from the dosage employed. Such effects may become evident immediately or over time, and are not necessarily directly related to the drug's main pharmacodynamic action. Secondary pharmacological actions can become the dominant clinical feature and thereby obscure the primary beneficial effect that is being sought. Alternatively, if the drug acts as an antigen, a complex series of immune-mediated (hypersensitivity) reactions may be precipitated that have no relationship to the original disease or the pharmacological effects of the drug. Finally, unexpected and bizarre drug-induced effects may occasionally occur that simply cannot be explained (idiosyncrasy).

Two basic types of adverse drug effects are recognized. Type A reactions reflect excess (or even diminished) but predictable, pharmacological actions of a drug that are generally dose dependent and rarely lead to mortality. The causes of this type of adverse drug effect include: 1) physiological factors such as species, breed, genetics, age, sex, body weight and surface area, diet, nutritional status, temperament, relative activity, circadian rhythms, and environmental conditions; 2) pharmacological factors such as dosage form, generic equivalence, dose rate and delivery route, time and frequency of administration, direct drug-drug interactions, pharmacokinetic interactions, pharmacodynamic interactions, and drug-diet interactions; 3) pathological states such as toxemia and pyrexia, shock, electrolyte and acid-base derangements, uremia and renal disease, hepatopathy, cardiovascular disease, anemia, respiratory disease, GI disorders, neurological disturbances, and impaired immunocompetence.

Type B adverse reactions lead to aberrant drug effects that are totally unrelated to any anticipated responses and are usually independent of the dose employed. Mortality rates may be quite high. The basic causes include: 1) Errors in drug formulation, or accidental contamination of the preparation with either toxic substances or pathogenic microorganisms. Neither of these possibilities is likely when modern commercially prepared products are utilized for medicating animals. However, crudely compounded drug formulations always represent a potential hazard. 2) Unique patient characteristics. Genetic differences between animals of the same species and even breed may be responsible for dramatic differences between the reactions encountered in various animal subpopulations. Pharmacogenetic variances have been well established in man. Another unique characteristic of an animal is its immune status and whether there has been previous exposure to a particular pharmacological agent that has been recognized as an antigen by the host's immune system. Drug allergy, or hypersensitivity, is the most common form of type B reaction in veterinary medicine.

PHYSIOLOGICAL FACTORS MODIFYING DRUG ACTION

Species: Although the basic mechanism of action of a drug may be the same, the intensity and duration of the effect produced in various animal species can vary considerably. However, in many cases, the range of therapeutic plasma levels correlate quite closely, even with those found in man. Thus, species variations in the responses elicited by a fixed dose of a drug can be attributed to differences in either pharmacokinetic processes (absorption, distribution, biotransformation, and excretion) or in the pharmacodynamic sensitivity of specific tissue receptors.

There are substantial anatomical and functional differences among the GI tracts of the various domestic and wild animal species. These unique characteristics can influence the disposition of drugs administered PO. The carnivorous species are periodic feeders that have relatively short GI tracts with transit times of ~6 hr. The pH of the gastric juice in these species is usually 1-3. The scope of the fermentation processes in the colon is not great. Carnivores have well-developed emetic reflexes and can vomit quite readily. Drug absorption in cats and dogs is relatively uncomplicated and occurs mainly in the upper GI tract. However, the systemic availability of the drug depends on the extent of the first-pass effect through the gut epithelium and liver. This can be sufficiently different between cats and dogs to reflect in variations in the fraction of an oral dose available systemically.

Monogastric herbivores, eg, equids, guinea pigs, and rabbits, have relatively voluminous ceca and colons in which active microbial degradation of cellulose and other insoluble carbohydrates occurs. These hindgut fermentation processes are sensitive to disruption by broad-spectrum antimicrobial agents—with fatal consequences in some instances. Microfloral metabolism of drugs can produce a metabolite profile that is very different from that in monogastrics. Horses tend to be continuous feeders, with the stomach serving as a temporary storage organ for ingested feed. The intragastric pH of horses varies considerably (range 1-7). The bioavailability of many preparations dosed PO in horses is often unpredictable. Feeding can markedly influence plasma-concentration time curves as well as the areas under the curves, eg, giving phenylbutazone PO before feeding or with the ration generally leads to good absorption with peak plasma levels in 2-3 hr. However, if phenylbutazone is administered PO after feeding, absorption may be delayed considerably and is often incomplete. The shortest intestinal transit time expected in adult horses is ~30 hr. Equidae, not having gallbladders, excrete bile constantly, and active biliary elimination of drugs with notable enterohepatic cycling is quite characteristic for these species. Horses are not capable of effective vomiting; in fact, emetic efforts may be disastrous.

Ruminants (pregastric fermenters) possess a large forestomach, consisting of the ruminoreticulum and omasum, which is never empty and in which active microbial growth and metabolism proceed in the form of continuous flow culture. There is a steady but intermittent delivery of ingesta, containing not only many of the end-products of microbial digestion but also the bacteria and protozoa themselves, into the abomasum for further utilization by the host animal.

Drug absorption from the ruminoreticulum is typically retarded because of dilution in ruminal fluid. Even though the ruminoreticulum and omasum are lined by stratified squamous epithelium, the basic principles that govern the diffusion of drugs from the GI tract into the systemic circulation remain the same as in other species, and depend mainly on the drug's lipid solubility and concentration gradient. With ruminal stasis, the rate of absorption is invariably decreased. Buffering systems maintain the usual pH of ruminal fluid between 6.0 and 6.8, but this depends on diet and the time of collection relative to feeding. Animals on high-grain diets tend to have intraruminal pH values of 5.5-6.0, whereas excess protein or nonprotein nitrogen intake produces higher than normal values, up to 8.0. Denial of feed for any length of time also leads to more neutral or even alkaline values for ruminal fluid pH. The bioavailability of drugs administered PO is variable, because of the complexity of the forestomach activity in these animals. In addition, the anaerobic microflora is capable of inactivating several drugs in the ruminoreticulum; chloramphenicol, trimethoprim, and the digitalis glycosides are well-known examples. However, the reverse is also possible: broad-spectrum antimicrobial agents destroy the ruminal microflora with resultant ruminal atony and disruption of other forestomach functions. Intestinal transit times in domestic ruminants are quite long, being ~40 hr or more in most species. Although rumination is a normal complex regurgitant reflex, ruminants are not capable of vomiting in the physiological sense.

In addition to the considerable variations between species with respect to the GI fate of drugs administered PO, there are also species differences related to the intracorporeal distribution of drugs. Depending on their physicochemical characteristics, pharmacological agents may or may not diffuse into the large voluminous compartments of the GI tracts of species such as the equids and ruminants. The weight of the content of the ruminoreticulum in cattle may constitute 10-15% of the body weight but may or may not represent a distribution compartment. Ion-trapping within the GI tract depends on the usual pH values in the various large compartments found in these species.

Drugs that are highly lipid soluble tend to accumulate over time in body fat depots. Thus, in animals such as fat pigs or lambs, and finished steers, adipose tissue may represent a large distribution compartment for those lipid-soluble agents that are slowly metabolized.

There are often notable interspecies variations in the degree of plasma-protein binding of drugs, both acidic and basic. Differences in the concentration of the plasma proteins are also recognized. Small changes in the degree of binding of drugs in the plasma and tissues may lead to significant redistribution of highly bound drugs between tissues and plasma. Frequently, the tissue distribution of drugs differs quantitatively between species.

The passage of drugs across the placenta is another facet of interspecies variation in drug distribution. Although not always predictable or consistent, it seems that species with less intimate placentations (epitheliochorial) tend to exclude drugs from the fetus more than do those with more intimate placentations (endotheliochorial, hemochorial, or hemoendothelial). The differences may be more quantitative than qualitative.

Most of the pharmacokinetic differences between species are due to varying rates or different pathways for the metabolic transformation of drugs. In addition, many environmental and nutritional factors can influence both phase 1 and phase 2 reactions in different species. As a general rule, carnivores tend to conjugate drugs and their metabolites slowly, whereas these reactions in omnivores tend to be faster and in herbivores more rapid yet. Domestic animals appear to be able to oxidize drugs more efficiently than man. The effect of GI microflora on the drug biotransformation process and the consequent variations observed among species must also be considered.

Marked differences in duration of blood concentrations of salicylate, chloramphenicol, phenylbutazone, amphetamine, phenol, and several other drugs are observed among horses, ruminants, pigs, dogs, cats, rodents, and man. This observation greatly influences dosage regimens; eg, the plasma half-life of salicylate is 38, 8, 6, ~5, 1, and 0.8 hr in cats, dogs, pigs, man, horses, and goats, respectively. The dosage interval recommended for man would poison a cat. Conversely, this regimen would not be adequate to treat fever in horses. Dogs and cats metabolize 85-90% of a dose of meperidine within 1 hr of administration. Because of its short duration of action, this drug is not very useful for the management of pain in those species. Because cats metabolize phenol slowly relative to other animals, they are much more readily intoxicated by this disinfectant.

Several specific differences exist with respect to drug-metabolizing enzymes. The cat is deficient in hepatic glucuronosyltransferase. This results in a dependence on different and slower pathways for biotransformation of certain compounds, with frequent increases in the duration of action and potential toxicity of these agents. Dogs have a deficiency of arylamine acetyltransferase and also possess a hepatic deacetylase that rapidly removes acetyl groups. Thus, acetylated derivatives of sulfonamides are not found in canine urine as they are in other species. Pigs are not capable of sulfate conjugation reactions.

Because of the complexity of the various biotransformation capabilities, and the number of metabolic pathways potentially available or not available, inherent danger exists in extrapolating information derived from studies in one species (including man) to another without due regard for possible differences in the pharmacokinetic fate of the agent in the second species.

There do not seem to be major deviations among mammals with respect to the mechanisms of drug excretion. However, the avian kidney may be less efficient in its ability to eliminate drugs such as the barbiturates. There also may be differences in the active tubular secretion of certain drug classes in particular species. If renal excretion of a drug is influenced by the pH of the urine, elimination will occur at different rates in ruminants (urinary pH 7-8), horses and pigs (urinary pH ~7), and carnivores (urinary pH usually 5-6.5).

The rate of biliary excretion and the presence or absence of an extensive enterohepatic cycle may represent the major reason for variations in the elimination half-life of a drug among species. Various animals utilize biliary excretion for different sized molecules; eg, rat >325 daltons, and man >500 daltons.

Lactating animals may excrete large quantities of drug in milk.

In addition to the differences between the pharmacokinetic patterns in the various animal species, in many instances, because of variations in biochemical, physiological, or integrative processes, unique responses may occur. A selection of these reactions is listed below to emphasize the variation in drug response.

Species	Drug	Reaction
Horses	Certain phenothiazine neuroleptics	Extreme excitement
	Phenothiazine neuroleptics	Permanent penile paralysis
	Tetracyclines, macrolides, lincosamides	Fatal colitis
	Monensin	Fatal cardiac failure
Donkeys	Etorphine/acepromazine (at horse dose rate)	Severe respiratory depression and cardiac irregularities
Cattle	Xylazine	Extreme sensitivity to depressant effects
	Morphine	Excitatory, aberrant behavior
Dogs	Iodochlorhydroxyquin	Fatal encephalitis
Cats	Acetaminophen (biotransformation dependent)	Fatal centrilobular hepatic necrosis
	Phenolic compounds	Marked sensitivity
	Morphine and other opioid analgesics (at usual doses)	Excitatory
	Aminoglycosides	Especially sensitive to neurotoxic effects

Genetic Factors: Certain genetic or breed characteristics may also alter the susceptibility of an animal to a particular pharmacological agent. Several pharmacogenetic factors have been elucidated in man, but this aspect of pharmacology has not been well studied in animals. The few examples of known unique breed responses include the following. Shetland and Welsh pony crosses seem to be more susceptible to the GI effects of phenylbutazone. The response of Thoroughbreds to CNS depressant drugs is sometimes unpredictable. Brahman cattle are more susceptible to the effects of xylazine than are the European breeds. Certain strains of sheep lack the esterase enzyme necessary for the inactivation of the organophosphate anthelmintic haloxon, which explains the sporadic neurotoxicity in lambs following drenching with haloxon. Greyhounds and similar breeds often show prolonged sleeping time after the administration of thiopental sodium, possibly due to limited redistribution in these lean dogs. Brachycephalic breeds, such as the Pug, Pekingese, and Bulldog, may exhibit syncope following administration of acepromazine because of sinoatrial block resulting from vagal overtone. Some Collies are much more sensitive to ivermectin than are others, presumably because of a difference in their blood brain barrier, or due to sequestration in the CNS.

Age: Neonates (up to ~1 mo) differ from older individuals of the same species in a number of significant ways. Toxicity as a result of drug therapy during the neonatal period is not uncommon. The blood-brain barrier that prevents the diffusion of many drugs and endogenous compounds into the brain of the adult is poorly developed in the fetus and the newborn of some species. Neonatal animals are susceptible to marked changes in environmental temperature because of a larger surface area to body weight ratio and a lesser capacity to limit heat loss. Drugs that impair temperature regulatory mechanisms can easily jeopardize a neonate's well-being. Fetal Hgb is different from adult Hgb, and the neonate undergoes the change early in life. Moreover, the fetal RBC are deficient in methemoglobin reductase, hence there is a sensitivity to oxidant drugs. Several classes of drugs, including sulfonamides, nitrofurans, methylene blue, acetylsalicylic acid, and the phenothiazines, may produce methemoglobinemia in the newborn.

Pharmacokinetic parameters may differ markedly in the newborn for a number of reasons. Little, if any, information is available regarding quantitative adjustments to dose rates or frequencies in the very young, but the differences in disposition kinetics make it imperative that dose rates be reduced in the neonate—at least for the first 4 wk of life. There is an increased permeability of the small intestine during the period immediately following birth, and the absorption of drugs usually retained in the intestine may be appreciable during this period. Milk, however, may retard the absorption of drugs such as the tetracyclines because of calcium chelation. The ruminant is essentially a monogastric animal until the ruminoreticulum is seeded with microflora and the fermentation processes begin by about the third or fourth week of life. Another difference is the body water compartments at this early age. Body water makes up a higher percentage of body weight at birth than late in infancy. Furthermore, the extracellular fluid volume is greater than the intracellular volume. This effectively reduces the concentration of drugs that are distributed in the extracellular space, and alterations in drug distribution patterns are frequent in neonates. Hypoproteinemia (mostly due to low albumin levels) is also quite common in neonates, and this in turn may increase the amount of drug available to diffuse into tissues. Because the body content of fat is low (2-3%) in neonates, adipose tissue cannot represent a significant distribution compartment. However, the greatest single factor altering pharmacokinetics during the neonatal period is the deficiency of hepatic microsomal enzyme function for the first 4 wk, and particularly during the first week. This limitation almost invariably leads to prolonged tissue levels and even toxic effects if adult dose regimens are followed. Drugs that have considerably longer half-lives in neonates, particularly within the first week, include phenytoin, phenobarbital, chloramphenicol, salicylates, and theophylline. Renal function is typically deficient at birth and develops fully only during the first 1-2 mo; thus, rates of elimination of drugs are slow. Also, neonates or young animals may be more susceptible to toxic effects of drugs on the kidneys. For example, foals are more susceptible to gentamicin-induced nephrotoxicity than are adult horses. However, in ruminants, within 5-7 days, renal function is adequate for excretion of xenobiotics, and seems to mature within 1-2 wk.

The stage of growth may also predispose young animals to certain adverse drug effects. Antianabolic or catabolic drugs delay growth, as will drugs that suppress or impair appetite. Agents that impede normal calcium absorption and deposition inhibit bone development. In addition, the administration of steroids with androgenic properties can lead to premature closure of the epiphyseal growth plates, with consequent lessening of the animal's anticipated adult size.

Appreciation for pharmacokinetic considerations in geriatric animals has increased during the past few years. Indications are that activity of hepatic microsomal drug enzymes declines with aging. The half-lives of some drugs may be increased by up to 50% in geriatric animals, and this is usually accompanied by a reduction in total plasma clearance. These differences are not reliably predictable and depend on the characteristics of the drug and the individual animal. The physiologic changes that occur with aging and that contribute to alterations in drug disposition include reductions in lean body mass, total body water, plasma albumin concentrations, cardiac output, hepatic mass, liver blood flow, glomerular filtration rate, and renal plasma flow. Few studies have been conducted in geriatric animals, and no fixed pharmacokinetic guidelines for dosage adjustments are available. However, when medicating old animals, caution should be exercised with regard to the dose rates selected.

The efficacy of bacteriostatic drugs depends on a competent immune system. Since neonates and very old animals usually are not fully immunocompetent, bactericidal drugs should be used to control bacterial infections in these animals.

Sex: The influence of sex on drug effects and the occurrence of adverse drug reactions relates principally to reproductive function. However, the rate of biotransformation and hence elimination of some endogenous and foreign compounds, eg, the sex steroids, may differ between male and female animals. Occasional variations are also observed in the response to specific drugs between males and females.

The main pharmacotherapeutic concerns associated with the drug treatment of females are the following: 1) potential effect on the reproductive organs and their function; 2) possible embryocidal, teratogenic, or abortifacient actions when administered to a pregnant animal; 3) potential influence on parturition—either to delay or to induce parturition; 4) possible effects on lactation—either inhibitory or stimulatory; 5) presence of a residue in the milk of a lactating animal—either because of possible harmful effects to the suckling young or because of public health considerations.

In males, possible adverse actions of drugs relate to the reproductive system, both the gonads and the accessory glands, particularly the prostate. Stimulatory or inhibitory effects may be induced by appropriate therapeutic agents.

Body Weight and Surface Area: An approximation of surface area is occasionally employed for determining the dose of very toxic drugs, eg, some of the antineoplastic agents, but usually body weight is the primary determinant. However, the use of body weight does have several limitations that need to be recognized when particularly powerful therapeutic agents are administered. Differences between body weight and "true" lean body weight become evident when dealing with the following states: obesity, starvation, ascites or generalized edema, fill of the GI tract in herbivores, severe dehydration, immaturity, old age, and the presence of large tumors.

Diet and Nutritional Status: Well-nourished animals normally cope with the disposition and elimination of drugs with little difficulty. In animals suffering from protein-caloric malnutrition, absorption, distribution, biotransformation, and excretion processes may all be impaired to a greater or lesser degree for many of the reasons discussed above.

Temperament: The temperament of an animal may influence its response to a drug—particularly the CNS-active agents. The response to neuroleptics and tranquilizers often depends in large measure on the animal's mental state before and following administration. Even placebo effects have been described in animals other than man under certain conditions.

Relative Activity and Circadian Rhythms: Many biological "rhythms" have been identified and characterized in domestic animals. These circadian cycles may have diurnal or nocturnal peaks. Their chronopharmacological importance relates to the desirability of designing therapeutic regimens to follow particular cycles rather than to disrupt or inhibit the controlling mechanisms that operate through feedback loops. This approach to restricting the adverse effects of drugs is well illustrated by the long-term use of alternate-day, early morning therapy with short-acting glucocorticoids to limit the potential suppression of the hypothalamic-pituitary-adrenal axis.

Environmental Conditions: In addition to the role of environmental factors in determining the forage available for herbivorous species, ambient conditions may directly influence the action of a number of drugs. Extreme heat and cold lead to peripheral vasodilation or vasoconstriction, respectively, with possible effects on drug disposition. High temperatures increase the rate of volatilization of the inhalant anesthetics and also increase the respiratory rate, thus facilitating inhalant anesthesia when open methods of administration are used. Extreme environmental temperatures may also influence the blood levels of several hormones such as epinephrine, thyroxine, triiodothyronine, and the glucocorticoids.

PHARMACOLOGICAL FACTORS MODIFYING DRUG ACTION

Drug Dosage and Administration: Typically a standard dose rate is furnished for a drug preparation, together with the required route of administration and the appropriate time interval between doses. These recommendations by the manufacturer are based on pharmacokinetic studies in the target species. However, because the test animals are often healthy, whereas it is diseased animals that are treated, some clinical judgement is often required with respect to the dose to be used. In most instances, administration at the recommended rate, frequency, and route produces an anticipated kinetic pattern and a satisfactory therapeutic response when used for a specifically indicated disease condition. However, several facets related to drug dosage forms and their administration may unexpectedly alter the drug response.

The absorption of a drug from the common parenteral injection sites, other than IV, is determined chiefly by the formulation of the drug, the vascularity of the tissue in which the preparation is deposited, and to a lesser extent by the degree of ionization and lipid solubility of the drug substance. An additional consideration is the anatomical site of the injection. In cattle, differences have been found between the peak plasma concentrations of oxytetracycline when injected IM in the neck, shoulder, and buttock; highest levels were found after injection in the shoulder region. Other considerations include tissue reaction at the injection site, and the influence this might have on absorption into the systemic circulation. Unintended drug delivery into relatively avascular tissues delays absorption, eg, into fascial sheaths between muscle bundles (intermuscular) or into subcut. adipose tissue. The base or salt form of the drug used, as well as the vehicles, solubilizers, stabilizers, buffers, and emulsifying agents included in the formulation, are all capable of modifying the rate of absorption of the drug from the site of injection. This should be considered when comparing different preparations of the same drug.

Many oral drug preparations are solid dosage forms, although suspensions, pastes, and even solutions are quite common. Any solid dosage form needs to disintegrate and dissolve before absorption can occur. Dissolution frequently controls the rate of drug absorption; thus, differences between the bioavailability of various pharmaceutical formulations of the same drug may be encountered, with consequent temporal and quantitative differences between their pharmacological effects. In all cases with both parenteral and oral administration, the greater the concentration of a drug in a preparation, the faster will be its rate of absorption into the systemic circulation, and the sooner its pharmacological effects will become evident.

Therapeutic Inequivalence: Although generic preparations of a drug manufactured by a variety of pharmaceutical companies may be expected to be equally effective at the same dosage, this is not always the case. The reasons for therapeutic or generic inequivalence between different products that contain the same amount of the same active principle (chemically equivalent) are often complex and obscure. There is usually some form of component reaction or interaction in solid dosage forms that is responsible for the reduced bioavailability of the less effective formulation. Excipient differences have been recognized as the cause of the inequivalence encountered between preparations that contain tetracyclines, phenobarbital, phenylbutazone, phenytoin, and several other drugs. Different particle sizes, which influence the rate of dissolution of the active principle, have led to discrepancies between products that contain digoxin, nitrofurantoin, griseofulvin, oxytetracycline, chloramphenicol palmitate, and ampicillin (ampicillin trihydrate versus ampicillin). Crystal polymorphism has been responsible for the therapeutic inequivalence evidenced between preparations containing chloramphenicol as well as those containing aluminum hydroxide. Several chemically equivalent formulations intended for parenteral administration have also revealed diminished bioavailability of the active principle, which can lead to unpredictable therapeutic responses. Once again, there may be several reasons for the ultimate differences in the blood levels that are obtained. The actual formulation with the particular vehicles and stabilizers used, the chemical form of the drug employed, and the tissue reactions that occur at the injection site may all be responsible for different rates of absorption. Drug preparations intended for parenteral administration that have evidence of therapeutic inequivalence include chloramphenicol, oxytetracycline, diazepam, and iron dextran.

The clinical significance of generic inequivalence and the possibility of resultant therapeutic failures has become less problematical in recent years; regulatory requirements for the licensing of a new product containing an already approved drug now demand that full bioequivalence of the new formulation be demonstrated. However, when changing from one product to another, the clinical response should be monitored to assure that the preparations are indeed equivalent.

Direct Drug-Drug Interactions: When pharmaceutical preparations are mixed indiscriminately before administration by virtually any route, interactions may occur between the active ingredients or between the active ingredients and formulation adjuncts. Incompatibilities that occur may result in precipitation; chemical inactivation; or changes in the color, taste, or physical form of the preparations. The occurrence of drug-drug interactions in the pharmaceutical phase is frequently unpredictable. Detrimental reactions may be obvious but are often subtle and not easily detected. Specific products vary considerably with respect to their potential incompatibilities. The constituents involved in such *in vitro* reactions could include the active principles, vehicles, stabilizers, correctives, preservatives, solubilizers, and antioxidants. Even the type of container or stopper (glass, plastic, or rubber) can play a role. Environmental factors such as temperature, humidity, agitation, and ultraviolet light may also initiate detrimental reactions in inappropriately mixed formulations. The time between the mixing of products and their subsequent PO, parenteral, or topical administration may also allow a degree of inactivation of incompatible ingredients.

Many drug incompatibilities have been recognized and described. A few select examples are listed below to emphasize the degree of caution that should be exercised whenever pharmaceutical preparations are mixed.

Drug	Incompatible Preparations
Atropine sulfate	Barbiturates, diazepam
Chloramphenicol sodium succinate	Hydrocortisone sodium succinate, heparin sodium, chlorpromazine hydrochloride, promethazine hydrochloride, gentamicin sulfate, penicillins, erythromycin, tetracyclines, vitamins B and C
Gentamicin sulfate	Carbenicillin (and other semisynthetic penicillins), cephalosporins, chloramphenicol sodium succinate, sulfonamides, heparin sodium
Tetracyclines	Salts of calcium, aluminum, magnesium, and other tri- and divalent cations, penicillins, cephalosporins, tylosin, chloramphenicol sodium succinate, hydrocortisone sodium succinate, sodium bicarbonate
Meperidine	Barbiturates, sodium bicarbonate, heparin sodium, methylprednisolone, sodium succinate
Calcium gluconate	Carbonate, phosphate and sulfate salts (eg, sodium bicarbonate, potassium phosphate, streptomycin sulfate), promethazine hydrochloride, tetracyclines, sulfonamide solutions
Semisynthetic penicillins Sodium benzylpenicillin Aminoglycosides Barbiturates Diazepam Phenothiazine neuroleptics Vitamin B complex	Many incompatibilities—should not be mixed with other drug preparations

In addition to the above, many drugs do not retain their integrity and activity over time when diluted in certain commonly used parenteral fluids—either if added alone or in combination with other drugs. Again, just a few examples of the many known are listed to illustrate this type of potential interaction.

Drug	Incompatible Parenteral Fluids
Ampicillin sodium	Glucose solution Dextran solutions
Oxytetracycline	Solutions containing Ca^{++} or Mg^{++} hydrochloride (eg, Ringer's solution) Glucose solutions
Gentamicin sulfate	Any fluid in which the concentration of gentamicin exceeds 1 g/L
Diazepam	Insoluble in most solutions
Methylprednisolone sodium succinate	Sodium lactate solutions
Sodium bicarbonate	Sodium lactate solutions Ringer's solutions Other Ca^{++}-containing solutions

The general rule to avoid direct drug-drug interactions is simply **not** to mix pharmaceutical preparations before or during their administration unless it is known that the respective formulations are completely compatible.

A few direct drug-drug interactions may even occur within the body after separate administration of the agents. Examples include: some aminoglycosides inactivate certain penicillins at sites of infection (eg, kanamycin and methicillin, gentamicin and carbenicillin); tetracyclines chelate di- and trivalent cations (Ca^{++}, Fe^{++}, Al^{+++}, etc); protamine inactivates heparin (used to reverse excess heparin effects on coagulation); calcium gluconate and sodium sulfonamide solutions, when administered simultaneously, can form gels in the vein with subsequent embolism and occlusion; kaolin binds rifampin and lincomycin in the GI tract.

Drug-Diet Interactions: A dietary component or the presence of food may influence the absorption of drugs, which in turn may impair the absorption of nutrients. However, in most cases the absorption of drugs administered PO is not particularly affected by dietary constituents, and they are well absorbed whether given either with or between meals. There are a few notable exceptions. Absorption of the tetracyclines is impaired by milk and milk products because of the presence of calcium ions. The presence of food may also substantially reduce the absorption of sulfisoxazole, ampicillin and some other semisynthetic penicillins (but not amoxicillin), cephalexin, tetracyclines, lincomycin, and rifampin. Conversely, the absorption of griseofulvin is markedly increased when given with fat, cream, or margarine. This represents a useful way of attaining high levels of griseofulvin in the keratin layers of the skin in dermatomycosis. The presence of food in the stomach may exert a nonspecific effect in reducing or slowing the absorption of some drugs, eg, the absorption of phenylbutazone in horses becomes somewhat unpredictable when it is administered after feeding. In ruminants, eating and the presence of fresh feed in the ruminoreticulum increases ruminal motility and enhances blood flow to the forestomach. Under these circumstances, the rate of absorption of drugs from the ruminoreticulum tends to increase.

Some drugs administered PO may interfere with the absorption of specific nutrients—especially with long-term administration. Chronic anticonvulsant therapy with phenytoin suppresses absorption of dietary folic acid, and daily administration of mineral oil impedes the absorption of the fat-soluble vitamins, which ultimately leads to a deficiency. Oral dosage of antibiotics, such as the tetracyclines and aminoglycosides, which reach effective antibacterial levels in the lower small intestine and large intestine, can lead to suppression of microbial synthesis of vitamin K and the vitamin B complex. In species that depend, at least in part, on the microbial production in their intestinal tracts of these essential nutrients, chronic administration of broad-spectrum antibiotics can lead to subclinical avitaminosis.

Pharmacokinetic Interactions: One or several drugs can interfere with the pharmacokinetic fate of concurrently administered drugs in several ways. Such interactions may involve the absorption, distribution, biotransformation, or excretion of drugs.

Drug Interactions Involving GI Absorption: There are many mechanisms through which the rate of absorption of drugs from the GI tract may be modified by a second drug. Antacids and H_2-blockers increase the intragastric pH and thereby may change the disintegration and dissolution rates of solid oral dosage forms, and also delay the absorption of weakly acidic drugs. Sodium bicarbonate typically reduces the absorption of the tetracyclines. Because the stomach is not a major site of absorption and most drugs are primarily absorbed from the proximal small intestine by virtue of its much greater surface area, the rate of gastric emptying and the degree of intestinal motility may markedly influence the rate of drug absorption. Agents such as anticholinergics, adrenergics, neuroleptics, antihistaminics, and opioid analgesics diminish GI motility. Conversely, cholinergics, metoclopramide, antacids, and some purgatives enhance GI movement. The net effect on the absorption rate of drugs administered PO when the GI tract is under the influence of motility modifiers depends largely on whether they are acids or bases, and whether they are normally rapidly or slowly absorbed. Drugs given PO may complex with each other in some fashion, eg, they may form ion pairs or chelates, and their absorption may then be diminished or enhanced. Tetracycline absorption is diminished by the formation of insoluble chelates with di- and trivalent cations such as Ca^{++}, Fe^{++}, and Al^{+++}. The absorption of dicumarol is increased by magnesium hydroxide because of the greater solubility of the chelate that is formed. Kaolin, activated charcoal, and cholestyramine reduce the GI absorption of many drugs concurrently administered PO because of their propensity to bind to other substances (adsorption). Malabsorption syndromes can result from toxic effects of certain drugs on intestinal mucosal cells. For example, chloramphenicol, neomycin, and tetracycline produce characteristic lesions in the intestinal mucosa of calves. The morphological changes include diffuse reduction in villous height and numbers, flattened mucosal epithelium, and multifocal villous fusion. Adrenergic agents with α activity induce pronounced splanchnic vasoconstriction which, in turn, deters the rapid absorption of drugs from the GI tract into the portal circulation. For as yet unknown reasons, high plasma concentrations of insulin facilitate the absorption of meperidine, salicylate, and chlorpromazine from the intestine.

Drug Interactions Involving Absorption From Injection Sites: The rate of absorption following parenteral administration is governed primarily by the anatomical site employed for the injection, the form of the drug and the vehicle used, and the regional blood flow. Interaction of inadvisedly mixed injections may lead either to an increased absorption rate if vasodilation occurs or to delayed absorption if a vasoconstrictive response results. This interaction may be deliberate, best illustrated by the combined use of epinephrine and local analgesics to prolong the duration of their effect at the site of administration.

Drug Interactions Involving Distribution: The concurrent administration of 2 or more drugs may alter their intracorporeal distribution pattern. Competition for plasma-protein binding sites is quite common. Acidic drugs that possess the greatest affinity displace less strongly bound agents, and the net excess of free drug may then lead to exaggerated or toxic responses. The few examples below serve to emphasize this sometimes dangerous form of pharmacokinetic interaction.

Strongly Bound Drug	Displaced Drug	Effect of Interaction
Phenylbutazone	Coumarins (especially warfarin)	Hemorrhage due to excess inhibition of the synthesis of vitamin-K-dependent clotting factors
Nonsteroidal anti-inflammatory drugs (NSAID)	Sulfonamides	Enhanced sulfonamide activity and toxicity
NSAID	Methotrexate	Increased methotrexate toxicity
Valproic acid	Phenytoin	Increased plasma phenytoin levels

In addition to the effects on drug disposition that may result from displacement from protein-binding sites, the pharmacodynamic effects of one drug may affect the tissue distribution of another. Examples include drug-induced alterations in cardiac output, blood shunts, and changes in capillary permeability.

Drug Interactions Involving Biotransformation: Of the pharmacokinetic factors that control drug action, the rate of metabolic transformation is one of the most important. Hence, interactions that result in changes in the rate of drug metabolism can be of great clinical significance. One drug can alter the metabolism of a second drug either by stimulating (inducing) or inhibiting the microsomal enzyme systems. The extent to which drug-metabolizing enzymes may be induced varies with the species and with the degree of previous exposure to inducing agents. The usual consequence of microsomal enzyme induction is an abbreviated effect of the second drug because it is biotransformed much more rapidly. However, in those cases in which pro-drugs are converted to active compounds by metabolic transformation, toxic effects may become evident because of the facilitation of the activation process. Inducing agents need to be administered repetitively over several days to stimulate microsomal enzyme activity maximally. In veterinary medicine, few therapeutic agents are administered for prolonged periods, but there are some important exceptions, such as anticonvulsants, nonsteroidal anti-inflammatory drugs, sex steroids, and antifungal agents. A selection of drugs that induce microsomal enzyme activity and the compounds with an increased rate of biotransformation are listed below.

Inducing Agent	Compounds with Increased Rates of Biotransformation	
Phenobarbital	Barbiturates	Cortisol
	Phenytoin	Testosterone
	Phenylbutazone	Progesterone
	Warfarin	Bilirubin
Phenylbutazone	Phenylbutazone	
	Corticosteroids	
	Sex steroids	
Phenytoin	Corticosteroids	
	Sex steroids	
Griseofulvin	Warfarin	

Phenothiazine neuroleptics, diazepam, diphenhydramine, mitotane, estradiol, progestogens, androgens, and other barbiturates can also induce microsomal enzyme activity.

Some drugs are capable of inhibiting the biotransformation of others. The mechanism usually involves competitive enzyme inhibition and, unlike induction, occurs immediately after the inhibitor reaches the enzyme. Although the effect may be observed quickly, in some cases it may take several days before the clinical evidence of microsomal (or other) enzyme inhibition of drug metabolism becomes apparent. Microsomal enzyme inhibitors that are of clinical importance include chloramphenicol, cimetidine, quinidine, and prednisolone. The suppression of barbiturate and phenytoin metabolism by chloramphenicol can have serious consequences. Allopurinol, a xanthine oxidase inhibitor, reduces the hepatic inactivation of several agents, including 6-substituted purines such as azathioprine and mercaptopurine.

Drug Interactions Involving Excretion: Drug interactions can affect the efficiency of the organs involved in the excretion of drugs and their metabolites. Several mechanisms may be responsible for such interactions. Any drug that modifies renal blood flow may alter the clearance of other drugs by changing both the glomerular filtration rate and the tubular transport process. Increased renal blood flow generally promotes the renal excretion of drugs and/or their metabolites. The reverse is true for renal ischemia induced by vasoconstrictive agents. Increased urine flow rates resulting from administration of diuretics may increase the renal excretion of concurrently administered drugs—although in some cases the diuretics themselves compete with other agents for tubular transport carriers, and this reduces their renal elimination. Alteration of urinary pH changes the rate of excretion via the kidneys, principally when the pK_a of the drug is within the range of the urine pH. Even minor deviations in urine pH then substantially modify the degree of ionization of either acids or bases, and hinder or facilitate their reabsorption from the tubules. Weak bases, such as morphine, meperidine, procaine, and several antihistamines, are excreted more rapidly at lower urine pH values, and more slowly at higher. The opposite applies for weak acids, such as nalidixic acid, nitrofurantoin, several sulfonamides, some barbiturates, and many nonsteroidal anti-inflammatory drugs (NSAID). Urinary alkalinizing agents that are capable of influencing the excretion rate of concurrently administered drugs include sodium bicarbonate, sodium citrate, and sodium acetate. The carbonic anhydrase inhibitors that act as diuretics also alkalinize the urine. Urinary acidifiers (with effects opposite those of the alkalinizing agents on the renal excretion of drugs) include ascorbic acid, methionine, sodium acid phosphate, and ammonium chloride. The carriers responsible for the tubular transport of drugs have a limited capacity, and competition for secretion can occur between similar organic ions. Anions compete with anions, and cations with cations for transport sites, although organic cations are generally potent molecules that are not given in doses high enough to saturate the transport mechanisms. Examples of drugs that are acidic in nature and undergo renal elimination by a shared carrier-mediated transport system include penicillins, cephalosporins, probenecid, sulfonamides, acetazolamide, furosemide, NSAID (eg, aspirin, phenylbutazone, naproxen, mefenamic acid, and ibuprofen), and phase II drug metabolites (eg, glucuronic acid, glycine, and sulfate conjugates). Basic drugs that utilize a tubular carrier-mediated transport process include procainamide, dopamine, trimethoprim, triamterene, thiamine, and several opioid agents, such as morphine and dihydrocodeine.

Drug interactions associated with biliary excretion seem to be relatively unimportant. Pharmacological agents that influence hepatic blood flow can affect the efficiency of bile production and flow. In addition, enterically active antimicrobial agents can modify normal enterohepatic cycling by preventing bacterial hydrolysis of drug conjugates in the GI tract.

Pharmacodynamic Interactions: Many pharmacodynamic interactions are recognized that occur when 2 or more drugs are administered simultaneously. In many instances the resultant effects are indeed desired and beneficial; eg, premedication with neuroleptics before induction of general anesthesia (functional potentiation), the reversal of narcosis with opioid antagonists such as naloxone (competitive antagonism), and the treatment of digitalis overdosage with propranolol (functional antagonism). However, in some cases, the combined effects of 2 or more drugs may induce or increase toxicity (additive effects or potentiation). Certain aspects of a few examples are discussed below. 1) Aminoglycoside antibiotics are ototoxic, nephrotoxic, and may precipitate acute peripheral vasodilation following IV administration. In addition, they have a curare-like effect at the neuromuscular junction and exert a negative inotropic effect on the heart. The ototoxic and nephrotoxic effects are potentiated by loop diuretics such as furosemide. The neuromuscular and cardiac effects are potentiated by most general anesthetics, especially halothane and thiopental. Calcium ions and short-acting acetylcholinesterase antagonists reverse these latter effects. 2) Lincomycin, clindamycin, and polymyxins exert a neuromuscular blocking effect, and caution is advised when any nondepolarizing neuromuscular blocking agent is used concurrently. 3) Tetracycline antibiotics also possess a neuromuscular blocking effect that may be potentiated by general anesthetics or hypocalcemia. 4) The toxicity of cardiac glycosides is enhanced by hypercalcemia, hypomagnesemia, hypokalemia, and hypothyroidism. Serum concentration and toxicity of digoxin are increased by coadministration of quinidine; at the same time, the inotropic effects of digoxin are lessened. Coadministration with furosemide results in elevation of serum digoxin. Propranolol ameliorates cardiac glycoside intoxication and also lessens the positive inotropic effect. 5) Halothane and methoxyflurane sensitize the myocardium to the arrhythmogenic effects of catecholamines. Fatal ventricular fibrillation can be reliably produced by the release or administration of epinephrine in halothane-anesthetized dogs. Induction of anesthesia with thiobarbiturates potentiates this effect. Premedication with acepromazine, lidocaine, or propranolol prevents this dangerous interaction. 6) Diamidines such as diminazene and phenamidine are inhibitors of acetylcholinesterase. If an animal is treated with one of these antiprotozoal agents soon after being dipped in an organophosphate insecticide, toxicity may occur. 7) Succinylcholine, the depolarizing muscle relaxant, is hydrolyzed *in vitro* by serum cholinesterases. Organophosphate and carbamate insecticides inhibit cholinesterase, and thus potentiate the action of succinylcholine. 8) Propranolol, a β-receptor blocker, precipitates hypoglycemia in insulin-dependent diabetics. 9) The antiarrhythmics quinidine and procainamide potentiate the action of muscle relaxant drugs. 10) Fatal renal failure following the combined use of methoxyflurane and tetracyclines has been reported. 11) When amphotericin B and digitalis glycosides are administered concurrently, the potential for cardiac arrhythmias is enhanced. 12) Long-term use of phenytoin and phenobarbital or primidone leads to cholestatic hepatopathy. 13) Verapamil and propranolol given together IV may cause a high degree of heart block. 14) Phenobarbital enhances digoxin toxicity, but the mechanism is not understood. 15) Diphemanil methylsulfate can precipitate fatal ventricular fibrillation in thiamylal-anesthetized dogs.

PATHOLOGICAL FACTORS MODIFYING DRUG ACTION

Pathological lesions in major organ systems, or pathophysiological changes within body fluids, can substantially alter both the pharmacokinetic fate and the pharmacological action of many drugs. However, the potential influence of the disease state on the fate and action of drugs administered to sick animals is rarely considered during therapeutic management. This is understandable simply because there is a dearth of experimental and clinical data to serve as a basis for rational dosage adjustments in pathological states; the clinical approach must still be empirical. Nevertheless, several pathological conditions are known to modify drug action in a number of species, especially in man.

Gastrointestinal Disease: Several conditions may alter the absorption rates of drugs administered PO. Increased, decreased, or even unpredictable absorption patterns may be evident, depending on the lesions and pathophysiological changes present. The following disease conditions or clinical signs could be responsible for deviations in the usual drug absorption processes—and the possibility should always be considered when treating such cases.

Vomiting (many causes)
Gastritis
Gastric ulceration
Achlorhydria or hypochlorhydria
Ruminoreticular stasis
Ruminal lactacidosis
Rumenitis
Diarrhea (many causes)
Enteritis (many forms)
Duodenal ulceration

Steatorrhea
Pancreatic disorders
Other malabsorption syndromes
Ileus
GI obstructions
Ulcerative colitis
Peritonitis
Post-laparotomy
Gastrotomy or enterotomy

Hepatic Disease: Either acute or chronic liver disease can alter several pharmacokinetic determinants and the disposition and elimination of many drugs. The most important facets of drug disposition and elimination affected by liver disease are the following: 1) impairment of the activity of drug-metabolizing enzyme systems due to hepatocyte damage; 2) limitation of the efficiency of the hepatobiliary secretory system due to hepatocellular failure; 3) changes in hepatic blood flow, particularly in circulatory shock, cirrhosis, and portosystemic venous shunting; 4) reduced synthesis of plasma proteins, especially albumin, and alteration in their drug-binding capacity; 5) development of ascites and peripheral edema with consequent enlargement of the volume of distribution for many drugs, which prolongs their elimination half-lives.

In addition to the influence of hepatic dysfunction on the kinetic fate of agents that usually undergo biotransformation, the reduced metabolic transformation of those drugs with a systemic bioavailability that is generally restricted by first-pass metabolism may be sufficient that serious toxic effects occur quickly.

Many disease states may affect the liver's role in drug clearance. Examples include viral, bacterial, and toxic hepatitis; cirrhosis due to a number of causes; liver abscessation; and derangements (congenital and acquired) in hepatic circulation. In treating cases with impaired hepatic blood flow or function, it is often necessary to reduce the doses of drugs that are usually metabolically transformed, and to increase the intervals between doses to avoid excess systemic accumulation. The clinical responses should be monitored carefully.

Renal Disease: If urinary excretion is an important route of elimination, renal failure results in decreased drug clearance and thus slower removal of the drug from the body. A usual dosage regimen in such cases leads to accumulation and, ultimately, to toxicity. In addition, animals with renal insufficiency often react abnormally to a number of drugs, irrespective of the alterations in elimination. This increased sensitivity may be due to changes in plasma-protein binding, increased receptor responsiveness, derangements of acid-base balance, uremia, hyper- and hypokalemia, hyper- and hyponatremia, dehydration, and hyper- and hypotension.

A number of disturbances may occur within failing kidneys, all of which may influence the excretion and renal clearance of drugs. Changes in the pH of the filtrate also alter the excretion rates of drugs with appropriate pK_a values. Renal ischemia, glomerular lesions, tubular damage, impaired intrarenal perfusion, functional disabilities of the tubular cells, and obstructive lesions (in the tubules, collecting ducts, and ureters) may all influence the effective renal clearance of drugs and/or their metabolites. The slower removal of the drug from the body results in accumulation and an increased likelihood of toxicity if the usual dosage regimen is followed. Drugs such as aminoglycosides, penicillins, cephalosporins, colistin, tetracyclines (except doxycycline), sulfonamides, nitrofurantoin, 5-fluorocytosine, methotrexate, procainamide, methenamine, digoxin, and barbiturates are examples of agents that are wholly or largely eliminated by the kidneys. Adjustment of dosage is necessary when using these drugs in animals with renal insufficiency.

There are several approaches to establishing a dose schedule. First, if feasible, a regimen may be individualized for a particular animal. Actual plasma concentrations may be used to control drug therapy, and the kinetic parameters discussed earlier can be calculated to determine optimal dose rates and frequencies. Second, when an agent has a fairly wide therapeutic index, halving the standard dose or doubling the usual dosage interval should be sufficient in uremic animals to maintain therapeutic plasma levels without serious danger of accumulation. Finally, when potentially toxic drugs (eg, gentamicin, kanamycin and other aminoglycosides, cephaloridine, sulfonamides, digoxin, and some antineoplastic agents) are administered and renal insufficiency is present, more refined modification of dosage regimens is necessary.

Since both renal clearance and the renal fractional rate constant are directly proportional to creatinine clearance, one approach is to calculate the fraction of the normal dose to be given at the usual dosage interval: $D_{(ri)} = \dfrac{D \times Cl_{cr} \text{ (patient)}}{Cl_{cr} \text{ (normal)}}$, in which $D_{(ri)}$ is the dose in the presence of renal insufficiency, D is the usual maintenance dose, and Cl_{cr} is the creatinine clearance.

Alternatively, the dose may be kept constant and the dosage intervals increased: $T_{(ri)} = \dfrac{T \times Cl_{cr} \text{ (normal)}}{Cl_{cr} \text{ (patient)}}$, in which $T_{(ri)}$ is the dosage interval in the presence of renal disease, and T is the usual dosage interval.

The term 1/serum creatinine (mg/dL) has been substituted for the creatinine clearance ratios when these were not obtainable. However, in man, the relationship between $t_{1/2}$ and serum creatinine is not linear above 4 mg/dL. Thus, the formulas may be somewhat less reliable at higher serum creatinine levels.

Diseases and Drug-protein Binding: In a number of pathological states, a decrease in the plasma-protein binding of drugs, usually acids, is observed. This may be due to many factors related either to the protein, the drug, or the binding conditions. A decrease in the extent of drug plasma-protein binding does not invariably lead to enhanced drug effects.

Hypoalbuminemia alters the binding capacity for many drugs. Common clinical conditions associated with hypoalbuminemia include aging, burns, neoplasia, cardiac failure, protein-losing enteropathy, inflammatory disease, injury, liver disease, nephrotic syndrome, renal failure, and nutritional deficiency. Conditions resulting in the modification of the albumin compartment volume may also lead to discrepancies in the anticipated distribution of drugs. The predominant disease states that result in sequestration of plasma proteins in the interstitial compartment include inflammatory states, pregnancy, septic shock, cardiogenic shock, and pulmonary edema.

In several diseases, there is decreased affinity of drugs for plasma albumin. There may be several reasons for this phenomenon, including the release of endogenous binding inhibitors, and metabolic acidosis. The pathological states associated with decreased affinity of drugs for albumin include liver disease, chronic renal failure with uremia, the nephrotic syndrome, malnutrition, and cardiac failure.

The plasma-protein binding of basic drugs differs somewhat from acidic drugs, which bind largely to albumin. Basic drugs interact with a number of plasma constituents including α_1-acid glycoprotein (an acute phase protein), lipoprotein, and albumin. Whereas the trend for albumin is almost always to decrease in concentration, α_1-acid glycoprotein and lipoprotein show large fluctuations due to physiological and pathological conditions. Associated with changes in the plasma levels of these specific proteins, both decreases and increases in the binding of basic drugs have been recorded.

Cardiovascular Disease: Cardiovascular insufficiency, due to either cardiac failure or circulatory shock, is often associated with disturbances in cardiac output, autonomic nervous system activity, central and systemic venous pressures, and sodium and water metabolism. These disturbances may in turn influence the extent and pattern of tissue perfusion and may lead to tissue hypoxia and visceral congestion. GI motility may also be altered. Cardiac failure potentially affects the disposition of drugs, which may then necessitate adjustment in dosage regimens for optimal therapy. However, no ready guidelines are available.

A few special features need emphasis. Redistribution of the cardiac output to preserve blood flow to the heart and brain leads to a diminished volume of distribution, as well as decreased renal and hepatic perfusion with resultant delay in drug elimination. Both of these factors tend to lead to increased plasma levels of any parenterally administered drug. Splanchnic vasoconstriction encountered in shock delays the GI absorption of any agent administered PO.

In congestive heart failure with marked ascites and dependent edema, the accumulated fluid may or may not represent a distribution compartment. If it does, the total weight of the animal can be used to calculate a dose rate, provided there is not a concurrent rapid loss of the fluid due to appropriate therapy. Moreover, in such cases, hypoalbuminemia and reduced binding capacity are often features that could alter the normal distribution patterns of a drug.

Generally, when cardiovascular dysfunction is present, loading doses should be conservative, and continued therapy monitored closely either by watching for clinical signs of overdosage or by measuring plasma levels of the drugs being employed.

Pulmonary Disease: Acute hypoxemia appears to decrease intrinsic hepatic clearance, while chronic hypoxia appears to increase it. The free fraction of some basic drugs is decreased in plasma taken from animals suffering from chronic hypoxemia. Blood-gas disturbances also can affect drug disposition by decreasing hepatic and renal perfusion.

Respiratory disease can significantly change drug disposition through a number of interacting mechanisms. These have not been adequately studied to provide a basis for clinical dosage adjustment. Drugs showing flow-dependent hepatic clearance (eg, lidocaine, meperidine, propoxyphene) and those with predominantly renal clearance (eg, aminoglycosides, digoxin) should be used with caution when respiratory disease is present. Theophylline doses should also be reduced on an empirical basis.

Neurological Disturbances: A large number of neurological disorders may potentially alter the effect of many drugs—both those with CNS activity as well as several that do not normally act within the CNS. Clearly, lesion-induced changes in

CNS functions influence an animal's response to CNS depressant agents. Moreover, in meningoencephalitis, many drugs that do not normally do so may penetrate the blood-brain barrier and produce unusual effects, eg, penicillin G may act as a convulsant. Damage to autonomic or vital medullary centers may also influence the response of specific target tissues to either stimulant or depressant drugs. In idiopathic canine epilepsy and epileptiform conditions in general, phenothiazine neuroleptics can precipitate seizures and should not be used as tranquilizers or for premedication before general anesthesia in affected animals.

Other Pathological States: Several other pathological states may influence either the pharmacokinetic fate or the pharmacodynamic effects of a number of specific drugs. A selection of these are listed below to emphasize the significant influence disease conditions can have on drug action. 1) Anemia. Tissues may be hyper- or hyporesponsive when anemia and hypoxemia are present. The myocardium may become especially sensitive to the action of positive inotropic and chronotropic agents. Biotransformation and excretion processes can also be seriously disrupted. 2) Toxemia. The disposition and elimination of many drugs, as well as their toxicity, may become altered in toxemic states. 3) Electrolyte disturbances. Even minor deviations from normal plasma electrolyte values can lead to significant changes in the response to certain drugs; hypocalcemia as well as hypo- and hyperkalemia are prime examples. The digitalis glycosides are much more toxic in hypokalemia. 4) Acid-base derangements. Alkalosis often enhances the response of excitable tissue to provocative drugs. Conversely, systemic acidosis tends to depress the reactions of excitable tissues such as nerves, skeletal muscle, the myocardium, and smooth muscle. Tissue acidosis limits the diffusibility of many local anesthetics to their site of action. The bactericidal action of the aminoglycoside antibiotics is less efficient in acidosis. Systemic acidosis also tends to change the plasma-protein binding of drugs. The pH of the urine can change during acid-base derangements with subsequent alterations in the usual renal excretion rates of many of those drugs with appropriate pK_a values. 5) Endocrine and metabolic disturbances. Several endocrine and metabolic derangements may be exacerbated by the administration of exogenous agents. For example, incipient diabetes mellitus may be precipitated by the administration of glucocorticoids and by the progestogen megestrol acetate. Hyperthyroidism often increases the responsiveness of an animal to a variety of drugs, and such cases should be managed carefully. 6) Impaired immunocompetence. When, for whatever reason, host defense systems are not fully functional, the successful clinical use of several antimicrobial drugs is placed in jeopardy. This is especially true for the bacteriostatic group of agents.

DRUG-INDUCED HYPERSENSITIVITY REACTIONS

Hypersensitivity or "allergic" reactions to drugs do not appear to have a high incidence in veterinary medicine (perhaps <10% of all drug-related adverse effects). Nevertheless, immune-mediated responses due to the antigenic properties of some drugs can lead to serious and even fatal consequences. Hypersensitivity in animals has been associated most frequently with penicillins and cephalosporins, but tetracyclines, chloramphenicol, sulfonamides, macrolides, lincosamides, nitrofurans, isoniazid, levamisole, corticosteroids, protein hormones, iodinated contrast media for use in radiography, and several other drugs may precipitate various forms and degrees of immune-based reactions. In addition, several carriers and solubilizers are also capable of effecting the sudden release or activation of autacoids such as histamine, serotonin, kinins, prostaglandins, leukotrienes, and platelet-activating factor, and lead to clinical signs associated with type I hypersensitivity. Examples of such substances capable of releasing autacoids include polysorbate 80 (surfactant used as an emulsifier and dispersing agent), carboxymethylcellulose (used as a carrier to prepare suspensions), certain diamidines (antiprotozoal agents), morphine, and tubocurarine.

Generally, hypersensitivity reactions cannot be anticipated unless the animal has a history of being sensitive to some drug or perhaps of being atopic. Unlike type A adverse drug reactions, allergic responses usually are not dose related, and severe manifestations can occur following exposure to very limited amounts of an antigenic drug.

Because most drug molecules are relatively small, they usually do not elicit an immune response of their own accord; to become immunogenic, they or their metabolites must form covalent bonds with macromolecules such as endogenous proteins, and to a lesser extent with polysaccharides or polynucleotides. This covalent binding of drugs (thus acting as haptens) to appropriate endogenous macromolecules is the exception rather than the rule, but does occur to a significant degree with some classes of drugs. Also, in hypersensitivity reactions following repeated administration of a drug preparation, several microbiological products (either contaminant proteins or polymeric complexes) may be present that can act as primary antigens. This particular problem has been encountered with penicillins, cephalosporins, polymyxin, amphotericin B, and several other antibiotic preparations. Cross-reactivity must also always be considered in an animal with a history of allergic drug reactions. In this instance, administration of closely related drugs may precipitate signs of hypersensitivity. Cross-reactivity may be encountered with the penicillins, cephalosporins, and sulfonamides. Because a sulfamyl group is common to all of them, cross-reactivity also occurs between sulfonamides, furosemide, thiazide diuretics, and the sulfonyl-urea group of oral hypoglycemic drugs.

Immunologic Mechanisms: Drug reactions mediated by immune mechanisms may be associated with any one of the 4 basic types of hypersensitivity (*see also* IMMUNE SYSTEM, p 421 *et seq*).

   Type I reactions (anaphylaxis) are initiated by antigen reaction with basophils and mast cells previously sensitized by IgE antibody, which leads to the sudden release of pharmacologically active substances (vasoactive amines, kinins, prostaglandins, leukotrienes, platelet-activating factor, and various chemotactic factors). General and local anaphylactic reactions due to drugs may occur.

   Type II reactions (antibody-mediated cytotoxicity or cell-stimulating) are initiated by IgG, IgM, or IgA antibodies reacting to antigenic substances on the surface of body cells (either a normal component or a foreign hapten) or associated structures, such as myoneural receptors, intracellular cement substance, etc. Complement also participates in this reaction as do certain kinds of mononuclear cells. Many types of body cells can be damaged, but blood cells seem to be especially susceptible to immune-mediated lysis and phagocytosis. Stimulation of secretor organs (eg, thyroid) or neutralization of biologically active molecules (eg, insulin) may lead to specific deficiency states. The types of allergic drug manifestations related to type II reactions (autoimmune responses) include hemolytic anemia, leukopenia, thrombocytopenia, glomerular nephritis, and resistance to insulin replacement therapy. Transfusion reactions are also a form of type II hypersensitivity.

   Type III reactions (immune-complex damage) are initiated when antigen reacts with precipitating antibody, which forms complexes of various sizes that may then localize in tissues, usually small blood vessel walls, and cause damage (vasculitis) and/or interfere with the function of the tissue membranes involved. The prerequisites for this type of reaction are a continuous source of circulating antigen and continuous production of specific antibody (IgM or IgG, although IgE may also play a role). The best example of a drug-induced type III reaction is serum sickness, which involves IgG and is a multisystem complement-dependent vasculitis. Drugs acting as haptens and capable of producing serum sickness include penicillins, lincomycin, erythromycin, sulfonamides, trimethoprim-sulfonamide combinations, and certain hormones.

   Type IV reactions (cell-mediated immune reactions or delayed hypersensitivity) are initiated by the specific response of active, sensitized lymphocytes (T-cells) to an allergen with the resultant release of lymphokines and/or the development of cytotoxicity without antibodies being involved. Activated macrophages (due to lymphokine release) also become cytotoxic. Cell-mediated hypersensitivity is the mechanism involved in allergic contact dermatitis, which may result from topically applied or locally injected drugs.

Clinical Manifestation of Drug-induced Hypersensitivity: Anaphylaxis is an acute, systemic, life-threatening reaction characterized in many species by hypotension, bronchospasm, angioedema, urticaria, erythema, pruritus, pharyngeal and/or laryngeal edema, cardiac dysrhythmias, vomiting, colic, and hyperperistalsis. Only one or many of these clinical signs may be present. Anaphylaxis most commonly follows parenteral administration of drugs, but also may occur after inhalation or oral exposure. Clinical signs usually develop within seconds to minutes and are at their peak in 10-30 min, but the onset may be delayed for ≥ 1 hr after administration of a relatively insoluble, repository dosage form such as benzathine penicillin. If the reaction is not fatal, the manifestations subside over hours. Death generally is attributable to cardiac arrest, shock, or asphyxia.

Treatment of drug-induced anaphylactic reactions should proceed as follows: epinephrine or other β-adrenoreceptor agonists; theophylline or other phosphodiesterase inhibitors; a glucocorticoid that will modify the effects of the released mediators on target tissues; and sodium chromoglycate, which inhibits the degranulation of mast cells. Antihistamines (H_1-blockers) are not particularly useful once histamine release has occurred; however, they will limit the adverse effects of histamine if administered prophylactically.

Serum sickness is a systemic reaction that occurs in response to certain drugs and is manifest by lymphadenopathy, neuropathy, vasculitis, nephritis, arthritis, urticaria, and fever. Generally, the onset of serum sickness in response to a drug is delayed until 10-20 days after inception of therapy. An accelerated form of the reaction (onset in 2-3 days) may occur in individuals that have been previously sensitized to the drug. Clinical signs often persist for several days after withdrawal of the drug.

Drugs that have been incriminated most frequently include the sulfonamides, penicillins, streptomycin, lincomycin, erythromycin, p-aminosalicylic acid, and certain anticonvulsants and hormones. Immediate withdrawal of the drug is necessary to reduce the severity of this form of type III reaction, although corticosteroids are also useful in attenuating severe serum sickness reactions.

Hematologic manifestations: Hemolytic anemia, thrombocytopenia, and agranulocytosis are occasional manifestations of immune-mediated adverse drug reactions. Several mechanisms and types of hypersensitivity reactions may be involved. Anemia may be due to frank hemolysis or to a shortened RBC life span because of antigen-antibody reactions involving the RBC membrane. Autoimmune hemolytic anemia is a special type of this case. Drugs that may produce immune-mediated hemolytic anemia in man include penicillin, α-methyldopa, dipyrone, quinine, quinidine, p-aminosalicylic acid, phenacetin, and rifampin. Estrogens are of particular significance in dogs.

Immune-mediated thrombocytopenia may result from mechanisms similar to those associated with RBC hemolysis. The drugs incriminated include sulfonamides, isoniazid, rifampin, estrogens, and phenylbutazone.

Agranulocytosis, a potentially fatal allergic drug reaction, is more common in man than in other animals. The contribution of immune-mediated reactions to drug-induced agranulocytosis remains obscure, but antileukocyte antibodies have been demonstrated in several instances. The immunologic effects may be on the stem cells in the bone marrow. Drugs most frequently associated with agranulocytosis in man are phenylbutazone, oxyphenbutazone, amidopyrine, sulfonamides, cephalothin, semisynthetic penicillins, chloramphenicol, p-aminosalicylic acid, phenothiazines, gold compounds, anticonvulsants, propylthiouracil, indomethacin, dipyrone, tolbutamide, barbiturates, antihistamines, and arsenicals.

Autoimmune reactions: In addition to hemolytic anemia and thrombocytopenia, drugs have been incriminated in the development of systemic lupus erythematosus (SLE), polymyositis, hepatitis, tubular nephropathy, and inhibition of coagulation factor VIII. Drug-induced SLE has been observed in animals treated with isoniazid, griseofulvin, and tetracycline. Autoimmune reactions to drugs usually subside within several months after the offending drug is withdrawn. Immunosuppressive therapy is warranted only when the autoimmune response is unusually severe.

Cutaneous manifestations: Contact dermatitis, initiated by local exposure to a drug that acts as a hapten, is a hypersensitivity reaction (type IV) that may be encountered in animals. The extent and severity of the lesion that develops depends on the area of application, its degree of penetration, and several other factors. Delayed hypersensitivity reactions may also develop at an injection site. Other cutaneous manifestations may result from immune-mediated responses to drugs. Examples include urticaria and angioedema (type I), cutaneous lesions of systemic lupus erythematosus (type III), and petechiae or purpura caused by thrombocytopenia or vasculitis (types II and III). Cutaneous drug eruptions may be expressed in a wide variety of pathological lesions. Drugs that have been reported to cause skin eruptions include tetracaine, chloramphenicol, penicillin G, ampicillin, tetracycline, gentamicin, streptomycin, neomycin, griseofulvin, thiabendazole, 5-fluorocytosine, phenytoin, quinidine, thiacetarsamide, prednisolone, acepromazine, estrogens, thyroid extract, benzoyl peroxide, and sulfonamides.

Diagnosis: If the need for diagnosis justifies the inherent risk to the animal, a clinical diagnosis of drug-induced hypersensitivity may be based on the following criteria. The reaction should: 1) be elicited by a small amount of the drug, 2) not resemble the normal pharmacological action of the drug, 3) occur only after a lapse of an induction period of 5-7 days following initial exposure to the drug, 4) include clinical signs considered characteristic of hypersensitivity, and 5) occur promptly following re-exposure to the drug.

SYSTEMIC PHARMACOTHERAPEUTICS

CARDIOVASCULAR SYSTEM

POSITIVE INOTROPES

Positive inotropes increase the strength of cardiac muscle contraction by increasing the quantity of intracellular calcium available for binding by muscle proteins. This, in turn, augments contractile protein interaction in the myocardial cell. Increased intracellular calcium can be achieved by increasing cyclic adenosine monophosphate (cAMP) production by stimulating adenylate cyclase, or decreasing cAMP degradation by inhibiting phosphodiesterases and altering the Na^+/Ca^{+2}-ATPase exchange pump.

CARDIAC GLYCOSIDES

The source of digitalis is the dried leaf of the foxglove plant (*Digitalis purpurea*). The active component of cardiac glycosides is an aglycone, which is released from attached sugars by hydrolysis.

The most probable mechanism of action for the inotropic effect of digitalis is inhibition of the membrane-bound Na^+/K^+-ATPase "pump"; when this occurs, Na^+ increases in the cell, the exchange of Na^+ for Ca^{+2} is augmented, and calcium influx is increased. The increased intracellular calcium in turn leads to increased release of Ca^{+2} from the sarcoplasmic reticulum and increased cardiac muscle contractility. Changes in the ratio of intracellular and extracellular electrolytes can result in increased automaticity and cardiac arrhythmias.

Digitalis also has a negative chronotropic effect due to decreased conduction velocity in the A-V node. In addition, digitalis potentiates vagal (cholinergic) activity in the heart. Changes in conduction can ultimately result in A-V nodal blockade. At toxic levels, digitalis also can directly slow sinus nodal activity due to increased sensitivity to acetylcholine. Since the atria are sensitive to acetylcholine, atrial conduction is also enhanced in the diseased heart, which can then lead to atrial arrhythmias.

Disposition: Digoxin and digitoxin are the 2 most widely used preparations. Disposition varies with the preparation. Oral absorption of digoxin is unreliable and depends on the preparation, varying from 40 to 90%. Absorption of the alcohol (elixir) form is best. Variation in bioavailability of tablets results from differences in dissolution between products. Absorption is retarded by food, although the absorption of digitoxin is much more complete because it is more lipid soluble. Both drugs are distributed slowly and are concentrated in cardiac tissues. Only 25% of digoxin is bound to plasma proteins, while ~90% of digitoxin is protein bound. Digoxin is primarily eliminated unchanged by the kidneys; its half-life (~1.7 days in dogs) is strongly influenced by renal function. Digitoxin is metabolized by the liver (one of the products is digoxin); its half-life in dogs is 8-12 hr.

Preparations: Digoxin is available for administration IV or PO. IV administration results in pharmacological effects in 5-30 min with a maximal effect in 2 hr. However, toxic drug concentrations are more difficult to avoid with this route. Digoxin should not be given IM because it causes pain and necrosis. Administration PO results in pharmacological effects in 1-2 hr.

Drug Interactions: The concurrent administration of quinidine will increase plasma concentrations of digoxin, probably due to displacement from tissue-binding sites. Interactions between digitalis and diuretics stem primarily from the effects on potassium (hypokalemia). Administration of β-adrenergic agonists increases the likelihood of arrhythmias. Amphotericin B may also cause hypokalemia and thus potentiate digitalis intoxication.

Toxicity: Toxic effects with digitalis glycosides are frequent and can be lethal. Cats are more sensitive to digoxin than dogs. Probably the most frequent cause of toxicity is overdosing. The potential for toxicity is increased with hypokalemia. Any cardiac arrhythmia may be induced by digitalis. The likelihood and severity of toxicity are related to the severity of cardiac disease. Other signs of toxicity include diarrhea, anorexia, and nausea and vomiting due to direct stimulation of the chemoreceptor trigger zone. Frequently, these are the earliest indications of toxicity. Neurological effects include malaise and drowsiness. Digitalis toxicity can be diagnosed (and avoided) by monitoring plasma drug concentrations. Treatment of intoxication includes 1) discontinuation of digitalis therapy; 2) discontinuation of potassium-depleting diuretics; and 3) administration of phenytoin (blocks A-V nodal effects of digitalis), and lidocaine (for ventricular arrhythmias) and potassium, if indicated (preferably PO). Atropine may be useful to treat sinus bradycardia, and second or third degree heart block induced by cholinergic augmentation.

Clinical Use: Digitalis is used for restoring adequate circulation in animals with congestive heart failure (ie, poor systolic function) or to slow the ventricular rate as a treatment of supraventricular arrhythmias, such as atrial fibrillation or flutter. Both syndromes require long-term treatment. Digoxin (dogs: 0.0055-0.011 mg/kg, PO, b.i.d.; cats: 0.001 mg/kg, PO, b.i.d.) is the cardiac glycoside drug of choice except in animals with renal disease; digitoxin should then be administered. Calculation of digoxin doses should be based on lean body weight, and dosages should be reduced in the obese animal in the presence of ascites. Electrolyte disorders should be corrected before dosage.

PHOSPHODIESTERASE INHIBITORS

Phosphodiesterases (PDE) inhibit the breakdown of cAMP and therefore increase intracellular cAMP concentrations. The result is an increase in myocardial contractility. Methylxanthine derivatives have been classified as PDE inhibitors but this is controversial. Of the methylxanthines, theophylline is the most cardiopotent. In addition to their cardiac effects, these drugs have significant CNS, renal, and smooth muscle effects. Their use for cardiac disease is limited to conditions that accompany respiratory disease that would benefit from bronchodilation.

The mechanism of action of amrinone and milrinone is probably inhibition of PDE and increased intracellular cAMP levels. These effects appear to occur without a dramatic rise in myocardial oxygen consumption. Milrinone is characterized by a toxic to therapeutic ratio of 100 in normal dogs, and is 20-30 times as potent as amrinone. Peripheral vasodilation is another major therapeutic benefit of these drugs. Administration IV or PO of milrinone results in marked positive inotropic effects in animals with congestive heart failure (CHF). Contractility increases up to 90% versus only 60% in animals receiving digitalis. Exacerbations of arrhythmias may occur in some animals. Milrinone may replace the cardiac glycosides as the first-choice positive inotrope in dogs with CHF.

β-ADRENERGIC AGONISTS

These drugs cause their positive inotropic effects by stimulation of adenyl cyclase and increased cAMP.

Dopamine is an endogenous catecholamine precursor with selective β 1 activity. However, it also stimulates the release of norepinephrine. At low doses, it stimulates renal dopaminergic receptors causing increased renal blood flow and diuresis. Dopamine is not effectively absorbed if given PO. It is rapidly metabolized by the body and has a half-life of <2 min. Dopamine is most commonly available as a solution, which is further diluted with saline or dextrose. The drug is administered IV, usually by constant infusion. Cardiac arrhythmias may occur due to β-adrenergic activity. Indications include cardiogenic or endotoxic shock, and oliguria.

Dobutamine is a synthetic drug similar to dopamine, but it does not cause release of norepinephrine and therefore has minimal effects other than β 1 activity. Dobutamine is a more effective positive inotrope than dopamine, although it does not dilate the renal vascular bed. Like dopamine, dobutamine is not effective PO and has a plasma half-life of ~2 min. Dobutamine is also prepared as a solution to be diluted with dextrose. It is the preferred drug for short-term therapy of refractory congestive heart failure. It is a potent vasopressor drug causing an immediate rise in blood pressure due to direct myocardial stimulation and peripheral vasoconstriction.

Compared to other inotropic drugs, epinephrine causes the greatest increase in the rate of energy usage and myocardial oxygen demand. This increase in oxygen need may be detrimental to the failing heart. Epinephrine is rapidly metabolized in the GI tract and is not effective after administration PO. Absorption is more rapid after IM versus subcut. administration because of local vasoconstriction. It is available in several preparations and is effective following IV, pulmonary, and nasal administration. However, because of the decreased efficiency of cardiac work, epinephrine is not used as a positive inotropic agent, but only for emergency therapy of cardiac arrest. Ventricular arrhythmias can be expected. In addition, CNS signs may occur.

Isoproterenol is a nonspecific β agonist that, like epinephrine, increases myocardial oxygen demand. Tachycardia and the potential for other arrhythmias excludes its use in the cardiac patient. Calcium is also a positive inotrope but must be given as a slow IV injection or infusion. Calcium must be administered carefully because it can cause cardiac rigor and standstill at high doses. The gluconate form is preferred to calcium chloride.

Glucagon is also a positive inotropic agent.

ANTIARRHYTHMICS

Antiarrhythmics have been grouped into 4 main classes according to their dominant electrophysiological effect on myocardial cells.

CLASS I DRUGS

Class I agents comprise the standard membrane-stabilizing drugs such as quinidine, procainamide, and lidocaine. These agents work by selectively blocking the fast Na^+ channels and depressing phase 0 of the action potential. This is caused by a direct membrane-stabilizing or "local anesthetic" effect. The decrease in phase 0 depolarization results in decreased conduction velocity. In addition, the class I drugs increase the threshold of excitability and decrease the rate of spontaneous phase 4 depolarization, thus reducing the emergence of ectopic foci. Some of these drugs also are useful in treating re-entrant arrhythmias.

Class I agents can be further subdivided based on their effects on the refractory period and the rate of repolarization. Class IA drugs include quinidine, procainamide, and disopyramide. **Quinidine** is related to the antimalarial drug quinine.

It has a broad spectrum of efficacy against supraventricular and ventricular arrhythmias. It is useful in the treatment of re-entrant arrhythmias such as atrial fibrillation. In the atria, quinidine also has indirect, anti-vagal ("atropine-like") effects.

The sulfate preparation of quinidine is absorbed rapidly following administration PO. The gluconate form is absorbed more slowly. It can be given IM but is painful. Although 90% is protein bound, distribution is rapid to most tissues. The half-life is ~6 hr.

Quinidine (dogs and cats: 10-20 mg/kg, PO, q6-8hr) can be used for acute and chronic treatment of supraventricular and ventricular arrhythmias. Individualized therapy is necessary because of moderate individual variation. Cardiotoxicity may result in A-V blockade or ventricular arrhythmias. The atropine-like effects of quinidine may result in increased impulse conduction through the A-V node to the ventricles and paradoxical acceleration. Quinidine, particularly in the sulfate form, can cause vasodilation and GI side effects.

Procainamide affects cardiac automaticity, excitability, responsiveness, and conduction similarly to quinidine. However, its effects on the autonomic nervous system are significantly weaker. It does not cause α-adrenergic blockade or paradoxical acceleration. Procainamide is rapidly and almost completely absorbed following administration PO. Only ~20% is protein bound. Procainamide is extensively biotransformed by the liver to metabolites that are generally inactive in dogs. The drug is available as oral capsules and tablets for chronic use. IV preparations are available for acute therapy and can also be administered IM.

Procainamide (dogs: 5-20 mg/kg, PO, q6-8hr; 2 mg/kg, IV, q5-10min) is a broad-spectrum antiarrhythmic. In general, its actions parallel those of quinidine, and it is useful in animals that have failed to respond to quinidine therapy. Toxicities include cardiotoxicity, similar to that induced by quinidine, hypotension with rapid IV administration (bolus), and GI signs (anorexia, nausea, vomiting, and diarrhea).

Disopyramide has pharmacological effects and a spectrum of activity that are similar to those of procainamide and quinidine, although its primary use is for ventricular tachyarrhythmias. Disopyramide is quickly absorbed following administration PO, but it undergoes rapid metabolism and clearance. Its half-life is <2 hr in dogs, which necessitates multiple daily administrations. This, coupled with the potential cardiotoxicities associated with disopyramide, limits its use in small animals.

Class IB drugs include lidocaine, tocainide, and phenytoin. **Lidocaine** is used predominantly for emergency treatment of ventricular arrhythmias. Lidocaine has minimal effect on the autonomic system. However, it counteracts arrhythmias in abnormal Purkinje and ventricular fibers without affecting normal cardiac tissues. Although well absorbed PO, lidocaine is subject to first-pass metabolism and only ⅓ of the drug reaches the systemic circulation. Absorption is complete following IM administration. Distribution of lidocaine to tissue is rapid. It is extensively metabolized by the liver; liver disease and reduced hepatic blood flow prolong the half-life, which is normally <1 hr in dogs.

Lidocaine is prepared for IV administration; no other drug should be included in the solution prepared for treatment of cardiac arrhythmias. It can be administered IV as a rapid bolus or as a continuous infusion (dogs: 1-2 mg/kg, IV bolus, followed by 30-50 mg/kg/min). A narrow-spectrum drug used solely for emergency management of ventricular arrhythmias, lidocaine has few undesirable effects. Toxicity is manifested in dogs primarily as CNS signs. Drowsiness or agitation may progress to muscle twitching and convulsions at higher plasma concentrations. In cats, which are more susceptible to toxicity, cardiac suppression may occur.

Tocainide is an analog of lidocaine that does not undergo extensive first-pass metabolism and thus is effective after administration PO. Tocainide has been used in dogs (17-30 mg/kg, PO, t.i.d.) for the long-term control of ventricular arrhythmias that respond to lidocaine.

Phenytoin has a limited spectrum of antiarrhythmic activity in the heart. Its primary usefulness in veterinary medicine is for the management of digitalis-induced arrhythmias because it significantly shortens A-V nodal and Purkinje refractory period in digitalized animals.

CLASS II DRUGS

Class II antiarrhythmic drugs are the β-adrenergic receptor blocking agents. **Propranolol**, the prototype β blocker, is a competitive nonselective β blocker, occupying both β-1 and β-2 receptors. As a β-1 blocker, propranolol exhibits a negative chronotropic effect in conditions of supraventricular tachycardia. Propranolol is also a negative inotrope. This pharmacological effect can be detrimental in the animal with small cardiac reserve (eg, the animal with congestive heart failure [CHF]) but is beneficial in cats with hypertrophic cardiomyopathy.

Clinical indications for propranolol include reduction of ventricular rate in cases of supraventricular tachycardias, hypertrophic and other forms of obstructive heart disease, and hyperthyroidism. Propranolol (dogs: 5-40 mg, PO, t.i.d.; cats: 2.5-5 mg, PO, t.i.d.) is used clinically as a negative chronotrope in dogs and cats with supraventricular arrhythmias and as a negative chronotrope and inotrope in cats with hypertrophic cardiomyopathy. Digitalization may be necessary before its use in dogs with CHF. Propranolol should be avoided in cats with evidence of respiratory disease (eg, asthma).

The toxic effects of propranolol are the result of β blockade and include bradyarrhythmias, hypotension, heart failure, bronchospasm, and hypoglycemia, particularly in diabetics. One should be particularly cautious in administering a β blocker when the animal has little myocardial reserve.

A variety of other β-blocking (specifically, β-2) agents are currently under investigation for clinical use. These newer β blockers include **timolol, nadolol, alprenolol**, and **metoprolol**. The pharmacological differences between these drugs relate to β-1 versus β-2 selectivity, and therefore their efficacy and safety.

CLASS III DRUGS

Class III drugs prolong the cardiac action potential and refractory period. They have no effect on the fast Na^+ conductance and do not cause β blockade. There are 2 members of this class: bretylium and amiodarone.

Bretylium affects primarily the Purkinje fibers and ventricles, hence it has a narrow spectrum of activity. It is not used clinically in veterinary medicine, but is used in human medicine for ventricular arrhythmias. It reportedly can cause defibrillation in cases of ventricular fibrillation in man and has been investigated for similar effects in dogs. Bretylium also causes the release of norepinephrine from adrenergic neurons and thus may be associated with undesirable side effects.

Amiodarone is presently used in Europe and has been under investigation in the USA but currently its use is limited in small animals.

CLASS IV DRUGS

Class IV antiarrhythmic drugs are variously referred to as Ca^{+2} agonists or Ca^{+2}-channel-blocking drugs. Those used in veterinary medicine include **verapamil** and **diltiazem**.

Although these drugs are also referred to as calcium antagonists, they do not directly antagonize calcium. Rather, they inhibit the entry of calcium into the cell or inhibit its mobilization from intracellular stores. Contraction of both cardiac and smooth muscle depends on Ca^{+2}; calcium blockers impair calcium-channels in both tissues. In the heart, specialized tissues capable of automaticity and A-V conduction tissues are particularly affected. The differences in pharmacological effects induced by these drugs often results from their effect on the ability of the slow calcium channel to recover from inhibition. Calcium-channel blockers that do not alter the rate of recovery have little effect on conducting tissues. Drugs that do delay recovery of the channels can also delay conduction. For example, verapamil decreases the rate of recovery of calcium channels; thus, it not only decreases the magnitude of the action potential but also slows conduction through the A-V node. The faster A-V nodal stimulation occurs, the more effective is the A-V nodal blockade induced by verapamil; thus, verapamil is useful for supraventricular arrhythmias.

Verapamil and diltiazem exert their greatest cardiac effects in the sinoatrial and A-V nodes. Sinus rate and A-V conduction is slowed and ventricular rate is reduced in animals with atrial fibrillation or flutter. Ventricular arrhythmias are generally unresponsive. While verapamil has a low bioavailability following administration PO due to first-pass metabolism, diltiazem is characterized by a high bioavailability in dogs. Diltiazem has shown therapeutic efficacy in the treatment of supraventricular arrhythmias in dogs and hypertrophic cardiomyopathy in cats.

Cardiac side effects of verapamil and diltiazem include hypotension, bradycardia, various degrees of heart block, and exacerbation of congestive heart failure due to negative inotropic effects. Verapamil is associated with more adverse effects than diltiazem, thus diltiazem is the preferred drug.

VASOACTIVE DRUGS

Vasodilator drugs can be categorized as afterload reducers or preload reducers according to the type of vessels that they dilate. Afterload reduction is achieved by dilation of arterioles (ie, resistance vessels), while preload reduction occurs with dilation of veins (ie, capacitance vessels).

ARTERIAL DILATORS

Hydralazine is a pure arterial vasodilator. It relaxes arteriolar smooth muscle by inhibiting calcium fluxes into the cell, or by increasing local prostacyclin concentrations. The result is a decrease in peripheral vascular resistance without decrease in myocardial contractility.

Hydralazine is bound to smooth muscle, which results in a biological half-life that is longer than plasma half-life. The drug is well absorbed following administration PO but (in man) is subject to first-pass metabolism. The incidence of toxicity caused by hydralazine may be significant. Hypotension may occur. Hydralazine frequently causes increased heart rate; this effect may prove to be detrimental to the animal with congestive heart failure (CHF) because of increased myocardial oxygen demands.

Indications for hydralazine (dogs and cats: 1-2 mg/kg, PO, b.i.d. to t.i.d.) include afterload reduction in animals with moderately early and late signs of CHF. The drug should be titrated to individual animal response.

Captopril is a commonly used arterial dilator (afterload reducer) in dogs and cats. Renin catalyzes the formation of angiotensin II from angiotensin I by angiotensin-converting enzyme in the lungs. Angiotensin is important in the pathogenesis of CHF because it initiates a series of events (including sodium retention) designed to increase blood volume but which often contribute to the development of CHF. Angiotensin II also directly stimulates peripheral vasoconstriction of resistance vessels, thus increasing systemic vascular resistance. Captopril is a highly specific inhibitor of the angiotensin-converting enzyme. Thus, captopril induces vasodilation (arterial), decreased systemic blood pressure, increased cardiac output, and reduced heart rate. Aldosterone secretion is reduced (not obliterated) and natriuresis occurs. Some venodilation may reduce preload.

Captopril (dogs: 1-2 mg/kg, PO, t.i.d.) is rapidly absorbed following administration PO. Its bioavailability is significantly reduced with food, and it should be administered 1 hr before feeding. The duration of effect in dogs is ~6 hr. Excretion is slower in animals with impaired renal function.

Marked hypotension may occur following captopril administration, especially in animals treated with diuretics. Treatment should be initiated in small increments and individualized to animal response. Potassium-sparing diuretics should not be used concurrently to avoid hyperkalemia.

Phentolamine is a potent arterial vasodilator. It is an α-adrenergic blocker and therefore primarily affects the resistance (arteriolar) vessels, but it does dilate the capacitance vessels as well. It is seldom used clinically because of expense.

Effects of **calcium-channel blockers** are primarily arterial in nature with little to no venodilator effects occurring. Coronary vasodilation is significant. The order of vasodilator potency of these drugs is: nifedipine > verapamil > diltiazem. Nifedipine causes vasodilation at concentrations that have little effect on the heart. The use of these drugs as hypotensive agents in small animals is limited.

ARTERIAL AND VENOUS DILATORS

Organic nitrates and nitrites relax all smooth muscle and thus cause arterial and venous smooth muscle dilation. These drugs directly dilate coronary vessels. At low concentrations, which are generally used clinically, venular dilation predominates and net systemic vascular resistance is usually not affected. Pharmacological effects occur rapidly. First-pass metabolism limits the use of these drugs to IV, sublingual, and topical (ointment) administration.

Nitroglycerin is not a nitro compound as the name suggests, but is a member of the organic nitrate group. As with other nitrates, nitroglycerin relaxes all smooth muscle. However, the dose of nitroglycerin used results in predominantly venous dilation and preload reduction. Pulmonary and systemic congestion and myocardial workload are reduced. Nitroglycerin is indicated for acute (emergency) treatment of congestive heart failure (CHF), particularly that associated with fulminant pulmonary edema. It is available for IV and sublingual use and as an ointment. The 2% ointment preparation is the most commonly used in veterinary medicine; it is applied ($\frac{1}{8}$ to $\frac{1}{2}$ in. [3-6 mm], t.i.d.) to the hairless portion of the animal's skin (abdomen or ear).

Nitroprusside is one of the most potent vasodilators available (*see also* phentolamine, above). As an organic nitrate, nitroprusside reduces preload and afterload. The advantages of this drug include its potency, its effect in both preload and afterload reduction, immediate hemodynamic effects, extremely short half-life, and low cost. The major disadvantage is that it must be administered by constant IV infusion. The drug is useful for emergency treatment of severe CHF. Hypotension is the major complication and necessitates close monitoring.

Prazosin is an α-adrenergic receptor blocker. However, prazosin is also a venous dilator (perhaps due to inhibition of cAMP) and is thus considered by many to be both a preload and afterload reducer. Prazosin is effective PO but tolerance develops rapidly. In addition, prazosin undergoes significant first-pass metabolism. However, it is an effective antihypertensive agent, particularly when used in combination with other drugs. This drug is not used clinically, probably because hydralazine affords a much better reduction in peripheral resistance and an increase in cardiac output.

DRUGS ACTING ON THE BLOOD AND/OR BLOOD-FORMING ORGANS

HEMATINICS

Anemia can be treated pharmacologically by: 1) providing components needed for RBC production, including Hgb synthesis, and 2) stimulating bone marrow formation of RBC.

Vitamin B_{12} is essential for DNA synthesis. Deficiency causes inhibited nuclear maturation and division. Maturation arrest of RBC in the bone marrow leads to megaloblastic or pernicious anemia. Vitamin B_{12}, a porphyrin-like compound consisting of a ring structure that contains a centrally located cobalt, is derived from the diet and microbial synthesis in the GI tract. However, except for ruminants, microbial production occurs in the large intestine, from which vitamin B_{12} is not readily absorbed. Dietary deficiency of B_{12} is rare; deficiency usually results from poor absorption from the GI tract.

Its absorption is complicated and depends on gastric acid, pepsin, and intrinsic factor secreted from parietal cells. Intrinsic factor binds to and protects vitamin B_{12} from digestion. In this form, B_{12} is absorbed to highly specific receptor sites in the brush border of the ileum, where it enters enterocytes by pinocytosis. Vitamin B_{12} is bound in the plasma to transcobalamin. Excessive B_{12} is stored in large quantities in the liver and is slowly released as needed. Vitamin B_{12} is excreted into the bile but undergoes enterohepatic cycling. Interference with its absorption by the ileum will result in continuous depletion, although many months of defective absorption are necessary before deficiency occurs.

Vitamin B_{12} (dogs: 100-200 μg/day; cats: 50-100 μg/day) is available in parenteral preparations such as cyanocobalamin or a more highly protein-bound form, hydroxocobalamin. There are no significant toxicities associated with therapy. Indications for B_{12} therapy are limited to cases of B_{12} malabsorption such as ileectomy, gastrectomy, or deficiency malabsorption syndromes. Chronic administration of cimetidine can also lead to B_{12} deficiency since an acid environment is necessary for B_{12} absorption.

Folic acid is needed for DNA and RNA synthesis. Its source is the diet, including yeast, liver, kidney, and green vegetables, although it can also be formed by microbes. Folic acid is stored in the liver, but not as avidly as B_{12}. Because it is destroyed by catabolic processes every day, serum levels fall rapidly in the presence of deficient diets. Absorption of folic acid is not as sensitive as that of B_{12}, although jejunal pathology can result in folate deficiency.

Folic acid (dogs: 5 mg/day, PO; cats: 2.5 mg/day, PO) is available in both oral and parenteral forms. Significant toxicity is not associated with therapy. Indications for therapy include inadequate intake due to administration of selected drugs (methotrexate, potentiated sulfa drugs, some anticonvulsants such as phenytoin), liver disease, malabsorption, or other chronic debilitating diseases.

Iron is necessary for Hgb formation. It is available in the diet either as a heme form, which is a small percent of the total but is readily absorbed, or a non-heme form. Absorption of the non-heme form is profoundly affected by diet. Iron is absorbed from the proximal jejunum, where it immediately combines in the enterocyte to the globulin transferrin. It is transported in the plasma in this form, but the binding is loose and iron can be easily transferred to tissues. Iron enters cells via specific receptors that interact with transferrin. In the cell, iron combines with the protein apoferritin to become ferritin, the soluble form of iron storage. Smaller quantities are also stored as the insoluble hemosiderin; the quantity of this storage form increases when the total quantity of iron in the body is much more than apoferritin can accommodate. There is no mechanism for the excretion of iron other than via the GI tract. GI elimination occurs by exfoliation of enterocytes containing iron, biliary elimination, and elimination of dietary iron that has not been absorbed.

Indications for iron therapy are limited to treatment or prevention of iron deficiency (eg, blood loss, pregnancy). Iron is available in both oral and parenteral preparations. Oral preparations should be ferrous salts such as sulfate (dogs: 100-300 mg/kg/day; cats: 50-100 mg/day), gluconate, and fumarate. Therapy can be continued for several months. Toxicities and side effects are dose related. Parenteral preparations are indicated if oral preparations cannot be tolerated or are not feasible (ie, neonatal pigs). Iron dextrans can be given as a single IM injection (100 mg) at 2-3 days of age in newborn piglets. Toxicity may occur and is manifested as pale skin, bloody diarrhea, and shock (*see also* p 1369). When comparing efficacy of parenteral preparations, dextran complexes and hydrogenated dextrans are more efficient than dextrins. Hgb formation requires pyridoxine and the trace elements copper and cobalt (necessary for ruminal microflora B_{12} synthesis). "Shotgun" preparations contain a combination of hematinic agents. The efficacy of such products is questionable. As with any hematinic preparation, provision of these compounds will be ineffective if the nutritional status of the animal is poor.

Anabolic steroids are compounds structurally related to testosterone and possessing similar protein-anabolic activity but with minimal androgenic effects such as masculinization. As part of their anabolic activity, these compounds increase the circulating RBC and possibly granulocytic mass. Their proposed mechanisms of action include: 1) increased erythropoietin (ERP) production via ERP-stimulating factor, 2) differentiation of stem cells into ERP-stimulating-factor-sensitive cells (eg, hemocytoblasts), and 3) direct stimulation of erythroid-progenitor cells. The effect of anabolic steroids requires functional RBC, adequate ERP levels, and sufficient cells in the bone marrow. Thus, the effectiveness of anabolic steroids in treating anemia may be limited, depending on the cause. The absorption and disposition of anabolic steroids depends on the type of preparation and the species to which it is administered. Most are eliminated following hepatic metabolism.

Anabolic steroids can be divided into 2 categories depending on the presence or absence of an alkyl (CH_3) group at the 17-carbon position. They are available as oral and parenteral preparations, including oil-base products intended for slow release. The alkylated products are the most effective bone-marrow stimulants, but are also more hepatotoxic than the non-alkylated products. The alkylated products are also more effectively absorbed when given PO. Alkylated anabolic steroids include oxymetholone (dogs and cats: 1 mg/kg, q18-24hr, PO) and stanozolol (dogs: 1-4 mg, PO, b.i.d.; 25-50 mg, IM, weekly; cats: 1 mg, PO, b.i.d.; 25 mg, IM, weekly; horses: 0.55 mg/kg, IM, weekly for 4 wk). Nonalkylated anabolic steroids include nandrolone decanoate (dogs: 1-1.5 mg/kg/wk, IM; cats: 1 mg/kg/wk, IM; horses and cattle: up to 200 mg, IM or subcut., every 7-10 days; sheep and pigs: up to 100 mg, IM or subcut., every 7-10 days). Oxymethalone and stanozolol are classified as schedule IV drugs.

Side effects of anabolic steroids include virilization and hepatotoxicity. Cholestatic liver damage occurs early and can be significant but apparently is reversible. Clinical indications for use of anabolic steroids include chronic, nonregenerative anemias. Response to therapy is variable and the time to clinical improvement is long, frequently $\geq$3 mo. Pulse doses may be better, and large doses should be avoided to prevent negative feedback inhibition.

HEMOSTATICS

Lyophilized concentrates of one or more clotting factors are available as topical or local hemostatics. Most act to provide an artificial factor or structural matrix that facilitates clotting. An intact hemostatic mechanism is necessary. These absorbable products are indicated for capillary oozing from small, superficial vessels. Concentrated factors include thromboplastin, thrombin (available as a powder, solution, or sponge), and fibrinogen. Artificial matrices include absorbable gelatin sponge and oxidized cellulose.

Astringents act locally by precipitating proteins. These agents do not penetrate tissues, thus are restricted to surface cells. They can be damaging to surrounding tissues. Examples include ferric sulfate, silver nitrate (eg, sticks), and tannic acid (eg, STA).

Epinephrine and norepinephrine are hemostatics by virtue of their vasoconstrictive effects. They may be included in topical medications to decrease blood flow to the tissues, or applied intranasally in tampons to decrease epistaxis.

Systemic hemostatics include fresh blood or blood components administered to animals suffering from coagulation factor deficiency. Examples include fresh plasma, fresh frozen plasma, cryoprecipitate and platelet-rich plasma. Vitamin K is a hemostatic only in instances of vitamin K deficiency. It is necessary for hepatic synthesis of coagulation factors II, VII, IX, and X. Vitamin K_1 (phytonadione) is a plant form of vitamin K that can be given PO (5 mg, b.i.d., or 2.5-5 mg/kg, q8-12hr) or parenterally (0.25 mg/kg, daily in 2 or 3 divided doses, IM or subcut.) It is more effective, and at a faster rate, than other analogs. It can be given IV (if administered not faster than 5-10 mg/min, although anaphylactic reactions have been reported) and IM. Vitamin K_3 (menadione) is usually absorbed too slowly to be used effectively in acute conditions. However, it can be used for chronic therapy.

ANTIHEMOSTATICS

Anticoagulants interfere either directly or indirectly with the clotting cascade.

Heparin is a heterogenous mixture of sulfated (anionic) mucopolysaccharides named because of its initial discovery in high concentrations in the liver. It is prepared from porcine intestinal mucosa and bovine lung. It acts indirectly to facilitate endogenous anticoagulants, specifically antithrombin III and heparin cofactor II. These molecules form stable complexes with and thus inactivate clotting factors, especially thrombin. Heparin is released in its active form after inactivation of the clotting factor and thus can interact with other molecules. The effect is greater with low concentrations of heparin.

Its absorption and distribution are limited by the large size and polarity of the heparin molecule. Oral absorption is poor, hence it is referred to as a "parenteral" anticoagulant. Although anticoagulant activity is first order, half-life of the drug is dose-dependent, and steady-state concentrations are difficult to achieve. Heparin is metabolized by heparinase in the liver and by reticuloendothelial cells. Metabolites of heparinase activity are excreted in the urine. The half-life is prolonged in renal or hepatic failure.

Heparin is a heterogenous mixture; only ~33% of the molecules in the drug preparation inhibit coagulation, and heparin plasma concentrations cannot be correlated with anticoagulant activity. Thus, the concentration of heparin is standardized by bioassay as units of activity (1 mg = 100 IU). Heparin is available as a sodium or lithium salt. The sodium salt is usually the preferred preparation for *in vivo* use. The drug is administered parenterally (100-250 IU/kg, subcut. or IV, t.i.d.); deep subcut. or intrafat injection prolongs persistence of therapeutic concentrations. Large hematomas can occur with deep IM injection. Heparin is administered IV, either intermittently or as a constant infusion. Blood coagulation times should be monitored during therapy. Side effects and toxicities of heparin are limited to potential hemorrhage, although as a foreign protein, allergic reactions are also possible. At high doses, heparin is also antithrombotic. Heparin is contraindicated in the bleeding animal, and in disseminated intravascular coagulopathy (DIC) unless replacement blood or plasma therapy is also given.

Heparin may interact with any other antithrombotic drug. Clinical indications for heparin therapy include the prevention or treatment of venous or pulmonary embolism, atrial fibrillation with embolization, and as an anticoagulant for diagnostic use and blood transfusions. Heparin is used in conjunction with blood and/or plasma for the treatment of DIC. Heparin has also been used to clear hyperlipidemia.

Vitamin K antagonists (oral anticoagulants) differ from heparin primarily in their duration of activity and magnitude of effect. Their primary importance in veterinary medicine has been because of their toxic rather than therapeutic effects. The vitamin K antagonists consist of 2 groups: the coumarin derivatives and the indanedione anticoagulants. Both interfere with the hepatic synthesis of vitamin-K-dependent clotting factors. They block the reduction of vitamin K following its use in factor synthesis, thus effectively reducing the concentration of vitamin K. Their anticoagulant activity (and therefore therapeutic or toxic effect) is delayed for 8-12 hr following administration or accidental ingestion because of the persistence of factors synthesized before administration. Factor VII has the shortest half-life and therefore is the first factor to become deficient.

The vitamin K antagonists are rapidly and completely absorbed following administration PO. Peak levels occur in 1 hr. They are almost totally protein bound in the plasma, and their volume of distribution is limited to the albumin space. They are metabolized by the liver to primary metabolites and then conjugated to glucuronides. They undergo an enterohepatic cycle. These drugs are prepared for therapeutic use as tablets and solutions (eg, warfarin). However, they are more commonly used as oral rodenticides. A variety of factors can increase the activity of these drugs, including hypoproteinemia, antimicrobial therapy, hepatic disease, hypermetabolic states, pregnancy, and the nephrotic syndrome. Drug interactions are significant only when used therapeutically for chronic treatment. Because they are highly protein bound, they will be displaced by other drugs that are protein bound (eg, acetylsalicylic acid and phenylbutazone) and their anticoagulant effects will be increased to the point of toxicity. This has been a significant problem in horses being treated for laminitis. Drug interactions also occur with other antihemostatics.

Clinical use of these drugs has been limited to prophylaxis of venous thrombosis and laminitis in horses. More recent studies suggest that they may be useful in the treatment of feline thromboembolic disease. Toxicity, manifest as hemorrhage, is the major concern with these drugs. Secondary poisoning resulting from the ingestion of a rodent that has eaten treated bait is the most common cause of toxicity. This is particularly likely to occur following ingestion of second-generation coumarin derivatives or indanediones since these drugs are potent and have long half-lives. Treatment for anticoagulant rodenticide toxicity is both symptomatic and specifc.

Specific therapy is vitamin K_1, which is an effective antidote but must be given as long as the anticoagulant is present in the body at toxic levels. This duration varies depending on the drug. Several weeks of therapy may be necessary following ingestion of long-acting rodenticides. Vitamin K_3 (menadione) is much less expensive than K_1 but is also far less effective and never should be used as the sole antidote in cases of severe coagulopathy.

Fibrinolytics (thrombolytics) increase the activity of plasmin (fibrinolysin), the endogenous compound that is responsible for dissolving clots. Streptokinase and streptodornase are synthesized by streptococci. They are used in the treatment of selected chronic wounds (eg, burns, ulcers, chronic eczemas, ear hematomas, otitis externa, osteomyelitis, chronic sinusitis, or other chronic lesions) that have not responded to other therapy. They are available as powders for local or systemic administration.

Antithrombotic drugs affect platelet activity, which is normally controlled by substances (such as prostaglandins) generated both outside and within the platelet. Modulation of platelet activity can be achieved by interacting with these substances. Nonsteroidal anti-inflammatory drugs inhibit the formation of cyclooxygenase, the enzyme responsible for the synthesis of prostaglandin products from arachidonic acid that has been released into cells and platelets. The formation of all prostaglandins will be inhibited, including that of thromboxane, a potent platelet aggregator and vasoconstrictor. In addition to its inhibitory effects on cyclooxygenase, aspirin irreversibly acetylates thromboxane synthetase, the specific enzyme responsible for the synthesis of thromboxane. Aspirin is a potent inhibitor of platelet activity; new platelets must be generated before the effects of aspirin on platelet activity disappear. At higher doses, aspirin inhibits prostacylin, a prostaglandin product that counteracts the thrombogenic effects of thromboxane. Thus, the drug must be used cautiously for antiplatelet effects.

FLUID THERAPY

Appropriate selection of replacement or maintenance fluids and how these fluids should be administered requires an understanding of the normal maintenance of water, electrolyte, and hydrogen ion balance in the body as well as of the various perturbations that can occur during disease. The principles of fluid therapy are addressed below, but specific indications and recommendations are in the discussions on clinical management of diseases.

PATHOPHYSIOLOGIC ASPECTS OF BODY WATER BALANCE

Total body water (TBW) represents ~60% of the body weight of an adult animal. At birth, TBW may be as high as 75%, and with old age as low as 55% of body wt. Obese animals have proportionately lower TBW, and males generally have higher levels of body water than do females.

TBW is made up of intracellular fluid (ICF), which represents ~60% of TBW or ~40% of the total body wt, and the extracellular fluid (ECF). The components of the ECF compartments are plasma water (5-8% of total body wt); interstitial fluid surrounding cells and in dense connective tissue and bone (15-20% of total body wt); transcellular fluids such as CSF, bile, synovial fluid, and water in the GI tract (~5% of total body wt except in ruminants and horses); and finally lymph (usually a small percentage of the total).

Water is absorbed from the GI tract through aqueous-filled pores in the enterocytes in response to osmotic pressure differences across the intestinal mucosa. Several complex mechanisms are responsible for the osmotic gradients necessary for the absorption of water. Basically, the balance of water between plasma and interstitial fluid is maintained by differences between colloidal and hydrostatic pressures in the interstitial and vascular compartments. Plasma colloidal osmotic pressure is the principal force that retains and attracts water into the vascular compartment through the capillary endothelium, while at the same time the higher hydrostatic pressure on the arteriolar side of the capillary beds drives water into the interstitial space. Colloidal osmotic pressure depends on the concentration of plasma proteins, with low concentrations (principally of albumin) allowing more water than normal to escape into the interstitial space. Capillary hydrostatic pressure increases with either increased arteriolar or increased venous pressure (usually due to failing cardiac function), which results in excessive outflow of plasma water into the interstitium. Although the concentrations of mono- and divalent ions differ between intra- and extracellular fluid, isotonicity prevails in each. The volume of intracellular water is mainly maintained by intracellular protein; when the volume of extracellular water declines, plasma proteins attract intracellular water into the vascular compartment, which leads to cellular dehydration.

Water balance is governed by intake of fluids or food containing water, as well as by generation of water due to metabolism of proteins, fats, and carbohydrates (5 mL/kg/day), versus loss through the urine, feces, respiratory tract, and skin. Drinking is controlled by thirst, which in turn is induced mainly by plasma hypertonicity or a contracted ECF volume, although several other mechanisms may be involved. If plasma become hypertonic because of water loss, osmoreceptors in the supraoptic nucleus are stimulated to release antidiuretic hormone (ADH or vasopressin) from the neurohypophysis. ADH increases the permeability of the distal renal tubules and collecting ducts to water only, so that the water that is then reabsorbed reduces ECF tonicity. ADH release also occurs via neural pathways when ECF volume is markedly reduced, such as from dehydration or hemorrhage. Another critical response to hypovolemia is activation of the renin-angiotensin-aldosterone system. This response is initiated by volume receptors in the renal juxtaglomerular apparatus, through which renin is released. Renin (an enzyme) promotes the formation of angiotensin I in the plasma, which in turn is converted to angiotensin II in the lungs. Angiotensin II results in the release of aldosterone from the adrenal cortex. Aldosterone promotes the reabsorption of sodium from the distal renal tubules in exchange for potassium (K^+) and hydrogen (H^+), which are then excreted. As plasma becomes hypertonic due to increasing sodium levels, ADH is released and water retention is facilitated. Angiotensin II is also an active vasoconstrictor and a potent dipsogen.

Water is normally lost from the body through several routes. Urinary loss, which may vary from 2 to 20 mL/kg/day, generally accounts for ~75% of TBW loss. Feces, which normally contain 50-60% water (depends on species), may account for 2-5% of daily water loss. Insensible water loss through the respiratory tract, mouth, and skin is responsible for ~20% of daily water loss, but environmental conditions can increase this significantly. Frank sweating and lactation can also contribute significantly.

Dehydration: The pathophysiologic responses to a water deficit are described above. Many disease states result in excessive loss of body water, eg, polyuria (due to several causes), vomiting, diarrhea, hyperhidrosis, and hemorrhage. Dysphagia or any other interference with water intake also quickly lead to depletion of TBW and signs of dehydration.

The signs associated with a water deficit are fairly characteristic for most species and are outlined below.

Dehydration	Clinical Signs
<5%	No abnormalities detectable.
5%	Slightly doughy inelasticity of skin, dry mucous membranes.
7-8%	Definite inelasticity of skin, capillary refill time 2-3 sec, slight depression of eye into orbit, cooling of extremities.
10-12%	Severe loss of skin elasticity, capillary refill time >3 sec, markedly sunken eyeballs, shock in debilitated animals, involuntary muscle twitching, cold extremities.
12-15%	Obvious shock, death imminent.

Diagnosis is based on the physical findings, loss of body weight (in an anorectic animal, weight loss of 0.1-0.3 kg/day/1000 calorie requirement can be expected, and anything above this may be attributed to fluid loss), elevated PCV, increased plasma protein concentration, increased plasma osmolarity, and hypernatremia. Except for the clinical signs, the above parameters can be used only in light of known pre-existing values. However, they are useful indicators of successful rehydration—particularly plasma osmolarity.

If feasible, the oral intake or administration of water is the preferred approach for treatment. Parenteral administration of a 5% dextrose solution will replete body water. The volume needed in liters can be calculated directly from the percent dehydration present. Plasma electrolyte levels should be monitored during rapid IV rehydration to prevent any marked dilutional effects.

Overhydration: Excess body water leads to hypotonicity of the ECF and consequent diffusion of water into cells, which produces an increase in cellular volume with a concurrent decrease in cellular electrolytes (cellular edema). Hypotonicity of the ECF leads to a reduction in ADH output and hence increased urinary water loss (diuresis).

The causes of excessive water retention include congestive heart failure, acute renal failure, inappropriate ADH secretion, and also the administration of excessive water (iatrogenic).

Clinical signs associated with water excess include abdominal and skeletal muscle cramping, stupor, or convulsions, and if severe, pulmonary and even peripheral edema. Hypertension and marked diuresis also may be evident. In addition, hyponatremia, hypochloremia, and reduced plasma and urine osmolarity suggest overhydration.

Denial of access to water or correction of fluids being administered are essential to correcting overhydration. Potent diuretics (eg, furosemide) are also indicated.

THE COMPOSITION OF PLASMA, INTERSTITIAL FLUID, AND INTRACELLULAR FLUID

To simplify comparisons, general average values for the composition of the 3 major fluid compartments of the body are used here rather than ranges, and only the solutes and electrolytes discussed below are listed in TABLE 1.

SODIUM BALANCE

Sodium ion (Na^+) is the most abundant ECF cation (145 mEq/L); <5 mEq/L is present intracellularly. The main functions of Na^+ in the body include maintenance of membrane potentials and initiation of action potentials in excitable membranes. The Na^+ concentration also largely determines ECF osmolarity and volume. The differential concentration of Na^+ is the principal force for the movement of water across cellular membranes. In addition, Na^+ plays an important role in the absorption of glucose and perhaps some amino acids from the GI tract.

Na^+ is ingested with food and water, and is lost from the body in urine, feces, and sweat. It is also present in almost all body secretions (tears, milk, etc). Most Na^+ secreted into the GI tract is reabsorbed. The excretion of sodium is regulated by the renin-angiotensin-aldosterone system. In the proximal renal tubule, 60-70% of filtered Na^+ is reabsorbed by osmotic, chemical, and electrical gradients. In the ascending loop of Henle, 20-25% more is absorbed with chloride. In the distal renal tubule, sodium is reabsorbed under the influence of aldosterone in exchange for either K^+ or H^+, depending on the acid-base status.

Hyponatremia: Sodium ion deficit may occur due to reduced intake of Na^+ (starvation or deficient diet); excessive loss via the urine, feces, or secretions; or because of dilution due to excessive water retention in the ECF.

Common causes include diarrhea (particularly secretory diarrhea), excessive use of diuretics, hypoadrenocorticism (Addison's disease), inappropriate secretion of antidiuretic hormone (occasionally encountered in neoplastic conditions as well as

Table 1. Concentrations of Major Solutes

	Plasma	Interstitial	Intracellular
			(depends on tissue)
Electrolytes (mEq/L)			
Cations: Na^+	145	155	<5
K^+	3.5-5	3.5-5	145
Ca^{++}	5	5	<1
Mg^{++}	2.5	2.5	35
Anions: Cl^-	106	116	5
HCO_3^-	27	30	0-10
$HPO_4^{-2}/H_2PO_4^-$	2	3	70-100
SO_4^{-2}	1	1	5-10
Organic acids	6	6	1
Protein (as anion)	16	2	40-60
Hydrogen ion			
H^+ (nmol/L)	40	40	100
pH	7.40 (A)	7.4	7.0
	7.35 (V)		
Non-electrolytes			
Protein (g/dL)	7.0	0.2	18.0
Albumin	3.5		
Globulins	3.2		
Fibrinogen	0.3		
Glucose (mg/dL)	50-110 (species differ)	50-110 (species differ)	0-20
Urea (mg/dL)	20-40	20-40	20-40
Blood gases (in tissues)			
pO_2 (mm Hg)	40	35	0-20
pCO_2 (mm Hg)	45 (V)	46	48-50
	40 (A)		

There is a balance between the cations and the anions in each compartment; the total is always the same and electrical neutrality is maintained.

A = arterial
V = venous

in pulmonary and CNS disease states), iatrogenic water load, and decreased dietary availability. Severe hypoproteinemia and hyperlipidemia may lead to spuriously low laboratory values for plasma Na^+ concentration.

Signs of hyponatremia may include fatigue and weakness, agitation and convulsions (due to cerebral edema), hemolysis and hemoglobinuria, colic, diarrhea, excessive salivation and lacrimation, and finally, depending on the cause, oliguria.

Diagnosis is based on a plasma Na^+ value <135 mEq/L and a urine specific gravity <1.010.

Following correction of the cause, administration of sodium in saline solution (0.9% NaCl) may or may not be indicated. Complications of saline infusion include volume overload (especially in those with congestive heart failure) and hyperchloremic metabolic acidosis.

Hypernatremia: Salt poisoning or lack of drinking water are common causes of sodium ion excess. Excessive hypotonic fluid loss leading to hypernatremia also occurs during advanced chronic renal disease. Hyperadrenocorticism (Cushing's disease) also produces excessively high plasma Na^+ concentrations.

Associated signs include pronounced thirst, dry mucous membranes, constipation, hyperpyrexia, CNS disturbances, and ultimately convulsions.

A plasma Na^+ concentration >150 mEq/L and a urine specific gravity >1.030 indicate a hypernatremic state.

Following correction of the cause, fluids containing low sodium levels should be administered PO and/or parenterally, eg, 5% dextrose or 2.5% dextrose in 0.45% saline. These fluids should be administered carefully, as too rapid reduction of plasma osmolarity can lead to cerebral edema.

POTASSIUM ION BALANCE

Potassium ion (K^+) is the major intracellular cation (145-150 mEq/L). Only 3.5-5 mEq/L is present in the ECF. K^+ is intimately associated with maintenance of membrane potentials and plays a key role in the repolarization of excitable membranes. It is also involved in many enzyme functions, particularly those associated with energy metabolism within cells. K^+ also has been linked to the absorption of several amino acids from the GI tract. As glucose is transported into cells, K^+ is also carried intracellularly; this is an important co-transport association.

K^+ is secreted in gastric and pancreatic juice, bile, and intestinal secretions, and is present in sweat. All the K^+ filtered through the glomerulus is reabsorbed but 60-90 mEq/L is secreted in the distal renal tubules. Elevated plasma K^+ concentrations lead to the secretion of aldosterone from the adrenal cortex, which then causes an increased excretion of K^+ in exchange for Na^+ in the distal tubule. When acidosis is present, K^+ leaves the cells in exchange for the excess H^+ entering them. Also, more H^+ and fewer K^+ are exchanged for Na^+ in the distal tubule. Hyperkalemia often results. When an alkalotic condition prevails, K^+ will move into cells in exchange for H^+. Hypokalemia may cause alkalosis because less K^+ is available for Na^+-K^+ exchange in the distal tubule, so H^+ replaces K^+ in the process. Excessive bicarbonate is then generated in the kidneys, which then returns to the systemic circulation leading to metabolic alkalosis. The urine is often acidic under these conditions because of the H^+ exchange; this leads to paradoxical aciduria in systemic alkalosis.

Hypokalemia: Potassium ion deficit may occur due to reduced intake (starvation, anorexia, or deficient diet) or to excessive K^+ loss in GI fluids (vomiting, diarrhea) or urine. Dilutional effects also can lead to hypokalemia, as can the translocation of K^+ into cells in association with glucose and under the influence of insulin. Since 97% of total body K^+ is intracellular, notable depletion can occur with little change, or even with an increase in plasma K^+ if metabolic acidosis is present.

Hypokalemia can occur under several conditions: poor diet; anorexia; administration of K^+-free fluids; metabolic alkalosis; administration of glucose and insulin; chronic vomiting or diarrhea; intestinal sequestration of fluids; and excessive urinary losses caused by primary or secondary hyperaldosteronism, renal disease, or the protracted use of diuretics. Potassium deficits also can occur following tissue destruction and the subsequent urinary loss of the released K^+.

Signs become evident when plasma K^+ concentrations fall to <2.5 mEq/L. These include weakness of skeletal muscles, reduced intestinal motor tone and activity, depression and lethargy, hypotension, weak pulse, and cardiac arrhythmias with characteristic ECG changes (flattening or inversion of the T wave, depressed S-T segment, increased amplitude of P and R waves, and prolonged P-Q and QRS intervals).

Diagnosis is based on a plasma K^+ value of <2.5 mEq/L. Importantly, this figure does not reflect the total body status of K^+ because of its principal intracellular location.

Following correction of the cause(s) of hypokalemia, K^+ administration can be instituted if prolonged fluid therapy is required, large K^+ loss has occurred, overt clinical signs of hypokalemia are present, or the plasma K^+ concentration remains <2.5 mEq/L. K^+ replacement should preferably be provided PO; parenteral routes may be useful but iatrogenic hyperkalemia should be avoided. The maximum rate of administration of K^+ should be 0.5 mEq/kg/hr, and the concentration in parenteral fluids should be 20 mEq/L—and should never exceed 40 mEq/L. The need to increase or decrease K^+ delivery should be based on laboratory results. Acid-base imbalances can dramatically affect K^+ concentrations in the ECF.

For parenteral use, a 15% KCl solution yields 2 mEq of K^+/mL. Available oral preparations include potassium citrate, potassium gluconate, potassium phosphate, KCl oral solution, and KCl in a wax matrix.

Hyperkalemia: This can result from a variety of causes such as excessive intake, diminished renal excretion, or excessive release from cells. Total body K^+ concentration may be decreased, increased, or within normal limits even with hyperkalemia present.

Increased intake of K^+ can be due to high doses of potassium-containing drugs (eg, potassium penicillin G [which contains 1.7 mEq K^+/million units of penicillin G]), rapid IV infusion of K^+-containing fluids, or the replacement of NaCl with KCl in sodium-restricted diets. Decreased renal elimination can result from oliguric acute renal failure, hypoadrenocorticism, urinary tract obstruction, rupture of the urinary tract or bladder, and excessive use of potassium-sparing diuretics. Diffusion of K^+ from the intracellular to the extracellular compartment can be caused by metabolic acidosis or the rapid release of K^+ from tissues following injury or during acute catabolic states.

The main signs are weakness, muscle twitching, irritability, colic, and characteristic cardiac arrhythmias (extrasystoles, intraventricular conduction blocks, high peaked T waves, shortened Q-T intervals, widened QRS intervals, decreased amplitude or disappearance of the P wave, depressed S-T segment, and ultimately ventricular asystole or fibrillation). A plasma K^+ concentration >6 mEq/L is cause for concern, particularly if the associated clinical signs of hyperkalemia are also present.

In a non-emergency with decreased renal function, K^+ intake should be restricted, and if necessary, peritoneal dialysis with K^+-free solutions implemented. In a non-emergency with normal renal function, alkalinizing fluids or mineralocorticoids such as desoxycorticosterone acetate (DOCA) should be administered. Sodium polystyrene sulfonate is an anion-exchange resin that can be administered PO or by enema to bind K^+ in the GI tract.

For life-threatening hyperkalemia, 0.5-1 mL/kg of a 10% calcium gluconate solution is injected over 5-10 min. This should be followed by a 10% glucose solution with 5 IU of insulin, plus 8-10 mEq bicarbonate added to each 100 mL, administered at a rate of 5-10 mL/kg, IV over 30-60 min.

CHLORIDE BALANCE

Chloride (Cl^-) is the major extracellular anion (103-110 mEq/L). It is ingested with food and drinking water and is freely absorbed from the GI tract. Although chloride readily follows the cationic Na^+ in a passive fashion when diffusion occurs across cellular membranes, in certain select sites such as the ascending loop of Henle, a specialized carrier transport system for Cl^- is present and in these cases it is Na^+ that follows passively. Cl^- is present in most secretions with Na^+ except in gastric juice in which Cl^- and H^+ are responsible for the acidity. In the ECF, Cl^- and bicarbonate (HCO_3^-) are inversely related to one another. For example, with a constant plasma anion gap (made up of organic acids, phosphates, sulfate and protein), if Cl^- decreases, HCO_3^- will increase proportionately, and vice versa. Depending on the body's need for HCO_3^-, more or less Cl^- is excreted in the urine as the ammonium salt. This permits Na^+ exchange for H^+ since the tubule secretes ammonia and H^+ into the lumen, and in exchange Na^+ and HCO_3^- return to the plasma. The regulation of Cl^- concentration in the ECF is directly but passively related to Na^+ concentration (all body fluids are electrically neutral).

Hypochloremia: This occurs with increased secretion and subsequent loss of gastric juice (eg, vomiting due to pyloric obstruction) or intestinal fluids (eg, secretory diarrhea), with increased renal elimination in chronic renal failure, and with an enhanced production of bicarbonate. Hypochloremia is a laboratory rather than a clinical diagnosis and is often a component of electrolyte imbalance. It is readily corrected by administering saline solutions parenterally or giving salt PO.

Hyperchloremia: This results from excessive salt intake, a decreased production of bicarbonate to compensate for respiratory alkalosis, diminished renal excretion due to inability of the tubules to produce HCO_3^- (eg, in renal tubular acidosis), and from dehydration due to a loss of water only. Reversal of hyperchloremia depends on correction of the primary disorder and, if necessary, administration of Cl^--free fluids such as 5% dextrose.

HYDROGEN ION, CARBON DIOXIDE, AND BICARBONATE BALANCE
(Acid-base balance)

Physiologic Considerations: Hydrogen ion (H^+) is constantly being produced in the body. Homeostatic mechanisms maintain the normal H^+ concentration (40 nmol/L or $10^{-7.4}$ mEq/L) in the ECF within a fairly narrow range, which avoids disruption of enzymatic and other vital physiologic functions such as membrane conduction. Several buffer systems assist in the process, but the role of the carbonic acid/bicarbonate buffer system is particularly important because it is readily controllable. The respective roles of H^+, carbon dioxide (CO_2), and bicarbonate (HCO_3^-) in acid-base balance are discussed below.

H^+, CO_2, and HCO_3^- are all produced directly or indirectly by cellular catabolism (unlike all of the other cations and anions, which are ingested). The end products of intermediary metabolism are H_2O, CO_2, and free or trapped energy. H^+ results from: 1) the oxidation of sulfur-containing amino acids and of phosphoproteins to sulfuric acid and phosphoric acid, respectively; 2) the incomplete oxidation of fats and carbohydrates to organic acids such as pyruvic, acetic, and many others; 3) lactic acid in the case of anaerobic glycolysis; and 4) the dissociation of carbonic acid formed from CO_2 and H_2O. The limits of H^+ concentration in the ECF to sustain life are 10^{-7} to 10^{-8} mEq/L or pH 7-8.

CO_2 is constantly produced from various decarboxylation reactions in cells. Most of this CO_2 is exhaled through the lungs. Transport of CO_2 in the blood occurs as dissolved or free CO_2 (7%), as carbamino moieties associated with Hgb or plasma proteins (23%), and as HCO_3^- (70%) formed in RBC under the drive of the carbonic-anhydrase-mediated reaction: $CO_2 + H_2O \rightleftarrows H_2CO_3 \rightleftarrows H^+ + HCO_3^-$
In the lungs, the reactions reverse to those that occur in the tissues occur swiftly to release CO_2 for exhalation.

Besides in RBC, HCO_3^- is formed in many tissues where it is needed, eg, in renal tubules and in digestive glands. The kidneys are a primary site of HCO_3^- production because of the abundance of carbonic anhydrase present. Renal reabsorption of Na^+ and H^+ occurs in association with HCO_3^- formation. At the normal ECF pH of 7.4, there is 20 times more HCO_3^- than H_2CO_3. This can be demonstrated by the Henderson Hasselbach equation: pH = pK + log $[HCO_3^-]$/$[H_2CO_3]$. If the pH is 7.4. and the pK_a of H_2CO_3 is 6.1, then the proportion of HCO_3^-/H_2CO_3 is 20:1. Since $NaHCO_3$ represents almost all of the HCO_3^- in the ECF, and arterial pCO_2 is principally responsible for the level of carbonic acid, this relationship can also be written as $[NaHCO_3]$/$[CO_2]$ = 20:1. Plasma HCO_3^- levels are either established accurately using direct pH and pCO_2 measurements and the Sigaard Anderson nomogram, or less accurately by determining "total CO_2" values (which include HCO_3^- and H_2CO_3 in one measurement). These results usually reflect somewhat higher levels (1.1-1.3 mEq/L) for plasma HCO_3^- but are clinically useful within reasonable physiologic limits.

Most H^+ is eliminated by conversion of HCO_3^- to carbonic acid and then (under the influence of carbonic anhydrase) to CO_2 and H_2O, with the CO_2 being exhaled. Elevated blood H^+ concentrations stimulate the respiratory center in the medulla to promote this elimination of CO_2. H^+ is also eliminated by secretion through the distal renal tubules in exchange for Na^+, and subsequent association with several anions and other substances such as ammonia, in which case NH_4^+ is formed. H^+ is also actively secreted by a complex energy-demanding process in association with Cl^- by oxyntic cells in the gastric mucosa.

HCO_3^- can be reconverted to H_2O and CO_2 in the lungs as described above. The HCO_3^- that is filtered through the glomerulus is almost totally reabsorbed from the tubules under normal conditions. HCO_3^- is also present in many secretions such as ruminant saliva, pancreatic juice, bile, and ileal secretions in horses.

The regulation of H^+, HCO_3^-, and CO_2 concentrations in the blood is governed by the respiratory center, the kidneys (which react somewhat more slowly to ionic balances and mineralocorticoid influences), and by various buffer systems in the body. Respiration controls CO_2 and thus H_2CO_3 levels, the respiratory centers being responsive to elevated pCO_2 and H^+ concentrations. Increased CO_2 elimination lowers the H_2CO_3 and hence H^+ concentrations in the ECF; decreased CO_2 elimination leads to increased H^+ levels in the ECF.

Acids in the body are principally neutralized by $NaHCO_3$ in the short term and by other buffer systems in the long term. The general reaction is: H^+A^- + $NaHCO_3 \rightleftarrows NaA + H_2CO_3$. Phosphates and the other buffers act in a similar fashion. H^+ that is derived from the H_2CO_3 is then eliminated in the kidneys by one of several mechanisms, all of which allow Na^+ reabsorption and the return of HCO_3^- to the ECF. When excessive HCO_3^- is present, these "recapturing" steps are depressed and HCO_3^- is excreted in the urine.

Other than the bicarbonate buffer system (HCO_3^-/H_2CO_3) and the phosphate buffer system ($HPO_4^{-2}/H_2PO_4^-$), several other buffer pairs exist. Plasma proteins act as extracellular H^+ acceptors and therefore as buffers. Intracellular buffer systems include protein, phosphates, Hgb, and oxyhemoglobin. Bone also accepts H^+ in a gradual fashion in exchange for Na^+ and K^+.

ACID-BASE DISTURBANCES

Although it is now recognized that mixed acid-base disturbances occur quite frequently in a number of diseases, only uncomplicated primary derangements are discussed below (to serve as a basis for the institution of appropriate fluid therapy).

Uncompensated Metabolic Acidosis: This occurs with an increased production or ingestion of organic acids, or with an excessive loss of HCO_3^-. Also, when the ability to excrete H^+ or to reabsorb HCO_3^- in the kidneys is lost, metabolic acidosis ensues.

Several common disease syndromes can lead to severe metabolic acidosis. Ketoacidosis can be caused by starvation, diabetes mellitus, pregnancy ketosis (toxemia), and lactation ketosis. Ketoacidosis results from incomplete metabolism of fatty acids that are then mobilized because of the lack of available glucose for the cells. Lactic acidosis can result from decreased tissue perfusion associated with hypovolemia and peripheral vasoconstriction (circulatory shock). It can also be due to hypoxemia resulting from poor pulmonary uptake or excessive use of O_2 (fever, seizures). Hepatic dysfunction or decreased hepatic blood flow also leads to decreased lactic acid metabolism and consequently lactic acidosis. In ruminants, excessive generation of lactic acid due to grain overload produces metabolic acidosis following the absorption of large amounts of lactic acid. Uremic acidosis can be caused by pre-renal effects such as a reduced glomerular filtration due to hypovolemic shock, renal dysfunction such as renal tubular acidosis, and post-renal lesions such as urinary tract obstruction. Diarrhea involving the small intestine results in HCO_3^- loss and consequent metabolic acidosis. Bicarbonate-rich intestinal secretions may also be sequestered with lower intestinal obstructions as well as in paralytic ileus. This too leads to hypobicarbonatemia and metabolic acidosis. Iatrogenic causes of metabolic acidosis include the administration of diuretics that act as carbonic anhydrase inhibitors and acidifying salts such as ammonium chloride.

Typically, hyperpnea is seen in cases of metabolic acidosis as efforts are made to compensate through CO_2 elimination. There is depression of the sensorium, progressing to coma. Motor responses become impaired, and respiratory muscle function is often depressed. Signs compatible with the specific etiology are also present.

Low plasma HCO_3^-, normal pCO_2, and low arterial blood pH (<7.3) are indicative of uncompensated metabolic acidosis. Calculation of the anion gap is helpful in determining whether the metabolic acidosis is due to acid excess or bicarbonate loss. The anion gap is equal to plasma $(Na^+ + K^+) - (Cl^- + HCO_3^-)$ and represents the concentration of unmeasured anions such as organic acids, phosphates, sulfates, and proteins. The normal anion gap is between 15 and 25 mEq/L. Metabolic acidosis with an increased anion gap occurs in lactic acidosis, diabetic ketoacidosis, azotemic renal failure (increased phosphates and sulfate), and intoxications with substances such as ethylene glycol and salicylates. Metabolic acidosis with a normal anion gap occurs in diarrhea, renal tubular acidosis, excessive use of carbonic anhydrase inhibitors, following ammonium chloride administration, and in expansion acidosis caused by excessive saline administration (increases plasma chloride while reducing bicarbonate concentrations).

Volume replacement is critical for the correction of many acid-base imbalances; in mild to moderate cases of metabolic acidosis, this may be the only treatment required. Management of severe uncompensated metabolic acidosis requires that plasma HCO_3^- concentration be returned to levels >20 mEq/L. Fluids for this purpose include those containing either bicarbonate or organic anions such as lactate, acetate, citrate, or gluconate (which are metabolized to yield CO_2, which in turn is converted to HCO_3^-). With respect to the effect on H^+ concentration, 1 mM of HCO_3^- is equivalent to 1 mM of lactate or any other organic anion provided that they are metabolized to CO_2 and H_2O. Bicarbonate is the preferred alkalinizing salt if hepatic blood flow or function is impaired, or when high concentrations of lactate are already present such as in grain overload syndromes in ruminants. Organic anion solutions are best when the alkalinizing agent is to be added to a calcium-containing solution because bicarbonate and calcium react over time forming a precipitate of $CaCO_3$. Volume deficits in acidotic animals should never be corrected utilizing solutions without bicarbonate or bicarbonate equivalents at least equal to normal plasma. Dilution of existing HCO_3^- levels could seriously aggravate the acidotic state in such instances.

The actual base deficit can be determined in a number of ways. Commonly, the following formula is used: 0.3 × body wt in kg × (25 mEq/L − measured plasma HCO_3^-) = base deficit in mEq/mL. Bicarbonate solutions administered to correct the base deficit in cases of metabolic acidosis can be given according to a number of strategies. One approach is to slowly administer $1/3$ to $1/2$ of the calculated need IV, and then follow with the remainder added to isotonic fluids over the next 12-24 hr. Alternately $1/3$ to $1/2$ of the calculated requirement can be administered during the first hour of fluid therapy, mixed with an isotonic fluid that already contains 20-24 mEq/L of HCO_3^-; the remainder can then be administered after evaluation of laboratory values. If the clinical signs are mild, a base deficit of ~5 mEq/L is generally present; in moderate cases, a deficit of 10 mEq/L is a reasonable figure; and in severe cases, a base deficit of as much as 15 mEq/L may be present. Excessive sodium bicarbonate infusion can result in ECF hyperosmolality and even intracranial hemorrhage. Rapid HCO_3^- infusions may also cause paradoxical CSF acidosis, acute hypokalemia, and decreased blood O_2 availability to tissues.

In metabolic acidosis, hyperkalemia commonly occurs because H^+ moves intracellularly, replacing K^+, and if K^+ cannot be effectively excreted, plasma K^+ levels will increase. Aldosterone release is triggered, which promotes K^+ excretion by the kidneys provided they are fully functional. Plasma K^+ concentrations are often an unreliable indicator of K^+ deficit in metabolic acidosis. Acidosis also increases urinary calcium excretion by decreasing renal tubular reabsorption of Ca^{++}, increasing Ca^{++} release from bone, and diminishing protein binding of Ca^{++}.

Compensated Metabolic Acidosis: Hyperventilation occurs when elimination of CO_2 via the lungs leads to a reduction in the pCO_2. H^+ enters cells in exchange for K^+ or even Na^+. More H^+ is secreted by the distal tubule. Urine pH is typically low. The excess H^+ is buffered by plasma protein and other buffers such as the phosphate and the Hgb systems. Skeletal Na^+ can also exchange for H^+.

The signs are the same as for primary uncompensated metabolic acidosis (*see* above). Hyperkalemia (acute) or hypokalemia with corresponding cardiac irregularities may occur.

Compensated metabolic acidosis is recognized by low plasma HCO_3^- levels, low arterial pCO_2, and low or low normal pH. Complete compensation rarely occurs. The anion gap depends on the cause of the acidosis.

Uncompensated Metabolic Alkalosis: Metabolic alkalosis occurs due to loss of acid, excessive ingestion or administration of base, and when hypokalemia prevails because H^+ then enters cells in exchange for K^+. The causes of uncompensated metabolic alkalosis include the loss of acid from the stomach due to vomiting, provided duodenal and pancreatic bicarbonate-rich secretions are not also lost. This generally occurs with vomiting in dogs. Sequestration of HCl-containing secretions also leads to metabolic alkalosis, eg, right abomasal displacement in cattle and gastric atony associated with duodenitis in horses. Systemic alkalosis occurs with H^+ and Cl^- loss because plasma HCO_3^- increases to replace Cl^-. Excessive ingestion or administration of base also leads to metabolic alkalosis. Primary hypokalemia produces a net renal retention of Na^+ and HCO_3^-, leading to metabolic alkalosis.

Metabolic alkalosis typically leads to hypopnea. Hyperreflexia and muscle hypertonicity, which can even progress to tetany and convulsions, are frequently encountered with severe metabolic alkalosis. This is because with an elevated plasma pH, ionized Ca^{++} levels are depressed due to the increased binding of Ca^{++} to plasma proteins. Alkalosis also leads to increased Ca^{++} movement into cells, and in the case of renal tubular cells, increased excretion of Ca^{++}. The net effect is a decreased fraction of ionized Ca^{++} in the plasma and consequent membrane hyperexcitability.

Increased plasma HCO_3^- levels together with an increase in the arterial blood pH (>7.4) indicate umcompensated metabolic alkalosis.

Other than for correction of the primary causes, the parenteral administration of isotonic saline, Ringer's solution, or half-normal saline with 20-30 mEq of KCl/L added (according to the calculated deficit) is indicated. Ammonium chloride administered PO or IV as a 0.9-2% solution also may be used as an acidifying solution, but hepatic function must be unimpaired (to detoxify the ammonium) and a Na^+ or K^+ deficit should not be present since the function of these cations is not replaced by NH_4^+.

Compensated Metabolic Alkalosis: Hypoventilation (decreased rate and depth) results in diminished CO_2 elimination and increased pCO_2 and carbonic acid levels in the plasma. The kidneys excrete increased amounts of HCO_3^- because distal tubular reabsorption is reduced with the decreased availability of H^+. If hypokalemia is present, H^+ is still exchanged for Na^+, which produces an alkalosis with a paradoxical aciduria.

The signs are the same as for primary uncompensated metabolic alkalosis (*see* above). Because complete compensation of acid base disorders rarely occurs, the following findings suggest a compensated metabolic alkalosis: increased plasma HCO_3^-, hypokalemia, hypochloremia, increased arterial CO_2, and increased arterial blood pH.

Uncompensated Respiratory Acidosis: Respiratory acidosis develops when the elimination of CO_2 is impaired, which then produces increased blood pCO_2 and H_2CO_3 levels in the plasma. Any condition that reduces alveolar ventilation untimately leads to respiratory acidosis. Examples include general anesthesia, overdosage with CNS-depressant drugs (especially opiate analgesics and barbiturates), airway obstruction, pneumothorax, pleural effusion, hydrothorax, atelectasis, pneumonia, emphysema, asthma, pulmonary edema, weak or paralyzed respiratory muscles, and abdominal distention.

The signs of a systemic acidosis are present (*see* METABOLIC ACIDOSIS, above). Cyanosis and loss of consciousness also ultimately occur in severe respiratory acidosis. The clinical signs and primary diagnosis will often suggest that respiratory acidosis must be present. Confirmatory laboratory findings show a decreased arterial blood pH (<7.3) and an elevated pCO_2.

Fluids are of secondary importance in the treatment of uncompensated respiratory acidosis. A patent airway must be established and ventilatory assistance instituted. O_2 is administered only if absolutely necessary. If pO_2 increases without correcting the pCO_2, cerebral blood flow is decreased, which may further depress CNS functions, including respiration. In acute respiratory failure, IV administration of a $NaHCO_3$ solution may be needed to temporarily raise the arterial pH from potentially life-threatening levels while steps are being taken to correct alveolar ventilation.

Compensated Respiratory Acidosis: The anticipated compensatory responses in cases of respiratory acidosis include an increased respiratory rate to promote the elimination of CO_2, and enhanced HCO_3^- resorption in the kidneys. The excess H^+ is excreted in combination with ammonia to form ammonium in the distal tubular fluid.

Signs of the primary disease are present. In most instances, chronic respiratory disease of some form, eg, emphysema, leads to partially compensated respiratory acidosis. In addition to the suggestive clinical signs, the laboratory findings reveal a moderately decreased arterial blood pH, an increased arterial blood pCO_2, and an increase in plasma HCO_3^-.

Fluid therapy is not helpful. Controlled O_2 therapy and ventilatory assistance are indicated while the primary condition is being corrected.

Uncompensated Respiratory Alkalosis: Respiratory alkalosis is induced by hyperventilation leading to exaggerated alveolar exchange and increased CO_2 elimination. Any cause of hyperventilation that is not due to hypercapnia or acidosis can lead to uncompensated respiratory alkalosis. Examples of such conditions include apprehension, fear, hysteria, pain, hyperthermia, septicemia, early aspirin and sulfonamide intoxication, encephalitis, and hypoxia—especially anemic hypoxia.

Hyperventilation should be an anticipated clinical sign. The other physical signs of a primary alkalosis may also become evident over time, eg, hyperreflexia. Tachycardia and hypotension may be present.

Marked hyperpnea suggests that primary respiratory alkalosis is present or imminent, provided that it is not an adaptive or compensatory response. The laboratory findings reveal an increase in arterial blood pH (>7.4) and a marked decrease in arterial pCO_2.

Treatment is based on treating the primary cause, after which physiologic correction will quickly occur.

Compensated Respiratory Alkalosis: The compensatory responses that occur when hyperventilation persists include the following: Bicarbonate is converted to H_2CO_3 by receiving H^+ from the buffer systems such as Hgb, plasma proteins, and ECF phosphates; therefore plasma HCO_3^- levels fall. Potassium moves into cells in exchange for H^+, and the concentration of H^+ increases in the ECF. The kidneys excrete increased amounts of HCO_3^- because less K^+ and H^+ are available to recapture tubular HCO_3^-.

The signs are the same as for primary respiratory alkalosis (*see* above). In addition to suggestive clinical signs, confirmatory laboratory findings show a moderate increase in arterial pH, a decrease in arterial pCO_2, and a compensatory decrease in HCO_3^-.

Treatment is the same as for uncompensated respiratory alkalosis.

EVALUATION OF THE ANIMAL BEFORE FLUID THERAPY

Before instituting fluid therapy, state of hydration, electrolyte balance, acid-base status, caloric needs, renal function, and effectiveness of alveolar ventilation need to be carefully considered.

Inquiries should concern evidence of diarrhea, vomiting, polydipsia, polyuria, anorexia, frequency of drinking, fever, excessive salivation, panting, abnormal behavior, and other physical signs. Duration and severity of the condition observed may assist in estimating the magnitude of fluid loss. Accurate knowledge of the body weight before the disease condition is also helpful in managing a case.

Texture and elasticity of the skin is important since dehydration causes loss of dermal moisture, which leads to a slow return of the skin to its normal position after it has been lifted (check over lumbar region with the animal standing). The skin of obese animals normally tends to retain elasticity in the presence of dehydration, and the skin of cachetic and geriatric animals has less elasticity as a result of loss of fat and protein. The temperature of the skin over the extremities should also be assessed.

Dry cool mucous membranes suggest a serious body fluid deficit. Capillary refill time should also be determined (usually <1.5 sec).

The position of the eyes in the orbits is important; "sunken eyes" or enophthalmos are strongly suggestive of dehydration.

Cardiovascular assessment is critical. Tachycardia with a weak thready pulse and marked hypotension are indications of vascular collapse due to a major fluid deficit.

Several laboratory tests are helpful in determining state of hydration, electrolyte balance, acid-base status, and renal function before institution of corrective fluid therapy. PCV may be useful to monitor rehydration. A reduction in plasma volume increases the PCV. Plasma protein concentration is also helpful but not necessary for the initial assessment. BUN is a good measure of renal function and, in this context, of glomerular filtration rate. The BUN and creatinine values depend on renal function before dehydration. The plasma concentrations of the electrolytes also should be measured and then monitored: Na^+, K^+, Ca^{++}, Mg^{++}, Cl^-, and HCO_3^-. The anion gap should be calculated. Measurement of plasma osmolality is an extremely useful indicator of the state of dehydration and a helpful guide during corrective rehydration. Arterial blood pH, HCO_3^- levels or total CO_2, base deficit, pCO_2, and pO_2 should be determined. Acid-base parameters ideally should be assessed in anaerobically collected arterial blood. Venous blood may yield useful results except in cases of anemia, stagnant hypoxia, or when collected with the animal struggling.

Urinalysis is critical for evaluation before institution of fluid therapy. If possible, urine production should be monitored. Urine specific gravity and preferably osmolality are important indicators of renal-concentrating ability. The presence of signs of renal disease (casts, leukocytes, etc) are important since the kidneys are the primary site of water and electrolyte regulation. If renal function is intact and no infection is present, urine pH can serve as a rough measure of acid-base balance, but only when the history and clinical signs are also considered.

FLUID VOLUME REPLACEMENT

The calculation of water and electrolyte deficits allows a standard approach to fluid therapy. Fluid therapy should correct existing deficits, satisfy maintenance needs, and replace continuing loss. Progress should be carefully monitored using clinical signs and laboratory values as they become available.

Correction of Existing Deficits: The volume of fluid needed can be judged from the history, physical examination, and laboratory data, eg, a 50-kg animal that is 10% dehydrated requires 5 L of fluid to simply replace an existing volume deficit. Electrolyte replacement needs also can readily be calculated, except for K^+.

Maintenance of Hydration and Electrolyte Balance: Maintenance fluid therapy is required when an animal does not voluntarily ingest sufficient food and water to replace normal losses via the urine, feces, respiratory tract, and skin. Maintenance water needs are usually 40-60 mL/kg/day but do depend on the animal's total surface area. These values change with stress, fever, and age (eg, very young animals require 135 mL/kg/day, and older animals often have a higher maintenance requirement due to polyuria associated with chronic renal disease). Certain drugs, such as corticosteroids and diuretics, may also influence maintenance fluid requirements.

The electrolyte composition of fluids used for maintenance differs from that of replacement fluids. Up to a half of daily fluid losses may be via insensible routes and this loss represents electrolyte-free water. Thus the electrolyte levels in maintenance fluids are typically lower than in replacement fluids, and the concentration of K^+ is usually higher than that of Na^+.

Continuing Losses: The volume and requirements of fluids needed to replace continuing losses depend in large measure on the clinical condition, eg, diarrhea, vomiting, polyuria, polypnea. These continuing losses need to be measured or estimated.

Available Fluids and Their Composition: The following fluids are most commonly used in veterinary medicine.

Polyionic solutions: Lactated Ringer's solution (LRS) is an isotonic fluid with a composition very similar to that of ECF. The lactate is rapidly metabolized to HCO_3^- in the body. LRS is the fluid of choice for restoring ECF volume. Ringer's solution is also isotonic but does not contain lactate. It is used for treating alkalosis. Maintenance polyionic solutions are low in Na^+ (40 mEq/L) but higher than LRS in K^+ (10-16 mEq/L).

Dextrose solutions: Because glucose is readily metabolized, administration of 5% dextrose is equivalent to administering free water. Concentrated dextrose solutions (20-50%) are available, and are used to correct hypoglycemia or to provide calories for total parenteral nutrition. Dextrose (5%) in saline and in half-strength saline are also available.

Parenteral nutrition solutions: Amino acid solutions, fat emulsions, and concentrated dextrose solutions are being used more and more in veterinary medicine for total parenteral nutrition (hyperalimentation).

Sodium chloride solutions: NaCl (0.9%) in water (saline) produces an isotonic solution (osmolality 308 mOsm/kg). Hypertonic saline solutions (7.5% and 2400 mOsm/kg) are being used to treat hypovolemic shock on an emergency basis.

Potassium chloride solutions: Commonly, a 15% solution of KCl (2 mEq/mL) is used to make additions of K^+ to fluids to treat hypokalemia. The maximum rate of administration to avoid toxicity should be 0.5 mEq/kg/hr. KCl solutions can be added to parenteral solutions at the rate of 20-40 mEq/L.

Sodium bicarbonate solutions: An 8.4% solution of $NaHCO_3$ yields 1 mEq/mL of HCO_3^-. A 1.3% $NaHCO_3$ solution is isotonic. $NaHCO_3$ solutions can be slowly administered IV or added to infusion fluids that do not contain Ca^{++}.

Calcium solutions: Several calcium solutions are available for IV use. They should always be administered carefully with constant monitoring of cardiac rhythm. A 10% calcium gluconate solution produces 0.45 mEq/mL of Ca^{++}, and a 10% $CaCl_2$ solution yields 1.36 mEq/mL.

For the electrolyte concentration of common parenteral solutions, *see* TABLE 2, below.

ADMINISTRATION OF FLUIDS

Routes of Administration: Several factors affect the choice of the route for the administration of replacement or maintenance fluids. Included among these are the rapidity with which the fluids need to be delivered; the availability of adequate patient restraint; and the presence of GI, respiratory, or renal disease.

Oral (PO) Route: The oral route is a safe, physiologic, and inexpensive route by which to administer fluids; however, severe hypovolemia or GI disease may preclude its use. In anorectic animals, a stomach tube or pharyngostomy tube is a good method for supplying both fluids and caloric requirements.

Table 2. Composition of Parenteral Fluids

	Sodium (mEq/L)	Potassium (mEq/L)	Calcium (mEq/L)	Magnesium (mEq/L)	Chloride (mEq/L)	Bicarbonate or equivalent (mEq/L)	Glucose	Osm (mOsm/kg)
Normal plasma	145	4.2	5	2.5	108	24	100 mg/dL	280-300
5% dextrose	0	0	0	0	0	0	5 g/dL	252
Saline	154	0	0	0	154	0	0	308
Ringer's solution	147	4	5	0	156	0	0	312
Lactated Ringer's	130	4	3	0	109	28 (lactate)	0	272
Acetated Ringer's	130	4	3	0	109	28 (acetate)	0	272
Equivalent solutions	140	5	0-5	0	98	50 (lactate or acetate)	0	296
Enriched K$^+$ solutions	138-140	10-12	5	3	102-108	47-56 (lactate or acetate)	0	308-316
Maintenance solutions	40	10-16	0-5	3	40	16-24 (lactate or acetate)	0.5 g/dL*	110-385

*if dextrose is to be added

Subcut. Route (Hypodermoclysis): Only isotonic and nonirritating fluids should be administered subcut. and then only in modest volumes at any one site. The absorption and distribution of fluids is relatively slow from subcut. sites; this is an advantage if rapid replacement is not required, since the intense diuresis that often follows IV delivery is avoided.

Intravenous: The major advantage of the IV route is that large fluid volumes can be administered rapidly in animals that are in hypovolemic crisis. Nonisotonic solutions can also be injected IV if necessary—although always slowly and carefully to avoid extravascular leakage. Indwelling IV catheters provide an ideal portal for repetitive or constant fluid administration. Hazards associated with the IV administration of fluids include volume overload if monitoring is inadequate; thrombophlebitis and subsequent valvular endocarditis if improper techniques are used; pyrogenic reactions if the fluid is contaminated; air embolism if fluids are being delivered under pressure and run out before being replaced; and hemorrhage through the catheter site, especially if excessive heparin has been employed to keep the catheter patent.

Other Routes: Occasionally the IP route is used for fluid administration but it is not a favored approach. The intraosseous route may be used in neonates when insertion of a needle into a vein is extremely difficult but it is possible to place a needle in the marrow of a long bone.

Rate of Administration: Slow administration of fluids IV is the preferred parenteral route of fluid replacement. A commonly used rate is 20-30 mL/kg/hr, although up to 90 mL/kg/hr has been used experimentally in acute shock cases. Once urine formation has been reestablished at a satisfactory level, 10 mL/kg/hr is probably an adequate rate. During surgery 5-10 mL/kg/hr is recommended. Hypertonic solutions, and certain electrolytes such as K^+, Ca^{++}, and Mg^{++}, as well as concentrated HCO_3^- should never be rapidly infused IV.

Monitoring Fluid Therapy: Intensive fluid therapy should be monitored using clinical signs, urine production, plasma electrolytes, blood gases and pH, BUN, and blood glucose. Central venous pressure (CVP) using a jugular catheter positioned at the level of the right atrium can be monitored to prevent overhydration and pulmonary edema. Normal CVP is 0-5 cm H_2O, and increases of >2 cm H_2O indicate a need to slow the infusion rate.

Possible Complications: Several complications may be associated with volume replacement. Circulatory overload should be prevented by avoiding the administration of excessive volumes. Certain disease states predispose to potential volume overload; these include myocardial failure and the inability to handle an increase in vascular volume, renal failure with anuria or oliguria, pulmonary disease or trauma (danger of pulmonary edema), Cushing's disease, and hyperaldosteronism (increased Na^+ and water retention).

A concern associated with intense prolonged diuresis induced by overhydration is iatrogenic renal medullary "wash-out" with resultant inability to concentrate urine. This corrects over time once fluid administration has ceased.

Overzealous infusion of crystalloid solutions also dilutes plasma proteins to the point that the intravascular colloidal pressure can no longer prevent excessive diffusion of water into the interstitial space or GI tract.

SHOCK

Many clinical conditions can result in a state of "shock". Although the initiating causes are diverse, the development of circulatory shock becomes progressively more uniform, and the final pathophysiologic changes are quite similar. General characteristics and approaches to the therapeutic management of circulatory shock are reviewed below. (The doses given below are for dogs.)

Circulatory shock is an acute circulatory insufficiency in which cardiac output is inadequate for normal tissue perfusion. The syndrome involves complex derangements in both physiologic and metabolic mechanisms. Metabolic and cellular changes are sequential, and their severity varies with time as well as with the degree of the initial disturbance. Once shock is evoked, the progression of events is largely independent of the initiating cause.

Diminished blood flow results in insufficient tissue oxygenation. Cellular functions, including basic cellular metabolism, decline and ultimately fail. Maintenance or loss of oxidative mechanisms determines the reversibility or irreversibility of shock. Therefore, the treatment of shock centers on prevention and correction of cellular hypoxia.

Circulatory shock is related, at least initially, to generalized excessive changes in peripheral vascular resistance, a diminished effective blood volume, or acute heart failure. The end result in each instance is similar: inadequate flow of blood to provide for sufficient tissue perfusion followed by multiorgan failure. The clinical signs generally reflect the direct effect of the initiating disturbance, the subsequent physiologic response to the perturbation, and the consequences of prolonged tissue hypoxia. Common signs include a weak rapid pulse, diminution of heart sounds, pale cold dry mucous membranes, prolonged capillary refill time (>3 sec), weakness, depressed sensorium, coldness of the skin (especially over the extremities), oliguria or anuria, prostration, and finally coma. Except in cardiogenic shock, the peripheral veins usually collapse. Arterial hypotension is a common feature of shock, but its significance is less vital than is the lack of peripheral perfusion and oxygen delivery to the tissues. Accordingly, therapy designed to improve arterial pressure should not do so at the cost of reducing tissue blood flow (eg, potent adrenergic vasoconstrictors).

CAUSES AND TYPES OF SHOCK

Circulatory shock may be grouped into 3 major types according to the primary etiology: hypovolemic, vasculogenic, and cardiogenic.

Hypovolemic Shock (shock due to reduction in blood volume): This follows severe volume loss from the circulation: the rapid loss of >20 mL of blood per kg body wt induces circulatory shock. Frequently, this is the result of major tissue trauma (internal bleeding) or severance of a large artery with external hemorrhage. Serious plasma loss can occur whenever increased capillary permeability develops over an extensive area, such as with superficial burns or in acute intestinal obstruction, in which transudation of plasma into the intestinal lumen and peritoneal cavity occurs. Significant depletion of plasma volume also occurs due to excessive sweating, prolonged diuresis, or persistent emesis and diarrhea. Such rapid reductions in plasma volume may induce hypovolemic shock similar to that induced by severe whole blood loss.

Vasculogenic Shock (shock due to changes in venous capacitance or peripheral resistance): Severe bacterial infections, particularly but not exclusively those caused by gram-negative organisms, are a significant cause of shock. Bacterial toxins may be a direct cause of shock due principally to their effect of producing widespread vascular endothelial and subsequent tissue damage ("septic shock"). Because of this vascular endothelial damage, endotoxin can activate the clotting cascade and cause disseminated intravascular coagulation. In septicemia, endotoxins from organisms such as *Escherichia coli*, *Proteus* spp, and *Klebsiella* spp may be introduced into the general circulation. These endotoxins may increase portal vein pressure because of hepatic vein constriction, and increase pulmonary arterial pressure because of pulmonary venoconstriction. Cardiac output falls progressively, and large quantities of blood are sequestered in venous capacitance vessels. The sequestration of large volumes of blood in the splanchnic area removes this fluid from the effective circulatory volume. In this regard, endotoxic or septic shock is similar to hypovolemic shock.

Vasomotor paralysis ensues from depression or trauma to special areas of the CNS, particularly the medulla and thoracolumbar spinal cord. Profound hypotension with inadequate tissue perfusion follows. Catecholamines and pharmacologic agents that produce prolonged sympathetically mediated vasoconstriction also may be involved in the genesis of circulatory shock because of impaired tissue perfusion. Anaphylaxis caused by the release of several vasoactive agents may induce circulatory shock if not treated expeditiously.

Cardiogenic Shock (shock due to acute changes in myocardial function): Circulatory shock resulting from sudden reduction in cardiac pumping capacity is less common in other animals than in man. In animals, cardiogenic shock results from the heart failing to fill properly, as in cardiac tamponade, constrictive pericarditis, hydropericardium, or excessive intrathoracic pressure during positive pressure ventilation. Cardiogenic shock may also be due to the heart failing to empty adequately. Incomplete emptying can be due to acute cor pulmonale, increased vascular resistance, rupture of the chordae tendinae, severe toxic depression of myocardial contractility, or the onset of certain cardiac dysrhythmias. Cardiogenic shock is characterized by low cardiac output, arterial hypotension, increased systemic resistance, and elevated central venous pressure. Pronounced jugular distention, often with pulsation, and evidence of cardiac failure on auscultation or electrocardiographic examination are common. Decrease in effective circulating blood volume occurs in cardiogenic shock. Myocardial depression is now recognized as often being a contributing factor to advanced shock due to other causes.

PATHOPHYSIOLOGY

The primary disorder in shock is a decrease in effective circulating blood volume, usually from severe hemorrhage or trauma. In septic shock, extensive vascular pooling, and thus effective sequestration of blood, also leads to decreased effective blood volume. Venous return is reduced markedly and the central venous pressure is low. Cardiac output and arterial pressure decrease, resulting in inadequate tissue perfusion and stagnant hypoxia.

Due to the hypoxia and arterial hypotension, reflex neuroendocrine responses occur. Pain accentuates these reactions. Intense sympathetic activity is induced. Catecholamine release at neuroeffector endings and from the adrenal medulla is enhanced, as is the pituitary release of adrenocorticotropic hormone and antidiuretic hormone. The renin-angiotensin-aldosterone system is also activated. Sympathetic cardiac stimulation results in greatly increased heart rate and contractility. Hepatic glycogenolysis results in hyperglycemia and some degree of hyperkalemia. Sympathetic vasoconstrictor tone continues to increase, particularly in the skin, mucous membranes, skeletal muscles, kidneys, and splanchnic areas. Weakness becomes evident. Mucous membranes become pale and dry, and the body surface, particularly on the extremities, becomes cool. Blood is redistributed so that the heart and brain are preferentially perfused. Reduced renal blood flow results in decreased glomerular filtration with resultant oliguria or anuria. Prolonged renal ischemia may lead to tubular necrosis, a process accentuated by hemoglobinemia or myoglobinemia, which may be present in trauma cases. Renal shutdown is marked by azotemia, hyperkalemia, and eventually pronounced metabolic acidosis.

With inadequate tissue perfusion, anaerobic glycolysis increases, with consequent increases in levels of blood pyruvate and lactate. Metabolic acidosis develops because of the lactic acidemia; in response to this, a decrease in pCO_2 indicates ventilatory compensation (if physiologically possible). Development of metabolic acidosis at the tissue level reduces the degree of arteriolar constriction, but the postcapillary venules often remain constricted; this results in extravasation of fluids from the capillaries into tissue spaces.

Cerebral depression may be attributed to the acidosis and to reduced cerebral blood flow due to the general arterial hypotension and to specific cerebral vasoconstriction in response to hypocapnia. The hypocapnia is caused by increased alveolar ventilation in response to metabolic acidosis. The compensatory hypocapnia may effect a partial correction of the bicarbonate buffer imbalance.

Other changes that may have profound effect on an animal in circulatory shock include progressive myocardial depression, microcirculatory sludging of blood and development of disseminated intravascular coagulation (DIC), generalized disruption of cells and their organelles, and GI ischemia with damage to the epithelium and loss of blood and fluids into the intestinal lumen. An increased absorption of intestinal toxins may also occur.

A number of additional endogenous mediators, eg, histamine, kinins, eicosanoids (prostaglandins, thromboxanes, and leukotrienes), platelet-activating factor, complement, β-endorphins, tumor necrosis factor, myocardial depressant factor, and oxygen-derived free radicals, are released during the genesis of shock. They may play important roles in precipitating many of the physiologic and metabolic alterations that occur. Several of these substances released in septic shock are often identical to those released during acute inflammatory processes. However, in septic shock they exert their actions systemically rather than locally, and cause vasodilation, endothelial damage, increased capillary permeability, activation of the complement system, and mobilization of leukocytes. Preventing or reversing the effects of these potent endogenous mediators is often an integral addition to the management of shock.

THERAPY OF SHOCK

Immediate correction of volume deficits by administration of fluid or blood to the hypovolemic animal is critical. Except in cases of severe external bleeding, the early need is not for RBC, but for fluid; the PCV often is high because of the loss of plasma and interstitial fluid. Restoration of the plasma volume frequently requires significantly greater quantities of fluid than can be accounted for by known or calculated losses, because of one or more of the following: 1) certain losses may be hidden or inapparent, eg, internal bleeding; 2) loss of vascular tone, particularly of the veins, necessitates a greater than normal filling volume; 3) impairment of capillary wall integrity results in the continuous loss of fluid into tissues; 4) moderate hypervolemia ensures optimal stroke volume and thus improved cardiac output if the heart is adequately competent; and 5) electrolyte solutions administered IV are distributed largely to the interstitial compartment and only ~25% may be retained in the vasculature.

Fluids may be administered according to predetermined dose rates, based on estimated need, or until the physical signs and the results of monitoring (especially central venous pressure) indicate that a satisfactory quantity has been given. The selection of fluids depends on the prevailing state of shock. Administration of **whole blood** may be indicated if hemorrhage or hemolysis has been significant and capillary sludging and DIC have not already occurred. The PCV may or may not be low, depending on the length of time since the loss of blood and on the degree of fluid shift from extravascular compartments. In general, blood should be administered IV at ~20-40 mL/kg, except when blood loss is continuing. Administration of whole blood should be accompanied by balanced electrolyte solutions in a ratio of one part blood to 2-6 parts fluid. This is especially true in traumatic shock and in advanced shock from any cause. The additional fluid volume is vital for replacement of fluid lost into extravascular spaces because of loss of capillary endothelial integrity. If there is a history of previous blood transfusion, cross-matching is required to decrease the risk of transfusion reactions.

Plasma, serum, and fractionated protein solutions should be considered whenever there is need to expand blood volume without RBC. Two to 5 mL of plasma per kg body wt may initially be given rapidly IV, then more slowly to a total quantity of 5-20 mL/kg. Principal limitations on the use of plasma are cost and availability.

Several types of **plasma expanders** for the management of shock are available. Those of most importance are dextran solutions. Low-molecular-weight dextran solutions (eg, dextran 40) enhance the shift of fluid into vascular beds and prevent capillary sludging and DIC. The initial dose rate of dextran 40 is 10-15 mL/kg, IV; the total dose should not exceed 20 mL/kg over 24 hr. The half-life of dextran 40 is 3.5 hr. Dextran 70 has a plasma half-life of 72 hr but may result in accentuated sludging of blood in microcirculatory vessels. Hydroxyethyl starch, composed of polymerized starch molecules, is another alternative to plasma. Electrolyte solutions should also be administered whenever dextrans or other colloid volume expanders are used; otherwise fluid shifts from tissues may be excessive and compensatory mechanisms become exhausted.

The early administration of sufficient quantities of **electrolyte solutions** is perhaps the most critical intervention in shock therapy. Treatment should be based on achieving volume expansion sufficient to effect satisfactory arterial pressure, peripheral perfusion, and adequate urine output without excessive elevation of central venous pressure (>5-10 cm H_2O).

Various types of electrolyte solutions are available, but lactated Ringer's solution (LRS) is preferred to normal saline whenever large quantities of fluid are administered. However, LRS should not be administered if there is pronounced hyperkalemia. The lactic acidemia associated with shock does not preclude administration of LRS except if hepatic function and/or blood flow are severely impaired. Because LRS may have a pH ≤ 7, it may be buffered by adding 0.75 g $NaHCO_3$ to each liter to raise the pH to 7.4. Additional steps to correct metabolic acidosis are often required. An 8.4% sodium bicarbonate solution contains 1 mEq/mL of $HCO_3{}^-$ and is particularly useful in correcting a bicarbonate deficit and thus the metabolic acidosis of shock. For methods of determining and correcting acid-base imbalances, see p 1362 et seq.

The dosage of fluids depends on the severity of shock and the circulatory response to the fluids received. In hypovolemic shock, 20-40 mL/kg is a conservative dose rate; up to 300 mL/kg may be required.

The use of intravenously administered **hypertonic saline solutions** with a tonicity 8 times that of plasma is a recent advance in shock therapy. Most commonly a 7.5% NaCl solution is employed. Hypertonic saline (HSL, 4 mL/kg), administered IV over an 8- to 10-min interval, is often effective in restoring cardiac output, tissue perfusion, and urine production irrespective of whether the precipitating cause of shock is trauma, hemorrhage, or sepsis. HSL may be especially useful when cranial trauma has occurred and development of cerebral edema is possible. Contraindications for HSL administration include dehydration with pronounced hypernatremia, and uncontrolled hemorrhage (which may worsen following the administration of HSL because of volume shifts to the extracellular compartment). A great advantage of hypertonic solutions is the small volume of fluid required for the emergency treatment of shock.

In most animals suffering from shock, the reduction in tissue oxygenation results primarily from reduced cardiac output or from arteriovenous shunting in poorly ventilated pulmonary capillaries. The latter condition is corrected most successfully by **improving alveolar ventilation** rather than by providing oxygen. However, if there is interference with the diffusion of gases across the alveoli, **oxygen** administered by mask, tent, or endotracheal tube may be highly beneficial.

Most **adrenergic drugs** have limited usefulness in the treatment of circulatory shock because they are vasoconstrictive, potentially arrhythmogenic, and increase tissue oxygen demands. An important exception is the use of epinephrine to treat anaphylaxis. In some shock states in which there is progressive loss of myocardial contractility, adrenergic inotropic agents may be essential for cardiac stimulation. Dopamine (2-5 mg/kg/min) and dobutamine (5-10 µg/kg/min) have only modest vasoactive properties but are potent inotropic drugs and can be used in an IV drip with greater safety than other catecholamines.

Although controversial, **corticosteroids** in massive doses may be indicated in shock, but only after repletion of fluid volume. If administered earlier, their vasodilatory action may induce a fall in arterial pressure and worsen venous pooling. An appropriate dose of dexamethasone phosphate is 4-6 mg/kg, or of prednisolone or methylprednisolone as the sodium succinate salts (these more water-soluble salts may act more rapidly), 25-30 mg/kg. Following volume repletion in shock, corticosteroids effectively promote tissue perfusion by precapillary sphincter dilation. Additional benefits in septic shock include disinhibition of gluconeogenesis, inhibition of prostanoid and leukotriene synthesis, improved GI perfusion, vascular and lysosomal membrane preservation, and inhibition of complement-induced granulocyte aggregation. The major disadvantages of corticosteroids are their potent immunosuppressive activity and their tendency to produce GI ulceration. They are most effective when given early in the development of septic shock.

Other Therapeutic Measures: Depending on the type of shock or the initiating cause, a number of agents have been used to correct or obtund specific aspects of the syndrome.

Broad-spectrum **bactericidal agents** should be employed whenever shock is due to sepsis or trauma. A broad-spectrum penicillin, cephalosporin, or aminoglycoside is usually a good selection. However, the potential cardiodepressant effects of the animoglycosides should be considered.

Administration of **heparin** should be restricted to those cases in which DIC has been demonstrated or is likely to occur. DIC may be ameliorated by correction of acidosis, volume expansion, vasodilator therapy, and the administration of heparin (250 IU/kg, IV, repeated q4hr).

Mannitol at 1-3 g/kg (as a 10% solution) may enhance urine flow in the hypotensive shock animal that has received adequate fluid replacement. Mannitol also minimizes cerebral edema in head trauma cases.

Nonsteroidal anti-inflammatory drugs are cyclooxygenase inhibitors that prevent the formation of prostaglandins, including prostacyclin and thromboxane A_2. They appear to be most beneficial when administered early, before septicemia or endotoxemia develops. Flunixin meglumine at 1 mg/kg, IV, has been used successfully.

Dimethyl sulfoxide (DMSO) is an oxygen-free radical scavenger that has prevented reperfusion injury to the vasculature following periods of ischemia. Because of this beneficial action, the possible usefulness of DMSO in the treatment of septic or hypovolemic shock is under review.

Endogenous opioids, such as β-endorphins, which are released during the genesis of shock (septic or hypovolemic) as well as when severe pain is present, have notable hypotensive effects. The opiate antagonist **naloxone** at dose rates of 1-10 mg/kg has reversed this effect in some cases. Although the mechanisms involved are not fully understood, in cases of septic shock naloxone has increased arterial blood pressure, myocardial contractility, and cardiac output, with a consequent improvement in clinical signs and even survival rates.

Metabolism enhancers such as glucose and high-energy phosphates (eg, ATP, administered as an ATP $MgCl_2$ complex) have been used as adjuvant therapy in the management of shock cases with equivocal results. A combination of 3 g glucose, 1 u insulin, and 0.5 mEq KCl/kg, infused IV over 4-5 hr, has been beneficial in some cases. Dichloroacetate, which has been used experimentally, increases the oxidation of pyruvate to acetyl-CoA, which then prevents the conversion of pyruvic acid to lactic acid and thus reduces the lactic acidemia associated with endotoxic shock.

The use of bacterial **endotoxin antisera** containing anti-lipopolysaccharide IgG for the treatment of septic shock has been successful in a number of species. The antiserum is prepared by hyperimmunizing horses. It facilitates the opsonization of bacteria and increases the complement-mediated destruction of gram-negative bacteria.

DIGESTIVE SYSTEM, MONOGASTRIC

Disease processes of the GI tract and associated organs probably are more prevalent than those of any other organ system. While there are notable species differences, digestive processes usually include prehension, ingestion, maceration, and solubilization of food, followed by further degradation of solubilized particles, either by host enzymes or by symbiotic microorganisms within the GI tract.

Involved are motility of the GI tract, glandular and epithelial secretions, enzymatic hydrolysis of macro- and micromolecules, absorption of end-products through the GI epithelium into the portal circulation or lymphatics, and elimination of the residue. Complex metabolic and electrophysiological reactions in epithelial, glandular, and visceral smooth muscle cells as well as normal hemodynamic responses in the splanchnic circulation are essential for optimal function. The GI tract may be modulated by the autonomic nervous system and also by central relays within the CNS. There are also several classes of hormones, both circulating (endocrine) as well as locally released and acting (paracrine), that influence GI motility and secretions. Several of these gut hormones are also found in the CNS where they may act as mediators in neurotransmission. These common neural and humoral mechanisms have lead to the concept of a "brain-gut axis" that controls food intake, digestion, absorption, and perhaps even metabolic utilization of nutrients. Various pharmacological agents modify these physiological functions and are utilized for the treatment of GI disturbances.

The changes that result from a variety of insults and lesions may interfere with prehension and deglutition or lead to an increase or decrease in exocrine secretions and bile flow, an increase or decrease in GI motility, alterations in blood flow, or loss of structural integrity. Protective reflexes such as ptyalism and vomiting may also be initiated. Pain is a frequent feature of GI dysfunction, and is best exemplified by colic in horses. Inappetence or anorexia are common sequelae of diseases affecting the digestive as well as other organ systems.

THERAPEUTIC OBJECTIVES, MONOGASTRIC DIGESTIVE DISORDERS

The general objective is to facilitate a quick return to normal of all functions (*see also* DIG, PRINCIPLES OF THERAPY, p 100). On this basis, treatment of GI diseases can be divided into 4 categories.

Supportive treatment, which consists of correcting fluid and electrolyte imbalances, and resting the GI tract, is especially important in acute disturbances when the restriction of food intake for 24-48 hr is critical for successful management. Such an approach allows time for enterocyte growth and replacement, reduces fluid and electrolyte losses, promotes the return of normal GI tone and motility, and reduces the possibility of secondary fermentative diarrhea due to the breakdown of undigested nutrients in the ileum and colon. In many GI diseases, dietary restriction and supportive care alone are often sufficient to allow restoration of normal function.

Symptomatic treatment is the use of agents to control or correct clinical signs. Antiemetics, motility modifiers, antacids, protectants and adsorbents, visceral analgesics, appetite stimulants, and choleretics and other digestants are used for this purpose. These agents reduce the frequency of vomiting and diarrhea (thus, fluid and electrolyte loss), reduce associated pain, promote food intake and digestion, and help restore normal GI function.

Specific treatment is aimed at the identified cause of the disorder. Classes of drugs used for such specific purposes include antibiotics, parasiticides, antisecretory drugs, anti-inflammatory agents, specific protectants, laxatives, and digestive enzyme replacements.

Dietary modification, often a dramatically successful treatment for specific digestive disorders, may also be viewed as supportive and symptomatic in most cases. It may be the single most important factor in the treatment of both acute and chronic GI disease. However, restriction or manipulation of dietary components in the management of digestive disease is not discussed here. (*See also* MHN, p 1088 *et seq.*)

DRUGS AFFECTING APPETITE

The control of appetite and its pharmacological modulation is complex, incompletely understood, and often equivocal (*see also* APPETITE, p 1093, and OBESITY, p 450). There are long- and short-term control mechanisms for food intake. Appetite is regulated by hypothalamic nuclei (hunger and satiety centers) and other components of the limbic system. The neurons involved are responsive to glucose concentration; amino acid levels and their balance; and neural input from receptors in the oropharynx, stomach, and duodenum. Long-term control may also depend on fat stores in the body.

Disorders of appetite are common; anorexia or inappetence accompanies many systemic diseases. Overeating associated with obesity occurs in companion animals and may be part of the cause of the fatty liver syndrome in cattle (qv, p 444).

Prevention or treatment of inappetence or overeating are important but often neglected facets of management. Drugs are available that modify appetite, but disorders affecting appetite are best approached by treating the underlying disease processes, regulating the diet, and educating the owner. Providing small quantities of highly palatable food at frequent intervals is often helpful in restoring the appetite of a sick or recovering animal.

Agents that have been used to promote appetite include B vitamins (especially hydroxocobalamin), glucocorticoids, anabolic steroids, benzodiazepines, and cyproheptadine. Little scientific evidence is available to support such use of these drugs, but some anorectic horses seem to respond to the B vitamins, and some cats to react favorably to benzodiazepines such as chlordiazepoxide and diazepam. Also, feed intake seems to be markedly enhanced by administration of glucocorticoids to cattle and other animals, perhaps because of steroid-induced euphoria. Cyproheptadine is both an H_1- and SHT_1-receptor blocker that promotes weight gain, growth, and appetite in people. Beta agonists also seem to have considerable potential. Bitters, such as nux vomica, quassia, and gentian, because of a stomachic effect, have been used as appetite stimulants in large animals but often with questionable results; they are still included in "tonics".

Appetite suppressants or anorectic agents are not used in veterinary medicine to treat obesity because it is usually simpler to reduce the caloric intake of an animal.

DRUGS AFFECTING THE MOUTH, PHARYNX, AND ESOPHAGUS

Salivary Stimulants (Sialogogues): Sialogogues increase the volume and fluidity of saliva. They are rarely used to specifically treat hypoptyalism or xerostomia, but bitters, which stimulate taste buds and thus salivary flow, are commonly incorporated into "tonic" preparations. There is little scientific evidence to support a beneficial role for bitters. Cholinergics stimulate the salivary glands directly and lead to a copious flow of serous saliva. Alpha-adrenergic drugs promote the secretion of scanty amounts of viscous saliva. Ptyalism is seen in cases of mercurialism and iodinism.

Salivary Inhibitors (Antisialogogues): These decrease the flow and fluidity of saliva, and usually respiratory and digestive secretions. Anticholinergics, such as atropine (horses, dogs, cats: 0.04 mg/kg, IV, IM, subcut.; cattle: 0.08 mg/kg, IV, IM, subcut.) or glycopyrrolate (dogs: 10 mg/kg, IV, IM, subcut.; cats: 10 mg/kg, IM), are routinely employed to reduce excessive salivation associated with administration of general anesthetics. Five to 10 times normal doses, administered repetitively, are required to control the extreme salivation encountered with organophosphate intoxication. Several neuroleptics, anticonvulsants, and antihistamines, when used in high doses, produce xerostomia as a side effect. Dehydration is an additional cause of dry buccal mucous membranes.

Alimentary Demulcents: These are a diverse group of usually water-soluble compounds that coat, lubricate, and mechanically protect irritated or abraded mucous membranes in the mouth, pharynx, and esophagus, and also frequently act as suspending agents. They are most often used as lubricants (eg, for stomach tubes) or to mask the taste of medications. Common examples include syrups, gums (acacia and tragacanth), glycerol, propylene glycol, egg albumin, gelatin, starch, and mineral oil.

DRUGS AFFECTING GASTRIC FUNCTIONS

Emetics: Vomiting is a complex protective reflex that occurs effectively only in certain animal species—mostly carnivores and omnivores. Emetic efforts in horses and ruminants can lead to fatal consequences. The act of vomiting is controlled through the emetic center in the medulla, which receives impulses from several different sources, including the pharynx, visceral organs (stomach, duodenum, small intestine, peritoneum, pancreas, liver, gallbladder, uterus, and heart), vestibulum auris and semicircular canals, the cerebral cortex, and the chemoreceptor trigger zone (CRTZ).

Emetics are mainly employed in dogs and cats, rarely in pigs and exotic species, and not in horses or cattle. They may be indicated following the ingestion of noncorrosive poisons—though gastric lavage is the preferred approach—and in cases when there may be ingesta in the stomach, which could be regurgitated during induction or recovery from general anesthesia. Emetics are contraindicated following ingestion of corrosive poisons or petroleum products, in comatose or semiconscious animals with medullary depression (danger of aspiration into the lungs), in esophageal obstruction, in the presence of hernias or prolapses, and following recent abdominal surgery. They should be administered only to animals fully capable of vomiting and in which vomiting will cause no harm.

Emetics may act either by stimulating peripheral receptors or the central centers. Those that act peripherally or by reflex induce vomiting by irritating the epithelium of the oropharynx, esophagus, stomach, or duodenum. Distention of these organs also contributes to the initiation of the emetic reflex. The more useful agents of this group include sodium chloride, sodium carbonate, copper sulfate, zinc sulfate, syrup of ipecac, and mustard seed. Sodium chloride, either in the crystalline form (dogs: $\frac{1}{2}$-1 tsp, deposited behind the tongue) or as a saturated or strong tepid solution (dogs: 30-60 mL, PO, depending on size of animal), generally produces emesis in 10-20 min. A large sodium carbonate crystal is less reliable than sodium chloride. One percent solutions of copper sulfate or zinc sulfate (dogs: 10-30 mL, PO) may produce vomiting in 30-45 min but are not especially reliable, and any undissolved crystals are caustic. Syrup of ipecac (cats: 2-6 mL, PO) contains the alkaloid emetine, which is a potent nauseant and emetic (locally and centrally acting), and most often produces a response in dogs or cats in ~15-30 min. Because emetine is potentially toxic when absorbed, it is important to induce vomiting successfully; otherwise, gastric lavage may be necessary to remove excess syrup of ipecac from the stomach. The response to freshly ground mustard seed (not prepared mustard or mustard powder) mixed in tepid water and given PO is variable.

Central-acting emetics directly stimulate either the emetic center or CRTZ. Many drugs may cause vomiting but only a few are used specifically for this purpose. Apomorphine, an opiate derivative that is a dopamine agonist, stimulates neurons in the CRTZ and is a reliable emetic in dogs (0.05 mg/kg, subcut.); vomiting generally occurs 3-10 min after administration. A half or whole soluble tablet (6 mg) placed in the conjunctival sac also is effective. The emetic center becomes unresponsive to repetitive doses of apomorphine; it produces a degree of CNS depression in dogs but quite marked excitement can occur in cats, in which it should not be used. It is not effective in pigs. Many of the opioid (narcotic) analgesics related to morphine produce vomiting initially but, because of their biphasic effect, medullary centers become depressed and unresponsive to repeated doses. This effect is useful when opioid analgesics are used for premedication in emergency surgery since emptying of the stomach before induction of general anesthesia can be assured. Xylazine is also an effective and reliable emetic when administered to cats (0.05-1 mg/kg, IM) but less so in dogs.

Although several classes of drugs are capable of causing vomiting, this is usually of little clinical consequence. However, it may be a significant sign when digitalis glycosides or nonsteroidal anti-inflammatory drugs are being administered. Because some dogs vomit voluntarily in response to orally dosed products, vomiting may occur without regard to the emetic properties of the product.

Antiemetic Drugs: Vomiting is an important response to the ingestion of harmful substances, but protracted vomiting leads to dehydration, acid-base and electrolyte disturbances, and ultimately physical exhaustion. Aspiration pneumonia and gastric rupture are also potential complications. The act of vomiting may be dangerous in esophageal obstruction, particularly when caused by sharp, pointed foreign bodies. In many instances, vomiting is a clinical sign associated with systemic disease, but once a diagnosis is made it is necessary to control excessive emetic episodes. Debilitating vomiting may also occur as a side effect following radiation therapy and cancer chemotherapy. Motion sickness and psychogenic vomiting may be prevented by use of appropriate antiemetic agents.

An etiological diagnosis should be established before use of antiemetic drugs, to avoid obscuring the diagnosis. In addition, fluid and electrolyte therapy, dietary management, and treatment of the primary cause are fundamental to the rational use of antiemetic drugs.

Antiemetics may act peripherally either to reduce afferent input from receptors, or to inhibit efferent components of the reflex response. They may also act centrally by blocking relays to and through the CRTZ and emetic center. Those that act peripherally may be useful to reduce vomiting associated with acute pharyngitis, esophagitis, gastritis, gastric ulceration, and gastroenteritis. Peripheral-acting antiemetics include anticholinergics, metoclopramide, and domperidone. Most anticholinergics that block muscarinic receptors do not cross the blood-brain barrier and thus do not inhibit cholinergic transmission in the emetic center. The peripheral-acting anticholinergics include glycopyrrolate, propantheline (dogs, cats: 0.25 mg/kg, t.i.d., PO), methscopolamine (do not use in cats; dogs: 0.3-1.5 mg/kg, t.i.d., PO), and isopropamide. Their ability to suppress vomiting is probably related to the inhibition of afferent vagal impulses and GI secretions, and relief of GI smooth muscle spasms. Side effects that may be seen with anticholinergics include xerostomia, mydriasis, tachycardia, urinary retention, ileus, and gastric retention. The delay in gastric emptying may itself cause vomiting, and anticholinergics should not be used for >3 days in the vomiting animal. Antimuscarinics are contraindicated in glaucoma, pyloric or intestinal obstruction, intestinal ileus, and urinary retention.

Local-acting agents include protectants, adsorbents, gastric antacids, and local anesthetics. Alimentary demulcents, eg, kaolin, pectin, and bismuth subsalicylate (dogs, cats: 2 mL of 8.75% solution/kg, t.i.d., PO), may provide a protective coating on inflamed mucosal surfaces. Gastric antacids such as magnesium hydroxide and aluminum hydroxide (dogs, cats: 10-30 mL/kg, t.i.d., PO) are indicated when gastric acidity contributes to the underlying pathogenesis of vomiting. Topical anesthetics such as benzocaine, which block receptors in the gastric mucosa, are occasionally included in oral preparations intended to suppress vomiting. Local-acting antiemetics are rarely particularly effective and may even induce emesis of their own accord because of initial irritation and gastric distention.

Metoclopramide possesses antidopaminergic activity. It depresses the CRTZ, but also promotes the release of acetylcholine and increases the sensitivity of visceral smooth muscle to it. Central control mechanisms may also be involved. Pharmacodynamic effects of metoclopramide include an increase in lower esophageal sphincter tone, an increase in the force and frequency of gastric contractions, facilitation of gastric emptying with enhanced coordination of pyloric relaxation and duodenal motility, and decreased transit time in the proximal small intestine. As an antiemetic, the main indications of metoclopramide include severe and intractable emesis due to chemotherapy as well as nausea and vomiting associated with delayed gastric emptying, gastroesophageal reflux, reflux gastritis, and peptic ulceration. It also has been advocated for the control of persistent vomiting caused by parvoviral enteritis. It is well absorbed orally but undergoes significant first-pass metabolism with a bioavailability of 50-70%. Tissue distribution is rapid, and excretion is both renal and hepatic; the plasma half-life in dogs is only 90 min. Side effects include nervousness, restlessness, listlessness, and depression. GI disorders may also be observed. Constipation is quite common with long-term use. Metoclopramide is contraindicated in GI obstruction or perforation, in epilepsy, and in animals receiving neuroleptics. Atropine and the opioid analgesics antagonize its action. The dose for dogs and cats is 0.1-0.3 mg/kg, t.i.d., PO, subcut., or IV. A satisfactory IV infusion rate is usually ~0.02 mg/kg/hr.

Domperidone (dogs: 0.1-0.5 mg/kg, IM; 0.5-1 mg/kg, PO) is another dopamine antagonist. It does not cross the blood-brain barrier, and its effect seems to be restricted to increasing gastric contractions.

Central-acting antiemetics possess variable ranges of activity. Sedatives, such as the barbiturates, and anxiolytics, such as diazepam, may control psychogenic and behavioral vomiting. Emesis due to excessive labyrinthine stimulations (motion sickness or vestibulitis) can be prevented by certain antihistaminic agents and on occasion by anticholinergic drugs. The antihistamines that prevent vomiting seem to influence neural pathways (H_1 and cholinergic) from the vestibular organs by mechanisms that remain obscure but are not directly related to their sedative actions. The main clinical differences between the various antihistamines in this group are the duration of their effects and the degree of sedation produced. Commonly employed agents include dimenhydrinate (dogs, cats: 8 mg/kg, t.i.d., PO), diphenhydramine (dogs, cats: 2-4 mg/kg, t.i.d., PO), cyclizine (dogs, cats: 4 mg/kg, t.i.d., IM), meclizine (dogs, cats: 4 mg/kg/day, PO), and promethazine (dogs, cats: 2 mg/kg/day, PO or IM). The principal side effects of the group include sedation (especially dimenhydrinate, diphenhydramine, and promethazine), incoordination, xerostomia, and blurred vision. Cyclizine and meclizine are potentially teratogenic and should not be administered to animals that may be pregnant.

Since muscarinic cholinergic fibers mediate central pathways of the vomiting center, anticholinergic drugs that penetrate the CNS could be useful. Such drugs include atropine, aminopentamide, and l-hyoscine or scopolamine. However, response to these agents is variable. Scopolamine has a particularly brief duration of action in animals and also leads to excitement in cats.

Central-acting antidopaminergic drugs (eg, phenothiazine derivatives, butyrophenones, diphenylbutylpiperidines, and metoclopramide) are frequently effective broad-spectrum antiemetics. Antiemetics in the phenothiazine group inhibit the CRTZ at low doses and depress the emetic center at higher doses. These agents are primarily dopaminergic and adrenergic antagonists, but they also possess antihistaminic and weak anticholinergic activity. Though they are generally effective in the control of emesis, especially if it is due to CRTZ stimulation, they are not useful when vomiting is due to labyrinthine stimulation or when GI disease is severe. In the latter case, blockade of afferent impulses from the GI tract with anticholinergic drugs used in combination with phenothiazine antiemetics may be more successful. Phenothiazine derivatives used as antiemetics include chlorpromazine (dogs, cats: 0.5 mg/kg, q6-8hr, IM or IV), promazine (dogs, cats: 0.13 mg/kg, t.i.d., IM), acepromazine (dogs, cats: 0.06-0.25 mg/kg, IM or subcut.; 1-3 mg/kg, PO), perphenazine (dogs, cats: 0.04 mg/kg, q6hr, IM), and thiethylperazine (dogs, cats: 0.13-0.44 mg/kg, t.i.d., IM). Hypotension due to α-adrenergic blockade is a potentially serious side effect that might occur, especially in dehydrated animals. Sedation and extrapyramidal signs also become evident at higher doses.

Butyrophenones have antiemetic effects that are similar to those of the phenothiazine derivatives, though their mechanisms of action are somewhat different. Droperidol and haloperidol (dogs: 0.02-0.1 mg/kg, every 2-4 days, PO or IM) are effective broad-spectrum antiemetics with haloperidol being long-acting (up to 4 days). Diphenylbutylpiperidines, used as antipsychotics in man, seem to affect only neurotransmission in the CRTZ relative to their antiemetic properties. Pimozide (dogs: 0.025-0.1 mg/kg, PO) is a diphenylbutylpiperidine with a particularly long duration of action (up to 6 days for drug-induced emesis).

Other central-acting antiemetic agents that are useful occasionally include trimethobenzamide, diphenidol, and opiates. The mechanism of action of trimethobenzamide (dogs: 3 mg/kg, t.i.d., IM) is unknown, but it seems to be effective for the control of vomiting caused by drug therapy, toxins (uremia), and metabolic imbalances. Diphenidol effectively controls emesis, including that caused by vestibular disorders, but since it induces hallucinations in man, it is not widely used. Opiates bind to receptors in the medullary vomiting center and though emesis often occurs initially, opioid analgesics such as fentanyl (dogs: 0.01 mg/kg, IM) can prevent vomiting due to other narcotics. Ondansetron is a serotonin-3 receptor antagonist that significantly reduces nausea and vomiting associated with cisplatin therapy in man.

Modulators of Gastric Motility and Secretion: Several agents promote the functional activity of the stomach by increasing motility and secretions. Cholinergic agents, such as neostigmine and bethanechol, produce a stomachic effect by stimulating gastric muscarinic receptors. Metoclopramide and domperidone exert a gastrokinetic effect by their antidopaminergic procholinergic actions. Bicarbonate and carbonate salts, when given PO to monogastric animals, induce gastric secretion due to the rapid genesis of carbon dioxide, which leads in turn to distention of the stomach and hyperemia of the mucosa. Gastric acid secretagogues used for diagnostic purposes in cases of suspected hypochlorhydria include pentagastrin (dogs: 6 mg/kg, subcut.), betazole (a histamine isomer [dogs: 1.7 mg/kg, subcut.]), and histamine acid phosphate (dogs: 0.04 mg/kg, subcut.), which stimulate acid secretion maximally. In the latter case, an H_1 antihistamine should be administered 30 min before histamine challenge to prevent serious side effects.

Gastric motility and secretion are reduced by agents with antimuscarinic activity such as atropine, glycopyrrolate, aminopentamide, propantheline, dicyclomine, and several others. This group of drugs is of lesser importance in animals other than man because gastric secretion is not as continuous. Adrenergics and some antihistamines, as well as several neuroleptics and opioid analgesics, also delay gastric emptying. In addition to the anticholinergics, gastric secretion is diminished by vasopressin, prostaglandins of the E and D series, omeprazole (which blocks the hydrogen ion carrier), and histamine H_2-receptor antagonists.

Cimetidine, ranitidine, and famotidine are reversible competitive antagonists of histamine at H_2 receptors, and inhibit histamine-evoked gastric acid secretion in a dose-dependent manner. They also diminish, to a greater or lesser degree, secretion induced by gastrin, acetylcholine, and the presence of food, suggesting some common mechanism. The main therapeutic indications for these gastric antisecretory agents are uremic gastritis, gastric and duodenal ulcers, stress-related erosive gastritis, and hypersecretory conditions. Cimetidine and ranitidine also appear to effectively control upper GI bleeding when hemorrhage is not due to erosion of major blood vessels. They also have been used in gastroesophageal reflux disorders, esophagitis, and duodenal gastric reflux. In exocrine pancreatic insufficiency, cimetidine or ranitidine, if given ~30 min earlier, prevent enzymatic and acid hydrolysis of replacement pancreatic enzymes in the stomach.

The oral dose of cimetidine in dogs is 5-10 mg/kg, q6-8hr; the IV dose is 10 mg/kg, q.i.d., preferably infused slowly over 30-40 min. The IV dose in foals is 5 mg/kg, q4-6hr. Ranitidine is given at 0.5 mg/kg, b.i.d. Cimetidine is rapidly absorbed from the GI tract, although food will delay the process. The drug is ~70% bioavailable and is excreted in the urine primarily unchanged. The plasma half-life is ~2 hr but may be prolonged by liver or kidney disease. The side effects seen with cimetidine are generally minor even at relatively high doses. Cimetidine is a microsomal enzyme inhibitor and impairs the metabolism of concurrently administered drugs. This effect may be useful in preventing acetaminophen intoxication in cases of known excessive ingestion. Ranitidine is a more potent inhibitor of gastric acid secretion than cimetidine. It also reduces hepatic blood flow by ~20%. About 50% is absorbed following administration PO, and the elimination half-life is ~3 hr. Unlike cimetidine, ranitidine has limited effects on the metabolism of other drugs. Although there have been a number of reported side effects in man, and false-positive urine protein may be seen in animals, limited veterinary experience has not indicated serious toxicity from this drug.

The secretion of mucus, an integral part of the gastric mucosal barrier, is of cardinal importance for the protection of gastric epithelium from autodigestion by hydrochloric acid and pepsin. The production of mucus by the neck cells of gastric glands is stimulated by hydrochloric acid, cholinergic drugs, serotonin, insulin, and prostaglandin E_1 and E_2 derivatives (such as misoprostol and enprostil, respectively). Mucus secretion is decreased by glucocorticoids, which are well known for their ulcerogenic action. The antiprostaglandin nonsteroidal anti-inflammatory drugs, eg, aspirin, phenylbutazone, and ibuprofen, decrease mucus secretion and reduce the concentration of the glycoproteins usually present—effects that also predispose to gastric ulceration.

Sucralfate (dogs: 1 g/25 kg, t.i.d., PO) is a disaccharide that binds to ulcer sites and inhibits bile and pepsin activity, thus promoting ulcer healing. Oral tetracycline, phenytoin, cimetidine, and ranitidine are bound locally by sucralfate; these drugs should not be given within 2 hr of sucralfate administration.

Antacids: In monogastric animals, antacids are used to neutralize hydrochloric acid and to inhibit the activation of pepsinogen by increasing the intragastric pH to >4. (In ruminants, their chief use is to counteract the acidity of grain overload [see DIGESTIVE SYSTEM, RUMINANT, p 1387].) Nonsystemic antacids neutralize gastric contents without causing systemic alkalosis. The compounds used clinically include calcium carbonate, aluminum hydroxide, and several magnesium salts (hydroxide, trisilicate, and carbonate), or combinations of these agents. Many antacids also possess adsorbent and complexing properties and can impair the absorption of concurrently administered drugs such as the tetracyclines, anticholinergics, cimetidine, and digoxin. The increase in intragastric pH also may alter the absorption rate of drugs co-administered with antacids. Nonsystemic antacids are useful in the treatment of acute gastritis, reflux esophagitis, chronic renal failure (uremia), gastric and duodenal ulceration, and in cases recovering from acute gastric dilation. The duration of action of the various antacids depends on gastric emptying time, the volume of acid secreted, and the respective neutralizing capabilities. Side effects include acid rebound, which occurs with carbonates and bicarbonates, osmotic diarrhea due to magnesium salts, and constipation from calcium and aluminum salts. Aluminum hydroxide impairs the absorption of phosphate from the GI tract, and this effect may lead to phosphate depletion and osteomalacia. Chronic administration of calcium carbonate should be avoided since it produces a slowly developing systemic alkalosis, gastric acid rebound, hypercalcemia, and calciuria with metastatic calcification and urolithiasis. The reduced frequency of administration of antacids (compared with man) is because the gastric acid secretion is intermittent rather than continuous.

The most frequently employed systemic antacid is sodium bicarbonate, although sodium citrate and sodium acetate are also systemic alkalinizing agents (see also FLUID THERAPY, p 1355). These agents are used to correct metabolic acidosis and to alkalinize urine. Sodium bicarbonate given PO is highly soluble and reacts almost instantly with hydrochloric acid to form carbon dioxide, salt, and water. The carbon dioxide is absorbed and reconverted to bicarbonate in the body. Metabolic alkalosis results if the bicarbonate is administered in excess. Rapid generation of carbon dioxide with gastric distention and increased secretion (acid rebound) is a potential side effect of sodium bicarbonate given PO.

Therapeutic Management of Gastric/Duodenal Ulceration: The following agents (discussed above) may be considered for the management of gastric or duodenal ulceration: gastric antacids, cimetidine or ranitidine, antimuscarinic agents, carbenoxolone, sucralfate, and prostaglandin E_1 and E_2 analogs (such as misoprostol and enprostil, respectively).

DRUGS AFFECTING INTESTINAL FUNCTIONS

Laxatives and Purgatives: Laxatives (aperients) promote the elimination of soft, formed feces; purgatives (cathartics) produce a more fluid evacuation. Although the difference between these may just be a matter of dose, this is not always the case. Elevated levels of fecal water are due either to diminished absorption or to net secretion of electrolytes and water into the lumen of the intestine. Electrolyte secretory processes are mediated within enterocytes by cyclic AMP, cyclic GMP, and calmodulin. Several intestinal secretagogues—both physiological and pharmacological—are capable of initiating intestinal secretion through one or more of these mechanisms. Fluid accumulation in the intestine seems to be a prerequisite for catharsis, whereas the role of intestinal motility as part of the response is equivocal. Diarrhea may be associated with intestinal hypomotility as well as hypermotility. Shortened intestinal transit times are usually due to intrinsic myenteric reflexes rather than general cholinergic stimulation mediated by the parasympathetic system.

The commonly employed laxatives and purgatives are used for the treatment of chronic constipation due to nondietary causes and movable intestinal foreign bodies such as hair balls. They also are used for the evacuation of the GI tract before surgery, radiography, or proctoscopy, and to facilitate defecation in animals in which excessive straining would be undesirable and to hasten the removal of unabsorbed toxin in cases of poisoning.

Undesirable effects associated with the excessive administration of purgatives include superpurgation, dehydration, loss of electrolytes, secondary hyperaldosteronism, osteomalacia, and metabolic acidosis. Contraindications for the use of potent cathartics include enteritis, colitis, intestinal obstruction, and late pregnancy. Several of the agents also distribute into milk and can adversely affect suckling young.

Lubricant and emollient laxatives (fecal softeners): The lubricant laxatives given PO act unchanged and are not appreciably absorbed. They simply soften and lubricate the fecal mass. Mineral oil (liquid paraffin) is a commonly employed bland, lubricant laxative (cats: 2-6 mL; dogs: 5-30 mL; horses: 250-1000 mL; cattle: 250-500 mL; pigs: 25-300 mL). Although safe, a few effects of mineral oil need to be emphasized: with persistent administration, it can impair the digestion and absorption of nutrients, particularly the fat-soluble vitamins; constipation may become a problem with protracted use because of diminished intestinal responsiveness to local mucosal irritation; pneumonitis following accidental delivery into the trachea or bronchi is a serious complication; prolonged use may produce granulomatous lesions in the intestinal wall and regional lymph nodes because limited absorption does occur; anal leakage in a house pet is a nuisance; and it can readily bypass a partial intestinal obstruction, which may be clinically misleading.

Raw linseed oil (horses, cattle: 500 mL, PO) possesses lubricant laxative properties, although it forms linoleates in the upper small intestine and thus also acts as an irritant cathartic.

Anionic surfactants such as docusate sodium (dioctyl sodium succinate, DSS) are given PO to soften feces. Docusate sodium dosages are: horses and cattle, 5-15 g; dogs and cats, 2 mg/kg. Dosages for docusate calcium are: horses and cattle, 7-22 g; dogs and cats, 3 mg/kg. Docusate facilitates the GI absorption and hepatic cell uptake of other drugs. It should not be used with mineral oil or the anthraquinone purgatives. Docusate is excreted in milk and can produce a laxative effect in the suckling young.

Poloxamer 188 (poloxalkol) is a nonionic surfactant that lowers the surface tension of intestinal fluids, thus softening the feces.

Simple bulk laxatives: These are not digested in the small intestine but they absorb water, swell, and form an emollient gel. The increased volume leads to distention with consequent reflex contraction and an increase in peristalsis. In the large intestine, microfloral fermentation of cellulose components leads to the formation of organic acids and other osmotically active products that then enhance the laxative effect. Meteorism and very fluid feces often follow. Methylcellulose (dogs: 0.5-5 g, PO; cats: 0.5-1 g, PO), carboxymethylcellulose sodium, psyllium or plantago seed (dogs: 3-10 g, PO; cats: 3 g, PO), agar, wheat bran, and prunes belong to this group of laxatives.

Osmotic cathartics (saline bulk purgatives): These are absorbed incompletely or not at all from the GI tract; they retain or attract water into the intestinal lumen. The increased volume stretches the mucosa and stimulates mechanoreceptors, which reflexly cause an increase in peristaltic activity. Adequate drinking water must always be provided. In horses, catharsis may be seen in 3-12 hr; in ruminants, within 12-18 hr. Magnesium salts are frequently used PO as saline purgatives. These include magnesium sulfate (Epsom salts [dogs: 5-25 g; cats: 2-5 g; horses: 30-100 g; cattle: 250-500 g; pigs: 25-125 g]), magnesium hydroxide suspension (milk of magnesia [dogs: 5-10 mL; cats: 2-6 mL; horses, cattle: 1-4 L]), magnesium oxide, and magnesium citrate. Only 20% of the magnesium ions are normally absorbed and subsequently eliminated in the urine. If excessive magnesium is absorbed or if renal elimination is impaired, CNS depression and other signs of hypermagnesemia may become evident. Calcium given IV reverses these effects. Magnesium sulfate should be used as a laxative in horses only at lower doses.

Orally administered sodium salts, such as sodium sulfate (Glauber's salt) as a 6% solution (dogs: 5-25 g; cats: 2-5 g; horses: 250-375 g; cattle: 500-750 g; pigs: 30-60 g), sodium phosphates, potassium sodium tartrate (Rochelle salt), and even sodium chloride in excess act as saline cathartics.

Sugar alcohols, such as mannitol and sorbitol, when given PO induce an osmotic laxative effect because they are poorly absorbed and are fermented in the terminal ileum and large intestine. Lactulose, a synthetic disaccharide, is also not hydrolyzed by host enzymes but undergoes fermentation in the large gut to produce acetic, lactic, and other organic acids; this in turn leads to lowering of the pH and an osmotic effect that produces diarrhea. Lactulose (dogs: 5-15 mL, t.i.d., PO) is used to treat chronic constipation as well as hepatic encephalopathy. In the latter case, acidification of the contents of the large intestine favors the formation of nonabsorbable ammonium ions and quaternary amines, thereby reducing the need for detoxification by the liver. Gas production may increase following administration of lactulose.

Irritant cathartics (contact purgatives): These act directly or indirectly, depending on whether a metabolic conversion is required before the product is active. Once believed to act by stimulating the mucosal lining of the GI tract, thereby initiating local reflexes that enhance intestinal transit, it seems that they also activate secretory mechanisms, thus provoking fluid accumulation in the lumen. The indirect group includes several vegetable oils, hydrolysis of which, by pancreatic lipase in the small intestine, releases irritant fatty acids. Castor oil is converted to highly irritant ricinoleates, raw linseed oil to less irritant linoleates, and olive oil to mild oliveates. Castor oil (dogs: 5-25 mL, PO; foals: 25-50 mL, PO) is used mainly in nonruminants and is often employed in calves (before the rumen is functional) and foals. The effect occurs in 4-8 hr in small animals and 12-18 hr in large animals.

Members of the diphenylmethane group, which appear to have a greater effect on the large intestine, are also classified as irritant cathartics although their mechanism of action is unclear. An effect is usually seen within 6-8 hr. Phenolphthalein is a potent purgative but only in primates and pigs. Bisacodyl (dogs: 5-20 mg, q12-24hr, PO; cats: 2.5-5 mg, q12-24hr, PO), another of the group, appears to inhibit glucose absorption and Na/K-ATPase activity and to alter the motor activity of the visceral smooth muscle. Used PO or by enema, only ~5% of any dose of bisacodyl is absorbed.

The anthraquinone cathartics (emodin purgatives) also act indirectly. Their action is principally on the large intestine, and they are not effective if transit through the small intestine is delayed. Danthron (1,8-dihydroxyanthraquinone [dogs: 25-45 mg/kg/day, PO; horses: 15-40 g, q24-36hr, PO]) is the prototype of the group. The others are precursor glycosides; they may be absorbed to some extent, but the unabsorbed part is hydrolyzed by bacterial enzymes in the large intestine to release the active aglycones known as emodins. The effect of danthron should be evident within 6-14 hr in small animals and 12-36 hr in large animals. Repeat dosing should be avoided in large animals, especially horses, because of the long latent period and the possibility of severe superpurgation. Sufficient anthraquinone can reach the milk to affect nursing young. Urine may show color changes. The naturally occurring anthraquinone glycosides include senna and sennosides, cascara sagrada, and aloin.

Purgatives so highly irritant that they may cause severe colic and superpurgation, are known as drastics and no longer used therapeutically. Examples include jalap, podophyllum, colocynth, croton oil, and barium chloride.

Neuromuscular purgatives: Neostigmine, physostigmine, bethanechol, and carbachol increase peristaltic activity within 10-30 min following parenteral administration and within 2-4 hr following administration PO. They initiate hypermotility and promote secretion in the GI tract. Colic may be precipitated, and these agents should be used carefully if a mechanical obstruction is present or the viability of the bowel is suspect. Neostigmine has fewer side effects than the others.

Several other substances, eg, vasopressin, oxytocin, and prostaglandin $F_{2\alpha}$ and other prostaglandin analogs, also stimulate visceral smooth muscle to contract, either directly or indirectly.

Enemas: Enemas are most useful for the relief of simple fecal impaction. Soapy water (soft anionic soap), isotonic or hypertonic saline, sorbitol, glycerol, docusate sodium, mineral oil, and vegetable oils have been used successfully. Commercially available enemas with phosphate salts as the active ingredients should not be used in cats since they can precipitate potentially fatal hyperphosphatemia, hypocalcemia, and hypernatremia.

Modulators of Intestinal Motility and Secretions (Antidiarrheal Agents): Dietary correction and fluid therapy (qv, p 1355) are probably the most important features of the clinical management of both acute and chronic diarrhea. However, several classes of drugs modify intestinal motility and secretion and may be therapeutically beneficial. In all diarrheal disease, there is an increased loss of fecal water because an overall net secretion of electrolytes and water in some part of the GI tract overwhelms the absorptive capacity distal to the site of secretion. Hypermotility is known to be contributory in several diarrheal syndromes (eg, in organophosphate poisoning), in which shortened intestinal transit time is associated with decreased resorption of electrolytes and water. However, in many forms of diarrhea, intestinal motility is decreased rather than increased. Several forms of coordinated movement occur in the small intestine and colon, which serve to mix the liquified contents and to propel the ingesta aborally. Rhythmic segmentations due to simple nonprogressive contractions of circular muscle serve mainly as mixing movements that also promote absorption of the end products of digestion. Peristaltic activity is mainly propulsive but also assures mixing and maximal absorption. Both longitudinal and circular smooth muscle are involved in peristaltic movements. Diminished rhythmic segmentation results in a decreased functional resistance to the flow of intestinal contents. Even weak peristaltic waves can then propel gut contents for long distances and cause excessive fluid to reach the colon and rectum. However, increased rhythmic segmentation slows aboral movement of ingesta and promotes absorption of fluid. Thus, an ideal motility modifier for the control of diarrhea should increase rhythmic segmentation but decrease peristalsis and intestinal secretions.

Opioid analgesics and derivatives decrease peristaltic activity in the GI tract. Specific opiate receptors are present not only in the CNS but also within the myenteric plexuses in the intestinal wall. The effect of opiates seems to be that they block acetylcholine release, perhaps by presynaptic inhibition, which in turn diminishes propulsive motility but enhances GI segmentation and tone (including that of the sphincters). Absorption of electrolytes and water is also promoted by these agents, secretion is reduced, and visceral pain is suppressed. Naloxone and the other narcotic antagonists reverse the effects of opiates on the GI tract; atropine partially abolishes the effect on intestinal smooth muscle but does little to reduce propulsive activity. Opiates used for their effects on the GI tract include the following: powdered opium, tincture of opium (laudanum), camphorated tincture of opium (paregoric—dogs: 2-15 mL, t.i.d., PO; foals and calves: 15-20 mL, PO), morphine, oxymorphone, codeine (dogs: 0.25-0.5 mg/kg, q6-8hr, PO), and meperidine.

Diphenoxylate (dogs, cats: 0.5-1 mg/kg, t.i.d., PO; horses, cattle: 0.5 mg/kg, PO) and difenoxin, which is an active metabolite of diphenoxylate, are used specifically to control diarrhea. Their action is largely dependent on a direct peripheral effect on the GI wall. They are often employed in combination with atropine-like compounds.

Loperamide (dogs: 2 mg/25 kg, PO) is effective in the symptomatic control of acute and chronic diarrhea. It has structural similarities to diphenoxylate, but does not cross the blood-brain barrier. Few side effects occur following administration PO. Side effects of the other opioid analgesics include constipation, sedation, and bloat. They are contraindicated in animals with invasive or toxigenic intestinal bacterial infections and severe hepatic dysfunction, and should be avoided in cats.

Anticholinergic agents diminish motor and secretory activity of the GI tract, and often relax spasms of visceral smooth muscle though other than acetylcholine mediators may also be involved. Such antimuscarinic drugs are then known as antispasmodics or spasmolytics. Although antimuscarinic agents are commonly used as spasmolytics in antidiarrheal mixtures, it is now clear that several forms of diarrhea may occur in the presence of drug-induced intestinal paralysis or ileus. Thus, this group of agents should not be used indiscriminately to control diarrhea, especially in horses. It may be that these drugs reduce diarrhea by an effect on fluid secretion and absorption rather than on motility.

The belladonna alkaloids (atropine and hyoscine), their congeners (atropine methonitrate, homatropine methobromide, hyoscine butylbromide, anisotropine methylbromide), and synthetic anticholinergic agents (aminopentamide, dicyclomine, and diphemanil methylsulfate) are antimuscarinic agents that may be used as spasmolytics. Possible side effects of anticholinergic agents are xerostomia, loss of accommodation, urinary retention, constipation, tachycardia, and CNS stimulation. The synthetic groups are mostly substituted quaternary amines and are devoid of central effects. Because most of the belladonna alkaloid derivatives are substituted tertiary amines, they may have CNS effects.

Anticholinergic agents combined with anxiolytic sedatives: When stress-related functional motility disturbances or other psychogenic causes of diarrhea are suspected, combinations of anticholinergic drugs (such as clidinium or isopropamide) with central-acting tranquilizers (such as chlordiazepoxide or prochlorperazine) are often used successfully.

Miscellaneous antisecretory drugs: A number of potentially useful drugs that have not been studied extensively have shown some evidence of clinical benefit. These include: glucocorticoids, adrenergics, calcium-calmodulin antagonists, and nonsteroidal anti-inflammatory drugs (NSAID). Glucocorticoids are beneficial in treating refractory chronic diarrhea and chronic GI inflammation. They stimulate active sodium absorption in the jejunum, ileum, and colon. However, because of undesirable side effects from prolonged use, they should be replaced by other drugs as soon as possible.

Adrenergics appear to act predominantly by increasing basal fluid absorption and do so at very low concentrations. The mechanisms involved are unclear. Alpha$_2$-adrenergic agonists (eg, clonidine) are potentially the most useful.

Calcium-calmodulin antagonists may act by stimulating active absorption as well as by inhibiting stimulated intestinal secretion, but the mode of action is not clear. Several drugs with this effect (eg, chlorpromazine, trifluperazine) are useful in the control of secretory diarrhea.

NSAID, eg, aspirin, indomethacin, and flunixin, inhibit the cyclooxygenase pathway of arachidonic acid metabolism and thereby suppress the formation of prostaglandin mediators. The roles of various prostaglandins in intestinal motility as well as in absorption and secretory processes is complex, and the inhibition of prostaglandin synthesis will not consistently influence secretory diarrheal states. However, in some acute and chronic diarrheal syndromes, NSAID may be beneficial.

Protectants and Adsorbents: These compounds are not absorbed from the GI tract. The protectants seem to coat the GI epithelium and prevent irritation or erosion. The adsorbents bind chemical compounds, which precludes their absorption. Many compounds possess both properties to varying degrees. The most frequently used are magnesium trisilicate, hydrated magnesium aluminum trisilicate (activated attapulgite), natural hydrated aluminum silicate (kaolin), aluminum hydroxide and phosphate, bismuth salts, calcium carbonate, pectin (natural polygalacturonic acids), and activated charcoal. Kaolin does not decrease fecal water in diarrhea and may actually enhance the intestinal secretion of sodium. The insoluble bismuth salts that are used include the salicylate form, which has antiprostaglandin synthetase effects that enhance its control of diarrhea. Because of its adsorptive activity and rapidity of action, activated charcoal (20-120 mg/kg body wt, mixed with water PO) is valuable for treatment of certain poisonings in many species. It forms a stable complex with these substances, which permits their evacuation from the body. An activated charcoal suspension may be used for gastric lavage.

GI astringents are no longer utilized frequently to treat diarrhea. They precipitate proteins, alter surface characteristics, and tend to form a protective layer on the mucosal surface, but many are caustic. Those most frequently encountered are tannic acid and catechu (gallotannic acid). Although tannic acid has been reported to reduce the severity of diarrhea, its effectiveness has not been proved, and it is dangerous when used in excess. Catechu is preferable because the slow release of catechutannic acid in the intestine reduces its toxicity.

Antimicrobial Agents: Several classes of antimicrobials (*see* p 1413 *et seq*) are employed for the treatment of specific and nonspecific forms of infectious intestinal disease. Motility modifiers, protectants, adsorbents, and antimicrobial agents are often used in combination to treat bacterial enteritis. Aminoglycosides (neomycin, spectinomycin), penicillins (ampicillin, amoxicillin), sulfonamides (succinylsulfathiazole, phthalylsulfathiazole), nitrofurans (nitrofurazone, furazolidone), and quinolones (diiodohydroxyquinolone, iodochlorhydroxyquinolone) are the groups most commonly employed.

If the diarrhea is not due to primary or secondary bacterial infection, antibiotics are unlikely to be useful. Additionally, antibiotics can alter the normal intestinal flora and allow superinfections to emerge. Antibacterials are indicated when there is severe mucosal damage, notable inflammatory reaction (acute or chronic), systemic involvement from the bacterial enteritis, or hepatic encephalopathy.

DRUGS FOR SPECIFIC INTESTINAL DISORDERS

Sulfasalazine (dogs: 15-20 mg/kg, t.i.d., PO, for 3-4 wk) has been useful for the treatment of chronic ulcerative colitis syndromes. Its specific mechanism of action is unknown. The salicylate fraction may be released in the hindgut to exert an antiinflammatory effect while the sulfonamide component suppresses local microflora.

Cholestyramine binds bile acids and endotoxin within the intestinal lumen. Its main use has been in man for control of hypercholesterolemic syndromes and treatment of intractable diarrhea.

Simethicone is a mixture of liquid dimethyl polysiloxanes with antifoaming and water-repellant properties. It is used as an adjunct in the treatment of flatulence, gastric bloating, and postoperative gaseous distention of the GI tract.

DRUGS AFFECTING DIGESTIVE FUNCTIONS

Gastric Digestion: Dilute hydrochloric acid can be used as a replacement for gastric juice but needs to be administered by stomach tube to avoid dissolution of tooth enamel. Pepsin preparations may be administered with hydrochloric acid to treat gastric achylia.

Pancreatic Digestion: Pancreatic extracts, eg, pancreatin obtained from pig pancreas, that simulate pancreatic exocrine secretions are supportive in animals suffering from chronic inflammation and degenerative atrophy of the pancreas, although lifelong treatment may be needed. Enteric-coated preparations are probably better than uncoated preparations because they are less likely to be destroyed in the stomach. Powder forms can be added to food, and the dosage adjusted to obtain normal feces. Although simultaneous administration of nonsystemic alkalinizing agents would seem to be necessary to maintain an optimal pH for enzyme activity, it does not seem to be necessary clinically. Cimetidine given 30 min before dosing with pancreatic extract prevents gastric inactivation of the enzymes. Dietary control is essential for the successful management of animals with pancreatic insufficiency.

Diastases are amylolytic enzymes that may be used for replacement of pancreatic amylase and to control flatulence.

Bile Flow: Bile acids and their salts promote the digestion of fats and the absorption of long-chain fatty acids and fat-soluble vitamins. Bile production is enhanced by stimulation of the vagus nerve and by the hormone secretin, but bile acid salts themselves are mainly responsible for bile secretion—the "bile-salt-dependent flow". Several natural bile salts and partially synthetic derivatives are used as choleretics. Included are naturally occurring bile acid conjugates such as glycocholate and taurocholate. Sodium dehydrocholic acid (dogs: 100 mg/kg, IV; cattle: 3 g, IV) is more potent. Chenodeoxycholic acid, ox bile extract (dogs: 100-300 mg, PO, after meals), florantyrone, and tocamphyl are also employed. Overdosage with these compounds causes diarrhea.

Clanobutin and methoxynaphthalene-oxybutyric acid are oxybutyric acid derivatives that have been used to treat several GI disorders in livestock; although solid supportive evidence is scarce, they are believed to aid digestion.

MANAGEMENT OF SEVERE VISCERAL PAIN

Pain is frequently associated with disturbances of the GI system. Distention, inflammation, or ischemia of the abdominal organs, and mechanical or chemical irritation of the parietal peritoneum may produce pain that is often diffuse and of high intensity. Signs of abdominal pain may be the first indication of a GI disturbance.

The peripheral-acting analgesics (eg, NSAID) and the aniline derivatives (eg, acetaminophen) are rarely effective in relieving severe visceral pain. Flunixin meglumine (dogs: 0.3-1 mg/kg, IM; horses: 1 mg/kg, IM or IV) is an exception in that this drug is useful in controlling some colic attacks for a short time. NSAID and related drugs may relieve intestinal spasms caused by certain inflammatory mediators and could reduce visceral pain.

Central-acting analgesics are much more powerful in alleviating visceral pain. The opioid analgesics and xylazine are used for this purpose. Morphine (dogs: 0.5-1 mg/kg, IM; cats: 0.1 mg/kg, IM) is the prototype of the opioid analgesics and is still the most versatile and inexpensive of the group. The duration of action is ~6 hr in dogs and cats. The dose for horses is 0.1 mg/kg, but the total dose should not exceed 60 mg. Higher doses produce excitement in cats and horses.

Meperidine (dogs and cats: 5-10 mg/kg, IM; horses: 1-6 mg/kg, IM or IV) is a safe opioid analgesic, but it is about a tenth as potent as morphine and has a short duration of action (horses, 20 min; dogs, 45 min; cats, 2 hr).

Oxymorphone (dogs: 0.1-0.2 mg/kg, IM; cats: 0.075 mg/kg, IM; horses: 0.02-0.03 mg/kg, IM) is ~10 times as potent as morphine but is less prone to produce excitement in horses.

Pentazocine (dogs: 1-2 mg/kg, IM; horses: 1-2 mg/kg, IM) is an opioid agonist-antagonist that possesses about a fourth of morphine's potency. The duration of action is generally ~2 hr in horses but is much shorter in dogs. Other opioid agonist-antagonists, such as butorphanol, are also useful for the control of visceral pain.

Xylazine (dogs, cats: 1 mg/kg, IM; horses: 2-3 mg/kg, IV; cattle: 0.1-0.2 mg/kg, IM), though short-acting in most cases, is useful for reducing visceral pain. The duration of analgesia in horses is only 30-40 min at a dosage of 1.1 mg/kg. The effect is even shorter in dogs and cats. In cattle, the duration of action is up to 2 hr, and xylazine is an excellent agent for this purpose in this species.

DIGESTIVE SYSTEM, RUMINANT

Despite interspecies differences, the digestive processes in most ruminants are quite similar. Other than the forestomach(s), the components of the ruminant GI tract are similar to those of monogastric mammals. The ruminant abomasum is a true glandular stomach, and functions as do monogastric stomachs. Ruminants differ significantly from other mammals in that much of their feed undergoes microbial predigestion in the forestomachs, chiefly in the rumen and reticulum. There is also postgastric fermentation in the cecum and colon, but this is much less important than in some other herbivores, eg, horses.

The forestomach may be regarded as a fermentation vat in which symbiotic bacteria and protozoa act in a favorable environment to reduce plant products, some of which (cellulose) would otherwise not be digestible, to forms that are. Sugars and starches are fermented rapidly, celluloses less so; the end products are chiefly volatile fatty acids (VFA), CO_2, energy, and water. By no means is all plant material "digested", but the ruminant can utilize a larger portion of much plant material than can most monogastrics. Considerable gas is produced, principally carbon dioxide and methane, most of which is removed by eructation. All protein is not altered by the fermentation processes; some passes through to the omasum and lower tract unchanged; also, as with starches and lipids, conversion of protein by the microbes results in nutrients digested by the host animal. Additionally, B vitamins and vitamin K are synthesized by the microbes.

The newborn ruminant is essentially monogastric; the forestomach develops and becomes functional over several weeks. The microbial population starts to establish early—as soon as the first milk is ingested—but requires time for anatomical development of the rumen and for exposure to older animals and "infected" feed. Young raised in complete isolation are unlikely to develop normal gut flora, a lack of protozoa being one likely result.

Interaction of host and gut flora obviously is inescapable. Upset of any one of the components can be detrimental to the interaction, eg, reduced salivary flow may allow pH to fall and the microbial population to be altered to an extent that is harmful to the animal. Proper feed and feeding intervals (fermentation is a continuous process); regurgitation, rechewing, and reswallowing; continuous mixing ("churning"); sufficient water; and unrestricted "outflow" to the rest of the GI tract are necessary, as is the proper microbial population.

Depression of ruminoreticular motility or fermentation, or both, occurs with many conditions: improper feeding (overload or deficiency of specific nutrients), lack of water, infectious diseases, intoxications, lesions of any part of the upper GI tract, or metabolic states (eg, hypocalcemia).

THERAPEUTIC OBJECTIVES, RUMINANT DIGESTIVE DISORDERS

The primary objectives are to remove the cause and to promote the return of normal digestive function. The aim is to meet or reestablish the requirements for optimal ruminoreticular function as quickly as possible. (*See also* DIG, PRINCIPLES OF THERAPY, p 100.)

Appropriate substrate for microbial fermentation: This is best achieved by providing a palatable balanced ration and encouraging the animal to eat. Soluble sugars, such as sucrose, initially provide a readily available energy source to stimulate ruminal digestion, but if administered in excess may lead to development of ruminal acidosis. Nonprotein nitrogen (NPN) compounds, such as urea, serve as a nitrogen source for microfloral synthesis of protein, but should be used judiciously and introduced gradually to the ration.

Co-factors necessary for microbial fermentative processes: A number of co-factors are required; they are rarely limiting, except for phosphate and perhaps sulfate, and are commonly included in commercially available ruminotoric mixtures. Co-factors deemed to be necessary include phosphorus, sulfur, calcium, magnesium, cobalt, copper, manganese, zinc, iron, and possibly iodine.

Removal of soluble end-products, undigested solid residues, and gas: This is achieved by active ruminoreticular motility, the release of free gas by eructation, and passage of ruminoreticular ingesta through the reticulo-omasal orifice during the reticular phase of primary contractions.

Maintenance of continual flow culture of ruminal microorganisms: Ruminoreticular dysfunction almost invariably leads to a disruption or even elimination of the established population of ruminal microorganisms. A satisfactory method for replacing microflora in such cases is to administer fresh ruminoreticular fluid collected from healthy animals that are on a diet similar to that of the sick animal. Appropriate readily digestible substrate should be provided at the same time. A large volume of fluid is also desirable.

Fluid medium: An important feature of the treatment of forestomach dysfunctions, especially ruminal atony, is to ensure that the contents of the ruminoreticulum are fluid (essential for normal ruminoreticular fermentation). Water, saline, Ringer's solution, artificial saliva, and ruminal fluid itself may be used for this purpose. Vegetable bitters such as gentian and nux vomica in ruminotoric mixtures have been used in attempts to stimulate salivary flow to provide the fluid environment in which fermentation can proceed.

Optimal intraruminal pH: Depending on the diet, the intraruminal pH may vary but is generally between 6 and 7, except when the animal is on a high-energy diet (lower pH) or unusually high protein or NPN intake (higher pH). Correction of intraruminal pH with alkalinizing or acidifying agents is important in the treatment of ruminoreticular dysfunctions.

Mixing cycles and eructation: Active ruminoreticular motility is an essential requirement for optimal forestomach function. Fermentation processes, absorption, the passage of digesta to the omasum and abomasum, and the removal of free gas by eructation are all enhanced by normal contractile activity. There are no ideal ruminotorics to stimulate ruminoreticular motility. The condition of the animal, the disease process, and other pharmacological actions of the drugs available tend to influence the effects of the agents that have been used for this purpose. Conditioned responses to the presence of feed and feeding itself are means by which physiological ruminoreticular motility can be notably enhanced. Enticing an animal to eat is a useful and practical way of inducing strong primary ruminoreticular contractions, though for a limited period of time.

DRUGS FOR SPECIFIC PURPOSES

Esophageal Groove Closure: The esophageal groove reflex (elicited by receptors in the mouth and pharynx) is well developed in suckling neonates but becomes less reliable in older animals. After ~2 yr in cattle and ~18 mo in sheep, provoked reticular groove closure is often irregular, incomplete, or absent. Bypassing the ruminoreticulum can have several advantages. Drugs administered directly into the ruminoreticulum are absorbed very slowly when compared with abomasal delivery. Moreover, drugs may be degraded by ruminal microflora (eg, chloramphenicol and digitalis glycosides) or the drugs may be harmful to the microbial system (eg, tetracyclines, penicillins, sulfonamides). Administration PO of medicaments intended for local intestinal effect (eg, purgatives, antidiarrheals, contrast media, and some anthelmintics) should be preceded by administration of an appropriate salt solution to close the reticular groove to avoid ruminoreticular dispersion.

In cattle, closure of the groove can be elicited with 2 oz (60 mL) of 5% copper sulfate, 5% zinc sulfate, 10% sodium bicarbonate, or 10% sodium sulfate; in sheep, 1-2% copper sulfate is effective. Onset of the reflex response takes ~5-10 sec, and the groove may remain closed for up to 60 sec. Suckling is a strong stimulus for this reflex even in adults. It is best to allow sick calves and lambs to drink medicated milk from a nipple to assure abomasal delivery and rapid absorption. Importantly, administration PO of liquid medications to ruminants may result in spontaneous closure of the reticular groove in a certain number of cases (up to 60%), which results in complete or partial ruminoreticular bypass.

Esophageal Obstruction: Esophageal obstruction due to a foreign body leads to severe discomfort and acute free-gas bloat. Physical removal of the object is often hampered by marked spasm of the surrounding muscle. Specific spasmolytic drugs such as aminopromazine (cattle: 1 mg/kg body wt, IV) or methindizate hydrochloride may be used. Acepromazine may also have some beneficial effect. The caudal esophageal sphincter has a role in the rate of ruminal gas eructation; ritanserin or ketanserin (5-hydroxytryptamine antagonists) may cause relaxation of this particular sphincter.

Ruminotorics: Agents and mixtures that promote forestomach function (fermentation and motility) are known as ruminotorics. Typically, such mixtures consist of bitters (eg, nux vomica, ginger, capsicum, gentian) to stimulate salivation and perhaps ruminal contractions, alkalinizing compounds (eg, magnesium oxide and hydroxide, calcium and ammonium carbonate, sodium bicarbonate) to elevate a low ruminal fluid pH—and the magnesium salts will also act as cathartics, glucogenic substrates (eg, sodium or calcium propionate, glycerol, propylene glycol), minerals (eg, cobalt, copper, manganese, iron, zinc, calcium) as co-factors for microbial enzyme function, and salts (eg, phosphates) as buffers and to maintain osmolarity. The effectiveness of commercially available ruminotoric preparations is questionable. Generally, a physiological approach as described under THERAPEUTIC OBJECTIVES, above, is much more satisfactory.

Mineral oil (1-2 L) or dioctyl sodium sulfosuccinate (DSS, 3-4 oz [90-120 mL] in 1-2 L of water) administered PO or via nasogastric tube followed by gentle ruminal massage can be helpful in promoting the dissolution and passage of impacted fibrous ruminal contents. DSS can markedly depress rumen protozoa; thus, ruminal transfaunation should follow the use of this agent if ruminal atony continues.

Ruminal Fluid Transfer: Fresh ruminal fluid is considered to be the best available "ruminotoric" since it contains viable ruminal bacteria (1×10^8-10^{11}/mL) and protozoa (1×10^5-10^6/mL) as well as many useful fermentation factors (volatile fatty acids [VFA], microbial protein, minerals, vitamins, buffers). Volumes of 5-20 L of strained fresh ruminal juice given PO or by tube are indicated in cattle with ruminoreticular stasis. Lesser volumes are used in small ruminants. Ruminal fluid can be aspirated through a stomach tube from the ruminoreticulum of normal animals using an extractor pump, or it can be collected at slaughterhouses. A rumen-cannulated donor animal is particularly convenient. It is best for the donor to be on a ration similar to that of the recipient, since the ruminal microflora will then be more appropriately adapted. Provided the initiating condition or lesion is responding favorably, improvement almost invariably follows the reestablishment of normal ruminal microflora, with consequent normalization of the fermentation process and ruminoreticular motility.

Antizymotics and Antifoaming Agents: The therapeutic approaches to the control of acute frothy bloat involve the administration of antifoaming agents to reduce foam stability and to promote release of free gas, which is then promptly eructated, and of antizymotics to depress ruminal fermentation. Antizymotic agents that are used include oil of turpentine (cattle: 15-30 mL in 300-600 mL of raw linseed oil, PO; sheep: 4-8 mL in 60-300 mL of raw linseed oil), formalin (cattle: 4 mL in 300 mL water, t.i.d., PO; sheep: 0.6-1 mL in 100 mL water, t.i.d., PO), and antibiotics, such as penicillin, PO.

Acute frothy bloat in cattle should be treated with 25-50 g (30-60 mL) poloxalene, administered by drench or stomach tube. The direct intraruminal injection of poloxalene often does not give satisfactory results. Two to 5% concentrations of polymerized methyl silicone (3.3% emulsion, cattle: 30-60 mL; sheep: 7-15 mL) are used in a similar manner as poloxalene, though direct intraruminal injection via a needle or cannula may be more satisfactory in this case. Vegetable oils (or emulsions of these oils) such as peanut oil, sunflower oil, or soybean oil (cattle: 60 mL; sheep: 10-15 mL) also relieve acute frothy bloat when given PO. Oil of turpentine (cattle: 15-60 mL; sheep: 10 mL) in a demulcent vehicle also has been used, but this volatile oil does taint flesh and milk for up to 4 or 5 days.

Ruminoreticular Antacids: Ruminal alkalinizing agents are principally used to treat ruminal lactic acidosis (pH <6) due to grain engorgement or soluble carbohydrate overload. The antacids that may be given PO, q8-12hr, include magnesium hydroxide (cattle: 100-300 g; sheep: 10-30 g), magnesium oxide (cattle: 50 g; sheep: 5 g), magnesium carbonate (cattle: 10-80 g; sheep: 1-8 g), aluminum hydroxide (cattle: 15-30 g; sheep: 1-2 g), ammonium carbonate (cattle: 15-30 g; sheep: 1-2 g), calcium carbonate (cattle: 60-360 g; sheep: 10-20 g), and sodium bicarbonate (cattle: 60-120 g; sheep: 40-60 g). The most useful ruminal antacids seem to be calcium hydroxide and magnesium carbonate. Magnesium oxide is chemically very active and may cause severe ruminal alkalosis. The alkalinizing ability of the other salts may be slow and even ineffective. The addition of sodium bicarbonate to highly acidic ruminoreticular content may also lead to the rapid release of carbon dioxide and a worsening of the pre-existing bloat often encountered in severe ruminal lactacidosis. Magnesium salts also exert cathartic effects for a few days.

Ruminoreticular Acidifying Agents: Ruminal acidifying agents are used to treat ruminal stasis or simple indigestion as well as acute urea poisoning. In ruminal stasis, the intraruminal pH often increases to >7.5 because of the constant inflow of bicarbonate-rich saliva in the absence of active ruminal fermentation and formation of VFA. In acute urea intoxication, the elevated intraruminal pH increases the activity of urease and facilitates much greater absorption of free ammonia (pK_a of ammonium is 9.1). Acidification in these cases returns the pH of ruminoreticular content toward physiological levels, promotes the uptake of VFA, depresses the absorption of ammonia, and inhibits excessive urease activity. Acetic acid (4-5%) or vinegar (cattle: 1-2 L; sheep: 250-500 mL) is the most common acidifying agent used. Lactic acid and orthophosphoric acid are also effective and safe but must first be diluted to a solution of ~5%. Propionic acid administered intraruminally inhibits rumen motility and reduces feed intake.

Modulators of Ruminoreticular Motility: Since most forestomach disorders result in ruminal atony, an essential component to reestablishing normal function is to facilitate and return the primary ruminoreticular contractions to their usual strength and frequency; parasympathomimetic agents (neostigmine, physostigmine, carbachol, and bethanechol) have been used for this purpose. All these drugs have cholinergic effects, which are potentially hazardous. Neostigmine (cattle: (0.02 mg/ kg, subcut.; sheep: 0.01-0.02 mg/kg, subcut.) generally produces the fewest side effects but tends to increase frequency of ruminoreticular contractions rather than their strength. This is particularly true in ruminal atony. The stimulatory effect of neostigmine is not always reliable, and some inhibition of motility can occur. This may be due to the adrenergic component associated with ganglion stimulation by cholinergic agents. Carbachol (cattle: 1-4 mg, subcut.; sheep: 0.1-0.2 mg, subcut.) tends to cause uncoordinated spastic and functionless contractions as well as paralysis of the reticulum. Spontaneous bloat may occur as the result of interference with eructation by carbachol.

Metoclopramide has been reported to be useful to correct disorders of ruminoreticular motility, but few definitive studies are available; it does produce powerful abomasal contractions. Conditioned responses to the presence of feed and feeding itself are 2 physiologic means by which ruminoreticular motility can be notably enhanced. Benzodiazepines have a transient appetite-enhancing effect in some ruminants (eg, diazepam at 0.15 mg/kg in cattle and 0.05-0.5 mg/kg in sheep) and may stimulate ruminal contractions.

Endotoxin-induced ruminal stasis can be prevented by opioid antagonists such as naloxone, naltrexone, and diprenorphine. Antihistaminic and antiserotonergic agents are not particularly useful in these cases. The antiprostaglandin nonsteroidal anti-inflammatories only partially antagonize endotoxin-induced ruminal stasis, though they do suppress the febrile reaction.

A number of factors may exert a detrimental influence on forestomach motility and result in ruminoreticular stasis or atony. Systemic and/or intraruminal alkalosis depresses motility, as does an intraruminal pH of <5. Sympathetic activity or adrenergic agents causes a transitory paresis of the forestomach. Fever also depresses motility. Ionic imbalances may disrupt forestomach motor activity (particularly marked in hypocalcemic states). Hyperglycemia causes inhibition of ruminoreticular motility. Histamine causes paralysis of the rumen and reticulum with marked depression of eructation. Bradykinin and serotonin seem to have similar inhibitory effects. Distention of the abomasum or cecum causes reflex inhibition of ruminal mixing cycles and paralysis of the reticulum. Excessive duodenal acidity, eg, from lactic acid, produces a similar effect. Gastrin, cholecystokinin, and secretin exert inhibitory effects on the frequency of ruminoreticular motility. Cholecystokinin may, however, increase the amplitude of ruminal contractions. Energy deficiency or prolonged fasting ultimately leads to rumen stasis. Excessive concentrations of VFA, particularly butyrate, also depress motility. Lesions involving the vagal nerve impair forestomach function depending on which nerve branch or portion of the ruminant stomach is involved. Several pharmacological agents such as anticholinergics, adrenergics, opiate analgesics, CNS depressants, and several toxic compounds (such as cyanide) are capable of producing ruminoreticular paresis. An important cause of ruminal atony is pain, and analgesics may well be helpful in such cases.

MUSCULAR SYSTEM

Drugs that affect skeletal muscle function fall into several therapeutic categories. There are those used during surgical procedures that produce paralysis (neuromuscular blockers), as well as those that reduce spasticity (skeletal muscle spasmolytics) associated with various neurological and musculoskeletal conditions. In addition, there are several therapeutic agents that influence metabolic and other processes in skeletal muscle. Included among these are the nutrients (see MHN, p 1088 et seq) that are required for normal muscle function and that are employed to prevent or mitigate degenerative muscular conditions. An example of this approach is the use of selenium and vitamin E to prevent and/or treat muscular dystrophies such as white muscle disease, and various forms of capture myopathy in wild animals. The steroidal, nonsteroidal, and various other anti-inflammatory agents, eg, dimethyl sulfoxide, are also commonly used to treat acute and chronic inflammatory conditions involving skeletal muscle. Anabolic steroids, with their ability to promote muscle growth and development, are administered in selected cases in which serious muscle deterioration has occurred as a complication of a primary disease syndrome.

The clinical pharmacology of the neuromuscular blockers, skeletal muscle spasmolytics, and anabolic steroids are discussed below.

NEUROMUSCULAR BLOCKING AGENTS

The peripherally acting skeletal muscle relaxants characteristically interfere with the transmission of impulses from motor nerves to skeletal muscle fibers at the neuromuscular junction, thus reducing or abolishing motor activity. The skeletal muscle paralysis that ensues is not associated with depression of the CNS. Animals are fully conscious throughout the period of immobilization unless an anesthetic or hypnotic agent is administered concurrently.

Modification of neuromuscular transmission can be instigated either at the axonal membrane (pre-junctional blockade) or at the cholinergic receptors in the sarcolemma (post-junctional blockade).

There are no clinically useful drugs that act pre-junctionally but a number of important substances can impair the synthesis, storage, and release of acetylcholine, thus resulting in pre-junctional blockade at the motor end-plate and consequently paralysis.

Examples of pre-junctional blocking agents include: 1) Biotoxins such as black widow spider venom (depletes acetylcholine stores), botulinum toxin (decreases acetylcholine release), tetradotoxin from the puffer fish and saxitoxin from shellfish (block Na^+-conducting channels), and grayanotoxin found in rhododendrons (facilitates excessive Na^+ entry through the sarcolemma leading to constant depolarization of the membrane). 2) Electrolytes such as Mg^{++} in excess (inhibits release of acetylcholine from the axon and uncouples the excitation-contraction process by competing with Ca^{++}) and depleted Ca^{++} levels (decreases release of acetylcholine and impairment of excitation-contraction coupling). 3) Drugs such as local anesthetics in high concentration (stabilize membrane by blocking both Na^+ and K^+ channels) and hemicholinium (inhibits synthesis of acetylcholine by blocking choline uptake into the nerve). 4) Antibiotics such as the aminoglycosides, polymyxins, tetracyclines, and lincosamides (appear to act by decreasing the availability of Ca^{++} at membrane-binding sites on the axonal terminal and perhaps by reducing the sensitivity of the nicotinic receptors to acetylcholine).

Post-junctional blocking agents are employed clinically and act either by blocking the nicotinic receptors in a competitive fashion (nondepolarizing agents), or by interacting with these receptors in a manner that does not allow the membrane to repolarize so that paralysis results (depolarizing agents). The mechanisms involved in the latter case are not fully understood. All of the neuromuscular blocking drugs are structurally similar to acetylcholine (actually 2 molecules linked end-to-end). The depolarizing agents are usually simple linear structures and the nondepolarizing agents are more complex bulky molecules. With a single exception (vecuronium), all possess a quaternary nitrogen in their structure, which makes these drugs poorly lipid soluble.

Competitive Nondepolarizing Agents: The members of this group of peripherally acting skeletal muscle relaxants are often referred to as curarizing agents because of their relationships with the curare alkaloids that were first used clinically. The currently available drugs, which interact with nicotinic cholinergic receptors on skeletal muscle cells and render them inaccessible to the transmitter function of acetylcholine (and thus produce a flaccid paralysis), include tubocurarine, metocurine (dimethyltubocurarine), gallamine, pancuronium, alcuronium, atracurium, vecuronium, and fazadinium.

As a general rule, nondepolarizing muscle relaxants are not absorbed from the GI tract and must be administered parenterally, usually IV. Plasma-protein binding is insignificant, and there is rapid equilibration but only within the extracellular fluid. The blood-brain and blood-placental barriers are rarely traversed. Tubocurarine, metocurine, and gallamine are not biotransformed to any extent and are excreted unchanged, principally in the urine but sometimes in bile. The other members of the group undergo metabolic transformation to some degree, and the metabolites are excreted by both renal and biliary routes in most instances. The elimination half-lives at standard doses range from 60-100 min and the duration of paralysis from 30-60 min, except in the case of atracurium and vecuronium, which have shorter actions of ~20-30 min.

Following IV administration of these agents, the skeletal muscles become totally flaccid and nonresponsive to neuronal stimulation. Muscles capable of rapid movement, such as those of the eye, are paralyzed before the larger muscles of the head and neck, which are followed by those of the limbs and body. Lastly, the diaphragm becomes paralyzed and respiration ceases. If ventilation is controlled (tracheal intubation and positive pressure ventilation), there are no adverse effects and full recovery occurs in reverse order, with the diaphragm regaining function first. All of the currently used nondepolarizing muscle relaxants produce cardiovascular effects, many of which are mediated by autonomic and histamine receptors. Tubocurarine and, to a much lesser extent, metocurine produce hypotension, which probably results from the liberation of histamine and, in larger doses, from ganglionic blockade. Premedication with an antihistamine will reduce tubocurarine-induced hypotension. Pancuronium causes a moderate increase in heart rate and, to a lesser degree, cardiac output. Gallamine increases heart rate by both a vagolytic action and sympathetic stimulation.

A number of agents can potentiate the activity of neuromuscular blockers. These include other peripherally acting skeletal muscle relaxants, inhalant anesthetics (halothane, methoxyflurane), antibiotics (aminoglycosides, polymyxins, tetracyclines, and lincosamides), and various other drugs (quinidine, procaine, lidocaine, diazepam, and barbiturates). Several states such as hyper- and hypomagnesemia, hypokalemia, acidosis, and hypothermia also prolong the action of this group of drugs. Animals suffering from myasthenia gravis are much more susceptible to the action of muscle relaxants.

Indications for the use of nondepolarizing neuromuscular blocking agents include muscle relaxation of the operative field, hypoxemic animals resisting mechanical ventilation, tracheal intubation, animals with unstable cardiovascular function that require anesthesia but cannot tolerate cardiac depression, cesarean section in toxic or high-risk animals, epileptiform convulsions not controllable with usual anticonvulsant agents, tetanus, strychnine poisoning, shivering animals in which the metabolic demand for oxygen should be reduced, and capture of certain exotic species (eg, gallamine used for immobilization of crocodiles). Animals should **always** be carefully monitored when under the influence of neuromuscular blocking drugs, and support of ventilation is essential.

The action of the competitive relaxants can be reversed by anticholinesterase drugs, especially neostigmine, following the administration of atropine, which eliminates excessive muscarinic responses. This attribute is a great advantage for this group of peripherally acting muscle relaxants.

The selection of IV dose rates given below serves only as general guidelines for the use of competitive blocking agents.

Tubocurarine chloride	horse: ≤0.22-0.25 mg/kg
	dog, cat: ≤0.4 mg/kg
Gallamine triethiodide	All species (except pig): 0.8-1 mg/kg
Pancuronium bromide	dog, cat: 0.6 mg/kg
Alcuronium chloride	dog, cat: 0.1 mg/kg
Atracurium besylate	dog, cat: 0.5 mg/kg

Antagonists

Neostigmine	0.04 mg/kg, with atropine at 0.04 mg/kg
Pyridostigmine	0.2-0.25 mg/kg, with atropine at 0.04 mg/kg
Edrophonium	0.125 mg/kg

Depolarizing Agents: Succinylcholine (suxamethonium) is the only commonly used peripherally acting muscle relaxant that is a depolarizing agent. Decamethonium, the other member of the group, is rarely employed clinically.

Depolarizing blocking drugs occupy the post-junctional cholinergic receptors and, by mechanisms that remain obscure, elicit prolonged depolarization of the end-plate region, which prevents the synaptic membrane from completely repolarizing—which renders the motor end-plate unresponsive to the normal action of acetylcholine. Characteristically, succinylcholine elicits transient muscle fasciculations before causing neuromuscular paralysis. The onset of action of succinylcholine is rapid following IV injection (20-50 sec), and the duration of the effect is usually 5-10 min in most species. Succinylcholine is rapidly hydrolyzed by pseudocholinesterases in the plasma and liver in most species, but substantial genetic differences exist.

Following IV administration of succinylcholine, transient muscle fasciculations are usually very evident although general anesthesia tends to attenuate them. Other pharmacological effects are associated with the depolarizing muscle relaxants. Succinylcholine-induced cardiac arrhythmias are many and varied. The drug stimulates all autonomic cholinergic receptors—both nicotinic and muscarinic. Sudden hyperkalemia may be precipitated by succinylcholine, and muscle pain occurs with the use of succinylcholine in the absence of anesthesia. Following recovery from succinylcholine-induced muscle paralysis, muscle damage and even myoglobinuria can occur. Malignant hyperthermia or clinical signs related to this syndrome may also follow the use of succinylcholine in susceptible animals.

The factors, discussed above, that can alter the activity of competitive blocking agents may also impact on the action of succinylcholine. In addition, previous (within 1 mo) or concurrent use of organophosphate anthelmintics or external parasiticides may have a significant impact on the recovery time from succinylcholine immobilization, because of prolonged inhibition of the pseudocholinesterase enzyme systems. A genetically mediated deficiency of pseudocholinesterases also has been identified in certain strains of sheep. Cattle are much more susceptible to the effects of succinylcholine.

The indications for the clinical use of succinylcholine are similar to those for the nondepolarizing agents. However, it must be emphasized that succinylcholine should **never** be employed as an agent for euthanasia or for immobilization for castration without local or general analgesia. The use of succinylcholine for game-cropping procedures is also highly undesirable.

No antagonists are available to reverse the action of the depolarizing muscle relaxants. Continued positive-pressure ventilation until recovery occurs is the only therapy in cases of overdosage.

The IV dose rates for succinylcholine are:

Horses:	0.125-0.20 mg/kg (~8 min recumbency)
Cattle:	0.012-0.02 mg/kg (~15 min recumbency)
Dogs:	0.22-1.1 mg/kg (~15-20 min paralysis)
Cats:	0.22-1.1 mg/kg (~3-5 min paralysis)

SKELETAL MUSCLE SPASMOLYTICS

Muscle spasticity is characterized by an increase in tonic stretch reflexes and painful flexor muscle spasms, often together with muscle weakness. Various clinical conditions such as trauma, myositis, muscular and ligamentous sprains and strains, intervertebral disk lesions, tetanus, strychnine poisoning, and even anxiety can be associated with acute muscle spasms. The mechanisms underlying clinical spasticity appear to involve not the stretch reflex arc itself but higher centers with involvement of descending pathways that result in hyperexcitability of motor neurons in the spinal cord. Drug therapy may ameliorate some of the clinical signs of spasticity by modifying the stretch reflex, or by interfering directly with the excitation-coupling process in the muscle itself. Agents used for therapeutic management of clinical syndromes in which acute, painful skeletal muscle spasms are an important feature are typically classified as centrally acting muscle relaxants. The efficacy of these agents has been difficult to assess for many reasons, but they do have some use in veterinary medicine.

Malignant hyperthermia (qv, p 448) is a fulminating to insidious hypermetabolic disorder of skeletal muscle. The syndrome has been recognized in susceptible breeds of pigs such as Pietrain, Poland China, and American Landrace, and less often in cats, dogs, and horses. In susceptible animals, hyperthermia and hypermetabolic episodes are initiated by the administration of potent halogenated anesthetic agents, depolarizing skeletal muscle relaxants, and amide local anesthetics. Stress from trauma, surgery, transportation, and other causes can initiate the syndrome in awake susceptible individuals. In addition, attacks may occur during recovery from general anesthesia. The underlying defect appears to be an idiopathic increase in myoplasmic calcium ion concentration in skeletal muscle. As a consequence, total body oxygen consumption increases 2-3 times more than for normal individuals. Core body temperatures can rise to as high as 109°F (43°C) at the rate of 1°C q5min. In progressive hypermetabolic states, muscle rigidity, pyrexia, tachypnea, respiratory and metabolic acidosis, hypoxia, hypercapnia, electrolyte disturbances, and enzymatic shifts develop. This particular form of muscle spasticity can be treated with a specific agent, dantrolene.

Centrally Acting Muscle Relaxants: A variety of drugs thought to be capable of blocking interneuronal pathways (polysynaptic reflexes) in the spinal cord and perhaps in the midbrain reticular activating system, but not of inhibiting the monosynaptic relay of the stretch reflex, have been used to treat acute episodes of skeletal muscle spasticity associated with several neurological and musculoskeletal disorders. The efficacy of these agents has not been reliably established but clinical success is not infrequent. The mechanisms involved may be more intricate than those set out above. The effect, in fact, may be central and due to sedation in some cases. The various agents in this class include: 1) Carbamate derivatives, eg, chlorphenesin carbamate, meprobamate, carisoprodol, and methocarbamol. These are regarded as typical centrally acting muscle relaxants. Methocarbamol has enjoyed the greatest use in veterinary medicine (dogs, cats: 44 mg/kg, PO, t.i.d., or in severe conditions, 55-220 mg/kg, IM or IV; horses: in moderate conditions, 4.4-22 mg/kg, IV, and in severe conditions, 22-25 mg/kg, IV). 2) Glyceryl ethers, eg, mephenesin and glyceryl guaiacol ether (glyceryl guaiacolate, guaifenesin). Guaifenesin is mainly used in horses as an adjunct to various general anesthetics. It has also been used successfully to reverse the clinical signs of strychnine intoxication in dogs. 3) Benzodiazepines, eg, diazepam. 4) Baclofen, which appears to act as an agonist at certain GABA receptors and may thereby exert presynaptic inhibitory effects reducing the release of excitatory neurotransmitters in the CNS, is as effective as diazepam in reducing muscle spasticity but causes much less sedation.

Intracellular Muscle Relaxant: Dantrolene is a unique drug that reduces skeletal muscle strength by inhibiting excitation-contraction coupling in the skeletal muscle fiber itself. The mechanism of action is based on interference with the release of activator calcium from the sarcoplasmic reticulum. Motor units that contract rapidly are more sensitive to dantrolene than are slowly contracting units. Cardiac and smooth muscle are much less responsive to the drug's effect. There are no central or neuromuscular junctional effects. Dantrolene is specifically used to treat or prevent malignant hyperthermia (MH) in animals, though it also may be of some benefit in certain cases of severe spasticity due to upper motor neuron lesions. Major adverse effects associated with dantrolene include generalized muscle weakness, sedation, GI disturbances, and a form of hepatitis that may become serious. Hepatic function should always be monitored. The following doses of dantrolene sodium have been used in affected animals:

Horses:	1-2 mg/kg, PO, q.i.d. (prophylactic)
	1-3 mg/kg, IV, repeated in 10 min (MH crisis)
Pigs:	2-3 mg/kg, IV
Dogs:	2.5 mg/kg, IV, q.i.d.

ANABOLIC STEROIDS

Compounds structurally related to testosterone but possessing protein anabolic activity with minimal androgenic (masculinizing) effects are classed as anabolic steroids. They are often used therapeutically in debilitated animals suffering from notable muscular atrophy (eg, with inanition).

The absorption, distribution, biotransformation, and excretion of anabolic steroids generally follow patterns similar to those of the parent androgens. Prolonged absorption following parenteral administration (IM) occurs with the longer chain fatty acid preparations, such as decanoate and undecylenate esters, requiring up to 4 wk for complete absorption to occur from injection sites. Excretion time for shorter-acting anabolic steroids is generally ~10-14 days.

The metabolic activities of the anabolic steroids include: protein anabolism and a positive nitrogen balance; increased muscle mass due to increased protein and glycogen content; high retention of calcium and phosphate; electrolyte balance "normalized" with appropriate assimilation of sodium, potassium, chloride, and water; promotion of renal and extrarenal erythropoietin production; stimulation of bone marrow stem cells (only certain anabolic steroids).

The therapeutic indications for this group of agents include: 1) growth promotion, 2) debility following illness or surgery, 3) muscular dystrophy, 4) geriatric cases, 5) osteoporosis and orthopedic conditions, 6) anemia—especially aplastic anemia (testosterone, nandrolone, and fluoxymesterone stimulate renal and extrarenal erythropoietin production as well as undifferentiated stem cells; other anabolic steroids possess only erythropoietin-stimulating properties), 7) renal failure (increase appetite and vigor, rate of gain, PCV, Hgb concentration, and RBC count, and may reduce BUN levels), 8) hepatic disorders, 9) mammary tumors, and 10) prolonged use of corticosteroids (iatrogenic Cushing's disease).

When an anabolic steroid is administered to an animal, it is important to assure adequate intake of protein, calories, vitamins (especially pyridoxine, folate, and hydroxocobalamin), iron, and copper. Beneficial hematological responses may not be evident until several weeks after a course of treatment is initiated. Sudden withdrawal of anabolic steroids should be avoided.

A number of potential side effects and contraindications are associated with the administration of the anabolic steroids. The more significant of these include: 1) androgenic effects with increased libido in males and abnormal sexual behavior in females; 2) azoospermia, anestrus, and other adverse reproductive side effects; 3) edema due to sodium and water retention; 4) icterus due to intrahepatic cholestasis; 5) increased levels of serum transaminase enzymes as well as triglycerides; 6) hepatic adenocarcinoma (rare); 7) steroid fever due to formation of pyrexigenic steroid metabolites; 8) exacerbation of prostatic hypertrophy or carcinoma; 9) epiphyseal plate closure leading to stunted growth; 10) decreased bone strength; 11) reduced tensile strength of tendons; 12) behavioral teratogenicity with alteration of endocrine balances in later years.

The anabolic steroids used in veterinary medicine include:

Parenteral forms

Nandrolone decanoate	Dog: 1-5 mg/kg/wk, IM (maximum 200 mg)
	Horse: 200 mg (maximum)
Nandrolone phenpropionate	Dog: 25-50 mg/2 wk, IM or subcut.
	Cat: 10-20 mg/2 wk, IM or subcut.
Stanozolol	Dog: 2-10 mg/kg/wk, IM
	Cat: 10-25 mg/wk, IM
	Horse: 0.55 mg/kg/wk, IM (up to 4 wk)
Boldenone undecylenate	Horse: 1.1 mg/kg, IM, q3wk

Oral forms

Oxymetholone	Dog: 1.1 mg/kg/day
Stanozolol	Dog: 0.25-3 mg/kg/day
	Cat: 0.5-2 mg/cat, b.i.d.
Ethylestrenol	Dog: 0.05 mg/kg/day (up to 2 wk)

NERVOUS SYSTEM

ANTICONVULSANTS

Treatment Protocols: During a seizure episode or status epilepticus, the route of administration for anticonvulsants is IV. The oral route is preferred for long-term maintenance therapy, although absorption may be limited or variable depending on the drug used. Subcut. or IM injections are seldom used because of the variability in drug absorption.

Maintenance anticonvulsant therapy should be initiated in animals that have >1 seizure monthly or >1 seizure on any particular day, if the first episode is protracted or severe, or during an episode of status epilepticus (as a follow-up to emergency treatment, *see* below). Treatment should begin with a single drug at the minimal required level for effect and with an interim period equal to the interval between past episodes. (Owners should keep a calendar to document the frequency and pattern of seizures as a guide for treatment strategy.) This regimen is maintained if seizures are controlled without toxic effects. If control is unsatisfactory, the dose should be increased over multiple steps before adding or switching to a new drug. Doses may be doubled in early stages and increased by 50% in later stages. To discontinue a drug, even when changing drugs, the dose should be tapered off gradually to avoid precipitating a seizure.

In status epilepticus, treatment is essential to prevent death from hyperthermia, acidosis, hypoperfusion, and hypoxia. A benzodiazepine should be used first, because its transient effect permits a rapid shift in the therapeutic approach. For dogs, an initial IV bolus of diazepam (0.5-2 mg/kg) or, alternatively, clonazepam (0.05-0.2 mg/kg) may be necessary to reduce motor activity to permit placement of an IV catheter. Fluids are then infused to correct any detectable metabolic disturbances and diazepam added at 5-20 mg/hr. Alternatively, IV boluses of diazepam may be repeated up to a total of 3 times before switching to phenobarbital, to begin the maintenance phase of therapy in dogs. Phenobarbital may be given as a 2-4 mg/kg, slow IV bolus q10min up to a total of 3-4 doses. As a safer alternative in dogs, phenobarbital may be infused IV to effect at 3-10 mg/hr. If phenobarbital is effective in controlling seizures, a maintenance regimen may be initiated with phenobarbital, discontinuing anticonvulsant infusion 2-4 hr later. In small breeds, the infusion with diazepam alone is continued after the oral administration of phenobarbital. Cats in status epilepticus are best treated with diazepam only (0.5-2 mg/kg, IV) and seldom need any other anticonvulsant. Diazepam is generally continued as maintenance treatment in cats, with oral doses ranging from 0.5 to 2 mg/kg divided into 3 daily doses. Phenobarbital is a second drug of choice for maintenance, 3-6 mg/kg divided into 2-3 daily doses. For foals with neonatal maladjustment syndrome, seizures are best treated with diazepam, 5-20 mg, given slowly IV. This dose may be repeated, and with a few doses, convulsions do not recur in some foals. However, if seizures are repeated, medication with diazepam or another anticonvulsant should be continued for 1-4 wk before a gradual withdrawal. After diazepam treatment, phenobarbital may be administered at doses of 5-20 mg by slow IV injection. The maintenance dose follows as 9 mg/kg, b.i.d. or t.i.d. Alternatively, treatment of foals can be initiated and later maintained with phenytoin (for doses, see below). In all species, if seizures are otherwise uncontrollable, sodium pentobarbital can be given at 2-4 mg/kg to the effect of sedation or anesthesia. Also, if cerebral edema is suspected, see PRINCIPLES OF THERAPY, NERVOUS SYSTEM, p 575.

Horses with seizures induced by toxins or drug adverse effects can be treated with diazepam (0.1-0.15 mg/kg, IV). Alternatively, a mixture of guaifenesin (5%) and thiamylal (2 mg/mL) may be given at 1 mL/kg to effect.

Anticonvulsant Drugs Commonly Used for Dogs, Cats, and Horses

	Maintenance Therapy	Status Epilepticus
Dog	Phenobarbital* Diphenylhydantoin Clonazepam Primidone	Diazepam* Phenobarbital Sodium pentobarbital
Cat	Diazepam* Phenobarbital	Diazepam* Sodium pentobarbital
Foal	Diazepam* Phenobarbital Diphenylhydantoin	Diazepam* Phenobarbital Sodium pentobarbital
Adult horse	Diazepam*	Diazepam* Guaifenesin and thiamylal

*Drugs of choice

Phenothiazine tranquilizers should be avoided in epileptic treatment in all species, because these drugs lower the seizure threshold. Also, xylazine should not be used during seizures, since it severely depresses cardiovascular and respiratory function; even at low doses, it can cause prolonged sedation and death.

Of the benzodiazepines, **diazepam** and **clonazepam** are most commonly used. Injectable solutions should not be left in plastic containers, including syringes, because of rapid inactivation (over minutes). Diazepam is not suitable for oral maintenance therapy in dogs, because it is absorbed poorly and eliminated rapidly, and a tolerance to anticonvulsant effects develops rapidly. However, it is a drug of choice for controlling canine status epilepticus, and continuous IV infusion (5-20 mg/hr) is preferred over repeated IV boluses (1-2 mg/kg). Diazepam is the anticonvulsant of choice for cats in either maintenance therapy (0.5-2 mg/kg/day, PO in 2-3 divided doses) or treating status epilepticus (0.5-2 mg/kg, IV). Not only is the elimination rate slower in cats, but cats do not develop a tolerance to its anticonvulsant effects. Diazepam also has a long elimination half-life in horses, and it is therefore the anticonvulsant of choice (5-20 mg/dose) in foals with neonatal maladjustment syndrome. Higher doses can be fatal to neonates. For seizures in adult horses, diazepam can be given at 0.1-0.15 mg/kg, IV.

Unlike diazepam, clonazepam can be used in dogs for oral maintenance therapy, because anticonvulsant tolerance develops less rapidly, the saturatability of its metabolism reduces the elimination rate at therapeutic concentrations, and it is more highly absorbed orally, particularly in micronized formulations. In maintenance therapy in dogs, it is best used as an adjunct to phenobarbital at doses of 0.1-0.5 mg/kg, t.i.d. Diarrhea sometimes develops with clonazepam, but this may be avoided by increasing the dose frequency from 1 to 3 times daily over a period of several days.

Phenobarbital is the preferred maintenance drug for dogs due to safety, efficacy, low cost, and convenience for monitoring serum concentrations. Because of a long half-life in all species, 2 wk are required to approach steady state in plasma concentration, and dosage adjustment should be attempted only at 2-wk intervals. In dogs, it is used as a follow-up to diazepam in status epilepticus by an IV infusion to effect (3-10 mg/hr) or a slow IV bolus (2-4 mg/kg), or IM injection (3-6 mg/kg). As in all species, caution is necessary in switching from diazepam to phenobarbital, because a potentiatation of their effects produces a risk of respiratory and cardiovascular collapse. For long-term maintenance in cats and dogs, phenobarbital may be dosed at 2-6 mg/kg/day, PO, divided in 2, sometimes 3, daily doses. In foals, phenobarbital may be started as a follow-up to diazepam with 5-20 mg administered IV over 20 min, and then maintained at a dose of 9 mg/kg, b.i.d. or t.i.d. In all species, extreme variation in oral absorption necessitates drug level monitoring, 3 wk from initiation of therapy and 2 wk after dosage changes. Therapeutic concentrations are 20-45 mg/dL. Sedation has a low incidence in dogs, disappearing within the first week of treatment. In the foal, however, the dose should be reduced if the animal becomes highly sedated.

Phenytoin (diphenylhydantoin) is no longer recommended for use in dogs or cats due to undesirable rates of metabolism: too rapid in dogs, reducing its effectiveness, and too slow in cats, increasing the risk for toxicity. In dogs, it may still be used in status epilepticus as a slow IV injection of 2-5 mg/kg. Foals with neonatal maladjustment syndrome can be started on phenytoin at 5-10 mg/kg, IV, with subsequent treatments of 1-5 mg/kg, IV, IM, or PO, q2-4hr for 12 hr. Afterwards, dosage should continue q6-12hr. The dose may need to be reduced if sedation is observed.

Primidone is less preferred than phenobarbital because most of its anticonvulsant activity is due to its metabolism to phenobarbital. It requires a t.i.d. versus b.i.d. administration, and it can be hepatotoxic. Nevertheless, one report indicates that dogs that are not well controlled by phenobarbital may respond better to primidone. ALT (SGPT), serum alkaline phosphatase, or BSP should be monitored to safeguard against hepatotoxicity. For use only in dogs, the initial dose is 10-15 mg/kg/day in 3 divided doses. The dose is increased over time to a maximum of 35 mg/kg/day. If treatment is switched to phenobarbital, the initial dose should be ⅕ the previous primidone dose to achieve a comparable concentration of phenobarbital. Primidone is not recommended for use in cats.

Sodium pentobarbital is generally reserved as a last resort for the treatment of uncontrollable status epilepticus in dogs and cats, when diazepam and phenobarbital have failed. In these species, it is administered at 2-4 mg/kg to effect for anesthesia. In foals, as an alternative to diazepam and phenobarbital, it may be given at 2-4 mg/kg, IV to effect for controlling convulsions; sedation is likely at these doses.

TRANQUILIZERS, SEDATIVES, AND ANALGESICS

Tranquilization by drug effect reduces anxiety and induces a sense of tranquility without drowsiness. Drug-induced sedation has a more profound effect, and produces drowsiness and hypnosis. Analgesia is the reduction of pain, which according to a drug's effect, may be more pronounced in either the viscera or the musculoskeletal system. Many drugs cannot be categorized by only one pharmacological effect, ie, as tranquilizers, sedatives, or analgesics; eg, many psychotropic drugs can either tranquilize or sedate according to the dose administered, and many sedatives are also analgesics. Also, drugs classified as tranquilizers, sedatives, and/or analgesics may have additional effects in behavioral modification, antiemesis, etc.

Listed below are drugs that are commonly used in dogs, cats, horses, cattle, and pigs for tranquilization, sedation, or analgesia. Drugs are omitted that may have some of these effects but are used mainly for other properties, eg, as antispasmodics, antiemetics, or preanesthetics. Single-use doses are emphasized, since many situations require only a brief duration of effect, but frequency of administration is also provided for drugs likely to be used for multiple-dose therapy. The doses listed apply to the use of each drug alone, as opposed to a combination for anesthesia or neuroleptanalgesia. No reference is made to schedule restrictions, extra-label use, or precautions in the use of these drugs. This presentation of doses serves only as a general guide. Package inserts and referenced texts should be consulted for information on the pharmacology and alternative applications of each drug.

Table 3. Tranquilizers or Sedatives without Analgesic Effects: Doses (mg/kg unless otherwise indicated), Route, and Frequency of Administration

Drug	Dogs	Cats	Horses	Cattle	Pigs
Benzodiazepine Diazepam	1 IV, PO		0.05-0.4 IV	0.5-1.5 IV	0.5-1.5 IV; 5.5 IM
Butyrophenone Azaperone			0.4-0.8 IM		2.2 IM
Phenothiazines Acepromazine maleate	0.05-0.1 IV, IM, subcut; 0.55-2.2 PO; q6-8hr	0.11-0.22 IV, IM, subcut; 1.1-2.2 PO; q8-12hr	0.04-0.1 IV, IM, subcut., PO; q24hr	0.05-0.1 IV, IM, subcut.	0.1-0.2 IV, IM, subcut.
Chlorpromazine hydrochloride	0.55-4.4 IV; 1.1-6.6 IM; 3.2 PO, q6-8hr, PRN*	0.55-4.4 IV; 1.1-6.6 IM; 3.2 PO, q6-8hr, PRN			
Ethylisobutrazine hydrochloride	2.2-4.4 IV; 4.4-11 IM, PO; q24hr				
Promazine hydrochloride	2-6 IV, IM, PO; q6-8hr	2-4.4 IV, IM, PO; q6-8hr	0.4-1 IV, IM; 1-2 PO	0.4-1 IV, IM; 1.6-2.8 PO	0.4-1 IV, IM
Triflupromazine hydrochloride	1.1-2.2 IV; 2.2-4.4 IM	4.4-8.8 IM	0.22-0.33 IV, IM (maximum 100 mg/ horse/day)		

*PRN = as needed

Table 4. Analgesics: Doses (mg/kg unless otherwise indicated), Route, and Frequency of Administration

Drug	Dogs	Cats	Horses	Cattle	Pigs
Opioid Analgesics**					
Butorphanol tartrate	0.05-0.1 IM, subcut.; 0.55 PO; q6-12hr	0.1-0.2 IV, subcut.	0.03-0.2 IV, IM		
Meperidine hydrochloride	5-10 IM; q6hr, PRN*	3 IM; q6hr, PRN	0.2-0.4 IV; 2.2-4 IM		
Morphine sulfate	0.22-0.88 IM, subcut.; q4-6hr, PRN	0.1 IM, subcut.; PRN	0.2 IV; 0.2-0.4 IM	500 mg/cow, IV	
Oxymorphone hydrochloride	0.1-0.2 IV, IM, subcut.; q24hr	0.1-0.2 IV, IM, subcut.; q24hr	0.02-0.03 IV, IM		
Pentazocine lactate	1.7-3.3 IM; b.i.d.	2.2-3.3 IV, IM, subcut.	0.33 IV, IM		
Nonopioid Sedative Analgesic					
Xylazine hydrochloride	0.05-0.1 IV; 1-2 IM, subcut.	0.5-1 IV; 1-2 IM, subcut.	0.5-1 IV; 2.2 IM	0.05-0.1 IV; 0.1-0.2 IM	2 IM
Nonpsychotropic Analgesics					
Acetaminophen	25-30 PO; q6hr, PRN	Contraindicated			
Aspirin	10 PO; b.i.d.	10 PO; q48hr	30-47.5 PO; q6-12hr	100 PO; b.i.d.	10 PO; q6hr, PRN
Dipyrone	28 IV, IM, subcut., PO; q8hr	28 IV, IM, subcut., PO; q8hr	5-10 g/horse IV, IM; q8hr PRN	50 IV, IM, subcut.	50 IV, IM, subcut.
Flunixin meglumine	0.55 IV; 2.2 PO; q24hr		1 IV, IM, PO; q24hr		
Meclofenamic acid	1.1 PO; q24hr		2.2 PO; q24hr		
Naproxen	5 PO initial; 1.2-2.8 PO, q24hr maintenance		5 IV; 10 PO, b.i.d.		
Phenylbutazone	22 IV: 15 PO; t.i.d. (maximum 0.8 g/dog/day)		4.4 PO, b.i.d., day 1; 2.2 PO, b.i.d. 4 days; 2.2 PO, q24hr or every other day	2-5 IV; 4-8 PO	2-5 IV; 4-8 PO

* PRN = as needed
**Recommended doses of opiates may produce excitement in cats and horses.

RESPIRATORY SYSTEM

Disease processes that affect the respiratory system generally impede ventilation and alveolar gas exchange in several different ways. (*See also* RESPIRATORY SYSTEM, INTRODUCTION, p 708.) Inflammation of the lung or airways is the most common cause of respiratory embarrassment. Pneumonia, bronchopneumonia, bronchitis, tracheitis, laryngitis, sinusitis, and rhinitis are conditions that are encountered at varying degrees of severity in most animals. The possible causes of these inflammatory lesions include chemical irritants, hypersensitivity reactions, viruses, bacteria including chlamydia and mycoplasmas, fungi, and helminths. In the early stages of acute inflammation, respiratory tract secretions often diminish in volume and become viscid, which produces a dry inflamed mucosa—which causes a harsh, debilitating, unproductive cough. Chronic inflammatory respiratory diseases are often complex from a therapeutic point of view. The possible presence of fibrosis, abscessation, bronchiectasis, emphysema, edema, impaired immune defense mechanisms, and secondary cardiovascular involvement add to the difficulty of managing chronic cases.

Constriction of the airways, which may be mediated by various inflammagens such as histamine, kinins, prostaglandins, and leukotrienes, or by cholinergic stimulation, is important in many respiratory diseases. Since tidal volume varies with airway diameter, bronchoconstriction, together with a buildup of mucus or exudate in the bronchi, can readily lead to hypoxemia, hypercapnia, and respiratory acidosis.

Pulmonary edema, involving the lung interstitium and septa or the alveoli themselves, is a serious problem. The pathogenesis often is multifaceted, depending on the etiology, but usually there is an increase in the permeability of the capillary-alveolar membranes or an imbalance of hydrostatic and oncotic pressures in the pulmonary capillary beds. The permeability of the capillary-alveolar membranes may be disrupted by bacterial or viral infections, endotoxins, inhaled noxious agents (phosgene, ammonia, sulfur dioxide, smoke, and others), systemic toxins (ANTU, organophosphates, snake venom, 3-methyl indole), uremia, anaphylaxis, disseminated intravascular coagulation, aspiration pneumonia, drowning, and excessive irradiation. Pulmonary hypertension (due to several clinical conditions, including excessive parenteral fluid therapy) and hypoalbuminemia are the major circulatory-related precipitants of pulmonary edema.

Respiratory rate and depth are controlled by medullary centers that respond reflexly to arterial pO_2, pCO_2, pH, lung volume, and several other factors. Any impediment of respiratory reflex functions can lead to hypoxemia and hypercapnia. Respiratory depression occurs during general anesthesia, with cranial trauma, following severe intoxication, and in association with systemic acidosis.

The mechanisms that protect the alveolar gas exchange surfaces and that should always be considered when treating respiratory disorders include the following:

1) Pulmonary clearance mechanisms
    a) Mucociliary system
           Warming and humidifying inspired air
           Aerodynamic filtration
           Mucociliary escalator system
    b) Cough and sneezing reflexes
    c) Alveolar macrophages
    d) Alveolar surfactant
    e) Epithelial vascular exchange
    f) Lymphatic drainage
2) Pulmonary defense mechanisms
    a) Interferon
    b) Lysozyme
    c) Local immunity
           Secretory antibodies (IgA and IgG)
           Cell-mediated immunity
    d) Humoral immunity
3) Physical reactions (caseation, sequestration, nodules)

THERAPEUTIC OBJECTIVES IN THE MANAGEMENT OF RESPIRATORY DISEASES

Specific objectives depend on the etiology and pathophysiology: 1) Support intrinsic pulmonary defense systems (eg, adequate nutrition, hydration, minimal stress, immunopotentiators, interferon, hyperimmune serum) and avoid impairing the clearance and inactivating mechanisms (eg, starvation, dehydration, chilling, acidosis, uremia, endotoxemia, corticosteroids, immunosuppressant drugs, poor lung perfusion, low oxygen tension, viral and secondary bacterial infections). 2) Promote tracheobronchial secretions to protect dry, inflamed mucosae or to facilitate clearance of mucus and purulent exudate (mucokinetic or expectorant agents following rehydration). 3) Increase the beat frequency of airway cilia to promote airway clearance (cilia augmentors). 4) Suppress excessive unproductive coughing, which is exhausting and disseminates infection (antitussive agents). 5) Enhance alveolar ventilation and ensure adequate oxygen delivery (bronchodilators, oxygen therapy, and respiratory analeptics [only if specifically indicated]). 6) Shrink swollen and hyperemic mucosae in the respiratory tract (decongestants, antihistamines, and corticosteroids). 7) Prevent the development of pulmonary edema. 8) Minimize the destructive effects of acute inflammation within the lungs or respiratory tract (nonsteroidal anti-inflammatory drugs [or corticosteroids—but only in extreme situations]). 9) Treat specifically identified infections with indicated chemotherapeutic agents (antibacterial, antifungal, antiviral, or antiparasitic drugs).

EXPECTORANTS/MUCOKINETIC AGENTS

Healthy cilia, adequate volumes of respiratory tract secretions, and a functional cough are necessary to effectively clear airway mucus; however, many diseases disturb these functions and promote retention and inspissation of respiratory tract mucus. Tracheobronchitis, bronchopneumonia, and chronic obstructive pulmonary disease are good examples of such pathological states. Several pharmacological agents have been used to mobilize and effectively evacuate exudates that impair ventilation. Many of these medications can alter the consistency and rheological behavior of airway mucus, but often only at higher than recommended doses. The clinical usefulness of mucokinetic agents remains obscure mainly because there are no reliable methods to quantitate and evaluate the nature of tracheobronchial secretions during therapy. Nevertheless, expectorants are almost always included as ingredients in cough medicines and are frequently used to treat respiratory disorders in large animals.

Tracheobronchial secretions can be modified and mobilized by increasing the sol (colloid solution) layer, the hydration of mucus, and the motility of cilia, and by decreasing the amount and viscosity of mucus. These effects can be achieved by direct local action on the tracheobronchial epithelial cells and the submucosal tubuloacinar glands, or by reflex action mediated by autonomic (especially vagal) pathways. Expectorant or mucokinetic agents are administered PO, parenterally, or by inhalation (vaporization or nebulization).

Mucokinetic Diluents: These substances dilute airway mucus after aerosol or systemic administration. Dehydration is common in animals with lung disease because of diminished water intake and excessive insensible water loss associated with pyrexia and hyperpnea. In this state, it is difficult to evacuate airway secretions. Thus, rehydration is essential for effective expectorant therapy. Water and saline solutions are the practical mucokinetic diluents used to liquify hyperviscous mucus; oral rehydration, administration of parenteral fluids, and inhalation of water vapor (vaporization or "steaming") or saline aerosols (nebulization) are the approaches used. Diluents also serve as convenient carrier vehicles in aerosol therapy. Several surface active agents, with a mode of action closely related to that of diluents, are also used to facilitate hydration, emulsification, and liquification of adhesive bronchial secretions. Commonly used surface active agents are propylene glycol

(2-5%), sodium bicarbonate (2-5%), and glycerin (5%). These agents may be administered by nebulization or, at lower concentrations, instilled directly into the respiratory tract.

Bronchomucotropic Drugs (Expectorants): These drugs increase the volume and fluidity of secretions from the airway mucosa by mechanisms that are not completely understood. The modes of action are most likely based on stimulation of the gastropulmonary vagal reflex, the vagal center, terminal cholinergic fibers, or the submucosal glands directly. Various classes of bronchomucotropic agents are used.

Aromatic Volatile Oils, Stearoptenes, and Balsams: Many of the traditional expectorants are volatile oils or their derivatives, and resin-containing balsams. These agents probably stimulate the tracheobronchial glands directly and produce an associated active hyperemia in the respiratory tree. The most frequently encountered compounds found in various cough remedies include oil of eucalyptus, oil of pine, terebene, camphor, menthol, benzoin, and terpin hydrate. These compounds may be dosed PO but are usually employed in vaporizers for inhalation. Essential oils are potentially toxic. They tend to produce GI and urinary tract irritation.

Secretory Expectorants: Several inorganic and organic salts (saline expectorants) seem to stimulate the gastropulmonary vagal reflex with subsequent activation of the submucosal bronchial glands. With iodide salts, direct stimulation occurs because iodides concentrate in the glands. The most frequently used saline expectorants are potassium-, calcium-, and sodium iodide (potassium iodide—horses, cattle: 2-20 g/day, PO; dogs: 50 mg/kg/day, PO), ethylenediamine dihydroiodide, ammonium chloride and carbonate (ammonium chloride—horses: 4-15 g/12-24 hr, PO; dogs: 50 mg/kg, b.i.d., PO), and sodium and potassium nitrate. The main adverse effects to be avoided with saline expectorants are iodinism with prolonged use of the iodides, and acute hyperammonemia with ammonium salts in animals with hepatic insufficiency.

A number of substances of plant origin that produce nausea and emesis at higher doses are occasionally used at lower levels to stimulate the vagus to produce reflex secretion by the tracheobronchial glands. These agents are found mostly in proprietary cough mixtures. Examples are ipecac, squill, balsam of tolu, and cocillana.

Glyceryl guaiacolate (guaifenesin), a derivative of guaiacol obtained from creosote, is a common secretory expectorant in cough medications. It is active as a centrally acting muscle relaxant and sedative when administered IV (*see also* p 1395). Carbon dioxide and certain sulfonamides also act as secretory expectorants.

Mucolytic Expectorants: Mucolytics are substances that interfere with the structural integrity (and thus alter the viscosity) of the constituents in mucoid or purulent airway secretions, which favors airway clearance via the mucociliary escalator. Depolymerization of glycoprotein molecules or hydrolysis of protein or nucleoprotein strands are the usual mechanisms involved.

Acetylcysteine and carbocysteine are mucolytic agents that are administered as aerosols or intratracheally. Acetylcysteine, one of the most effective mucolytic drugs of this type, is generally used as a 10 or 20% solution b.i.d. to t.i.d. Two features of concern are its tendency to cause bronchospasm, ciliary inhibition, and severe coughing, and its propensity to inactivate antibiotics, particularly penicillins.

Bromhexine is another mucolytic expectorant that increases bronchial secretions and decreases their viscosity. It also results in an increase in immunoglobulin levels in airway secretions. It may be administered either PO or parenterally and has been used as ancillary therapy in the management of bronchopneumonia in horses, cattle, and pigs, as well as for the treatment of amniotic fluid aspiration in newborn calves and piglets (horses: 0.1-0.25 mg/kg, daily for 7 days; calves: 0.5-1 mg/kg, daily; dogs, cats: 1 mg/kg, b.i.d.).

Dembrixine enhances serous glandular secretions and diminishes the viscosity of tracheobronchial mucus. This drug has been used in horses at 0.3-0.5 μg/kg, b.i.d. for 10 days.

Several types of enzymes have been administered by inhalation or instillation into the bronchi to dissolve components of mucopurulent bronchial secretions. Included among these preparations are deoxyribonuclease, streptokinase, streptodornase, and trypsin. The response to these medications remains equivocal, and side effects, including airway irritation, are not uncommon.

CILIA AUGMENTORS

These are substances that increase, directly or indirectly, the beat frequency of airway cilia. The precise mechanisms involved remain unclear.

Expectorants: Potassium iodide and ammonium chloride are probably the most effective.

Adrenergic agents with prominent β_2 activity are the most effective cilia augmentors. Examples include isoproterenol, metaproterenol, salbutamol, terbutaline (cats: 1.25 mg/day, divided b.i.d.), fenoterol, albuterol, and clenbuterol (horses: 0.8 µg/kg, IV or PO, b.i.d. for 10 days).

In addition to their ability to relax smooth muscle of airways, the **methylxanthines**, especially aminophylline, increase the beat frequency of cilia.

Cholinergic agents such as neostigmine directly stimulate ciliary activity and bronchial secretions, but their airway-constricting effects preclude their therapeutic use for this purpose.

ANTITUSSIVE AGENTS

These agents diminish the frequency of coughing, and are indicated only when coughing is painful, unproductive, distressing, exhausting, or likely to exacerbate lung damage. They should not be used for productive coughs since this would allow the collection of fluids and exudate in the bronchial tree, nor should they be employed symptomatically in the absence of a diagnosis since indiscriminate inhibition of the coughing reflex could have disastrous consequences. This group of drugs acts by interfering with the cough reflex, either at the sensory receptors in the pharynx or larynx or by inhibition of the cough center in the medulla.

Locally Acting Antitussives: Locally acting antitussives are either demulcents, such as glycerin, syrup, or honey, which coat and soothe inflamed mucosae (rarely of much use in animals); or local anesthetics that block sensory impulses from the pharynx and larynx. Benzonatate acts both peripherally and centrally.

Centrally Acting Antitussives: Opiates and several of their derivatives are potent inhibitors of the medullary cough center at subanalgesic doses and are used specifically as antitussives. Two groups are recognized: those that retain narcotic properties, and a modified group known as the non-narcotic antitussives that tend not to produce euphoria or dependency.

Examples of **narcotic antitussives** include the following: morphine and camphorated tincture of opium (paregoric), codeine (dogs, cats: 1-2 mg/kg, b.i.d., PO), hydromorphone (dihydromorphinone), hydrocodone (dihydrocodeinone), and butorphanol (a narcotic agonist-antagonist; dogs: 0.25 mg/kg, IM; cats: 0.055-0.11 mg/kg, subcut.).

Examples of **non-narcotic antitussives** include the following: dextromethorphan (dogs, cats: 2 mg/kg, q.i.d., PO), pholcodine, benzonatate, and noscapine (tends to result in histamine release in dogs). Both the narcotic and non-narcotic antitussives tend to produce sedative effects, respiratory depression, occasional vomiting, and constipation with continued use.

BRONCHODILATORS

Bronchoconstriction produced by chemical mediators in hypersensitivity and inflammatory reactions often is a significant component of respiratory disease. Minor reductions in airway diameter have a marked effect on expiratory effort. To correct or prevent this, various bronchodilators are commonly used in cough mixtures, asthma preparations, or in regimens to treat acute bronchitis and pulmonary edema.

Several **adrenergic agents** have been used to elicit bronchodilation through β-receptor action and the cAMP mechanism. Those with both β_1 and β_2 activity include epinephrine (used for severe anaphylaxis), ephedrine (used in cough mixtures), isoproterenol, and orciprenaline. Selective β_2 activity produces bronchodilation without significant cardiostimulatory effects. This desirable property is evident in such longer-acting adrenergic agents as salbutamol, fenoterol, hexoprenaline, clenbuterol, terbutaline, and others. Common side effects observed with β_2 selective adrenergic drugs include nervousness, sweating, muscle tremors, weakness, and vomiting with high doses.

Epinephrine, ephedrine (dogs, cats: 1-3 mg/kg, q8-12hr, PO), and pseudoephedrine also possess α-agonistic properties that are beneficial because the induced vasoconstriction in the bronchi reduces mucosal swelling.

Methylxanthines such as caffeine, theophylline, and theobromine possess the ability to inhibit phosphodiesterase and thereby to increase the levels of cAMP within cells. The effect on the bronchi is to relax contracted bronchial smooth muscle cells. Since β_2 agonists promote the synthesis of cAMP through adenylate cyclase, and the methylxanthines prevent the inactivation of cAMP by phosphodiesterase, it is rational to use bronchodilators from both classes when dealing with a refractory case. The methylxanthines may also possess other pharmacological effects that promote bronchodilation.

Theophylline and several of its derivatives are the most useful methylxanthine bronchodilators. Theophylline itself can be administered PO only, whereas theophylline ethylenediamine (aminophylline—horses: 9-15 mg/kg, b.i.d., PO; dogs: 10 mg/kg, b.i.d., PO, IM, or IV; cats: 5 mg/kg, b.i.d., PO or IV), theophylline sodium glycinate, and choline theophyllinate (oxtriphylline) are also available in dosage forms suitable for injection.

Anticholinergic agents decrease vagal tone in bronchiolar smooth muscle, and may be useful in certain cases of bronchoconstriction. Atropine has been used for many years for the palliative relief of chronic obstructive pulmonary disease (heaves) in horses. Atropine and other anticholinergic drugs, such as glycopyrrolate, ipratropium, and deptropine, augment the bronchodilator effects of the adrenergic agents. The reduction in tracheobronchial secretions with an increase in mucus viscosity is a disadvantage of the anticholinergic agents when they are used to treat bronchoconstrictive states. Ipratropium delivered by aerosol is said not to have these side effects.

Corticosteroids (see ANTI-INFLAMMATORY AGENTS, p 1502) are very beneficial in cases of severe crippling asthma that are not responsive to the standard bronchodilator therapy. Due to the ability of corticosteroids to inhibit phospholipase enzymes in cell membranes, they prevent the formation of prostaglandins and leukotrienes—powerful endogenous bronchoconstrictive substances. The corticosteroids also counteract the effect of histamine and other inflammagens, and enhance the bronchodilator effects of sympathomimetics. Though they should not be used routinely as bronchodilators, the corticosteroids may produce successful responses in chronic refractory allergic respiratory conditions or in life-threatening bronchoconstrictive episodes.

DECONGESTANTS

Adrenergic agents with α-agonistic activity produce vasoconstriction in mucous membranes, which reduces swelling and edema. These drugs are used topically as nasal decongestants in allergic and viral rhinitis, and systemically as respiratory tract decongestants. The use of decongestants in veterinary medicine is not common. Examples of α-adrenergic agents used for this purpose include ephedrine, pseudoephedrine, phenylephrine, phenylpropanolamine, and naphazoline.

ANTIHISTAMINIC AND OTHER ANTIALLERGIC AGENTS

Antihistaminic agents that block H_1 receptors are commonly included in cough mixtures and cold remedies, and have been employed in the treatment of acute respiratory infections. The role of histamine in hypersensitivity reactions and as an inflammagen is well known, but the routine use of antihistamines for the treatment of disorders of the respiratory system, other than allergic manifestations, remains of questionable benefit. Several of these agents, however, do exert some central action on the cough center and may reduce bronchospasm; examples include promethazine and diphenhydramine.

Cromolyn sodium (sodium cromoglycate) is used to control asthmatic attacks in man. It acts by preventing antigen-induced release of histamine and other mediators from sensitized mast cells. Because it is available only as an aerosol of fine particles to be administered by inhalation, it is not often used in veterinary medicine. However, when it is administered to horses using a special nebulizer (80 mg/day for 1-4 days), clinically normal horses will be protected for 3-20 days.

RESPIRATORY ANALEPTICS

Respiratory analeptics (or medullary stimulants), such as doxapram and bemegride, are occasionally used to stimulate the respiratory centers in the medulla. Their use is mostly limited to cases of drug-induced medullary depression and apnea in the neonate. A number of therapeutic short-comings are associated with their use.

OXYGEN THERAPY

When alveolar ventilation is critically compromised, for whatever reason, the primary goal is to provide an adequate supply of oxygen. Oxygen should be delivered by means of a mask, endotracheal tube, nasal catheter, respirator, or an oxygen cage. It is advisable to administer a mixture of 95% oxygen and 5% carbon dioxide. Oxygen tends to increase the viscosity of respiratory secretions and, if administered alone for any length of time, may damage pulmonary endothelial cells and lead to pulmonary edema and generalized atelectasis (oxygen toxicity). The addition of carbon dioxide promotes hyperemia of the respiratory tract and an increase in the volume and fluidity of secretions and, more importantly, provides a physiological stimulation of the respiratory centers. A concentration of 40-60% oxygen in the inspired air is regarded as optimal; flow rates of 2-5 L/min for small animals, and ~12 L/min for large animals are used.

MANAGEMENT OF ACUTE PULMONARY EDEMA

Pulmonary edema often constitutes an acute life-threatening condition that requires prompt and diligent attention. A selection of the following therapeutic interventions may be appropriate to manage a case, depending on the etiology and pathophysiology: oxygen therapy—with a volume respirator and positive end-expiratory pressure (5-20 cm H_2O); bronchodilators—adrenergic agents and aminophylline; narcotic analgesic—morphine (small doses) decreases respiratory rate, diminishes anxiety, and dilates splanchnic vessels; diuretics—preferably a loop-acting agent such as furosemide; colloidal solutions—plasma or whole blood to correct hypoalbuminemia (6% gelatin or 6% dextran-70 in saline); corticosteroids and dimethyl sulfoxide—may limit transcapillary effusion in the presence of pulmonary insult; ethanol nebulization (or other nonionic surfactants such as propylene glycol and glycerol)—limits foaming within the bronchial tree and promotes effective alveolar ventilation and gaseous exchange; inotropic agents—when pulmonary edema is caused or aggravated by left ventricular failure; and antibiotics—used prophylactically to prevent secondary bacterial infection.

URINARY SYSTEM

This discussion focuses on small animals, in which urinary tract diseases are more prevalent than they are in large animals. However, the principles of approach are applicable to all species. For more information on specific diseases, see the URINARY SYSTEM, p 869 *et seq* (and also the INDEX).

Diseases of the canine and feline urinary tract are common; the urinary tract is second only to the skin in developing bacterial infections. Acute or chronic problems in renal function may be life-threatening, especially in geriatric cats. Since the primary function of the kidneys is to maintain the body's electrolyte and fluid balance, diseases of other systems are often reflected in renal dysfunction. Many of these diseases are treated by management, not cure. Therefore, understanding the therapeutics of these diseases is crucial.

ACUTE RENAL DISEASE (ARD)

Acute renal dysfunction can be subdivided into 3 main categories: anuric, oliguric, and nonoliguric. It is critical that urine production be measured to decide correctly which therapy to employ, and to monitor its effect. Acute failure can be precipitated by prerenal, renal, and postrenal causes. Prerenal causes are the most common and amenable to treatment. Acute tubular necrosis (ATN) from ischemic or toxic insults is less common, and often difficult to treat. Detection of azotemia (or uremic signs) in the presence of a concentrated urine specific gravity (>1.030) indicates a prerenal etiology or early ATN. If prerenal causes can be ruled out, ATN should be considered and urine output monitored. Dogs producing <0.25-5 mL of urine/kg/hr in the face of normal hydration should be considered to be in acute renal failure.

Fluid Therapy: (*See also* p 1355.) Rehydration is accomplished best with isotonic IV fluids. However, the exact type of fluid depends on electrolyte imbalances present and the acid-base status. If the animal has normal cardiovascular function, volume diuresis should be tried by giving an excess of fluid equal to 1-3% of the body weight. Fluids should not be delivered rapidly, particularly if the animal is oliguiric or anuric, but be given over 4-6 hr.

Diuretics/Vasodilators: In the oliguric animal not responding to volume diuresis, furosemide may be used; however, its effectiveness is unclear. It should not be used in anuric animals due to lack of efficacy and potential toxicity. A standard protocol is an initial IV dose of 2 mg furosemide per kg body wt, followed by increasing the dose by 2 mg/kg/hr until diuresis follows or until a total dose of 6-8 mg/kg is reached. If diuresis results, furosemide is continued t.i.d. as needed. Furosemide does not "flush" the kidneys, improve renal function, nor increase the glomerular filtration rate; it may however, improve renal blood flow, decrease resorption of sodium and chloride, and increase free water excretion.

Mannitol is efficacious in experimental models of ATN, acting as a protectant against further tubular damage and initiating an osmotic diuresis. Doses of 0.25-0.5 g/kg of a 20% (0.2 g/mL) solution of mannitol should be given over 15-20 min. If diuresis begins, mannitol can be repeated q6hr.

In animals with oliguric or anuric renal failure, dopamine is valuable. It is an adrenergic neurotransmitter with specific receptors in the renal vasculature. Doses of 2-4 µg/kg/min can increase renal blood flow and glomerular filtration. The drug has a very short half-life, and the dose can be adjusted easily by decreasing or increasing the infusion rate. A significant increase in heart rate suggests that the drug is activating β receptors that will actually decrease renal blood flow, and indicates the dose should be lowered. Development of an arrhythmia also indicates the dose should be lowered.

CHRONIC RENAL DISEASE (CRD)

Fluid Therapy: In chronic renal failure, fluid homeostasis is most affected and dehydration often precipitates an acute crisis. Rehydration and correction of acid-base disturbances are a priority. The same principles used in ARD are used in this disorder, but in general are more successful.

Antacids/H$_2$ Antagonists: Common sequelae of CRD involve electrolyte imbalances, particularly in calcium-phosphate and uremic gastritis. Hyperphosphatemia is responsible for many long-term sequelae of CRD by causing an increase in parathyroid hormone (PTH). Thus, treatment is best accomplished by using a diet that is restricted in protein and phosphorus. Some animals may also require aluminum-containing antacids, which bind phosphorus in the intestine and thus decrease its absorption. The antacid should contain aluminum hydroxide, carbonate, or oxide. Aluminum hydroxide gel is commonly used and its dose must be individualized by monitoring serum phosphorus concentrations. Optimally, the fasting serum phosphorus should be 3-5 mg/dL.

Uremic gastritis can occur in both ARD and CRD. Specific H_2 antagonists, eg, cimetidine or ranitidine, reduce stomach acidity and are helpful in reducing the extent of tissue injury and pain. Both block the histamine receptor, which (when stimulated by acetylcholine, histamine, or gastrin) causes acid secretion. Cimetidine can be given at 5-10 mg/kg, IV, q8-12hr and when possible switched to a similar dose PO. Ranitidine is more potent and has a longer biological half-life and therefore has a lower dose rate: 0.5-2.5 mg/kg, b.i.d. Sucralfate is commonly used with an H_2 blocker, but it should be noted that this combination is not logical. Sucralfate is a complex sugar that forms a thick, sticky polymer if pH is <4. This sticky material adheres to denuded gastric mucosa and protects the surface from acid and further destruction. H_2 antagonists increase the pH of the stomach, which decreases their usefulness. Comparative clinical trials in man have found sucralfate equal to cimetidine; one or the other should be used to treat uremic gastritis. Cimetidine has the added clinical advantage of decreasing serum PTH concentrations.

GLOMERULAR DISEASE

A variety of glomerulonephropathies are found in dogs and cats, and the term is used to describe a heterogeneous group of diseases that affect primarily the glomeruli. Most are caused by an immune-mediated mechanism; therefore, treatment is directed at alleviating the underlying disease (eg, pyometra, *Dirofilaria immitis* infection, or bacterial sepsis). Prognosis for these diseases is good. When the cause is unknown, neoplasia, or amyloid deposition, the prognosis is guarded because a single effective treatment regime has not been established. Glucocorticoids, immunosuppressive therapy, dimethyl sulfoxide, and protein-restricted diets have been used with variable results. (Note: Steroids are of no benefit in dogs or cats with renal amyloidosis, and may be harmful.)

DIABETES INSIPIDUS (DI)

Nephrogenic DI is not a specific disease but represents a physiologic condition in which the kidneys fail to concentrate urine despite adequate (or excessive amounts of) antidiuretic hormone (ADH, vasopressin). This is in contrast to central or pituitary-dependent DI, in which the lack of ADH production causes excessive polydipsia and polyuria. The diuretic chlorothiazide (20-40 mg/kg, b.i.d.) combined with a low-salt diet is a moderately effective treatment of both forms of DI (qv, p 278). The mechanism is not completely understood but probably involves the natriuretic effect of chlorothiazide; this in turn depletes the body of sodium, which stimulates the atrial natriuretic factor (ANF). ANF increases the absorption of sodium (and water) in the proximal tubule, which leaves less filtrate to go to the distal tubule where ADH works, and thus reduces urine production.

In central DI, vasopressin (pitressin tannate in oil) can be given as an injectable starting at 1-2 u, subcut. every 2-3 days and adjusted until the polydipsia decreases. Alternatively, desmopressin acetate can be given intranasally or subconjunctivally starting with a dose of 1 drop, t.i.d.

URINARY TRACT INFECTIONS (UTI)

UTI in dogs are common, and often respond to a multitude of antibiotic regimes. There are, however, many cases of nonresponding or recurring infection that require a more systematic approach to therapy. This involves a simple process defining duration, clinical severity, and location, and identification of the UTI as a relapsing or recurring infection. Based on these factors, therapeutic approaches and clinical expectations can be developed, improving the chances of resolving these often frustating cases. Signs of UTI vary with its location and duration. Simple urethrocystitis can be acute, or an acute exacerbation of a chronic condition. The animal has the classical signs of pollakiuria, dysuria, and gross or occult hematuria. *Escherichia coli* and *Staphylococcus* spp account for over two-thirds of acute UTI regardless of geographical location. *Escherichia coli* has been identified as having a predilection for colonizing the urogenital tract of dogs. This predilection may explain why UTI are so common in dogs and why dogs with a lack of appropriate defenses are continually reinfected.

Many animals, however, have either no clinical signs but bacteriuria, or clinical signs but no culturable bacteria. Urinalysis is particularly important in animals with a previous history of UTI or with medical risk factors for developing subclinical bacteriuria. Risk factors are diabetes mellitus, CRD, hyperadrenocorticism, or chronic steroid treatment. Animals with evidence of bacteria on urinalysis but with negative cultures may be infected with mycoplasma, and reculturing for this pathogen is indicated.

Recurring versus a relapsing infection is important to identify. Recurring infections imply a bacteriological cure from the previous infection, with subsequent recolonization of the urinary tract. These animals are often predisposed to infections due to anatomical or systemic diseases that alter their normal defenses. A relapsing infection is one that was not completely eradicated with the last treatment. The importance in differentiating these 2 conditions is in the approach to treatment and therapeutic expectations.

The common approach to therapy has been reduced to simply choosing a correct antibiotic, but this simplistic approach, when unsuccessful, implies that failure was a result of using the wrong antibiotic. Thus, the simple objective of antimicrobial therapy fails to consider the complex environment in which some infections exist. The goal of antimicrobial therapy is to help the body eliminate infectious organisms. The natural defense mechanisms are of primary importance in preventing or controlling infection. Development of uropathogens or opportunistic infections is prevented by hypertonicity and pH of the urine, complete voiding, and lack of substantial nutrients (sugars, protein). Once microbial invasion has occurred, several host responses may combat the invading organisms.

Therapeutic objectives are necessary to modify treatment efficiently. What clinical or laboratory signs indicate successful treatment and how long into therapy are they expected? When should therapy be reevaluated and what criteria used to decide when to change antibiotics and to which one? Also, antimicrobial therapy is sometimes expected to do more than kill pathogens. Clinical signs may not all be caused by the pathogen: successful antibiotic therapy does not ensure an improvement in the animal's clinical status.

Simple, Acute Urethrocystitis: The therapeutic plan should include a 2- to 3-wk course of an antibiotic with a good to excellent probability of success against the most likely pathogens involved: *Escherichia coli*, staphylococci, and streptococci. Bacterial infection may be eradicated with trimethoprim/sulfadiazine at 30 mg/kg, once daily or divided b.i.d., or with amoxicillin/clavulanic acid at 5-7.5 mg/kg, b.i.d. Clinical signs, if present, should decrease within a few days. If signs are still present after 4 days, then the urine should be cultured (the antibiotic in the urine will not be a problem if the bacteria are resistant).

Simple, Relapsing Urethrocystitis: The therapeutic plan should include a urinalysis, culture and sensitivity, abdominal radiographs, and serum chemistries. Expectations depend on finding a possible etiology for the relapse. If none is found, the prognosis can still be good, but not for 100% success. Subsequent antibiotic therapy should be started only if unacceptable clinical signs are present, and the antibiotic should be of a different family than that of the previous treatment. Enrofloxacin and ciprofloxacin at 2.5-5 mg/kg and 5-10 mg/kg, b.i.d., respectively, are both fluoroquinolones that can be effective in these cases. If the cause cannot be identified, then an antibiotic (identified as effective in a culture and sensitivity) should be used in a treatment regime of 3-4 wk with a urine culture done during the second week. A culture should be performed 1 wk and 1 mo following the last dose to ensure complete resolution.

Simple, Recurring Urethrocystitis: The therapeutic plan is the same as for relapses (*see* above). The expectations of cure, however, are less since ability to prevent colonization of the urinary tract may be deficient. An initial plan should involve 2-3 wk of an appropriate antibiotic (chosen from susceptibility testing), followed by a culture and sensitivity 3 days after cessation of antibiotic therapy to ensure eradication. In cases of multiple episodes of recurring urethrocystitis, antibiotic therapy should continue once daily (at night) with bimonthly urine cultures for 3-6 mo to ensure success. Amoxicillin (2.5-5 mg/kg) or tetracycline (5 mg/kg) can be effective in these cases. Once-a-day therapy may have to be continued indefinitely depending on the degree of immunocompetence. Emergence of resistance during this period is not uncommon and if it occurs will require changing antibiotics and lowering expectations of cure.

Complicated Urinary Tract Infections: Pyelonephritis, prostatitis, emphysematous cystitis, or relapsing or recurring urethrocystitis in animals with a systemic cause for the infection may be described as complicated. The therapeutic plan may involve surgery. Antibiotic therapy before a culture and sensitivity test is warranted only if the animal is systemically infected, or if surgery must be done before results of the test are known. In severely debilitated, renally compromised animals, cefoxitin at 2.5-5 mg/kg, IV, b.i.d. to t.i.d., is recommmeded because of its excellent efficacy and potency against *Escherichia coli*, the most common UTI pathogen. In less compromised animals, able to tolerate oral drugs, enrofloxacin (2.5-5 mg/kg, b.i.d.) or ciprofloxacin (5-10 mg/kg, b.i.d.) combined with amoxicillin (2.5-5 mg/kg) provides broad and potent antibacterial coverage. Both should be administered a few hours before surgery to ensure adequate absorption. If a urinary catheter is required, no antibiotic should be used until it is removed since catheters inhibit normal defense mechanisms.

FELINE UROLOGICAL SYNDROME (FUS)

FUS is more likely to be a lower urinary tract disease of diverse origins than a specific disease entity. Identifiable infectious causes of FUS are uncommon in cats; ~95% are sterile cystitis. Feline bacterial cystitis is treated as in dogs. There are no known treatments of the more common form of the disease, but dietary management to lower the chance of recurrence and symptomatic relief of the discomfort of micturation is commonly used.

There is no indication for antibiotic use in nonobstructed, sterile FUS. It is usually a self-limiting disease with a clinical course of 5-7 days. Low-magnesium diets have proliferated in commercial feline diets based on the correlation between high magnesium content and urethral obstruction of male cats. Propantheline (as well as a host of other quaternary anticholinergics) is an antimuscarinic antagonist similar to atropine but more potent and without CNS effects. The drug blocks the parasympathetic control of the bladder and theoretically decreases its sphincter spasticity due to irritation. A dose of 7.5 mg/cat every 3 days is suggested in nonobstructed cats. The efficacy of this treatment is unclear. A short course (3-5 days) of short-acting glucocorticoids (prednisone or prednisolone) may alleviate bladder irritation.

UROLITHIASIS

Urolithiasis (qv, p 885) is common in both dogs and cats. Most uroliths are secondary to bacterial infections (*Staphylococcus* sp, *Proteus* sp) causing an alkaline pH. However, some (eg, cystine uroliths) are due to genetic metabolism errors and require a different therapeutic approach.

Antibiotics: Antibiotic selection should be based on a culture from the urolith if possible, or if not, from the urine. Appropriate antibiotics should be initiated after surgical removal and culture. Starting antibiotic therapy while uroliths are present may improve the acute signs of cystitis but may not resolve the infection. If an antibiotic is used while on a calculolytic diet, the antibiotic should be used for the entire length of treatment unless urine culture and sensitivity indicate a change in sensitivity. These animals should be monitored carefully since the recurrence of uroliths is high due to recurrent urinary tract infection, which may require chronic antibiotic therapy.

Diet: Feeding a commercial calculolytic diet exclusively can be an effective non-surgical treatment of these types of uroliths. Such diets have low amounts of high-quality protein to decrease urea and therefore ammonium ion excretion. They are reduced in magnesium and phosphorus and have increased quantities of sodium chloride to stimulate water intake. They should produce a polydipsia-polyuria and encourage the dog to drink. The diet should not be supplemented, and should be continued ≥1 mo after radiographic evidence of dissolution.

Urinary Acidifiers: Uroliths not responding to diet may be helped by acidifying the urine. Ammonium chloride is an effective urinary acidifier at 600 mg/kg/day, but it does increase the concentration of available ammonium ions. DL-Methionine at 0.2-1 g/day is less effective but better tolerated and not a component of uroliths.

Other Agents: Acetohydroxamic acid (AHA) at 25 mg/kg/day can be used successfully as an adjuvant to prevent recurrence in those dogs with struvite uroliths due to urease-producing bacteria (those that increase the pH of the urine). AHA is a urease inhibitor that prevents these bacteria from breaking down urea to ammonium ions, a major component of struvite. Allopurinol at 10 mg/kg, t.i.d., is recommended in dogs with urate crystals due to an inability to process purines.

URINARY INCONTINENCE

Urinary incontinence can be from estrogen or testosterone deficiencies, neurogenic dysfunction (urethral sphincter hypotonus), anatomical abnormalities (eg, ectopic ureters), or paradoxical obstruction from urethral calculi or neoplasia. The latter 2 must be treated surgically.

Hormones: Estrogen-responsive incontinence is a well-described phenomena in female dogs, yet the role estrogen plays in maintaining urethral sphincter tone is unknown. Treatment with synthetic estrogens (diethylstilbestrol [DES]) for all cases of incontinence has fallen out of favor due to other successful approaches and the high frequency of bone marrow toxicity induced by estrogens. However, for those female dogs with estrogen-responsive incontinence, DES is recommended at 0.1-0.3 mg/kg, daily for 7-10 days, followed by a similar dose once a week. Some of these dogs may require less DES and should be maintained at the lowest possible dose. Testosterone-responsive incontinence is less common in castrated male dogs. Injectable testosterone cypionate has had long-term effects (months) after a single dose of 5 mg/kg. Synthetic methylated testosterones should be avoided as they not uncommonly cause hepatic toxicity.

Adrenergic Agonist: Phenylpropanolamine (PPA) is a weak α agonist used in cold medications and over-the-counter diet pills. The muscles controlling the urethral muscle tone are under adrenergic control; thus, PPA increases sphincter tone. The dose is 12.5-50 mg/kg, b.i.d. to t.i.d. The effect is short-lived and the dose needs to be titrated to effect. As with any adrenergic agonist, side effects are excitability and restlessness. Skipping a single dose and restarting at half of the previous dose should be sufficient in cases of an overdose. In addition to the above agents, PPA may be used in either male or female dogs as an alternative to DES or testosterone to obtain optimal control.

URINARY RETENTION

Disorders of micturition are characterized by abnormalities in either the voiding or storage of urine, and may be non-neurogenic (eg, urolithiasis, prostatitis) or neurogenic in nature. Neurogenic disorders are usually divided into 3 categories. Upper motor neuron lesions involve the spinal cord cranial to the sacral segments, the brain stem, the cerebellum and the cerebrum; lesions of these areas are characterized by lack of voluntary control of urination, partial bladder emptying, increased urethral sphincter tone, and large residual volume. The second category of lower motor neuron (LMN) injuries involves the pelvic nerve, the sacral spinal cord segments, cauda equina, and the bladder. LMN damage results in a large residual urine volume and is characterized by involuntary urine leakage when abdominal pressure is increased. Breakdown of the tight junctions between detrusor muscle cells of the bladder (postobstruction) prevents normal depolarization and contraction of the detrusor muscles, resulting in an atonic bladder. The bladder is easily expressed in all LMN conditions. The third category is reflex dyssnergia, which is characterized by increased sphincter tone opposing detrusor muscle contraction, which functionally obstructs the bladder.

Management: When the urethral sphincter tone is normal or hypotonic, manual expression 3-4 times daily is usually sufficient. Urinary tract infection in these dogs is common and likely to recur following treatment. Antibiotics should be used as needed, and continued treatment is unwarranted since it will likely select for a resistant organism to colonize the bladder.

Anti-adrenergic: When the sphincter muscle tone is excessive and manual expression nonproductive, an antiadrenergic agent is recommended. Phenoxybenzamine is an irreversible α-adrenergic blocking agent that has been used with some success. Initial doses are 10 mg/dog/day, with the dose doubled every 4-6 days until the bladder can be expressed manually or the dog is voiding on its own. This drug is a potent α blocker that can cause hypertension and weakness. The biologic effect is independent of its half-life since new receptors have to be made before the effect is decreased.

Muscle Relaxers: Diazepam is a benzodiazepine that is usually used to reduce anxiety. However, at higher doses it is a central muscle relaxant. The drug is unspecific and relaxation sufficient to allow micturation may cause sedation. Dogs metabolize diazepam 20-30 times faster than man and can tolerate much higher doses. Doses can be started at 2-10 mg/day/dog and increased as needed until effective, or excessive sedation develops. The animal should be encouraged to urinate or the bladder expressed ~30 min after administration.

Cholinergics: In dogs with detrusor hyporeflexia or atony, bethanecol chloride may be of some benefit. This cholinergic agonist stimulates the initiation of the detrusor muscle concentration but does not work at the motor nerve end-plates. Therefore, in dogs with weak contractions, bethanecol at 5-25 mg/kg, PO, t.i.d., may increase contractions. In dogs with total areflexia, however, this drug has no effect.

CHEMOTHERAPEUTICS

When an animal is treated with a chemotherapeutic agent, 3 entities are involved: the host animal, the pathogen, and the drug. This relationship is called the chemotherapeutic triangle, and the key features are illustrated below.

The chemotherapeutic armamentarium includes antibacterial, antiviral, antifungal, antiparasitic, and antineoplastic compounds. The basic mechanisms through which many of these agents exert their destructive effects against pathogens are known. More importantly, the methods by which harmful organisms may protect themselves against the action of specific drugs are also becoming better understood. The pharmacological modulation of these processes has added new dimensions to modern chemotherapeutics.

Chemotherapeutic agents may be selectively toxic for invading micro- or macroorganisms, but in many cases they are also capable of producing adverse effects in the host animal. To avoid toxic manifestations, the dose rate often becomes critical; additionally, the clinical condition of the animal and concurrently administered drugs also can be responsible. Chemotherapeutic agents that are absorbed or

Figure 3.   Chemotherapeutic Triangle

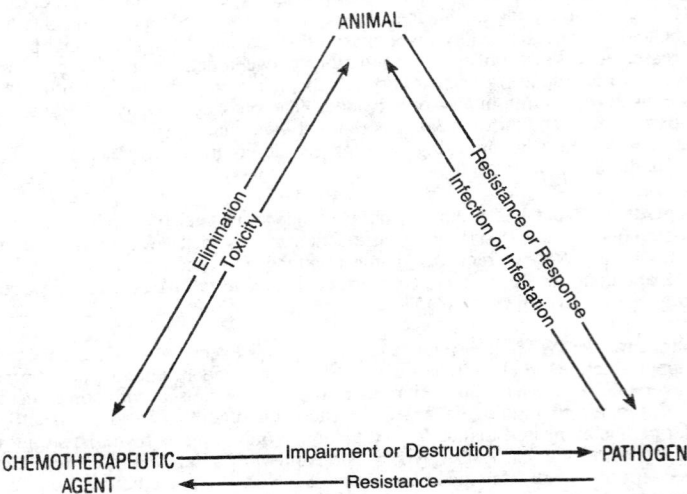

injected into the body are eliminated by the same processes that are discussed above for all xenobiotics. The effect that disease may have on the absorption, distribution, biotransformation, and excretion of a therapeutic agent may be of notable clinical significance.

The effect of the pathogen on the host and its response to infection are also important components of the chemotherapeutic triangle. The pathogenesis of the disease, the pathophysiological reactions, and the resultant lesions may have important bearings on clinical management; in addition to appropriate chemotherapy, supportive and adjunctive treatment may be crucial for success. Therapeutic measures such as fluids, blood transfusion, antisera, anti-inflammatory drugs, positive inotropic agents, and bronchodilators could well be life-saving, depending on the particular case.

Also, nonspecific and specific immune mechanisms play a vital role as part of the animal's response to an invading pathogen. Host defense mechanisms should be sustained by whatever means possible when treating an infectious or parasitic disease; otherwise, protracted recovery or relapses are almost inevitable. Minimizing stress, furnishing quality nutritional support, administering specific immunoglobulins, and using immunopotentiators are some of the approaches that may be employed. These general principles apply to the use of each class of chemotherapeutic agent that is discussed below.

GUIDELINES FOR CLINICAL USE OF
ANTIMICROBIAL AGENTS

The rational therapeutic management of infection is based on selection of an appropriate antimicrobial agent and course of treatment that will inhibit or destroy the specific pathogens without compromising the animal's response. The pathogen should be destroyed, or at least inhibited swiftly, to permit the host to begin recovery without relapse, and to avoid emergence of microbial resistance and drug-induced toxicity. Factors related to the animal, the antimicrobial agent, and the pathogenic organism all play significant roles.

Successful antimicrobial therapy is based on 4 objectives. 1) Identify and characterize the pathogen(s), including its antimicrobial sensitivity, and select a drug based on the sites of infection and the lesions. 2) Achieve effective concentrations of the indicated antimicrobial agent for a sufficient period at the site(s) of infection. 3) Select a dose rate, frequency, and route of administration of the antimicrobial agent, as well as the duration of therapy, that will ensure a cure and prevent relapse without causing any harmful drug-induced effects in the animal. 4) Provide specific as well as appropriate supportive therapy to enhance the animal's ability to overcome the infection and associated disease conditions.

The ideal is to know the minimal inhibitory concentration (MIC) or even the minimal antibiotic concentration (MAC) of an antibacterial agent for a particular pathogen, and then to employ dose rates that provide at least 4-5 times the MIC in the infected tissues or fluids. (For aminoglycosides, 8 times the MIC is optimum, but this is near the toxic range for most agents in this class.) However, the reported MIC for a particular bacterial species is not always constant. Methodology, different strains (regional), media used, rate of drug diffusion in the media, time (regrowth), bacteriostatic versus bactericidal concentrations, and degree of bacterial inhibition actually required for effective therapy are all significant considerations. It may not even be necessary to maintain inhibitory concentrations of antimicrobial drugs at all times during treatment. Persistent antibacterial effects at subinhibitory concentrations (postantibiotic effects), which facilitate removal of affected bacteria by host defense mechanisms, have been demonstrated for penicillins, cephalosporins, macrolides, tetracyclines, aminoglycosides, and several other antibacterial agents. Organisms damaged by antibiotics are more susceptible to leukocidal activity.

The immunocompetence of the animal should always be appraised, recognizing that extraneous factors, stress, disease, malnutrition, and the effects of concurrently administered drugs may influence the animal's ability to resist infection. Host defense systems are seriously compromised in bone marrow depression, hypogammaglobulinemia, incapacitated alveolar macrophages, tracheobronchitis, necrotic enteritis, starvation, and other conditions. In addition, immunosuppressants (eg, corticosteroids and antineoplastics) compromise immune response. Any impediment of immune capabilities can be expected to modify the effectiveness of many antimicrobial agents, especially those with only bacteriostatic activity.

The use of combinations of antibacterial drugs (*see* below) to treat or prevent infections is widespread and may be beneficial. However, many factors may confound the synergistic or additive effects of antimicrobial agents, and antagonism does occur between specific drugs, both *in vitro* and *in vivo*. As a rule, antibacterial agents should not be used in combination indiscriminately or without justification.

REQUIREMENTS FOR SUCCESSFUL ANTIMICROBIAL THERAPY

1) Clinical diagnosis. Successful chemotherapy usually requires a specific diagnosis, even though a reasonable preliminary diagnosis is often all that is possible, at least initially.

2) Microbiological diagnosis. Treatment should be aimed at a specific pathogen whenever feasible. However, polymicrobial infections often occur. The ideal is a conclusive microbiological diagnosis, but frequently this must be presumptive (at least initially), and treatment must be based on experience. Rational deduction may be necessary under field conditions. The examination of a direct smear stained with Wright's or Gram's stain may prove to be helpful to at least establish what types of pathogens are involved (gram-positive or gram-negative rods or cocci).

3) Culture and sensitivity testing. Isolation and characterization of the causative pathogen, sensitivity testing, and determination of the MIC provide a sound foundation from which to select the antimicrobial drug as well as dosage regimen. However, under field conditions, it is often difficult to attain laboratory support for antimicrobial therapy.

4) Appropriate selection of antimicrobial agents. Among the factors to be considered are the causative microorganism(s), results of sensitivity tests, pathogenicity of organisms, pathological lesions, acuteness of infection, kinetics of the drug(s)

indicated, expense, potential drug toxicity, organic dysfunctions (especially kidney and liver function), and possible interactions with co-administered drugs.

5) Correct dosage and route of administration. The dose selected should result in adequate therapeutic concentrations at the site(s) of infection for sufficient time without causing side effects or toxicity. For bactericidal drugs, therapeutic success appears to be greater if the concentration remains above the MIC for about one-half to two-thirds of the dosage interval. The advocated dosage schedules should be carefully followed for 3-5 days, or longer if needed, to ensure elimination of the pathogen and to prevent relapse or reinfection.

6) Ancillary treatment, nutritional support, and nursing care. Supportive treatment, optimal nutrition, and general nursing care are often critical for successful management of infectious disease. Ancillary treatment might include the use of anti-inflammatory agents, antidiarrheal preparations, expectorants, bronchodilators, inotropic agents, urinary acidifiers and alkalinizers, immunopotentiators, and fluid and electrolyte replacement. Attention should be given to caloric and nutrient intake, especially of protein and vitamins. These nutrients play a cardinal role in immune responsiveness.

COMBINATION THERAPY

Treatment with antimicrobial combinations may be necessary in certain cases. The administration of 2 or more agents may be beneficial to: 1) treat mixed bacterial infections in which the organisms are not susceptible to a common agent, 2) achieve synergistic antimicrobial activity against particularly resistant strains (eg, *Pseudomonas aeruginosa*), 3) overcome bacterial tolerance, 4) prevent the emergence of drug resistance, 5) minimize toxicity, or 6) prevent inactivation of an antibiotic by enzymes produced by other bacteria that are present.

Additive or synergistic effects do occur when antibacterial agents are used in combination, but antagonism may also emerge, sometimes with serious consequences. Generally, bacteriostatic agents act in an additive fashion, whereas bactericidal agents are often synergistic. However, the effects of several bactericidal antibiotics are substantially impaired by simultaneous use of a bacteriostatic agent. This is a general guideline only; many exceptions are known, and many confounding factors also play a role. A general classification of some common antimicrobials as bactericidal or bacteriostatic is listed below:

Bactericidal (at **usual** concentrations)	Bacteriostatic
penicillins	tetracyclines
cephalosporins	chloramphenicol
aminoglycosides	macrolides
trimethoprim/sulfonamides	lincosamides
nitrofurans	spectinomycin
metronidazole	sulfonamides
quinolones	

Examples of combination therapy for mixed infections include the use of clindamycin, metronidazole, or the semisynthetic penicillins for their anaerobic coverage in combination with aminoglycosides for their gram-negative efficacy. Synergism against certain bacterial pathogens frequently can be achieved with combinations of penicillins or cephalosporins and aminoglycosides. The combined use of trimethoprim with selected sulfonamides also has a synergistic effect.

Preventing the development of resistance with combination antimicrobial therapy is best exemplified by the use of carbenicillin or ticarcillin together with gentamicin or tobramycin for the treatment of *Pseudomonas* infections.

Bacterial enzymatic inactivation of β-lactam antibiotics such as the penicillins and cephalosporins can be prevented by concurrent administration of a β-lactamase inhibitor such as clavulanic acid or sulbactam.

MECHANISMS OF ACTION

Antimicrobial agents affect susceptible organisms in various ways. Details are covered under each class later. The following is a general listing of the various mechanisms of action. 1) Inhibition of cell wall synthesis: penicillins, cephalosporins and cephamycins, vancomycin, bacitracin, cycloserine. 2) Impairment of cell membrane function: polymyxin B, colistin, tyrocidin, amphotericin, nystatin. 3) Inhibition of protein synthesis: tetracyclines, aminoglycosides, spectinomycin, chloramphenicol, macrolides, lincosamides. 4) Inhibition of DNA synthesis and replication: novobiocin, quinolones, griseofulvin. 5) Inhibition of DNA-dependent RNA polymerase: rifamycins. 6) Inhibition of folinic acid and consequently DNA synthesis: sulfonamides, trimethoprim.

Bacteria, in turn, sometimes protect themselves from these destructive effects by a variety of means as outlined below and discussed in more detail under each class of antimicrobial agents.

REASONS FOR FAILURE OF ANTIBACTERIAL THERAPY

1) The diagnosis was incorrect, eg, viral and not bacterial infection. 2) The organisms were not susceptible to the action of the antibiotic that was selected, or they were in static phase and therefore refractory ("persisters"). 3) Although originally susceptible, the bacteria developed resistance. 4) The antibiotic(s) was insufficient for multiple pathogens. 5) A combination of incompatible antibiotics was administered. 6) Superinfection by a resistant opportunistic pathogen occurred. 7) Reinfection by the original or by other pathogenic bacteria occurred. 8) Drainage was inadequate in surgical infections, or a foreign body was present. 9) Perfusion and penetration to the site of infection was impaired because of inflammation, cellular debris, tissue destruction, abscessation, etc. 10) Defense mechanisms (specific and nonspecific) of the animal were compromised by disease, malnutrition, or concurrent therapy. 11) Detrimental changes, such as hypoxia, acidosis, or accumulation of tissue debris, occurred in infected tissue, which reduced the effectiveness of the antibiotic or sulfonamide. 12) An inappropriate route of administration was selected or an incorrect dosage regimen was followed because the pharmacokinetic characteristics of the antimicrobial drug were not appreciated. 13) Expired or substandard products were used. 14) The selected agent had to be withdrawn because of adverse side effects. 15) Interaction of the selected antimicrobial agent(s) with other concurrently administered drugs occurred, which diminished the antimicrobial effect or altered the pharmacokinetics of the agent(s). 16) The prescribed dosage regimen was not reliably followed (lack of owner compliance). 17) Supportive therapy was inadequate. 18) Nutritional deficits were not corrected. 19) Nursing care was substandard, and the stress associated with the disease process was not obtunded. 20) Predisposing management factors were not rectified.

RESISTANCE OF MICROORGANISMS TO ANTIBACTERIAL AGENTS

The emergence of bacteria resistant to antimicrobial agents within an animal population or during therapy is a matter of great concern. Resistance requires that a previously successful therapeutic approach be discarded, especially if suitable alternative antimicrobial drugs are available; additionally, there frequently is alarm from an epidemiological and public health point of view.

There are differences in use of the term "antibiotic resistance". Natural resistance implies an intrinsic property in an organism that confers resistance, whereas acquired resistance suggests that an organism has obtained, by one mechanism or another, the means to survive exposure to an antimicrobial agent. Chromosomal, extrachromosomal, and transpositional resistance are terms used when the genetic determinants are on chromosomes, plasmids, or transposons, respectively. Phenotypic resistance, due to differences in physical and functional characteristics, is best exemplified by the bacterial-wall-defective variants such as L-forms, spheroblasts, and protoplasts, and by the impermeability of the cell walls of some gram-negative bacteria due to very narrow conduits or porins. Microbiological resistance implies an increase in the usual MIC range to levels that are too high to be reached at standard therapeutic dose rates. Clinical resistance, for which there may be many causes, is a general term used to describe unexpected lack of response to treatment in a clinical case.

Causes of conditional resistance include the physiological state of the organism (eg, quiescent, as in "persisters"), antagonism or inactivation by a second agent, inactivation of the drug by enzymes produced by other bacteria at the site of infection, antagonism of the effect of the antimicrobial agent due to tissue debris or a foreign body, and inhibition of antibacterial action because of a low pH or hypoxia.

Resistance may also be classified in terms of the mechanisms of acquisition. Examples include selection of resistant clones, chromosomal mutation, phage transduction, and R-factor acquisition by conjugation.

The biochemical basis for microbial resistance to antibacterial agents permits a further approach to distinguishing various forms of resistance. Examples include the synthesis of destructive enzymes, altered receptor site or enzyme specificity, alternate metabolic pathways, modified carrier systems, and various barriers to penetration.

The means by which bacteria can protect themselves against antimicrobials include: 1) Increased production of inactivating enzymes, which may be constitutive or inducible, eg, penicillins, cephalosporins, aminoglycosides, chloramphenicol. 2) Defective production of autolytic enzymes ("tolerance"), eg, penicillins and cephalosporins. 3) Alteration of the specific configuration of target sites, eg, oxacillin, cloxacillin, macrolides, lincomycin, streptomycin. 4) Decreased enzyme affinity, eg, trimethoprim. 5) Induction of membrane transport systems to remove the antibacterial, eg, tetracyclines. 6) Inhibition or changes in membrane transport systems to prevent entry of the antibacterial, eg, aminoglycosides. 7) Utilization of alternate metabolic pathways, eg, sulfonamides, trimethoprim. 8) Increased synthesis of a key metabolic intermediate, eg, para-aminobenzoic acid in sulfonamide resistance. 9) Development of impermeable cell walls with extremely narrow porins, eg, *Pseudomonas aeruginosa* in response to many antibiotics.

In each of these cases, a modification of protein synthesis and enzyme activity is necessary to confer resistance, thus this adaptation is genetically determined.

Bacteria have 2 types of genetic structures that may confer resistance—chromosomes and plasmids. Both consist of double-stranded DNA, and both are associated with the bacterial inner cell membrane at some time. Plasmids are not essential for survival but do carry genetic determinants that confer both antibiotic resistance and virulence on bacteria. There is always only one plasmid of its type in a cell (called "incompatibility").

Chromosomal resistance to antibacterial agents depends on a mutation in the bacterial genes that leads to resistance to particular antimicrobial agents. In this case, the antibacterial drugs act only as selective agents that allow the resistant mutants to emerge either by a single step or sequential mutations. Their genesis is independent of the presence of the agent. Mutated bacteria are often metabolically deranged and are at a selective growth disadvantage, and usually disappear with time in the absence of the antimicrobial agent.

Plasmid-mediated resistance (R-factor or acquired resistance) is far more complex. Plasmids may contain from 20-500 genes that can carry resistance to a number of different antibacterial agents (3-6 is quite a common number; up to 9 have been recorded) as well as specific virulence factors. Many specific plasmids have been isolated, characterized, and identified. The 3 possible mechanisms by which plasmids may migrate from one bacterium to another are transformation, transduction, and conjugation. In **transformation**, naked DNA seems to pass from the donor to the recipient through the growth medium. This process appears to be confined to a limited range of bacteria. In **transduction**, the transfer is mediated by a bacteriophage that makes use of its specialized molecular equipment adapted for inserting DNA into recipient bacteria. Normally, it is phage DNA that is transferred; in certain cases, however, some DNA from the episome in the bacterial cell replaces the proper phage nucleic acid sequence. Phage-mediated transduction occurs in some gram-positive (especially *Staphylococcus aureus*) as well as gram-negative species. In **conjugation**, the DNA passes from the donor cell to the recipient via a bridge formed during direct cell-to-cell contact. This is the most sophisticated form of transmission since, for transfer to occur at all, the donor must have the necessary surface appendage (sex pilus) to form the bridge. This pilus is coded for by a resistance transfer factor (RTF) on the plasmid and is called a conjugative sequence (vs a nonconjugative plasmid without an RTF).

General facets of conjugation make it an important process as far as gene transfer under natural conditions is concerned. Many types of bacteria can act as recipients, and resistance can pass freely from organisms normally saprophytic in the gut of animals to pathogenic bacteria. Transfer among *Pasteurella* and *Pseudomonas* spp seems to be less efficient. In general, transfer occurs more frequently between gram-negative bacteria, and only rarely between gram-positive organisms. Conjugation allows the passage of a number of distinct genes at one time. Thus, resistance to several antibiotics, all mediated by different biochemical means, may be acquired in a single step. The great efficiency of the conjugation process makes the probability of gene transfer to a super-infecting pathogen high.

Genetic sequences capable of coding for resistance can migrate from a plasmid to a chromosome and then back to the plasmid. These sequences are then transpositional and are known as "transposons". A number of transposons responsible for the transfer of R-factor resistance also have been isolated, characterized, and identified.

The clinical relevance of plasmid-mediated resistance in veterinary medicine principally concerns: 1) intestinal infections, in which the reservoir of R-factors may be carried by saprophytic flora in the gut; 2) the use of low levels of antibiotics (as in animal feeds), which may lead to a high incidence of R-factors in a given population; and 3) the indiscriminate use of antibiotics, which may eliminate the effectiveness of many antimicrobial agents in the future.

The following guidelines will help to minimize the emergence of bacterial resistance. 1) Do not use a broad-spectrum antibacterial agent if a narrow-spectrum agent is also active against the causative organism(s). 2) Regularly seek and use information regarding endemic infections and sensitivity patterns when choosing an antibiotic. 3) Always follow appropriate dose rates. 4) When a combination regimen is used to prevent the development of resistant strains, use the individual agents in full dosage. 5) Select antibacterials for topical application from those against which development of resistance is uncommon. 6) For prophylaxis, use an antibacterial agent that prevents colonization of a specific organism or eradicates it shortly after it has become established. 7) To the extent that it is consistent with reasonable practice, make every effort to use antibiotics only when the medical indications are clear, and to avoid overuse of newer agents when already available agents are effective.

ANTIBACTERIAL AGENTS

PENICILLINS

The penicillins are a large and commonly used class of β-lactam antibiotics that share many features, such as their chemistry, mechanism of action, pharmacological properties, clinical effects, and immunological characteristics.

CLASSES

Several subclassifications of the penicillins, based mainly on differences in antibacterial spectra, are recognized:

Narrow-spectrum β-Lactamase-sensitive Penicillins: This group includes naturally occurring penicillin G (benzylpenicillin) in its various pharmaceutical forms, and a few biosynthetic acid-stable penicillins intended for oral use (penicillin V [phenoxymethyl-penicillin] and phenethicillin [phenoxyethyl-penicillin]). Penicillins in this class are active against many gram-positive and a limited number of gram-negative bacteria, but they are susceptible to β-lactamase (penicillinase) hydrolysis.

Narrow-spectrum β-Lactamase-resistant Penicillins: This group, through substitution on the penicillin nucleus (6-aminopenicillanic acid [6-APA]), is refractory to a greater or lesser degree to the effects of various β-lactamase enzymes produced by resistant gram-positive organisms, particularly *Staphylococcus aureus*. However, penicillins in this class possess lower activity against many gram-positive bacteria than does penicillin G, and are inactive against almost all gram-negative bacteria. Acid-stable members of this group (that are used PO) include isoxazolyl penicillins such as oxacillin, cloxacillin, dicloxacillin, and flucloxacillin. Methicillin and nafcillin are available as parenteral preparations. Temocillin is a semisynthetic penicillin that is β-lactamase stable but also active against nearly all isolates of gram-negative bacteria except *Pseudomonas* spp.

Broad-spectrum β-Lactamase-sensitive Penicillins: Penicillins in this class are derived semisynthetically from 6-APA and are active against many gram-positive and gram-negative bacteria. However, they are readily destroyed by the β-lactamases (produced by many bacteria). Many members of the group are acid stable and are administered either PO or parenterally. Of those used in veterinary medicine, aminopenicillins, eg, ampicillin and amoxicillin, are the best known. Several ampicillin precursors that are more completely absorbed from the GI tract also belong to this class (eg, hetacillin, pivampicillin, and talampicillin). Mecillinam is less active than ampicillin against gram-positive bacteria but is highly active against many intestinal organisms (except *Proteus* spp) that do not produce β-lactamases.

Broad-spectrum β-Lactamase-sensitive Penicillins with Extended Spectra (newer generations of penicillins): Several semisynthetic broad-spectrum penicillins also possess activity against *Pseudomonas aeruginosa*, certain *Proteus* spp, and even strains of *Klebsiella, Shigella*, and *Enterobacter* spp in certain cases. Examples of this class include carboxypenicillins (carbenicillin, its acid-stable indanyl ester, and ticarcillin), ureido-penicillins (azlocillin and mezlocillin), and piperazine penicillins (piperacillin).

β-Lactamase-protected Broad-spectrum Penicillins (potentiated penicillins): Several naturally occurring and semisynthetic compounds are capable of inhibiting many of the β-lactamase enzymes produced by penicillin-resistant bacteria. When used in combination with broad-spectrum penicillins, there is a notable synergistic effect since the active penicillin is protected from enzymatic hydrolysis—and thus is fully active against a wide variety of previously resistant bacteria. Examples of this novel chemotherapeutic approach include clavulanate-potentiated amoxicillin and ticarcillin as well as sulbactam-potentiated ampicillin.

GENERAL PROPERTIES

The penicillins are somewhat unstable, being sensitive to heat, light, extremes in pH, heavy metals, and oxidizing and reducing agents. Also, they often deteriorate in aqueous solution, and thus require reconstitution with a diluent just before injection. Penicillins are poorly soluble, weak organic acids that are administered parenterally as suspensions in water or oil, or as water-soluble salts. For example, sodium or potassium salts of penicillin G are highly water soluble and are absorbed rapidly from injection sites, whereas organic salts in microsuspension such as procaine penicillin G or benzathine penicillin G are gradually absorbed over 1-3 (or even more) days, respectively. The trihydrate forms of the semisynthetic penicillins possess greater aqueous solubility than the parent compounds and are usually preferred for both parenteral and oral use.

Penicillins contain a β-lactam nucleus that when cleaved by a β-lactamase enzyme (penicillinase) produces penicilloic acid derivatives that are inactive, but which may act as the antigenic determinants for penicillin hypersensitivity. β-lactamases are produced by gram-positive organisms (*Staphylococcus aureus, S epidermidis*), and 5 of the 6 types of β-lactamases are produced by gram-negative organisms. Modification of the 6-aminopenicillanic acid nucleus, either by biosynthetic or semisynthetic means, has produced the array of penicillins used clinically. These differ in their antibacterial spectra, pharmacokinetic characteristics, and susceptibility to microbial enzymatic degradation.

ANTIMICROBIAL ACTIVITY

Mode of Action: Penicillins impair the development of bacterial cell walls by interfering with transpeptidase enzymes responsible for the formation of the cross-links between peptidoglycan strands. These enzymes are associated with a group of proteins in both gram-positive and gram-negative bacteria called the penicillin-binding proteins (PBP). During bacterial cell growth, while the peptidoglycan structure is being formed, autolysins continuously cleave the lattice to provide acceptor sites for new strands. Normal bacterial growth depends on a balance between cell wall deposition and autolysis. When a penicillin interacts with PBP and inhibits the synthetic enzymes, defective cell walls are formed, which lead to abnormal elongation of cells, formation of spheroplasts, or osmotic lysis. The effect of the penicillins is generally bactericidal, although bacteriolysis may also occur. However, at levels lower than minimal inhibitory concentrations (at so-called minimal antibiotic concentrations), β-lactam antibiotics do exert residual effects on bacterial structure and function that, in turn, promote phagocytosis.

β-lactam antibiotics have little influence on formed bacterial cell walls, and even susceptible organisms must be actively multiplying or growing: penicillins are most active during the logarithmic phase of bacterial growth. They also tend to be somewhat more active in a slightly acidic environment (pH 5.5-6.5), perhaps because of enhanced membrane penetration.

Bacterial Resistance: Only microorganisms that have cell walls are susceptible to the action of penicillins and other β-lactam antibiotics. Within this range of bacteria, resistance to penicillins is well recognized and takes a number of forms.

Permeability Barrier: In gram-positive organisms, capsular materials may hinder access to the cytoplasmic membrane, but this rarely limits the diffusion of the cell wall inhibitors. Gram-negative bacteria possess a restricting sieving mechanism in their outer membranes, which reduces the penetration of several types of antibiotics. Different species of gram-negative bacteria exhibit varying permeability barriers to β-lactam antibiotics, and these impair access of the antibiotics to the membrane-associated binding proteins. For example, the permeability barrier of *Haemophilus influenzae* is readily traversed by β-lactam antibiotics; *Escherichia coli* presents a greater obstacle to these agents; and the outer membranes of *Pseudomonas aeruginosa* are penetrated with great difficulty by most β-lactam compounds. The chemical nature of β-lactams (penicillins, cephalosporins, and the β-lactamase inhibitors) as well as their concentration gradients also greatly influence their penetration of bacteria to their targets at the surface of the cytoplasmic membrane, giving rise to the differences between antibacterial spectra of the various classes of penicillin. Penicillins are also often used in combination with other antibiotics that disrupt the integrity of the membranes and thereby facilitate access by penicillins. The genetic loci controlling permeability generally have been considered to be chromosomally located, but they also may be plasmid-specified genes.

Specific Bacterial Binding Proteins: Resistance to β-lactam antimicrobial agents can be acquired by alterations in the PBP targets of these drugs. A loss or decrease in affinity of crucial PBP can lead to a significant increase in penicillin resistance.

L-forms of Bacteria: A phenotypic form of resistance can occur when spheroplasts (incomplete cell wall) or protoplasts (absence of cell wall) are present. These so-called "L-forms" must be present in a hyperosmotic environment, eg, the renal medulla, to survive; otherwise they will lyse. The clinical significance of this form of resistance is unclear.

Quiescent Organisms: In any bacterial population, a few organisms will always be quiescent, and since the penicillins are active only against growing bacteria, the static organisms are unaffected and may persist. These "persisters" may then develop normally after the antibiotic is removed.

Tolerance: Some bacterial isolates, when treated with inhibitors of cell-wall synthesis, undergo inhibition of growth but not lysis at usual concentrations. These "tolerant" organisms are defective in their production or use of autolytic enzymes and can survive exposure to β-lactam antibiotics. Clinically, relapses and failures in serious infections due to tolerant organisms may be prevented by the frequently synergistic effect of the aminoglycosides with β-lactam antibiotics.

β-Lactamase (Penicillinase) Resistance: The most important mechanism of bacterial resistance to penicillins and the other β-lactam antibiotics is enzymatic inactivation. There are at least 6 major types of β-lactamase enzymes that are capable of cleaving the β-lactam ring, which renders the drug inactive. Some of these enzymes are active exclusively against penicillins, others are principally active against cephalosporins, and several types hydrolyze both equally. The type and concentration of β-lactamases are also bacterial species specific. Gram-positive β-lactamases are generally excreted into the external environment as exoenzymes, are produced in large quantity, are plasmid-mediated (single determinant), are usually inducible (rarely constitutive), are unable to initiate self-transmission (rely principally on transduction), and are active primarily against penicillins. Staphylococcal strains are the main gram-positive bacteria in which β-lactamase resistance develops, often very quickly. Gram-negative β-lactamases are generally heterogenous (wide range), retained within the periplasmic space, produced in small quantity, often constitutive (less often inducible), able to initiate self-transmission (conjugation mechanisms), and active against both penicillins and cephalosporins. Gram-negative bacteria capable of resistance as a result of β-lactamase production include *Escherichia, Haemophilus, Klebsiella, Pasteurella, Proteus, Pseudomonas,* and *Salmonella* spp; resistance may take longer to develop in some of these strains.

β-lactamase-induced resistance is widespread. Of veterinary isolates, ~50-60% of *Staphylococcus* spp strains and 40-70% of *E coli* strains are resistant to penicillin G; 15-40% of *E coli* strains from farm animals may also be resistant to ampicillin.

Antibacterial Spectra: Penicillin G and its oral congeners such as penicillin V, are active against both aerobic and anaerobic gram-positive bacteria and, with a few exceptions (*Haemophilus* and *Neisseria* spp and strains of *Bacteroides* other than *B fragilis*), are inactive against gram-negative organisms at usual concentrations. Organisms usually sensitive *in vitro* to penicillin G include streptococci, penicillin-sensitive staphylococci, *Corynebacterium pyogenes, Clostridium* spp, *Erysipelothrix rhusiopathiae, Actinomyces ovis, Leptospira canicola, Bacillus anthracis, Fusiformis nodosus,* and *Nocardia* spp.

The semisynthetic β-lactamase-resistant penicillins, such as oxacillin, cloxacillin, floxacillin, and nafcillin, have spectra similar to those noted above (though often at higher MIC) but also include many of the β-lactamase-producing strains of staphylococci (especially *S aureus* and *S epidermidis*).

A large number of gram-positive and gram-negative bacteria (but not β-lactamase-producing strains) are sensitive to the semisynthetic broad-spectrum penicillins (ampicillin and amoxicillin). Susceptible genera include *Staphylococcus, Streptococcus, Corynebacterium, Clostridium, Escherichia, Klebsiella, Shigella, Salmonella, Proteus,* and *Pasteurella.* While bacterial resistance is widespread, the combination of β-lactamase inhibitors and broad-spectrum penicillins markedly enhances the spectrum and efficacy against both gram-positive and gram-negative pathogens. Clavulanate-potentiated amoxicillin is an excellent example of such a synergistic association.

The anti-*Pseudomonas* and other extended-spectrum penicillins are active against most of the usual penicillin-sensitive bacteria, often have a degree of β-lactamase resistance, and usually possess activity against one or more characteristic penicillin-resistant organisms. Examples include the use of carbenicillin and ticarcillin against *Pseudomonas aeruginosa* and several *Proteus* strains; and of piperacillin against *Pseudomonas aeruginosa,* several *Shigella* and *Proteus* strains, and some *Citrobacter* and *Enterobacter* spp. *Streptococcus faecalis* is often resistant to these new extended-spectrum penicillins.

PHARMACOKINETIC FEATURES

There are substantial differences in the pharmacokinetic fates of the many penicillins; only a few general guidelines are presented to emphasize singularly significant aspects.

Absorption: Most penicillins in aqueous solution are rapidly absorbed from parenteral sites. Delayed absorption occurs when the inorganic penicillin salts are suspended in vegetable oil vehicles or when the sparingly soluble repository organic salts, eg, procaine penicillin G and benzathine pencillin G, are administered parenterally. These latter preparations should never be injected IV. Only some penicillins are acid stable and can be administered PO at standard doses. Absorption occurs from the upper GI tract, but the degree and rate of absorption differs greatly among the various penicillins. Peak serum concentrations are generally achieved within 2 hr of PO administration. Absorption of penicillins may also occur following intrauterine infusion.

Distribution: Following absorption, penicillins are widely distributed in body fluids and tissues. The volume of distribution tends to reflect extracellular compartmentalization, although some penicillins, such as amoxicillin, do penetrate into tissues quite well. Significant levels of the various penicillins are generally encountered in the liver, bile, kidneys, intestines, muscle, and lungs, but only very low concentrations occur in poorly perfused areas such as the cornea, cartilage, and bone. The diethylamino salt of penicillin G produces particularly high levels in pulmonary tissue. The penicillins usually do not readily traverse the normal blood-brain, placental, mammary, or prostatic barriers; however, massive doses or inflammation often allow diffusion to occur into the respective fluids. Inflammation also permits effective levels of some penicillins to be reached in abscesses (except when very chronic) as well as pleural, peritoneal, and synovial fluids. Penicillins are reversibly and loosely bound to plasma proteins. The extent of this binding varies with particular penicillins and their concentration, eg, ampicillin is usually ~20% bound, and cloxacillin may be ~80% bound. Pregnancy increases the volume of distribution, which has the effect of lowering the concentration of drug produced by a given dose.

Biotransformation: Penicillins are generally excreted unchanged, but fractions of a given dose may undergo metabolic transformations by unknown mechanisms (usually <20% metabolized). Penicilloic acid derivatives that are formed tend to be allergenic.

Excretion: Sixty to 90% of a parenterally administered penicillin is eliminated in the urine within a short time (eg, up to 90% of penicillin G within 6 hr), which results in high levels in urine, often sufficient to suppress not only gram-positive but also many gram-negative bacteria. About 20% of renal excretion occurs by glomerular filtration and ~80% by tubular secretion—a process that may be deliberately inhibited (to prolong effective levels in the body) by probenecid and other weak organic acids. Anuria may increase the half-life of penicillin G (normally ~30 min) to 10 hr. The biliary route also may be a major excretory pathway for the broad-spectrum semisynthetic penicillins. Clearance values for penicillins are considerably lower in neonates than in adults. Penicillins are also eliminated in milk, although often only in trace amounts in the normal udder, and may persist for up to 90 hr. Penicillin residues in milk also have been found following intrauterine infusion of the antibiotic.

Pharmacokinetic Values: Selected pharmacokinetic values for some penicillins in a few species are listed below. Dosage modifications may be necessary because of age or disease.

Elimination, Distribution, and Clearance of Penicillins

Penicillin	Species	Elimination half-life (min)	Volume of distribution (mL/kg)	Clearance (mL/kg/min)
Penicillin G	Dogs	30	156	3.6
	Horses	38	301	5.5
Ampicillin	Dogs	48	270	3.9
Amoxicillin	Cattle	84	493	4.0
Ticarcillin	Dogs	48	347	4.9
Carbenicillin	Cattle	122	330	5.5

THERAPEUTIC INDICATIONS

The penicillins are commonly used to treat or prevent local and systemic infections caused by susceptible bacteria. There are several acute infectious disease syndromes that are specifically responsive. Penicillins are also used topically in the eye and ear as well as on the skin, and intramammary administration to treat or prevent bovine mastitis is widespread.

SPECIAL CLINICAL CONCERNS

Side Effects and Toxicity: Organ toxicity is rare. Hypersensitivity reactions do occur (particularly in cattle)—skin reactions, angioedema, drug fever, serum sickness, vasculitis, eosinophilia, and anaphylaxis are common manifestations. Cross-sensitivity between penicillins is well recognized. Intrathecal administration may result in convulsions. Guinea pigs, chinchillas, birds, snakes, and turtles are sensitive to procaine penicillin. The use of broad-spectrum penicillins may lead to superinfection, and GI disturbances may occur following PO administration of ampicillin. Potassium penicillin G should be administered IV with some caution, especially if hyperkalemia is present. The sodium salt of penicillin G may also contribute to the sodium load in congestive heart failure.

Interactions: Displacement of penicillins from plasma-protein binding sites and delayed tubular secretion occurs when drugs such as salicylates, phenylbutazone, sulfonamides, and other weak acids are administered concurrently. Gut-active penicillins potentiate the action of anticoagulants by depressing vitamin K production by gut flora. Absorption of ampicillin is impaired by the presence of food. Carbenicillin and ticarcillin interact chemically with the aminoglycosides and should not be mixed *in vitro*. Ampicillin and penicillin G are incompatible with many other drugs and solutions and should not be mixed.

Effects on Laboratory Tests: Alterations in laboratory determinations may occur, depending on the penicillin used. Alkaline phosphatase, AST (SGOT), ALT (SGPT), and eosinophil count may be elevated. A false positive Coombs' test may also result following penicillin therapy. A positive test for urine glucose and protein is also possible. Procaine is detectable in the urine of horses for several days following the administration of procaine penicillin; the pre-race withdrawal time may be up to 6 days.

Drug Withdrawal and Milk Discard Times: Pre-slaughter withdrawal times for food animals and milk discard times are determined by the regulatory agencies in each country. These must be followed carefully to prevent food residues and consequent public health implications. The selection of times listed below can serve only as general guidelines.

Penicillin	Species	Withdrawal time (days)	Milk discard time (days)
Procaine penicillin G (IM)	Cattle	10 (label dose) 30 (20,000 IU/kg, b.i.d.)	3
	Sheep	9	
	Pigs	7	
Benzathine penicillin G (IM)	Cattle	30	
Ampicillin (IM)	Cattle	6	
	Preruminant calves	15	
Amoxicillin (IM)	Cattle	30	2

DOSE RATES OF COMMONLY USED PENICILLINS

The following is a selection of general dosages for some penicillins. The dose rate and frequency should be adjusted as needed for the individual animal.

Penicillin	Dosage	Route	Frequency (hr)
Sodium penicillin G	10,000-20,000 IU/kg	IV,IM	6
Potassium penicillin G	25,000 IU/kg	PO	6
Procaine penicillin G	10,000-30,000 IU/kg	IM, subcut.	12-24
Benzathine penicillin G	10,000-40,000 IU/kg	IM (horses), subcut. (cattle)	48-72
Penicillin V	15,000 IU/kg or 8-10 mg/kg	PO	8
Cloxacillin	10 mg/kg	IM, PO	6
Ampicillin	5-10 mg/kg	IV,IM,subcut.	8-12
	10-25 mg/kg	PO	6-12
Amoxicillin	4-7 mg/kg	IM	12-24
	11 mg/kg	PO	dog, 12 cat, 12 or 24
Sodium carbenicillin	10-20 mg/kg	IV, IM	8-12
Potassium clavulanate: amoxicillin (1:4)	10-20 mg/kg (amoxicillin) 2.5-5 mg/kg (clavulanate)	PO	12
Probenecid (prolongs blood levels of penicillins that have short plasma half-lives or that are costly)	1-2 mg/1000 IU penicillin G (dogs)	PO	6

CEPHALOSPORINS AND CEPHAMYCINS

The cephalosporins, and the closely related cephamycins, are a class of β-lactam antibiotics that has proliferated rapidly. They are similar to the penicillins in several respects, and also share many pharmacological features as a group. Because of cost, their use in veterinary medicine has been limited, but increasing numbers are now being utilized.

CLASSES

The early cephalosporins differed mainly with respect to pharmacokinetic characteristics; the newer generations have much broader ranges of activity, and the modern classification of the group is based mainly on antibacterial spectra.

First-generation Cephalosporins: This group includes cephalothin, cephaloridine, cephapirin, cefazolin, cephalexin, cephradine, and cefadroxil. Cephalosporins in this group are usually quite active against many gram-positive bacteria but are only moderately active against gram-negative organisms. They are relatively susceptible to β-lactamases (cephalosporinases) and are not as effective against anaerobes as are the penicillins.

Second-generation Cephalosporins: This group includes cefamandole, cefoxitin (a cephamycin), cefotiam, cefachlor, cefuroxime, and ceforanide. These agents are generally active against both gram-positive and gram-negative bacteria. Moreover, they are relatively resistant to β-lactamase. They are ineffective against enterococci, *Pseudomonas aeruginosa, Actinobacter* spp, and many obligate anaerobes.

Third-generation Cephalosporins: This group includes ceftiofur, ceftriaxone, cefsulodin, cefotaxime, cefoperazone, moxalactam (not a true cephalosporin), and several others. Typically, these have only moderate activity against gram-positive bacteria but are active against a wide variety of gram-negative bacteria, including in certain instances *Pseudomonas* spp, *Proteus vulgaris, Enterobacter* spp, and *Citrobacter* spp. They are usually highly resistant to β-lactamase enzymes. Third-generation cephalosporins are often able to penetrate the blood-brain barrier and are frequently indicated in bacterial meningitis caused by susceptible pathogens. Ceftiofur has been specifically approved for use in cattle with bronchopneumonia, especially if caused by *Pasteurella haemolytica* or *P multocida*.

GENERAL PROPERTIES

The physical and chemical properties of the cephalosporins are similar to those of the penicillins, although they are somewhat more stable to pH and temperature changes. Cephalosporins are weak acids derived from 7-aminocephalosporanic acid. They are used either as the free base form for PO administration (if acid stable) or as sodium salts in aqueous solution for parenteral delivery (sodium salt of cephalothin contains 2.4 mEq sodium/g). Cephalosporins also contain a β-lactam nucleus that is susceptible to β-lactamase (cephalosporinase) hydrolysis. These β-lactamases may or may not also attack penicillins. Modifications of the 7-aminocephalosporanic acid nucleus and substitutions on the sidechains by semisynthetic means have produced differences among cephalosporins in antibacterial spectra, β-lactamase sensitivities, and pharmacokinetic fates.

ANTIMICROBIAL ACTIVITY

Mode of Action: This is similar to that of the penicillins. Cephalosporins also bind to penicillin-binding proteins located beneath the cell wall and thereby interfere with the action of transpeptidase and other cell-wall enzymes. A residual antibacterial effect is also evident with the cephalosporins. As a group, these antibiotics are most stable and effective at a pH of 6-7.

Bacterial Resistance: Resistance to the cephalosporins may be mediated in several ways that are basically comparable to those associated with penicillin resistance.
  Permeability Barrier: There may be lack of bacterial permeability to the particular cephalosporin. First-and second-generation cephalosporins are not capable of penetrating the outer membrane of *Pseudomonas aeruginosa*.
  Specific Bacterial Binding Proteins: Alteration in structure of target sites mediated by genetic mechanisms identical to those of penicillin resistance may lead to reduced sensitivity to the cephalosporins.

β-Lactamase (Cephalosporinase) Resistance: Cephalosporins generally are stable against the plasmid-mediated β-lactamases produced by gram-positive bacteria such as *Staphylococcus aureus.* Several types of inducible β-lactamases produced by gram-negative organisms may be mediated either by plasmids or chromosomally, and may hydrolyze either or both penicillins and cephalosporins (cross-resistance). Second- and particularly third-generation cephalosporins have greater stability against gram-negative β-lactamases.

L-forms, Persisters, and Tolerance: These also are forms of resistance encountered against the cephalosporins (*see* PENICILLINS, above).

Antibacterial Spectra: The first-generation cephalosporins are generally effective against most gram-positive aerobic cocci and several of the gram-negative bacteria, including *E coli*, and *Proteus, Klebsiella, Salmonella, Shigella*, and *Enterobacter* spp. Cephalosporinase-producing organisms are not susceptible. The second-generation cephalosporins have greater activity against gram-negative organisms but are somewhat less active against gram-positive species. This trend continues with the third-generation cephalosporins, which may even be active against *Pseudomonas aeruginosa.* The newest members of this group are also highly resistant to β-lactamase. The cephalosporins may be effective against anaerobic bacteria except *Bacteroides fragilis*, which is susceptible only to certain cephalosporins.

PHARMACOKINETIC FEATURES

Not much information is available on the fate of the cephalosporins in animals; many of the recommendations are based on extrapolation from human data.

Absorption: Only a few cephalosporins are acid stable and thus effective when administered PO (cephalexin, cephradine, cefadroxil, and cefachlor). They are usually well absorbed, and bioavailability values are 75-90%. The others are administered either IV or IM, with peak plasma concentrations occurring ~30 min following injection.

Distribution: Cephalosporins are widely distributed through most body fluids and tissues, including kidneys, lungs, joints, bone, soft tissues, and the biliary tract, but in general, the volume of distribution is <0.3 L/kg. However, poor penetration into the CSF, even in inflammation, is a notable feature of the standard cephalosporins. The third-generation cephalosporins (eg, moxalactam) may achieve good penetration into the CSF. The degree of plasma-protein binding is variable (eg, 20% for cefadroxil and 80% for cefazolin).

Biotransformation: Several cephalosporins (such as cephalothin, cephapirin, cephacetrile, and cefotaxime) are actively deacetylated, primarily in the liver but also in other tissues. The deacetylated derivatives are much less active. Few of the other cephalosporins are metabolized to any appreciable extent.

Excretion: Most cephalosporins are excreted by renal tubular secretion, though glomerular filtration is important in some cases (cephaloridine, cephalexin, and cefazolin). In renal failure, dose rates should be reduced. Biliary elimination of the newer cephalosporins (eg, cefoperazone) may be significant. Generally, these β-lactam antibiotics maintain effective blood levels for only 6-8 hr.

Pharmacokinetic Values: Plasma half-lives are often 30-120 min, but there are exceptions. Third-generation cephalosporins tend to have longer plasma half-lives in man, but this is not always the case in other animals—substantial species differences exist. A selection of pharmacokinetic values for cephalosporins is listed to serve as a guide. Dosage modifications are often required in hepatic and renal disease.

Elimination, Distribution, and Clearance of Cephalosporins

Cephalosporin	Species	Elimination half-life (min)	Volume of distribution (mL/kg)	Clearance (mL/kg/min)
Cefazolin	Horses	45	188	5.5
Cefotaxime	Sheep	25	134	9.0
Cephalexin	Dogs	84	—	—
Cefadroxil	Dogs	120	—	—
	Cats	150-180	—	—
Ceftiofur	Cattle	~360	—	—

THERAPEUTIC INDICATIONS

The cost of cephalosporins has limited their use in veterinary medicine. They are particularly useful for treating infections of soft tissue and bone due to bacteria that are resistant to other commonly employed antibiotics. Because of their favorable pharmacokinetic characteristics and effectiveness, they are often administered IV, 1 hr before surgery. Because of their ability to penetrate tissues and fluids so readily (the CSF being an exception for most), they are often effective in the management of osteomyelitis, prostatitis, and arthritis. Oral cephalosporins are also usually effective in the management of urinary tract infections, except those due to *Pseudomonas aeruginosa*. Cephapirin benzathine is employed for dry-cow therapy and cephapirin sodium is used in treatment of mastitis. Ceftiofur is used to treat bovine respiratory disease principally caused by *Pasteurella* spp.

SPECIAL CLINICAL CONCERNS

Side Effects and Toxicity: The cephalosporins are relatively nontoxic, though cephaloridine may be nephrotoxic in some species. IM injections can be painful, and repeated IV administration may lead to local phlebitis. Nausea, vomiting, and diarrhea may occasionally occur. Hypersensitivity reactions of several forms have been encountered, particularly in animals with a history of acute penicillin allergy. Superinfection may arise with the use of cephalosporins, and *Pseudomonas* or *Candida* spp are likely opportunistic pathogens. Prolonged treatment with cephalosporins in man has been associated with interstitial nephritis, hepatitis, thrombocytopenia, and neutropenia. These drugs should be used with caution in animals with renal disease. Chronic administration of cephaloridine may lead to anemia in cats.

Interactions: *In vitro* incompatibilities are quite common for cephalosporin and cephamycin preparations. Potential pharmacokinetic interactions are similar to those of the penicillin group. Aminoglycosides may enhance cephaloridine nephrotoxicity, but there is some doubt about this particular interaction. Furosemide and ethacrynic acid, however, do appear to potentiate the nephrotoxic action of cephaloridine.

Effects on Laboratory Tests: Several laboratory determinations may be altered by the cephalosporins. Alkaline phosphatase, AST (SGOT), ALT (SGPT), LDH, and BUN may be elevated. A false-positive Coombs' test and a false-positive urine glucose may also be present. Hypernatremia may be caused by the sodium salts of various cephalosporins.

Drug Withdrawal and Milk Discard Times: Although prolonged tissue residues for most cephalosporins are not anticipated, withdrawal times are not available for most of the cephalosporins since they are not approved for use in food animals in most countries.

Cephalosporin	Withdrawal time	Milk discard time
Ceftiofur	0 days	
Sodium cephapirin (intramammary)	4 days before slaughter	4 days
Benzathine cephapirin (dry-cow treatment)	42 days after latest infusion	3 days after calving—milk not used for food

DOSE RATES

The following is a selection of general dosages for some cephalosporins. The dose rate and frequency should be adjusted as needed for the individual animal.

Cephalosporin		Dosage (mg/kg)	Route	Frequency (hr)
Cephalothin	(sm an)	20-35	IM, IV	6-8
Cephapirin	(sm an)	30	IM, IV	4-6
Cefazolin	(sm an)	20-25	IM, IV	6-8
Cephalexin	(sm an)	10-30	PO	6-8
Cefadroxil	(sm an)	22	PO	12
Ceftiofur	(cattle)	1.1	IM	24

AMINOGLYCOSIDES
(Aminocyclitols)

These are mostly bactericidal drugs that share chemical, antimicrobial, pharmacologic, and toxic characteristics.

CLASSES

Specific Aminoglycoside Antibiotics—Narrow-spectrum Aminoglycosides: Included in this group are streptomycin and dihydrostreptomycin, which are mainly active against aerobic, gram-negative bacteria.
Broad-spectrum Aminoglycosides: Neomycin, framycetin (neomycin B), paromomycin (aminosidine), and kanamycin possess broader spectra than streptomycin that often include several gram-positive as well as many gram-negative aerobic bacteria. Gentamicin, tobramycin, amikacin, sisomicin, and netilmicin are broad-spectrum aminoglycosides with extended spectra that include *Pseudomonas aeruginosa*.

Miscellaneous Aminoglycoside Antibiotics: The chemical structure of apramycin differs somewhat from that of the typical aminoglycosides but is similar enough to be included in this class. The structure of spectinomycin is unusual but it is fairly comparable to other aminocyclitols with regard to its mechanism of action and antibacterial spectrum.

GENERAL PROPERTIES

Chemically, the aminoglycoside antibiotics are characterized by an aminocyclitol group, with aminosugars attached to the aminocyclitol ring in glycosidic linkage. Because of minor differences in the position of substitutions on the molecules, there may be several forms of a single aminoglycoside; eg, gentamicin is a complex of gentamicins C_1 and C_2, and neomycin is a mixture of neomycins B, C, and fradiomycin. The amino groups contribute to the basic nature of this class of antibiotics, and the hydroxyl groups on the sugar moieties to high aqueous solubility and poor lipid solubility. If these hydroxyl groups are removed (eg, tobramycin), antibiotic activity is markedly increased. Differences in the substitutions on the basic ring structures within the various aminoglycosides account for the relatively minor differences in antimicrobial spectra, patterns of resistance, and toxicities. Aminoglycosides are typically quite stable. When the water solubility of an aminoglycoside is marginal, it is usually the sulfate salt that is used for PO or parenteral administration.

ANTIMICROBIAL ACTIVITY

Mode of Action: Aminoglycosides are more effective against rapidly multiplying organisms; they possess several mechanisms by which they affect and ultimately destroy bacteria. They need only a short contact with bacteria to kill them. Their main site of action is the membrane-associated bacterial ribosome through which they interfere with protein synthesis. To reach the ribosome, they must first cross the bacterial cell wall and then the cell membrane. Because of the polarity of these compounds, a specialized transport process is required. The first concentration-dependent step requires binding of the aminoglycoside to anionic components in the cell membrane. The subsequent steps are energy-dependent and involve the transport of the polar, highly charged aminoglycoside across the cytoplasmic membrane followed by interaction with the ribosomes. The driving force for this transfer is probably the membrane potential. These processes are much more efficient if the energy utilized is aerobically generated.

Several features of these mechanisms are of clinical significance: 1) The antibacterial activity of the aminoglycosides depends on an effective concentration of antibiotic outside the cell. 2) Anaerobic bacteria and induced mutants are generally resistant because they lack appropriate transport systems. 3) With low oxygen tension, as in hypoxic tissues, transfer into bacteria is diminished. 4) Divalent cations, eg, calcium and magnesium, are capable of antagonizing transport into bacteria because they can combine with the specific anionic sites and exclude the cationic aminoglycosides. 5) Transport of aminoglycosides across bacterial cell membranes is facilitated by an alkaline pH; a low pH may increase membrane resistance >100-fold. 6) Changes in osmolality also can alter the uptake of aminoglycosides. 7) Some aminoglycosides are transported more efficiently than others, and thus tend to possess greater antibacterial activity. 8) Synergism is common when aminoglycosides and β-lactam antibiotics (penicillins and cephalosporins) are used in combination. The cell-wall injury induced by the β-lactam compounds allows increased uptake of the aminoglycoside by the bacterial cell because of easier accessibility to the cell membrane.

The intracellular site of action of the aminoglycosides is the ribosome, which has binding sites at both the 30 S and 50 S subunits, although they bind particularly to the former. There is some variation between aminoglycosides with respect to their affinity and degree of binding. A number of steps in protein synthesis appear to be affected, but this too varies among aminoglycosides. Spectinomycin lacks the capacity to produce misreading of the mRNA and often is not bactericidal, in contrast to the other members. At low concentrations, all aminoglycosides may be only bacteriostatic.

A cell-membrane effect is also seen. The functional integrity of the bacterial cell membrane is lost during the late phase of the transport process, and high concentrations of aminoglycosides may cause nonspecific membrane toxicity, even to the point of bacterial cell lysis.

Bacterial Resistance: Several mechanisms of resistance to the aminoglycoside antibiotics have been described. These may be plasmid-mediated or due to mutation.

One mechanism of nonplasmid-mediated resistance is **impaired transport** across the cell membrane. Because the transport process is active and oxygen-dependent, anaerobic bacteria (eg, *Bacteroides fragilis* and *Clostridium perfringens*) and facultative anaerobes (eg, enterobacteria and *Staphylococcus aureus*) are more resistant to the aminoglycosides when in an anaerobic environment. Resistance due to impaired transport can be induced by exposure to sublethal concentrations of these antibiotics. Examples of this form include streptomycin resistance among strains of *Pseudomonas aeruginosa*, low-level aminoglycoside resistance among enterococci, and gentamicin resistance in *Streptococcus faecalis*.

Impaired ribosomal binding may not be a clinically important form of resistance. Examples include *Escherichia coli* strains in which a single step mutation prevents the binding of streptomycin to the ribosome. The same mechanism has been described in *Pseudomonas aeruginosa*.

Enzymatic modification of aminoglycosides may be plasmid-encoded as well as chromosomally mediated. The enzymes are encountered in both gram-negative and gram-positive bacteria. There are 3 major types of enzymes involved, with several subclasses in each case. The main groups are acetylating enzymes (acetyltransferases), adenylating enzymes (nucleotidyltransferases), and phosphorylating enzymes (phosphotransferases). The susceptibility of the aminoglycosides to specific enzymatic attack is quite variable, and the substrate profiles differ for each subclass. This explains the common incidence of cross-resistance yet the frequent differences in susceptibility patterns. Chemical alteration of an aminoglycoside may render it relatively stable to enzymatic hydrolysis, eg, kanamycin modified to amikacin is relatively resistant to inactivating enzymes.

Several **other mechanisms of resistance** are recognized: 1) Increasing the concentration of divalent cations in the media (especially Ca^{++} and Mg^{++}) increases resistance in *Pseudomonas aeruginosa*. 2) Mutants of *P aeruginosa* produce an excess of outer cell membrane protein, called H1, that confers relative resistance to gentamicin. 3) A low pH, as found in acidic urine or in abscess cavities, leads to persistent viability of microorganisms even with relatively high concentrations of aminoglycosides.

Antibacterial Spectra: Streptomycin and dihydrostreptomycin possess relatively narrow spectra, and bacterial resistance is becoming prevalent. However, some staphylococci and a number of gram-negative bacilli are still susceptible, among which are strains of *Actinomyces bovis*, *Pasteurella* spp, *E coli*, *Salmonella* spp, *Campylobacter fetus*, *Leptospira* spp, and *Brucella* spp. *Mycobacterium tuberculosis* is also sensitive to streptomycin.

Neomycin, framycetin, and kanamycin possess broader spectra than streptomycin, and their clinical use is most often directed against gram-negative species such as *E coli*, and *Salmonella*, *Klebsiella*, *Enterobacter*, *Proteus*, and *Acinetobacter* spp. The aminoglycosides with broad spectra that include *P aeruginosa* (gentamicin, tobramycin, amikacin, sisomicin, and netilmicin) are often highly effective against a wide variety of aerobic bacteria. Anaerobic bacteria and fungi are not appreciably affected; streptococci are usually only moderately sensitive or quite resistant.

PHARMACOKINETIC FEATURES

The pharmacokinetic features of the aminoglycosides are similar in most species.

Absorption: Aminoglycosides are poorly absorbed (usually <10%) from the normal GI tract. However, enteritis and other pathological changes may allow significantly greater absorption to occur and, in renal failure, toxic levels can accumulate. Absorption from IM injection sites is rapid and nearly complete (>90% availability), except in severely hypotensive animals. Peak blood levels are usually achieved within 30-90 min after IM administration. Absorption following subcut. injection may be protracted. Absorption following IP administration can be rapid and substantial, and has the potential to produce serious side effects. Aminoglycosides can be administered IV by bolus injection, or by intermittent or continuous infusions. However, bolus injections and continuous infusions have a high risk of toxicity; intermittent infusions are safer. Serum levels of aminoglycosides may reach bactericidal levels following repeated intrauterine infusion, particularly in endometritis.

Distribution: Because of their polarity at physiological pH, the aminoglycosides distribute into the extracellular fluid space with minimal penetration into most tissues except the kidneys (where they accumulate in the renal cortex) and the endolymph of the inner ear. The extracellular fluid compartment approximates 25% of body weight, but this volume can change substantially and significantly influence the concentration of an aminoglycoside. Contraction of the extracellular fluid space occurs with dehydration due to any cause, and during gram-negative sepsis. An increase in aminoglycoside distribution volume can occur in animals with congestive heart failure or ascites. Neonates also have a large extracellular fluid compartment relative to body weight. Although aminoglycosides are not appreciably bound to plasma proteins (usually <20%), they do attain therapeutic concentrations in the synovial, pleural, and even peritoneal fluids, especially if inflammation is present. However, effective levels are not reached in CSF, bronchial secretions, ocular fluids, milk, intestinal fluids, or prostatic secretions. Fetal tissue and amniotic fluid concentrations are very low in most species.

Biotransformation/Excretion/Pharmacokinetic Values: The aminoglycosides are not metabolized in the body. They are eliminated unchanged in the urine by glomerular filtration, with 80-90% of administered drug being recoverable from the urine within 24 hr of IM administration. A variable fraction of filtered aminoglycoside is absorbed onto the brush border of the proximal tubule and loop of Henle cells. After binding, they are transported into the cell and sequestered in lysosomes, and subsequently redistributed into the cytosol. Excessive accumulation (mainly in the renal cortex) leads to a characteristic tubular cell necrosis. Glomerular filtration rates differ between species and are often less in neonates, which may explain the greater sensitivity to aminoglycosides in newborn foals and puppies.

Elimination depends on cardiovascular and renal function, age, volume of distribution (Vd), fever, and several other factors. The Vd is usually represented by the volume of the extracellular fluid compartment. The aminoglycosides have relatively short plasma half-lives—about 1 hr in carnivores and 2-3 hr in herbivores. The elimination kinetics often follow those of a 3-compartment model. About 90% of the injected drug is excreted unchanged through the kidneys during the β phase of elimination. The remainder is excreted over a protracted period, or γ phase, probably due to the gradual release of the antibiotic from renal intracellular binding sites (terminal elimination half-life often 20-200 hr). The limited selection of pharmacokinetic values for 2 typical aminoglycosides listed below serves as a basis for any required dosage modifications that may be necessary due to age or renal insufficiency. The best way to alter a dosage regimen of aminoglycosides is to monitor plasma concentrations.

Elimination, Distribution, and Clearance of Aminoglycosides

Aminoglycoside	Species	Elimination half-life (min)	Volume of distribution (mL/kg)	Clearance (mL/kg/min)
Gentamicin	Dogs	75	335	3.10
	Horses	110	190	1.23
	(foals)	200	300	1.04
Kanamycin	Dogs	60	255	3.05
	Horses	85	174	1.43
	Sheep	100	217	1.52

THERAPEUTIC INDICATIONS

The aminoglycosides are commonly used to control local and systemic infections caused by susceptible aerobic bacteria (generally gram-negative). Examples include septicemia; tracheobronchitis; pneumonia; osteoarthritis; and infections of the urinary tract, GI tract, and skin and wounds. Several aminoglycosides are also employed topically in the ears and eyes. Intrauterine infusion to treat endometritis is also frequent. Occasionally, they are infused into the udder to treat mastitis.

SPECIAL CLINICAL CONCERNS

Side Effects and Toxicity: Ototoxicity, neuromuscular blockade, and nephrotoxicity are reported most frequently; these effects may vary with the aminoglycoside and dose used, but all members of the group are potentially toxic. Nephrotoxicity is of major concern and may result in renal failure due to acute tubular necrosis with secondary interstitial damage. Aminoglycosides accumulate in proximal tubular epithelial cells, where they are sequestered in lysosomes and interact with ribosomes, mitochondria, and other intracellular constituents to cause cell injury. Nonoliguric renal failure is the usual observation; it is generally reversible, although recovery may be prolonged. Any failure in glomerular filtration results in excessively high concentrations of aminoglycoside, which in turn result in further renal damage. Renal function should be monitored during therapy. Polyuria, decreased urine osmolality, enzymuria, proteinuria, cylindruria, and increased fractional sodium excretion are indicative of aminoglycoside nephrotoxicity. Later, blood urea and creatinine concentrations may be elevated. Early changes or evidence of nephrotoxicity can be detected in 3-5 days with more overt signs in 7-10 days. Several factors predispose to aminoglycoside nephrotoxicosis: these include age (with young [especially the newborn foal and puppy] and old animals being sensitive), compromised renal function, total dose, duration of treatment, dehydration and hypovolemia, aciduria, acidosis, severe sepsis or endotoxemia, concurrent administration of furosemide, and exposure to other potential nephrotoxins (eg, methoxyflurane, amphotericin B, cis-platinum, and perhaps some cephalosporins). In renal insufficiency, either the dose rate or interval (*see* below) must be adjusted accordingly to prevent toxicity.

Aminoglycosides may result in ototoxicity, manifest by auditory or vestibular dysfunction. Vestibular injury leads to nystagmus, incoordination, and loss of the righting reflex. The lesion is often irreversible, although physiological adaptation can occur. Cats are particularly sensitive to the toxic vestibular effects. Hearing impairment is produced by permanent damage and loss of the hair cells in the organ of Corti. High-frequency hearing is impaired first, and deafness may not be complete, depending on the dosage used. Such an impediment could be of enormous importance, eg, in guide dogs, and aminoglycosides should not be administered to these animals except under extenuating circumstances. Aminoglycosides should not be instilled into the ear unless the tympanic membrane is intact, lest the drug diffuse into the inner ear where it could cause damage. Several risk factors may predispose to vestibular and cochlear damage by aminoglycosides in addition to those mentioned above under nephrotoxicity, including pre-existing acoustical or vestibular impairment and previous treatment with potentially ototoxic drugs or loop-acting diuretics (furosemide and ethacrynic acid). The ototoxic potential is highest for gentamicin, sisomicin, and neomycin, and is lowest for netilmicin.

All aminoglycosides, when administered in doses that result in high plasma levels, have been associated with muscle weakness and respiratory arrest attributable to neuromuscular blockade. Neomycin, kanamycin, amikacin, gentamicin, and tobramycin represent a decreasing order of potency of these neuromuscular effects. The effect is due to the chelation of calcium and competitive inhibition of the prejunctional release of acetylcholine in most instances (there are some differences among aminoglycosides). The blockade is antagonized by calcium gluconate and somewhat less consistently by neostigmine.

Other forms of toxicity and side effects include CNS disturbances and even convulsions; collapse, following rapid IV administration; superinfection when used topically or PO; a malabsorption syndrome due to allocation of intestinal villous function, when used PO in neonates; occasional hypersensitivity reactions; contact dermatitis; cardiovascular depression; and inhibition of some WBC functions, such as neutrophil migration and chemotaxis and even bactericidal activity at high concentrations.

Interactions: Enhanced nephrotoxicity may become evident with concurrent administration of aminoglycosides and other potentially nephrotoxic agents. Neuromuscular blockade is more likely when aminoglycosides are administered at the same time as skeletal muscle relaxants. Aminoglycoside ototoxicity is enhanced by the loop-acting diuretics, especially furosemide. Cardiovascular depression may be aggravated by aminoglycosides when administered to animals under halothane anesthesia. High concentrations of carbenicillin, ticarcillin, and piperacillin inactivate aminoglycosides both *in vitro* and *in vivo* in the presence of renal failure.

Effects on Laboratory Tests: BUN, serum creatinine, serum transaminases, and alkaline phosphatase values may be elevated. Proteinuria is a significant laboratory finding.

Drug Withdrawal and Milk Discard Times: Withdrawal times for food animals and milk discard times are determined by regulatory agencies in each country. These must be followed carefully to prevent food residues and public health concerns. The general times listed below serve only as broad guidelines for the aminoglycoside antibiotics.

Route	Approximate withdrawal time (days)
Oral	20-30 (3 for neonatal pigs)
Parenteral	100-120 (40 for neonatal pigs [often not approved for food animals])
Udder infusion	2-3* (often not approved for food animals)

*milk discard time

DOSE RATES

The following is a selection of general dosages for some aminoglycosides. The dose rate and frequency should be adjusted as needed for the individual animal (*see* below).

Aminoglycoside	Dosage	Route	Frequency (hr)
Gentamicin	1-2 mg/kg	IM, subcut.	8
Kanamycin	4-5 mg/kg	IM, subcut.	8
Streptomycin/ dihydrostreptomycin	7.5-12.5 mg/kg	IM, subcut.	12
Amikacin	5-7.5 mg/kg	IM, subcut.	12
Netilmicin	1-2 mg/kg	IM, subcut.	8
Neomycin	5 mg/kg	PO	8-12
	0.5-1 g/quarter	intramammary	24

While a nomogram based on creatinine clearance values or the creatinine clearance values themselves could be used to calculate appropriate dosage modifications in renal insufficiency, such an approach is rarely practical. The ideal is to monitor both plasma amminoglycoside concentrations and renal function during therapy. As a precaution, the following general guidelines may be followed in cases of renal failure that have elevated plasma creatinine values.

Plasma creatinine (mg/dL)	Dose	Interval
<1	Full	Standard
2	Full	2 × standard
3	Full	3 × standard
4	Half or full	2 or 4 × standard, respectively
>5	Aminoglycosides contraindicated	

Dose rates should be reduced or treatment interval increased in neonates (especially puppies and foals), in renal failure, and in obese animals. Doses may be increased in animals with edema, hydrothorax, or ascites, provided their renal function is unimpaired.

MISCELLANEOUS AMINOCYCLITOL ANTIBIOTICS

Apramycin is used to control gram-negative infections, particularly *Escherichia coli* and salmonellae in calves and piglets. It also posesses activity against *Proteus, Klebsiella, Treponema*, and *Mycoplasma* spp. There is little cross-resistance within the aminoglycosides, and plasmid-mediated resistance is yet to be confirmed. Apramycin is poorly absorbed after administration PO (<10%). It is rapidly absorbed from parenteral injection sites. Peak plasma levels occur within 1-2 hr of IM administration. It distributes only into the extracellular fluid and is excreted unchanged in the urine (95% within 4 days). The elimination half-life in calves is ~4-5 hr. Apramycin is toxic in cats but is considered safe in most other species (3-6 times the recommended oral dose rarely produces toxicity). The oral dose rate is 20-40 mg/kg, once daily for 5 days. The parenteral dose rate is 20 mg/kg, b.i.d. The withdrawal time in pigs and calves (Europe) is 28 days following oral use.

The structure of spectinomycin differs from that of the aminoglycosides, but it also binds to bacterial ribosomes and interferes with protein synthesis. However, the effect is bacteriostatic rather than bactericidal. Spectinomycin can be inactivated by an enzyme coded for by an R factor, but mutant resistance due to diminished ribosomal binding is perhaps more common. It is active against several strains of streptococci, a wide range of gram-negative bacteria, and *Mycoplasma* spp; most *Chlamydia* spp are resistant. It is poorly absorbed from the GI tract but is rapidly absorbed after IM administration, with peak blood levels occurring within 1 hr. Like aminoglycosides, this antibiotic also penetrates tissues rather poorly, and its distribution is principally extracellular. Metabolic transformation of spectinomycin is limited, and 80% can be recovered unchanged in the urine over 24-48 hr. About 75% is eliminated by glomerular filtration in ~4 hr. At usual doses, no major toxic reactions have been reported. It is administered both PO at 20 mg/kg, b.i.d., and IM at 5-10 mg/kg, b.i.d. Withdrawal time for pigs is usually ~3 wk.

TETRACYCLINES

The tetracyclines are broad-spectrum antibiotics with similar antimicrobial features, but they do differ somewhat from one another in terms of their spectra and pharmacokinetic disposition.

CLASSES

There are 3 naturally occurring tetracyclines (oxytetracycline, chlortetracycline, and demethylchlortetracycline) and several that are derived semisynthetically (tetracycline, rolitetracycline, methacycline, minocycline, doxycycline, lymecycline, and others). Elimination times permit a further classification into short-acting (tetracycline, oxytetracycline, chlortetracycline), intermediate-acting (demethylchlortetracycline and methacycline), and long-acting (doxycycline and minocycline).

GENERAL PROPERTIES

All of the tetracycline derivatives are crystalline, yellowish, amphoteric substances that, in aqueous solution, form salts with both acids and bases. They characteristically fluoresce when exposed to ultraviolet light. The most common salt form is the hydrochloride, except for doxycycline, which is available as doxycycline hyclate. The tetracyclines are stable as dry powders but not in aqueous solution, particularly at higher pH ranges (7-8.5). Preparations for parenteral administration need to be carefully formulated, often in propylene glycol or polyvinyl pyrrolidone with additional dispersing agents, to provide stable solutions. Tetracyclines form poorly soluble chelates with bivalent and trivalent cations, particularly calcium, magnesium, aluminum, and iron. Doxycycline and minocycline exhibit the greatest liposolubility and better penetration of bacteria such as *Staphylococcus aureus* than does the group as a whole.

ANTIMICROBIAL ACTIVITY

Mode of Action: The exact site involved in their antimicrobial activity has not been clarified, but these antibiotics bind reversibly to bacterial 30 S ribosomes and inhibit protein synthesis, perhaps by several mechanisms. Mainly, the binding of aminoacyl-tRNA to the acceptor site on the mRNA-ribosome complex seems to be impaired. This effect also is evident in mammalian cells, although microbial cells are selectively more susceptible because of the greater concentrations that occur. Tetracyclines enter microorganisms in part by diffusion and in part by an energy-dependent, carrier-mediated system that is responsible for the high levels achieved in susceptible bacteria. The tetracyclines are generally bacteriostatic, and a responsive host defense system is essential for their successful use. At high concentrations, as may be attained in urine, they become bactericidal because the organisms seem to lose the functional integrity of the cytoplasmic membrane. Tetracyclines are more effective against multiplying microorganisms and tend to be more active at a pH of 6-6.5.

Bacterial Resistance: Microbial resistance to tetracyclines is based almost exclusively on decreased penetration of the drug into previously susceptible organisms. Two forms are recognized: 1) impaired uptake into bacteria, seen in mutant strains that do not possess the necessary transport system, and 2) plasmid-mediated resistance, which confers the property of either diminished uptake or active efflux of tetracycline from the bacterial cell. The genomes for these capabilities may be transferred either by transduction (as in *Staphylococcus aureus*) or by conjugation (as in many enterobacteria). Resistance develops slowly in a multistep fashion but is widespread because of the extensive use of low levels of tetracyclines.

Antimicrobial Spectra: All tetracyclines are about equally active and typically possess about the same broad spectrum, which comprises both aerobic and anaerobic grampositive and gram-negative bacteria, mycoplasmas, rickettsiae, chlamydiae, and even some protozoa (amebae). Strains of *Pseudomonas aeruginosa, Proteus, Serratia, Klebsiella,* and *Corynebacterium* spp frequently are resistant, as are many pathogenic *E coli* isolates. Even though there is general cross-resistance among tetracyclines, doxycycline and minocycline usually are more effective against staphylococci.

PHARMACOKINETIC FEATURES

Absorption: After usual oral dosage, tetracyclines are absorbed primarily in the upper small intestine. Chlortetracycline is poorly absorbed (~35%) compared with most of the others (usually ~60-80%), and minocycline and doxycycline are well absorbed (~90%). Effective blood levels are reached in 2-4 hr. GI absorption can be impaired by sodium bicarbonate, aluminum hydroxide, magnesium hydroxide, iron, calcium salts, milk, and milk products. For doxycycline and minocycline, the latter only applies to a lesser extent. Tetracyclines at therapeutic levels should not be administered PO to ruminants: they are poorly absorbed and can substantially depress ruminal microfloral activity. Specially buffered tetracycline solutions can be administered IM and IV.

Through chemical manipulation (especially choice of carrier and high magnesium content), the absorption of oxytetracycline from IM sites may be delayed, which produces a long-acting effect. Tetracyclines can cause tissue necrosis at injection sites, in which residues may remain for several weeks. Absorption of tetracyclines also may occur from the uterus and udder, though plasma levels remain low.

Distribution: Tetracyclines distribute rapidly and extensively in the body, particularly after parenteral administration. They enter almost all tissues and body fluids; high concentrations are found in the kidneys, liver, bile, lungs, spleen, and bone. Lower levels occur in serosal fluids, synovia, CSF, ascitic fluid, prostatic fluid, and vitreous humor. The more lipid-soluble tetracyclines (doxycycline and minocycline) readily penetrate tissues as well as the blood-brain barrier, and CSF levels reach ~30% of the plasma concentrations. They also are present in saliva and tears. Because tetracyclines tend to chelate calcium ions (less so for doxycycline), they are deposited irreversibly in the growing bones and in dentine and enamel of unerupted teeth of young animals, or even the fetus if transplacental passage occurs (*see* SPECIAL CLINICAL CONCERNS, below). Because of this property, they may serve as markers in developing bone or in proliferating bone tissue. Tetracyclines are bound to plasma proteins to varying degrees (eg, oxytetracycline, 30%; tetracycline, 60%; doxycycline, 90%).

Biotransformation: Biotransformation of the tetracyclines seems to be limited in most domestic animals, and generally about one-third of a given dose is excreted unchanged. Rolitetracycline is metabolized to tetracycline. Doxycycline and minocycline may be more extensively biotransformed than other tetracyclines (up to 40% of a given dose).

Excretion: Tetracyclines are excreted via the kidneys (glomerular filtration) and the GI tract (biliary elimination and directly). Generally 50-80% of a given dose is recoverable from the urine, although several factors may influence renal elimination, including age, route of administration, urine pH, glomerular filtration rate, renal disease, and the particular tetracycline used. Intestinal elimination is always significant, commonly ~10-20%, even with parenteral administration; for doxycycline and its metabolites, this is the major route of excretion. Tetracyclines are also eliminated in milk; peak concentrations occur 6 hr after a parenteral dose, and traces are still present up to 48 hr. Levels in milk usually attain ~50-60% of the plasma concentration, and are often higher in mastitic milk.

Pharmacokinetic Values: The plasma half-lives of tetracyclines are 6-12 hr and even longer depending on age (slow elimination in animals <1 mo old), disease, and the tetracycline itself. In large animals, daily injections of standard dosages usually are sufficient to maintain effective inhibitory concentrations. Long-acting formulations of oxytetracycline, when injected IM, generally produce plasma concentrations >0.5 μg/mL for ~72 hr. Tetracyclines usually are administered PO q8-12hr, or q12-24hr for doxycycline and minocycline.

Elimination, Distribution, and Clearance of Tetracyclines

Tetracycline	Species	Elimination half-life (hr)	Volume of distribution (mL/kg)	Clearance (mL/kg/min)
Oxytetracycline	Dogs	6	3000	4.23
	Calves (<3 mo)	10-13	1500-2400	3.45
	Cattle	7-10	800-1000	3.33
	Horses	8-10	1100	2.89
Minocycline	Dogs	7	2000	3.21

THERAPEUTIC INDICATIONS

The tetracyclines are used to treat both systemic and local infections. General organ infections include bronchopneumonia, bacterial enteritis, urinary tract infections, cholangitis, metritis, mastitis, prostatitis, and pyodermatitis. Specific conditions include bovine pinkeye, chlamydiosis, heartwater, anaplasmosis, actinomycosis, actinobacillosis, nocardiosis (especially minocycline), ehrlichiosis (especially doxycycline), eperythrozoonosis, and haemobartonellosis. Minocycline and doxycycline are often effective to a somewhat lesser degree against resistant strains of *Staphylococcus aureus.*

In addition to antimicrobial chemotherapy, the tetracyclines are employed for other purposes. As additives in animal feeds, they serve as growth promoters. Because of the affinity of tetracyclines for bones, teeth, and necrotic tissue, they can be used to delineate tumors by fluorescence. Demethylchlortetracycline has been used to inhibit the action of antidiuretic hormone in cases of excessive water retention.

SPECIAL CLINICAL CONCERNS

Side Effects and Toxicity: Because several diverse effects may result from the administration of the tetracyclines, caution should be exercised. Superinfection by nonsusceptible pathogens such as fungi, yeasts, and resistant bacteria is always a possibility when broad-spectrum antibiotics are used. This may lead to GI disturbances following either PO or parenteral administration, or "persistent infection" when they are applied topically, eg, in the ear. Severe and even fatal diarrhea can occur in horses receiving tetracyclines, especially if they are severely stressed or critically ill.

High doses administered PO to ruminants seriously disrupt microfloral activity in the ruminoreticulum, eventually producing stasis. Elimination of the gut flora in monogastric animals reduces the synthesis and availability of the B vitamins and vitamin K from the large intestine. With prolonged therapy, vitamin supplementation is a useful precaution.

Tetracyclines chelate calcium in teeth and bones; they become incorporated into these structures, inhibit calcification (eg, hypoplastic dental enamel), and cause yellowish then brownish discoloration. At extremely high concentrations, the healing processes in fractured bones is impaired.

Rapid IV injection of a tetracycline can produce hypotension and sudden collapse. This appears to be related to the ability of the tetracyclines to chelate ionized calcium, though a depressant effect by the propylene glycol carrier itself may also be involved. This effect can be avoided by slow infusion of the drug (>5 min) or by pretreatment with IV calcium gluconate.

The IV administration of undiluted propylene-glycol-based preparations leads to intravascular hemolysis, which results in hemoglobinuria, and possibly other reactions such as hypotension, ataxia, and CNS depression.

Because tetracyclines interfere with protein synthesis even in host cells and therefore tend to be catabolic, an elevation in BUN can be expected. The combined use of glucocorticoids and tetracyclines often leads to a significant weight loss, particularly in anorectic animals.

Hepatotoxic effects due to large doses of tetracyclines have been reported in pregnant women and in other animals. The mortality rate is high.

The tetracyclines are also potentially nephrotoxic and are contraindicated (except for doxycycline) in renal insufficiency. Fatal renal failure has been reported in septicemic and endotoxemic cattle given high doses of oxytetracycline. The administration of expired tetracycline products may lead to acute tubular nephrosis.

Swelling, necrosis, and yellow discoloration at the injection site almost inevitably occur. Phototoxic dermatitis may be seen in human patients treated with demethylchlortetracycline and other analogs, but this reaction is rare in other animals. Hypersensitivity reactions do occur; eg, cats may show a "drug fever" reaction often accompanied by vomiting, diarrhea, depression, inappetence, and eosinophilia.

The tetracyclines are capable of inhibiting WBC chemotaxis and phagocytosis when present in high concentrations at sites of infection. This clearly hinders normal host defense mechanisms. The addition of glucocorticoids to the therapeutic regimen would impair immunocompetence even further.

Interactions: The absorption of tetracyclines from the GI tract is decreased by milk and milk products (less so for doxycycline and minocycline), antacids, kaolin, and iron preparations. Tetracyclines gradually lose activity when diluted in infusion fluids and exposed to ultraviolet light. Vitamins of the B-complex group, especially riboflavin, hasten this loss of activity in infusion fluids. Tetracyclines also bind to the calcium ions in Ringer's solution.

Methoxyflurane anesthesia combined with tetracycline therapy may be nephrotoxic. Microsomal enzyme inducers such as phenobarbital and phenytoin shorten the plasma half-lives of minocycline and doxycycline. Except for minocycline and doxycycline, the presence of food can substantially delay the absorption of tetracyclines from the GI tract. The tetracyclines are less active in alkaline urine, and urine acidification can increase their antimicrobial efficacy.

Effects on Laboratory Tests: Tetracyclines may elevate amylase, BUN, BSP, eosinophil count, AST (SGOT), and ALT (SGPT). Tetracyclines used in combination with diuretics are often associated with a marked rise in the BUN. Decreases may be evident for cholesterol, glucose, potassium, and prothrombin time. A false-positive urine glucose test is also possible.

Drug Withdrawal and Milk Discard Times: Withdrawal times for food animals and milk discard times are determined by regulatory agencies in each country. These must be followed carefully to prevent food residues and public health concerns. The times listed below serve only as broad guidelines for the tetracycline antibiotics.

Tetracycline	Species	Withdrawal time (days)
Oxytetracycline	Cattle*	15-22
long-acting	Cattle*	28
Oxytetracycline	Pigs	22
Oxytetracycline	Poultry	5
Chlortetracycline	Cattle	10
Chlortetracycline	Pigs	1-7

*Not for use in lactating dairy cows.

DOSE RATES

The following is a selection of general dosages for some tetracyclines. The dose rate and frequency should be adjusted as needed for the individual animal.

Tetracycline	Species	Dosage (mg/kg)	Route	Frequency (hr)
Tetracycline	Cats, Dogs	7	IM, IV	12
		20	PO	8
Oxytetracycline	Cats, Dogs	7	IM, IV	12
		20	PO	8
	Cattle, Sheep, Pigs	5-10	IM, IV	24
	Calves, Foals, Lambs, Piglets	10-20	PO	8-12
	Horses	5	IV	12-24
Doxycycline	Dogs	5-10	PO	24
		5	IV	24

CHLORAMPHENICOL AND CONGENERS

Chloramphenicol is a highly effective and well-tolerated broad-spectrum antibiotic. However, it does have several features that demand careful use in companion animals; in several countries, including the USA and Canada, they have led to prohibition of its use in food-producing animals.

CLASSES

Chloramphenicol is a unique antimicrobial agent; however, because of its tendency to cause blood dyscrasias in man, 2 related drugs have been developed. Thiamphenicol is less effective but safer than chloramphenicol; florfenicol, a thiamphenicol derivative, is significantly more active *in vitro* than chloramphenicol against many pathogenic strains of bacteria. Neither of these analogs has been used to any extent in veterinary medicine as yet.

GENERAL PROPERTIES

Chloramphenicol is a relatively simple neutral nitrobenzene derivative with a bitter taste. It is highly lipid soluble and is used either as the free base or in ester forms (eg, the neutral-tasting palmitate for administration PO and the water-soluble sodium succinate for parenteral injection). Chloramphenicol is a relatively stable compound and is unaffected by boiling, provided that a pH of 9 is not exceeded.

ANTIMICROBIAL ACTIVITY

Mode of Action: Chloramphenicol inhibits microbial protein synthesis by binding to the 50 S subunit of the 70 S ribosome and impairing peptidyl transferase activity. The binding of aminoacyl-tRNA to the active site of peptidyl transferase is also prevented. The effect is usually bacteriostatic but, at high concentrations, chloramphenicol may be bactericidal for some species. The inhibition of protein synthesis by chloramphenicol occurs in both prokaryotic and eukaryotic (mitochondrial) ribosomes.

Bacterial Resistance: Resistance against chloramphenicol develops slowly and in a step-wise fashion. In clinical bacterial isolates, resistance is generally plasmid-mediated and is due to the production of chloramphenicol acetyltransferase, though other inactivating enzymes also may be involved. In resistant gram-negative bacteria, chloramphenicol acetyltransferase is a constitutive enzyme; in gram-positive organisms, the enzyme is inducible. In *Pseudomonas aeruginosa* and in strains of *Proteus* and *Klebsiella* spp, resistance is also nonenzymatic and is based on an inducible permeability block that is both chromosomal and plasmid-mediated. Resistance to chloramphenicol often occurs together with resistance to tetracycline, erythromycin, streptomycin, ampicillin, and other antibiotics.

Antimicrobial Spectrum: Many genera of gram-positive and gram-negative bacteria and several anaerobes such as *Bacteroides fragilis*, as well as *Rickettsia* and *Chlamydia* spp are susceptible. Of special note is the efficacy against many *Salmonella* spp and the resistance of most strains of *Pseudomonas aeruginosa*.

PHARMACOKINETIC FEATURES

Absorption: Absorption occurs promptly and rapidly from the upper GI tract when chloramphenicol base is administered PO to nonruminant animals. Maximum blood levels usually occur in 1-3 hr. Because ruminal microflora readily reduce the nitro group, chloramphenicol is inactivated in the ruminoreticulum and is not available for absorption. The larger ester forms of chloramphenicol require hydrolysis by lipases to release the antibiotic for absorption from the GI tract; thus, the systemic availability of chloramphenicol is delayed when the palmitate and other ester preparations are used. Generic inequivalence has been encountered with oral dosage forms. The presence of food and intestinal protectants does not interfere with the absorption of chloramphenicol, though drugs that depress GI motility do.

Chloramphenicol sodium succinate may be injected both IV and IM. However, hydrolysis is required in the body because only free chloramphenicol base is active. The kinetics of this hydrolysis reaction may be slow and incomplete, with considerable individual and species variability. The absorption of chloramphenicol base itself from IM injection sites is notably restricted; eg, in horses, the therapeutic blood concentration of 5 μg/mL is achieved at a dose of 50 mg/kg body wt, IM, only after 6-8 hr. Chloramphenicol base is absorbed following IP injection.

Distribution: About 40-60% of chloramphenicol in plasma is reversibly bound to albumin, and the free fraction readily diffuses into almost all tissues (including the brain); highest concentrations are reached in the kidneys, liver, and bile. Substantial levels (~50% of plasma values) are also reached in many body fluids such as the CSF and aqueous humor. Milk concentrations are ~50% those of plasma but may be higher in mastitis. Transplacental diffusion occurs in all species, with levels of ~75% being reached in the fetus as compared with the dam. Chloramphenicol does not attain effective concentrations in normal synovial fluid, but does so in septic arthritis. The blood-prostate barrier is an exception to chloramphenicol's extensive intracorporeal distribution: levels in the inflamed gland are low to nil. About 15-20% of peak serum concentrations occur within abscesses.

Biotransformation: Unlike many other antibacterial agents, chloramphenicol undergoes extensive hepatic metabolism. Though some nitroreduction and other phase I reactions occur, free chloramphenicol is biotransformed primarily by glucuronide conjugation. Urinary products following administration of chloramphenicol sodium succinate include inactive forms, mainly the unhydrolyzed sodium succinate and the glucuronide; only 5-15% appears as biologically active chloramphenicol. There are several clinical concerns with respect to chloramphenicol's biotransformation. In cats, a characteristic genetic deficiency in glucuronyl transferase activity leads to plasma half-lives that are often considerably longer than those in other species (eg, cats, 5.1 hr; ponies, 54 min), and dosages need to be adjusted accordingly. Very young animals frequently do not have full microsomal enzyme capabilities, and the plasma half-lives of chloramphenicol in the young (<4 wk) of many species are often much longer than those of adults. Foals appear to be a notable exception to this generalization. Liver disease also prevents chloramphenicol from undergoing normal metabolic degradation, and active antibiotic accumulates in the body.

Excretion: The principal route of excretion is renal. Free chloramphenicol and the chloramphenicol sodium succinate dosage form undergo glomerular filtration (5-10%), whereas the glucuronide metabolite is eliminated by tubular secretion (90-95%). Only 5-15% of chloramphenicol is present in the urine in the active, unchanged form. The biliary route also plays a part in its excretion, but enterohepatic cycling is often pronounced, and usually only a small amount of chloramphenicol is recoverable in feces. Enterohepatic cycling prolongs blood levels to some degree in herbivores.

Pharmacokinetic Values: The plasma half-life of chloramphenicol varies among species and depends on age in some species. The specific volumes of distribution usually reflect the extensive diffusion into tissues. Dose rates and frequencies are typically adjusted for the species and age of the animal (*see* below). The pharmacokinetic values are approximately as follows:

Species	Elimination half-life (hr)	Volume of distribution (mL/kg)
Cats	5.1	2360
Dogs	4.2	1700
Calves (<1 wk)	5.0	1080
Cattle	3.0	1580
Horses	0.9	950

THERAPEUTIC INDICATIONS

Chloramphenicol is used to treat both systemic and local infections. Chronic respiratory infections, bacterial meningoencephalitis, brain abscesses, ophthalmitis and intraocular infections, pododermatitis, dermal infections, and otitis externa represent forms of bacterial infection often responsive to chloramphenicol. Salmonellosis and *Bacteroides* sepsis are fairly specific indications. Urinary tract infections are often successfully treated with chloramphenicol, notwithstanding the fairly low concentration of active antibiotic present in the urine. Hematogenous delivery of chloramphenicol to the site of infection may play a role in these cases.

SPECIAL CLINICAL CONCERNS

Side Effects and Toxicity: In man, chloramphenicol may produce 2 distinctive syndromes of bone marrow suppression. One form is characterized by nonregenerative anemia (with or without thrombocytopenia or leukopenia), increased serum iron, bone marrow hypocellularity, cytoplasmic vacuolization of blast cells and lymphocytes, and maturation arrest of erythroid and myeloid precursors. This suppression is dose dependent and reversible. Daily doses of 50 mg/kg for 3 wk can produce similar effects in cats. Milder hematologic effects are evident in dogs at much higher daily doses (225 mg/kg). Such blood dyscrasias may also be seen in susceptible neonatal animals given standard adult doses of chloramphenicol. This toxic effect is postulated to be due to interference with mRNA and protein synthesis in rapidly multiplying cells.

The second form of bone marrow suppression is much more serious. It is a non-dose-related aplastic anemia that usually is irreversible and often appears after the drug has been discontinued. The peripheral blood shows pancytopenia, and the bone marrow may be hypoplastic or aplastic. Usually, a hemorrhagic diathesis and secondary infection are also evident. The incidence is ~1:25,000-40,000. The aplastic anemia may result from toxic intermediates associated with the nitro group; thiamphenicol, without the nitro group, does not produce aplastic anemia, an observation that supports the theory. Due to the possibility that tissue residues in food animals might induce aplastic anemia in man, use of chloramphenicol in food animals has been banned in the USA and several other countries. A form of aplastic anemia, apparently a type of hypersensitivity reaction to chloramphenicol, has been recognized in dogs.

GI disturbances can occur in all nonruminant animals. Oral use in neonatal calves leads to a malabsorption syndrome associated with ultrastructural and functional changes of the small intestinal enterocytes. Anorexia and depression have been observed in cats treated for >1 wk.

Because chloramphenicol can suppress anamnestic immune responses, animals should not be vaccinated while being treated with this antibiotic. Because of its ability to inhibit protein synthesis, excessive topical application on wounds may delay healing.

In both male and female rats, chloramphenicol has adversely affected the structure and functions of the gonads. In large animals, adverse signs are most often associated with propylene-glycol-based preparations which, when infused rapidly IV, may result in collapse, hemolysis, and death.

Notwithstanding the severity of the chloramphenicol-associated side effects noted above, this antibiotic is relatively safe, provided overdosage is avoided, courses of therapy are limited to 1 wk, the dose is reduced for newborn animals and animals with impaired liver function, and there is no evidence of a pre-existing bone marrow depression.

Interactions: Chloramphenicol is a potent noncompetitive microsomal enzyme inhibitor that can substantially prolong the duration of action of a number of co-administered drugs. Frank toxic effects are likely if administration is repeated. Examples of such drugs include pentobarbital, codeine, phenytoin, nonsteroidal anti-inflammatory drugs, and coumarins.

In combination with sulfamethoxypyridazine, chloramphenicol can cause hepatic damage. Chloramphenicol also delays the response of anemia to iron, folic acid, and vitamin B_{12}. It will interfere with the actions of many bactericidal drugs such as the penicillins, cephalosporins, and aminoglycosides: such combinations should not be used under most circumstances. Aqueous solutions of chloramphenicol sodium succinate should not be mixed with other preparations before administration because of a high incidence of incompatibility.

Chloramphenicol should not be administered concurrently with other antibacterial agents (such as the macrolides and lincosamides) that bind to the 50 S ribosomal subunit.

Effects on Laboratory Tests: Chloramphenicol may cause elevated alkaline phosphatase levels and may increase prothrombin times. A reduction in WBC and thrombocyte counts may also be seen. Anemia becomes evident in extreme cases. A false glucosuria test is possible.

Drug Withdrawal and Milk Discard Times: The use of chloramphenicol in food animals is prohibited in several countries; in others, withdrawal times vary considerably and may be as long as 2 wk.

DOSE RATES

The following are general dosages for chloramphenicol, which may be used parenterally, PO, or topically. The dose rate and frequency should be adjusted as needed for the individual animal.

Species	Dosage (mg/kg)	Route	Frequency (hr)
Cat	45-60	PO, IV, IM	12
Dog	45-60	PO, IV, IM	6-8
Horse	50	PO	6-8
		IV	2-4

MACROLIDES

The macrolide antibiotics typically have a large lactone ring in their structure, and are much more effective against gram-positive than against gram-negative bacteria. They are also active against mycoplasmas and some rickettsiae. (*See also* POLYENE MACROLIDE ANTIBIOTICS, p 1465.)

CLASSES

Macrolides fall into 3 classes, depending on the size of the lactone ring. None of the 12-membered ring group is used clinically. Erythromycin and the closely related oleandomycin and troleandomycin belong to the 14-membered ring group. Of the 16-membered ring type, spiramycin, josamycin, and tylosin are used clinically.

GENERAL PROPERTIES

A macrolide is actually a complex mixture of closely related antibiotics that differ from one another with respect to the chemical substitutions on the various carbon atoms in the structure, and in the aminosugars and neutral sugars. For example, erythromycin is mostly erythromycin A, but B, C, D, and E forms may also be included in the preparation. The macrolide antibiotics are colorless, crystalline substances. They contain a dimethylamino group, which makes them basic. Although they are poorly water soluble, they do dissolve in more polar organic solvents. Macrolides are often inactivated in both basic (pH >10) as well as acidic environments (pH <4 for erythromycin). The multiple functional groups make it possible for them to undergo a large number of chemical reactions. More stable ester forms are commonly used in pharmaceutical preparations—eg, acetylates, estolates, lactobionate, succinates, propionates, and stearates.

ANTIMICROBIAL ACTIVITY

Mode of Action: The antimicrobial mechanism seems to be the same for all members of the group. They interfere with protein synthesis by reversibly binding to the 50 S subunit of the ribosome. They appear to bind at the donor site, thus preventing the translocation necessary to keep the peptide chain growing. The effect is essentially confined to rapidly dividing bacteria and mycoplasmas. Macrolides are regarded as being bacteriostatic, but at high concentrations erythromycin is bactericidal. Macrolides are significantly more active at higher pH ranges (7.8-8).

Bacterial Resistance: Resistance to macrolides in gram-positive organisms results from alterations in ribosomal structure and loss of macrolide affinity. The resistance may be intrinsic or plasmid-mediated, constitutive or inducible, and may develop rapidly (erythromycin) or slowly (tylosin). Cross-resistance between macrolides is common. Gram-negative organisms are probably resistant because macrolides cannot penetrate their cell walls. There are a few exceptions, and gram-negative forms without cell walls are usually sensitive.

Antimicrobial Spectra: Macrolides are active against most aerobic and anaerobic gram-positive bacteria, although there is considerable variation as to potency and activity. In general, macrolides are not active against gram-negative bacteria, although some strains of *Pasteurella, Haemophilus,* and *Neisseria* spp may be sensitive. *Bacteroides fragilis* strains are moderately susceptible. Macrolides are active against atypical mycobacteria, *Mycobacterium, Mycoplasma, Chlamydia,* and *Rickettsia* spp but not against protozoa or fungi. *In vitro* synergism is encountered with cefamandole (against *Bacteroides fragilis*), ampicillin (against *Nocardia asteroides*), and rifampin (against *Rhodococcus equi*).

PHARMACOKINETIC FEATURES

Absorption: Macrolides are readily absorbed from the GI tract if not inactivated by gastric acid. Oral preparations are often enteric-coated, or stable salts or esters, such as stearate, lactobionate, glucoheptate, propionate, and ethylsuccinate are used. Peak plasma levels occur within 1-2 hr in most cases, although absorption patterns may be erratic due to the presence of food and may depend on the salt or ester used. Absorption from the ruminoreticulum is usually delayed and is unreliable. Erythromycin and tylosin may also be administered IV or IM. Absorption is rapid, but pain and swelling occur at the injection sites.

Distribution: Macrolides become widely distributed in tissues, and concentrations are about the same as in plasma, or even higher in some instances. They actually accumulate within many cells, including macrophages, in which they may be 20 times the plasma concentration. With spiramycin, the tissue concentrations remain especially high even though plasma concentrations are rather low. Macrolides tend to be concentrated in the spleen, liver, kidneys, and particularly the lungs. They enter pleural and ascitic fluids but not the CSF (only 2-13% of plasma concentration unless the meninges are inflamed). They concentrate in the bile and milk. Up to 75% of the dose is bound to plasma proteins, and they bind to α-1-acid glycoproteins rather than albumin.

Biotransformation: Metabolic inactivation of the macrolides is usually extensive, but the relative proportion depends on the route of administration and the particular antibiotic. Following administration PO, 80% of an erythromycin dose undergoes metabolic inactivation, whereas tylosin appears to be eliminated in an active form.

Excretion: Macrolide antibiotics and their metabolites are excreted mainly in bile (>60%), and often undergo enterohepatic cycling. Urinary clearance is often slow and variable (often <10%) but may represent a more significant route of elimination following parenteral administration. The concentration of macrolides in milk often is several times greater than in plasma, especially in mastitis.

Pharmacokinetics: The plasma half-lives of macrolides usually are 1-3 hr, and apparent volumes of distribution of 1000-2000 mL/kg reflect the extensive tissue distribution. Effective inhibitory concentrations are maintained for ~8 hr following administration PO and for ~12-24 hr following IM injection. Dosage frequencies are commonly 2-3 times/day, PO, or 1-2 times/day, parenterally.

THERAPEUTIC INDICATIONS

The macrolides are used to treat both systemic and local infections. They are often regarded as alternatives to penicillins for the treatment of streptococcal and staphylococcal infections. General indications include upper respiratory tract infections, bronchopneumonia, bacterial enteritis, metritis, pyodermatitis, urinary tract infections, arthritis, and others. Formulations for treating mastitis are also available and often have the advantage of a short withholding time for milk.

SPECIAL CLINICAL CONCERNS

Side Effects and Toxicity: Toxicity and side effects are uncommon, although pain and swelling may occur at injection sites. Hypersensitivity reactions have occasionally been observed. Erythromycin estolate may be hepatotoxic and cause cholestasis; it may also induce vomiting and diarrhea, particularly when high doses are administered. Horses are sensitive to macrolide-induced GI disturbances that can be serious and even fatal. In pigs, tylosin may cause edema of the rectal mucosa, mild anal protrusion with diarrhea, and anal erythema and pruritus. After 5 mg/kg/day, dogs had a greater tendency to develop ventricular tachycardia and fibrillation during acute myocardial ischemia.

Interactions: Macrolide antibiotics probably should not be used with chloramphenicol or the lincosamides since they may compete for the same 50 S ribosomal binding site, although the *in vivo* significance of this potential interaction is unclear. An acidic environment depresses macrolide activity. Macrolide preparations for parenteral administration are incompatible with many other pharmaceutical preparations. Erythromycin and troleandomycin are microsomal enzyme inhibitors that depress the metabolism of some drugs.

Effects on Laboratory Tests: Alkaline phosphatase, bilirubin, BSP, total WBC count, eosinophil count, AST (SGOT), and ALT (SGPT) may increase. Cholesterol levels may decrease.

Drug Withdrawal and Milk Discard Times: Withdrawal times and milk discard times are determined by the regulatory agency in each country. These should be followed carefully to prevent food residues and public health concerns. The times given below serve only as general guidelines.

Macrolide	Species	Withdrawal time (days)	Milk discard time (hr)
Erythromycin	Cattle	14	36-72
	Pigs	7	
Tylosin	Cattle	21	96
	Pigs	14	

DOSE RATES

The following is a selection of general dose rates for some macrolides. The dose rate and frequency should be adjusted as needed for the individual animal.

Macrolide	Species	Dosage (mg/kg)	Route	Frequency (hr)
Erythromycin	Cattle	8-15	IM	12-24
	Cats	15	PO	8
	Foals	25	IM	8
Tylosin	Cattle	10-20	IM	12-24
	Pigs	10	IM	12-24
		7-10	PO	8
	Cats	10	IM	12

LINCOSAMIDES

GENERAL PROPERTIES

Lincosamides are derivatives of an amino acid and a sulfur-containing octose. They are monobasic and more stable in salt forms (hydrochlorides and phosphates).

ANTIMICROBIAL ACTIVITY

Mode of Action: Lincomycin and clindamycin bind exclusively to the 50 S subunit of bacterial ribosomes and suppress protein synthesis. Lincosamides, macrolides, and chloramphenicol, though not structurally related, seem to act at this same site. The lincosamides are bacteriostatic or bactericidal depending on the concentration. Activity is enhanced at an alkaline pH.

Bacterial Resistance: Resistance to lincosamides appears slowly, perhaps as a result of chromosomal mutation. Plasmid-mediated resistance has been found in strains of *Bacteroides fragilis*. Resistance appears to be due to an alteration in the 50 S ribosomal subunit. Cross-resistance with other antibiotics has been shown *in vitro* but not *in vivo* with erythromycin.

Antimicrobial Spectra: Lincomycin has a limited spectrum against aerobic pathogens but a fairly broad spectrum against anaerobes. Clindamycin is a more active analog with somewhat different pharmacokinetic patterns. Many gram-positive cocci are inhibited by lincosamides, but most gram-negative organisms are resistant, as are most mycoplasmas. *Bacteroides* spp and other anaerobes are usually susceptible. *Clostridium difficile* strains appear to be regularly resistant.

PHARMACOKINETIC FEATURES

Absorption: Lincomycin is incompletely absorbed from the GI tract, especially if administered soon after feeding; peak plasma levels occur within 2-4 hr. Absorption from IM injection sites is good; peak plasma levels are reached in 1-2 hr. About

90% of an oral dose of clindamycin is absorbed, and effective plasma concentrations are achieved more rapidly than with lincomycin. Absorption is not significantly affected by the ingestion of food. Clindamycin palmitate is used PO and clindamycin phosphate IM; the latter reaches peak plasma concentration in 1-3 hr.

Distribution: Lincosamides are widely distributed in many fluids and tissues, including bone, but significant concentrations are not attained in the CSF even when the meninges are inflamed. They diffuse across the placenta in many species. About 90% of clindamycin is bound to plasma proteins. It also accumulates in polymorphonuclear WBC and alveolar macrophages, but the clinical relevance of this phenomenon is unclear.

Biotransformation: Following administration PO, ~50% of a dose of lincomycin and 80-90% of a clindamycin dose are metabolically altered in the liver. Metabolites often retain activity. Liver disease impairs the biotransformation of lincosamides.

Excretion: Unchanged antibiotic and several metabolites may be excreted in bile and urine. The proportions depend on the route of administration. Levels remain high in the feces for some days, and growth of sensitive microorganisms in the large intestine may be suppressed for up to 2 wk. Milk is also an important excretory route.

Pharmacokinetics: The elimination half-life of lincosamides is frequently >3 hr and the apparent volume of distribution ≥1 L/kg. They are usually administered b.i.d.

THERAPEUTIC INDICATIONS

The lincosamides are indicated for infections caused by susceptible gram-positive organisms, particularly streptococci and staphylococci, and those caused by anaerobic pathogens.

SPECIAL CLINICAL CONCERNS

Side Effects and Toxicity: No serious organ toxicity has been reported, but GI disturbances do occur. Clindamycin-induced pseudomembranous enterocolitis (caused by toxigenic *Clostridium difficile*) is a serious adverse reaction encountered in man. Lincosamides are contraindicated in horses because severe and even fatal colitis may develop. Skeletal muscle paralysis may occur at high concentrations. Hypersensitivity reactions occasionally occur. These antibiotics should be avoided in neonates because of their limited capacity to metabolize drugs.

Interactions: Lincosamides have additive neuromuscular effects with anesthetic agents and skeletal muscle relaxants. Kaolin-pectin prevents their absorption from the GI tract. They should not be combined with bactericidal agents or with the macrolides.

Effects on Laboratory Tests: Alkaline phosphatase, AST (SGOT), and ALT (SGPT) may be elevated.

Drug Withdrawal Times: In several countries, there is a 2-day withdrawal time for pigs.

DOSE RATES

The following is a selection of general dosages for some lincosamides. The dose rate and frequency should be adjusted as needed for the individual animal.

Lincosamide	Species	Dosage (mg/kg)	Route	Frequency (hr)
Lincomycin	Cattle	10	IM	12
	Pigs	10	IM	12
		7	in feed	
	Dogs	20	PO	24
	Cats	10	IM	12
		25	PO	12
Clindamycin	Cats	10	IM or PO	12

MISCELLANEOUS ANTIBIOTICS

A number of antibiotics are used periodically for several diverse purposes. Several of these are discussed below.

POLYMYXINS

Of this group of polypeptide antibiotics, polymyxin B and polymyxin E, or colistin, are most commonly used topically and PO. Colistimethate is a form of colistin intended for parenteral administration. Polymyxins are bactericidal; they interact strongly with phospholipids in bacterial cell membranes and radically disrupt their permeability and function. The polymyxins are more effective against gram-negative than gram-positive bacteria. Their rather narrow spectrum includes *Enterobacter, Klebsiella, Salmonella, Pasteurella, Bordetella,* and *Shigella* spp, and *Escherichia coli.* Most *Proteus* spp are not susceptible. Although intrinsic bacterial resistance to polymyxins is recognized, resistance is uncommon and is chromosome-dependent only. Polymyxins act synergistically when combined with potentiated sulfonamides, tetracyclines, and some other antibacterials; they also reduce the activity of endotoxins in body fluids, and may be beneficial in endotoxemia. Their action is inhibited by divalent cations, unsaturated fatty acids, and quaternary ammonium compounds.

Polymyxins are not absorbed following PO or topical administration; peak plasma levels are reached ~2 hr after parenteral administration. Blood levels usually are low because polymyxins bind to cell membranes as well as tissue debris and purulent exudates. They undergo renal elimination mostly as degradation products and their plasma half-lives are 3-6 hr. The polymyxins are notably nephrotoxic and neurotoxic. Neuromuscular blockade can occur at higher concentrations. Intense pain at sites of injection and hypersensitivity reactions also can be expected. Polymyxin B is a potent histamine releaser. The main indication for parenteral use of polymyxins is life-threatening infection due to gram-negative bacilli or *Pseudomonas* spp that are resistant to other drugs. Polymyxins are also used PO against susceptible intestinal infections. Topical application is common, eg, for otitis externa.

Recommended dose rates for polymyxins vary considerably. A general guideline is 20,000 u/kg, PO, b.i.d.; 5000 u/kg, IM, b.i.d.; 50,000-100,000 u by intramammary infusion; 100,000 u intrauterine in cattle. IV administration of polymyxins is potentially dangerous.

BACITRACINS

Bacitracins are branched, cyclic, decapeptide antibiotics. Bacitracin A is the most active of the group and the main component of the commercial bacitracin preparations that are used either topically or PO. These antibiotics are bactericidal. They interfere with cell membrane function, suppress cell wall formation by preventing the formation of peptidoglycan strands, and they inhibit protein synthesis. Bactericidal activity requires the presence of divalent cations such as zinc. The spectrum of bacitracins is similar to that of penicillin G and is mostly limited to gram-positive and a few gram-negative bacteria, as well as some spirochetes.

Most gram-negative organisms are not susceptible, probably due to lack of penetration of the drug through the outer membrane. Resistance is rare. Bacitracins are often used in combination with neomycin and polymyxins to enhance the antibacterial spectrum. Bacitracins are not appreciably absorbed from the GI tract and are not employed systemically because of their pronounced nephrotoxicity. However, they are used locally in wound powders and ointments, dermatological preparations, eye and ear ointments, and as feed additives in swine and poultry rations for growth promotion. In antibiotic-associated pseudomembranous colitis caused by *Clostridium difficile* cytotoxin, bacitracin (given PO) is considered an alternative to vancomycin. Hypersensitivity reactions to bacitracins occur occasionally.

VANCOMYCIN

Vancomycin is a complex glycopeptide that binds to precursors of the peptidoglycan layer in bacterial cell walls. This effect prevents cell wall synthesis and produces a rapid bactericidal effect in dividing bacteria. Vancomycin is active against most gram-positive bacteria but is not effective against gram-negative cells because of their large size and poor penetrability. Resistance to vancomycin does not readily occur. The drug is widely distributed in the body. Excretion (in active form) is via the kidneys; in renal insufficiency, striking accumulations may occur. The plasma half-life in dogs is 2-3 hr. The only indication for the use of parenteral vancomycin is serious infection due to methicillin-resistant *Staphylococcus aureus*. Although poorly absorbed, oral vancomycin is used to treat antibiotic-associated enterocolitis, especially if caused by *Clostridium difficile*. Febrile reactions and thrombophlebitis (because of tissue irritation) at injection sites may occur. Hypersensitivity reactions are observed infrequently. Ototoxicity and nephrotoxicity were fairly common in the past, but are rare today because of fewer impurities in the final form.

SODIUM FUSIDATE

Fusidic acid and its salts are highly active against gram-positive bacteria, especially *Staphylococcus aureus*. Fusidate inhibits bacterial protein synthesis and may be bacteriostatic or bactericidal. This steroid antibiotic is well absorbed from the GI tract and is widely distributed throughout the body, though it does not diffuse into the CSF. About 95% of sodium fusidate in the circulation is bound to plasma proteins. The drug is inactivated by biotransformation, which is extensive. Bile is the primary route of excretion. Staphylococcal infections have become the primary clinical indication for sodium fusidate, and it may be administered topically, PO, or IV. However, IV administration must be into a large vein and done with caution.

NOVOBIOCIN SODIUM

Novobiocin is a narrow-spectrum antibiotic that may be bacteriostatic or bactericidal at higher concentrations. It is mostly active against gram-positive bacteria, but a few gram-negative strains also are in the spectrum. There is a synergistic effect with tetracyclines. Many species of bacteria are capable of developing resistance to novobiocin. Adverse reactions are quite frequent when this antibiotic is administered, and currently its main use is in combination with other agents for the treatment of bovine mastitis.

TIAMULIN FUMARATE

Tiamulin is active against gram-positive bacteria, mycoplasmas, and anaerobes including *Treponema hyodysenteriae*. It is also clinically effective in the treatment of swine dysentery and mycoplasmal arthritis. Tiamulin is well absorbed when administered PO. The dose is 8.8 mg/kg body wt, daily for 3-5 days, in either food or water. The parenteral dosage for mycoplasmal pneumonia in pigs is 15 mg/kg. In poultry, tiamulin interferes with monensin and salinomycin metabolism, and if the drugs are fed together, they become toxic. Generally, however, tiamulin has few side effects.

RIFAMYCINS

Several semisynthetic derivatives (rifamycin SV, rifampin [rifampicin], rifamide) of natural rifamycins have enjoyed some use as extended-spectrum antibiotics. Rifamycins interfere with the synthesis of RNA in microorganisms by binding to subunits of sensitive DNA-dependent RNA polymerase. They are active against gram-positive organisms, some mycobacteria, a few strains of gram-negative bacteria (mostly cocci; bacilli are more resistant), some anaerobes, and chlamydiae; at high concentrations they are also active against several viruses. Fungal and yeast infections resistant to rifampin alone often respond when a rifamycin is added to an antifungal agent such as amphotericin B. Resistance to rifamycins may develop rapidly as a one-step process. For this reason, they are often administered in combination with other antimicrobials such as penicillins, erythromycin, miconazole, and amphotericin B. Though the primary use of the rifamycins in man has been directed toward the treatment of tuberculosis, rifampin has been employed in foals to control *Rhodococcus-equi*-induced pneumonia. Because rifamycins penetrate tissues and cells to a substantial degree, they are particularly effective against intracellular organisms. Rifampin is readily but incompletely (~40%) absorbed from the GI tract, and peak plasma levels occur within 2-4 hr. Concurrent feeding may reduce or delay absorption. Rifampin may also be administered IM or IV. About 75-80% of rifampin is bound to plasma proteins. It is widely distributed in body tissues and fluids because of its high lipid solubility. Rifampin is biotransformed to several metabolites, some of which are active, and is primarily excreted in bile (used for cholangitis in man) and to a lesser degree in urine. Enterohepatic cycling of the parent drug and its main metabolite (desacetylrifampin) commonly occurs. The elimination half-life of rifampin is dose-dependent: in horses, it is ~6 hr; in dogs, ~8 hr. The plasma half-life progressively shortens by ~40% during the first 2 wk of treatment due to the induction of hepatic microsomal enzymes; conversely, it is increased with hepatic dysfunction. Rifampin is usually well tolerated and produces few side effects. GI disturbances and abnormalities in liver function (icterus) have been reported in man. Hypersensitivity reactions can also result from rifampin administration, and renal failure is a possible consequence when intermittent dosage schedules are followed. Partial, reversible immunosuppression of lymphocytes occurs. Urine, feces, saliva, sputum, sweat, and tears are often colored red-orange by rifampin and its metabolites. CNS depression after IV administration and temporary inappetence occur in horses. The dose range for rifampin in horses is 10-25 mg/kg body wt, daily, PO or parenterally.

SULFONAMIDES AND SULFONAMIDE COMBINATIONS

Despite the availability of the antibiotic drugs reviewed above, sulfonamides remain among the most widely used antibacterial agents in veterinary medicine, chiefly because of low cost and their relative efficacy in some common bacterial diseases. The synergistic action of sulfonamides with specific diaminopyrimidines has added a significant dimension to sulfonamide therapy.

CLASSES

The many sulfonamides and sulfonamide derivatives available for clinical use can be categorized into several types, based mainly on their indications and duration of action in the body.

Standard use sulfonamides: In most species, members of this large group are administered 1-4 times a day, depending on the drug, to control systemic infections caused by susceptible bacteria. In some instances, administration of the sulfonamide every second or even third day may be sufficient to maintain blood levels if the drug is eliminated particularly slowly in the species being treated. Sulfonamides included in this class are sulfathiazole, sulfamethazine (sulfadimidine), sulfamerazine, sulfadiazine, sulfapyridine, sulfabromomethazine, sulfaethoxypyridazine, sulfamethoxypyridazine, sulfadimethoxine, and sulfachlorpyridazine.

Highly soluble sulfonamides used for urinary tract infections: a few very water-soluble sulfonamides, eg, sulfisoxazole (sulfafurazole) and sulfasomidine, are rapidly excreted via the urinary tract (>90% in 24 hr) mostly in an unchanged form; because of this, they are primarily employed for the treatment of urinary tract infections.

Poorly soluble sulfonamides used for intestinal infections: Some sulfonamide derivatives, such as sulfaguanidine, are so insoluble that they are not absorbed from the GI tract (<5%). Phthalylsulfathiazole and succinylsulfathiazole undergo bacterial hydrolysis in the lower GI tract with the consequent release of active sulfathiazole. Salicylazosulfapyridine (sulfasalazine) is also hydrolyzed in the large intestine to sulfapyridine and 5-aminosalicylic acid, an anti-inflammatory agent. This drug is used for the management of ulcerative colitis in dogs.

Potentiated sulfonamides (qv, p 1455): Certain diaminopyrimidines when used in combination with sulfonamides cause a sequential blockade of microbial tetrahydrofolate synthesis, which ultimately kills the organism. Sulfonamides are used in combination with pyrimethamine to treat protozoal diseases such as leishmaniasis and toxoplasmosis.

Sulfonamides used topically: Several sulfonamides are used topically for specific purposes. Sulfacetamide is not highly efficacious, but is occasionally used to treat ophthalmic infections. Mafenide and silver sulfadiazine are used on burn wounds to prevent invasion by many gram-negative and gram-positive organisms. Sulfathiazole is commonly included in wound powders for the same purpose.

GENERAL PROPERTIES

The sulfonamides are derivatives of sulfanilamide. All have the same nucleus to which various functional groups have been added to the amido group or in which various substitutions on the amino group are made. These changes produce compounds with varying physical, chemical, pharmacological, and antibacterial properties. Although amphoteric, sulfonamides generally behave as weak organic acids and are much more soluble in an alkaline than in an acidic environment. Those of therapeutic interest have pK_a values between 4.8 and 8.6. Water-soluble sodium or disodium salts are used for parenteral administration. Such solutions are highly alkaline, somewhat unstable, and readily precipitate out with the addition of polyionic electrolytes. In a mixture of sulfonamides (eg, the sulfapyrimidine group), each component drug exhibits its own solubility; therefore, a combination of sulfonamides is more water-soluble than a single drug at the same total concentration. This is the basis of triple sulfonamide mixtures used clinically. The N-4 acetylated sulfonamides, except for the sulfapyrimidine group (sulfamethazine, sulfamerazine, sulfadiazine), are less water-soluble than their nonacetylated forms. This has bearing in the development of sulfonamide crystalluria. The highly insoluble sulfonamides (phthalylsulfathiazole and succinylsulfathiazole) are retained in the lumen of the GI tract for prolonged periods and are known as "gut-active" sulfonamides.

ANTIMICROBIAL ACTIVITY

Mode of Action: The sulfonamides are structural analogs of para-aminobenzoic acid (PABA) and competitively inhibit an enzymatic step (dihydropterate synthetase) during which PABA is incorporated into the synthesis of dihydrofolic acid (folic acid). Because dihydrofolate synthesis is reduced, the levels of tetrahydrofolate (folinic acid) formed from dihydrofolate diminish. Tetrahydrofolate is an essential component of the coenzymes responsible for single carbon metabolism in cells. Acting as antimetabolites to PABA, sulfonamides eventually block, in a complex fashion, the enzymes needed for the biogenesis of purine bases, for the transfer of desoxyuridine to thymidine, and for the biosynthesis of methionine, glycine, and formylmethionyl-transfer-RNA. This results in suppression of protein synthesis, impairment of metabolic processes, and inhibition of growth and multiplication of those organisms that cannot utilize preformed folate. The effect is bacteriostatic, although a bactericidal action is evident at the high concentrations that may occur in urine.

Sulfonamides are most effective in the early stages of acute infections when organisms are rapidly multiplying. They are not active against quiescent bacteria. Typically, there is a latent period before the effects of sulfonamide therapy become evident. This lag period occurs because the bacteria utilize existing stores of folic acid, folinic acid, purines, thymidine, and amino acids. Once these stores are depleted, bacteriostasis occurs. Bacterial growth can resume when the concentration of PABA increases or the level of sulfonamide falls below an enzyme-inhibitory concentration. Adequate cellular and humoral defense mechanisms are critical for successful sulfonamide therapy.

Although all of the sulfonamides possess the same mechanism of action, differences are evident with respect to activity, pharmacokinetic fate, and even antimicrobial spectrum at usual concentrations. The differences are due to the variety of physiochemical characteristics encountered among the sulfonamides.

The bacteriostatic efficacy of sulfonamides can be reduced radically by excess PABA, folic acid, thymine, purine, methionine, plasma, blood, albumin, tissue autolysates, and endogenous protein degradation products.

Bacterial Resistance: Both chromosomal and R-factor-mediated resistance to sulfonamides have been attributed to altered forms of dihydropterate synthetase for which sulfonamides have a lowered affinity. Another mechanism of resistance is the hyperproduction of PABA, which will overcome the metabolic block imposed by the inhibition of dihydropterate synthetase. Cross-resistance between sulfonamides is the general rule. Resistance does emerge gradually and is widespread in many animal populations; continued use of sulfonamides will increase the incidence. Plasmid-mediated sulfonamide resistance in intestinal gram-negative bacteria is often linked with ampicillin and tetracycline resistance.

Antimicrobial Spectrum: Different sulfonamides may show quantitative but not necessarily qualitative differences in antimicrobial activity. Sulfonamides inhibit both gram-positive and gram-negative bacteria, a few *Chlamydia, Nocardia,* and *Actinomyces* spp, and some protozoa such as coccidia and *Toxoplasma* spp. More active sulfonamides may include several species of *Streptococcus, Staphylococcus, Salmonella, Pasteurella,* and even *Escherichia coli* in their spectra. Strains of *Pseudomonas, Klebsiella, Proteus, Clostridium,* and *Leptospira* spp are most often highly resistant, as are rickettsiae.

PHARMACOKINETIC FEATURES

There are notable differences among the many sulfonamides with respect to their pharmacokinetic fate in the various species. The standard classification of short-acting, medium-acting, and long-acting sulfonamides that is used in human therapeutics is usually inappropriate in veterinary medicine because of species differences in disposition and elimination.

Absorption: Sulfonamides may be administered PO, IV, IP, IM, intrauterine, or topically, depending on the specific preparation. Except for the poorly absorbed sulfonamides intended for intestinal use, most are rather rapidly and completely absorbed from the GI tract of monogastric animals. Absorption from the rumino-reticulum is delayed, especially if ruminal stasis is present. Therapeutic doses of sulfonamides are usually administered PO except in acute life-threatening infections when IV infusions are used to establish adequate blood levels as rapidly as possible. Sulfonamides are frequently added to drinking water or feed either for therapeutic purposes or to improve feed efficiency. A few highly water-soluble preparations may be injected IM, eg, sodium sulfadimethoxine, or IP (some irritation of the peritoneum can occur). Absorption is rapid from these parenteral sites. Generally, sulfonamide solutions are too alkaline for routine parenteral use.

Distribution: Sulfonamides are distributed throughout all body tissues. The distribution pattern depends on the ionization state of the sulfonamide, the vascularity of specific tissues, the presence of specific barriers to sulfonamide diffusion, and the fraction of the administered dose bound to plasma proteins. The unbound drug fraction is freely diffusible. Plasma-protein-bound to a greater or lesser extent, sulfonamides may occur at 50-90% of the blood level in pleural, peritoneal, synovial, and ocular fluids. Concentrations in the kidneys exceed plasma levels, and those in the skin, liver, and lungs are only slightly less than the corresponding plasma levels. Concentrations in muscle and bone are ~50% those in the plasma, and in the CSF may be 20-80% of blood levels, depending on the particular sulfonamide. Low levels are encountered in adipose tissue. Following parenteral administration, sulfamethazine is found in jejunal and colonic contents at about the same concentration as in blood. Passive diffusion into milk also occurs; although the levels achieved are usually inadequate to control infections, sulfonamide residues may be detected in milk.

Biotransformation: Sulfonamides are usually extensively metabolized, mainly by several oxidative pathways, acetylation, and conjugation with sulfate or glucuronic acid. Species differences are marked in this regard. The acetylated, hydroxylated, and conjugated forms have little antibacterial activity. Acetylation (poorly developed in dogs) reduces the solubility of most sulfonamides except for the sulfapyrimidine group. The hydroxylated and conjugated forms are less likely to precipitate in urine.

Excretion: Most sulfonamides are excreted primarily in the urine. Bile, feces, milk, and sweat are excretory routes of lesser significance. Glomerular filtration, active tubular secretion, and tubular reabsorption are the main processes involved. The proportion reabsorbed is influenced by the inherent lipid solubility of individual sulfonamides and their metabolites and by urinary pH. Urinary pH, renal clearance, and the concentration and solubility of the respective sulfonamides and their metabolites determine whether solubilities are exceeded and crystal precipitation occurs. This can be prevented by alkalinizing the urine, increasing the fluid intake, reducing dose rates in renal insufficiency, and using triple-sulfonamide combinations.

Pharmacokinetic Considerations: There are great differences between the pharmacokinetic values of various sulfonamides in animals. Extrapolation of these values is rarely appropriate, eg, the plasma half-life of sulfadiazine is 10.1 hr in cattle and 2.9 hr in pigs. The recommended dose rates and frequencies reflect this disparity in elimination kinetics.

THERAPEUTIC INDICATIONS

The sulfonamides are commonly used to treat or prevent acute systemic or local infections. Disease syndromes treated with sulfonamides include actinobacillosis, coccidiosis, mastitis, metritis, colibacillosis, pododermatitis, polyarthritis, respiratory infections, and toxoplasmosis.

Principles of Sulfonamide Therapy: Sulfonamides are more effective when administered early in the course of a disease. Chronic infections, particularly with large amounts of exudate or tissue debris present, often are not responsive. In severe infections, the initial dose should be administered IV to reduce the lag time between dose and effect. In many instances, the initial dose should be double the maintenance dose. Adequate drinking water should be available at all times and urine output monitored. Concurrent administration of urinary alkalinizers prevents crystalluria. A course of treatment should not exceed 7 days under usual circumstances, but a favorable response within 72 hr is a requirement to continue sulfonamide therapy. Treatment should be continued for 48 hr after remission to prevent relapse and the emergence of resistance. The ability to mount an immune response must be intact for successful sulfonamide therapy.

SPECIAL CLINICAL CONCERNS

Side Effects and Toxicity: Adverse reactions to sulfonamides may be due to hypersensitivity or direct toxic effects. Possible hypersensitivity reactions include urticaria, angioedema, anaphylaxis, skin rashes, drug fever, polyarthritis, hemolytic anemia, and agranulocytosis. Crystalluria with hematuria, and even tubular obstruction, can occur but is not common in veterinary medicine. Sulfonamides with prolonged plasma half-lives and high solubilities tend not to cause crystalluria, particularly if water intake is high and the urine is alkaline. Acute toxic manifestations may be observed following too rapid IV administration or if an excessive dose is injected. Clinical signs include muscle weakness, ataxia, blindness, and collapse. GI disturbances, in addition to nausea and vomiting, may occur when sulfonamide levels are sufficiently high in the tract to disturb normal microfloral balance and vitamin B synthesis. Sulfonamides depress the cellulolytic function of ruminal microflora, but the effect is usually transient (unless excessively high levels are reached). Several adverse effects have been reported following prolonged treatment. Included among these are bone marrow depression (aplastic anemia, granulocytopenia, thrombocytopenia), hepatitis and icterus, peripheral neuritis and myelin degeneration in the spinal cord and peripheral nerves, photosensitization, stomatitis, conjunctivitis, and keratitis sicca (especially with sulfadiazine). Mild follicular thyroid hyperplasia may be associated with prolonged administration of sulfonamides to sensitive species such as dogs. Several sulfonamides may lead to decreased egg production and growth. Topically, the sulfonamides retard healing of uncontaminated wounds.

Interactions: Sulfonamide solutions are incompatible with calcium- or other polyionic-containing fluids as well as many other preparations. Sulfonamides may be displaced from their plasma-protein-binding sites by other acidic drugs with higher binding affinities. Antacids tend to inhibit the GI absorption of sulfonamides. Alkalinization of the urine promotes sulfonamide excretion, and urinary acidification increases the risk of crystalluria. Some sulfonamides act as microsomal enzyme inhibitors, which may lead to toxic manifestations of concurrently administered drugs such as phenytoin.

Effects on Laboratory Tests: Bilirubin, BUN, BSP, eosinophils, LE cells, methemoglobin, AST (SGOT), and ALT (SGPT) may be elevated. Platelet, RBC, and WBC counts are often decreased. Urinalysis may show a change in color, glucose, porphyrins, and urobilinogen. Sulfonamide crystals may also be found.

Drug Withdrawal and Milk Discard Times: Preslaughter withdrawal times for food animals and milk discard times are determined by the regulatory agencies in each country, and are currently (as this was being written) under review in the USA. These must be followed carefully and responsibly to prevent food residues and consequent public health implications. The times listed below serve only as general guidelines, and are not to be regarded as substitutes for approved labeling.

Sulfonamide	Species	Withdrawal time (days)	Milk discard time (hr)
Sulfamethazine	Cattle	10 (or 28, slow-release bolus)	96
	Pigs	14	
Sulfabromethazine	Cattle	10	96
Triple sulfonamide solution (8% sodium sulfamethazine, 8% sodium sulfapyridine, 8% sodium sulfathiazole)	Cattle	10	96
Sulfadimethoxine	Cattle	7	60

DOSE RATES

The following is a selection of general dosages for some sulfonamides (*see* notes under withdrawal and milk discard times). The dose rate and frequency should be adjusted as needed for the individual animal.

Sulfonamide	Species	Dosage (mg/kg)		Route	Frequency (hr)
		Initial	Maintenance		
Sulfathiazole	Horses	66	66	PO	8
	Cattle,	66	66	PO	4
	Sheep, Pigs				
Sulfamethazine	Cattle	220	110	PO, IV	24
Sulfadiazine	All	50	50	PO	12
Sulfadimethoxine	All	55	27.5	PO	24
Sulfaethoxypyridazine	Cattle	55	55	PO	24
	Pigs	110	55	PO	24
Sulfapyridine	Cattle	132	66	PO	12
Succinylsulfathiazole	All	160	80	PO	12

POTENTIATED SULFONAMIDES

A group of **diaminopyrimidines** (trimethoprim, methoprim, ormetoprim, aditoprim, pyrimethamine) inhibit dihydrofolate reductase in bacteria and protozoa far more efficiently than in mammalian cells. Used alone, these agents are not particularly effective against bacteria, and resistance develops rapidly. However, when combined with sulfonamides, a sequential blockade of microbial enzyme systems occurs with bactericidal consequences. Examples of such potentiated sulfonamide preparations include trimethoprim/sulfadiazine (co-trimazine), trimethoprim/sulfamethoxazole (co-trimoxazole), trimethoprim/sulfadoxine (co-trimoxine), and ormetoprim/sulfadimethoxine.

General Properties: Trimethoprim and ormetoprim are basic drugs that tend to accumulate in more acidic environments such as acidic urine, milk, and ruminal fluid.

Antimicrobial Features: In susceptible bacteria, the sulfonamide component blocks the synthesis of dihydrofolic acid and the particular diaminopyrimidine used in combination inhibits the next enzyme in the sequence (dihydrofolate reductase) to prevent the formation of tetrahydrofolic acid (folinic acid). Folinic acid is required for the synthesis of DNA. This sequential blockade produces a bactericidal rather than bacteriostatic effect under usual conditions, but in the presence of thymidine, only bacteriostasis is evident because the block is circumvented.

The optimal ratio *in vitro* for the combination of trimethoprim or ormetoprim and a sulfonamide depends on the type of microorganism but is usually ~1:20. However, the commercially available preparations employ a ratio of 1:5 because of pharmacokinetic considerations.

Bacterial resistance to trimethoprim readily occurs, but resistance to the combination is not common: the presence of a sulfonamide appears to delay the emergence of bacterial resistance. Resistance may take 2 forms: mutant resistance, with bacteria becoming dependent on exogenous folinic acid or thymidine; and plasmid-mediated resistance, based on enzyme modification.

Antibacterial Spectrum: Sulfonamide-diaminopyrimidine combinations are active against gram-negative and gram-positive organisms, including *Actinomyces, Bordetella, Clostridium, Corynebacterium, Fusobacterium, Haemophilus, Klebsiella, Pasteurella, Proteus, Salmonella, Shigella,* and *Campylobacter* spp, as well as *Escherichia coli,* streptococci, and staphylococci. Some streptococcal strains are only moderately sensitive, as are *Brucella, Erysipelothrix, Nocardia,* and *Moraxella* spp. The antibacterial spectrum does not include *Pseudomonas* or *Mycobacterium* spp.

Pharmacokinetic Features: Trimethoprim is rapidly absorbed following administration PO (peak plasma levels in ~2-4 hr) except in ruminants, in which it tends to be trapped in the ruminoreticulum and appears to undergo a degree of microbial degradation. Absorption occurs readily from parenteral injection sites; effective antibacterial concentrations are reached in <1 hr, and peak levels in ~4 hr. Trimethoprim diffuses extensively into tissues and body fluids. Tissue concentrations are often higher than the corresponding plasma levels, especially in lungs, liver, and kidneys. About 30-60% of trimethoprim is bound to plasma proteins. The extent of metabolic transformation of trimethoprim has not yet been established, although there is a suggestion that hepatic biotransformation can be extensive, at least in ruminants. This may not be the case in all species; >50% of a dose is excreted unchanged in many instances. Trimethoprim is largely excreted in the urine by glomerular filtration and tubular secretion. A substantial amount may also be found in the feces. The concentrations in milk are often 1-3.5 times higher than those in plasma. The plasma half-life of trimethoprim is quite prolonged in most species; effective levels may be maintained for >12 hr, with the result that the frequency of administration is usually 12-24 hr. The elimination rates of trimethoprim in sheep seem to be much shorter than for monogastric species.
Elimination of ormetoprim appears to be prolonged.

Side Effects and Toxicity: Side effects due to the potentiated sulfonamides are quite rare, although adverse reactions to the sulfonamide components still occur. Up to 10 times the recommended dose of trimethoprim has been given with impunity. Prolonged administration of trimethoprim at reasonably high levels leads to maturation defects in hematopoiesis due to impaired folinic acid synthesis. This effect is readily reversible by supplementation with folinic acid.

Dose Rates: The following is a selection of general dosages. The dose rate and frequency should be adjusted as needed for the individual animal.

Combination	Dosage (mg/kg)	Route	Frequency (hr)
Trimethoprim/	15	PO	12
sulfadiazine:	15-60	PO, IV, IM	24
Trimethoprim/	16-24	IV, IM	24
sulfadoxine:			
Ormetoprim/	55	PO	24 (initial dose)
sulfadimethoxine:	27.5	PO	24 (subsequent doses)

Drug Withdrawal and Milk Discard Times: Preslaughter withdrawal times for food animals and milk discard times are determined by the regulatory agencies in each country. These must be followed carefully and responsibly to prevent food residues and consequent public health implications. The times given here serve only as guidelines.

Combination	Withdrawal time (days)	Milk discard time (days)
Trimethoprim/ sulfadiazine:	3	7
Trimethoprim/ sulfadoxine:	5 (PO) 28 (parenteral)	

QUINOLONES

Quinolone carboxylic acid derivatives are synthetic antimicrobial agents that are becoming more important in veterinary medicine. Nalidixic acid and its congener oxolinic acid have been employed for treatment of urinary tract infections for some years, while flumequine has been used sucessfully in several countries to control intestinal infections in livestock. Recently, a number of broad-spectrum antimicrobial agents have been produced by modification of the various 4-quinolone ring structures.

CLASSES

Known generically as quinolones or 4-quinolones, these drugs are derived from several closely related ring structures that possess certain common features. The major classes are presented below with several clinically useful examples of each.
Quinolone carboxylic acids: enrofloxacin, norfloxacin, ciprofloxacin, pefloxacin, danofloxacin, rosoxacin, acrosoxacin, and oxolinic acid.
Naphthyridine carboxylic acids: enoxacin and nalidixic acid.
Cinnoline carboxylic acids: cinoxacin.
Pyridopyrimidine carboxylic acids: pipemidic acid, piromidic acid.
Quinolizine carboxylic acids: ofloxacin, flumequine.

GENERAL PROPERTIES

Within the diversity of their various ring structures, the quinolones have a number of common functional groups that are essential for their antimicrobial activity. In addition, various modifications have produced compounds with differing physical, chemical, pharmacokinetic, and antimicrobial properties. For example, substitution at position 6 with a fluorine moiety markedly enhances activity against both gram-negative and gram-positive bacteria, as well as mycoplasmas and chlamydiae. These so-called fluoroquinolones, which will probably prove to be the most efficacious within each class, include enrofloxacin, norfloxacin, ciprofloxacin, ofloxacin, danofloxacin, flumequine, and other newer experimental drugs. In addition, substitution with a piperazine ring at position 7 significantly increases tissue and bacterial penetration with consequent enhancement of activity; substitution with an oxygen atom at position 8 improves activity against gram-positive and anaerobic organisms without affecting the bactericidal profile.

The quinolones are amphoteric and, with a few exceptions, generally exhibit poor water solubility between pH 6 and 8. In concentrated acidic urine, such as may be found in dogs and cats, some quinolones form needle-shaped crystals. Liquid formulations of various quinolones for PO or parenteral administration usually contain freely soluble salts in stable aqueous solutions. Solid formulations, eg, tablets, capsules, or boluses, contain the active ingredient either in its betaine form or, occasionally, as the hydrochloride salt.

ANTIMICROBIAL ACTIVITY

Mode of Action: The quinolones inhibit the bacterial enzyme DNA-gyrase (topoisomerase) that is responsible for the supercoiling of DNA so that the DNA can twist in a number of chromosomal domains and seal around an RNA core. To do this, the chromosome also must be transiently nicked before sealing. When DNA-gyrase is inhibited by quinolones, a reduction in the supercoiling occurs with a consequent disruption of the spatial arrangement of DNA. The exposed nicks induce exonucleases that degrade chromosomal DNA into small fragments. Mammalian topoisomerases with nicking activity exist, but these enzymes are fundamentally different from bacterial gyrase and are not susceptible to quinolone inhibition. The quinolones are usually bactericidal; susceptible organisms lose viability within 20 min of exposure to optimal concentrations of the newer fluoroquinolones. Typically, clearing of cytoplasm at the periphery of the affected bacterium occurs and is followed by lysis. Affected bacteria are then recognizable only as ghosts.

Quinolones are known to produce a postantibiotic effect in a number of bacteria (eg, *Escherichia coli, Klebsiella pneumoniae, Pseudomonas aeruginosa*). The effect generally lasts 4-8 hr after exposure. Ideal bactericidal concentrations of the quinolones are often between 0.1 and 10 μg/mL; efficacy tends to diminish at higher concentrations. This unusual biphasic effect is thought to be due to suppression of RNA synthesis at higher quinolone concentrations.

The fluoroquinolones often have significant antibacterial activity at extraordinarily low concentrations, eg, the minimum inhibitory concentrations (μg/mL) for enrofloxacin against some common veterinary pathogens are: *E coli*, <0.01-0.5; *Klebsiella* spp, <0.03-0.5; *Salmonella* spp, 0.003-0.5; *P aeruginosa*, 0.25-2; *Pasteurella haemolytica*, <0.008-0.12; *Staphylococcus aureus*, 0.03-1; *Streptococcus* spp, 0.06-4; and *Mycoplasma* spp, 0.01-1.

Bacterial Resistance: Although resistance develops quite rapidly to nalidixic acid and some other older quinolones, only low-frequency chromosomal mutational resistance to the newer quinolones has been recognized, and it is not regarded as a significant problem. Resistance is due to modification of the target gyrase enzyme. Plasmid-mediated resistance is rare. Fortunately, the virulence of refractory mutants diminishes substantially, and these bacterial populations tend to disappear because of growth deficiencies. Cross-resistance does occur between some closely related quinolones.

Antimicrobial Spectrum: The fluoroquinolones, eg, enrofloxacin and ciprofloxacin, are active against a wide range of gram-negative and a number of gram-positive aerobes. They are highly effective against all intestinal bacterial pathogens as well as several intracellular pathogens, eg, *Brucella* spp. These newer quinolones also possess significant activity against *Mycoplasma* and *Chlamydia* spp. Obligate anaerobes tend to be resistant to most quinolones, as are most enterococcal group D *Streptococcus* spp (*S faecalis* and *S faecium*).

The older quinolones, eg, nalidixic acid and oxolinic acid, and the nonfluorinated quinolones, eg, cinoxacin, tend to have only a moderately extended gram-negative spectrum.

A synergistic effect of quinolones with the β-lactams, aminoglycosides, clindamycin, and metronidazole has been demonstrated *in vitro*.

PHARMACOKINETIC FEATURES

Among the few quinolones that have been studied to any degree in domestic animals, pharmacokinetic differences are significant. Because of the physicochemical nature of the group, this is to be expected. A general overview follows, but some diversity should be anticipated.

Absorption: Quinolones are commonly administered PO, although forms of enrofloxacin and ciprofloxacin are available for IV, IM, and subcut. administration. Absorption into the blood following IM or subcut. delivery is rapid; following administration PO, peak blood concentrations are usually attained within 1-3 hr. Bioavailability is often >80% for most quinolones, except in ruminants with functional forestomachs, in which bioavailability may be as low as 20%. The presence of food may delay absorption in monogastric animals.

Distribution: The quinolones, with few exceptions (eg, cinoxacin), penetrate all tissues well and quickly. Particularly high levels are encountered in the kidneys, liver, and bile, but levels found in prostatic fluid, bone, endometrium, and CSF are also quite notable. Most quinolones also cross the placental barrier. The apparent volume of distribution of most quinolones is large. The degree of plasma-protein binding is extremely variable, from ~10% for norfloxacin to >90% for nalidixic acid.

Biotransformation: Some quinolones are eliminated unchanged (eg, ofloxacin), some are partially metabolized (eg, cinoxacin, ciprofloxacin, enrofloxacin), and a few are completely degraded (eg, acrosoxacin, pefloxacin). Characteristically, phase I reactions produce a number of primary metabolites (up to 6 have been described for some quinolones) that retain some antibacterial action. Conjugation with glucuronic acid then ensues, followed by excretion.

Excretion: Renal excretion is the major route of elimination for most quinolones. Both glomerular filtration and tubular secretion are involved. Urine concentrations are often high for 24 hr after administration, and crystals may form in concentrated acidic urine. The clinical significance of this finding is unclear. In renal failure, clearance is impaired and reductions in dose rates are essential. Biliary excretion of parent drug, as well as conjugates, is an important route of elimination in some cases (eg, ciprofloxacin, pefloxacin, nalidixic acid). Quinolones appear in the milk of lactating animals, often at high concentrations that persist for some time.

Pharmacokinetic Considerations: The plasma half-lives are quite variable among species and the different quinolone classes: 3-6 hr are common, but prolonged plasma half-lives are encountered, eg, 10 hr for pefloxacin in man. Plasma concentrations attained are usually directly proportional to the dose administered. Although somewhat lower, the plasma drug concentration following administration PO is not greatly different from that following subcut. injection. The elimination patterns are also quite similar for PO and parenteral routes.

THERAPEUTIC INDICATIONS

Quinolones are indicated for the treatment of local and systemic infections caused by susceptible microorganisms, particularly against deep-seated infections and intracellular pathogens. Therapeutic success has been obtained in respiratory, intestinal, urinary, and skin infections; and in bacterial prostatitis, meningoencephalitis, osteomyelitis, and arthritis.

SPECIAL CLINICAL CONCERNS

Side Effects and Toxicity: Although side effects with the older quinolones (nalidixic and oxolinic acids) were relatively common, the newer ones seem to be tolerated well. The group tends to be neurotoxic, and convulsions can occur at high doses. Vomiting and diarrhea occur rarely with fluoroquinolones. Dermal reactions and photosensitization have been described in man, but the occurrence seems low. Hemolytic anemia has also been encountered. Administering large doses of quinolones for any length of time during pregnancy has resulted in embryonic loss and maternotoxicity. Because high prolonged dosages in growing dogs has produced cartilagenous erosions leading to permanent lameness, excessive use of quinolones should be avoided in immature animals. The safety of quinolones (especially enrofloxacin) has been established in laboratory animals, calves, pigs, dogs, cats, and poultry. Quinolone administration in horses has not yet been extensively studied, but there is some indication that damage to the cartilage in weight-bearing joints may occur.

Interactions: The likelihood of interactions has not yet been clearly established. Antacids probably interfere with the GI absorption of this group of drugs. It also seems that nitrofurantoin impairs the efficacy of quinolones if used concurrently for urinary tract infections. Quinolones do inhibit the biotransformation of theophylline, leading to prolonged and potentially toxic plasma levels.

Effects on Laboratory Tests: AST (SGOT), ALT (SGPT), alkaline phosphatase, and BUN may be elevated. Urinalysis may reveal needle-shaped crystals.

DOSE RATES

The following is a selection of general dosages for some quinolones. The dose rate and frequency should be adjusted as needed for the individual animal.

Quinolone	Species	Dosage (mg/kg)	Route	Frequency (hr)
Nalidixic acid	Cats/Dogs	3	PO	6
Norfloxacin	Dogs	10-20	PO	12
Ciprofloxacin	Dogs	5-15	PO	12
Enrofloxacin	Cats/Dogs	2.5	PO, subcut.	12
		5	PO, subcut.	24
	Pigs	2.5-5	PO, IM	24
	Preruminant calves	2.5-5	PO, subcut.	24

MISCELLANEOUS ANTIMICROBIAL AGENTS

In addition to the antibiotics and sulfonamides, several other types of antimicrobial agents are employed in veterinary medicine to treat specific infectious diseases. Three of these classes are discussed here: nitrofurans, nitroimidazoles, and hydroxyquinolines.

NITROFURANS

Nitrofurans are synthetic chemotherapeutic agents with a broad antimicrobial spectrum; they are active against both gram-positive and gram-negative bacteria, including *Salmonella* and *Giardia* spp, trichomonads, amebae, and some coccidial species. However, when compared with other antimicrobial chemotherapeutic agents, their potency is not particularly great. The nitrofurans appear to inhibit a number of microbial enzyme systems, including those involved in carbohydrate metabolism, and they also block the initiation of translation. However, their basic mechanism of action has not yet been clarified. Their primary action is bacteriostatic, but at high doses they are also bactericidal. They are much more active in acidic environments (pH 5.5 is optimal for nitrofurantoin activity). Resistant mutants are rare and clinical resistance emerges slowly. Among themselves, nitrofurans show complete cross-resistance, but there is no cross-resistance with any other antibacterial agents. Because of very slight water solubility, the nitrofurans are used either PO or topically. No nitrofuran is effective systemically. They are either not absorbed at all from the GI tract or are so rapidly eliminated that they reach inhibitory concentrations only in the urine. Toxic signs encountered with excessive doses of nitrofuran derivatives include CNS involvement (excitement, tremors, convulsions, peripheral neuritis, GI disturbances, poor weight gain, and depression of spermatogenesis. Various hypersensitivity reactions can also occur. Some nitrofurans are carcinogenic, and their future use is in doubt.

Nitrofurantoin: Nitrofurantoin is used to treat urinary tract infections caused by susceptible bacteria, such as *Escherichia coli, Staphylococcus aureus, Streptococcus pyogenes,* and *Aerobacter aerogenes. Proteus* spp, *Pseudomonas aeruginosa,* and *Streptococcus faecalis* are usually resistant. Following administration PO, nitrofurantoin is rapidly and completely absorbed (the macrocrystal form takes longer) and is swiftly eliminated by the kidneys, mainly by tubular secretion (~40% in the unchanged form). Serum concentrations are low, and little unbound drug is available for diffusion into the tissues. The plasma half-life is only ~20 min. Nitrofurantoin is concentrated in acid urine. When the pH reaches ~5, the drug becomes supersaturated without precipitation and achieves maximal antibacterial action. Nitrofurantoin can be administered both PO and parenterally. The dose for dogs and cats is 4.4 mg/kg body wt, PO, t.i.d. for 4-10 days. Side effects are not common at usual dosages, but nausea, vomiting, and diarrhea can occur. CNS disorders have been observed, and polyneuropathy is a serious effect that occurs in man. Animals with decreased renal function have a predisposition for polyneuritis. Various manifestations of hypersensitivity reactions can occur. Yellow discoloration of teeth occasionally has been reported in very young animals.

Nitrofurazone: Nitrofurazone is only slightly soluble in water but, in general, corresponds to nitrofurantoin in terms of its mechanism of action, antimicrobial spectrum, potency, and physicochemical characteristics. Its main indications include the treatment of bovine mastitis, bovine metritis, and wounds (pus, blood, and milk reduce the antibacterial activity). This nitrofuran is also used as a feed additive (0.05%) to control intestinal bacterial and coccidial infections. The withdrawal time for nitrofurazone in pigs is 5 days.

Furazolidone: This is a nitrofuran with a wide range of antimicrobial activity that includes *Clostridium, Salmonella, Shigella, Staphylococcus,* and *Streptococcus* spp, and *E coli.* It is also active against *Eimeria* and *Histomonas* spp. It is usually administered PO to treat intestinal infections but may also be applied topically. The usual oral dose of furazolidone in calves is 10-12 mg/kg body wt, b.i.d. for 5-7 days. Caution should be exercised when treating small calves (eg, Jersey breed) to avoid excessive dose rates, lest neurotoxicity result—signs include head tremors, ataxia, visual impairment, and convulsions.

Miscellaneous Nitrofurans: Nifuraldezone, like furazolidone, is used to control bacterial enteritis in calves. Nifurprazine is used only topically as an antibacterial agent. Furaltadone is used both PO to prevent intestinal infections, and directly into the teat to treat mastitis.

NITROIMIDAZOLES

The 5-nitroimidazoles are a group of drugs that have both antiprotozoal and antibacterial activity. Antitrichomonal and anti-amebic nitroimidazoles include metronidazole, tinidazole, nimorazole, flunidazole, and ronidazole. Metronidazole and nimorazole are effective in the treatment of giardiasis, while dimetridazole, ipronidazole, and ronidazole control histomoniasis in poultry. Several nitroimidazoles possess antitrypanosomiasis activity. Metronidazole and ronidazole and other nitroimidazoles are active against anaerobic bacteria. Metronidazole is the compound that has been the most studied and is discussed as the prototype of the group.

Metronidazole: This has been used for many years in the therapeutic management of trichomoniasis, giardiasis, and amebiasis, and is active against obligate anaerobic bacteria. It is not active against facultative anaerobes, obligate aerobes, or microaerophilic bacteria other than *Campylobacter fetus* and *Corynebacterium vaginalis.* At concentrations readily attained in serum after PO or parenteral administration, metronidazole is active against *Bacteroides fragilis, B melaninogenicus, Fusobacterium* spp, *Clostridium perfringens,* and other *Clostridium* spp. It is generally less active against nonsporeforming, gram-positive bacilli such as *Actinomyces, Propionibacterium, Bifidobacterium,* and *Eubacterium* spp. Metronidazole is also somewhat less active against gram-positive cocci such as *Peptostreptococcus* and *Peptococcus* spp, but the less sensitive strains are usually not obligate anaerobes.
   Metronidazole is bactericidal at concentrations equal to or slightly higher than the minimal inhibitory concentration. The precise mode of action is unclear, but it seems that after the drug enters a susceptible organism it is first reduced and then binds to DNA, causing loss of the helical structure, strand breakage, and impairment of DNA function. Only susceptible organisms (bacteria and protozoa) appear to be capable of metabolizing the drug.
   The pharmacokinetic pattern of metronidazole generally follows that expected of a highly lipid-soluble basic drug. It is readily but variably absorbed from the GI tract (bioavailability 60-100%), with peak serum concentrations occurring within 1-

2 hr, and becomes widely distributed in all tissues. Metronidazole penetrates the blood-brain barrier and also attains therapeutic concentrations in abscesses and in empyema fluid. It is only slightly bound to plasma proteins. Biotransformation is quite extensive, and excretion of parent drug and metabolites occurs by both the renal and biliary routes. The elimination half-life in dogs is ~4.5 hr, and in horses, 1.5-3.3 hr.

The principal clinical indications for metronidazole include the treatment of specific protozoal infections (amebiasis, trichomoniasis, giardiasis, and balantidiasis) and anaerobic bacterial infections such as those that may be encountered in abdominal abscesses, peritonitis, empyema, genital tract infections, periodontitis, otitis media, osteitis, arthritis, and meningitis, and in necrotic tissue. Metronidazole has been successfully employed to prevent infection after colonic surgery. Nitroimidazoles also act as radiosensitizers, and metronidazole has been used as an adjunct to the radiotherapy of solid tumors.

Side effects are not commonly associated with metronidazole. High doses may induce signs of neurotoxicity in dogs, such as tremors, muscle spasms, ataxia, and even convulsions. Reversible bone marrow depression has been reported. The drug should not be used in pregnant animals, particularly during the first trimester, though the evidence for carcinogenicity and mutagenicity is still tenuous. Metronidazole may produce a reddish brown discoloration of the urine due to unidentified pigments.

Recommended dose rates for metronidazole in dogs are: for anaerobic infections, 44 mg/kg body wt, PO, followed by 22 mg/kg, q.i.d.; for giardiasis, 25 mg/kg, PO, b.i.d.; for trichomoniasis, 66 mg/kg, PO, daily. Courses of therapy are generally 5-7 days. Both PO and IV preparations are available.

HYDROXYQUINOLINES

The 8-hydroxyquinolines are a group of synthetic compounds with antibacterial, antifungal, and antiprotozoal activity. The best known compounds of this class are iodochlorhydroxyquin (clioquinol), diiodohydroxyquin (iodoquinol), broxyquinoline, and hydroxyquinoline. Their main use in veterinary medicine, because they are not absorbed from the GI tract to any degree, has been for the treatment of intestinal infections caused by bacteria or by protozoa such as *Giardia*. Hydroxyquinolines are also used topically for skin infections caused by bacteria and fungi. Hydroxyquinolines are potentially neurotoxic when used for prolonged periods. The dose for a 455-kg horse is 10 g, PO, daily, using a decreasing dosage regimen to end medication.

ANTIVIRAL DRUGS AND INTERFERON

The conventional approach to the control of virus-induced diseases is to develop effective vaccines, but this is not always possible. Because viruses are obligate intracellular parasites that use the host's genetic machinery to produce new virus particles, drugs that could impair the process also will have narrow therapeutic indices. Only a few agents have been found to be reasonably safe and effective against a limited number of viral diseases—mostly in man. Widespread clinical use of antiviral drugs is not common in veterinary medicine. Only a selection of the more promising agents and their purported attributes are briefly discussed.

PYRIMIDINE NUCLEOSIDES

A variety of pyrimidine nucleosides (both halogenated and nonhalogenated) effectively inhibit the replication of herpes simplex viruses with limited host cell toxicity. The exact mechanism of action of these compounds has not been fully elucidated, but their selectivity seems to depend on the impediment of one or more virally specified enzymes because of altered viral protein synthesis. Idoxuridine (IDU) is effective for the treatment of herpesvirus infection of the superficial layers of the cornea (herpesvirus keratitis) and of the skin, but is toxic when administered systemically. Trifluridine, also an analog of deoxythymidine, is currently the agent of choice for the treatment of herpesvirus keratitis in man. The other antiviral pyrimidine nucleosides have not been employed clinically to any notable extent.

PURINE NUCLEOSIDES

Certain purine nucleosides have proved to be effective antivirals and are used as systemic agents. Two of these antiviral drugs deserve special mention. Vidarabine, or ara-A, is used topically for ocular herpes and systemically for herpetic encephalitis as well as for neonatal herpesvirus infections. This drug acts as an antimetabolite and, once it has been phosphorylated to the ara-ATP form, appears to inhibit the viral DNA polymerase. Vidarabine is administered IV in large volumes of fluid and is rapidly inactivated. It may produce bone marrow suppression and CNS side effects when high blood levels are reached.

Acyclovir (acycloguanosine) represents a new generation of antiviral agents, mainly because of its unique mechanism of action. This purine nucleoside is phosphorylated more efficiently by virus-induced thymidine kinase and then, when ultimately in the triphosphate form, is a better substrate and inhibitor of viral rather than cellular DNA polymerase. Acyclovir is relatively safe and is useful against a variety of infections caused by DNA viruses, especially the herpesvirus family. However, resistance can occur. It is available as an ophthalmic ointment, a topical ointment and cream, an IV preparation, and various oral formulations. The prodrug, deoxyacyclovir, is more readily absorbed from the GI tract than acyclovir. Other antiviral purine nucleoside analogs are currently under study.

RIBAVIRIN

Ribavirin is a synthetic triazole nucleoside (an analog of guanosine) with a broad spectrum of activity against many RNA and DNA viruses, both *in vitro* and *in vivo*. Susceptible viruses include adenoviruses, herpesviruses, orthomyxoviruses, paramyxoviruses, poxviruses, picornaviruses, rhabdoviruses, rotaviruses, and retroviruses. Viral resistance to ribavirin is rare. The action of ribavirin involves specific inhibition of viral-associated enzymes, inhibition of the capping of viral mRNA, and inhibition of viral polypeptide synthesis. It is well absorbed, widely distributed in the body, eliminated by both renal and biliary routes as both parent drug and metabolites, and has a plasma half-life of 24 hr in man. It does not have a wide margin of safety in domestic animals. Toxicity is manifest by anorexia, weight loss, bone marrow depression and anemia, and GI disturbances. It has been successfully administered by topical, parenteral, oral, and aerosol routes. Efficacy depends on the site of infection, method of treatment, age of the animal, and the infecting dose of virus. Human influenza studies with ribavirin have produced equivocal results to date.

AMANTADINE

Amantadine, and its derivative rimantadine, are synthetic antiviral agents that appear to act on an early step of viral replication after attachment of virus to cell receptors. The effect seems to lead to inhibition or delay of the uncoating process that precedes primary transcription. Amantadine may also interfere with the early stages of viral mRNA transcription. Amantadine at usual concentrations inhibits replication of different strains of influenza A virus, influenza C virus, Sendai virus, and pseudorabies virus. It is almost completely absorbed from the GI tract, and ~90% of a dose administered PO is excreted unchanged in the urine over several days (human data). The main clinical use has been to prevent infection with various strains of influenza A viruses. However, in man, it also has been found to produce some therapeutic benefit if taken within 48 hr after the onset of illness. Amantadine and its derivatives may be given by the PO, intranasal, subcut., IP, or aerosol routes. It produces few side effects, most of which are CNS related; stimulation of the CNS is evident at very high doses.

INTERFERON AND ITS INDUCERS

Interferons are a group of inducible cellular glycoproteins that interact with cells and render them resistant to infection by a wide variety of RNA- and DNA-containing viruses. In addition, interferons have numerous other effects on target cells, including a reduction in the rate of cell proliferation and alterations in the structure and function of the cell surface, the distribution of cytoskeletal elements, and the expression of several differentiated cellular functions. Interferons induce the synthesis of new proteins that are responsible for the activation of cellular endonucleases that degrade viral mRNA. Human interferons are classified as α, β, or γ, depending on their physical stability, immunologic neutralization properties, host range, and homology in amino acid sequence. Those used in clinical trials have been produced by induction of synthesis by human WBC, fibroblasts, lymphoblasts, and more recently by recombinant DNA techniques in bacteria. Numerous modes of antiviral action have been proposed: in addition to their ability to establish an antiviral state in host cells, they also appear to modulate the immune system of the host.

Interferons inhibit the replication of a wide variety of viruses. Among the RNA-containing viruses, the togaviruses, rhabdoviruses, orthomyxoviruses, paramyxoviruses, reoviruses, and several strains of picornaviruses and oncornaviruses are sensitive to inhibition by interferons. Among the DNA-containing viruses, the poxviruses, and several strains of herpes simplex types 1 and 2 viruses, as well as cytomegalovirus are inhibited by interferons. Adenoviruses are generally resistant. There are extreme variations in sensitivity to interferon among different types and even strains of virus. In addition, the responses in different model and test systems can be extraordinarily variable. Interferons appear not to be as useful in the therapy of viral infections as was hoped for initially. A native human lymphokine preparation containing α interferon has been useful against infectious bovine rhinotracheitis (IBR) virus in feeder calves under some circumstances; it appears to reduce virus excretion during infection, tempers the pyrexia associated with IBR, and may improve average daily weight gain. Interferons are usually administered parenterally but recently also have been used PO with some success. Though rare at recommended dosages, side effects may be seen at higher levels.

Several substances induce interferon and have been tested for the prevention and treatment of viral infections and for treatment of neoplastic diseases. Though effective in some model systems, interferon inducers have not yet been found to be clinically useful because of their toxicity. High-molecular-weight inducers include polyriboinosinic acid/polyribocytidylic acid or poly (I)/poly (C); low-molecular-weight inducers include tilorone, amino-bromo-phenyl-pyrimidinol (ABPP), and amino-iodo-phenyl-pyrimidinol (AIPP).

MISCELLANEOUS ANTIVIRAL AGENTS

Several drug classes continue to be investigated mainly because of their *in vitro* antiviral activities. Their potential clinical usefulness remains obscure in most instances. Included among these agents are thiosemicarbazones, guanidine, zidovidine (azidothymidine), benzimidazoles, arildone, phosphonoacetic acid, rifamycins and antibiotics, and several natural products.

ANTIFUNGAL AGENTS

Topical infections caused by a large variety of fungi may become established on the skin and adnexa or mucous membranes (buccal, GI, ruminal, vaginal). The external auditory canal and cornea may also be invaded by yeasts and fungi that are opportunistic pathogens. Locally active antifungal drugs (qv, p 1472) are used to treat such topical infections.

A number of serious systemic fungal diseases are well recognized in several parts of the world. Antifungal agents have greatly reduced earlier mortality rates due to systemic mycoses in man. A relatively narrow selection of drugs is used in these cases.

POLYENE MACROLIDE ANTIBIOTICS

A number of polyene antifungal antibiotics has been isolated from various strains of *Actinomyces*, but only amphotericin B, nystatin, and pimaricin (natamycin) are used in veterinary medicine. The polyenes are poorly soluble in water and the common organic solvents. They are reasonably soluble in highly polar solvents such as dimethylformamide and dimethyl sulfoxide. In combination with bile salts, such as sodium deoxycholate, amphotericin B is readily soluble (micellar suspension) in 5% glucose. This colloidal preparation is used for IV infusion. The polyenes are quite unstable in aqueous, acidic, or alkaline media but in the dry state, in the absence of heat and light, they remain stable for indefinite periods. They should be administered parenterally as freshly prepared aqueous suspensions (stable for 1 wk if refrigerated).

ANTIFUNGAL ACTIVITY

Mode of Action: The polyenes bind to sterol components in the phospholipid-sterol membranes of fungal cells to form complexes that induce physical changes in the membrane. The number of conjugated bonds and the molecular size of a particular polyene macrolide influence its avidity for different sterols in fungal cell membranes. Amphotericin B, because of its greater affinity, binds to ergosterol, the major sterol in fungal membranes, rather than the cholesterol in host cells. The disruption of membrane function produces potassium ion efflux from the fungal cell and hydrogen ion influx, producing internal acidification and a halt in enzymatic functions. Sugars and amino acids also eventually leak from an arrested cell. Fungistatic effects are most often evident at usual polyene concentrations. High drug concentrations and pH values between 6.0 and 7.3 in the surrounding medium may lead to fungicidal rather than fungistatic action. In addition to these direct effects on susceptible yeasts and fungi, evidence suggests that amphotericin B may also act as an immunopotentiator (both humoral and cell-mediated), thus enhancing the host's ability to overcome mycotic infections.

Fungal Resistance: Resistance to the polyene antifungal macrolides is rare—both clinically and *in vitro*. Resistance develops slowly and does not reach high levels, even after prolonged treatment.

Antimicrobial Spectra: The polyene antibiotics possess broad antifungal activity against organisms ranging from yeasts to filamentous fungi and from saprophytic to pathogenic fungi, but there are great differences between the sensitivities of the various species and strains of fungi. *In vitro* sensitivities (both resistant and highly susceptible) do not always correlate well with the clinical response, which suggests that host factors may also play a role. Many algae and some protozoa (*Leishmania, Trypanosoma, Trichomonas,* and *Entamoeba* spp) are sensitive to the polyenes but these compounds have no significant activity against bacteria, actinomycetes, viruses, or animal cells. Amphotericin B is effective against yeasts (eg, *Candida* spp, *Rhodotorula* spp, *Cryptococcus neoformans*), diamorphic fungi (eg, *Histoplasma capsulatum, Blastomyces dermatitidis, Coccidioides immitis*), dermatophytes (eg, *Trichophyton, Microsporum* and *Epidermophyton* spp), and molds. The drug also has been used successfully to treat disseminated sporotrichosis, pythiosis, and zygomycosis, though it may not always be effective. The main use of nystatin is for the treatment of mucocutaneous candidiasis, but it is effective against other yeasts and fungi. The antimicrobial activity of pimaricin is similar to that of nystatin, though it is mainly employed for the local treatment of candidiasis, trichomoniasis, and mycotic keratitis.

PHARMACOKINETIC FEATURES

Absorption: The polyene macrolide antibiotics are poorly absorbed from the GI tract, though amphotericin B has reached reasonable blood levels in some experimental animals. Amphotericin B is usually administered IV (occasionally intrathecally or intraocularly) or topically. Nystatin and natamycin are mostly applied topically. Nystatin is given PO to treat intestinal candidiasis. Minimal absorption occurs from sites of local application.

Distribution: Amphotericin B becomes widely distributed in the body following IV infusion. It appears to become associated with cholesterol-containing membranes in many different tissues from which it is slowly released into the circulation. Penetration into the CSF, saliva, aqueous humor, vitreous humor, and hemodialysis solutions is generally poor. Amphotericin B becomes highly bound to plasma lipoproteins (~95%).

Biotransformation and Excretion: About 5% of a total daily dose is excreted unchanged in the urine. Over a 2-wk period, ~20% of the drug may be recovered in the urine. The hepatobiliary system accounts for 20-30% of the excretion process. The fate of the remainder of amphotericin B is unknown.

Pharmacokinetics: Amphotericin B has a biphasic elimination pattern. The initial phase lasts 24 hr, during which levels fall rapidly (70% for plasma and 50% for urine). The second elimination phase has a 15-day half-life, during which plasma concentrations decline very slowly. Amphotericin B is usually infused IV, q48-72hr, until the total cumulative dosage has been reached.

THERAPEUTIC INDICATIONS

Amphotericin B is used principally in the treatment of systemic mycotic infections; nystatin is primarily indicated for the treatment of mucocutaneous (skin, oropharynx, vagina) or intestinal candidiasis; pimaricin is mainly used in therapeutic management of mycotic keratitis.

SPECIAL CLINICAL CONCERNS

Side Effects and Toxicity: Oral administration of nystatin can lead to anorexia and GI disturbances. The IV infusion of amphotericin B is potentially harmful, but the main concern is nephrotoxicity. Within 15 min of IV administration, renal arterial vasoconstriction occurs and lasts for 4-6 hr. This leads to diminished renal blood flow and glomerular filtration. Because amphotericin B binds to the cholesterol component in the membranes of the distal renal tubules, a change in permeability occurs in these cells, leading to polyuria, polydipsia, concentration defects, and acidification abnormalities. The net result is a distal renal tubular acidosis syndrome. The metabolic acidosis leads to bone buffering, the excessive release of calcium into the circulation, and ultimately, nephrocalcinosis due to calcium precipitation in the acidic environment of the distal tubules. Almost every animal treated with amphotericin B suffers some degree of renal impairment, which may become permanent depending on the total cumulative dose. The administration of amphotericin B can lead to a number of other side effects, including anorexia, nausea, vomiting, hypersensitivity reactions, drug fever, normocytic normochromic anemia, cardiac arrhythmias and even arrest, hepatic dysfunction, CNS signs, and thrombophlebitis at the injection site.

The incidence of the serious side effects of amphotericin B therapy can be reduced. Pretreatment with anti-emetic, antihistaminic agents prevents the nausea, vomiting, and hypersensitivity reactions. Giving corticosteroids IV also limits severe hypersensitivity reactions. Mannitol (1 g/kg, IV) with each dose of amphotericin B, and sodium bicarbonate (2 mEq/kg, IV or PO, daily) may help prevent acidification defects, metabolic acidosis, and azotemia. Saralasin (6-12 μg/kg/min, IV) and dopamine (7 μg/kg/min, IV) infusions have prevented amphotericin-B-induced oliguria and azotemia in dogs. IV fluids or furosemide administered before amphotericin B administration prevent pronounced decreases in renal blood flow and glomerular filtration rate.

Interactions: Amphotericin B may be combined with other antimicrobial agents with synergistic results. This often allows a reduction in both the total dose of amphotericin B and the length of therapy. Examples include 5-flucytosine and amphotericin B combinations for the treatment of cryptococcal meningitis, minocycline and amphotericin B for coccidioidomycosis, and imidazole and amphotericin B combinations for several systemic mycotic infections. Rifampin may also potentiate the antifungal activity of amphotericin B.

Drugs to be avoided during amphotericin B therapy include aminoglycosides (nephrotoxicity), digitalis drugs (increased toxicity), curarizing agents (neuromuscular blockade), mineralocorticoids (hypokalemia), thiazide diuretics (hypokalemia, hyponatremia), anticancer drugs (cytotoxicity), and cyclosporin (nephrotoxicity).

Effects on Laboratory Tests: Plasma bilirubin, CPK, AST (SGOT), ALT (SGPT), BUN, and eosinophil count increase. Plasma potassium and platelet count decrease. Urine protein increases.

DOSE RATES

The following is a selection of general dosages for some polyene macrolide antibiotics. The dose rate and frequency should be adjusted as needed for the individual animal.

Polyene Antifungal	Dosage	Route	Frequency
Amphotericin B (0.1 mg/mL in 5% dextrose)	0.1-0.5 mg/kg Total dose: 4-11 mg/kg	IV, slowly	3 times/wk
Nystatin (dogs)	50,000-150,000 u	PO	8 hr
Pimaricin 5% ophthalmic solution	1 drop	eye (topical)	1-2 hr

IMIDAZOLES

Imidazoles may possess antibacterial, antifungal, antiprotozoal, and anthelmintic activity. Several distinct phenylimidazoles are therapeutically useful antifungal agents with wide spectra against yeasts and filamentous fungi responsible for either superficial or systemic infections. The anthelmintic thiabendazole is also an imidazole with antifungal properties. Clotrimazole, miconazole, econazole, and ketoconazole are the most clinically important members of this group.

All 4 imidazoles are relatively insoluble in water but can be dissolved in organic solvents such as chloroform, propylene glycol, and polyethoxylated castor oil (preparation for IV use but dangerous in dogs). They are weak dibasic agents. Alterations in side-chain structure determine antifungal activity as well as the degree of toxicity.

ANTIFUNGAL ACTIVITY

Mode of Action: Imidazoles alter the cell membrane permeability of susceptible yeasts and fungi by blocking the synthesis of ergosterol (demethylation of lanosterol is inhibited), the primary cell sterol of fungi. Other enzyme systems are also impaired, such as those required for fatty acid synthesis. Because of the drug-induced changes of oxidative and peroxidative enzyme activities, toxic concentrations of hydrogen peroxide occur intracellularly. The overall effect is cell membrane and internal organelle disruption and cell death. The cholesterol in host cells is not affected by the imidazoles.

Fungal Resistance: Sensitivity to the imidazoles varies greatly between various strains of yeasts and fungi, but neither natural nor acquired resistance appears to be prevalent.

Antimicrobial Spectra: The antifungal imidazoles also possess some antibacterial action but are rarely used for this purpose. Miconazole has a wide antifungal spectrum against most fungi and yeasts of veterinary interest. Sensitive organisms include *Blastomyces dermatitidis, Paracoccidioides brasiliensis, Histoplasma capsulatum, Candida* spp, *Coccidioides immitis, Cryptococcus neoformans,* and *Aspergillus fumigatus.* Some *Aspergillus* and *Madurella* spp are only marginally sensitive. Ketoconazole has an antifungal spectrum similar to miconazole, but it is more effective against *Coccidioides immitis* and some other yeasts and fungi. Ketoconazole is the most active of the antifungal imidazoles. Clotrimazole and econazole are used for superficial mycoses (dermatophytosis and candidiasis); econazole also has been used for oculomycosis. Thiabendazole is effective against *Aspergillus* and *Penicillium* spp.

PHARMACOKINETIC FEATURES

Because ketoconazole is the only imidazole commonly used systemically, the pharmacokinetic fate of this antifungal agent is discussed.

Absorption and Distribution: Ketoconazole is rapidly but sometimes erratically absorbed from the GI tract; plasma levels peak within 2 hr after administration PO. An acidic environment is required for the dissolution of ketoconazole, and a decrease in gastric acidity can reduce its bioavailability. The rate of absorption appears to be increased when the drug is given with meals, but reports are conflicting. Ketoconazole appears to be widely distributed in the body with detectable concentrations in saliva, milk, and cerumen. CSF penetration is poor. Of ketoconazole in the circulation, >95% is bound to plasma proteins, mostly albumin. The highest concentrations are found in the liver, adrenal glands, lungs, and kidneys.

Biotransformation and Excretion: Hepatic metabolism of ketoconazole by oxidative pathways is extensive. Only ~2-4% of an orally administered dose appears unchanged in the urine. The biliary route is the major excretory pathway (>80%); ~20% of the metabolites are eliminated in the urine.

Pharmacokinetics: The rate of elimination of ketoconazole appears to be dose dependent—the greater the dose, the longer the elimination half-life. There is also a biphasic elimination pattern with rapid elimination in the first 1-2 hr, then a slower decline over the next 6-9 hr. Ketoconazole is usually administered b.i.d.

THERAPEUTIC INDICATIONS

1) Dermatomycoses: ketoconazole, PO; miconazole, clotrimazole, or econazole, topically. 2) Mucocutaneous candidiasis: ketoconazole, PO. 3) Nasal aspergillosis and penicilliosis: thiabendazole, PO. 4) Systemic blastomycosis, coccidioidomycosis, histoplasmosis, cryptococcosis, and aspergillosis: ketoconazole, PO (often in addition to amphotericin B).

SPECIAL CLINICAL CONCERNS

Side Effects and Toxicity: Ketoconazole produces few side effects, but nausea, vomiting, and hepatic dysfunction can occur. Altered testosterone and cortisol metabolism as well as blunted adrenal responsiveness to ACTH have been reported. Reproductive disorders related to ketoconazole administration may occur in dogs. The other antifungal imidazoles are now used topically only.

Interactions: Ketoconazole may be used concurrently with amphotericin B or 5-flucytosine to potentiate its antifungal activity. The absorption of ketoconazole is inhibited by concurrent administration of cimetidine, ranitidine, anticholinergic agents, or gastric antacids. Rifampin decreases the serum levels of active ketoconazole because of microsomal enzyme induction. There is an increased risk of hepatoxicity if ketoconazole and griseofulvin are administered together.

Effects on Laboratory Tests: AST (SGOT), ALT (SGPT), plasma bilirubin, and plasma cholesterol increase. Adrenal responsiveness is altered.

DOSE RATES

The following are general dosages for the antifungal imidazoles. The dose rate and frequency should be adjusted as needed for the individual animal.

Antifungal Imidazole	Dosage (mg/kg)	Route	Frequency (hr)
Ketoconazole (dogs)	5-20	PO	12
Thiabendazole	44	PO	24
	or 22	PO	12

FLUCYTOSINE

Flucytosine (5-fluorocytosine) is a fluorinated pyrimidine related to fluorouracil that was initially developed as an antineoplastic. It should be stored in airtight containers protected from light. Solutions for infusion are unstable and should be stored between 15° and 20°C. Usually it is given PO in capsules.

ANTIFUNGAL ACTIVITY

Mode of Action: Flucytosine is converted by cytosine deaminase in fungal cells to fluorouracil, which then interferes with RNA and protein synthesis. Fluorouracil is metabolized to 5-fluorodeoxyuridylic acid, an inhibitor of thymidylate synthetase. DNA synthesis is then also halted. Mammalian cells do not convert large amounts of flucytosine to fluorouracil, and thus are not affected at usual dose levels.

Fungal Resistance: Resistance to flucytosine can develop rapidly even during the course of treatment; this has restricted its use as the sole treatment for mycotic infections. The mechanisms of resistance are not completely understood.

Antimicrobial Spectrum: The following are the main organisms usually sensitive to flucytosine: *Cryptococcus neoformans, Candida albicans,* other *Candida* spp, *Torulopsis glabrata, Sporothrix schenckii, Aspergillus* spp, and agents of chromoblastomycosis (*Phialophora, Cladosporium*). The other fungi responsible for systemic mycoses are resistant to flucytosine.

PHARMACOKINETIC FEATURES

Absorption and Distribution: Flucytosine is rapidly and well absorbed from the GI tract with peak plasma levels being reached in 1-2 hr in animals that have received the drug for several days. The drug is widely distributed in the body with a volume of distribution approximating the total body water. Flucytosine is minimally bound to plasma proteins. There is excellent penetration into body fluids such as the CSF, synovial fluids, and aqueous humor.

Biotransformation and Excretion: Nearly all of an oral dose (85-95%) is excreted unchanged. Flucytosine is principally excreted by glomerular filtration (>80%). The clearance of flucytosine is approximately equivalent to that of creatinine. In renal failure, elimination of flucytosine is markedly impaired.

Pharmacokinetics: With normal renal function, the plasma half-life of flucytosine is usually 2-4 hr, but may be up to 200 hr with oliguria. Serum levels of 50-100 μg/mL are usually in the therapeutic range.

THERAPEUTIC INDICATIONS

The following are the more common indications for flucytosine: 1) cryptococcal meningitis (used together with amphotericin B): ~30% of the isolates develop resistance during the course of treatment; 2) candidiasis: ~90% of isolates are usually sensitive; 3) aspergillosis: some strains are sensitive at <5 μg/mL; 4) chromomycosis: some strains are very sensitive; 5) sporotrichosis: some cases may respond.

SPECIAL CLINICAL CONCERNS

Side Effects and Toxicity: Flucytosine is often well tolerated over long periods, but toxic effects may be observed when serum levels are high (>100 μg/mL). These include GI signs (nausea, vomiting, diarrhea) and reversible hepatic and hematological effects (increase of liver enzyme levels, anemia, neutropenia, thrombocytopenia). In dogs, erythemic and alopecic dermatitis may be observed but subside on withdrawal of the drug.

Interactions: There is synergistic antifungal activity between amphotericin B and ketoconazole, and the combination may retard the emergence of strains resistant to flucytosine. The renal effects of amphotericin B prolong elimination of flucytosine. If flucytosine is used together with immunosuppressive drugs, severe depression of bone marrow function is possible.

Effects on Laboratory Tests: Alkaline phosphatase, AST (SGOT), ALT (SGPT), and other liver leakage enzymes increase. RBC, WBC, and platelet counts decrease.

DOSE RATES

General dosages for flucytosine are 25-50 mg/kg and 30-40 mg/kg, PO, q6-8hr in dogs and cats, respectively. The dose rate and frequency should be adjusted as needed for the individual animal. Dosage modification is essential in renal failure. Flucytosine serum levels should be monitored if possible.

GRISEOFULVIN

Griseofulvin is a systemic antifungal agent that is effective against the common dermatophytes. It is practically insoluble in water and only slightly soluble in most organic solvents. Particle sizes of griseofulvin vary from 2.7 μm (ultramicrosized) to up to 10 μm (microsized).

ANTIFUNGAL ACTIVITY

Mode of Action: Dermatophytes concentrate griseofulvin by an energy-dependent process. The drug then causes disruption of the mitotic spindle by interacting with the polymerized microtubules in susceptible dermatophytes. This leads to the production of multinucleate fungal cells. The inhibition of nucleic acid synthesis as well as the formation of hyphal cell wall material may also be involved in the action of griseofulvin. The effect is to produce distortion, irregular swelling, and spiral curling of the hyphae. Griseofulvin is fungistatic rather than fungicidal, except in young active cells.

Fungal Resistance: Dermatophytes can be made resistant to griseofulvin *in vitro*.

Antifungal Spectrum: Griseofulvin is active against the various species of dermatophytes: *Microsporum, Epidermophyton,* and *Trichophyton* spp. It has no effect on bacteria, other fungi, yeasts, or *Actinomyces* or *Nocardia* spp.

PHARMACOKINETIC FEATURES

Absorption: Administration PO produces peak plasma levels in ~4 hr, but absorption from the GI tract continues over a prolonged period. Absorption is highly variable, being influenced by a number of factors. The rates of disaggregation and dissolution in the GI tract limit the bioavailability of griseofulvin; thus, microsized and ultramicrosized particles are usually used. High-fat meals, margarine, or propylene glycol significantly enhance GI absorption of griseofulvin.

Distribution: Griseofulvin is deposited in keratin precursor cells within 4-8 hr of administration PO. Sweat and transdermal fluid loss appear to play an important role in griseofulvin transfer in the stratum corneum. When these cells differentiate, griseofulvin remains bound and persists in keratin, making it resistant to fungal invasion. For this reason, new growth of hair, nails, or horn is the first to become free of fungal infection. As the fungus-containing keratin is shed, it is replaced by normal skin and hair. Only a small fraction of a dose of griseofulvin remains in the body fluids or tissues.

Biotransformation and Pharmacokinetics: Depending on the species, 10-50% of a griseofulvin dose is excreted almost exclusively as metabolites in the urine, and the remainder in the feces for ~4-5 days following administration. The elimination half-life of griseofulvin is ~24 hr in several species. The drug can be detected in 48-72 hr at the base level of the skin, in 6-12 days in the lower quarter, and in 2-19 days in the middle section of the horny layer.

THERAPEUTIC INDICATIONS

Griseofulvin is used for dermatophyte infections in dogs, cats, calves, horses, and other domestic and exotic animal species. Most dermatophytes are sensitive, but certain species do present greater therapeutic challenges than others. Several may require higher dose rates for satisfactory control.

SPECIAL CLINICAL CONCERNS

Side Effects and Toxicity: Side effects induced by griseofulvin are rare. Nausea, vomiting, and diarrhea have been observed. Hepatotoxicity has also been reported. Animals with impaired liver function should not be given griseofulvin, since its biotransformation will be reduced and toxic levels may be reached. Idiosyncratic toxicity in cats has been reported. It is contraindicated in pregnant animals (especially mares and queens) because it is teratogenic.

Interactions: Lipids increase the GI absorption of griseofulvin. Barbiturates decrease its absorption and antifungal activity. Griseofulvin is a microsomal enzyme inducer and promotes the biotransformation of many concurrently administered drugs. The combined use of ketoconazole and griseofulvin may lead to hepatotoxicity.

Effects on Laboratory Tests: Alkaline phosphatase, AST (SGOT), and ALT (SGPT) increase. Proteinuria may be detected.

DOSE RATES

The following are general dosages for griseofulvin. The dose rate and frequency should be adjusted as needed for the individual animal.

Species	Dosage (mg/kg)	Route	Frequency
Dogs, Cats	25 (microsized)	PO	Once daily for 3-6 wk, but up to 12 wk may be required.
	12.5 (ultramicrosized)	PO	Once daily for 3-6 wk, or longer if required.
Horses, Cattle	5-10	PO	Once daily for 3-6 wk, or longer if required.

IODIDES

Sodium and potassium iodide have both been employed to treat selected bacterial, actinomycete, and fungal infections, though sodium iodide is preferred. The *in vivo* effects of iodides against fungal cells are not well understood. Iodide is readily absorbed from the GI tract and distributes freely into the extracellular fluid and glandular secretions. Iodide concentrates in the thyroid gland (50 × corresponding plasma level) and to a much lesser degree in salivary, lacrimal, and tracheobronchial glands. Long-term use at high levels leads to accumulation in the body, and iodinism. Clinical signs of iodinism include lacrimation, salivation, increased respiratory secretions, coughing, inappetence, dry scaly skin, and tachycardia. Cardiomyopathy has been reported in cats. There is also impediment of host defense systems such as decreased immunoglobulin production and reduced leukocyte phagocytic capability. Iodinism may also lead to abortion and infertility.

Sodium iodide has been used successfully to treat cutaneous and cutaneous/lymphadenitis forms of sporotrichosis; attempts to control various other mycotic infections with iodides often have produced equivocal results.

The dosage (PO, once daily) for sodium iodide (20% solution) is 44 mg/kg body wt for dogs, and 22 mg/kg for cats. The dose for horses is 125 mL of 20% sodium iodide solution, IV, daily for 3 days, then 30 g, PO, daily for 30 days after clinical remission. The dose rate for treating actinomycosis and actinobacillosis in cattle is 66 mg/kg body wt, IV slowly, repeated weekly. Potassium iodide should **never** be injected IV.

LOCAL ANTIFUNGAL AGENTS

A large number of agents that possess antifungal activity are applied topically, either on the skin, in the ear or eye, or on mucous membranes (buccal, nasal, vaginal) to control superficial mycotic infections. Concurrent systemic therapy with griseofulvin is often helpful for therapeutic management of dermatophyte infections. The hair should be clipped from affected areas and the nails trimmed to fully expose the lesions before application of antifungal preparations. Bathing the animal may also be helpful. Isolation or restricted movement of infected animals is wise, especially when dealing with zoonotic fungi.

The preparations used may be in the form of solutions, lotions, sprays, powders, creams, or ointments for dermal application, or in the form of irrigant solutions, ointments, tablets, or suppositories for intravaginal use. The concentration of the active principle in these preparations varies and depends on the activity of the specific agent.

The clinical response to local antifungal agents is unpredictable. Resistance is common to many of the available drugs. Spread of infection and reinfection add to the difficulty of controlling superficial infections. Perseverance is often an essential element of therapy.

Some topical antifungal agents that have been used with success in various conditions and species include:

Iodine preparations:	tincture of iodine, potassium iodide, iodophors
Copper preparations:	copper sulfate, copper naphthenate, cuprimyxin
Sulfur preparations:	monosulfiram, benzoyl disulfide
Phenols:	phenol, thymol
Fatty acids and salts:	propionates, undecylenates
Organic acids:	benzoic acid, salicylic acid
Dyes:	crystal (gentian) violet, carbolfuchsin
Hydroxyquinolines:	iodochlorhydroxyquin
Nitrofurans:	nitrofuroxine, nitrofurfurylmethyl ether
Imidazoles:	miconazole, ticonazole, clotrimazole, econazole, thiabendazole
Polyene antibiotics:	amphotericin B, nystatin, pimaricin, candicidin, hachimycin
Miscellaneous agents:	tolnaftate, acrisorcin, haloprogin, ciclopirox olamine, dichlorophen, hexetidine, chlorphenesin, triacetin, polynoxylin

ANTIPROTOZOAL AGENTS

ANTICOCCIDIALS

Coccidiosis occurs as an acute or subacute disease in a wide range of avian and mammalian hosts. See AVIAN COCCIDIOSIS, p 1551, MAMMALIAN COCCIDIOSIS, p 103, and COCCIDIOSIS IN RABBITS, p 1063. In poultry, the adverse effects on flock performance are a primary concern. The following discussion relates primarily to the use of anticoccidials in poultry.

There are 2 distinct classes of anticoccidials: 1) coccidiostats, which arrest or inhibit growth of intracellular coccidia and give rise to latent infection after drug withdrawal, and 2) coccidiocides, which destroy coccidia during their development. Some anticoccidial drugs may be initially coccidiostatic but eventually coccidiocidal. Most anticoccidials currently used in poultry production are coccidiocides.

Anticoccidials are generally given to poultry in the feed to prevent acute disease and the economic loss often associated with subacute infection. Producers may use one anticoccidial continuously through succeeding flocks, rotate anticoccidials q4-6mo, or change anticoccidials during a single growout. The latter, called a shuttle program, usually involves a change between the starter and grower rations.

The natural development of immunity to coccidiosis can be slowed down, or possibly prevented, by use of some highly effective anticoccidials. In the production of broiler birds during a short growout of 37-44 days, this may be of little consequence. However, a natural immunity is important in replacement birds since they are likely to be exposed to coccidial infections for extended periods while not on anticoccidial drugs. Anticoccidial programs for replacement birds are usually designed to allow immunizing infection to occur without the severe effects of acute outbreaks.

Anticoccidials are commonly withdrawn from broiler birds 3-5 days before slaughter. This is done to meet regulatory requirements, in some instances, and to reduce production costs. Occasionally the anticoccidial is withdrawn >5 days before slaughter. Because broiler birds have varying susceptibility to infection at this point, the risk of coccidiosis outbreaks is increased under these circumstances.

MODES OF ACTION

Not all modes of action are well understood. Some of the better defined and more common agents are described briefly below.

Amprolium: Amprolium is structurally similar to thiamine (vitamin B_1) and is a competitive antagonist. Because of the relatively high requirement of rapidly dividing coccidia for thiamine, the drug has a safety margin of ~8:1 when used at the highest recommended level in feed. Maximal effect occurs about day 3 of the life cycle of coccidia. Poor activity of amprolium against some *Eimeria* spp has resulted in its use in mixtures, usually with the folic acid antagonists, particularly ethopabate and sulfaquinoxaline.

Clopidol: This pyridinol halts development of the sporozoites or trophozoites of *Eimeria* spp. A coccidiostat only, it must be given before or soon after exposure to be effective. Development of resistance is a problem.

Folic Acid Antagonists: Sulfonamides and ethopabate are structural antagonists of para-aminobenzoic acid (PABA), which is incorporated into folic acid. The host has no requirement for PABA and uses preformed folic acid. The efficacy of these compounds arises from the need of coccidia for nucleic acids, especially at the later second schizont stage. Because of their activity only at later stages of coccidial growth, these drugs are not ideal as anticoccidials. Although resistance to these compounds is widespread, they are effective when used in mixtures (often with amprolium), especially when clinical signs are already evident. Their action at the second schizont stage also allows a degree of immunity to develop.

Diaveridine, ormetoprim, and pyrimethamine are relatively selective in their activity against the protozoan enzyme dihydrofolate reductase. They have synergistic activity with sulfonamides, and often are used in mixtures with these compounds.

Halofuginone Hydrobromide: This is related to the antimalarial drug febrifuginone, and is effective against most asexual stages of *Eimeria* spp. It has both coccidiostatic and coccidiocidal effects.

Ionophores (monensin, salinomycin, lasalocid, narasin, maduramicin): The ability of the ionophores to form complexes with various ions, principally sodium, potassium, and calcium, and transport these into and through biological membranes accounts for their activity. *In vitro* and *in ovo* studies have shown that both extra- and intracellular stages of the parasite are affected by ionophores. Their principal activity is exerted during the early, asexual stages of parasite development. Drug tolerance has been slow to emerge and variable in occurrence, probably because of the biochemically nonspecific way these natural products of fermentation (*Streptomyces* and *Actinomadura*) act on the parasite.

Some ionophores depress weight gain when given at or slightly above the recommended levels in the absence of coccidial infection. Primarily, this is the result of reduced feed consumption, but it is often offset by improved feed conversion.

Nicarbazin: While not completely understood, the mode of action is via inhibition of succinate-linked nadide reduction and the energy-dependent transhydrogenase, and the accumulation of calcium in the presence of ATP. Nicarbazin must not be used in layers, and a 4-day withdrawal period is required in broilers. Medicated birds are at increased risk of heat stress in hot weather.

Nitrobenzamides (eg, dinitolmide): Activity, chiefly against *E tenella* and *E necatrix*, is greatest against the asexual stages by arresting parasite development, ie, a static effect.

Table 5. Anticoccidials for Prophylactic Use in Poultry

	Use Level (% in feed)		Withdrawal Time (days)
	Chickens	Turkeys	
Amprolium	0.0125-0.025	0.0125-0.250	0
Amprolium + ethopabate	0.0125-0.025 + 0.0004-0.004	—	0
Chlortetracycline	0.022	—	0
Clopidol or meticlorpindol	0.0125-0.025	—	0-5
Decoquinate	0.003	—	0
Dibutyltin dilaurate (Butynorate)	—	0.0375	28
Dinitolmide (Zoalene)	0.004-0.0125	0.0125-0.01875	0
Furazolidone	0.0055	—	5
Halofuginone hydrobromide	0.0003	0.00015-0.0003	4-7
Lasalocid sodium	0.0075-0.0125	—	3
Maduramicin ammonium	0.0005-0.0006	—	5
Monensin sodium	0.01-0.0121	0.006-0.01*	0
Narasin	0.006-0.008	—	5
Narasin + nicarbazin	0.003-0.005 (of the combination)		5
Nicarbazin	0.0125	—	4
Nitrofurazone	0.0055		5
Nitromide + sulfanitran + roxarsone	0.025 + 0.03 + 0.005	—	5
Oxytetracycline	0.022	—	3
Robenidine hydrochloride	0.0033	—	5
Salinomycin sodium	0.0044-0.0066	—	0
Sulfadimethoxine + ormetoprim	0.0125 + 0.0075	0.00625 + 0.003755	
Sulfaquinoxaline	0.015-0.025	0.0175	10

* Up to 10 wk of age.
Compiled from various sources including the *Feed Additive Compendium*, The Miller Publishing Co., 1988.

Quinolones (eg, buquinolate, decoquinate, nequinate): These act on the sporozoite stage by disrupting electron transport in the mitochondrial system. Their main use is in shuttle programs and withdrawal feeds. Toxicity is low. Rapid emergence of resistance to these compounds has been their major weakness.

Robenidine: A guanidine derivative, robenidine allows initial intracellular development of coccidia, but prevents formation of mature schizonts. It is both coccidiostatic and coccidiocidal. There have been problems with drug resistance, and a 5-day withdrawal period is needed to avoid altering flavor of the poultry meat.

DRUGS USED FOR PREVENTION OF COCCIDIOSIS

Drugs approved in the USA for use in poultry are listed in TABLE 5 (see above). Anticoccidials not approved in the USA, but available in various other countries include the purine derivative arprinocid, and a combination of clopidol plus methylbenzoquate. Globally, the anticoccicials most widely used today for coccidiosis prevention in chickens, in alphabetical order, are amprolium (and combinations), clopidol (and combinations), dinitolmide, halofuginone, lasalocid, monensin, nicarbazin, and salinomycin.

ANTICOCCIDIALS FOR THERAPEUTIC USE IN POULTRY

Most anticoccidials used for treatment of established disease are given via the drinking water. Those drugs approved for use in chickens in the USA are listed in TABLE 6 (see below). Care must be taken to observe drug withdrawal times, which may be >10 days.

Anticoccidial Drugs for Coccidiosis in Turkeys: Many large turkey producers have experienced problems with outbreaks of coccidiosis and have resorted to use of a preventive anticoccidial for birds up to 8-10 wk of age. Greater bird concentration associated with confinement rearing has increased the need for such programs. Drugs approved for use in feed are summarized in TABLE 5 (see above).

Table 6.   Drugs for Treatment of Coccidiosis in Chickens

	Feed or Water	Active Ingredient: Treatment, Duration	Withdrawal Time (days)
Amprolium	water	0.012-0.024%, 3-5 days; 0.006%, 1-2 wk	0
Chlortetracycline	feed	0.022% + 0.8% calcium; not more than 3 wk	0
Furazolidone	feed	0.011%, 5-7 days followed by 0.0055% for 2 wk	5
Nitrofurazone, soluble	water	0.0082%, 5 days	5
Oxytetracycline	feed	0.022% + 0.18-0.55% calcium; not more than 5 days	3
Pyrimethamine + sulfaquinoxaline	water	0.0015% pyrimidine compound + 0.005% sulfaquinoxaline; 2-3 days on, 3 off, 2 on	5
Sodium sulfachloropyrazine monohydrate	water	0.03%, 3 days	4
Sulfadimethoxine	water	0.05%, 6 days	5
Sulfamethazine (sulfadimidine)	water	0.1%, 2 days; 0.05%, 4 days	10
Sulfaquinoxaline	feed	0.1%, 2-3 days on, 3 off; followed by 0.05%, 2 on, 3 off, 2 on	10

MAMMALIAN ANTICOCCIDIALS

In mammals, the objective usually is therapy rather than prophylaxis as in poultry; in most situations only clinical outbreaks receive attention (affected animals, and those of similar age and in the same pen). Usually, the same compounds used in poultry are used in mammals, although few are approved for this use.

Anticoccidials approved in the USA include amprolium (5-10 mg/kg, cattle), decoquinate (0.5 mg/kg, cattle and goats), lasalocid (1 mg/kg to a maximum of 360 mg/head/day, cattle; 15-70 mg/head/day, sheep), and monensin (in the feed—0.00055-0.0033%, cattle; 0.0022%, goats). Sulfonamides are of some benefit as therapy (presumably in all host species) if administered early enough. Specific sulfonamides include sulfamerazine (65-130 mg/kg), sulfaquanidine (0.1 mg/kg), and sulfaquinoxaline (8-70 mg/kg) in bolus or water-soluble formulations. Diiodohydroxyquinoline has been approved as an anticoccidial in cattle in some countries.

OTHER ANTIPROTOZOALS

Chemotherapy, chemoprophylaxis, and chemoimmunization are important in the control and management of the arthropod-transmitted hemoparasitic diseases of domestic animals. Drug resistance, tissue residues, drug toxicity, and cost are factors that must be considered. Therapeutic control in the future may be influenced by the expense and difficulty of developing new replacement compounds.

TRYPANOSOMIASIS

(See TABLE 7, p 1480).

Chemotherapy and chemoprophylaxis are essential in the control of trypanosomiasis, particularly in view of the lack of effective vaccines and the problems associated with vector control. Treatment of trypanosomiasis frequently is complicated by development of drug resistance, toxicity, and the damaging dermonecrosis produced by some of the trypanocidal agents. The development of few, if any, commercially available compounds since 1955 has led to reliance on the same drugs which, in turn, has exacerbated the resistance problem. The widely used compounds are: quinapyramine, homidium, pyrithidium, isometamidium, diminazene, and suramin. To overcome or reduce resistance, these compounds are often used in sequence and in combination.

Quinapyramine sulfate remains the most effective drug for treatment of *Trypanosoma brucei* and *T evansi* in horses, even though it is poorly tolerated. Quinapyramine as a complex with suramin has shown good prophylactic properties for *T evansi* in horses and *T simiae* in pigs, depending on the dose level and severity of challenge. Dogs infected with *T brucei* are successfully treated with quinapyramine (5 mg/kg, subcut.), diminazene (7 mg/kg, subcut.), or suramin (7-10 mg/kg, IV). Pigs infected with *T brucei* may be treated successfully with either homidium or quinapyramine, but *T simiae* infections proceed so rapidly that treatment is often ineffective. *Trypanosoma simiae* in pigs may be prevented by prophylactic administration of isometamidium (12.5-35 mg/kg, IM), or quinapyramine (7.5 mg/kg, subcut.) plus diminazene (5 mg/kg, subcut.).

Problems of resistance to quinapyramine led to temporary withdrawal of the drug from the market, but it is now available again and is the only alternative drug for the treatment of suramin-resistant strains of *T evansi* in camels.

Infections of *T brucei* in cattle are often mild, and may be treated effectively with either quinapyramine or diminazene; *T vivax* and *T congolense* infections can be treated successfully with isometamidium or diminazene, and often with both. When trypanosomes are encountered, herd treatment should be considered since the infection probably is not limited to sick animals, nor to those with positive blood smears. In high-exposure tsetse fly areas, regular periodic chemoprophylaxis is often required. At present, alternate treatments with isometamidium and diminazene are preferred, with the latter drug being used for strategic therapy. Infections that relapse after treatment should always be treated with a drug different from the one used initially.

BABESIOSIS

(See TABLE 8, p 1480).

Drug selection and dosage in the treatment of babesiosis is influenced by the objectives of treatment: these may be to moderate clinical signs, eliminate the infectious organism, or prevent infection. The compound selected and its dose are also influenced by the *Babesia* spp causing the infection and the drug tolerance of the host.

Numerous chemical compounds have been used with varying success. If specific and effective chemotherapy is given early, before the onset of severe anemia or nervous system disorders, recovery without supportive treatment is the rule; however, if delayed, supportive treatment becomes important. Some babesiacidal drugs are so effective that one treatment eliminates the causative agent. Under some circumstances this is desirable in that reservoirs of infection are eliminated, but it may be undesirable if the animal is to be kept in an endemic zone where re-exposure is likely.

Most babesiacidal compounds are toxic to the host, so caution is required in their use. Drug-resistant *Babesia* organisms can be developed experimentally and probably occur in nature, but this problem has not yet evolved as a major constraint. Generally, the large species, eg, *Babesia bigemina, B canis,* and *B caballi,* respond more readily to treatment, frequently at lower drug levels than their smaller counterparts, *B bovis, B gibsoni,* and *B equi.*

Trypan blue probably was the first compound used successfully to treat babesiosis in cattle. An IV injection at 2-3 mg/kg body wt is effective against *B bigemina* but ineffective against *B bovis.* It is also effective against *B caballi* (but not *B equi*) of horses and *B canis* of dogs. At present, its use is usually limited to dogs, and then only under special circumstances.

The quinoline derivatives are effective in the treatment of bovine babesiosis. These drugs, however, have a low therapeutic index and may produce transient side effects, including excessive salivation, rapid and labored breathing, frequent urination, and general restlessness. Such reactions are usually transient and may be moderated by atropine.

Quinuronium used at 1 mg/kg, given once or twice with a 24-hr interval between doses, is effective against *B bigemina, B bovis,* and *B divergens*; however, at this level it does not eliminate infection. A less soluble salt of quinuronium given as an implant (1 g) has prevented *B bovis* and *B divergens* infections for >3 wk. Quinuronium may be used to treat *B canis* infections, but is not recommended for *B gibsoni* infections.

Acridine derivatives are also effective, but they appear to have been largely replaced by the diamidine derivatives. Acriflavine is reportedly effective against *B bigemina* and *B bovis* at 2.2 mg/kg, IV, given as a 5% solution.

Many diamidine derivatives, eg, diminazene, imidocarb, amicarbalide, phenamidine, and pentamidine, have proved effective and safe for treatment of babesiosis. Diminazene is effective against *B bigemina, B bovis, B ovata,* and *B divergens* in cattle at 3-5 mg/kg, IM. In horses, *B caballi* is susceptible to diminazene at 5 mg/kg, given twice with a 24-hr interval, but 6-12 mg/kg is required for *B equi.* Strain or isolate difference in susceptibility to treatment occurs. In dogs, diminazene at as little as 2.5-3.5 mg/kg has been effective in *B canis* infection, but 5-7 mg/kg is required for *B gibsoni.* Diminazene at 7.5-10 mg/kg, IM, has produced severe CNS disorders in dogs. Toxicity can be minimized by extending the time interval between doses.

Pentamidine, at 0.5-2 mg/kg, subcut., is therapeutically effective in cattle, but even at 5 mg/kg has failed to eliminate carrier infections. Pentamidine has been recommended for chemoimmunization, in which induction of carrier infections is desirable, while avoiding severe clinical reactions.

Phenamidine at 8-13 mg/kg, IM, is generally successful in treating *B bigemina, B caballi,* and *B canis.* Two doses of 10 and 5 mg/kg, given 3 days apart, were reported to be effective against *B gibsoni* infection.

Amicarbalide at 10 mg/kg, IM, has been effective against *B divergens, B bigemina,* and *B bovis* in cattle. Two doses of 8.8 mg/kg, IM, at a 24-hr inter al eliminated *B caballi* infections in horses, but 11 mg/kg, IM, given 4 times at 24- and 48-hr intervals did not eliminate *B equi*. Only 4 of 8 horses became free of *B equi* infections when treated by injection of 22 mg/kg, daily for 1 wk.

Imidocarb is highly effective in the treatment and prevention of babesiosis. An early formulation using the dihydrochloride salt has been replaced by a dipropionate formulation. Imidocarb is not recommended for IV use. In cattle, imidocarb is used safely for treatment of *B bigemina*, *B bovis*, and *B divergens* at 1-3 mg/kg, subcut. or IM, and generally eliminates the infection. The simultaneous administration of 0.15 mg of imidocarb/kg and attenuated *B bovis* vaccine has allowed carrier infection to occur without serious clinical signs, but an even lower dose may be required if vaccine strains are highly attenuated. Imidocarb at 2 mg/kg, given before exposure effectively prevents *B bigemina* for up to 60 days, and *B divergens* and *B bovis* for up to 21 days. This prophylactic effect has been utilized for the temporary protection of cattle being shipped from *Babesia*-free areas to endemic zones of the tropics. Ideally, prophylactic treatment should be given ~7 days after exposure to infection. Imidocarb is slowly metabolized, resulting in persistent tissue levels and, for this reason, its use is restricted in some countries to nonfood animals. It is also toxic under some conditions, notwithstanding its generally high therapeutic index. Transient side effects of excessive salivation, lacrimation, increased frequency of defecation, and tachypnea may be noticed for 30-40 min after injection. Fatal toxicosis in cattle may result with doses >15 mg/kg. Death due to imidocarb is associated with hyperemia, enlargement, and necrosis of the kidneys; pulmonary congestion; edema; hydrothorax; and hydroperitoneum.

Babesia equi and *B caballi* in horses are treated successfully with imidocarb. One injection of 2.4 mg/kg usually brings about a clinical remission of infection due to *B caballi*, and 2 injections 24 hr apart usually clear the infection. *Babesia equi* is more refractory to treatment, usually requiring 2 doses of 4.8 mg/kg, 48 hr apart. To clear *B equi* infections, imidocarb at 4 mg/kg, given 4 times at 72-hr intervals, is recommended. Since transient toxic side effects (extreme restlessness, sweating, and abdominal pain) are seen in horses, it may be desirable to divide the 4 mg/kg dose, giving 2 injections 1 hr apart; also, pretreatment with atropine sulfate, the specific antidote, may be helpful. Imidocarb (3-5 mg/kg) has been used to treat *B canis* infections in dogs, and there is some indication that it also has prophylactic activity. It is effective in the treatment of *B ovis* infection of sheep at 1.2 mg/kg, although a second similar dose may be necessary after ~2 wk to control recrudescence of the infection.

Over-reliance on these highly effective babesiacidal drugs may have led to some neglect of supportive and symptomatic treatment. With the increasing incidence of babesiosis in companion animals, greater emphasis is being given to supportive treatment, and the extrapolation of these techniques to food-producing animals is indicated in selected cases and probably should receive greater attention in the future.

THEILERIOSIS

(*See* TABLE 9, p 1481).

Until a few years ago, there was no effective specific treatment for acute theileriosis; however, the tetracyclines have been used successfully in cases caused by *Theileria parva*, although large doses given very early in the course of infection are required. The number of treatments required following *T parva* infection has been reduced as improved tetracycline formulations have been developed. Methods of chemoimmunization have been developed in which inoculations of infective *T parva* stabilates were followed by daily injections for 4-6 days of oxytetracycline at 5-10 mg/kg. A long-acting oxytetracycline formulation requires only a single injection of 20 mg/kg, IM, on the day of stabilate exposure.

Tetracyclines have both therapeutic and prophylactic activity against theileriosis due to *T annulata*. Rolitetracycline moderated clinical infection when administered daily for 4 days at 4 mg/kg, IM, beginning on the day of stabilate inoculation. Results were similar following a single injection of a long-acting oxytetracycline formulation at 20 mg/kg, IM.

Parvaquone has high therapeutic activity against both *T parva* and *T annulata*. It may be given either as a single injection at 20 mg/kg, or divided into 2 doses of 10 mg/kg, given 48 hr apart. Another member of the same series, buparvaquone, is also available. A single injection of 2.5 mg/kg, IM, usually cures clinical infections of *T parva, T lawrencei, T annulata,* or *T orientalis* (*sergenti*), but in severe cases, a second treatment 48-72 hr after the first may be required. Treatment rapidly reduces the fever and produces a marked degeneration of macroschizonts and intraerythrocytic piroplasms.

The anticoccidial compound halofuginone also has marked antitheilerial activity. Cattle showing active clinical infections of *T parva, T annulata,* and *T lawrencei* recovered following treatment with halofuginone (1.2 mg/kg, PO). Within 12 hr, temperature was normal; within 24 hr, schizont degeneration was evident. Treatment of *T mutans* was not as effective. The therapeutic index of halofuginone is low; the oral administration of 2 mg/kg causes a transient diarrhea, and ≥3 mg/kg produces more severe effects, including profuse diarrhea, cachexia, and subnormal temperature. The water-soluble halofuginone lactate is somewhat better tolerated than the insoluble hydrobromide. Halofuginone does not appear to be effective against *Theileria* spp during incubation and has little effect on intraerythrocytic piroplasms.

Table 7. Compounds Commonly Used to Treat Trypanosomiasis in Domestic Animals
(*See also* TABLE 9, p 82.)

Generic name	Dose (mg/kg) and Route	Susceptible Trypanosomes
Quinapyramine dimethyl sulfate or chloride	5, subcut.	*brucei, congolense, equiperdum, evansi, simiae(?), vivax*
Homidium chloride or bromide	1, IM	*brucei, congolense, vivax*
Diminazene aceturate	3.5-7, IM	*brucei, congolense, evansi, vivax*
Isometamidium chloride	0.5-2, IM	*congolense, vivax*
Pyrithidium bromide	2, IM	*congolense, vivax*
Suramin	7-10, IV	*brucei, equiperdum, evansi*

Table 8. Compounds Commonly Used to Treat Babesiosis in Domestic Animals

Generic name	Dose (mg/kg) and Route	Susceptible *Babesia* spp
Trypan blue	2-3, IV	*bigemina, caballi, canis*
Quinuronium sulfate	1-2, subcut. or IM	*bigemina, bovis, caballi, divergens, motasi*
Acriflavine hydrochloride	2.2, IV	*bigemina, bovis*
Diminazene diaceturate	3-7, IM	*bigemina, bovis, caballi, canis, divergens, equi, gibsoni, motasi, ovata, perroncitoi*
Pentamidine isethionate	2-16, subcut. or IM	*bigemina, canis, gibsoni*
Phenamidine isethionate	8-13, subcut.	*bigemina, caballi, canis, gibsoni*
Amicarbalide diisethionate	5-10, IM	*bigemina, bovis, caballi, divergens, ovata*
Imidocarb dipropionate (and dihydrochloride)	1-5, subcut.	*bigemina, bovis, caballi, canis, divergens, equi, motasi, ovata, ovis*

Table 9.   Compounds Commonly Used to Treat Theileriosis in Domestic Animals

Generic name	Dose (mg/kg) and Route
Oxytetracycline	
50 mg/mL	5-15, IV, 4-6 times daily after initial exposure, or early in infection
200 mg/mL (long-acting form)	20, IM, 1-2 times after initial exposure
Chlortetracycline	1.5, PO, daily for 28 days
Rolitetracycline	4, IM, 4 times daily, beginning on day of exposure
Parvaquone	20, IM, 1 time, curative
Buparvaquone	2.5, IM, 1-2 times, curative
Halofuginone lactate	1.2, PO, 1 time, curative

ANTHELMINTICS

Research has provided an array of highly effective and selective anthelmintics, but they must be used correctly and judiciously if a favorable clinical response is to be obtained. It is impossible to list all claims and precautions regarding all drugs in all countries in a discussion such as this; the label should be read before using any drug. Additional information is found under relevant disease headings.

Modern drugs possess a wide margin of safety, considerable activity against immature or larval stages of parasites, and a broad spectrum of activity. Nonetheless, the usefulness of any anthelmintic is limited by the inherent efficacy of the drug itself, its mechanism of action, its pharmacokinetic properties, features relating to the host animal (eg, operation of the esophageal groove reflex), or features relating to the parasite (eg, its location in the body, its degree of hypobiosis, or whether it has developed anthelmintic resistance).

The "ideal" anthelmintic should: 1) have a broad spectrum of activity against mature and immature parasites (including hypobiotic larvae), 2) be easy to administer to a large number of animals, 3) have a wide margin of safety and be compatible with other compounds, 4) not require long withholding periods because of residue(s), and 5) be economical.

MECHANISMS OF ACTION

Anthelmintics must be selectively toxic to the parasite. This is usually achieved by 1) inherent pharmacokinetic properties of the compound, which cause the parasite to be exposed to higher concentrations of the anthelmintic than are the host cells, or 2) inhibiting metabolic processes vital to the parasite. While the primary physiological mode of action of anthelmintics is not fully understood, general sites of action and biochemical mechanisms of many of them are known. Parasitic helminths must maintain an appropriate feeding site, and nematodes and trematodes must actively ingest and move food through their digestive tracts to maintain an appropriate energy state, which requires proper neuromuscular coordination. The pharmacological basis of the treatment for helminths generally involves interference with one or both of the energy processes, which cause subsequent starvation of the parasite; or neuromuscular coordination, which leads to paralysis and subsequent expulsion of the parasite.

Energy Processes: There are several classes of anthelmintics that directly or indirectly impair energy processes.

Inhibitors of Tubulin Polymerization: benzimidazoles and probenzimidazoles (which are metabolized *in vivo* to active benzimidazoles and thus act in the same manner).

Uncouplers of Oxidative Phosphorylation: salicylanilides and substituted phenols.

Inhibition of Enzymes in the Glycolytic Pathway: clorsulon.

The benzimidazoles inhibit tubulin polymerization; it is believed that the other observed effects, including inhibition of transport and energy metabolism, are consequences of the failure in microtubule function. Inhibition of these secondary events appears to play an essential role in the lethal effect on worms. Since they progressively deplete energy reserves, an important factor in efficacy of the benzimidazoles is prolongation of contact time between drug and parasite. These compounds have a broad spectrum of activity and are often effective against adults, larvae, and eggs. Since they are chemically similar and affect the same metabolic pathway in the parasite, cross-resistance frequently exists among the group.

Uncoupling of oxidative phosphorylation processes has been demonstrated for a number of compounds, especially the fasciolicides. Although isolated nematode mitochondria are susceptible, many fasciolicides are ineffective against nematodes *in vivo*, apparently due to a lack of drug uptake. Because these compounds are general uncouplers of oxidative phosphorylation, their safety indexes are not as high as are those of the benzimidazoles, although they are adequate if used as directed. Loose feces and slight loss of appetite may be seen in some animals after treatment at recommended dose rates. High dosages may cause blindness, hyperthermia, convulsions, and death—classical signs of uncoupled phosphorylation.

Clorsulon is rapidly absorbed into the bloodstream, and when *Fasciola hepatica* ingest it (in plasma and bound to RBC), they are killed because enzyme inhibition disrupts their primary source of energy.

Neuromuscular Coordination: Interference with this process may occur by inhibiting the breakdown or mimicking the action of excitatory neurotransmitters, and result in spastic paralysis of the parasite. Other mechanisms include mimicking the action of the inhibitory transmitter or causing hyperpolarization, which causes flaccid paralysis of the parasite. Either spastic or flaccid paralysis of an intestinal helminth allows it to be expelled by the normal peristaltic action of the host.

Cholinesterase Inhibitors: organophosphates—coumaphos, crufomate, dichlorvos, haloxon, naftalofos, trichlorfon.

Cholinergic Agonists: 1) imidazothiazoles—levamisole, tetramisole; 2) pyrimidines—morantel, pyrantel.

Muscle Hyperpolarization: piperazine.

Potentiation of Inhibitory Transmitters: avermectins.

Thus, anthelmintic modes of action are closely related to the life-support requirements of the parasites. Differential toxicity between host and parasite is based on a unique parasite life system or on an effective concentration of drug that inhibits the parasite's system without interfering with the host's comparable system (selective toxicity).

ADMINISTRATION

Anthelmintics can be administered in various ways. In general, drench, paste, and injectable preparations allow a greater degree of control over the amount of anthelmintic administered than in-feed or medicated block preparations. Whichever method of administration is selected, the manufacturer's instructions should be read with particular regard to: 1) the spectrum of activity, 2) the class of animal for which the product is recommended and any limitations of its use that may be advised, 3) the dose rate and any increase in dosage that may be recommended to deal with different developmental stages or different species or types of worm, and 4) the withholding period (in food-producing animals).

The solubility of a compound (and nature of the solvent) largely governs the route of administration. Insoluble anthelmintics usually must be given PO in the form of suspensions, pastes, or granules. The more soluble compounds may be given PO as a solution, topically as a "pour-on" (organophosphates, levamisole), or as an injectable solution (nitroxynil, rafoxanide, levamisole). Particle size has a significant effect on efficacy or toxicity of an agent administered PO. In general, small particle size increases the rate and extent of dissolution in, and absorption from, the GI tract, and may increase the efficacy of a compound.

Drench and Paste Preparations: Many anthelmintics, particularly the benzimidazoles and certain fasciolicides, are available as suspensions. Their containers should be well shaken before use to ensure that the chemical is adequately dispersed. Others, usually for equine use, are in paraffin-based, oral-dosing syringes; the paste is deposited on the tongue.

Injectable Preparations: Certain soluble anthelmintics (notably levamisole, diethylcarbamazine, netobimin) or anthelmintics that may be formulated to "behave" like an aqueous solution (eg, ivermectin and nitroxynil) are available as injectable preparations. With some anthelmintics, the formulation or route of administration may alter efficacy and/or spectrum, but frequently they do not change. In some situations, notably with cattle and pigs, injectable formulations have an added advantage of ease of administration. Local reactions at the injection site may occasionally be noticed, but generally are of little consequence, provided the site is not an area from which prime cuts of meat are taken.

Topical Preparations: Currently available pour-on preparations include levamisole and ivermectin, and are licensed only for use in cattle. In these preparations, the drug is contained within a liquid or vehicle that is thoroughly absorbed through the skin after application.

In-feed Preparations: Many of the benzimidazoles are available for mass medication in the feed. In-feed preparations allow limited control over the amount of anthelmintic that individual animals consume, unless they are fed separately or in small supervised groups. Therefore, some animals may receive more or less than the recommended dose. However, with a safety margin such as that of the benzimidazoles, this should not be a problem.

Sustained-release Formulations: These are a new approach to administration of anthelmintics. The objective is to provide a long period of chemoprophylaxis and/or therapy without the need for repeated treatment and handling of animals. Erodible matrices, degradable polymers, and controlled-release glasses (CRG) have helped focus on the possibilities for continuous release or programmed release surges of drugs at pre-set time intervals. This "pulsed-released" approach creates a new dimension in the manipulation of animal production and disease control.

The unique anatomy of the ruminant GI tract facilitates the entrapment of controlled-release devices. Ruminal retention is based on the density or shape of the device. Although sustained-release rumen devices for mineral or trace element supplementation have been used for years, reliable methods of delivering organic drugs such as anthelmintics are relatively recent. Controlled release of anthelmintics provides a useful alternative to repeat dosing with conventional products; continuous anthelmintic output can protect animals from overwintered pasture infestation and prevent a subsequent pasture buildup of eggs and infective larvae.

Weight, size, integrity of the material, and density of the device are critical for bolus retention. When density is used to prevent regurgitation, it should be >2.5 g/mL. If a formulation is of low density, an expanded configuration may be used to hinder regurgitation; the device is administered in compact form and expands within the rumen.

Macromolecules of organic anthelmintics can be enclosed within a sintered block of phosphate glass, which gives a constant release rate as the glass dissolves in the ruminal fluids. The physical properties of CRG also facilitate the development of "pulsed-release" systems. Variations in dissolution rates can be utilized to govern release of active constituents within an assembly of glass tubules. The interval between release pulses can be controlled by modifying the shape of the tubular assembly and the dissolution rate of the various tubules. Alternatively, a sequential arrangement of cells of active ingredients enclosed in relatively insoluble glass may be separated by cores of CRG of high solubility. Pulse intervals are a function of the size of the spacer cores and their dissolution rate. Anthelmintic ruminal devices are exemplified by the morantel tartrate sustained-release bolus. The ends of the cylinder were capped with 2 microporous, sintered polyethylene disks impregnated with hydrogel. The bolus was designed to deliver an efficacious level of anthelmintic over the grazing season (90 days). A disadvantage is that the metallic shell remains in the rumen for the life of the animal.

A biodegradable bolus has recently been developed. After the ruminal fluid breaks down a retaining tape, a sheet of plastic laminate unravels and releases morantel tartrate over a 90-day period. With time, the plastic degrades and is naturally eliminated.

The cylindrical pulsed-release system for oxfendazole consists of a steel end weight from which extends a magnesium alloy core rod. Six plastic segments are arranged sequentially along this core, 5 of which hold an annular tablet containing 750 mg oxfendazole. In the rumen, corrosion of the central core initiates the release of an encapsulated oxfendazole segment. In one version, the first dose is released soon after administration; in another, the first dose is released ~3 wk after administration and 4 more doses at regular predetermined intervals according to the core corrosion rate. The anthelmintic life span of the system is up to 130 days.

Less sophisticated sustained-release formulations of parasiticides utilize impregnated resin pellets as the controlling device, eg, dichlorvos in the form of resin pellets provides a stable slow release following administration PO. As the pellets traverse the gut, the dichlorvos is gradually released from the plasticized pellets, which provides maximum anthelmintic activity while protecting the host animal from sudden and excessively high exposure levels.

Controlled-release delivery formulations have several potential advantages over conventional types of single- or repeat-dose treatment: 1) extended duration of drug action, 2) the need for frequent and repeat dosing is avoided, 3) side effects associated with peak blood levels or fluctuating levels are minimized, 4) more desirable and more effective kinetic profiles are obtained, 5) premature inactivation and elimination of the drug dose is avoided, and 6) targeting of drugs to specific sites and selectivity of action is possible.

ABSORPTION AND DISTRIBUTION

Following administration, anthelmintics are usually absorbed into the bloodstream and transported to different parts of the body, including the liver, where they are metabolized, and eventually excreted in the feces and urine. With some anthelmintics, eg, probenzimidazoles, antiparasitic activity lies not with the original compound, but with its metabolites. The speed with which an anthelmintic is metabolized and excreted determines the length of the withdrawal time; this speed can vary among species, and may also be affected by the route of administration and the dose.

While many GI parasites reside in the lumen or close to the mucosa, others dwell at sites other than the gut, eg, liver and lungs; for action against these, absorption of orally administered drug from the gut is essential. Intestinal parasites come in contact not only with the unabsorbed drug passing through the GI tract but also with the absorbed fraction in the blood as they feed on the intestinal mucosa, and with any that is recycled into the gut. This is an important aspect of efficacy of many of the benzimidazoles.

Route of administration influences persistence in the body, and thus efficacy. In ruminants, administration directly into the abomasum, via the esophageal groove, may increase the rate of absorption (and thus of excretion, which may reduce efficacy). Operation of the ruminal bypass acts to reduce the efficacy of certain benzimidazole anthelmintics, eg, immediate arrival of oxfendazole in the abomasum following dosing reduces its efficacy from 91% to 45% against thiabendazole-resistant strains of *Haemonchus contortus*. The rumen acts as a drug reservoir from which plasma concentrations can be sustained for long periods, and slows the passage of unabsorbed drug through the GI tract. In general, the benzimidazoles are most effective if deposited directly into the rumen, less so if injected into the abomasum.

The absorption of levamisole is not affected by the route of administration since it is highly soluble and is unaffected by ruminal bypass.

In a number of situations, animals deliberately or inadvertently are given less than the recommended dose. The result is likely to be lowered efficacy.

METABOLISM AND EXCRETION

Metabolism of an anthelmintic may alter activity; eg, albendazole is rapidly oxidized to its sulfoxide, which is active, and then further oxidized to its sulfone, which is inactive. Similarly, fenbendazole and oxfendazole (fenbendazole sulfoxide) are active, but the oxidation product fenbendazole sulfone is inactive. In the case of fasciolicides, such as diamfenetide, metabolism within the GI tract may be important for full efficacy. Because rumen bacteria metabolize and destroy the activity of nitroxynil, it must be injected. The more usual site of metabolism is the liver, in which oxidation and cleavage reactions commonly occur. Thiabendazole is rapidly metabolized in the liver to hydroxythiabendazole, with the sulfate and glucuronide conjugates of this metabolite being more soluble in water than the parent drug, and rapidly excreted by the kidneys. Frequently, active metabolites are resecreted back into the GI tract. Many of the more modern benzimidazoles and their metabolites reenter the GI tract by passive diffusion. The biliary route may also be important in recycling benzimidazoles such as albendazole to the GI tract. However, resecretion via the liver and bile is especially important for drugs active against adult *Fasciola* spp. Many fasciolicides, such as the salicylanilides and the substituted phenols, appear to bind strongly to plasma proteins. The fasciolicidal effects of salicylanilides, such as rafoxanide, in sheep were found to depend on persistence of the drug in plasma, which influences their transport throughout the body and also the rate of elimination from the host. Associated with persistence, however, is the need for longer withholding periods. Oxyclozanide also is bound to plasma protein and then metabolized in the liver to the anthelmintically active glucuronide and excreted in high concentration in the bile duct where it encounters the mature flukes. Immature flukes in the liver parenchyma ingest mainly liver cells, which contain little anthelmintic; plasma-protein binding limits entry of the drug into the tissue cells. As the flukes grow and migrate through the liver, they cause extensive hemorrhaging and come into contact with plasma-protein-bound anthelmintic. When they reach the bile ducts, they are in the main excretory channels for the active metabolites of the fasciolicides and thus exposed to toxic concentrations. This may explain why mature flukes are more vulnerable to most fasciolicides than immatures. The higher concentrations of fasciolicides and their metabolites in feces than in urine suggest that the bile ducts are their main excretory pathways.

Diamfenetide is metabolized in the gut, and to a greater extent in the liver, to an active metabolite that can enter the hepatic cells and exert its antiparasitic effect against very young stages of the fluke. The low plasma-protein binding of this compound, coupled with the rapid excretion of its active metabolite, necessitates only a short withdrawal time.

WITHHOLDING PERIODS

Most anthelmintics have withdrawal times if milk or meat from treated animals is intended for human consumption; it is important to observe the specific requirements for each. Modern benzimidazoles are retained in the body for much longer periods than earlier ones and have correspondingly longer withholding periods. Thiabendazole is absorbed and excreted most quickly; fenbendazole, oxfendazole, and albendazole are absorbed and excreted over a longer period, which necessitates withholding periods of 8-14 days before slaughtering for meat, and 3-5 days before milking for human consumption. Other members of the group have withholding periods between these extremes.

A similar relationship between the rate of metabolism and activity against immature parasites also exists with certain fasciolicides. Rafoxanide, nitroxynil, and brotianide bind more strongly to blood proteins than does oxyclozanide, and therefore remain in the blood for longer periods. While this greater persistence is associated with greater activity against immature liver flukes, the penalty is a longer withholding period: 21-30 days before slaughter for rafoxanide, nitroxynil, and brotianide, compared with 14 days for oxyclozanide.

Levamisole and morantel are rapidly excreted; thus, withholding periods for meat are short, and frequently there is no, or only a short withholding period for milk. Ivermectin is excreted in milk, and is not recommended when milk is intended for human consumption; commensurate with its long period of activity, it has a significant withholding period before slaughter, which varies with the formulations (and local regulations).

SAFETY

Most modern anthelmintics have wide safety margins, ie, the dose that can be given to an animal before adverse effects are induced is much higher than the dose recommended for use. For all benzimidazoles the safety index (SI) is wide. It is not so wide for levamisole (SI = 6) nor for most of the chemicals active against liver flukes (SI = 3-6). Also, if for any reason the dose rate of an anthelmintic is increased, the safety margin is correspondingly decreased; eg, if the dose rate is doubled, the SI is halved.

RESIDUES

Total residues can be divided into 1) extractable residues—the fraction that includes all compounds and metabolites in free form or loosely bound in tissues, and 2) residues not readily extracted by solvents—nonextractable or bound residues.

Bioavailability and toxicity of **bound residues** often differ from those of the parent compound. Bound residues may contain the parent compound or degradation products of the parent compound covalently bound to endogenous macromolecules.

When benzimidazoles undergo biotransformation, electrophilic reactants are formed; these metabolites may undergo nonextractable binding. Although the basic benzimidazole ring structure is relatively stable for thiabendazole and cambendazole, products of thiazole ring metabolism are incorporated into hepatic tissue protein. Albendazole, mebendazole, and cambendazole also form bound residues. Measurements of residues depend on the type and sensitivity of the test system. Bound residues of parbendazole found in the liver of sheep after 15 days have been attributed to incorporation into amino acids. With thiabendazole, radiolabeled metabolites are found in proteins, lipids, nucleic acids, and glycogen in the liver.

Toxicological assessment of the bound fraction is difficult; bioavailability studies and relay toxicity methods may be tried. With cambendazole and albendazole, bound-residue bioavailability is low. In rats administered calf liver treated with radiolabeled cambendazole, only 15% of total radioactivity was absorbed. Relay embryotoxicity studies for these 2 benzimidazoles in rats following feeding of liver residue tissue revealed no toxicity. Bioavailability of albendazole-bound residues from beef liver is 4-5%.

Bound residues, although potentially toxic, may also be considered relatively nontoxic for a number of reasons. Once bound, the fixed residue may no longer possess biological reactivity and become "unbound". However, when the risk involves allergenicity, bound residues may possess the potential to trigger hypersensitivity reactions. It is difficult to distinguish between drug-related residues bound to macromolecules and fractions that have entered the normal metabolic pool. Current evidence suggests that because of the low residue levels in target animal tissues and the observed low bioavailability, covalently bound residues do not present a major hazard. In light of current scientific knowledge, their toxicological significance is speculative.

Extractable residues from benzimidazoles undoubtedly constitute toxicological risk. Concern regarding extractable residues is related to the established toxicological properties of this group.

ANTHELMINTIC COMPOUNDS

See also the discussions of specific helminthiases, including those in the poultry section.

BENZIMIDAZOLES

The benzimidazoles comprise the largest chemical family used to treat endoparasitic diseases in domestic animals. They are characterized by a broad spectrum of activity and a wide safety margin. Their high degree of efficacy is related both to their pharmacodynamic and pharmacokinetic characteristics. Those of current interest are thiabendazole, cambendazole, parbendazole, mebendazole, fenbendazole, oxfendazole, oxibendazole, albendazole, thiophanate, febantel, netobimin, and triclabendazole. Both albendazole and triclabendazole possess activity against liver flukes. However, unlike all the other benzimidazoles, triclabendazole has no activity against roundworms.

The group includes thiabendazole analogs and benzimidazole carbamates; substitution of various side chains and radicals on the parent benzimidazole nucleus produces the individual members. Newer benzimidazole carbamates are characterized by novel substituents on the benzimidazole nucleus and replacement of the thiazole ring by methylcarbamate. Such modifications have spawned a new benzimidazole generation with much slower rates of elimination, higher potencies, broader spectra, and complex metabolic pathways. Inherent in these developments is the potential of greater biological reactivity of their metabolites.

A number of benzimidazoles, eg, febantel, thiophanate, and netobimin, exist in the form of pro-drugs, active because they are metabolized in the animal body to the biologically active benzimidazole carbamate nucleus. Synthesis of benzimidazole carbamates depends on a cyclization process: metabolic or chemical modification generates an active anthelmintic *in vivo* from an inactive pro-drug precursor. Febantel is hydrolyzed to the active metabolite fenbendazole. Netobimin undergoes processes of reduction, cyclization, and oxidation to yield albendazole sulfoxide. All these substances have low toxicity in mammals. Some of the benzimidazoles are teratogenic and, depending on the dose rate, are contraindicated in early pregnancy, and require withholding periods.

Being sparingly soluble in water, most benzimidazoles are given PO as a suspension, paste, or powder. Differences in the rate and extent of absorption from the GI tract depend on such factors as species, dosage, formulation, solubility, and operation of the esophageal groove reflex.

Benzimidazoles bind to tubulin, a structural protein, and block polymerization of tubulin into microtubules. This damages the integrity and transport functions of the absorptive cells within the parasite. Enzymes of electron transport, such as fumarate reductase, are also inactivated by benzimidazoles, which interferes with absorption and utilization of foodstuffs by the parasite. Accordingly, the antiparasitic effect is a lethal, but relatively tardy, process.

Binding of benzimidazoles to tubulin is reversible and saturable. Antimitotic effects have been documented for a number of benzimidazoles, and some experimental work has revealed effects such as chromosome doubling, due to malfunctioning of the mitotic spindle caused by depolymerization of microtubules.

The wide safety margin of benzimidazoles is due to their greater selective affinity for parasitic tubulin than for mammalian tissues. Nonetheless, this selective toxicity is not absolute; some toxic effects based on antimitotic activity (teratogenicity/embryotoxicity) can occur in target species.

The most effective of the group are those with the longest half-life in the body, such as oxfendazole, fenbendazole, albendazole, and their pro-drugs, because they are not rapidly metabolized to inactive products. Effective concentrations are maintained for an extended period in the plasma and gut, which increases efficacy against immature and arrested larvae and adult nematodes.

The following generalities apply to this group: 1) They are more effective in ruminants and horses, in which their rate of passage is slowed by the rumen or cecum. 2) Divided doses are more effective than a single dose because the nature of their antiparasitic action depends on prolongation of contact time. 3) The most effective benzimidazoles are less readily metabolized to inactive soluble products than earlier compounds, ie, their kinetics are slowed.

In the case of oxfendazole, absorbed drug is at least as important in achieving efficacy against nematodes in the abomasum and small intestine as the unabsorbed drug passing down the GI tract. Once in the bloodstream, it recycles across the gut wall between the vascular system and the GI tract. Worms in the mucosa of the abomasum and small intestine may be exposed to this recycling anthelmintic to a greater extent than to drug contained in the passing ingesta in the GI tract.

Albendazole is oxidized to the sulfoxide, and both possess anthelmintic and embryotoxic properties. The sulfoxides of albendazole and fenbendazole (oxfendazole) are further oxidized to the sulfones. Activity is associated with both the sulfide and sulfoxide, which are metabolically interconvertible.

The principal route of metabolism for fenbendazole, oxfendazole, and albendazole appears to be oxidation of the sulfide to the sulfoxide and sulfone metabolites. Ruminal fluid can cause reduction of the sulfoxide to the sulfide. Fenbendazole, oxfendazole, and febantel follow similar metabolic patterns. Fenbendazole and oxfendazole are interconvertible.

The metabolism and excretion of thiabendazole is more extensive in cattle than in sheep, and cattle seem to possess greater capacity for oxidative metabolism for benzimidazole parasiticides. Systemic anthelmintic activity of thiabendazole is greater in sheep than in cattle, eg, although ineffective against lungworm infection in cattle, it does possess useful activity against the ovine lung parasite.

Residues of albendazole, oxfendazole, fenbendazole, febantel, and thiabendazole concentrate primarily in the liver in cattle and sheep, and persist longest in this tissue. Residues are more persistent for fenbendazole, oxfendazole, and febantel than for albendazole or thiabendazole. Although residues are detectable in milk for these drugs, their presence is relatively short-lived. The persistence of high blood concentrations of such active benzimidazoles is important for activity against both tissue-dwelling parasites, such as arrested *Ostertagia ostertagi* larvae, and parasites in the gut, such as *Haemonchus* and *Trichostrongylus* spp.

In ruminants, oral dosing with the benzimidazoles removes most of the major adult GI parasites and many of the larval stages. Albendazole, fenbendazole, oxfendazole, and febantel possess activity against inhibited fourth-stage larvae of *Ostertagia* spp. The degree of efficacy of these compounds in the prophylaxis of ostertagiasis type II may be related to the degree of hypobiosis of the larvae (ie, those with low metabolic rate have a low energy requirement, and thus are not very susceptible to disruption by the benzimidazoles) and also to the esophageal groove bypass effect. Efficacy against *Dictyocaulus viviparus* has also been noted for these insoluble benzimidazoles.

Parbendazole is the primary benzimidazole for which teratogenic effects (skeletal malformations) have been demonstrated in sheep. Cambendazole, oxfendazole, albendazole, and febantel are also teratogenic in sheep, whereas fenbendazole, mebendazole, and oxibendazole are not. Teratogenic effects occur at dosages much lower than those associated with acute toxicity in target species. Teratogenicity varies among animal species; dose rate, specific benzimidazole, and stage of embryonic development are major influencing factors. Cattle seem to be unaffected by most benzimidazoles that are teratogenic in sheep. A similar relationship exists between rats and rabbits. Many benzimidazoles teratogenic in sheep are also teratogenic in rats.

Although benzimidazoles all possess similar pharmacodynamic effects (antitubulin), species differences in sensitivity to embryotoxic effects are attributable to metabolic and pharmocokinetic disposition factors. Benzimidazoles can be classified as: those that are not teratogenic *per se* and have no teratogenic metabolite (eg, oxibendazole), those that are not teratogenic but give rise to a teratogenic metabolite (eg, albendazole), those that seem to be teratogenic *per se* and have no teratogenic metabolite (eg, oxfendazole), and those that are possibly teratogenic *per se* and have additionally a metabolite that seems to be more toxic than is the parent compound (eg, mebendazole).

In horses, the benzimidazoles are characterized by effective removal (90-100%) of almost all mature strongyles, but third- and fourth-stage larvae are more difficult to eliminate. High levels and repeated administration may be necessary for extraintestinal migrating stages of large strongyles, and for small-strongyle larvae embedded or encysted in the wall of the intestine.

Repeated doses are thought to be advantageous because the lethal effect of benzimidazoles is a slow process, hence, their recent incorporation into feed supplements. Ascarid removal in horses varies with various members of the benzimidazole group; frequently an increased dosage is required. Activity against *Strongyloides* sp varies also, but *Oxyuris equi* is usually removed by any of the benzimidazoles at the recommended dose.

In dogs and cats, mebendazole is used for treatment of roundworms, hookworms, and tapeworms. However, treatment must be given b.i.d. for 3 days. Fenbendazole has been utilized in a divided dose regimen in the bitch against tissue-dwelling larvae of *Toxocara canis* and *Ancylostoma caninum*; daily administration of 50 mg/kg to bitches from day 40 of pregnancy through day 14 after parturition resulted in the birth of pups free of both parasites.

In cattle and sheep, at 10 mg/kg, PO, triclabendazole is highly effective against immature *Fasciola hepatica* infections in the liver parenchyma, and against the mature stage in the bile ducts. The maximum tolerated dose in the target species is 200 mg/kg, thus, the safety margin is 20. Of the other benzimidazoles and probenzimidazoles used for nematode control, some possess marginal efficacy at elevated dose rates against liver flukes; albendazole and netobimin are active against mature *F hepatica*. Because of the lack of efficacy against the immature stages, most benzimidazoles are not indicated for treatment of acute fascioliasis and have limited value in control of the disease.

IMIDAZOTHIAZOLES

The anthelmintic activity of tetramisole, a racemic mixture, resides almost entirely in the L-isomer, levamisole; the dosage can be reduced by one half using the L-isomer alone. Reducing the dosage also appreciably increases the margin of safety. Levamisole is widely used as an anthelmintic, and some preparations of tetramisole are still available. Levamisole possesses a broad spectrum of activity against GI helminths and lungworms. It is commonly used in cattle, sheep, pigs, goats, and poultry. It lacks efficacy against some arrested larvae, such as those of *Ostertagia ostertagi*, and has no activity against flukes and tapeworms. It is normally administered PO or by subcut. injection; generally the 2 routes are considered equivalent in efficacy. Levamisole slow-release boluses are available in some countries. Topical preparations for cattle have recently been developed.

Levamisole stimulates nematode ganglia, and leads to neuromuscular paralysis of the parasites. (Hexamethonium, a ganglionic blocker, inhibits the action of levamisole.) It acts on the roundworm nervous system, and is not ovicidal. Its broad spectrum of activity, ease of use (being water soluble), reasonable safety margin, and lack of teratogenic effects have allowed it to be used successfully in a wide range of hosts. Because of its mechanism of action, the peak blood concentration is more relevant to its antiparasitic activity than the duration of concentration. Subcut. administration should provide better efficacy against lungworms than oral, by virtue of the higher plasma (and therefore lung) concentrations achieved. In addition, because of its different mechanism of action, levamisole possesses activity against benzimidazole-resistant parasites.

In cattle, peak blood levels of levamisole occur in <1 hr after subcut. administration. These concentrations then decline rapidly and 90% of the total dosage is excreted in 24 hr, largely in the urine. After oral dosing in cattle, levamisole residues are present in muscle, fat, liver, and kidney 2 hr after medication, but by 48 hr after treatment are below the limits of assay detectability (0.1 ppm). Blood and urine levels of levamisole peak 2-6 hr after, but are below the limit of detectability at 36 and 72 hr after treatment, respectively. Highest residue levels appear in the liver. No residues are detectable in the tissues, blood, or urine 7-8 days after injection.

Excretion is rapid, and the consequent withholding periods are shorter than for the insoluble benzimidazoles. Mammalian toxicity with levamisole or especially with tetramisole is usually greater than for the benzimidazoles, although toxic signs are unusual unless the normal therapeutic dosage is exceeded. Levamisole toxicity in the host animal is largely an extension of its antiparasitic effect, ie, cholinergic-type signs of salivation, muscle tremors, ataxia, urination, defecation, and collapse. In fatal levamisole poisoning, the immediate cause of death is asphyxia due to respiratory failure. Atropine sulfate can alleviate such signs. Levamisole may cause some inflammation at the site of subcut. injection, but usually this is transient.

Levamisole possesses immunostimulant effects, and has been used in man and to a limited extent in other animals in several diseases (see p 1521).

TETRAHYDROPYRIMIDINES

Pyrantel was first introduced as a broad-spectrum anthelmintic against GI parasites of sheep, and subsequently has been used in cattle, horses, dogs, and pigs. It is prepared for use as a tartrate, embonate, or pamoate salt.

Aqueous solutions are subject to isomerization on exposure to light, with a resultant loss in potency; therefore, suspensions should be kept out of direct sunlight. It is not recommended for use in severely debilitated animals because of its levamisole-type pharmacological action.

Pyrantel tartrate is well absorbed by pigs and dogs, less well by ruminants. Metabolism is rapid, and the metabolites are excreted rapidly in the urine (40% of the dose in dogs); some unchanged drug is excreted in the feces (principally in ruminants). Peak blood levels are usually attained 4-6 hr after administration PO. The pamoate salt of pyrantel is poorly soluble in water; this offers the advantage of reduced absorption from the gut and allows the drug to reach and be effective against parasites in the lower end of the large intestine, which makes it useful in horses and dogs. Pyrantel is used PO as a suspension, paste, drench, or tablets. It is effective against ascarids, large and small strongyles, and pinworms.

Morantel is the methyl ester analog of pyrantel and, in ruminants, it tends to be somewhat safer and more effective than pyrantel. It is absorbed rapidly from the abomasum and upper small intestine of sheep, metabolized rapidly in the liver, and ~17% of the initial dose is excreted in the urine as metabolites within 96 hr after dosing.

Both pyrantel and morantel have a higher efficacy against adult gut worms and larval stages that dwell in the lumen or on the mucosal surface than against the stages found in the mucosa such as arrested Ostertagia larvae. A sustained-release ruminal bolus for use in cattle (qv, p 1483), which releases the morantel over 60-90 days, has been introduced. No withdrawal period (at least in some countries) is required for the biodegradable morantel bolus for cattle.

ORGANOPHOSPHATES (OP)

A number of OP have been used as anthelmintics. Originally they were employed extensively as insecticides, then as ectoparasiticides: dichlorvos is now used frequently as an anthelmintic in horses, pigs, dogs, and cats; trichlorfon in horses and dogs; and coumaphos, crufomate, haloxon, and naftalofos in ruminants. OP inhibit many enzymes, especially acetylcholinesterase, by phosphorylating their esterification site. This blocks cholinergic nerve transmission in the parasite, which results in spastic paralysis. The cholinesterases of host and parasite and those of different species of parasites vary in their susceptibility to OP. Such variations are considered in development and production of OP. The susceptibility of its cholinesterase enzymes to the OP, the rate at which the inhibition can be reversed, and the rate of inactivation of the various OP in the host animal largely determine the relative toxicity to different animals.

OP tend to be labile to varying extents in alkaline media and may be partially hydrolyzed and inactivated in the alkaline region of the small intestine, eg, the oral dose rate for trichlorfon in cattle is 4.5 times the subcut. dose. In ruminants, OP generally have satisfactory efficacy for nematode parasites of the abomasum (especially *Haemonchus* spp) and small intestine but lack satisfactory efficacy for parasites of the large bowel. OP usually are rapidly oxidized and inactivated in the liver. Their margin of safety is generally less than that of the benzimidazoles, and strict attention to dosage is necessary.

Because of its high volatility, dichlorvos is a particularly versatile OP that can be incorporated as a plasticizer in vinyl resin pellets; it is released slowly from the inert pellets as they pass through the GI tract, which provides a therapeutic concentration along the tract. This controlled release governs the concentration available to the host as well as the parasites, and thereby increases the safety margin. When passed in the feces, the pellets still contain ~45-50% of the original drug. Dichlorvos is rapidly absorbed and metabolized in the body. It is particularly useful in pigs against all major parasites and was one of the first broad-spectrum anthelmintics to be used in this species. It is also effective against helminths and bots in horses.

Trichlorfon (metrifonate) is used in horses because of its high degree of activity against bots, ascarids, and oxyurids. It also has been used in ruminants and small animals. As with other OP, trichlorfon tends to have a narrow margin of safety.

Dichlorvos and trichlorfon are particularly effective against bots and ascarids, and are effective against a broad-spectrum of other GI helminths also. Their principal problem is adverse reactions due to cholinesterase inhibition. Contraindications, in general, are respiratory disease; parturition within 1 mo; evidence of diarrhea or other GI problems; and use or contemplated use of insecticides, muscle relaxants, phenothiazine-derived tranquilizers, or CNS depressants.

Haloxon is probably the safest OP anthelmintic for use in ruminants, even though some sheep may be hypersensitive (*see* p 595). The concentration required to inhibit cholinesterase activity of the parasite is extremely low; in addition, mammals possess cholinesterase that forms unstable complexes with haloxon. Its primary action is against parasites of the abomasum and small intestine. It may be administered PO as a paste, bolus, or drench, and displays efficacy against adult *Haemonchus*, *Trichostrongylus*, *Cooperia*, and *Strongyloides* spp. Its activity is somewhat less, but still good, against *Ostertagia*, *Bunostomum*, and *Nematodirus* spp. Haloxon is rapidly absorbed from the gut, metabolized fairly rapidly, and excreted in the urine.

Certain precautions should be followed when using OP. Generally, their toxicity is additive; thus, concurrent use of other cholinesterase-inhibiting drugs should be avoided. Atropine and 2-PAM are used as antidotes to OP toxicity (*see also* p 1669).

OP can be hazardous to man. Being lipid soluble, they are absorbed well through unbroken skin. They also have the propensity to interact with many other drugs. OP are relatively rapidly degraded in the animal body, and tissue residues are unlikely to pose a serious consumer hazard if specified withholding periods are enforced. Perhaps the major risk arises from contamination of the environment through fecal excretion or accidental drug spillage. Fish are particularly susceptible, and many instances of serious water pollution and fish kills have been attributed to careless disposal of OP pesticides. Sprays, collars, and washes of OP used for small animals can present significant hazards to young infants following ingestion, inhalation, or transcutaneous absorption.

AVERMECTINS

The avermectins, which are products, or chemical derivatives thereof, of *Streptomyces avermitilis*, have a potent, broad, antiparasitic spectrum at low dose levels. They are active against many immature and mature nematodes and arthropods. Ivermectin, which is comprised of ≥80% 22,23 dihydroavermectin B_{1a} and ≤20% of the B_{1b} homolog, is active against many parasites including arrested and developing larvae and adults of the important cattle and sheep nematodes. Abamectin, a closely related compound, has a similar spectrum of activity but has not been as widely utilized.

Structurally related compounds have recently been approved in some countries: moxidectin for use in cattle, milbemycin oxime for dogs. Also, approval is expected for doramectin.

There is substantial evidence that the activity of the avermectins results from an increased release of the neurotransmitter γ-aminobutyric acid (GABA) and enhanced binding of GABA to its postsynaptic receptors, which leads to consequent opening of chloride ion channels and decreased cell function. However, there is also evidence that ivermectin affects chloride channels independently of GABA. The precise mode of action is unclear, but the result is paralysis and, eventually, death of the parasite.

Although paralysis is the most evident effect of ivermectin in parasites, suppression of reproductive function also has been observed in ticks. Ivermectin displays no activity against cestodes or trematodes, presumably because these parasites do not utilize GABA as a neurotransmitter. It is well absorbed when administered PO, parenterally, or as a pour-on. The route of administration and the formulation affect its disposition profile. High levels are reached in the lungs and skin regardless of the route of administration. Efficacies >95% have been achieved against parasites of the skin, respiratory system, and blood after PO treatment. Concentrations of ivermectin are maintained in body fluids for prolonged periods. In cattle dosed subcut. with ivermectin at 0.3 mg/kg, a half-life of 70 hr of radioactive residue in plasma was reported. Following IV delivery of ivermectin at 0.2 mg/kg in sheep, a terminal half-life of 178 hr was detected. This relatively long half-life is related to the high potency of the compound, as studies with other anthelmintics have indicated that efficacy is profoundly affected by the kinetic profile. In sheep, low plasma levels were reported when ivermectin was administered into the rumen; however, its anthelmintic activity was not affected.

Most ivermectin is excreted in the feces, the remainder in the urine. Minimal residues are present in the muscle and kidneys, and highest concentrations are detected in the liver and fat tissues. Residues in all tissues are largely extractable with little or no macromolecularly bound drug or metabolites present. The major single component in the edible tissues of cattle, sheep, and pigs is the unaltered parent drug. Ivermectin is also excreted in the milk of lactating animals.

Although mammals utilize GABA as a central neurotransmitter, generally they are not adversely affected by ivermectin, probably because, being a macrolide of large molecular weight, ivermectin does not readily cross the blood-brain barrier of the mammal to affect the GABA receptors of the CNS. There have been a number of cases of CNS depression in purebred and crossbred Collies (*see also* p 1493). Ivermectin in feces or soil degrades at a slow but significant rate. In a winter environment, decomposition is slow (half-life of 91-217 days); when exposed to an outdoor summer environment, ivermectin in soil has a half-life of 7-14 days.

Avermectins cause little adverse effect on freshwater algae, and virtually none on germination or growth of plants. Studies have shown that residues in feces of animals treated with avermectin B_1 inhibit the development of dung beetle larvae. Larval development of the buffalo fly in fresh feces of treated cattle is prevented for up to 14 or more days after treatment.

Peak concentrations of ivermectin and metabolites in the accumulated waste of cattle and sheep is ~18-19 ppb. Assuming that the dung is evenly spread over the pasture, concentration of dung and metabolites in soil is estimated to be <0.1 ppb. From laboratory experiments, exposure levels of 300 mg/kg of soil (ppm) are necessary for toxicity to earthworms. Thus a margin of 3 million exists between anticipated pasture/soil levels and the toxic levels for earthworms.

In cattle at subcut. doses of 0.2 mg/kg, ivermectin is highly effective against most GI nematodes, including the adult and larval stages of *Ostertagia* (including the inhibited fourth-stage larvae), *Trichostrongylus, Oesophagostomum*, and *Haemonchus* spp, as well as the lungworm *Dictyocaulus viviparus*.

A useful feature of parenteral treatment in cattle is the persistent efficacy against the immature stages of certain nematodes. This period of protection varies with the nematode species, but can be up to 21 days for lungworms. Ivermectin also displays activity against a number of economically important arthropod parasites of cattle (*see* p 1499).

Although the 2 formulations have somewhat different spectra of activity, given PO or subcut. to sheep, ivermectin at 0.2 mg/kg is effective against immature and adult stages of common endoparasites. The injectable formulation is also effective against several of the ectoparasites of sheep.

In pigs, ivermectin is given subcut. at 0.3 mg/kg body wt. The spectrum of activity includes the adults and larvae of *Ascaris suum, Hyostrongylus rubidus, Oesophagostomum* spp, and the lungworm *Metastrongylus apri*, in addition to the mange mite and sucking louse. The treatment of pregnant sows can block the transcolostral transmission of *Strongyloides ransomi* to piglets. Efficacy against *Trichuris suis* is ~80%.

As paste or liquid given PO to horses at 0.2 mg/kg, ivermectin is highly effective against *Trichostrongylus axei, Parascaris equorum, Oxyuris equi, Strongylus vulgaris, S edentatus, Dictyocaulus arnfieldi*, and adults of *S equinus, Triodontophorus* spp, *Habronema muscae*, and *Strongyloides westeri*, and bots (*Gasterophilus* spp). It is also effective against larvae of *Habronema muscae, Draschia megastoma*, and *Onchocerca* sp (dermatoses). Although an IM formulation was originally employed, the oral formulations are now the only preparations approved for use in horses.

Arterial larval stages of *Strongylus* spp tend to be refractory to most anthelmintics, although intensive therapy with certain members of the benzimidazole class has been useful against these migratory pathogenic strongyle stages. Many studies with ivermectin at the standard dosage have indicated 100% efficacy against these arterial larvae. Such treatment has prevented vascular damage following experimental infection, reduced the size of cranial mesenteric aneurysms, and increased circulation to arteries distal to the aneurysm. With time, resolution of arteritis and thrombosis and a return to the smooth contour of the arteries follows such treatments. The ubiquitous but less pathogenic "small strongyles" are also susceptible to ivermectin.

Many canine parasites are susceptible to ivermectin at the dosages used in other animals; however, since some dogs are adversely affected at these levels, only one dosage for one parasite is recommended in dogs: 6 μg/kg body wt, given at 1-mo intervals, prevents development of *Dirofilaria immitis*, the cause of heartworm disease. At higher doses (>50 μg/kg), some Collies are adversely affected by ivermectin; at much higher doses (200 μg/kg), these idiosyncratic reactions included depression, muscle weakness, blindness, coma, and death. Many cases of ataxia progress to paralysis and decreased consciousness. Relatively higher brain concentrations of ivermectin are found in sensitive Collies than in other dogs or host species, which indicates greater penetration across the blood-brain barrier (or sequestration).

Ivermectin is teratogenic in rats, rabbits, and mice but only at or near maternotoxic dose levels. Mice are the most sensitive species at a dosage of 0.2-0.4 mg/kg/day. Reproduction and multigeneration studies have demonstrated that neonatal rats are more susceptible to the toxic effects of ivermectin than adult rats. From mouse teratogenicity studies and from multigeneration studies in rats, the no-effect levels (NEL) of 0.2 mg/kg/day have been established.

Based on the relationship of these NEL to residue levels in edible tissues from pharmacokinetic studies, the current withdrawal times for sheep and cattle have been established. However, due to their high potency and elimination through milk, ivermectin preparations are contraindicated for use in animals that produce milk for human consumption. Year-round parasite control programs can involve 3-4 treatments per year in young stock. The primary impact on the environment from use of ivermectin in farm animals is excretion of the drug by treated animals via their feces and urine (*see* p 1492).

SALICYLANILIDES, SUBSTITUTED PHENOLS, AROMATIC AMIDE

Salicylanilides: brotianide, clioxanide, closantel, niclosamide, oxyclozanide, rafoxanide.

Substituted Phenols: bithionol, disophenol, hexachlorophene, niclofolan (menichlopholan), nitroxynil.

Aromatic Amide: diamfenetide (diamphenethide).

All members of these chemical groupings possess efficacy against liver flukes. Diamfenetide is unique in that it possesses exceptionally high activity against the youngest immature stages of the liver fluke in sheep, with a diminution of its activity as the flukes mature. Nitroxynil is normally administered subcut.; the rest of the group are given PO. The salicylanilides and substituted phenols act to uncouple or disconnect the mitochondrial reactions involved in electron-transport-associated events from ATP generation. This uncoupling is lethal to *Fasciola hepatica* and other blood-sucking helminths. *In vivo*, mainly the adult flukes are affected, with variable activity against the immature flukes in the liver parenchyma. The lowered efficacy of a number of the salicylanilides and substituted phenols against the immature flukes may be due to the high protein binding of these drugs in the blood. A number of these compounds, however, appear to possess activity against 6-wk-old flukes in cattle and sheep, affecting them either at the time of administration or, more probably, by persisting in blood until the flukes start to ingest blood and become exposed to higher drug concentrations. Metabolism may affect the pharmacological activity of various fasciolicides, and some of this metabolism may occur in the GI tract. For diamfenetide, which is given PO, this metabolism may be important for full efficacy. Nitroxynil is metabolized by ruminal bacteria, which destroys its activity and restricts administration to injection. Following absorption, diamfenetide is further metabolized in the liver to an amine metabolite that is active against flukes; it is not active against liver flukes *in vitro* unless incubated in the presence of enzymatically functional liver cells. Oxyclozanide is metabolized in the liver to the active glucuronide, which is excreted in the bile in high concentrations in the vicinity of the adult fluke. Most of the available fasciolicides are administered as oral suspensions or occasionally as solutions by subcut. injection.

Niclosamide is poorly absorbed from the GI tract; the bulk of the dose remains in the lumen of the gut where it exerts its taeniacidal effect by inhibiting oxidative phosphorylation in the parasite. It is used primarily in dogs, and in eastern Europe, in ruminants infected with *Moniezia* spp.

Increasing the dosage of these compounds frequently results in increased activity against the later parenchymal stages of *Fasciola* spp, but when such elevated dosages are employed, the inherent safety margin of the particular drug in use must be recognized. The bile ducts are important in the excretion of many of these phenol-based compounds, as evidenced by the high proportion of these and their metabolites excreted in the feces rather than the urine. The increased susceptibility of the developing flukes is largely related to the long plasma half-lives of the compounds, which require lengthy withdrawal times. The fasciolicidal activity of salicylanilides in sheep depends on the extent to which they persist in plasma; eg, rafoxanide is fully absorbed, and plasma levels of $\sim$29 μg/mL are found 24 hr after dosing. The plasma half-life is $\sim$4 days, and it binds to plasma proteins with a very high affinity. Plasma can dissolve up to 2 mg/mL, but it is virtually insoluble in water. Relatively high levels of residues are found in plasma even 42 days after dosing, but residues in other tissues are negligible. The plasma half-life of disophenol is even longer, being 7-14 days in dogs, and >30 days in sheep. The penalty for high efficacy associated with long plasma half-life is the need for long withholding periods.

The high efficacy of many salicylanilides and substituted phenols against blood-ingesting parasites, eg, *Haemonchus contortus* and hookworms, may be related to their attachment to plasma proteins. Presumably they are released to poison the parasite after it ingests blood.

Pharmacokinetic data for many modern fasciolicides is sparse. Peak plasma levels, which may be an indicator of efficacy, are reached in 12-24 hr for salicylanilides and 3-4 days for bithionol sulfoxide. The absorption of fasciolicides given parenterally (nitroxynil) is rapid and complete—peak plasma levels are reached 30-60 min after dosing. The relatively high residues of nitroxynil found in milk are due to the relatively high dose rate, parenteral administration, and the tendency to form stable complexes with serum and body proteins.

Nitroxynil is retained in the liver and plasma of sheep at detectable levels (>0.1 ppm) for 66 days after a single dose of 10 mg/kg. Although binding to serum albumin occurs, long-term exposure to the drug is critical for antiparasitic activity.

Plasma levels associated with activity against the mature fluke are >55 ppm. Closantel, rafoxanide, and oxyclozanide have long terminal half-lives in sheep (14.5, 16.6, and 6.4 days, respectively), which are related to the high plasma-protein binding of these 3 drugs (>99%), and residues in liver are detectable for weeks following administration.

Because these drugs, with the possible exception of diamfenetide, are general uncouplers of oxidative phosphorylation, their safety indexes are not as high as for many other anthelmintics, but nonetheless, are more than adequate if used as directed. Adverse effects are most commonly seen in animals severely stressed, in poor condition nutritionally or metabolically, or with severe parasitic infections. Commonly, a slight loss of appetite and looseness of feces may be seen following treatment at recommended dosages. High dose rates may cause blindness and classical signs of uncoupled phosphorylation, viz, hyperventilation, hyperthermia, convulsions, tachycardia, and ultimately death. Consumer concerns arise because of narrow safety margins, pharmacodynamic effects, long half-lives, high binding to plasma protein, deposition in the liver, and excretion in detectable quantities in milk. However, because these fasciolicides are used no more than 2-3 times/yr, residues are unlikely to occur in milk with any great frequency. Nonetheless, safe levels could possibly be exceeded in infants or small children consuming ≥1 L of milk/day, even at the end of the withholding period.

MISCELLANEOUS ANTHELMINTICS

Phenothiazine was discovered to have anthelmintic activity in 1938, and for years was used extensively in livestock, but has been largely replaced by drugs with broader spectra of activity. It is still used, primarily in ruminants, in prophylactic, low-level, in-feed programs; and in horses, in mixtures with other drugs. It is not used in pigs, dogs, or cats. The mode of action is not well understood. Toxicity within host species is variable, but the safety margin is narrow in comparison with most of the newer anthelmintics. Its efficacy is best against *Haemonchus* and *Oesophagostomum* spp in ruminants, and small strongyles in horses.

Piperazine and its derivative diethylcarbamazine (DEC) were first introduced as anthelmintics in 1947. Piperazine is rapidly absorbed from the GI tract, and piperazine base can be detected in the urine as early as 30 min after administration. The excretion rate is maximal at 1-8 hr, and excretion is practically complete within 24 hr. Piperazine acts to block neuromuscular transmission in the parasite by hyperpolarizing the nerve membrane, which leads to flaccid paralysis. It also blocks succinate production by the worm. The parasites, paralyzed and depleted of energy, are expelled by peristalsis. The spectrum of activity of piperazine is largely against ascarid parasites in all species and also *Oesophagostomum* spp. There is variable activity against hookworms and strongyles, and little effect against whipworms or flat worms. The safety margin is wide.

DEC also acts to paralyze nematodes by interfering with nerve function. It is widely used for heartworm prophylaxis in dogs. In existing infection, the dogs must first be cleared of adults and microfilariae to avoid reaction, then are given DEC daily PO throughout the mosquito season. DEC is also used to treat prepatent hoose (lungworm disease) in cattle, although it is relatively ineffective against the mature form of *Dictyocaulus viviparus*. It is routinely given IM at 22 mg/kg body wt for 3 consecutive days, although it is reported that one injection at 44 mg/kg gives better respiratory relief.

Praziquantel has high efficacy against cestode parasites at a relatively low dose rate, but no effect on nematodes. In dogs, it is rapidly absorbed, and maximal blood levels are reached as early as 30-60 min after administration. After absorption it is believed to be re-excreted back into the intestinal lumen via the mucosa, which may explain the extremely high efficacy even against 3-day-old *Echinococcus granulosus*. Cestodes buried in the crypts of Lieberkühn surrounded by mucus and inflammatory exudate are usually rather inaccessible to anthelmintics in the lumen of the gut. Delivery to the sites of infection from the bloodstream makes for more effective action. Re-secretion into the gut is rapid; studies have identified the active drug in the ileum within 8 min of administration when the bulk of the administered dose still remained far higher up the GI tract. Praziquantel exerts its antiparasitic effects in many ways, impairing both motility and function of the suckers of the cestode. *In vivo* studies have indicated that it induces spastic paralysis of the parasite; thus, praziquantel acts, as many anthelmintics, primarily on neuromuscular coordination. It also influences the permeability of the integument of the worm, which can lead to excessive calcium and glucose loss. Its margin of safety is wide.

Clorsulon is a sulfonamide given PO as a suspension for liver fluke infection in cattle. Immature flukes (8 wk old) require a higher dose (7 mg/kg) than adult flukes (3.5 mg/kg). In plasma, clorsulon is bound to protein, which when ingested by liver flukes, inhibits enzymes of the glycolytic pathway. Although the safety margin is wide, it should not be used in dairy cows of breeding age, and withdrawal time before slaughter is 8 days.

Bunamidine is another anticestodal compound, used in small animals. It is most effective if given after fasting. It is absorbed and metabolized in the liver, and leads to digestion of the tapeworms in the gut of the host. Vomiting and mild diarrhea may be seen, and exercise or excitement should be avoided in dogs soon after dosage.

Nitroscanate, like the substituted phenols, probably acts by uncoupling oxidative phosphorylation. It is one of the newer broad-spectrum anthelmintics introduced for use in small animals against *Toxocara, Toxascaris, Taenia, Dipylidium, Ancylostoma, Uncinaria*, and *Echinococcus* spp. Vomiting occasionally occurs after dosage.

RESISTANCE

The development by nematodes of resistance to various chemical groups of anthelmintics is now recognized as a problem with a major potential. Until relatively recently, resistance to anthelmintics in nematodes had been slow to develop under field conditions (in comparison with antibiotic resistance in bacteria). However, resistance is likely to become more widespread because relatively few chemically dissimilar groups of anthelmintics have been introduced over the past decade. Most of the commonly used anthelmintics belong to 2 or 3 chemical classifications, within which all individual compounds act in a similar fashion. Thus, resistance to one particular compound is accompanied by resistance to other members of the group.

Continued application of a highly effective anthelmintic selectively removes most susceptible genotypes, with the resultant progeny of succeeding generations being composed of resistant strains. Resistance to an anthelmintic is expressed by passage of increased numbers of parasite eggs, higher establishment rates of adults in the host, and greater numbers of larvae on the pasture after treatment than would occur if the parasites were susceptible to the drug. While resistance of *Haemonchus* spp is becoming a global problem, resistance of *Trichostrongylus* and *Ostertagia* spp, to date, is mainly confined to sheep in Australia and South America. Resistance of small strongyles in horses is also a problem in several areas.

The development of significant resistance seems to require 9-10 generations of helminths, and studies indicate that anthelmintics of different chemical groupings or of differing modes of action should be used in alternate years to prolong their worthwhile therapeutic existence. Care should be taken to use the anthelmintic no more often than is needed to control the parasites; emphasis should be placed on husbandry methods to minimize exposure to the helminths. Also, selection for resistance may be expected to be minimized by using an appropriate anthelmintic at a dose rate not less than that recommended by the manufacturer.

Cross-resistance is frequently seen between members of the benzimidazole group because of their similar mechanisms of action. Control of benzimidazole-resistant parasites by, eg, levamisole, can be expected because of its different mode of action. Although there is no cross-resistance between levamisole and benzimidazoles, this does not mean that worms resistant to both kinds of drugs will not evolve. In addition, cross-resistance between levamisole and morantel can occur due to the similarities of their mechanisms of action.

In summary, emphasis should be placed on management practices designed to reduce exposure to parasites, and to minimize the frequency of anthelmintic use. Also, evolution of anthelmintic resistance may be delayed by using chemicals with different modes of action. The current recommendation is for a slow rotation of the different chemical groups; ie, the anthelmintic should be changed (rotated) between the generation intervals of the parasites, rather than within a single generation interval. The latter usage may, in fact, hasten the development of resistance to more than one chemical. This means that no individual worm should be repeatedly subjected to anthelmintics from more than one chemical group. Since, with important exceptions, such as *Haemonchus contortus*, there are usually only 1-2 generations of parasites per annum, anthelmintics from different groups probably should be rotated annually between dosing seasons. In the control of parasites, there is no doubt that long-term economic benefit is obtained only by planned treatment of a whole flock or herd and considering the biology of the parasite(s). Good results should be obtained provided that correct control measures are directed against the parasitic phase in the body of the host at the appropriate time, and attention is given to the free-living, nonparasitic stages in the environment.

EXTERNAL PARASITICIDES

EXTERNAL PARASITICIDES, LG AN

To maintain health and to prevent losses in production, animals may require treatment with various drugs to reduce or eliminate arthropod parasites. Accurate identification of the pest or correct diagnosis based on clinical signs is necessary for selection of the appropriate drug. The selected agent can be administered or applied directly to the animal, or introduced into the environment to reduce the arthropod population to a level that is no longer of economic or health consequence. (This level varies with the parasite.)

Certain pest arthropods, such as lice, keds, and mange mites, live continuously on the skin and are controlled only by treating the host. Because mange mites burrow into the skin, they are more difficult to control with sprays or dips than are lice and keds, which are found on the surface of the skin. Other arthropods, such as ticks and poultry mites, stay on the host long enough to feed, which may be as short as 30 min in the case of nymphs and adults of soft ticks, or as long as 21 days in the case of all feeding and molting stages of 1-host species of hard ticks. Biting flies, such as the horn fly, can be found continuously on the backs and undersides of cattle, where they suck blood ≥20 times a day; other biting flies, such as stable flies and horse flies, and mosquitoes feed to repletion and leave the animal to lay eggs. Nonbiting flies, such as the face fly or the house fly, can be very annoying and may cause eye problems by their feeding or by transmission of pinkeye or eyeworms. Larvae of certain blowflies live on the skin or in tissues of sheep and other animals and cause cutaneous myiasis; larvae of other flies, such as sheep nose bot, horse bot, and cattle grubs, spend several months inside animals—in nasal passages, stomach, or tissues (back or esophagus), respectively.

METHODS OF TREATMENT

Various techniques are available. When pasture or lot conditions and management systems are favorable, or when prescribed by law, animals may be dipped in insecticides. Dipping vats are constructed so that animals are thoroughly immersed in the vat fluid, and the liquid that drains from the animals returns to the vat. Vat construction can vary from large rectangular plunge vats (that contain >2500 gal. [~10,000 L]) to small circular vats used for dipping sheep and goats. A cage vat consists of a metal cage to hold the animal that is lowered mechanically into the dip. Because of unique requirements for stability and safety, only a few formulations of insecticides are approved for use in dipping vats. Vats are advantageous in that, with proper management and care, treatment of large animals is very thorough.

However, there are disadvantages: 1) vats are usually permanent structures (although portable vats are available) and animals must be moved to the vat location; 2) because of the large amount of insecticide needed to charge vats, the cost of initial charge is high; and 3) vats must be managed properly so that the insecticide is maintained at the appropriate concentration. All parasiticides deplete from the vat faster than the carrier fluid and, to maintain therapeutic or prophylactic concentrations, the vat must be topped up with a higher than initial concentration of dip. A number of systems are now available for the automatic replenishment of parasiticide and carrier in the desired proportions. When the vat contents are no longer usable (contaminated with dirt and manure, or do not contain sufficient insecticide), they are considered to be hazardous wastes and must be disposed of in accordance with applicable laws.

A more common method of application of aqueous emulsions or suspensions is spraying. Sprayers are portable and may be hand-or motor-driven, and only enough insecticide to treat a specific number of animals need be prepared. A spray treatment is only as effective as the equipment and operator permit. A thorough spraying (1½-2½ gal. at 300 psi [6-10 L at 20 atmospheres]) of all parts of an animal's body is necessary to control certain pests (eg, mites, ticks); in contrast, a less thorough spraying (1-2 quarts [1-2 L] at low pressure) may adequately control horn flies. In countries that have eradication policies for ectoparasites such as *Psoroptes ovis* (sheep scab mite), spray treatment may not be acceptable since regulations may require complete immersion.

The portable spray-dip machine combines certain aspects of dipping vats and sprayers. The machine consists of a metal treatment chamber, which confines the animal, situated over a metal sump that collects the runoff. The chamber contains pipes fitted with a number of nozzles that direct a high-volume, low-pressure spray to all parts of the animal while it is confined in the treatment chamber. After spraying is complete, the animal is held in the chamber so that the runoff is collected for respraying. A spray-dip machine must be operated correctly, managed continuously, and maintained sufficiently to ensure that animals are treated thoroughly.

Insecticides may be applied by hand to a few animals at a time as washes, ointments (especially to skin or wounds to control cutaneous myiasis), dusts, mist sprays, spray foams, aerosols, etc. Ear ticks may be controlled by insecticides applied directly into the ears. Other hand-applied treatments include the pour-on method, which consists of applying a water-diluted, emulsifiable concentrate or a ready-to-use formulation. The liquid should be poured along the backline from the shoulders to the hip bones. Pour-on treatments are used to apply insecticides for the control of cattle grubs (with systemically active parasiticides), horn flies, lice, and other arthropods. The spot-on treatment method consists of applying a small volume of concentrated insecticide to a single spot on the animal's back. Spot-on treatments are used to apply insecticides for control of cattle grubs and lice on cattle and goats, and as an aid in the control of both biting and nuisance flies on cattle. They are also used for the control of sucking lice on pigs, and head flies, lice, keds, and ticks on sheep.

Cattle may be treated individually with insecticide-impregnated tags or strips attached to the ears, or tags and tapes attached to tails. Horses may be treated with such tags attached to halters or with strips attached to halters or to tails. These devices slowly release insecticide and can provide long-term control of horn flies and aid in the control of nuisance flies. Unfortunately, in a number of areas, especially in the southern and midwestern USA, horn flies have become resistant to the pyrethroid insecticides that are commonly used in insecticide-impregnated ear tags. Such tags are highly effective in controlling Gulf Coast and ear ticks.

In addition, cattle may be treated individually with ivermectin (subcut. injection or pour-on), which is systemically active against cattle grubs, sucking lice, and mites (plus nematodes).

To avoid gathering range animals for treatment, cattle owners may use self-treatment devices, such as back rubbers or dust bags. Back rubbers consist of burlap or other cloth material wrapped around wire, chain, or cable suspended between 2 posts or a post and the ground. The material is charged with an insecticide diluted with oil; when cattle rub against the charged material, insecticide is transferred to their bodies. Burlap or canvas bags can be suspended between posts so that animals can apply insecticide to their faces and bodies. Back rubbers or dust bags can be placed in pastures so that cattle can use them, or can be placed in aisles or at openings to areas that contain salt, feed, water, etc, so that cattle must pass under them daily or more frequently. This "forced use" situation allows for more certain treatment than the "free choice" situation. To protect them from the elements (especially rain), dust bags are usually hung under shelters. Back rubbers and dust bags, if used sufficiently, can apply enough insecticide to cattle to control horn flies and lice, and may aid in the control of face flies and other arthropods that are on cattle for short periods.

Range cattle may be treated for horn fly control with ultra-low volumes of insecticides applied by low-flying airplanes. Flies on stanchioned dairy cattle or dairy cattle and beef cattle confined in drylots may be controlled by daily mist applications of insecticides as emulsions or as ready-to-use products over the backs of the animals.

A variety of flies, especially the horn fly and face fly, breed in undisturbed cow manure; others, especially the stable fly and house fly, breed in horse or cow manure mixed with straw, hay, and spilled feed, and in other filth and debris around structures. Fly larvae that breed in manure can be controlled by allowing cattle or horses to consume daily a mineral mixture or feed additive that contains an insecticide that is effective against larvae of all 4 species of flies, or an insect growth regulator that is effective only against horn fly larvae. Minimal amounts of active ingredient must be consumed daily for the treatment to be effective. Such treatments do not control the adult flies that migrate to treated cattle or horses from nearby animals; thus, even though no flies are produced from the manure of the treated animals, nonisolated cattle and horses can be parasitized by moderate to large numbers of immigrant flies. This is often distressing to owners who expect to see treated animals free of flies. Care must also be taken so as not to upset the delicate ecological balance by contaminating the environment with insecticides.

Horses are generally difficult to treat with conventional power sprayers because usually they are frightened by the noise of the machinery and the spray. Insecticides and repellents can be applied to the skin of horses by hand-activated mist sprayers, foggers, pressurized aerosols, wipe-on cloths, sponges, or stick rub-ons. Individual horses may be treated PO with paste or liquid formulations or with feed-additive powders or pellets to control bot larvae.

CHEMOTHERAPEUTIC AGENTS

Most chemotherapeutic agents registered and labeled for use as external parasiticides for large animals are organophosphates or pyrethroids. A limited number of organochlorines and, for some ectoparasites, ivermectin are also available. Because approved usages vary from country to country, and with time, the label should be read before use of any specific product.

Only those products that are not excreted in the milk are approved for use on lactating dairy cattle. A few products that contain coumaphos, fenvalerate, methoxychlor, permethrin, or pyrethrins may be applied directly to lactating dairy cattle. These external parasiticides may be applied as whole body, full coverage sprays or as mist sprays, dusts, in backrubbers or face rubbers, dust bags, or aerosols directly onto the cattle. Tags impregnated with chlorpyrifos or stirofos (organophosphates), or permethrin or fenvalerate (pyrethroids) may be attached to the ears of lactating dairy cows. Feed-through-treatments (treatments given in the feed to control parasites that utilize the feces) that contain stirofos or methoprene can be given to lactating dairy cattle.

A larger variety of external parasiticides can be applied to beef or nonlactating dairy cattle. Labels of all external parasiticides contain specific information on approved periods before slaughter or freshening during which application is permissible. These periods are necessary to permit metabolization and excretion of the parasiticide, and may be as short as zero days (ie, cattle could freshen or be slaughtered immediately after treatment) or as long as 60 days. All parasiticides approved for lactating dairy cattle may also be used on nonlactating dairy cattle and beef cattle. In addition, products containing chlorpyrifos, dioxathion, fenthion, ivermectin, lindane, phosmet, or trichlorfon may be used on beef and nonlactating dairy cattle.

The same restrictions that apply to the use of chemotherapeutic agents on lactating dairy cattle also apply to their use on lactating dairy goats. Sheep (except when their milk is being used for human consumption) and nonlactating goats may be treated with products that contain the following: coumaphos, dioxathion, fenvalerate, lindane, methoxychlor, permethrin, or pyrethrins. Minimum time from treatment to slaughter varies from 0 to 60 days.

Horses that are not to be used as food for human consumption may be treated with products that contain coumaphos, crotoxyphos, dioxathion, fenvalerate, ivermectin, malathion, methoxychlor, permethrin, phenothrin, phosmet, pyrethrins, tetrachlorvinphos, or trichlorfon.

Pigs may be treated with products that contain coumaphos, dioxathion, fenthion, fenvalerate, ivermectin, lindane, methoxychlor, permethrin, phosmet, or pyrethrins. In pigs, the minimum time from treatment to slaughter varies from 0 to 60 days.

SAFETY RESTRICTIONS

It is important to be aware of and follow safety restrictions to prevent poisoning or damaging of treated animals. All organophosphates available for use on animals are cholinesterase inhibitors. They should not be used simultaneously or within a few days before or after treatment or exposure to other cholinesterase-inhibiting drugs, pesticides, or chemicals. They should not be applied to sick, convalescent, or stressed animals, or animals <3 mo old.

The number and use of organochlorine insecticides approved for use on animals are limited. Generally, animals <3 mo old should not be treated, nor should animals in cold stormy weather, or those that are overheated or sick.

The few pyrethroid insecticides available for use on large animals are considered safe, but have general precautionary statements on their labels.

Some parasiticides may be used only by or under the supervision of a veterinarian; others are available to the general public. Approvals vary from country to country. Labels for pesticides contain explicit information on hazards to animals, man, and the environment; storage of unused insecticide; and disposal of the container. For each insecticide, the label is the primary source of information on uses and safety instructions.

EXTERNAL PARASITICIDES, SM AN

Fleas and ticks on dogs and cats have a widespread prevalence. A wide variety of ectoparasiticides is available and brand switching is frequent, which is an indication of the problems faced in achieving acceptable parasite control. The veterinarian is uniquely qualified to provide key advice on host/parasite interrelationships (such as resistance and life cycles) and selection of the most suitable control program. Unfortunately, many small animal owners purchase their parasiticides in supermarkets or pet supply shops where professional advice is not available. Many veterinarians now merchandise insecticidal products and encourage client education by their staff; to do so they must be alert to technological improvements in both insecticidal chemistry and delivery systems, and also must be aware of new findings that pertain to existing products.

Many factors influence the choice of product: active chemical ingredient, target parasite, efficacy, safety, regulatory status of the product, convenience, and aesthetic acceptability.

ACTIVE CHEMICAL INGREDIENTS

Nomenclature can be confusing if the shorter approved name is not used and the full chemical name is written (eg, O,O-diethyl O-[3,5,6-trichloro-2-pyridyl] phosphorothioate vs chlorpyrifos). The use of chemical trade names can cause added confusion (eg, Dursban = chlorpyrifos). Although most commercial products contain only one active ingredient, it is not uncommon for ≥2 to be combined. All labels should be read carefully for ingredients and directions for use.

Cholinesterase Inhibitors: Two groups of compounds, organophosphates and carbamates, share the same mechanism of action—inhibition of acetylcholinesterase. They are popular for their rapid action and potency. Before treatment, it should be determined that the animal's cholinesterase levels are not depressed due to recent application of the same or related product to the animal or premises. Those approved for small animal therapy include the following:

   Organophosphates: chlorpyrifos, dichlorvos, malathion, diazinon, phosmet, coumaphos, fenthion, chlorfenvinphos, ronnel, stirofos, cythioate.

   Carbamates: carbaryl, propoxur.

Chlorinated Hydrocarbons: These compounds are becoming less popular because of their persistence in the environment, although this factor brought the benefit of prolonged action. Lindane (γ-benzene hexachloride), DDT, and chlordane are no longer approved by most government regulatory authorities. Bromocyclen and methoxychlor are still occasionally used.

Pyrethrins and Pyrethroids: Natural pyrethrins are extracted from chrysanthemum flowers, and are notable for their rapid but brief action and relative lack of toxicity in dogs and cats. To enhance their efficacy, they are often mixed with synergists such as piperonyl butoxide.

   Synthetic pyrethroids are pyrethrum-like compounds that possess greater potency and residual effects. They include permethrin, resmethrin, allethrin, fenvalerate, tetramethrin, and cypermethrin.

Rotenone: Obtained from derris and cube roots, rotenone is a naturally occurring insecticide that has been largely superseded but sometimes is still used in mixtures with other active ingredients. Its primary use is against ear mites and demodectic mange.

Formamidines: This group of acaricidal compounds, which kill by inhibiting monoamine oxidase, offers a useful alternative for treatment of ticks and mange mites on livestock when resistance to cholinesterase inhibitors has developed. Amitraz is the only one approved for use against generalized demodicosis in dogs.

Synergists: Piperonyl butoxide and N-octyl bicycloheptene dicarboxamide inhibit the microsomal enzyme systems of insects, and thus can prolong the activity of a wide variety of insecticidal compounds. They are often included in the formulations of topical preparations, particularly those containing pyrethrins.

Growth Regulators: Methoprene is the first compound of this interesting new class of low toxicity "biorational approach" chemicals. It is not directly insecticidal but prevents metamorphosis of larvae into adults. It is used for sustained flea control on premises, and is often combined with conventional insecticides. Its direct use on animals is relatively new and is claimed to sterilize newly laid flea eggs. New insect growth regulators (IGR) being developed include diflubenzuron, phenoxycarb, and pyriproxyfen.

Repellents: Dimethyl phthalate and deet (N-N-diethyl-m-toluamide) are often used in fly and mosquito repellent products. Their role in flea and tick control is unsupportable, and may present toxicity problems associated with their solvent action on other compounds in formulations. Citrus and herbal oils are sometimes included in insecticidal products for purported repellent activity. Some are effective, but others probably provide aromatic value only.

Miscellaneous: Benzyl benzoate is an inexpensive acaricide useful as an adjunct in the treatment of sarcoptic mange in dogs. It is toxic to cats. Sulfur is still used, though infrequently, in the form of lime-sulfur solution for the treatment of notoedric mange in cats. Use of sulfur in the diet of dogs for purported flea control belongs in the realm of "folk medicine" along with household ultrasound generators, garlic, and cider vinegar.

TARGET PARASITE EFFICACY

Due to specific formulation and drug delivery technology, it is possible for certain insecticides to be used in a wide variety of ectoparasite control products. In general, ticks and fleas are usually controlled by the same active compounds, but resistance may reduce efficacy locally for both groups. Care should be taken when treating mite infestations, however, to choose products that contain compounds specifically active against the target parasite.

Duration of activity (ie, "knockdown" or sustained effects) are often the prime concern in product choices. Some products allow for parasite recovery, while others are so slow that parasite loads on the host are not reduced because the rate of reinfestation exceeds the kill rate.

SAFETY

Because animal toxicity can be modified by formulation technology, active ingredients are not the sole guide to safety assessment. Most commercial products have undergone adequate safety evaluation for regulatory approval, and the label remains the best source of information. Care should be taken not to multiply cholinesterase inhibition by using simultaneous treatments of animal and premises with organophosphate or carbamate products. Because cats are sensitive to many insecticides, use on or near them requires caution. Human and environmental safety also should be considered, especially for usage in treatment of premises. The safety of older insecticidal compounds is sometimes questioned: the compound may break down into more toxic components, or regulatory approval may be withdrawn due to new testing data (eg, carcinogenicity or environmental concerns). Scientific controversies of this nature are not easily resolved. Formulations that are generally safe may induce skin reactions, or even fatal reactions in certain sensitive breeds of dogs and cats.

DELIVERY SYSTEM CONVENIENCE

Consumer convenience is an important factor in product choice, especially for flea and tick control. A bewildering array of systems is now available—powders, aerosols, sprays, foams, shampoos, rinses, pour-ons, mousses, oral tablets or liquids, and impregnated collars or medallions. All have their uses according to the individual situation and parasite problem. Possible flammability of solvent-containing products should not be overlooked for indoor use.

AESTHETIC ACCEPTABILITY

For dogs and cats that live closely with their owners, aesthetic acceptability is important. Product odor, staining, effect on hair coat, noises of pressurized packages, and irritation of skin, eyes, and mucous membranes may affect the temperament of both animals and their owners.

ANTI-INFLAMMATORY AGENTS AND TREATMENT OF INFLAMMATION

Inflammation is common to almost all diseases that involve microbiological, chemical, or physical injury to living tissues. Acute inflammation may be defined as the microcirculation response to injury; the cardinal signs are heat, redness, pain, swelling, and loss of function. The accompanying microcirculatory changes comprise arteriolar vasodilation, increased small vein permeability, formation of edema fluid, and WBC migration to the site of injury. The desirable outcome of this process, which at least initially is protective and homeostatic, is isolation and destruction of the injurious agent and resolution of the inflammatory lesion so that normal tissue conditions are fully restored. If, however, the challenging stimulus persists, the inflammation may become chronic and the microcirculatory changes characteristic of acute inflammation are replaced by lesions typical of the chronic disease, including tissue destruction and fibrous tissue formation.

Although anti-inflammatory drugs are used extensively to treat both acute and chronic inflammatory conditions, none is curative. In general, they suppress rather than abolish inflammatory reactions, thereby providing symptomatic relief. The sometimes limited efficacy reflects the complexity and multifactorial nature of inflammatory processes. Proposed mediators of acute inflammation include histamine, 5-hydroxytryptamine (5-HT, serotonin), bradykinin, prostaglandin E_2 (PGE_2), prostacyclin (PGI_2), platelet activating factor (PAF), leukotriene B_4, and interleukin 1. Proteolytic and other tissue-destructive enzymes become involved in chronic inflammation, but much less is known about both these mediators and those substances concerned with tissue repair. The difficulties in designing new anti-inflammatory agents, and in achieving clinical response, are due to: 1) the large number of mediators that exist, eg, a specific antihistamine will antagonize only those components of the reaction (mainly restricted to the early vascular changes occurring in acute inflammation) for which histamine is responsible; 2) species differences in mediator roles; 3) synergistic interactions between mediators, eg, prostaglandins markedly enhance the vasodilator effects of histamine and the pain-inducing actions of bradykinin; and 4) the continuing discovery of new "mediators", such as interleukin 6 and lipoxin A. The precise roles of these newer putative mediators have yet to be defined, and although, in some instances, antagonists of their formation or action have been studied, they are not generally available for clinical use in anti-inflammatory therapy.

Mediators are central to a discussion of anti-inflammatory agents, since almost all of the drugs in clinical use are known or presumed to act by inhibiting the action, synthesis, or release of one or more mediators. Therefore, their sources and roles are reviewed briefly. Histamine is stored in mast cell granules and platelets, and is released by inflammatory and immunological stimuli. It plays an important role in acute inflammation, exerting a dilator action on arterioles and increasing the permeability of small venules to plasma proteins. Serotonin is found in platelets and in mast cells of some rodent species, in which it may be involved in early microvascular changes in acute inflammation. However, the generally poor clinical efficacy of antihistamine and antiserotonin drugs suggests that the role of both serotonin and histamine as mediators in nonimmune inflammation is limited. Plasma kinins such as bradykinin are not stored but are released by the action of kininogenase from plasma α-2-globulins. Bradykinin is a potent vasodilator and causes pain by stimulating peripheral receptors, but it has a short half-life.

Prostanoids, such as PGE_2 and PGI_2, like the kinins, also are synthesized *de novo* from arachidonic acid. These compounds are potent arteriolar dilators, but their more important role in inflammation probably is indirect. Small amounts markedly enhance the actions of other mediators (histamine and bradykinin) in producing microvascular dilation, increased permeability, and pain (hyperalgesia). The complement fragments C_{3a} and C_{5a} are potent chemoattractants, which also induce mast cell degranulation.

Leukotriene B_4 (LTB_4), a potent chemoattractant formed by the action of lipoxygenase enzymes on arachidonic acid, may be involved in mediating WBC passage into inflammatory exudate. Inhibitors of LTB_4 synthesis such as BW540C have been evaluated experimentally, but their place in therapy has not yet been determined. PAF, like prostanoids and leukotrienes, is derived from cell membrane phospholipid by the action of phospholipase A_2, which is activated by cell membrane perturbation. PAF can be released by most cell types in the body, and its actions are equally diverse. It produces all the important components of acute inflammation (vasodilation, edema, hyperalgesia, and WBC extravasation), and is currently the subject of research as a putative mediator of immune and nonimmune inflammatory conditions (eg, heaves in horses).

Tissue damage induces a systemic reaction in the form of the acute phase response (APR). The complex changes in serum protein concentrations, which comprise the APR, lead to both tissue necrosis and reparative healing processes. Fundamental to induction of the APR is the release of a range of cytokines, including interleukins, interferons, and tumor necrosis factor. The roles of specific cytokines is still the subject of much research, but it is clear that the 2 forms of interleukin 1 (IL-1α and IL-1β) are important inflammatory mediators as well as inducers of the APR and the pyrexia that accompanies infectious conditions.

Interleukins (eg, IL-1 and IL-6) are also thought to play important roles in cartilage degeneration in joint diseases. Cartilage degeneration itself cannot be classified as an 'inflammatory'' reaction, since cartilage is an avascular and aneural tissue. However, cartilage loss may be attributable to or associated with soft-tissue inflammation (synovitis, capsulitis) in joint diseases. The role of interleukins in both inflammatory and noninflammatory joint diseases is ill defined, but much experimental evidence demonstrates their ability to stimulate synovial cells and chondrocytes to release pain-inducing mediators (eg, PGE_2) and cartilage-degrading enzymes (eg, collagenase and stromelysin). Some of the newer agents with chondroprotective properties (discussed below) probably act through inhibition of such degrading enzymes.

Anti-inflammatory drugs act by several mechanisms, some of which are ill defined. They may be classified as nonsteroidal anti-inflammatory drugs (NSAID), steroids, or miscellaneous agents. Steroids with anti-inflammatory properties comprise the natural glucocorticoid hormone, cortisol, and many more potent and specific synthetic derivatives. NSAID include numerous compounds of diverse chemical structure; most are believed to share a common mechanism of action, and almost all are weak organic acids.

NONSTEROIDAL ANTI-INFLAMMATORY DRUGS (NSAID)

This large group of compounds can be divided into 2 main subgroups, carboxylic acids (R-COOH) and enolic acids (R-COH). Further divisions, based on chemical structure, can be made. The main subgroups of enolic acids are the pyrazolones such as phenylbutazone, oxyphenbutazone, dipyrone, and isopyrin, and the oxicams, which include piroxicam, isoxicam, and miloxicam. Carboxylic acid subgroups comprise the salicylates (eg, acetylsalicylate [aspirin]), propionic acids (eg, ibuprofen, ketoprofen, naproxen, and carprofen), anthranilic acids (eg, meclofenamic acid), phenylacetic acids (eg, acetaminophen), aminonicotinic acids (eg, flunixin), and indolines (eg, indomethacin).

Nature and Mode of Action: Despite widely differing chemical structures, most NSAID share 3 basic properties: they are anti-inflammatory by their local actions, and antipyretic and analgesic by their effects on the CNS. Potency for each property can vary from drug to drug. For example, phenylbutazone is more effective peripherally (anti-inflammatory) than centrally, while isopyrin is an effective analgesic with weak anti-inflammatory actions; therefore, there is some logic in using these drugs in combination. Acetaminophen has weak peripheral actions and does not produce significant GI irritation, nor does it have significant anti-inflammatory activity, although it acts centrally as an analgesic.

These differences in activity are explicable in terms of the basic mode of action of NSAID, which is to inhibit cyclooxygenase, the enzyme that converts arachidonic acid to the cyclic endoperoxides, PGG_2 and PGH_2. By the actions of further specific enzymes, these compounds are converted to a major group of inflammatory mediators, the eicosanoids, which includes PGE_2 and PGI_2. However, the cyclooxygenase structure varies among tissues, and NSAID differ in their ability to combine with them, which explains differences in potency, and in species response. For example, plasma levels of phenylbutazone required for efficacy in treatment of joint disease in man are within 100-150 μg/mL, but horses require only 10-30 μg/mL.

In addition to cyclooxygenase, a second enzyme (lipoxygenase) can use arachidonic acid as a substrate. This gives rise to the leukotriene family of compounds, one of which, LTB_4, may be an important mediator of WBC passage into sites of inflammation. Agents such as BW755C and timegadine, which inhibit both cyclooxygenase and lipoxygenase, have been studied. Although they are not in general clinical use, such compounds may eventually provide a broader spectrum of anti-inflammatory activity than NSAID, comparable to that of steroids, since experimentally they have been shown to block both cellular and vascular components of the acute inflammatory reaction.

Administration and Pharmacokinetics: Throughout the GI tract, particularly in the stomach of monogastric animals, the pH is normally more acid than the plasma. An acid environment promotes the absorption of NSAID which, as weak organic acids, are more ionized in plasma and therefore absorbed by the mechanism of ionic or diffusion trapping. A similar mechanism arising from drug binding to plasma protein also promotes the absorption of most NSAID; however, other factors are involved. The low solubility in acidic media of some NSAID, eg, aspirin, leads to precipitation in the stomach, which delays absorption and increases local irritation. In horses and ruminants, diet may be important. *In vitro* studies with phenylbutazone, meclofenamate, and flunixin have shown that these drugs bind to hay (and nuts), and this may explain why peak concentrations in plasma can be delayed for up to 18 hr in horses. Possibly, these drugs first become adsorbed onto hay and later are released by fermentative digestion to become available for absorption in the large intestine. This mechanism could also explain why high doses of phenylbutazone exert their main ulcerogenic effects caudally in horses.

In ruminants, closure of the esophageal groove can cause orally administered sodium meclofenamate to bypass the rumen. High abomasal and plasma concentrations of this drug soon after oral dosing confirm that a variable portion of the dose may bypass the rumen, but this mechanism may not apply to all NSAID. In spite of the many variables affecting NSAID absorption in ruminants and monogastric species, absorption is generally good, with bioavailability values up to 100%.

Some drugs (phenylbutazone, dipyrone, isopyrin, carprofen, and flunixin) are available in parenteral formulations for IV dosing. Flunixin is less irritating than phenylbutazone and is the only drug recommended for IM as well as IV administration to horses and cattle. In spite of some irritation, phenylbutazone is well absorbed from IM sites in cattle, and has a bioavailability approaching 100%. In horses, however, extravascular administration can cause sloughing and abscess formation.

Plasma-protein binding for most NSAID is high (>90%); for phenylbutazone and flunixin it is >99%, although salicylate is exceptional, with binding of ~50%. The high degree of protein binding limits renal excretion of most NSAID, although some metabolites may be actively secreted by the proximal tubular cells. Salicylate, with its lower degree of protein binding, is excreted in urine in higher concentrations than other NSAID and the rate of excretion depends on pH. Whereas alkaline urine traps salicylate molecules in the nonpermeable ionized form (which can be utilized in treating acute salicylate overdosage), acid urine favors reabsorption of the drug.

Plasma-protein-binding levels >90% may also limit the distribution of NSAID from plasma to body fluids and tissues. However, this does not necessarily limit therapeutic efficacy in acute inflammation, since protein leaks from the vascular compartment into inflamed tissues, and drug concentrations in inflammatory exudate commonly exceed the levels in plasma. However, protein binding does limit penetration into fluids such as saliva and milk; for phenylbutazone, concentrations are ~1% of the plasma levels, corresponding to the non-bound plasma concentration.

Another important excretory route for some NSAID and their glucuronide metabolites is active secretion in bile. This does not necessarily lead to curtailment of the drug's action, since glucuronic acid can be hydrolyzed in the intestine, and the parent drug may then be reabsorbed via an enterohepatic shunt.

The usual effect of biotransformation of NSAID is to yield metabolites that are less active and more polar than the parent compounds. Such metabolites are readily excreted in urine or bile, or both, although other metabolites with significant anti-inflammatory actions (eg, salicylate from aspirin, and oxyphenbutazone from phenylbutazone) can be formed. The NSAID most studied in animals, phenylbutazone and aspirin, show marked species differences in plasma clearance. Reported half-life elimination values for salicylate are 0.5 hr in cattle, 1-3.7 hr in horses, 6 hr in pigs, 9 hr in dogs, and up to 38 hr in cats. Half-life values for phenylbutazone are 3 hr in rabbits, 4-6 hr in horses, dogs, pigs, and guinea pigs, 15-19 hr in goats, 32-60 hr in cattle, and 72 hr in man. For naproxen, reported values are 2 hr in monkeys, 4-5 hr in pigs and horses, 14 hr in man, and up to 92 hr in dogs. In dogs, there are apparently breed differences in half-life, with reported values of 72 hr in mongrels and 35 hr in Beagles. These species differences in clearance profoundly affect the dosing interval and toxicity. Thus, for aspirin, a dose of 25 mg/kg, given t.i.d. in dogs, and once daily in cats, is likely to provide effective and safe plasma and tissue levels; fatalities due to naproxen have been reported in dogs receiving the drug at equivalent human or equine dosages, whereas oral dosing with 5 mg/kg on day 1, and 2 mg/kg/day thereafter seems to be safe over several weeks.

For most drugs, half-life is independent of dose rate, since clearance mechanisms are not saturated when clinical dose levels are administered. However, for phenylbutazone and aspirin in some species, elimination is dose dependent, so that cumulation to toxic levels in plasma and tissues readily occurs with high doses; adherence to recommended doses is important, especially for phenylbutazone in horses and for aspirin in cats.

Other factors in addition to half-life must be considered in determining safe and effective dose levels of NSAID; a very short half-life value does not necessarily preclude use of a given drug. There may be several reasons why actions can be longer than would be predicted from half-life. One drug, aspirin, binds irreversibly to cyclooxygenase, while most others are reversible antagonists, and the former may have more persistent actions. This is true for the anti-thrombotic actions of aspirin, which are due to irreversible blockage of platelet cyclooxygenase, but not for the analgesic and anti-inflammatory effects, which are attributable primarily to the metabolite salicylate (a reversible inhibitor of cyclooxygenase). NSAID tend to accumulate in inflammatory exudate, from which they are cleared more slowly than from plasma. After oral administration, absorption continues as the drug is being metabolized and excreted, so that even drugs possessing short half-lives (eg, meclofenamate and flunixin with IV half-lives of 0.9 and 1.6 hr in horses) can achieve effective levels from once-daily dosing. Also, some drugs are converted to active metabolites.

Biotransformation is generally the main factor that terminates NSAID activity, and species differences in rates of biotransformation account for the species differences in half-life described above. Differences in biotransformation, hence, half-lives, also occur within species, and age and sex differences have been demonstrated in man. Fewer animal studies have been done, but since hepatic biotransformation and renal excretory mechanisms develop gradually over the first month of life in mammals, longer dosing intervals are likely to be appropriate for all neonates. In old animals, hepatic and renal clearance mechanisms also are less efficient, and longer dosing intervals or lower doses should be used.

Residues: Limited studies indicate that NSAID do not accumulate in high concentrations in tissues in food-producing animals. Milk concentrations are limited by both plasma-protein binding and the pH of milk, which is more acidic than plasma. Tissue levels of meclofenamate and phenylbutazone are lower than plasma levels and, for phenylbutazone, tissue and plasma concentrations decrease in parallel. Phenylbutazone, and especially its metabolite oxyphenbutazone, can be detected in equine urine for several days after the last dose.

Salicylate metabolites are frequently detected in the urine of horses in the absence of salicylate medication. Salicylates are natural ingredients of many forages and the levels are quite high in some legumes (eg, alfalfa).

Side Effects: NSAID can affect many enzymes and biochemical pathways at high dose levels, but the toxic effects probably are mainly due to inhibition of cyclooxygenase. This ubiquitous enzyme is present in all cell types except for RBC, and it subserves many roles; therefore, it is not surprising that NSAID usage may lead to diverse side effects.

The most common side effect is irritation and possibly ulceration of the GI mucosa. All NSAID exert this action to varying degrees. Relative to anti-inflammatory activity, ulcerogenicity is generally high for aspirin, intermediate for naproxen and phenylbutazone, and low for salicylate and sulindac. However, many factors, including diet, nutritional status, age, species, sex, and even time of day seem to be important in determining the degree of damage, and generalizations can be dangerous. In particular, toxicity data cannot be transposed between species. In addition, high NSAID concentrations in the bile may also expose distal sections of the gut to high concentrations in some species. This could account for the greater ulcerogenic action of indomethacin in the dog, which has an efficient enterohepatic circulation, than in poorly recycling species like the monkey.

The mechanism that produces GI ulcers is uncertain. Severe ulceration can occur in all parts of the gut, and damage can occur following IV as well as oral dosing. Prostacyclin is a vasodilator prostanoid that may function as a local hormone and regulate blood flow to the gut mucosa; inhibition of its synthesis by NSAID leads to ischemia, and hypoxia may be the mechanism of erosion that leads to ulceration. Severe erosion causes bleeding into the gut or a plasma protein-losing enteropathy. With toxic doses of phenylbutazone (only moderately greater than therapeutic doses), ulceration in horses has been sufficiently severe to cause hemoconcentration and death from hypovolemic shock. All horses seem to be particularly susceptible. Whereas daily oral dose rates of phenylbutazone of 10-14 mg/kg may be lethal within 2 wk in horses, amounts 10 times greater have failed to induce ulcers in dogs when administered over 1 mo, yet the elimination half-life is similar (4-8 hr) in the 2 species. Other factors, eg, drug formulation and aging of animals, also have been implicated in causing toxicity, but dose rate is probably of overriding significance. For most NSAID in most species, low to moderate doses with continuous daily doses over many months have proved clinically acceptable.

Several approaches have been adopted to minimize the incidence and severity of GI lesions, notably for aspirin; these include development of slow-release formulations, enteric coating, and water-soluble salts, but none has been wholly successful. Lysine-acetylsalicylate, a water-soluble salt, reduces the incidence of emesis, anorexia, and ulceration in dogs, and is also well tolerated when given IM.

High doses of NSAID can produce renal tubular nephritis. Renal papillary necrosis has been described in horses that received standard clinical doses of NSAID. However, this lesion may arise only when animals under treatment have restricted access to water. Fluid retention and edema may occur during NSAID therapy, but these effects are uncommon. Both cytological and cholestatic forms of hepatotoxicity have been reported in man and suspected in other animals. Because of possible liver damage, it is important to adhere to recommended doses with NSAID. Such damage may lead to impaired drug metabolism and a vicious cycle of cumulation and further toxicity.

In man, blood dyscrasias following long-term treatment with NSAID are not uncommon. Similar findings in dogs, horses, and cats have been reported, but from the available data, it is unclear whether particular drugs or certain species are implicated; although dyscrasias can occur with recommended doses, the incidence does not seem to be high. In cats, acetaminophen poisoning is common, usually as a result of owner administration of the drug, and probably because of formation of the reactive, electrophilic metabolite N-acetyl-p-benzoquinoneimine. Potentially fatal Heinz body anemia, methemoglobinemia, liver failure, and facial edema occur. N-acetylcysteine is given PO by gavage as an antidote; it acts by providing sulfhydryl groups with which the toxic acetaminophen metabolites can combine. Inhibition of platelet aggregation with NSAID can lead to impaired blood clotting, and prolonged use may predispose to hemorrhage. Because of its irreversible mode of action, and because of the inability of platelets to synthesize new cyclooxygenase, aspirin is likely to present greater problems in this regard than other NSAID.

The life-threatening cardiovascular and respiratory effects that occur with high doses of NSAID are not encountered with therapeutic doses. However, doses of phenylbutazone only 3 times greater than therapeutic doses cause dilatation and degeneration of the walls of small veins in horses.

Drug Interactions: In general, the administration of 2 NSAID confer no advantage over higher doses of a single drug. However, if one agent possesses good central analgesic activity (eg, isopyrin) and the other is more effective as an anti-inflammatory agent (eg, phenylbutazone), clinical efficacy may be enhanced. However, when using these drugs together, both half-lives are greater than when administered singly, so that toxic cumulation can occur if the dosing interval is <24 hr. A similar interaction between phenylbutazone and oxyphenbutazone has been described. A different type of drug interaction can occur with NSAID that are highly bound to plasma protein. If administered with other agents that are highly protein bound, competition for binding sites may lead to displacement of one or both compounds and to raised plasma concentrations of unbound drugs. For this reason, the combined use of the anticoagulant warfarin and phenylbutazone in the therapy of equine navicular disease is contraindicated except with extreme caution.

Uses: By their central actions, NSAID are analgesic, but this response is weaker than that attainable with narcotic analgesic agents of the morphine type. Central analgesia may contribute to the clinical efficacy of NSAID only to a limited extent, and their value in severe pain normally is limited. The more important peripheral analgesic action derives from inhibition of synthesis of prostanoids such as PGE_2, which are hyperalgesic as a consequence of their synergism with inflammatory mediators such as bradykinin.

NSAID are used to treat many forms of acute inflammation of the musculoskeletal system, including traumatic injury, and routine use for their analgesic and antiedematous actions following surgery is increasing. They also are used for long-term therapy of chronic inflammation of both soft and hard tissues. In this circumstance they provide symptomatic relief through their analgesic actions, but the progress of disease is not slowed. Indeed, experimental studies on canine stifle cartilage have shown that some, but not all, NSAID reduce cartilage proteoglycan synthesis. Such an action *in vivo* would be expected to exacerbate degenerative changes in joint diseases. However, proof that this occurs in clinical cases is lacking.

NSAID such as meclofenamic acid have been used effectively in treating nonimmune inflammation and in suppressing anaphylactic responses in cattle.

NSAID (notably flunixin) available as solutions are administered parenterally for their analgesic actions in equine spasmodic colic, but suppression of clinical signs may obscure the diagnosis. Some of the cardiovascular and metabolic changes arising in endotoxic shock are caused by increased circulating levels of eicosanoids, such as prostacyclin and thromboxane A_2, and the IV administration of NSAID to inhibit the synthesis of these compounds represents a rational approach to therapy. However, preformed eicosanoids are not affected, and this limits the effectiveness of treatment.

Endotoxemias associated with equine colic, acute and peracute bovine mastitis, and canine septic peritonitis have been treated with NSAID such as flunixin.

Viral and bacterial infections of the GI tract have been treated with NSAID. The inflammatory component of these diseases is suppressed, and reduced scouring times and lowered mortality have been reported in calves and piglets.

PGE_2 is a potent endogenous pyretic agent; it acts on the anterior hypothalamus to affect the thermoregulatory centers. Inhibition of its synthesis provides the basis for the antipyretic action of NSAID in infections associated with fever. Symptomatic relief is afforded when body temperature is lowered, but NSAID do not possess antimicrobial properties; they may even affect adversely the course of viral diseases, since interferon production is greater when body temperature is raised. In spite of this, NSAID have proved useful in the treatment of acute respiratory disease caused by parainfluenza type 3 virus in calves, and also in fog fever, and in acute interstitial pneumonia caused by *Ascaris suum*. In these instances, however, it is the local anti-inflammatory action rather than the central antipyretic action that is useful.

Newer Drugs: A number of newer NSAID, previously used in man, have been investigated for their toxicological and pharmacokinetic properties in other animals, particularly dogs and horses, and several have also been subjected to clinical trials. Among these are carprofen, piroxicam, eltenac, and CERM 10202. Not all of the agents investigated have proved to be acceptable; eg, when administered PO in effective doses to dogs, ibuprofen caused repeated and consistent vomiting even when used in enteric-coated formulations. There remains, moreover, a dearth of information on both newer and existing drugs for use in species other than horses and dogs, and this is particularly true for cats. Aspirin is still the only NSAID for which pharmacokinetic information is available in cats.

STEROIDS

The main steroid hormones secreted by the adrenal cortex, the corticosteroids, are divisible into 2 general classes, mineralocorticoids and glucocorticoids. The former group includes aldosterone, the physiological effects of which are exerted on water and electrolyte balance. The glucocorticoids affect carbohydrate, lipid, and protein metabolism; some possess weak mineralocorticoid properties as well, and they are potent anti-inflammatory agents when administered locally or systemically. The main glucocorticoid hormone, cortisol (hydrocortisone), is used as an anti-inflammatory agent, but a number of synthetic steroids with increased glucocorticoid potency and reduced mineralocorticoid activity are also available. For example, prednisone and prednisolone are 3-4 times more potent than cortisol as glucocorticoids, but have only half the mineralocorticoid activity. Anti-inflammatory activity runs in parallel with glucocorticoid potency. Therefore, in clinical use, prednisone and prednisolone produce less disturbance to electrolyte balance than cortisol. Methylprednisolone and triamcinolone are ~5 times more potent than cortisol as glucocorticoids and are virtually devoid of mineralocorticoid activity. Dexamethasone and betamethasone similarly lack effects on electrolyte balance, but are 30-35 times as potent as cortisol as anti-inflammatory agents. For a discussion of the principal actions of cortisol and the control of its secretion, *see* THE ADRENAL GLANDS, p 260. Cortisol and other glucocorticoids are gluconeogenic, enhancing the release of amino acids from muscle, skin, and connective tissue, and increasing amino acid conversion to glucose. They cause hyperglycemia, particularly in ruminants, and the storage of glucose in the liver as glycogen is increased, although glucose uptake and utilization by other tissues is suppressed. The rate of lipolysis is increased, and fatty acids and glycerol are released from adipose tissue; the glycerol so formed may be converted to glucose. Intestinal absorption of calcium is decreased while renal excretion is increased; parathormone secretion is increased and osteoclast stimulation occurs. These effects, in combination, promote the mobilization of calcium from bone, and bone strength is thereby reduced. Glucocorticoids promote diuresis by increasing glomular filtration rate and depressing distal tubular water reabsorption.

The principal effect on blood is to cause leukocytosis due to an increase in the number of circulating neutrophils. Numbers of circulating lymphocytes and eosinophils are reduced, and glucocorticoids generally depress the activity of lymphoid tissues; when high doses are given to some species, a decrease in thymus weight and shrinkage of the spleen and lymph nodes occur. The immunosuppressant action of glucocorticoids is manifest by a reduction in cell-mediated immunity and decreased antibody production. In some species, these effects occur even with low doses of steroid. Although lymphoid tissue depression is undesirable, this action can be utilized in the treatment of some neoplastic conditions such as lymphosarcoma.

Nature and Mode of Action: The exact mechanisms by which steroids act are unknown, but it is clear that (unlike NSAID) they suppress all aspects of acute and chronic inflammatory processes. Microvascular dilation, increased permeability, and edema, hyperalgesia, and fibrin deposition are inhibited. The early migration of polymorphonuclear WBC and the later extravasation of monocytes are reduced, and phagocytic activity is depressed. In the later stages, capillary growth, fibroblast proliferation, and collagen deposition are inhibited, and wound healing and cicatrization are delayed.

Anti-inflammatory steroids have a general stabilizing action on biological membranes. Cell, lysosomal, and mitochondrial membrane stabilization appears to reduce the release or synthesis of acute inflammatory mediators and diminishes the tissue degradative effects produced by lysosomal enzyme release in chronic inflammation. However, this hypothesis is not universally accepted and does not explain how steroids act at the molecular level.

One important biochemical pathway that is blocked by steroids is the arachidonic acid cascade. Liberation of arachidonic acid from the phospholipid component of cell membranes depends on phospholipase A_2. Steroids indirectly inhibit this enzyme by inducing synthesis of endogenous polypeptides, the lipocortins, which possess anti-phospholipase activity. This indirect mode of action explains the latent period of up to 5 hr between administration and effect, and it also means there is no simple relationship between effect and drug concentration in plasma or at the site of action at a given time.

Arachidonic acid acts as substrate for 2 enzyme systems, cyclooxygenase (which is blocked by aspirin-like drugs, ie, NSAID) and lipoxygenase (which is not blocked by normal clinical doses of NSAID). Steroids, by acting more proximally in the biochemical pathway than NSAID, therefore block the synthesis of a greater number of putative inflammatory mediators. Cyclooxygenase-derived compounds, such as PGE_2 and PGI_2, are important mediators of acute inflammatory responses, while lipoxygenase generates the leukotriene group of compounds. At least one of the latter, LTB_4, is a potent chemotactic agent that may stimulate WBC migration into exudate, while others (LTC_4 and LTD_4) are released in allergic airway diseases. They may be concerned with mediation of responses in conditions such as fog fever in cattle, chronic obstructive pulmonary disease in horses, and many other forms of immune and nonimmune inflammation.

Administration and Pharmacokinetics: Topical application to the skin or mucous membranes is a common method of administration and achieves high drug concentrations at the site of action while reducing the risks of systemic side effects. However, most steroids are readily absorbed and, if the animal is able to lick sites of application, absorption from the gut occurs as well. Thus, systemic effects can occur following local usage. Compounds have been developed in which topical activity is high, but absorption is low and systemic activity therefore reduced. They include betamethasone-17-valerate and beclomethasone dipropionate.

Corticosteroids are well absorbed if given orally, and this route is commonly used for medium- to long-term treatment. The risks of undesirable suppression of the hypophyseal-pituitary axis (HPA) should be considered with such therapy, and means to minimize it adopted. A short-acting preparation can be given at twice the normal dose on alternate days in place of the normal single dose once daily. HPA suppression subsides on nontreatment days, but therapeutic effects persist since drug action outlasts the period for which detectable circulating levels occur (*see* above). Dogs should be dosed in the morning and cats in the evening, so that peak blood levels coincide with maximal concentrations of endogenous cortisol. This suppresses the HPA for the shortest possible time in each 24-hr period.

Corticosteroids also are administered frequently by parenteral routes, and although oral dosing is simpler, parenteral therapy provides more predictable blood levels and a more rapid onset of action for short- to medium-term treatment. IV administration of water-soluble preparations (succinates, phosphates, and m-sulfobenzoates) can be used in emergency cases. Pharmacokinetic parameters have been established for IV dosing with some steroids. The half-life values for dexamethasone, eg, given IV, are 53 min in horses, 110-130 min in dogs, and 290-335 min in cattle. Very high doses can be given on a single occasion without risk of toxicity, eg, for animals in shock, 10 times the normal dose is required for clinical efficacy. Water-soluble preparations are also rapidly absorbed from IM sites, and esters (eg, acetate, adamantoate, phenylpropionate, acetonide, isonicotinate) with limited water solubility are available as suspensions for slower IM absorption and a more sustained action. Some depot preparations, eg, acetonide and adamantoate esters, provide effective levels over several days and even weeks, but the convenience of using such products should be weighed carefully against the unavoidable HPA suppression arising from the long-term maintenance of high circulating steroid concentrations.

For the treatment of chronic joint diseases, eg, arthritis, intra-articular injection is sometimes used after removal of an equal volume of synovial fluid. By this means, the risks of systemic side effects are reduced—but not abolished, since some formulations can be absorbed rapidly. Therefore, long-acting preparations that persist locally for several days may be used. With all intra-articular injections, a careful aseptic technique is required. Steroids reduce soft-tissue inflammation (synovitis and capsulitis) and alleviate stiffness and pain, which permits freer joint movement. However, they interfere with natural repair processes, eg, suppression of chondrocyte metabolism; their use also can reduce proteoglycan content and induce atrophathy in horses. In addition, they may induce osteoporosis and osseous metaplasia; consequently, intra-articular usage is controversial.

Side Effects: The side effects that may occur during treatment are related to the physiological effects described above. Compounds with mineralocorticoid activity, such as prednisolone and prednisone, tend to cause retention of sodium and water, hence, edema; urinary potassium increases, which leads to hypokalemia and metabolic alkalosis. Side effects related to glucocorticoid actions include polyuria and compensatory polydipsia in the early stages of treatment, hyperglycemia and, if renal threshold for glucose absorption is exceeded, glucosuria. Protein catabolism leads directly to muscle wasting and indirectly to delayed wound healing. The lipolytic effect of steroids is accompanied by redistribution of body fats and the characteristic "moonface" appearance in man. Similar effects have been reported in dogs. Altered calcium metabolism can, with prolonged treatment, lead to osteoporosis and bone fractures. Reduced GI motility, thinning of the gastric mucosa, and reduced mucus production may arise, but glucocorticoids are rarely ulcerogenic. Nevertheless, it is clear that spinal cord trauma may predispose to steroid-induced ulceration, and steroids may also potentiate the ulcerogenicity caused by some NSAID. The immunosuppressant actions are mentioned above. Reversible hepatomegaly with medium- or long-term therapy has been described, and teratogenicity may occur when steroids are administered in pregnancy, but the latter effect is not well established.

On cessation of steroid therapy, the HPA recovers slowly over several weeks, and the animals are particularly vulnerable to stress if treatment is terminated abruptly. Restoration of normal HPA function is best achieved by gradually reducing the dose rate while increasing the interval between doses.

Uses: Anti-inflammatory steroids are used extensively to treat many immune and nonimmune inflammatory conditions. Both allergic (eg, sweet itch in horses and flea-bite allergy in cats) and nonspecific eczemas respond to therapy, and steroids are commonly incorporated in preparations for otitis externa and inflammatory conditions of the eye. They are useful in breaking the itch-scratch cycle in canine dermatoses. Local allergies respond to steroid therapy, but in acute anaphylaxis, onset of action is too slow to be of practical value. Steroids have been recommended for all forms of shock (endotoxic, hemorrhagic, anaphylactic), but again, the slow onset of action is disadvantageous. Absorption from subcut. and IM sites in animals in shock is slow, so that treatment should be given IV. Moreover, the high doses required render such treatment impractical and expensive in large animals. In shock, steroids diminish blood stasis and promote tissue perfusion.

When bacterial infection is the cause of an inflammatory reaction, steroids are commonly administered with appropriate antibacterial agents. They may be incorporated in intramammary products for use in bovine mastitis. They may reduce the local irritancy of such products, and their anti-inflammatory actions can shorten the period of clinical signs. However, they also are likely to suppress normal defense mechanisms in the mammary gland. In acute mastitis associated with endotoxemia, IV steroids help to suppress the circulatory and metabolic effects of endotoxins.

Disorders of the musculoskeletal system for which steroids have been used include traumatic arthritis and myositis, bursitis, tendonitis, eosinophilic myositis, osteoarthritis, and canine immune-mediated diseases such as rheumatoid arthritis. In the arthritides, transient relief is usually obtained, but the use of steroids may be contraindicated (*see* above) since they interfere with natural repair processes. Repeated injections or long-acting preparations may induce degenerative changes in cartilage (steroid arthropathy). In laminitis, treatment should be restricted to the first 24 hr of the syndrome. (Thereafter, steroids may hasten pedal bone rotation and perforation of the sole.)

Respiratory conditions, allergic and nonallergic, in which there is an inflammatory component, include acute respiratory distress syndrome in cattle and chronic obstructive pulmonary disease in horses. Both may be treated with steroids, but they are perhaps best reserved for life-threatening situations when high doses of water-soluble preparations may be given IV. Other indications include ulcerative colitis, autoimmune hemolytic anemia, and cerebral edema.

Because of the risks of serious side effects, it is worth reiterating the guidelines for steroid use: 1) Because of variations in patient response and disease severity, dosing schedules should be established individually. 2) Neither single large doses nor short-term therapy is likely to produce serious side effects. 3) The incidence and severity of toxicity increase with the duration of treatment. 4) Corticosteroid treatment is palliative and not curative. 5) The abrupt termination of dosing after a prolonged course of treatment may reveal a life-threatening degree of adrenal insufficiency. 6) The immunosuppressive actions of corticosteroids increase the risks of infection in the absence of antimicrobial therapy.

Contraindications: Glucocorticoids are direct antagonists to insulin; therefore, they exacerbate diabetes mellitus and should not be used in animals with this disease. Their use should be avoided in acute infections in view of their immunosuppressive actions and, when used in nonacute bacterial infection, bactericidal antibiotics should be used in preference to bacteriostats. In general, steroids are contraindicated in viral infections, in animals with corneal ulcers (because of their effects on wound healing), and in late pregnancy, when they may induce parturition. Intra-articular administration should not be done when: there is sepsis within or around the joint, there is intra-articular fracture, the articular cartilage is damaged, there are extensive degenerative bony lesions, previous injections have been ineffective, or there is a possibility that the joint will be over-exercised.

MISCELLANEOUS ANTI-INFLAMMATORY AGENTS

Hyaluronic Acid: Hyaluronic acid, a normal constituent of connective tissue matrix and synovial fluid, is a large-molecular-weight mucopolysaccharide produced by type A synoviocytes and chondrocytes; it accounts for the high viscosity and thixotropic properties of synovial fluid. In joint injury, synovial fluid viscosity decreases as the amount of hyaluronic acid present decreases, and depolymerization of the hyaluronic acid occurs. In articular cartilage, hyaluronic acid is linked to proteoglycan molecules to form the aggregated proteoglycan matrix that entraps water molecules. This confers on cartilage its protective biomechanical function. In the early stages of arthritis, articular cartilage degradation occurs with the loss of proteoglycans, hyaluronate, and later, collagen.

The roles of hyaluronic acid in normal joint function provide the basis for the local, intra-articular administration of sodium hyaluronate in degenerative joint diseases. The precise mode of action is unknown, but binding of hyaluronate to cartilage proteoglycans may slow cartilage degradation, and increased synovial fluid viscosity may be implicated. However, hyaluronate possesses other properties: it reduces leukocyte migration, inhibits lymphocyte activation, suppresses phagocytic activity, and reduces the permeability of synovial membranes.

Excellent clinical responses (although much of the evidence is based on anecdotal reports rather than on well-controlled trials) have been reported following the intra-articular injection of sodium hyaluronate in equine joint disease. Some forms of canine synovitis and arthritis, particularly those involving the shoulder joint, also have been treated with sodium hyaluronate; although there are no serious side effects, local swelling has been described in some horses.

Orgotein: This compound, a water-soluble metalloprotein that contains copper and zinc, occurs in all mammalian tissues and is almost devoid of toxicity. The precise mode of action is unknown. It does not possess analgesic, antipyretic, or immunosuppressant actions, but it does exhibit superoxide dismutase activity; therefore, it is a free radical scavenger. It combines with the superoxide radicals generated by phagocytosing polymorphs and released into the surrounding tissues to form hydrogen peroxide. Free radicals, such as superoxide, may act in several ways to produce tissue and joint damage, eg, they cause depolymerization of hyaluronic acid. Prevention of such depolymerization in synovial fluid and articular cartilage may constitute the mechanism of action of orgotein.

Orgotein has been used, principally in horses, in the treatment of joint, tendon, and soft-tissue injuries, including septic arthritis. Intra-articular injection is generally used. Transient side effects in ~5% of cases include increased lameness and swollen joint capsules. Soft-tissue injuries have been treated with deep IM injection.

Copper-containing Compounds: Copper deficiency can exacerbate some inflammatory conditions, and it has been suggested that normal levels of copper tend to suppress inflammation. Hypotheses that attempt to explain the anti-inflammatory actions of copper-containing compounds include direct free radical scavenging activity, induction of superoxide dismutase or ceruloplasmin, and reduced prostaglandin synthesis; however, the mode of action is unknown. Some products also contain known anti-inflammatory agents of other classes, eg, copper salicylate and copper phenylbutazone, and some products for topical application contain dimethyl sulfoxide.

Chondroprotective Agents: Two compounds with complex and unknown modes of action, but that have the property of slowing cartilage breakdown and promoting new cartilage synthesis, have been used as chondroprotective agents. Polysulfated glycosaminoglycan (PSGAG) has been used by intra-articular injection (and more recently IM) in the therapy of traumatic and degenerative (but not septic) arthritis in horses. The related compound, sodium pentosan polysulfate, has been used similarly by intra-articular injection in horses and also intra-articularly and IM in dogs.

PSGAG, a polymer based on repeating units of hexosamine and hexuronic acid, is extracted from bovine tracheal tissue. Its structure is similar to heparin and the aggregated proteoglycan molecules that form cartilage matrix. PSGAG and pentosan bind to cartilage, and exhibit particular affinity for osteoarthritic cartilage. Binding leads to reduced cartilage breakdown and increased synthesis of new matrix, but how these effects are achieved is unknown. A range of pharmacological effects for PSGAG has been clearly demonstrated. They include inhibition of clotting and complement cascades, reduced superoxide radical generation, delayed "de-differentiation" of chondrocytes in culture, protection of chondrocytes from steroid-enhanced death rates, increased hyaluronic acid synthesis and decreased breakdown, and inhibition of a wide range of lysosomal and non-lysosomal enzymes (including collagenase, cathepsins, and metalloproteinases). For example, concentrations of PSGAG achievable in equine joints following intra-articular injection of therepeutic doses inhibit stromelysin (proteoglycanase), an important enzyme that breaks down cartilage matrix by "disaggregating" the aggregated proteoglycan molecules. This would seem to provide a likely basis for the drug's therapeutic effects.

Side effects of chondroprotective agents seem to be minimal. High, but not therapeutic, doses inhibit clotting through heparin-like actions. Transient synovial effusion and arthralgia have been reported following intra-articular PSGAG in horses, and experimentally, PSGAG has potentiated a subinfective dose of *Staphylococcus aureus* in equine carpal joints. Chondroprotective agents are contraindicated in the presence of joint sepsis, but provided careful aseptic precautions are taken in their administration, the risk of joint infections should not be increased.

Disease-modifying Agents: In human rheumatoid arthritis, therapy in the early stages of the disease is based on one of the many NSAID available, but as the disease progresses, additional treatment with one of the so-called disease-modifying agents is instituted. These include gold salts (gold sodium thiomalate, aurothioglucose, auranofin), penicillamine, and the anti-malarial drugs chloroquine and hydroxychloroquine. These drugs have a number of properties in common: although several actions have been described (eg, gold salts are toxic to macrophages, immunosuppressive, and inhibitory to a number of enzymes; penicillamine has a stabilizing action on collagen), the mechanisms of actions are unknown; the onset of action is slow (in the case of gold salts favorable responses may not be seen until 5-6 mo after commencing therapy); and all are relatively toxic. These properties make the clinical use of the disease-modifying agents difficult and consequently uncommon. Nevertheless, gold has been used in canine rheumatoid arthritis; weekly IM injections of gold sodium thiomalate have been given for up to 16 wk.

Nonsteroidal Immunosuppressants: Another class of agents for which limited use has been found in immune-based joint diseases, such as immune-mediated canine arthritis, are the immunosuppressants. They include methotrexate, azathioprine, chlorambucil, 6-mercaptopurine, and cyclophosphamide. All are cytotoxic and must be used with care, although client acceptance of the risks of toxicity can permit a more aggressive approach than is generally possible in human patients. Therapy to induce remission usually involves combined treatment with an immunosuppressant and a steroid. Toxicity potential can be minimized by giving the immunosuppressant on alternate days, by periods of nontreatment, and by alternating the choice of drug for a given animal.

IMMUNOTHERAPY

The immunologic defenses of the body respond to antigen stimulation by production of antibodies and/or by activation of cell-mediated immunity. Administration of a specific antigen (as in a vaccine) may result in development of a specific immune response to the inducing antigen only. A nonspecific immunostimulant stimulates the immune system as a whole and either reduces immunosuppression or provokes a general increase in disease resistance. Although vaccines can provoke effective, and often specific, long-term immunity, nonspecific immunostimulation is of shorter duration and less effective, and probably is best used only for diseases in which it has proved to be beneficial.

SPECIFIC IMMUNOTHERAPY

ACTIVE IMMUNIZATION

Active immunization involves administration of antigen derived from an infectious agent so that an animal mounts a specific immune response and achieves resistance to that agent. Several criteria determine whether a vaccine should be used. First, the actual cause of the disease must be determined. Although this appears self-evident, it has not always been followed in practice; eg, in the bovine respiratory disease complex (BRD), although *Pasteurella haemolytica* can be isolated consistently at necropsy, these bacteria are not the sole cause of this syndrome. Second, it must be established that an appropriate immune response can protect against the disease in question. In some viral diseases, eg, equine infectious anemia, feline infectious peritonitis, and Aleutian disease in mink, an immune response is part of the disease, and vaccination may make it more severe. Finally, the risks of vaccination must not exceed those caused by the disease itself. The BRD complex also provides an example of this; experimental and epidemiological data show that *Pasteurella* vaccines that depend on antibody formation may increase, not reduce, the severity of lung disease. Also, unnecessary use of vaccines may complicate diagnosis based on serology and perhaps make final eradication of a disease impossible.

When vaccines are used to control disease in a population rather than in individuals, the concept of herd immunity must be considered. Herd immunity refers to increased resistance of a group because of the presence of some immune animals within the group, which reduces the probability of a susceptible animal countering an infected one. As a result, spread of infectious disease is slowed or blocked.

An ideal vaccine for active immunization should confer prolonged, strong immunity in both the vaccinated animal and its fetus. It should be free of adverse side effects, inexpensive, stable, adaptable to mass vaccination, and should stimulate an immune response distinguishable from that due to natural infection so that vaccination and eradication may proceed simultaneously.

Unfortunately, 2 of these requirements, high antigenicity and absence of adverse effects, tend to be incompatible. Live vaccines may stimulate a good immune response, but pose risks of residual virulence or contamination; inactivated vaccines are usually much safer but may be weaker immunogens.

Vaccines that contain killed organisms are safe with respect to residual virulence and contamination, and relatively easy to store. Some live vaccines may possess residual virulence, not only for the vaccinated animal but also for others, and may possibly revert to a fully virulent type and spread to unvaccinated animals. Live vaccines always run the risk of contamination with unwanted organisms, eg, outbreaks of reticuloendotheliosis in chickens in Japan and Australia have been traced to contaminated Marek's disease vaccines. It has been suggested, but not yet proved, that poultry adenovirus and canine parvovirus may have been distributed in contaminated vaccines, and bovine viral diarrhea virus may contaminate vaccines that contain cells of bovine origin. Finally, live vaccines require considerable care in their preparation, storage, and handling to avoid inactivating the organisms.

Because of these disadvantages, concern is growing about the long-term consequences of seeding the environment with modified-live organisms that may be able to become virulent, and a perceptible trend is toward use of inactivated products.

The disadvantages of inactivated vaccines correspond to the advantages of live vaccines. Thus, the use of adjuvants to increase effective antigenicity may cause local reactions, and multiple doses or high individual doses of antigen increase the risks of producing hypersensitivity and increasing costs.

INACTIVATION OF ORGANISMS USED IN VACCINES

Inactivated organisms should be as similar to living organisms as possible. Crude methods of killing, eg, heating, are usually unsatisfactory; if chemicals are used, it is essential that they produce little change in the antigens. This can be accomplished by destroying the nucleic acids of the agent while leaving the protein antigens intact. Compounds used in this way include formaldehyde, acetone, alcohol, ethylene oxide, ethyleneimine, acetylethyleneimine, and β-propiolactone. Photoinactivation using psoralens is an emerging technology.

Attenuation: Killed organisms are commonly much less immunogenic than living ones. As a compromise, the virulence of an organism can be reduced (attenuated) to the point that it is able to replicate, but is no longer pathogenic. Attenuation commonly involves adapting organisms to unusual conditions, or culturing in unfavorable media or at an unfavorable temperature. Bacteria can be rendered avirulent by culture under abnormal conditions, and viruses can be attenuated by growth in species to which they are not naturally adapted; eg, rinderpest virus was first attenuated by growth in goats, then further attenuated in rabbits, and finally, adapted to tissue culture to produce a safe vaccine. Other examples are adaptation of African horse sickness virus to mice and of canine distemper virus to ferrets.

An alternative method of virus attenuation is multiple passages in eggs, which has been done for canine distemper, bluetongue, and rabies vaccines. The most common method is prolonged tissue culture. Usually, cells from the species to be vaccinated are used to reduce the risk of side effects induced by the administration of foreign tissue. In these cases, virus attenuation may be accomplished by growing the organism in cells that it would not normally infect; eg, canine distemper virus normally infects lymphoid cells, but for attenuation the virus is repeatedly cultured in canine kidney cells.

The desired result of attenuation is development of a genetically stable avirulent agent. This may be difficult to achieve, and reversion to virulence is a serious risk. However, it has become increasingly possible to modify the genes of organisms so that they become irreversibly attenuated, eg, a swine pseudorabies vaccine is available in which the thymidine kinase gene has been removed from the virus. Herpesvirus requires thymidine kinase to replicate. Viruses from which this gene has been removed can infect neurons but cannot replicate and cause disease; this vaccine not only confers effective protection, but blocks cell invasion by virulent pseudorabies virus, and prevents development of a persistent carrier state. It is also possible to alter surface antigens so a virus induces an antibody response distinguishable from that caused by wild strains.

For some diseases, related organisms normally adapted to another species can impart immunity; eg, measles virus can protect dogs against distemper, and bovine viral diarrhea virus can protect against hog cholera.

Under some circumstances, fully virulent organisms can be used in vaccination procedures, eg, vaccination against contagious ecthyma (orf) of sheep. Lambs are vaccinated by rubbing dried, infected scab material into scratches made on the inner thigh, which produces local infection with no untoward effect on the lambs; they become solidly immune. Because the vaccinated animals may spread the disease, however, they must be separated from unvaccinated stock for a few weeks.

Subunit Vaccines: When the immunogenic portion of an organism can be identified positively, it can be used in a vaccine by itself. Thus, purified tetanus toxin, inactivated by treatment with formalin (tetanus toxoid) is used for active immunization against tetanus. The attachment pili of enteropathogenic *Escherichia coli* can be isolated and the purified pilus proteins incorporated into vaccines. The antipilus antibodies thus provoked protect animals by preventing bacterial attachment to the intestinal wall.

If quantities of purified antigen cannot be produced economically by fractionation, genetic material that codes for antigens can be isolated by recombinant DNA techniques. This DNA can then be placed in a bacterium, yeast, or other cell in which it codes for that protein. Gene cloning to prepare a veterinary vaccine began with genetic material taken from the foot-and-mouth disease virus. Gene coding for a major viral antigen was cloned into *E coli*; the bacteria synthesized the antigen that was then purified and used in a vaccine for cattle.

Another example of a subunit vaccine is one directed against the cloned β subunit of *E coli* enterotoxin. β subunits are immunogenic and function as effective toxoids. The β gene has been cloned, linked with a powerful promoter, and transfected into a nonpathogenic strain of *E coli*.

Recombinant DNA techniques are useful when protein antigens need to be synthesized in large, pure quantities. Unfortunately, such pure proteins are often poor protective antigens because they are not faithful copies of the native antigen or are not glycosylated properly. An alternative method is to clone the gene of interest into an attenuated living carrier organism such as vaccinia virus or *Salmonella* bacterium. Unfortunately, the use of attenuated carrier organisms has some intrinsic limitations and all the disadvantages of modified live vaccines.

Synthetic Peptides: Although antigens may be large, they usually possess only a small number of sites (epitopes) that are important in inducing protective immunity. If the structure of a protective antigen is known, its important epitopes may be identified, their structure analyzed and then artificially synthesized. These synthetic epitopes may then be used in a vaccine if they are large enough to be immunogenic.

ADMINISTRATION OF VACCINES

Subcut. or IM injection is the simplest and most common method; it is an excellent approach for relatively small numbers of animals, and for diseases in which systemic immunity is important. However, local immunity is sometimes more important than systemic immunity, and in these cases, it is more appropriate to administer the vaccine at the site of microbial invasion; eg, intranasal vaccines are effective in protecting cattle against infectious bovine rhinotracheitis, cats against feline rhinotracheitis and calicivirus infections, and poultry against infectious bronchitis and Newcastle disease. Unfortunately, these techniques require handling of each individual animal. Aerosolization of vaccines enables them to be inhaled by all the animals in a herd, an obvious advantage when the herd is large. This method is used to vaccinate mink against canine distemper and mink enteritis, and poultry against Newcastle disease. Alternatively, a vaccine may be administered in feed or drinking water; eg, erysipelas vaccination of pigs, and vaccination of poultry for Newcastle disease, infectious laryngotracheitis, and avian encephalomyelitis. Fish and shrimp may be vaccinated by adding antigen to the water in which they live.

Mixed Vaccines: Because of the complexity of many disease syndromes, it is common to use mixtures of organisms in single vaccines; eg, for bovine respiratory disease complex, combined vaccines are available for bovine respiratory syncytial virus, infectious bovine rhinotracheitis, bovine viral diarrhea, parainfluenza 3, and *Pasteurella haemolytica*. Such a mixture may be used to protect animals against several different agents with economy of effort, but it may be wasteful to use vaccines against organisms that are not causing problems.

Mixed vaccines that save considerable time and effort are also available for dogs and cats. Manufacturers recognize that when a mixture of different antigens is inoculated simultaneously, competition may occur between them, and modify their vaccine accordingly. Vaccines should never be mixed indiscriminately, since one component may dominate and interfere with responses to the other components.

Vaccination Schedules: Although it is impossible to give exact schedules for each vaccine, certain principles are common to all methods of active immunization. Since newborn animals may be passively protected by maternal antibodies, vaccination usually is not successful early in life. If stimulation of immunity is deemed necessary at this stage, the dam may be vaccinated during the later stages of pregnancy, the doses being timed so that peak antibody levels are reached at the time of colostrum formation. Successful active vaccination is usually possible only after passive immunity has waned. Since the exact time of maternal immunity loss cannot be predicted, young animals must be vaccinated at least twice to ensure successful immunization.

The interval between doses varies; some vaccines may require administration q6mo, whereas others, which produce a long-lasting immunity, may be given only once q2-3yr. The interval between doses is also determined by the disease. Some diseases are seasonal and vaccines may be given before expected disease outbreaks. Examples include lungworm vaccine given in early summer before lungworm season, anthrax vaccine given in spring, and *Clostridium chauvoei* vaccine given to sheep before turning them out to pasture. Because bluetongue of lambs is spread by midges *(Culicoides varipennis)* and thus is a disease of summer and early fall, vaccination in spring will protect during the susceptible period.

FAILURES IN VACCINATION

There are many reasons why a vaccine may fail. In some cases it may actually be ineffective, possibly because it contains the wrong strain of organisms or the wrong antigens. The method of manufacture may have destroyed the protective epitopes or there may simply be insufficient antigen. Such problems are relatively uncommon and generally can be avoided by using vaccines from reputable manufacturers. An effective vaccine may fail due to unsatisfactory administration;

eg, a live vaccine may be inactivated as a result of improper storage, use of antibiotics in conjunction with a live bacterial vaccine, chemical sterilization of syringes, or excessive use of alcohol on the skin. Administration by nonconventional routes may also affect efficacy. When vaccine is administered to poultry or mink by aerosol or in drinking water, the aerosol may not be evenly distributed throughout a building, or some animals may not drink adequate amounts. Also, chlorinated water may inactivate vaccine.

If an animal is incubating the disease before vaccination, the vaccine will not be protective; it is not possible to vaccinate against an already contracted disease.

The immune response, being a biological process, never confers absolute protection nor is equal in all members of a vaccinated population. Since the response is influenced by many factors, the range in a random population tends to follow a normal distribution: the response of most animals will be "average", a few will be excellent, and a small portion will be poor. Those with a poor response may not be protected by an effective vaccine; it is difficult to protect 100% of a random population by vaccination. The size of this unresponsive population varies among vaccines, and its significance depends on the nature of the disease. For highly infectious diseases in which herd immunity is poor and infection is rapidly and efficiently transmitted, eg, foot-and-mouth disease, the presence of unprotected animals can permit the spread of disease and disrupt control programs. Problems also can arise if the unprotected animals are individually important, as in the case of companion animals or breeding stock. In contrast, for diseases that are inefficiently spread, eg, rabies, 60-70% protection in a population may be sufficient to effectively block disease transmission within that population and therefore may be satisfactory from a public health perspective.

The most important cause of vaccine failure is the presence of passively derived maternal antibodies in young animals. Vaccine failures also can occur when the immune response is suppressed, eg, heavily parasitized or malnourished animals may be immunosuppressed and should not be vaccinated. Stress, including pregnancy, extremes of cold and heat, and fatigue or malnourishment may reduce a normal immune response, probably due to increased glucocorticoid production.

ADVERSE CONSEQUENCES OF VACCINATION

The more common risks associated with vaccines include residual virulence and toxicity, contamination with other pathogens, allergic responses, disease in immunodeficient hosts (modified live vaccines), neurological complications, and harmful effects on the fetus. For example, lesions of mucosal disease may be seen in calves vaccinated against bovine viral diarrhea. Vaccines that contain killed gram-negative organisms may also contain endotoxins, which stimulate release of interleukin 1, and can cause stress with pyrexia and leukopenia. Although such a reaction is usually only a temporary inconvenience to males, it may be sufficient to provoke abortion in females. In general, it is prudent to avoid vaccinating pregnant animals unless the risks of not vaccinating are greater. Bluetongue vaccine has been reported to cause congenital anomalies when given to pregnant ewes. The stress from a vaccination reaction may be sufficient to activate latent infections, eg, activation of equine herpesvirus has been demonstrated following vaccination against African horse sickness. One other adverse reaction is the "sting" that occurs when some vaccines are administered. This can cause problems for the vaccinator if the vaccinated animal objects strenuously. Some vaccines cause mild immunosuppression, eg, modified live parvovirus vaccines may suppress the immune response in puppies to the point that they succumb to distemper when vaccinated with modified live distemper virus.

In addition to potential virulence or toxicity, vaccines, like any antigen, may provoke hypersensitivity reactions. For example, type I hypersensitivity may occur in response to any of the antigens found in vaccines, including those from eggs or tissue culture cells. All forms of hypersensitivity are more commonly associated with multiple injections of antigen; therefore, they tend to be associated with use of inactivated products. Type III hypersensitivity reactions are also potential hazards of vaccination. These may cause an intense local inflammatory reaction or a generalized vascular disturbance such as purpura. An example of a type III reaction is clouding of the cornea in dogs vaccinated against infectious canine hepatitis. Type IV hypersensitivity reactions expressed as granuloma formation may occur at the site of inoculation in response to the use of depot adjuvants.

Amyloidosis is a problem seen in horses used for antiserum production, although it usually does not result from normal vaccination procedures. It is associated with excessive stimulation of interleukin 1 production.

PRODUCTION, PRESENTATION, AND CONTROL OF VACCINES

In most countries, the production of veterinary biologicals is regulated by government authorities. In general, regulatory authorities have the right to license establishments that produce vaccines and to inspect those premises to ensure that the facilities and the methods employed are satisfactory. All vaccines are checked for safety and potency. Safety tests include confirmation of the identity of the organism used and of the freedom of the vaccine from extraneous organisms as well as tests for toxicity. Because the living organisms found in vaccines normally die over time, it is necessary to ensure that they will be effective even after storage. Although properly stored vaccines may still be potent after the expiration of their designated shelf life, this should never be assumed; expired vaccines should not be used.

PASSIVE IMMUNIZATION

Passive immunization involves the production of antibodies in one animal by active immunization and transfer of these antibodies to susceptible animals to confer immediate protection. The transfer of maternal antibody to offspring via the placenta or colostrum is the natural (and very important) form of passive immunization. Antisera may be produced in cattle against anthrax, in dogs against distemper, and in cats against panleukopenia. Their most important role is in protection against toxigenic organisms, eg, *Clostridium tetani* or *C perfringens*. Such antisera are known as immune globulins and are generally produced in young horses by a series of immunizing inoculations.

To check the potency of preparations of immune globulin, comparison is made with an international biological standard. An International Unit (IU) of tetanus immune globulin is the specific neutralizing activity contained in 0.03384 mg of the international standard. The US Standard Unit (AU) is twice the IU.

Tetanus immune globulin (tetanus antitoxin) is given to animals to confer immediate protection against tetanus. At least 1500-3000 IU of immune globulin should be given to horses and cattle; at least 500 IU to calves, sheep, goats, and pigs; and at least 250 IU to dogs. The exact amount varies with the amount of tissue damage, degree of wound contamination, and time elapsed since injury. Tetanus immune globulin is of little use once clinical signs appear, although massive doses of up to 300,000 IU may help.

To reduce their antigenicity for other species, immune globulins of horse origin are usually treated with pepsin.

Monoclonal Antibodies: Antibodies produced by the normal immune response are derived from many different plasma cells. As a result, although they will combine with a specific antigen, they are a heterogeneous mixture. Homogeneous antibodies can be generated through the use of cell lines called hybridomas; these, called monoclonal antibodies, represent an alternative source of passive protection. Currently, however, these are mainly made by mouse hybridomas and thus consist of mouse antibodies, and may sensitize other animal species. Nevertheless, mouse monoclonal antibodies against the K99 pilus antigens of *E coli* can be given PO to calves to protect them against diarrhea caused by this organism.

Monoclonal antibodies also are used in diagnosis. Because they are homogeneous and specific, they have the ability to differentiate between closely related infectious agents in a manner that is impossible with conventional antibodies, eg, they can differentiate between the rabies viruses obtained from skunks, bats, or dogs.

NONSPECIFIC IMMUNOTHERAPY

In many situations, it is desirable to enhance the activity of an animal's immune system; this may include stimulation of the normal immune response to enhance protection, and treatment of immunosuppressive conditions. The several different types of immunopotentiators vary according to their origin, mode of action, and use.

Adjuvants: Materials that enhance an immune response when administered with an antigen are called adjuvants. The simplest are those that function by slowing the release of antigen into the body and thereby prolong the immune response. Some antigen/adjuvant mixtures form depots from which the antigen is slowly released; examples of depot-forming adjuvants include aluminum hydroxide, aluminum phosphate, and potassium aluminum sulfate (alum). The antigen is adsorbed onto the salt crystals before inoculation. Upon injection, the salt/antigen mixture forms a small nodule in the tissues that slowly leaks antigen into the body and provides a prolonged antigenic stimulus. Antigens that normally persist for only a few days may be retained in the body for several weeks by this technique. Depot adjuvants enhance only the primary immune response and have little effect on secondary reactions. Other slow-release adjuvants include beryllium sulfate, silica, kaolin, and carbon. Although many other adjuvants have been administered experimentally, few have been accepted for use in domestic animals. Recently, several new adjuvants have been licensed for use in animal vaccines; most are unidentified because the products are proprietary.

Immunostimulants: In contrast to adjuvants, immunostimulants need not be administered together with antigen to enhance immunity. They are generally given to induce a nonantigen-specific enhancement of the immune system. They appear to be most useful when treating chronic diseases in which there is good evidence of immunosuppression. They are used in the therapy of equine sarcoid, of chronic skin diseases such as staphylococcal pyoderma or demodicosis, and in immunosuppressive viral diseases such as feline leukemia.

Many bacteria have been employed as immunostimulants. The most potent of these is BCG, the live attenuated vaccine strain of *Mycobacterium bovis.* BCG produces a generalized enhancement of both B- and T-cell-mediated responses, and of phagocytosis, graft rejection, and resistance to infection. Because BCG causes tuberculin sensitivity, these organisms must be fractionated to remove the reactive material. Thus, mycobacterial cell wall fractions, muramyl dipeptide (MDP), and trehalose dimycolate have all been used as immunostimulants. MDP, the most potent factor from mycobacteria, enhances antibody production and stimulates and activates macrophages.

Another organism, *Propionibacterium acnes,* also promotes a generalized enhancement of nonspecific immunity. The cell wall of this organism contains MDP and lipid compounds that are immunostimulatory. Administered into the circulatory system, this material has a complex activity since it stimulates: 1) phagocytosis by macrophages and neutrophils; 2) increased activity of natural killer cells; 3) development of T and B lymphocytes; and 4) increased production of interleukin 1, interferons, and tumor necrosis factor. *Propionibacterium acnes* also increases resistance to infection by many pathogenic bacteria and viruses. It is used in therapy of dogs with pyoderma and horses with respiratory disease.

Endotoxins from gram-negative bacteria enhance antibody formation if given at about the same time as the antigen. They have a general immunostimulatory activity reflected in a nonspecific resistance to bacterial infections. Endotoxins may also enhance immune reactivity by promoting release of interferons from cells. Crude bacterial mixtures have been used to stimulate immunity to tumors in animals.

Certain complex carbohydrates, eg, zymosan, glucan, dextran sulfate, and lentinans, are immunostimulants and can activate macrophages.

Other immunostimulants may be derived from natural mediators of the immune system. Some thymic hormones have significant stimulatory effects on the immune system. Very low doses of interferons may be useful in treating retrovirus-induced immunosuppression such as occurs in feline leukemia.

One drug that may stimulate the immune system is levamisole. A broad-spectrum anthelmintic, levamisole functions in a manner similar to the thymic hormone thymopoietin, ie, it stimulates T-cell differentiation and response to antigens. Thus, it enhances bovine lymphocyte blastogenesis and interferon production, and increases phagocytic activity in macrophages and neutrophils. It probably also enhances cell-mediated cytotoxicity, lymphokine production, and suppressor cell function. The effects of levamisole are greatest in animals with depressed T-cell function, and it has little or no effect on the immune system of normal animals; therefore it may help in the treatment of chronic infections and neoplastic diseases, but may exacerbate disease caused by excessive T-cell function.

ANTINEOPLASTIC CHEMOTHERAPEUTIC AGENTS

The fundamental biochemical differences between cancer cells and normal cells are not well understood. None of the empirically developed antineoplastic drugs appears to act on a process or component that is unique to cancer cells. Clinically useful drugs achieve a degree of selectivity on the basis of certain characteristics of cancer calls that can be used as pharmacological targets. These characteristics include: rapid rate of malignant cell division and growth, variations in the rate of drug uptake or in the sensitivity of different types of cells to particular drugs, and retention in the malignant cells of hormonal responses characteristic of the cells from which the cancer is derived, eg, responsiveness of certain breast carcinomas.

Aspects of normal cell growth and the cell cycle provide the rationale for antineoplastic chemotherapy. In particular, the S phase, in which DNA synthesis occurs; the M phase, beginning with mitosis and ending with cytokinesis; and the G_0 phase, a dormant or nonproliferative phase of the cell cycle, are of major importance in the successful application of antineoplastic chemotherapy. Tumor doubling time is related to the length of the cell cycle and the portion of cells undergoing cell division. Antineoplastic agents can be classified according to a number of schemes relative to effects at different stages of the cell cycle. In the simplest sense, cycle nonspecific agents are considered to be lethal to cells in all phases of the cell cycle. Cells are killed exponentially with increasing drug levels, and the dose-response curves follow first order kinetics. Phase-specific agents exert their lethal effects exclusively or primarily during one phase of the cell cycle, usually S or M. The greater the rate of cell division, the more effective are these drugs. The G_0 phase of the cell cycle is important, not as a target for chemotherapeutic agents, but as a sanctuary in which dormant tumor cells can escape the effects of drug therapy.

GENERAL CLINICAL CONSIDERATIONS

The decision to utilize antineoplastic chemotherapy depends on the type of tumor to be treated, the stage of malignancy, and the condition of the animal. Chemotherapy can be used as an adjuvant to surgery and irradiation and can be administered immediately after or before the primary treatment. Adjuvant therapy administered before surgery or irradiation is termed neo-adjuvant therapy and is intended to improve the effectiveness of the primary therapy by possibly decreasing tumor size, stage of malignancy, or presence of micrometastatic lesions. Responses to cancer chemotherapy can range from palliation (remission of secondary signs, generally without increase in survival time) to complete remission (in which clinically detectable tumor cells and all signs of malignancy are absent). The percentage and duration of complete remissions are criteria for the successfulness of a particular chemotherapeutic protocol.

Effective clinical use of antineoplastic drugs depends on the ability to balance the killing of tumor cells against the inherent toxicity of many of these drugs to host cells. Because of their narrow therapeutic indices, dosages for antineoplastics are frequently calculated based on body surface area (see p 48) rather than body mass. Antineoplastic agents are commonly administered in various combinations referred to as protocols. One advantage of combination therapy is enhanced destruction of tumor cells when drugs with different target sites or mechanisms of action are used. If the side effects of the component agents are different, the combination may be no more toxic than the individual agents given separately. Combinations that include a cycle-nonspecific drug administered first, followed by a phase-specific drug, may offer the advantage that cells surviving the first drug are provoked into mitosis and are therefore more susceptible to the second drug. Another advantage of combination therapy is the decreased possibility of development of drug resistance.

Special considerations associated with administration of antineoplastic drugs include evaluation of the quality of life provided to the animal, medical and nutritional support, control of pain, and psychological comfort for the owner. Many owners who choose to treat neoplasia in their pets have experienced cancer themselves or have been involved with individuals or family members who have had cancer. Discussion of neoplasia in pets therefore must be handled tactfully and provide the owners with appropriate information for decision-making.

RESISTANCE TO ANTINEOPLASTIC CHEMOTHERAPY

Failure to respond, or resistance, can occur for several reasons. Pharmacokinetic resistance occurs when the concentration of a drug in the target cell is below that required to kill the cell. This may be due to altered rates of drug absorption, distribution, biotransformation, or excretion. In addition, marginal blood flow to a tumor may result in poor drug delivery that causes inadequate concentrations and creation of a population of quiescent, less susceptible cells. Cytokinetic resistance occurs when complete eradication of the tumor cell population is not accomplished; this may occur as a result of dormant tumor cells, dose-limiting host toxicity associated with drug therapy, and the inability to achieve a 100% tumor-cell kill rate even at therapeutic drug dosages. An additional cause of tumor-cell resistance can be attributed to biochemical mechanisms developed within the tumor cell that: 1) block transport mechanisms for drug uptake, 2) alter target receptors or enzymes critical to drug action, 3) increase concentrations of normal metabolites antagonized by the antineoplastic drug, or 4) cause genetic changes that result in protective gene amplification or altered patterns of DNA repair.

PATTERNS OF TOXICITY

Antineoplastic agents that act primarily on rapidly dividing and growing cells produce several common patterns of toxicity including bone marrow suppression, GI complications, and immune suppression. Bone marrow suppression can be particularly life-threatening due to increased incidence of infection associated with leukopenia, increased risk of hemorrhage associated with thrombocytopenia, and anemia. GI complications can include nausea and vomiting, ulcerative enteritis, stomatitis, and diarrhea. Additional toxicities associated with antineoplastic drug therapy may include inhibition of spermatogenesis, teratogenesis, carcinogenesis, alopecia, and tissue necrosis due to extravasation of certain drugs.

ANTINEOPLASTIC AGENTS

Chemotherapeutic antineoplastic agents can be grouped by biochemical mechanism of action into the following general categories: alkylating agents, antimetabolites, vinca alkaloids, antineoplastic antibiotics, hormonal agents, and miscellaneous agents. Each category is discussed below, with specific examples of clinically relevant veterinary drugs.

Alkylating Agents: These form highly reactive intermediate compounds that are able to transfer alkyl groups to DNA. Monofunctional alkylating agents transfer a single alkyl group and usually result in miscoding of DNA, strand breakage, or depurination. These reactions can result in cell death, mutagenesis, or carcinogenesis. Polyfunctional alkylators typically cause DNA strand crosslinking and inhibition of mitosis with consequent cell death. Resistance to one alkylating agent often implies resistance to other similar drugs and can be caused by increased production of nucleophilic substances that compete with target DNA for alkylation. Decreased permeation of alkylating agents and increased activity of DNA repair systems are also considered common mechanisms of resistance.

Individual alkylating agents are generally cell-cycle nonspecific and can be subgrouped according to chemical structure into nitrogen mustards, ethylenimines, alkyl sulfonates, nitrosoureas, and triazene derivatives. The most common subgroup used in veterinary medicine is the nitrogen mustard group. Mechlorethamine hydrochloride is the prototype of the nitrogen mustards and has been used to treat Hodgkin's disease in man, mycosis fungoides, lymphoreticular neoplasia, and pleural and peritoneal effusions. Because of the highly unstable nature of mechlorethamine and its extremely short duration of action, it is not widely used in veterinary medicine. Derivatives of mechlorethamine that are commonly used include cyclophosphamide, chlorambucil, and less frequently, melphalan.

Cyclophosphamide is a cyclic phosphamide derivative of mechlorethamine that requires metabolic activation by the cytochrome P_{450} oxidation system in the liver. Given PO or IV, dose-limiting leukopenia associated with bone marrow suppression is the primary toxicity. Sterile hemorrhagic cystitis caused by acrolein, a metabolite of cyclophosphamide, can occur and should be treated by active diuresis and intravesicular administration of N-acetylcysteine. Nausea, vomiting, and alopecia may also be observed with use of cyclophosphamide. This drug is used to treat hemolymphatic neoplasms, sarcomas, lung and mammary carcinomas, other carcinomas, and multiple myeloma.

The slowest acting nitrogen mustard, chlorambucil, achieves effects gradually and often can be used in animals with compromised bone marrow. It can cause bone marrow suppression, but this is usually late in onset and rapidly reversible. This drug is given PO and is most commonly used in treatment of chronic well-differentiated lymphocytic leukemias, macroglobulinemias, mycosis fungoides, and polycythemia vera; it is considered ineffective in rapidly proliferating tumors.

Melphalan, a 1-phenylalanine derivative of mechlorethamine, is given PO or IV and used to treat multiple myeloma and, infrequently, ovarian and mammary carcinomas, lymphoreticular neoplasia, and lung tumors.

One alkylating agent, triethylenethiophosphoramide, is used to treat carcinomas of the mammary gland, lungs, GI tract, head and neck, prostate, kidneys, liver, biliary tract, and pancreas. It may also be used intravesicularly in the treatment of transitional cell carcinoma of the bladder. Busulfan, an alkyl sulfonate, is used specifically in the treatment of chronic myelocytic leukemia. Leukopenia is common and may be severe; additional side effects may include diarrhea, pulmonary fibrosis, and an increased frequency of leukemia. Streptozotocin, a naturally occurring nitrosourea, is used to treat malignant pancreatic islet-cell tumors or insulinomas. Nephrotoxicity and hepatotoxicity may be seen.

Antimetabolites: Antimetabolites resemble normal cellular metabolites and so can subvert normal metabolic pathways in a toxic manner. Three subgroups of antimetabolites, folic acid, and pyrimidine and purine analogs, are used in veterinary medicine.

The prototype folic acid analog is methotrexate, an inhibitor of dihydrofolate reductase (DHFR), the enzyme that catalyzes conversion of folic acid to tetrahydrofolate. Tetrahydrofolate deficiency blocks reactions requiring folate coenzymes and so disrupts both DNA and RNA synthesis. Methotrexate is an S-phase specific drug that must be actively transported across cell membranes and can be given PO, IV, IM, or intrathecally if required for treatment of CNS neoplasia. The drug is excreted in the urine and at high doses may precipitate in renal tubules. Side effects may include leukopenia, nausea, vomiting, alopecia, delayed hepatotoxicity, and pulmonary infiltrates. Folinic acid can be used to bypass the metabolic blockade produced by folic acid analogs and thus result in rescue of treated cells. Since tumor cells appear less efficient at transport of folinic acid, some degree of selectivity is achieved in the rescue. Resistance to methotrexate may develop due to impaired transport of the drug into cells, production of altered forms of DHFR, or increased concentrations of DHFR. Methotrexate is used to treat lymphoreticular neoplasia, myeloproliferative disorders, metastatic transmissible venereal and Sertoli cell tumors, and has been tried at high doses in the treatment of osteosarcoma.

Two pyrimidine analogs, 5-fluorouracil and cytarabine, are commonly used in veterinary medicine. 5-Fluorouracil must be converted to an active 5-fluoro-2'-deoxyuridine-5'-phosphate form (F-dUMP) to bind the enzyme thymidylate synthetase and block or inhibit DNA and RNA synthesis. This drug is considered S-phase specific and is used IV but is also available for topical use. Metabolism is via the liver and the drug readily enters CSF. Acute side effects include nausea, vomiting and diarrhea, with delayed GI and oral ulceration and bone marrow suppression possible. Occasional CNS reactions have been reported in dogs, and severe irreversible neurotoxicity and sudden death have been described in cats. Although thought to be effective in treatment of squamous cell carcinoma in cats, toxicity appears to preclude its use in this species. Resistance may develop by decreased activation of the drug or acquisition of altered thymidylate synthetase that is not inhibited. 5-Fluorouracil is used to treat GI, liver, skin, and mammary carcinomas, and solar keratoses.

Cytarabine (cytosine arabinoside) is an analog of 2'-deoxycytidine and must be activated by conversion to a 5'-monophosphate nucleotide. The nucleotide analog, AraCTP, causes inhibition of DNA synthesis by substitution of arabinose for deoxyribose in the sugar moiety of DNA; cytarabine may also inhibit DNA repair enzymes. This drug is S-phase specific, and its effectiveness is directly proportional to exposure of cells to the drug; continuous infusion or repeated injections are usually required. The most common toxicity is leukopenia with megaloblastic changes. Nausea, vomiting, and diarrhea may occur acutely, while GI disturbances, stomatitis, alopecia, and hepatotoxicity can be seen as delayed side effects. Inhibition of conversion to AraCTP or increased degradation of AraCTP can account for development of resistance. Cytarabine is used to treat lymphoreticular neoplasia, myeloproliferative disease, and CNS lymphoma.

Two purine analogs, 6-mercaptopurine (6-MP) and 6-thioguanine (6-TG), have been used occasionally in veterinary medicine. 6-Mercaptopurine is a sulfhydryl-substituted analog of hypoxanthine that must be converted to an active 6-thioinosine-5'-phosphate (T-IMP) form by hypoxanthine-guanine phosphoribosyltransferase (HGPRT). The active drug inhibits purine nucleotide synthesis and metabolism and thus disrupts DNA and RNA synthesis and function. This S-phase specific drug can be administered PO or IV and undergoes rapid metabolic degradation and some renal excretion. Bone marrow suppression is gradual and infrequent with 6-MP; acute GI disturbances are also infrequent but do occur. Resistance may develop by diminished activation of the drug by HGPRT. 6-MP is used to maintain remission in acute lymphocytic leukemia and has been used to treat granulocytic leukemia.

6-TG is a sulfhydryl-substituted analog of guanine and, like 6-MP, is converted by HGPRT to an active form capable of altering purine nucleotide synthesis and metabolism and DNA and RNA synthesis and function. This is also an S-phase specific drug. 6-TG is given PO and has side effects and mechanisms of resistance similar to 6-MP except that leukopenia may be more severe and GI disturbances less common. This drug is used to treat acute lymphocytic and granulocytic leukemia.

Vinca Alkaloids: These are large and complex molecules derived from the periwinkle plant. Binding to tubulin, the major component of cellular microtubules, accounts for the antineoplastic effects of these drugs. As a result of tubulin binding, the mitotic spindle apparatus is disrupted and segregation of chromosomes in metaphase is arrested. These effects account for the primary M-phase action of these drugs, although other anti-tubulin effects related to cytoskeletal maintenance and protein trafficking may occur.

The 2 drugs of importance in this class are vincristine and vinblastine. Both are given IV, and both cause severe local vesication if injected perivascularly; serious complications include deep, indolent ulceration exposing underlying tendons and bone. The vinca alkaloids are metabolized primarily in the liver but may be partially excreted in an unchanged form in the urine. Although related structurally, resistance to one vinca alkaloid does not imply resistance to all drugs in this category. Vincristine use is limited by neurologic toxicity that may include a slowly reversible sensorimotor peripheral neuropathy and muscle weakness. Constipation and alopecia may also occur. In comparison, the dose-limiting toxicity associated with vinblastine use is related to bone marrow suppression and leukopenia, with neurologic toxicity occurring only at high doses. Mild nausea and vomiting may also be observed with vinblastine use. Vincristine is used to treat a variety of lymphoreticular neoplasms, carcinomas, sarcomas, and transmissible venereal tumors. Vinblastine is likewise used to treat lymphoreticular neoplasia and some carcinomas.

Antineoplastic Antibiotics: The antineoplastic antibiotics are products of *Streptomyces*. The important veterinary drugs in this group include actinomycin D (dactinomycin), doxorubicin, and bleomycin. Additional drugs less commonly used in veterinary medicine include daunorubicin, mithramycin, and mitomycin.

Actinomycin A was the first *Streptomyces* antibiotic isolated and was followed by related antibiotics including actinomycin D. Actinomycin D binds with double-stranded DNA and blocks the action of RNA polymerase, thus preventing DNA transcription. This drug is considered cell-cycle nonspecific and is given IV. Nausea, vomiting, and phlebitis are indications of acute toxicity, while bone marrow suppression, in particular leukopenia, may be the most common delayed side effect. Alopecia and stomatitis may also occur. Resistance to actinomycin D may develop due to decreased cellular uptake of the drug. This drug is used to treat lymphoreticular neoplasms, methotrexate-resistant choriocarcinoma, testicular carcinoma, and rhabdomyosarcoma.

The anthracycline antibiotics, daunorubicin and doxorubicin, have become important newer antineoplastic antibiotics. Both intercalate and bind to DNA between base pairs on adjacent strands, which causes an uncoiling of the DNA helix. Uncoiling destroys the DNA template and inhibits RNA and DNA polymerases. Scission of DNA is thought to be mediated by either the enzyme topoisomerase II or by generation of free radicals. Intracellular interactions of anthracycline antibiotics result in the formation of semiquinone radical intermediates capable of generating hydrogen peroxide and hydroxyl radicals. Considered cell-cycle nonspecific because of the damage associated with radical formation, these drugs probably have their maximum effect during the S phase of the cell cycle. Given IV, the anthracycline antibiotics are severe vesicants if administered perivascularly and may cause a serious, delayed phlebitis. Urticaria may be seen in the area of anthracycline injection; shortly after administration, erythematous areas may appear along the vein. Recurrence of this response may be prevented by premedication with corticosteroids and antihistamines. The anthracycline antibiotics are metabolized in the liver to a variety of less active and inactive products.

Doxorubicin toxicity can be manifested in a variety of acute and delayed reactions. Acute toxicities include nausea, vomiting, transient ECG changes, arrhythmias, and even cardiovascular collapse. Generalized erythema, head-shaking, and urticaria have been described in dogs. Red urine not associated with hematuria may also occur. Delayed toxicities can be severe, the major problem being cardiac toxicity associated with binding of drug to cardiac DNA and free radical damage to myocardial membranes. A nonspecific decrease in cardiac fibrils occurs, which leads to digitalis-unresponsive congestive heart failure. Cardiac toxicity can occur weeks to months following treatment and appears to be dose-related. In addition to cardiac toxicity, bone marrow suppression with leukopenia and thrombocytopenia, vomiting, stomatitis, and alopecia may occur. Doxorubicin is used widely in the treatment of many tumors, including soft-tissue and bone sarcomas, lymphoreticular neoplasms, and various carcinomas. If doxorubicin is used in conjunction with radiation therapy, damage by radiation may be augmented. This radiation recall effect may necessitate reduction in radiation and/or drug dosages. Because of the significant toxicity associated with the use of doxorubicin, newer generation drugs specifically aimed at reduction of cardiac toxicity have become available in human medicine; 2 of these, idarubicin and epirubicin, may become useful in veterinary medicine.

Bleomycin represents another group of antineoplastic antibiotics relevant to veterinary medicine. The drug designated bleomycin is actually a mixture of bleomycin glycopeptides that differ only in their terminal amine moiety. The cytotoxic action of these glycopeptides depends on their ability to cause chain scission and fragmentation of DNA molecules. Cells accumulate in the G_2 phase of the cell cycle, which accounts for the designation of this drug as a G_2- and M-phase specific agent. Bleomycin may also affect DNA repair enzymes. Given IV or subcut., a large portion of the drug is excreted via the kidneys. Acute side effects include nausea, vomiting, fever, and allergic reactions including anaphylaxis. Bleomycin has minimal myelosuppressive and immunosuppressive activities but does have an unusual delayed pulmonary toxicity, which may begin as a nonspecific pneumonitis that progresses to pulmonary fibrosis. Dangers from pulmonary complications are especially important in older animals with preexisting pulmonary disease. Mucocutaneous reactions including alopecia, stomatitis, hyperpigmentation, and skin ulceration may also be seen as delayed toxicity syndromes. Bleomycin may be used to treat testicular tumors, squamous cell carcinoma, lymphoma, and seminoma.

Hormonal Agents: Hormonal therapy for neoplasia in veterinary medicine commonly involves the use of glucocorticoids. Direct anti-tumor effects are related to their lympholytic properties; these drugs can inhibit mitosis, RNA synthesis, and protein synthesis in sensitive lymphocytes. Glucocorticoids are considered cell-cycle nonspecific and are often used in chemotherapeutic protocols following induction by another agent. Unfortunately, resistance to a given glocorcorticoid may develop rapidly and typically extends to other glucocorticoids. Toxic effects of glucocorticoid therapy can include peptic ulceration, glucose intolerance, polydipsia/polyuria, immunosuppression, necrotizing pancreatitis, osteoporosis, hypokalemia, cataracts, muscle atrophy, and Cushing's disease. Indirect benefits of glucocorticoid therapy in cancer include symptomatic improvements in appetite and attitude, suppression of noninfectious fevers, management of hypercalcemia of malignancy, and relief of edema associated with spinal cord and brain tumors.

Prednisone and prednisolone are commonly used to treat lymphoreticular neoplasms in combination with other chemotherapeutic agents. Dexamethasone, prednisone, and prednisolone are especially useful in treatment of leukemias and lymphomas of the CNS since they readily enter the CSF.

Other steroid hormones utilized in veterinary cancer therapy include estrogenic treatment of prostatic hyperplasia, perianal glandular neoplasms, and palliation of advanced prostatic carcinoma. Complications of estrogen therapy can include thrombocytopenia, feminization, fluid retention, and life-threatening bone marrow suppression and aplastic anemia. Anti-estrogen therapy with drugs such as tamoxifen citrate may also be utilized in estrogen-receptor-positive mammary carcinomas to block growth-stimulatory hormonal activities in these cells. In addition, anti-estrogens have been used in the treatment of endometrial carcinomas.

Progestins have been used to oppose growth stimulatory effects of hormones in endometrial, prostatic, breast, renal cell, and ovarian carcinomas. Toxic side effects of the progestins can include fluid retention, hypercalcemia, thromboembolism, and cholestatic jaundice.

Androgens have been used in the treatment of breast carcinoma but are not commonly used in veterinary medicine. Anti-androgens, such as flutamide and cyproterone acetate, have been used experimentally in the treatment of prostatic and perianal neoplasia.

Miscellaneous Antineoplastic Agents: Three drugs commonly used as antineoplastics in veterinary medicine that do not fall into any of the categories mentioned above include L-asparaginase, cisplatin, and mitotane (o,p'DDD).

L-asparaginase is an enzyme derived from *Escherichia coli* that catalyzes hydrolysis of asparagine. Because some tumor cells are unable to produce asparagine, treatment with this drug deprives these cells of exogenously supplied asparagine and ultimately limits protein synthesis. Since protein synthesis is active in the G_1 phase of the cell cycle, L-asparaginase is considered to be a G_1-phase specific drug. L-asparaginase may be given IV, subcut., IM, and by intraperitoneal injection. Acute toxic effects include nausea, vomiting, abdominal pain, and hypersensitivity reactions. Anaphylaxis on repeated administration may occur as a result of host anti-asparaginase antibody production; pre-treatment of animals with antihistamine helps preclude this acute toxic reaction. Anti-asparaginase antibody production may also account for the development of tumor resistance, as can a decreased tumor cell requirement for asparagine. Delayed side effects of L-asparaginase therapy generally do not include bone marrow suppression or GI effects, but can involve hepatic and renal toxicity, pancreatitis, CNS effects, and alterations in clotting mechanisms. L-asparaginase is commonly used to treat lymphoreticular neoplasms.

Cisplatin functions primarily as a bifunctional alkylator and has an unusual structure. It (cis-diamine-dichloroplatinum) is a platinum ion complexed to 2 chloride ions and 2 ammonium molecules. This drug causes inter- and intrastrand DNA crosslinking that disrupts DNA helices and prevents DNA synthesis. Cisplatin is cell-cycle nonspecific and is administered by IV drip in combination with fluids and mannitol to promote diuresis. Excretion of the drug is prolonged, with a half-life of up to 5 days. Acute toxic responses to cisplatin can include intense nausea and vomiting and anaphylaxis. Extreme, dose-limiting, proximal tubular renal necrosis is the most serious delayed side effect. Other responses may include ototoxicity, mild to moderate bone marrow suppression, peripheral neuropathy, and renal potassium and magnesium wasting. In veterinary medicine, cisplatin has been used in the treatment of osteosarcoma and for management of transitional cell carcinoma. Because of the extreme toxic side effects of cisplatin, newer generation derivatives such as carboplatin and iproplatin have been developed and may become useful in veterinary medicine.

Mitotane (o,p,'DDD), a derivative of the insecticides DDT and DDD, causes selective destruction of normal neoplastic adrenal cortical cells. It may act by inhibiting adrenocorticotropic-hormone-induced steroid production, which causes atrophy of the inner zones of the adrenal cortex. Mitotane is administered PO with plasma concentrations detectable for several weeks. In man, as much as 60% of an oral dose may be excreted in the feces. Nausea and vomiting are the major side effects with little observed toxicity in the kidneys, liver, or bone marrow. Delayed toxicities may include somnolence, dermatitis, and hemorrhagic cystitis. Mitotane is used to treat adrenal cortical hyperplasia and for palliation of inoperable adrenal cortical neoplasia.

ANTISEPTICS AND DISINFECTANTS

Antiseptics and disinfectants are nonselective, anti-infective agents, applied topically. Their activity ranges from a simple reduction in the numbers of microorganisms to keep them within safe limits for public health (sanitization), to a complete destruction of microbes (sterilization) on the applied surface. In general, antiseptics have a -static or -cidal effect on organisms and are applied on tissues to suppress or prevent microbial infection. Disinfectants are germicidal compounds usually applied to inanimate surfaces. Sometimes the same compound may act as an antiseptic or as a disinfectant, depending on the drug concentration, conditions of exposure, and numbers of organisms, etc. To achieve maximum efficiency, it is essential to use the proper concentration of the drug for the purpose intended. However, the logic that "if a little is good, twice as much is better" is not only uneconomical, but often has toxicological implications.

Topical anti-infective agents are extensively used in surgery for the antisepsis of the surgical area and surgeon's hands, and to disinfect surgical instruments, apparel, and hospital premises. Other common uses are as disinfectants for home and farm premises, in water treatment, in public health sanitation, and as antiseptics in soaps, teat dips, and dairy sanitizers. Antiseptics have also been used for treating local infections. However, in most cases, systemic chemotherapeutic agents are now preferred because they often penetrate better into the foci of infection and are less likely than the topical anti-infectives to lose their potency when in contact with body fluids and debris in the infected area.

Ideally, antiseptics and disinfectants should possess a broad spectrum and potent germicidal activity, with rapid onset, and long-lasting effect. They must retain this activity even in the presence of pus, necrotic tissue, and other organic material. High lipid solubility and good dispersibility increase their effectiveness. Antiseptics should not be toxic to the host tissues, and should not impair healing. Disinfectants should be nondestructive to applied surfaces. Offensive odor, color, and staining properties should be absent or minimal.

Most of these compounds exert their antimicrobial effect by denaturation of intracellular protein, alteration of cellular membranes (often through extraction of membrane lipids), or enzyme inhibition. Chemical classes of a few of the commonly used disinfectants and antiseptics are briefly characterized below:

ACIDS AND ALKALIES

Acids: Hydrogen ion is bacteriostatic at pH ~3-6 and bactericidal at pH <3. Strong mineral acids (HCl, H_2SO_4, etc) in concentrations of 0.1 to 1N have been used as disinfectants; however, their corrosive action limits their usefulness. However, unionized weak organic acids can readily penetrate and disrupt bacterial cell membranes. Acids are used as food preservatives (eg, benzoic acid), antiseptics (eg, boric acid, acetic acid, etc), fungicides (eg, salicylic acid, benzoic acid), spermatocides (eg, acetic acid, lactic acid), and cauterizing agents (strong mineral acids).

Boric acid is bacteriostatic with very weak, if any, germicidal capability. A 2-5% aqueous solution can be applied to a variety of skin lesions as an antimicrobial agent. It does not irritate the tissues or mucous membranes.

Acetic acid, 1%, can be used in surgical dressings, and 0.25% acetic acid is a useful antibacterial agent for irrigation of the urinary tract. At 5% it is bactericidal to many bacteria, and has been used to treat otitis externa caused by *Pseudomonas, Candida, Malassezia,* or *Aspergillus* spp.

Alkalies: Hydroxyl ion also exerts antimicrobial activity. A pH >9 will inhibit most bacteria. Hydroxides of sodium and calcium are employed as disinfectants. Their irritant/caustic property usually precludes their application on tissues.

Sodium hydroxide: A 2% solution of soda lye (contains 94% NaOH) in hot water is used as a disinfectant against many common pathogens such as those causing fowl cholera and pullorum disease. It is a potent caustic and must be handled with care.

Calcium hydroxide (hydrated or air-slaked lime): Lime (CaO) soaked in water produces $Ca(OH)_2$. Aqueous suspensions of slaked lime are used to disinfect premises.

ALCOHOLS

Primary aliphatic alcohols are germicidal. Their potency increases but water solubility decreases with chain length until amyl alcohol is reached. Antimicrobial effect is related to their lipid solubility (damages bacterial membrane) and their capacity to precipitate protoplasmic proteins. However, they do not destroy bacterial spores. Ethyl alcohol (ethanol) and isopropyl alcohol (isopropanol) are the most widely used alcohols. They can be used in concentrations ranging from 30 to 90% in aqueous solutions; however, best results are usually obtained with 70% ethanol or 50% isopropanol. Higher concentrations tend to be less effective. Isopropanol is slightly more potent than ethanol due to its greater depression of surface tension. "Rubbing alcohol" is a mixture of alcohols with isopropanol as its principal ingredient. It is used as a skin disinfectant and rubefacient.

ALKYLATING AGENTS

Alkylating agents like formaldehyde, glutaraldehyde, ethylene oxide, and propylene oxide are active against bacteria, viruses, fungi, and (unlike many other disinfectants) also against spores.

Ethylene and propylene oxides are gaseous fumigants used for sterilizing animal feed, human food, surgical equipment that cannot be autoclaved, and laboratory equipment, etc. Both are noncorrosive. However, ethylene oxide has better penetrability than propylene oxide, and therefore is more commonly used.

Formaldehyde is a gas, whereas glutaraldehyde is an oil at room temperatures. However, both are readily soluble in water. Their solutions are irritant/caustic to tissues. However, they possess potent germicidal properties against all organisms including spores. Their solutions do not appreciably lose antimicrobial properties in the presence of organic matter, and are noncorrosive to metals, paints, and fabric. Both are used as disinfectants. Formalin contains ~40% formaldehyde gas in aqueous solution with variable amounts of methyl alcohol to prevent polymerization. A 1-10% solution of formaldehyde is commonly employed as a disinfectant. Glutaral (glutaraldehyde), a 1-2% alkaline solution (pH 7.5-8.5) in 70% isopropanol, is a more potent germicide than 4% formaldehyde. It is often used to sterilize surgical and endoscopic instruments and plastic and rubber apparatus.

BIGUANIDES

Chlorhexidine is the most popular antiseptic of this group. It has potent antimicrobial activity against most gram-positive and some gram-negative bacteria, but not against spores. A 0.1% aqueous solution is -cidal against *Staphylococcus aureus, Escherichia coli,* and *Pseudomonas aeruginosa* in 15 sec. It is somewhat less active against other gram-negative organisms and most viruses. Nosocomial infections by *Pseudomonas* sp have occurred from the use of contaminated chlorhexidine solutions in which the bacteria persisted. In susceptible organisms, it disrupts the cytoplasmic membrane. Its activity is enhanced by alcohols and alkaline pH, and is somewhat depressed by high concentrations of organic matter (pus, blood, etc), soap, hard water, and contact with cork. However, it is not appreciably affected by small quantities of organic matter. It is one of the most commonly used surgical and dental antiseptics. A 4% emulsion of chlorhexidine gluconate is used as a skin cleanser, a 0.5% w/v in 70% isopropanol as a general antiseptic, and a 0.5% w/v in 70% isopropanol with emollients as a hand rinse. Chlorhexidine is incorporated in shampoos, ointments, skin and wound cleansers, teat dips, surgical scrubs, etc, for its antimicrobial properties. A 1% chlorhexidine acetate ointment is used as a topical antiseptic in treatment of external wounds in dogs, cats, and horses. Chlorhexidine has low potential for systemic or dermal toxicity. It can be effectively combined with other disinfectants, surfactants, and vehicles (eg, cetrimide).

HALOGENS AND HALOGEN-CONTAINING COMPOUNDS

Iodine and chlorine are used as topical antimicrobial agents. They owe their activity to high affinity for protoplasm, where they are believed to oxidize proteins and interfere with vital metabolic reactions.

Elemental **iodine** is a potent germicide with a wide spectrum of activity, and low toxicity to tissues. A solution containing 50 ppm iodine kills bacteria in 1 min and spores in 15 min. It is poorly soluble in water but readily dissolves in ethanol, which enhances its antibacterial activity.

Preparations: Iodine tincture contains 2% iodine with 2.4% potassium iodide (KI) dissolved in 50% ethanol. It is used as a skin disinfectant. Strong iodine tincture contains 7% iodine and 5% KI dissolved in 85% ethanol. It is more potent but also more irritant than tincture of iodine. Iodine solution contains 2% iodine and 2.4% KI dissolved in aqueous solution. It is used as a nonirritant antiseptic on wounds and abrasions. Strong iodine solution contains 5% iodine and 10% KI in aqueous solution.

Iodophores (eg, povidone-iodine) are water-soluble combinations of iodine with detergents, wetting agents, solubilizers, and other carriers. They slowly release iodine as an antimicrobial agent, and are widely employed as skin disinfectants, particularly before surgery. They do not sting or stain, and are nontoxic to tissues, but may be corrosive to metals. They are effective against bacteria, viruses, and fungi but less so against spores. Iodophor solutions retain good bactericidal activity at pH <4 even in the presence of organic matter, and often change color when the activity is lost. Phosphoric acid is often mixed with iodophores to maintain an acidic medium. They have been used in teat dips to control mastitis, as dairy sanitizers, and as a general antiseptic/disinfectant for various dermal and mucosal infections.

Chlorine exerts a potent germicidal effect against most bacteria, viruses, protozoa, and fungi, through formation of undissociated hypochlorous acid (HOCl) in water at acid to neutral pH. It is effective against most organisms at a concentration of 0.1 ppm, but much higher concentrations are required in the presence of organic matter. Alkaline pH ionizes chlorine and decreases its activity by reducing its penetrability. Chlorine has a strong acrid smell and is irritant to the skin and mucous membranes. It is widely used to disinfect water supplies and inanimate objects (eg, utensils, bottles, pipelines) in dairies, creameries, and milk houses.

Preparations: Inorganic chlorides include sodium hypochlorite solutions. A 5% NaOCl solution decomposes on exposure to light. A 2-5% NaOCl solution can be used as a disinfectant, and a more diluted form (0.5%) can be used for irrigating suppurating wounds, but it dissolves blood clots and delays clotting. Calcium hypochlorite is used as a disinfectant.

Organic chlorides contain chlorine weakly bonded to nitrogen, which is slowly released for germicidal activity. They are generally less irritant, more stable, and more convenient to use than hypochlorite solutions.

HEAVY METALS

Mercury: Mercuric bichloride, one of the early antiseptics, was later replaced by the less irritant and less toxic organic mercurials, eg, merbromin, thimerosal, nitromersol, phenylmercuric nitrate. At moderate concentrations, they are bacteriostatic and act by inhibiting the bacterial enzymes through their affinity for the sulfhydryl groups. This effect can be reversed by sulfur-containing compounds, eg, cysteine, glutathione. Mercurials are not effective against spores. Due to potential persistence of mercury in the environment as a contaminant, use of mercurial antiseptics or disinfectants has largely tapered off.

Silver compounds can produce caustic, astringent, and antibacterial effects. Silver ions combine with sulfhydryl, amino, phosphate, and carboxyl groups, and thus precipitate proteins and also interfere with essential metabolic activities of microbial cells.

A 0.1% aqueous solution of silver nitrate is bactericidal and somewhat irritant, whereas a 0.01% solution is bacteriostatic. A 0.5% solution is sometimes applied as dressing on burns to reduce infection and induce rapid eschar formation. Colloidal silver compounds, which release silver ions slowly, are bacteriostatic and have a more sustained effect. They do not irritate the tissues and have little astringent or caustic effect. They are generally used as mild antiseptics and in ophthalmic preparations.

OXIDIZING AGENTS

These compounds generally exert a short-acting germicidal effect on most organisms through release of nascent oxygen, which irreversibly alters their proteins. They have little or no action on spores. Nascent oxygen is rendered inactive when it combines with organic matter.

Hydrogen peroxide solution (3%) liberates oxygen when in contact with catalase present on wound surfaces and mucous membranes. The effervescent action mechanically helps remove pus and cellular debris from the wounds and is valuable for cleaning and deodorizing infected tissue. The antimicrobial action is of short duration and is limited to the superficial layer of the applied surface as there is no penetration of the tissues.

Potassium permanganate occurs as dark crystals that dissolve in water to produce deep purple solutions, which stain tissues and clothing brown. A 1:10,000 solution kills many microorganisms in 1 hr. Higher concentrations tend to irritate the tissues. Old solutions turn chocolate brown in color and lose their activity.

PHENOLS AND RELATED COMPOUNDS

Phenols include pure phenol and substitution products with halogens and alkyl groups. They all denature proteins and are general protoplasmic poisons.

Phenol (carbolic acid) is bacteriostatic at concentrations of 0.1-1%, and is bactericidal/fungicidal at 1-2%. A 5% solution kills anthrax spores in 48 hr. The bactericidal activity is enhanced by EDTA and warm temperatures, and is decreased by alkaline medium (through ionization), lipids, soaps, and cold temperatures. Concentrations >0.5% exert a local anesthetic effect, whereas a 5% solution is strongly irritant and corrosive to the tissues. Oral ingestion or extensive application to skin can cause systemic toxicity, manifested by CNS and cardiovascular effects; death may result. It has also been implicated as a carcinogen.

Phenol has good penetrating power into organic matter and is mainly employed for disinfection of inorganic equipment and organic materials that are to be destroyed (eg, infected food and excreta). Because of its irritant and corrosive properties and potential systemic toxicity, it has not found much use as an antiseptic except to cauterize infected areas, eg, infected umbilicus of neonates. It is also incorporated in cutaneous applications for pruritus, stings, bites, burns, etc, because of its local anesthetic/antibacterial properties, to relieve itching and control infections.

Cresol (cresylic acid) is a mixture of ortho-, meta-, and para-cresols and its isomers. It is a colorless liquid, but after exposure to light and air turns pink then yellowish and finally dark brown. A 2% solution of either pure or saponated cresol in hot water is commonly used as a disinfectant for inanimate objects.

Hexachlorophene has a strong bacteriostatic action against many gram-positive organisms (including staphylococci) but only a few gram-negative ones. It is used widely in medicated soaps. Frequent washings every day with hexachlorophene sustain sufficient residue on the skin to provide prolonged bacteriostatic action. Washing with other soaps promptly removes these residues. Repeated exposure of skin to high concentrations of hexachlorophene may lead to sufficient absorption of the antiseptic to cause spongiform degeneration of the white matter in the brain causing nervous disorders. To prevent such neurotoxicity, products containing >0.75% hexachlorophene are available only on prescription. Accidental oral ingestion of hexachlorophene results in acute poisoning.

Pine tar is a viscid blackish brown liquid, used primarily for antiseptic bandaging of wounds of the hoof and horn. Pine tar contains phenol derivatives that provide antimicrobial properties.

SURFACE-ACTIVE COMPOUNDS

Surfactants lower the surface tension of an aqueous solution and are used as wetting agents, detergents, emulsifiers, antiseptics, and disinfectants. As antimicrobials, they alter the energy relationship at interfaces. Based on the position of the hydrophobic moiety in the molecule, they are classified as anionic and cationic surfactants.

Anionic Surfactants: Soaps are dipolar anionic detergents with the general formula RCOONa/K, which dissociate in water into hydrophilic K^+ or Na^+ ions and the lipophilic fatty acid ions $RCOO^-$. Since NaOH and KOH are strong bases (whereas most fatty acids are weak acids), most soap solutions are alkaline (pH 8-10) and may irritate sensitive skin and mucous membranes. Soaps emulsify lipoidal secretions of the skin and remove them along with most of the accompanying dirt, desquamated epithelium, and bacteria, which are then rinsed away with the lather.

The antibacterial potency of soaps is often enhanced by inclusion of certain antiseptics, eg, hexachlorophene, phenols, carbanilides, potassium iodide. They are incompatible with cationic surfactants.

Cationic Surfactants: These are mostly quaternary ammonium compounds, eg, benzalkonium chloride, benzathonium chloride, cetylpyridinium chloride. The major site of action of these compounds appears to be the cell membrane, where they become adsorbed and cause changes in permeability. Their activity is reduced by porous or fibrous materials (eg, fabrics, cellulose sponges, which adsorb them), and is inactivated by anionic substances (eg, soaps, proteins, fatty acids, phosphates). Therefore, they are of limited value in the presence of blood and tissue debris. They are effective against most bacteria, some fungi (including yeasts), and protozoa, but not against viruses and spores. An aqueous solution of 1:1000 to 1:5000 exhibits good antimicrobial activity, especially at slightly alkaline pH. When applied to skin, they form a film under which microorganisms can survive, which makes these compounds unreliable.

OTHER AGENTS

Antibacterial activity of **dyes** was first reported in 1913; subsequently, discovery of sulfonamides as chemotherapeutic agents ensued from the antibacterial activity observed in the dye protosil.

Azo dyes (eg, scarlet red and phenazopyridine HCl) are most active in an acidic medium and effective against gram-negative organisms. Scarlet red is often used as a 5% ointment on sores, ulcers, and wounds. Pyridium is often incorporated as an analgesic with sulfonamides for the treatment of urinary tract infections.

Acridine dyes (eg, acriflavine HCl) are more active against gram-positive bacteria. Their activity is enhanced in an alkaline medium, and antagonized by hypochlorites.

Nitrofurazone is used as a 0.2% powder or ointment for the treatment of superficial bacterial infections of wounds, burns, cutaneous ulcers, and eczema.

GROWTH PROMOTANTS

The growth of animals can be affected by hormones (natural or synthetic) that bind to specific receptors in the target tissue, or by antimicrobial compounds that change the population of microorganisms in the GI tract of healthy animals, resulting in improved animal performance.

Since the ear is discarded at slaughter, implants should be inserted in the ear to avoid the possibility of residues and their effects being carried to the consumers of treated animals. No growth promotant should be used unless it has been officially approved and local regulations are followed.

STEROID HORMONES

Endogenous Steroids: Steroid hormones are produced in the gonads, and the major compounds used for anabolic purposes are estradiol, progesterone, and testosterone. The sexual status of an animal influences growth rate and body composition; eg, bulls grow 8-12% faster than steers, have better feed efficiency (eat less feed per unit gain in body wt), and produce a leaner carcass. These beneficial effects are due to the sex steroids produced in the testes (mainly testosterone and estradiol—which in ruminants, is also anabolic and produced in relatively large quantities by the testes). The naturally produced endogenous steroids are not orally active, require relatively large doses to be administered for physiological effects, and can adversely affect the behavior of treated animals (*see* TABLE 10).

Estradiol: A potent anabolic agent in ruminants at blood concentrations of 5-100 pg/mL, it is administered as an ear implant, either as a compressed tablet or a silastic rubber implant. When administered in compressed tablets, a second steroid (usually testosterone or progesterone) should be present in a ratio of ~1 part estradiol to 10 parts of the other steroid, to slow down the release rate of estradiol and prolong the effective life span of the implant to 100 days.

Use of silastic rubber as the vehicle to administer estradiol enhances the effective life span of the implant. Estradiol, on its own, increases 1) nitrogen retention, 2) growth rate by 10-20% in steers, 3) lean meat content by 1-3%, and 4) feed efficiency by 5-8%. It can be used in steers to best advantage, but has some anabolic effects in heifers and veal calves. It works best in lambs in conjunction with androgens, and is not effective as an anabolic agent in pigs.

Testosterone: A potent anabolic agent at the relatively high serum concentrations of 1-5 ng/mL, testosterone is not used on its own as an anabolic agent in farm animals. It is generally used as the propionate formulation with 20 mg estradiol benzoate (EB) in a compressed tablet implant, in which its major role may be to slow down the release rate of estradiol. In high concentrations in blood, it induces male secondary sexual characteristics such as aggression and mounting, but this is not a problem with the current formulations; the behavior resulting from use of 20 mg EB and 100 mg progesterone is not different from that following the use of 20 mg EB + 200 mg testosterone propionate.

Progesterone: There is no clear evidence to suggest progesterone on its own is anabolic in farm animals. Its major use is to slow down the release of estradiol from compressed pellet implants. However, melengestrol acetate (MGA), a synthetic progestogen, suppresses estrus and increases growth rate in heifers.

Synthetic Steroids: In addition to natural steroids, synthetic steroids, which are generally more potent and have less androgenicity and thus less adverse effects on behavior, are also used (*see* TABLE 11). The synthetic steroids used are either androgens, eg, trenbolone acetate (TBA, which binds to androgen receptors and stimulates the effects of testosterone on growth), or progestogens, eg, MGA.

Synthetic steroidal androgens are not commonly used as anabolic agents. TBA is currently the most common synthetic androgen used for growth promotion in cattle, to a lesser extent in sheep, and is not used in pigs or horses. It has weak androgenic activity but has greater anabolic activity than testosterone.

It has no obvious side effects, and is a strong anabolic agent on its own in female cattle and sheep, but in castrated males it gives maximum response when used in conjunction with estrogens (*see* TABLE 12). It is administered as a pellet-type implant containing 200-300 mg TBA in heifers and cull cows, and can be used with estradiol in doses ranging from 140 to 200 mg TBA either as a combined or as separate implants.

Synthetic Nonsteroidal Estrogens: There are 2 major types of compounds in this class. **Stilbene estrogens** (either diethylstilbestrol [DES] or hexestrol) are currently banned in most countries as anabolic agents because they are genotoxic, have high oral activity, are not easily metabolized, and are excreted mainly as the parent compound in feces.

An analog of a naturally occurring plant estrogen (zearalenone), **zeranol** is estrogenic and has a weak affinity for the uterine estradiol receptor. It is used in animal production as a subcut. ear implant at a dose of 36 mg for cattle and 12 mg for sheep, with a duration of activity of 90-120 days. In steers, it increases nitrogen retention, growth rate by 12-15%, and feed conversion by 6-10%; lower responses are seen in heifers. Its effects are additive to those of androgens (generally TBA).

RATIONALE OF USING GROWTH PROMOTANTS

Hormones: In general, the principle that dictates the type of hormone to be used is the need to supplement or replace the particular hormone type that is deficient in the animals to be treated. Females produce estrogens normally, so better results are obtained from the administration of male androgens, eg, TBA. However, in some cases anabolic responses are obtained by giving supplemental estrogens, eg, to cull cows. Maximum anabolic responses are obtained in steers from a combination of an estrogen and an androgen. Bulls produce high quantities of androgens, therefore estrogens are the hormones of choice to use in beef bull production. Estrogens suppress gonadotropic output (LH and FSH secretion) from the anterior pituitary gland, which results in suppression of testicular growth; in beef production this can be an advantage, but the corollary is that estrogens should not be used in males, or indeed androgens in females, retained for breeding purposes.

Feed Additives: These can be fed once the rumen is functioning, although some compounds can be fed to calves.

Use in Calves: Calves have a high conversion of feed into animal tissue. Therefore, their responses to the use of anabolic agents are variable. Responses of 0-10% have been obtained when zeranol was given to 3-mo-old castrated male calves. No significant response has been obtained from TBA. Bull calves in an intensive bull beef system can be given an estrogen implant at 1-2 mo of age to suppress testicular development, which may lead to subsequent reduction in mounting and aggression. A growth response of 5-8% is also sometimes obtained from this implant. These young bulls need to be reimplanted every 100 days if compressed pellet implants are used. It is doubtful if it is worth implanting heifer calves due to the low and variable responses obtained.

Use in Weanlings: A major limitation to the use of anabolic agents in weanlings is the low liveweight gain they may achieve due to poor feeding. Hence, anabolic agents should only be considered if the weanlings are expected to gain >0.5 kg/day. Zeranol can be used in male castrates. Alternatively, a feed additive can be given to both male and female weanlings. Dairy heifer replacements can also be given a feed additive at this time.

Use in Yearlings: Higher and more consistent responses are obtained in yearling and older cattle than in calves or weanlings. This is partly related to age and partly to the higher plane of nutrition. In the case of pellet-type implants, the effectiveness of which is 90-100 days, consideration can be given to re-implanting cattle in mid-summer provided gains in excess of 0.5 kg/day are maintained. A 20-30% increase in daily gain has followed implantation of male castrates with an estrogen and an androgen. Less research has been done in yearling heifers so a definite recommendation cannot be given. However, on present knowledge, TBA could be considered for use in these animals.

Use in Finishing Beef Cattle: The choice of implant to use in the finishing phase is governed to some extent by which implants, if any, have been previously used. Feed additives can also be used during housing. Responses are good when animals are on a high plane of nutrition. Feed conversion efficiency is improved and lean meat content of the carcass is generally improved by hormone implants. Feed additives do not affect carcass composition. Although less clear, conformation of implanted cattle tends to improve.

In steers, an androgen plus an estrogen hormone combination can be used. Pellet-type implants are effective for 90-100 days; in a 4- to 5-mo finishing period, a silastic implant or re-implanting cattle after 70-80 days should be considered, as the response from the pellet-type implants is decreasing at this stage. Of course, in a prolonged finishing phase, long-acting implants can be used, which obviate the need to re-implant the estrogen component of the combination treatment. The other major alternative is to use a hormonal implant and a feed additive.

Heifers should be given TBA or a feed additive. They can be given estradiol, but the probability that 20-40% of the heifers will show mammary development is a serious drawback and can result in some heifers being classified as "cow heifers" after slaughter.

Cull cows can be given TBA or estradiol or a feed additive. Mammary development is obviously of no concern in cull cows. TBA may play some role in drying off cull cows still in milk.

Use in Beef Bull Systems: Should it be recommended that a farmer implant bulls used for beef production? In some trials in which bulls were treated with estrogens, the following have been achieved: increase in growth rate of 2-10%, and suppression of testicular growth with a consequent reduction in mounting and aggression. This would make them easier to manage on the farm and less subject to "dark cutting" following slaughter.

The mechanism involved appears to be the reduction of gonadotropic hormones (LH and FSH) from the pituitary gland by estrogen, which has a stong negative feedback effect on LH and FSH secretion. This reduction in LH and FSH results in decreased testicular size and lower testosterone levels with a consequent reduction in aggressive behavior. However, there appears to be sufficient testosterone secreted to maintain an anabolic effect. Therefore, the repeated use of estrogens in bulls beginning at 1-3 mo of age may lead to a hormonal castration-type effect with increased growth rate.

POSSIBLE COMPLICATIONS

If given to pregnant heifers, TBA will result in increased incidence of severe dystocia, masculinization of female genitalia of the fetus, increased calf mortality, and reduced milk yield in the subsequent lactation.

Any hormonal implant will have a negative feedback effect on pituitary gonadotropins, thereby reducing LH and FSH secretion. Therefore, they can affect the regularity of estrous cycles and reduce conception rate in females, and reduce testicular development and thus sperm output in males. This means that hormonal growth promotants should never be used in animals that are or may be used for breeding purposes, nor to increase growth in yearling thoroughbreds or pedigree bulls for show purposes.

FACTORS AFFECTING RESPONSE

Plane of Nutrition: Animals should be gaining a minimum of 0.5 kg/day before an economic response is obtained. Implants are best used in animals on a high plane of nutrition and under good husbandry conditions. They are an aid to, but not a substitute for, good husbandry. Consequently, there is no point in implanting cattle destined for a 3- to 4-mo "store period"

Sex and Age of Animal: Steers give maximum response. Minimal responses are obtained in calves, and good responses are obtained from yearlings and older animals. Maximum responses are probably obtained in older beef cattle at the beginning of an intensive winter finishing period.

Prior Implantation: This does not affect the response to the next implantation. Also, once the implant effect has ceased, the rate of gain reverts back to the rate that was obtained before implantation, assuming the level of feeding has not changed. Also, extra weight induced by implants in early life is transferred through to extra carcass weight at slaughter.

ANIMAL BEHAVIOR FOLLOWING IMPLANTS

In general, no undue side effects have been reported following the use of either zeranol or TBA alone or in combination in cattle. However, implanted cattle may succumb to stress more easily than nonimplanted cattle. The major problem arises from the use of estradiol as a growth promotant. Its use in the various implants outlined in TABLE 11 has been associated with increased mounting behavior and aggression. These effects generally last for 1-10 days after implantation and then subside. In some cases, the size of rudimentary teats can be increased. In extreme circumstances, however, there has been a small number of reports of undesirable behavior in steers, which has lasted for 4-10 wk. The cause of this unpredictable adverse behavior is not clear, but it is generally more severe in dairy cattle used for beef production. To minimize the adverse behavior after implantation, it is important to avoid crushing the pellet-type implants when inserting them, and mixing strange cattle with implanted animals. If the problem is severe, the buller steers should be identified and removed; if very severe, removal of the implants or administration of 50-100 mg progesterone in oil for a number of days to suppress behavior should be considered.

Pigs: In pigs, the growth responses from the use of estradiol, progesterone, and zeranol are variable but generally low. TBA does seem to increase lean meat content of pig carcasses.

Sheep: In sheep (*see* TABLE 12), the responses to anabolic agents parallel those obtained in cattle. The most consistent responses have been obtained in lambs finished on high-concentrate diets; a 10-15% increase in daily gain can be expected. Anabolic steroids should not be used in lambs that are destined to be retained for breeding. The reasons for this are the same as those discussed above for cattle. Also, implantation with zeranol reduces testicular development in ram lambs, and delays the onset of puberty and reduces the ovulation rate in female sheep. Moreover, the short finishing period and the extensive nature of some production systems militate against widespread practical use of growth pomotants in sheep.

GROWTH HORMONE (GH)

The most common peptide affecting growth is GH. Its structure is species-specific, and it has a short half-life (20-30 min), is not orally active, and is rapidly metabolized and cleared by gut, liver, and kidneys. When administered to cattle, GH increases growth rate (5-10%), feed conversion efficiency, and lean meat in the carcass. Recombinant GH in pigs has improved performance dramatically, resulting in 20% increased daily gain, 5% decrease in feed intake, and a 20% decrease in the quantity of feed required per kg liveweight gain. The effects on the carcass are ~10% increase in lean content, and decrease in fat of up to 35%. When a daily dose of 25 mg or suitable slow-release preparations that elevate GH for 2-4 wk are given, it is also a potent stimulator of milk production, and increases milk yield of dairy cows by 20%. GH is not commercially approved in most countries.

β ADRENOCEPTOR AGONISTS

β adrenoceptor agonists are catecholamines and are chemically similar in structure to epinephrine and norepinephrine, and have paracrine, neurotransmitter, and endocrine (hormonal) effects. They act by binding to specific $\beta 2$ receptors in target tissues such as adipocytes or muscle. The major use of β adrenoceptor agonists in animal production is to induce change in body composition leading to decreased fat and increased lean meat content. Side effects include marked short-term effects on the cardiovascular system, including an increase in heart rate for a number of days after treatment.

The effects of certain β agonists are to increase growth rate, and improve feed efficiency and lean meat content of beef cattle, sheep, pigs, and poultry. Lean meat content of steers was increased by 10% and fat content decreased by 7%, but organoleptic quality of meat may be adversely affected. Dose level of compound used affects the response obtained, and the optimum dose often varies for different production parameters measured. The most consistent effects are the decreased fat content and increase in lean meat, but their effects on meat quality are not clear.

ANTIMICROBIAL FEED ADDITIVES

There are a number of compounds that can improve growth rate and feed conversion efficiency in healthy livestock on an optimal plane of nutrition, which are often referred to as growth promotants (or promoters). Most of these are antimicrobial compounds, administered in the feed at low dose rates, in comparison to the high doses required for therapeutic effects. There are other compounds known as "probiotics", which are described as organisms and compounds that influence the balance of intestinal microbial population and thus increase growth and efficiency of livestock. Probiotics may help to overcome the negative effects of certain conditions that detrimentally modify the gut flora. Thus, they are useful in some cases to minimize GI upsets or to help overcome stress due to weaning or transport of livestock. The unicellular yeast fungus may also have beneficial effects on rumen fermentation and thereby improve digestion and feed efficiency.

The manipulation of rumen fermentation to improve animal production by decreasing methane yield is important because of the high energy loss in the run en

Table 10. Natural Steroid Hormones for Consideration as Growth Promotants in Farm Animals

Hormone	Type of Implant	Content of Implant	Duration of Effect (days)	Animal	Growth Response (%)	Potential Side Effects
Estradiol 1	Pellet	20 mg EB* + 200 mg progesterone	100-120	Steers	10-15	Abnormal behavior
2	Pellet	20 mg EB + 200 mg testosterone propionate	100-120	Heifers Cull cows	5-15	Udder development
3	Pellet	10 mg EB + 100 mg progesterone	100-120	Veal calves		
4	Silastic rubber	45 mg estradiol	365	Steers	10-15	Abnormal behavior
5	Silastic rubber	24 mg estradiol	200	Steers	10-15	Abnormal behavior
6	Polylactic Acid	28 mg estradiol	365	Steers	10-15	Abnormal behavior
Progesterone	See 1 and 3 above					
Testosterone	See 2 above					

*estradiol benzoate

Table 11. Some Synthetic and Nonsteroid Hormone Compounds for Consideration as Growth Promotants in Farm Animals

Hormone	Administration	Content of Implant	Duration of Effect (days)	Animal	Growth Response (%)	Potential Side Effects
TBA[1]	Pellet implant	200 or 300 mg	60-90	Heifers Cull cows Steers	5-12	
TBA + EB[2]	Pellet implant	140 mg TBA + 20 mg EB	60-100	Steers Veal calves	10-20	Behavioral problems
Zeranol	Pellet implant	36 mg zeranol	90-120	Cattle	10-15	
Zeranol	Pellet implant	12 mg zeranol	90-120	Lambs	10-15	
MGA[3]	In feed	0.25 to 0.5 mg, PO, per day	As long as it is given	Heifers Cull cows	5-10	Long-term administration may result in increased mammary development

[1]trenbolone acetate
[2]estradiol benzoate
[3]melengestrol acetate

Table 12. Effects of Some Growth Promotants on the Performance of Lambs
(Performance of Controls = 100)

| Treatment | Daily Liveweight Gain | | | Feed Efficiency |
	Weaned lambs at pasture	Weaned concentrate-fed lambs	Young suckling lambs	Weaned concentrate-fed lambs
Zeranol	115	119	109	86
Zeranol + TBA*	-	111	-	89
Estradiol + TBA	-	113	113	82
Estradiol + TBA + progesterone	-	121	113	78
Estradiol + progesterone	-	117	-	80

*Trenbolone acetate

Table 13. Some Antibacterial Growth Promotants Used in Livestock Production

Compound	Class	Absorption	Effects
Zinc bacitracin	Peptide	Not absorbed	Growth promotion in poultry
Flavomycin	Phosphoglycolipid	Not absorbed	Increase feed efficiency, growth promotion in poultry, cattle
Virginiamycin	Peptide	Not absorbed	Growth promotion in poultry
Avoparcin	Glycopeptide	Not absorbed	Increase feed efficiency, growth promotion in poultry, pigs, and cattle
Lasalocid Na	Ionophore	Poorly absorbed	Increase feed efficiency, growth promotion in cattle
Monensin Na	Ionophore	Poorly absorbed	Increase feed efficiency, growth promotion in cattle

from methane production. A second approach is to change energy metabolism in the rumen and the proportion of volatile fatty acids produced with increased production of propionic acid. Other compounds can alter rumen fermentation by modification of nitrogen and protein metabolism.

The antimicrobial growth promotants commonly used in livestock are listed in TABLE 13. Ionophores, in general, increase feed conversion efficiency in ruminants on a high-concentrate diet, while they also increase growth rate in ruminants on a high-roughage diet. Antibiotic compounds, in general, increase growth rate 5-10% and feed conversion efficiency by 5-7%. They can be used in both males and females without any adverse effects on ovarian or testicular development or function since they do not affect gonadotropin secretion. Unlike anabolic steroids, they do not affect carcass composition. They can be used in conjunction with various chemical messengers, and generally their combined effects are additive. These compounds can be subdivided as follows:

Ionophore Antibiotics: The ionophore-type feed additives (eg, monensin and lasalocid) modify the movement of ions across biological membranes, modify rumen microflora, decrease acetate and methane production, may improve nitrogen utilization, and can increase dry-matter digestibility in ruminants. Administration of monensin to cattle results in: 2-10% improvement in liveweight gain (in animals on a high-roughage diet), an increase of 3-7% in feed conversion efficiency, and up to a 6% decrease in feed consumption.

Initially, it was used only as a feed additive, but following the recent introduction of a controlled-release intra-ruminal bolus, the use of monensin has been extended to animals at pasture. Other ionophores generally have similar effects.

Non-ionophore Antibiotics: Narrow-spectrum glycoprotein antibiotics (eg, avoparcin) and phosphoglycolipid antibiotics (eg, flavophospholipol) can alter the rumen flora by inhibiting the action of some gram-positive gut microorganisms and peptoglycan formation, giving similar production responses to those from using ionophores. In addition to yearling and finishing cattle, these compounds can also be administered to calves, either in milk replacer or in supplemental concentrates. The means by which these compounds exert their antimicrobial effect differ for various products.

Gut-active Growth Promotants: This category of growth promotants includes enzymes and probiotics. Examples of enzymes that are supplemented in the diet are amylase, lipase, and protease. The probiotic feed additives consist of selected strains of lactobacilli and streptococci that alter the microbial species present in the GI system, to the benefit of the treated animal. Unicellular yeasts are also used.

The net effect of these feed additive compounds is to increase the metabolizable energy available for production and growth.

PART VII
DISEASES OF POULTRY

POU

BLOOD-BORNE ORGANISMS

Avian blood may contain various disease agents. Some are within blood cells: *Plasmodium, Haemoproteus, Leucocytozoon, Atoxoplasma (Toxoplasma, Lankesterella),* and rickettsiae. Others are free in the plasma: spirochetes, trichomonads, trypanosomes, and microfilariae. Some of these are motile and easily detectable when viewed in wet-smear with darkfield or reduced-light microscopy. (Other microorganisms, eg, *Pasteurella multocida* or *Erysipelothrix insidiosa*, may be seen in blood smears.)

Table 1.　Blood-borne Organisms in Poultry

Agent	In RBC	In WBC	Free	Schizonts In Blood	Motile Forms	Spread By
Aegyptianella	yes	no	no	no	no	T
Atoxoplasma	**	***	?	no	no	F,D
Borrelia	no	no	yes	no	yes	F,I,T,M
Haemoproteus	yes	no	*	no	*	H,C
Leucocytozoon	yes	yes	*	no	*	S,C
Microfilariae	no	no	yes	no	yes	S,C,L
Plasmodium	yes	no	*	yes	*	M,I
Trichomonas	no	no	yes	no	yes	F
Trypanosoma	no	no	yes	no	yes	H,D,S,M

　* = As blood cools, microgametes produced, freed in blood.
　** = Sometimes.
*** = Usually.
　T = Ticks, F = Feces, D = Mites, I = Blood injection, M = Mosquito,
　H = Hippoboscids, C = *Culicoides*, S = Simulids, L = Lice.

AEGYPTIANELLOSIS

Aegyptianella spp are rickettsiae seen in RBC as "signet-ring" bodies (0.5-4 μm). Affected avian species include domestic chickens, turkeys, ducks, and geese, along with passerines and psittacines. Transmission is by various ticks or blood inoculation.

Ruffled feathers, anorexia, droopiness, diarrhea, and hyperthermia are found. Anemia, enlargement of liver and spleen, yellow-green kidneys, and punctiform hemorrhage of the serosa are seen.

Tetracyclines are said to be effective in treatment. Control of ticks (qv, p 1622) is important.

ATOXOPLASMOSIS

Passerine birds, such as canaries, mynah birds, and finches, may be fatally affected by what is apparently a 2-host coccidial protozoan, variously called *Atoxoplasma, Toxoplasma, Lankesterella, Isospora, Encephalitozoon,* or *Haemogregarina.* The parasite is reported to be spread by oocysts in the droppings, and/or arthropod vectors, such as the red mite. Acute deaths occur in young birds; older birds may have a chronic course of infection.

Hepatomegaly, detectable by observing the abdomen after wetting the belly wall with alcohol, is common. Smears from the blood (or better, the buffy coat from a capillary tube) reveal mononuclear cells with the parasite in a clear notch in the nucleus. Some have reported parasitism of RBC; overstaining is usually necessary for detection. Droppings contain oocysts.

In acutely affected young birds, usually the liver and spleen are enlarged and necrotic. In chronic cases, the lesions of the liver and spleen resemble lymphoid leukosis tumors.

Anticoccidial drugs, such as a mixture of pyrimethamine and sulfaquinoxaline (or other sulfonamide), can be used as part of a preventive program for nestlings. Detection and treatment of mite infestations are also important.

FILARIASIS

Wild birds often have microfilariae in the blood. Many avian filarial species exist. Sometimes, nearly all of a common grackle flock carry microfilariae; the adult worms are under the dura mater over the posterior dorsum of the cerebrum. The American robin and the English sparrow may have larvae in the blood. Pet birds, such as Java sparrows, Cordon Bleu finches, cockatoos, and other psittacines, and others may have these parasites.

The adults may be in various organs (eg, in small vessels, the lungs, under the serosa of air sacs) usually peculiar to the species. Spread is usually by blood-sucking insects, which are hosts for part of the life cycle.

Not much is known about the effect of these filarids on the hosts. Adult grackles seem to be unaffected, but possibly nestlings have signs and lesions. *Splendidofilaria passerina*, pathogenic in English sparrows, causes thickening, necrosis, and stenosis of pulmonary vessel walls. *Diplotriaena tricuspis* in jays causes pneumonia with lung consolidation.

The microfilariae can be seen in thin wet smears with darkfield or reduced-light microscopy, or in stained thin smears.

There is no recognized treatment. It is likely that drugs effective against *Dirofilaria immitis* (qv, p 73) would be useful.

HAEMOPROTEUS INFECTION

An infection that seems not to be troublesome in many birds, although signs have been reported in quail, pigeons, turkeys, and some psittacines. Gamonts are the only stages of *Haemoproteus* seen in the blood. The infection is not transferred by injection of infected blood except when stray infected endothelial cells are present. Vectors are usually hippoboscid flies, although biting midges (*Culicoides* spp) are vectors for some species. Congestion of the lungs is the most common pathological change.

Antimalarial drugs may be used for treatment. Efforts to eliminate the vector should be made; since they live on the host, a housed flock once cleared of them should remain so, unless new birds are introduced.

LEUCOCYTOZOONOSIS

A disease caused by arthropod-borne protozoa that resemble *Plasmodium* (*see* below and also p 1007), except that they lack meronts (schizonts) in circulating blood cells and do not have pigment granules. *Leucocytozoon* meronts, some very large, are found in various organs. Gamonts, which enlarge and distort the host cell so that it is unrecognizable, are seen in RBC or WBC. Of the numerous species of *Leucocytozoon*, many are restricted to a certain species or order of birds. In North America, important species in poultry include *L smithi* in turkeys and *L simondi* in waterfowl. *Leucocytozoon andrewsi*, thought by some to be a mild strain of *L caulleryi*, was originally described in chickens in South Carolina.

Nondomestic birds have many *Leucocytozoon* spp, eg, blood smears from red-tailed hawks often contain gamonts. Several species produce serious losses in Asian countries, eg, *L caulleryi* causes a lethal hemorrhagic disease of chickens.

"Aberrant" leucocytozoonosis is a disease of psittacines apparently caused by *Leucocytozoon* spp that usually are parasitic in some other avian host (7 of 9 psittacine genera reported with this are of Australian origin, one is from South America, and one from Africa). Gamonts are not seen in the blood; diagnosis depends on finding the meronts in the heart and other musculature. Carcasses may be in good condition with full crops.

Wild birds are reservoirs in some areas, and are responsible for initiation of infection in domestic flocks. Wild bird parasitemia often increases dramatically (called "spring rise") in late April and early May, just before dipterous vectors, blackflies (*Simulium* spp), or biting midges (*Culicoides* spp) increase. Ducks recovered from *L simondi* infection relapse when light cycles are manipulated to increase egg production.

Acute disease is seen more often in the young, especially in fly season; parasitemia is usually high in these. Subacute or chronic disease is seen in the young outside fly season, and in older birds at any season; parasitemia is usually low. Mortality may approach 100% but varies greatly with species and strain of parasite, breed of host, and other factors.

Clinical Findings, Lesions, and Diagnosis: Acutely affected birds usually are listless and have anemia and leukocytosis, tachypnea, diarrhea with green droppings, and often CNS signs. Feed consumption is below normal. These signs are evident ~1 wk after infection, and coincide with the start of parasitemia. Visibly affected birds die after 7-10 days, or may recover with sequelae of poor growth and egg production.

Death results from occlusion of vital blood vessels by the large meronts, or from respiratory distress consequent to blockage of lung capillaries by the numerous parasites and to the anemia caused by hemorrhages. Hemorrhages, splenomegaly, and hepatomegaly are seen. Grossly visible white dots in many organs are the meronts.

In thin blood smears, gamonts may be seen along the edges and the "tail" of the smear. The shape of the gamont varies with the species—some are elongated with long tapering extremities, while others are rounded. There are no pigment granules. Serology may detect prior infection.

Treatment and Control: Treatment usually is not effective. Prophylactic medication with combined pyrimethamine (1 ppm) and sulfadimethoxine (10 ppm) in the feed controls *L caulleryi*; clopidol (1.25-2.5 ppm) controls *L smithi*.

PLASMODIUM INFECTION

Plasmodium spp, often not species-specific, cause disease in birds similar to malaria in man. Infections in North American domestic birds occur in pigeons and canaries (nestlings severely affected), and in turkeys (no mortality reported). Zoo penguins are notably susceptible, and die. The disease has been reported in falcons. The bald eagle and the cliff swallow are reported to share *Plasmodium polare* infection.

As in human malaria, mosquitoes are vectors of avian plasmodiosis. *Plasmodium* differs from *Leucocytozoon* and *Haemoproteus* in having meronts in RBC as well as in other cells of the body. Susceptible birds can be infected by injection of infected blood.

Clinical Findings, Lesions, and Diagnosis: Affected birds are droopy and weak; severely affected birds have a protruding abdomen. Usually, the liver and spleen are enlarged and discolored (chocolate to black). There may be ocular hemorrhage. Blood smears usually have numerous gamonts and meronts. Infected cells also have dark pigment granules (digested Hgb). As liquid blood samples cool, changes occur—microgamonts produce microgametes that enter the plasma, leaving the host cell altered in appearance. Microgametes of *Plasmodium* and related hematozca, when moving in a wet smear, can be mistaken for *Borrelia* spirochetes (qv, p 1565).

Treatment and Control: Chemotherapy is effective in treating affected individuals or flocks. Chloroquine, 250 mg/120 mL (4 oz) of drinking water, may be used. Grape or orange juice may be used to disguise the drug's bitterness. In penguins, 5 mg/kg body wt daily, in fish, is used for prevention. Pyrimethamine is said to be the best suppressive drug. Any antimalarial drug may be tried; however, strain differences in drug susceptibility are found.

In mosquito areas, canary breeder houses and pigeon breeder lofts should be screened as a preventive measure.

SPIROCHETOSIS

Several *Borrelia* spp have been found in birds. *See* p 1565.

TRICHOMONADEMIA

Trichomonads (*Tetratrichomonas [Trichomonas] gallinarum*) have been observed in the blood of sick chickens. Such birds have blackhead-like lesions of the ceca and liver.

TRYPANOSOMIASIS

Trypanosomes have been reported from chickens and pigeons, but are not a problem in commercial flocks. They are widespread in wild birds. Passerines, such as canaries and finches, and psittacines have been reported to be affected. Some report that trypanosomes are found in the blood only in the summer. These protozoans are said to be spread by blood-sucking arthropods, such as hippoboscid flies, red mites, simulids, and mosquitoes.

Droopiness and inappetence are generally reported; death has occurred when parasitemia is high.

Darkfield or reduced-light microscopy of very thin wet smears of blood and bone marrow reveals the motile protozoa. Stained thin smears are useful for showing the morphology of the parasite. Marrow smears are more often positive.

Since pamaquine naphthoate is no longer marketed, there is no known treatment. Metronidazole or amphotericin B might be tried.

CHICK ANEMIA VIRUS (CAV) INFECTION
(Avian anemia virus infection, Blue wing disease, Anemia dermatitis syndrome, Hemorrhagic aplastic anemia syndrome)

A transient, acute, infectious, immunosuppresive disease of young chickens characterized by anorexia, lethargy, depression, anemia, atrophy or hypoplasia of lymphoid organs, hemorrhages (cutaneous, subcut., and IM), and increased mortality rates.

Etiology, Epidemiology, and Pathogenesis: The cause is a small, heat-resistant, chloroform-resistant virus. Final taxonomic classification of this virus has not been made. Antibody to CAV occurs worldwide, and the disease has been described in most countries with a developed chicken industry. CAV is not known to infect birds other than chickens.

CAV is transmitted horizontally by direct contact, contaminated fomites (fecal-oral/nasal route), and vertically through the embryonated egg. Most breeder flocks become infected and develop CAV antibody before they begin to lay fertile eggs. If egg-producing seronegative breeder flocks are infected, CAV will be vertically transmitted: as long as the hen is viremic (1-3 wk), hatched chicks will be CAV-infected. If hens are seropositive, maternally derived antibody generally protects progeny from disease but not from infection. Chicks <1 wk old without maternal antibody to CAV can become infected and develop disease.

Age resistance to disease (not infection) begins at ~1 wk, and is complete 2 wk after hatching. However, the protective effects of maternal antibody and age resistance can be overcome by CAV co-infection with immunosuppressive agents such as infectious bursal disease virus, herpesvirus (Marek's disease), and reticuloendotheliosis virus.

Many flocks of SPF chickens have antibody to CAV. Spread of infection by CAV-contaminated embryo- or cell-culture-derived vaccines and biologicals is possible but has not been shown to occur.

When 1-day-old susceptible chicks are inoculated IM with CAV, viremia occurs within 24 hr. Virus can be recovered from most organs and rectal contents up to 35 days after inoculation. Anemia probably results from decreased erythropoiesis. Neutralizing antibody is detectable 21 days after infection, and clinical, hematologic, and pathologic parameters return to normal ~35 days after infection.

Clinical Findings and Lesions: Signs of illness or adverse effects on egg production do not occur when susceptible adult chickens become CAV-infected. Clinical disease occurs 12-17 days after infection. Chicks are anorectic, lethargic, depressed, and pale. PCV are low (in chickens, anemia is defined as a PCV of <27), and blood smears often reveal anemia, leukopenia, or pancytopenia depending on the stage of the disease. Blood may be watery and clot slowly. Mortality rates usually are ~10%, but may be >50%.

Organs are pale, and the thymus and bursa of Fabricius are small. Bone marrow is pale or yellow. Hemorrhage may be present in or under the skin, skeletal muscle, and other organs. Histologically, depletion of lymphoid cell populations is seen in primary and secondary lymphoid organs. Granulocytic and erythrocytic compartments in the bone marrow are atrophic or hypoplastic. Purulent or granulomatous lesions seen in these or other organs usually are associated with bacteria or protozoa.

Diagnosis: A tentative diagnosis is based on history, signs, and gross and clinicopathologic findings. Final diagnosis requires virus isolation. To isolate CAV, laboratories must maintain MDCC-MSB1 cultures (a Marek's-disease-tumor-derived lymphoblastoid cell line) or have susceptible (antigen- and antibody-negative) day-old chicks or chick embryos. Electron microscopy may be used to find CAV particles in plasma from viremic chicks. A presumptive diagnosis can be made if paired indirect immunofluorescence or virus-neutralization tests detect seroconversion to CAV.

Treatment and Prevention: There is no specific treatment. Secondary bacterial infections may be treated with antibiotics. No vaccines currently are available for use in the USA, although one is available in Germany. In some areas, transfer of litter to noncontaminated premises and the addition of crude homogenates of tissues from affected chickens to the drinking water have been used to ensure infection and seroconversion of parent flocks before they begin to lay eggs, thereby diminishing the risk of egg transmission. These procedures are not without risk and cannot be unreservedly recommended. Because severe clinical disease is the result of interaction between CAV and other immunosuppressive viruses, control of each of these pathogens is probably equally important.

DISSECTING ANEURYSM
(Aortic rupture, Internal hemorrhage)

A fatal disease of turkeys, and less frequently of chickens, characterized by massive internal hemorrhage resulting from rupture of aneurysms formed in various parts of the vascular system. The frequency with which the posterior aorta is affected has given rise to the term "aortic rupture". The disease has been reported in the USA, Canada, and the UK. Most breeds of turkeys are susceptible, and th;

largest and most rapidly growing males, 8-24 wk old are affected most often; females are also affected, but at a lower incidence. It usually occurs only in rapidly growing birds.

Etiology: The exact cause is unknown. Probably several factors contribute to the development of fatal cases in turkeys. For the disease to occur, birds must be fed and managed in such a way that they are growing rapidly, and they must have a genetic susceptibility. A prolonged lipemia generally develops during the period of rapid growth, and the period of greatest mortality typically corresponds to a sharp rise in blood pressure with dissecting aneurysms developing at the site of arteriosclerotic plaques. The lipemia may result from a high dietary intake of fat or the effects of hormonal factors, such as high dietary concentrations of estrogens. Although β-aminopropionitrile, the toxic agent in *Lathyrus odoratus*, is capable of producing the disease, there is no evidence that this or other nitriles are responsible for dissecting aneurysms in turkeys under natural conditions.

Clinical Findings: Affected birds that had shown no premonitory signs are found dead with marked pallor of the head and neck. Occasionally, a caretaker observes an apparently healthy bird die within a few minutes. The incidence is usually <1%, but may be as great as 10%. Formerly, when male turkeys were implanted with stilbestrol, the incidence was as great as 20%.

Lesions: The carcass is markedly anemic with large quantities of clotted blood in the peritoneal cavity and over the kidneys, or in the pericardial sac. Sometimes, massive hemorrhages are present in the lungs, kidneys, and leg muscles. The rupture in the ventral wall of the posterior aorta at about the position of the testes, or in the cardiac atrium, can be located readily by carefully washing away the blood clot. The aortic lumen may contain an organized adherent thrombus at the site of rupture. Ruptures in smaller blood vessels are more difficult to locate. Almost always, an intimal thickening or a large, fibrous plaque is present in the region of the rupture. Marked accumulation of lipids in the thickened intima and in the fibrous plaques can be identified by stains.

Control: There is no known treatment; coagulants and vitamin K are useless, since there is no defect in the clotting mechanism. Losses sometimes may be reduced during the critical period between 16 and 23 wk of age by limiting feed intake. High-fat diets should not be fed during this period. Reserpine (0.0001% in the ration for not more than 5 days, and 0.00002% when fed continuously) in birds >4 wk old reduced losses, probably by reducing blood pressure. Some studies have indicated that the incidence of aortic rupture can be reduced by adding 240 ppm of copper to the diet.

HYPERTENSIVE ANGIOPATHY (HA) IN TURKEYS

A common condition associated with sudden death in rapidly growing male turkeys. The incidence (1-2% in most flocks) varies with the strain of turkey.

Etiology: No infectious agents have been incriminated; ventricular arrythmias secondary to severe hypertension may be the cause. Turkeys dying of HA have heavier heart weights, especially of the left ventricle. The incidence can be altered by changing the environment.

Clinical Findings, Lesions, and Diagnosis: Sudden death ("apparent heart attack") in apparently healthy, rapidly growing, 7- to 15-wk-old male turkeys is observed. Mortality of 6% has been reported.

Most lesions are referable to the cardiovascular system. The most consistent gross lesion is subcapsular perirenal hemorrhage of varying degrees; a common finding is pulmonary congestion and edema. Others include congestion of the intestinal vasculature, and a swollen, dark red, mottled spleen. Histological changes are not dramatic, although renal and pulmonary perivascular edema and/or hemorrhage are often prominent. Hypertensive changes in arterioles, especially in the spleen and kidney, are usually detected, but whether this change is significantly different from age-matched controls is questionable.

Diagnosis is based on the history, typical distribution of lesions, and absence of any detectable agents. (*See also* FLIP-OVER DISEASE, p 1573.)

Control: There is no specific medication to prevent or treat HA. Activities that increase stress on the cardiovascular system (eg, moving, increased environmental temperatures, and noise) should be minimized, especially between 7 and 15 wk of age. Reducing growth rate by lowering protein and energy levels in the feed decreases the incidence, and using a "step-up" lighting program appears to do so.

INCLUSION BODY HEPATITIS (IBH)

An acute disease of young chickens, associated with anemia and hemorrhagic disorders, that has been observed in many areas of the world. A similar disease has been reported in turkeys and quail. Once considered common, IBH is now rarely diagnosed.

Etiology, Transmission, and Pathogenesis: Adenoviruses have been considered to be the cause. Birnavirus (the cause of infectious bursal disease [IBD]) and chick anemia virus (CAV, one cause of infectious anemia) have been associated with adenovirus infections; both of these cause immunosuppression and contribute greatly to the severity of disease caused by adenoviruses.

Adenoviruses are ubiquitous and are transmitted horizontally and vertically. Infections are common and widespread in chickens. Chicks and young chickens are affected most commonly. Infection by adenovirus usually results in minimal hepatic disease. Anemia does not occur. However, if CAV- or IBD-infected birds are infected with adenovirus, clinical disease becomes evident.

Clinical Findings, Lesions, and Diagnosis: Sudden mortality usually is seen in chickens <6 wk old. Mortality is seldom >7%. Signs associated with diseases caused by other pathogens (eg, bacteria, fungi, or viruses) commonly occur if birds have been immunosuppressed. In these cases, mortality rates may be >30%. Bone marrow, livers, and other organs usually are pale. Congestion and multifocal areas of light or dark discoloration and fluid are seen in livers or skin. Hemorrhage may occur in any organ. The bursa of Fabricius usually is small. Microscopically, solitary prominent basophilic inclusion bodies are seen in hepatocyte nuclei.

A tentative diagnosis is based on typical microscopical findings and confirmed by isolating adenovirus from portions of liver. Immunosuppression resulting from IBD or CAV infections usually is the predisposing event that culminates in clinical IBH.

Treatment and Prevention: Treatment consists of nursing care. Antibiotics may help prevent secondary bacterial infections. Sulfonamides are contraindicated if evidence of hematologic disease or immunosuppression is seen.

Broiler-breeder flocks should have high levels of IBD antibody before they begin to lay fertile eggs. Vaccines against IBH or CAV are not commercially available.

ROUND HEART DISEASE

A spontaneous cardiomyopathy of young turkeys, characterized by sudden death due to cardiac arrest. It has been suggested that the condition should be called spontaneous cardiomyopathy to distinguish it from round heart disease of chickens, a different syndrome that is rarely recognized today.

The etiology is unknown. A genetic predisposition is involved in at least some instances. Possibly some outbreaks have been associated with hypoxia during incubation of the eggs. Excess furazolidone in the diet produces an identical syndrome. Implication of a possible inherited serum trypsin inhibition or a viral myocarditis has not been confirmed.

Most deaths occur during the first 4 wk of life, with mortality peaking at 2 wk. Many poults die suddenly, but some may have ruffled feathers, drooping wings, a general unthrifty appearance, and show labored, gasping breathing before death. After 3 wk of age, mortality is sporadic. Characteristically, the affected poult in the first 4 wk of life has a greatly enlarged heart due to dilatation of both ventricles, congested lungs, and a swollen liver. Ascites, anasarca, pulmonary edema, and hydropericardium may or may not be present. In older poults, the enlarged hearts are due to marked hypertrophy of ventricles in addition to dilatation. Histologically, lesions in abnormal hearts are nonspecific and include congestion, minor degeneration of fibers, and focal infiltration by lymphocytes.

Generally, diagnosis is based on history and gross findings at necropsy; although the ECG can be used, it is of little practical use. Feed should be checked for excess furazolidone. Sodium and polychlorinated biphenyls or related compounds may produce similar syndromes.

No treatment is available. Good brooding practices may reduce mortality. Any toxins should be eliminated and incubation conditions reviewed.

COCCIDIOSIS

A parasitic disease caused by protozoa of the phylum Apicomplexa, family Eimeriidae. In poultry, the species belong to the genus *Eimeria* and occur in the intestine except for *E truncata*, which occurs in the goose kidney. The infectious process is rapid (4-7 days) and is characterized by parasite replication in host cells with extensive damage to the intestinal mucosa. Generally, the parasites are strictly host-specific, and the different species have a predilection for different parts of the intestine. Coccidia are distributed worldwide, and have been found in jungle fowl, the ancestors of domestic chickens. (*See also* CRYPTOSPORIDIOSIS, p 1554.)

Etiology: The life cycle of the genus *Eimeria* is summarized under COCCIDIOSIS in mammals (qv, p 103). Coccidia are almost universally present in poultry-raising operations, but clinical disease occurs only after ingestion of relatively large numbers of sporulated oocysts by susceptible birds. Both clinically infected and recovered birds shed oocysts in their droppings, which contaminate feed, dust, water, litter, and soil. Oocysts may be transmitted by mechanical carriers, eg, equipment, clothing, insects, and other animals. Fresh oocysts are not infective until they sporulate; under optimal conditions (70-90°F [21-32°C] with adequate moisture and oxygen), this requires 1-2 days. The prepatent period is 4-7 days. Sporulated oocysts may survive for long periods, depending on environmental factors. Oocysts are resistant to most disinfectants, but are killed by ammonia gas and methyl bromide.

Pathogenicity is influenced by host genetics, nutritional factors, concurrent diseases, and strain of the coccidium. *Eimeria necatrix* and *E tenella* are the most pathogenic in chickens because schizogony occurs in the lamina propria and crypts of Lieberkühn of the small intestine and ceca, respectively, and extensive hemorrhage occurs. With most species, development occurs in epithelial cells lining the villi. A useful level of immunity usually develops promptly in response to moderate and continuing infection. True age-immunity does not occur, but older birds are usually more resistant than young birds because of earlier exposure to disease.

Clinical Findings: Signs are highly variable in flocks, and range from decreased growth rate to a high percentage of visibly sick birds, severe diarrhea, and high mortality. Usually, feed and water consumption decrease. Weight loss, development of culls, decreased egg production, and increased mortality are observed. Mild infections of intestinal species, which would otherwise be classed as subclinical, may cause depigmentation. Survivors of severe infections recover in 10-14 days but may require more time to return to normal production. The degree of immunity acquired before development of clinical disease may influence severity and course of a flock infection.

Chickens: In *E tenella* infection, involvement of the ceca rather than the small intestine is a distinguishing characteristic, and can be recognized by accumulation of blood in the ceca and by bloody droppings. Cecal cores, which are accumulations of clotted blood, tissue debris, and oocysts, may be found in birds surviving the acute stage.

Eimeria necatrix produces major lesions in the anterior and middle portions of the small intestine. Small white spots, usually intermingled with rounded, bright- or dull-red spots of various sizes, can be seen on the serosal surface. The white spots are diagnostic for this species if clumps of large schizonts can be demonstrated microscopically. In severe cases, the intestinal wall is thickened, and the infected area dilated to 2-2½ times the normal diameter; blood may be in the lumen. Fluid loss may result in marked dehydration; the crop is often concurrently distended with water. Although the damage is in the small intestine, the sexual phase of the life cycle is completed in the ceca where the oocysts are found. Oocysts of all other species can be recovered from the area of major lesions.

Eimeria acervulina infection is characterized by numerous gray or whitish transverse patches in the upper half of the small intestine, and may not be easily distinguished on gross examination. The clinical course in a flock is usually protracted. Poor growth, development of culls, and low mortality are often observed.

Eimeria maxima develops in the small intestine, where it causes dilatation and thickening of the wall. Some hemorrhage occurs, which tends to result in a grayish, brown, or pink mucous exudate. The oocysts and gametocytes (particularly microgametocytes), which are present in the lesions, are distinctly large.

Eimeria brunetti occurs in the lower small intestine, rectum, ceca, and cloaca. In moderate infections, there is a catarrhal enteritis and thickening of the intestinal wall. In severe infections, extensive coagulative necrosis and sloughing of the mucosa occurs throughout most of the small intestine.

Eimeria mitis is now recognized as pathogenic in the lower small intestine. Formerly, it was confused with *E mivati*, but there is now doubt as to validity of the latter species name.

Eimeria praecox is parasitic in the upper half of the intestine and may decrease rate of growth, but is of less economic importance than the other species.

Eimeria hagani, although rare and of little or no pathogenicity, develops in the anterior part of the small intestine.

Turkeys: Only 4 of the 7 species of coccidia in turkeys (*Eimeria adenoeides, E dispersa, E gallopavonis,* and *E meleagrimitis*) are considered pathogenic; *E innocua, E meleagridis,* and *E subrotunda* are thought to be relatively nonpathogenic. Oocyst sporulation occurs within 1-2 days after expulsion from the host; the prepatent period is 4-6 days.

Eimeria adenoeides and *E gallopavonis* infect the lower ileum, ceca, and rectum. The developmental stages are found in the epithelial cells of the villi and crypts. The affected portion of the intestine may be dilated and have a thickened wall. Thick, creamy material or caseous casts that contain enormous numbers of oocysts are found. *Eimeria meleagrimitis* chiefly infects the upper small intestine. The lamina propria or deeper tissues may be parasitized, which results in necrotic enteritis (qv, p 1561). *Eimeria dispersa* occurs in the upper small intestine and causes a creamy, mucoid enteritis that fills the entire intestine, including the ceca. Large numbers of gametocytes and oocysts are associated with the lesions.

Common signs in infected flocks include reduced feed consumption, rapid weight loss, droopiness, ruffled feathers, and severe diarrhea. Bloody droppings do not occur, but wet droppings with mucus are common. Clinical infections are seldom observed in poults >8 wk old. Morbidity and mortality may be high.

Ducks: A large number of specific coccidia have been reported in both wild and domestic ducks, but validity of some of the descriptions is questionable. Presence of *Eimeria, Wenyonella,* and *Tyzzeria* spp has been confirmed. *Tyzzeria perniciosa* is a known pathogen, which balloons the entire small intestine with mucohemorrhagic material that later becomes caseous. Other species apparently produce hemorrhagic enteritis with a characteristic anatomic distribution. *Eimeria* spp also have been described as pathogenic; the other coccidia of domestic ducks are considered relatively nonpathogenic. A number of coccidia have been reported in wild ducks. Infrequent but dramatic outbreaks occur in 2- to 4-wk-old ducklings. Morbidity and mortality may be high.

Geese: The most striking coccidial infection of geese is that produced by *Eimeria truncata,* in which the kidneys are enlarged and studded with poorly circumscribed, yellowish white streaks and spots. The tubules are dilated with masses of oocysts and urates. Mortality may be high. At least 5 other *Eimeria* spp have been described as parasitizing the intestine.

Diagnosis: Coccidial infections are readily confirmed by demonstration of oocysts in feces or intestinal scrapings. Responsible diagnosis can demand much skill, since the presence of oocysts has little relationship to current or impending clinical disease; knowledge of flock appearance, morbidity, mortality, feed intake, characteristic odor, and growth rate or rate of lay is often critical. Necropsy of several representative specimens is advisable. Classical lesions of *E tenella* and *E necatrix* may be diagnostic. Familiarity with the lesions, site parasitized by different species, and the size, shape, and location of oocysts allow a reasonably accurate differentiation of the coccidial species in most instances. Mixed coccidial infections are common.

A diagnosis of coccidiosis is warranted if oocysts, merozoites, or schizonts are demonstrated microscopically and if lesions and flock history are compatible. The frequency of subclinical coccidial infections in some individuals in a population demands care in eliminating other possible flock disorders.

Control: Practical methods of management cannot be expected to completely prevent infection. Maintaining poultry at all times on wire floors to separate birds from droppings usually prevents all but minor infections; clinical coccidiosis is observed only rarely under such circumstances. Other methods of control are designed to allow development of immunity or to minimize infection, usually by use of drugs. Since coccidiosis may cause serious problems for chickens throughout life, methods of control in this species are discussed in detail.

Immunity: A species-specific immunity develops, the degree of which largely depends on the extent of infection that occurs following initial exposure. Repeated infection with small numbers of oocysts produces greater immunity than that obtained with single exposure to greater numbers, and is less damaging to the host.

A "vaccine" in the form of standardized doses of sporulated oocysts of the various coccidial species is available. It is administered in the drinking water during the first 2 wk of life. Since the "vaccine" serves only to introduce infection, the litter must be managed to allow oocyst sporulation; spraying the litter may be necessary to keep it moist but not wet.

Drug Use When Immunity Is Needed: Immunity depends on stimulation by subclinical infection. Clinical disease is prevented by the interaction of the environment and one or more of the many anticoccidial drugs that are available. Failures occur if the suppression is either inadequate or too great. Drugs vary in their ability to interfere with development of immunity.

Drug Use When No Immunity Is Needed: No immunity is necessary in chickens reared for meat production, or in floor-reared layers to be moved to cages; for these, exposure and infection should be minimized. Litter should be dry to minimize oocyst sporulation, and highly effective anticoccidial drugs at relatively high levels may be used continuously. Drug withdrawal is usually necessary to avoid residues in meat or eggs.

Anticoccidial Drugs: Many drugs are available for prevention and treatment of coccidiosis in chickens, and a smaller number for use in turkeys. These are listed in TABLES 5 and 6, pp 1475 and 1476.

All are provided by the manufacturer in premixes with detailed instructions for prophylactic use, which is preferred since most of the damage occurs before signs become apparent and delayed treatment may not benefit the entire flock. Only a few of the prophylactic drugs are also effective therapeutically. Water medication is generally preferred over feed medication for treatment. Increased levels of vitamins A and K or antibiotics are sometimes used in the ration to improve rate of recovery.

Correct drug concentrations depend on governmental approvals and management considerations. Relatively low dosages may be used continuously for prevention or if development of immunity is desired. Higher dosages may be used over short periods of time for treatment or if a high level of exposure is anticipated. Recommended dosage varies with the species of coccidia involved. All manufacturer's warnings should be carefully observed.

Continuous use of anticoccidial drugs may result in selection for and survival of drug-resistant strains of coccidia. Fortunately, there is little cross-resistance to anticoccidials with different modes of action. Change of drug may be beneficial when resistance has been established; however, little benefit may be expected from frequent changing of drugs. "Shuttle programs", in which one group of chickens is treated sequentially with different drugs, is a common practice used in an attempt to reduce selection for resistance.

CRYPTOSPORIDIOSIS

A parasitic disease caused by protozoa (phylum Apicomplexa) that are related to coccidia of the genera *Eimeria*, *Isospora*, *Sarcocystis*, and *Toxoplasma*, but are members of the family Cryptosporidiidae. It was thought that the genus *Cryptosporidium* had ≥19 species, but recent research has thrown much doubt on this because of transmission of human isolates to calves and rodents. Cryptosporidia are parasitic in the intestine of mammals (*see* p 108); in birds, they are commonly in the bursa of Fabricius and respiratory tract. The disease is more severe in turkeys than in chickens, and is frequently fatal in quail.

The life cycle of *Cryptosporidium* is similar to that of other coccidia, involving asexual and sexual phases, and culminates in oocyst production. In the host, the oocyst forms 4 sporozoites without sporocysts. It is generally accepted that the life cycle is not self-limiting because some oocysts are thin-walled and release sporozoites after trypsin/bile stimulation, with immediate invasion. The endogenous cycle is short (4-7 days), the endogenous stages are small (4-7 μm), and the parasites are just beneath the epithelial cell membranes.

In turkeys and chickens, the parasites are reported to occur in the sinuses, trachea, bronchi, cloaca, and bursa of Fabricius. The respiratory disease causes coughing, gasping, and airsacculitis. Lungs become gray and wet. Signs last several weeks, and death may occur.

Examining tissue scrapings from the bursa of Fabricius, cloaca, and trachea, and finding the characteristic small (5 μm) oocysts can be diagnostic. Concentration using saturated sugar solution with examination by phase-contrast and/or interference-contrast microscopy is preferred.

There are no satisfactory control measures except isolation and good sanitation. All known anticoccidial drugs are ineffective against *Cryptosporidium* spp.

CORONAVIRAL ENTERITIS OF TURKEYS
(Bluecomb, Transmissible enteritis)

An acute, highly contagious disease of turkeys characterized by sudden onset, marked depression, anorexia, diarrhea, dehydration, and weight loss. Mortality may be high, particularly in poults, but loss of condition in growing and adult birds may be more important economically.

Etiology and Epidemiology: The causative agent is a coronavirus, but the clinical disease is complicated by other intestinal viral and bacterial infections. Bluecomb spreads by direct or indirect contact with infected birds or contaminated premises. Droppings of infected birds are rich in virus, and recovered birds may continue to shed virus for months. Environmental factors do not appear to influence the occurrence; however, the stress of adverse environment may contribute to the severity of the disease. Cold weather, especially freezing, increases survival of the virus.

Clinical Findings: A short incubation period, often 48-72 hr, is followed by general depression, anorexia, and diarrhea in the flock. Young poults appear cold, chirp constantly, and seek heat. Feed and water consumption drop markedly, and poults lose weight rapidly. Morbidity and mortality may approach 100% in uncontrolled outbreaks. Young birds have few lesions other than flaccid, distended intestines that contain excess fluid and gas. The ceca are distended with foamy, pale brown, fetid fluid.

Morbidity and mortality are variable in growing and adult turkeys. Profuse diarrhea, with mucoid threads or casts in the droppings, is common. Dehydration and weight loss are often pronounced, and recovery may require several weeks to regain lost weight. Cyanosis of the head is common. Breeder hens experience a severe drop in egg production and produce abnormal eggs with chalky shells.

Lesions in older birds are more extensive. Body musculature is dehydrated, and petechial hemorrhages may be seen on the viscera. Kidneys commonly are swollen and contain an excess of urates, and the pancreas may have multiple chalky white areas. Severe catarrhal enteritis is common, and mucoid casts may be present. The crop may be distended and contain sour-smelling fluid. The spleen is often small and pale gray.

Diagnosis: Although clinical findings and lesions are suggestive, definitive diagnosis requires laboratory techniques. Among these are demonstration of coronaviral antigen in intestines of affected birds by direct FA techniques, detection of coronavirus particles in intestinal contents by electron microscopy, reproduction of the disease in SPF poults with bacteria-free intestinal filtrates, and negative findings for common bacterial and protozoal infections. Disorders of poults that may produce similar signs include hexamitiasis (qv, p 1560), salmonellosis (qv, p 1596), inanition, and water deprivation. Other intestinal viruses (which are common in commercial flocks, including rotavirus, reovirus, astrovirus, and possibly others) can cause disease that resembles mild coronaviral enteritis. In older birds, septicemias such as fowl cholera (qv, p 1574) and erysipelas (qv, p 1571) may cause diagnostic confusion.

Prophylaxis and Treatment: Management and sanitation practices to minimize introduction of virus should be employed. Depopulation of problem premises followed by thorough cleaning and disinfection of buildings and equipment is effective in breaking the cycle of infection. Such farms are best cleaned during summer and should be left vacant for ≥1 mo.

Commercial biologics are not available. "Controlled" exposure programs have been used with variable success on some problem farms, but such procedures are not recommended except in unusual circumstances.

The course of disease outbreaks may be altered by good nursing care and judicious use of antibiotics and other drugs to combat secondary bacterial infections and dehydration. Affected birds in the brooder house should be given supplemental heat, and birds on range should be protected from adverse environmental conditions. The selection of an antibiotic is empiric at best, but tetracyclines, neomycin, streptomycin, penicillin, and bacitracin are among those used with variable success. Antibiotics may be added to drinking water in combination with calf milk-replacer and electrolyte, eg, 25 lb (11.4 kg) calf milk-replacer, 450 g of potassium chloride, and 100 g of antibiotic to 100 gal. (380 L) of water. Birds should be medicated for 7-10 days. During and after treatment, birds should be observed closely for secondary intestinal mycosis, a common sequela of antibiotic therapy.

DUCK VIRAL ENTERITIS
(DVE, Duck plague)

An acute, highly contagious infection of ducks, geese, and swans of all ages, characterized by sudden death, high mortality, and hemorrhages and necrosis in internal organs. It has been reported in domestic and wild waterfowl of Europe, Asia, North America, and Africa, and has resulted in serious or limited economic losses in the duck industries and massive and limited die-offs of wild waterfowl.

Etiology: The causal herpesvirus is nonhemagglutinating and nonhemadsorbing, and produces intranuclear inclusion bodies in infected tissues and tissue cultures. All strains are antigenically similar, but vary in virulence. Egg transmission probably does not occur in domestic ducks, but has been demonstrated in infected carrier wild waterfowl. Infection can be transmitted by parenteral, intranasal, or oral administration of infected tissues. Recovered birds may remain carriers.

Clinical Findings: The incubation period is 3-7 days. Sudden high and persistent mortality is often the first sign of the disease. Mortality may be 5-100% depending on the virulence of the virus; more adults die than young ducks. Mature ducks die in good flesh. Dead males may evidence prolapse of the penis. In laying flocks, egg production may drop sharply. Photophobia, inappetence, extreme thirst, droopiness, ataxia, nasal discharges, soiled vents, and a watery or bloody diarrhea may be seen. Ducklings evidence dehydration, weight loss, blue beaks, and blood-stained vents.

Lesions: There are tissue hemorrhages, free blood in the body cavities, destruction of lymphoid tissues, and degenerative changes in the parenchymatous organs. Petechial and ecchymotic hemorrhages are found on the heart, liver, pancreas, mesentery, and other organs. In the GI tract, specific enanthematous lesions may occur; these are macular mucosal hemorrhages that progress to yellowish white encrusted plaques, which can be found on the longitudinal mucosal folds of the esophagus, at the esophageal-proventricular junction, on the surface of the intestinal annular lymphoid bands, and in the cloaca. In young ducks, hemorrhages and degenerative changes may be found in the thymus and bursa. Ruptured yolk and free blood may be found in the abdominal cavity of laying ducks.

Diagnosis: A presumptive diagnosis may be based on the history and lesions. Isolation of the virus on the chorioallantoic membrane of susceptible embryonating duck eggs or in duck-embryo fibroblastic tissue culture, and neutralization of the virus with specific antiserum confirm the diagnosis. The disease should be reported to the appropriate regulatory agency.

Prophylaxis and Treatment: Contact with wild, free-flying waterfowl, or introduction of infected waterfowl must be avoided. Strict isolation of susceptible ducks is required. Control and eradication can be effected by depopulation, sanitation, and disinfection of premises. An effective chick-embryo-adapted, modified live vaccine has been approved for use in domestic ducks and zoological aviaries and by private aviculturists. It is most commonly used in domestic breeder ducks and is administered subcut. in the back of the neck in 0.5 mL doses; a booster is recommended 1 yr later. The live virus vaccine is not recommended for wild ducks.

DIGESTIVE TRACT HELMINTHIASIS
(Nematode and cestode infections)

Of the thousands of worm species extant, ~100 have been recognized in wild and domestic birds in the USA. Nematodes (roundworms) are the most significant in number of species and in economic impact.

Generally, nematodes have separate sexes with morphologic differences, eg, males of *Tetrameres* spp are elongate and slender, gravid females are globe-shaped.

The size and shape of nematode species vary widely; ascarids are sturdy and long (up to 4.5 in. [116 mm]), capillarids are slender and long (2.3 in. [60 mm]), but other nematodes are much shorter (0.08-0.48 in. [2-12 mm]). Cestodes (tapeworms) also vary in size. *Raillietina* spp may be >12 in. (30 cm), while *Davainea proglottina* often is <0.16 in. (4 mm). The proglottids of individual tapeworms are hermaphroditic. Tapeworms have been recovered in thousands from individual chickens or turkeys.

Transmission: Modern confinement rearing of poultry has reduced the frequency and variety of these endoparasite infections, which were common earlier in range birds and in backyard flocks. However, severe parasitism still may occur in floor-reared layers, breeders, or pen-reared game birds; contributing factors may be the use of built-up litter (which fosters the propagation of intermediate hosts), or the parasites' resistance to therapeutic drugs, or both.

Nematodes have either a species-specific direct life cycle with bird-to-bird transmission by ingestion of infective eggs or larvae, or an indirect cycle that requires an intermediate host (eg, insects, snails, or slugs). Eggs of many nematode species are resistant to low temperatures and disinfectants.

Cestodes require an intermediate host (eg, insects, crustaceans, earthworms, or snails). Floor layers, breeders, and broilers are infected with *R cesticillus* by ingestion of the intermediate host, small beetles that breed in contaminated litter. Cage layers in unscreened houses may become infected with *Choanotaenia infundibulum* by eating its intermediate host, the housefly.

Pathogenesis and Clinical Findings: *Ascaridia*, *Heterakis*, and *Capillaria* spp are widely distributed and cause such nonspecific signs as general unthriftiness, inactivity, depressed appetite, and retarded growth; death may result. A mere few ascarids may depress weight, and larger numbers may block the intestinal tract. This parasite, via the cloaca, may migrate up the oviduct to become enshelled later within the egg (an aesthetic, but not a public health problem, avoidable by careful egg-candling before the release of eggs to market).

Heterakis gallinarum, a mild pathogen, in large numbers may cause thickening, inflammation, or nodulation in the cecal walls. *Heterakis isolonche*, highly pathogenic in pheasants, may cause 50% mortality. *Heterakis gallinarum* carries *Histomonas meleagridis*, the blackhead organism (qv, p 1576).

Capillaria contorta in the mucosae of the crop and esophagus, and *C obsignata* in the wall of the small intestine, cause marked thickening and inflammation of the organs. Birds harboring large numbers of these thread-like worms become weak and emaciated, and may die.

Among other nematodes, *Amidostomum anseris* attacks the gizzard lining of ducks and geese, and causes dark discoloration, necrosis, and sloughing at the parasites' loci. *Dispharynx nasuta* causes ulceration, thickening, and maceration of the proventriculus; heavily infected birds may die. *Tetrameres americana*, a bright red worm discernible through the proventricular wall, causes diarrhea, emaciation, and with heavy infection, death. *Trichostrongylus tenuis* causes inflamed ceca, weight loss, anemia, and death, especially in young birds. *Ornithostrongylus quadriradiatus*, a bloodsucking parasite, causes pigeons to regurgitate bile-stained fluid mixed with food; greenish mucoid diarrhea from hemorrhagic intestines, emaciation, and death follow.

Most pathogenic tapeworms are found in the small intestine; the scolex, usually buried in the mucosa, generally causes mild lesions. *Davainea proglottina* may cause weight loss. *Raillietina tetragona* causes weight loss and decreased egg production; *R echinobothrida* produces granulomata at its attachment sites ("nodular disease").

Diagnosis: A reliable diagnosis can be made only by accurate identification of the individually recovered parasites; careful and complete necropsy techniques are essential. Only by specific recognition of the parasite can meaningful recommendations be made on flock therapy and management.

Table 2. Common Helminths in the Digestive Tract of Poultry

Parasite	Host	Intermediate Host or Life Cycle	Organ Infected	Pathogenicity
NEMATODES				
Amidostomum anseris	Duck, goose, pigeon	Direct	Gizzard	Severe
Ascaridia dissimilis	Turkey	Direct	Small intestine	Moderate
Ascaridia galli	Chicken, turkey, duck, quail	Direct	Small intestine	Moderate
Capillaria caudinflata (columbae)	Chicken, turkey, duck, game birds, pigeon	Earthworms	Small intestine	Moderate to severe
Capillaria contorta (annulata)	Chicken, turkey, duck, game birds	None or earthworms	Mouth, esophagus, crop	Severe
Capillaria obsignata	Chicken, turkey, goose, pigeon, quail	Direct	Small intestine, ceca	Severe
Cheilospirura hamulosa	Chicken, turkey, game birds	Grasshoppers, beetles	Gizzard	Moderate
Cyrnea colini	Turkey, game birds	Cockroaches	Proventriculus	Mild
Dispharynx nasuta	Chicken, turkey, game birds, pigeon	Sowbugs	Proventriculus	Moderate to severe
Gongylonema ingluvicola	Chicken, game birds	Beetles, cockroaches	Crop, esophagus, proventriculus	Mild
Heterakis gallinarum	Chicken, turkey, duck, game birds	Direct	Ceca	Mild, but transmits agent of histomoniasis
Ornithostrongylus quadriradiatus	Pigeon, dove	Direct	Small intestine	Severe
Subulura brumpti	Chicken, turkey, duck, game birds	Earwigs, grasshoppers, beetles, cockroaches	Ceca	Mild
Tetrameres americana	Chicken, turkey, duck, game birds, pigeon	Grasshoppers, cockroaches	Proventriculus	Moderate to severe
Trichostrongylus tenuis	Chicken, turkey, duck, game birds, pigeon	Direct	Ceca	Severe
CESTODES				
Choanotaenia infundibulum	Chicken	House flies	Upper intestine	Moderate
Davainea proglottina	Chicken	Slugs, snails	Duodenum	Severe
Metroliasthes lucida	Turkey	Grasshoppers	Intestine	Unknown
Raillietina cesticillus	Chicken	Beetles	Duodenum, jejunum	Mild
Raillietina echinobothrida	Chicken	Ants	Lower intestine	Severe, nodules
Raillietina tetragona	Chicken	Ants	Lower intestine	Severe

Treatment and Control: Improvement of sanitary practices and application of approved insecticides to soil and litter when premises are unoccupied may interrupt the parasite's life cycle by destroying its intermediate host. When the premises are restocked, groups of birds of different species or ages should be widely separated to avoid intergroup spread of parasites.

Only approved drugs may be used in birds producing eggs or meat for market. Because decisions on the acceptance and propriety of approved drugs are changed frequently, current information on any drug's regulatory status should be obtained before its use; label directions and recommended doses should be followed precisely.

Piperazine compounds are relatively nontoxic and widely used against ascariasis. Several piperazine salts are available; because only the piperazine moiety is efficacious, doses should be calculated based on mg of active piperazine/bird. Piperazine should be consumed by birds within a few hours because only relatively high concentrations of the drug eliminate worms; it may be given to chickens as a single dose, 50-100 mg/bird, or at 0.2-0.4% in their feed or at 0.1-0.2% in their drinking water; to turkeys at 100 mg/bird <12 wk old, 100-400 mg/bird ≥12 wk old, or in feed or water concentrations as for chickens.

Phenothiazine controls cecal worms in chickens at 0.5 g/bird, in turkeys at 1 g/bird, given in 1 day. Combined in drinking water, 1-day treatment, phenothiazine (0.5-0.56%) and piperazine (0.11%) remove both heterakids and ascarids.

Hygromycin B, 0.00088-0.00132% in feed, controls ascarids, cecal worms, and capillarids. Coumaphos, 0.004% in feed for 10-14 days for replacements, or 0.003% in feed for 14 days for layers, is used more commonly against capillarids. Butynorate, 0.07-0.14% in feed, is effective against tapeworms. Several other compounds are effective for helminth control, but currently are not approved for use: pyrantel tartrate and mebendazole against *A anseris*; levamisole against *Subulura brumpti*; mebendazole, thiabendazole, pyrantel tartrate, and citarin against *Trichostrongylus tenuis*; and hexachlorophene and niclosamide against tapeworms.

HEMORRHAGIC ENTERITIS OF TURKEYS

A widely distributed acute infection of turkeys >4 wk old, characterized by splenomegaly and intestinal hemorrhage.

Etiology: The causative virus, a type II avian adenovirus, is morphologically and serologically indistinguishable from the virus that causes marble spleen disease of pheasants (qv, p 1580). It can be propagated in B-lymphoblastoid cell lines of turkey origin. It is readily transmitted by oral contact with contaminated matter and remains infective for several weeks in the litter, but is inactivated by various disinfectants as well as drying. Primary viral replication occurs in reticuloendothelial cells, particularly in the spleen.

Clinical Findings and Lesions: The disease is characterized by acute onset, depression, bloody droppings, and death. Flock mortality may be 1-60% over a 2-wk period, although the usual mortality is 0.5-3%. An early age resistance to clinical disease, regardless of maternal antibody status, is recognized. Pathogenic strains of the virus can cause depression of both B- and T-cell immune responses, which may last up to 5 wk after exposure to the virus. Increased susceptibility to colibacillosis is often seen following outbreaks of the disease.

Specific lesions are confined to the spleen and intestines; the most obvious is severe hemorrhage into the intestine, with the upper parts being most involved. The spleen is enlarged and mottled, but may be small and pale if hemorrhage has been extensive.

Diagnosis: The lesions are characteristic, and can differentiate the disease from acute septicemias such as fowl cholera and erysipelas. Prominent reticuloendothelial hyperplasia with type II avian adenovirus intranuclear inclusion bodies in the spleen is diagnostic. *In vitro* tests for isolation, propagation, and neutralization of the virus are available, but require use and manipulation of special turkey B-lymphoblastoid cell lines. The ELISA is more sensitive than the agar-gel-precipitin test in identifying viral antigen and antibody.

Control: For years, control was based on vaccination by turkey-spleen-propagated avirulent strains of hemorrhagic enteritis virus or marble spleen disease virus of pheasants. Recently, vaccines produced in a turkey B-lymphoblastoid cell line have been developed and are being used in many areas. The vaccine is administered via the drinking water at 4-5 wk of age; however, age at vaccination may vary, depending on status of maternal antibody. In some cases, maternal antibody may interfere with vaccination until 5 wk of age. Immunity induced by vaccination or exposure to disease seems to be long lasting. Convalescent serum can be injected to prevent or reduce flock mortality during an outbreak.

HEXAMITIASIS

An acute, catarrhal enteritis of turkeys, pheasants, quail, chukar partridges, and peafowl, now rare in North America. The highest mortality occurs in 1- to 9-wk-old birds. Natural infection has not been observed in chickens. Pigeons are susceptible to another species of *Hexamita*.

Etiology: The causative protozoan parasite, *Hexamita meleagridis*, is spindle-shaped, averages 8 μm by 3 μm, and has 6 anterior and 2 posterior flagella. It has not yet been cultured in artificial media, although it has been grown in the allantoic cavity of developing chicken and turkey embryos. It is transmitted directly by ingestion of infected feces. Encysted hexamitids may be more important in transmission than free flagellates. Many survivors become carriers and shed parasites in their droppings.

Clinical Findings and Lesions: The nonspecific signs include watery diarrhea, dry unkempt feathers, listlessness, and rapid weight loss although the birds continue to eat. Birds may die in convulsions. Bulbous dilatations of the small intestine (especially duodenum and upper jejunum) filled with watery contents are characteristic. The crypts of Lieberkühn contain myriad *H meleagridis*, which attach to the epithelial cells by their posterior flagella.

Diagnosis: Diagnosis depends on finding the flagellates by microscopical examination of scrapings of the duodenal and jejunal mucosa. *Hexamita* sp move with a rapid, darting motion (in contrast to the jerky motion of trichomonads). To avoid contamination of instruments with other cecal protozoa, the duodenum should be opened first. *Hexamita* sp may be demonstrated in poults that have been dead for several hours if the scrapings are placed in a drop of warm (104°F [40°C]), isotonic saline solution on the slide. Finding a few *Hexamita* in birds >10 wk old does not justify a diagnosis.

Prophylaxis and Treatment: Because many birds remain carriers, breeder turkeys and poults should be raised on separate premises if possible, preferably with separate attendants. Wire platforms should be used under feeders and waterers. Pheasants and quail may also be carriers.

Furazolidone (0.0055% in the feed continuously), oxytetracycline (0.22% in the feed for 2 wk), chlortetracycline (0.022-0.044% in the feed for 2 wk), and butynorate have been used to prevent and treat hexamitiasis. Treatment does not substitute for adequate sanitation and management programs.

NECROTIC ENTERITIS

An acute enterotoxemia, characterized by sudden onset, explosive mortality, and confluent necrosis of the mucosa of the small intestine, that primarily affects 2- to 12-wk-old broilers. It also has been reported in other avian species in the same age range.

Etiology, Transmission, and Pathogenesis: Necrotic enteritis has been associated with *Clostridium perfringens* Type C, and with toxigenic strains of Type A. It occurs most frequently in broiler houses with old, built-up litter.

Enterotoxemia is likely to occur only when the gut microecology is altered drastically. Such alterations may result from changes in the gut contents due to variation in the quality or quantity of feed ingested, depressed motility, damage of the intestinal mucosa by aggressive pathogens (eg, salmonellae or coccidia), or toxins. These changes may promote clostridial colonization with subsequent toxin production. Necrotic enteritis has been reproduced experimentally by infusing numerous clostridial cells and preformed toxin directly into the duodenum.

Clinical Findings, Lesions, and Diagnosis: Infected chickens are depressed and may have diarrhea. Clinical features progress rapidly; death occurs within a few hours. The disease persists in a flock for 5-10 days and mortality is 2-50%. The breast is dehydrated and darkened; the liver is usually swollen and congested; the small intestine is ballooned and friable and contains foul-smelling, brown fluid; the mucosa is covered with a brownish, diphtheritic membrane.

Large numbers of short, thick, gram-positive rods observed in a stained smear of a mucosal scraping help to make a presumptive diagnosis. Histological findings consist of coagulative necrosis of one-third to one-half the thickness of the intestinal mucosa, and masses of short, thick, rod-like bacteria in the fibrinonecrotic debris. *Clostridium perfringens* can be cultured anaerobically from intestinal contents. All toxigenic types of *C perfringens* (A, B, C, D, and E) are culturally identical and can be distinguished only by a toxin-neutralization test. Lesions produced by *Eimeria brunetti* can be similar to those in necrotic enteritis, but uncomplicated coccidiosis (qv, p 1551) is seldom as acute or severe. Ulcerative enteritis (qv, p 1563) can resemble necrotic enteritis clinically, but the intestinal lesions are usually focal and located in the ileum, ceca, and rectum.

Treatment and Control: Strict sanitation and efforts to prevent coccidiosis, salmonellosis, and other intestinal infections minimize the risk of necrotic enteritis. Drastic changes in feed should be avoided, and feed and water should be monitored for contaminants that alter intestinal motility or devitalize intestinal mucosa. Bacitracin methylene disalicylate is effective for preventing and treating necrotic enteritis. The preventive level is 50 g/ton (55 ppm) in the feed; therapeutic levels are 100-200 g/ton (110-220 ppm). Penicillin, erythromycin, and the tetracyclines at 20 ppm in the feed also are said to be effective.

ROTAVIRAL INFECTIONS IN CHICKENS, TURKEYS, AND PHEASANTS

A viral disease characterized by enteritis and diarrhea in young birds. Rotaviral infections in chickens without clinical signs have also been described. Mortality is variable and is usually due to dehydration and emaciation.

Avian rotaviruses consist of 4 distinct serotypes (A-D): Group A rotaviruses share a common group antigen with mammalian rotaviruses; group D rotaviruses have been identified only in avian species. The relationships of the other 2 avian serotypes to mammalian serotypes have not yet been established. Transmission is horizontally by the oral route. Egg transmission has not been reported.

Early signs of diarrhea (wet litter), depression, and poor or abnormal appetite can be observed 2-5 days after infection. Dehydration occurs rapidly, and mortality can be as high as 30-50% in pheasants and turkeys. The survivors appear healthy but smaller than normal. Lesions consist of dilated intestines filled with yellowish watery contents with gas bubbles. Often, the carcass is dehydrated.

Early diarrhea and inappetence that sometimes ends with death is indicative but not pathognomonic of rotaviral infection. Fecal samples or intestinal contents can be examined directly or after ultracentrifugation by electron microscopy with negative staining. Numerous rotaviral particles can be observed, ~70 nm in diameter, with double-shelled capsids, and are distinguishable from reovirus by their more sharply defined outer edges. For viral isolation in chicken-embryo liver cells or chick kidney cells, fecal material must be treated with trypsin. Isolated rotaviruses belong mostly to serotype A, and in general do not cause cytopathic effects on primary isolation. The presence of virus can be demonstrated 2-3 days postinoculation by immunofluorescent staining.

No commercial vaccines are available; thorough cleaning and disinfection of infected houses is advisable to limit infection. There is no specific treatment.

THRUSH
(Candidiasis, Moniliasis, Sour crop)

A mycotic disease of the digestive tract of chickens and turkeys caused by *Candida (Monilia, Oidium) albicans*. Lesions are most frequently found in the crop and consist of thickened mucosa and whitish, raised, circular ulcers. The mouth and esophagus may show the same lesions. Hemorrhagic spots, necrotic debris, and pseudomembranes are not uncommon. Depression and emaciation may be the only clinical signs. An accurate diagnosis may be established by demonstrating tissue invasion histologically and by culture of the organism. Young chicks and poults are most susceptible, and malabsorption of feed occurs, which leads to a variety of secondary nutritional problems. This disease commonly occurs following use of therapeutic levels of various antibiotics.

Minimizing use of antibiotics in poultry feed helps reduce the incidence of thrush, however nystatin (110 ppm) in the feed gives significant protection against it. Affected birds can be treated successfully with copper sulfate at a dilution of 1:2000 in the drinking water, or nystatin (220 ppm) in the feed.

TRICHOMONIASIS

A disease of domestic fowl, pigeons, doves, and hawks characterized, in most cases, by caseous accumulations in the throat and usually accompanied by weight loss. It has been termed "canker", "roup", and, in hawks, "frounce" (qv, p 1006). Falconers have known the disease for centuries.

Etiology: The causative organism is a flagellated protozoan, *Trichomonas gallinae*, which lives in the sinuses, mouth, throat, esophagus, and other organs. It is more prevalent among domestic pigeons and wild doves than among chickens or turkeys, although severe outbreaks have been reported in domestic fowl. Some strains of *T gallinae* are highly fatal in pigeons and doves. Hawks may become diseased after eating infected birds, and commonly show liver lesions, with or without throat involvement. Parent pigeons and doves transmit the infection to their offspring in contaminated pigeon milk. Contaminated water probably is the most important source of infection for chickens and turkeys.

Clinical Findings: The disease course is rapid. The first lesions appear as small, yellowish areas on the oral mucosa. They grow rapidly and coalesce to form masses that frequently completely block the esophagus, and may prevent the bird from closing its mouth. Much fluid may accumulate in the mouth. There is a watery ocular discharge and, in more advanced stages, exudate about the eyes may result in blindness. Birds lose weight rapidly and become weak and listless. Death usually ensues within 8-10 days. In chronic infections, birds appear healthy, although trichomonads usually can be demonstrated in scrapings from the mucous membranes of the throat.

Lesions: The bird may be riddled with caseous necrotic foci. The mouth and esophagus contain a mass of necrotic material that may extend into the skull and sometimes through the surrounding tissues of the neck to involve the skin. In the esophagus and crop, the lesions may be yellow, rounded, raised areas, with a central conical caseous spur, often referred to as "yellow buttons". The crop may be covered by a yellowish diphtheritic membrane that may extend to the glandular stomach. The gizzard and intestine are not involved. Lesions of internal organs are most frequent in the liver; they vary from a few small, yellow areas of necrosis to almost complete replacement of liver tissue by caseous necrotic debris. Adhesions and involvement of other internal organs appear to be contact extensions of the liver lesions.

Diagnosis: Lesions of *T gallinae* infection are quite characteristic, but not pathognomonic; those of pox and other infections can be similar. Diagnosis should be confirmed by laboratory demonstration of the causative trichomonad. This is accomplished readily by microscopical examination of a smear of mucus or fluid from the throat. The organisms can be cultured easily on various artificial media such as 0.2% Loeffler's dried blood serum in Ringer's solution, or in saline-bicarbonate solution; or a 2% solution of pigeon serum in isotonic salt solution. Good growth is obtained at 98.6°F (37°C). Antibiotics may be used to reduce bacterial contamination.

Control: Because *T gallinae* infection in pigeons is so readily transmitted from parent to offspring in the normal feeding process, chronically infected birds should be removed at once. In pigeons, recovery from infection with a less virulent strain of *T gallinae* appears to provide some protection against subsequent attack by a more virulent strain. Metronidazole PO at 60 mg/kg body wt has prevented mortality. Dimetridazole PO at 50 mg/kg body wt or in the drinking water (0.05% for 5-6 days) is reported to suppress the disease. These 2 drugs are not registered for use in the USA but are available in other countries.

ULCERATIVE ENTERITIS
(Quail disease)

An acute or chronic enteritis primarily in bobwhite quail (*Colinus virginianus*), but frequently seen in 5- to 7-wk old chickens, and also reported in young turkeys, pheasants, grouse, and other gallinaceous birds. It occurs worldwide.

Etiology, Epidemiology, and Pathogenesis: *Clostridium colinum* is a fastidious and difficult-to-culture, spore-forming, anaerobic rod, ~1 μm wide by 3-4 μm long. The spores are oval and subterminal.

The organism is shed in the feces of infected birds. Quail and chickens that develop chronic disease remain carriers. To induce experimental infection in quail, $\geq 10^6$ organisms given PO are required; chickens require $\geq 10^9$ organisms. Outbreaks of ulcerative enteritis in chickens may follow outbreaks of coccidiosis, infectious bursal disease, and inclusion body hepatitis. After oral infection, the organism produces enteritis and ulcers in the lower third of the intestinal tract. Some organisms may pass to the liver via the portal circulation and produce diffuse or focal liver necrosis. Although large numbers of bacteria resembling *C colinum* can be seen in the ulcerative lesions of the gut and necrotizing lesions of the liver, histological features of these lesions suggest that in addition to bacterial invasion, a toxin also may be involved in the pathogenesis of this disease. However, no toxin has yet been identified.

Clinical Findings: In susceptible quail, the disease is acute, and mortality may be 100% in a few days. In chickens, signs are usually less dramatic, and mortality is ≤10% during the clinical course of the disease (≥2-3 wk). Some affected quail or chickens may die without obvious signs of disease or weight loss. Infected birds discharge characteristic droppings that are streaked with urates surrounded by a watery ring. Chronically affected birds are listless and anorectic; they appear humped-up, with the neck retracted and eyes partially closed.

Lesions: The primary lesions are found in the lower third of the small intestine, ceca, and liver. Lesions in the intestine and ceca vary from punctate hemorrhages to ulceration. The well-defined ulcers vary in size and may be 5 mm in diameter. The larger ulcers may show yellow diphtheritic membranes with a depressed center and raised edges. Perforating ulcers are frequent and cause local or diffuse peritonitis. Liver lesions appear as yellow isolated foci or irregularly shaped yellow areas in the parenchyma. The only other organ that may show lesions is the spleen; it may be enlarged and either hemorrhagic or necrotic.

Diagnosis: Although histomoniasis (qv, p 1576) and inclusion body hepatitis (qv, p 1550) may superficially resemble ulcerative enteritis, coccidiosis (qv, p 1551) causes the greatest problem in differential diagnosis. Often, both infections occur simultaneously. In ulcerative enteritis, the spore-forming rods that resemble *C colinum* can be demonstrated in gram-stained blood, liver, and spleen in septicemic birds. *Clostridium colinum* can be isolated from infected livers and spleens cultured under strict anaerobic conditions on pre-reduced anaerobic blood agar plates.

Treatment and Control: Bacitracin and streptomycin are the most effective drugs; bacitracin is used in the feed at 0.005-0.01%, streptomycin at 0.006%. Either drug can be given in the drinking water prophylactically or therapeutically. In addition, the tetracyclines and furazolidone at 0.02% in the feed are also effective.

Medicated flocks often have little resistance against reinfection. Therefore, contaminated litter should be removed, and treatment may need to be continued or repeated periodically. Because bobwhite quail are highly susceptible, they should be raised on wire or slat floors as a prophylactic measure.

AVIAN PARAMYXOVIRUS TYPE 3 IN TURKEYS

Uncomplicated infections of laying turkeys with avian paramyxovirus type 3 (PMV-3) may severely decrease egg production.

Etiology and Epidemiology: Newcastle disease (ND) virus is a prototype paramyxovirus, but numerous serologically distinct viruses that fulfill the criteria of that genus have been isolated from avian species. These have been placed in 9 serotypes, PMV-1 to PMV-9. ND viruses (a PMV-1) represent the most important paramyxovirus pathogens for poultry. However, PMV-3 viruses frequently have been demonstrated to infect turkeys and have been associated with respiratory and egg production problems. Turkey PMV-3 isolates have been differentiated from those of other birds by use of monoclonal antibodies.

Turkeys and imported exotic birds appear to be the 2 predominant sources of PMV-3 viruses. Evidence suggests that in the imports, the viruses are associated primarily with psittacines, although they have been isolated from passerines in quarantine. PMV-3 viruses have not been isolated from feral birds and, although chickens are susceptible experimentally, turkeys are the only poultry known to be naturally infected. The method of transmission between turkeys is unclear. Primary introduction into a flock or geographical area presumably results from contact with infected feral birds. Spread within a flock is usually slow. PMV-3 infections of turkeys have been reported from North America and Europe.

Clinical Findings: In uncomplicated infections in turkeys, the first sign is often a drop in egg production. However, early mild respiratory signs have been reported, which suggests the respiratory tract may be the initial site of infection. The drop in egg production varies considerably with the age of the birds and secondary infections. In complicated infections of birds a few weeks into lay, the effective loss may be ~1-2 eggs/bird/wk for 5-6 wk, after which production returns to expected levels. Production problems are associated with a high level of white-shelled eggs, and the hatchability and fertility of the eggs produced are also reduced. Infection at, or just before, the point of lay may result in more serious losses, with the flock failing to reach target production throughout the laying period. Far more serious respiratory disease and egg production problems have been recorded when dual infection with ND virus, influenza viruses, chlamydiae, mycoplasmas, or other bacteria has occurred. There have been no reported studies on the lesions associated with PMV-3 infections of turkeys.

Diagnosis: Most diagnoses have been by clinical signs and serology. Antibodies to PMV-3 may be detected by hemagglutination inhibition (HI) tests. ND virus and PMV-3 viruses cross-react in HI tests, which causes diagnostic problems in vaccinated birds. ND-vaccinated birds show a rise in HI titers to both viruses if subsequently infected with PMV-3 virus. PMV-3 virus can be isolated from tracheal or fecal swabs or tissue samples from infected birds by inoculation of 8- to 10-day-old embryonating chicken eggs via the allantoic cavity. Confirmation of the virus as PMV-3 can be done by HI testing with specific antiserum; proper controls are important because of the cross-reaction with ND viruses. PMV-3 viruses are not readily isolated from infected turkeys, which suggests the excretion period may be limited.

Prophylaxis and Control: PMV-3 viruses appear to spread slowly. Good hygiene, including careful disinfection and time between restocking, has not always prevented infection in subsequent flocks. Inactivated, oil-emulsion vaccines are available in the USA, the UK, and other European countries for use in turkey breeding flocks. These are injected twice, 4 wk apart, before the birds begin to lay (usually when 20-24 wk old).

AVIAN SPIROCHETOSIS
(Avian borreliosis)

An acute, febrile, septicemic, bacterial disease of a wide variety of birds. The causal organism, a blood-inhabiting, actively motile spirochete, *Borrelia anserina*, is ~0.2-0.3 μm wide and 8-20 μm long and consists of 5-8 loosely arranged coils. No reliable data are available concerning *in vitro* cultivation. It can be propagated in embryonating duck or chick embryos, or young ducks or chicks.

The disease is found worldwide, but generally in temperate or tropical regions, wherever the biological vectors are found. The notable worldwide vector is *Argas (Persicargas) persicus*, the "cosmopolitan" fowl tick, but other *Argas* spp transmit the disease in different geographic areas. In the western USA, a highly efficient vector is *A (P) sanchezi*.

Diverse immunological and serological types of *B anserina* have been demonstrated in many areas. Recovery from one type confers solid immunity against the homologous types for ≥1 yr, but none against heterologous strains. Relapses, such as occur with some human *Borrelia* infections, are unknown in *B anserina* infection of birds; any reinfection can be attributed to a heterologous type.

Transmission: Generally, an infected *Argas* tick can transmit the disease at every feeding, and maintains the infection throughout larval, nymphal, and adult stages. The ticks also transmit the infection transovarially, ie, the F_1 larvae are infective. *Borrelia*-infected ticks remain infected despite feeding on chicks hyperimmune to *Borrelia anserina*, or on chicks with high blood levels of anti-*Borrelia* chemotherapeutic agents, such as the penicillins. Other vectors (lice, mosquitoes, some species of ticks, inanimate objects) can transmit the spirochete mechanically to a susceptible host whenever the piercing apparatus becomes contaminated with *Borrelia*-positive blood. Ingestion of bile-stained fecal droppings containing the spirochete, as well as acts of cannibalism during spirochetemia can result in infection. Following the bite of an infected tick, the incubation period is ~4-7 days.

Clinical Findings: Signs are highly variable, depending on the virulence of the spirochete, and thus are not pathognomonic. They include listlessness, depression, somnolence, moderate to marked shivering, and increased thirst. Young birds are affected more severely than older ones. During the initial stages of the disease, there is usually a greenish yellow diarrhea with increased urates. The course of the disease is 1-2 wk. Mild strains are not unusual. However, in many tick-infested geographical areas, morbidity can approach 100% and mortality >90% has been recorded.
Lesions: An enlarged spleen with petechial or ecchymotic hemorrhages is the most notable gross lesion. This "mottled" or "marbled" appearance is not unlike spleens in marble spleen disease of pheasants (qv, p 1580). However, a contrasting situation may be observed in Mongolian pheasants, in which the spleen is reported to be small and pale. Occasionally, the liver may be swollen and contain focal areas of necrosis. Kidneys may be enlarged and pale. A green, catarrhal enteritis can often be observed.

Diagnosis: Diagnosis rests on demonstration of *Borrelia* in the blood, either as actively motile *Borrelia* during darkfield microscopy, or as stained spirochetes in Giemsa-stained blood smears. In young birds, the *Borrelia* may reach vast numbers per oil-immersion field and persist for several days. Older birds usually have low numbers of *Borrelia* that are detected only with difficulty, or not at all, and that persist for only 1-2 days. Anemia is common and results in increased numbers of immature RBC. Agar-gel diffusion and various serological tests have been described, but are of questionable value due to diverse serotypes that exist in some localities. Specific agglutinins clump the spirochetes in successively larger clumps during the terminal stages of the disease. Agglutination-lysis then begins to disintegrate these clumps; spirochetal degradation products are liberated, and they may result in pyrexia. Death occurs most often 1-3 days after *Borrelia* disappear from the bloodstream.

Treatment and Control: Several chemotherapeutic agents are effective. The most widely used are penicillin derivatives, but the streptomycins and tetracyclines are also effective. The antibiotics can be completely efficacious if the regimen is instituted when the number of spirochetes per oil-immersion field is low or moderate; however, if large numbers of spirochetes are present in the bloodstream when chemotherapy is begun, the sudden liberation of large quantities of spirochetal degradation products can result in more deaths than no treatment.
Control must first be directed against the biological vector. *Argas* ticks are notable for their long life span, ability to survive for extended periods without a blood meal, efficiency in transmitting the spirochete, and an ability to remain securely hidden in cracks and crevices often beyond the effective reach of pesticides. Accordingly, control is difficult. A combination of tick eradication and immunization offers the most effective means of control.
Immunization can be highly successful and, next to eradication of the biological vector, is the preferred method of control. Bacterins prepared from infective blood have been used with success. The most widely used bacterins are egg-propagated products composed of yolk material containing the spirochetes, but whole-egg propagated bacterins have been used successfully; usually 1-2 IM injections suffice. Formalin (0.2%) is usually used to inactivate the spirochetes. Extreme care must be employed to use the appropriate serotype(s) of the spirochete in any given locality. Little if any cross-protection is afforded to different serotypes.

CAMPYLOBACTERIOSIS
(Avian vibrionic hepatitis, Avian infectious hepatitis)

A contagious, primarily intestinal, bacterial infection of various birds and mammals including man (qv, p 102). Subclinical infection is common in chickens and turkeys. Clinical infection in chickens characterized by a major decline in egg production, morbidity, and mortality is now rarely seen.

Etiology: The causal agent, *Campylobacter fetus* subsp *jejuni* (*Vibrio hepaticus*), resembles a *Vibrio* and can be isolated on 10% blood agar under reduced oxygen tension or by yolk-sac inoculation of 5- to 8-day chicken embryos. The embryos die in ~4 days, and the bacterium can be demonstrated in stained yolk smears or by culture of the yolk on blood agar. Isolates vary in their biochemical, serological, and pathogenic properties.

Clinical Findings: Infection in chickens typically is subclinical and confined to the intestinal tract. In clinical infections, only a few birds in a flock appear affected at any one time, but occasionally the disease is acute, with sudden deaths. In subacutely affected pullet flocks, egg production lags, while in older flocks, egg production may decrease as much as 35% over extended periods. Severely affected birds lose weight; have shriveled, dry, and scaly combs; are listless; and roost or stand apart from the rest of the flock. Less severely affected birds may appear normal, but their egg production fluctuates.

Lesions: Older chickens exhibit variable hemorrhagic and necrotic changes in the liver. Some have many small hemorrhages, with occasional bubble-like hematocysts under the capsule; this sometimes ruptures and releases blood into the body cavity. Other livers have a few pinhead-sized, grayish white necrotic foci, or are enlarged and mahogany-brown, or firm and friable and have irregular asterisk- or cauliflower-shaped necrotic areas up to 1 cm in diameter. Other findings include a bile-stained liver, ascites and hydropericardium, enlarged and pale kidneys, and catarrhal enteritis. In young chickens, the heart lesions are more severe and consistent than in mature birds.

The histological lesions in the liver range from early fatty metamorphosis and vascular changes to lymphocytic and heterophilic infiltration of the portal triad and focal necrosis of the parenchyma. Inflammatory cells may infiltrate the liver capsule, and the kidneys may have focal accumulations of heterophils and lymphocytes. The numbers of heterophils, thrombocytes, and total WBC are increased; Hgb, PCV, RBC, and lymphocytes are decreased.

Diagnosis: A presumptive diagnosis can be made from a typical history of low egg production, an increased number of culls, and characteristic lesions. A rapid technique for confirming diagnosis is the examination of bile by phase-contrast microscopy. *Campylobacter* sp also can be isolated from the bile or liver using the technique described above; typical "*Vibrio*" forms appear in a stained smear or in a wet-mount with phase-contrast microscopy. The bacterium can be isolated from feces with appropriate selective media. Other bacterial infections such as fowl cholera, pullorum, and typhoid may produce similar liver lesions.

Treatment: Dihydrostreptomycin sulfate (25 mg/lb [55 mg/kg] body wt, once IM) or furazolidone (0.02% in mash on an all-mash diet for 2 wk and 0.01% for a further 2 wk) gives good control, if given early in an outbreak. Since exposure apparently confers little immunity, reinfection sometimes occurs. Since most strains of *Campylobacter* sp have been found highly susceptible to erythromycin in sensitivity tests, this drug may be of value in treating infected flocks.

CHLAMYDIOSIS
(Psittacosis, Ornithosis)

An inapparent to peracute to chronic infection of wild and domestic birds, characterized by intestinal, respiratory, or systemic infection. It is transmissible to other animals including man. The disease occurs worldwide and is particularly important in colonial nesting species, domestic poultry (turkeys, pigeons, and ducks), and in caged birds (primarily psittacines), both captured and aviary-bred (*see also* p 1002).

Disease in man usually follows exposure to air- or dust-borne organisms when infected birds are processed at dressing plants, confined in breeding aviaries, or there is close proximity to even a single infected pet bird. Some individuals, especially those with impaired cell-mediated immunity, are more susceptible than others. Simple precautions are to use a detergent disinfectant to wet the feathers of dead birds, wear a dust mask or plastic face shield and gloves, and use a fan-exhausted examining hood.

Etiology and Epidemiology: The cause is any avian strain of *Chlamydia psittaci*, an obligate intracellular bacterium. All chlamydial strains contain an identical genus-specific antigen but may differ in the antigenic specificity of their cell-wall antigens.

Respiratory discharges or feces from infected birds contain infective elementary bodies; airborne particles and dusts may spread the organism. Infected nestlings in colonies or breeding aviaries may become carriers and shed the organism for an extended time if they survive. Environmental stress may provoke a recurrence of frank disease in carriers, which may result in transmission of the organism. Unusually virulent chlamydial strains that produce high mortality have been found in gulls, egrets, turkeys, and some psittacines. Less virulent strains are usually found in psittacines, pigeons, and ducks. All strains appear to be infectious to man.

Clinical Findings and Lesions: Nasal and ocular discharges, conjunctivitis, sinusitis, diarrhea, dullness, weakness, inappetence, and weight loss are often seen. Airsacculitis, pericarditis, perihepatitis, and peritonitis with serofibrinous exudate, focal necrosis in liver and spleen, and hepatosplenomegaly are common in acutely affected birds. Chronic infections, seen frequently in Psittacidae and Columbidae, may be characterized only by an enlarged spleen, an enlarged, discolored liver, or both. Lesions are often absent in inapparent infections even though birds are shedding the organism.

Diagnosis: A tentative diagnosis may be made by detection of intracytoplasmic groups of chlamydiae in impression smears of diseased organs stained by the Gimenez, Giemsa, or Macchiavellos method. Confirmation should be made by a laboratory prepared to isolate and identify chlamydiae. Freshly collected heart, pericardial sac, air sacs, and spleen should be shipped in a chlamydia-transport medium. Freezing is often detrimental to the organism; refrigeration and prompt delivery are preferred. Antibiotics should be added to transport media to reduce bacterial contamination. When the disease is suspected in nonexpendable birds, isolation attempts should be made, preferably from choanal or cloacal swabs. Cotton swabs, if used, must be properly discarded after expressing material collected into chlamydia-transport medium for shipment. Because of intermittent shedding of organisms, several samples from the same bird or from several birds may be needed. Serological testing is of value, particularly by complement fixation.

Thyroid enlargement (from iodine deficiency) or mites (*Sternostoma* sp) may cause respiratory difficulty in pet birds. Swollen spleen and liver along with severe respiratory distress may result from hemosporidial (*Plasmodium, Leucocytozoon* spp), systemic bacterial, toxic, or acute viral diseases. Aspergillosis is common in birds. Influenza and mycoplasmosis produce respiratory signs and lesions. Fowl cholera and colibacillosis may produce similar lesions in turkeys.

Prophylaxis and Treatment: Chlamydiosis is relatively rare in poultry. Why outbreaks are sporadic is not clear. Preventive measures, such as screening houses against wild bird entry, are justified, but drug prophylaxis, in the absence of cases in the area, is unwarranted. Effective vaccines are not available. On tentative diagnosis, treatment with chlortetracycline (CTC) should be initiated. Poultry flocks should be given 400 g of CTC/ton of mash feed without supplemental calcium. In confirmed cases, treatment should be continued 2 wk. Such treatment usually stops losses and allows birds to be marketed, after a 2-day withdrawal, without danger to processing plant workers or consumers. However, there have been reports of persons contracting chlamydial infections during the further processing of infectious turkey products. Birds should not be retained for future production. Outbreaks should be reported to public health and regulatory officials.

COLIBACILLOSIS
(Colisepticemia, *Escherichia coli* infection)

A common systemic disease of worldwide economic importance in poultry. It occurs as acute fatal septicemia or subacute pericarditis and airsacculitis.

Etiology: *Escherichia coli* is a gram-negative, rod-shaped bacterium normally found in the intestines of poultry and most other animals; although most are nonpathogenic, a limited number produce extraintestinal· infections. Pathogenic strains are most commonly of the 02, 078, 01, 035, and 036 serotypes, but a large number of others also produce disease. Virulence factors include the capacity to resist phagocytosis, utilization of highly efficient iron acquisition systems, resistance to killing by serum, and adherence to respiratory epithelium. The capacity to bind Congo red dye when grown on special media has been used in some laboratories as an *in vitro* phenotypic marker for pathogenic strains.

Pathogenesis: Large numbers of *E coli* are maintained in the poultry house environment through fecal contamination. Initial exposure to pathogenic *E coli* may occur in the hatchery from infected or contaminated eggs, but systemic infection usually requires predisposing environmental or infectious causes. Mycoplasmosis, infectious bronchitis, Newcastle disease, hemorrhagic enteritis, and turkey bordetellosis are often complicated by colibacillosis. Poor air quality and other environmental stresses may also predispose to *E coli* infections.

Systemic infection occurs when large numbers of pathogenic *E coli* gain access to the bloodstream from the respiratory tract or possibly intestine. Bacteremia progresses to septicemia and death, or extends the infection to serosal surfaces, pericardium, joints, and other organs.

Clinical Findings and Lesions: Signs are nonspecific and vary with age, organs involved, and concurrent diseases. Young birds dying of acute septicemia have few lesions except for enlarged, hyperemic liver and spleen with increased fluid in body cavities. Birds that survive septicemia develop subacute fibrinopurulent airsacculitis, pericarditis, perihepatitis, and lymphocytic depletion of bursa and thymus. (Unusually pathogenic salmonellae produce similar lesions in chicks.) Although airsacculitis is a classic lesion of colibacillosis, whether it results from primary respiratory exposure or extension of serositis is unclear. Sporadic lesions include pneumonia, arthritis, osteomyelitis, and salpingitis.

Diagnosis: Isolation of a pure culture of *E coli* from heart blood, liver, or typical visceral lesions in a fresh carcass indicates primary or secondary colibacillosis. Consideration should be given to predisposing infections and environmental factors. Pathogenicity of isolates is established when parenteral inoculation of young chicks or poults results in fatal septicemia or typical lesions within 3 days.

Control: Treatment strategies include attempts to control predisposing infections or environmental factors, and early use of antibacterials indicated by susceptibility tests. Commercial bacterins, administered to breeder hens or chicks, have provided some protection against homologous *E coli* serotypes.

DUCK VIRAL HEPATITIS

An acute, highly contagious, viral disease of young ducklings, characterized by a short incubation period, sudden onset, high mortality, and characteristic liver lesions. Three distinct types of duck hepatitis virus (DHV) have been isolated from diseased ducks. The disease is of economic importance in all duck-raising areas of the world. A natural outbreak of DHV Type I has been reported in mallard ducklings. Experimental Type I infections have been produced in goslings, turkey poults, young pheasants, quail, and guinea fowl.

Etiology: The originally described and most virulent DHV, Type I, is a picornavirus and is readily propagated in chick and duck embryos. It does not produce hemagglutinins. Field experience with Type I indicates that egg transmission does not occur. It can be transmitted experimentally by parenteral or oral administration of infected tissues.

Viruses differing from classic DHV Type I have been recognized as causes of hepatitis in ducklings. Of these, DHV Type II is considered to be an astrovirus; DHV Type III is a picornavirus, antigenically distinct from Type I virus, and cannot be propagated in chick embryos.

Clinical Findings, Lesions, and Diagnosis: The incubation period for Type I virus is 18-48 hr. Affected ducklings become lethargic, paddle spasmodically, and die within minutes, typically with opisthotonos. Although adults may become infected, clinical signs have not been seen in ducks >7 wk old. Mortality may be as high as 95% in ducklings. Practically all deaths occur within 1 wk after onset of signs. Inadequate nutrition and intoxications may increase duckling susceptibility.

The clinical course of DHV Type II infection has been reported to be similar to that of Type I, and can occur in ducklings immune to Type I infection. DHV Type III infections occur in ducklings <2 wk old despite immunity to Type I virus. The clinical course of Type III infection is less severe, and mortality rarely is >30%.

The lesions caused by all 3 types of DHV are similar. The principal pathognomonic lesion is an enlarged liver covered with hemorrhagic foci up to 1 cm in diameter. The spleen may be enlarged and mottled. Kidneys may be swollen, and renal blood vessels congested.

A presumptive diagnosis is based on the history and lesions. Virus isolation or serum neutralization tests may be used for positive identification. Types II and III viruses are not neutralized by classic Type I antiserum.

Prophylaxis and Treatment: Prophylaxis is by strict isolation, particularly during the first 5 wk of age. Contact with wild waterfowl should be avoided. Rats have been reported as a reservoir host of the virus; therefore, pest control is indicated.

Immunization of breeder ducks with modified live virus vaccines, employing Types I, II, and III viruses, provides parenteral immunity that effectively prevents high losses in young ducklings. The Type I virus vaccine is administered subcut. in the neck to breeder ducks at 16, 20, and 24 wk of age and q12wk thereafter throughout the laying period. The 3 initial immunizations are advisable for passive protection of ducklings.

The chick-embryo origin, modified live Type I virus vaccine also can be employed for early vaccination of Type-I-susceptible ducklings (progeny of nonimmune breeders). This vaccine is administered subcut. or by foot web stab method in a single dose to day-old ducklings. These ducklings rapidly develop an active immunity over 3-4 days.

Antibody against Type I virus, prepared from the eggs of hyperimmunized chickens, administered subcut. in the neck, at the time of initial loss, is an effective flock treatment.

ERYSIPELAS

A worldwide disease generally manifest in poultry as an acute septicemia; 1 or 2 birds are found dead, but in ensuing days, mortality increases dramatically. The disease is most important in turkeys; however, there have been economically significant outbreaks in chickens, ducks, and geese. It is also found in other avian species, mammals (qv, p 335), and slime on fish. There have been no documented cases of human infection resulting from consumption of poultry processed through regulated food channels; however, man is at risk of infection (**erysipeloid**) when handling infected birds.

Etiology: The non-host-specific cause is *Erysipelothrix rhusiopathiae*, a gram-positive, pleomorphic, extracellular rod. It can be cultivated on artificial media supplemented with blood or serum of various animals. It grows on solid surfaces at 35-37°C in air or preferably in 5-8% carbon dioxide. It is not readily destroyed by the usual laboratory disinfectants, and disinfection of premises is difficult because of its survival in the litter and soil for various lengths of time. It is inactivated by a 1:1000 concentration of bichloride of mercury, 0.5% sodium hydroxide solution, 3.5% liquid cresol compound, or 5% solution of phenol; it is resistant to formalin.

The many serotypes of *E rhusiopathiae* vary in pathogenicity and virulence, and certain ones are more frequently isolated, but the relationship of serotype to infection is not absolute. There is no pattern among the strains whether they cause the septicemic, urticarial, or endocardial forms of the disease, or are avirulent. All pathogenic strains have at least one protective antigen in common; therefore, bacterins can be prepared.

Epidemiology: The disease occurs sporadically in poultry of all ages. The incidence is reported to be higher in males, but this is not supported by experimental data. Infection results from entrance of the bacteria through breaks in the skin, through the mucous membranes such as during artificial insemination, by ingestion of contaminated foodstuffs, and possibly by mechanical transmission by biting insects. Since poultry are cannibalistic, the infection can spread quickly within a flock when the viscera of a septicemic bird are eaten. Although the soil may be a source, it is most likely due to contamination by feces or foodstuffs rather than by the organism multiplying there. Carrier animals, including poultry, should be considered as a source of this pathogen.

In nonvaccinated birds, morbidity and mortality can be 1-50%; adjacent groups may not be affected. In vaccinated flocks, some birds may be depressed for a short period and recover. Depending on time after vaccination, mortality may be 0-15%. Mortality in vaccinated and nonvaccinated poultry is influenced by the virulence of the organism; in turkeys, a genetic-induced resistance is probably involved.

Clinical Findings: This is primarily an acute infection that results in sudden death. In an affected flock, a few birds may be depressed but easily aroused; within 24 hr, a few birds will be dead. Chronic clinical disease is not usual in a flock, but individuals may have cutaneous lesions and swollen hocks. Turkeys with vegetative endocarditis usually do not have clinical signs and may die suddenly. Erysipelas should be suspected in flocks that have been artificially inseminated 4-5 days before an episode of death without clinical signs. In laying hens, egg production may drop markedly.

At necropsy, a generalized darkening of the skin or various sized areas of diffuse darkening is common. Usually, the liver and spleen are enlarged and friable. There may be other gross lesions such as peritonitis, pericarditis, catarrhal exudate in the GI tract, and degeneration of fat associated with the thigh and heart.

Diagnosis: Differential diagnoses for acute erysipelas in a flock should include other bacterial infections, poisoning, stampede injuries, and predators. A presumptive diagnosis can be based on an impression smear of the liver or spleen, or a smear of cardiac blood or bone marrow that shows gram-positive, slender, pleomorphic rods, singly and in microcolonies. In partially decomposed specimens, bone marrow is the specimen of choice. Other bacterial pathogens that may mimic *E rhusiopathiae* infection are *Pasteurella* spp, most often *P multocida*. Isolation and identification of *E rhusiopathiae* is necessary for a definitive diagnosis.

Treatment and Control: At present, antibiotic resistance of *E rhusiopathiae* apparently is not a problem. The antibiotic of choice is a rapid-acting penicillin. As soon as a presumptive diagnosis is made, potassium or sodium penicillin should be administered IM at 10,000 u/lb (0.5 kg) body wt simultaneously with a full dose of erysipelas bacterin. When it is impractical to handle each bird, penicillin (10,000,000 u/gal. [4 L]) in drinking water for 4-5 days greatly reduces losses. Sulfonamides and oral oxytetracycline are not effective. Broad-spectrum antibiotics, eg, erythromycin, are effective. Any antibiotic should be given according to recommendations, and the withdrawal time observed. Antibiotic in feed or water treats only those in the flock that are still eating and drinking at a normal rate, and may not have dramatic results. Vaccination with a bacterin helps protect those birds in the flock not yet infected. Antibiotic therapy or vaccination does not eliminate the production of carriers or the carrier state.

Vaccination will control erysipelas. Use of bacterins in flocks used for meat is useful, but is labor intensive. In breeders, the bacterin should be given q2-4mo. A problem with live vaccines is contamination of the premises, which probably mandates future use of the vaccine. Vaccines used in drinking water have given protection for short periods. Vaccines for pigs have been used successfully to immunize turkeys; however, efficacy of a vaccine in an animal other than poultry does not necessarily translate from that animal to poultry.

There are no specific husbandry recommendations other than sound management practices for the control of erysipelas.

FATTY LIVER SYNDROME

A noninfectious disease of chickens, primarily of cage layers, characterized by enlarged fat-infiltrated livers, with or without subcapsular hemorrhages and excessive abdominal fat deposits. Excessive caloric intake is thought to be one causative factor. The disease occurs frequently after molting, when caloric intake is high. Cage layers move less, using less energy, which may contribute to the problem. Fatty liver syndrome without excessive body fat is thought to be associated with mycotoxins (eg, aflatoxins) in feed.

Decreased egg production can be observed. Low mortality (2-5%) from internal liver hemorrhage can occur. Affected birds may appear overweight with heavy abdominal fat. The primary gross lesion is an enlarged, greasy, yellowish, friable liver. Frequently, petechial hemorrhages can be found on the liver surface; internal hemorrhage from liver rupture is common, and large blood clots can be found in the abdominal cavity. Such birds have pale combs and wattles. Microscopic lesions are confined to fatty infiltration and sometimes degeneration of hepatocytes. Excessive abdominal fat is common.

In mycotoxicosis ("lean bird fatty liver"), livers are yellowish with petechial hemorrhages, but not swollen; they have microscopic lesions of centrilobular necrosis and bile duct hyperplasia, and no excessive abdominal fat is found.

High-protein feeds (up to 20%) have been tried with variable success. Addition of 6% oat hulls to the feed has been successful at times. Addition of 1000 g of choline, 10,000 IU of vitamin E, 12 mg of vitamin B_{12}, and 2 lb (1 kg) of inositol per ton of feed also has been suggested as a treatment.

FLIP-OVER DISEASE

(Sudden death syndrome, Heart attack, Acute death syndrome, Fatal syncope,
Lung edema, Lung congestion, Dead in good condition)

Young, healthy, fast-growing broiler chickens die suddenly with a short, terminal, wing-beating convulsion. Many affected broilers just "flip-over" and die on their backs; 60-80% are males. Flip-over has been recognized as a disease entity for >30 yr. It has been reported in most intensive-broiler-growing areas of the world. It is uncommon or unrecognized when low-density feed is used and the ratio of feed intake to weight gain is >2.5 at 6 wk, or when broilers take 8 wk to reach 2 kg. The cause is unknown but probably it is a metabolic disease related to carbohydrate metabolism, cell membrane integrity, and intracellular electrolyte balance. Death likely results from ventricular fibrillation. The modern broiler tends to eat to its physical capacity rather than to meet its energy requirement, and continues to grow rapidly while maintaining a low feed-to-gain ratio. Flip-over appears to be related to high carbohydrate intake and good feed conversion. It is not known whether all broilers are susceptible or whether the low incidence suggests a genetic predisposition.

Incidence has been increasing since the condition was first recognized, likely at least in part because of improved feed conversion in broilers. Mortality may now average 2% in North America; in some all-male flocks, the loss is >4%. In flocks with good management and disease control, it may be the most important cause of death, producing up to 70% of the flock mortality.

Clinical Findings: Broilers show no premonitory signs. They appear healthy and may be feeding, sparring, walking, or resting, but suddenly extend their necks, gasp or squawk, and die rapidly with a short period of wing beating and leg movement, during which they frequently flip themselves onto their backs. They also may be found dead on their sides or breasts.

Flip-over may occur as early as day 3 and may continue until 10-12 wk in roaster flocks. The time of peak mortality varies, but usually is between days 14-32, although it can be as early as day 9. It is most likely to occur after day 28, particularly if growth is restricted in young broilers. Mortality of 0.25%-0.5% per day can occur for 1-3 days.

Lesions: Confirmation is difficult since no specific lesions are present. Dead birds are well fleshed, have an empty or partially filled crop containing normal ingesta, and feed in the gizzard. The abdomen is distended because the bird is fat and because the intestines are dilated and filled with semisolid digesta and mucus (as in any broiler that dies with the intestine full of feed). There is no evidence of stasis. The muscles are mottled red and white with congestion of the dependent muscles. Organs are moderately to severely congested. There may be small hemorrhages in the liver and kidney. The ventricles of the heart are contracted (but not hypertrophied), and the atria are dilated and blood filled. (If autolysis is advanced, the ventricles may be dilated.) The lungs are congested and frequently edematous; however, pulmonary edema increases with time after death and is not prominent in broilers that are examined within a few minutes after death. The gallbladder may be small or empty (as it is in many broilers on full feed). There are no specific histological lesions.

Diagnosis: Good broilers found dead on their backs may be assumed to have died of flip-over since that position is rare in death from other causes except cardiac tamponade, asphyxia, and ascites syndrome (pulmonary hypertension, qv, p 1628). Good birds on their sides or breasts, scattered in a random fashion in the pen also usually are classed as flip-over. The full GI tract (particularly the full intestine), the large pale liver, the large normal bursa, the contracted ventricles and dilated blood-filled atria, the lung congestion and edema, along with the lack of pathological lesions help support the diagnosis.

The condition called sudden death syndrome in Australia in broiler breeders coming into production is a different disease; it is reported to be caused by potassium and phosphorous deficiency. Similar mortality caused by a combination of high environmental temperature and hypophosphatemia or by acute hypocalcemia has been reported in North America.

Sudden death in turkeys can be caused by choke, aortic rupture, and by acute (possibly hypertensive) lung congestion and edema with splenomegaly and splenic and perirenal hemorrhage.

Prevention and Control: It has been suggested that activity caused by bright light (particularly sunlight), noise, and other disturbances may increase the incidence. After the first 3-4 days, low-intensity or low-intensity-intermittent lighting should be used, and broilers should be disturbed as little as possible. Long dark periods (18 hr dark for 3-4 wk) after the first 3-4 days reduces flip-over. Raising the feed conversion by feeding a less dense ration or reducing feed intake by 15-20% does not appear to be justified.

FOWL CHOLERA

A contagious, widely distributed disease affecting domestic and wild birds. It usually occurs as a septicemia of sudden onset with high morbidity and mortality, but chronic and asymptomatic infections also occur.

Etiology: *Pasteurella multocida*, the causal agent, is a small, gram-negative, nonmotile rod that may exhibit pleomorphism after repeated subculture. In freshly isolated cultures or in tissues, the bacteria have a bipolar appearance when stained with Wright's stain. Although this organism may infect a wide variety of animals, strains isolated from nonavian hosts generally do not produce fowl cholera. Strains that cause fowl cholera represent a number of immunotypes, which complicates prevention of the disease by using bacterins. The organism is susceptible to ordinary disinfectants, sunlight, drying, and heat. Turkeys are more susceptible than chickens, older chickens are more susceptible than young ones, and some breeds of chickens are more susceptible than others.

Clinical Findings, Lesions, and Diagnosis: These vary greatly, depending on the course of disease. In acute cholera, dead birds may be the first indication of disease. Fever, depression, anorexia, mucoid discharge from the mouth, ruffled feathers, diarrhea, and increased respiratory rate are usually seen. Many of the lesions are related to vascular disturbances. Hyperemia is especially evident in the vessels of the abdominal viscera. Petechial and ecchymotic hemorrhages are common, particularly in subepicardial and subserosal locations. Increased amounts of peritoneal and pericardial fluids are frequently observed. Livers may be swollen and often develop multiple, small, necrotic foci. Pneumonia is particularly common in turkeys.

The signs and lesions of chronic fowl cholera are generally related to localized infections. Sternal bursae, wattles, joints, tendon sheaths, and footpads are often swollen because of accumulated fibrinosuppurative exudate. Exudative conjunctivitis and pharyngitis may occur. Torticollis may result when the meninges, middle ear, or cranial bones are infected.

A presumptive diagnosis may be based on the characteristic signs and lesions, and demonstration of gram-negative, bipolar organisms in blood and other tissues; a more conclusive diagnosis requires isolation and identification of *P multocida*.

Prophylaxis: Good management practices are essential to prevention. Adjuvant bacterins (water-in-oil) are widely used and generally effective; autogenous bacterins are recommended when polyvalent bacterins are found to be ineffective. Attenuated vaccines are available for administration in drinking water to turkeys and by wing-web inoculation to chickens. These live vaccines can effectively induce immunity against different serotypes of *P multocida*. They are recommended for use in healthy flocks only.

Treatment: Sulfonamides and antibiotics are commonly used; early treatment and adequate dosages are important. Sensitivity testing often aids in drug selection. Sulfaquinoxaline sodium in feed or water usually controls mortality, as do sulfamethazine, sulfadimethoxine, and sodium sulfamerazine. (Sulfas should be used with caution in breeders.) High levels of tetracycline antibiotics in the feed (0.04%) or parenterally may be useful. Penicillin administered IM is often effective for sulfa-resistant infections.

GOOSE VIRAL HEPATITIS
(GVH, Derzsy's Disease)

An acute, highly fatal, parvovirus infection of wild and domestic goslings characterized by tissue hemorrhages, liver lesions, ascites, hydropericardium, feather loss, and anorexia. Limited outbreaks have also been reported in Muscovy ducklings. It occurs worldwide and is economically important to goose and Muscovy duck producers.

Etiology: The disease can be reproduced by a Type I goose parvovirus, although adenoviruses also have been isolated from affected goslings. The parvovirus, ~25-27 nm in diameter, is highly resistant, and can be propagated in susceptible goose and Muscovy duck embryos and tissue cultures. Egg transmission occurs in contaminated hatcheries and pens.

Clinical Findings: Experimentally, the incubation period is 4-7 days. Deaths usually occur at 9-14 days of age. During early stages of the disease, goslings manifest inappetence, thirst, crowding, conjunctivitis, and nasal discharge. Food and water are refused entirely before death. In more chronic forms, the skin becomes reddened, the feathers are lost or become necrotic at their tips, and survivors become stunted. Age resistance is marked, and the disease is absent in goslings >4 wk old. In Muscovy ducks up to 12 wk old, sudden molt followed by stunting has been observed. Recovered birds are immune. Recovered females transfer maternal antibodies to the progeny through the egg yolk.

Lesions: At necropsy, the most characteristic change is a swollen and occasionally firm liver with petechial hemorrhages on the surface. Tissue hemorrhages in other organs, hydropericardium, ascites, and fibrinous pseudomembranes on the epithelial lining of the oral cavity and tongue are common. The thyroid may be enlarged. Histological lesions include focal hepatic and myocardial degeneration, necrosis, and hemorrhage. Heterophilic cell infiltrations, bile duct proliferations, and fatty infiltrations are observed in the liver. Intranuclear inclusions are present in hepatocytes and Kupffer's cells.

Diagnosis: A presumptive diagnosis can be based on the characteristic clinical course, age incidence, and gross and histological lesions. Diagnosis is confirmed by isolation of the virus in susceptible goose embryos and tissue cultures; neutralization of the virus by specific antiserum; and immunofluorescence of the virus in tissue cultures, tissue sections, or smears.

Differential diagnoses include duck plague (which may infect geese or Muscovy ducks), adenovirus infections, avian influenza, and hemorrhagic nephritis and enteritis. Bacterial infections due to *Pasteurella anatipestifer* and *Escherichia coli* also should be considered.

Prophylaxis and Treatment: Strict isolation of GVH-free goslings during their first 4 wk prevents the disease. Immunization of breeder geese to increase parenteral humoral antibody levels of newly hatched goslings is indicated for infected flocks. The virus can be attenuated by the 40th-passage culture in goose-fibroblast tissue cultures, which can be employed as a breeder vaccine. Since it is weakly immunogenic, it should be injected with an adjuvant. Breeders should be vaccinated twice, 3-6 wk apart, at least 3 wk before the laying season. The vaccination should be repeated twice yearly to insure adequate protection throughout the entire growing season. Intensively reared Muscovy ducklings exposed to GVH should be vaccinated at 3 wk of age. Hyperimmune or convalescent serum (1 mL) administered subcut. to day-old goslings is indicated to prevent or treat the disease in exposed flocks.

HISTOMONIASIS
(Blackhead, Infectious enterohepatitis)

A protozoal disease affecting turkeys, peafowl, ruffed grouse, quail, and occasionally chickens. Turkeys of all ages are susceptible, but greatest mortality occurs in birds ~12 wk old.

Etiology: The protozoan parasite *Histomonas meleagridis* is transmitted most often in embryonated eggs of the cecal nematode *Heterakis gallinarum*, and sometimes directly by ingestion of infected feces. A large percentage of chickens harbor this worm, which in itself is not pathogenic, and histomonads have also been located in adult worms of both sexes. Three species of earthworms can harbor *H gallinarum* larvae containing *H meleagridis*, which are infective to both chickens and turkeys. *Histomonas meleagridis* survives for long periods within *Heterakis* eggs, which are resistant and may remain viable in the soil for years. Histomonads are released from *Heterakis* larvae in the ceca a few days after entry of the nematode, and replicate rapidly in cecal tissues. The parasites migrate into the submucosa and muscularis mucosa, and cause extensive and severe necrosis. Histomonads reach the liver either by the vascular system or via the peritoneal cavity, and rounded necrotic lesions quickly appear on the liver surface.

Traditionally, this disease has been thought of as affecting turkeys, while doing little damage to chickens. However, the disease in chickens has an early cecal involvement. Mild liver lesions occur occasionally. Mortality is low, but morbidity can be high in young chickens, especially broilers. Tissue responses to infection may resolve in 4 wk, but birds may be carriers for another 6 wk.

Clinical Findings: Signs are apparent 7-12 days after infection and include listlessness, drooping wings, unkempt feathers, and sulfur-colored droppings. The head may be cyanotic, hence the name "blackhead". Young birds have a more acute disease and die within a few days after signs appear. Older birds may be sick for some time and become emaciated before death.

Lesions: The primary lesions are in the ceca, which exhibit marked inflammatory changes and ulcerations, causing a thickening of the cecal wall. Occasionally, these ulcers erode the cecal wall, causing peritonitis and involvement of other organs. The ceca contain a yellowish green, caseous exudate or, in later stages, a dry, cheesy core. Liver lesions are circular, yellowish green, and characteristically depressed. In turkeys, they may be up to 4 cm in diameter. The liver and cecal lesions together are pathognomonic. However, the liver lesions must be differentiated from those of tuberculosis, leukosis, avian trichomoniasis, and mycosis, which are raised and grayish or gray-yellow. In some cases, especially in chickens, histopathological examination is helpful. Histomonads are intercellular, although they may be so closely packed as to appear intracellular. The nuclei are much smaller than those of the host cells, and the cytoplasm less vacuolated. Scrapings from the liver lesions or ceca may be placed in isotonic saline solution for direct microscopical examination; *Histomonas* sp must be differentiated from other cecal flagellates.

Prophylaxis and Treatment: Strict sanitation is indicated. Use of large wire platforms for feeders and waterers reduces the danger of infection. Since healthy chickens often carry infected cecal worms, the practice of ranging chickens with turkeys should be avoided. Grouse and quail also may carry the infection to turkey yards. Since *H gallinarum* ova can survive in soil for many months, turkeys should not be put on ground contaminated during the past 1-2 yr. A rotation system, in which the turkeys are moved q3-5wk, helps to reduce the chances of infection.

The following drugs are used for the control of histomoniasis: nitarsone (prophylaxis)—0.01875% of feed until 5 days before marketing; furazolidone (prophylaxis)—0.011% of feed, continuously, (treatment)—0.022% of feed for 2-3 wk; carbarsone—turkeys (prophylaxis)—0.025-0.0375% of feed, continuously until 5 days before marketing. Dimetridazole has been used prophylactically at 0.015-0.02% of feed, continuously until 5 days before marketing, and for treatment at 0.06-0.08% (soluble powder) in feed limited to 7 days or 0.05% in water for 6 days, followed by preventive feed medication, but it is no longer approved.

INFECTIOUS BURSAL DISEASE
(IBD, Gumboro disease)

An acute, highly contagious, birnavirus infection of young chickens that occurs worldwide. Infections before 3 wk of age are normally subclinical but cause immunosuppression due to widespread destruction of undifferentiated lymphocytes. In recent years, "variant" strains of IBD virus have been identified that cause immunosuppression but do not induce clinical disease in older chickens. These strains have major antigenic differences from the "standard" strains.

Etiology and Transmission: The causal virus (IBDV) is most readily isolated from the bursa of Fabricius, but may be isolated from any organ. It is shed in the feces and is transferred from house to house by fomites. It is very stable and difficult to eradicate from premises.

IBDV may be isolated in 8- to 11-day-old "clean" chicken embryos with inocula from birds in the early stages of disease. The chorioallantoic membrane is more sensitive to inoculation than is the allantoic sac. Generally, embryos die within 3-7 days with virus titers of 10^2-10^5. The virus also may be isolated in cell cultures derived from the cloacal bursa, and some strains may be isolated in chicken-embryo fibroblasts. Cell-culture-adapted strains of IBDV produce a cytopathic effect, and such assays may be used for quantitative serological tests. Two serotypes of IBDV have been identified, and there is considerable antigenic variation between strains within a serotype. Serotype 2 is associated primarily with turkeys but does not cause significant clinical disease or immunosuppression.

Clinical Findings: Results of infection depend on age, breed of chicken, and virulence of the virus, and may be divided into subclinical and clinical infections. The age most susceptible to clinical disease is 3-6 wk, but severe infections have occurred in Leghorn chickens up to 18 wk of age.

Subclinical Infections: Due to economic losses, the early subclinical infection is the most important form of the disease; it causes severe, long-lasting immunosuppression due to destruction of immature lymphocytes in the bursa of Fabricius, thymus, and spleen. The humoral (B cell) immune response is most severely affected; however, the cell-mediated (T cell) immune response also is impaired. Chickens immunosuppressed by early IBDV infections do not respond well to vaccination against Newcastle disease, infectious bronchitis, or Marek's disease. Infections with normally nonpathogenic viruses and bacteria may be exacerbated and precipitate inclusion body hepatitis (adenovirus), necrotic dermatitis (*Clostridium* sp), and other syndromes. IBDV also makes the cells that line the intestine more vulnerable to damage due to coccidiosis. Subclinical infections by the newer "variant" strains occur in immature birds of all ages. Severe long-term immunosuppression results from early infections with these strains, and severe bursal atrophy occurs in immature birds of all ages.

Clinical Infections: Onset of the disease is sudden after an incubation of 3-4 days. Chickens exhibit severe prostration, incoordination, watery diarrhea, soiled vent feathers, vent picking, and inflammation of the cloaca. Losses range to >20%. Recovery occurs in <1 wk, delaying broiler weight gains by 3-5 days. The presence of parental antibody will modify the clinical course of the disease. Virulence of field strains of the virus appears to vary considerably.

Lesions: Necropsy reveals primary lesions in the cloacal bursa and the pectoral, thigh, and leg muscles. The bursa is swollen, edematous, yellowish, and occasionally, hemorrhagic, especially in birds that have died of the disease. Congestion and hemorrhage of the pectoral, thigh, and leg muscles is common. Initial descriptions of this disease described lesions of the kidney (swelling and urate deposits); however, these were found to be a result of either concurrent infectious bronchitis infections or severe dehydration, or both. Chickens recovered from IBDV infections have small, atrophied, cloacal bursas due to the nonregenerative destruction of the bursal follicles.

Control: There is no treatment. Depopulation and rigorous disinfection of contaminated farms have achieved limited success. Live IBD vaccines of chick-embryo or cell-culture origin and of varying virulence can be administered by eye drop, drinking water, or subcut. routes at 1-21 days of age. The immune response can be altered by parental immunity, and the more virulent vaccine strains can override higher levels of antibody.

Chicks in broiler flocks (and in some commercial layer operations) should carry high levels of parental immunity to provide protection during early brooding, which would minimize early infection and subsequent immunosuppression or infection, or both. Breeder flocks should be vaccinated one or more times during the growing period, first with a live vaccine and again just before egg production with an oil-adjuvanted, inactivated vaccine. The latter vaccines induce higher and more uniform levels of antibody that persist longer than do live vaccines. The immune status of breeder flocks should be monitored periodically with a quantitative serological test such as virus neutralization or ELISA. If antibody levels fall, hens should be revaccinated to maintain adequate immunity in the progeny.

LISTERIOSIS

A quite rare disease of birds that usually occurs as a septicemia and sometimes as a localized encephalitis. Encephalitis combined with septicemia has been observed in young geese. Chickens, turkeys, geese, ducks, canaries, and parrots appear to be the most commonly affected avian species.

In workers at poultry-processing plants, conjunctivitis due to *Listeria monocytogenes* has been linked to handling of apparently normal but infected chickens. Abortions and congenitally infected babies have been associated with handling of *L monocytogenes*-positive birds or those that have died with the disease, but these cases were not confirmed.

Etiology and Epidemiology: *Listeria monocytogenes* is a gram-positive, coccoid to bacillus-shaped nonsporeformer that tends to form long filaments, particularly in older cultures. Based on somatic and flagellar antigens, several serotypes have been described. *Listeria monocytogenes* can be cultured on blood and tryptose agar or brain heart infusion. It is widely distributed among avian species. The organism is common in soil, with concentrations increasing in late winter and early spring. Since it has been isolated from apparently normal birds and from birds dying from causes other than uncomplicated listeriosis, it is possible that carrier birds play an important role in the perpetuation of the disease in birds and mammals. The largely opportunistic character of infections is demonstrated by its common association with concurrent diseases such as coccidiosis, infectious coryza, salmonellosis, and parasitic infections.

Clinical Findings and Lesions: Young birds appear to be more susceptible than mature ones. Transmission and subsequent infections occur by ingestion of contaminated nasal secretions, feces, and soil. In most avian species, the incubation period has not been documented; in turkeys, it is 16 hr to 52 days. Frequently, *L mono-cytogenes* infections are subclinical. However, signs of infection are suggestive of a septicemia and include depression, listlessness, and peracute death. In this form, it is common to find only dead birds. In the subacute and chronic forms, signs are related to encephalitis, and include torticollis, stupor, paresis, and paralysis. Adult birds may die suddenly with septicemia, while young birds tend to have chronic infections.

In uncomplicated listeriosis, lesions include multiple areas of degeneration and necrosis of the myocardium with congestion, increased pericardial fluid, and pericarditis. Petechial hemorrhages can be observed in the proventriculus and heart. Splenomegaly and hepatomegaly with bile retention and focal areas of necrosis are common. With the encephalitic form, no gross brain lesions are observed; microscopically, however, there is infiltration of macrophages, plasma cells, lymphocytes, and a few heterophils within the necrotic foci of the affected tissue.

Diagnosis: Listeriosis can be suspected based on the history, clinical signs, necropsy lesions, and microscopic observation of the bacteria in the myocardial fibrils and/or hepatocytes. The disease can be confirmed by isolation from the blood, liver, heart, spleen, or brain of a gram-positive, nonacid-fast, nonsporeforming bacillus that is catalase-positive, motile, aerobic, and ferments sugars. Isolation by direct culture from the affected tissues may not be successful because of low concentration of organisms in the tissues; however, recovery increases significantly if a portion of the specimen is refrigerated for 4-8 wk and subcultured weekly.

Differential diagnoses include colibacillosis, pasteurellosis, erysipelas, velogenic viscerotropic Newcastle disease, and many of the acute and chronic bacterial diseases.

Treatment and Control: The tetracyclines are efficacious in both the acute and subacute forms when given at 5-10 mg/kg body wt daily for 1 wk. Treatment of the chronic form is usually unsuccessful. Rigid sanitation and disinfection procedures with culling and isolation of affected birds may be helpful.

MALABSORPTION SYNDROME
(Runting syndrome, Pale bird syndrome)

A disease of growing chickens; meat type or broilers are affected most commonly. The condition is frequently characterized by stunted growth and a lack of skin pigmentation; it has been identified in virtually all countries in which intensive poultry production occurs.

Etiology and Transmission: Mycotoxins and several viruses, including parvoviruses, astroviruses, caliciviruses, and reoviruses have been implicated. Although the etiology is believed to be complex, only reoviruses have thus far been identified as major pathogens. This group of viruses is prevalent worldwide in all commercially produced poultry as well as many other avian species. Avian reoviruses tend to be species-specific, and those isolated from chickens share a common, group-specific, soluble antigen that can aid in recognition and diagnosis.

Transmission occurs via both the oral and respiratory routes; the latter is most common. In addition, in persistently infected hens, the virus can be transmitted in the eggs for long periods. Increased viral persistence and transmissibility are generally associated with increased virulence.

Clinical Findings: The disease is typically recognized in 1- to 6-wk-old broiler chicks, and is characterized by stunted growth, lack of pigmentation in the skin and unfeathered areas, feathering abnormalities, undigested feed in the feces, and a reluctance to walk because of arthritis, tenosynovitis, or osteoporosis. Diarrhea is not uncommon during the initial phases. Mortality rates are generally higher than those for unaffected flocks, but a definitive pattern has not been demonstrated. Severely affected birds do not respond to changes in feed or management practices and are usually culled before processing. Arthritic changes may occur (*see* VIRAL ARTHRITIS, p 1607).

Lesions: The severity and type of lesions resulting from both field and laboratory infections vary with the particular reovirus involved and age of the bird. In birds infected during the first week of life with a highly pathogenic reovirus, lesions include arthritis, osteoporosis, hepatitis, myocarditis, pancreatitis, and atrophy and necrosis of the intestinal villi. Other digestive tract lesions, including atrophied gizzards, proventriculitis, and enteritis, have been reported in older, commercially grown birds. Additionally, encephalomalacia may be observed occasionally, presumably as a result of nutrient malabsorption or malutilization.

Diagnosis: Clinical signs and lesions permit a presumptive diagnosis, although a similar syndrome may be caused by a retrovirus (*see* RETICULOENDOTHELIOSIS, p 1588). More conclusive evidence can be provided by isolation of the virus in the yolk sac of 5- to 7-day-old chicken embryos or primary cultures of chicken-embryo kidney or liver cell cultures. Isolated virus should be inoculated intratracheally into day-old chicks to verify pathogenicity. Virus neutralization and agar-gel-precipitin tests can be used to verify infection on a flock and individual bird basis.

Control: Several commercial vaccines are available. Active immunization can be accomplished by vaccinating with attenuated virus at 1 day of age. Alternatively, passive immunization of broilers is achieved by vaccinating breeding stock with either live or inactivated vaccines, or both. There is no effective treatment for severely affected birds.

MARBLE SPLEEN DISEASE OF PHEASANTS (MSD)

The causal virus is apparently antigenically similar, if not identical, to the adenovirus of hemorrhagic enteritis of turkeys (qv, p 1559), but characterization is incomplete. MSD is sometimes called lung edema, but the primary lesions are seen in the spleen. MSD is usually seen in semimature or mature birds. Depression is noted, and the death loss is variable. Frequently, however, sudden death occurs with no premonitory signs as a consequence of massive pulmonary edema.

Generally, the spleen is enlarged and mottled giving a marbling effect. Histologically, necrosis of the splenic lymphoid cells and hyperplasia of the white pulp are common. Basophilic intranuclear inclusion bodies are often present in the reticuloendothelial cells. Infective spleen tissue may be used as an antigen in the agar-gel-precipitin test with specific antiserum to confirm a diagnosis of MSD. However, typical gross splenic lesions are generally diagnostic in the absence of known bacterial pathogens. Methods to control and prevent hemorrhagic enteritis in turkeys appear to be equally effective in preventing MSD in pheasants.

MYCOPLASMOSIS

Several pathogenic *Mycoplasma* spp have been isolated from avian hosts; *M gallisepticum, M iowae, M meleagridis,* and *M synoviae* are the most important. Mycoplasmas are fastidious bacteria, 0.3-0.8 μm in diameter, lack a cell wall, and require a rich growth medium with serum. They do not survive for more than a few hours or days outside the host and are vulnerable to common disinfectants. Each has distinctive epidemiological and pathological characteristics.

MYCOPLASMA GALLISEPTICUM (MG) INFECTION
(PPLO infection, Chronic respiratory disease [CRD], Infectious sinusitis)

MG infection is commonly designated as CRD in chickens, and infectious sinusitis in turkeys. Infection may also occur in pheasants, chukar partridges, and peafowl. Infection in pigeons, quail, ducks, geese, and psittacine birds should be considered. Passerine-type birds are quite resistant. The disease is worldwide. Its effects are most severe in large commercial operations during winter.

MG is the most pathogenic avian mycoplasma; however, strains may differ markedly in virulence. Primary isolation is made in enriched broth medium that contains 10-15% serum, then plated on agar. Typical colonies are identified by immunofluorescence.

Transmission, Epidemiology, and Pathogenesis: In the USA, most breeder flocks are MG-free, and outbreaks are due to lateral transmission from infected chickens; however, in some parts of the world, egg transmission is a major source of infection. The incidence of egg transmission is highly variable, ranging up to 30-40% during the first 2 mo (approximately) after infection of susceptible birds in production. The transmission rate then lessens and is inconsistent (0-5%) until the end of production. Birds infected before the onset of production transmit through the egg at a much lower rate, if at all. The infection may be dormant in the infected chick for days to months, but when the flock is stressed, aerosol transmission occurs rapidly and infection spreads through the flock. Live virus vaccination, natural virus infection, cold weather, or crowding may initiate the spread. In addition, the infection may be carried by personnel (especially from an infected to a clean flock), fomites, or introduction of infected birds. In many flocks, the source of infection cannot be determined.

The epithelium of the upper air passages is most susceptible; however, in severe, acute disease the infection is also found in the lower respiratory tract. There is a marked interaction between respiratory viruses, *Escherichia coli*, and MG in the pathogenesis of CRD. Once infected, birds remain permanent carriers.

Clinical Findings: In chickens, uncomplicated infections may be inapparent. Affected birds have varying degrees of respiratory distress: slight to marked rales, difficulty in breathing, coughing, and sneezing. Morbidity is high and mortality low in uncomplicated cases. Nasal discharge and frothiness about the eyes may be present. In turkeys, the disease is generally more severe than in chickens, and swelling of the paranasal sinus is common. Feed efficiency and weight gains are reduced. Broilers and market turkeys may suffer high condemnations at processing due to airsacculitis. In laying flocks, birds may fail to reach peak egg production.

Lesions: Uncomplicated MG infections in chickens result in relatively mild sinusitis, tracheitis, and airsacculitis. *Escherichia coli* infections are often concurrent and result in severe air sac thickening and turbidity, with exudative accumulations, fibrinopurulent pericarditis, and perihepatitis, particularly in broilers. Turkeys develop severe mucopurulent sinusitis and varying degrees of tracheitis and airsacculitis. The mucous membranes are thickened, hyperplastic, necrotic, and infiltrated with inflammatory cells. Lymphofollicular areas occur in the submucosa.

Diagnosis: Most commonly, agglutination reactions are used for diagnosis. It should be confirmed by isolation and identification of the organism or by hemagglutination-inhibition because nonspecific false agglutination reactions are common, especially following the inoculation of inactivated, oil-emulsion vaccines or *M synoviae* infection. Isolates should be identified, since birds may also be infected with nonpathogenic *Mycoplasma* spp. Newcastle disease, infectious bronchitis, influenza, and other respiratory pathogens may offer problems in differential diagnosis.

Treatment and Control: In the field, many cases of MG infection are complicated by other pathogenic bacteria; thus, effective treatment must also attack the secondary invader. Most strains of MG are sensitive to antibiotics, eg, chlortetracycline, erythromycin, oxytetracycline, spectinomycin, tiamulin, tylosin, or enrofloxacin. Antibiotic is usually given in the feed or water for 5-7 days; however, in turkeys antibiotic may be given by injection initially, followed by feed or water medication. Although antibiotic medication may alleviate signs and lesions, it does not eliminate infection.

Eradication of MG from chicken and turkey breeding stock is well advanced in the USA and several other countries. Control may be based on identifying breeders without serum agglutination titers, and the most effective control method is to maintain seronegative stock. In valuable breeding stock, treatment of eggs, usually with tylosin or heat, may be utilized to eliminate egg transmission to progeny. Medication is not a good long-term control method, but is of value in treating individual infected flocks.

The use of MG-free birds is desirable; however, infection in multiple-age commercial egg farms where depopulation is not feasible presents a problem. An inactivated, oil-emulsion bacterin is available in most countries and is effective in preventing egg production losses, but does not prevent infection. More recently, a live vaccine has been licensed in the USA for use in infected, multiple-age layer flocks. It may be used only with the permission of the State Veterinarian. The vaccine consists of a mild strain of MG, and is usually given at ~10-14 wk of age. Vaccinated birds remain carriers, and immunity lasts through the laying season.

MYCOPLASMA IOWAE (MI) INFECTION

Originally thought to be of low pathogenicity in producing air-sac lesions in chickens and turkeys, MI is a potentially important cause of reduced hatchability in turkeys. MI was originally designated as the IJKNQR group of avian mycoplasmas. An enriched medium similar to those used for other avian mycoplasmas is suitable. It is resistant to 1% bile salts. There is considerable variation in antigenicity and pathogenicity among MI strains.

Infection is common in turkey flocks in Europe and has been reported in North America. It is relatively uncommon in chickens. MI is egg-transmitted, but little is known of other aspects of its epidemiology.

Many strains of MI are lethal to turkey embryos. After experimental inoculation of young poults, stunting, poor feathering, and various skeletal deformities such as tenosynovitis and chondrodystrophy are observed, but the mechanism is unknown. These effects have not been recognized in the field, probably because most infected individuals die before hatching. Older birds appear to be quite resistant.

Clinical Findings, Lesions, and Diagnosis: Affected turkey breeder flocks show no signs other than reduced hatchability (usually 2-5%). In many flocks, the hatchability returns to normal after 1-2 mo.

Most embryos die during the later stages of incubation. Dead turkey embryos are edematous, congested, and stunted, and may have clubbed down. Poults challenged *in ovo* or at 1 day of age may develop various deformities, eg, rotated tibia, deviated toes, chondrodystrophy, or erosion of the articular cartilage of the hock joint. Feathers may be poorly developed. Chicks challenged at 1 day of age may develop tenosynovitis and ruptured tendons.

Turkeys apparently have a poor antibody response; no reliable serological test is available. Diagnosis relies on isolation and identification of the causative agent.

Treatment and Control: The best method of control is to maintain flocks free of MI; however, because serology is unreliable, this may be difficult. Dipping hatching eggs in solutions of enrofloxacin has significantly reduced losses in hatchability.

MYCOPLASMA MELEAGRIDIS (MM) INFECTION

A widespread, egg-transmitted, infectious disease of turkeys in which the primary lesion in the progeny is airsacculitis. The organism is commonly found in the respiratory and reproductive tract of turkeys. MM is thought to be a specific pathogen for turkeys; however, the organism may occur in quail, peacocks, and pigeons.

The infection is found worldwide. MM has been eradicated in most basic breeders and many commercial flocks.

MM was recognized as a pathogen of turkeys following widespread elimination of *M gallisepticum* from breeding stock. Earlier publications refer to MM as the N strain or the H serotype of avian mycoplasma.

Transmission and Pathogenesis: Infection is established primarily through egg transmission, which can be as high as 30-50% or higher early in the production cycle. However, transmission in adult turkeys is unique and is related to genital contact. Early infections usually become quiescent at sexual maturity. In toms, the phallus and adjacent tissues retain infection and contaminate semen, thus infecting the vagina. Hens may retain infection in the bursa of Fabricius; this serves as a source of infection of the reproductive tract following rupture of the cloacal-vaginal occluding membrane at puberty. Infection ascends through the reproductive system and may reach the surface of the ovary. The high rate of egg transmission is from infection of the reproductive tract being incorporated into the egg following ovulation. Infection of the respiratory tract leads to transmission between birds in young flocks, and may be a factor in the spread to flocks previously free of the infection.

The marked difference in the pathogenicity of various strains of MM results in variable clinical manifestations. The high incidence of air-sac infection in turkey poults suggests a symbiotic host-parasite relationship. MM is involved in crooked necks and leg deformities, but the pathogenesis of this syndrome is not clear. The vaginas of naturally infected hens are free of infection 1-3 mo after removal of the source of infection. Immunity is not permanent, and hens can be reinfected with contaminated semen.

Clinical Findings: Embryo infection appears to reduce hatchability, poult quality, and growth rate. Superimposed stress may cause considerable poult mortality during the first few weeks. Infection during early rapid growth of hock joints, periarticular tissues, cervical vertebrae, and adjacent bone may produce major bone deformities such as crooked necks and hocks. Rales may develop in flocks 3-8 wk old and persist for several weeks without significant mortality or serious interference with growth.

Lesions: One-day-old poults have thoracic airsacculitis with thickening, turbidity, and marked caseous exudate. In 1-3 wk, the lesions may extend to the abdominal air sacs. These lesions recede with age. The air-sac lesions of roaster and mature birds are probably related to other factors. Tracheitis may be present. Sinusitis does not occur. Microscopic lesions in hens consist of lymphocytic foci in the fimbria, uterus, and vagina. In young poults, inflammatory lesions occur in the air sacs and lungs.

Diagnosis: A high incidence of air-sac lesions in day-old poults suggests MM infection. The plate and tube agglutination tests may be used, but antibody may not be detectable in birds with localized infection. In these cases, MM must be isolated. *Mycoplasma gallisepticum*, chlamydiae, bacteria, and respiratory viruses such as influenza must be eliminated as causes of air-sac infection.

Treatment and Control: The commercial use of MM-free flocks should be monitored by examining pipped embryos or cull poults for airsacculitis. Semen used for insemination must be MM free. Tylosin dip of eggs reduces the incidence of transmission in infected flocks, and improves weight gains and feed conversion ratios. Subcut. inoculation of a suitable antibiotic at 1 day of age, or water medication for the first 5-10 days, appears to reduce MM-caused airsacculitis and may improve weight gain.

MYCOPLASMA SYNOVIAE (MS) INFECTION
(Infectious synovitis)

First recognized as an acute to chronic infection of chickens and turkeys that produced an exudative tendonitis and bursitis, MS now occurs most frequently as a subclinical upper respiratory tract infection. MS infection also is a complication of airsacculitis in association with Newcastle disease or infectious bronchitis. MS occurs primarily in chickens and turkeys. Ducks, geese, guinea fowl, parrots, pheasants, and quail also may be susceptible. Serum (preferably swine serum) and an enzyme, nicotinamide adenine dinucleotide (NAD), are required for growth on artificial media.

Transmission, Epidemiology, and Pathogenesis: MS is egg-transmitted, but the rate is low (probably <5%), and some hatches of progeny of infected flocks may be free of MS. Egg transmission is greatest during the first 1-2 mo after infection of susceptible breeders. Lateral transmission is similar to *M gallisepticum*, but the rate of spread is more rapid.

MS isolates vary widely in pathogenicity. Isolates from cases of airsacculitis are more apt to produce air-sac lesions than those from synovial fluid or membranes. Some strains produce the typical clinical disease of synovitis. The paucity of natural outbreaks of infectious synovitis in chickens in recent years may be related to the adaptation of MS to the respiratory tract; however, clinical synovitis in turkeys is still relatively common.

Clinical Findings: Although slight rales may be present in birds with respiratory infection, usually no signs are noticed. Younger birds, especially those under stress or suffering concurrent infections, are more likely to be affected. Outbreaks of infectious synovitis occur most commonly in chickens at 4-6 wk, and in turkeys at 10-12 wk. Lame birds tend to sit. The more severely affected birds are depressed and are found around the feeders and waterers. Swellings of the hocks and foot pads are seen. Morbidity is 2-15% and mortality 1-10%. The effect on egg production appears to be minor or nil.

Lesions: In the respiratory syndrome, airsacculitis occurs when the bird is stressed from Newcastle disease, infectious bronchitis, or improper ventilation. In many cases, air-sac lesions resolve after 1-2 wk. Early in synovitis, the liver is enlarged and sometimes green. The spleen is enlarged and the kidneys are enlarged and pale. A yellow-to-gray, viscid exudate is present in almost all synovial structures; it is most common in the keel bursa, hock, and wing joints. In chronic cases, this exudate may become inspissated and orange.

Diagnosis: A presumptive diagnosis can be based on the lesions and clinical signs, but laboratory confirmation is necessary. Skeletal abnormalities must be eliminated as the cause of lameness. The disease must be differentiated from viral tenosynovitis and staphylococcal and other bacterial infections.

The serum plate agglutination test is used to detect infected flocks, but cross-reactions with *M gallisepticum* and other nonspecific reactions may occur. Reactors are confirmed by hemagglutination-inhibition or by isolation and identification of the organism. In turkeys, the agglutination test for MS may not be reliable, and isolation and identification of the causative agent is necessary.

Treatment and Control: Serological testing and isolation similar to those for *M gallisepticum* have resulted in eradication of the infection in most primary breeder flocks of chickens and turkeys. Administration of a tetracycline antibiotic in the feed may be beneficial in treatment or prevention of synovitis. When airsacculitis is a problem, preventive antibiotic therapy during the time of respiratory reaction to Newcastle disease and infectious bronchitis vaccine may be helpful. Medication of breeder flocks is of little value in preventing egg transmission.

MYCOTOXICOSIS
(Turkey X disease, Aflatoxicosis)

Disease caused by ingestion of aflatoxin, which is produced by *Aspergillus flavus* or *A parasiticus* growing on the feed (groundnut [peanut] meal, cereals, etc). (*See also* TABLE 3, MYCOTOXICOSES IN DOMESTIC ANIMALS, p 1680.)

Depression; ataxia; convulsions; opisthotonos; inappetence; reduced growth rate; loss of condition; bruising; decreased egg production, fertility, and hatchability; and increased mortality are common. Turkey poults and ducklings are particularly susceptible, as are pheasant chicks to a lesser degree. There may be a membranous glomerulonephritis and hyaline droplet nephrosis, and some degree of ascites and visceral edema may be apparent. The liver is pale and mottled with widespread necrosis. Excessive bile production is common. A marked catarrhal enteritis is characteristic, especially in the duodenum.

Aspergillus flavus may be isolated from feed, but this is not confirmatory of the disease without further tests. Biological assays for the toxin are available, in which ducklings or poults are used. Chemical assays are available that use fluorescent or chromatographic techniques. The disease should be suspected if histopathological examination of the liver reveals bile duct hyperplasia. The hepatic cells are enlarged with some necrotic foci.

Mold inhibitors should be used to control the growth of *A flavus* in the feed. Gentian violet (500-1500 ppm [0.5-1.5 g/kg]), propionic acid (500-1500 ppm [0.5-1.5 g/kg]), and thiabendazole (100 ppm [100 mg/kg]) have been used to prevent mold growth in feed.

No specific treatment is known. Affected poultry should be fed a high-energy, good-quality-protein diet fortified with increased levels of both water- and fat-soluble vitamins. The addition of low levels of antibiotics minimizes the effect of aflatoxicosis.

NEOPLASMS

The economically important neoplasms in poultry are 1) Marek's disease, 2) lymphoid leukosis, 3) a runting disease and chronic lymphoma caused by a nondefective reticuloendotheliosis virus, and 4) lymphoproliferative disease of turkeys. Several other neoplasms caused by viruses or other factors are of incidental importance.

Marek's disease is caused by a herpesvirus. Lymphoid leukosis, reticuloendotheliosis, and lymphoproliferative disease are each caused by retroviruses that are antigenically distinct from each other.

MAREK'S DISEASE

Chickens are the only important natural host, but quail and turkeys can be infected experimentally. Turkeys are commonly infected with turkey herpesvirus, an avirulent strain related to Marek's disease virus. Other birds and mammals appear to be refractory to the disease or infection.

Marek's disease is one of the most ubiquitous avian infections; it is identified among chicken flocks worldwide. Every flock except for those maintained under strict pathogen-free conditions may be presumed to be infected. Although clinical disease is not always apparent in infected flocks, a subclinical decrease in growth rate and egg production may be economically important.

Etiology: Three serotypes of the cell-associated herpesvirus are recognized: serotypes 1 and 2 designate virulent and avirulent chicken isolates, respectively; serotype 3 designates the related avirulent turkey herpesvirus. Serotypes 2 and 3, as well as attenuated serotype 1 viruses have been used as vaccines. Serotype identification is accomplished by reaction with type-specific monoclonal antibodies or by biological characteristics such as host range, pathogenicity, growth rate, and plaque morphology.

Transmission and Epidemiology: The disease is highly contagious and readily transmitted among chickens. The virus matures into a fully infective, enveloped form in the epithelium of the feather follicle, from which it is released into the environment. It may survive for months in poultry house litter or dust. Dust or dander from infected chickens is particularly effective in transmission. Infection usually occurs via aerosol exposure through the respiratory tract. Once infected, chickens continue to be carriers for long periods and act as sources of infectious virus. Shedding of infectious virus can be reduced, but not prevented, by prior vaccination. Unlike viruses of serotypes 1 and 2 that are highly contagious, turkey herpesvirus is not readily transmissible among chickens (although it is among turkeys, its natural host). Attenuated serotype 1 viruses vary greatly in their ability to be transmitted among chickens; the most attenuated are not transmitted. Marek's disease virus is not vertically transmitted.

Pathogenesis: Three types of virus/host cell interactions are recognized *in vivo*: productive infection, latent infection, and neoplastic transformation. Productive infection occurs transiently in lymphocytes, mainly of B-cell origin, within 1 wk after infection and is characterized by antigen production leading to cell death. Productive infection also occurs in the feather follicle epithelium, in which enveloped virions are produced. Latent infection of T cells is responsible for the long-term carrier state. No antigens are expressed, but virus can be recovered from such lymphocytes by co-cultivation with susceptible cells in tissue cultures. Some lymphocytes, latently infected with oncogenic serotype 1 virus strains, undergo neoplastic transformation. These transformed cells, provided they escape the immune system of the host, may multiply to form characteristic lymphoid neoplasms. Immune responses are both cell-mediated and humoral and are directed against viral and tumor-associated host antigens. Of these, cell-mediated immunity directed against viral antigens probably is the most important.

Clinical Findings and Lesions: Paralysis is sometimes noted, but more typically, affected birds show only depression before death. A transient paralysis syndrome has been associated with Marek's disease; chickens become ataxic for periods of several days, then recover. This syndrome is rare in immunized birds.

Enlarged nerves are one of the most consistent gross lesions in affected birds and, when present, have diagnostic significance. Various peripheral nerves, but particularly the vagus, brachial, and sciatic, become enlarged and lose their striations. Diffuse or nodular lymphoid tumors may be seen in various organs, particularly the liver, spleen, gonads, heart, lung, kidney, muscle, and proventriculus. Enlarged feather follicles (commonly termed skin leukosis) may be noted in broilers during processing and are a cause for condemnation. The bursa is only rarely tumorous and more frequently is atrophic. Histologically, the lesions consist of a mixed population of small, medium, and large lymphoid cells plus plasma cells and large anaplastic lymphoblasts. These cells represent a pleomorphic mixture of tumor cells and reactive inflammatory cells. When the bursa of Fabricius is involved, the tumor cells typically appear in interfollicular areas.

Diagnosis: Usually, diagnosis is based on enlarged nerves and lymphoid tumors in various viscera. The absence of bursal tumors helps distinguish this disease from lymphoid leukosis (*see* below); also, Marek's disease occurs at any age >3 wk. A diagnosis may be confirmed histologically or by demonstrating the tumor-associated surface antigen on some of the individual cells by immunofluorescence. Furthermore, T cells are more frequent than B cells in Marek's disease tumors; cells containing IgM are rare.

Control: Vaccination is the principal method of control. The efficacy of vaccines can be improved, however, by strict sanitation to reduce or delay exposure, and by breeding for genetic resistance. The most popular vaccine consists of turkey herpesvirus. Recently, a bivalent vaccine consisting of turkey herpesvirus and the SB-1 strain of serotype 2 Marek's disease virus has been used to provide additional protection against challenge with virulent serotype 1 isolates. Additional types of vaccines are used outside the USA. Because all vaccines are administered at hatching and require 1-2 wk to produce an effective immunity, exposure of chickens to virus should be minimized during the first few days after hatching. Cell-associated vaccines are generally more effective than cell-free vaccines because they are neutralized less by maternal antibodies. Vaccine efficacy is usually ≥90%. Since the advent of vaccination, losses from Marek's disease have been reduced dramatically in broiler and layer flocks. However, disease is occasionally noted in individual flocks. Of the many causes proposed for these so-called vaccine failures, exposure to very virulent virus strains appears to be among the most important. Use of the bivalent vaccine is designed to specifically counteract such strains.

LYMPHOID LEUKOSIS

Lymphoid leukosis occurs naturally only in chickens. Experimentally, some of the viruses of the leukosis/sarcoma group can infect and produce tumors in other species of birds or even mammals. The infection is known to occur in virtually all chicken flocks except for some SPF flocks from which it has been eradicated. The frequency of infection recently has been reduced substantially in the primary breeding stocks of several commercial poultry breeding companies. Should this control program continue, infection may become infrequent or totally absent in certain commercial flocks. The frequency of lymphoid leukosis tumors in infected flocks is typically low (<4%); disease is often inapparent.

Etiology: The disease is caused by certain members of the leukosis/sarcoma group of avian retroviruses. Isolates that can induce lymphoid leukosis in chickens are commonly called avian leukosis viruses, and belong to subgroups A, B, C, and D. Subgroups A and B are most prevalent in western countries. A fifth subgroup (E) designates nononcogenic endogenous viruses produced by viral genes integrated into the host cell DNA. The subgroups have distinct antigenicities and cellular host ranges that are determined by viral envelope glycoproteins. Viruses within a subgroup cross-neutralize to varying extents. All field strains of lymphoid leukosis virus are oncogenic, although some differences in oncogenicity and replicative ability have been recognized.

Transmission and Epidemiology: Avian leukosis virus is shed by the hen into the albumen or yolk, or both; infection probably occurs after the onset of incubation. Congenitally infected chickens usually remain viremic for life and fail to produce neutralizing antibodies. Horizontal infection after hatching is also important, especially when chicks are exposed immediately following hatching to high doses of virus, eg, in feces of congenitally infected chicks, or in contaminated vaccines. Horizontally infected chickens experience a transient viremia followed by antibody production. The earlier the infection, the more likely it is to lead to tolerance, persistent viremia, and to tumors. Thus, tumors are more frequent in congenital than in horizontal infections, but many more chickens are exposed horizontally than congenitally. Rates of embryo transmission typically are 1-10%; virtually all chicks in an infected flock are exposed by contact. Congenital and, in some cases, early horizontal infection can induce permanent carrier states characterized by shedding of virus or antigen into the environment and into eggs. Late infection (ie, inoculation at 12-20 wk of age) is unlikely to lead to virus shedding and has been used by some to reduce the level of shedding in flocks. Avian leukosis virus is not highly contagious in comparison to other viral agents and is readily inactivated by disinfectants. Transmission can be reduced or eliminated by strict sanitation. Following eradication of infection, standard disease control and sanitation practices can keep chicken flocks free of the disease.

Pathogenesis: Lymphoid leukosis is a clonal malignancy of the bursal-dependent lymphoid system. Transformation invariably occurs in the intact bursa of Fabricius, often as early as 4-8 wk after infection. Tumors require some time to develop. Mortality rarely occurs before 14 wk of age, and is more frequent around the time of sexual maturity. The disease can be prevented, even up to 5 mo of age, by treatments that destroy the bursa. The tumors are composed almost entirely of B lymphocytes that, in many instances, have IgM on their surfaces. No anti-tumor immune response has been recognized.

A subclinical disease syndrome characterized by poor growth, anemia, and depressed egg production in the absence of tumor formation is probably even more important economically than are deaths from lymphoid leukosis. Chickens with such subclinical disease usually shed virus or viral antigen into the albumen of eggs. The pathogenic mechanisms are poorly understood.

Clinical Findings and Lesions: Lymphoid leukosis has few typical clinical signs. Infected birds become depressed before death. Palpation often reveals an enlarged bursa, and sometimes an enlarged liver. Infected birds may not necessarily develop tumors, but they may lay fewer eggs.

Diffuse or nodular lymphoid tumors are common in the liver, spleen, and bursa, and occasionally in the kidneys, gonads, and mesentery. Involvement of the bursa is considered virtually pathognomonic. Sometimes the bursal tumors are small and observed only after careful examination of the mucosal surface of the organ. No involvement of the peripheral nerves is apparent. Microscopically, the tumor cells are uniform, large lymphocytes. Mitotic figures are frequent.

Diagnosis: Gross characteristics of diagnostic significance include the tumorous involvement of the liver, spleen, or bursa in the absence of peripheral nerve lesions. The tumors occur in birds ≥ 14 wk old. Histologically, the lymphoid cells are uniform in character, large, and contain IgM and B-cell markers (but not tumor-associated surface antigen) on their surface. The tumor can be differentiated from those of Marek's disease by gross and microscopic pathology and by examination of tumor cells for surface antigens. It cannot easily be differentiated from some B-cell lymphomas caused by reticuloendotheliosis virus; however, such tumors probably are extremely rare in the field.

Control: Lymphoid leukosis appears to be controlled best by reduction and eventual eradication of the causative virus. Breeder flocks are evaluated for viral shedding by testing for viral antigens in the albumen of eggs with complement-fixation or enzyme immunoassays. Eggs from shedder hens are discarded, so that progeny flocks typically have reduced levels of infection. If raised in small groups, infection-free flocks may be derived with relative ease. At present, these control measures are mainly used by primary breeding companies. Reduction of viral infection has reduced lymphoid leukosis mortality and improved egg production. Although it is not clear whether eradication will be adopted by the commercial industry, such a program seems feasible. Some chickens have specific genetic resistance to infection with certain subgroups of virus. However, this is unlikely to replace the need for reduction or eradication of the virus. Thus far, vaccination has not been promising.

RETICULOENDOTHELIOSIS

The host range of reticuloendotheliosis virus (REV) is much broader than that of Marek's disease or lymphoid leukosis. Chickens, turkeys, ducks, geese, and quail have experienced natural infection and disease, and probably many species of birds can be infected. Mammals appear refractory, although certain mammalian cell cultures are susceptible.

REV is not ubiquitous but is more widely distributed than once believed. It appears to be particularly prevalent in Israel, Australia, Japan, and the southern USA in chicken and turkey flocks.

Etiology: REV is a retrovirus unrelated to the viruses of the leukosis/sarcoma group. The isolates all belong to a single serotype, but differ in pathogenicity. The isolates can be classified as either nondefective or defective. Most field isolates appear to be nondefective for replication in cell cultures and contain no viral oncogene. One unique laboratory strain (strain T) is defective for replication in cell cultures and contains a viral oncogene, v-rel, that is responsible for an acute reticulum cell neoplasia in experimentally inoculated chicks; this neoplasm does not occur commonly in the field.

Transmission and Epidemiology: Horizontal transmission is probably more important than vertical, although both have been documented in chickens and turkeys. Transmission by mosquitoes and other blood-sucking insects is suspected. The virus has been isolated from litter. Congenital infection may occur, but probably is rare. The virus has been transmitted accidentally through use of contaminated vaccines. Contact transmission does occur, but the virus is not highly contagious, nor is it highly stable in the environment. More work is needed to determine the means by which it is maintained and transmitted.

Pathogenesis: The nondefective subgroups in strains of REV produce 3 distinct syndromes: non-neoplastic runting, acute neoplastic disease, and chronic neoplastic disease. Typically, the runting syndrome is seen 4-10 wk after administration of contaminated vaccines to day-old chicks. Chronic neoplastic disease has been induced experimentally in chickens, turkeys, and ducks; one type occurs in chickens after latent periods of >4 mo and appears identical to lymphoid leukosis. As in lymphoid leukosis, these tumors are composed of B cells, are bursal-dependent, and have IgM on their surface. Acute neoplasia, which occurs after a latent period of 6-8 wk, also has been observed in chickens, turkeys, ducks, and quail. This is a reticuloendotheliosis which, in chickens, may be confused with Marek's disease.

Clinical Findings and Lesions: The runting syndrome is characterized by weight loss, paleness, occasional paralysis, and abnormal feathering. Death from neoplasia is preceded by depression and occasionally by some of the same changes described for the runting syndrome.

Lesions include bursal and thymic atrophy, enlarged nerves, anemia, and abnormal feathering. Of these, the abnormal feathering, in which the barbules are compressed to the shaft over a small part of its length, may be of diagnostic value. The neoplasms typically involve the liver, spleen, and heart. The bursa is involved in the chronic B-cell lymphomas of chickens in a manner similar to that of lymphoid leukosis. Nonbursal lymphomas with shorter latent periods and lesions superficially resembling Marek's disease also are recognized in chickens. In turkeys, prominent lesions include enlarged livers and nodular lesions on the intestines; the bursa is only rarely tumorous. The tumors, regardless of type or host species, are usually composed of uniform, large, lymphoreticular cells.

Diagnosis: The lesions induced by REV are so diverse that diagnosis at gross necropsy is difficult; virus isolation or antibody detection is useful in confirmation. The nerve lesions are less extensive and contain more plasma cells than in Marek's disease. The runting syndrome is easily confused with immunosuppressive syndromes caused by a variety of other viral agents (eg, MALABSORPTION SYNDROME, qv, p 1579). The chronic B-cell lymphomas induced experimentally in chickens cannot be distinguished from those of lymphoid leukosis except by virus studies. The chronic lymphomas that occur in turkeys must be differentiated from lymphoproliferative disease of turkeys based on histology, virus isolation, and characterization of the virus-associated reverse transcriptase for activity in the presence of manganese or magnesium ions.

Control: No control measures are being practiced currently.

LYMPHOPROLIFERATIVE DISEASE IN TURKEYS

The natural disease has been described only in turkeys, commercial hybrid strains of which appear to differ in susceptibility. Chickens can be infected experimentally, but are less susceptible than turkeys. Ducks and geese are refractory to experimental infection. The disease has been identified in England and Israel, and probably has occurred in several European countries. Its presence in the USA has not been confirmed.

Etiology: The etiological agent probably is a retrovirus that is antigenically and genetically distinct from those causing lymphoid leukosis and reticuloendotheliosis. This virus has not been cultivated *in vitro*, but virus particles can be observed in tissues of infected turkeys; plasma is a good source of infective material.

Transmission, Epidemiology, and Pathogenesis: Contact transmission has been demonstrated among turkeys. Although vertical transmission has not yet been proved, this possibility also should be considered. The incidence of infection is far greater than the incidence of disease; high rates of infection can be demonstrated in certain flocks with no mortality. Infected turkeys often develop a persistent viremia that can be detected by the presence of a reverse transcriptase in the plasma. No satisfactory test for antibodies is available.

In natural outbreaks, up to 25% of turkeys die from neoplastic disease when 7-18 wk old. Males may be more susceptible than females. Poults are more susceptible to experimental inoculation at 4 wk than at hatching. Lesions appear first in the spleen and thymus, and can be recognized as early as 2 wk after infection.

Clinical Findings and Lesions: Affected birds die suddenly; some may be depressed before death. The most characteristic lesion is a greatly enlarged spleen, which is often pale or marbled. Gray-white tumor foci can be observed in the liver, thymus, gonad, pancreas, kidney, intestine, lung, and heart. In some cases, the peripheral nerves are enlarged. The tumor lesions are composed of a pleomorphic mixture of lymphoid cells, reticulum cells, and plasma cells.

Diagnosis: Diagnosis depends on the presence of characteristic gross and microscopic lesions. The tumors differ in their pleomorphic cellular composition from those of reticuloendotheliosis, which are composed of uniform lymphoreticular cells. The presence of reticuloendotheliosis virus should be excluded by appropriate tests for virus or antibodies. The plasma of turkeys with lymphoproliferative disease often contains a virus-associated reverse transcriptase that has a higher activity in the presence of magnesium ions than manganese ions; whereas with reticuloendotheliosis virus, the opposite is true.

Control: No control methods have been developed.

OTHER TUMORS

Of the numerous other transmissible and nontransmissible tumors known to occur in poultry, a few have limited importance. Most strains of leukosis/sarcoma viruses also induce nonlymphoid tumors (including sarcomas), erythroblastosis, myeloblastosis, hemangiomas, nephroblastoma, osteopetrosis, and related neoplasms. The nature of the tumors and their frequency depend on virus strain, chicken strain, and age, dose, and route of infection. Occasional outbreaks of predominantly one type of tumor are seen in the field. The Rous sarcoma virus, a member of this group, has been widely studied in the laboratory. Each strain usually causes a predominantly neoplastic disease and can be distinguished on the basis of pathogenicity. Some, eg, Rous sarcoma and erythroblastosis viruses, contain a viral oncogene that is responsible for their ability to induce neoplasms within a short incubation period, but such viruses are rare in the field. Others are defective for replication and require a nondefective helper virus.

Squamous cell carcinomas occur at relatively high frequencies in some broiler flocks and are a cause of condemnations. Typically, the lesions are observed during processing as crater-like eruptions on the defeathered skin. Transmissibility of this tumor has neither been demonstrated nor ruled out. An etiological agent has not yet been identified.

Adenocarcinomas of the ovary or oviduct are relatively common incidental tumors in mature chickens. These neoplasms often are characterized by multiple miliary implant tumors on the mesentery and other visceral surfaces, frequently accompanied by ascites. These tumors are not known to be virus induced or to be transmissible.

NEWCASTLE DISEASE
(Avian pneumoencephalitis)

An acute, rapidly spreading, viral disease of domestic poultry and other birds worldwide, characterized by rapid onset and variable mortality. Respiratory signs (coughing, sneezing, rales) are often accompanied or followed by nervous manifestations and, in infections with some strains, by diarrhea and swelling of the head.

Although Newcastle disease virus can produce a transitory conjunctivitis in man, the condition has been limited primarily to laboratory workers and vaccination teams exposed to large quantities of virus, before vaccination was widely practiced, to crews eviscerating poultry in processing plants. The disease has not been reported in individuals who rear poultry or consume poultry products.

Etiology and Epidemiology: The cause is an RNA virus, paramyxovirus-1 (PMV-1), which can be categorized into 3 groups: the **velogenic** strains are highly pathogenic and easily transmitted, the **mesogenic** strains are intermediate, and the **lentogenic** strains show low pathogenicity in chickens. Isolates that cause the respiratory-nervous syndrome, even those that are highly pathogenic, usually produce few or no distinctive gross lesions; however, isolates that cause the viscerotropic syndrome often do. Velogenic and mesogenic virus isolates kill 10-day-old chicken embryos in 2-4 days, lentogenic isolates usually in 4-6 days or not at all.

Virus is shed during incubation, during the clinical stage, and for a varying but limited period during convalescence. It is present in exhaled air, respiratory discharges, feces, eggs layed during clinical disease, and all parts of the carcass during acute infection and at death. Chickens are readily infected by aerosols and by ingesting contaminated water or food. While the primary source of virus is the chicken, other domestic birds and certain wild birds are susceptible and may be sources. Parrots, mynahs, and such caged birds as pittas that moved in commercial channels were the principal source of infection during the 1970-72 pandemic (USA) of the velogenic viscerotropic form of Newcastle disease. An outbreak of PMV-1 occurred in pigeons in the USA and the UK during 1984. This pigeon paramyxovirus is lentogenic for chickens and occurs worldwide in some pigeon populations.

Clinical Findings: Respiratory or nervous signs, or both, occur in the most widespread forms of the disease and are common in the USA. Signs appear almost simultaneously throughout the flock 2-15 days (av 5) after exposure. Young chickens are more susceptible and show signs sooner than older ones. Respiratory signs are gasping and coughing. Nervous signs include drooping wings, dragging legs, twisting of the head and neck, circling, depression, inappetence, and complete paralysis, and may accompany but usually follow the respiratory signs. Clonic spasms are seen in moribund birds. Laying flocks may have partial or complete cessation of production and not recover. Eggs from infected flocks may be abnormal in color, shape, or surface, and have watery albumen.

Viscerotropic signs, which predominate in the peracute disease, include watery and greenish diarrhea, and swelling of the tissues around the eyes and in the neck. Mortality depends on virulence of the virus strain, environmental conditions, and condition of the flock. In general, mortality is higher in young flocks (but 100% mortality may occur in adult flocks as well).

Lesions: Lesions are highly variable, reflecting the variation in tropism and pathogenicity of the virus. Petechiae may be seen on the serous membranes; hemorrhages of the proventricular mucosa and intestinal serosa occur, and are accompanied by necrotic areas on the mucosal surface. Congestion and mucoid exudates may be seen in the respiratory tract, with opacity and thickening of the air sacs.

Diagnosis: Tentative diagnosis of a rapidly spreading, respiratory-nervous disease may be confirmed by isolation of the hemagglutinating virus identified by inhibition with Newcastle disease antiserum. Paired serum samples showing a rise in hemagglutination-inhibition antibodies also confirm the disease. The acute form should be differentiated from highly pathogenic avian influenza (qv, p 1618) by virology and serology. Although it is difficult to differentiate between Newcastle strains other than by the rapidity with which they kill embryonating chicken eggs and adult chickens, grouping strains according to their geographic and temporal appearance using monoclonal antibodies has had some success. Oligonucleotide "fingerprinting" of the viral RNA has been used to differentiate between strains similar in all other respects.

Prophylaxis and Treatment: Live virus vaccines are widely used. (*See* tables on vaccination programs, poultry, p 1261 *et seq.*) Lentogenic strains, chiefly B1 and LaSota in the New World, are administered in drinking water or in spray or dust. Sometimes, administration is by nose or eye drop route. Healthy chicks are vaccinated as early as day 1-4 of life. However, delaying vaccination until the second or third week avoids partial blockage of the active immune response by maternal antibody. Mycoplasma and some other bacteria, if present, may act synergistically with some vaccines to aggravate the vaccine reaction. This effect may be potentiated by mass-vaccination methods. Failure to follow instructions (eg, use of sprays in windy houses or use of chemically treated water to dilute the virus) may result in incomplete or no protection after vaccination.

When other infections are present in the flock, and where required by law, killed vaccines should be used. Vaccines with oil adjuvants give the longest protection. Whether killed vaccines, lentogenic mass vaccines, wing-web, or IM-injected mesogenic strains are used, repeated vaccination is required to protect chickens throughout life. The frequency of revaccination largely depends on the risk of exposure and virulence of the field virus.

Disease control officials in the USA and some other countries use import restrictions and eradication methods to prevent establishment of the highly virulent, viscerotropic form of the disease. Other countries depend on vaccination. Proper administration of a high-titered vaccine is essential for induction of a good immune response.

OMPHALITIS
(Navel ill, "Mushy chick" disease)

A condition characterized by infected, unhealed navels in chicks, poults, and other young fowl. This noncontagious disease is associated with excessive humidity and marked contamination of the incubator. The navels fail to close. Opportunistic bacteria (coliforms, staphylococci, *Pseudomonas* spp, and *Proteus* spp) are often recovered. Proteolytic anaerobes are prevalent in outbreaks. Losses may be increased by chilling or overheating during shipment.

The affected chicks or poults usually appear normal until a few hours before death. Depression, drooping of the head, and huddling near the heat source usually are the only signs. The navel is inflamed and a scab may be present. The yolk sac is not absorbed and often is highly congested or broken; peritonitis may be extensive. Edema of the sternal subcutis may occur. Mortality often begins at hatching and continues to 10-14 days of age, with losses up to 15% in chickens and 50% in turkeys. Persistent, unabsorbed, infected yolks often produce stunted chicks or poults.

Careful control of temperature, humidity, and sanitation in the incubator prevents the disease. Only clean, uncracked eggs should be set. If eggs are washed, a sanitizing detergent must be used according to directions. Time, temperature, and frequent changes of water are as critical as the concentration of sanitizer in both wash and rinse water. The rinse should be warmer than the wash water but not >140°F (60°C).

The incubator should be cleaned and fumigated thoroughly between hatches and before the hatching season. Fumigation must be done with closed vents at high temperature and humidity. Thirty mL of 40% formaldehyde and 15 g of potassium permanganate per 20 cu ft (0.6 m³), or paraformaldehyde (in the strength recommended by the manufacturer) in a heating device should be used. Contamination of the machines may readily occur following fumigation unless the exterior of the machines and the rooms in which they are located are cleaned and disinfected.

There is no specific treatment.

PASTEURELLA ANATIPESTIFER INFECTION
(New duck disease, Infectious serositis)

A contagious, widely distributed disease that primarily affects young ducks and turkeys. Other waterfowl, chickens, and pheasants also may be affected. The epidemiology and pathogenesis are not understood. Ducks are believed to be infected when *P anatipestifer* is introduced into toenail scratches of the webbed foot. Turkeys may be infected by injuries or by the respiratory route when another pathogen disrupts the respiratory epithelium.

Affected ducks, usually 2-7 wk old, often have ocular and nasal discharges, mild coughing and sneezing, tremors of the head and neck, and incoordination. Stunting may occur, and mortality is usually 2-30%. Fibrinous exudate in the pericardial cavity and over the surface of the liver is the most characteristic lesion. Fibrinous airsacculitis is common, and infection of the CNS can result in fibrinous meningitis. The spleen and liver may be swollen. Pneumonia may occur.

In turkeys, usually 5-15 wk old, it has resulted in 5-60% mortality and condemnations of 3-13%. Affected turkeys often exhibit dyspnea, droopiness, hunched back, lameness, and a twisted neck. Fibrinous pericarditis and epicarditis are the most pronounced lesions. There may also be fibrinous perihepatitis, airsacculitis, and purulent synovitis. Osteomyelitis, meningitis, and focal pneumonia are observed occasionally.

Diagnosis is based on signs, lesions, and isolation and identification of the causative organism, since other diseases, particularly colibacillosis (qv, p 1569) and chlamydiosis (qv, p 1568), may produce similar lesions. Chocolate agar medium is recommended for isolation, although blood agar is also used, with incubation at 37°C in a candle jar or under 5% carbon dioxide. The isolate should be serotyped since the information may be needed for vaccine selection and epidemiology. Biochemical characteristics can be used to differentiate this organism from other bacteria that cause important diseases of ducks and turkeys, particularly *Escherichia coli* and *P multocida*. Impression smears help to rule in or rule out chlamydia.

Careful management practices are important for prevention of infection. Rigid sanitation and depopulation are necessary for elimination. A bacterin and, more recently, a live vaccine, which include the 3 most common immunotypes of *P anatipestifer* are available for use in ducks. An autogenous oil-emulsion bacterin can be used in turkeys. A combination of penicillin and streptomycin, or sulfaquinoxaline can be used for initial treatment, but an antibiotic sensitivity test should be performed.

POISONINGS

See also the TOX section, p 1632 *et seq*. Generally, birds are less susceptible to poisoning than are mammals, and instances of toxicity usually indicate departure from label recommendations. However, the possibility of residues of toxic substances in eggs or poultry meat is of concern. Label recommendations regarding withdrawal times for all potentially toxic substances should be followed scrupulously.

INORGANIC SOURCES

Carbon Monoxide: This poisoning commonly arises from exhaust fumes when chicks are being transported by truck or from improper ventilation in hatchers. Mortality may be high unless fresh air is provided immediately. At necropsy, the beak is cyanotic, and a characteristic bright pink color is noted throughout the viscera, particularly the lungs. Diagnosis can be confirmed by a spectroscopic analysis of the blood.

Copper: Copper sulfate in a single dose of >1 g is fatal. The signs are watery diarrhea and listlessness. A catarrhal gastroenteritis and burns or erosions in the lining of the gizzard, accompanied by a greenish, seromucous exudate throughout the intestinal tract, are found at necropsy.

Lead: Lead poisoning usually is caused by paint or orchard-spray material. Metallic lead in amounts of 7.2 mg/kg body wt is lethal. Signs are depression, inappetence, emaciation, thirst, and weakness. Greenish droppings are commonly observed within 36 hr. As poisoning progresses, the wings may be extended downward. Young birds may die within 36 hr after ingestion. Diagnosis of acute lead poisoning may be made from the history and necropsy findings of a greenish brown gizzard mucosa, enteritis, and degeneration of the liver and kidney. Chronic poisoning results in emaciation, and atrophy of the liver and heart. The pericardium is distended with fluid, the gallbladder is thickened and enlarged, and urate deposits are usually found in the kidneys. Ingestion of lead shot often occurs in wild waterfowl on heavily gunned feeding grounds. Retention of only a few lead pellets in the gizzard can kill a duck.

Mercury: Poisoning occurs from mercurial disinfectants and fungicides, including mercurous chloride (calomel) and bichloride of mercury (corrosive sublimate). Clinical signs are progressive weakness and incoordination. Diarrhea may occur, depending on the amount ingested. The caustic action of the chemical may produce gray areas in the mouth and esophagus, which usually ulcerate if the bird lives >24 hr. Catarrhal inflammation of the proventriculus and intestines may occur; if a large amount of mercury is ingested, extensive hemorrhage may occur in these organs. The kidneys are pale and studded with small white foci. The liver shows fatty degeneration.

Salt: The addition of 0.5% salt (NaCl) to the ration of chickens and turkeys is recommended, but amounts of >2% are usually considered dangerous. Rations for chicks have contained as much as 8% without injurious effect, but in poults, rations containing 4% were harmful and levels of 6-8% have resulted in mortality. The addition of 2% NaCl to the feed, or 4000 ppm in the water, depresses growth in young ducks and lowers the fertility and hatchability of the eggs in breeding stock.

Salt levels high enough to produce poisoning may be reached when salty protein concentrates (eg, fish meal) are added to rations already fortified with salt or when the salt is poorly incorporated in the feed. Sporadic poisoning also has been reported from accidental ingestion of rock salt or salt provided for other livestock. Necropsy findings are not diagnostic; enteritis and ascites are common. Watery droppings and wet litter often are suggestive of a high salt intake.

Selenium: Ingestion of feeds containing >5 ppm of selenium decreases the hatchability of eggs because of deformities of the embryos, which are unable to emerge from the shell because of beak anomalies. Eyes may be missing, and feet and wings may be deformed or underdeveloped. Selenium at 10 ppm, as in seleniferous grains in the laying ration, usually reduces hatchability to zero.

Mature birds seem to tolerate more selenium in their feed than pigs, cattle, or horses, without exhibiting signs of poisoning other than poor hatchability of their eggs. Starting rations containing 8 ppm selenium have reduced the growth rate of chicks, but 4 ppm had no noticeable effect. Rations containing as little as 2.5 ppm have resulted in meat and eggs with concentrations of selenium in excess of the suggested tolerance limit in foods. Sodium arsenite and some of the organic arsenicals, when administered to laying hens with selenium, have increased hatchability.

ORGANIC SOURCES

Various organic chemicals are dangerous, especially those used to treat seed grain.

Coffee Weed Seed: *Cassia obtusifolia* seeds are frequently found in corn and soybeans. When present at ≥2%, they cause reduced feed intake with lowered body weights, elevated feed conversion in broilers, and significant depression of egg production in laying birds. Necropsy lesions are absent.

Crotalaria: Seeds of many species are toxic to chickens. Concentrations of >0.05% in the feed produce signs of toxicosis. At 0.2%, weight gain is reduced markedly; 0.3% causes death in 18 days. Lesions consist of ascites, swelling or cirrhosis of the liver, and hemorrhages. Resistance to the toxin increases with age.

Gossypol: Cottonseed meal contains appreciable amounts of gossypol, which produces severe cardiac edema that results in dyspnea, weakness, and anorexia. Gossypol also causes egg-yolk discoloration when fed to laying hens.

Monensin: This ionophore coccidiostat is widely used in the broiler industry. At levels of >120 ppm, it reduces feed intake and weight gains; in layers, egg production is reduced. Signs of toxicity include a characteristic paralysis in which the legs are extended backward. Mortality occurs in turkeys if they are switched to a feed that contains monensin. They become paralyzed with the legs extended backward; no lesions are seen at necropsy.

Nicarbazin: This coccidiostat is used in broilers. It should not be fed to layers, in which it can cause discoloration and reduced hatchability of eggs (although the effect is reversible once the nicarbazin is withdrawn). It also may result in reduced heat tolerance in birds exposed to high temperature and humidity.

Nitrofurazone: This is used to treat several bacterial diseases in poultry. When fed at 0.022%, it causes hyperexcitability manifest by rapid movements, loud squawking, and frequent falling forward. In turkeys, which are more sensitive to nitrofurazone than chickens, it produces cardiac dilatation, ascites, and, when fed at 0.033%, mortality.

3-Nitro-4-hydroxyphenylarsonic Acid: When this compound, widely used in the feed to improve weight gains and feed efficiency, is improperly mixed or fed at a level 2-3 times higher than normal, it induces a high-pitched chirp and a "duck-walking" stance. Cervical paralysis is frequently seen in chickens that consume excessive amounts. Clinical signs are usually reversible in a few minutes.

Polychlorinated Biphenyls (PCB): Residues have been reported in the fatty tissue of chickens and turkeys in excess of the 5 ppm permitted in edible tissue, and in egg products in excess of the permitted 0.5 ppm. (*See also* PCB TOXICITY, p 1654.) PCB depress egg production and hatchability, and levels of 50 ppm produce cirrhosis of the liver and ascites in broilers and a drop in egg production and hatchability in hens.

Quaternary Ammonia: Quaternary-ammonia-based compounds are widely used as disinfectants. Turkeys are very sensitive; levels of 150 ppm result in substantial mortality. Clinical signs include reduced water intake, nasal and ocular discharge, facial swelling, and gasping. Necropsy lesions include caseous ulcers at the base of the tongue and commissures of the mouth.

Sulfaquinoxaline: Sulfonamides are widely used for treatment of several bacterial and protozoal infections in poultry. Sulfaquinoxaline, when fed at 0.25%, results in severe anemia. Hemorrhages are common on the legs, breast muscle, and in virtually all the abdominal organs. The bone marrow is pale, and the blood is slow to clot. Toxicity is frequently seen in hot weather when sulfaquinoxaline is used as a water medication. Water consumption increases rapidly as the temperature increases, which leads to increased drug intake. This toxicity usually is responsive to vitamin K therapy.

Thiram: This substance, used to treat seed corn, is toxic to chicks at 40 ppm and goslings at 150 ppm; it causes leg deformities and weight loss. At 10 ppm, it causes soft-shelled eggs, and at 40 ppm, egg production and hatchability are reduced. Turkey poults tolerate up to 200 ppm.

Toxic Fat: A crystalline halogen has been identified as the "toxic fat" factor in some feed. In young pullets, it reduces growth, retards sexual development, and increases mortality. Hatchability is lowered. Turkeys and ducks are less susceptible than chickens. Signs of intoxication include ruffled feathers, droopiness, and dyspnea. Lesions include ascites and hydropericardium, liver necrosis, subepicardial hemorrhage, and bile duct hyperplasia. Although the amount of toxin varies in feeds from different sources, 0.25-0.5% fed for 35-150 days produced typical lesions.

AUTOINTOXICATION

Self-poisoning due to the retention of metabolic waste products or the absorption of decomposition products, including bacterial toxins, that occur within the intestine. Signs include cyanosis, sluggishness, and diarrhea. Congestion of the muscles and viscera with kidney congestion, swelling, and blockage may be noted. Catarrhal enteritis is usually present. Antibiotics (eg, chlortetracycline, oxytetracycline) given at 0.01% in the mash and combined with a laxative may be helpful.

SALMONELLOSES

These may be divided into those caused by: 1) 2 *Salmonella* spp highly host-adapted to the chicken and turkey (*S pullorum* and *S gallinarum*); 2) *S arizonae*, containing a few serotypes commonly called paracolons; important in turkeys and, in a few countries, in chickens; and 3) the remaining ~2000 nonhost-adapted species. The latter group (paratyphoid) may be transmitted to almost all animals (*see* SALMONELLOSIS, p 148). Salmonelloses have major public health significance because contaminated food can infect man.

PULLORUM DISEASE

Infections by *S pullorum* usually cause high mortality in young chickens and turkeys and occasionally in adult chickens. A once common disease, it has been eradicated from most commercial stock. It usually occurs in other avian species only if they are in close contact with infected chickens or turkeys. Infection in mammals is rare.

Transmission is chiefly directly through the egg, but also occurs by direct or indirect contact. Infection transmitted via egg or hatchery usually results in mortality during the first few days of life and up to 2-3 wk of age. Affected birds huddle near a source of heat, do not eat, appear sleepy, and show whitish fecal pasting around the vent. Survivors frequently become asymptomatic carriers with localized infection of the ovary. Some of the eggs laid by such hens hatch and produce infected progeny.

Lesions in young birds usually include unabsorbed yolk sacs, focal necrosis of the liver and spleen, and grayish nodules in the lungs, heart, and gizzard muscle. Firm, cheesy material in the ceca and raised plaques in the mucosa of the lower intestine are sometimes seen. Occasionally, synovitis is prominent. Adult carriers sometimes have no gross lesions but usually have pericarditis, peritonitis, or distorted ovarian follicles with coagulated contents. Acute infections in mature chickens produce lesions that are indistinguishable from those of fowl typhoid (*see* below).

Lesions may be highly suggestive, but diagnosis should be confirmed by isolation and identification of *S pullorum*. It is readily isolated by direct plating on most nonselective, aerobic, solid media. Infections in mature birds can be identified by serological tests, followed by necropsy and culturing for confirmation.

Several antibacterials are effective in reducing mortality, but none eliminates the infection from a flock. Furazolidone at 0.022% in the feed is one of the most effective treatments. Control is based on routine testing of breeding stock to assure freedom from infection. Chickens are tested by a tube-agglutination or whole-blood method. The latter method is not dependable for testing turkeys, and either a tube-agglutination or serum-plate test is used. Variant or polyvalent antigens are sometimes necessary.

FOWL TYPHOID

The causal agent, *S gallinarum*, is very similar to *S pullorum*, and many consider them as one. Infection is rare in many countries, including the USA and Canada, but is a major problem in others. Although *S gallinarum* is egg-transmitted and produces lesions in chicks and poults similar to those produced by *S pullorum*, it has a much greater tendency to spread among growing or mature flocks. Mortality at all ages usually is high.

The older bird may be dehydrated and have a swollen, friable, and often bile-stained liver, with or without necrotic foci; enlarged spleen and kidneys; anemia; and enteritis. Diagnosis is by isolation and identification of the causal agent.

Treatment and control are as for pullorum disease (*see* above) except that a vaccine made from a rough strain of *S gallinarum* (9R) is useful in controlling mortality. Usually, it is most effective if administered at 9-10 wk of age, before natural exposure occurs. The standard serological tests for pullorum disease are equally effective in detecting fowl typhoid.

ARIZONA INFECTION
(Paracolon infection)

An acute or chronic egg-transmitted infection, chiefly of turkeys, by any of the serotypes of *S arizonae (Arizona hinshawii)*. Classification of this organism has been a matter of discussion, but it is now considered to be a *Salmonella* sp.

More than 100 serotypes have been identified from various birds, mammals, and reptiles. Serotype 18:Z4, Z32 accounts for most isolates from turkeys; food-borne infections of man occur occasionally, but usually are caused by other serotypes. One or more *S arizonae* serotypes are present in a large percentage of turkey flocks. Reptiles captured in the vicinity of turkeys frequently are infected and are thought to act as a reservoir of infection. Clinical infection in other birds and mammals is relatively rare.

Clinical Findings and Lesions: Neither signs nor lesions are distinctive. Mortality is usually confined to the first 3-4 wk of age. Some flocks are extensively infected without developing appreciable mortality. Infection tends to persist in a flock. Poults are unthrifty, and in some flocks, a considerable percentage develop eye opacity and blindness. Incoordination due to infection of the brain is common.

Yolk sacs are slowly absorbed, and livers may be enlarged and mottled. Some birds develop peritonitis, salpingitis, or local ovarian infections, but infections of the intestinal tract are more common.

Diagnosis: This is based on isolation and identification of the organism. The same culture methods as those used for paratyphoids (*see* below) are satisfactory. Affected eyes and brain are excellent sites for isolation. Environmental samples also may be used for detecting infection. Since egg transmission levels are often high, cultural examination of dead embryos, eggshells, and cull poults may identify infected breeding stock.

Treatment and Control: Various drugs are used to minimize mortality in poults. Streptomycin, spectinomycin, gentamicin, or other antibiotics are commonly injected at the hatchery; furazolidone at 0.011-0.022% in the feed is often used during the first few weeks. Early fumigation of hatching eggs and rigorous hatchery sanitation aid in reducing transmission.

PARATYPHOID INFECTIONS

These may be caused by any one of the many nonhost-adapted salmonellae. Several species may infect a bird or flock concurrently. *Salmonella typhimurium* is most common, but the prevalence of other species varies widely by geographic location and strain of bird. In the USA, most infections are produced by 10-20 species; some species or strains are more pathogenic than others. All birds may be susceptible, and infections are common in all species of domestic birds. Usually, the incidence is higher in young flocks. The public health significance of the infections warrants serious attention to control.

Clinical Findings: Infections are often subclinical. Mortality is usually confined to the first few weeks of age, and is higher in ducks and turkeys than in chickens. Shipping, delayed feeding, chilling, or overheating increases mortality. The clinical signs are not distinctive. Depression, poor growth, weakness, diarrhea, and dehydration may occur. Phage type 4 *S enteritidis* is widespread in parts of Europe and may cause mortality up to 20% in the first 3 wk of life. This and some other strains of this serotype may cause a substantial incidence of infection of the reproductive tract of hens, with true vertical transmission and important public health implications.

Lesions: These may include an enlarged liver with or without areas of focal necrosis, unabsorbed yolk sac with coagulation, and cecal cores. Infections occasionally localize in the eye or synovial tissues. Often, there are no lesions.

Diagnosis: Isolation and identification of the causal agent is essential. Direct culture from liver and yolk sac onto almost any standard type of aerobic medium is adequate for isolation. Either a selenite or tetrathionate enrichment broth transferred in 24-48 hr to brilliant green agar may be used to isolate the organism from intestinal or environmental samples.

Treatment and Control: Several antibacterial agents are of value in preventing mortality; none is capable of eliminating flock infection. Furazolidone at 0.022% in the feed is commonly used. Turkeys, in particular, are generally injected with one or more antibiotics after hatching.

Dependable control methods have not been developed. Strict sanitation in all hatching processes helps prevent transmission between successive lots of birds in a house. Early fumigation of hatching eggs is recommended to prevent shell-surface penetration by salmonellae. Washing should be undertaken only under strictly controlled conditions. Infection resulting from true egg transmission is rare, and no method has been devised to destroy the pathogens in the egg.

The heat of pelleting is reasonably effective in destroying salmonellae in feed ingredients. Maintenance of poultry in confinement and exclusion of all pets, wild birds, and rodents help prevent introduction of infection. The water source should be free of contamination. Early colonizing of the gut with selected normal microflora results in significant resistance to subsequent exposure.

Several methods of determining the *Salmonella* status of breeding flocks have been devised. Periodic culturing of environmental samples from litter, dust, water, hatchery debris, and cull chicks can be reasonably accurate for detecting infection. Serology is not highly dependable but has been of value in detecting *S typhimurium* infection in turkey flocks.

STAPHYLOCOCCOSIS
(Synovitis)

Staphylococcal infections occur in all types of poultry.

Etiology: *Staphylococcus aureus*, the predominant cause of staphylococcosis in poultry, appears to be an opportunistic infection. It may remain viable on inanimate objects for months. Phage typing has shown most isolates from poultry to be distinct from those isolated from man or other mammals. *Staphylococcus aureus* are gram-positive, coagulase-positive, facultative anaerobic cocci that grow readily on common types of culture media. Clinical isolations are best made on such selective media as mannitol salt agar or tellurate glycine agar.

The external tissues of poultry are also heavily colonized with nonvirulent staphylococci, most prominently with *S epidermidis* and *S simulans*. These coagulase-negative species also can be isolated in low concentrations from the liver and synovial fluid of some healthy birds. Thus, the coagulase reaction of isolates from a bird should be determined when making a diagnosis. Coagulase-negative species are nonpathogenic and may even act as interfering agents to help protect the bird from colonization by the virulent *S aureus*.

Pathogenesis and Epidemiology: Coagulase-positive staphylococci have been isolated from tracheae, lungs, livers, and hock joints of normal market-age turkeys; colonization rates vary markedly from flock to flock. Some flocks have no detectable *S aureus*; in others, ≥30% of the birds have infected livers and hock joints. Almost all laying hens are colonized by 50 wk of age.

It has been assumed that any type of injury that breaks the epithelial surfaces offers a potential site of entry. However, recent studies indicate that the respiratory tract may be the major natural route of infection since *S aureus* preferentially adhere to tissues of the respiratory tract, which can be readily colonized by the aerosolized bacteria. *Staphylococcus aureus* are apparently able to pass from the respiratory tract into the blood or lymphatic systems. Colonization of liver, spleen, and synovial fluid results from systemic spread, but may not necessarily lead to clinical disease. Clinical disease results when birds are first colonized with virulent *S aureus* and are then subjected to conditions that lower or impede their defense mechanisms. Varying degrees of virulence are seen among different isolates.

Turkeys raised on range with minimal protective housing had 5 times more staphylococcal synovitis than did turkeys raised in confinement or semiconfinement. Cage-reared chickens are reported to have a higher incidence of staphylococcal infections than if floor-reared. Staphylococcosis in chickens may, in some cases, be secondary to a reovirus infection.

Clinical Findings, Lesions, and Diagnosis: The staphylococci localize in the joints and tendon sheaths, which results in inflammation and lameness. Signs include reluctance to walk, droopiness, emaciation, and diarrhea, sometimes stained green with bile, and with tail feathers having chalky deposits. Affected birds are unable to reach food and water, and eventually die. Clinical disease is most frequent in 9- to 10-wk-old turkeys, and most often occurs following stress caused by other disease or by adverse environmental conditions; mortalities range from <1% to >15% and vary widely from flock to flock. Staphylococcosis may occur at any age in chickens, and in some areas is most often observed in laying hens and broiler-breeders after they come into egg production. It has also been seen in ducks, geese, pheasants, and pigeons.

Either hock joints or foot pads may be swollen and contain serous to caseous exudate. Synovial membranes are thickened and edematous with a heterophilic inflammatory response. The liver is swollen, congested, and greenish. Swollen kidneys and splenomegaly are usually seen; sometimes, the sternal bursa is involved.

Diagnosis is based on clinical signs and is confirmed by isolating coagulase-positive staphylococci from the involved tissues. Infections of synovial tissues by *Escherichia coli*, *Mycoplasma synoviae*, *M gallisepticum*, and *Pasteurella multocida* are of major importance in differential diagnosis.

Prophylaxis and Treatment: Vaccines directly against staphylococci are of no value. Vaccination against reovirus infection may help reduce the incidence of secondary staphylococcal disease. Bacterial interference has been used in local areas to reduce the incidence of staphylococcal synovitis in turkeys by ≥50%. This interference is accomplished by exposing poults to concentrated aerosols of a selected strain of *S epidermidis*, which colonizes the same tissues as pathogenic *S aureus* and also secretes a bacteriocin that kills *S aureus*. Proper housing, nutrition, and handling conditions that prevent injury or stress are major factors in reducing the prevalence of staphylococcosis. Antimicrobial agents may be of value in treatment and control, but sensitivity testing of the *S aureus* isolated from the flock should be done first, as many strains are resistant to commonly used agents.

STREPTOCOCCOSIS

A worldwide, acute septicemic or chronic infection that can affect chickens, turkeys, ducks, geese, pigeons, and numerous caged and wild birds. Mortality may be 0.5-50%.

Etiology and Epidemiology: *Streptococcus* spp are gram-positive, catalase-negative cocci that occur singly, in pairs, or in short chains. Poultry diseases are caused by many streptococci including *S faecalis*, *S faecium*, *S avium*, and *S durans* of the Lancefield serotype D; and *S zooepidemicus* of the Lancefield serotype C. Serotype D streptococci are normal intestinal microflora in avian species and mammals, including man, and are referred to as enterococci or "fecal streps". Streptococci are ubiquitous in the environment and are considered opportunistic organisms. *Streptococcus zooepidemicus* and *S faecalis* are considered the most pathogenic in avian species; however, all are capable of causing severe disease. Transmission is via the oral or aerosol route.

Clinical Findings and Lesions: After an incubation period of one day to several weeks, 2 distinct clinical forms can result. In the acute form, the signs are related to septicemia and include depression, lethargy, lassitude, pale combs and wattles, and a decrease in or cessation of egg production; many times, dead birds are the only finding. Necropsy lesions include an enlarged spleen, liver, and kidney. The spleen may be 2-3 times larger than normal, and dark red to purple. With hepatomegaly, hemorrhagic to necrotic foci may be on the serosal surface; these may extend into the parenchyma. Sanguineous pericardial and subcut. fluid with peritonitis is not uncommon.

Lameness, swollen hock and wing joints, conjunctivitis, and depression with emaciation are typical of chronic streptococcosis. The associated lesions include fibrinous arthritis and synovitis, salpingitis, pericarditis, perihepatitis, necrotic myocarditis, and valvular (vegetative) endocarditis. Well-circumscribed, pale areas of infarction in the liver due to emboli from the valvular lesions are common with vegetative endocarditis.

Diagnosis: Streptococci can be isolated on blood agar from the blood, or from lesions in the liver, spleen, or elsewhere; species can be differentiated by growth characteristics on MacConkey's agar and fermentation of sorbitol: *S zooepidemicus* does not grow on MacConkey's agar but ferments sorbitol, *S faecalis* grows on MacConkey's agar and ferments sorbitol, *S durans* and *S faecium* grow on MacConkey's agar but do not ferment sorbitol. Isolation of *S zooepidemicus* or *S faecalis* from affected avian tissue or lesions confirms the diagnosis.

Treatment: Penicillin and oxytetracycline are effective during the acute phase of the disease. Other effective antibiotics and antibacterials include erythromycin, bacitracin, novobiocin, and the nitrofurans. Isolates in clinical cases should be tested for drug sensitivity for optimal results.

TOXOPLASMOSIS

For etiology and general characteristics, *see* p 365. In chickens, clinical signs include anorexia, emaciation, paleness and shrinkage of the comb, drop in egg production, whitish feces, and sometimes diarrhea and ataxia. Some birds walk in circles, and exhibit torticollis, muscle spasms, paralysis, and blindness. The course may be rapid or protracted (2-3 wk), and is often fatal. In turkeys and geese, infections are mild and may be undetected. Characteristically, CNS lesions, such as necrosis of the midbrain and optic chiasm, are accompanied by pericarditis, myocarditis, necrotic hepatitis, and ulceration of the proventriculus and intestines. The pericardial sac is distended and contains reddish, serous fluid; subpericardial nodules may be present.

Since the Sabin-Feldman dye test is negative or only slightly positive, the diagnosis is confirmed by histological examination and isolation. An ELISA test is available. Neither prophylactic nor therapeutic treatments have been established.

TUBERCULOSIS

A slowly spreading, chronic, granulomatous bacterial infection, characterized by gradual weight loss. All birds appear to be susceptible, although to variable degrees; pheasants seem to be highly susceptible; the disease is uncommon in turkeys; it is more prevalent in captive than in wild birds. (*See also* TUBERCULOSIS in mammals, p 367.)

Etiology and Epidemiology: *Mycobacterium avium* serovars 1 and 2 are the usual cause, although *M tuberculosis* has been isolated from parrots and canaries. *Mycobacterium avium* is very resistant, and can survive in soil for up to 4 yr, in 3% hydrochloric acid for ≥2 hr, and in 4% sodium hydroxide for ≥30 min. The disease occurs worldwide, most commonly in small, barnyard flocks and in zoo aviaries; it is rarely found in young flocks. Wild birds, such as cranes, sparrows, starlings, and raptors, have been found infected.

Infected birds with advanced lesions excrete the organism in their feces. Cadavers and offal may infect predators and cannibalistic flockmates. Rabbits, pigs, and mink are readily infected. Cattle exposed to contaminated feces may respond to mammalian tuberculin and to johnin. *Mycobacterium avium* may cause disease in man: serovar 1, often isolated from tuberculous chickens, has been isolated from people with acquired immunodeficiency syndrome.

Clinical Findings and Diagnosis: Signs usually do not develop until late in the infection when birds become thin and sluggish, and lameness may be observed. In chickens, granulomatous nodules of varying size are usually found in the liver, spleen, bone marrow, and intestine. Some exotic species may have liver and spleen lesions without intestinal involvement, but bone marrow and small mesenteric nodules may be found. Lesions are not calcified.

Live birds may be tested with avian tuberculins, although these are of little value in "non-wattled" birds. Large numbers of acid-fast bacteria in smears from lesions provide a tentative diagnosis.

Control: Chemotherapy is ineffective. In commercial poultry flocks, relatively rapid turnover of populations, together with improved general sanitation, has largely eliminated this once common infection. Infected poultry should be destroyed, and any housing facilities thoroughly cleaned and disinfected using cresylic compounds. Dirt-floored houses should have several inches of the floor removed and replaced with dirt from a place where poultry have not been maintained. All openings should be screened against wild birds. It is best not to re-use ranges where tuberculous poultry have been kept. Avian tuberculosis in zoos is difficult to eradicate. New additions to the aviary should be quarantined for 2-3 mo.

VIRAL HEPATITIS OF TURKEYS

An acute, highly contagious, frequently subclinical infection that produces hepatic and pancreatic lesions in turkeys.

Etiology and Incidence: A picorna-like virus has been reported to cause a similar syndrome but may not represent the usual etiologic agent. The causal virus has not been classified. It is isolated without difficulty from the liver or other tissues of poults, but is isolated less consistently from older birds. It grows readily in the yolk sac of 5- to 7-day-old chick or turkey embryos and in chick-kidney-cell cultures. It is thermostable; ether-, phenol-, and creolin-resistant; and is susceptible to a high, but not low pH. The infection is widespread and common in some areas. Mortality has been reported only in poults.

Clinical Findings and Lesions: Usually the disease is subclinical and becomes apparent only when the birds are stressed. Morbidity and mortality vary according to the severity of stress. In poults <6 wk old, morbidity may reach 100% and mortality 10-15%. Breeder flocks may suffer from decreased production, fertility, and hatchability.

In the liver, foci of necrosis are 1-3 mm in diameter and may be confluent, as may hemorrhage or congestion that may nearly obscure the degenerative changes. Occasionally, the liver is bile-stained. The liver lesions resemble those of blackhead, but the absence of cecal lesions in hepatitis helps to differentiate the 2 diseases. Basophilic intranuclear inclusion bodies are seen rarely in the hepatocytes. The pancreas frequently exhibits relatively large, circular, gray areas of degeneration.

In the subclinical form, the lesions are less extensive and hepatic hemorrhage or congestion is seldom prominent. Affected tissues return to normal in 3-4 wk.

Diagnosis: Paratyphoid and paracolon infections produce necrotic areas in the liver that may be confused with those of viral hepatitis. These and other bacterial and mycotic infections must be differentiated by appropriate culturing techniques. Granulomas may be identified grossly or histologically. Blackhead usually produces concurrent cecal lesions unless modified by medication. In the latter case, histopathologic examination or demonstration of the respective etiologic agents is necessary.

Control: There is no known treatment. Secondary bacterial invasion does not appear to be important, but if it does occur, it should be treated on the basis of specific etiology. Although recovered birds possess demonstrable resistance to reinfection, no circulating antibodies have been found. Sanitation may be of value in preventing dissemination of the agent.

DISORDERS OF THE SKELETAL SYSTEM

This discussion is of disorders of genetic or unknown etiology. Disorders due to specific infectious diseases are discussed elsewhere in this section (POU), while those due to nutritional deficiencies are discussed on p 1267 et seq. (See also MYOPATHIES, below, and OTHER TUMORS, p 1590.)

Crooked Toes: A common developmental anomaly in both young growing turkeys and chickens, affecting a few birds in most flocks. Toes are bent either laterally or medially in a horizontal plane. Careful examination reveals twisting of the phalanges. This condition must be differentiated from curled toes due to a riboflavin deficiency, in which the toes are curled downwards and the primary lesion is in the nervous system. Crooked toes impair mobility and probably production efficiency. The cause is not understood, but may be related to tendon tension, which curls the toes around the perch when the hock is flexed. Infrared brooding and wire floors appear to increase the incidence. Use of roosts of the proper size reduce the incidence.

Epiphyseal Separation: When the legs of normal, young, rapidly growing broiler chickens are disarticulated at necropsy, the articular cartilage is often pulled off the femoral head and trochanters by the joint capsule, leaving the smooth, shiny growth plate. Occasionally part of the growth plate also pulls away, leaving rough, irregular, necrotic-looking, subchondral bone. This may occur spontaneously in turkeys with osteochondrosis.

Femoral Head Necrosis, Long Bone Necrosis: Spontaneous separation of the articular cartilage of the femoral head in turkeys with osteochondrosis results in femoral head necrosis. Osteochondrosis usually occurs because of hypoxia-induced thickening of the articular cartilage in rapidly growing turkeys. Osteomyelitis or avascular necrosis of a large dyschondroplastic mass also results in necrosis of the femoral head or other long bone. The term is also used (incorrectly) for cartilage separation of the femoral head (*see* above) and fracture of the top of the femur in chickens with osteoporosis (fragile bones, brittle bone disease).

Osteomyelitis: Infection of bone by pyogenic organisms causes osteomyelitis, followed by caseous and liquefactive necrosis. It occurs when bacteria enter the bone during a bacteremia and form a focus of infection in the subchondral area, a place that is susceptible to infection in both mammals and birds because gaps in the endothelial wall of the vascular tunnels under the growth plate allow bacteria to escape into the surrounding tissue, where they are inaccessible to mononuclear phagocytes. Bacteria may occasionally pass through the growth plate in transphyseal vessels, resulting in infection in the articular cartilage, and spread into the joint. Osteomyelitis is a common cause of long-bone necrosis and lameness in turkeys and is common in chickens, particularly broiler breeders. Osteomyelitis also occurs in the vertebrae, particularly T_6. The staphyloccal bacteremia that precedes osteomyelitis may enter through the respiratory or intestinal system; reducing numbers of staphylococci in the environment is important in prevention. Antibiotics (eg, novobiocin) are also used in prevention and treatment.

Rotated Tibia: A rotation of the shaft of the tibiotarsus that results in the metatarsus pointing laterally. The hock joint is normal with neither displacement of the gastrocnemius tendon nor bending of the distal tibiotarsal bone. The lesion is unilateral and the affected leg is often abducted, giving a "spraddle-legged" posture. Turkeys 2-14 wk old are primarily affected, and an incidence in some flocks of 15% has been reported. The etiology is obscure. Affected birds should be culled.

Shaky-Leg Lameness, Shaky-Leg Syndrome: A severe lameness, mainly of male turkeys 8-18 wk old, in which the turkeys are reluctant to rise and walk. When forced to rise, they stand with their bodies tipped forward and quiver with pain. The specific etiology is not clear, but it probably is caused by tendon or muscle pain. It is associated with wet or sticky litter conditions that cause foot-pad dermatitis and make walking painful. As a result, the turkeys spend much of their time squatting. They become stiff, develop muscle pain, and are increasingly reluctant to move. Once the cycle has been initiated, the stiffness and pain are self-perpetuating. Most turkeys recover as bone growth slows, but the extended time spent squatting on the floor frequently induces secondary foot, hock, and hip lesions. Good litter conditions and management strategies that promote activity are important in preventing turkey lameness and leg problems.

Spondylolisthesis (Kinky Back): A developmental anomaly of the spinal column of broiler chickens; vertebra T_6 is deformed with downward rotation of the anterior end. Compression of the spinal cord at the junction of T_6 and T_7 causes posterior paralysis. A few birds affected with clinical spondylolisthesis are found in many 3- to 6-wk-old broiler flocks, and an incidence of 1% has been reported in some flocks. Affected birds typically sit with the weight on their hocks and tail, and their feet off the ground. If disturbed, the only movement they are capable of making is to struggle backwards on their hocks. Some fall on their sides and usually are incapable of righting themselves. Careful observation will reveal earlier or less severely affected broilers. There is some evidence that genotype and growth rate are important in development of spondylolisthesis. Clinically affected birds should be culled. A mass of cartilage impinging on the cord produces similar signs. Subclinical spondylolisthesis without damage to the spinal cord and without clinical signs is common in broiler chickens.

Tibial Dyschondroplasia: A persistent mass of hypertrophic cartilage in the proximal end of the tibiotarsal bone in growing broiler chickens and turkeys. In many birds, the abnormal cartilage is restricted to the posterior medial portion of the proximal tibiotarsal bone, and birds are clinically normal. An incidence of 10-30% of subclinical dyschondroplasia is common in many flocks. In more severe cases, the abnormal cartilage occupies the whole metaphysis of the proximal tibiotarsal bone and also develops in the proximal tarsometatarsal bone. Birds with these more severe lesions may be lame, with bowing of the proximal metatarsus or backward bending of the proximal tibiotarsus. In some instances, fractures or avascular necrosis have occurred below the abnormal cartilage. The incidence of tibial dyschondroplasia is affected by genotype, and the calcium/phosphorus ratio and acid-base balance of the diet. A similar defect has been produced experimentally with grain contaminated with the fungus *Fusarium roseum* and with rations containing the fungicide thiram.

Valgus and Varus Deformation of the Intertarsal Joint: An outward or inward bending and twisting of the leg of chickens and turkeys. The deformity is generally unilateral, and the main deformation occurs in the distal tibiotarsal and to a lesser extent in the proximal tarsometatarsal bone. The gastrocnemius tendon may be displaced laterally. A few affected birds are found in most broiler-chicken and turkey flocks; in some flocks, incidence may be increased. The etiology is poorly understood. Genotype and brooding conditions may influence the incidence, which is increased when broiler chickens are raised in batteries. Reducing the growth rate, particularly during wk 1-3, reduces the incidence. Affected birds should be culled.

This condition superficially appears similar to perosis (qv, p 1269). In perosis, shortening of long bones due to degenerative changes in growth plates occurs before deformation of the leg.

MYOPATHIES

Degenerative changes and replacement of muscle by fat and connective tissue have been noted on microscopical examination of skeletal muscle of rapidly growing meat-type chickens and turkeys for several years. Focal or scattered fiber hyalinization, mineralization, and necrosis are common. Proliferation of connective and fatty tissue has also been reported. These lesions in "normal" meat-type poultry may interfere with the interpretation of the more extensive myopathies described below.

Deep Pectoral Myopathy of Turkeys (Degenerative myopathy, Green muscle disease): A condition involving degeneration, necrosis, and fibrosis of the deep pectoral (supracoracoideus) muscle in heavy meat birds (chickens, turkeys), most often turkey breeder hens. Flock incidence as high as 25% has been reported with few individuals developing the disease before 24 wk of age. The major loss is from downgrading or condemnation at processing.

The myopathy may occur uni- or bilaterally with the central one- to two-thirds of the muscle affected. Early, the involved muscle is pale, swollen, and edematous. Later, affected tissue is sharply demarcated from adjacent, viable muscle; eventually it is encapsulated, resulting in dry, green, necrotic muscle enclosed in a thick fibrous capsule. The defect can be identified by a depression of the breast over affected muscles or by transillumination of carcasses at slaughter.

The deep pectoral muscle functions to elevate the wing. Although well-developed in modern meat birds, it is little used. Following episodes of prolonged wing flapping (such as occurs during handling), when lame birds use their wings to assist ambulation, or if the bird is placed on its back, the muscle swells within its dense, fascial covering, becomes ischemic, and undergoes necrosis. The lesion can be produced artificially by stimulating the deep pectoral muscle to contract, and prevented by surgically opening the fascial sheath covering the muscle.

Occurrence can be reduced through careful handling of susceptible birds to prevent excessive wing flapping. The condition is heritable; selective breeding may provide a long-term method to decrease occurrence. Supplementing rations with selenium, vitamin E, or methionine has not influenced incidence.

Exertional Myopathy: Muscle-activity-induced myopathy occurs when local muscle hypoxia, and/or metabolic by-products of muscle metabolism (lactic acid) exceed the capacity of the vascular system to remove them, and they accumulate locally, causing muscle and vascular damage. This activates the mediators of inflammation, which increase the edema and vascular response.

Exertional myopathy can be caused by both isometric muscle activity (eg, transport, capture, or restraint myopathy as with turkey leg edema syndrome) or kinetic muscle activity (eg, deep pectoral myopathy [*see* above], which quickly becomes a compartment syndrome). Early gross lesions include pallor with edema or blood-stained transudate. There is swelling, degeneration, necrosis, and mineralization of muscle fibers, with edema, hemorrhage, and infiltration of heterophils and macrophages.

Mechanically Induced Myopathy: Avascular necrosis caused by pressure in heavy birds that are down because of lameness or leg deformity is seen occasionally and occurs most frequently in the breast muscle. On gross examination the tissue is firm and pale. Histological examination reveals swelling, hyalinization, and necrosis of fibers with edema, heterophils, and macrophages at the periphery.

Rupture of the gastrocnemius tendon is common in meat-type chickens, particularly in roasters and breeders. The rupture is usually primary and caused by excessive weight on tendons that have inadequate tensile strength. Damage by viral or bacterial agents, causing tendonitis may be predisposing. Rupture of the tendon of one leg puts stress on the other tendon, and bilateral rupture is frequent. Affected birds are lame or "down on their hocks" (creepers). Hemorrhage from the injury is visible as red, blue, or green discoloration in the tissue above the hock on the back of the leg, and results in condemnation of the affected part at processing (red-leg, green-leg). The ruptured tendon can be palpated as a hard mass on the back of the leg above the hock. Rupture of the gastrocnemious tendon is rare in turkeys. (*See also* RUPTURE OF THE PERONEUS LONGUS MUSCLE, below, and VIRAL ARTHRITIS, p 1607.)

Nutritional Myopathy: Nutritional muscular dystrophy (NMD) in poultry and waterfowl is selenium-responsive. Cysteine also may have a beneficial effect in chicks. Lesions of NMD have been reported in skeletal, heart, and smooth (gizzard and intestine) muscle of ducks, turkeys, and chickens. Arsenic, zinc, copper, and other metals are antagonistic and may precipitate outbreaks of NMD. Gross lesions are similar to those of NMD in mammals, with pale foci or streaking. Microscopic changes include focal or widespread swelling, edema, hyalinization, mineralization, degeneration, and lysis with infiltration of macrophages and heterophils. Hypercellularity from proliferation of sarcolemmal nuclei may be prominent if regeneration is occurring. Poultry feeds in many parts of the world contain added selenium at 0.1-0.4 ppm.

Rupture of the Peroneus (Fibularis) Longus Muscle: The origin of the peroneus muscle is on the proximal end of the tibiotarsus and patellar tissue, with attachments to other muscles in that area. In turkeys, the insertion appears to be in 3 places. A small band of tissue from the medial side of the muscle runs to the lateral tibial condyle area. The main muscle tendon crosses the lateral side of the hock and joins other tendons that extend the hock and may affect foot and toe movement. The muscle is thin and wide, covering the anterior and lateral surface of the leg. It has a heavy aponeurosis in which the tendon is imbedded. Rupture of the aponeurosis and muscle occurs as a 1-2 cm horizontal wound on the anterior surface of the muscle. It occurs above the middle of the tibiotarsus at the top of the ossifying tendon where the tendon attaches to the muscle. It occurs at 10-14 wk, the age at which turkey leg tendons become ossified, which reduces the elasticity of the tissue in that location.

Incidence appears to be increasing. It is most frequent in females and may affect up to 5% of the flock. The separation of the muscle likely occurs slowly, caused by activity such as repeated springing, in turkeys that are becoming heavier and maturing earlier each year. The attachments of this muscle suggest that antagonistic activity is possible. Affected birds are not lame, but the resulting hemorrhage causes a red, blue, or green discoloration under the skin on the anterior of the drumstick ventral to the rupture. The affected portion is trimmed at processing.

Toxic Myopathy: Ionophore toxicity causes muscle damage with depression, weakness, and inability to rise. Respiratory signs may be seen depending on the extent and severity of the muscle lesions. Stunting may also occur. Type I (red or fat-metabolizing) fibers are most susceptible. Lesions may also be found in heart muscle. Gross and histologic changes are similar to those of NMD (*see* above). Toxicity has also occurred when ionophore anticoccidials were used in conjunction with other drugs, particularly related products.

Cassia (coffee bean) toxicity can produce clinical signs and gross and histologic changes in muscle similar to those seen in ionophore toxicity.

Transport Myopathy of Turkeys (Leg Edema Syndrome): Heavy toms are primarily affected, although the condition also has occurred in hens, especially in flocks in the upper Midwest (USA). About 5% of all flocks have the condition, and morbidity within the flock is 2-70%. It occurs sporadically but is most commonly seen during fall and early winter. A high incidence has occurred in sequential flocks from the same farm. The cause is unknown. It is associated with increased body size and weight, increased transport time to processing plant, cool ambient temperatures, and valgus leg deformities. Flocks raised in confinement are likely to have a higher incidence than range flocks.

The pathogenesis is presumed to be due to impaired circulation; the resulting muscle ischemia and acute necrosis lead to edema that tends to be manifest in the large potential space in the subcutis of the medial thigh. Signs are rarely seen on the farm.

Often, only one leg is affected. No evidence of external trauma is seen. Skin over edematous subcut. tissue is pale, feather follicles are less visible, and the skin slips easily over underlying muscle when moved. Occasionally, there is crepitation. Affected areas are dark when the edematous areas contain blood. Typically, when lesions are cut, the edematous subcutis is a few to several mm thick, and is amber, occasionally green, or rarely red. Purulent exudate is absent, which distinguishes transport myopathy from cellulitis. If hemorrhage is present, the adductor muscle usually is torn. Removal of affected legs at processing results in carcass downgrading and economic loss. Microscopically, acute multifocal muscle necrosis is found, primarily in the adductor muscles. Sometimes, subacute or chronic lesions also are seen, which suggest earlier episodes of myopathy. Serum CPK increases sharply between farm and processing.

Programs designed to improve leg strength and conformation, and reduce trauma during transportation help reduce the incidence. Supplemental vitamin E also may be useful. If possible, flocks with a high incidence of valgus leg deformities should be marketed early at a nearby processing plant.

VIRAL ARTHRITIS
(Reoviral infection, Tenosynovitis)

Reovirus is ubiquitous in chickens and turkeys; some strains become viremic and localize in the large joints, resulting in arthritis, tendonitis, and synovitis. Most birds are thought to be susceptible to respiratory-intestinal strains of reovirus; chickens and turkeys are susceptible to viral arthritis, which is seen worldwide. Reoviruses also have been associated with pericarditis and myocarditis, hydropericardium, pasting, malabsorption, and femoral head necrosis. Further study is needed to define the role of reovirus strains in each of these clinical entities. (*See also* MALABSORPTION SYNDROME, p 1579.)

Transmission and Pathogenesis: The disease is egg-transmitted and is of short duration except when lateral transmission in a flock is prolonged. Respiratory and digestive infections may occur but are of short duration; however, the virus survives in tendon sheaths for extended periods. Spread occurs via aerosols, fomites, and mechanical means. The virus is resistant to heat and chemical inactivation.

Several serotypes of avian reoviruses have been identified; however, there appears to be cross-protection between some of the serotypes. Pathogenicity of the isolates varies widely. Serious outbreaks of viral arthritis are followed by a decreased incidence in later hatch groups of birds from the same parent flock. This may be related to decreased egg-transmission and development of parental immunity. Day-old chicks are more susceptible than older birds when exposed by natural means. The earlier in life the chick is infected, the longer the virus persists in the tissues.

Clinical Findings: The arthritic form (tenosynovitis) usually occurs in 4- to 8-wk-old broilers as bilateral swellings of the tendons of the shank and above the hock. The birds walk with a stilted gait. In severely affected flocks, rupture of the gastrocnemius tendon is frequent, and many cull birds are seen around the feeders and waterers. Mortality is 2-10%, and morbidity 5-50%. Severely affected birds rarely recover; those less severely affected do so in 4-6 wk. The infection is inapparent in many birds. Feed efficiency and rate of gain are lowered.

Lesions: An acute, fulminating infection is occasionally seen in young chicks and embryos with cardio-, hepato-, and splenomegaly with necrotic foci. Edema of the tendons of the leg is marked; petechial hemorrhages occur in the synovial membranes above the hock; fusion and calcification of the tendon bundles are common. Blood clots and hemorrhages occur with rupture of the gastrocnemius tendon; pitted erosions of the cartilage of the distal tibiotarsus occur with flattening of the condyles. Histologically, the synovial cells are hypertrophied, hyperplastic, and infiltrated with lymphocytes and macrophages. The synovia contains heterophils and macrophages. Infiltration of heterophils and/or lymphocytes between myocardial fibers is a constant finding. However, the infiltrating heterophils are difficult to distinguish from the clusters of young, proliferating heterophils (ectopic myelopoiesis) that are present in the heart muscle of all young, rapidly growing broiler chickens.

Diagnosis: A presumptive diagnosis can be based on bilateral swelling of the tendons of the shank and tendon bundle above the hock, and the inflammatory changes in the tendons and synovia described above. Virus isolation from affected tissues can be made in primary kidney, liver, or lung cells, or in the yolk sac or chorioallantoic membrane of embryonating chicken eggs. The agar-gel-precipitin test is usually positive, and most birds are positive early in the infection. Virus neutralization tests are used to detect the specific serotype. Culture procedures should be used to differentiate mycoplasmal and bacterial infections. Adenovirus is eliminated by culture of the synovia on embryo fibroblasts in cell culture. Other causes of lameness should be considered.

Treatment and Control: There is no treatment. Parental antibody prevents early infection in chicks, and should reduce or prevent egg-transmission. Since egg-transmission is the principal means of spread, it is desirable to have the breeder flock immune. Such a program should be directed to the serotypes present in the flock. Adult birds are resistant to clinical disease if exposed by natural routes.

BOTULISM
(Limberneck, Western duck sickness)

An intoxication due to ingestion of feed that contains *Clostridium botulinum* toxin, or to absorption of toxin elaborated in the intestine (toxicoinfection).

Etiology: Types A, C, and E toxins of *C botulinum* are the most common causes of botulism in poultry and waterfowl. The anaerobic spore-forming bacterium occurs commonly in soil, and in a suitable environment, may contaminate feedstuffs and grow and produce toxin. The conditions necessary to produce the type C toxicoinfections, which occasionally develop in chicken broiler flocks and may produce mortality of >10%, are not understood, but absence or disruption of the normal microflora of the gut may be a necessary precondition.

Sporadic episodes of botulism with massive mortality in wild waterfowl have occurred in the western USA and Canada and many other parts of the world. More recently, botulism due to Group E toxin has occurred in waterfowl in the Lake Michigan area. It occurs around lakes and marshes where there is relatively shallow water with decaying vegetation from fluctuating shore lines. Dead invertebrates in such material may be a major source of toxin for birds that feed in these areas.

Clinical Findings and Diagnosis: No characteristic lesions develop. There may be a slight enteritis and an enlarged spleen. Not all affected birds exhibit the flaccid paralysis of the neck that is well described by the common name "limberneck". The feathers may be removed easily. Death is usually due to respiratory paralysis.

A presumptive diagnosis can be made from clinical signs and lack of significant postmortem lesions. A positive diagnosis requires demonstration of the toxin in ingesta, serum, or the liver. Serum or filtrates of ingesta or liver from suspect birds are injected IP into 2 sets of mice, one of which is protected by simultaneous injection with botulinum antitoxin of the suspect type or types.

Control: Type-specific antitoxin is effective in treating affected birds but is usually not practical. Epsom salts may be useful to flush unabsorbed toxin from the intestinal tract. Fresh water should be supplied. Collection and disposal of dead birds is important to help limit an outbreak. Wild waterfowl should be dispersed from an affected area if possible. Stabilizing water levels, particularly in shallow waters, is a major method of prevention.

Field evidence indicates that the recurrent toxicoinfections that occur in some broiler houses can be prevented by cleaning and disinfecting followed by distributing sodium bisulfite on the floor and litter at 1 lb/1000 sq ft (1 kg/200 sq m). Prophylactic use of type C antitoxin is also effective but not economical.

EASTERN ENCEPHALITIS IN PHEASANTS

An acute viral disease of pheasants characterized by neurological signs, high morbidity, and often high mortality; it can be responsible for serious economic loss unless adequate control measures are taken. The infective agent is the virus of eastern equine encephalomyelitis (qv, p 599). Infection is normally transmitted by mosquitoes (*Culiseta melanura*), but once established in a flock, transmission is facilitated by the birds' pecking one another. Serological and other data clearly indicate that many other species of birds carry an inapparent infection. The virus has been isolated from mice, rats, foxes, dogs, and other mammals.

Clinical Findings and Diagnosis: The lesions are typical of the viral encephalitides. Signs include inappetence, staggering, and paralysis. Surviving birds may be blind, have unilateral or bilateral paralysis of various muscle groups, and have difficulty in holding up the head.

Morbidity may reach 90% and, in some outbreaks, mortality in individual pens has been as high as 90%. While birds in some pens are affected, those in adjacent pens may show no signs. Diagnosis may be confirmed by inoculation of guinea pigs or mice, or by chick-embryo tissue-culture methods. Prophylaxis may be accomplished in some instances by effective mosquito control or by confining birds ≥100 yards (100 m) from swampy *C melanura* habitats, and by husbandry practices designed to reduce injuries from pecking, eg, debeaking the birds at regular intervals and providing adequate space for exercise. Vaccination has not been uniformly successful but may be useful, particularly in flocks with a history of previous outbreaks. The dose is one-tenth the equine dose of either an eastern or bivalent eastern and western vaccine injected into the pectoral muscles, preferably at 5-6 wk of age, or when the birds are released from brooder houses. In northeastern USA, efforts should be made to have most birds vaccinated by the first week in July because outbreaks usually commence about the third week in July.

ENCEPHALOMYELITIS
(Epidemic tremor)

A worldwide viral disease of Japanese quail, turkeys, chickens, and pheasants, marked by ataxia and tremor of the head, neck, and limbs. Ducklings, pigeons, and guinea fowl are susceptible to experimental infection. The causative picornavirus can be grown in chicken embryos from nonimmune hens. It is transmitted for ~1 wk through a portion of eggs laid by infected hens, and then spreads laterally in the hatcher or brooder to susceptible hatch-mates.

Clinical Findings: Signs commonly appear at 7-10 days of age, although they may be present at hatching or delayed for several weeks. The main signs are unsteadiness, sitting on hocks, paresis, and even complete inability to move. Muscular tremors are best seen after exercising the bird; holding the bird on its back in the cupped hand helps in detection. About 5% of the flock may be affected, although morbidity and mortality may be much higher. The disease in adult birds is inapparent, except for a transient drop in egg production. The disease in turkeys is often milder than in chickens.

Lesions: No gross lesions of the nervous system are seen. Lymphocytic accumulations in the gizzard muscle may be visible as grayish areas. Lens opacities may occur weeks after infection. Microscopic lesions consist of lymphocytic foci in the pancreas, liver, gizzard, proventriculus, and CNS (perivascular cuffing), along with neuronal degeneration, endothelial hyperplasia, and gliosis.

Diagnosis: Avian encephalomyelitis must be differentiated from avian encephalomalacia (vitamin E deficiency), rickets, vitamin B_1 or B_2 deficiency, Newcastle disease, eastern encephalitis in pheasants, Marek's disease, and encephalitis caused by bacteria, fungi (eg, aspergillosis), or mycoplasmas. Diagnosis is based on history, signs, and histological study of brain, spinal cord, proventriculus, gizzard, and pancreas. Virus isolation in eggs free of avian encephalomyelitis antibody is sometimes necessary for confirmation. Serological testing may be helpful. Microscopic lesions are sparse and difficult to find in infected adults.

Prophylaxis and Treatment: Immunization of breeder pullets 10-15 wk old with a commercial vaccine is advised. Vaccination of table-egg flocks is sometimes advisable. Affected chicks and poults are ordinarily destroyed since few recover.

ARTIFICIAL INSEMINATION (AI)

Low fertility in turkeys, caused by unsuccessful mating as a consequence of large, heavily muscled birds or reduced libido is a serious and costly problem in the production of hatching eggs. AI is widely used to overcome this problem. In chickens, the practice has not found wide application, but it is routinely used in special breeding work.

Chicken and turkey semen are collected by stimulating the male to protrude its copulatory organ by massaging the abdomen and the back over the testes. This is followed quickly by pushing the tail forward with one hand and, at the same time, using the thumb and forefinger of the same hand to "milk" semen from the ducts of this organ. Semen flow response is quicker and easier to stimulate in the chicken than in the turkey. The semen may be collected with an aspirator or in a small tube or any cup-like container. The volume averages ~0.20-0.25 mL in the turkey, with a spermatozoon concentration of 6 to ≥8 billion/mL. In the chicken, volume is 2-3 times that of the turkey, but the concentration is about one-half.

Chicken and turkey semens begin to lose fertilizing capacity when stored >1 hr. Several commercial semen extenders are available and are routinely employed, particularly for turkeys. Extenders enable more precise control over inseminating dose, as well as facilitate filling of tubes. Results may be comparable to those using undiluted semen when product directions are followed.

For insemination, pressure is applied to the abdomen around the vent. This causes the cloaca to evert and the oviduct to protrude so that a syringe or plastic straw can be inserted ~1 in. (2.5 cm) into the oviduct and the correct amount of semen delivered. As the semen is expelled by the inseminator, pressure around the vent is released, which assists the hen in retaining cells in the vagina of the oviduct. Due to the high sperm concentration of turkey semen, 0.025 mL of undiluted pooled semen gives optimal fertility. For maximal fertility, turkeys must be inseminated at regular intervals of 10-14 days. In chickens, due to the lower spermatozoon concentration and shorter duration of fertility, 0.05 mL of undiluted pooled semen, at intervals of 7 days, is required to maintain fertility. The turkey hen's squatting behavior indicates receptivity and the time for making the first insemination. Initial inseminations may be performed before the initial oviposition. Fertility tends to decrease later in the season; therefore, it may be justified to inseminate more frequently or to cull the poorer layers.

Chicken and turkey semen may be frozen, but reduced fertility limits usage to special breeding projects. Under experimental conditions, fertility levels of 90% have been obtained for hens inseminated at 3-day intervals with 400-500 million frozen-thawed chicken spermatozoa.

DISORDERS OF THE REPRODUCTIVE SYSTEM

Cystic Right Oviduct: An abdominal cyst 1-15 cm in diameter, full of clear fluid and attached to the right side of the cloacal wall. It is a common incidental finding in the chicken and represents abnormal development of embryonic right urogenital tissue.

False Layer: A hen that ovulates normally but in which the yolk is dropped into the abdominal cavity rather than being collected by the oviduct. The yolk is absorbed from the abdominal cavity within 24 hr. The hen acts like a normal layer but does not produce eggs, is generally fat, and has free yolk in the abdominal cavity. The malfunction has been associated with damage to the oviduct by infectious bronchitis infection at an early age or with *Mycoplasma gallisepticum* infection.

Internal Layer: An aberration in which partially formed or fully formed eggs are found in the abdominal cavity. Such eggs probably reach the cavity by reverse peristalsis of the oviduct and are often misshapen due to partial absorption of the contents. No control or treatment is known.

Impacted Oviduct: The oviduct is distended with several partially formed eggs and much caseous material. The eggs are often misshapen and may have ruptured. The cause is unknown. Often the bird dies from peritonitis.

Prolapse of the Oviduct: In modern poultry operations this condition generally results in cannibalism (qv, p 1630). The prolapsed organ is picked by others in the flock, and the complete oviduct and parts of the adjacent intestinal tract are pulled from the abdominal cavity. The hen dies from hemorrhage and shock and is often referred to as a "blowout" or "pickout". Often it is difficult to determine whether blowouts are due to prolapse of the oviduct or eversion of the oviduct at egg laying. Generally, the ensuing cannibalism can be prevented by beak trimming. A high incidence has been associated with starting laying at too early an age or when too fat, or with very large eggs.

Salpingitis: An inflammation of the oviduct, which is generally distended with caseous exudate. In young pullets, this is often due to either *Mycoplasma gallisepticum* or *Escherichia coli* infection, and can result in reduced egg production. In mature hens, it is generally secondary to oviduct impaction or air-sac infection.

Yolk Peritonitis: This is characterized by yolk with a cooked appearance among the abdominal viscera and is a common cause of sporadic mortality in layers. Regression of the ovary results in free yolk in the abdominal cavity. If this yolk becomes infected, the bird dies from yolk peritonitis. Sporadic cases are often due to *Escherichia coli* infection, which may have entered the abdomen through the oviduct. If a high incidence is encountered in a flock, a bacterial septicemia such as fowl cholera or salmonellosis should be suspected.

EGG DROP SYNDROME (EDS)

A disease, first reported in 1976, characterized by production of soft-shelled and shell-less eggs in apparently healthy birds, that has been recognized worldwide, except in the USA.

Etiology: The causal adenovirus is widely distributed in both wild and domestic ducks and geese. The adenovirus group antigen cannot be demonstrated by conventional means, and EDS virus also differs from other avian adenoviruses by strongly agglutinating avian RBC. The virus grows to high titers in embryonating eggs or cell cultures of duck or goose origin. It also replicates well in chick kidney or chick-embryo liver cells and to a lesser degree in chick-embryo fibroblasts. It does not grow in chick embryonating eggs or in mammalian cells.

The resistant virus has at least 3 genotypes. One is associated with classical EDS, one with ducks in the UK, and one with EDS in Australia.

Epidemiology: The natural hosts for EDS virus are ducks and geese. Three types of disease are recognized in chickens. Classical EDS probably was due to contamination of a vaccine for Marek's disease grown in duck-embryo fibroblasts and subsequent adaptation of the virus to the chicken. Basic breeding stock was infected, and the virus was transmitted vertically through the egg. The virus often remained latent until the chick reached sexual maturity, when it was excreted in the eggs and droppings, to infect susceptible contacts. Because the virus is vertically transmitted and is reactivated around peak egg production, there was an apparent breed and age susceptibility. However, all ages and breeds of chickens are susceptible, although the disease tends to be most severe in heavy broiler-breeders or brown-egg producers.

Arising from the classical form, endemic EDS has been reported in many areas. Usually, it is seen in commercial egg producers. Flocks become infected at any stage in lay. The virus is spread mainly horizontally by contaminated egg collection

(Keyes) trays, and outbreaks are often associated with a common egg-packing station.

Rare sporadic EDS has been recognized in isolated flocks. It appears to be due either to contact with domestic ducks or geese or, more often, to water contaminated with wildfowl droppings. The risk is that these introductions could become endemic.

The main method of lateral spread is through contaminated eggs. Droppings also are infective, and man and contaminated fomites such as crates or trucks can spread virus. It also can be transmitted by needles when vaccinating and drawing blood. Insect transmission is possible, but not proved.

Pathogenesis: Following lateral or experimental infection, the virus grows to low titers in the nasal mucosa. This is followed by viremia, virus replication in lymphoid tissue, and then massive replication for ~8 days in the oviduct, especially in the pouch shell gland region. Changes in the eggshell occur coincidentally. Both the exterior and interior of eggs produced between 8 and ~18 days following infection contain virus. A copious exudate in the lumen of the oviduct is rich in virus, and this contaminates the droppings. Unlike conventional fowl adenoviruses, there is little, if any, growth in the epithelial cells of the intestine.

Chicks hatched from infected eggs may excrete virus and develop antibody. More often, the virus remains latent, and antibody does not develop until the bird starts to lay, at which time the virus is reactivated, grows in the oviduct, and the cycle repeats.

Clinical Findings and Lesions: In flocks without antibody, the first signs are loss of color in pigmented eggs, quickly followed by soft-shelled and shell-less eggs. Since birds tend to eat the shell-less eggs, they may be missed unless a search is made for the membranes. Mainly because of the shell-less eggs, egg production falls 10-40%. In flocks in which there has been some spread of virus and some of the birds have antibody (usually 10-20%), the condition is seen as a failure to achieve predicted production targets. Careful examination shows that these flocks are experiencing a series of small EDS episodes. Birds with antibody slow the spread of virus.

There is no effect on fertility or hatchability of those eggs suitable for setting. Diarrhea and a transient dullness may be observed before the eggshell changes occur.

The major pathological changes occur in the pouch shell gland. Surface epithelial cells develop intranuclear inclusion bodies and degenerate, and are replaced by squamous, cuboidal, or undifferentiated columnar cells. There is moderate to severe inflammatory infiltration of the mucosa.

Diagnosis: In classical EDS, the combination of poor eggshell quality at peak production in healthy birds is almost diagnostic. With endemic or sporadic EDS, disease can occur in any age of bird in lay. In cage units especially, spread can be slow and the clinical signs may be overlooked, the problem being perceived as a small depression (2-4%) of egg yield.

EDS can be distinguished from Newcastle disease and influenza virus infections by the absence of illness, and from infectious bronchitis by the eggshell changes that occur at or just before the fall in egg production and absence of ridges and malformed eggs sometimes seen in infectious bronchitis.

Virus can be isolated by inoculating embryonating duck eggs or duck- or chick-embryo liver cell cultures. While it is important to select birds producing abnormal eggs, this can be difficult, especially if the birds are on litter. An easier method is to feed affected eggs to antibody-free hens. Virus isolation from the pouch shell gland of these hens is attempted when the first abnormal eggs are produced.

The hemagglutination inhibition test (high levels of hemagglutinins are produced) using fowl RBC or the ELISA test are the serological tests of choice, and the serum neutralization test can be used for confirmation. The double immunodiffusion test also has been used. When selecting birds for diagnosis, especially in cage units, it is important to bleed only birds that are producing or have produced affected eggs.

Prophylaxis and Treatment: There is no treatment. The classical form has been eradicated from primary breeders. The endemic form can be controlled by washing and disinfecting plastic Keyes trays before reuse. The sporadic form can be prevented by separating chickens from other birds, especially waterfowl. General sanitary precautions are indicated, and potentially contaminated water should be chlorinated before use.

Inactivated vaccines with oil adjuvant are available and, if properly made, control the disease. They reduce but do not prevent virus shedding. These vaccines are given during the growing phase, usually at 14-18 wk old. They can be combined with other vaccines such as for Newcastle disease.

AIR SAC MITE

Cytodites nudus is a small mite occasionally noticed as white spots on the bronchi, lungs, and air sacs of chickens, turkeys, pheasants, pigeons, and canaries. (*See also* p 1006.) These mites are readily transmissible between birds but are rarely found in commercial industries. The life cycle and methods of transfer are unknown. Opinions vary as to the importance of the mite and damage it causes to the hosts. Destroying affected and exposed birds has been the recommended method of control.

ASPERGILLOSIS
(Brooder pneumonia, Mycotic pneumonia, Pneumomycosis)

A disease, usually of the respiratory system, of chickens, turkeys and less frequently ducklings, pigeons, canaries, geese, and many other wild and pet birds. In chickens and turkeys, the disease may be endemic on some farms; in wild birds, it appears to be sporadic, frequently affecting only an individual bird. It is usually seen in birds 7-40 days old. (*See also* pp 341 and 1004.)

Etiology and Epidemiology: *Aspergillus fumigatus* is a cause of the disease. However, several other *Aspergillus* spp, as well as other genera, eg, *Penicillium*, may be incriminated.

Chicks and poults may become infected during hatching as a result of inhaling large numbers of spores in heavily contaminated hatching machines or from contaminated litter. In older birds, infection is caused primarily by inhalation of spore-laden dust from contaminated litter or feed.

Clinical Findings and Lesions: Dyspnea, hyperpnea, somnolence and other signs of nervous system involvement, inappetence, emaciation, and increased thirst may be observed. The encephalitic form is most common in turkeys. In chicks or poults up to 6 wk old, the lungs are most frequently involved. Pulmonary lesions are characterized by cream-colored plaques a few millimeters to several centimeters in diameter; occasionally mycelial masses may be observed grossly within the air passages. The plaques also may be found in the syrinx, air sacs, liver, intestines, and occasionally the brain. An ocular form, in which large plaques may be expressed from the medial canthus, has been observed in chickens and turkeys.

Diagnosis: The fungus can be demonstrated by culture or by microscopical examination of fresh preparations. One of the plaques is teased apart and placed on a suitable medium, usually resulting in a pure culture of the organism. Histopathological examination using a special fungus stain reveals granulomas containing mycelia. Pathogenicity of the isolate is confirmed by injecting it into the air sacs of susceptible 3-wk-old chicks.

Differential diagnoses include infectious bronchitis, Newcastle disease, and laryngotracheitis.

Prophylaxis and Treatment: Strict adherence to sanitation procedures in the hatchery minimizes early outbreaks. Grossly contaminated eggs should not be set for incubation since they may explode and disseminate spores throughout the hatching machine. Contaminated hatchers should be fumigated with formaldehyde or thiabendazole (120-360 g/m³). Avoiding moldy litter or ranges serves to prevent outbreaks in older birds. Pens should be sprayed with nystatin and all equipment cleaned and disinfected.

Treatment of affected birds is considered useless.

GAPEWORM INFECTION

The gapeworm *Syngamus trachea* inhabits the trachea and lungs of many domestic and various wild birds. Infection may occur directly by ingestion of infective eggs or larvae; however, severe field infection is associated with ingestion of transport hosts (such as earthworms, snails, slugs, and arthropods [eg, flies]). Many gapeworm larvae may encyst and survive within a single invertebrate for years. Range infection is favored by seasonal climatic abundance of specific invertebrate hosts, eg, great numbers of earthworms brought to the surface by spring rains. Although gapeworms are not a problem in confinement-reared poultry, they are in game-farm pens, and cause serious economic losses in range-reared chickens, pheasants, turkeys, and peacocks. *Cyathostoma bronchialis* is the causative agent of the disease in geese and ducks.

Clinical Findings: Young birds are affected most severely. Sudden death and verminous pneumonia characterize early outbreaks. Signs of gasping, choking, shaking of the head, inanition, emaciation, and suffocation may follow. Necropsy reveals adult gapeworms obstructing the lumina of the trachea, bronchi, and lungs. Respiratory inflammation may be present. The blood-red female gapeworm is usually found in copulation with a much smaller, paler male with its head embedded deep in the host tissue. The joined pair have a "Y"-shaped, or forked appearance. The female worm may become detached from the male and feed freely within the lumen, or be coughed up and discharged from the body.

Prophylaxis and Treatment: To prevent wild birds from introducing infection, pens should be isolated by overhead and lateral screening. After infection occurs, pens should be "rested" and preferably rotated with crops; however, poultry and game birds should not be placed on newly plowed fields. Earthworm populations can be reduced before introduction of range-reared birds by soil treatments such as ethylene dibromide, rotenone, and chlordane. Various molluscicides, such as copper sulfate or pentachlorophenate, destroy slugs and snails.

Thiabendazole at 0.05% in the feed continuously for 2 wk effectively eliminates gapeworms from pheasants, and when given continuously for ≥4 days is said to help prevent and control infections. Tetramisole has been reported to be effective at 1.6 mg/lb (3.6 mg/kg) for 3 consecutive days in the drinking water. Poultry treated while larvae are migrating in the body develop immunity to gapeworms even though therapy may abort larval maturation.

INFECTIOUS BRONCHITIS

An acute, rapidly spreading, viral disease of chickens, characterized by infection of respiratory, urogenital, and GI tract tissues.

Etiology and Epidemiology: The causal coronaviruses are found worldwide and exist as numerous serotypes. Two or more serotypes may occur simultaneously in one geographic region.

A disease of chickens only, the virus is present in respiratory discharges and feces, and on contaminated eggshells. It is spread by droplets through the air; by ingestion of contaminated feed and water; and by contact with infected chickens, contaminated equipment, and clothing of caretakers. Chickens infected with some strains excrete virus in the feces for ≥1 mo after clinical recovery. Virus infections in layers and breeders occur cyclically as immunity declines, or on exposure to different serotypes.

Clinical Findings: Signs occur following an incubation period of 18-48 hr, and morbidity may be nearly 100%. Spread to other birds is rapid. The nature and severity of the disease are influenced by the age and immune status of the flock and virulence of the causal strain. Young chickens have coughing, sneezing, and tracheal rales for 10-14 days. Wet eyes and dyspnea may be observed. Facial or head swelling is seen occasionally, particularly in concurrent coliform infections of the sinus and turbinate mucosa. Nephrogenic strains can produce interstitial nephritis with high mortality (up to 60%) in young chickens. In most outbreaks, however, mortality is <5%, although secondary bacterial infections cause higher losses in meat-type chickens.

In layers, egg production may drop 5-50%, and eggs are often misshapen, thin-shelled, and contain watery albumen. Egg production and quality generally return to near normal levels in most birds on recovery. Poor-producing birds are culled.

Lesions: Respiratory tract lesions include mucoid exudate in the trachea and bronchi, generally without hemorrhage. A caseous plug may be found in the trachea of a young bird. Air sacs are thickened and opaque. Secondary bacterial infections in meat-type birds produce caseous airsacculitis, perihepatitis, and pericarditis. Nephrogenic strains produce swollen, pale kidneys, with tubules and ureters distended with urates. In layers, urolithiasis is associated with virus infection and certain dietary factors.

Diagnosis: Diagnosis cannot be based solely on clinical signs because of similarities to mild respiratory forms of Newcastle disease and infectious laryngotracheitis. Isolating and identifying the virus or showing a rise in serum antibodies by the ELISA, virus neutralization, or hemagglutination inhibition tests can confirm the diagnosis given a history of respiratory disease or reduced egg production.

The non-hemagglutinating and lipid-solvent-sensitive virus is isolated by inoculation of 9- to 11-day-old chicken embryos. Respiratory tissues and kidney are the best sources for isolations. Several blind passages of the virus may be necessary for isolation of some field strains. The virus produces embryo stunting, curling, and urate deposits in the mesonephros, with variable mortality.

Control: No available medication alters the course of the disease, although antibiotic therapy may reduce mortality due to secondary infections. Increasing the temperature in the house and under the hover by 5-10°F (3-4°C) may lower mortality.

Attenuated vaccines used for immunization may produce relatively mild respiratory signs. Live vaccines are initially given to 1- to 14-day-old chicks by spray, drinking water, or eyedrop. Revaccination is common. Adjuvanted killed vaccines are sometimes used in breeders and layers to prevent egg production losses.

Many serotypes are recognized, and a number of new or variant serotypes have been reported, which pose problems in immunization and diagnosis. Vaccination with selected variant serotypes is practiced in some areas. Outbreaks with mortality due to nephritis have been associated with several variant strains in Australia and the USA. Variant serotypes have been associated with egg production losses in vaccinated layer flocks.

INFECTIOUS CORYZA

An acute or subacute respiratory disease of worldwide distribution characterized by nasal discharge, sneezing, and swelling of the face under the eyes. It is quite important in tropical and temperate climates. Although it also occurs in pheasants, guinea fowl, and turkeys, the disease is primarily one of chickens, mainly of older growing pullets and young layers; it is occasionally seen in broilers in tropical climates. It is present in "backyard flocks" and "fancy breed" establishments throughout the USA, and in commercial flocks in California and the southeast.

Etiology: The causative bacterium, *Haemophilus paragallinarum (gallinarum)*, is a gram-negative, pleomorphic, nonmotile, catalase-negative, microaerophilic rod that tends to grow in filament formation. When grown on blood agar with a staphylococcal nurse colony, the satellite colonies appear as dewdrops, growing adjacent to the nurse colony. The filamentous rods can be demonstrated in stained nasal exudate smears from infected sinuses. The several serovars of *H paragallinarum* are grouped into 3 immunotypes.

Epidemiology and Transmission: Chronically ill or healthy carrier birds are the reservoir of infection. Chickens become susceptible at 4 wk, and their susceptibility increases with age. The incubation period is 1-3 days, and duration of the disease usually ~2 wk. Under field conditions, the disease may run up to several weeks in the presence of complicating diseases, eg, mycoplasmosis.

Once a flock has been infected, it is a constant threat to uninfected flocks. Transmission is by direct contact, airborne droplets, and contamination of drinking water. "All-in/all-out" management has essentially eradicated the disease from commercial poultry establishments in the USA. Commercial farms that have multiple-age flocks tend to perpetuate the disease.

Clinical Findings: In its mildest form (usually seen in young Leghorns or broilers), the only signs may be depression, with a serous nasal discharge and, occasionally, slight facial swelling. In the more severe form (usually young adult Leghorns or heavy breeders), there is severe swelling of one or both infraorbital sinuses with edema of the surrounding tissue, which may close one or both eyes. In adult birds, especially males, the edema may extend to the intermandibular space and wattles. The swelling usually abates in 10-14 days; however, if secondary infection occurs, the swelling can persist for months. There may be varying degrees of rales depending on the extent of infection. Egg production may be delayed in young pullets and severely reduced in producing hens.

Lesions: In acute cases, lesions may be limited to the infraorbital sinuses. There is a tenacious, copious, grayish, semifluid exudate. As the disease becomes chronic or other pathogens become involved, the sinus exudate may become consolidated and turn yellowish. Other lesions may include conjunctivitis, tracheitis, bronchitis, and airsacculitis.

Diagnosis: Isolation of a catalase-negative, nurse-colony-dependent organism from chickens in a flock with a history of a rapidly spreading coryza is diagnostic. Production of typical signs following inoculation with nasal exudate from infected into susceptible chickens is also reliable diagnostically. Antibodies may be detected by agglutination, agar-gel precipitation, or hemagglutination-inhibition ~2-3 wk after infection. Swelling of the face and wattles must be differentiated from fowl cholera (qv, p 1574). Other diseases that must be considered are mycoplasmosis, laryngotracheitis, Newcastle disease, infectious bronchitis, avian influenza, and vitamin A deficiency.

Control and Treatment: Prevention is the only sound method of control. "All-in/all-out" farm programs with sound management and isolation methods are the best way to avoid the disease. The poultryman should raise his own replacements or get them from clean flocks. If replacement pullets are to be placed on a farm that has a history of infectious coryza, bacterins are available to help prevent and control the disease. USDA-licensed bacterins are available, and bacterins also are produced within states for intrastate use; they also are produced in many other countries. The immunization should be given ~3 wk before infectious coryza usually breaks out on the individual farm. Antibodies detected by the hemagglutination-inhibition test after bacterin administration correlate with protective immunity. Controlled exposure to live organisms also has been used to immunize layers in endemic areas.

Because early treatment is important, water medication is recommended immediately until medicated feed is available. Erythromycin and oxytetracycline are usually beneficial. Various sulfonamides, and sulfonamide-trimethoprim, have been successful but must not be used in layers. In more severe outbreaks, although treatment may result in improvement, the disease may recur when medication is discontinued.

Preventive medication may be combined with a vaccination program where started pullets are to be reared or housed on infected premises.

INFECTIOUS LARYNGOTRACHEITIS

An acute, highly contagious, herpesvirus infection of chickens and pheasants characterized by severe dyspnea, coughing, and rales; or a subacute disease with lacrimation, tracheitis, conjunctivitis, and mild rales. It has been reported from most of the intensive-poultry-rearing sections of the USA and many other countries.

Clinical Findings: In the acute form, gasping, coughing, rattling, and extension of the neck during inspiration are seen 6-12 days after natural exposure. Reduced productivity is a varying factor in laying flocks. Affected birds lose their appetite and become inactive. The mouth and beak may be bloodstained from the tracheal exudate. Mortality varies, but may reach 50% in adults, and is usually due to occlusion of the trachea by hemorrhage or exudate. Signs usually subside after ~2 wk, although some birds may cough for 1 mo. Strains of low virulence produce little or no mortality with slight respiratory signs and lesions and a slight decline in egg production.

Following recovery, some birds remain carriers. Infection also may be spread mechanically. Several epidemics have been traced to the transport of birds in contaminated crates.

Diagnosis: The clinical signs and finding blood, mucus, and yellow caseous exudate, or a hollow caseous cast in the trachea, characterize the acute disease. Microscopically, a desquamative, necrotizing tracheitis is characteristic. In the subacute form, punctiform hemorrhagic areas in the trachea and larynx, and conjunctivitis with lacrimation permit a presumptive diagnosis. In uncomplicated cases, the air sacs usually are not involved. A conclusive diagnosis may be made by 1) demonstrating intranuclear inclusion bodies in the tracheal epithelium early in the course of the disease; 2) isolating and identifying the specific virus in chick embryos, tissue culture, or chickens; or 3) inoculating the infraorbital sinus or vent of known immune and susceptible birds. Neutralization of virus is less dependable but has been used.

Prophylaxis and Treatment: Some relief from signs is obtained by keeping the birds quiet, lowering the dust level, and using mild expectorants, being careful that they do not contaminate feed or water. Vaccination should be practiced in endemic areas and on farms where a specific diagnosis is made. Immediate vaccination of adults in the face of an outbreak shortens the course of the disease. Vaccination is best done with modified strains of low virulence applied to the conjunctiva (eye drop). Mass methods of vaccination such as spray or drinking water administration are less consistent in their results. Broiler flocks in some areas must be vaccinated when young, but this is unlikely to be effective if done under 4 wk of age. Some vaccine producers recommend revaccination when birds are to be held to maturity.

INFLUENZA
(Fowl plague)

A viral disease of domestic and wild birds with signs ranging from almost no clinical disease to high mortality. The incubation period also is highly variable, and ranges from a few days to 1 wk.

Etiology, Epidemiology, and Distribution: The causal orthomyxoviruses are type A influenza viruses. Both virulent and avirulent viruses with any of 13 known surface hemagglutinins are known to infect avian species. The viruses grow readily in embryonating chicken eggs and agglutinate RBC. Specific inhibition of this hemagglutination is the basis for the serological test for influenza antibodies. The viruses have a worldwide distribution and frequently are recovered from clinically normal sea birds, migrating waterfowl, imported pet birds, and live bird markets.

Clinical Findings and Lesions: Respiratory signs are most common, but other signs range from only a slight decrease in egg production or fertility to a fulminating infection with CNS involvement. In severely affected birds, greenish diarrhea; cyanosis and edema of the head, comb, and wattle; ecchymotic discoloration of the shanks and feet; and bloodstained oral and nasal discharges are common. Sinusitis is not uncommon in ducks, quail, and turkeys.

The location and severity of gross lesions are also highly variable and may consist of hemorrhages, transudation, and necrosis in the respiratory, GI, integumentary, and urogenital systems.

Diagnosis: Isolation of the virus in embryonating chicken eggs results in allantoic fluid that agglutinates RBC. The hemagglutination is not inhibited by Newcastle disease antiserum. A crude antigen prepared by grinding the chorioallantoic membrane of infected chicken embryos gives positive results with a gel-precipitation test using known positive influenza A antiserum. In its severe forms, the disease resembles acute fowl cholera and velogenic, viscerotropic Newcastle disease. In milder forms, it may be confused with other respiratory diseases.

Prophylaxis and Treatment: The use of nonviable oil-emulsion vaccine, while effective, is complicated by the 13 antigenically distinct hemagglutinin subtypes that may be responsible for the disease; to be effective, the autogenous virus or a virus of similar hemagglutinin type must be used in vaccine production. The other major viral surface antigen, neuraminidase, is not as important in influenza immunity as the hemagglutinin (but is useful for identification). Treatment of affected flocks with broad-spectrum antibiotics to control secondary bacterial invaders, and increased house temperatures may help reduce mortality. Amantadine hydrochloride, approved for treatment of influenza A in man, is effective in reducing the severity of influenza in some avian species, but amantadine-resistant virus frequently emerges. Suspected outbreaks should be reported to regulatory authorities.

QUAIL BRONCHITIS

An infectious, contagious disease of bobwhite quail observed in the wild and in captivity. It is a serious disease on certain farms where the birds are pen-reared, and particularly when birds of different ages are maintained on the same premises. It appears to occur worldwide.

The cause is an adenovirus, generally regarded as avian serotype 1, which can be isolated readily from the respiratory tract of acutely affected birds, and from the intestinal tract of mildly affected birds. It is highly contagious, and other avian species may be carriers. It spreads rapidly through multiple-age units.

Respiratory distress, coughing, sneezing, rales, lacrimation, and conjunctivitis are common. Loose, watery droppings are common in subacutely affected older birds. Mortality may be 100% in birds <2 wk old, usually <25% in birds >4 wk old. The disease often is self-limiting. Mild to severe tracheitis (the trachea may be completely filled with mucus), airsacculitis, conjunctivitis, mucoid enteritis, and gaseous distention of the intestines may be seen.

There is no specific treatment, but increasing the brooder temperature by 3-5°F (1.5-3°C), preventing "piling up", and strict isolation and sanitation are of value, as is avoiding multiple-age units. Recovered birds should be retained for breeders. Immunity is long lasting, possibly for life. New birds should not be introduced to premises without a 30-day quarantine.

SWOLLEN HEAD SYNDROME
(SHS, Dikkop [Thick head], Facial cellulitis)

An acute, infectious respiratory disease of chickens characterized by periorbital swelling, swollen lacrimal glands, sneezing, and variable mortality. SHS affects broiler chickens at 4-6 wk of age, broiler parents, and commercial layers. The disease has been reported in southern Africa, the Netherlands, the UK, and other countries.

Etiology: There is strong evidence that SHS is caused by a mixed infection of the avian pneumovirus responsible for turkey rhinotracheitis (qv, p 1621) and secondary adventitious bacteria, usually *Escherichia coli*, which invade the subcut. facial tissues resulting in the swollen head. There is also, however, evidence that the primary cause, at least in some areas, is a coronavirus serotypically distinct from other infectious bronchitis serotypes. Also, other respiratory agents including Newcastle disease, paramyxovirus-3, avian influenza, and infectious bronchitis virus may cause respiratory disease and egg production problems that are not dissimilar.

Clinical Findings and Lesions: The initial signs of SHS are sneezing followed by reddening and swelling of the lacrimal glands and swelling of the periorbital tissues, which extend over the head and down to the intermandibular wattle area over the next 24-36 hr. Birds scratch the face with the feet. Mortality may occur at this stage, or later after progression to a generalized polyserositis. SHS has a course of 5-10 days. Affected birds show petechiation to severe congestion of the turbinate mucosa and lacrimal glands, and when skin is removed from the swollen head, purulent and edematous subcut. cellulitis is revealed. Generally, the trachea is unaffected.

Adult chickens may also be affected but the signs are less severe—mild respiratory disease followed by a small portion of the affected flock showing markedly swollen heads. Other signs include torticollis, disorientation, and general depression. In laying birds, a significant drop in egg production usually occurs.

Diagnosis: This is based on typical signs supported by identification of the virus from the trachea, lungs, viscera, nasal exudate, and scrapings of the sinus tissue. Samples must be taken from birds showing early signs of infection to ensure successful recovery of the virus. Primary isolation is best performed in tracheal organ culture or embryonated turkey or chicken eggs; subsequently the virus can be cultivated in cell cultures.

The virus can be identified by electron microscopy or serology. Similar clinical signs have been seen with other respiratory viruses such as Newcastle disease and avian coronaviruses. Viral and bacterial isolation can differentiate between these diseases.

Treatment and Control: At present, no vaccine is commercially available. The disease is exacerbated by poor management practices such as inadequate ventilation, overstocking, poor litter conditions, and poor general hygiene. Antibiotics reduce the severity of the disease somewhat, presumably by controlling secondary bacteria.

TURKEY BORDETELLOSIS
(*Bordetella* rhinotracheitis, Turkey coryza)

A highly contagious upper respiratory disease of young turkeys, with high morbidity and low mortality. Broilers and commercial layer chickens are also susceptible. Infection is spread via direct contact and drinking water.

Etiology and Pathogenesis: The causal bacterium is gram negative, nonfermenting, and motile, and is highly resistant in the environment. Once designated *Alcaligenes faecalis*, *Bordetella avium* is now the accepted name.

Infection by *B avium* provides a favorable environment for secondary invaders. In the complicated disease, as usually seen in the field, the upper respiratory tract is heavily populated by bacteria, mainly *Escherichia coli*. Once *E coli* become established, a serious disease with high morbidity and mortality develops. Although *E coli* are always present in the turkeys' environment, they cause respiratory disease only if a primary agent damages the mucosa. As with many other respiratory diseases, environmental conditions and management factors play an important role: dust, ammonia, overcrowding, use of live vaccines, and temperature extremes are common problems that can aggravate the disease.

Clinical Findings and Lesions: The disease is most severe in turkey poults and mild or absent in layer chicks; older birds may show no clinical signs. In uncomplicated cases, there is accumulation of mucus at the nares, swelling of the submaxillary region, mouth breathing, excessive lacrimal secretion, and a sneezing sound called a snick. Morbidity is 100% and mortality is low, but mortality rises when the disease is complicated. Infection persists in the host for several weeks.

Gross and histological lesions are limited to the turbinates, sinuses, and trachea. A mild to severe mucoid rhinitis is observed. Transient periorbital subcut. edema, congestion of turbinate mucosa, accumulation of mucus in the pharynx and trachea, and occasional tracheal collapse are observed. Histological changes vary from shortening of the cilia and patchy to complete deciliation, to loss of pseudostratified columnar epithelial and goblet cells. Exudate consisting of sloughed cells, mucus, and occasional heterophils is present.

Diagnosis: Diagnosis is based on clinical signs, lesions, and isolation of the causative agent. *Bordetella avium* is relatively easy to isolate on common laboratory media from sinus and tracheal exudates of affected birds, but not necessarily easy to identify. Various bacteria that infect the respiratory tract, particularly other *Bordetella* spp, have characteristics similar to *B avium* and can complicate identification. *Bordetella avium* produces small, glistening, colorless colonies and agglutinates RBC from different species; most isolates fail to grow in broth containing 6.5% sodium chloride. *Bordetella-avium*-like isolates, which are not pathogenic, produce large opaque colonies, do not agglutinate RBC, and most are capable of growth in media containing 6.5% sodium chloride.

A microagglutination test is commonly used to detect serum antibodies and an ELISA is also described. A similar disease in Europe, turkey rhinotracheitis (*see* below), is caused by a virus, but serological studies indicate that the disease is not present in the USA.

Prevention and Treatment: Thorough cleaning and disinfection to eliminate the causative bacteria from houses that held infected flocks is important. Security measures to prevent introduction of the infection include control of traffic, rodents, and free-flying birds. Use of broad-spectrum antibiotics in the early stages of the disease may be helpful. A commercial live vaccine and a commercial bacterin are available for use in susceptible flocks. An experimental pilus vaccine is reported to induce protection and reduce the level of infection.

TURKEY RHINOTRACHEITIS

A viral disease clinically similar to turkey bordetellosis (*see* above) which, in uncomplicated infections, produces high morbidity and low mortality, and may cause losses in egg production.

Etiology and Epidemiology: There has been some confusion over the etiology of the disease due to its similarity with turkey bordetellosis; in the UK, France, and many other countries a virus, probably a pneumovirus, is recognized as the cause. Swollen head syndrome of chickens (qv, p 1619) may be caused by the same virus, with *Escherichia coli* as a secondary organism.

Although the virus has been isolated from the trachea, lungs, and viscera of infected poults, the most frequent source has been the nasal secretions or tissue scraped from the sinuses. Only contact spread of the disease has been confirmed, but contaminated water, movement of affected or recovered poults, movement of equipment and personnel, airborne virus, and vertical transmission have all been implicated in outbreaks.

Clinical Findings: Descriptions of disease vary greatly and may reflect differences in the secondary organisms involved. Respiratory signs in poults include snicking, rales, sneezing, nasal discharge (often frothy), foamy conjunctivitis, swelling of the infraorbital sinuses, and submandibular edema. In laying birds, there may be slight respiratory distress and subsequent drops in egg production of up to 70%. Serological evidence of the virus has occurred in some flocks without related clinical signs. Mortality is usually highest in poults; generally, mortality of 5-10% may be expected, but a range of 0.4-90% has been recorded.

Lesions: Deciliation of the trachea begins within 48 hr of experimental infection and is completed within 96 hr. Mucosal thickening, congestion of the tissues and infiltration with lymphocytes, plasma cells, and heterophils also occur. In natural infections, more severe pathological changes appear to be due to secondary organisms.

Diagnosis: Diagnosis may be confirmed by viral isolation in embryonating chicken eggs by yolk-sac inoculation, chick tracheal organ cultures, or chick embryo cells, and serological identification of the virus. However, more frequently, diagnosis is reached by clinical signs and serological evidence. Antibodies to the virus may be detected by virus neutralization in cell or tracheal organ culture, immunofluorescence, or immunodiffusion, but the most frequently used has been the ELISA test.

Prophylaxis and Control: At present no commercial vaccines are available. The response to treatment with various antibiotic regimens aimed at secondary organisms has not been uniform. Good management practices, such as adequate ventilation, good litter conditions, strict hygiene, and prevention of excessive heat or parasite buildup, have helped control the disease. Although the procedure is potentially hazardous and is not permitted in some areas, deliberate exposure of turkeys to the virus during the rearing period has been used successfully to control drops in egg production in some countries.

ECTOPARASITISM

BEDBUGS

Cimex lectularius is a common bloodsucking parasite in temperate and subtropical climates that attacks poultry, man, and most other mammals. It is rare in modern laying operations, but breeding houses and pigeon lofts may become heavily infested. The life cycle may be completed in 4-6 wk or extend much longer since nymphs can withstand fasting for ~70 days, and adults for up to 12 mo. Feeding usually occurs at night. The bugs become engorged within 10 min, then hide in cracks and crevices. If attacked by large numbers of bugs, birds may become ane-mic. Bites are usually followed by swelling and itching due to the injection of saliva into the wound.

Control is best accomplished by thorough cleaning of the houses, reducing hiding places for the bugs, and thorough high-pressure spraying of the houses as for the control of fowl ticks (*see* below).

FLEAS

The **sticktight flea** (*Echidnophaga gallinacea*) is unique among poultry fleas in that the adults become sessile parasites and usually remain attached to the skin of the head for days or weeks. The adult females forcibly eject their eggs so that they reach surrounding litter. The larvae develop best in sandy, well-drained litter. Hosts of the adult flea include chickens, turkeys, pigeons, pheasants, quail, man, and many other mammals. Irritation and blood loss may cause anemia and death, particularly in young birds.

The **western hen flea**, *Ceratophyllus niger*, seems to be confined to the Pacific coast area (USA). This flea actually breeds in the droppings and only feeds on birds occasionally. The **European chick flea**, *C gallinae*, is widespread in the USA. It breeds in nests and litter, and only goes on the birds to feed. It attacks many other birds besides chickens. The most important control measures are removing infested litter and dusting the litter surface with carbaryl, coumaphos, or malathion to kill immature fleas.

FLIES AND GNATS

Black Flies: *Simulium* spp (Simuliidae), also known as buffalo gnats and turkey gnats, are bloodsuckers and transmit leucocytozoonosis (qv, p 1545) to ducks, turkeys, and other birds. They are most abundant in the north temperate and subarctic zones, but many species occur in tropical areas. They often attack in swarms and cause anemia and death of birds either directly or through disease transmission. Black-fly control is extremely difficult since immature stages are restricted to running water, which is often some distance from the poultry farm. Larval control can be achieved with applications of temephos during early spring before adults emerge. Screens of 24 mesh per in. (2.54 cm) or smaller are required for adult control. Measures recommended for mosquito control in houses (*see* p 1625) are applicable to black-fly control. (*See also* p 797.)

Biting Midges: *Culicoides* spp (Ceratopogonidae) transmit a malaria-like organism, *Haemoproteus nettionis*, to wild and domestic ducks.

The Pigeon Fly: *Pseudolynchia canariensis* (Hippoboscidae) is an important parasite of pigeons in warm or tropical areas. It may transmit *Haemoproteus columbae*, which causes pigeon malaria. It may also cause heavy losses in squabs. The pigeon loft should be cleaned every 20 days, and the squabs can be dusted with pyrethrum powder.

FOWL TICKS

Argas persicus occurs worldwide in tropical and subtropical countries and is the vector of *Borrelia anserina* (spirochetosis, qv, p 1565). In the USA, the *A persicus* complex has been divided to include *A sanchezi* and *A radiatus*, as well as *A persicus*. These ticks are particularly active in poultry houses during warm dry weather. All stages may be found hiding in cracks and crevices during the day. Larvae can be found on the birds since they remain attached and feed for 2-7 days. Nymphs and adults feed at night in ~15-30 min. Nymphs feed and molt several times before reaching the adult stage. Adults feed repeatedly, and the females lay 50-100 eggs after each feeding. Adult females may live ≥4 yr without a blood meal.

In addition to being vectors of some poultry diseases (avian spirochetosis, aegyptianellosis, fowl cholera), fowl ticks produce anemia (most important), weight loss, depression, toxemia, and paralysis. Egg production decreases. Red spots can be seen on the skin where the ticks have fed. Since the ticks are nocturnal, the birds may show some uneasiness when roosting. Death losses are rare, but production may be severely depressed.

After houses are cleaned, walls, ceilings, cracks, and crevices should be treated thoroughly (using a high-pressure sprayer) with carbaryl, coumaphos, malathion, stirofos, or a mixture of stirofos and dichlorvos.

LICE

Avian lice, which belong to the order Mallophaga, have a life cycle of ~3 wk and normally feed on bits of skin or feather products. Lice may live for several months on the host but remain alive only for ~1 wk off the host. Man and other mammals may harbor avian lice, but only temporarily.

In intensive poultry systems, the most common and economically important louse to both chickens and turkeys is *Menacanthus stramineus*, the chicken body louse. It punctures soft quills near their base, or gnaws the skin at the base of the feathers and feeds on the blood. Chickens are less commonly infested with *Menopon gallinae* (on feather shafts), *Lipeurus caponis* (mainly on the wing feathers), *Cuclotogaster heterographa* (mainly on the head and neck), *Goniocotes gallinae* (very small, in the fluff), *Goniodes gigas* (the large chicken louse), *Goniodes dissimilis* (the brown chicken louse), *Menacanthus cornutus* (the body louse), *Menacanthus pallidulus* (the small body louse), or *Oxylipeurus dentatus*. Turkeys may also be infested with *Chelopistes meleagridis* (the large turkey louse), *Oxylipeurus polytrapezius* (the slender turkey louse), or *M stramineus* (the chicken body louse).

Because lice transfer from one bird species to another when the hosts are in close contact, other domestic and caged birds may be infested with species of Mallophaga that are usually host-specific.

Heavy populations of the chicken body louse lower reproductive potential in males, egg production in females, and weight gain in growing chickens. The skin irritations are also sites for secondary bacterial infections. Other species of lice are not highly pathogenic to mature birds, but may be fatal to chicks. Examination of birds, particularly around the vent and under the wings, reveals eggs or moving lice on the skin or feathers.

Lice are usually introduced to a farm through infested equipment, such as crates and egg flats, or by galliform birds. Lice are best controlled on caged chickens or turkeys by spraying with pyrethroids, carbaryl, coumaphos, malathion, or stirofos. Birds on the floor are more easily treated by scattering carbaryl, coumaphos, malathion, or stirofos dust on the litter.

MITES

The most economically important of the many external parasites of poultry are mites of the families Dermanyssidae (northern fowl mite, tropical fowl mite, and chicken mite) and Trombiculidae (turkey chigger).

COMMON CHIGGER

Trombicula alfreddugesi and other chigger species (harvest mites, red bugs) infest birds as well as man and other mammals. Heavily parasitized birds become droopy, refuse to eat, and may die from starvation and exhaustion. Larvae may be found either singly or in clusters on the ventral portion of the birds. Control on the range is aided by keeping the grass cut short and dusting with sulfur or malathion.

CHICKEN MITE

Dermanyssus gallinae (also called red mite, roost mite, or poultry mite) attacks chickens, turkeys, pigeons, canaries, and various wild birds. Rare in modern commercial cage-layer operations, it is found in breeder and small farm flocks. Chicken mites are nocturnal feeders that hide during the day under manure, on roosts, and in cracks and crevices of the chicken house, where they deposit eggs. Populations develop rapidly during the warmer months and more slowly in cold weather; the life cycle may be completed in only 1 wk. A house may remain infested for 6 mo after birds are removed.

Transmission of the northern fowl mite (NFM), the tropical fowl mite (*see* below), and the chicken mite is by mite dispersion, or by contact with infested birds, animals, or inanimate objects. In the integrated poultry industry, mites are dispersed most frequently on inanimate objects such as egg flats, crates, coops, or by personnel going from house to house or farm to farm.

Heavy infestations of either NFM or the chicken mite reduce reproductive potential in males, egg production in females, and weight gain in young birds. NFM are found either on the eggs or by parting feathers in the vent area. Chicken mites may be found in the chicken houses during the day, particularly in cracks or where roost poles touch supports, or on the birds at night.

Obtaining mite-free birds, and sanitation are important in preventing a buildup of mite populations. Once poultry have been infested with NFM, control may be achieved by spraying or dusting the birds and litter with carbaryl, coumaphos, malathion, stirofos, or a pyrethroid compound in areas where the parasites have not developed resistance to these chemicals. Miticide spray treatments must be applied with sufficient force to penetrate the feathers in the vent area. Nicotine sulfate is an effective fumigant for mites but is particularly hazardous. Pyrethrins and piperonyl butoxide are initially active, but have poor residual killing power. For chicken mite control, in addition to treating the birds, the inside of the house and all hiding places for the mite, such as roosts, behind nest boxes, and cracks and crevices, must be treated thoroughly using a high-pressure sprayer. Dimethoate and fenthion may be used as residual house sprays when poultry are not present.

DEPLUMING MITE

Cnemidocoptes gallinae burrow into the epidermis at the base of feather shafts and cause intense irritation and feather pulling in chickens, pheasants, pigeons, and geese in spring and summer. To control the depluming mite, affected birds should be isolated and treated by dipping individual birds in a mixture of sulfur (2 oz [60 g]), soap (1 oz [30 g]), and warm water (1 gal. [4 L]).

FEATHER MITE

Most feather mites belong to the families Analgidae (Analgesidae), Pterolichidae, and Proctophyllodidae and are rare on modern poultry ranches. They do little economic damage but may reduce egg production via malnutrition, feather loss, and dermatitis. No specific control method has been described.

NORTHERN FOWL MITE (NFM)

Ornithonyssus sylviarum is the most important parasite of caged layers and breeding chickens in the USA, and is a serious pest of chickens throughout the temperate zone of other countries. On turkeys, it is second in importance only to the turkey chigger in areas where the turkey chigger exists. It has been reported from many species of birds, and from rats, mice, and man; however, fertile populations are reported only on birds. The NFM is an obligate bloodsucking parasite that normally spends its entire life cycle (~1 wk) on the host. Off the host, it may live up to 2 mo, depending on temperature and relative humidity. In heavy infestations, the feathers, particularly in the vent area, are blackened. The mites, their eggs, cast skins, and excrement can be seen on the feathers and skin of the host when the feathers are parted, and the skin may be scabbed and cracked. Poultrymen often diagnose NFM infestations by seeing the mites on eggs.

For clinical findings and control, *see* CHICKEN MITE, above.

SCALY LEG MITE

Cnemidocoptes mutans is a small, spherical, sarcoptic mite that usually tunnels into the tissue under the scales of the legs. It is rare in modern poultry facilities, but when found, it is usually on older birds on which the irritation and exudation cause the legs to become thickened, encrusted, and unsightly. This mite may occasionally attack the comb and wattles. The entire life cycle is in the skin; transmission is by contact.

For control, affected birds should be culled or isolated, and houses cleaned and sprayed frequently as recommended for the chicken mite (*see* above). Individual bird legs may be dipped twice (10-day interval) in kerosene, crude oil, mineral oil, or linseed oil (not boiled), or coated with warm vaseline.

SUBCUTANEOUS MITE

Laminosioptes cysticola is a small parasite that is most often diagnosed by observing white-to-yellowish caseocalcareous nodules ~1-3 mm in diameter in the subcutis. Careful examination of the skin and subcutis of birds under a dissecting microscope frequently reveals the mites. Destroying the bird is the best control for this parasite.

TROPICAL FOWL MITE

Ornithonyssus bursa is distributed throughout the warmer regions of the world and has been reported from Texas, Florida, Illinois, Indiana, Maryland, and New York. It closely resembles the northern fowl mite in its biology and habits, but lays a greater proportion of its eggs in the nest. Hosts include chickens, turkeys, ducks, pigeons, sparrows, starlings, myna birds, and man. Western equine encephalomyelitis virus has been recovered from this mite.

For clinical findings and control, *see* CHICKEN MITE, above.

TURKEY CHIGGER

The larvae of *Neoschongastia americana* are parasitic on numerous birds. Across the southern USA they are the major pest of turkeys ranged on heavy clay soils in the summer. The chigger feeds in groups of up to 100 mites per lesion for 8-15 days. Turkeys may have 25-30 lesions each. One lesion, 3 mm in diameter, may cause significant downgrading at market time. To prevent downgrading, turkeys must be protected for ≥4 wk before marketing.

Sprays or dusts of malathion or chlorpyrifos on turkey ranges control chiggers. A preventive measure now utilized in many turkey-growing areas includes a shift from range to confinement rearing, or use of sheds to provide shade.

MOSQUITOES

Mosquitoes that feed on poultry usually belong to the genera *Culex, Aedes,* or *Psorophora.* Although mosquitoes are not as significant to poultry as to man, they may transmit several diseases, and large numbers reduce egg production or cause death.

Removal of mosquito-breeding habitats by emptying water-filled containers, clearing pool and pond edges of emergent vegetation, draining swampy areas, and filling low areas that collect water are the best control measures. Screening to prevent mosquito entry, residual wall sprays, or fogging within poultry houses also aids in control.

FOWLPOX

A worldwide, slow-spreading viral infection of chickens and turkeys characterized by proliferative lesions in the skin (cutaneous form) that progress to thick scabs, and by lesions in the upper GI and respiratory tracts (diphtheritic form).

Etiology and Epidemiology: The large DNA virus (an avipoxvirus, family Poxviridae) is highly resistant and may survive for several years in dried scabs. Field and vaccine strains have only minor differences in their genomic profiles, although the strains can be differentiated by electrophoresis. The virus is present in large numbers in the lesions and is usually transmitted by contact to pen mates through abrasions of the skin. Mosquitoes and other biting insects may serve as mechanical vectors. Transmission within flocks is rapid when mosquitoes are plentiful. Some affected birds may become carriers, and the disease may be reactivated by stress, such as moulting or by immunosuppression due to other infections.

Clinical Findings: Only a few birds develop lesions at one time. Lesions are prominent in some birds, and may significantly decrease flock performance. The cutaneous form is characterized by nodular lesions on various parts of the unfeathered skin of the chicken, and head and upper neck of the turkey. Generalized lesions of the feathered skin may also occur. In some cases, lesions are limited chiefly to the feet and legs. The lesion is initially a raised, blanched, nodular area that enlarges, becomes yellowish, and progresses to a thick, dark scab. Multiple lesions usually develop and often coalesce. Lesions in various stages of development may be found on the same bird. Localization around the nostrils may cause nasal discharge. Cutaneous lesions on the eyelids may cause complete closure of one or both eyes.

In the diphtheritic form, lesions occur on the mucous membranes of the mouth, esophagus, pharynx, larynx, and trachea (wetpox or fowl diphtheria). Occasionally, lesions occur almost exclusively in one or more of these sites. Caseous patches firmly adherent to the mucosa of the larynx and mouth or proliferative masses may develop. Tracheal lesions cause difficulty in respiration and may simulate infectious laryngotracheitis in chickens. Mouth lesions interfere with feeding.

Often the course of the disease in a flock is protracted. Extensive infection in a layer flock results in a decline in egg production. Cutaneous infections alone ordinarily cause low or moderate mortality, and these flocks generally return to normal production following recovery. Mortality is usually high in the generalized or diphtheritic form.

Diagnosis: Cutaneous infections usually produce characteristic gross and microscopic lesions. When only small lesions are present, it is often difficult to distinguish them from abrasions caused by fighting. Microscopical examination of affected tissues stained with H&E reveals eosinophilic cytoplasmic inclusion bodies. Elementary bodies can be detected in smears from the lesions stained by the Gimenez method. Laryngeal and tracheal lesions in chickens must be differentiated from infectious laryngotracheitis (qv, p 1617).

Prophylaxis and Treatment: Where pox is prevalent, chickens and turkeys should be vaccinated with live-embryo or cell-culture-propagated virus. The most widely used vaccines are attenuated fowlpox virus and pigeonpox virus isolates of high immunogenicity and low pathogenicity. In high-risk areas, vaccination with an attenuated vaccine of cell-culture origin in the first few weeks of life and revaccination at 12-16 wk is often sufficient. Health of birds, extent of exposure, and type of operation determine the timings of vaccinations. Because the infection spreads slowly, vaccination is often useful in limiting spread in affected flocks if administered when <20% of the birds have lesions. Since passive immunity may interfere with multiplication of vaccine virus, progeny from recently vaccinated or recently infected flocks should be vaccinated only after passive immunity has declined. Vaccinated birds should be examined 1 wk later for swelling and scab formation "take" at the site of vaccination. Absence of "take" indicates lack of potency of vaccine, passive immunity, or improper vaccination. Revaccination with another serial lot of vaccine is indicated.

POX IN OTHER AVIAN SPECIES

Infections with avian poxvirus have been recorded from a variety of wild and pet birds. Some isolates are primarily infectious for only the homologous host, whereas others are infectious for one or more additional species. Classification is usually based on host pathogenicity studies. Canarypox infection is usually severe, and mortality sometimes approaches 100%. Cutaneous lesions may develop, as may systemic infection with cytoplasmic inclusion bodies detected in lesions on histological examination. No effective vaccine for canaries is available in the USA. Poxvirus infection in psittacines may also be severe, especially in blue-fronted Amazon parrots. Poxviruses isolated from psittacines appear to be unrelated to poxviruses of other avian species.

Genomic profiles of canarypox, mynahpox, and quailpox viruses show marked differences from fowlpox virus when their DNA is compared after restriction endonuclease digestion. Quailpox virus shows marked antigenic differences from fowlpox virus, although some cross-reacting antigens are present, and provide limited or no cross-protection against fowlpox virus. A quailpox virus vaccine is available commercially.

Recently, a turkeypox vaccine has been developed to control pox in turkey flocks in which fowlpox vaccine is ineffective. The commercially available vaccine contains a turkeypox virus immunologically unrelated to fowlpox virus.

NECROTIC DERMATITIS
(Clostridial dermatomyositis, Gangrenous dermatitis, Gangrenous cellulitis)

An infectious disease characterized by sudden onset, sharp increase in mortality, and gangrenous necrosis of the skin over the thighs and breast. It occurs sporadically in 4- to 16-wk-old chickens, affects broiler and layer replacement stocks, and occasionally causes outbreaks in turkeys.

Etiology, Transmission, and Epidemiology: *Clostridium septicum* is isolated most frequently, but *C perfringens* and *C novyi* also may be present. In addition, other bacteria, particularly staphylococci and *Escherichia coli*, almost always accompany the clostridia in culture.

Young chicks immunosuppressed by infectious bursal disease (IBD, qv, p 1577) are predisposed. Skin lesions due to trauma, moist litter, bacterial infection (staphylococcosis), or selenium deficiency also may be predisposing factors. The disease has been induced by subcut. or IM inoculation of *C septicum* and a chemical irritant (calcium chloride). Inoculated chickens develop gangrenous necrosis of the skin and underlying musculature and can die within 12-48 hr. Systemic effects arise from both invading organisms and their elaborated exotoxins.

Clinical Findings and Lesions: The first sign usually is a sudden drastic increase in mortality in the affected flock. Overall mortality is 10-60%. Affected chickens show signs of extreme depression, lameness, and prostration, and die within 8-24 hr. Patches of red-to-black gangrenous skin are seen over the breast and thighs. Feather loss or sloughing of the epidermis occurs frequently. Palpation of the affected areas often reveals crepitation due to gas bubbles in the subcutis and musculature. At necropsy, an accumulation of bubbly serosanguineous fluid is seen in the subcutis. The underlying musculature has a cooked appearance. The liver and spleen are enlarged and may contain large necrotic infarcts. The kidneys usually are swollen, and the lungs are congested and edematous. Atrophy of the bursa of Fabricius may be found in chickens that were exposed to IBD virus in the first few weeks after hatching.

Diagnosis: Histopathological demonstration of gas gangrene and/or numerous, large, gram-positive rods, with or without spores in affected tissues is sufficient to confirm a clinical diagnosis. Isolation of *C septicum*, together with the history and clinical findings, differentiate necrotic dermatitis from exudative diathesis (selenium deficiency), staphylococcosis, and other diseases involving the skin.

Treatment and Control: This disease can be prevented by maintaining proper litter condition, minimizing mechanical injury, and controlling cannibalism. A breeder vaccination program against IBD to establish healthy, immunocompetent replacement stock has been useful in preventing this infection. Administration of oxytetracycline at 0.02% in the feed rapidly reduces mortality in field outbreaks.

MISCELLANEOUS CONDITIONS

AMMONIA BURN

A keratitis of domestic poultry due to excessive ammonia in the air. It is characterized by clouding and ulceration of the cornea, and ultimately, blindness. The excess ammonia is generally the result of bacterial fermentation in wet litter, compounded by poor ventilation. If the ammonia levels are reduced at an early stage, birds recover very slowly. The condition should be differentiated from keratoconjunctivitis due to infection or vitamin A deficiency.

ASCITES SYNDROME
(Waterbelly, Right ventricular failure, Pulmonary hypertension syndrome)

Ascites is an accumulation of noninflammatory transudate in one or more of the peritoneal cavities or potential spaces. The fluid, which accumulates most frequently in the 2 ventral hepatic, the peritoneal, or the pericardial spaces, may contain yellow protein clots. Ascites may result from 1) vascular damage, 2) increased vascular hydraulic pressure, 3) increased tissue or decreased vascular oncotic (usually colloidal) pressure, or 4) blockage of lymph drainage.

Increased vascular hydraulic pressure is the most common cause of ascites. In mammals and birds, the 2 most common causes of the increased pressure are right ventricular failure and hepatic fibrosis. In man, liver damage and the resultant hypertension is the most common cause.

In poultry, right ventricular failure (RVF) is usually secondary to valvular insufficiency and may result from inflammatory (valvular endocarditis) or degenerative (furazolidone-induced) disease of the myocardium or valves, or from congenital heart disease. In turkeys, spontaneous dilatory cardiomyopathy is a common cause of ascites. However, the most common cause of ascites in meat-type chickens is RVF in response to increased pulmonary arterial resistance. Pulmonary hypertension occurs frequently in chickens secondary to the hypoxia of high altitude by causing polycythemia and increased blood viscosity. It also occurs frequently secondary to the hypervolemia of sodium toxicity and less frequently from lung pathology. When the disease occurs at low altitudes in meat-type chickens, which have a high metabolic oxygen requirement, it is usually caused by primary or spontaneous pulmonary hypertension because of insufficient pulmonary capillary capacity.

In poultry, liver damage may be caused by aflatoxin, or toxins from plants such as *Crotalaria*. In broiler chickens, obstructive cholangiohepatitis (possibly caused by *Clostridium perfringens* infection) is the most common cause of the liver damage, which results in ascites. In both meat-type ducks and breeders, amyloidosis of the liver frequently causes ascites.

Pathogenesis and Epidemiology of Pulmonary Hypertension Syndrome (PHS)—Ascites Caused by Right Ventricular Failure (RVF): PHS is caused by increased pressure in the pulmonary arteries when the heart tries to pump more blood through the lungs to meet the body's oxygen requirement. The resultant volume and pressure overload on the right ventricle cause dilatation and hypertrophy of the right ventricular wall and RVF.

Bird lungs are rigid and fixed in the thoracic cavity. The small capillaries can expand very little to accommodate increased blood flow. Lung size in proportion to body weight, and particularly to muscle mass, decreases as meat-type chickens grow. Increased blood flow results in primary pulmonary hypertension and cor pulmonale with sporadic cases of RVF and ascites in fast-growing broilers. Predisposing factors that increase oxygen demand (cold), reduce oxygen-carrying capacity of the blood (carbon monoxide), increase blood volume (sodium), or interfere with blood flow through the lung (by lung pathology which narrows or occludes capillaries, by increased RBC size or rigidity, or by polycythemia with increased blood viscosity) may result in flock outbreaks of PHS with or without ascites.

The incidence of PHS is >2% in some broiler and many roaster flocks, and is occasionally 15-20% in other roaster flocks. Right ventricular hypertrophy is the response to an increased workload and eventually leads to RVF if the volume or pressure load persists. Hypertrophy of the right ventricular wall is directly related to pulmonary hypertension, and the ratio of the right ventricle to the total ventricular mass can be used as a measure of the increased pressure load on the right ventricle.

Clinical Findings: Occasionally, young broilers develop PHS, particularly if increased sodium or lung pathology (eg, aspergillosis) is involved, but in primary pulmonary hypertension, mortality is greatest after 5 wk of age. Clinical signs are not seen until RVF occurs and ascites develops. Clinically affected broilers have a pale head and a shrunken comb, and in white chickens the feathers lose their sheen. The abdominal skin may be red, and peripheral vessels congested. Since growth stops as RVF develops, affected broilers are smaller than their pen mates. The ascites increases the respiratory rate and reduces exercise tolerance. Affected broilers frequently die on their back and must be differentiated from flip-over disease (qv, p 1573). Not all broilers that die from PHS have ascites. Death may occur suddenly before clinical signs are observed.

Lesions: Most lesions are the result of increased hydraulic pressure secondary to RVF. There is a variable amount of clear yellow fluid and clots of fibrin in the abdomen. The liver may be swollen and congested, or firm and irregular with edema, and have clotted protein adherent to the surface; it may be nodular or shrunken; it may be white with edema and fibrosis under the capsule, or have large or small blobs of edema in the hepatoperitoneal sacs. There is mild to marked hydropericardium and, occasionally, there is pericarditis with adhesions. There is right ventricular dilatation and mild to marked hypertrophy of the right ventricular wall. The right atrium and vena cava are very dilated. Occasionally, there is thinning of the left ventricle. The lungs are extremely congested and edematous. The intestine may or may not be empty.

Diagnosis: Broilers that die from ascites or suddenly as the result of RVF or pulmonary hypertension can be identified by the enlarged heart; enlarged, thickened right ventricle; or fluid in the body cavities and heart sac. If the heart sac is enlarged or thickened, the broiler has probably died from PHS, even if there is no fluid in the body or heart sac.

Control: Ascites caused by PHS can be prevented by reducing the birds' oxygen requirement; slowing growth or reducing feed lowers the metabolic oxygen requirement. Environmental temperature, humidity, and air movement should be controlled to prevent excessive body heat loss. Ascites caused by other factors (sodium, lung damage, liver damage, etc) can be prevented by avoiding the etiologic agents involved. Altitudes >6000 ft (1850 m) are unsatisfactory for meat-type chickens, and growth must be slowed to prevent mortality. More care to prevent chilling is also necessary at higher altitudes.

BREAST BLISTERS

Sternal bursitis associated with thickening of the skin of the breast overlying the sternum. The bursa contains clear to bloody fluid and has a fibrous wall. If there is secondary infection, the bursa may contain cloudy fluid and caseous debris. It is primarily a problem in turkeys and meat-type chickens, and results in downgrading of the carcass. Predisposing factors include poor feather development, caked or wet litter, wire floors, and leg weakness. If the lesions are infected, staphylococcosis or infectious synovitis may be involved.

CANNIBALISM

A vice of chickens, turkeys, and game birds reared in captivity, characterized by varying degrees of tissue loss from picking of the vent, toes, feathers, or around the head. Predisposing factors include overcrowding, excessive light and temperature, insufficient or improperly placed feeder or drinking space, nutritional imbalances including mineral deficiencies, feeding only pelleted or concentrated feed, feeding high-caloric diets heavy in corn or low-fiber grains, or injuries. Feather picking, which may be so severe as to cause fatal hemorrhage, can occur in birds of any age. Toe picking generally occurs in young chicks started on paper, while head picking occurs in older birds in cages. Nose picking can be a serious problem in young quail. Vent picking can cause serious losses due to hemorrhage in young turkeys; in laying chickens it may extend to evisceration (*see also* PROLAPSE OF THE OVIDUCT, p 1611).

The incidence can be reduced by proper husbandry, but under some conditions and with some strains of birds, it can be prevented only by beak trimming. For proper control, half of the upper beak and the tip of the lower beak should be removed. Cautery is generally necessary to prevent excessive bleeding. Beak trimming is stressful and should be done with care. It can be done at 1 day of age or later; if done during laying it may reduce production.

FLUKE INFECTIONS

Modern poultry production methods have diminished the incidence of fluke infections, although the parasites persist where poultry are less stringently restricted and in some wild birds.

Prosthogonimus macrorchis invades birds after they consume infective metacercariae in developing or mature dragonflies, the secondary host. The piriform fluke matures in ~2 wk in the bursa of Fabricius or, in gallinaceous birds without a functional bursa (eg, chickens, turkeys, pheasants), in the oviduct.

Light infections without clinical signs appear in ducks and other birds with a functional bursa. In gallinaceous birds, heavy infections in the oviduct cause inappetence, droopiness, weight loss, calcareous cloacal discharge, and depressed or suppressed egg production (the eggs being soft-shelled). Lesions range from mild inflammation to distention or rupture of the oviduct due to exudate and egg components, and may lead to death. Diagnosis by fecal examination is unreliable since fluke eggs are not consistently present. Adult flukes may appear in the bird's eggs, or necropsy may reveal flukes in the oviduct.

To prevent fluke transmission, birds must be kept from feeding on dragonflies. Individual birds have been treated with carbon tetrachloride (1-5 mL PO), but the chemical is highly toxic to birds, especially chickens.

Collyriclum faba appear anywhere on the body as subcut. cysts 4-6 mm in diameter (usually containing 2 adults), but more frequently near the vent in turkeys, chickens, and other birds; the cysts ooze exudate, which attracts flies and predisposes to bacterial infection. Signs in young birds include locomotor difficulty and inappetence; heavy infections may be fatal. The parasites can be removed surgically. The life cycle is unknown but probably involves snails and insects such as dragonflies or mayflies. Prevention of infection requires restricting birds from areas frequented by aquatic insects.

GOUT

An abnormal accumulation of urates in the tissue. It occurs in 2 forms, articular and visceral. Articular gout is generally restricted to individual birds and may be due to a genetic defect in metabolism of uric acid. Some flock problems have been associated with abnormally high protein levels in the diet. It is characterized by accumulations of semisolid, white, pasty urates around joints, particularly those of the feet. Visceral gout may be a problem in individuals or in flocks; it is characterized by white chalky deposits of urates on serosal surfaces, particularly the epicardium and the surface of the liver, and within organs, particularly the kidney. It can be due to kidney damage, blockage of ureters, or water deprivation. Nephrotoxic strains of infectious bronchitis virus (qv, p 1614) may cause gout during or after the infection due to reduced kidney function.

MANSON'S EYEWORM INFECTION

Oxyspirura mansoni, Manson's eyeworm, is a slender nematode, 12-18 mm, that is found beneath the nictitating membrane of chickens and other fowl in tropical and subtropical regions. The parasite causes various degrees of inflammation, lacrimation, corneal opacity, and disturbed vision. Worm eggs deposited in the eye reach the pharynx via the nasolacrimal duct, are swallowed, passed in the feces, and ingested by the Surinam cockroach, *Pycnoscelus surinamensis*. Larvae reach the infective stage in the roach. When infected intermediate hosts are eaten, liberated larvae migrate up the esophagus to the mouth, then through the nasolacrimal duct to the eye, where the cycle is completed. Strict sanitary measures, including the use of approved insecticides on roach-infested premises, provide efficient control. Surgical removal of the nictitating membrane is reported to be a useful prophylactic measure. As a treatment, a local anesthetic is applied to the eye, and the worms in the lacrimal sac are exposed by lifting the nictitating membrane. A 5% cresol solution (1-2 drops) placed in the lacrimal sac kills the worms immediately. The eye should be irrigated with sterile water immediately to wash out the debris and excess solution. The eyes improve within 48-72 hr, and gradually become clear if the destructive process caused by the parasite is not too far advanced.

PENDULOUS CROP

A disease of chickens and turkeys characterized by a greatly enlarged, pendulous crop distended with food. The cause is unknown, but it has been suggested that it may be due to injury to the vagal nerve, or abnormal fermentation in the crop, which results in atony of the muscles. Surgical removal of crop contents and parts of the crop has been successful in treating valuable birds.

PART VIII
TOXICOLOGY

TOXICOLOGY, INTRODUCTION

Toxicology is the study of poisons on biological systems, including their properties, actions, and effects. The toxic agent is referred to as a **toxicant**. The term **toxin** is reserved for poisons produced by a biological source (eg, venoms, plant toxins); the redundant term biotoxin is occasionally used. **Toxicosis**, poisoning, and intoxication are synonymous terms for the disease produced by a toxicant. **Toxicity** (sometimes incorrectly used instead of poisoning) refers to the amount of a toxicant necessary to produce a detrimental effect. **Hazard** describes the likelihood of poisoning under conditions of use.

If 2 poisons act through similar mechanisms on the same organs, their combined effects may be **additive** (2 + 2 = 4) or **synergistic** (2 + 2 = >4). **Antagonism** is the inhibition or elimination of the effect of one agent by another (2 + 2 = <4). Antagonism may be chemical or functional.

Toxicant **accumulation** or **biomagnification** occurs when absorption exceeds the capacity of the body to destroy or excrete a xenobiotic (foreign) compound. Likewise, the terms are applied to the environment, an ecosystem, species, etc, when a compound increases because of increased application and/or decreased destruction or disappearance. These elements are used with **ecotoxicology**, the study of the relation of potentially toxic chemicals in living organisms and their environment. When residual compounds are introduced into plant or animal species early in the ecosystem food chain, the levels tend to be successively higher in the next species that feeds on the contaminated plant or animal; eg, predatory birds, which are at the "end" of the food chain, often have the highest levels of certain residual chemicals.

Tolerance is the ability of an organism to show less response to a specific dose of a chemical than it demonstrated on a prior exposure; it refers to acquired, not innate resistance.

Dose Expressions: Probably all toxic effects are dose dependent. (By usual standards, allergens or inducers of idiosyncratic reactions may appear to be exceptions, although even with these, presumably some dose is too small to cause detectable effects.) A dose may cause undetectable, therapeutic, toxic, or lethal effects. Further, the effective dose may differ from molecule to cell to organ, or to body level (or fetus versus mother). Usually, a dose is expressed as the amount of compound per unit of body wt; and the toxicant concentration as ppm or ppb. These quantitative expressions are usually reserved for levels in feedstuffs, water, air, tissue, etc.

The LD_{50} is the dose that is lethal to 50% of a test sample. It is the most common expression used to rate the potency of toxicants. Other expressions of dose are necessary to predict illness or lethality in an individual, eg, maximum nontoxic dose (MNTD), maximum tolerated dose (MTD), approximate lethal dose (ALD).

Elimination Expressions: The elimination or disappearance (by metabolic change) of a compound from an organ or the body is expressed in terms of **half-life ($t_{1/2}$)**, the amount of time required for disappearance of half the compound. The rate of elimination usually depends on the concentration of the compound: a constant fraction is eliminated per unit of time (first order kinetics); or a metabolic reaction may dictate the rate of elimination, and a constant amount is eliminated per unit of time (zero order kinetics). Different body compartments likely have different elimination rates. A 2-compartment system describes elimination that is initially rapid (from the central or plasma component), and subsequently slower (from the peripheral component, eg, liver, kidney, or fat) following IV administration.

Acute toxicosis refers to effects during the first 24 hr. Effects produced by prolonged exposure (3 mo or more) are referred to as **chronic toxicosis**. Subacute and subchronic are terms applied to the large gap between acute and chronic. Regardless of terms, the duration of exposure can greatly affect the toxicity of an agent; this is reflected by the **chronicity factor** (CF), the ratio of the acute to chronic LD_{50}. The biological system may tolerate a higher dose after prolonged exposure (eg, potassium cyanide, CF = 0.04). Other compounds are metabolized and eliminated in much the same manner regardless of the duration of exposure, and the lethal dose does not change appreciably (eg, caffeine, CF = 1.3). However, due to increased sensitization or cumulative effects, prolonged exposure to a toxicant may cause the chronic lethal dose to be much lower than the acute lethal dose (eg, warfarin, CF = 20).

METABOLISM OF POISONS

Absorption occurs via the GI tract, skin, lungs, eye, mammary gland, or uterus, or from sites of injection. Toxic effects may be local, but the poison must be dissolved and absorbed to some extent to affect the cell. The primary factor affecting absorption is solubility. Insoluble salts and ionized compounds are poorly absorbed, while lipid-soluble substances are generally readily absorbed, even through intact skin. For example, barium is toxic, but barium sulfate can be used for GI contrast radiography because of low absorption.

Hematogenous distribution or translocation carries the toxicant to reactive sites, including storage depots. The liver receives the portal circulation and is the organ most commonly involved with intoxication (and detoxification). The selective deposit of xenobiotic compounds in various tissues depends on receptor sites. The ease of chemical distribution depends largely on its water solubility. Aqueous-soluble agents tend to be excreted by the kidney; lipid-soluble chemicals are more likely to be excreted via the bile and accumulate in fat depots. The highest concentration of a poison within an animal is not necessarily found in the organ or tissue on which it exerts its maximal effect, ie, the target organ; eg, lead may be found in highest concentrations in bone, which is neither a site for toxic effects nor a reliable tissue for toxicological analysis. Knowledge of the translocation characteristics of poisons is necessary for proper selection of organs for analysis.

Metabolism or biotransformation of toxicants occurs in most cases and is an "attempt to detoxify". The metabolized xenobiotic can be more toxic than the original compound; this may be referred to as **lethal synthesis**, eg, many organophosphorous insecticides produce metabolites more toxic than the initial (or "parent") compounds (eg, parathion to paroxan).

Of the 2 phases of metabolism, Phase I includes oxidation, reduction, and hydrolysis mechanisms. These reactions, catalyzed by hepatic enzymes, generally convert foreign compounds to derivatives for Phase II reactions, although the products of Phase I may be excreted as such if polar solubility permits translocation. Phase II principally involves conjugation or synthesis reactions. Common conjugates include glucuronides, acetylation products, and combinations with glycine. Metabolism of xenobiotic agents seldom follows a single pathway. Usually, a fraction is excreted unchanged and the rest is excreted (or stored) as metabolites (often many different metabolites). Significant differences in metabolic mechanisms exist between species; eg, because cats lack forms of glucuronyl transferase, their ability to conjugate compounds such as morphine and phenols is compromised. In some cases, subsequent tolerance is due to enzyme induction initiated by the previous exposure.

Excretion of most xenobiotics and their metabolites is via the kidneys. Many polar and high-molecular-weight compounds are excreted via the bile. An enterohepatic cycle occurs when these products are excreted from the liver via bile, reabsorbed from the intestine, and returned to the liver. Milk is also an excretion pathway for some toxicants—a reason for public health concern. The excretion rate may be of primary concern because some toxicants can cause violative residues in food-producing animals. Excretion rates can be profoundly affected by the route of administration, dose, and condition of the animal, as well as other factors.

The mechanism of action of most poisons at the molecular level is still poorly understood. Most toxicants interfere with enzyme systems by denaturing the enzyme protein or by binding to the enzyme molecule and inhibiting its activity.

FACTORS AFFECTING THE ACTIVITY OF POISONS

Poisoning usually is determined more by the multitude of related factors than by the actual toxicity of the poison. Exposure-related, biological, or chemical factors regulate absorption, metabolism, and elimination, and accordingly, influence the clinical consequences (if any).

Factors Related to Exposure: The dose is a primary concern; however, it is seldom known. Duration and frequency of exposure are important (*see* CHRONICITY FACTOR, above). Necessary trace elements (Se, Cu, Zn, F, etc) often become toxic as the dose and exposure increase. The route of exposure affects absorption, translocation, and perhaps metabolic pathways. The time of administration relative to stress or food intake, etc, may also be a factor; eg, following ingestion of some toxicants, emesis may occur if the stomach is empty, but if partly filled, the toxicant is retained and poisoning can occur. Environmental factors, eg, temperature, humidity, and barometric pressure, affect rates of consumption and even the occurrence of some toxic agents. Many mycotoxins and poisonous plants are correlated with seasonal or climatic changes; eg, the ischemic effects of ergot poisoning are observed more often during cold weather, and plant nitrate levels are affected by rainfall.

Biological Factors: Various species and strains within species react differently to a particular poison because of variations in absorption, metabolism, or elimination. Functional differences may also affect the likelihood of poisoning (eg, because the rat does not vomit, it is more sensitive to the rodenticide red squill).

Age and size of the animal are primary factors in poisoning. Metabolism and translocation of xenobiotic agents are compromised by the underdeveloped microsomal enzyme system in young animals; membrane permeability and hepatic and renal clearance capabilities vary with age. Generally, the amount of toxicant required to cause poisoning is correlated to body weight, but with greater body weight, a disproportionate increase in toxicity (per unit body weight) of a compound often occurs. Body surface area may correlate more closely with the toxic dose; no measurement parameter is consistent for every situation.

The sex and hormonal status of the animal may affect the metabolism of a toxicant and thus alter the outcome; eg, females are more susceptible to several organophosphorous insecticides than males, presumably because lethal synthesis occurs more readily in females.

Nutritional and dietary factors, health status, organ pathology, and stress all affect poisoning. Nutritional factors may directly affect the toxin (by altering absorption) or indirectly affect the metabolic processes or availability of receptor sites. (The copper-molybdenum-sulfate interaction is an example of both.)

Chemical Factors: The chemical nature of a toxicant determines solubility, which in turn influences absorption. Nonpolar or lipid-soluble substances tend to be more readily absorbed than polar or ionized substances. The vehicle or carrier of the toxic compound also affects absorption. Isomers, including optical isomers, vary in their toxicity (eg, the γ isomer of benzene hexachloride [hexachlorocyclohexane] is much more toxic than other isomers).

Adjuvants are formulation factors used to alter the toxic effect of the active ingredient (eg, piperonyl butoxide enhances the insecticidal activity of pyrethrins). Binding agents, enteric coating, and sustained-release preparations influence absorption of the active ingredient. Generally, as absorption is delayed, toxicity decreases. Flavoring agents affect palatability, and thus the amount ingested.

Droplet size is an important consideration in sprays and dips because the dose increases with larger droplet size. This is one of many reasons to adhere closely to label instructions and recommended applications. Only formulations intended for animals should be used.

Contaminants and impurities may affect poisoning or be the primary toxicant (eg, dioxins, qv, p 1654).

DIAGNOSIS

As with any disease, diagnosis is based on history, clinical signs, lesions, laboratory examinations, and in some cases, bioassay (animal inoculation) procedures. Circumstantial evidence is valuable and should be carefully noted, but should never replace a thorough clinical and postmortem examination. Much of a case history may have no direct bearing on the diagnosis, but may be important in differential diagnosis. Anamnestic data from owners may overly stress obvious factors and omit subtle, important details. "Sudden death" is often actually "tardy observation".

Pertinent data and samples should be submitted to the diagnostic laboratory. A complete history is necessary for developing the scheme of laboratory investigation and may be valuable in case of litigation. Information should be detailed: eg, "CNS signs" is insufficient; most animals exhibit some type of CNS signs before death. Rather, exact actions and signs should be described. Examples of pertinent information include: 1) number of animals exposed/sick/dead, age, weight, and a chronology of morbidity and mortality; 2) clinical signs, course of the disease; 3) any prior disease; 4) lesions observed at necropsy, with careful examination of ingesta; 5) response to treatment (medication should be listed to avoid analytical confusion); 6) related events, eg, feed change, water source, other medications, feed additives, pesticide applications; and 7) description of facilities (a drawing may be helpful), access to refuse, machinery, etc, recent past locations and when moved. (*See also* COLLECTION AND SUBMISSION OF SAMPLES, p 934.)

PRINCIPLES OF THERAPY

At initial examination, immediate life-saving measures may be needed. Beyond this, treatment for poisoning includes 3 basic principles: 1) prevention of further absorption, 2) supportive/symptomatic treatment, and 3) specific antidotes.

Prevention of Further Absorption: Topically applied toxicants usually can be removed by thorough washing with soap and water; clipping of the hair or wool may be necessary. Emesis is of value in dogs, cats, and pigs if done within a few hours of ingestion. Emesis is contraindicated when the swallowing reflex is absent; the animal is convulsing; or if corrosive agents, volatile hydrocarbons, or petroleum distillates are involved. Oral emetics include syrup of ipecac (10-20 mL in dogs), sodium chloride (1-3 tsp in a cup of warm water), and hydrogen peroxide (5-25 mL). Apomorphine can be used in dogs parenterally at 0.05-0.1 mg/kg.

Gastric lavage, using an endotracheal tube and the largest bore stomach tube possible, is done on the unconscious or anesthetized animal. The head is lowered to a 30° angle and 10 mL of lavage fluid (water or saline) per kg body wt is gently flushed into the stomach, then removed—several times—until returned fluid is clear. Cathartics and laxatives may be indicated for more rapid elimination of the toxicant from the GI tract. A gastrotomy or rumenotomy may be necessary when lavage techniques are insufficient (or too slow in ruminants).

When the poison cannot be physically removed, certain agents administered orally can adsorb it and prevent its absorption. Activated charcoal is effective in adsorbing a wide variety of compounds and usually is the adsorbent and detoxicant of choice when poisoning is suspected.

Supportive Therapy: This often is necessary until the toxicant can be metabolized and eliminated. The type of support required depends on the animal's clinical condition, and may include control of seizures, maintenance of respiration, treatment for shock, correction of electrolyte and fluid loss, control of cardiac dysfunction, and alleviation of pain.

Specific Antidotes: Antidotes (when known) are listed for each toxicant. Some form complexes with the toxicant (eg, the oximes bind with organophosphorous insecticides, EDTA chelates lead), others block or compete for receptor sites (eg, vitamin K competes with the receptor for coumarin anticoagulants), and a few affect metabolism of the toxicant (eg, nitrite and thiosulfate ion release and bind cyanide).

ALGAL POISONING

Usually an acute and highly fatal condition caused by drinking water that contains high concentrations of toxic blue-green algae. Fatalities and severe illness of livestock, pets, and wildlife including birds have been associated with algal blooms in many countries worldwide.

Etiology, Epidemiology, and Pathogenesis: Toxic strains of *Microcystis, Anabena (Anabaena),* and *Aphanizomenon* are most commonly responsible for algal intoxication, although other genera also have been implicated. Both neurotoxic alkaloids and hepatotoxic peptides have been isolated from toxic algal blooms.

Poisoning usually does not occur unless there is a dense bloom. Factors contributing to such blooms are warm, sunny weather and eutrophic water. Wind concentration of the algae against the shore where livestock drink augments the problem. Experiments with *Microcystis* have revealed a sharp dose-response curve; up to 90% of the lethal dose of bloom could be ingested by sheep without measurable effect. The sensitivity of different species may also vary; monogastric animals are less sensitive to a toxin produced by a strain of *Anabena* than are ruminants and ducks.

The pathogenesis varies according to the toxin produced by the predominant species and strain of algae involved. *Microcystis aeruginosa* produces cytolytic peptide hepatotoxins that cause breakdown of the sinusoidal endothelium, damage to hepatocyte membranes, and necrotic changes in hepatocyte cytoplasm. Death is considered to be related to shock following massive liver necrosis and hemorrhage. Generalized hemorrhages are thought to result from depletion of coagulation factors. Strains of *Anabena flos-aquae* may produce toxins that are physiologically distinct—a secondary amine that acts as a strong depolarizing agent at nicotinic and muscarinic receptors (that causes death from respiratory paralysis) and an irreversible anticholinesterase toxin. Both have been isolated from different strains of this species. *Aphanizomenon flos-aquae* produces neurotoxins similar to the marine "red-tide" shellfish poisons.

Clinical Findings and Lesions: Toxic signs may appear within 1 hr, and death may occur in <24 hr after ingestion of the poisonous material. The most commonly reported sequence of events is rapid prostration, convulsions, and death. Abdominal pain, anorexia, vomiting, muscular tremors, dyspnea, cyanosis, and salivation are common; less common are icterus, diarrhea, and bloody feces. Photosensitization frequently occurs in animals that survive for several days.

Animals dying peracutely may show congestion of the CNS and fluid accumulation in the lungs and thorax. *Microcystis* toxicity results in a markedly enlarged and often hemorrhagic liver, fluid accumulation in the body cavities, and widespread petechiae and ecchymoses. Microscopical examination reveals centrilobular to near massive hepatic necrosis. In chronic cases, hepatic cirrhosis and ascites may be present.

Diagnosis: Diagnosis is based on history (recent contact with an abundance of potentially toxic freshwater algae), clinical signs, and postmortem findings. Samples of the algae should be collected as soon as possible to confirm the toxicity of the strain in the laboratory. In *Microcystis* poisoning, marked rises in serum concentrations of liver enzymes and bilirubin, and changes in coagulation parameters have been reported.

Control: Removal of animals from the affected water supply is essential. Algal growth may be suppressed with copper sulfate or other algicidal treatment, but this does not remove the toxin already present in the water. If no other water supply is available, animals should be allowed to drink only from the shore kept free of dense algae by the prevailing wind.

Animals dying from algal poisoning must not be used for food since the toxic principle is stable. The liver is the target organ for accumulation and excretion of the toxin of *Microcystis*.

Treatment: Following removal from the contaminated water supply, affected animals should be placed in a protected area out of direct sunlight. Ample quantities of water and good-quality feed should be made available. Administration of activated charcoal slurry and a laxative dose of heavy mineral oil has proved useful in removing the toxin from the GI tract. Affected animals usually are weak, and heroic procedures should not be employed.

In surviving animals, a long recuperative period is to be expected. Antibiotics, glucose, and calcium and magnesium supplementation have been used.

ARSENIC POISONING

In arsenic poisoning, the effects produced by the phenylarsonic feed additives and other organic or inorganic arsenic compounds must be distinguished.

ARSENICALS OTHER THAN PHENYLARSONIC DERIVATIVES

These include arsenic trioxide, arsenic pentoxide, sodium and potassium arsenate, sodium and potassium arsenite, monosodium methanearsonate (MSMA), disodium methanearsonate (DSMA), and copper acetoarsenite.

Etiology: Due to diminishing use of these substances, poisoning is now relatively infrequent. Sources are preparations used as rodenticides, wood preservatives, weed killers, baits, and insecticides. Arsenites are used to some extent as dips for tick eradication. Lead arsenate is sometimes used as a taeniacide in sheep. MSMA and DSMA are still used as cotton defoliants.

Clinical Findings: Poisoning is usually acute, with the major action on the GI tract and cardiovascular system. Profuse watery diarrhea, sometimes tinged with blood, is characteristic, as are severe colic, dehydration, weakness, depression, and weak pulse. The underlying cause of these effects is increased capillary permeability and cellular necrosis. Animals inadvertently sprayed with soluble arsenites may exhibit massive skin necrosis. The onset is rapid, and the course runs from hours to several weeks. In peracute poisoning, animals may simply be found dead.

Lesions: Inflammation of the GI tract is followed by edema, rupture of blood vessels, and necrosis of epithelial and subepithelial tissue. The necrosis may progress to perforation of the gastric or intestinal wall. Contents of the gut are fluid and blood tinged, and may contain shreds of epithelial tissue. There is diffuse inflammation of the liver and other abdominal viscera.

Diagnosis: Chemical determination of arsenic in tissues and ingesta provides confirmation. Liver and kidney tissue of normal animals rarely contain >1 ppm arsenic (wet wt); toxicity is associated with concentrations of >3 ppm. The determination of arsenic in ingesta is of value if exposure occurred within the previous 24-48 hr. High concentrations of arsenic can be found in the urine for several days following ingestion.

Treatment: Thioctic acid alone (IM, 23 mg/lb [50 mg/kg] body wt, t.i.d. as a 20% solution [50 g of dl-6,8-thioctic acid dissolved in 100 mL warm 5N NaOH, cooled, adjusted to pH neutrality with 1N HCl and brought to volume with distilled water]) or in combination with dimercaprol (IM, 1.4 mg/lb [3 mg/kg] body wt, q4hr for the first 2 days, q.i.d. on the third day, and b.i.d. for the next 10 days or until recovery is complete) may be beneficial in cattle. In other large animals, dimercaprol can be administered, but its efficacy is questionable. Oral sodium thiosulfate (20-30 g in 300 mL of water in adult horses and cattle; one-fourth of this dose in sheep and goats) has also been used. Treatment in small animals consists of dimercaprol (IM, 2.7-3.2 mg/lb [6-7 mg/kg] body wt, t.i.d.). The water-soluble derivative, 2,3-dimercaptopropane-1-sulfonate (DMPS), is said to be superior to dimercaprol, but is unavailable for clinical use in the USA. Supportive therapy may be of even greater value, particularly when cardiovascular collapse is imminent, and should be directed toward restoration of blood volume and correction of the massive dehydration with extracellular electrolyte solutions.

PHENYLARSONIC COMPOUNDS

These arsenicals include several derivatives used in pigs and poultry to improve production and, in the case of pigs, to treat dysentery. The major compounds in this class are arsanilic acid, roxarsone, and carbarsone.

Etiology: This form of toxicosis results from an excess of arsenic-containing additives in pig and poultry diets. Severity and rapidity of onset are dose-related. Signs may be delayed for weeks following incorporation of 2-3 times the recommended levels, or may occur within days when the excess is ≥10-fold recommended levels.

Clinical Findings and Diagnosis: The earliest sign in pigs may be a reduction in weight gain. This is followed by incoordination and posterior paralysis. Animals remain alert and maintain good appetites. Blindness is characteristic of arsanilic acid intoxications, but not of that of other organic arsenicals. Phenylarsonic toxicosis in ruminants is similar to that of classical arsenic toxicosis. An analysis of the feed for either total arsenic content or the suspect compound is indicated if doubt exists.

Treatment and Prognosis: There is no specific treatment, but the neurotoxic effects are usually reversible if the offending feed is withdrawn within 2-3 days of onset of ataxia. The nerve damage is irreversible once paralysis occurs. Blindness due to arsanilic acid is often irreversible, but appetite is retained and weight gains are good if competition for food is eliminated. Doubt exists as to the reversibility of the other neurotoxic effects when the onset of intoxication is slow and the exposure prolonged.

BRACKEN FERN POISONING

Bracken fern (*Pteridium aquilinum [Pteris aquilina]*) is widely distributed in upland and marginal areas throughout the world, including North and South America, Europe, Australia, and Japan. Ingestion of significant quantities produces signs of acute poisoning related to thiamine deficiency in monogastric animals, and bone marrow depletion (aplastic anemia) in ruminants. The toxic effects appear to be cumulative and may require 1-3 mo to develop, depending on the species of the animal, quantity consumed, time of year, and other factors. Both leaves and rhizomes contain the toxic principles, which vary in concentration with the seasons. Most acute poisonings are seen after periods of drought when grazing is scarce, but the plant is toxic even when present as a contaminant in hay—cases have occurred in stabled animals.

Long-term, low-level consumption has been associated with other clinical syndromes. **Enzootic hematuria** with hemorrhages or tumors in the bladder is seen in cattle in many areas of the world, and similar tumors have been observed in sheep. **Bright blindness** with retinal degeneration and hyperreflectivity of the tapetum is found in hill sheep in parts of England, and a similar condition has been recognized in cattle grazing bracken in Wales. Ingestion of bracken fern has been implicated in the occurrence of upper GI tract tumors in cattle in areas of Brazil and Scotland.

Some epidemiological evidence suggests that regular consumption of untreated milk from cattle with access to bracken may be associated with an increased risk of human esophageal or gastric cancer, but this is still under investigation. The greater risk to man is probably from direct consumption of the fern itself, a practice that continues in various countries throughout the world.

Etiology: Bracken fern contains a number of toxic factors, some of which are not yet fully characterized. Poisoning in non-ruminants is due to a thiaminase; the effects are essentially those of vitamin B_1 deficiency. Horses seem to be particularly susceptible, while disease in pigs is rare. Thiamine deficiency is generally not a problem in ruminants since the vitamin is synthesized in the rumen, but polioencephalomalacia associated with impaired thiamine metabolism in sheep has been attributed to consumption of bracken fern and rock fern (*Cheilanthes sieberi*) in Australia.

The nature of the bone marrow toxin (aplastic anemia factor) to which cattle are particularly susceptible has not been defined, although the compound ptaquiloside has been suggested. The toxin causes death of precursor cells in the marrow so that elements with a shorter life span are affected first. There is granulocytopenia and thrombocytopenia with resultant susceptibility to infection and tendency to spontaneous hemorrhage.

Bladder tumors in naturally occurring enzootic hematuria suggest that bracken fern may act as a carcinogen, and this has been confirmed experimentally: inclusion of bracken fern in the diet of rats, mice, guinea pigs, quail, and Egyptian toads has resulted in tumors at various sites depending on the species and duration of feeding. Identical tumors can be produced by feeding ptaquiloside. Epidemiological studies suggest that upper GI tract tumors in cattle may be due to the combined action of bracken fern and a bovine papilloma virus.

Clinical Findings: Signs of bracken-induced thiamine deficiency in horses (bracken staggers) include anorexia, incoordination, and a crouching stance with arched neck and feet placed wide apart. In severe cases, tachycardia is present, and death is preceded by convulsions, clonic spasms, and opisthotonus. The rectal temperature is usually normal, but may reach 104°F (40°C).

In pigs, signs of thiamine deficiency are less distinct and may resemble heart failure. Affected animals show anorexia and weight loss. Death can occur suddenly following terminal recumbency and dyspnea.

Acute bracken poisoning in cattle causes an acute hemorrhagic syndrome or, in some cases, sudden death. Affected animals are weak, pyrexic (106-110°F [41-43°C]), and have pale mucosae with petechiae. Clots of blood may be passed in the feces, and there is often bleeding from body orifices. The blood frequently fails to clot normally; where tabanid flies are abundant, the skin of affected cattle is marked by streaks of blood where the insects have fed. The disease is almost always fatal, and necropsy reveals multiple hemorrhages throughout the carcass. Necrotic ulcers may be present in the GI tract.

Chronic enzootic hematuria in cattle is characterized by intermittent hematuria and ultimate death due to anemia. The bladder contains small hemorrhages, dilated vessels, or tumors, which can be vascular, fibrous, or epithelial. In many cases, a mixture of lesions is found.

Bright blindness in sheep is a progressive retinal atrophy that derives its name from the hyperreflectivity of the tapetum in affected animals. Affected sheep are permanently blind and adopt a characteristic alert attitude. The pupils respond poorly to light, and ophthalmoscopy of advanced cases reveals narrowing of arteries and veins, and a pale tapetum nigrum with fine cracks and spots of gray.

Diagnosis: Other plants, such as horsetail (*Equisetum arvense*) and turnip (*Beta vulgaris*), can induce thiamine deficiency. In horses, the condition must be distinguished from other neurological disorders, including rabies or poisoning due to *Crotalaria* sp or ragwort (*Senecio jacobea*). Blood thiamine levels decrease from an average normal of 8.5 to 2.5 μg/dL, while blood pyruvate levels increase from a normal of ~2 to 8.5 mg/dL. In pigs, the signs and lesions may indicate heart failure. Definitive diagnosis is established by demonstrating reduced blood thiamine levels or a rise in blood pyruvate with a fall in RBC transketolase activity.

The acute hemorrhagic syndrome in cattle is distinctive, but signs may be confused with those of any of the acute septicemias including anthrax, or of other forms of poisoning such as mycotoxicosis, or poisoning by sweet clover or trichloroethylene-extracted soybean meal. In Australia, the rock or mulga fern, *C sieberi*, is highly toxic to cattle (and toxic to sheep), and induces the same signs as bracken fern.

Chronic enzootic hematuria must be distinguished from other causes of "red water", eg, the hemoglobinemia of babesiosis. Occasional cases are complicated by coexisting chronic pyelonephritis.

The retinal changes of bright blindness in sheep are characteristic but subtle, so diagnosis requires the exclusion of other causes of blindness including pregnancy toxemia, infectious keratoconjunctivitis, and cataracts.

Treatment: Treatment of thiamine deficiency is highly effective if diagnosis is made early. Injection of a solution of the vitamin at 5 mg/kg body wt is suggested, given initially IV q3hr, then IM for several days. Oral supplementation may be required for an additional 1-2 wk, although subcut. injection of 100-200 mg daily for 6 days has been successful in some cases.

.In acutely affected cattle, mortality is usually >90%, and the platelet count is the best prognostic indicator. Animals should be removed from contaminated pasture, but it is often difficult to convince farmers that the plant is poisonous because the disease can appear ≥2 wk after livestock are removed from the fern-infested area. Treatment with d-l-batyl alcohol to stimulate the bone marrow is of doubtful value. Antibiotics may be useful to prevent secondary infections. Blood or even platelet transfusions from a donor not grazing bracken may be appropriate, but large volumes are required (minimum of 2-4 L blood).

The other syndromes are essentially untreatable and must be controlled by denying access to the fern.

Prophylaxis: Bracken is usually grazed for want of more suitable food, although individual animals may develop a taste for the plant, particularly the young tender shoots and leaves. The disease has been prevented in ruminants and horses by improved pasture management and fertilization, or by alternating bracken-contaminated and non-contaminated pasture at 3-wk intervals.

Fern growth can be retarded by close grazing or trampling the stand in an alternate grazing system. In time, a pasture can be freed of bracken using this approach or by regular cutting of the mature plant or, if the land is suitable, by deep plowing. Herbicide treatment using asulam or glyphosate can be an effective (but expensive) method of control, especially if combined with cutting before treatment. Biological control by the use of microorganisms or insects has been considered, but the long-term implications are not clear.

CANTHARIDIN (BLISTER BEETLE) POISONING

Observed most often in horses, although sheep and cattle are affected occasionally, reports originate primarily from the central and southwestern USA. The blister beetles (*Epicauta* spp), which swarm in alfalfa hay during harvesting, contain a potent irritant and vesicant, cantharidin, which can produce nephritis, cystitis, and hyperemia and ulceration of the oral, esophageal, and GI mucosa. Signs include colic, salivation, shock, pollakiuria, and occasionally, synchronous diaphragmatic flutter. Hematuria, hemoconcentration, hypocalcemia, or neutrophilic leukocytosis may be present, but are not diagnostic. Most horses that die from cantharidin do so within 48 hr of onset of signs. Detection of blister beetles in alfalfa hay and of cantharidin in the urine or stomach contents by chromatography is necessary to confirm the diagnosis. There is no specific treatment, although administration of analgesics, fluids (IV, including calcium solutions), and mineral oil (PO) is often useful.

CHOCOLATE POISONING

Chocolate is derived from the roasted seeds of *Theobroma cacao* and contains theobromine (3,7-dimethylxanthine) and small amounts of caffeine (1,3,7-trimethylxanthine). Although many species are susceptible, chocolate poisoning occurs most commonly in dogs, in which it may be associated with the pharmacokinetics of theobromine. Contributing factors may include voracious and sometimes indiscriminate eating habits, and the availability of various chocolate products, eg, candy and other food items. In addition, *Theobroma cacao* shells, which are sometimes used in landscaping, reportedly have been responsible for a canine death.

Etiology: The theobromine content of unsweetened (baker's) chocolate is 450 mg/oz (15 mg/g), while milk chocolate contains 44 mg/oz (1.5 mg/g). Cacao meal and cacao shells contain 1-3% and ~0.2-3% theobromine, respectively. Chocolate-flavored dog treats contain negligible amounts of theobromine and are safe; white chocolate is also low enough in both theobromine and caffeine to be unlikely to cause poisoning. The therapeutic dose of theobromine in dogs is 20 mg/kg; fatalities have been reported at doses >200 mg/kg. Several deaths in dogs were reported following consumption (b.i.d. for 1-2 days) of a commercial dog food derived from cocoa by-products, which contained 0.2% theobromine.

Although wide variations occur, ingestion of ~0.04 oz (~1.3 mg) baker's chocolate or 0.4 oz (~13 mg) milk chocolate/kg body wt may cause signs if eaten by a dog, and doses 10 times higher may be fatal unless treated.

Pathogenesis: Relative to other methylxanthines, theobromine is pharmacologically weak and without CNS activity. However, large amounts have a diuretic effect, relax smooth muscles, and stimulate the heart and CNS. The diuretic effect appears to be due to inhibition of reabsorption of solutes in the proximal tubule and the diluting segment of the nephron. Smooth-muscle effects are most evident as relaxation of the bladder.

Theobromine produces dilation of the peripheral vessels and coronary arteries, but constricts the cerebral vasculature. Small amounts of methylxanthines decrease the heart rate via a vagal mechanism; however, high doses stimulate the heart directly and produce tachycardia. The overall effect is a mild increase in blood pressure. Premature ventricular contractions may occur.

The CNS effects of high doses of theobromine include nervousness, restlessness, insomnia, tremor, and clonic seizures. It may also stimulate the medullary respiratory center of the brain by producing an increased sensitivity to carbon dioxide. In addition, nausea and vomiting appear to be centrally mediated.

Clinical Findings: Signs of chocolate poisoning may not be observed for some time after ingestion and may be due to delayed absorption. In acute cases, signs most commonly develop after 8 hr, and death typically occurs 12-24 hr after ingestion. Occasionally in dogs, few clinical signs are exhibited until the animal dies abruptly of cardiac failure. For this reason, an animal known to have ingested a potentially toxic amount of chocolate should be observed closely for any evidence of cardiac dysrhythmias. More commonly, signs progress from thirst, vomiting, diarrhea, urinary incontinence, and agitation to nervousness, clonic muscle spasms, seizures, and coma.

Lesions: Gross evidence of chocolate is usually present in the GI tract at necropsy. Lesions may include hyperemia of the gastric and proximal duodenal mucosa, diffuse organ congestion, and petechial and ecchymotic hemorrhages in the thymus.

Microscopic changes may include pyknotic nuclei in the distal renal tubular epithelium, and cytoplasmic hyaline droplets with pyknosis and karyorrhexis in the epithelium of the renal convoluted tubules. In chronic feeding studies, dogs fatally poisoned with theobromine developed fibrotic changes in the right atrium of the heart.

Treatment: Emetics are indicated, and may be of benefit for at least 6-8 hr after ingestion due to the delayed absorption of chocolate. Activated charcoal (1 g/kg) effectively limits absorption of theobromine from the gut, and its benefits are enhanced with saline cathartics. Based on human data with the related methylxanthine theophylline, repeated doses of activated charcoal q4hr may significantly shorten the serum half-life of theobromine. Because of the risk of fluid and electrolyte imbalance, cathartics should be employed only with alternate doses of charcoal. Fluid and electrolyte status should be monitored carefully.

COAL-TAR POISONING

A variety of coal-tar derivatives induce acute to chronic disease in animals. Clinical effects are acute to chronic hepatic damage with attendant signs of icterus, ascites, anemia, and death. Coal-tar pitch poisoning has been reported from Canada, Germany, Ireland, Poland, and the USA. Toxicosis has been reported for common domestic food animals and pets.

Etiology: The distillation of coal tar yields a variety of compounds, 3 of which are notably toxic: cresols (phenolic compounds), crude creosote (composed of cresols, heavy oils, and anthracene), and pitch. Tars are also produced from crude petroleum or wood. Creosote contains less volatile liquid and solid aromatic hydrocarbons of coal tar and some phenols. Cresols, composed mainly of hydroxytoluenes, are used as disinfectants. Coal-tar and pine-tar pitch are the brown-to-black, amorphous, polynuclear hydrocarbon residues left after coal tar is redistilled. Access of animals to coal tars is often by direct chewing on or consumption of product, rather than inclusion in feed or water. Clay pigeons, tar paper, creosote-treated wood and bitumen-based flooring are typical sources.

Cresols, which are used as disinfectants, are readily absorbed through the skin. The lethal dose is 100-200 mg/kg body wt except in cats, which are especially sensitive. Because coal-tar-derived creosote is toxic to wood-destroying fungi and insects, it is used as a wood preserver. Sows confined to wooden farrowing crates treated with 3 brush applications of creosote were reported to have stillborn pigs, and the surviving pigs grew slowly. Other species are less susceptible, eg, the lethal dose of creosote in calves is 4 g/kg body wt. Pitch is used as a binder in clay pigeons, road asphalt, insulation, tar paper and roofing compounds, and to cover iron pipes and line wooden water tanks. Pigs that consume 15 g of "clay pigeons" over a 5-day period will die. Floor slabs with one-third lignite pitch reduced growth rate in pigs ~25%.

Clinical Findings: The cresols are locally corrosive; they stimulate the CNS and depress the heart, which results in vascular collapse. Death may occur from 15 min to several days after exposure. The first sign of pitch poisoning often is several dead pigs. Other pigs are depressed, which may progress to weakness, ataxia, sternal recumbency, icterus, coma, and death. Secondary anemia may develop. Coal-tar products may alter absorption of vitamin A; associated problems have included still-births in pigs, and hyperkeratosis in calves. Blood glucose is reduced terminally, while thymol turbidity, and serum chloride and phosphorus are elevated.

    Lesions: Except for contact irritation, cresols and creosote do not produce distinctive morphological lesions. Pitch poisoning causes a markedly swollen liver with a diffuse, mottled appearance. The lobules are clearly outlined by a light-colored zone, and their centers contain deep-red dots the size of a pinhead. There is centrilobular liver necrosis, with blood replacing the lost cells and filling the center of the lobule. The blood clots slowly or not at all. The carcass is icteric. Excessive fluid is found in the peritoneal cavity.

Diagnosis: Differential diagnoses include toxic plant poisonings (*Crotalaria, Senecio,* cocklebur), aflatoxicosis, gossypol toxicosis, yellow phosphorus poisoning, and vitamin E/selenium deficiency. Fragments of clay pigeons, tar paper, or other sources of coal tars found in the GI tract, or chemical detection of coal-tar products in tissues aid in confirming the diagnosis.

Treatment: There is no known treatment for animals with frank signs. Oral antibiotics and high-quality-protein diets may aid recovery.

COPPER POISONING

    Acute or chronic copper poisoning is encountered in most parts of the world. Sheep are affected most often, although other animals are also susceptible. In various breeds of dogs, especially the Bedlington Terrier, an inherited sensitivity to copper toxicosis (qv, p 26) similar to Wilson's Disease in man has been identified. Acute poisoning is usually observed after accidental administration of excessive amounts of soluble copper salts, which may be present in anthelmintic drenches, mineral mixes, or improperly formulated rations. Many factors that alter copper metabolism influence chronic copper poisoning by enhancing its absorption or retention. Low levels of molybdenum or sulfate in the diet are important examples. Primary chronic poisoning is seen most commonly in sheep when excessive amounts of copper are ingested over a prolonged period. The toxicosis remains subclinical until the copper that is stored in the liver is released in massive amounts. Blood copper concentrations increase suddenly, which causes severe intravascular hemolysis. The hemolytic crisis may be precipitated by many factors, including transportation, lactation, strenuous exercise, or a deteriorating plane of nutrition.

    Phytogenous and hepatogenous factors influence secondary chronic copper poisoning. Phytogenous chronic poisoning is observed following ingestion of plants such as subterranean clover (*Trifolium subterraneum*) that produce a mineral imbalance and result in excessive copper retention. The plants that are not hepatotoxic contain normal amounts of copper and low levels of molybdenum. The ingestion of plants such as *Heliotropium europaeum* or *Senecio* spp (qv, p 1698) for several months may cause hepatogenous chronic copper poisoning. These plants contain hepatotoxic alkaloids, which result in excessive copper retention in the liver.

Acute poisoning may follow intakes of 20-100 mg of copper/kg body wt in sheep and young calves, and 200-800 mg/kg in mature cattle. Chronic poisoning of sheep may occur with daily intakes of 3.5 mg of copper/kg body wt when grazing pastures that contain 15-20 ppm (dry matter) of copper, and when eating pelleted feeds that contain 50 ppm of copper. Clinical disease may occur in sheep that ingest cattle rations, which normally contain higher levels of copper, or when their water is supplied via copper plumbing; cattle are more resistant to copper poisoning than sheep, and thus are not affected in these instances. Copper is used as a feed additive for pigs at 125-250 ppm; levels >250 ppm are dangerous—although as for sheep, other factors may be protective, eg, high levels of protein, zinc, or iron. Chronic copper toxicosis is more apt to occur with low dietary intake of molybdenum and sulfur.

Clinical Findings: Acute copper poisoning produces severe gastroenteritis characterized by abdominal pain, diarrhea, anorexia, dehydration, and shock. Hemolysis and hemoglobinuria develop after 3 days if the animal survives the GI disturbances. The sudden onset of clinical signs in chronic copper poisoning is associated with the hemolytic crisis. Affected animals exhibit depression, weakness, anorexia, thirst, hemoglobinuria, and jaundice, but no additional GI disturbances. Several days or weeks before the hemolytic crisis, liver enzymes, including ALT (SGPT) and AST (SGOT), are usually elevated. During the hemolytic crisis, methemoglobinemia, hemoglobinuria, and reductions in PCV and blood glutathione are usually observed. Morbid animals often die within 1-2 days. Herd morbidity is often <5%, though usually >75% of affected animals die. Losses may continue for up to 2 mo after the dietary problem has been rectified. Severe hepatic insufficiency is responsible for early deaths. Animals that survive the acute episode may die of subsequent renal failure.

Lesions: Acute copper poisoning produces severe gastroenteritis with erosions and ulcerations in the abomasum of ruminants. Icterus develops in animals that survive >24 hr. Tissues discolored by icterus and methemoglobin are characteristic of chronic poisoning. Swollen, gunmetal-colored kidneys, port-wine-colored urine, and an enlarged spleen with dark brown-black parenchyma are manifestations of the hemolytic crisis. The liver is enlarged and friable. Histologically, there is centrilobular hepatic and renal tubular necrosis.

Diagnosis: Evidence of blue-green ingesta, and elevated fecal (8000-10,000 ppm) and kidney (>15 ppm, wet wt) copper levels are considered significant in acute copper poisoning. In chronic poisoning, blood and liver copper concentrations are elevated during the hemolytic period. Blood levels often rise to 5-20 μg/mL, as compared to normal levels of ~1 μg/mL. Liver concentrations >150 ppm (wet wt) are significant in sheep. The concentration of copper in the tissue must be determined to eliminate other causes of hemolytic disease.

Treatment and Control: Often, treatment is not successful. GI sedatives and symptomatic treatment for shock may be useful in acute toxicity. Penicillamine or calcium versenate may be useful if administered in the early stages of disease. Experimentally, ammonium tetrathiomolybdate (IV) has proved effective for the treatment and prevention of copper poisoning. Daily administration of ammonium molybdate (100 mg) and sodium sulfate (1 g) reduces losses in affected lambs. Plant eradication or reducing access to plants that cause phytogenous or hepatogenous copper poisoning is desirable. Primary chronic or phytogenous poisoning may be prevented by top-dressing pastures with 1 oz of molybdenum per acre (70 g/hectare) in the form of molybdenized superphosphate, or by molybdenum supplementation, or restriction of copper intake.

CYANIDE POISONING

Cyanide inhibits cytochrome oxidase and causes death from histotoxic anoxia. *See also* SORGHUM POISONING, p 1730.

Etiology: Cyanides are found in plants, fumigants, soil sterilizers, fertilizers, and rodenticides (eg, calcium cyanomide). Toxicity can result from improper or malicious use, but in the case of livestock, the most frequent cause is ingestion of plants that contain cyanogenic glycosides: these include *Triglochin maritima* (arrow grass), *Hoecus lunatus* (velvet grass), *Sorghum* spp (Johnson grass, Sudan grass, common sorghum), *Prunus* spp (apricot, peach, chokecherry, pincherry, wild black cherry), *Sambucus canadensis* (elderberry), *Pyrus malus* (apple), *Zea mays* (corn), and *Linum* spp (flax). The seeds (pits) of several plants such as the peach have been the source of cyanogenic glycosides in many cases. *Eucalyptus* spp, kept as ornamental house plants, have been implicated in deaths of small animals. Cyanogenic glycosides in plants yield free hydrocyanic acid (HCN) when hydrolyzed by β-glycosidase and when other plant cell structure is disrupted or damaged, eg, by freezing, chopping, or chewing. Microbial action in the rumen can further release free cyanide.

Apple and other fruit trees contain prussic acid glycosides in leaves and seeds, but little or none in the fleshy part of the fruits. In *Sorghum* spp forage grasses, leaves usually produce 2-25 times more HCN than do stems; seeds contain none. New shoots from young, rapidly growing plants often contain high concentrations of prussic acid glycosides. Cyanogenic glycoside potential in plants can be increased by heavy nitrate fertilization, especially in phosphorus-deficient soils. Spraying of cyanogenic forage plants with foliar herbicides such as 2,4-D can increase their prussic acid concentrations for several weeks after application.

Drought-stricken plants containing mostly leaves are slow to decrease their cyanogenic glycoside potential. Grazing stunted plants during drought is the most common cause of poisoning of livestock by prussic-acid-producing plants.

Frozen plants may release high concentrations of prussic acid for several days. After wilting, prussic acid release from plant tissues declines. Dead plants have less free prussic acid. When plant tops have been frosted, new shoots may regrow at the base; these can be dangerous because of glycoside content, and because livestock selectively graze them.

Ruminants are more susceptible than monogastric animals, and cattle slightly more so than sheep. Hereford cattle have been reported to be less susceptible than other breeds.

Clinical Findings: Signs can occur within 15-20 min to a few hours after animals consume toxic forage. Excitement can be displayed initially, accompanied by rapid respiration rate. Dyspnea follows shortly, with tachycardia. Salivation, excess lacrimation, and voiding of urine and feces may occur. Vomiting may occur, especially in pigs. Muscle fasciculation is common and progresses to generalized spasms before death. Animals stagger and struggle before collapse. Mucous membranes are bright red, but may become cyanotic terminally. Death occurs during severe asphyxial convulsions. The heart may continue to beat for several minutes after struggling and breathing stop. The whole syndrome usually does not exceed 30-45 min. Most animals that live 2 hr after onset of clinical signs recover.

Lesions: In acute or peracute cyanide toxicoses, blood may be bright cherry red initially, but can be dark red if necropsy is delayed; it may clot slowly or not at all. Mucous membranes may also be pink initially, then become cyanotic after respiration ceases. The rumen may be distended with gas, and the odor of "bitter almonds" may be detected after opening. Agonal hemorrhages of the heart may be seen. Liver, serosal surfaces, tracheal mucosa, and lungs may be congested or hemorrhagic; some froth may be seen in respiratory passages. Neither gross nor histologic lesions are consistently seen.

Multiple foci of degeneration or necrosis may be seen in the CNS of dogs chronically exposed to sublethal amounts of cyanide. These lesions have not been reported in livestock.

Diagnosis: Appropriate history, clinical signs, postmortem findings, and demonstration of HCN in rumen (stomach) contents or other diagnostic specimens support a diagnosis of cyanide poisoning. Specimens recommended for cyanide analyses include the suspected source (plant or otherwise), rumen or stomach contents, heparinized whole blood, liver, and muscle. Antemortem whole blood is preferred; other specimens should be collected as soon as possible after death, preferably within 4 hr. Specimens should be sealed in an airtight container, refrigerated or frozen, and submitted to the laboratory without delay. When cold storage is unavailable, immersion of specimens in 1-3% mercuric chloride has been satisfactory.

Differential diagnoses include poisonings by nitrate/nitrite, urea, organophosphate, carbamate, chlorinated hydrocarbon pesticides, and toxic gases (carbon monoxide and hydrogen sulfide); as well as infectious diseases or noninfectious diseases that cause sudden death.

Treatment: Immediate treatment is necessary. Sodium nitrite (10 g/100 mL of distilled water or isotonic saline) should be given IV at 20 mg/kg body wt, followed by sodium thiosulfate (20%) IV at ≥500 mg/kg; the latter may be repeated as needed with little hazard. Sodium nitrite therapy may be carefully repeated at 10 mg/kg body wt, q2-4hr or as needed.

Sodium thiosulfate alone is also an effective antidotal therapy at ≥500 mg/kg body wt, IV, plus 30 g/cow, PO, to detoxify any remaining HCN in the rumen. Oxygen may be helpful in supplementing nitrite or thiosulfate therapy, especially in small animals.

Caution: Many clinical signs of nitrate and prussic acid poisoning are similar, and injecting sodium nitrite induces methemoglobinemia identical to that produced by nitrate poisoning. If in doubt of the diagnosis, methylene blue, IV at 4-22 mg/kg, may be used to induce methemoglobin. Since methylene blue can serve as both a donor and acceptor of electrons, it can reduce methemoglobin in the presence of excess methemoglobin or induce methemoglobin when only hemoglobin is present (but sodium nitrate is the more effective treatment for cyanide poisoning if the diagnosis is certain).

ETHYLENE GLYCOL POISONING

All animals are susceptible, but it is most common in dogs and cats. The primary source is automotive antifreeze (~95% ethylene glycol). Other sources include heat-exchange fluids sometimes used in solar collectors and ice-rink freezing equipment, and some brake and transmission fluids, as well as diethylene glycol used in color film processing. Animals consume it voluntarily even when water is available. Toxicoses occur especially in fall, winter, and early spring, reflecting peak usage. High mortality (88%) has been reported in dogs and cats. Often, a history of exposure is not available, and poisoned animals are diagnosed postmortem or after renal damage has occurred.

Metabolism and Pathogenesis: Peak blood concentrations occur in dogs 1-3 hr after ingestion. Initial signs may appear ~1 hr after ingestion. Of the ingested dose, >50% is excreted unchanged in the urine, especially in the first 12 hr, and for up to 48 hr. Degradation occurs in the liver and kidneys. The first of 2 important rate-limiting steps is the oxidation of ethylene glycol by alcohol dehydrogenase to glycoaldehyde. Glycoaldehyde is readily metabolized to glycolic acid, which causes severe metabolic acidosis in dogs and cats. Urinary glycolate concentrations correlate with the clinical signs, including mortality.

The conversion of glycolic acid to glyoxylic acid is the second rate-limiting reaction. Slow degradation allows time for the glycolate to cause acidosis and nephrosis. Although glyoxylic acid is highly toxic, its short half-life prevents significant effects. Formic acid, carbon dioxide, glycine, serine, and oxalate are metabolites of glyoxylic acid. Oxalate is not further metabolized, but readily

Table 1. Ethylene Glycol Toxicity

Species	Minimum Lethal Dose, Undiluted	Minimum Lethal Dose, Diluted (50:50, Antifreeze:Water)
Cats	1.5 mL/kg body wt	For a 5-kg cat, 0.5 oz (15 mL)
Dogs	6.6 mL/kg body wt	For a 10-kg dog, 4.5 oz (132 mL)
Poultry	7-8 mL/kg body wt	
Cattle	2-10 mL/kg body wt (Younger animals appear to be more susceptible)	

combines with calcium to form a soluble complex, which is excreted by glomerular filtration. Calcium oxalate crystals frequently form in the renal tubules as the concentration of the filtrate increases and its pH decreases. The crystals are birefringent when viewed under polarized light and are usually 6-sided, elongated, and prism-shaped in urine. They are most prevalent in urine and kidney tissue, but may be observed in blood vessels of the brain and other tissues. The renal tubular damage associated with ethylene glycol ingestion is thought to be due primarily to glycolate and oxalate and not the presence of calcium oxalate crystals.

Clinical Findings: The signs in dogs and cats can be divided into acute (<12 hr of ingestion) and subacute (24-96 hr after ingestion). The acute signs are similar to those of alcohol intoxication. Most dogs and cats exhibit polydipsia, polyuria, knuckling, ataxia, vomiting, dehydration, depression, and possibly tachycardia and tachypnea. Coma and death may occur when large doses are ingested, but this is rare. Animals may appear to recover transiently from the acute stage before the onset of renal failure. Subacute clinical signs occur secondary to oliguric renal failure and uremia, and commonly include depression, anorexia, gastroenteritis, encephalopathy, coma, and death.

Pigs become depressed, weak, and reluctant to move. Knuckling and posterior ataxia may be followed by trembling, collapse, abdominal distention, pulmonary edema, and muffled heart sounds. Poultry may experience drowsiness, ataxia, dyspnea, and torticollis, followed by ruffled feathers, watery droppings, recumbency, and death. Cattle may exhibit tachypnea, ataxia, paraparesis, depression, and later, recumbency and death. Hemoglobinuria and epistaxis may be observed in cattle that ingest large doses.

Diagnosis: This is difficult because of the nonspecific multisystemic signs, which may mimic head trauma, encephalitis, drug overdose, acute gastroenteritis, pancreatitis, ketoacidotic diabetes mellitus, and acute renal failure from other causes. When ingestion is not witnessed, diagnosis is based on other history, clinical signs, and laboratory data.

Hypothermia is occasionally present in severely depressed animals housed outdoors. Abdominal palpation may cause pain due to renal edema. Oral ulcers and salivation secondary to uremia are often noted in dogs and cats with oliguric renal failure. These animals are usually in good flesh and not anemic, which helps to rule out chronic renal failure.

Within 3 hr of ingestion of toxic doses, the following laboratory findings usually provide the key to the correct diagnosis: normochloremic metabolic acidosis, an increased anion gap, minimally concentrated or isosthenuric urine with a low pH, and serum hyperosmolality. Serum osmolality can be increased as much as 100 mOsm/kg above normal (280-310 mOsm/kg) within 3 hr of ingestion and is a valuable diagnostic aid. Measurement of serum osmolality is inexpensive and readily available at referral laboratories or human hospitals. Calcium oxalate crystalluria may be absent or observed as early as 5 hr after ingestion in dogs and 3 hr in cats. Decreased renal excretory capacity and renal azotemia usually are not observed in cats and dogs until ~12 and 48 hr after ingestion, respectively. Hyperphosphatemia has been observed in dogs early after ingestion of commercial antifreeze solutions, before the onset of acute oliguric renal failure, probably because phosphate-containing rust inhibitors are incorporated into many antifreeze solutions.

Ethylene glycol in serum or urine can be analyzed in a specific test, but it usually is not detectable until after 24 and 48 hr, respectively.

Lesions: Dogs and cats usually exhibit renal edema and pulmonary congestion and hyperemia; those that die after the onset of renal failure often have hemorrhagic gastroenteritis. Pigs often develop perirenal edema as well as straw-colored fluid in the peritoneal and pleural cavities and sometimes in the abdominal wall; their kidneys may be pale, with scattered, superficial petechiae and ecchymoses; and pulmonary edema is common. Cattle also develop perirenal edema with swollen kidneys that are tan or black. Chickens usually do not develop gross lesions.

Calcium oxalate crystals usually can be seen in the kidneys. Renal tubules are usually dilated and filled with proteinaceous debris. Generally, there is little inflammatory reaction to the crystals, and tubular healing may occur in their presence. In surviving animals, renal lesions generally resolve, but occasionally, chronic fibrosing renal damage occurs.

Prognosis and Treatment: The prognosis worsens with the amount of time between ingestion and therapy. When coordination and postural and gag reflexes are intact, and an animal is seen within 2 hr of exposure, an emetic should be given. Activated charcoal and a saline cathartic should be given by stomach tube up to 3 hr after ingestion. Fluid therapy is essential to correct dehydration and promote urinary excretion of ethylene glycol and its metabolites. Urine output should be monitored to prevent fluid overload. When oliguria or anuria is not correctable, or when life-threatening toxicosis exists, peritoneal dialysis with a high bicarbonate/low acetate dialysate may be used.

When animals are treated within 12 hr of exposure, ethanol or 4-methylpyrazole (4MP) will inhibit ethylene glycol metabolism, which facilitates its excretion in the urine and reduces development of acidosis and cytotoxicity. Sodium bicarbonate will correct the metabolic acidosis and ion-trap metabolites, thereby enhancing urinary excretion. Classical therapy for dogs includes 5.5 mL of 20% ethanol in saline per kg body wt, IV; and 8 mL of 5% bicarbonate per kg, IP, each given q4hr for 5 treatments, then q.i.d. for 5 treatments. In cats, 20% ethanol is given IV at 5 mL/kg body wt, and bicarbonate at 6 mL/kg, IV, q.i.d. for 5 treatments, then t.i.d. for 4 treatments. Bicarbonate should be used judiciously in an effort to maintain the urine pH at ~7.5.

Lower-dose infusions of ethanol seem as effective as high-dose treatments. A solution of 30% ethanol and 1% sodium bicarbonate in 0.9% saline is given by rapid infusion at 1.3 mL/kg; the infusion rate is then reduced to 0.42 mL/kg/hr. The goal is to maintain blood ethanol at 50 mg/dL for 48 hr. Dogs are allowed to eat and drink during courses of therapy.

An alternative alcohol dehydrogenase inhibitor, 4MP, has been used with excellent results in dogs. Unlike ethanol, 4MP does not contribute to CNS depression or renal concentrating disorders. For dogs, a 5% solution of 4MP in propylene glycol should be given IV as follows: 20 mg/kg initially, followed by 15 mg/kg at 12 hr, 10 mg/kg at 24 hr, and 5 mg/kg at 30 hr after the first dose. The solution is filtered with a 0.22 μm filter before use. In cats, 4MP is not recommended because ethanol is more effective in preventing ethylene glycol biotransformation.

After hydration is reestablished, osmotic diuretics such as 20-25% mannitol may be used to promote excretion of ethylene glycol and reduce intrarenal edema. Overhydration should be avoided, especially in oliguric animals. Placement of a urinary catheter is of value in monitoring urine output, and measurement of central venous pressure may help avoid pulmonary edema.

Treatment with ethanol or 4MP is not indicated in animals that are in oliguric renal failure; in these, fluid, electrolyte, and acid-base abnormalities should be corrected, and diuresis initiated and maintained.

Vigorous supportive care is necessary to maintain the animal during the period of renal regeneration and compensation, which may take 3-4 wk. Peritoneal dialysis may be useful; however, in many cases the renal tubular damage is severe and irreversible.

FLUORIDE POISONING
(Fluorosis)

Fluorides are widely distributed in the environment. One to 2 ppm of fluorine in the ration is considered adequate. The maximal tolerable level varies with the species, from 40-50 ppm for cattle and horses, to 200 ppm for chickens.

Etiology: Toxic quantities of fluorides occur naturally in some feed products, eg, certain raw rock phosphates, the superphosphates produced from them, partially defluorinated phosphates, and the phosphatic limestones. High-fluorine phosphate rocks are one of the major sources of this element. Feed-grade phosphates must contain no more than 1 part of fluorine to 100 parts phosphorus. In certain areas, the drinking water, usually from deep wells, contains high levels of fluorides. Fluorine-containing gases and dusts from some chemical factories may contaminate forage crops. Factories that produce acid phosphate from rock phosphates, electrolytically produce aluminum, manufacture bricks from fluorine-bearing clays, calcine ironstone, or perform certain enameling processes are potentially dangerous. Contamination of the surrounding area, particularly in the direction of the prevailing wind, may extend 5-6 miles. Furthermore, forage crops grown on high-fluorine soils have elevated values due to mechanical contamination with soil particles.

In general, there is a correlation between solubility of a fluoride and its toxicity, eg, sodium fluoride is the most toxic, and calcium fluoride the least toxic of the common fluorides. The fluorides of rock phosphates and most cryolites are intermediate between these 2; industrial residues approach sodium fluoride in toxicity. When the fluorides are in soluble form or originate from industrial fumes or dusts, the tolerance levels are less than for fluoride in rock phosphate. Acute fluoride toxicosis is relatively rare and usually has resulted from accidental ingestion of compounds such as sodium fluosiliate, used as a rodenticide, or sodium fluoride, which has been used as an ascaricide in pigs.

Clinical Findings: Ingestion of excessive fluoride induces characteristic lesions of the skeleton and teeth, which results in intermittent lameness, excessive tooth wear, reduced feed and water intake, and decreased weight gain. Developing teeth and bone are particularly sensitive, and excessive exposure in early postnatal life is especially damaging.

Acute poisoning can result from inhalation of fluorine-containing gases or ingestion of large amounts of fluoride, and is manifest as gastroenteritis accompanied by nervous signs, usually followed within a few hours by collapse and death. However, fluoride poisoning is usually chronic. The criteria for recognizing a developing fluoride toxicosis have been placed in the following order of reliability: 1) chemical analyses to determine the amount of fluorine in the diet, urine, bones, and teeth; 2) tooth effects, such as chalkiness or mottling, erosion of enamel, enamel hypoplasia, and excessive wear; 3) lameness as the result of fluoride accumulation in bone (severely diseased cattle may move around on their knees due to spurring and bridging of the joints in the late stages); and 4) systemic evidence as reflected by anorexia, inanition, cachexia, exostoses, and bone changes. The normal levels of fluorine in plasma, urine, bones, and teeth for livestock are considered to be, respectively, <0.2, 1-8, 200-600, and 200-500 ppm. With exposure, urinary excretion rises promptly to its maximum, and retained fluoride is deposited in the skeleton until it becomes saturated. This point is ~30-40 times that of normal bone content, beyond which "flooding" of the soft tissues occurs, which causes a rise in plasma fluorides and metabolic breakdown.

Lesions: Mottling, staining, and excessive wearing occurs in teeth that develop during the time of excessive ingestion. Teeth that are fully formed before exposure are largely unaffected. A more advanced stage of fluorosis is marked by skeletal abnormalities: the bones become chalky white, soft, thickened, and in the extreme, develop exostoses that may be palpated, especially along the long bones and on the mandible. These osseous lesions can develop in animals exposed at any age. Degenerative changes in the kidneys, liver, and several endocrine organs, and anemia have been reported but are not pathognomonic.

Diagnosis: Casual observation of affected animals may suggest osteoporosis or deficiency of calcium, phosphorus, or vitamin D. The lameness, in advanced cases, may be wrongly attributed to an accident. The nonspecific staining often seen in cattle teeth may be confused with incipient fluorosis. Accurate diagnosis depends on demonstrating elevated fluorine in plasma, urine, and bone, and ultimately discovering the source of the element.

With elevated intake, the urinary fluoride levels increase quickly to 15-30 ppm and may reach upper limits of 70-80 ppm. Normal cattle have been shown to excrete <5 ppm, those with borderline toxicity excrete 20-30 ppm, and those showing systemic signs of toxicity excrete >35 ppm. In pigs, the bones appear normal with upwards of 3000-4000 ppm fluorine, and levels <4500 ppm in compact bones from cattle are considered innocuous. In dairy cattle, toxicosis is associated with levels >5500 ppm in compact bone and >7000 ppm in cancellous bone, with a "saturation" point of ~15,000-20,000 ppm. Levels of 4500-5500 ppm fluorine indicate a marginal zone. The toxic thresholds for fluorine in bones of sheep are believed to be lower, viz, 2000-3000 ppm in bulk cortical bone and 4000-6000 ppm in bulk cancellous bone. Another report indicated that chemical bone fluorosis, bone mottling, and abnormal bone could be characterized respectively as <2500 ppm, 2500-5000 ppm, and 5000-6000 ppm.

Treatment and Control: Control, other than by removal of animals from affected areas, is difficult. It has been suggested that affected areas may be utilized for production of animals having a relatively short economic life, eg, pigs, poultry, or finishing cattle and sheep. Feeding calcium carbonate, aluminum oxide, aluminum sulfate, magnesium metasilicate, or boron has either reduced absorption or increased excretion of fluoride, and thus could offer some control of chronic fluorosis under some conditions. However, no drug or chemical has yet been shown to cure the chronic effects of fluorine toxicity.

GOSSYPOL POISONING

Usually a subacute to chronic, cumulative, and sometimes insidious condition that follows consumption of cottonseed or cottonseed products that contain excess free gossypol. It is of most concern in domestic livestock, especially immature ruminants and pigs.

Etiology: Gossypol, the predominant pigment and probably the major toxic ingredient in the cotton plant (*Gossypium* spp), and other polyphenolic pigments are contained within small discrete structures called pigment glands, found in various parts of the cotton plant. Gossypol content of cottonseeds varies from a trace to >6%, and is affected by plant species/variety and environmental factors such as climate, soil type, and fertilization; it is a natural component of all but the rarely produced "glandless" variety of cotton.

Cottonseed is processed into edible oil, meal, linters (short fibers), and hulls. Cottonseed meal (CSM) is marketed with 50-90% protein, depending on intended use. Cottonseed oil soapstock (foots) is the principal by-product of cottonseed oil refining. Cottonseed and CSM are widely used as protein supplements in animal feed. Cottonseed soapstocks are being increasingly used as animal feed additives; cottonseed hulls are used as a source of additional fiber in animal feeds, and usually contain much lower gossypol concentrations than do whole cottonseeds.

All animals are susceptible, but monogastrics, immature ruminants, and poultry appear to be most frequently affected. Pigs, guinea pigs, and rabbits are reported to be sensitive, and dogs and cats to have intermediate sensitivity. Holstein calves seem to be the most sensitive of cattle breeds. Horses are relatively unaffected.

Clinical Findings: Signs may relate to cardiac or reproductive effects, or to effects on other systems. Prolonged exposure can cause acute heart failure. Pulmonary effects and chronic dyspnea are most likely secondary to cardiotoxicity.

Hepatotoxicity can be a primary effect, or secondary to congestive heart failure. Hematologic effects include increased RBC fragility, decreased oxygen release from oxyhemoglobin, and reduced oxygen-carrying capacity of blood.

Reproductive effects include reduced libido with decreased spermatogenesis (which may be reversible) in males, and irregular cycling, luteolytic disruption of pregnancy, and direct embryotoxic action in females. Green discoloration of egg yolks and decreased egg hatchability have been reported in poultry.

Signs of prolonged excess gossypol exposure in many animals are weight loss, weakness, anorexia, and increased susceptibility to stress. Young lambs, goats, and calves may suffer a cardiomyopathy and sudden death, or a more chronic course with depression, anorexia, and pronounced dyspnea. Adult dairy cattle may also have gastroenteritis, hemoglobinuria, and reproductive problems. Acutely exposed monogastric animals may have sudden circulatory failure, while subacute exposure may result in pulmonary edema secondary to congestive heart failure; anemia may be another common sequela. Violent dyspnea ("thumping") is the outstanding clinical sign in pigs.

Lesions: Some animals have no obvious gross postmortem lesions, but copious amounts of red-tinged fluid with fibrin clumps are frequently found in abdominal, thoracic, and pericardial cavities. Icterus and an enlarged, flabby, pale, streaked, and mottled heart with dilated ventricles and valvular edema may be evident. Skeletal muscles may also be pale. A froth-filled trachea and edematous, congested lungs are common, as is an enlarged, mottled or golden, friable liver with distinct lobular patterns. The kidneys, spleen, and other splanchnic organs may be congested, and possibly with petechiae. Hemoglobinuria, and edema and hyperemia of the visceral mucosa may occur.

Diagnosis: This is based on: 1) a history of dietary exposure to CSM or cottonseed products over a relatively long period; 2) signs, especially sudden death or chronic dyspnea, affecting multiple animals within a group; 3) lesions consistent with the reported syndrome and associated cardiomyopathy and hepatopathy, with increased amounts of fluids in various body cavities; 4) no response to antibiotic therapy; and 5) the presence of significant free gossypol in the diet. Free gossypol at >100 mg/kg (100 ppm) of feed in the diet of pigs or young ruminants <4 mo old supports a presumptive diagnosis. Adult ruminants can detoxify higher concentrations of gossypol, but intake should still be <1000 ppm in the diet. Gossypol can accumulate in liver and kidney, which are additional postmortem specimens for analyses. In sheep, gossypol concentrations (both free and/or bound) >10 ppm in the kidney and >20 ppm in the liver suggest excess gossypol exposure. However, background and significantly elevated tissue gossypol concentrations have not been determined in all animal species, so tissue analyses may be of limited diagnostic value.

Differential diagnoses include: poisonings by cardiotoxic ionophoric antibiotics (eg, monensin, lasalocid) and ammonia, nutritional/metabolic disorders (eg, selenium/vitamin E or copper deficiency), infectious diseases, noninfectious diseases (eg, pulmonary adenomatosis, emphysema), mycotoxicoses caused by *Fusarium-*

contaminated grain, and toxicoses caused by plants with cardiotoxic and other effects.

Prophylaxis and Control: There is no effective treatment. If gossypol toxicity is suspect, all cottonseed products should be removed from the diet immediately; however, severely affected animals may still die up to 2 wk later. Recovery depends primarily on extent of toxic cardiopathy. Mild to moderate myocardial lesions may be reversible with time if stress is minimized and animals are carefully handled. However, poor weight gains in affected livestock and increased susceptibility to stress may persist for several weeks after cottonseed products are removed from the diet.

A high intake of protein, calcium hydroxide, or iron salts appears to be protective in cattle. Cattle should also be given ≥40% of dry matter intake from a forage source. Added iron of up to 400 ppm in swine diets and up to 600 ppm in poultry diets was reported to be effective in preventing signs and tissue residues of dietary gossypol exposure when used in ratios of 1:1 to 4:1 of iron to free gossypol.

Prevention of tissue residues in animal organ meats consumed by man is an important public health consideration for those individuals already consuming cottonseed oil and cottonseed flour products in their daily diets. Until pharmacokinetic parameters of gossypol are more completely characterized in all food animal species, immediate salvage and consumption of animals surviving excess gossypol exposure is not recommended. Only those animals living for ≥1 mo after exposure should be considered safe for human food sources.

HALOGENATED CYCLIC HYDROCARBON POISONING
(PCB, PBB, Dioxins, and others)

The halogenated cyclic hydrocarbons (HCH), such as polychlorinated biphenyls (PCB), polybrominated biphenyls (PBB), and dioxins, are structurally related compounds that have become widespread environmental contaminants. PCB and PBB are mixtures of randomly halogenated congeners once commonly used in industry as lubricants and fire retardants. Dioxins, as well as chlorinated dibenzofurans, are unwanted by-products formed during high temperature manufacture of chlorophenoxy herbicides (*see* HERBICIDES, p 1655) and pentachlorophenol (qv, p 1696). Tetrachlorodibenzodioxin (TCDD), 1 of ~70 dioxins, is one of the most poisonous substances known. Chlorinated naphthalenes are HCH compounds once used in industry as wood preservatives and lubricants. Naphthalenes caused bovine hyperkeratosis (X-disease), which is now primarily of historical interest.

PCB, PBB, and dioxins are chemically stable, lipid-soluble chemicals that concentrate in biological organisms (bioaccumulate) and thereby present a hazard in the food chain of animals and man. Livestock also have been exposed as a result of contamination during feed preparation, exposure to building materials, or subsequent to other industrial or agricultural usage. These chemicals are rapidly absorbed by all routes of exposure and are stored in adipose tissue from which they are gradually eliminated. Because of slow excretion, meat and milk may contain residues for many years after exposure.

Although the production of PCB and PBB was halted before 1979, many PCB- and PBB-containing products are still in use. It is estimated that >400,000 tons of PCB have been lost into the environment since 1932.

Comparative studies indicate a similarity in the toxic responses displayed by animals exposed to PCB, PBB, and dioxins. Both the degree and position of halogenation affect relative potencies and persistence. Although there are species, age, sex, and dose differences, the toxic responses include: a wasting syndrome—weight loss that may not be directly related to decreased food consumption; skin disorders—chloracne, edema, alopecia, and hyperkeratosis;

immunosuppression—thymic and splenic atrophy and lymphoid involution; reproductive disorders—abnormal cycling, reduced conception, fetotoxicity, and testicular atrophy; endocrine disorders—altered steroid and thyroid hormones; hematological dyscrasias—bone marrow depression, porphyria; liver enzyme induction and liver enlargement; teratogenesis—eg, cleft palate; and carcinogenesis—eg, hepatic carcinoma. Young animals and, often, females are more susceptible.

Diagnosis is aimed at detecting PCB or PBB in milk fat, body fat, fresh liver samples, feed, or other suspected sources. Specimens of milk and other fluids should be collected in clean glass jars with caps lined with aluminum foil. Tissues may be shipped frozen in aluminum foil.

No useful treatment has been identified; the long-term residue problems and the apparent long-term damage to affected animals make treatment in livestock uneconomical.

HERBICIDE POISONING

Herbicides are used commonly to control noxious plants. Most of these chemicals, particularly the more recently developed organic synthetic herbicides, are quite selective for specific plants and have low toxicity for mammals; other less selective compounds (eg, arsenicals, chlorates, dinitrophenols) are more toxic to animals. Most animal health problems result from exposure to excessive quantities of herbicides because of improper or careless use or disposal of containers. Very few problems occur when these chemicals are used properly.

In most cases, at proper application levels, herbicide-treated vegetation will not contain sufficient concentration of the chemical to be hazardous. Particularly after the herbicides have dried on the vegetation, only small amounts can be dislodged. When herbicide applications have been excessive, damage to lawns, crops, or other foliage is often evident.

The residue potential for most of these agents is low. However, the possibility of residue of a specific agent should be explored if significant exposure of food-producing animals occurs.

This discussion includes some of the more commonly used herbicides. More specific information is available from the manufacturer (the label should be checked), cooperative extension service, or poison control center.

Amides (bensulide, CDAA, diphenamid, propanil): Some members of this group are more toxic than other plant-growth-regulator-type herbicides. Ruminants can be poisoned by diphenamid at ~440 mg/kg body wt, and CDAA at 22 mg/kg body wt. A lethal dose of bensulide for dogs is ~200 mg/kg. The prominent clinical sign is anorexia; other signs and lesions are not definitive and are similar to the chlorophenoxy acids (*see* below).

Ammonium Sulfamate: Ruminants apparently can metabolize this chemical to some extent and, in some studies, have made better gains than control animals. However, sudden deaths have occurred among cattle and deer that consumed treated plants. Large doses (>1.5 g/kg body wt) induce ammonia poisoning in ruminants. Treatment is designed to lower rumen pH by dilution with copious amounts of water to which weak acetic acid (vinegar) has been added.

Arsenicals: The use of inorganic arsenicals (sodium arsenite and arsenic trioxide) as herbicides has been reduced greatly because of livestock losses and environmental persistence. These compounds can be hazardous to animals when used as recommended. Ruminants (even deer) are apparently attracted to and lick plants poisoned with arsenite. The highly soluble arsenicals can concentrate in pools in toxic quantities after a rain has washed them from recently treated plants. Arsenicals are used as desiccants or defoliants on cotton. Residues of cotton harvest fed to cattle may contain toxic amounts of arsenic.

Signs and lesions caused by organic arsenical herbicides (cacodylic acid, DSMA, MSMA) resemble those of inorganic arsenical poisoning. Single toxic oral doses for cattle and sheep are 22-55 mg/kg body wt. Poisoning may be expected from smaller doses if consumed on successive days. Dimercaprol (3 mg/kg for lg an, and 2.5-5 mg/kg for sm an, IM q4-6hr) is the recommended therapy. Sodium thiosulfate also has been used (lg an, 20-30 g, PO in ~300 mL of water; one-fourth this dose for sheep); however, a rationale for its use is not established and it may be unrewarding. (*See also* ARSENIC POISONING, p 1639.)

Borax: This has been used as a herbicide, an insecticide, and as a soil sterilant, and is toxic to animals if consumed in moderate to large doses (>0.5 g/kg). Poisoning has not been reported when this material was used properly, but has occurred when it was accidentally added to livestock feed, and when borax powder was scattered openly for cockroach control. Principal signs with acute poisoning are diarrhea, rapid prostration, and perhaps convulsions. An effective antidote is not known. Balanced electrolyte fluid therapy with supportive care is indicated.

Carbamate and Thiocarbamate Compounds (barban, CDEC, chlorpropham, diallate, EPTC, pebulate, propham, terbutol, triallate, vernolate): These herbicides are moderately toxic; however, they are used at low concentrations. Poisoning problems would not be expected from normal use. Alopecia may be seen in animals for some time after ingestion.

Chlorobenzoic Acids (chloramben, dicamba, 2,3,6-TBA): The herbicides in this group are of a low order of toxicity to domestic animals, and poisoning following normal use has not been reported. Environmental persistence and toxicity to wildlife is also low for this group. The signs and lesions are similar to those described for the chlorophenoxy acids (*see* below).

Chlorophenoxy Compounds (2,4-D [2-4-dichlorophenoxyacetic acid], 2,4,5-T [2,4,5-trichlorophenoxyacetic acid], 2,4-DB, dalapon, MCPA, silvex): These acids and their salts and esters are the most common chemicals used to control undesirable plants. As a group, they are essentially nontoxic to animals exposed to properly treated forage. When large doses are fed experimentally, general depression, anorexia, weight loss, general tenseness, and muscular weakness, particularly of the hindquarters, are noted. Large doses in cattle may interfere with rumen function. Dogs may demonstrate myotonia, ataxia, and posterior weakness, and develop vomiting, diarrhea, and metabolic acidosis. (The oral LD_{50} for 2,4-D in dogs is ~100 mg/kg body wt. Silvex is unusual for this group in that as little as 2.6 mg/kg may cause ill effects in dogs.) Even large doses, up to 2 g/kg, have not been shown to leave chemical residues in the fat of animals. These compounds are plant growth regulators, and treatment may result in increased palatability of some poisonous plants as well as increased nitrate and cyanide content.

The use of 2,4,5-T was curtailed because extremely toxic contaminants, collectively called dioxins (qv, p 1654), were found. Dioxins are considered to be carcinogenic and cause teratogenic and reproductive damage, as well as other toxic effects. Although manufacturing methods have reduced the level of the contaminants, use of these herbicides remains limited.

Dinitro Compounds (dinoseb, dinitramine, DNOC): The dinitrophenol and dinitrocresol compounds are highly toxic to all classes of animals (eg, LD_{50} at 20-40 mg/kg body wt). Poisoning can occur if animals are sprayed accidentally or have immediate access to herbage that has been sprayed, partially because these compounds are readily absorbed through skin or lungs. Dinitrophenolic herbicides produce a marked increase in oxygen consumption and depletion of glycogen reserves. Clinical signs include fever, dyspnea, acidosis, tachycardia, and convulsions, followed by coma and death with a rapid onset of rigor mortis. Cataracts can occur in animals with chronic dinitrophenol intoxication. Exposure to dinitro compounds may cause yellow staining of the skin or hair. An effective antidote is not known. Affected animals should be cooled and sedated to help control hyperthermia. Phenothiazine tranquilizers may potentiate toxic effects, and atropine sulfate is contraindicated. Administration (IV) of large doses of carbohydrate solutions and parenteral vitamin A may be useful.

Dipyridyl Compounds (diquat, paraquat): The dipyridyl compounds are nonvolatile desiccant herbicides used at rather low rates of ~2 oz/acre (150 mL/hectare). These compounds act rapidly, are inactivated on soil contact, and rapidly decompose in light. They produce toxic effects in tissues by development of free radicals. Tissue irritation can occur following contact (eg, mouth lesions following recent spraying of pastures). Skin irritation and corneal opacity occur on external exposure to these chemicals, and inhalation is dangerous. Deaths have occurred in animals, including man, as a result of drinking from contaminated containers.

Paraquat and diquat have somewhat different mechanisms of action. Diquat exerts most of its harmful effects in the GI tract. Animals drinking from an old diquat container showed anorexia, gastritis, and severe loss of water into the lumen of the GI tract. Signs of renal impairment and CNS excitement occurred in severely affected individuals.

Paraquat has a biphasic toxic action after ingestion. Immediate effects are GI tract irritation and perhaps some renal involvement. This is followed in 1-2 wk by pulmonary lesions as a result of destruction of the alveolar pneumocytes, evidently due to lipid-membrane peroxidation. Signs of poisoning include gastroenteritis, and finally respiratory difficulty due to pulmonary edema, hyaline membrane deposition, and alveolar fibrosis. Toxicity of paraquat is enhanced by selenium/vitamin E deficiency, oxygen, and low tissue glutathione peroxidase activity.

Due to slow absorption of these chemicals, intensive oral administration of adsorbents in large quantities, and cathartics is advised. Bentonite is preferred, but activated charcoal will suffice. In conjunction with supportive therapy, eg, vitamin E and selenium, excretion is accelerated by forced diuresis induced by mannitol infusion and furosemide administration. Oxygen therapy should not be used.

Glyphosate: This is a widely used herbicide with low toxicity, although fish and pond life have been killed experimentally. Sprayed forage is preferred by cattle for 5-7 days after application with little or no problem. Acute LD_{50} in rats is >5 g/kg.

A few dogs and cats show eye, skin, and upper respiratory tract signs when exposed during or subsequent to an application to weeds or grass. A few cases of nausea, vomiting, staggering, and hindleg weakness have been seen in dogs and cats that were exposed to fresh chemical on treated foliage. The signs, although of considerable concern to some pet owners, usually disappear when exposure ceases, and minimal symptomatic treatment is needed. Washing the chemical off the skin, evacuating the stomach, and tranquilization are usually sufficient.

Methyluracil Compounds (bromacil, isocil, terbacil): These compounds can cause mild toxic signs at levels of 50 mg/kg body wt in sheep, 250 mg/kg in cattle, and 500 mg/kg in poultry when given for 8-10 daily doses. Signs include bloat, incoordination, depression, and anorexia. Application rates of over 5 lb/acre (5.6 kg/hectare) can be hazardous, especially for sheep, but no field cases of toxicity have been reported.

Phenyl or Substituted Urea Compounds (diuron, fenuron, linuron, monuron, norea): Exposure to toxic amounts of these herbicides is unlikely with recommended application and container-handling methods. Signs and lesions are similar to those described for the chlorophenoxy herbicides (*see* above). The substituted urea herbicides induce hepatic microsomal enzymes and may alter metabolism of other xenobiotic agents.

Sodium Chlorate: This is now seldom used as a herbicide. Treated plants and contaminated clothing are highly combustible and constitute fire hazards. Additionally, many cases of chlorate poisoning of livestock have occurred both from the ingestion of treated plants and from accidental consumption of feed to which it was mistakenly added as salt. Cattle sometimes are attracted to foliage treated with sodium chlorate. Considerable quantities must be consumed before signs of toxicity appear. The minimum lethal dose is 1.1 g/kg body wt for cattle, 1.54-2.86 g/kg for sheep, and 5.06 g/kg for poultry. Ingestion results in the conversion of Hgb to methemoglobin. Treatment with methylene blue must be repeated frequently because, unlike the nitrites, the chlorate ion is not inactivated in the conversion of Hgb to methemoglobin and is capable of producing an unlimited quantity of methemoglobin as long as it is present in the body. Blood transfusions may help reduce some of the tissue anoxia caused by methemoglobin; IV isotonic saline can hasten the elimination of the chlorate ion.

Triazine Compounds (atrazine, cyanazine, prometryn, propazine, simazine): Although these herbicides are widely used, incidents of poisoning are uncommon. Occasionally, accidental exposure of animals to large dosages (eg, open containers, spills) can cause toxic effects and even death. (Doses of 500 mg of simazine/kg or 30 mg atrazine/kg for 36-60 days were lethal to sheep.) Generally, single doses >100-200 mg/kg body wt can be detrimental; repeat administration may reduce the toxic dose to <100 mg/kg body wt. Deaths have been reported in sheep and horses grazing triazine-treated pastures 1-7 days after spraying. Cumulative effects are not evident. The signs and lesions are similar to those described for the chlorophenoxy compounds (*see* above).

HOUSE/ORNAMENTAL PLANTS TOXIC TO COMPANION ANIMALS

Plants are an important part of the decor of homes, thus, toxicoses in pets chewing on or ingesting these plants can be expected. Inquiries to Poison Control Centers on plants ingested by children <5 yr old are estimated at 5-10% of all inquiries. Similar estimates (though not documented) could be made for pets.

Little research has been done on the toxicity of house plants. Most of them are hybrids, and selecting for growth outside their natural environment could affect their degree of toxicity. Age of the pet, boredom, and changes in the surroundings are factors that may affect the incidence of poisoning. Puppies and kittens are very inquisitive, and almost everything they come in contact with reaches the mouth. Pets (especially single household pets) may become bored or restless if left alone or confined for too long at any one time, and chewing on objects for relief is common in pets of all ages. Pets of all ages explore changes in their environment, such as occurs when potentially poisonous plants are placed in the home during holidays. A common response is to chew on the leaves or ripe berries of these plants. TABLE 2, pp 1659-1664, gives more detail on the potential toxicity of some of these plants.

INSECTICIDE AND ACARICIDE (ORGANIC) TOXICITIES

Under present regulations, pesticide labels must carry warnings against use of many compounds on certain animals or under certain circumstances. These warnings may pertain to acute or chronic toxicity, or to residues in meat, milk, or other animal products. Since label changes may arise from state or federal legislative action, changes in executive interpretation, or changing ecological interests, it is important that current label directions are **always** read and followed—each and every time a new container is purchased.

Each exposure, no matter how brief or small, results in some of the compound being absorbed and perhaps stored. Repeated short exposures may eventually result in intoxication. Every precaution should be taken to minimize human exposure. This may include the use of rubber gloves, respirators, rain gear, or frequent changes of clothing, with bathing at each change. Respirators must have filters approved for the type of insecticide being used; ordinary dust filters will not protect the operator from phosphorous fumes. Such measures are generally sufficient to guard against intoxication. Overexposure to chlorinated hydrocarbon insecticides is difficult to measure except by the occurrence of signs of poisoning.

The cholinesterase-inhibiting property of the organophosphates may be used to indicate degree of exposure if the activity of the blood enzyme is determined frequently. In man, serum esterase is usually inhibited first and, in the absence of declining RBC activity, indicates a recent exposure of only moderate degree. Depression of the RBC-enzyme activity indicates a severe acute exposure or a chronic exposure. (Normal cholinesterase activity values vary from individual to individual, and a determination of activity has significance only when it can be compared with the normal value for that particular individual.) *Continued* on p 1665.

Table 2. House/Ornamental Plants Toxic to Companion Animals

Scientific Name (Family)	Common Name	Important Characteristics	Remarks and Toxic Principles and Effects	Treatment
Caladium spp (Araceae)	Caladium, Angel wings	Perennial herbs with simple, heart-shaped, thin, highlighted veins, variegated leaves; yellow-green spathe; grown from rhizomes.	Calcium oxalate crystals and unknowns found in all parts, especially the rhizomes. Ingestion causes immediate intense pain, local irritation to mucous membranes, excess salivation, swollen tongue and pharynx, diarrhea, and dyspnea.	Symptomatic.
Chlorophytum spp (Liliaceae)	Spider plant, St. Bernard's lily, Airplane plant	Rhizomatous herbs with leaves slightly glossy, succulent, narrow, strap-like, green—some with a broad yellow or white band down the middle; long cream hanging stems with small white flowers developing into plantlets. Often grown in hanging baskets.	Unknown toxin(s) found in the leaves and plantlets. Vomiting, salivation, retching, and transient anorexia observed in cats within hours of ingestion. Deaths and diarrhea have not been reported.	Symptomatic.
Cyclamen spp (Primulaceae)	Cyclamen, Snowbread, Shooting star	Herbaceous plants, grown from rhizomes or tubers; petioled, heart-shaped, deep green intermixed with lighter green coloration (same leaf), serrated leaves; stems upright, with a terminal pink or white butterfly-like flower.	Triterpinoid saponins found in the tuberous rhizomes. GI problems, convulsions, and paralysis. Toxins cause local irritation and are therefore well absorbed from the GI tract.	Symptomatic.

Table 2. House/Ornamental Plants Toxic to Companion Animals (continued)

Scientific Name (Family)	Common Name	Important Characteristics	Remarks and Toxic Principles and Effects	Treatment
Dieffenbachia spp (Araceae)	Dumbcane	Fairly tall, erect, unbranched, fleshy plant, the stem girdled with leaf scars; leaves large, thickly veined, sheath-like petioles, blade with white or yellow spots.	Calcium oxalate crystals and unknown toxic proteins (possible asparagine or protoanemonin) in all parts, including sap. On ingestion, there is immediate intense pain, burning and inflammation of the mouth and throat, anorexia, vomiting, and possibly diarrhea, with tongue extended, head shaking, excessive salivation, and dyspnea. Immediate pain limits amount consumed. Death infrequent.	Symptomatic.
Digitalis purpurea (Scrophulariacae)	Foxglove	An erect biennial with simple, petioled (long on lower, short or sessile on upper), alternate, toothed, hairy, ovate to lanceolate leaves; purple, pink, red, white, or yellow tubular flowers (with spots) in terminal racemes; fruit is a capsule with many seeds.	Cardiac glycosides (digitoxin, digitalin, digoxin, and others), saponins, and alkaloids found throughout plant. Potency not affected by drying. Generally, acute abdominal pain, vomiting, bloody diarrhea, frequent urination, irregular slow pulse, tremors, convulsions, and rarely death.	Symptomatic.
Dracaena spp (Agavaceae)	Dragon tree	Robust palm-like house plant with lance-shaped, thin, variegated, alternate, nonpetioled leaves. Yellow, red, or green stripes along leaf margins in some species. Lower leaves are lost, leaf scars remain and clearly demarcated, terminal leaves are retained as the plant matures.	Alkaloids, saponins, and resin found in the leaves. Vomiting and severe diarrhea indicative of GI irritation expected. Clinical cases have not been reported.	Symptomatic, to correct fluid and electrolyte imbalance.

Scientific Name (Family)	Common Name	Important Characteristics	Remarks and Toxic Principles and Effects	Treatment
Euphorbia pulcherrima (Euphorbiaceae)	Poinsettia, Christmas flower, Christmas star	A perennial shrub with a milky white sap throughout; leaves are alternate, petioled, distinctly veined, entire or lobed, and conspicuously bright red, pink, or white (terminal leaves), lower leaves remain green; flowers small and inconspicuous.	Milky sap contains unknown toxic principle(s); irritates mucous membranes and causes excessive salivation and vomiting, but not death. Toxicity (hybrid species) has not been supported experimentally. Toxic diterpenes (ingenol derivatives) found in other *Euphorbia* spp have not been found in this species.	Symptomatic. Gastric lavage, activated charcoal, and saline cathartics should be considered.
Ilex aquifolium (Aquifoliaceae)	English holly, European holly	Evergreen shrub with leaves leathery, glossy upper surface, spiny toothed, alternate, and petioled; fruits are red to yellow berries with many seeds and an aromatic taste.	Saponins; an alkaloid (theobromine), triterpene compounds, and unknown compounds with digitalis-like cardiotonic activity have been found in leaves, fruits, and seeds. Abdominal pains, vomiting, and diarrhea observed following ingestion of ≥2 berries. Death rare.	Symptomatic, at best.
Kalanchoe spp (Crassulaceae)	Kalanchoe, Air-plant, Cathedral-bells	Winter flowering, herbaceous, succulent, nonhardy annuals or perennials; fleshy, serrate or crenate, opposite, petioled leaves; bright red, orange, or pink flowers in umbel. Stems become woody and untidy with age.	Unknown toxic compound(s) found in the leaves. Within hours of ingesting a toxic dose, depression, rapid breathing, teeth grinding, ataxia, paralysis, opisthotonus (rabbit), and death (rat).	Symptomatic; atropine has been effective in rabbits.

Table 2. House/Ornamental Plants Toxic to Companion Animals (continued)

Scientific Name (Family)	Common Name	Important Characteristics	Remarks and Toxic Principles and Effects	Treatment
Narcissus spp (Amaryllidaceae) and *Hyacinthus* spp (Liliaceae)	Daffodils and hyacinths	Garden ornamentals that grow from bulbs (close resemblance to onion bulbs) and flower in early spring. Bulbs harvested and stored in fall for replanting in spring.	Calcium oxalate crystals and alkaloids (their toxic potential yet to be defined) are found in the bulbs. Following ingestion of a toxic dose (bulbs), vomiting, diarrhea, and rare deaths are reported. Bulbs in storage may be accessible to pets.	Symptomatic.
Philodendron spp (Aracea)	Philodendron	Climbing vines with aerial roots; leaves (major attraction as a house plant) are large, unlobed or pinnately lobed and heart-shaped; rarely flowering.	Calcium oxalate crystals and unidentified proteins throughout the entire plant. On ingestion, there is immediate pain, local irritation to mucous membranes, excessive salivation, edematous tongue and pharynx, dyspnea, and renal failure. Excitability, nervous spasms, convulsions, and occasional encephalitis have been reported in cats.	Symptomatic.
Phoradendron flavescens (Viscaceae)	Mistletoe	Perennial parasitic shrub that grows on deciduous trees. Evergreen, ovoid, opposite leaves on round, highly branched, green stem. White berries with single seed. Brought into homes during Christmas season.	Amines (β-phenylethylamine, acetylcholine, choline, and tyramine), toxic proteins (viscotoxins), and unknowns found in all parts. Vomiting, profuse diarrhea, dilated pupils, rapid labored breathing, shock, and death from cardiovascular collapse within hours of ingesting toxic dose.	Symptomatic.

Scientific Name (Family)	Common Name	Important Characteristics	Remarks and Toxic Principles and Effects	Treatment
Rhododendron spp (Ericaceae)	Azalea, Rhododendron	Evergreen or deciduous shrub with simple, alternate, entire, leaves; funnel-shaped flowers in terminal umbel-like clusters or solitary and of various colors; fruits are capsules with many seeds.	Andromedotoxins (gray-anotoxins) found in all parts, including the pollen and nectar. Within hours of ingestion of a toxic dose (1 g/kg), salivation, lacrimation, vomiting, diarrhea, dyspnea, muscle weakness, convulsions, coma, and death. Signs may last several days, but the toxin is not cumulative.	Symptomatic. Gastric lavage, activated charcoal, saline cathartics, calcium injection, and antibiotics to control possible pneumonia suggested.
Sansevieria spp (Agavaceae)	Sansevieria, Snake plant, Mother-in-law's tongue	Hardy, succulent house plant; leaves erect, elongate, lanceolate, and flat or cylindrical, dark green with or without a yellow stripe along the margins, and horizontal gray bands throughout; many yellow starlike flowers on a tall central raceme or spike.	Hemolytic saponin and organic acids found in the leaves and flowers. Vomiting, salivation, diarrhea, and hemolysis related to the GI activity of these compounds.	Symptomatic. Fluids and electrolytes may be necessary.
Schefflera spp (Araliaceae)	Schefflera, Umbrella tree	Fast-growing evergreen with glossy, palmately compound leaves that hang and spread, appearing like an umbrella; depending on the species, leaflets increase with plant maturity and are more compact; veins are pronounced; margins entire to slightly crenate.	Oxalate found in the leaves. Mucous membrane irritation, salivation, anorexia, vomiting, and if severe enough, diarrhea.	Symptomatic.

Table 2. House/Ornamental Plants Toxic to Companion Animals (continued)

Scientific Name (Family)	Common Name	Important Characteristics	Remarks and Toxic Principles and Effects	Treatment
Solanum pseudocapsicum (Solanaceae)	Jerusalem cherry	A shrub with simple, lanceolate, entire or slightly serrated leaves; small star-shaped white flowers; ripe fruits are red, shiny berries with many white seeds.	Solanocapsine and related alkaloids found in the leaves and fruits. Anorexia, abdominal pain, vomiting, hemorrhagic diarrhea, salivation, progressive weakness or paralysis, dyspnea, bradycardia, circulatory collapse, dilated pupils, and convulsions are reported.	Symptomatic. Gastric lavage, activated charcoal, electrolytes and fluids, and anticonvulsants suggested.
Taxus spp (Taxaceae)	Yew	Evergreen tree or small erect shrub with alternate, needle-like, glossy (upper surface), dull (lower surface) leaves; seeds (generally one per fruit), black-brown or green, nearly enclosed in a cup-shaped, fleshy, red covering (aril).	The alkaloids (taxines and ephedrine), cyanide, and volatile oils found throughout the plant except the fleshy aril. Nervousness, trembling, ataxia, dyspnea, collapse; bradycardia progressing to cardiac standstill and death without struggle. Empty right heart, dark tarry blood in left heart, limited nonspecific postmortem lesions.	Symptomatic at best; usually futile once clinical signs appear. Atropine may be helpful.

In addition to their effect on man, organic pesticides may have deleterious effects on fish and wildlife as well as domestic species. In no event should amounts greater than those specifically recommended be used, and maximum precautions must be taken to prevent drift or drainage to adjoining fields, pastures, ponds, streams, or other premises outside the area in which the treatment is essential.

The day-to-day and month-to-month legislative changes that will occur will be primarily the result of pressure from environmentalists, consumers, and others, rather than from toxicologists concerned with safety of livestock and other domestic animals. The safety of these compounds for these animals has been rather carefully established in the past. It is of utmost importance that changing recommendations and regulations be treated with respect and full compliance. Prosecution of individuals, including veterinarians, for failure to follow label directions or to heed label warnings and for failure to warn animal owners of the necessary precautions, has occurred.

An ideal insecticide or acaricide should be efficacious without risk of injury to livestock or persons making the application, and without leaving residues in the tissues, eggs, or milk. While many compounds meet some of these requirements, few satisfy all of them.

Poisoning by organic insecticides and acaricides may be caused by direct application, by ingestion of the compounds on feed or forage treated for the control of plant parasites, or by accidental exposure. This discussion does not cover all materials currently used as insecticides or acaricides, but is limited to those organic compounds most frequently hazardous as toxicants to livestock or as residues in animal products.

Chemical synthesis rarely yields 100% of the product of interest. In any compound, be it natural or man-made, there will be, in variable proportions, related compounds that may have biological effects different from the compound sought. A prime example is TDE ("Rhothane", DDD): the p,p'-isomer is an effective insecticide of low toxicity for most mammals; the o,p-isomer causes necrosis of the adrenal glands of man and dog and is employed to treat certain adrenal malfunctions. There is evidence that p,p'-DDT and o,p-DDT have a similar relationship.

Products stored under temperature extremes or held in partially emptied containers for unusually long periods may deteriorate. Storing a chemical in anything but the original container is hazardous. Some consumers continue to mix their own combinations, often to the disadvantage of the animals treated.

CARBAMATE INSECTICIDES

Carbaryl: The oral LD_{50} in rats is 307 mg/kg body wt and >500 mg/kg, dermally. A 2% spray is nontoxic to calves; 4% is nontoxic to mature cattle when applied dermally.

Carbofuran: The oral LD_{50} in rats is 8 mg/kg body wt. The minimum toxic dose in cattle and sheep is 4.5 mg/kg, becoming lethal at 18 and 9 mg/kg, respectively. The oral LD_{50} in dogs is 19 mg/kg. Pigs have been poisoned after drinking water contaminated by this compound.

Methomyl: The oral LD_{50} in rats is 17 mg/kg body wt. Cattle have been reported to be poisoned after consumption of forage inadvertently sprayed by this compound.

Propoxur: The oral LD_{50} in rats is 95 mg/kg body wt. In goats, the oral LD_{50} was found to be >800 mg/kg.

Clinical Findings: The carbamate insecticides act similarly to the organophosphates (OP) in that they inhibit cholinesterase at nerve junctions. However, the inhibiting bond is much less durable. Frequently, the inhibition cannot be seen in the laboratory because of this reversibility. Signs include hypersalivation, GI hypermotility, abdominal cramping, vomiting, diarrhea, sweating, dyspnea, cyanosis, miosis, muscle fasiculations (in extreme cases, tetany followed by weakness and paralysis), and convulsions. Death usually results from hypoxia due to bronchoconstriction.

Diagnosis: This usually depends on history of exposure to a particular carbamate and response to atropine therapy. However, when a history of carbamate poisoning is not provided but cholinergic signs suggest carbamates or OP, cholinesterase activity levels can be determined in serum, RBC, or brain tissue. Screening GI contents for carbamate insecticides may be helpful.

Treatment: Treatment of carbamate poisoning is similar to that of OP in that atropine sulfate injections readily reverse the effects of inhibition. Recommended dosages for atropine are as follows. **Dogs, cats:** dosed to effect (repeated as needed); usually 0.2-2 mg/kg, parenterally ($\frac{1}{4}$ of the dose given IV and the remainder given subcut.). Cats should be dosed at the lower end of the range. **Cattle, sheep:** 0.6-1 mg/kg, $\frac{1}{4}$ of the dose IV and the remainder subcut., repeated as needed. **Horses, pigs:** 0.1-0.2 mg/kg, IV, repeated as needed.

CHLORINATED HYDROCARBON COMPOUNDS

Due to tissue residues and chronic toxicity, use of most of these agents has been drastically curtailed. Only lindane, methoxychlor, and toxaphene are now approved for use on or around livestock.

Aldrin is a potent insecticide and a near relative of dieldrin. It is of the same order of toxicity, and the statements pertaining to dieldrin (*see* below) apply, in general, to aldrin. The use of aldrin has been banned in the USA except for termite control.

Benzene hexachloride (BHC, hexachlorocyclohexane) is a useful insecticide for large animals and for dogs, but is highly toxic to cats in the concentrations necessary for parasite control. Only the γ isomer is insecticidal. Because isomers other than the γ are stored excessively and for long periods in body tissues, it is best that **lindane**, which contains $\geq$99% of the γ isomer, be used in preference to the technical grade of BHC, which contains several isomers.

Cattle in good condition have tolerated 0.2% lindane applications, but stressed emaciated cattle have been poisoned from spraying or dipping in 0.075% material. Horses and pigs appear to tolerate 0.2-0.5% sprays, thereby leaving an adequate margin of safety for those species. Ordinarily, sheep and goats tolerate 0.5% applications. Emaciation and lactation are known to increase the susceptibility of animals to poisoning by lindane; therefore, such animals should be treated with extreme caution. Very young calves are poisoned by a single oral dose of lindane at 4.4 mg/kg body wt. Mild signs appear in sheep given 22 mg/kg, and death occurs at 100 mg/kg. Adult cattle have tolerated 13 mg/kg without signs. BHC is stored in the body fat and excreted in the milk.

Livestock exposure to **chlordane** occurs by consumption of treated plants or through carelessness and accidents. Very young calves have been killed by doses of 44 mg/kg, and the minimum toxic dose for cattle is ~88 mg/kg. Cattle fed chlordane as 25 ppm of their diet for 56 days showed 19 ppm in their fat at the end of the feeding. Emulsions and suspensions have been used safely on dogs at concentrations up to 0.25%, provided freshly diluted materials were used. In dry powders, it has been safely used in concentrations up to 5% on dogs. Pigeons and Leghorn cockerels and pullets suffered no effects after 1-2 mo exposure to vapors emanating from chlordane-treated surfaces.

Dieldrin is not recommended for use on livestock. Residues limit its application, and it is one of the most toxic chlorinated hydrocarbon insecticides. Young dairy calves are poisoned by 8.8 mg/kg body wt, PO but tolerate 4.4 mg/kg, while adult cattle tolerate 8.8 mg/kg and are poisoned by 22 mg/kg. Pigs tolerate 22 mg/kg and are poisoned by 44 mg/kg. Horses are poisoned by 22 mg/kg. Because of its effectiveness against insect pests on crops and pasture and consequent low dosage per acre, dieldrin is not likely to poison livestock grazing the treated areas. Diets containing 25 ppm of dieldrin have been fed to cattle and sheep for 16 wk without harmful effects other than residues in the fat. Residues in animal fat are slow to disappear. Considerable judgment must be exercised in marketing animals that have grazed treated areas or consumed products from previously treated areas, since the residue in edible tissue should be zero. The use of dieldrin has been banned in the USA except for termite control.

Statements pertaining to dieldrin (*see* above) apply, in general, to **endrin**, the most toxic of the 3 chlorinated cyclodiene insecticides.

Heptachlor is not recommended for use on livestock in the USA, but since it is very effective against certain plant-feeding insects, it is encountered from time to time in areas grazed by livestock. Young dairy calves can tolerate doses as high as 13 mg/kg body wt but are poisoned by 22 mg/kg. Sheep tolerate 22 mg/kg but are poisoned by 40 mg/kg. Diets containing 60 ppm of heptachlor have been fed to cattle for 16 wk without harmful effect other than the residues in the fat. It is converted by animals and stored in the body fat as heptachlor epoxide. For this reason, a specific analysis performed for heptachlor usually yields negative results, while the epoxide method reveals storage.

Methoxychlor is one of the safest chlorinated hydrocarbon insecticides. Young dairy calves tolerate 265 mg/kg body wt; 500 mg/kg is mildly toxic. While 1 g/kg produces rather severe poisoning in young calves, sheep are not affected. One dog was given 990 mg/kg daily for 30 days without showing signs. Six applications to cattle of a 0.5% spray at 3-wk intervals produces a residue in the fat of 2.4 ppm, and ~0.4 ppm of methoxychlor may be found in milk 1 day after spraying a cow with a 0.5% spray; methoxychlor sprays are not approved for use on animals producing milk for human consumption. Cattle and sheep store essentially no methoxychlor when fed at the rate of 25 ppm in the total diet for 112 days. If used as recommended, the established tolerance for methoxychlor in fat will not be exceeded.

Toxaphene can be used with reasonable safety if recommendations are followed, but can cause poisoning when applied or ingested in excessive quantities. Dogs and cats are particularly susceptible. Young calves have been poisoned by 1% toxaphene sprays, while all other farm animals except poultry can withstand 1% or more as sprays or dips. Chickens have been poisoned by dipping in 0.1% emulsions, and turkeys have been poisoned by spraying with 0.5% material. Toxaphene is primarily an acute toxicant and does not persist unduly in the tissues. Adult cattle have been mildly intoxicated by 4% sprays and severely by 8%. Adult cattle have been poisoned from being dipped in emulsions that contained only 0.5% toxaphene, an amount ordinarily safe, because the emulsions had begun breaking down, allowing the fine droplets to coalesce. The large droplets readily adhere to the hair of cattle, and the resultant dosage becomes equivalent to that obtained by spray treatments of much higher concentration. Toxaphene is lethal to young calves at 8.8 mg/kg body wt but not at 4.4 mg/kg. The minimum toxic dose for cattle is ~33 mg/kg, and for sheep between 22 and 33 mg/kg. Spraying Hereford cattle 12 times at 2-wk intervals with 0.5% toxaphene produced a maximum residue of 8 ppm in the fat. Cattle fed 10 ppm of toxaphene in the diet for 30 days had no detectable toxaphene tissue residues, while steers fed 100 ppm for 112 days stored only 40 ppm in their fat. This amount was eliminated in 2 mo after the feeding of toxaphene had been discontinued.

Clinical Findings: The chlorinated hydrocarbon insecticides are general CNS stimulants. They produce a great variety of signs, most of which are neuromuscular. The affected animal generally is first noted to be more alert or apprehensive. Fasciculation of the muscles is then observed, which commences in the facial region and extends backward until all the body musculature is involved. In poisoning by DDT, DDD, and methoxychlor, progressive involvement leads to trembling or shivering that is followed by convulsions and death. With the other chlorinated hydrocarbons, the muscular twitchings are followed by convulsions, usually without the intermediate trembling. Convulsions may be clonic, tonic, or both, and may last from only a few seconds to several hours, or may be brief and frequent. High fever may accompany the convulsions. The animal may become comatose. Abnormal postures, such as resting the sternum on the ground while remaining upright in the rear, or keeping the head down between the forelegs, is often seen. Some animals stand with their head pressed against a wall or fence. Many animals exhibit almost continual chewing movements. Occasionally, an affected animal becomes belligerent and attacks other animals or moving objects. Usually, there is a copious flow of thick saliva and urinary incontinence. Vocalizations of various sorts also are common. Some animals show none of these active signs, but are depressed, almost oblivious to their surroundings, and do not eat or drink. Such animals may live several days longer than those showing the more violent manifestations. In certain cases, the clinical signs alternate, the animal first being extremely excited and then severely depressed. The severity of the signs observed at a given time is not a sure prognostic index. Some animals have only a single convulsion and die, while others suffer innumerable convulsions but subsequently recover. Not infrequently, animals showing acute excitability have body temperatures ≥106°F (41°C). The signs of poisoning by these insecticides are highly suggestive, but are not sufficiently definitive to be diagnostic. Encephalitis or meningitis often presents similar signs.

Signs of acute intoxication by chlordane in birds are nervous chirping, collapse on hocks or side, excitability, and mucous exudates in the nasal passages. Signs of subacute and chronic intoxication are molting, dehydration and cyanosis of the comb, weight loss, and cessation of egg production.

Lesions: If death has occurred suddenly, there may be nothing more than cyanosis. More definite lesions occur as the duration of intoxication increases. Usually, there is congestion of various organs, particularly the lungs, liver, and kidneys, plus a blanched appearance of all organs if the body temperature was high before death. The heart generally is in systole, and there may be many hemorrhages of varying size on the epicardium. The appearance of the heart and lungs may suggest a peracute pneumonia and, if the animal was affected for more than a few hours, there may be pulmonary edema. The trachea and bronchi may contain a blood-tinged froth. In many cases, the CSF volume is excessive, and the brain and spinal cord frequently are congested and edematous.

Diagnosis: Chemical analysis of appropriate samples is necessary to confirm the poisoning: brain, liver, kidney, fat, stomach or rumen contents, and a sample of the suspected source should be analyzed. Brain levels of the insecticide are the most useful information. Whole blood, serum, and urine from live animals may be analyzed. In food-animal poisoning, fat samples, perhaps including fat biopsies from survivors, are necessary to estimate the residue potential.

Treatment: There are no known specific antidotes. When exposure has been by spraying, dipping, or dusting, a thorough bathing without brushing the skin, using detergents and copious quantities of cool water is recommended. If exposure was by ingestion, gastric lavage and saline purgatives are indicated. The use of digestible oils such as corn oil is contraindicated; however, heavy-grade mineral oil plus a purgative hastens the removal of the chemical from the intestine. Activated charcoal appears to be useful in preventing absorption from the gut.

When signs are excitatory, a barbiturate, chloral hydrate, or diazepam is indicated. All disturbing elements of the environment should be reduced or removed. If the animal shows marked depression, anorexia, and dehydration, therapy should be directed toward supplying appropriate nourishment either IV or by stomach tube. Residues in the exposed animal may be reduced by giving a slurry of activated charcoal or providing charcoal in feed. Feeding 5 g of phenobarbital per day may accelerate residue removal.

INSECTICIDES DERIVED FROM PLANTS

Most of the insecticides derived from plants traditionally have been considered safe for use on animals. Derris (rotenone) and pyrethrum are examples of such materials. **Nicotine** in the form of nicotine sulfate is an exception. Unless it is carefully used, poisoning may result; affected animals show tremors, incoordination, nausea, and disturbed respiration, and finally become comatose and die. Necropsy lesions include pale mucous membranes, dark blood, hemorrhages on the heart and in the lungs, and congestion of the brain. Treatment consists of removing the material by washing or by gastric lavage with tannic acid, administering activated charcoal, artificial respiration, and treating for cardiac arrest and shock. Mildly affected animals recover rapidly and spontaneously.

Pyrethrins are a group of closely related, naturally occurring compounds that are the active insecticidal ingredients of pyrethrum. Pyrethrum is extracted from the flowers of *Chrysanthemum cinerariaefolium* and has been an effective insecticide for many years. Synergists, such as piperonyl butoxide, sesamex, piperonyl cyclonene, etc, are added to increase stability and effectiveness. This is accomplished by microsomal oxidation. By inhibiting mixed function oxidases, synergists also potentiate mammalian toxicity, as has been observed in rodent studies.

Pyrethroids are synthetic derivatives of natural pyrethrins and include: allethrin, cypermethrin, decamethrin, fenvalerate, fluvalinate, permethrin, and tetramethrin. Generally, these compounds are more effective insecticides and are less toxic to mammals than the natural pyrethrins; they appear to be not well absorbed from the skin (however, allergic manifestations from skin contact and inhalation are common in man). Mildly affected animals as well as those in early stages of toxicosis often display hypersalivation, vomiting, diarrhea, mild tremors, hyperexcitability, or depression. This syndrome may be confused with organophosphate or carbamate toxicosis. More severely affected animals can have hyperthermia, hypothermia, dyspnea, severe tremors, disorientation, and seizures. Death is due to respiratory failure. Generally, clinical signs begin within a few hours of exposure. However, the onset of signs may be significantly delayed due to grooming behavior or delayed dermal absorption.

Generally, treatment is not required after ingestion of a dilute pyrethrin/pyrethroid preparation. Because the chief hazard may be the solvent, induction of emesis may be contraindicated. A slurry of activated charcoal at 2-8 g/kg may be administered, followed by a saline cathartic (magnesium or sodium sulfate [10% solution] at 0.5 mg/kg). Oils and fats, which promote the intestinal absorption of pyrethrum, should be avoided. In the case of dermal exposure, the animal should be bathed using a mild detergent. Initial assessment of the animal's respiratory and cardiovascular integrity is important. Further treatment involves institution of basic life-support measures, including control of seizures, and symptomatic and supportive care. Seizures should be controlled with either diazepam (administered to effect at 0.2-2 mg/kg, IV) or methocarbamol (55-220 mg/kg, IV, not exceeding 200 mg/min). Phenobarbital or pentobarbital can be used if diazepam or methocarbamol are unsuccessful or transient in their effects.

ORGANOPHOSPHOROUS COMPOUNDS (OP)

These pesticides have now replaced the banned organochlorine compounds and subsequently have become a major cause of animal poisoning. A large number have been developed for plant and animal protection, and they vary greatly in toxicity, residue levels, and excretion. In general, they offer a distinct advantage by producing little or no tissue and environmental residues.

Many of the OP now used as pesticides are not potent inhibitors of esterases until activated in the liver by microsomal oxidation enzymes; they are generally less toxic, and intoxication occurs more slowly. Certain OP preparations are prepared by microencapsulation, thus releasing the active compound slowly. This increases the duration of effectiveness and reduces toxicity; however, the toxic properties are still present.

Azinphos-methyl (or -ethyl): The maximum nontoxic oral dose for calves is 0.44 mg/kg body wt, for cattle and goats 2.2 mg/kg, and for sheep 4.8 mg/kg.

Carbophenothion: Dairy calves <2 wk of age sprayed with water-based formulations showed poisoning at 0.05% and higher concentrations. Adult cattle have been poisoned by concentrations of 1%. Sheep and goats have been poisoned by 22 mg/kg body wt, PO, but not at 8 mg/kg. The LD_{50} for rats is ~31 mg/kg; a daily dosage of 2.2 mg/kg for 90 days produced poisoning. Dogs tolerated a diet containing 32 ppm for 90 days.

Chlorfenvinphos: Adult cattle were poisoned by ≥0.5% sprays, while young calves were poisoned only when the concentration was raised to 2%. The minimum oral toxic dose appears to be ~22 mg/kg for all ages of cattle. The acute oral LD_{50} for rats is 10-39 mg/kg.

Chlorpyrifos: The LD_{50} in goats was 500 mg/kg body wt, PO; in rats, it was 97 mg/kg. In comparison to calves, steers, and cows, bulls (particularly of the exotic breeds) are highly susceptible to a single dose of chlorpyrifos.

Coumaphos is used against cattle grubs and a number of other ectoparasites, and for treatment of premises. The maximum concentration that may be safely used on adult cattle, horses, and pigs is 0.5%. Young calves and all ages of sheep and goats must not be sprayed with concentrations of >0.25%; 0.5% concentrations may be lethal. Adult cattle may show mild signs at 1% concentrations.

Crotoxyphos is of rather low toxicity; however, Brahman cattle are markedly more susceptible to poisoning than are the European breeds. Cattle (except as above), sheep, goats, and pigs all tolerate sprays containing crotoxyphos at 0.5% levels or higher. The toxic dose appears to be in the 2% range except for Brahmans, in which 0.144%-0.3% may be toxic.

Demeton: The LD_{50} dose in goats was 8 mg/kg body wt, PO, while rats showed an LD_{50} of 2 mg/kg, PO, and 8 mg/kg on dermal application.

Diazinon: When sprayed, young calves appear to tolerate 0.05%, but are poisoned by 0.1% concentrations. Adult cattle may be sprayed repeatedly at weekly intervals with 0.1% concentrations without inducing poisoning. Diazinon appears to be tolerated by young calves at 0.44 mg/kg body wt, PO, but poisoning results at 0.88 mg/kg. Adult cattle tolerate 8.8 mg/kg, PO, but are poisoned by 22 mg/kg. Sheep tolerate 17.6 mg/kg but are poisoned by 26 mg/kg.

Dichlorvos has many uses on both plants and animals. Because it is rapidly metabolized and excreted, residues in meat and milk are not a problem if label directions are followed. Dichlorvos is of moderate toxicity, with a minimum toxic dose of 10 mg/kg body wt in young calves and 25 mg/kg in horses and sheep. The LD_{50} in rats is 25-80 mg/kg, PO. A 1% dust was not toxic to cattle. Flea collars that contain this compound may cause skin reactions in some pets.

Dimethoate: When administered PO, the minimum toxic dose for young dairy calves was ~48 mg/kg body wt, while 22 mg/kg was lethal for cattle 1 yr old. Daily doses of 10 mg/kg for 5 days in adult cattle lowered blood cholinesterase activity to 20% of normal but did not produce poisoning. Horses have been poisoned by doses of 60-80 mg/kg, PO. When applied topically, 1% sprays have been tolerated by calves, cattle, and adult sheep.

Dioxathion is a mixture of cis- and trans-isomers (70%) and reaction products (30%). It is used for both plant and animal protection. It is rapidly metabolized and is not likely to produce residues in meat greater than the 1 ppm official tolerance. Concentrations ≤0.15% are generally employed on animals. The minimum toxic dose in calves is 5 mg/kg body wt, PO, while the oral LD_{50} in rats is 19-45 mg/kg. Sprays of 0.5% have not been toxic in cattle or sheep, and sprays of 0.25% are nontoxic in goats and pigs. Dioxathion has killed young calves at 8.8 mg/kg, PO, and produced intoxication at 4.4 mg/kg.

Disulfoton: The maximum nontoxic oral dose for young calves is 0.88 mg/kg body wt; for cattle and goats, 2.2 mg/kg; and for sheep, 4.8 mg/kg. Several occurrences of intoxication have occurred in cattle following consumption of harvested forages previously sprayed with this insecticide.

EPN is related to parathion (*see* below). It is approximately one-half as toxic when externally applied, but when given PO, it is of approximately equal toxicity. The oral LD_{50} in rats is 7-36 mg/kg body wt, while the dermal LD_{50} is 22-230 mg/kg. Dogs were not poisoned at doses >100 mg/kg.

Famphur: The maximum nontoxic dose found in calves was 10 mg/kg body wt, and 50 mg/kg in cattle, sheep, and horses. This compound is effective against warbles in cattle, but (as for all grubicides) directions must be followed as to time limits on application; larvae killed while migrating in the body may elicit a reaction.

Fenthion: The minimum toxic dose for cattle was 25 mg/kg body wt, PO; 50 mg/kg, PO, killed sheep.

Malathion is one of the safest OP and is roughly equivalent to toxaphene. Young calves tolerate 0.5% sprays, but 1% sprays are toxic; adult cattle tolerate 2% sprays. Given PO, malathion is toxic at 100 mg/kg but not at 55 mg/kg body wt; young calves tolerate 11 mg/kg but are poisoned by 22 mg/kg. Malathion is excreted in the milk of cattle.

Methyl Parathion: The LD_{50} in rats from a single oral dose is 9-25 mg/kg body wt compared to 3-13 mg/kg for ethyl parathion. Microencapsulation of this compound decreases its toxicity, and the lethal dose in cattle has thus been increased from a 0.5% spray to a 2% spray.

Mevinphos: The LD_{50} in rats is 3 mg/kg body wt, PO or topically.

Naled: The oral LD_{50} in rats is 430 mg/kg body wt.

Oxydemeton-methyl: The maximum nontoxic oral dose was 0.88 mg/kg body wt for young calves, 2.2 mg/kg for cattle, and 4.8 mg/kg for sheep and goats.

Parathion, widely used for control of plant pests, is approximately one-half as toxic as TEPP (*see* below). It has been used as a dip and spray for cattle in some countries (not in the USA). Most cases of poisonings (occupational) in man by insecticides thus far reported have been attributed to parathion or its degradation products. As a spray, it produces definite signs of poisoning in young calves at a 0.02% concentration and occasional transitory signs at 0.01%. Parathion is lethal to sheep at 22 mg/kg body wt, PO, but not at 11 mg/kg. Young dairy calves are poisoned by 0.44 mg/kg, while 44 mg/kg is required to poison older cattle. Parathion is used extensively in the control of mosquitoes and insects in the orchard and on truck crops. Normally, because so little is used per acre, it presents no particular hazard to livestock. Because of its potency, particular care should be taken to prevent accidental exposure. Parathion is not stored in animal tissues in appreciable amounts.

Phorate: The minimum toxic dose was 0.25 mg/kg body wt in calves, 0.75 mg/kg in sheep, and 1 mg/kg in cattle. The oral LD_{50} in rats is 1-4 mg/kg.

Phosmet: The minimum oral toxic dose is 25 mg/kg body wt in cattle and calves, and 50 mg/kg in sheep. The oral LD_{50} in rats is 147-316 mg/kg.

Ronnel (fenchlorphos) produces mild signs of poisoning in cattle at 132 mg/kg body wt, but severe signs do not appear until the dose is increased to ~440 mg/kg. The minimum toxic dose in sheep is 400 mg/kg. The acute oral LD_{50} in rats is 906-1740 mg/kg. Concentrations as high as 2.5% in sprays have failed to produce poisoning of cattle, young dairy calves, or sheep. Poisoning usually occurs in 2 stages. The animal first becomes rather weak and, although moving about normally, may be placid. Diarrhea also may appear at this time; the feces are often flecked with blood. Later, salivation and dyspnea appear if the dose is high. At the lower dosages, the salivation and dyspnea probably will not be seen. Blood cholinesterase activity declines slowly over 5-7 days. Ronnel produces residues in meat and milk, therefore, strict adherence to label restrictions is essential. The residues may be removed by giving the animal activated charcoal for several days.

Ruelene is active both as a systemic and contact insecticide in livestock, has some anthelmintic activity, and is of rather low toxicity. Dairy calves have been poisoned by ≥44 mg/kg body wt, PO, while adult cattle required 88 mg/kg for the same effect. Sheep have shown moderate intoxication by 176 mg/kg; Angora goats were about twice as sensitive. Pigs have been poisoned by 11 mg/kg and horses by 44 mg/kg. Most livestock tolerate a 2% topical spray. The acute oral LD_{50} in female rats is ~770 mg/kg.

Temephos: The oral LD_{50} for rats is 1 g/kg (or more) body wt while the dermal LD_{50} is >4 g/kg.

Terbufos is a soil insecticide used to control corn rootworms. The minimum oral toxic dose is ~1.5 mg/kg body wt for sheep and cattle. Several occurrences of intoxication in cattle have occurred. Ingestion of 7.5 mg/kg was lethal to heifers.

The oral LD_{50} of **tetrachlorvinphos** in rats is 4 g/kg body wt, while the minimum toxic dose in pigs is 100 mg/kg.

Tetraethyl pyrophosphate (TEPP) probably is one of the most acutely toxic of all insecticides. Although it is not used on animals, accidental exposure occurs occasionally. One herd of 29 cattle ranging in age from calves to adults was accidentally sprayed with 0.33% TEPP emulsion; all were dead within 40 min.

Trichlorfon: As a spray, this is tolerated by adult cattle at a 1% concentration. When given PO, it is tolerated by young dairy calves at 4.4 mg/kg body wt, but produces poisoning at 8.8 mg/kg. Adult cattle, sheep, and horses appear to tolerate 44 mg/kg, while 88 mg/kg produces poisoning. Dogs were unaffected when fed 1000 ppm of trichlorfon for 4 mo. Trichlorfon is metabolized rapidly.

Clinical Findings: In general, OP pesticides have a narrow margin of safety, and the dose-response curve is quite steep. Signs of OP poisoning are those of cholinergic overstimulation of the parasympathetic nervous system, which can be grouped under 3 categories: muscarinic, nicotinic, and central. Muscarinic signs, usually first to appear, include hypersalivation, miosis, frequent urination, diarrhea, vomiting, colic, and dyspnea due to increased bronchial secretions and bronchoconstriction. Nicotinic effects include muscle fasciculations and weakness. The central effects include nervousness, ataxia, apprehension, and seizure activity. Cattle and sheep more commonly show severe depression. Stimulation in dogs and cats usually progresses to convulsions. Some OP (eg, amidothioates) do not enter the brain easily, so that CNS signs are mild. Onset of signs after exposure is usually within hours but may be delayed for ≥ 2 days. Severity and course of intoxication is influenced principally by the dosage and route of exposure. In acute poisoning, the primary clinical signs may be respiratory distress and collapse followed by death due to respiratory muscle paralysis.

Diagnosis and Lesions: An important diagnostic aid is the cholinesterase activity in blood and brain. Unfortunately, the depression of blood cholinesterase does not necessarily correlate with the severity of poisoning; signs are observed when nerve cholinesterase is inhibited, and the enzyme in blood reflects, only in a general way, the levels in the nervous tissue. The key factor appears to be the rate at which the enzyme activity is reduced. Results of analyses performed after exposure may be negative, since OP do not remain long as the parent compound in tissues. Chlorinated OP compounds appear to have more tissue residue potential. Frozen stomach and rumen samples should be analyzed for the pesticide since OP are generally more stable in acids.

Animals with acute OP poisoning have nonspecific or no lesions. Pulmonary edema and congestion, hemorrhages, and edema of the bowel and other organs may be found. Animals surviving >1 day may become emaciated and dehydrated.

Treatment: Drugs used to treat OP poisoning can be categorized into 1) muscarinic blocking agents, 2) cholinesterase reactivators, and 3) emetics, cathartics, and adsorbants to decrease further absorption. The central and peripheral muscarinic effects of OP are blocked with atropine sulfate administered to effect, usually at a dose rate, in dogs and cats, of 0.2-2 mg/kg body wt (cats should be dosed at the lower end of the range), q3-6hr or as often as clinically indicated. For horses and pigs, the dose is 0.1-0.2 mg/kg, IV, repeated q10min as needed; for cattle and sheep, the dose is 0.6-1 mg/kg, one-third of the dose given IV, the remainder IM or subcut., repeated as needed. Adequate atropinization exists when the pupils are dilated, salivation ceases, and the animal appears more alert. Animals initially respond well to atropine sulfate; however, the response to continued treatment becomes less apparent. Overtreatment with atropine should be avoided. Nicotinic cholinergic effects, muscle fasciculations, and muscle paralysis are not alleviated by atropine, so that death from massive overdoses of OP will still occur.

An improved treatment combines atropine with the cholinesterase-reactivating oxime, 2-pyridine aldoxime methchloride (2-PAM, pralidoxime chloride). The dose of 2-PAM is 20-50 mg/kg body wt, given as a 10% solution IM or by slow IV injection, repeated as needed. Response to cholinesterase reactivators decreases with time after exposure; therefore, treatment with oximes must be instituted as soon as possible (within 24-48 hr). The rate at which the enzyme/organophosphate complex becomes unresponsive to activators varies with the OP encountered.

Removal of the poison from the animal also should be attempted. If exposure was dermal, the animal should be washed with detergent and water but without scrubbing. Induction of emesis is indicated if oral exposure of <2 hr is suspected; emesis is contraindicated if the animal is depressed. Oral administration of mineral oil decreases absorption of pesticide from the gut. Activated charcoal (3-6 g/kg as a water slurry) adsorbs OP and helps elimination in the feces. This is particularly recommended in cattle. Continued absorption of OP from the large amount of ingesta in the rumen has caused prolonged toxicosis in cattle. Artificial respiration or administration of oxygen is advantageous. Phenothiazine tranquilizers should be avoided. Succinylcholine should not be used for at least 10 days after OP exposure.

DELAYED NEUROTOXICITY FROM TRIARYL PHOSPHATES

For some time, compounds known as triaryl phosphates (eg, triosthocresyl phosphate) have been used as flame retardants, plasticizers, lubricating oils, and hydraulic fluids. These compounds are weak cholinesterase inhibitors. More significant, however, is their ability to inhibit "neurotoxic esterase", which is located in the brain and spinal cord. A form of delayed neurotoxicity results from the inhibition of neurotoxic esterase. Triaryl phosphates have caused accidental poisonings in man and others (mostly cattle). Some OP insecticides (eg, PEN, leptophos) can also cause delayed neurotoxicity. However, field cases have been rare. The lesions associated with delayed neurotoxicity include demyelination of peripheral and spinal motor tracts due to loss of neurotoxic esterase function. Clinical signs associated with delayed neurotoxicity include muscle weakness and ataxia that progresses to flaccid paralysis of the hindlimbs. Signs of toxicity are usually not manifest until 8-21 days after exposure to a neurotoxic OP. There are no specific antidotes for neurotoxic triaryl phosphates.

SOLVENTS AND EMULSIFIERS

Solvents and emulsifiers are required in most liquid preparations of insecticides. Usually they are of low toxicity, but like the petroleum products (which many are), they must be considered as possible causes of poisoning. In direct treatment with pesticides, emulsification must be thorough with an average droplet size of ~5 μm (preferably smaller), lest excessive amounts be applied to treated animals. Treatment should be as for the petroleum products (qv, p 1696).

Acetone: GI irritation, narcosis, and kidney and liver damage are the main signs. Treatment consists of gastric lavage, oxygen, and a low-fat diet. Additional supportive treatment may be given as the signs dictate.

Isopropyl Alcohol: The signs are GI pain, cramps, vomiting, diarrhea, and CNS depression (dizziness, stupor, coma, death from respiratory paralysis). The liver and kidneys are reversibly affected. Dehydration and pneumonia may occur. Treatment consists of emetics, gastric lavage, milk, CNS stimulants, oxygen, and artificial respiration.

Methanol: Nausea, vomiting, gastric pain, reflex hyperexcitability, opisthotonos, convulsions, fixed pupils, and acute peripheral neuritis are typical. Toxic effects are due in part to the alcohol itself, and in part to formic acid produced by its oxidation. Treatment should include emetics (apomorphine) followed by gastric lavage with 4% sodium bicarbonate, saline laxative, oxygen therapy, sodium bicarbonate solution IV, and analgesics; however, the prognosis is poor. Intensive and prolonged alkalinization is the mainstay of treatment. Ethanol retards the oxidation of methanol and may be given as an adjunct therapy.

SULFUR AND LIME-SULFUR

Sulfur and lime-sulfur are 2 of the oldest insecticides. Elemental sulfur is practically devoid of toxicity, although poisoning has occurred occasionally when large amounts were mixed in cattle feed. Specific toxic dosages are not known, but probably exceed 4 g/kg body wt. Lime-sulfur, which is a complex of sulfides, may cause irritation, discomfort, or blistering, but rarely causes death. Treatment consists of removing the residual material and applying bland protective ointments plus any supportive measures that may be indicated.

IRON TOXICITY IN NEWBORN PIGS

Reports of toxicity following subcut. or IM injection of iron preparations in newborn piglets are sporadic, and the risk is not high. However, 3 forms of toxicity may occur. In some litters, death occurs quickly from 30 min to 6 hr after injection; in others, death is delayed for 2-4 days. (*See also* ANEMIAS OF DECREASED HEMOGLOBIN PRODUCTION, p 18.)

In the first form, damage to the muscles around the injection site causes potassium, among other substances, to be released; the blood potassium level rises and interferes with the heart's action. Affected piglets become weak, cannot stand, and have muscle tremors followed by convulsions. Respiratory distress may be observed. Usually, the whole litter is affected; piglets may appear anemic, and there is swelling at the injection site. On necropsy, skin and muscles may appear pale, and there is edema and a brownish black discoloration at the injection site. Waxy degeneration of skeletal and heart muscle may be seen; there may be hemorrhages in the heart and necrosis of the liver and kidneys.

In the second, less acute, form of toxicity, the excess iron appears to block the body's defense mechanisms by overwhelming the phagocytic cells, which increases the likelihood of infection. Death occurs after ~2-4 days. In young piglets, the most likely infection is an *Escherichia coli* enteritis and, although at necropsy some of the changes seen in the first form occur, they are less obvious, and the enteritis contributes markedly to any mortality.

The most important precipitating factor is vitamin E/selenium deficiency of the sow, which results in deficiency in the piglets; such iron toxicity can be prevented by raising the levels of vitamin E and selenium by feed supplementation (50 IU vitamin E/kg feed) or injection of the sow during pregnancy.

A third, more rare, form of toxicity is associated with the massive mobilization of calcium following injection of iron preparations, both in the presence and absence of supplementary vitamin D. Calciphylaxis, as it is called, occurs within several days of iron injection, and is associated with the development of hard swellings at injection sites. Death may occur, and calcification in other parts of the body may be seen at necropsy.

LEAD POISONING

One of the most frequently diagnosed poisonings in veterinary medicine worldwide, it has been reported in all domestic and several zoo animal species. It occurs most commonly in cattle and dogs, probably because of their indiscriminate eating habits and relative susceptibility to lead. Pigs, goats, horses, and chickens are comparatively resistant. The incidence of clinical lead poisoning may decline since lead is now used sparingly in paint, and use of leaded gasoline is diminishing. However, pasture contamination, junkpiles containing lead items, and old batteries continue to exist and present a potential hazard for livestock.

Etiology: Examples of acute exposure include ingestion by cattle of paint, plates from storage batteries, grease, or used motor oil. Dogs may receive an acute exposure by ingesting a large lead object (eg, a curtain weight or a shotgun slug) that remains in the stomach. Chronic exposures that culminate in clinical lead poisoning have occurred in cattle, horses, and sheep following ingestion of vegetation and soil contaminated by atmospheric fallout from smelters and mining operations, or from contaminating particles blown from trucks hauling old batteries for recycling. Chronic exposure from ingestion of lead-contaminated feed also can occur. Dogs may be chronically exposed by ingesting materials found in the home, such as linoleum, crumbling plaster, or peeling paint. When lead poisoning in a dog is diagnosed, the owner should be advised that any young children in the same dwelling should be examined, since the sources of lead for dogs would also be available to children. Lead poisoning is rare in cats, probably because of their fastidious eating habits. Wild ducks frequently are poisoned by ingested lead pellets (qv, p 1594).

Clinical Findings: Young animals usually are more severely affected than older ones. Although the hematopoietic systems of some species are highly sensitive to lead, the major clinical signs are neurological and/or GI in origin. Signs in cattle usually commence 2-3 days following ingestion of a fatal dose. The animal may bellow, stagger, show maniacal excitement, crash into objects, and appear blind. Death may occur within 2 hr, or convulsive episodes may be interspersed with periods of depression, ataxia, circling, and leaning and pushing on objects. Muscle twitching, "snapping" of the eyelids, and grinding of the teeth are common. In some cases, dullness and anorexia, along with signs of colic, predominate. Often, constipation persists for several days. Occasionally, more frequently in older cattle and sheep, there is diarrhea. Chronic ingestion of contaminated forage for weeks or months, during which cattle are asymptomatic, may suddenly culminate in a seizure and death. Thus, the clinical manifestations of acute or chronic ingestion of lead in cattle are similar.

A chronic syndrome is characteristic in horses. Signs include anorexia, weight loss, depression, weakness, stiffness, colic, diarrhea, laryngeal paralysis ("roaring"), and often, anemia.

The initial signs in dogs may consist of anorexia, emesis, colic, and diarrhea or constipation. The occurrence of neurological signs, which may be expressed as either depression or excitation, usually alert the owner to seek veterinary assistance. Excitatory signs include hyperesthesia, hysterical barking, champing fits, short seizures, and muscular spasms.

Lesions: Animals may die with no observable gross lesions. Ingested lead-containing material may be found in the GI tract. There may be gastritis, hyperemia, petechiae or ecchymoses in various organs, and brain edema. Horses sometimes die as a result of aspiration pneumonia secondary to laryngeal paralysis.

Diagnosis: Lead poisoning should be included in the differential diagnosis whenever animals with no prior history of neurological problems have an acute onset of neurological abnormalities. The concentration of lead in the renal cortex, liver, or whole blood provides definitive confirmation of lead exposure; values of >4, 4, and 0.2 ppm (wet wt) for these tissues, respectively, indicate abnormal lead accumulation. Levels at least twice these are usually found in fatal cases. Nucleated RBC and basophilic stippling are associated with lead poisoning in dogs, but is not confirmatory; these findings also occur with autoimmune hemolytic anemia. Measurements of blood δ aminolevulinic acid dehydratase and/or free erythrocyte protoporphyrin also are useful in the diagnosis of lead intoxication. However, these tests require collection and sample care that make them difficult to use in the field. They also require elaborate testing equipment and clinical expertise.

Treatment: Effectiveness depends on the extent of injury to tissues, especially nervous tissue; extensive and prolonged injury makes treatment of little value. Intestinal lavage or a cathartic, such as sodium or magnesium sulfate (PO, 160-205 mg/lb [350-450 mg/kg], 20% solution), may be employed to remove lead remaining in the GI tract. Administration of edetate calcium disodium (CaEDTA: cattle, horses—IV or subcut., 50 mg/lb [110 mg/kg] body wt, 2 doses 6 hr apart every other day for 3 treatments; dogs—subcut., 50 mg/lb [110 mg/kg] body wt of a 1% solution [diluted with 0.9% saline or 5% dextrose solution], divided into 4 doses, every other day for 3 treatments) is indicated, since it mobilizes lead from tissues and enhances its urinary excretion. Treatments may have to be repeated, but a 1-wk rest period without exposure to CaEDTA should be interposed between treatments. (CaEDTA is not as readily available as it once was; it is best to identify a source and periodically check to see that it is still available.)

Thiamine, at 2-4 mg/kg, b.i.d., subcut., in conjunction with CaEDTA, has been reported to alleviate signs of lead poisoning in cattle.

D-penicillamine (an oral chelating agent) can be used in dogs. It should be given on an empty stomach at 110 mg/kg, daily for 2 wk. This drug may produce unpleasant side effects, so the dog should be monitored closely during treatment. It should not be used in cattle, horses, or sheep.

Whenever chelating agents are used, water intake and urine output should be monitored closely. Good nursing and supportive care should be provided.

MERCURY POISONING

The dissimilarities of the toxic effects of the alkyl mercury compounds and elemental mercury as compared to other organic or inorganic mercurials necessitate a separate discussion of these groups.

ALKYL MERCURIAL DERIVATIVES AND ELEMENTAL MERCURY

These include the elemental form of the substance and various mercurial fungicides once used to treat seeds stored for planting. Poisoning results from the inadvertent use of treated seed as livestock feed. Elemental mercury may cause poisoning by inhalation of its vapor. Contaminated fish are a concern where mercury pollutes the waters; methylmercury is readily formed from inorganic mercury by aquatic microorganisms, and fish accumulate the methylmercury. Commercial cat food (tuna) has been shown to contain 5-6 ppm mercury, and neurological disturbances have been reported in cats on an exclusive tuna diet for 7-11 mo. The neurological signs associated with alkyl mercurials and elemental mercury are accompanied by degenerative lesions of the CNS. Treatment in such circumstances is useless.

ORGANIC AND INORGANIC MERCURIALS OTHER THAN THE ALKYL DERIVATIVES OR ELEMENTAL MERCURY

These include mercuric chloride (corrosive sublimate), a disinfectant; mercurous chloride (calomel), a cathartic; aryl mercurial compounds; and mercurial diuretic drugs. Poisoning in animals is usually due to accidental ingestion of mercuric chloride or its solutions. Mercurous chloride may be toxic when retained in the GI tract for prolonged periods. Aryl mercurials, used as fungicides to treat seeds stored for planting, are a potential source of animal poisoning.

In overwhelming doses, death may occur rapidly due to ventricular fibrillation. More commonly, the severe corrosive GI effects manifest as vomiting and bloody diarrhea. In such cases, severe renal damage also occurs, with anuria, or polyuria in less severe cases. In the rare case of chronic poisoning due to inorganic mercury, the major action is on the CNS and resembles alkyl mercury poisoning (*see* above). In acute poisoning due to excessive oral intake, severe degenerative (necrotic) and inflammatory lesions of the GI tract are observed.

Laboratory analysis should differentiate between normal concentrations of mercury in tissues and feed (<1 ppm) and concentrations associated with acute poisoning. The organ of choice for toxicological examination is the kidney, which selectively accumulates mercury.

Sodium thiosulfate (20% solution IV, 10 mL/100 lb [45 kg] body wt, q8hr) given together with dimercaprol (IM, 1.4 mg/lb [3 mg/kg] body wt, q4hr for the first 2 days, q6hr on the third day, and q12hr for the next 10 days or until recovery is complete) may be of benefit. The water-soluble derivative, 2,3 dimercaptopropane-l-sulfonate (DMPS), is superior to dimercaprol in promoting the excretion of mercurial compounds, but this drug is unavailable for clinical use in the USA. Dimercaprol is an effective antidote for mercurial diuretics. Binding of mercury still in the GI tract to protein such as eggs and milk, or by the oral administration of sodium thiosulfate may be beneficial. Alternatively, gastric lavage with sodium formaldehyde sulfoxalate (100-250 mL, 5% solution) is useful. This serves to reduce divalent mercury to the less toxic monovalent form. The use of electrolyte solutions to combat dehydration should be monitored carefully to avoid overhydration in the presence of anuria.

METALDEHYDE POISONING

A molluscicide commonly used in domestic gardens, especially during the wet season, usually metaldehyde is combined with bran, either as flakes or pellets, and is palatable to dogs and farm animals. Some products also contain arsenic or carbamate insecticides, which are usually less toxic at the dosage used than the metaldehyde. All species are susceptible to metaldehyde (toxic dose 0.3-0.8 mg/kg); dogs are the species most frequently poisoned. Metaldehyde is hydrolyzed in stomach acid to acetaldehyde polymers that readily enter the brain. Poisoning reduces brain serotonin and norepinephrine levels.

Clinical signs of toxicosis are similar in all mammals. Nervous signs are prominent and include hyperesthesia, nystagmus, muscle tremors, and incoordination, followed by opisthotonos and continuous tonic convulsions. Nystagmus is most severe in cats. Nervous signs are less exaggerated by stimulation as in strychnine poisoning (qv, p 1732), which may appear similar clinically. Hypersalivation, polypnea, dyspnea, tachycardia, and fever (profuse sweating in horses) are also seen. Severe acidosis develops in all species. Cholinergic signs (especially pupillary constriction) may occur if the product contains a carbamate. Early death is from respiratory failure, while survivors may develop liver failure. Postmortem lesions include congestion and edema of the liver, kidneys, and lungs, and intestinal hemorrhage. A mild formaldehyde-like odor may be present on opening the stomach or rumen. Stomach content is the preferred sample for analysis due to the rapid loss of acetaldehyde from tissue.

An emetic (if signs are mild), or gastric lavage with sodium bicarbonate is recommended. Diazepam is preferred to reduce excitement and convulsions. Barbiturates are indicated only if the animal does not respond.

Activated carbon or high doses of mineral oil are recommended since metaldehyde is oil soluble. Fluids with sodium lactate to reduce acidosis are required. Cold water rinses are recommended when fever is severe.

MOLYBDENUM POISONING

In ruminants, the dietary intake of excessive molybdenum causes, in part, a secondary hypocuprosis. Ruminants are much more susceptible to molybdenum toxicity than nonruminants.

Etiology: The metabolism of copper, molybdenum, and inorganic sulfate is a complex and incompletely understood interrelationship. It appears that the ruminal interaction of molybdates and sulfides gives rise to thiomolybdates. These compounds decrease the availability of dietary copper, and when absorbed, impede the metabolism of tissue copper and inhibit copper enzymes. Therefore, the susceptibility of ruminants to a high intake of molybdenum depends on a number of factors: 1) the copper content and intake of the animal—tolerance to molybdenum decreases as the content and intake of copper fall; 2) the inorganic sulfate content of the diet—high dietary sulfate with low copper exacerbates the condition, low dietary sulfate causes high blood molybdenum levels due to decreased excretion; 3) the chemical form of the molybdenum—water-soluble molybdenum in growing herbage is most toxic, while curing decreases toxicity; 4) the presence of certain sulfur-containing amino acids; 5) the species of animal—cattle are less tolerant than sheep; 6) the age—young animals are more susceptible; 7) the season of year—plants concentrate molybdenum beginning in spring (maximum level reached in fall); and 8) the botanic composition of the pasture—legumes take up more of the element than other plant species.

Molybdenosis associated with copper deficiency has been observed in areas with peat or muck soils, where plants grow in alkaline sloughs (eg, western USA), as a result of industrial contamination, where excess molybdenum-containing fertilizer has been applied, and where applications of lime appeared to increase plant molybdenum uptake.

In the diet, copper:molybdenum ratios of 6:1 are considered ideal; 2:1-3:1, borderline; and <2:1, toxic. Dietary molybdenum of >10 ppm can cause toxicity regardless of copper intake; as little as 1 ppm may be hazardous if copper content is <5 ppm (dry-weight basis).

Clinical Findings and Diagnosis: Molybdenosis in cattle is characterized by persistent, severe scouring with passage of liquid feces full of gas bubbles (**peat scours** or **teart**). Nonspecific signs may include unthriftiness, anemia, emaciation, joint pain (lameness), osteoporosis, and fading of the coat color. Depigmentation is most noticeable in black animals and especially around the eyes, which gives a spectacled appearance. Sheep, and young animals in particular, show stiffness of the back and legs with a reluctance to rise. Joint and skeletal lesions appear to be due to defects in connective-tissue and growth-plate development. Clinical signs appear within 1-2 wk of grazing affected pasture.

A provisional diagnosis can be made if the diarrhea stops within a few days of oral dosing with copper sulfate, and is strengthened if other causes of diarrhea and unthriftiness (including GI parasites) are ruled out. Diagnosis is confirmed by demonstrating abnormal concentrations of molybdenum and copper in blood or liver and by a high dietary intake of molybdenum relative to copper.

The disease may be confused with many other enteritides and is commonly mistaken for internal parasitism, especially in young cattle. In pastured animals, it is not uncommon for the 2 diseases to occur simultaneously.

Prophylaxis and Treatment: In areas where the molybdenum content of the forage is <5 ppm, the use of 1% copper sulfate ($CuSO_4 \cdot 5H_2O$) in salt has provided satisfactory control of molybdenosis. With higher levels of molybdenum, 2% copper sulfate has been successful; up to 5% has been used in a few regions where the molybdenum levels are very high. In areas where, for various reasons, cattle do not consume mineral supplements, the required copper may be supplied as a drench given weekly, as parenterally administered repository copper preparations, or as a top-dressing to the pasture. (*See also* NUTRITIONAL DISEASES OF CATTLE AND SHEEP, p 1194).

MYCOTOXICOSES

Acute or chronic intoxications due to exposure to feed or bedding contaminated with toxins that may be produced during growth of various saprophytic or phytopathogenic fungi or molds on cereals, hay, straw, pastures, or any other fodder. A few principles characterize mycotoxic diseases: 1) the cause may not be immediately identified; 2) they are not transmissible from one animal to another; 3) treatment with drugs or antibiotics has little effect on the course of the disease; 4) outbreaks are usually seasonal because particular climatic sequences may favor fungal growth and toxin production; 5) study indicates specific association with a particular feed; and 6) examination of feedstuff may reveal large numbers of fungi, but this does not necessarily indicate that toxin production has occurred.

Often, a number of mycotoxins with different toxic properties may be present in feedstuffs, and clinical signs and lesions may not conform to those seen when animals are dosed experimentally with pure, single mycotoxins. Several mycotoxins are immunosuppressive, which may allow viruses, bacteria, or parasites to create a secondary disease that is more obvious than the primary.

There is no known treatment; removal of the source of the toxin (ie, the moldy feedstuff) appears to be the only effective method. If financial circumstances do not allow for disposal of the moldy feed, it can be blended with unspoiled feed just before feeding to reduce the toxin concentration, or fed to less susceptible species.

Important mycotoxic diseases that occur throughout the world are summarized in TABLE 3, pp 1680-1683.

Sampling and Submitting Feeds for Laboratory Analysis: Much of the error in detecting mycotoxins in feed results from sampling or subsampling rather than analytical methodology. Samples can be taken at various stages—from growing crops or during transport or storage. Whenever possible, samples should be taken after particulate size has been reduced (eg, by shelling or grinding) and soon after blending has occurred (as in harvesting, loading, or grinding). Sampling is most effective if small samples are taken at periodic, predetermined intervals from a moving stream of grain or feed. These individual stream samples should be combined and mixed thoroughly, after which a subsample of 10 lb (4.5 kg) should be taken.

Probe sampling is acceptable when grain has been recently blended, but is less reliable since different microenvironments within the storage facility may cause areas of mold or mycotoxin concentration. A suggested method of probe sampling is to sample at 5 locations, each 1 ft (30 cm) from the periphery of a bin, plus once in the center. This should be done for each 6 ft (2 m) of bin depth. Thus, taller bins would require more samples and the total weight should be >10 lb.

Dry samples are preferable for transport and storage. Samples should be dried at 176-194°F (80-90°C) for ~3 hr to reduce moisture to 12-13%. If mold studies are to be done, drying at 140°F (60°C) for 6-12 hr should allow preservation of fungal activity.

Containers should fit the nature of the sample. For dried samples, paper or cloth bags are recommended. Plastic bags should be avoided unless grain is dried thoroughly. Plastic bags are useful for high-moisture samples only if refrigeration, freezing, or chemicals are used to retard mold growth during transport or storage. Once a sample has cooled or frozen, warming may induce condensation and allow mold growth. Thus, any refrigerated sample must be maintained that way until analysis is performed.

AFLATOXICOSIS

Aflatoxins are produced by toxigenic strains of *Aspergillus flavus* and *A parasiticus* on peanuts, soybeans, corn (maize), and other cereals either in the field or during storage when moisture content and temperatures are sufficiently high for mold growth. Aflatoxicosis in mammals and poultry presents a diverse pattern of toxic response and disease in relation to species, sex, age, nutritional status, and the duration of intake and level of aflatoxins in the rations. Earlier recognized disease outbreaks called "moldy corn toxicosis", "poultry hemorrhagic syndrome", and "*Aspergillus* toxicosis" may have been caused by aflatoxins.

Aflatoxicosis occurs in many parts of the world and affects growing poultry, especially ducklings and turkey poults, young pigs, pregnant sows, calves, and dogs. Adult cattle, sheep, and goats are relatively resistant to the acute form of the disease, but show susceptibility to toxic diets fed over long periods. Experimentally, all species of animals tested have shown some degree of susceptibility. Dietary levels of aflatoxin (in ppb) generally tolerated are: young poultry, ≤50; adult poultry, ≤100; weaner pigs, ≤50; finishing pigs, ≤200; calves, <100; cattle, <300. Metabolites of aflatoxin (aflatoxin M_1 and M_2) are excreted in milk; feedstuffs that contain aflatoxins should not be fed to dairy cows.

Aflatoxins bind to macromolecules, especially nucleic acids and nucleoproteins. Their toxic effects include mutagenesis due to alkylation of nuclear DNA, carcinogenesis, teratogenesis, and immunosuppression. The liver is the principal organ affected. High doses of aflatoxins produce severe hepatocellular necrosis; prolonged low dosage produces reduced growth rate and liver enlargement.

Clinical Findings: In acute outbreaks, deaths occur after a short period of inappetence. Subacute outbreaks are more usual, and unthriftiness, weakness, anorexia, and sudden deaths can occur. Frequently, there is a high incidence of concurrent infectious disease, often respiratory, that responds poorly to the usual chemotherapy.

Lesions: In acute cases, there are widespread hemorrhages and icterus. Microscopically, the liver shows marked fatty accumulations and massive centrilobular necrosis and hemorrhage. In subacute cases, the hepatic changes are not so pronounced, but there is some liver enlargement and an increased firmness. There may be edema of the gallbladder. Microscopically, the liver shows proliferation and fibrosis of the bile ductules and an increase in the size of hepatocytes and their nuclei (megalocytosis). The GI mucosa may show glandular atrophy and associated inflammation. In the kidneys, there may be tubular degeneration and regeneration. Prolonged feeding of low concentrations of aflatoxins may produce diffuse liver fibrosis (cirrhosis) and cholangio- or hepatocellular carcinoma.

Table 3. Mycotoxicoses in Domestic Animals

Disease	Toxins (when known)	Fungi or Molds	Regions Where Reported	Contaminated Toxic Foodstuff	Animals Affected	Signs and Lesions
Aflatoxicosis	Aflatoxins	Aspergillus flavus, A parasiticus	Widespread (warmer climatic zones)	Moldy peanuts, soybeans, cottonseeds, rice, sorghum, corn (maize), other cereals	All poultry, pigs, cattle, sheep, dogs	See also p 1679, and POULTRY MYCOTOXICOSIS, p 1585.
Diplodiosis	Unknown	Diplodia zeae	South Africa	Moldy corn (maize)	Cattle, sheep	Nervous system disorders, cold and insensitive limbs. Recovery usual on removal of source.
Ergotism	Ergot alkaloids	Claviceps purpurea	Widespread	Seedheads of many grasses, grains	Cattle, horses, pigs, poultry	See also p 1684.
	Paspalinine and paspalitrems, tremorgens	C paspali, C cinerea	Widespread	Seedheads of paspalum grasses	Cattle, horses, sheep	See PASPALUM STAGGERS, p 1689.
Estrogenism and vulvovaginitis	Zearalenone	Fusarium graminearum (roseum) Perfect state: Gibberella zeae	Widespread	Moldy corn (maize) and pelleted cereal feeds, standing corn, corn silage, other grains	Pigs, cattle, sheep, poultry	Vulvovaginitis in pigs, estrogenism in cattle and sheep, reduced egg production in poultry. See also p 1685.
Facial eczema (Pithomycotoxicosis)	Sporidesmins	Pithomyces chartarum (Sporidesmium bakeri)	Widespread	Toxic spores on pasture litter	Sheep, cattle, farmed deer	See also p 1686.
Leukoencephalomalacia	Fumonisin B_1	Fusarium moniliforme	Egypt, USA, South Africa, Greece	Moldy corn (maize)	Horses, other Equidae, pigs	Depends on degree and specific site of brain lesion. See also p 1684.

Disease	Toxins (when known)	Fungi or Molds	Regions Where Reported	Contaminated Toxic Foodstuff	Animals Affected	Signs and Lesions
Moldy corn poisoning	See aflatoxicosis, estrogenism and vulvovaginitis, ochratoxicosis, trichothecene toxicosis, leukoencephalomalacia					
Mold nephrosis	See ochratoxicosis (below)					
Mycotoxic lupinosis (as distinct from alkaloid poisoning)	Phomopsins	Phomopsis leptostromiformis	Widespread	Moldy seed, pods, stubble, and haulm of several Lupinus spp affected by Phomopsis stem blight	Sheep, occasionally cattle, horses, pigs	Lassitude, inappetence, stupor, icterus, marked liver injury. Usually fatal. See also p 1689.
Ochratoxicosis	Ochratoxin; also citrinin	Aspergillus ochraceus and others; Penicillium viridicatum, P citrinum	Widespread	Moldy barley, corn (maize), wheat	Pigs, poultry	Perirenal edema, enlarged pale kidneys with cortical cysts, and tubular degeneration and fibrosis. Immunosuppression.
Perennial ryegrass staggers	Lolitrems	Acremonium loliae, an endophyte fungus confined to Lolium perenne	Australia, New Zealand, Europe, USA	Endophyte-infected ryegrass pastures	Sheep, cattle, horses, deer	Tremors, incoordination, collapse, convulsive spasms. See RYEGRASS STAGGERS, p 1725.

(continued)

Table 3. Mycotoxicoses in Domestic Animals (continued)

Disease	Toxins (when known)	Fungi or Molds	Regions Where Reported	Contaminated Toxic Foodstuff	Animals Affected	Signs and Lesions
Poultry hemorrhagic syndrome	Probably aflatoxins and rubratoxins	Probably *Aspergillus flavus, A clavatus, Penicillium purpurogenum, Alternaria* sp	USA	Moldy grain and meal	Growing chickens	Depression, anorexia, no weight gain, widespread internal hemorrhages, sometimes aplastic anemia, death. *See* MYCOTOXICOSES, p 1678.
Pulmonary edema, emphysema	4-Ipomeanol	*Fusarium solani (javanicum)*	USA	Moldy sweet potatoes	Cattle	Pulmonary edema, leading to interstitial pneumonia and emphysema.
Slobbers	Slaframine (and swainsonine)	*Rhizoctonia leguminicola*	USA	Blackpatch-diseased legumes (notably red clover) eaten as forage or hay	Sheep, cattle	Salivation, bloat, diarrhea, sometimes death. Recovery usual when removed from clover. *See* SLAFRAMINE TOXICOSIS, p 124.
Sweet clover poisoning	Dicumarol	*Penicillium* spp, *Mucor* spp, *Aspergillus* spp	North America	Sweet clover (*Melilotus* spp)	Cattle, horses, sheep	*See also* p 1733.
Tremorgen ataxia syndrome	Penitrems, verruculogen, paxilline, fumitremorgens, aflatrems, roquefortine	*Penicillium crustosum, P puberulum, P verruculosum, P roqueforti, Aspergillus flavus, A clavatus, A fumigatus, A clavatus* and others	USA, South Africa, probably worldwide	Moldy feed	All species	Tremors, polypnea, ataxia, collapse, convulsive spasms.

Disease	Toxins (when known)	Fungi or Molds	Regions Where Reported	Contaminated Toxic Foodstuff	Animals Affected	Signs and Lesions
Trichothecene toxicosis (Fusariotoxicosis) (Vomiting and feed refusal in pigs)	Non-macrocyclic trichothecenes (deoxynivalenol, T-2 toxin, diacetoxyscirpenol, many other trichothecenes)	*Fusarium sporotrichioides, F culmorum, F graminearum, F nivale*; other fungal species	Widespread (except for deoxynivalenol, more likely in temperate to colder climates)	Cereal crops, moldy roughage	Pigs, cattle, horses, poultry	Vomiting, feed refusal, loss of appetite and milk production, diarrhea, staggers. Skin irritation. Immunosuppression. Recovery on removal of contaminated feed. *See also* p 1690.
(Stachybotryotoxicosis)	Macrocyclic trichothecenes (satratoxin, roridin, verrucarin)	*Stachybotrys atra (alternans)*	USSR, southeast Europe	Moldy roughage, other contaminated feed	Horses, cattle, sheep, pigs	Stomatitis and ulceration, anorexia, leukopenia. Extensive hemorrhages in many organs, inflammation and necrosis in the gut. Immunosuppression.
(Myrotheciotoxicosis, Dendrodochiotoxicosis)	Macrocyclic trichothecenes (verrucarins, roridins, etc)	*Myrothecium verrucaria, M roridum*	Southeast Europe, USSR	Moldy rye stubble, straw	Sheep, cattle, horses	Acute: diarrhea, respiratory distress, hemorrhagic gastroenteritis, immunosuppression, death. Chronic: ulceration of GI tract, unthriftiness, gradual recovery.
(Fescue foot)	Macrocyclic trichothecenes (baccharinoids)	*Myrothecium verrucaria*	Brazil	Plants of *Baccharis* spp that contain the toxins	Cattle, other herbivores	Epithelial necrosis of GI tract.
			USA, Australia, New Zealand, Italy	Tall fescue grass	Cattle	Lameness, weight loss, hyperthermia, dry gangrene of extremities. *See also* p 1687.

Diagnosis: Disease history, necropsy findings, and microscopical examination of the liver should indicate the nature of the hepatotoxin, but senecio poisoning (qv, p 1698) may show hepatic changes that are somewhat similar. The presence and levels of aflatoxins in the feed should be determined. Aflatoxin M_1 can be detected in urine if intakes of the toxin are high.

Control: Avoidance of contaminated feeds by monitoring batches for aflatoxin content is suggested. Young, newly weaned, and pregnant and lactating animals require special protection from suspected toxic feeds. Dilution with noncontaminated feedstuff is one possibility to cope with the problem. Ammoniation of grain reduces contamination but is not currently approved for use in food animals.

Hydrated sodium calcium aluminosilicates (HSCAS) recently have shown promise in reducing effects of aflatoxin when fed to pigs or poultry; at 10 lb/ton (5 kg/tonne), they provided substantial protection against dietary aflatoxin. HSCAS reduced, but did not eliminate, residues of aflatoxin M_1 in milk from dairy cows fed aflatoxin B_1.

EQUINE LEUKOENCEPHALOMALACIA

A mycotoxic disease of the CNS that affects horses, mules, and donkeys. It occurs sporadically in North and South America, South Africa, Europe, and China. It is associated with the feeding of moldy corn, usually over a period of several weeks. The causative fungus is *Fusarium moniliforme*, and the toxin has been classified as fumonisin B_1.

The same toxin has been reported to cause acute epidemics of disease in pigs, usually adults, characterized by pulmonary edema and hydrothorax.

Signs include apathy, drowsiness, pharyngeal paralysis, blindness, circling, staggering, and recumbency. The clinical course is usually 1-2 days but may be as short as several hours or as long as several weeks. Icterus may be present if the liver is involved. The characteristic lesion is liquefactive necrosis of the white matter of the cerebrum. The necrosis is usually unilateral but may be asymmetrically bilateral. Some horses may have hepatic necrosis similar to that seen in aflatoxicosis.

No treatment is available. Avoidance of moldy corn is the only prevention, although this is difficult since the corn may not be grossly moldy or it may be contained in a mixed feed.

ERGOTISM

A worldwide disease of farm animals that results from continued ingestion of sclerotia of the parasitic fungus, *Claviceps purpurea*, which replaces the grain or seed of rye and other small grains or forage plants, such as the bromes, bluegrasses, and ryegrasses. The hard, black, elongated sclerotia may contain varying quantities of ergot alkaloids of which the levorotatory alkaloids, ergotamine and ergonovine (ergometrine), are pharmacologically most important. Cattle, pigs, sheep, and poultry are involved in sporadic outbreaks, and most species are susceptible.

Etiology: Ergot causes vasoconstriction by direct action on the muscles of the arterioles, and repeated dosages injure the vascular endothelium. These actions initially result in reduced blood flow and, eventually, complete stasis with terminal necrosis of the extremities due to thrombosis. A cold environment predisposes the extremities to gangrene. In addition, ergot has a potent oxytocic action and also causes stimulation of the CNS, followed by depression.

Clinical Findings and Lesions: Cattle may be affected by eating ergotized hay or grain or occasionally by grazing seeded pastures that are infested with ergot. Lameness, the first sign, may appear 2-6 wk or more after initial ingestion, depending on the concentration of alkaloids in the ergot and the quantity of ergot in the feed. Hindlimbs are affected before forelimbs, but the extent of involvement of a limb and the number of limbs affected depends on the daily intake of ergot. Body temperature and pulse and respiration are increased. **Epidemic hyperthermia** and hypersalivation may occur in cattle poisoned with *C purpurea* (*see also* FESCUE LAMENESS, p 1687).

Associated with the lameness are swelling and tenderness of the fetlock joint and pastern. Within ~1 wk, sensation is lost in the affected part, an indented line appears at the limit of normal tissue, and dry gangrene affects the distal part. Eventually, one or both claws or any part of the limbs up to the hock or knee may be sloughed. In a similar way, the tip of the tail or ears may become necrotic and slough. Exposed skin areas, such as teats and udder, appear unusually pale or anemic. Abortion does not occur.

The only constant lesions at necropsy are in the skin and subcut. parts of the extremities. The skin is normal to the indented line, but beyond, it is cyanotic and hardened in advanced cases. Subcut. hemorrhage and some edema occur proximal to the necrotic area.

In pigs, ingestion of ergot-infested grains may result in reduced feed intakes and reduced weight gains. If fed to pregnant sows, ergotized grains result in lack of udder development with agalactia at parturition, and the birth of small litters of weak, undersized piglets of which few survive. No other clinical signs or lesions are seen.

Sheep with ergotism show clinical signs similar to those of cattle. Additionally, the mouth may be ulcerated, and marked intestinal inflammation may be seen at necropsy. A convulsive syndrome has been associated with ergotism in sheep.

Diagnosis: Diagnosis is based on finding the causative fungus in grains, hay, or pastures provided to stock showing signs of ergotism. Extraction and detection of ergot alkaloids may be done in suspect ground grain meals.

Identical signs and lesions of lameness, and sloughing of the hooves and tips of ears and tail are seen in fescue foot in cattle grazing in winter on tall fescue grass infected with an endophyte fungus. In gilts and sows, lactation failure not associated with ergot alkaloids is prevalent.

Control: Ergotism can be controlled by an immediate change to an ergot-free diet. Under pasture feeding conditions, frequent grazing or topping of pastures prone to ergot infestation during the summer months reduces flower-head production and helps to control the disease. Grain that contains even small amounts of ergot should not be fed to pregnant or lactating sows.

ESTROGENISM AND VULVOVAGINITIS
(*Fusarium* estrogenism)

Fusarium spp molds are extremely common, and often contaminate growing plants and stored feeds. *Fusarium graminearum* produces zearalenone, one of the resorcyclic acid lactones (RAL). Zearalenone (formerly called F_2 toxin) is a potent nonsteroidal estrogen and is the only known mycotoxin with effects that are primarily estrogenic. Under controlled administration, zearalanol, a closely related RAL, is widely used in cattle as an anabolic agent. Zearalenone-contaminated grains and fodders can produce reproductive disorders when animals consume them.

Estrogenism due to zearalenone was first clinically recognized as vulvovaginitis in prepubertal gilts fed moldy corn (maize), but zearalenone is occasionally reported as a disease-causing agent in sporadic outbreaks in dairy cattle, sheep, chickens, and turkeys. Extremely high dosages are required to produce disease in poultry.

Etiology: Zearalenone has been detected in corn, oats, barley, wheat, and sorghum (both fresh and stored); in rations compounded for cattle and pigs; in corn ensiled at the green stage; and in hay. It has been detected occasionally in samples from pastures in temperate climates at levels thought to be sufficient to cause reproductive failure of grazing herbivores. In cattle, dietary concentrations >10 ppm may cause reproductive dysfunction.

Clinical Findings: The condition cannot be distinguished from excessive estrogen administration. In pigs, zearalenone primarily affects weaned and prepubertal gilts, in which it causes hyperemia and enlargement of the vulva. There is hypertrophy of the mammary glands and uterus, with occasional prolapse of the latter in severe cases. In multiparous sows, effects of zearalenone include diminished fertility, anestrus, reduced litter size, smaller offspring, and probably fetal resorption; others exhibit either constant estrus or pseudopregnancy.

Dairy heifers may show a range of clinical signs in relation to severity. These include weight loss, vaginal discharge, nymphomania, uterine hypertrophy, and in pregnant heifers, abortion 1-3 mo after conception—usually followed by multiple returns to service. These effects are probable at dietary concentrations of >10 ppm. Young males may become infertile, with atrophy of the testes.

Ewes may show reduced reproductive performance (reduction in ovulation rates and numbers of fertilized ova, and markedly increased duration of estrus) and abortion or premature live births.

Lesions: Lesions in pigs include ovarian atrophy and follicular atresia, uterine edema, cellular hypertrophy in all layers of the uterus, and a cystic appearance in degenerative endometrial glands. The mammary glands show ductal hyperplasia and epithelial proliferation. Squamous metaplasia is seen in the cervix and vagina.

Diagnosis: This is based on reproductive performance in the herd or flock, together with clinical signs and history of diet-related occurrence. Examination of suspect feed for zearalenone and careful examination of reproductive organs at necropsy are required.

Differential diagnoses include reproductive tract infections and other causes of impaired fertility such as diethylstilbestrol in the diet of housed stock. In grazing herbivores, especially sheep, the plant estrogens (eg, isoflavones associated with some varieties of subterranean and red clovers, and coumestans in certain medic [eg, alfalfa] fodders) should be considered.

Treatment: Unless stock are severely or chronically affected, recovery of reproductive functions and regression of signs are usual 1-4 wk after the intake of zearalenone stops. However multiparous sows may remain anestrous up to 8-10 wk.

FACIAL ECZEMA
(Pithomycotoxicosis)

A mycotoxic disease of grazing livestock in which the toxic liver injury commonly results in photodynamic dermatitis. In sheep, the face is the only site of the body that is readily exposed to ultraviolet light, hence the common name. Most common in New Zealand, the disease also occurs in Australia, France, South Africa, several South American countries, and probably North America. Sheep, cattle, and farmed deer of all ages can contract the disease, but it is most severe in young animals.

Etiology and Pathogenesis: Sporidesmins are secondary metabolites of the saprophytic fungus, *Pithomyces chartarum*, which grows on dead pasture litter. The warm ground temperatures and high humidity required for rapid growth of this fungus restrict disease occurrence to hot summer and autumn periods shortly after warm rains. By observing weather conditions and estimating toxic spore numbers on pastures, danger periods can be predicted and farmers alerted.

The sporidesmins are excreted via the biliary system, in which they produce severe cholangitis and pericholangitis as a result of tissue necrosis. Biliary obstruction may occur, which restricts excretion of bile pigments and results in jaundice. Similarly, failure to excrete phylloerythrin in bile leads to photosensitization.

Previous ingestion of toxic spores causes potentiation, thus a succession of small intakes of the spores can lead to subsequent severe outbreaks.

Clinical Findings, Lesions, and Diagnosis: Few signs are apparent until photosensitization and jaundice appear ~10-14 days after intake of the toxins. Animals frantically seek shade. Even short exposure to the sun rapidly produces the typical erythema and edema of photodermatitis in unpigmented skin. The animals suffer considerably, and deaths occur from one to several weeks after photodermatitis appears.

Characteristic liver and bile duct lesions are produced in all affected animals whether photosensitized or not. In acute cases showing photodermatitis, livers are initially enlarged, icteric, and have a marked lobular pattern. Later, there is atrophy and marked fibrosis. The shape is distorted and large nodules of regenerated tissue appear on the surface. In subclinical cases, livers often develop extensive areas in which the tissue is depressed and shrunken below the normal contour, which distorts and roughens the capsule. Generally, these areas are associated with fibrosis and thickening of corresponding bile ducts. Bladders commonly show hemorrhagic or bile-pigment-stained ulcerative erosions of the mucosa with circumscribed edema.

The clinical signs together with characteristic liver lesions are pathognomonic. In live animals, high levels of hepatic enzymes may reflect the extensive injury to the liver.

Control: To minimize intake of pasture litter and toxic spores, short grazing should be avoided. Feeding other feedstuffs during danger periods and encouraging clover dominance in pastures help to provide a milieu unsuited to growth and sporulation of *P chartarum* on litter.

The application of benzimidazole fungicides to pastures considerably restricts the buildup of *P chartarum* spores and reduces pasture toxicity. A pasture area calculated at 1 acre (0.45 hectare)/15 cows or 100 sheep should be sprayed in midsummer with a suspension of thiabendazole, and animals admitted to and maintained on the sprayed areas only when predicted danger periods of fungal activity prevail. The fungicide is effective within 4 days after spraying, provided that no more than 1 in. (2.5 cm) of rain falls within 24 hr during the 4-day period. After this time, heavy rainfall does little to reduce the effectiveness of spraying since the thiabendazole becomes incorporated within the plants. Pastures will then remain safe for ~6 wk. After this period, spraying should be repeated to ensure protection over the entire dangerous season.

Sheep and cattle can be protected from the effects of sporidesmin if given adequate amounts of zinc. Zinc may be administered by drenching with zinc oxide slurry, spraying pastures with zinc oxide, or adding zinc sulfate to drinking water.

Sheep may be selectively bred for natural resistance to toxic effects of sporidesmin. The heritable trait for resistance is high. Ram sires are now being selected in stud and commercial flocks for resistance to the disease either by natural field challenge or by low-level controlled dosage of ram lambs with sporidesmin.

FESCUE POISONING

FESCUE LAMENESS
(Fescue foot)

A condition of cattle, resembling ergot poisoning, caused by a toxic substance in tall fescue (*Festuca arundinacea*). It commences with lameness in one or both hindfeet and may progress to necrosis of the distal part of the affected limb(s). The tail and ears also may be affected independently of the lameness. In addition to gangrene of these extremeties, affected animals may show loss of body mass, an arched back, and a rough coat. Outbreaks have been confirmed in cattle, and similar lesions have been reported in sheep.

Tall fescue is a cool-season perennial grass adapted to a wide range of soil and climatic conditions; it is used in Australia and New Zealand for stabilizing the banks of watercourses. It is the predominant grass in the transition zone in the eastern and central USA. Reliable reports of fescue lameness have come from Kentucky, Tennessee, Florida, California, Colorado, and Missouri, as well as from New Zealand, Australia, and Italy.

The causative toxic substance has actions similar to those produced by sclerotia of *Claviceps purpurea*. Ergot poisoning (*see* above), however, is not the cause of fescue lameness. Ergotism is most prevalent in late summer when the seed heads of grass mature. Fescue lameness is most common in late fall and winter, and has been reproduced in cattle by feeding dried fescue free of seed heads and ergot. Three fungi from toxic pastures have been implicated in fescue foot. *Fusarium sporotrichioides* produces a butenolide *in vitro*, which is capable of inducing some of the lesions of the disease. In addition, 2 clavicipitaceous endophytes, *Balansia epichloe* and *Acremonium coenophialum (Epichloe typhina)*, can synthesize ergot alkaloids in culture. Unequivocal evidence that any of these fungi can cause fescue foot, however, is lacking. The etiology of fescue foot remains unresolved.

Some reports indicate an increased incidence of fescue lameness as the age of the plants increases, and following severe droughts. Strains of tall fescue vary in their toxicity (eg, Kentucky-31 is more toxic than Fawn) due to variation in infection level with the fungus, and high variability within a strain. In some Kentucky-31 fescues, infection levels cannot be detected. High nitrogen applications appear to enhance the toxicity. Susceptibility of cattle is subject to individual variation. Low environmental temperature is thought to exacerbate the lesions; however, high temperatures increase the severity of other toxic problems. One of the causes of **epidemic hyperthermia**, in which a high proportion of a herd of cattle exhibits hypersalivation and hyperthermia, is tall fescue poisoning. It appears that the toxin is a vasoconstrictor that induces hyperthermia in hot weather and results in cold extremities during cold weather. Another cause of this is poisoning with *Claviceps purpurea*.

For clinical findings and control, *see* FESCUE LAMENESS (in cattle), p 497.

SUMMER FESCUE TOXICOSIS

A warm season condition characterized by a reduction in feed intake and weight gains or milk production. The toxin(s) affects cattle, sheep, and horses during the summer when they are grazing or being fed tall fescue forage or seed. The severity of the condition varies from field to field and year to year.

The toxin(s) is present in tall fescue forage or seed contaminated with the endophytic fungus, *Acremonium coenophialum*.

In addition to reduced performance, other signs may appear within 1-2 wk after fescue feeding is started, and include fever, tachypnea, rough coat, lower serum prolactin levels, and excessive salivation; the animals seek wet spots or shade. Lowered reproductive performance also has been reported. Agalactia has been reported for both horses and cattle. (*See also* PERITONEAL FAT NECROSIS, p 222.) Thickened placentae and birth of weak foals have been reported in horses. The severity increases when environmental temperatures are >75-80°F (24-27°C) and if high nitrogen fertilizer has been applied to the grass.

To obtain control, toxic tall fescue pastures must be destroyed and reseeded with seed that does not contain endophytic fungus, since transfer of the fungus from plant to plant is primarily, if not solely, through infected seed. Not using pastures during hot weather, diluting tall fescue pastures with interseeded legumes, or offering other feedstuffs helps reduce severity.

MOLDY CORN POISONING

In the past, disease outbreaks were labeled according to the major source of feed employed at the time of the beginning of disease, eg, moldy corn. As analytical and other laboratory tests improved, the toxins causing the disease are more often than not identified. For these reasons, the term "moldy corn poisoning" has become somewhat meaningless, because the term may refer to aflatoxicosis (qv, p 1679), estrogenism (p 1685), ochratoxicosis (p 1681), trichothecene toxicosis (p 1683), or leukoencephalomalacia (p 1684).

MYCOTOXIC LUPINOSIS

Lupines (*Lupinus* spp) cause 2 distinct forms of poisoning in livestock, viz, lupine poisoning and lupinosis. The former is a nervous syndrome caused by alkaloids present in bitter lupines; the latter is a mycotoxic disease characterized by liver injury and jaundice, which results mainly from the feeding of sweet lupines. Lupinosis is important in Australia and South Africa and also has been reported from New Zealand and Europe. There is increasing use of sweet lupines, either as forage crops or through feeding of their residues after grain harvest as strategic feed for sheep in Mediterranean climate zones. Sheep, and occasionally cattle and horses, are affected, and pigs also are susceptible.

Etiology and Pathogenesis: The causal fungus is *Phomopsis leptostromiformis*, which causes *Phomopsis* stem-blight, especially in white and yellow lupines; blue varieties are resistant. It produces sunken linear stem lesions that contain black stromatic masses, and also affects the pods and seeds. The fungus is also a saprophyte and grows well on dead lupine material, eg, haulm, pods, and stubble, under favorable conditions. The fungus produces phomopsins as secondary metabolites on infected lupine material, especially after rain.

Clinical changes are mainly attributable to toxic hepatocyte injury, which causes mitotic arrest in metaphase, isolated cell necrosis, and hepatic enzyme leakage, with loss of metabolic and excretory function.

Clinical Findings, Lesions, and Diagnosis: Early signs in sheep and cattle are inappetence and listlessness. Complete anorexia and jaundice follow, and ketosis is common. Cattle may show lacrimation and salivation. Sheep may become photosensitive. In acute outbreaks, deaths occur in 2-14 days.

In acute disease, icterus is marked. Livers are enlarged, orange-yellow, and fatty. More chronic cases show bronze- or tan-colored livers that are firm, contracted in size, and fibrotic. Copious amounts of transudates may be found in the abdominal and thoracic cavities and the pericardial sac.

Feeding of moldy lupine material, together with clinical signs and elevations of serum liver enzyme levels, strongly indicate lupinosis.

Control: Frequent surveillance of sheep, and of lupine fodder material for characteristic black spot fungal infestation, especially after rains, is advised. The utilization of lupine cultivars, bred and developed for resistance to *P leptostromiformis* is advocated. Oral doses of zinc ($\geq$0.5 g/day) have given useful protection from phomopsin-induced liver injury to sheep.

PASPALUM STAGGERS

An incoordination resulting from eating paspalum grasses infested by *Claviceps paspali*. The life cycle of this fungus is similar to that of *C purpurea* (*see* ERGOTISM, p 1684). The yellow-gray sclerotia, which mature in the seed heads in autumn, are round and 2-4 mm in diameter. Ingestion of sclerotia causes nervous signs in cattle most commonly, but horses and sheep also are susceptible. Guinea pigs can be affected experimentally. The toxicity is not ascribed to ergot alkaloids; paspalinine and paspalitrem A and B, tremorgenic compounds from the sclerotia, are thought to be the toxic principles.

A sufficiently large single dose causes signs that persist for several days. Animals display continuous trembling of the large muscle groups. If they attempt to move, their action is jerky, and limb movements are incoordinated. If they attempt to run, they fall over in awkward positions. Condition is lost after prolonged exposure, and complete paralysis can occur. The time of onset of signs depends on the degree of the infestation of seed heads and the grazing habits of the animals. Experimentally, early signs appear in cattle after ~100 g of sclerotia per day has been administered for >2 days. Although the mature ergots are toxic, they are most dangerous just when they are maturing to the hard, black (sclerotic) stage.

Recovery follows removal of the animals to feed not contaminated with sclerotia of *C paspali*. Topping of the pasture to remove affected seed heads has been effective in control.

TRICHOTHECENE TOXICOSIS

The trichothecene mycotoxins are a group of closely related secondary metabolic products of several families of imperfect, saprophytic, or plant pathogenic fungi such as *Fusarium, Trichothecium, Myrothecium, Cephalosporium, Stachybotrys, Trichodesma, Cylindrocarpon,* and *Verticimonosporium* spp. The first trichothecenes were isolated in the 1940's and 1950's during the search for antibiotic metabolites of fungi, but only during the last 2 decades have efforts been made to characterize the effects of trichothecenes on mammals and other organisms. On the basis of molecular structure, the trichothecenes are classed as non-macrocyclic (eg, deoxynivalenol or vomitoxin, T-2 toxin, diacetoxyscirpenol, and others) or macrocyclic (satratoxin, roridin, verrucarin).

The trichothecene mycotoxins are highly toxic at the subcellular, cellular, and organic system level. They swiftly penetrate cell lipid bilayers, thus allowing access to DNA, RNA, and cellular organelles. At the subcellular level, these toxins inhibit protein synthesis and covalently bond to sulfhydryl groups.

Trichothecene mycotoxins are generally cytotoxic to most cells, including neoplastic cells; they are not mutagenic. Toxicity of the trichothecenes is based on direct cytotoxicity, and is often referred to as a radiomimetic effect. The cutaneous cytotoxicity that follows administration of these compounds is a nonspecific, acute, necrotizing process with minimal inflammation of both the epidermis and dermis. Stomatitis, hyperkeratosis with ulceration of the esophageal portion of the gastric mucosa, and necrosis of the GI tract have been seen following ingestion of trichothecenes.

Given in sublethal toxic doses via any route, the trichothecenes are highly immunosuppressive in mammals; however, long-term feeding of high levels of T-2 toxin does not seem to activate latent viral or bacterial infections. The main immunosuppressive effect of the trichothecenes is at the level of the T suppressor cell, but the toxins may affect function of helper T cells, B cells, or macrophages, or the interaction between all of these cells.

Hemorrhagic diatheses may occur following thrombocytopenia, or defective intrinsic or extrinsic coagulation pathways. It appears that hemorrhage results from depression of clotting factors, thrombocytopenia, inhibition of platelet function, or possibly a combination of these.

Refusal to consume contaminated feedstuff is the typical sign, which limits development of other signs. If no other food is offered, animals may eat reluctantly, but in some instances, excessive salivation and vomiting may occur. In the past, the ability to cause vomiting had been ascribed to deoxynivalenol only, hence the common name, **vomitoxin**. However, other members of the trichothecene family also can induce vomiting. Irritation of the skin and mucous membranes and gastroenteritis are another set of signs typical of trichothecene toxicosis. Hemorrhagic diatheses can occur, and the radiomimetic injury (damage to dividing cells) is expressed as lymphopenia or pancytopenia. Paresis, seizures, and paralysis occur in almost all species. Eventually, hypotension may led to death.

Due to the immunosuppressive action of trichothecenes, secondary bacterial, viral, or parasitic infections may mask the primary injury. The lymphatic organs are smaller than normal, and may be difficult to find on necropsy.

Until now, no specific name has been given to most non-macrocyclic trichothecene-related diseases, although the term **fusariotoxicosis** is often used. Some other names used are: moldy corn poisoning in cattle, bean hull poisoning of horses, and feed refusal and emetic syndrome in pigs. A condition in chickens, referred to as "rickets in broilers", is also thought to be caused by trichothecenes.

Macrocyclic trichothecene-related disease have received a number of specific names. The best known is **stachybotryotoxicosis** of horses, cattle, sheep, pigs, and poultry, first diagnosed in the USSR, but occurring also in Europe and South Africa. Cutaneous and mucocutaneous lesions, panleukopenia, nervous signs, and abortions have been encountered. Death may occur in 2-12 days.

Myrotheciotoxicosis and **dendrodochiotoxicosis** have been reported from the USSR, and New Zealand. The signs resemble those of stachybotryotoxicosis, but death may occur in 1-5 days.

Diagnosis: Because the clinical signs are so nonspecific, or masked by secondary infections and disease, diagnosis is difficult. Analysis of feed sample is often costly and time consuming, but should be attempted. Interim measures are careful examination of feedstuff for signs of mold growth or caking of feed particles, and switching to an alternate feed supply. Change of feed supply often results in immediate improvement, and thus may provide one more clue that the original feed was contaminated.

Control: Symptomatic treatment and feeding of uncontaminated feed are probably the best choice. (Steroidal antishock and anti-inflammatory agents, such as methylprednisolone, prednisolone, and dexamethasone, have been used successfully in trials.) Poultry and cattle are more tolerant of trichothecenes than pigs.

NITRATE AND NITRITE POISONING

Many species are susceptible to nitrate/nitrite poisoning, but cattle are affected most frequently. Ruminants are especially vulnerable because the ruminal flora reduces nitrate to ammonia, with nitrite, which is ~10 times more toxic than nitrate, as an intermediate product. Nitrate reduction (and nitrite production) also occurs in the cecum of equids, but not to the same extent as in ruminants. Young pigs also have GI microflora capable of reducing nitrate to nitrite, but mature monogastric animals (except equids) are more resistant to nitrate toxicosis because this pathway is age limited.

Acute intoxication is manifest primarily by methemoglobin formation (nitrite ion in contact with RBC reacts with Hgb to form a stable methemoglobin) and resultant anoxia. Secondary effects due to vasodilatory action of the nitrite ion on vascular smooth muscle may occur. The nitrite ion may also alter metabolic protein enzymes. Ingested nitrates may directly irritate the GI mucosa, and produce abdominal pain and diarrhea.

Though usually acute, the effects of nitrite or nitrate toxicity may be subacute or chronic, and include retarded growth, lowered milk production, vitamin A deficiency, minor transitory goitrogenic effects, abortions, and increased susceptibility to infection.

Etiology: Nitrates and/or nitrites are used in pickling and curing brines for preserving meats, certain machine oils and antirust tablets, gunpowder and explosives, and fertilizers, and may serve as therapeutic agents for certain noninfectious diseases, eg, cyanide poisoning. Toxicoses occur most commonly in unacclimated domestic animals from ingestion of plants that contain excess nitrate, but also from accidental ingestion of fertilizer or other chemicals. Nitrate levels may be hazardous in ponds that receive extensive feedlot or fertilizer runoff; these types of waters may also contaminate shallow, poorly cased wells. Although nitrate concentrations are increasing in groundwater in the USA, well water is rarely the sole cause of excess nitrate exposure.

Water with high nitrate levels and significant coliform contamination has greater potential to affect health adversely and lower productivity than do either nitrate or bacteria alone. Livestock losses have occurred during cold weather due to the concentrating effect of freezing, which increases nitrate content of remaining water in stock tanks.

Crops that readily concentrate nitrate include cereal grasses (especially oats, millet, and rye), corn (maize), sunflower, and sorghums. Weeds that commonly have high nitrate concentrations are pigweed, lamb's quarter, thistle, Jimson weed, fireweed (*Kochia*), smartweed, dock, and Johnson grass. Anhydrous ammonia and nitrate fertilizers and soils naturally high in nitrogen tend to increase nitrate content in forage.

Excess nitrate in plants is generally associated with damp weather conditions and cool temperatures (55°F [13°C]), although high concentrations are also likely to develop when growth is rapid during hot, humid weather. Drought conditions, however, particularly if occurring when plants are immature, may leave the vegetation with high nitrate content. Decreased light, cloudy weather, and shading associated with crowding conditions can also cause increased concentrations of nitrates within plants. Well-aerated soil with a low pH, and low or deficient amounts of molybdenum, sulfur, or phosphorus in soil tend to enhance nitrate uptake, whereas soil deficiencies of copper, cobalt, or manganese tend to have opposing effects. Anything that stunts growth increases nitrate accumulation in the lower part of the plant. Phenoxy acid derivative herbicides, eg, 2,4-D and 2,4,5-T, applied to nitrate-accumulating plants during early stages, cause increased growth and a high nitrate residual (10-30%) in surviving plants, which are lush and eaten with apparent relish even though previously avoided.

Nitrate, which does not selectively accumulate in fruits or grain, is found chiefly in the lower stalk. Nitrate in plants can be converted to nitrite under the proper conditions of moisture, heat, and microbial activity after harvesting.

Clinical Findings: Signs of nitrite poisoning usually appear suddenly due to tissue hypoxia and low blood pressure as a consequence of vasodilation. Rapid weak heart beat, subnormal body temperature, muscular tremors, weakness, and ataxia are early signs of toxicosis. Brown, cyanotic mucous membranes develop rapidly. Rapid difficult breathing, and anxiety and frequent urination are common. Some monogastric animals, usually because of excess nitrate exposure from non-plant sources, exhibit salivation, vomiting, diarrhea, abdominal pain, and gastric hemorrhage. Affected animals may die suddenly without appearing ill, in terminal anoxic convulsions within 1 hr, or after a clinical course of 12-24 hr or longer. Under certain conditions, adverse effects may not be apparent until animals have been eating nitrate-containing forages for days to weeks. Some that develop marked dyspnea recover, but then develop interstitial pulmonary emphysema and continue to suffer respiratory distress; most of these recover fully within 10-14 days. Abortion and stillbirths may occur in some cattle. Prolonged excess nitrate exposure coupled with cold stress and inadequate nutrition may lead to the alert downer cow syndrome in pregnant beef cattle; sudden collapse and death can result.

Lesions: Blood that contains methemoglobin usually has a chocolate-brown color, although dark red hues may also be observed. Pinpoint or larger hemorrhages on serosal surfaces may be seen. Dark brown discoloration evident in moribund or recently dead animals is not pathognomonic however, and other methemoglobin inducers must be considered. If necropsy is postponed too long, the brown discoloration may disappear with conversion back to Hgb.

Diagnosis: Excess nitrate exposure can be assessed by laboratory analysis for nitrate in both antemortem and postmortem specimens. High nitrate and nitrite values in postmortem specimens may be an incidental finding, and indicative only of exposure and not toxicity. Plasma is the preferred antemortem specimen, since some plasma-protein-bound nitrate could be lost in the clot if serum was collected. Additional postmortem specimens from either toxicoses or abortions include ocular fluids, fetal pleural or thoracic fluids, fetal stomach contents, and maternal uterine fluid. All specimens should be frozen in clean plastic or glass containers before submission, except when whole blood is collected for methemoglobin analysis. Because the amount of nitrate in rumen contents is not representative of concentrations in the diet, evaluation of rumen contents is not recommended.

Methemoglobin analysis alone is not a reliable indicator of excess nitrate/nitrite exposure except in acute toxicosis, because 50% of methemoglobin present will be converted back to Hgb in ~2 hr, and alternate forms of nonoxygenated Hgb that may be formed by reaction with nitrite are not detected by methemoglobin analysis.

Field tests for nitrate include diphenylamine blue (1% DPB in concentrated sulfuric acid) and nitrate test strips. All field tests are presumptive and should be confirmed by standard analytical methods at a qualified laboratory. The DPB test is more suitable to determine presence or absence of nitrate in suspected forages. Nitrate test strips (dipsticks) are effective in determining nitrate values in water supplies, and can be used to evaluate nitrate and nitrite content in serum, plasma, ocular fluid, and urine.

Differential diagnoses include poisonings by cyanide, urea, pesticides, toxic gases (eg, carbon monoxide, hydrogen sulfide), chlorates, aniline dyes, aminophenols, drugs (eg, sulfonamides, phenacetin, and acetaminophen), infectious or noninfectious diseases (eg, grain overload, hypocalcemia, hypomagnesemia, pulmonary adenomatosis, or emphysema), and any sudden unexplained deaths.

Treatment: Slow IV injection of 1% methylene blue in distilled water or isotonic saline should be given at 4-22 mg/kg body wt, or more, depending on severity of exposure. Lower dosages may be repeated in 20-30 min if the initial response is not satisfactory. Lower dosages of methylene blue can be used in all species, but only ruminants can safely tolerate higher ones. If additional exposure or absorption occurs during therapy, retreating with methylene blue q6-8hr should be considered. Rumen lavage with cold water and antibiotics may stop the continuing microbial production of nitrite.

Control: Animals may adapt to higher nitrate content in feeds, especially when grazing summer annuals such as sorghum-sudan hybrids. Multiple, small feedings help animals adapt. Trace mineral supplements and a balanced diet may help prevent nutritional/metabolic disorders associated with long-term excess dietary nitrate consumption. Feeding grain with high-nitrate forages may reduce nitrite production.

High-nitrate forages may also be harvested and stored as ensilage rather than dried hay or green chop; up to half the nitrate content in forages may be lost. Raising cutter heads of machinery during harvesting operations selectively leaves the more hazardous stalk bases in the field.

Hay appears to be more hazardous than fresh green chop or pasture with similar nitrate content. Heating may assist bacterial conversion of nitrate to nitrite; feeding high-nitrate hay, straw, or fodder that has been damp or wet for several days, or stockpiled, green-chopped forage should be avoided. Large round bales with excess nitrate are especially dangerous if stored outside; rain or snow can leach and subsequently concentrate most of the total nitrate present into the lower third of these bales.

Water transported in improperly cleaned liquid fertilizer tanks can be extremely high in nitrate. Young unweaned livestock, especially neonatal pigs, can be more sensitive to nitrate in water.

NONPROTEIN NITROGEN POISONING
(Ammonia toxicosis)

Usually an acute, rapidly progressing, highly fatal condition caused by ingestion of excess urea or other sources of nonprotein nitrogen (NPN). Sources of NPN have different toxicities in various species, but mature ruminants are affected most commonly. After ingestion, NPN undergoes hydrolysis and releases excess ammonia (NH_3) into the GI tract, which is absorbed and leads to hyperammonemia.

Etiology: The most common sources of NPN in feeds are urea, urea phosphate, and ammonia (anhydrous) and salts such as monoammonium- and diammonium phosphate. Because feed-grade urea is unstable, it is formulated (usually pelleted) to prevent degradation to NH_3. Biuret, a less toxic source of NPN, is now used less than in the past. Natural protein sources such as rice hulls, cottonseed meal, and straw or other low-quality forages may be treated with anhydrous ammonia to increase available nitrogen in supplemented livestock diets. Most sources of NPN are usually provided to ruminants by direct addition of dry supplement to a complete mixed or blended diet, free-choice access to NPN-containing range blocks or cubes, or lick tank systems combined with molasses as a supplement. NPN poisoning is a common sequela of abrupt change to urea or other NPN in the diet when only natural protein was previously fed. Also, farm animals sometimes drink liquid fertilizers or ingest dry granular fertilizers that contain ammonium salts or urea.

Ruminants are most sensitive because urease is normally present in the functional rumen after 50 days of age. Dietary exposure of unacclimated ruminants to 0.3-0.5 g of urea/kg body wt may cause adverse effects; doses of 1-1.5 g/kg are usually lethal. Urease activity in the equine cecum is ~25% that of the rumen, and horses may receive NPN as a feed additive; however, horses are more sensitive to urea than other monogastrics, and doses ≥4 g/kg can be lethal. Ammonium salts at 0.3-0.5 g/kg may be toxic in all species and ages of farm animals; doses ≥1.5 g/kg usually are fatal. Pigs and neonatal calves are generally unaffected by ingestion of urea except for a transient diuresis.

Livestock may require days or weeks for total adaptation before rumen microflora can utilize the gradually increasing amounts of urea or other NPN in the diets; however, adaptation is lost relatively quickly (1-3 days) once NPN is removed from the diet.

Diets low in energy and high in fiber are more commonly associated with NPN toxicosis, even in acclimated animals. Highly palatable supplements, such as liquid molasses or large protein blocks crumbled by precipitation, may lead to consumption of lethal amounts of NPN, as may improperly maintained lick tanks.

Clinical Findings: The period from urea ingestion to onset of clinical signs is 20-60 min in cattle, 30-90 min in sheep, and longer in horses. Early signs include muscle tremors (especially of face and ears), exophthalmia, abdominal pain, frothy salivation, polyuria, and bruxism. Tremors progress to incoordination and weakness. Pulmonary edema leads to marked salivation, dyspnea, and gasping.

Horses may exhibit head pressing; cattle are often agitated, hyperirritable, violent, and belligerent as toxicosis progresses; sheep usually appear depressed. An early sign in cattle is rumen atony; as toxicosis progresses, ruminal tympany is usually evident, and violent struggling and bellowing, a marked jugular pulse, severe twitching, tetanic spasms, and convulsions may be observed. The PCV, and serum levels of NH_3, glucose, lactate, potassium, phosphorus, AST (SGOT), ALT (SGPT), and BUN usually are significantly increased.

As death nears, animals become cyanotic, dyspneic, anuric, and hyperthermic, and blood pH decreases from 7.4 to 7.0. Regurgitation may occur, especially in sheep. Death related to excess NPN usually occurs within 2 hr in cattle, 4 hr in sheep, and 3-12 hr in horses. Survivors recover in 12-24 hr with no sequelae.

Lesions: Carcasses of animals dying of NPN poisoning appear to bloat and decompose rapidly, with no specific characteristic lesions. Frequently, pulmonary edema, congestion, and petechial hemorrhages may be observed. Mild bronchitis and catarrhal gastroenteritis are often reported. Regurgitated and inhaled rumen contents are commonly found in the trachea and bronchi, especially in sheep. The odor of NH_3 may or may not be apparent in ingesta from a freshly opened rumen or cecum. A ruminal or cecal pH ≥7.5 from a recently dead animal is highly suggestive of NPN poisoning. The ruminal pH remains stable for several hours after death under most circumstances, but continues to rise in NPN toxicosis.

Diagnosis: NPN poisoning is suggested by signs, lesions, history of acute illness, and dietary exposure. Exposure to excess NPN may be evaluated through laboratory analysis for the ammonia nitrogen (NH_3-N) in both ante- and postmortem specimens, and for urea or other NPN in suspected feeds and other dietary sources. Specimens for NH_3-N analysis include ruminal-reticular fluid, serum, whole blood, and urine. All specimens should be frozen immediately after collection and thawed only for analysis; alternatively, ruminal-reticular fluid may be preserved with a few drops of saturated mercuric chloride solution to each 100 mL of specimen.

Animals dead more than a few hours in hot ambient temperatures or 12 hr in moderate climates probably have undergone too much autolysis to be of diagnostic value.

The amount of urea or the equivalent NPN in biological specimens is meaningless; however, urea and NPN should be determined in representative feeds and other dietary sources. Values for urea and NPN in feed permit calculation of the protein equivalent (1 part protein = 0.34 parts urea; 1 part urea = 2.92 parts protein) in feed as well as the total estimated dose of NPN ingested.

Concentrations of $\geq$2 mg/100 mL NH_3-N in blood or serum indicate excess NPN exposure. The concentration of NH_3-N in ruminal-reticular fluid is >80 mg/100 mL in most cases of NPN poisoning, and may be >200 mg/100 mL. Acclimated ruminants fed diets high in legume hay, soybean meal, cottonseed meal, linseed meal, fish meal, or milk by-products may have rumen fluid NH_3-N concentrations approaching 60 mg/100 mL with no apparent toxicity. The pH of ruminal-reticular fluid should also be determined; a pH of 7.5-8 (at time of death) is indicative of NPN toxicity.

Differential diagnoses include: poisonings by nitrate/nitrite, cyanide, 4-methylimidazole, lead, pesticides, and toxic gases (carbon monoxide, hydrogen sulfide, nitrogen dioxide); acute infectious diseases; and noninfectious diseases such as encephalopathies (leukoencephalomalacia, hepatic encephalopathy, polioencephalomalacia, and others), enterotoxemia/rumen autointoxication, protein engorgement, grain engorgement, rumen tympany, and pulmonary adenomatosis. Nutritional/metabolic disorders related to hypocalcemia, hypomagnesemia, and other elemental aberrations should also be considered.

A CNS disorder in cattle fed ammoniated hay, silage, molasses, and protein blocks is thought to be caused by the formation of 4-methylimidizole through the action of NH_3 on soluble carbohydrates (sugars) in these feedstuffs. Elevated blood NH_3 concentrations are not thought to be responsible for the toxic manifestations. Affected cattle have wildly aberrant behavior, causing the syndrome to be called "bovine bonkers". Since nursing calves are affected, the toxic principle apparently is excreted in milk.

Treatment: Examination and treatment may be difficult because of violent behavior. Animals that are recumbent and moribund usually do not respond favorably to treatment.

If possible, affected animals should be treated by ruminal infusion of 5% acetic acid/vinegar at 0.5-2 L in sheep and goats, and 2-8 L in cattle (ruminal-reticular fluid specimens for analysis should be taken before acetic acid therapy). Concomitant infusion of iced (0-4°C) water (up to 40 L in adult cattle, proportionally less in sheep and goats) is also recommended. Acetic acid lowers rumen pH and prevents further NH_3 absorption; administration may have to be repeated if affected animals again show clinical signs. Acetic acid also inactivates existing NH_3 in the GI tract and rapidly forms ammonium acetate, which can be utilized by rumen microflora but does not release NH_3. Cold water lowers the rumen temperature and dilutes the reacting media, which slows urease activity. In valuable animals, removed rumen contents should be replaced with a hay slurry, and a transfer of some rumen contents from a healthy animal may serve as an inoculum to restore normal function, although severely affected animals may not survive. Ruminal tympany should be corrected if indicated, and a trochar may be installed to prevent recurrence.

Pulmonary edema is difficult to treat, although lowering blood pressure, as with α-adrenergic blocking agents such as ergotamine, may help.

Supportive therapy is also indicated: isotonic saline solutions IV to correct dehydration, and calcium gluconate and magnesium solutions IV to relieve tetanic seizures.

Prevention and Control: Urea should not be fed at a rate exceeding 2-3% of the concentrate or grain portion of ruminant diets, and should be limited to ≤1% of the total diet. Additionally, NPN should constitute no more than one-third of the total nitrogen in the ruminant diet. Once the decision is made to feed NPN, animals must be slowly adapted to, and maintained on, a consistent dietary NPN content with no significant deviation. Temporary absences of NPN from the diet should be avoided at all costs. While properly adapted adult cattle can tolerate up to 1 g urea/kg body wt/day, a safer feeding rate is no more than half that amount.

PENTACHLOROPHENOL POISONING
(Penta poisoning)

Penta has been used as a fungicide, molluscicide, insecticide, and as a wood preservative, and is still used for outdoor wood treatment. It should never be used indoors. It can be absorbed through the intact skin and lungs, and it is an intense irritant to the skin and mucous membranes. When absorbed, it increases metabolism by uncoupling cellular phosphorylation. Animals fed in troughs made of lumber treated with penta may salivate and have irritated oral mucosa. Vaporization or leaching of penta in pens, enclosures, homes, and barns has caused illness and death. Signs of poisoning include nervousness, rapid pulse and respiratory rate, weakness, muscle tremors, fever, and convulsions, followed by death. Chronic poisoning results in fatty liver, nephrosis, and weight loss. Additional problems reported with contaminated shavings include "off flavors" in broilers, impaired immune response in chickens, and possibly decreased fertility in boars. Penta can cause residues in animal tissues. Also, a significant amount of hexachlorobenzene is metabolized in animal tissues to penta.

Whole blood analysis for penta may aid in the diagnosis of poisoning. There is no known antidote. Termination of exposure, bathing dermally exposed animals, oral administration of activated charcoal, and supportive therapy may be indicated. Recently, many commercial lots of technical grade penta were shown to contain small but biologically significant amounts of highly toxic impurities (dioxins and furans). Cattle, pigs, and chickens exposed to wood treated with commercial grade penta that contained these contaminants have shown increased mortality, decreased productivity, and other less specific herd health problems. (*See* HALOGENATED CY-CLIC HYDROCARBON POISONING, p 1654.) Antipyretics, eg, aspirin and acetaminophen, should not be used. Treatment involves cooling the animal and removing it from the source of poison, and administering fluids, electrolytes, and anticonvulsants.

PETROLEUM PRODUCT POISONING

Ingestion of petroleum, petroleum condensate, gasoline, diesel fuel, kerosene, or other hydrocarbon mixtures may cause illness or death. Cattle, and less frequently sheep or goats, may ingest such products because they are curious, water is not available, food or water is contaminated, or when seeking salt or other nutrients; a cow may consume several gallons at one time.

Petroleum fractions have been used as insecticides and acaricides for many years, either alone or as part of formulations. Small quantities of these may be applied to the skin with little or no harmful effects, but large quantities can induce severe reactions. Pipeline breaks, accidental release from storage tanks, and tank car accidents may contaminate land and water supplies. Animals may have access to open or leaky containers of fuel or other hydrocarbon materials. The toxicity of a hydrocarbon mixture is related primarily to its highly volatile, low molecular weight components; however, crude petroleum that has lost much of its lighter components through weathering is still hazardous. Variation in composition of petroleum and petroleum-derived hydrocarbon mixtures explains some of the differences in toxic effects. Mixtures of low viscosity, eg, gasoline, naphtha, and kerosene, have a high aspiration hazard and irritant activity on pulmonary tissues. Gasoline and naphtha fractions may induce vomiting, which contributes to aspiration hazard. Fractions more viscous than kerosene are less likely to be inhaled, and even if aspirated produce a less fulminating pneumonia. Lubricating oils and greases are hazardous more because of toxic additives or contaminates (eg, highly chlorinated naphthalenes, lead) than because of natural petroleum constituents. On occasion, waste oils have contained highly toxic substances such as tetrachlorodibenzodioxin (TCDD).

Clinical Findings: Petroleum hydrocarbon toxicity may involve the respiratory, GI, or central nervous systems, and/or the skin. Pneumonia due to aspiration of hydrocarbons and rumen contents into the lungs is usually the most serious consequence of ingestion of these materials. Acute bloat may cause death shortly following consumption of highly volatile hydrocarbons, eg, gasoline, naphtha. CNS effects consistent with the anesthetic-like action of low-molecular-weight hydrocarbons and cerebral anoxia are sometimes present, and are usually associated with aspiration. Signs range from sudden death due to bloat to no observable effect. Anorexia, decreased rumen motility, and mild depression may begin in ~24 hr and last 3-14 days depending on dose and content. Hypoglycemia may occur several days after ingestion. These signs and weight loss may be the only responses seen in animals that do not bloat or aspirate oil. Some fail to reestablish normal rumen function and develop a chronic wasting condition.

Oil may not affect the feces for several days following ingestion, at which time the feces become dry and formed when kerosene or lighter hydrocarbon fractions are ingested; in contrast, heavier hydrocarbon mixtures tend to be cathartic. Regurgitated or vomited oil may be seen on the muzzle and lips. Signs attributable to pulmonary adsorption of hydrocarbons or cerebral anoxia include excitability, depression, shivering, head tremors, apparent visual dysfunction, and incoordination. Acute pneumonia and possibly pleuritis (coughing, rapid shallow respiration, reluctance to move, head held low, weakness, oily nasal discharge, dehydrated appearance) occur in some animals that aspirate highly volatile mixtures; death usually occurs within days. Respiratory signs may be limited to dyspnea shortly before death in animals that aspirate heavier hydrocarbons. Increased PCV, Hgb, and BUN, indicating mild to moderate hemoconcentration, are associated with development of pneumonia. Neutropenia, lymphopenia, and eosinopenia occur initially, and are followed by a relative increase in neutrophils. The WBC count may remain low, return to normal, or be moderately elevated near-term. Abortion several days following exposure is occasionally seen in oil-field cases.

When larger quantities (eg, 60 g of xylene per adult cow) are applied to the skin, severe reactions may occur: anorexia, depression, dyspnea, salivation, vomiting, dizziness, trembling, and even death.

Lesions: Aspiration pneumonia is the most consistent postmortem finding in animals that did not die of bloat. This may be accompanied by tracheitis, pleuritis, and hydrothorax if highly volatile fractions such as gasoline or naphtha are involved. Lung lesions are usually bilateral and found in the caudoventral apical, cardiac, cranioventral diaphragmatic, and intermediate lobes. Affected portions are dark red and consolidated, and may contain multiple abscesses. Encapsulated pulmonary abscesses may be found in cattle surviving up to several months following aspiration. Skin lesions may be obvious following topical application/exposure, and include drying, cracking, or blistering.

Diagnosis: Hydrocarbon odor may be in lungs, ruminal contents, and feces. Despite ingestion of large doses, hydrocarbons may not be visible in ruminal contents after ~4 days. Adding warm water to the GI contents may cause any oily contents to collect at the surface, but finding oil in the GI tract does not in itself justify a diagnosis of poisoning; most oils have low toxicity if not aspirated. Samples of GI contents, lung, liver, kidney, and the suspected source should be collected for chemical analysis to demonstrate presence of hydrocarbons in tissue (particularly lung) and GI contents, and to match those found in tissues and ingesta with the suspected source. Samples must be carefully protected from cross-contamination during necropsy and transportation to the laboratory. Positive chemical findings together with appropriate clinical and pathologic findings are confirmatory. Diagnosis in oil-field situations is often complicated by involvement of other toxicants, eg, explosives, lead from grease and "pipe dope", arsenicals, organophosphate esters, caustics (acids or alkalis), and saltwater.

Treatment: Bloat pressure should be released by passing a stomach tube; using a trocar risks forcing oil into the peritoneal cavity and results in peritonitis. In the absence of bloat, the prime objectives are to prevent aspiration and to mitigate GI dysfunction. Ruminal lavage via stomach tube increases the risk of aspiration; rumenotomy to remove ruminal contents and replace them with healthy ruminal material is safer. More chronic cases involving primarily hypofunction of the rumen may also respond to this procedure. Cathartics, if used, should be of the saline type.

Because secondary infection may be important, broad-spectrum antimicrobials should be given for ≥7 days to animals known or suspected to have consumed oil. The use of steroids in hydrocarbon aspiration is questionable and may be harmful. Treatment of aspiration pneumonia (qv, p 709) is rarely effective; prognosis is poor. However, because signs of aspiration may not appear for several days, prognosis based on initial clinical findings may be misleading.

Treatment of poisoning or damage due to cutaneous exposure should be directed at removal of the material from the skin with the aid of soap or detergents and copious amounts of cool water, but without brushing or abrading the skin. Further treatment depends on the clinical signs, and is largely restricted to supportive therapy.

Petroleum hydrocarbon poisoning can be avoided only by preventing access to these materials.

PYRROLIZIDINE ALKALOIDOSIS
(Seneciosis, Senecio poisoning, Ragwort toxicity)

Typically, a chronic poisoning that results in hepatic failure. It is caused by many toxic plants, most commonly of the genera *Senecio, Crotalaria, Heliotropium, Amsinckia, Echium, Cynoglossum,* and *Trichodesma.* These plants grow mainly in temperate climates, but some (eg, *Crotalaria* spp) require tropical or subtropical climates. The plants most commonly responsible are ragwort (*S jacobea*), woolly groundsel (*S redellii, S longilobus*), rattleweed (*Crotalaria retusa*), and seeds of yellow tarweed (*A intermedia*).

Cattle, horses, farmed deer, and pigs are most susceptible. Poisoning in sheep and goats requires ~20 times more plant material than in cattle. Individual susceptibility varies greatly within species; young growing animals are most susceptible.

Etiology and Pathogenesis: More than 30 toxic factors (alkaloids with a pyrrolizidine base) have been found in the plants. It is likely that their toxic effects are unique. *Senecio jacobaea* contains jacobine; retrorsine, seneciphylline, and monocrotaline are other pyrrolizidine alkaloids frequently incriminated in toxicities.

Under normal conditions these plants are avoided by grazing animals, but during drought conditions they may be eaten; an occasional animal will become habituated to the plant, even when good forage is available. Animals are also poisoned by eating the plant material in hay or silage. Seeds from *Crotalaria, Amsinckia,* and *Heliotropium* spp, which have been harvested with grain, have been responsible for the disease in horses, cattle, pigs, and poultry. Some animals may eat these plants preferentially as roughage when they are available on extremely lush pasture.

The toxic alkaloids are metabolized to highly reactive pyrroles, which produce cytotoxic effects on target sites, most commonly nuclei of hepatocytes. There is an antimitotic effect, the precise mechanism of which is unknown. Other target sites are renal and pulmonary vascular and fibrous tissues. Alkaloids of *Crotalaria* affect the widest range of tissues in most species.

Clinical Findings: The signs and pathological effects are similar in all animal species regardless of the species of plant involved or the toxic pyrrolizidine alkaloids it contains. The acute form, characterized by sudden death from hemorrhagic liver necrosis and visceral hemorrhages, is rare. Effects on the liver of repeated low intake of toxic plants are cumulative and progressive; clinical signs may not be seen for several weeks or months (often after consumption of the plant has ceased). In *Heliotropium* poisoning, severe losses are produced in sheep only after they have grazed the plants for a second season. In sheep, the liver may store excess copper, which eventually may lead to the hemolytic crisis of chronic copper poisoning (qv, p 1645).

In horses and cattle, some of the signs are loss of condition, anorexia, dullness, and constipation or diarrhea. Tenesmus and passing of blood-stained feces may be followed by rectal prolapse, especially in cattle. Ascites and icterus may be present, and cattle and sheep sometimes show intermittent photosensitization. Some animals become progressively weaker and rarely move, while others wander aimlessly with an awkward gait, either stumbling against or actively pushing headlong into fences or other structures. Still others may become frenzied and dangerously aggressive. Pica may be observed. Death may occur suddenly or following prolonged recumbency with hepatic coma and high blood-ammonia levels.

Lesions: In acute cases the liver may be enlarged, hemorrhagic, and icteric; in chronic cases it is atrophied, fibrous, finely nodular, and usually pale with a glistening surface due to fibrous thickening of the capsule. Other livers are markedly icteric. The gallbladder is often edematous and grossly distended with thick, mucoid bile. Edema of the abomasum and segments of the bowel, mesentery, and associated lymph nodes is common, and much ascitic fluid may be found in the abdominal cavity. In some cases, numerous small hemorrhages are present in the abdominal serous membranes.

Characteristic histological changes occur in the liver. Irreversible enlargement of individual hepatocytes (megalocytosis) is unique, and is conspicuous in horses and sheep, but less pronounced in cattle. In cattle, marked perivenous fibrosis of sublobular veins is usually present, but this is not a consistent finding in horses and sheep. In all species there are marked increases in connective tissue, both within and around the lobules. Bile duct hyperplasia is variable, but may be the most striking microscopic change seen in some affected livers. Pigs may show pulmonary congestion, hemorrhage, septal fibrosis, alveolar epithelialization, and emphysema. Renal tubule, lining cells, and glomerular epithelial cells also may be individually enlarged.

Diagnosis: A diagnosis based on history, clinical signs, and gross necropsy findings can usually be confirmed by histological examination of liver and renal tissue. When liver cirrhosis is extensive, hypoalbuminemia and hyperglobulinemia develop, and serum levels of fibrinogen, bilirubin, γ glutamyl transferase, and glutamate dehydrogenase are generally elevated. Effects of other plant and fungal hepatotoxins and nephrotoxins, and chronic fascioliasis, must be ruled out.

Treatment and Control: Further intake of toxic plant material must be prevented. Animals showing signs rarely recover, and lesions present in asymptomatic animals may progress and result in further losses over several months. Since high protein intake may prove harmful, rations high in carbohydrates are indicated. Methionine in 10% dextrose solution, IV, is said to be of value in treating horses.

The diminished ability of the liver to regenerate after pyrrolizidine alkaloid poisoning suggests a guarded prognosis. Factors in preventing further outbreaks should be stressed.

Sheep are commonly used for grazing control of *S jacobaea, H europaeum,* and *E plantagineum,* although the practice carries risks unless sheep destined for early slaughter are used. Biological control of plants with predator moths, flea beetles, and seed flies is being attempted and has met with variable success. Control of *Senecio* and related toxic species in pastures by annual herbicide applications, preferably in spring before hay or silage conservation, gives satisfactory control of the plants. Measures that enhance destruction of the alkaloids in the rumen of sheep also have shown some promise.

POISONOUS PLANTS OF TEMPERATE NORTH AMERICA

INTRODUCTION

See also p 1658.

Poisonous plants are among the important causes of economic loss to the livestock industry; they should be considered when evaluating livestock illness and decreased productivity. Poisonous plants affect animals in many ways: death, chronic illness and debilitation, decreased weight gain, abortion, birth defects, increased parturition interval, and photosensitization. In addition to these more obvious losses, loss of forage, additional fencing, increased labor and management costs, and frequently, interference with proper harvesting of forage must be considered.

Most poisonous range plants fall into 2 general categories: 1) those that are indigenous to a range and increase with heavy grazing, and 2) those that invade after overgrazing or disturbance of the land. Among those not in these categories are certain locoweeds and larkspurs, both of which form part of the normal range plant community. Poisonous plants can be found in most plant communities, and should be considered in most grazing situations.

Livestock poisoning by plants often can be traced to problems of management or range condition, or both, rather than simply to the presence of poisonous plants. Usually, animals are poisoned because hunger or other conditions cause them to graze abnormally. Overgrazing, trucking, trailing, corraling, or introducing animals onto a new range tend to induce hunger or change behavior, and poisoning may occur.

Not all poisonous plants are unpalatable, nor are they restricted to overgrazed ranges and pastures. Furthermore, poisonous plants do not always kill or otherwise harm animals when consumed. Many plants can be useful forage or toxic, eg, plants such as lupine and greasewood may be part of an animal's diet, and the animal is poisoned only when it consumes too much of the plant too fast. To prevent poisoning, it is important to understand the factors involved when a useful forage becomes a poisonous plant.

Definitive diagnosis of suspect plant poisonings is difficult. Most individuals need not concern themselves with large numbers of poisonous plants; they need only be acquainted with those growing in the area where they are involved with livestock, but they should be acutely aware of those plants and the conditions under which livestock may be poisoned. A tentative diagnosis is possible if one knows of: 1) any local soil deficiencies or excesses (which may complicate plant toxicities or simply confuse as to cause of a syndrome), 2) the syndromes associated with each of the poisonous plants in the area, 3) the time of year during which each is most likely to cause problems, 4) the detailed history of the animal(s) over the last 6-8 mo, and 5) any change of management or environmental condition that may cause an animal to change its diet or grazing habits. Indeed, in some cases, eg, locoism, this may be all that is required in addition to identification of the plant involved. Identification of the plant is important, whatever its stage of growth—and is especially useful if it can be identified in the stomach contents of the poisoned animal. Chemical analysis of toxicants often is not useful. Metabolic profiles are useful for some toxicities, and in some, the postmortem lesions are distinctive.

Table 4. Poisonous Plants of Temperate North America

Dangerous Season	Scientific Name	Common Name	Habitat and Distribution	Affected Animals	Important Characteristics	Toxic Principle and Effects	Remarks and Treatment
SPRING and FALL	*Cicuta* spp	Water hemlock	Open, moist to wet environments; throughout.	All	White flower, umbels. Veins of leaflets ending at notches. Stems hollow except at nodes. Tuberous roots from chambered rootstock.	Resinoids (cicutoxin, cicutol) in roots, stem base, young leaves. Toxicity retained when dry, except in hay. Rapid onset of clinical signs, with death in 15-30 min. Salivation, muscular twitching, dilated pupils. Violent convulsions, coma, death. Human poisoning common.	Sedatives to control spasm and heart action. Prognosis good if alive 2 hr after ingestion.
	Hymenoxys odorata	Bitterweed	Roadways, lakebeds, flooded areas, overgrazed range; southwest.	Sheep, rarely cattle	Multibranched annual or perennial up to 2 ft high. Yellow flower head. Leaves divided into narrow glandular segments.	Sesquiterpene lactone (hymenovin) in the fresh or dry plant. Salivation, vomiting, green nasal discharge, depression, anorexia, abdominal pain. Lesions: inflammation of GI tract, foreign body pneumonia, renal degeneration.	Toxin cumulative. Avoid overgrazing. Remove from pasture.
	Hymenoxys richardsonii	Pingue, also Colorado rubberweed	Arid foothills (6000-8000 ft [1800-2400 m]); western.	Sheep, also cattle, goats	Perennial herb. Leaves bright green, divided into narrow glandular segments.	Same as for *H odorata* (above).	Same as for *H odorata*.
SPRING	*Nolina texana*	Sacahuista, Beargrass	Open areas on rolling hills and slopes; southwest.	Sheep, cattle, goats	Perennial with many clustered, long narrow leaves. Stem mostly underground. Several flower stems with many small, white flowers in clusters.	Unidentified hepatotoxin (buds, flowers, fruit). Photosensitization, anorexia, icterus, prostration. Dark urine, yellowish discharge from eyes, nostrils. Lesions: hepatic and renal degeneration, GI inflammation.	Remove animals from area where plant grows during blooming season. See PHOTOSENSITIZATION, p 820.
	Peganum harmala	African rue	Arid to semiarid ranges; southwest.	Cattle, sheep, probably horses	Multibranched, leafy, perennial, bright green, succulent herb. Leaves divided. Flowers white, single.	Alkaloids (seeds, leaves, stems; seeds more toxic). Anorexia, hindleg weakness, knuckling of fetlock, listlessness, excess salivation, subnormal temperature, pollakiuria. Lesions: gastroenteritis, with hemorrhages on heart and under liver capsule.	Unpalatable. Eaten only under drought conditions.

Table 4. Poisonous Plants of Temperate North America (continued)

Dangerous Season	Scientific Name	Common Name	Habitat and Distribution	Affected Animals	Important Characteristics	Toxic Principle and Effects	Remarks and Treatment
	Phytolacca americana	Pokeweed, Poke	Disturbed rich soils such as recent clearings, pastures, waste areas; eastern.	Pigs, also cattle, sheep, horses, man	Tall (to 9 ft), glabrous, green, red-purple, perennial herbs. Berries black-purple, staining, in drooping racemes.	Oxalic acid, a saponin (phytolaccotoxin), and an alkaloid (phytolaccin) in all parts; roots most toxic. Vomiting, abdominal pain, bloody diarrhea, hemolytic anemia, drop in production (dairy cattle). Terminal convulsions, death from respiratory failure. Lesions: ulcerative gastritis, mucosal hemorrhage, dark liver.	Oils and protectants (GI tract). Dilute acetic acid PO, stimulants. Blood transfusion (hemolytic anemia).
	Quercus spp	Oaks	Most deciduous woods; throughout.	All grazing animals, mostly cattle	Mostly deciduous trees, rarely shrubs, with 2-4 leaves clustered at tips of all twigs.	Gallotannin thought to be the toxin (young leaves and sprouting acorn). Anorexia, rumen stasis, constipation, followed by dark tarry diarrhea, dry muzzle, frequent urination, rapid weak pulse, death. Lesions: perirenal edema, nephrosis, gastroenteritis.	Diet must consist of >50% oak buds and young leaves for a period of time. Elevated BUN with diet history diagnostic. Treatment symptomatic. Oral ruminatorics helpful. *See also* p 1720.
(may be year round)	Sarcobatus vermiculatus	Greasewood	Alkaline or saline bottom soils, not in higher mountains; arid west.	Sheep, cattle	Large deciduous shrub with spiny stems. Fleshy, alternate, round in cross-section. Flowers inconspicuous.	Oxalates (sodium and potassium). Dyspnea, weakness, depression, some salivation, atony of GI tract, coma, death. Hyperkalemia, hypocalcemia, increased BUN. Lesions: hemorrhage and edema of rumen wall, ascites, swollen kidneys (renal tubular necrosis and dilation).	Toxic when large quantity consumed in short time. Do not allow hungry animals to graze plant.
(and occasionally FALL)	Xanthium spp	Cocklebur	Fields, waste places, exposed shores of ponds or rivers; throughout.	All animals, more common in pigs	Coarse annual herb. Fruit covered with spines, 2 beaked, with 2 compartments.	Carboxyatractyloside (seeds and young seedlings). Anorexia, depression, nausea, vomiting, weakness, rapid weak pulse, dyspnea, muscle spasms, convulsions. Lesions: GI inflammation, acute hepatitis, nephritis.	Seedlings or grain contaminated with seeds. Oils and fats PO may be beneficial; warmth, stimulants IM.

Dangerous Season	Scientific Name	Common Name	Habitat and Distribution	Affected Animals	Important Characteristics	Toxic Principle and Effects	Remarks and Treatment
	Zygadenus spp	Death camas	Foothill grazing lands, occasionally boggy grasslands, low open woods; throughout.	Sheep, cattle, horses	Perennial, bulbous, unbranched herbs with basal, flat, grass-like leaves. Flowers greenish, yellow, or pink; in racemes or panicles. No onion odor.	Steroidal alkaloids, glycoalkaloids, and ester alkaloids (all parts). Salivation, vomiting, muscle weakness, ataxia or prostration, fast weak pulse, coma, death. No distinctive lesions.	Seeds most toxic. Leaves and stems lose toxicity as plant matures. Atropine sulfate and picrotoxin subcut.
SPRING and SUMMER	*Aesculus* spp	Buckeye	Woods and thickets; eastern USA and California.	All grazing animals	Trees or shrubs. Leaves opposite and palmately compound. Seeds large, glossy brown, with large white scar.	Glycoside, aesculin; also alkaloids and saponins in all parts, especially seeds and leaves. Depression, incoordination, twitching, paralysis, inflammation of mucous membranes.	Young shoots and seeds especially poisonous. Stimulants and purgatives.
	Amianthium muscaetoxicum	Fly poison, Staggergrass, Crow poison	Open woods, fields, and acid bogs; eastern.	All grazing animals	Bulbous perennial herb. Leaves basal, linear. White flowers in a compact raceme, the pedicels subtended by short, brownish bracts.	Unidentified alkaloid, similar to those with *Zygadenus* (all parts). Salivation, vomiting, rapid and irregular respiration, weakness, death from respiratory failure.	No practical treatment. Especially dangerous for animals new to pasture. Keep animals well fed.
	Cassia obtusifolia	Coffeepod, Sicklepod	Found in cultivated (corn, soybean, or sorghum) and abandoned fields, along fences, roadsides; naturalized in eastern USA.	All grazing animals, mostly cattle, and poultry (qv, p 1595)	Annuam shrub frequently found in same fields as *C occidentalis*. Distinguishing features: leaflets fewer in number and more rounded; seed pods long, round to 4-sided and more curved; seeds shiny, brown, and rhomboid.	Toxic principles thought to be the same as in *C occidentalis*. Clinical signs, though similar, are less severe with *C obtusifolia*.	Treatment ineffective in down animals; salvaging most economical. Remove animals from source.

Table 4. Poisonous Plants of Temperate North America (continued)

Dangerous Season	Scientific Name	Common Name	Habitat and Distribution	Affected Animals	Important Characteristics	Toxic Principle and Effects	Remarks and Treatment
	Cassia occidentalis	Coffee senna, Coffeeweed, Styptic weed, Wild coffee	Common along roadsides, waste areas and pastures; naturalized in eastern USA.	Cattle, horses, chickens, goats, sheep, rabbits	Annual herb >3 ft tall, with glandular, alternate pinnately compound (8-12 ovate to lanceolate leaflets, terminal pair the largest) leaves. Flowers yellow, axillary, solitary, or in short racemes. Long, flat, straight to slightly curved pods with clearly outlined seed contents. Of the pods, seeds, and wilted foliage, the seeds are most toxic.	The anthraquinones (emodinglycosides and oxymethylanthraquinone), chrysarobin and lectin (toxalbumins), and alkaloids are associated with GI dysfunction and myodegeneration. Afebrile, ataxic, with diarrhea and coffee-color urine, recumbent but eat and are alert shortly before death. Increased serum CPK and isocitric dehydrogenase activities, hyperkalemia and myoglobinuria frequent. Lesions: cardiac and skeletal muscle degeneration. Congestion, fatty degeneration and centrilobular necrosis (liver) in addition to tubular degeneration (kidneys) have been reported also. Death probably due to hyperkalemic heart failure.	No specific treatment known. Although gross lesions similar to those of vitamin E/selenium deficiency, this therapy contraindicated. Mineralocortical hormone therapy may facilitate potassium excretion. Remove animals from source. Symptomatic treatment may help, but salvaging more economical.
(also seeds in FALL)	*Delphinium* spp	Larkspurs	Either cultivated or wild, usually in open foothills or meadows and among aspen; mostly western.	All grazing animals, mostly cattle	Annual or perennial erect herbs. Flowers each with one spur, in racemes. Perennial with tuberous roots. Leaves palmately lobed or divided.	Polycyclic diterpenoid alkaloids (eg, delphinine) in all parts, fresh or dry. Straddled stance, arched back, repeated falling, forelegs first. Constipation, bloat, salivation, vomiting. Death (respiratory and cardiac failure). Most often no lesions.	Young plants and seeds more toxic. Toxicity decreases with maturity.

Dangerous Season	Scientific Name	Common Name	Habitat and Distribution	Affected Animals	Important Characteristics	Toxic Principle and Effects	Remarks and Treatment
	Descurainia pinnata	Tansy mustard	Dense stands especially in wet years; arid southwest.	Cattle	Annual to 2 ft tall, stem and leaves covered with fine pubescence. Leaves alternate, deeply pinnately dissected. Inflorescence on elongated raceme. Flower small with 4 spreading yellow to yellow-green petals. Fruit-copula with 2 carpels and long waxy seeds in 2 rows.	Toxic principle unknown; must be grazed over relatively long period. Partial or complete blindness, inability to use tongue or swallow, "paralyzed tongue", "blind staggers", wandering, head pressing, emaciation, death if not treated.	Administer 2-3 gal. (8-12 L) water b.i.d. with stomach tube. Include nourishment if animal weak. Prognosis good if treatment started early. Possibly mustards cause the same condition
	Lantana spp	Lantana	Ornamentals and wild; in lower coastal plain of southeast USA, and southern California.	All grazing animals	Shrubs. Young stems 4-angled. Leaves opposite. Flowers in flat-topped clusters, yellow, pink, orange, or red. Berries black.	Triterpenes (lantadene A and B) and unknowns in all parts, especially leaves and green berries. Anorexia, jaundice, watery feces, photosensitization. Lesions: degenerative change in liver and kidney. Death due to liver insufficiency, renal failure, myocardial damage.	Remove plants from pasture. Keep animals out of light sources after eating plant.
	Tetradymia spp	Horsebrush	Arid foothills and higher desert and sagebrush ranges, dense stands along trails; western.	Sheep	Shrubs with yellow flowers in spring, not later. Leaves spiny, silvery white. Early deciduous.	Furanoeremophilanes (tetradymol and others). Photosensitization, "big head", loss of hair and wool, skin ulcerations, blindness, secondary infections. Lesions: dermal necrosis and edema, hepatic and renal degeneration. Abortions may occur.	Animal must be consuming black sagebrush (*Artemisia nova*) to show toxic effects. Remove animal from sunlight; antihistamines, topical antibiotics, and parenteral corticosteroids beneficial.
	Veratrum spp	False hellebore, Skunk cabbage	Low, moist woods and pastures, and high mountain valleys; throughout.	Sheep, cattle	Erect herbs. Leafy throughout, leaves large and plaited. Flowers small and white or greenish.	Steroidal alkaloids. Vomiting, excess salivation, cardiac arrhythmia, bradycardia, dyspnea, muscle weakness and paralysis, coma, congenital cyclops in lambs from ewes exposed to *V californicum* (qv, p 650).	Respiratory and heart stimulants.

Table 4. Poisonous Plants of Temperate North America (continued)

Dangerous Season	Scientific Name	Common Name	Habitat and Distribution	Affected Animals	Important Characteristics	Toxic Principle and Effects	Remarks and Treatment
SUMMER and FALL	*Acer rubrum*	Red maple	Moist land and swamps; eastern.	Horses	A large tree at maturity. Leaves opposite, 2-6 in. across, palmately 3- or 5-lobed each, roughly triangular, and coarsely toothed. Red to yellow polygamous flowers. Fruit, a pair of one-seeded winged units connected at base.	Unknown toxic principle(s) in wilted leaves. Methemoglobinemia, Heinz body anemia, and intravascular hemolysis; weakness, polypnea, tachycardia, depression, icterus, cyanosis, brownish discoloration of blood and urine.	Not common. Methemoglobinemia a prognostic indicator. Isotonic fluids, oxygen, and blood transfusion can be helpful. Methylene blue therapy not rewarding.
	Apocynum spp	Dogbanes	Open woods, roadsides, fields; throughout.	All	Erect, branching, perennial herb with milky sap arising from creeping underground root stock. Leaves opposite. Flowers white to greenish white in terminal clusters. Fruit long, slender, paired, with silky-haired seeds.	A resinoid and glucoside with some cardioactivity found in leaves and stems of green or dry plants. Increased temperature and pulse, dilated pupils, anorexia, discolored mucous membranes, cold extremities, death.	IV fluids and gastric protectants suggested.
	Centaurea repens	Russian knapweed	Waste areas, roadsides, railroads, and overgrazed rangeland; not common on cultivated or in irrigated pastures; mostly western and upper midwestern USA.	Horses	Perennial weed with slender rhizomes. Stems erect and well branched. Leaves pinnately lobed to entire, not spiny, narrowed basally but not petioled and of decreasing length up the plant. Thinly pubescent or glabrous. Blue, pink, or white flowers. One-seeded fruit with whitish, slightly ridged attachment scar.	Unidentified alkaloid in fresh or dried plant. Chronic exposure; acute onset of signs. Inability to eat or drink, facial dystonia, chewing, yawning, standing with head down, severe facial edema, gait normal, head pressing, aimless walking or excitement most severe the first 2 days, become static thereafter. Death from starvation, dehydration, aspiration pneumonia.	More toxic than *C solstitialis* (see below) but with similar pathology and prognosis. Some relief with massive doses of atropine but not an effective treatment. Euthanasia recommended.

Dangerous Season	Scientific Name	Common Name	Habitat and Distribution	Affected Animals	Important Characteristics	Toxic Principle and Effects	Remarks and Treatment
	Centaurea solstitialis	Yellow star thistle, Yellow knapweed	Waste areas, roadsides, pastures; mostly western.	Horses	Annual weed. Leaves densely covered with cottony hair. Terminal spreading cluster of bright yellow flowers with spines below. Branches winged.	Unidentified alkaloid. Involuntary chewing movements, twitching of lips, flicking of tongue. Mouth commonly held open. Unable to eat; death from dehydration, starvation, aspiration pneumonia.	Horses graze because of lack of other forage. Extended period of consumption essential for toxicity. Liquefactive necrosis of substantia nigra and globus pallidus (brain) pathognomonic. No treatment. Euthanasia recommended.
	Eupatorium rugosum	White snakeroot	Woods, cleared areas, waste places, usually the moister and richer soils; eastern.	Sheep, cattle, horses	Erect perennial herb. Tremetol leaves, opposite, simple, serrated. Flowers small, white, and many. Often grows in large patches.	Complex benzyl alcohol (tremetol in the leaves and stems). Excreted via the milk; cumulative. Weight loss, weakness, trembling (muzzle and legs) prominent following exercise, constipation, acetone odor, fatty degeneration of liver, partial paralysis of throat, death in 1-3 days.	"Milk sickness or trembles". Treatment symptomatic. Heart and respiratory stimulants and laxative may be necessary. Remove animal from access to plant, discard milk (hazardous to man).
	Oxytenia (Iva) acerosa	Copperweed	Arid, alkaline soils in foothills, sagebrush plains; southwest.	Cattle, sheep	Tall, perennial herb with narrow leaflets. Flowers in many heads resembling goldenrod.	Unknown; all above-ground parts, green or dry. Anorexia, marked depression, weakness, coma; death without struggle within 1-3 days.	Supplement diet or change pasture.
	Perilla frutescens	Perilla mint, Beefsteak plant	Ornamental originally from India, escaped to moist pastures, fields, roadsides, and waste places; eastern.	Cattle primarily, horses and other livestock susceptible	Annual, freely branched, squared stems. Opposite, purple or green, coarsely serrated leaves. White to purple flowers. Strong pungent odor when crushed.	Green or dry, 3-substituted furans: perilla ketone, egomaketone, isoegomaketone. Two-10 days following exposure: dyspnea (especially on exhaling), open-mouth breathing, head lowered, reluctant to move, death on exertion. Lesion: pulmonary emphysema and edema.	Treatment ineffective once clinical signs severe. Parenteral steroids, antihistamines, and antibiotics may help. Handle gently (prevents exertion and death). Seeds produce edible oil.

Table 4. Poisonous Plants of Temperate North America (continued)

Dangerous Season	Scientific Name	Common Name	Habitat and Distribution	Affected Animals	Important Characteristics	Toxic Principle and Effects	Remarks and Treatment
	Prosopis glandulosa (juliflora)	Mesquite	Dry ranges, washes, draws; southwest.	Primarily cattle, also goats; sheep resistant	Deciduous shrub or small tree with smooth or furrowed gray bark, paired spines. Leaves divided. Legume pod long, constricted between seeds.	Unknown principle in the beans. Chronic wasting with rumen atony, excess salivation, continuous chewing. Partial paralysis of tongue, facial muscle tremor, submandibular edema, anemia. Lesions: emaciation, small firm kidneys and liver, gastroenteritis, filled rumen.	High sucrose content of beans alters rumen microflora, inhibiting cellulose digestion and B vitamin synthesis if grazed for extended period. Combined stocking of cattle and sheep reduces cattle loss.
	Robinia pseudoacacia	Black locust, False acacia, Locust tree	Open woods, roadsides, pinelands, on clay soils preferably; eastern USA.	All grazing animals, mostly horses	Tree or shrub. Deciduous, alternate, pinnately compound (>10 elliptic to ovate leaflets) leaves. Pair of spines at the base of each leaf. Flowers in loose, fragrant, white to cream, drooping racemes. Flattened, brown pods containing 4-8 seeds persist throughout winter.	The glycoside robitin, a lectin (hemagglutinin), and the phytotoxins robin and phasin found throughout the plant, although the flowers have been suggested as the toxic principles. Diarrhea, anorexia, weakness, posterior paralysis, depression, mydriasis, cold extremities, frequently laminitis and weak pulse. Death infrequent; recovery period extensive. Postmortem lesions restricted to GI tract.	Laxatives and stimulants suggested. Treatment symptomatic.
	Solanum spp	Nightshades, Jerusalem cherry, Potato, Horse nettle, Buffalo bur	Fence rows, waste areas, grain and hay fields; throughout.	All	Fruits small; yellow, red, or black when ripe; structurally like tomatoes; clustered on stalk arising from stem between leaves.	Glycoalkaloid solanine (leaves, shoots, unripe berries). Acute hemorrhagic gastroenteritis, weakness, excess salivation, dyspnea, trembling, progressive paralysis, prostration, death.	Pilocarpine, physostigmine, GI protectants. Seeds may contaminate grain.
FALL and WINTER	*Daubentonia (Sesbania) punicea*	Rattlebox, Purple sesbane	Cultivated and escaped, in waste places; southeastern USA coastal plain.	All	Shrub. Flowers orange. Legume pods longitudinally 4-winged.	Rapid pulse, weak respiration, diarrhea, death.	Seeds poisonous. Remove animal from source. Saline purgatives.

Dangerous Season	Scientific Name	Common Name	Habitat and Distribution	Affected Animals	Important Characteristics	Toxic Principle and Effects	Remarks and Treatment
	Halogeton glomeratus	Halogeton	Deserts, overgrazed areas, winter ranges, alkaline soils; western.	Sheep, cattle	Annual herb. Leaves fleshy, round in cross-section, tip with stiff hair. Axillary flowers inconspicuous. Fruits bracted and conspicuous.	Oxalic acid, oxalate. Acute course. Rapid labored respiration, depression, weakness, coma, death. Lesions: hemorrhages and edema of rumen wall, swollen kidneys, oxalate crystals in kidneys and rumen wall.	Toxic dose consumed over short period. Increase water consumption.
	Haplopappus heterophyllus	Rayless goldenrod, Burroweed	Dry plains, grasslands, open woodlands, and along irrigation canals; southwest.	Cattle, sheep, horses	Bushy perennial 2-4 ft tall, with many yellow flower heads. Leaves alternate, linear, sticky.	Complex benzyl alcohol (tremetol); resin acid; primarily nursing young and nonlactating animals. Reluctance to move, trembling, weakness, vomiting, dyspnea, constipation, prostration, coma, death.	"Milksickness". Remove young and discard milk (hazardous to man).
	Juglans nigra	Black walnut	Native to eastern USA; now from eastern seacoast, west to Michigan and most of the Midwest, south to Georgia and Texas.	Horses	Tree with deciduous, alternate, pinnately compound leaves (numerous lanceolate leaflets with serrated margins; leaflets in middle are largest. Male and female flowers on same tree but different inflorescence. Thick husk nut does not open when ripe. Twigs have chambered pith.	Juglone, phenolic derivative of naphthoquinone. Shavings with <20% black walnut toxic within 24 hr of exposure. Reluctance to move; depression; increased temperature, pulse, respiration rate, abdominal sounds, digital pulse, hoof temperature; distal limb edema; lameness. Severe laminitis with continued exposure.	Nonfatal; laminitis and edema of the lower limbs. Remove shavings promptly. Treat for limb edema and laminitis. Improvement observed in 24-48 hr with no sequelae.

Table 4. Poisonous Plants of Temperate North America (continued)

Dangerous Season	Scientific Name	Common Name	Habitat and Distribution	Affected Animals	Important Characteristics	Toxic Principle and Effects	Remarks and Treatment
	Melilotus officinalis and *M. alba*	Sweet clover, White sweet clover	Commonly found on alkaline soils, fields, roadsides, and waste places; forage crop in southern and northern USA.	Most commonly cattle, also horses and sheep	Annual or biennial herb 3-6 ft tall. Leaves alternate, pinnately compound with 3 obovate leaflets, serrated margins. Yellow or white flowers borne on racemes. Small one-seeded pods.	See SWEET CLOVER POISONING, p 1733.	See p 1734.
	Notholaena sinuata var *cochisensis*	Jimmy fern, Cloak fern	Dry rocky slopes and crevices, chiefly limestone areas; southwest.	Sheep, goats, cattle	Evergreen, perennial, erect fern with divided leaves, folding when dry. Leaflets about as wide as long, scaly on back.	Unknown (excreted in milk). Nervous syndrome, incoordination, arched back, trembling, increased respiratory rate and pulse. Death when not allowed to rest.	Avoid driving during danger period. Provide ample watering, placed to avoid long walks. Allow rest if signs occur.
	Sesbania (Glottidium) vesicaria	Bladder pod, Rattlebox, Sesbane, Coffee bean	Mostly open, low ground, abandoned cultivated fields; southeastern USA coastal plain.	All	Tall annual. Legume pods flat, tapered at both ends, 2-seeded. Leaves pinnate, divided. Flowers yellow.	Unknown (green plant and seeds). Ruminants: hemorrhagic diarrhea, shallow rapid respiration, fast irregular pulse, coma, death. Lesions: hemorrhages in abomasum and intestines, dark tarry blood.	Green seeds are more toxic. Remove animal from source immediately. General supportive treatment—saline purgatives, rumen stimulants, IV fluids.
	Sophora secundiflora	Mescal bean, Frijolito, Mountain laurel	Hills and canyons, limestone soils; southwestern Texas into Mexico.	Cattle, sheep, goats	Evergreen shrub or small tree. Leaves alternate, divided, and leathery. Flowers violet-blue, fragrant. Seeds large and bright red with hard seed coat, in legume pod.	Quinolizidine alkaloid (seeds and probably leaves). Violent trembling, stiff gait, falling on exercise, recumbent for a few minutes, becoming alert and eating.	Toxic effect not cumulative, consume large amounts quickly. Seeds more dangerous when crushed.

Dangerous Season	Scientific Name	Common Name	Habitat and Distribution	Affected Animals	Important Characteristics	Toxic Principle and Effects	Remarks and Treatment
FALL, WINTER, and SPRING	*Melia azedarach*	Chinaberry	Fence rows, brush, waste places; southeast.	Pigs and sheep, others less susceptible	Small to medium deciduous tree. Fruit cream or yellow with a furrowed globose stone, persisting on tree through winter. Large amount required for intoxication.	Several alkaloids and a saponin (all parts), fruit most toxic. Restlessness, vomiting, constipation, cyanosis, rapid pulse, dyspnea, death within 24 hr.	Gastroenteritis usual. Recovery may be spontaneous. Laxatives and GI protectants suggested.
ALL SEASONS	*Acacia berlandieri*	Guajillo	Semiarid range lands; southwestern Texas into Mexico.	Sheep, goats	Deciduous shrub or small tree. Leaf divided. Flowers white to yellowish in dense heads. Fruit a legume with margins thickened.	Amine, N-methyl-β-phenyl-ethylamine. Chronic course. Ataxia of hindquarters (limberleg), marked excitation, prostration, remain alert, death from starvation.	Dominates vegetation in some areas. Valuable to sheep industry due to high nutritive value and dominance. Supplement during drought to reduce possibility of poisoning.
(especially SPRING)	*Agave lecheguilla*	Lecheguilla	Low limestone hills, dry valleys, and canyons; southwest.	Sheep, goats, cattle, usually during drought	Perennial, stemless, with thick, fleshy, tapered leaves having sharply serrated margins. Flowers infrequently with tall terminal panicle.	Unidentified hepatotoxin (causing photosensitivity) and a toxic saponin (abortifacient action). Subacute course. Listlessness, anorexia, icterus, yellow discharge from eyes and nostrils, photosensitization, coma, death.	Remove animals from range and provide shade. *See* PHOTOSENSITIZATION, p 820.
	Agrostemma githago	Corn cockle	Weed, grain fields, and waste areas; throughout.	All	Green winter annual with silky-white hairs, opposite leaves, purple flowers, black seeds.	Saponin (githagenin) in seeds. Acute course. Profuse watery diarrhea, vomiting, dullness, general weakness, tachypnea, hemoglobinuria, death.	Oils and GI protectants. Neutralize toxin (dilute acetic acid PO). Blood transfusions may be necessary.
	Asclepias spp	Milkweeds	Dry areas, usually waste places, roadsides, streambeds.	All	Perennial erect herbs with milky sap. Seeds silky-hairy from elongated pods.	Steroid glycosides and toxic resinous substances (all parts), green or dry. Staggering, tetanic convulsions, bloating, dyspnea, dilated pupils, rapid and weak pulse, coma, death.	Sedatives, laxatives, and IV fluids suggested.

Table 4. Poisonous Plants of Temperate North America (continued)

Dangerous Season	Scientific Name	Common Name	Habitat and Distribution	Affected Animals	Important Characteristics	Toxic Principle and Effects	Remarks and Treatment
	Astragalus spp, *Oxytropis* spp, (certain species only)	Locoweed	Mostly western.	All grazing animals	Stemmed or stemless perennial herbs. Leaves alternate and pinnately compound. Flowers leguminous. Chronic intoxication.	Swainsonine. Depression, emaciation, incoordination, dry lusterless hair. Abortions. Neurovisceral cytoplasmic vacuolation. Congestive right heart failure in cattle grazing at high altitudes.	Avoid grazing of source. Both green and dry plants are toxic.
	Astragalus spp (certain species only)	Milkvetch, etc (many common names)	Nearly all.	All grazing animals	As above.	Miserotoxin, other aliphatic nitro compounds. Posterior paralysis, goose-stepping, depression, rough coat, pulmonary emphysema, acute death, cord demyelination.	Avoid grazing of pre-flower stage.
	Astragalus spp (certain species only — selenium accumulators)	Many common names	Seleniferous areas, mostly western and midwestern.	All grazing animals	As above.	Selenium (chronic). Slow growth, reproductive failure, loss of hair, sore feet, acute death.	Avoid grazing seleniferous plants for extended periods. *See* SELENIUM POISONING, p 1727.
	Baccharis spp	Silverling, Baccharis, Yerba-de-pasmo	Open areas, often moist; eastern and southwestern.	Cattle	Shrubs. Numerous small, whitish flowers. Leaves resin-dotted, and persistent southward.	Unidentified. Acute course. Bloat, staggering, trembling, restlessness, polypnea, tachycardia, death.	Most dangerous in early growing stage. Toxin concentrated in leaves and flowers. No specific treatment.
	Brassica, *Raphanus*, *Descurainia* spp	Mustards, Crucifers, Cress	Fields, roadsides; throughout.	Cattle, horses, pigs	Annual herbaceous weeds with terminal clusters of yellowish flowers and slender, elongated seed pods.	Glucosinolates (isothiocyanate, thiocyanates, nitrites) in seeds and vegetative parts, fresh or dry. Acute/chronic course. Anorexia, severe gastroenteritis, salivation, diarrhea, paralysis, photosensitization, hemoglobinuria.	Remove from source. Administer GI protectants (mineral oil).

Dangerous Season	Scientific Name	Common Name	Habitat and Distribution	Affected Animals	Important Characteristics	Toxic Principle and Effects	Remarks and Treatment
	Conium maculatum	Poison hemlock	Roadside ditches, damp waste areas; throughout.	All	Purple-spotted hollow stem. Leaves resemble parsley, parsnip odor when crushed. Tap root. Flowers white, in umbels.	Piperidine alkaloids (coniine and others) in the vegetative parts. Acute course. Dilated pupils; weakness; staggering gait; slow pulse, progressing to rapid and thready. Slow, irregular breathing; death from respiratory failure. Teratogenic in cattle.	Coniine excreted via lungs and kidneys, mousy odor of breath and urine (diagnostic). Administer saline cathartics; neutralize alkaloids with tannic acid, together with stimulants.
	Crotalaria spp	Crotalaria, Rattlebox	Fields and roadsides; eastern and central USA.	All	Annual or perennial legume. Yellow flowers in racemes, pods inflated. Bracts at base of pedicels of flowers and fruits persistent. Leaves simple or divided. Seeds in harvested grain.	Pyrrolizidine alkaloid (monocrotaline) and other unidentified alkaloids (all parts, especially seeds). Chronic course. Chickens — diarrhea, pale comb, ruffled feathers; horses — unthriftiness, ataxic, walking in circles, icterus; cattle — bloody diarrhea, icterus, rough coat, edema, weakness; death may occur from a few weeks to months after ingestion.	Cumulative, fresh or dry. No treatment.
	Cynoglossum officinale	Hound's tongue	Native to Europe; throughout USA.	Horses, cattle, sometimes sheep	Annual or biennial herbaceous plant, 16-40 in. tall. Alternate, simple, elliptic, velvety leaves. Blue or purple flowers in racemes. Fruits are 4 conspicuous, spiny, flattened nutlets.	Pyrrolizidine alkaloids (heliosupine and echinatine) throughout the fresh or dry plant. Clinical signs similar to those of *Senecio* spp. Unpleasant odor of the fresh plant (but not when found in hay) discourages consumption.	Pyrrolizidine alkaloids carcinogenic; milk, liver, and kidneys from cattle ingesting toxic amounts of these plants hazardous for human consumption. See *Senecio* spp, p 1718.
	Datura stramonium	Jimson weed, Thorn apple	Fields, barn lots, trampled pastures, and waste places on rich bottom soils; throughout.	All	Leaves wavy. Flower large (4 in.), white, tubular. Fruit a spiny pod, 2 in. (5 cm) long.	Tropane alkaloids (atropine, scopolamine, hyoscyamine) in all parts, seeds in particular. Acute course. Weak rapid pulse and heartbeat, dilated pupils, dry mouth, incoordination, convulsions, coma.	All parts, mainly in hay or silage. Urine from animal dilates pupils of laboratory animals (diagnostic). Treatment nonspecific; cardiac and respiratory stimulants: physostigmine, pilocarpine, arecoline.

Table 4. Poisonous Plants of Temperate North America (continued)

Dangerous Season	Scientific Name	Common Name	Habitat and Distribution	Affected Animals	Important Characteristics	Toxic Principle and Effects	Remarks and Treatment
	Drymaria pachyphylla	Inkweed, Drymary	Heavy alkaline clay soil in low areas or dry, overgrazed pastures; southwest.	Cattle, sheep, goats	Multibranched, succulent, prostrate annual. Opposite leaves. Small white flowers.	Unknown toxin. Diarrhea, restlessness, depression, coma, death. Lesions: gastroenteritis with congestion of liver, kidneys, spleen. Petechial hemorrhages on heart.	Dangerous during drought, after rain, or at night. Avoid overstocking to improve range.
	Festuca arundinacea	Tall fescue	A coarse, hardy, drought-resistant grass; Pacific Northwest, Missouri, Oklahoma, and Kentucky; the major pasture grass in Southeastern USA.	Mostly cattle and horses	Coarse, deeply rooted perennial grass. Broad, dark-green, ribbed, rough upper surface, and smooth sheathed leaves. Grows in clumps.	*See* FESCUE POISONING, p 1687.	*See* p 1687.
	Gelsemium sempervirens	Yellow jessamine, Evening trumpet flower, Carolina jessamine	Open woods, thickets; southeast.	All	Climbing or trailing vines. Evergreen, entire, opposite leaves. Yellow tubular flowers, very fragrant.	Alkaloids (gelsemine and others, related to strychnine) in all parts. Acute course. Weakness, incoordination, dilated pupils, convulsions, coma, death within 48 hr. Limberneck in fowl.	No specific treatment. Relaxants and sedatives suggested.
	Gutierrezia (Xanthocethalum) microcephala	Broomweed, Snakeweed, Slinkweed, Turpentine weed	Widespread over dry range and desert; primarily southwest.	Cattle, sheep, goats, pigs	Multibranched, perennial, resinous shrub. Yellow-flowered heads.	Unknown. Acute poisoning, anorexia, listlessness, hematuria, diarrhea followed by constipation. In cattle, abortions with retained placenta, stillbirths or premature and weak calves.	Supplementing diet will help but not entirely prevent abortion in cattle.

Dangerous Season	Scientific Name	Common Name	Habitat and Distribution	Affected Animals	Important Characteristics	Toxic Principle and Effects	Remarks and Treatment
	Helenium (Dugaldia) hoopesii	Orange sneezeweed	Moist slopes and well-drained mountain meadows; western.	Sheep, rarely cattle	Perennial herb. Orange sunflower-like heads or yellow flowers. Leaves alternate.	Sesquiterpene lactones (helenalin, hymenoxin). Subacute course (spewing sickness). Depression, weakness, restlessness, stiff gait, salivation, pronounced vomiting, emaciation, eventual death.	Cumulative. Aspiration pneumonia frequent. Remove from access to plant. Graze sneezeweed areas for only short periods of time. Can graze intermittently with some success.
	Helenium microcephalum	Smallhead sneezeweed	Moist ground; southern.	Cattle, sheep, goats	Annual, erect herb, simple-stemmed below, bushy above. Stem winged. Narrow leaves throughout. Flowers in small heads; disk pale red-brown, rays yellow.	Sesquiterpene lactone (helenalin) in flowering stage. Depression, weakness, restlessness, stiff gait, salivation, vomiting.	Cumulative. Remove from pasture. Cathartics may help.
	Hypericum perforatum	St. John'swort, Goatweed, Klamath weed	Dry soil, roadsides, pastures, ranges; throughout.	Sheep, cattle, horses, goats	Perennial herb or woody below. Leaves opposite, dotted. Flowers many, yellow, with many stamens.	Photodynamic pigment (hypericin). Subacute course. Photosensitization, pruritus and erythema, blindness, convulsions, diarrhea, hypersensitivity to cold water contact, death.	Remove animals from source and sunlight. Corticosteroids parenterally, topical broad-spectrum antibiotics.
(especially WINTER and SPRING)	Kalmia spp	Laurel, Ivybush, Lambkill	Rich moist woods, meadows, or acid bogs; eastern and northwestern.	All, often sheep	Woody shrub. Evergreen, glossy leaves. Flowers pink to rose, showy.	Resinoid (andromedotoxin) and a glucoside (arbutin) in vegetative parts. Acute course. Incoordination, excess salivation, vomiting, bloat, weakness, muscular spasms, coma, death.	Undigested rumen contents and ingesta in lungs at necropsy. Laxatives, demulcents, nerve stimulants, atropine.
	Kochia scoparia	Kochia	Throughout.	Cattle	Annual to 5 ft tall. Many branched stems give a bushy appearance. Leaves are petiolate, lanceolate, thin, and flat. Fruit has 5 wedge-shaped wings.	An alkaloid has been suggested. This plant may also accumulate nitrate and oxalate. Photosensitization, polioencephalomalacia. Slow growth, sulfates seem to intensify the polio.	Harvested foliage is the source of toxin. Protect from sun in case of photosensitization; for polio, treat with vitamin B.

Table 4. Poisonous Plants of Temperate North America (continued)

Scientific Name	Common Name	Habitat and Distribution	Affected Animals	Important Characteristics	Toxic Principle and Effects	Remarks and Treatment
Ligustrum spp	Privet, Ligustrum, Hedge plant	An ornamental; common as hedge; found at abandoned farm home sites, along fences, and in bottom lands.	All livestock	Shrubs up to 15 ft tall. Simple, opposite, short-petioled, evergreen or deciduous leaves. Numerous small, white flowers in panicles. Fruit is a 1- to 2-seeded, black or dark blue berry, which persists throughout winter.	Ligustrin, ligustron, syringin, syringopictrin, and other unknown compounds in the leaves and fruit. Primarily GI irritants—diarrhea, abdominal pain, incoordination, paresis, weak pulse, hypothermia, convulsions, sometimes death.	Treatment symptomatic and supportive; correct dehydration.
Lupinus spp	Lupines, Bluebonnet	Dry to moist soils, roadsides, fields, and mountains; throughout, but poisoning mostly western.	Sheep, cattle, goats, horses, pigs	Perennials. Leaves simple or palmately divided. Flowers blue, white, red, or yellow in terminal raceme.	Quinolizidine alkaloids (20 known) concentrated in the seeds (fresh and dry); some piperidine alkaloids. Acute course. Inappetence, dyspnea, struggle, convulsions, death from respiratory paralysis. Some species teratogenic in cattle.	Do not disturb sick animals; remove from source as they begin to recover. No effective treatment, but survivors recover completely. *See also* p 1689.
Nandina domestica	Nandina, Heavenly bamboo, Chinese sacred bamboo	Common ornamental in southern USA.	All grazing animals, especially ruminants	Upright, unbranched, and multistemmed, evergreen shrub, 3-7 ft tall. Alternate, bi- to tripinnately compound leaves; leaflets are subsessile, elliptic-lanceolate, half as wide as long, entire, leathery, metallic bluish-green becoming purple in fall. Small, white flowers; 2-seeded, bright red berries in large panicles persist throughout fall and winter.	Cyanogenic glycosides in the foliage and fruits, hydrolyzed in GI tract to free cyanide thereby affecting cellular respiration. *See* CYANIDE POISONING, p 1647. Prognosis good if survives for 1 hr after signs begin.	Acute outcome precludes effective treatment for most; IV sodium nitrite/ sodium thiosulfate treatment of choice. Picrate test indicates plant's toxic potential. *See* CYANIDE POISONING, p 1647.

Dangerous Season	Scientific Name	Common Name	Habitat and Distribution	Affected Animals	Important Characteristics	Toxic Principle and Effects	Remarks and Treatment
	Nerium oleander	Oleander	Common ornamental in southern regions.	All	Evergreen shrub or tree. Leaves whorled and prominently, finely, pinnately veined beneath. Flowers showy, white to deep pink.	Digitoxin-type glycosides (oleandroside, nerioside, and others) in all parts, fresh or dry. Acute course. Severe gastroenteritis, vomiting, diarrhea, increased pulse rate, weakness, death.	No specific treatment. Atropine in conjunction with propranolol reported helpful.
	Photinia fraseri, P serrulata, P glabra	Fraser's photinia, Chinese photinia, Red leaf photinia, Red tip photinia	Common ornamental (hedge or screen) in southern USA.	All grazing animals, mostly ruminants	Evergreen shrubs, 10-15 ft tall. Alternate, oblong-ovate serrated leaves, copper-red (when young) turning dark green in 2-4 wk. Prominent, whitish flowers in spring; showy, red berries in fall.	Same as for *N domestica* (above).	Same as for *N domestica.*
(especially WINTER)	*Pinus ponderosa*	Western yellow pine	Coniferous forests of Rocky Mountains at moderate elevations; western.	Cattle	Tree, 150-180 ft. Leaves in groups of 3, yellowish green, 7-11 in. long. Bark platy, reddish orange.	Unknown toxin. Chronic course. Abortions in late gestation, stillbirths or weak calves, depressed, edema of vulva and udder, retained placenta.	Pine-needle ingestion during last half of gestation — may abort following single exposure. Keep pregnant cows away from source.
(especially WINTER and SPRING)	*Prunus caroliniana*	Laurel cherry, Cherry laurel	Woods, fence rows, and often escaped from cultivation; southern regions.	All grazing animals	Leaves evergreen, shiny, leathery. Broken twigs with strong cherry bark odor. Fruit black.	Hydrocyanic acid (wilted leaves, bark, and twigs). Peracute course. Difficult breathing, bloat, staggering, convulsions, followed by prostration and death. Mucous membranes and blood bright red.	*See* CYANIDE POISONING, p 1647.
	Prunus spp	Chokecherries, Wild cherries, Peaches	Waste areas, fence rows, woods, orchards, prairies, dry slopes.	All grazing animals, mostly cattle and sheep	Large shrubs or trees. Flowers white or pink. Cherries or peaches. Crushed twigs with strong odor.	Glycoside-yielding cyanide (rumen hydrolysis). Excitement leading to depression, dyspnea, incoordination, convulsions, prostration; death may occur in 15 min from asphyxiation.	Mucous membranes, bright pink color; blood, bright red color. *See* CYANIDE POISONING, p 1647.

Table 4. Poisonous Plants of Temperate North America (continued)

Scientific Name	Common Name	Dangerous Season	Habitat and Distribution	Affected Animals	Important Characteristics	Toxic Principle and Effects	Remarks and Treatment
Psilostrophe spp	Paperflowers		Open range lands and pastures; southwest.	Sheep	Perennial composite. Erect, woolly stems branching from base. Many small heads of yellow flowers.	Sesquiterpene lactone. Depression, incoordination, anorexia, weakness, trembling, rapid irregular pulse and respiration, coughing, vomiting, aspiration pneumonia, death.	Antimicrobial actions of sesquiterpene lactone in rumen affect metabolism. Supplement diet with sodium sulfate and high protein.
Pteridium aquilinum	Bracken fern		Dry poor soil, open woods, sandy ridges.	All grazing animals	Leaves firm, leathery, 3-pinnate.	*See* BRACKEN FERN POISONING, p 1641.	*See* p 1641.
Ricinus communis	Castor bean		Cultivated in southern regions.	All	Large, palmately lobed leaves. Seeds resembling engorged ticks, usually 3 in somewhat spiny pod.	Phytotoxin — ricin in all parts (seeds are especially toxic). Acute to chronic course (death or recovery). Violent purgation, straining with bloody diarrhea, weakness, salivation, trembling, incoordination.	Diagnosis: presence of seeds, RBC agglutination, precipitin test. Specific antiserum, ideal antidote; sedatives, arecoline hydrobromide, followed by saline cathartics suggested.
Senecio spp	Groundsel, Senecio		Grassland areas; mostly western.	Cattle, horses, sheep to a limited extent in the USA	Perennial or annual herbs. Heads of yellow flowers with whorl of bracts below.	Pyrrolizidine alkaloids, volatile oils, and nitrogen oxides (fresh or dry). Acute poisoning not common. Dullness, aimless walking, increased pulse, rapid respiration, weakness, colic, delayed death (days to months). Cattle: prolapsed rectum from persistent straining. Horses: nervous signs evident in later stages.	Liver biopsy diagnostic in early stages. Liver function test of value for subclinical condition in cattle. No general treatment. *See also* p 1698.
Sorghum halepense	Johnson grass		Weed of open fields and waste places; southern and scattered north to New York and Iowa.	All grazing animals	Coarse grass with large rhizomes and white midvein on leaf. Topped by large, open panicle.	Same as for *S vulgare* (below).	Same as for *S vulgare*.

Dangerous Season	Scientific Name	Common Name	Habitat and Distribution	Affected Animals	Important Characteristics	Toxic Principle and Effects	Remarks and Treatment
	Sorghum vulgare	Sorghum, Sudan grass, Kafir, Durra, Milo, Broomcorn, Schrock, etc	Forage crops and escapes; throughout.	All	Coarse grasses with terminal flower cluster. Some to 8 ft tall.	Hydrocyanic acid (drought, trampling, frost, second growth) and nitrate (heavy fertilization, drought) in vegetative parts. Acute course. Difficult breathing, bloat, staggering, convulsions, death. Blood bright red (cyanide) or chocolate brown (nitrate).	Hay: Safe for cyanide (volatile), not safe for nitrate (analyze). *See* CYANIDE POISONING, p 1647, and NITRATE/NITRITE POISONING, p 1691.
	Taxus spp	Yew	Most of North America; Japanese and English yew common ornamentals.	All	Evergreen perennial tree or shrub. Bark reddish brown then flaking in scales. Leaves linear, 0.5-1 in. (1.5-2.5 cm) long, 2 ranked on twig, upper surface dark green, lower yellow-green, mid ribs prominent. Flowers unisexual, inconspicuous. Fruit single stony seed. Bright scarlet color.	Toxic alkaloids in bark, leaves, seeds. Gaseous distress, diarrhea, vomiting, tremors, dyspnea, dilated pupils, respiratory difficulty, weakness, fatigue, collapse, coma, convulsions, bradycardia, circulatory failure, death. Death may be rapid.	Poisoning usually results when branches and trimmings fed to livestock either intentionally or inadvertently.
(especially dry season)	*Triglochin* spp	Arrowgrass	Salt marshes, wet alkaline soils, lake shores.	Sheep, cattle	Grasslike, except leaves are thick. Heads of fruits globular on erect raceme. Flowers inconspicuous.	Hydrocyanic acid in leaves. Salivation, dyspnea, excitement followed by depression, incoordination, prostration, convulsions followed by death from anoxia.	Often, animals found dead. *See* CYANIDE POISONING, p 1647.

QUERCUS POISONING
(Poisoning by oak buds or acorns)

Most animals are susceptible, although cattle and sheep are most often affected. Most species of oak (*Quercus* spp) found in Europe and North America are considered toxic. Consumption of large quantities of young oak leaves in the spring or green acorns in the fall produces clinical signs several days later. The toxic principle, which appears to be gallotannins or their metabolites, causes GI and renal dysfunction. Signs include anorexia, depression, emaciation, rumen stasis, serous nasal discharge, polydypsia, polyuria, and constipation followed by mucoid to hemorrhagic diarrhea. Renal insufficiency may be evidenced by elevated BUN and creatinine, proteinuria, hyperphosphatemia, hypocalcemia, and urine with a low specific gravity. Pale swollen kidneys, perirenal edema, subcut. edema, ascites, and hydrothorax are common necropsy findings. Edema and reddening of intestinal mucosa and ulceration of the esophagus and rumen may be seen. Diagnosis is based on clinical findings, necropsy, history, and histopathology of the kidney (ie, nephrosis). Other common diseases that resemble oak poisoning include pigweed (*Amaranthus* spp) poisoning and aminoglycoside antibiotic poisoning.

Calcium hydroxide comprising 10% of the ration may be used as a preventive measure if exposure to acorns or oak leaves cannot be avoided. Calcium hydroxide, ruminatorics, and purgatives may be effective antidotes if administered early in the course of disease. Fluid therapy and transplantation of ruminal microflora may be beneficial. Recovery is rare once renal dysfunction is advanced.

RODENTICIDE POISONING

Many poisons have been used against rodent pests. Farm animals, pets, and wildlife often gain access to these poisons via the baits or the destroyed pests, or by malicious intent. This discussion covers only the rodenticides that are in most common use. Strychnine poisoning (qv, p 1732) is discussed separately.

Anticoagulant Rodenticides (Warfarin and Congeners): Potentially dangerous to all mammals and birds, these are the most frequent cause of poisoning in pets. Pets and wildlife may be poisoned directly from baits or indirectly by consumption of poisoned rodents. Intoxications in domestic animals have resulted from contamination of feed with anticoagulant concentrate, malicious use of these chemicals, and feed mixed in equipment used to prepare rodent bait.

All anticoagulants have the basic coumarin or indanedione nucleus. The "second-generation" anticoagulants brodifacoum and bromadiolone are highly toxic to nontarget species (dogs, cats, and potentially livestock) after a single feeding. The "first-generation" anticoagulants, warfarin, pindone, coumafuryl, coumachlor, isovaleryl indanedione, and others less frequently used, are multiple-dose poisons requiring frequent feedings, which greatly reduces their toxicity. The "intermediate" anticoagulants, chlorophacinone and in particular diphacinone, require fewer feedings than "first-generation" chemicals, and thus are more toxic to nontarget species than the "first-generation" group.

The anticoagulants antagonize vitamin K, which interferes with the normal synthesis of coagulating proteins (clotting factors I, II, VII, IX, and X) in the liver; thus adequate amounts are not available to convert prothrombin into thrombin. A latent period, dependent on species, dose, and activity, is required, during which clotting factors already present are used up. New products have a longer biological half-life, and therefore have prolonged effects and require prolonged treatment, eg, the half-life in canine plasma of warfarin is 15 hr, diphacinone is 5 days, and bromadiolone is 6 days, with the maximum effect estimated at 12-15 days. Brodifacoum may continue to be detectable in serum for up to 24 days.

Clinical signs generally reflect some manifestation of hemorrhage, including anemia, hematomas, melena, hemothorax, hyphema, epistaxis, hemoptysis, and hematuria. Signs dependent on hemorrhage, such as weakness, ataxia, colic, and polypnea, may be seen. Depression and anorexia occur in all species even before bleeding occurs.

A diagnosis of anticoagulant rodenticide toxicosis is usually made based on history of ingestion of the substance. Other diseases that should be ruled out when massive hemorrhage is encountered include disseminated intravascular coagulation, congenital factor deficiencies, von Willebrand's disease, platelet deficiencies, and canine ehrlichiosis. A prolonged prothrombin, partial thromboplastin, or thrombin time in the presence of normal fibrinogen, fibrin degradation products, and platelet counts is strongly suggestive of anticoagulant rodenticide toxicosis, as is a positive therapeutic response to vitamin K_1.

Vitamin K_1 is antidotal. Recommended dosages vary from 0.25 to 2.5 mg/kg in warfarin (coumarin) exposure, to 2.5 to 5 mg/kg in the case of long-acting rodenticide intoxication (diphacinone, brodifacoum, bromadiolone, etc). Vitamin K_1 is administered subcut. (with the smallest possible needle to minimize hemorrhage) in several locations to speed absorption. IV administration of vitamin K_1 is contraindicated as anaphylaxis may result. The oral form of K_1 may be used daily after the first day, commonly at the same level as the loading dose, and divided b.i.d. Fresh or frozen plasma (9 mL/kg) or whole blood (20 mL/kg) IV is required to replace needed clotting factors and RBC if bleeding is severe. One week of vitamin K_1 treatment is usually sufficient for first-generation anticoagulants. For intermediate and second-generation anticoagulants or if anticoagulant type is unknown, treatment should continue for 4-6 wk to control long-term effects. Administration of vitamin K_1 with a fat-containing ration such as canned dog food increases the bioavailability 4-5 times as compared with vitamin K_1 given alone.

Coagulation should be monitored weekly until values remain normal for 5-6 days after cessation of therapy. Vitamin K_3 given as a feed supplement is ineffective in the treatment of anticoagulant rodenticide toxicosis. Additional supportive therapy may be indicated, including thoracocentesis to relieve dyspnea due to hemothorax, and supplemental oxygen if needed.

ANTU (α-Naphthylthiourea): ANTU causes local gastric irritation; when absorbed, it increases permeability of the lung capillaries in all animals, although there is a marked species variability in dose response. Properties of ANTU, when compared with those of warfarin, have led to near abandonment of its use. Dogs and pigs are occasionally poisoned, ruminants are resistant. Animals with an empty stomach readily vomit after ingestion of ANTU; however, food in the stomach decreases the stimulation to vomit, and fatal quantities of the chemical may be absorbed. Signs include vomiting, hypersalivation, coughing, and dyspnea. Animals prefer to sit. Severe pulmonary edema, moist rales, and cyanosis are present. Dependent signs include weakness, ataxia, rapid weak pulse, and subnormal temperature. Death from hypoxia may occur within 2-4 hr of ingestion, while animals that survive 12 hr may recover.

The lesions are suggestive. The most striking findings are pulmonary edema and hydrothorax. Hyperemia of the tracheal mucosa, mild to moderate gastroenteritis, marked hyperemia of the kidneys, and a pale mottled liver are found in most cases. Tissue for chemical analysis must be obtained within 24 hr.

Emetics should be used only before respiratory distress is evident. Prognosis is grave when severe respiratory signs occur. Agents providing sulfhydryl groups, eg, n-amyl mercaptan or sodium thiosulfate (10% solution), are beneficial. Positive-pressure oxygen therapy, an osmotic diuretic (eg, mannitol), and atropine (0.02-0.25 mg/kg) may help to relieve the pulmonary edema.

Bromethalin: A new non-anticoagulant, single-dose rodenticide, which is a neurotoxin that appears to uncouple oxidative phosphorylation in the CNS. CSF pressure increases, placing pressure on nerve axons, resulting in decreased nerve impulse conduction, paralysis, and death. The minimum toxic dose for dogs is 1.67 mg/kg; the minimum lethal dosage is 2.5 mg/kg (25 g of bait/kg body wt).

Bromethalin can cause either an acute or a chronic syndrome. The acute effects follow consumption of ≥ 5 mg bromethalin/kg body wt. Signs, which include hyperexcitability, muscle tremors, grand mal seizures, hindlimb hyperreflexia, CNS depression, and death, may appear ~10 hr after ingestion. Chronic effects are seen with lower dosage and may appear 24-86 hr after ingestion. This syndrome is characterized by tremors, depression, ataxia, vomiting, and lateral recumbency. These effects may be reversible if exposure to bromethalin is discontinued. Bromethalin toxicosis should be considered when cerebral edema or posterior paralysis is present.

Treatment should be directed at blocking absorption from the gut and reducing cerebral edema. Use of mannitol as an osmotic diuretic and corticosteroids have been suggested, but have shown little effect in bromethalin-poisoned dogs. Use of a super-activated charcoal, perhaps for several days, may increase recovery rate.

Cholecalciferol: A relatively new rodenticide, this was introduced with claims that it was less toxic to nontarget species than to rodents. However, clinical experience has shown that cholecalciferol-containing rodenticides are a significant health threat to dogs and cats; cholecalciferol produces hypercalcemia, which results in renal failure, cardiac abnormalities, hypertension, central depression, and GI upset.

Signs generally develop within 18-36 hr of ingestion and can include depression, anorexia, polyuria, and polydipsia. As serum calcium concentrations rise, clinical signs become more severe. Serum calcium concentrations >16 mg/dL are not uncommon. GI smooth muscle excitability decreases, and is manifest by anorexia, vomiting, and constipation. Hematemesis and hemorrhagic diarrhea may develop as a result of dystrophic calcification of the GI tract, and should not lead to a misdiagnosis of anticoagulant rodenticide toxicosis. Loss of renal concentrating ability is a direct result of hypercalcemia. As hypercalcemia persists, mineralization of the kidneys results in progressive renal insufficiency.

Diagnosis is based on history of ingestion, clinical signs, and hypercalcemia. Other causes of hypercalcemia, such as hyperparathyroidism, normal juvenile hypercalcemia, paraneoplastic hypercalcemia, hemoconcentration (hyperproteinemia), and diffuse osteoporosis should be ruled out. Gross lesions associated with hypercalcemia include pitted, mottled kidneys; diffuse hemorrhage of the GI mucosa; and roughened, raised plaques on the great vessels and on the surface of the lung and abdominal viscera.

Recommended therapy includes gastric evacuation, generally followed by administration of activated charcoal at 2-8 g/kg in a water slurry. Calciuresis is accomplished with 0.9% sodium chloride solution and administration of furosemide (initial bolus of 5 mg/kg, IV, followed by a constant rate IV infusion of 5 mg/kg/hr) and corticosteroids (prednisolone 1-2 mg/kg, b.i.d.). Furosemide and prednisolone should be continued for 2-4 wk, and the serum calcium concentration monitored at 24 hr, 48 hr, and 2 wk after cessation of treatment. Additionally, salmon calcitonin can be used at 4-6 IU/kg, subcut. q2-3hr, until the serum calcium stabilizes at <12 mg/dL. The dose of prednisolone should be tapered if it is administered for >2 wk to prevent acute adrenocortical insufficiency. Continuous peritoneal dialysis may be considered if the animal is in renal failure. A low-calcium diet should be provided in all cases of significant exposure to cholecalciferol rodenticides.

Phosphorus: In its white (or yellow) form, phosphorus is hazardous to all domestic animals but infrequently used as a rodenticide today. It is locally corrosive, and hepatotoxic when absorbed. The onset of signs of poisoning is sudden. Early signs include vomiting, severe diarrhea (often hemorrhagic), colic, and a garlic-like odor to the breath. Apparent recovery may occur up to 4 days after ingestion, but additional signs of acute liver damage usually develop, including hemorrhages, abdominal pain, and icterus. Hepatic encephalopathy is followed by convulsions and death. Lesions include severe gastroenteritis, fatty liver, multiple hemorrhages, and black tarry blood that fails to clot; the corpse may be phosphorescent, and the gastric contents have a garlic odor. Death is due to hepatic and renal failure.

Prognosis is grave unless treatment is instituted early. A 1% solution of copper sulfate is an effective emetic, and it also forms a nonabsorbable copper phosphide complex. Gastric lavage with a 0.01-0.1% solution of potassium permanganate or a 0.2-0.4% solution of copper sulfate should be followed by a saline cathartic and activated charcoal adsorbent. Any fat in the diet must be avoided for 3-4 days or longer because fats favor the absorption of phosphorus. Mineral oil has been recommended since it dissolves phosphorus and prevents absorption.

Red Squill: A plant (*Urginea maritima*)-derived cardiac glycoside, this is a rodenticide of limited current use. Since the rat is incapable of vomiting, red squill is more toxic to that species. It is considered relatively safe because it is unpalatable to domestic animals and, when eaten, usually induces vomiting in dogs and cats, and requires large quantities for toxicity in farm animals. However, dogs, cats, and pigs have been poisoned. Signs are vomiting, ataxia, and hyperesthesia followed by paralysis, depression, or convulsions. Bradycardia and cardiac arrhythmias may end in cardiac arrest. The clinical course seldom is longer than 24-36 hr.

Treatment consists of supportive therapy and evacuation of the GI tract using gastric lavage and saline cathartics. Atropine sulfate subcut. at 6- to 8-hr intervals may prevent cardiac arrest. Phenytoin at 16 mg/lb (35 mg/kg), t.i.d., should be given to dogs to suppress arrhythmias.

Sodium Fluoroacetate (1080): 1080 is a colorless, odorless, tasteless, water-soluble chemical that is highly toxic (0.1-8 mg/kg) to all animals, including man. (Its use is thus heavily restricted to certain commercial applications.) Fluoroacetate is metabolized to fluorocitrate, which blocks the tricarboxylic acid cycle—a mechanism necessary for cellular energy production. It produces its effects by 2 general mechanisms: 1) overstimulation of the CNS, resulting in death in convulsions; and 2) alteration of cardiac function that results in myocardial depression, cardiac arrhythmias, ventricular fibrillation, and circulatory collapse. CNS stimulation is the main reaction in dogs, while the cardiac effect predominates in horses, sheep, goats, and chickens. Pigs and cats appear to be about equally affected by both.

A characteristic lag phase of ≥ 30 min after ingestion occurs before the onset of nervousness and restlessness. Marked depression and weakness follow in all species except dogs and pigs. Affected animals rapidly become prostrate, and the pulse is weak and 2-3 times the normal rate. Death is due to cardiac failure. Usually, dogs and pigs rapidly develop tetanic convulsions similar to those of strychnine poisoning. Many exhibit signs of severe pain. Vomiting is prominent in pigs; dogs usually have urinary and fecal incontinence and exhibit frenzied running. The course is rapid; affected animals die within hours after signs appear. Few animals that develop marked signs recover. Congestion of organs, cyanosis, subepicardial hemorrhages, and a heart stopped in diastole are common postmortem findings.

Emetics are contraindicated if clinical signs are present. Gastric lavage and adsorbents (activated charcoal, 0.5 g/kg) are recommended. Prognosis is grave if clinical signs are severe. Barbiturates are preferred for controlling seizures. Glyceryl monoacetate (monacetin) has been used as a competitive antagonist of fluoroacetate. The recommended dose is 0.25 mL/lb (0.55 mL/kg), IM, or IV in 5 parts of sterile isotonic saline solution, q30min for several hours.

The danger of secondary poisoning due to ingestion of killed rodents is high, which has led to severe restrictions on use of fluoroacetate (and fluoroacetamide) in the USA; use of 1080 has been banned on all federal land. A black dye must be mixed with 1080 for identification; only certified, insured exterminators can purchase it.

Sodium Fluoroacetamide (1081): 1081 causes signs similar to those of 1080 (*see* above), and requires the same treatment.

Thallium Sulfate: Banned for use as a rodenticide, this is a general cellular poison that affects all species. Onset of clinical signs is delayed 1-3 days and although all body systems are affected, the most severe signs refer to the GI, respiratory, integumentary, and nervous systems. Signs include gastroenteritis (occasionally hemorrhagic), abdominal pain, dyspnea, blindness, fever, conjunctivitis, gingivitis, and tremors or seizures. After an apparent recovery or after repeated small doses, chronic dermatitis characterized by alopecia, erythema, and hyperkeratosis occurs. Necrosis of many tissues is a common necropsy finding.

Treatment of acute thallium poisoning includes emetics, gastric lavage with a 1% solution of sodium iodide, and IV administration of a 10% solution of sodium iodide. Diphenylthiocarbazone is antidotal. Symptomatic treatment of the diarrhea and convulsions is indicated with particular attention to fluid and electrolyte balance. Sodium diethyldithiocarbamate has been recommended in small animals with variable success.

Zinc Phosphide (and occasionally aluminum phosphide): This has been used extensively around farms and barns because affected rats tend to die in the open. Toxicity of zinc phosphide is due to liberation of phosphine gas at acid pH in the GI tract. The gas results in direct irritation of the tract along with cardiovascular collapse. The toxic dose is ~40 mg/kg, and onset is rapid in animals with a full stomach. Clinical signs include vomiting, abdominal pain, aimless running and howling, followed by depression, dyspnea, and convulsions (which may suggest strychnine or fluoroacetate poisoning). Death is due to respiratory arrest. The odor of acetylene is present in vomitus or stomach contents. Less frequent lesions include visceral congestion and pulmonary edema. Diagnosis is based on history of exposure to zinc phosphide, suggestive clinical signs, and detection of zinc phosphide in stomach contents. Zinc levels in the blood, liver, and kidneys may be elevated. Treatment must include supportive therapy, calcium gluconate, and appropriate fluids to reduce acidosis. Sodium bicarbonate (cattle: 2-4 L of 5%) PO to neutralize stomach acidity is recommended.

RYEGRASS TOXICITY

ANNUAL RYEGRASS STAGGERS

An often fatal neurotoxic disease that occurs in livestock of any age and either sex that graze on pastures in which annual ryegrass (*Lolium rigidum*) is present and in the seedhead stage of growth. It occurs in western and southern Australia and in South Africa in November-March. Hay of *Festuca rubra* var *commutata* (Chewing's fescue) with *Clavibacter*-infected seedhead galls has caused a similar disease in cattle and horses in Oregon.

In Australia, the responsible corynetoxins are produced in seedhead galls induced by the nematode *Anguina funesta* and colonized by a *Clavibacter* sp. These bacteria-infested galls are present in infected annual ryegrass pastures from early spring onward, but animals show no signs of toxicity until early summer. Spread of bacteria-infested nematodes to adjacent healthy annual ryegrass pastures is slow.

The corynetoxins are highly toxic glycolipids that inhibit specific glycosylation enzymes and therefore deplete or reduce activity of essential glycoproteins. Experimentally, the corynetoxins deplete fibronectins and cause failure of the hepatic reticuloendothelial system.

Outbreaks occur 2-6 days after animals graze a paddock that contains annual ryegrass infected at a toxic level; deaths occur within hours, or up to 1 wk after onset of signs. Characteristic neurological signs are similar to those of perennial ryegrass staggers (*see* below). However, mortality from annual ryegrass toxicity is commonly 40-50%, occasionally greater. The lesions include congestion, edema, and hemorrhage of the brain and lungs, and degeneration of the liver and kidneys.

Diagnosis is based on the characteristic neurological signs of tremors, incoordination, rigidity, and collapse when stressed, with animals often becoming apparently normal again when left undisturbed. When animals are severely affected, nervous spasms supervene, and convulsions in recumbency are soon followed by death. Close regard to the history and contents of the pastures grazed will assist in differentiation of staggers caused by perennial ryegrass, phalaris, and the ergots of paspalum and other grasses; polioencephalomalacia and enterotoxemia are other differential diagnoses.

No specific treatment is practicable. Losses can be minimized by early recognition of signs and removal to safe grazing or by reducing grazing pressure. Grazing of hay aftermath should be avoided. Burning toxic annual ryegrass paddocks in the fall destroys most of the galls colonized by bacteria and minimizes the risk of toxicity in the following season.

PERENNIAL RYEGRASS STAGGERS

A neurotoxic condition of grazing livestock of all ages, this occurs only in summer and fall and only on pastures in which perennial ryegrass (*Lolium perenne*) or hybrid ryegrasses are the major components. It occurs sporadically in parts of North America, Europe, and Australia; in New Zealand, a high incidence each year causes considerable loss and seriously disrupts management procedures and stock movement. Sheep, cattle, horses, and farmed deer of either sex are susceptible.

The tremorgenic neurotoxins responsible are lolitrems, mainly lolitrem B. These indole toxins are produced in perennial and hybrid ryegrasses infected with the endophytic fungus *Acremonium loliae*. The amounts of fungal hyphae and lolitrem B in infected plants increase to toxic levels in summer and fall, and decrease again to safe levels in the cooler seasons. Mycelia of the fungus are present in all the aboveground parts of infected plants but are especially concentrated in leaf sheaths, flower stalks, and seed. Infected plants exhibit no signs, and the fungus is spread only through infected seed. Viability of the endophyte gradually declines when infected seed is stored at ambient temperatures and moderate humidity so that few seeds contain viable endophytes after 2 yr. Neurotoxic tremorgens are believed to produce incoordination of movement by interference with neuronal transmission in the cerebral cortex through the production of a reversible biochemical lesion; no specific histological lesion is recognized.

Signs develop gradually over a few days. Fine tremors of the head and nodding movements are the first signs noted in animals approached quietly and watched carefully. Noise, sudden exercise, or fright elicits more severe signs of head nodding with jerky movements and incoordination when first moved. Running produces stiff, bounding movements with marked incoordination, and often results in collapse in lateral recumbency with opisthotonos, nystagmus, and flailing of stiffly extended limbs. The attack soon subsides, and within minutes the animal regains its feet and rejoins the group. If again forced to run, the episode is repeated. The signs are most severe when animals are heat stressed.

Within flocks and herds, individual susceptibility varies greatly, and this trait is heritable. In outbreaks, morbidity may reach 80-90%, but mortality is low (0-5%). Deaths are usually accidental or due to the inability to forage for food and water.

The strict seasonal occurrence of characteristic tremors, incoordination, and collapse in several or many animals grazing predominantly perennial ryegrass pastures strongly implicates this disease. Reference to the botanical composition of the pastures will exclude annual ryegrass toxicity (*see* above) and paspalum staggers (qv, p 1689), which have similar clinical signs and seasonality. Microscopical examination of the ryegrass sward will reveal the extent of endophyte infection.

Since movement and handling of animals exacerbates signs, individual treatment is generally impractical. Recovery is spontaneous in 1-2 wk if animals are moved to nontoxic pastures or crops.

Because the endophyte and the lolitrems are not uniformly distributed within ryegrass plants, control by grazing management can help prevent the disease. Well-controlled leafy swards, not allowed to bolt to seed, nor overgrazed down into the leaf sheath zone, are likely to provide safe grazing during the dangerous season, even when a high proportion of ryegrass plants are endophyte infected. Encouragement of growth of other grass species and clovers in established swards also reduces the intake of toxic ryegrass.

Safe new pastures can be established using ryegrass seed with little or no endophyte infection. Alternatively, seed that has been stored for 18-24 mo probably contains few viable endophytes and would produce nontoxic pastures.

SALT POISONING

Salt (sodium chloride, NaCl) may be toxic when excessive quantities are ingested and intake of potable water is limited. "Salt poisoning" is a misnomer because the condition usually occurs with concomitant water deprivation. Deaths have been attributed to salt poisoning in cattle, pigs, sheep, horses, dogs, and poultry in various parts of the world. In the USA, pigs, cattle, and chickens are affected most frequently.

Etiology: Toxicity of the sodium ion is directly related to water consumption. With water deprivation, sodium propionate, acetate, carbonate, etc, produce the same toxicosis as NaCl.

Feeder pigs on feed containing only 0.25% salt have had sodium ion toxicosis when water intake was limited, yet even 13% salt in the feed may not produce poisoning if adequate fresh water is consumed. Optimally, with fresh water fully available, pig feeds should contain 0.5-1% salt. Feeding whey or brine that contains 3-4% salt can result in toxicosis of most livestock and poultry species. Ingestion of copious amounts (1-3 kg) of salt by deprived animals may result in toxicosis, even when water is available, especially in cattle.

Chickens are susceptible to sodium ion toxicosis when water intake is restricted in hot weather, or in cold weather when the water supply freezes. Chickens tolerate up to 0.25% salt in drinking water. Wet mash that contained 2% salt caused poisoning in ducklings. Salt in wet mash seems more toxic than it is in dry feeds, probably because birds eat more wet mash and caretakers then are less careful to provide another source of water.

Cattle and sheep on range may develop salt poisoning when a high percentage of mineral supplement is provided, and the water intake is limited or saline. Sheep tolerate 1% salt in drinking water but 1.5% may be toxic. Some recommend that drinking water should contain ≤0.5% total salts for any species of livestock. High concentrations of salt can cause gastroenteritis and dehydration.

Clinical Findings: In pigs, early signs (rarely observed) may be increased thirst, pruritus, and constipation. Affected animals may be blind, deaf, and oblivious to their surroundings; will not eat, drink, or respond to external stimuli; or may wander aimlessly, push against objects, and circle or pivot around a single front or rear limb. After 1-5 days of limited water intake, intermittent seizures occur with the pig sitting on its haunches, jerkily drawing its head backward and upward, finally falling on its side in clonic-tonic seizures and opisthotonos; terminally, pigs lie on their sides, paddling in a coma, and die within a few to 48 hr.

In pigs (but not other species) during the first 48 hr, circulating eosinophils disappear and are attracted to the cerebrovascular and meningeal areas, and collect around the vessels within the cerebral cortex and adjacent meninges. After 3-4 days, the eosinophils leave the cerebral area; cortical laminar necrosis and even cavitation usually follow if the animal lives another 10-12 hr.

Cattle show vomiting, diarrhea, abdominal pain, anorexia, and mucus in the feces; there may be continuous polyuria and a nasal discharge. Neurological signs include blindness and seizures followed by partial paralysis. A characteristic sequela of salt poisoning in cattle is dragging of the hindfeet while walking and, in more severe cases, knuckling of the fetlock joints.

Lesions: In pigs, blood-filled pinpoint ulcers are found on a markedly congested and inflamed gastric mucosa. Cattle have gastric inflammation or ulceration, or both, edema of the skeletal muscles, and hydropericardium. Sometimes no gross necropsy lesions are evident.

Diagnosis: Plasma and CSF concentrations of sodium of >160 mEq/L, especially when CSF has a greater concentration than plasma, are indicative of salt poisoning. In the cerebrum, >1800 ppm sodium (wet wt) is compatible with toxicosis. Confirmation of a diagnosis depends on finding characteristic microscopic lesions in the cerebral cortex.

Treatment: Immediate removal of the offending feed or liquid is imperative. Fresh water must be provided to all animals, initially in small amounts at frequent intervals. Ingestion of a large amount of water at this stage, however, may exacerbate neurologic signs due to brain edema. Severely affected animals unable to find water or to drink it should be given water cautiously via stomach tube. Usually, ~50% of affected animals die regardless of treatment.

SELENIUM POISONING

Trace amounts of selenium (0.1-0.3 ppm) in the diet are required to prevent deficiency diseases such as white muscle disease in cattle and sheep, hepatosis dietetica in pigs, and exudative diathesis in chicks. The maximum tolerable level for all livestock has been considered to be 2 ppm but may be as high as 5 ppm (although some believe that levels as low as 4-5 ppm can inhibit growth).

Evidence of selenium toxicity in grazing animals was first identified in the Great Plains of the USA. Localized seleniferous areas also have been identified in Ireland, Israel, Canada, Australia, the USSR, China, and South Africa.

There are 3 distinct forms of selenium poisoning: acute; chronic, of the blind-staggers type; and chronic, of the alkali-disease type. In animals suffering from toxicity, blood selenium levels are generally >1.5 g/mL and their hair contains >5 ppm selenium. A "garlicky" odor of an animal's breath is a good clue of selenium toxicity.

Etiology: Chronic selenium poisoning ("alkali disease") results when animals consume naturally seleniferous forages and grains that contain 5-40 ppm of selenium. Soils capable of supporting seleniferous plants have been found only in regions where the mean annual rainfall is <20 in. (50 cm). Certain plants known as "accumulators" require selenium for growth and often contain several thousand ppm. When consumed by animals, these accumulator plants may produce a poisoning commonly called "blind staggers". Seleniferous plants that are not removed from the land may decay, become incorporated in the topsoil, and thus become a source of selenium for nonseleniferous plants, which in turn may then be a toxic hazard; hence, the reason for the alternative name of "converter" plants.

Since the selenium in soils comes from certain geological formations, the areas that produce highly seleniferous vegetation are spotty and localized. Vegetation with high selenium has been found consistently in the western plains of Canada, and in Mexico. Most of the selenium poisoning in livestock in the USA has been reported from Colorado, Nebraska, South Dakota, and Wyoming. Occasionally, toxicity develops in dogs following use of selenium-containing shampoos, and in pets given excess selenium tablets as medication. Selenium toxicity has occurred in man and other animals in China following the use of high-selenium coal to cook food over an open flame and to fertilize fields.

CHRONIC SELENIUM POISONING

"ALKALI DISEASE" TYPE

Gross lesions in chronic selenium poisoning of the "alkali disease" type usually include erosion of the joints of long bones, atrophy and cirrhosis of the liver, atrophy of the heart, anemia, and ascites. Hgb concentrations decrease in the early stages and may be an aid in early diagnosis.

Blood levels of selenium are usually 1-2 ppm in animals with alkali disease, whereas in those with blind staggers, they are 1.5-4 ppm. Other changes in blood due to excess selenium intake include decreased fibrinogen levels and prothrombin activities; elevated serum alkaline phosphatase, ALT (SGPT), AST (SGOT), and succinic dehydrogenase activities; and increased content of oxidized glutathione with a concomitant decrease of reduced glutathione. Content of selenium in the hair and/or urine may be indications of toxicity.

Clinical Findings: Chronic poisoning in cattle, horses, and pigs develops when seleniferous grains or forages containing 5-40 ppm are consumed over weeks or months. The signs common to these species include cracking of the hooves, lameness, stiffness of joints, dullness and lack of vitality, emaciation, and loss of hair. In horses, the loss of long hair from the mane and tail usually is the first clinical sign and is followed by cracking of the hoof at the coronary band. New growth of the hoof pushes the dead tissue downward and, if interruption of growth has been prolonged, the old portion of the hoof may separate and slough. In cattle, a series of interruptions of growth may result in deformed hooves, 6-7 in. (15-18 cm) long and turned upward at the ends. Pigs show breaks in the hoof similar to those in cattle. Sows have a lowered conception rate and an increase in the number of pigs born dead. Chronic selenium poisoning of the "alkali disease" type is not common in sheep; death losses occur from acute poisoning soon after sheep are moved onto seleniferous range forage. Eggs with ≥2.5 ppm selenium from birds in high selenium areas show low hatchability, and the embryos are usually deformed, without beaks, and with "ropy" feathers. This has been a problem with waterfowl in southern California.

Treatment and Control: Three possibilities exist for the prevention or treatment of selenium poisoning in animals: 1) treatment of the soil so that selenium uptake by plants is reduced and maintained at nontoxic levels; 2) treatment of the animals so that selenium absorption is reduced or excretion increased, thus preventing toxic accumulations in the tissues; and 3) including in the animal's diet substances that antagonize or inhibit the toxic effects of selenium within body tissues and fluids. However, none of these effectively eliminates selenium toxicity under field conditions. The most effective method is to remove the source of selenium—identified seleniferous areas of the USA have been removed from production. High dietary protein, linseed oil meal, sulfur, arsenic, silver, mercury, copper, and cadmium have reduced selenium toxicity in laboratory animals, but the practical use of these to reduce toxicity is limited. Bromobenzene has enhanced urinary loss of selenium in rats and dogs. A high-protein ration helps to control chronic selenium poisoning, and use of salt containing arsenic at 0.00375% may reduce the incidence of chronic selenium poisoning in cattle that graze seleniferous range. Stiffness in cattle and horses may be relieved by the oral administration of compounds such as naphthalene and bromobenzene, which form mercapturic acids. The usual treatment is 4-5 g of naphthalene daily for 5 days, repeated after a 5-day interval.

"BLIND STAGGERS" TYPE

This develops in animals that consume highly seleniferous plants or grains (usually containing >30 ppm) for weeks or months. In cattle, blind staggers is manifest in 3 stages: 1) The animal tends to wander and may walk into objects in its path. Body temperature is normal, but vision is impaired and appetite is poor. 2) The wandering increases, the front legs become weak, and vision becomes further impaired. 3) The throat and tongue become paralyzed, temperature is subnormal, and death follows from respiratory failure. In sheep, the 3 stages are less clearly differentiated. Congestion and necrosis of the liver, congestion of the renal medulla, epicardial petechiae, hyperemia and ulceration in the abomasum and small intestine, and erosion of the articular surfaces (particularly of the tibia) are the usual lesions observed at necropsy.

There is no specific antidote; supportive therapy, eg, forced fluids, may be useful.

ACUTE SELENIUM POISONING

Acute poisoning under field conditions is rare, since animals usually avoid these plants. However, when pasture is limited, accumulators may be almost the only food available, and large losses among sheep and cattle have occurred. When sufficient highly seleniferous (accumulator) plants are consumed to cause severe acute intoxication, death usually follows within a few hours. The gait is uncertain, the temperature elevated, the respiration labored with frothing from the nostrils, and the pupils are dilated. Prostration occurs before death from respiratory failure. Losses in sheep grazing seleniferous vegetation may be high. In one outbreak, 340 mature sheep died within 24 hr of consuming highly seleniferous *Astragalus bisulcatus.* There is no known treatment.

SNAKEBITE

Venomous snakes fall into 2 classes: the elapines, which include the cobra, mamba, and coral snakes; and the 2 families of viperines, the true vipers (eg, puff adder, Russell's viper, and common European adder) and the pit vipers (eg, rattlesnakes, cottonmouth moccasin, copperhead, and fer-de-lance). Poisonous North American snakes include pit vipers and coral snakes.

Elapine snakes have short fangs and tend to hang on and "chew" venom into their victims. Their venom is neurotoxic and paralyzes the respiratory center; animals that survive these bites seldom have any sequelae. Viperine snakes have long, hinged, hollow fangs; they strike, inject venom (a voluntary action), and withdraw. Many bites by vipers reportedly do not result in injection of substantial quantities of venom. Viperine venom is typically hemotoxic, necrotizing, and anticoagulant, although a neurotoxic component is present in the venom of some species, eg, the Mojave rattlesnake (*Crotalus scutulatus scutulatus*).

Fatal snakebites are more common in dogs than in any other domestic animal. Due to the relatively small size of some dogs in proportion to the amount of venom injected, the bite of even a small snake may be fatal. Because of their size, horses and cattle seldom die as a direct result of snakebite, but fatalities may follow bites on the muzzle, head, or neck when dyspnea results from excessive swelling. Serious secondary damage sometimes occurs; livestock bitten near the coronary band may slough a hoof.

Snakebite, with envenomation, is a true emergency. Owners should not waste time in efforts at first aid other than to keep the animal quiet and limit its activity. Rapid examination and appropriate treatment are paramount.

Diagnosis: In many instances, the bite has been witnessed, and diagnosis is not a problem. However, many conditions thought by the owner to be snakebites are actually fractures, abscesses, spider envenomations, or allergic reactions to insect bites or stings. Owners should be instructed, when possible, to bring the **dead** snake along with the bitten animal; they should be warned not to mutilate the snake's head since identification may depend on the head's morphology. Many snakebites do not result in envenomation, or are made by nonpoisonous snakes.

Typical pit viper bites are characterized by severe local tissue damage that spreads from the bite site. Marked discoloration of the tissue occurs within a few minutes, and dark, bloody fluid may ooze from the fang wounds if not prevented by swelling. Frequently, the epidermis sloughs when the overlying hair is clipped or merely parted. Hair may hide the typical fang marks. Sometimes only one fang mark or multiple punctures are present. In elapine snakebites, pain and swelling are minimal; systemic neurological signs predominate.

Treatment: This should be instituted as soon as possible because irreversible effects of venom begin immediately after injection. After ascertaining that envenomation has occurred, the course of treatment is determined by several factors.

Elapine snakebites may be treated with antivenin (which may be available on an as-needed basis through larger hospital emergency rooms) and supportive care, including anticonvulsants if necessary. A polyvalent, horse-serum-origin antivenin against North American pit vipers is readily available and should be used in all cases of substantial pit viper envenomation.

The progression of events following pit viper envenomation can be divided into 3 phases: the first 2 hr, the ensuing 24 hr, and a variable period (usually ~10 days) afterwards. The first phase is the acute stage in which untreated, severely enve-nomized animals usually die. If death does not occur during this period, and the untreated animal is not in shock nor depressed, the prognosis usually is favorable. The acute phase can be prolonged for several hours by use of corticosteroids and, if administered, prognostication should be withheld. If the animal is active and alert after 24 hr, death due to the direct effects of the venom is unlikely. The third phase is a convalescent period in which infection (possibly anaerobic) may be of concern. If necrosis has been extensive, sloughing occurs and may be so severe as to involve an entire limb.

Although not always completely correct, it is prudent to consider both the size of the snake as an indicator of the quantity of venom injected, and the size of the snake relative to that of the victim. In dogs and cats, bites to the thorax or abdomen generally have a higher mortality than those to the head or extremities. However, this may relate to the size and vulnerability of the victim since smaller animals are more likely to be bitten on the body. Domestic animals vary in their sensitivity to the venom of pit vipers. In decreasing order, sensitivity is reportedly: horse, sheep, goat, dog, rabbit, pig, and cat. If there has been a previous bite, the victim may have developed some degree of active humoral immunity and be less vulnerable to the toxic effects of the venom.

Treatment for pit viper envenomation should be directed toward preventing or controlling shock, neutralizing venom, minimizing necrosis, and preventing sec-ondary infection. Any dog or cat presented within 24 hr of a snakebite showing signs of pit viper envenomation requires intensive treatment, starting with IV fluids to combat hypotension. The use of corticosteroids is being seriously questioned, principally because they alone do not alter the ultimate outcome. They do, however, prolong the clinical course, and therefore may "buy time" in which to effect cura-tive measures. Rapidly active corticosteroids may help to control shock, protect against tissue damage, and minimize the likelihood of allergic reactions to antive-nin. Antivenin is essential to treatment because its action is the only direct and specific mechanism for neutralizing snake venom. Smaller animals probably receive a larger dose (per unit body wt) of venom than more massive animals and, accord-ingly, require larger doses of antivenin. Up to 100 mL of antivenin may be neces-sary for small dogs bitten by a large snake; 5-10 mL may be injected into the tissues around the bite, and the remainder given IV. The efficacy of antivenin is diminished if the bite occurred >24 hr ago. In the event of an anaphylactoid reaction to the heterologous (horse) serum components in antivenin, 0.5-1 mL of 1:1000 epineph-rine should be administered subcut.

Broad-spectrum antibiotics should be given to prevent wound infection and other secondary infections. Several potential pathogens, including *Pseudomonas aeruginosa, Clostridium* spp, *Corynebacterium* spp, and staphylococci have been isolated from rattlesnakes' mouths. Antibiotics should be continued until all superfi-cial lesions have healed.

Tetanus antitoxin also should be administered; other supportive treatment (eg, blood transfusion in the case of hemolytic or anticoagulant venoms) is administered as needed. In most cases, surgical excision is impractical and/or unwarranted. Anti-histamines were reported to be contraindicated, but diphenhydramine hydrochloride is frequently given along with antivenin to treat snakebite in man.

Procedures to neutralize venom (high-voltage, low-amperage electric shock and trypsin) have not proved effective in controlled studies.

SORGHUM POISONING
(Sudan grass poisoning)

Reported almost exclusively in horses, though a similar syndrome has been re-ported in sheep and cattle, it has been observed primarily in the southwestern USA. Lathyrogenic agents, and cyanogenic glycosides and nitrates, have been suggested as causes. The syndrome develops in horses after they have grazed hybrid sudan pastures for weeks to months, and produces axonal degeneration and myelomalacia in the spinal cord. (*See* CYANIDE POISONING, p 1647.)

Sorghum poisoning is characterized by posterior incoordination and ataxia, cystitis, urinary incontinence, and alopecia on the hindlegs due to urine scald. The incoordination and ataxia may progress to flaccid paralysis. Deformities of the fetal musculoskeletal system may occur. Access to sorghum grasses should be restricted if the syndrome is likely to appear. Affected horses often die from pyelonephritis. Although recovery is rare, treatment with antibiotics may be helpful.

SPIDER BITES

Envenomation of animals by spiders is relatively uncommon and difficult to recognize. It may be suspected on clinical signs, but confirmatory evidence is rare. Spiders of medical importance in the USA do not inflict particularly painful bites, so it is unusual for a spider bite to be suspected until clinical signs appear. It is also unlikely that the offending spider will remain in close proximity to the victim for the time (0.5-6 hr) required for signs to develop. Almost all spiders are venomous, but few possess the attributes necessary to cause clinical envenomation in mammals: mouth parts of sufficient size to allow penetration of the skin, and toxin of sufficient quantity and/or potency to produce consequential morbidity.

The spiders in the USA that are capable of causing clinical envenomation belong to 2 groups, widow spiders (*Latrodectus* spp) and brown spiders (mostly *Loxosceles* spp).

WIDOW SPIDERS

Widow spiders usually bite only when accidental skin contact occurs. The most common species is the black widow, *L mactans*, characterized by the red hourglass on her ventral abdomen. In the western states, the western black widow, *L hesperus*, predominates, while the brown widow, *L bishopi*, is found in the south, and the red widow, *L geometricus*, is found in Florida.

Latrodectus venom is one of the most potent biologic toxins. The most important of its 5 or 6 components is a neurotoxin that causes release of the neurotransmitters norepinephrine and acetylcholine at synaptic junctions, which continues until the neurotransmitters are depleted. The resulting severe, painful cramping of all large muscle groups account for most of the clinical signs.

Unless there is a history of a widow spider bite, diagnosis must be based on clinical signs, which include restlessness with apparent anxiety or apprehension; rapid, shallow, irregular respiration; shock; abdominal rigidity and/or tenderness; and painful muscle rigidity, sometimes accompanied by intermittent relaxation (which may progress to clonus, and eventually to respiratory paralysis). Partial paresis also has been described.

An equine origin antivenin is commercially available but is usually reserved for confirmed bites of high-risk individuals (very young or very old). Symptomatic treatment is usually sufficient, but may require a combination of therapeutic agents. Calcium gluconate IV (10 mL of a 10% solution is the usual human dose) is reportedly helpful. Demerol or morphine, also given IV, provides relief from pain and produces muscle relaxation. Muscle relaxants and diazepam are also beneficial. Tetanus antitoxin also should be administered. Recovery may be prolonged; weakness and even partial paralysis may persist for several days.

BROWN SPIDERS

There are at least 10 species of *Loxosceles* spiders in the USA, but the brown recluse spider (BRS), *L reclusa*, is the most common, and envenomation by it is typical of that by the others. These spiders have a violin-shaped marking on the cephalothorax, but it may be indistinct or absent in some species. In the northwestern USA, the unrelated spider *Tegenaria agrestis*, reportedly causes a clinically indistinguishable dermonecrosis in man, and presumably in other animals. BRS venom has vasoconstrictive, thrombotic, hemolytic, and necrotizing properties. It contains several enzymes, including a phospholipase (sphingomylinase D), which attacks cell membranes. Pathogenetic mechanisms of the characteristic dermal necrosis are poorly understood, but activation of complement, chemotaxis, and accumulations of neutrophils affect (or amplify) the process. Medical authorities claim that not all BRS bites result in severe localized dermal necrosis. Systemic signs sometimes accompany BRS envenomation.

A history of a bite by a "fiddlebacked" brown spider is useful but rare. A presumptive diagnosis may be based on presence of a discreet, erythematous, intensely pruritic skin lesion that may have irregular ecchymoses. Within 4-8 hr, a vesicle develops at the bite wound, and sometimes a blanched zone circumscribes the erythematous area, imparting a "bull's-eye" appearance to the lesion. The central area sometimes appears pale or cyanotic. The vesicle may degenerate to an ulcer, which, unless treated in a timely manner, may enlarge and extend to underlying tissues, including muscle. Sometimes a pustule follows the vesicle, and on its breakdown, a black eschar remains. The final tissue defect may be extensive and indolent, and require months to heal.

Systemic signs, including hemolysis, thrombocytopenia, and disseminated intravascular coagulation are more likely to occur in cases with severe dermal necrosis, and also may not appear for 3-4 days after the bite. Fever, vomiting, edema, hemoglobinuria, hemolytic anemia, renal failure, and shock may result from systemic loxoscelism.

In known bites, early treatment can be successful, but unfortunately, many cases are not recognizable until cutaneous necrosis has become extensive; treatment at that stage is less rewarding (but still of value). Immediate application of cold packs is beneficial, and if administered early, corticosteroids protect against cutaneous necrosis by stabilizing cell membranes and suppressing chemotaxis. Corticosteroids also tend to protect against systemic involvement. Radical excision has been advocated, but its value is questionable. Dapsone, an inhibitor of leukocyte function, which is frequently used in the treatment of leprosy, is currently considered the drug of choice for BRS bites. In man, it is administered at 100 mg, b.i.d. for 14-25 days. Broad-spectrum antibiotics are useful in preventing secondary infection, and tetanus immunoprophylaxis should be considered.

STRYCHNINE POISONING

An alkaloid from the plant *Strychnos nux-vomica*, strychnine is used as a rodenticide and occasionally as a ruminatoric. It is highly toxic to most domestic animals. The oral LD_{50} in dogs, cattle, horses, and pigs is 0.5-1 mg/kg; in cats, 2 mg/kg. Deliberate or accidental poisoning occurs more frequently in dogs, occasionally in cats, and rarely in livestock.

Strychnine stimulates the CNS, especially the spinal cord and medullary centers. The principal mode of action is believed to be by competitive inhibition of the inhibitory neurotransmitter glycine. This results in uninhibited stimulation of motor neurons, which affects all the striated muscles. However, since the extensors are more powerful than the flexors, they predominate to produce symmetrical and generalized rigidity and tonic seizures.

Strychnine is readily absorbed from the GI tract. It is metabolized in the liver and excreted in urine. With treatment, most of a toxic dose is eliminated within 24 hr. Acidification of urine promotes ion-trapping and urinary excretion of the alkaloid.

Clinical Findings: Following oral administration, signs normally appear within 1 hr, but can be somewhat delayed if food is in the stomach. Early signs are apprehension, nervousness, tenseness, and muscle stiffness. Severe tetanic seizures may appear spontaneously or be initiated by stimuli such as touch, sound, or a sudden bright light. The extreme and often overpowering extensor rigidity causes the animal to assume a "sawhorse" stance. The violence of the spasm may throw an animal off its feet. Breathing may cease momentarily. The tetanic convulsion lasts from a few seconds to ≥ 1 min. Periods of relaxation are intermittent and become less frequent as the clinical course progresses. During convulsions, the pupils are dilated and the mucous membranes cyanotic. Frequency of the seizures increases and death eventually occurs from exhaustion or hypoxia during a seizure. The entire syndrome, if untreated, may be less than 1-2 hr. There are no characteristic lesions. In cases that have prolonged convulsions before death, agonal hemorrhages of the heart and lungs, and cyanotic congestion due to anoxia may be seen.

Diagnosis: Tentative diagnosis is usually based on evidence of ingestion, clinical signs, and lack of lesions. For differential diagnosis, other convulsive disorders may be considered. Several other poisons (eg, chlorinated hydrocarbons, zinc phosphide, nitrophenide, fluoroacetate, organophosphates, carbamates, nicotine, 4-aminopyridine), tetanus toxin, and pathological conditions (eg, massive hepatic necrosis) are reported to produce signs that resemble those of strychnine poisoning.

Unequivocal diagnosis is by recovery of strychnine from the stomach contents and visceral organs, and also vomitus if available.

Treatment: Treatment is directed at: 1) expulsion of the substance from the GI tract, and detoxification of that which remains, and 2) maintaining relaxation and preventing asphyxia by assisting respiration. Stomach contents can be removed by emesis and gastric lavage. Emesis should not be induced in hyperesthetic, anesthetized, or convulsing animals. Detoxification of the remaining strychnine is attempted by oxidizing it with potassium permanganate ($KMnO_4$), precipitating it with tannic acid, or adsorbing it with activated charcoal; the latter is probably most effective. Before signs appear, the stomach may be evacuated by apomorphine at 0.1 mg/kg in dogs, or by xylazine at 0.44 mg/kg in cats.

Gastric lavage, using warm hypertonic saline solution, 1:1000 $KMnO_4$, strong tea, or a 2% tannic acid solution, should be attempted. A high enema with warm saline may be advantageous. Use of activated charcoal (5 g/kg body wt, PO) is strongly recommended after gastric lavage. If convulsions are present or imminent, pentobarbital sodium IV is the drug of choice in small animals; chloral hydrate may be used in larger animals, but either must be given to effect and repeated as often as necessary. Methocarbamol, diazepam, and xylazine also have been used to control strychnine seizures in dogs, but with variable success. Administration of 5% dextrose in isotonic saline solution helps to maintain kidney function.

SWEET CLOVER POISONING

An insidious hemorrhagic disease occurring in animals that consume toxic quantities of spoiled sweet clover (*Melilotus officinalis* and *M alba*) hay or silage.

Etiology: During the process of spoiling, the harmless natural coumarins in sweet clover are converted to toxic dicumarol. Any method of hay storage that allows molding of sweet clover promotes the likelihood of formation of dicumarol in the hay. Weathered, large round bales, particularly the outer portion, usually contain the highest levels of dicumarol. When toxic hay or silage is consumed, hypoprothrombinemia results, presumably because dicumarol combines with the proenzyme to prevent formation of the active enzyme required for synthesis of prothrombin. It probably also interferes with synthesis of factor VII, and other coagulation factors. (*See* HEMOSTATIC DISORDERS, p 52.) The toxic agent crosses the placenta in pregnant animals, and newborn animals may be affected at birth. All species of animals studied are susceptible, but instances of poisoning have involved mainly cattle and, to a limited extent, sheep, pigs, and horses.

Clinical Findings and Lesions: All clinical signs are referable to hemorrhages, which result from faulty blood coagulation. The time of appearance of clinical disease after consumption of toxic sweet clover varies greatly and depends on the dicumarol content of the particular specimen of sweet clover fed, age of the animals, and amount of feed consumed. If the dicumarol content of the ration is low or variable, animals may consume it for months before signs of disease appear.

Initial signs may be stiffness and lameness, due to bleeding into the muscles and joints. Hematomas, epistaxis, or GI bleeding may be observed. Death may occur suddenly with little preliminary evidence of disease and is caused by massive hemorrhage or bleeding after injury, surgery, or parturition. Neonatal deaths rarely occur without signs in the dam.

Hemorrhage is the characteristic necropsy finding; large extravasations of blood are commonly found in the subcut. and connective tissues.

Diagnosis: This is based on a history of continuous consumption of sweet clover hay or silage over relatively long periods, compatible signs and lesions, and markedly prolonged blood clotting time or demonstration of reduced prothrombin content of the plasma. Most diseases with hemorrhagic manifestations, such as blackleg, pasteurellosis, bracken fern poisoning, and aplastic anemia, can be readily differentiated based on clinical, pathological, and hematological findings. This is the only commonly acquired disease, except purpura hemorrhagica (common only in horses), in which such large hemorrhages occur, but *see also* RODENTICIDE POISONING, p 1720.

Congenital or inherited diseases affecting coagulation factors or blood platelets such as hemophilia A may be characterized by large hemorrhages.

Treatment: The hypoprothrombinemia and anemia can be immediately corrected, to a degree, by IV administration of 2-4 L of whole blood per 1000 lb (450 kg) body wt (from an animal not being fed sweet clover). This procedure should be applied to all animals with marked signs, and repeated if necessary. In addition, parenteral administration of synthetic vitamin K_3 (menadione) is reported to increase prothrombin production. All severely affected animals should receive this drug until their blood clotting time returns to normal. Either synthetic vitamin K or a blood transfusion is sufficient to correct mild cases of intoxication if feeding toxic hay is stopped. Vitamin K_1 (phytonadione) is more effective than vitamin K_3, and while it is more costly, in experimentally induced cases, it was effective when given IM once at 1.1-3.3 mg/kg body wt, which suggests it may be the preferred treatment.

Prophylaxis: Cultivars of sweet clover, low in coumarin and safe to feed, have been developed. If one of these is not available, the only certain way to prevent the disease is to avoid feeding sweet clover hay or silage. Although well-cured sweet clover is not dangerous, the absence of visible spoilage is insufficient evidence of safety. There is no quick chemical test for dicumarol. Suspected feed may be fed to rabbits, which require a shorter feeding period to produce fatal hemorrhage; periodic determination of prothrombin time in the rabbits further reduces the test period. However, some rabbits are refractory to dicoumarin, making negative tests suspect. Dicumarol levels of 20-30 mg/kg of hay are usually required to cause poisoning in cattle.

TOAD POISONING

Dogs and, less frequently, cats may be poisoned by oral exposure to many types of toads that occur throughout the world. Severity varies greatly, depending on extent of contact and type of toad. Venom is produced by all toads, but its potency varies with species, and apparently between geographical locations within individual species. Toad venom, a defensive mechanism, is secreted by glands located dorsal and posterior to the eyes, and by other dermal structures, including warts. The venom, a thick, creamy-white, highly irritating substance, can be expelled quickly by the contraction of periglandular muscles in the skin. Its many components include bufagins, which have digitalis-like effects, catecholamines, and serotonin. The most toxic species in the USA appears to be the giant or marine toad,

Bufo marinus, an introduced species that is established in Florida, Hawaii, and Texas. Mortality is 20-100% in untreated cases, depending on venom potency.

Diagnosis: Encounters with toads are most common in warm or mild weather. Signs of poisoning are variable, and range from local effects to convulsions and death. Severity depends on host factors, extent of exposure, length of time since exposure, and species of toad. Local effects (profuse, sometimes frothy salivation, accompanied by vigorous head shaking, pawing at the mouth, and retching) are immediate, probably because the venom is extremely irritating. Vomiting is not unusual, especially in severe cases, and although it may persist for several hours, this may be as far as poisoning by the common indigenous toads progresses. With more severe intoxication, as from *B marinus*, cardiac arrhythmias, dyspnea, cyanosis, and seizures are characteristic. Both cardiac and CNS involvement are potentially life-threatening.

Treatment: A specific antidote for the toxins in toad venom is not available. Therapy is therefore directed at minimizing absorption of the venom and controlling the associated clinical signs. Where less toxic toads prevail, minimal treatment may be required. The mouth should be immediately and thoroughly flushed with copious amounts of water. The victim should be prevented from inhaling aerosols of saliva or water that contain toad venom. Atropine may be effective in reducing the volume of saliva and the risk of aspiration. More severely affected animals require more extensive therapeutic approaches. Cardiac arrhythmias should be identified and controlled using standard treatment protocols. Atropine or dopamine should be considered if bradyarrhythmias exist, while tachyarrhythmias should be treated with lidocaine, phenytoin, propranolol, or procainamide hydrochloride. CNS excitation, if present, should be controlled by pentobarbital anesthesia, diazepam, or a combination of the two. Thiamylal, halothane, and other forms of anesthesia may be contraindicated since they may predispose the myocardium to ventricular fibrillation. Supplemental oxygen and mechanical ventilation may also be needed if cyanosis and dyspnea are prominent.

PART IX
ZOONOSES

This abbreviated list of zoonoses attempts to mention those diseases that are more important in terms of their likelihood to infect man, and in terms of their severity. For these diseases that may be a hazard to those who work with animals, an indication of when the risk exists (and thus how to reduce it) is given. In most instances, those diseases important to animal health are discussed in more detail elsewhere in the MANUAL (consult the index).

Disease	Causative Organism	Principal Animals Involved	Known Distribution	Probable Means of Spread to Man
BACTERIAL DISEASES				
Anthrax	*Bacillus anthracis*	Warm-blooded animals	Worldwide	Human infections usually through the skin; may be inhaled or ingested. Spores in soil or animal products are resistant.
Brucellosis	*Brucella abortus* *B melitensis* *B suis* *B canis*	Cattle Goats, sheep Pigs, caribou Dogs	Worldwide	Direct contact with excretions or secretions, including milk of infected animals.
Campylobacteriosis	*Campylobacter* spp	Many animals	Worldwide Incidence appears to be increasing	Most species or subspecies appear to be reasonably host-specific but cross-infection is possible, usually via fecal contamination of food.
Cat scratch fever	Unidentified bacillus	Cats, dogs, others (little or no effect other than in man)	Northern Hemisphere Common	Scratches, "licks", bites.

Disease	Organism	Animals affected	Distribution	Transmission
Clostridial diseases (*see also* Tetanus, below)	*Clostridium* spp	Mammals, birds, fish	Worldwide	Wound infection from spores in soil (gas gangrene) is chief hazard for man, but food poisoning occurs. Little danger of direct cross-species transmission.
DF-2 infection	Dysgonic Fermenter (DF-2)	Dogs, other mammals	USA	Unknown, but dogs and their bites are suspect.
Erysipeloid (Erysipelas in animals other than man)	*Erysipelothrix rhusiopathiae*	Pigs, turkeys, pigeons, sea mammals, fish	Worldwide	Wound infection (in man).
Glanders	*Pseudomonas mallei*	Equidae, also Felidae, man, others	Rare except for Southern Asia, Mongolia, Iran	Nasal discharges and necropsy exposure.
Leptospirosis	*Leptospira* spp (many serovars)	Domestic and wild animals, especially rodents	Worldwide	In man, by direct contact with an infected animal's urine or tissue (or aborted fetus), or from contaminated soil or water.
Listeriosis	*Listeria monocytogenes*	Numerous animals and birds	Worldwide	Food-borne among domestic animals; routes of infection in man not well defined.
Lyme disease (Borreliosis)	*Borrelia burgdorferi*	Deer, dogs, horses, rodents, raccoons, opossums	USA (endemic in NE), Europe, Australia	Tick bite, and possibly urine and tissues.
Melioidosis	*Pseudomonas pseudomallei*	Rodents, sheep, goats, horses, pigs, nonhuman primates, kangaroos	Asia, Australia, East Indies, South America, USA	Soil or water contamination of wounds, ingestion, inhalation; not from animal to animal.
Plague	*Yersinia pestis*	Rodents, cats, dogs, others	Western USA, Central and South America, SE Asia, Southern Africa	Fleas, contact with infected animals, inhalation.

(continued)

ZNS

ZOONOSES (continued)

Disease	Causative Organism	Principal Animals Involved	Known Distribution	Probable Means of Spread to Man
Psittacosis (Ornithosis)	*Chlamydia psittaci*	Parakeets, pigeons, parrots, turkeys, ducks, geese, etc	Worldwide	Usually by inhaling dust from feces or feathers. Other isolates from cattle, sheep, goats, opossums, etc, rarely cause disease in man. However, pregnant women are at risk around aborting sheep.
Rat bite fever	*Streptobacillus (Actinobacillus) moniliformis Spirillum minus*	Rodents	Worldwide	Bites of rodents, ingestion, wounds.
Salmonellosis	*Salmonella* spp (2000 serotypes)	Poultry, pigs, cattle, horses, dogs, cats, wild mammals and birds, reptiles, amphibians, crustaceans	Worldwide	Usually via ingestion of undercooked food contaminated with feces; handling diseased animals.
Tetanus	*Clostridium tetani*	Herbivores	Worldwide	Wound infection from soil, especially if contaminated with feces.
Tuberculosis	*Mycobacterium bovis*	Cattle, nonhuman primates	Worldwide, except for countries that have eliminated the disease in cattle	Ingestion, inhalation.
	M tuberculosis	Monkeys and other nonhuman primates; rarely dogs, cats, other domestic animals	Worldwide	Exposure to animals infected with human tuberculosis (uncommon).
Tularemia	*Francisella tularensis*	Rabbits, dogs, cats, rodents, sheep	Circumpolar in Northern Hemisphere	Ingestion, exposure to infected animals (eg, skinning rabbits), arthropod bites.

Disease	Organism	Reservoir	Distribution	Transmission
Vibriosis	Vibrio parahaemolyticus, V alginolyticus	Saltwater fish, shellfish	Pacific basin, shores of Asia, Australia, and North America; Atlantic and Gulf of Mexico coasts and elsewhere	Ingestion of undercooked contaminated food.
Yersiniosis	Yersinia pseudotuberculosis, Y enterocolitica	Animals and birds	Northern Hemisphere	Contaminated food or water.

FUNGAL DISEASES

Many fungal diseases occur in man and other animals, but most are uncommon to rare, and most are the result of environmental exposure rather than of cross-species contagion. Ringworm is a "true zoonosis".

Disease	Organism	Reservoir	Distribution	Transmission
Ringworm	Microsporum spp, Trichophyton spp	Many mammals, also birds	Worldwide	Direct contact with infected animals and fomites.

PARASITIC DISEASES

Protozoan Diseases

Several genera of protozoans may infect man and other animals, but risk of human infection from contact with other animals is low. Most such infections are acquired by ingestion of material contaminated with human feces; some are transmitted by biting insects. Those listed below are more common or could be considered "true zoonoses".

Disease	Organism	Reservoir	Distribution	Transmission
Chagas' disease	Trypanosoma cruzi	Dogs, cats, pigs, armadillos, other mammals	Western Hemisphere, southern USA to central Argentina	Fecal material of triatoma bug (Reduviidae) into bite wounds, blood transfusion.
Sarcosporidiosis	Sarcocystis spp	Pigs, cattle, sheep, ducks	Worldwide	Ingestion of meat.
Toxoplasmosis	Toxoplasma gondii	Mammals, especially cats, birds	Worldwide	Ingestion of oocysts shed in feces of infected cats, and meat that contains cysts.

(continued)

ZOONOSES (continued)

Disease	Causative Organism	Principal Animals Involved	Known Distribution	Probable Means of Spread to Man
Trypanosomiasis, African sleeping sickness	*Trypanosoma brucei*	Wild and domestic ruminants	Africa	Bite of infected tsetse fly.

Trematode (Fluke) Infections

Man shares several fluke infections with other animals. Some of these may be acquired by eating raw or undercooked fish, crustaceans, or contaminated plants. Others are acquired if the skin is exposed to water that contains infective cercariae.

Cestode (Tapeworm) Infections

Man shares several tapeworm infections with other host species. Infection with the adults is undesirable but of much less significance than is infection with the larval stages (via ingestion of worm eggs).

Beef tapeworm, Cysticercosis	*Taenia saginata*	Cattle, buffalo, giraffe, llama	Worldwide	Ingestion of "measly" beef.
Echinococcosis, Hydatid disease	*Echinococcus granulosus*	Dogs, wild carnivores, sheep, cattle	Worldwide	Ingestion of eggs shed in feces of carnivores.
	E multilocularis	Canidae, domestic cats, small rodents	Northern Hemisphere	Ingestion of eggs shed in feces of carnivores.
Fish tapeworm	*Diphyllobothrium* spp	Dogs, fish-eating animals	Worldwide	Ingestion of raw or partially cooked infected fish.
Pork tapeworm, Cysticercosis	*Taenia solium*	Pigs, others	Worldwide	Ingestion of "measly" pork, autoinfection.

Sparganosis	*Spirometra* spp	Dogs, cats, raccoons, amphibians	Worldwide	Direct contact or ingestion of raw tissues of crustaceans (*Cyclops* spp); ingestion of undercooked feral pigs; use of infected frog or snake meat as wound dressing.

Nematode (Roundworm) Infections

Some of these diseases occur in man and other animals, although most are reasonably host-specific. Rarely, people may become infected with parasites of other host species through insect bites, ingestion of infected tissue, or contact with infective larvae. The following are of considerable importance.

Cutaneous larva migrans	*Ancylostoma brasiliense*, *A caninum*	Dogs, cats	Worldwide	Skin penetration by infective larvae.
Trichinosis	*Trichinella spiralis*, other *Trichinella* spp	Pigs, bears, other carnivores, rodents	Worldwide	Ingestion of undercooked infected meat.
Visceral larva migrans	*Toxocara canis*, *T cati*	Dogs, cats	Worldwide	Ingestion of eggs shed in feces of dogs, cats.

DISEASES CAUSED OR BORNE BY ARTHROPODS

It is not uncommon for persons handling animals infested with mites (usually *Sarcoptes* spp) or fleas (eg, from dogs or birds) to become infested, although usually the infestation on the abnormal host is short-lived. This can, however, lead to significant discomfort or, on occasion, to transmission of other diseases, eg, plague. Rarely, screwworms or bot flies infest man. Various ticks infest man as well as other animals, and the consequences may be serious. Some ticks cause paralysis of their hosts (including man) via envenomization. The greatest dangers lie not in the arthropod infestation itself, but in the diseases for which the arthropods may serve as vectors. Several encephalitides, hemorrhagic fevers, rickettsioses, and protozoal blood parasitoses are transmitted by arthropods. Arthropod-borne bacterial diseases include Lyme disease, plague, and tularemia.

(continued)

ZOONOSES (continued)

RICKETTSIAL DISEASES

Some rickettsial diseases may be transmitted by bites of ticks or mites (*see* above). These are uncommon in man but serious, eg, Rocky Mountain Spotted Fever, Boutonneuse Fever. Q-fever is of little or no importance in other animals but occasionally is a problem in man; transmission is via aerosols, ticks, or handling aborted and newborn animals.

VIRAL DISEASES

Most of those listed are rare in man, but a few, eg, the poxes and rabies, are important and "true zoonoses".

Disease	Causative Organism	Principal Animals Involved	Known Distribution	Probable Means of Spread to Man
African green monkey disease	Marburg virus	African Green Monkey (*Cercopithecus aethiops*)	Central Africa	Contact with infected tissues.
Argentinian hemorrhagic fever	Arenavirus group (Junin virus)	Rodents	Argentina	Rodent excretions and secretions, inhalation.
Bat salivary gland (Rio Bravo) fever	Flavivirus/Group B	Bats	Western USA	Laboratory infections in man, and bat bites.
Bolivian hemorrhagic fever	Arenavirus group (Machupo virus)	Rodents	Bolivia	Rodent excretions and secretions, inhalation.
California encephalitis	Bunyavirus	Hares, rabbits, squirrels	Western and central USA	Mosquitoes—*Aedes* spp.
Cocal	Vesicular stomatitis group	Equidae, pigs, cattle	Trinidad	Mites, mosquitoes.
Colorado tick fever	Orbivirus	Squirrels, porcupines, small rodents	Western USA	Ticks—*Dermacentor* spp.

Disease	Agent	Animal hosts	Distribution	Transmission
Contagious ecthyma (Orf)	Parapoxvirus	Sheep, goats	Worldwide	Contact exposure.
Cowpox	Poxvirus	Cattle	Worldwide	Contact exposure.
Crimean-Congo hemorrhagic fever	Crimean Congo virus group	Cattle, rodents	Southern USSR, Africa, Asia	Ticks—*Hyalomma* and *Ornithodoros* spp; handling diseased tissues.
Equine encephalomyelitis (EEE, WEE, VEE)	Alphaviruses	Wild birds, domestic fowl, horses, mules, donkeys	Western Hemisphere	Mosquitoes—several genera.
Foot-and-mouth disease	Rhinovirus Types A, O, C, SAT, and Asia	Cattle, pigs, related species	Europe, Asia, Africa, South America	Contact exposure; man has been affected.
Simian herpesvirus (B virus)	Herpesvirus	Rhesus monkeys	Widespread in Africa and Asia	Bites of monkeys, occupational exposure.
Infectious hepatitis (human)	A-virus	Nonhuman primates	Worldwide	Contact exposure.
Influenza and Parainfluenza	Myxoviruses	Pigs, rodents, dogs, possibly birds	Worldwide Common	Contact exposure. Animals rarely source for man
Japanese B encephalitis	Flavivirus/Group B	Wild birds, pigs, horses (incidentally)	Asia and Pacific Islands Rare	Mosquitoes—*Culex* spp, *Aedes* spp.
Lassa fever	Arenavirus	Rodents, others	Africa	Rodents, urine or contaminated dust, possibly man to man.
Louping ill	Flavivirus/Group B	Sheep; less often cattle, sheepdogs. Rodents, deer, shrews, and red grouse may be carriers	Great Britain, Northern Ireland	Ticks—*Ixodes ricinus*.

(continued)

ZOONOSES (continued)

Disease	Causative Organism	Principal Animals Involved	Known Distribution	Probable Means of Spread to Man
Lymphocytic choriomeningitis	Arenavirus	Monkeys, dogs, mice, hamsters, guinea pigs	Worldwide	Host excretions and secretions.
Monkeypox	Poxvirus	Nonhuman primates	West Africa	Contact.
Murray Valley encephalitis	Flavivirus/Group B	Wild birds	Australia, New Guinea	Mosquitoes—*Culex annulirostris*.
Nairobi sheep disease	Ganjam group	Sheep, goats	Kenya, Uganda, Congo, Mozambique, South Africa	Ticks—*Rhipicephalus appendiculatus*.
Newcastle disease	Paramyxovirus	Fowl	Worldwide Common	Occupational exposure. Uncommon in man.
Pseudocowpox	Poxvirus	Cattle	Worldwide Common	Contact.
Rabies	Lyssavirus	Carnivores and Chiroptera (bats)	Worldwide except Australia, New Zealand, Britain, Scandinavia, Japan, Taiwan; a number of smaller islands are also free	Bites of diseased animals. Possibly inhalation.
Rift valley fever	Bunyavirus	Sheep, goats, cattle	Africa	Mosquitoes—*Aedes* and *Eratmopodies* spp. Contact on necropsy or handling fresh meat.
Russian spring-summer encephalitis	Flavivirus/Group B	Birds, small mammals, sheep	Central Asia, USSR	Ticks—*Ixodes persulcatus, Haemaphysalis* spp.

Disease	Virus	Reservoir	Distribution	Vector
St. Louis encephalitis	Flavivirus/Group B	Wild birds and domestic fowl	USA, Caribbean, northern South America, Central America, Canada	Mosquitoes—*Culex* spp.
Tick-borne encephalitis (Central European)	Flavivirus/Group B	Rodents, hedgehogs, birds, cattle, sheep, goats	Sweden, Finland, Poland, Austria, Hungary, Yugoslavia, USSR, Czechoslovakia	Ticks—*Ixodes ricinus*. (May be milk-borne.)
Wesselsbron disease	Flavivirus/Group B	Sheep, cattle	South Africa, Uganda, Cameroons, Thailand	Mosquitoes—*Aedes, Mansonia, Culex* spp.
West Nile fever	Flavivirus/Group B	Wild birds, domestic quadrupeds	Africa, Middle East, South Asia, Europe, USSR Common	Mosquitoes—*Culex* spp.
Yellow fever	Flavivirus/Group B	Monkeys	Tropical Central and South America, Africa	Mosquitoes—*Aedes* spp, *Haemagogus* sp.

INDEX

Page numbers in **bold type** indicate principal references

A

NOTES

NOTES

NOTES

NOTES

NOTES

NOTES

NOTES

NOTES

NOTES

NOTES

NOTES

NOTES

NOTES

NOTES

NOTES

NOTES

NOTES

NOTES

NOTES